SECOND EDITION

PHARMACOLOGY *for* WOMEN'S HEALTH

Edited by

Mary C. Brucker, CNM, PhD

Editor
Nursing for Women's Health
Washington, DC
Assistant Professor, Adjunct
Nurse-Midwifery/WHNP Program
Georgetown University
Washington, DC

Tekoa L. King, CNM, MPH

Health Sciences Clinical Professor
School of Nursing
University of California, San Francisco
San Francisco, California
Deputy Editor
Journal of Midwifery & Women's Health

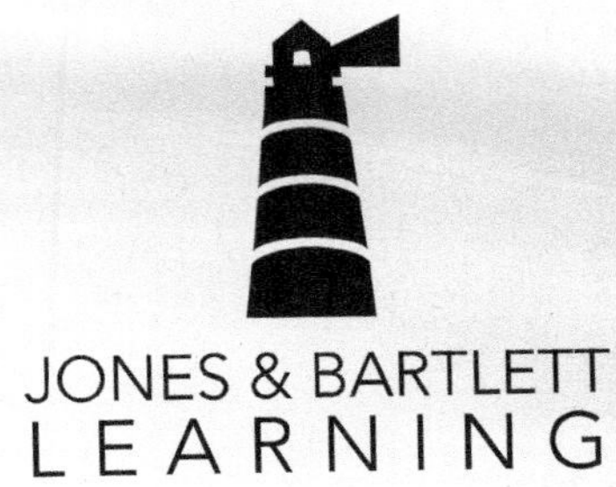

JONES & BARTLETT
LEARNING

World Headquarters
Jones & Bartlett Learning
5 Wall Street
Burlington, MA 01803
978-443-5000
info@jblearning.com
www.jblearning.com

Jones & Bartlett Learning books and products are available through most bookstores and online booksellers. To contact Jones & Bartlett Learning directly, call 800-832-0034, fax 978-443-8000, or visit our website, www.jblearning.com.

Substantial discounts on bulk quantities of Jones & Bartlett Learning publications are available to corporations, professional associations, and other qualified organizations. For details and specific discount information, contact the special sales department at Jones & Bartlett Learning via the above contact information or send an email to specialsales@jblearning.com.

07887-9

Production Credits
VP, Executive Publisher: David D. Cella
Executive Editor: Amanda Martin
Acquisitions Editor: Teresa Reilly
Editorial Assistant: Danielle Bessette
Production Manager: Carolyn Rogers Pershouse
Production Editor: Vanessa Richards
Production Assistant: Juna Abrams
Marketing Communications Manager: Katie Hennessy
VP, Manufacturing and Inventory Control: Therese Connell
Composition: CAE Solutions Corp.
Cover Design: Kristin E. Parker
Rights & Media Research Assistant: Wes DeShano
Media Development Editor: Shannon Sheehan
Cover Image: © Sofimanning/Shutterstock
Printing and Binding: LSC Communications
Cover Printing: LSC Communications

Library of Congress Cataloging-in-Publication Data
Pharmacology for women's health / [edited by] Mary C. Brucker, Tekoa L. King. — Second edition.
p. ; cm.
Order of names reversed on previous edition.
Includes bibliographical references and index.
ISBN 978-1-284-05748-5 (paperback)
I. Brucker, Mary C., editor. II. King, Tekoa L., editor.
[DNLM: 1. Pharmacological Processes. 2. Genital Diseases, Female—drug therapy. 3. Pregnancy Complications—drug therapy. 4. Women's Health. QV 37]
RG131
615'.1082--dc23

2015018277

6048

Printed in the United States of America
25 24 23 10 9 8 7 6 5

Contents

Introduction

"My drug rep brings great pizza. I always support her by prescribing her products."

Women's Healthcare Provider in Practice

"As long as a student knows the name, dose, and contraindications for at least one or two drugs for a specific condition, they can practice safely."

Faculty Teaching a Graduate Clinical Pharmacology Course

"I can always look it up when I'm in practice."

Student

The above comments can be found in the beginning of the *First Edition*. However, they remain true today and illustrate why this book is needed. As the amount of drug information available explodes, providers find themselves overwhelmed and sometimes unprepared to identify the appropriate intervention for a particular clinical situation.

Most books about drugs fall into one of two categories—they either focus on basic pharmacology, rich with information about pharmacokinetics and pharmacodynamics, or they address pharmacotherapeutics with an emphasis on conditions and indicated treatments. The former provides in-depth information that, unfortunately, is often detached from actual practice, making it difficult for a healthcare professional to retain and later use. The pharmacotherapeutics approach helps the clinician link a condition and drug together, but frequently does not provide enough information for future decision making, especially as postmarketing adverse effects become apparent or new agents emerge.

Pharmacology for Women's Health is specifically designed for all healthcare providers who care for women. This book combines both basic pharmacology and pharmacotherapeutics and is divided into six distinct but complementary sections. The first section, "Introduction to Pharmacology," begins with an overview of modern pharmacology and continues with chapters that provide the basic framework needed by a clinician. For some readers, this content may be new; for others it will provide a review.

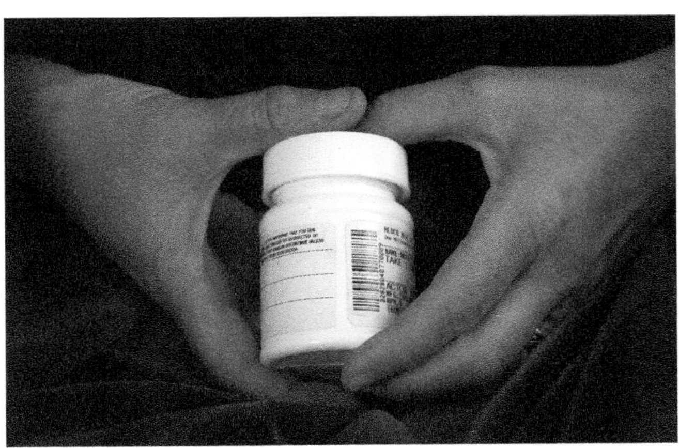

Recognition that some agents are used for reasons other than treating women with pathologic conditions is the rationale for clustering chapters into the second section, "Lifestyle and Preventive Healthcare Practices." The chapters in this section explore drugs used to prevent disease, such as vitamins and immunizations. This section also includes chapters that review drugs used to aid smoking withdrawal and those used to treat obesity. In addition, this section has chapters that address use of drugs involved in treating substance abuse.

Some drugs such as antimicrobials or hormonal agents are used to treat a wide variety of conditions. Medications in these drug categories can be prescribed for their primary therapeutic effects or even for their side effects (e.g., the use of antihistamines for sedation). Discussion of the use of the same antibiotic that is indicated for a woman with a respiratory, urinary, or dermatologic infection would be redundant information for readers if addressed in each separate chapter. Therefore, selected drug classifications, namely antimicrobials, analgesics and anesthetics, antihistamines, and steroidal hormones, comprise the chapters in the third section. Although few in number, these chapters include a large amount of essential material about these classes of drugs, and when specific ones are mentioned for pharmacotherapeutic reasons in other chapters, the reader will be able to refer to this section for detailed information. Due to the common use of these types of agents, this section is titled "Essential Drug Categories."

The largest number of chapters is found in the next section, "Pharmacotherapeutics for Common Conditions." In these chapters, evidence-based information about treatment of women with conditions ranging from the common cold to cancer can be found. All chapters are focused on care provided by primary care professionals. When appropriate, agents with indications that vary based on gender, age, or reproductive state, are so discussed.

Reproduction, contraception, and gynecologic conditions, as well as pregnancy and breastfeeding are addressed in the last two sections, "Gynecology" and "Pregnancy and Lactation." Women experience profound physiologic changes over the course of adult life. These changes affect pharmacotherapeutics and are therefore a primary consideration prior to prescribing medications for women. Thus, it is appropriate that we honor these transitions with separate chapters.

All the chapters in this book begin with a glossary of terms used in that chapter and a description of the underlying physiology so the reader can better understand use of pharmacologic agents. This book does not provide detailed physiology of pathologic conditions, diagnosis, or nonpharmacologic treatments. Readers are referred to other texts for additional information on those subjects. Most chapters include cases that illustrate clinical use of the agents reviewed. Every effort has been made to verify that the information presented is current and accurate. This book is not intended to be a replacement for appropriate health care.

Acknowledgments

This text is dedicated to women, with the hope that they all receive the care that they need and deserve, especially when pharmacologic agents are indicated.

Many colleagues cautioned us upon undertaking the editing of this text. More than once we heard that writing a textbook was as onerous as a prolonged labor and a second edition was just as difficult, if not more so. Yet for us, this continues to be a labor of love. The process remained stimulating, probably in large part because of our editing partnership. By this time, we have adopted each other and each other's families. We also benefited from a wide network of old and new friends and colleagues. We were fortunate to have a fabulous group of authors and colleagues who shared their time and expertise so liberally. The University of California at San Francisco and Georgetown University enabled us to obtain the needed resources and obscure references.

Family members provided support and understanding. Our heartfelt thanks to Bill Fawley, Nancy Jo Reedy, Cathy Rosser, Kya, Tim, and Simon Barounis, Linda Cady, Todd Fawley and Deepa Patel, and Ted Brucker. These family members all saw more of our backs as we sat at computers than they ever anticipated. For the one who said, "What, again?" when the computer emerged one evening in the midst of a vacation at Disney, and for the one who said, "And what year will that book be done?" . . . here it is.

Contributors

Susan A. Albrecht, CRNP, PhD
Associate Dean
University of Pittsburgh School of Nursing
Pittsburgh, PA

Ivy M. Alexander, PhD, APRN, ANP-BC, FAAN
Clinical Professor
Director of Advanced Practice Programs
University of Connecticut
Storrs, CT

Teresa E. Baker, MD
Associate Professor
Department of Obstetrics and Gynecology
Texas Tech University Health Sciences Center
Amarillo, TX

Sharon M. Bond, CNM, PhD
Staff Midwife
Dept. of Obstetrics and Gynecology
Medical University of South Carolina
Charleston, SC

Esther R. Ellsworth Bowers, CNM/WHNP, MSN, MS, MEd
Staff Midwife
Flagstaff Birth & Women's Center
Flagstaff, AZ

Mary C. Brucker, CNM, PhD
Editor
Nursing for Women's Health
Associate Professor, Adjunct
Nurse-Midwifery/WHNP Program
Georgetown University
Washington, DC

Cheryl A. Carlson, PhD, APRN, NNP-BC
Neonatal Nurse Practitioner
Medical University of South Carolina
Charleston, SC

Donna D. Caruthers, RN, PhD
Associate Vice President of Academic Affairs
Interim Director of Institutional Research
Title IX Coordinator
Westmoreland County Community College
Youngwood, PA

Patricia W. Caudle, DNSc, CNM, FNP-BC
Associate Professor
Frontier Nursing University
Hyden, KY

Austin J. Combest, PharmD, BCOP, MBA
Sr. Clinical Scientist & Director, UNC/PPD Drug Development Fellowship
PPD Worldwide Headquarters
Wilmington, NC

Wendell L. Combest, PhD
Professor
Shenandoah University
Winchester, VA

Robin Webb Corbett, PhD, FNP-C, RNC
Associate Professor
East Carolina University College of Nursing
Greenville, NC

Dawn Durain, CNM, MPH
Associate Director, Nurse-Midwifery Program
School of Nursing, University of Pennsylvania
Philadelphia, PA

Nicole K. Early, PharmD, BCPS, CGP
Assistant Professor
Midwestern University College of Pharmacy, Glendale
Glendale, AZ

Christina E. Elmore, CNM, MSN
Clinical Instructor
University of Utah
Salt Lake City, UT

William P. Fehder, CRNA, PhD
Clinical Associate Professor
Boston College William F. Connell School of Nursing
Chestnut Hill, MA

Katie Ferraro, MPH, RD, CDE
Assistant Clinical Professor
Hahn School of Nursing and Health Science
University of San Diego
San Diego, CA

Juliana van Olphen Fehr, CNM, PhD
Professor
Shenandoah University
Winchester, VA

Alexa A. Gorwoda, PharmD
Pharmacist
Albuquerque, NM

Barbara W. Graves, CNM, MPH, MN
Staff Nurse-Midwife
Baystate Medical Center
Springfield, MA

Thomas W. Hale, RPh, PhD
Professor
Texas Tech University School of Medicine
Amarillo, TX

Jennifer G. Hensley, CNM, WHNP-BC, LCCE, EdD
Associate Professor
Specialty Director, Nurse-Midwifery and Women's Health Nurse Practitioner Programs
University of Colorado, Denver
Aurora, CO

Cecilia M. Jevitt, CNM, PhD, FACNM
Associate Professor, Midwifery Specialty Coordinator
Yale University School of Nursing
New Haven, CT

Padma Kandadai, MD, MPH
Assistant Professor
Boston University School of Medicine
Boston, MA

Samantha A. Karr, PharmD, FCCP, BCPS, BCACP, BC-ADM
Associate Professor
Midwestern University
Glendale, AZ

Kristi Watson Kelley, PharmD, FCCP, BCPS, CDE, BC-ADM
Associate Clinical Professor, Pharmacy Practice and Clinical Pharmacist
Auburn University Harrison School of Pharmacy and Continuity of Care Clinic
Baptist Health, Inc.
Birmingham, AL

Joyce L. King, FNP, CNM, PhD
Associate Professor, Clinical and Director of the Nurse-Midwifery Program
Emory University School of Nursing
Atlanta, GA

Tekoa L. King, CNM, MPH
Health Sciences Clinical Professor
School of Nursing, University of California, San Francisco
San Francisco, CA
Deputy Editor
Journal of Midwifery & Women's Health

Nicole T. Lassiter, CNM, MSN, WHNP
Faculty
Frontier Nursing University
Hyden, KY

Judith A. Lewis, PhD, RN, FAAN
Professor Emerita
Virginia Commonwealth University
Richmond, VA

Frances E. Likis, DrPH, NP, CNM, FACNM, FAAN
Associate Director
Vanderbilt University Evidence-Based Practice Center
Editor-in-Chief
Journal of Midwifery & Women's Health
Nashville, TN

Judy Wright Lott, NNP-BC, PhD, FAAN
Dean Emeritus
Baylor University (Retired)
Waco, TX

Nancy K. Lowe, CNM, PhD
Professor
College of Nursing University of Colorado
Editor
Journal of Obstetric, Gynecologic, & Neonatal Nursing
Aurora, CO

Laura E. Manns-James, MSN, CNM, WHNP-BC
Faculty
Frontier Nursing University
Hyden, KY

Hayley Mark, RN, PhD, FAAN
Director, Baccalaureate Program
Associate Professor
Johns Hopkins University School of Nursing
Millersville, MD

William F. McCool, CNM, PhD
Director, Midwifery Graduate Program
School of Nursing, University of Pennsylvania
Philadelphia, PA

Rebekah Jackowski McKinley, PharmD
Assistant Professor
Midwestern University College of Pharmacy, Glendale
Glendale, AZ

Cindy L. Munro, PhD, RN, ANP-BC, FAANP, FAAN, FAAAS
Associate Dean for Research and Innovation, Professor
University of South Florida College of Nursing
Tampa, FL

Patricia Aikins Murphy, CNM, DrPH
Professor
University of Utah College of Nursing
Salt Lake City, UT
Deputy Editor
Journal of Midwifery & Women's Health

Michael W. Neville, PharmD, BCPS, FASHP
Assistant Dean for Students, Professor
Wingate School of Pharmacy
Wingate, NC

Katharine K. O'Dell, CNM, NP, PhD
Associate Professor of OB/GYN
University of Massachusetts Medical School
Worcester, MA

Maria Openshaw, CNM, MS
Instructor
Boston University School of Medicine
Boston, MA

Kathryn M. Osborne, RN, CNM, PhD
Associate Professor
Rush University College of Nursing
Chicago, IL

Laura W. Owens, PharmD, AAHIVP
Chief of Pharmacy Services
Carolina Family Health Centers, Inc.
Wilson, NC

Nancy Jo Reedy, CNM, MPH
Adjunct Instructor and Clinical Faculty Advisor
Georgetown University
Washington, DC

Mary Ann Rhode, CNM, MS
Nurse-Midwife
St. Joseph Hospital
Denver, CO

Rebekah L. Ruppe, CNM, DNP
Assistant Professor of Nursing
Columbia University School of Nursing, Graduate Midwifery Program
New York, NY

Paul L. Sacamano, MPH, ANP-BC, ACRN
Research Assistant
Johns Hopkins Bloomberg School of Public Health
Baltimore, MD

Maureen T. Shannon, CNM, FNP, PhD
Associate Professor
School of Nursing and Dental Hygiene, University of Hawaii, Manoa
Honolulu, HI

Barbara Peterson Sinclair, MN, RNP
Professor Emerita, Consultant
California State University, Los Angeles
Los Angeles, CA

Barbara VanDersarl Slocum, MSN, CNM, WHNP-BC
Lone Tree OB/GYN
Lone Tree, CO

Margaret S. Stemmler, CNM, MPH, PhD
Lecturer
California State University, Dominguez Hills
Carson, CA

Marianne (Teri) Stone-Godena, CNM, MSN
Assistant Professor
Rhode Island College
Providence, RI

Nell L. Tharpe, CNM, CRNFA, MS, FACNM
Adjunct Faculty
Philadelphia University
Philadelphia, PA

Laura V. Tsu, PharmD, BCPS, CGP
Clinical Assistant Professor
Chapman University School of Pharmacy
Irvine, CA

James R. Walker, CRNA, DNP, FNAP, FAAN
Associate Professor, DNP Program Director
Baylor College of Medicine
Houston, TX

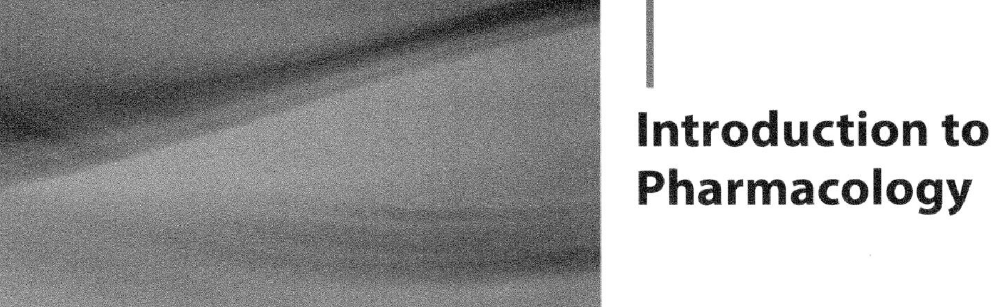

I

Introduction to Pharmacology

Pharmacologic agents are ubiquitous in today's society, and pharmacotherapeutics is an essential component of primary care practice. The four chapters in this section are dedicated to basic information about drugs. The chapter titled *Modern Pharmacology* reviews the clinical context that prescribing takes place in today, including regulation, taxonomy, and general use. *Principles of Pharmacology* describes the pillars in the foundation of pharmacology, including pharmacokinetics and pharmacodynamics. The chapter *Pharmacogenetics* introduces a twenty-first-century approach that will soon be an essential consideration prior to prescribing many drugs. This chapter reviews information about genetics that influence the clinical effects of pharmacologic agents The future may well encompass a genetic assessment for an individual prior to customized prescribing. The last chapter in this section, *Drug Toxicity*, addresses adverse effects of drugs in more detail, including toxic effects and poisonings associated even with commonly used agetns. All of the chapters in this section have clinical examples to illustrate the importance of the pharmacologic principles in practice.

1 Modern Pharmacology

Mary C. Brucker

Chapter Glossary

Adverse drug event (ADE) Untoward medical occurrence that may present during treatment with a pharmaceutical product but that does not necessarily have a causal relationship with the pharmacologic treatment.

Adverse drug reaction (ADR) Response to a drug that is noxious and unintended and that occurs at doses normally used for prophylaxis, diagnosis, or therapy.

Approved drug Substance that has been evaluated by the Food and Drug Administration (FDA) and allowed to be marketed as a drug in the United States.

Behind-the-counter (BTC) Descriptor for drugs that are sold without prescription, but that are subject to restrictions such as proof of identity because of potential risks. For example, pseudoephedrine is BTC because it may be used as an ingredient in the production of methamphetamine.

Black box warning Warning that appears on the package insert of a drug that notes harms associated with use of this drug. Black box warnings are mandated by the FDA and are often added to package inserts after postmarketing studies reveal unexpected adverse drug reactions or adverse drug events.

Brand names Trademarked names assigned to drugs by manufacturers. Some brand names are similar to the generic name (e.g., pseudoephedrine/Sudafed); others suggest their indications for use (e.g., Tamiflu is indicated for treatment of influenza).

Breakthrough therapy/breakthrough drugs Agents whose approval by the FDA are expedited after evidence shows that the drugs, either alone or in combination with other treatments, provide superior outcomes for individuals with specific serious conditions or diseases.

Chemical name Name that describes the chemical composition of the agent. The chemical name is rarely used by prescribers and consumers.

Clinical trials Research studies using human subjects to answer specific questions about new therapies, or new ways of using known treatments. Clinical trials are used to determine whether new drugs are both *safe* and *effective*.

Compounding Mixing or combining ingredients to produce a pharmaceutical agent.

Contraindications Situations in which an agent should *not* be used.

Controlled substances Pharmaceuticals listed in schedules found in U.S. Law 21 U.S.C. §802(32)(A). These drugs include both opiates and nonopiates, but generally all controlled substances have a high risk of addiction.

Counterfeit drugs Pharmaceuticals that are produced and sold in a deceptive manner so that they appear to be authentic drugs.

Designer drugs Drugs directed toward a specific biologic target that bind to and inhibit key molecules involved in a disease or pathologic event.

Direct-to-consumer (DTC) Advertisements for selected drugs placed in popular media and directed to the general public as opposed to being directed to providers.

Dispense (furnish) Process of giving a drug or drug prescription to a consumer.

Drug Chemical substance that brings about changes in a biologic system through its chemical action(s). Also called a *medication* or *pharmaceutical*.

Drug recall Removal of a pharmaceutical agent from the marketplace. It may be either voluntary or mandated by the FDA.

Effectiveness Ability of a drug or treatment to produce a result in real-life circumstances.

Food and Drug Administration (FDA) Regulatory body responsible for approving and monitoring most pharmaceuticals and devices marketed in the United States.

Formulary List of approved or available drugs. A formulary is often used by insurance companies to identify agents that will be reimbursed or paid for by the insurer.

Generally recognized as safe and effective (GRAS/E) Phrase used to describe why an agent has been determined to be safe to sell over the counter.

Generic name Formulation that contains the same active ingredients found in a brand-name formulation and is bioequivalent to that brand-name drug.

High-alert drugs Pharmaceuticals that are associated with significant harm if used in error.

Investigational new drug (IND) Designation for an agent that may be evaluated in clinical trials under regulation by the FDA.

Medication errors Mishaps that occur during prescribing, transcribing, dispensing, administering, adhering to, or monitoring a drug.

Multiple-drug intake (MDI) Synonym for polypharmacy.

New drug application (NDA) Application through which a potential agent is registered as part of the FDA's drug approval process. For example, a company must file an NDA with the FDA to study a drug in clinical trials.

Off-label uses Uses or prescriptions of a drug for conditions other than those approved by the FDA.

Orphan drugs Agents that are prescribed for rare conditions and, therefore, have limited and infrequent use.

Over-the-counter (OTC) Pharmaceuticals sold without prescriptions; if some restrictions are placed on the drug's sale, then the OTC agent also may be called a behind-the-counter (BTC) drug.

Pharmacoeconomics Field of study that identifies, measures, and evaluates the costs of drug therapy to healthcare systems and society.

Polypharmacy Practice of treating individuals with multi-drug regimens; this term generally is accepted to mean administration of five or more drugs. It may also be referred to as multiple-drug intake (MDI) or, in the case of lethal poisonings and overdoses, as combined-drug intoxication (CDI).

Precautions Situations listed on the package insert that can be associated with an adverse drug event (e.g., concomitant ingestion of alcohol with an agent; use of a contraceptive by women weighing more than 200 pounds). The evidence of association or the potential adverse drug event is not deemed important enough to contraindicate use of the agent or issue a black box warning.

Pregnancy categories FDA drug classification system to identify the fetal risks of drugs when used during pregnancy.

Prescriptive authority Privilege afforded by law to healthcare providers that allows them to order the dispensing of prescription medications.

Safety Plasma level or dose at which a drug's known adverse effects are not apparent.

Side effects Expected physiologic responses unrelated to the desired drug effect.

Warnings FDA identification and dissemination of information about potential conditions associated with major adverse effects. Warnings include black box warnings, or serious information one step away from removal of the drug from the marketplace.

Society and Health

All societies have major concerns, both collectively and among individual members, about the maintenance of health and treatment of conditions or diseases. Over the millennia, a wide variety of interventions have been used for either or both of these objectives. Even today, interventions such as spiritual care, manipulation of body positions, variations in nutrition, and types of exercise remain the primary treatments for some conditions; are first-line interventions in many cultures; and are often are the topics of research studies. However, the use of pharmaceuticals has become one of the most—if not *the* most—common treatment for health conditions today.

Pharmacology and Drugs

Pharmacology is a word derived from the Greek word *pharmakon*, which means medicine or poison. Most sources define pharmacology more precisely as the study of how drugs interact with a living organism to produce a change in physiologic function. Any agent, substance, or medication that is used for medicinal purposes is a pharmaceutical.

Although there is general consensus on the definition of the word *pharmacology*, one of the great difficulties in the discussion of modern pharmacology is the existence of multiple meanings of the term *drug*. Within one context, *drug* connotes use of an illegal substance (e.g., cocaine) and is associated with substance abuse. Not all drugs are illicit, however, and drugs such as marijuana that were previously illicit currently may be approved for medical use in some states. Prescriptive pharmaceuticals as well as **over-the-counter (OTC)** agents are also termed drugs. Nutritional supplements are viewed as drugs by most consumers, although they are not regulated as such by the **Food and Drug Administration (FDA)**.[1] Therefore, it is wise to clarify the meaning of terms used. In this text, a **drug** is a chemical substance that brings about changes in a biologic system through its chemical action. The terms *pharmaceuticals, medications,* and *drugs* will be used interchangeably. Illicit or recreational drugs will be noted as such to promote clarity.

History of Pharmaceuticals

Details of the historical origins of the use of botanicals, herbals, or other types of medications are shrouded in the past. Early records suggest that traditional Chinese medicine practices included liberal use of such agents. From the Indian subcontinent, Ayurvedic medicine combined medications with surgical procedures as early as 1000 BC. Hippocrates, the great Greek physician, was also a herbologist, advocating multiple botanical treatments, many of which still can be found on the market today.

During the Middle Ages in Europe, some of the spices and herbs brought back from the Crusades were said to have attributes of magical healing. By the 1500s, apothecaries were found in various European towns. In the 1600s, botanists and herbalists, such as the Englishman Nicholas Culpeper, were codifying use of herbs and publishing findings and recommendations. Gradually, the use of botanicals became an expected intervention when health was threatened or disease was evident.

In the 1800s, a new industry was born with the advent of patent medicines and potions.[2] Ironically, patent medicines were not copyrighted, but rather were composed of secret ingredients under a trademarked name. Lydia Pinkham's Vegetable Compound included a number of herbs in alcohol.[3] Pinkham marketed the product to women for treatment of menstrual pain and disorders and accrued a personal fortune from widespread sales. The soft drink Coca-Cola was originally marketed as a nerve tonic patent medicine. Use of patent medicines was a logical strategy to treat common diseases in an era in which healthcare providers were unregulated and many provider-prescribed strategies had harmful effects (e.g., those associated with the liberal use of heavy metals). Most patent medicines were not harmful in regular doses, although their effectiveness could be subject to debate. Some older remedies continue to live in today's over-the-counter market, albeit with different ingredients, including Carter's Little Liver Pills, Luden's Cough Drops, and Fletcher's Castoria.

The nineteenth century was midwife to the birth of today's major pharmaceutical houses. Between 1830 and the turn of the twentieth century, the following groups began wholesale production of drugs: Schering and Merck in Germany; Hoffman-LaRoche in Switzerland; Burroughs Wellcome in England; and Abbot, Smith Kline, Parke-Davis, Eli Lilly, Squibb, and Upjohn in the United States. Other important companies such as Bayer (Germany), Ciba-Geigy and Sandoz (Switzerland), and Pfizer (United States) were first founded as producers of organic chemicals during the same time frame, and later moved into the area of pharmaceuticals.[4]

The Twentieth Century

If the nineteenth century was one of creation and growth of the modern pharmaceutical industry, the twentieth century was one of explosion and controversy. Pharmaceuticals became treatments for health promotion as well as treatments for disease. Vaccines were lauded as an example of primary prevention of disease. Immunizations, including the controversies regarding their current use, are discussed in detail in the *Immunizations* chapter.

During the 1900s, it became clear that pharmaceuticals could have adverse effects. Reports of adverse effects, allergic reactions, drug–drug interactions, and resistance to microbes began to populate the literature, especially in the last half of the century. Inadvertent or intentional overdoses involving prescription drugs became infamous because of the deaths of celebrities such as Marilyn Monroe, Elvis Presley, and Michael Jackson. The ready availability of medications with clinically significant **side effects** is a current topic in the pharmaceutical literature and popular press. Combining different agents has become such a common problem, it is referred to by some as **polypharmacy** or **multiple-drug intake (MDI)**.

Thus, it was predictable that regulation of pharmaceuticals came of age in the 1900s. This was the century in which laws were passed in the United States in an attempt to protect the public in a variety of areas.

The United States Food and Drug Administration

In the United States, the regulatory agency whose mission is to protect the public by assuring that drugs, biologic products, medical devices, the national food supply, cosmetics, and products that emit radiation are safe, effective, and secure is the Food and Drug Administration (FDA). The U.S. Federal Food, Drug, and Cosmetic Act was passed in 1938, establishing the FDA as a governmental body regulating all aspects of pharmaceuticals. This act has undergone many modifications ranging from changes in minor rules to major revisions of the act itself, changes that continue today as Congress oversees the work of the FDA.

The origins of the FDA date back to 1906, with the passage of the Pure Food and Drug Act, also known as the Wiley Act. This legislation was designed to provide regulatory oversight to prevent manufacture, sale, and transportation of adulterated, misbranded, or poisonous foods, drugs, medicine, or liquors. In 1938, the Wiley Act was replaced with the Federal Food, Drug, and Cosmetic Act.

The Kefauver-Harris Amendment of 1962 was passed in response to the discovery of the teratogenic effects of thalidomide. This amendment put into place the requirement that drugs show evidence of **safety** and **effectiveness** before being approved for marketing in the United States. Evidence of safety and effectiveness is the essence of the FDA standards today.[5] Drug safety is paramount for the FDA. Included among the myriad activities of the FDA are monitoring drug claims, especially those advertised to consumers; establishing standards for drug testing; and awarding approval for new pharmaceuticals, as well as approval for the prescription medications that companies desire to move to over-the-counter status. The *Drug Toxicity* chapter discusses these activities in more detail.

In 1997, an amendment to the Federal Food, Drug, and Cosmetic Act was passed that established an open website registry that required drugs used for life-threatening conditions to be registered (www.ClinicalTrials.gov) for clinical trials. However, in other ways, the 1997 amendment eased FDA oversight of drugs. Drug approval could be based on one randomized controlled trial (RCT) and confirmatory evidence, a fast-track approval process was established whereby drug approval could be granted based on surrogate endpoints, and pharmaceutical companies were allowed to disseminate information about **off-label uses** of their drugs to healthcare providers.[6] Recent additions to the Federal Food, Drug, and Cosmetic Act include authorization for regulation of bioterrorism agents, requirements for enrollment into **clinical trials**, and expansion of FDA authority to assess postmarketing safety of drugs. This type of assessment is the purview of pharmacoepidemiology—the discipline that provides information about the health and cost outcomes of drugs, devices, and biologics after their approval for clinical use. Pharmacoepidemiology is defined as the study of the use of and effects of drugs in large numbers of people. Pharmacoepidemiology monitors reports of adverse effects, morbidity, or mortality following use of drugs after they are marketed. As a result of such monitoring, some drugs are withdrawn for use after being approved by the FDA.

After the 1999 publication of the Institute of Medicine's *To Err Is Human* report, prevention of **medication errors** took center stage in the efforts to provide safe health care.[7] Experts from many disciplines have promoted strategies that include methods for patient identification when a person is hospitalized; incorporation of "time-outs" during procedures, including those involving anesthesia; promotion of electronic prescribing to decrease the risk of misreading the drug name or the dose on handwritten prescriptions; recommendations to avoid sound-alike **brand names** (Box 1-1); simplification of packaging; and education of individuals so that they know their medications and can personally advocate for the correct administrations.

Box 1-1 High-Risk Sound-Alikes

The most common brand name for fosphenytoin, an antiepileptic drug, is *Cerebyx*. Cerebyx is an example of a drug that is considered to be a high-risk sound-alike due to its similarity to other frequently prescribed agents. Other pharmaceuticals that are similar to Cerebyx include Celebrex, a common brand of celecoxib, a nonsteroidal anti-inflammatory often used as a treatment for arthritis; Celexa (citalopram hydrobromide), an SSRI; and a botanic, huperzine A, now marketed under the brand name of Cerebra and suggested for treatment/prevention of Alzheimer's disease, although data are lacking on effectiveness.

Since these names are so similar, extra caution must be taken when caring for individuals who report taking these agents, as they, too, can become confused about which drug is being used. The FDA has a program within its organization, the Office of Surveillance and Epidemiology, formerly Office of Drug Safety, which periodically conducts meetings and publishes findings to promote clearer and unique naming options in an attempt to decrease accidental medication errors.

Table 1-1 The 2007 Amendments to the Federal Food, Drug, and Cosmetic Act

Amendment Provision	Description
Clinical trial registries expanded to include new drugs	All clinical trials evaluating any drug or biologic or medical device must be registered with www.ClinicalTrials.gov. The information on this website is available to the public, and the drug manufacturer is required to update information about the status of the clinical trial.
Required disclosure of study results	All clinical trials must disclose study results to the registry and results data bank section of www.ClinicalTrials.gov.
Postapproval safety studies may be required	In the past, postapproval studies were voluntary. Now, if the FDA has information about possible safety concerns, the agency can require that a postapproval study be conducted.
Safety labeling changes	The 2007 amendment gives the FDA authority to mandate a change to a drug label that describes safety information.
Risk evaluation and mitigation strategy (REMS)	The FDA may require that a drug manufacturer submit a REMS plan that specifies how a drug will be monitored to determine whether the benefits continue to outweigh the risks as the drug is more widely disseminated.
Technologies to ensure safety in the drug supply chain	The FDA is required to develop standards and methods to identify and validate effective technologies that will ensure the safety of the drug supply chain. These measures are intended to ensure that drugs marketed in the United States are free of contaminates, adulteration, or misbranding.

Abbreviations: FDA = Food and Drug Administration.

In 2006, the Institute of Medicine published a report titled *The Future of Drug Safety*. This report included 25 recommendations for improving the process of overseeing drug development from the preapproval process through postmarketing evaluations and strongly advocated that FDA authority be expanded and strengthened to protect the public from **adverse drug events (ADE)**.[8] Building on this work, the Food and Drug Administration Amendments Act of 2007 (H.R. 3580) expanded the FDA's authority in several ways (Table 1-1).

Today, the FDA has expanded authority to monitor and regulate the safety of marketed drug products by requiring drug manufacturers to conduct postapproval studies or clinical trials if the FDA becomes aware of new safety information. In addition, the FDA can require postapproval changes to drug labels that address safety issues such as the risk for an **adverse drug reaction (ADR)**. The 2007 amendment produced several other major changes in pharmaceutical regulation, including giving the FDA authority to review **direct-to-consumer (DTC)** television advertisements prior to their dissemination; the FDA can now assign civil monetary penalties if such advertisements are determined to be false or misleading. More recent changes have focused on tobacco and the definition of **orphan drugs**.[9] The FDA has been attempting to label tobacco as a drug for purposes of regulation.[8-10]

This new ability to mandate postapproval changes to drug labels is well intended, albeit often difficult to implement. To allow informed decision making, comprehensive information must be available about the benefits and adverse effects of the medication in question. Knowledge of beneficial effects often is more likely to be available than knowledge of adverse effects. Most drug studies use an RCT methodology that is particularly useful to demonstrate if an intervention is beneficial, but RCTs are less useful for identifying rare adverse effects and not all publications report all ADEs.[11,12] RCTs tend to be small in terms of the number of participants; they are also limited to enrollees who are either healthy, as in the case of contraceptive studies, or to those who have a single diagnosis. In addition, they are conducted for a relatively short period of time. In reality, the effects of drugs women use are rarely completely evaluated in RCTs. Therefore, agents may come into the market, only to be removed within a few years as unexpected adverse drug reactions emerge when the drug is used by a larger population, including individuals who have additional disorders or who are taking additional medications. Large observational studies facilitate the identification of adverse drug reactions. Although they do not have the rigor of an RCT, their findings can be combined with the results of RCTs to help providers obtain more complete information about risks and benefits necessary for the person being informed.

The United States Pharmacopeia

The United States Pharmacopeia (USP) works closely with the FDA. The mission of the USP is to establish public standards to assure consumers of the quality, safety, and benefit of medicines and foods through a unique process of public involvement and use of volunteers. Unlike the FDA, which is a federal agency, the USP is a nongovernment, not-for-profit, public health organization. This organization is approximately a century older than the FDA. Indeed, by the end of the 1800s, all state boards of pharmacy had mandated that pharmaceutical companies use the USP standards. USP standards as used when drugs are assessed for purity, potency, and consistency. Although the USP standards are U.S. based, they are recognized and used in more than 100 countries. USP standards are published in the *United States Pharmacopeia—National Formulary* and applied to prescription and over-the-counter medications. Should a dispute arise regarding a drug's purity or identity, the methods found in the USP for evaluation of purity, potency, assay/bioassay, and other properties would be the legally binding ones.

Although the development of standards and the verification of purity and quality are the most well known of USP's activities, this organization engages in several other activities. These additional functions include development of healthcare information that is unbiased about drugs; administration of the Medication Errors Reporting Program (MedMark), an online program for the reporting of medication errors and adverse drug effects; and support of a drug quality and information project to promote international drug safety.

Although the FDA is essential to pharmaceutical regulation and scrutiny, the sheer number of other organizations involved in aspects of drug development, use, and prescription illustrates the complexity involved in the use of pharmaceuticals today. The private sector, as exemplified by pharmaceutical companies and manufacturers of medical goods, is a major stakeholder in this activity. The USP belongs to the public sector, and is a nongovernmental organization. Other governmental bodies intimately involved with drugs in the United States include the Centers for Disease Control and Prevention (CDC), which publishes recommendations for treatments of disorders and diseases; the Drug Enforcement Administration (DEA), which regulates **controlled substances**; the Federal Communications Commission (FCC), which regulates advertising for over-the-counter drugs; and state governments, which control prescriptive authority for providers.

Categories of Drugs

The Naming of Drugs

Every drug has multiple names. Each agent has a **chemical name**, or a precise term describing it. The chemical name often is abbreviated or truncated into the **generic name**. Today, suffixes often are shared with other pharmaceuticals in the same drug category in an attempt to simplify relationships. For example, the names of angiotensin-converting enzyme (ACE) inhibitors used for hypertension tend to end in *pril*, such as captopril and lisinopril. In addition to chemical names and generic names, patented trade names and brand names are used for drugs. These brand names are the ones most frequently remembered by consumers due to advertising and skillful choices in assigning a brand name. For example, some brands specific for women include Evista, Evra, and Sarafem. Sometimes brand names sound alike, which may contribute to consumer confusion. For example, the brand Celebrex is an analgesic, whereas the sound-alike Celexa is an antidepressant. The various categories of drugs include over-the-counter, generic, orphan, and compounded agents.

Over-the-Counter Drugs

As opposed to drugs that require a legal prescription prior to purchase, over-the-counter (OTC) agents are pharmaceuticals that may be purchased by a consumer without a prescription. Originally, prescription drugs were available only at the counters of pharmacies or apothecaries. Over-the-counter drugs, in contrast, were found at the counters of general stores—hence the name. OTC agents are most commonly used for conditions that are considered minor and not an indication for medical consultation. Such products should not have significant adverse effects, need detailed drug monitoring, or have a major risk of addiction. Both OTC and prescription drugs are regulated by the FDA, although advertising of OTC agents is regulated by the FCC rather than the FDA. More than 80 drug categories of OTC agents exist, and millions of dollars are spent on these pharmaceuticals annually.

In the early 1970s, the FDA called together panels of experts to evaluate the OTC agents available at that time.[13] The FDA desired to reassure the public that all OTC drugs were both safe and effective. This was a major undertaking because more than 300,000 products were available as OTC products and the ingredients in them numbered more than 1000. Eventually it was decided that only the ingredients would be assessed. An OTC monograph system was devised so that the drugs determined to be **generally recognized as safe and effective (GRAS/E)** could remain on the market and not need to obtain a **new drug application (NDA)** for the purpose of being submitted to the FDA for approval. Few pharmaceutical companies choose to expend the time and financial commitment associated with filing an NDA. Therefore, most of the OTC products available today are well-established pharmaceuticals. All OTC agents are subject to specific labeling regulations, including requirements governing their names, indications, dosing, **warnings**, and information for healthcare providers.

After a drug has been available by prescription and has an established record of safety, and usually when its patent is about to expire, the manufacturer may seek to obtain permission to move the agent to the OTC market. The last few decades have seen a number of pharmaceuticals that have moved from prescription-only to OTC status. Although the manufacturer ultimately may sell a drug for less money on the OTC market than by prescription, a greater volume of the drug is sold overall when the drug is OTC and has an opportunity to develop a brand following. Antisecretory antihistamines originally used for ulcer treatment and marketed for OTC treatment of heartburn (pyrosis) such as cimetidine (Tagamet) moved from prescription-only status to OTC in 1995. Other popular drugs that are now OTC include nonsedating antihistamines like loratadine (Claritin) and cetirizine hydrochloride (Zyrtec). Discussion has ensued regarding the possibility of more agents being switched, especially statins, because some other countries have already done so or are considering such a change.[9,14,15]

Because of either the length of time on the market and wide availability of the OTC agents or the scrutiny involved with prescription agents before they became OTC, few problems have been noted with OTC drugs. One notable exception was the FDA mandate in 2000 to withdraw phenylpropanolamine (PPA), a common ingredient in both cold remedies and weight loss agents. PPA was found to be associated with hemorrhagic stroke, and this risk is higher in women compared to men. In 2007, manufacturers voluntarily withdrew several OTC cough and cold remedies for infants after the FDA released information about both the ineffectiveness of the agents and the risk of overdose.

Another OTC agent, pseudoephedrine, led to a new variation of OTC drugs—that is, **behind-the-counter (BTC)** drugs. Pseudoephedrine remains an OTC agent. However, this drug can be added to other substances to produce methamphetamine for illicit use. Moving it from an easily accessible open shelf to a location behind the pharmacy counter allows a pharmacist or designee to obtain identification and record each purchase. The intention is that abuse could be tracked, yet consumers who legitimately wish to use the drug can continue to do so.

Generic versus Brand Drugs

Generic drugs are pharmaceuticals that contain the same active ingredients found in an original brand formulation. More than 60% of prescriptions are filled with generic drugs.[16,17] Generics must be demonstrated to be bioequivalent to the brand-name formulation; that is, they must be between 80% and 125% equal in bioavailability. These drugs usually emerge after patent protections for the original brands have expired, usually 7–12 years after first commercial production or 20 years after the first application for FDA consideration. Under the 1984 Drug Price Competition and Patent Term Restoration Act (Hatch-Waxman Act), an applicant desiring to market a generic agent must file an abbreviated new drug application (ANDA) with the FDA. Scientific materials that support the bioequivalence of the generic drug compared to the branded product are presented, and when the ANDA is approved, the **approved drug** is added to the FDA Approved Drug Products list (sometimes called the *Orange Book*) with an annotation to illustrate the equivalency.

In the majority of states, a pharmacist may substitute a generic drug for the equivalent brand-name product. Although generics are bioequivalent, some prescribers choose to note that no substitution is allowed; in such a case, the pharmacist must furnish the brand-name agent. This action is sometimes necessary because, although generic drugs and brand-name agents are bioequivalent, sometimes they have different effects in an individual, secondary to minor changes in product ingredients such as fillers and binders or differences in individual metabolism.

Orphan Drugs

Occasionally there is a relatively rare medical condition (affecting fewer than 200,000 individuals) that can be treated by a pharmaceutical agent. The development and marketing of the drugs used to treat these rare conditions, called orphan drugs, may cost too much for these agents to be of interest to most pharmaceutical houses. Incentives are therefore provided to companies that develop and manufacture orphan drugs, including selected federal grants, as well as a 7-year period of exclusivity for selling the drug in the U.S. market.

Breakthrough Drugs

In 2012, the FDA Safety and Innovation Act was signed into law.[18] This act identified a new category of **breakthrough therapy**, encompassing agents colloquially called **breakthrough drugs**. These medications are used to treat individuals with serious or life-threatening conditions. Breakthrough drugs can be used alone or in combination with one or more other drugs. Some early evidence based on clinically significant metrics that the drug is superior to current therapies is required to warrant this status. The advantage of drugs being classified into this category is that they are awarded an expedited review by the FDA, specifically receiving a decision on their approval within 60 days of the request.

Compounded Drugs

In years past, pharmacists mixed together pharmaceutical compounds instead of filling a prescription with pills sealed in blister packs. The process of mixing a pharmaceutical remedy, especially for a specific individual, is known as **compounding**. Although compounding remains uncommon today, the number of pharmacists practicing compounding appears to be growing. Some of the reasons for this growth are consumers' desire to avoid the inactive ingredients found in pills or creams that may be allergens (e.g., gluten) or to transform solid formulations into more easily swallowed liquids. Another reason for compounding is to produce bioidentical hormones, which are formulations of hormones that have varying potencies.

Compounding pharmacies generally are regulated by local jurisdictions, such as the states in which they are located, rather than by federal authorities. Traditional compounding pharmacies produce agents such as hormone therapy for a specific woman. However, today many compounding pharmacies produce quantities of a single agent such as steroids in sterile injectable forms and legally send them to other states. In 2012, one such pharmacy in the New England area inadvertently disseminated contaminated steroids to multiple sites in several states, which resulted in more than 700 individuals suffering harm and more than 50 persons dying.[19,20] This event fueled the argument that large compounding pharmacies are becoming indistinguishable from pharmaceutical companies, yet by calling themselves a "compounding pharmacy," they can avoid more rigorous FDA regulations. Based on that argument, proponents of tightening oversight of these pharmacies advocate that the compounds they produce should be evaluated in the same way that new drugs are assessed. To date, no regulatory changes regarding compounding pharmacies have been made.

High-Alert Drugs

High-alert drugs are pharmaceuticals associated with significant harm if they are used in error. Agents commonly labeled with this term include anticoagulants, adrenergic agents, chemotherapeutic drugs, and opiates. Oxytocin, for example, is a high-alert drug.[21] Designation of a drug as high alert does not indicate that errors are more likely with the medication; rather, it signals that when such errors occur, the results can be seriously injurious to the individual. Special strategies to reduce the risk of medication errors when high-alert drugs are used have been advocated, including consumer education about the drugs, use of auxiliary labels and electronic alerts, and use of redundancies such as double checks.[22]

Counterfeit Drugs

Counterfeit drugs are illegal agents that may be adulterated, past their expiration date, or mislabeled. Mislabeling includes having less or none of the expected active ingredient and/or having ingredients not listed on the label. Counterfeiting of drugs is a global problem, and one to which the United States is not immune.

Although a large number of medications—both branded and generic agents—have been found to be fake, it is likely that the majority of counterfeit drugs are lifestyle drugs (e.g., Viagra) that are advertised through the Internet. The FDA's Office of Criminal Investigation expends major time and energy attempting to protect the public from these counterfeit drugs, which are often shipped from other countries to the United States. Not only are many of these agents ineffective, but some of them contain harmful ingredients.[23,24]

Designer Drugs

New drugs have been developed to affect specific biologic targets. Some sources call these **designer drugs**, although confusion with this term may exist: In the drug abuse lexicon, the same descriptor is used to designate the combination of a variety of agents to create a new illicit or recreational drug. Designer drugs are toward a specific biologic target where they bind to and inhibit key molecules involved in a disease or pathologic event. For example, the selective estrogen receptor modulator raloxifene (Evista) is chemically similar to tamoxifen citrate (Nolvadex), but does not have the latter's risk for inducing endometrial cancer. Designer drugs are described in more detail in the *Pharmacogenetics* chapter.

Drug Development and Approval

Originally, drugs were developed largely based on empirical observations of the effects purported to occur after ingestion of plant substances. Today, many drugs are derived synthetically. However, drugs can also be formed from constituents of plants or botanicals, animal derivations, and humans, for such agents as insulin. Often new drugs are developed using anecdotal information about the effects of older drugs. Some agents used for one disorder have been found to have side effects that are advantageous when those drugs are used as a treatment for another disorder. For example, antihistamines are FDA approved for treatment of motion sickness or insomnia, not because of their basic therapeutic effect to treat allergic reactions but because of their side effect as antinausea agents. Similarly, the drug terbutaline (Brethine) was originally developed as a treatment for asthma, but is also used as a uterine tocolytic because it interferes with uterine contractility.

Drug testing and approval are regulated at the federal level.[25] Figure 1-1 provides a visual overview of this process. The FDA has several centers, including the Center for Drug Evaluation and Research (CDER); it is through CDER that the FDA regulates the drug testing and approval processes. The following is a general description of how a new drug is studied, although some exceptions may occur.

An **investigational new drug (IND)** application is a legal method by which federal approval may be obtained to transport pharmaceuticals or medical devices to areas in which they may be used in clinical trials. Optimally, clinical trials are randomized, double blinded, and placebo controlled. Upon completion of the trials, the study results may be presented to the FDA in an NDA form with a request for approval. In the past, there has been criticism that companies might undertake multiple clinical trials to study one drug and release data only from those that successfully demonstrated effectiveness or safety. Today, clinical trials have to be registered with the FDA before data are obtained in an attempt to promote transparency.

Clinical Drug Trials

Several distinct phases of clinical testing are required for any NDA. Phase 1 trials are designed to determine the basic pharmacokinetics (i.e., how the drug behaves in the body with regard to absorption, metabolism, and excretion) of the new drug. When established drugs are being proposed for new indications, previous studies may be used for this purpose. Animal testing and in vitro models are still in active use. However, computer modeling and other technological modalities for evaluating the metabolism or toxicity of a drug have also been developed. Application of genomics, proteomics (the study of the structure and functions of proteins), and computational approaches now allow scientists to predict the metabolites of molecules. These techniques enable the drug developer to more accurately predict the pharmacodynamic (i.e., how the body responds to the drug with regard to duration of exposure and drug dose) activity of the drug and its metabolites, and integrate these predictions with human cell signaling and metabolic processes and networks. Toxicogenomic data can be included in this process.[26]

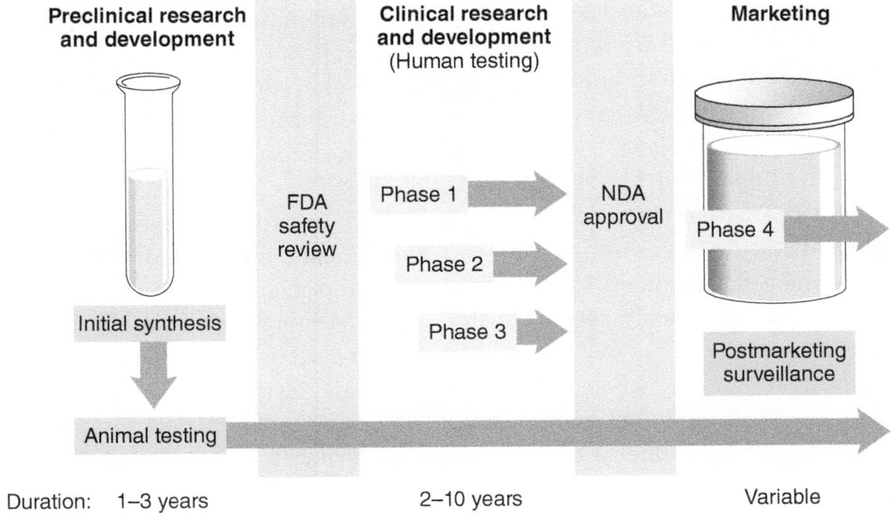

Figure 1-1 Steps required by the FDA for reviewing a new drug.

Source: Hanson GR, Venturelli PJ, Fleckenstein AE. *Drugs and Society.* 11th ed. Burlington, MA: Jones & Bartlett; 2012.[13]

Once a promising pharmaceutical agent has been identified, its toxic and therapeutic doses are determined.[27] Animal testing initially is performed to evaluate drug safety, including determination of the dose range that results in adverse or toxic side effects. Animal testing protocols typically use two or more species in an attempt to control for interspecies differences in pharmacokinetics. Animal testing is undertaken to determine the doses used in preliminary human testing, and its results may be described in the drug product labeling or human trial documents. Unfortunately, cross-species pharmacokinetics are not consistent, and the results of animal testing are not always predictive of human response to a pharmaceutical agent.

Dose–response relationships describe the required dose and frequency of dosing based on the therapeutic index for a drug in a specific population (such as pregnant women, neonates, or nonpregnant reproductive-age women). The therapeutic index is the dose range between the minimum therapeutic dose and the dose that initiates a toxic dose. Identification of the therapeutic index determines the potential therapeutic value and safety of a drug. Increasing the dose of a drug with a narrow therapeutic index (e.g., theophylline [Theo-Dur]) increases the probability of drug toxicity. Factors such as body mass index, metabolic rates, and genetics may all affect the therapeutic index for an individual.

Phase 1 clinical trials seek to determine the distribution, metabolism, and pharmacologic actions of drugs in humans; to determine the side effects associated with increasing doses; and to evaluate for evidence of effectiveness. Human participants are healthy individuals, usually adults of average weight and without chronic diseases. Persons younger than 18 years are excluded from most trials except those that are pediatric focused—a limitation for contraceptive studies because women in this age range frequently need and use contraceptive products.

Phase 2 clinical trials are conducted to evaluate the effectiveness of the drug for a particular indication or indications among individuals with the disease or condition under study, and to determine the common short-term side effects and risks. These studies usually have a small number of participants.

Phase 3 trials are undertaken after the smaller Phase 2 studies indicate the drug may be effective. Larger numbers of participants are involved in Phase 3 clinical trials, and risks and benefits are established through such studies. The basic information needed for drug labeling is determined during Phase 3. Collectively, Phases 1–3 are called preapproval studies.

Phase 4 trials are known as postmarketing studies. No matter how rigorous the Phase 1–3 studies are, wide postmarketing may reveal unexpected results. Untoward events or responses identified during the drug preapproval process are considered adverse drug reactions (a type of adverse drug event) when there is a reasonable possibility of association between the adverse event and the pharmaceutical agent. More recently, there has been an emphasis on the postmarking period because adverse events are more likely to be found in larger populations and within a real-life environment. For example, if a Phase 3 trial included 3000 participants, but a major adverse drug reaction associated with the drug occurs only once in 10,000 individuals, postmarketing may be the only venue in which this drug effect will be revealed. Also, drug–drug interactions may be first identified in postmarketing studies that include individuals who are taking other drugs as well as the one being evaluated. The 2007 FDA Amendment Act mandated increased reporting of drug adverse effects, and it is anticipated that additional attention will be paid to this area in the future. The *Drug Toxicity* chapter provides more detailed information on adverse drug reactions and events.

Regulation of Approved Pharmaceuticals

Legal Requirements for the Package Insert (Label)

Package inserts were first standardized in the late 1960s. One of the first package inserts written was for combination oral contraceptives, in which specific risks and benefits were required to be included. The FDA determines which information is to be provided in the package insert, and on occasion will mandate changes based on newer studies.

Although there is a standard format for the package insert, some manufacturers deviate from it slightly, such as by replacing some of the titles with lower-literacy versions. Among the required components are the brand and generic names of the drug; description of chemical structure, formulation, route of administration, and inactive ingredients; clinical pharmacology, usually containing a synopsis of the clinical trials; approved indications; **contraindications**; warnings, including serious side effects; **precautions**, especially for drug–drug interactions; adverse drug reactions, including those that might be considered minor side-effects; drug abuse and dependency potential;

overdose potential; recommended dose; and how the agent is supplied, including constraints for storage. Since 2006, package inserts also must include "Highlights," a section that summarizes risks and benefits; a table of contents; the date of initial approval; and contact information (web address and toll-free telephone number) to promote easier reporting of adverse effects.[28,29]

FDA Contraindications, Precautions, Warnings, and Other Actions

Precautions may appear on package inserts and are distinct from contraindications. A contraindication specifies who should not take the drug. Persons who are allergic to a drug have a contraindication to its use because adverse reactions are likely. However, precautions indicate that specific individuals who may be at a higher risk for an adverse drug reaction than the general population should use the drug carefully. For example, the transdermal contraceptive patch, marketed as Ortho Evra, has a precaution for women who weigh more than 90 kg (198 pounds).[30] This precaution exists because there is evidence that contraception is less effective among women who have a higher body mass index (BMI), although the strength of this association is difficult to assess from the original studies, because participation was limited to women who were of a healthy weight or at least no more than 35% heavier than the optimal weight. Therefore, currently data are not strong enough to mandate labeling weight of 90 kg or more a contraindication, but the precaution is included, which means the provider should review the evidence with a woman who weighs more than 90 kg and is considering using the contraceptive transdermal patch.

FDA warnings notify prescribers and the public about adverse effects that may be adverse drug reactions. After a drug is approved and marketed, the FDA continues to have a role in monitoring use of the drug. The manufacturer is legally required to review and report any adverse drug reaction to the FDA that is reported to the company. Unexpected serious reactions are to be reported within 15 days; other reactions may be reported on a quarterly basis as long as the drug is marketed. The FDA also solicits direct reports from consumers and providers through a program called MedWatch. This system includes an online voluntary reporting form, which can be completed on the FDA website. Based on reports received, the FDA may choose to issue a warning and require that it be added to or substituted for the existing package insert warnings. When warnings are issued, they are placed on the FDA website and publicized through press releases; they may also be explained in letters directly sent to prescribers and included in the package inserts.

On a postmarketing basis, drugs are used in real-life situations that include the possibility of potential drug–drug, drug–food, or drug–herb interactions.[31] Additional unexpected hazards may become evident via more research using the drug or via reports of adverse drug reactions noted by consumers. For example, in 1999, Merck and Company received approval to market rofecoxib (Vioxx), a nonsteroidal anti-inflammatory drug (NSAID). This agent did not induce gastrointestinal irritation, a side effect common with the other NSAIDs available at the time, but subsequent studies suggested rofecoxib was associated with an increased risk of heart attacks and strokes.[32] A flurry of editorials were published questioning details about the original clinical trials. One trial in particular, sponsored by Merck, was conducted with the intention of assessing rofecoxib (Vioxx) for the additional indication of prevention of colorectal polyps, but it was terminated prematurely when it became apparent that the relative risk for myocardial infarction and stroke was increased almost 100% among individuals using rofecoxib compared to those taking the placebo (relative risk [RR] = 1.92; 95% CI, 1.19–3.11; $P = .008$).[32] Although the FDA was in discussion with the manufacturer about the implications of these findings, Merck withdrew the drug from the marketplace, making any potential FDA warnings moot.

When a prescription drug is found to be associated with serious adverse reactions, including life-threatening risks, the FDA can issue its strongest warning, known as a **black box warning**. A black box warning is so named because a black border surrounds the text of the warning in both the package insert and on the FDA website/publications. An example of a black box warning is the one mandated by the FDA for medroxyprogesterone acetate in oil (Depo-Provera). In 2004, a black box warning was added to the label for this contraceptive agent, advising women and providers that there were sufficient data to identify a relationship between prolonged use of the drug and loss of bone density. The new recommendation contained within the black box stated that women should not use the agent for more than 2 years continuously unless other contraceptive methods were inadequate.

The most severe action that the FDA can take is to issue a **drug recall** order. Drug recalls or withdrawals from the market are almost exclusively secondary to the drug being determined to be unsafe; these removals can be either voluntary or mandatory.[33] A report in 2001 by the

U.S. General Accounting Office noted that the majority of drugs withdrawn between 1997 and 2001 had more pronounced adverse effects for women than men.[34] Some drugs may be withdrawn from the U.S. market, yet remain available in other countries.

Regulation of Direct-to-Consumer Advertising

Prior to 1997, the vast majority of pharmaceutical marketing in the United States consisted of educating healthcare professionals directly through visits by pharmaceutical representatives and exhibits at conferences, or indirectly through advertisements in journals. However, controversies about marketing existed even at that time. A 1992 study carried out by a group of experts using the FDA criteria of the time evaluated more than 100 drug ads and found that more than 40% contained misleading claims and 44% were deemed inadequate to be the sole source of information.[35]

Direct-to-consumer advertisements are often seen today. They are required to follow recently established FDA criteria because this federal agency has regulatory power over the content of advertising that addresses prescription drugs. Three types of DTC advertisements are allowed. The most common type is product claim advertisements, which include the drug's brand name, indications, risks, and benefits. This type of DTC must conform to FDA criteria. Help-seeking advertisements discuss the condition but do not name any particular drug and, therefore, are not regulated by the FDA. The third type, reminder advertisements simply list the brand name, dose, or cost. Because they do not make claims or discuss indications, such ads are also exempt from FDA regulation. Advertising for over-the-counter drugs is under the purview of the Federal Trade Commission.

DTC advertising initially was advocated as an attempt to better educate consumers and ultimately promote appropriate use of medications among consumers. A review of a decade of such advertising found that DTC communications were firmly entrenched in U.S. media, with the average American seeing an estimated 16 hours of these ads every year just on television.[36] Unfortunately, DTC advertising is also associated with problems such as overuse of medications, medicalization of common discomforts, and expenditures of more than $40 billion annually.[37] Over the years, the FDA has required selected ads to be withdrawn. For example, the manufacturer of terbinafine (Lamisil) had to change one of its ads that implied the drug was always a totally successful treatment for nail infection.

Prescriptive Authority

During the 1900s, **prescriptive authority** was afforded by law to physicians, veterinarians, dentists, and podiatrists in all states, and pharmacists were authorized to fill prescriptions and dispense drugs. In the last few decades, physician assistants, certified nurse-midwives, certified midwives, nurses in advanced practice, and psychologists have received full or limited prescriptive authority in most states. In addition, some other classes of prescribers have emerged. Pharmacists have presented claims that they can be safe prescribers and should be integral members of the healthcare team. The burgeoning array of psychoactive agents has led to some governmental agencies recognizing psychologists and other mental health professionals as prescribers.

Prescriptive authority is regulated by the state in which the prescriber works. Although physicians have no limits on the types of prescriptions that they can write, the prescriptive authority for other providers—such as podiatrists, certified nurse-midwives, and certified midwives—usually is limited to that person's professional scopes of practice. In some states, the prescriptive authority is delegated, indicating the authority is held by a prescribing physician and delegated to others, often a limited number of healthcare professionals.

Discussion has occurred regarding the state-based approach to prescriptive authority.[39] In the mid-1900s, it was logical to assume that a written prescription would be hand-carried to the local pharmacy, where it was filled. Today, it is common for a prescriber to electronically transmit a new prescription to a pharmacy, even if the pharmacy is just a few blocks away. That pharmacy, however, is likely to be a branch of a large conglomerate whose span of operations stretches across several states. Although the prescriber is authorized in one state, the individual may pick up the medication at a pharmacy branch located in another state. Moreover, the role of Internet-based pharmacies has raised legal issues regarding prescribing authority. U.S. pharmacies can operate online assuming the drugs they are dispensing are FDA approved and a legal prescription is available. Other Internet pharmacies are based outside the United States; they may not require a prescription and may illegally mail pharmaceuticals, including those that are not FDA approved, to individuals in the United States. Under these circumstances, such transport of drugs is considered illegal. These issues add to the debate about whether it is time for a federal prescriptive authority to be developed.

Regulation of Controlled Substances

Controlled substances are drugs, both opiates and nonopiates, that have a high risk of addiction. Controlled substances are regulated by the Drug and Enforcement Administration (DEA) of the U.S. federal government. These agents generally are categorized according to schedules (Table 1-2).[25] Prescribers of controlled substances must have legal state authority to prescribe and must obtain an identification number from the DEA for this purpose. Originally, prescribers were provided DEA numbers that began with the letter A; those numbers have been exhausted, so that now most of these identifiers start with the letter B. It is anticipated that the letter C will be used as the prefix in the near future. For physician assistants, nurses in advanced practice, midwives, and others, the DEA number begins with the letter M. The types of drugs that these healthcare professionals prescribe may be limited by a state according to state-devised schedules. A complex system to generate unique DEA numbers was developed in an attempt to identify forged prescriptions for controlled substances, but the equation can now be found on the Internet, and busy pharmacists have little time to do the necessary calculations. Nevertheless, this system persists.[39]

Table 1-2 Schedules for Controlled Substances

Schedule	Description	Example
I	The drug or other substance has a high potential for abuse. The drug or other substance has no currently accepted use in treatment in the United States. There is lack of accepted safety for use of the drugs or other substance under medical supervision.	Heroin
II	The drug or other substance has a high potential for abuse. The drug or other substance has a currently accepted medical use in treatment in the United States. Abuse of the drug or other substance may lead to severe psychological or physical dependence.	Methadone, morphine
III	The drug or other substance has less potential for abuse than the drugs or other substances in Schedules I and II. The drug or other substance has a currently accepted medical use in treatment in the United States. Abuse of the drug or other substance may lead to moderate or low physical dependence or high psychological dependence.	Products with < 90 mg of codeine per dose unit (Tylenol with codeine [Vicodin])
IV	The drug or other substance has a low potential for abuse relative to the drugs or other substances in Schedule III. The drug or other substance has a currently accepted medical use in treatment in the United States. Abuse of the drug or other substance may lead to limited physical dependence or psychological dependence relative to the drugs or other substances in Schedule III.	Phenobarbital (Luminal)
V	The drug or other substance has a low potential for abuse relative to the drugs or other substances in Schedule IV. The drug or other substance has a currently accepted medical use in treatment in the United States. Abuse of the drug or other substance may lead to limited physical dependence or psychological dependence relative to the drugs or other substances in Schedule IV.	Cough preparation containing < 200 mg of codeine per 100 mL or 100 g (Robitussin AC)

Source: United States Public Law, Title 21, Code of Federal Regulations (CFR) Part 1300 to 21 CFR §1308.[25]

The Role of the Pharmacist

During the Middle Ages, the role of the apothecary was well established. Such a healthcare professional was the forerunner of today's pharmacist. Apothecaries received prescriptions and filled them with the appropriate remedy. Many of the treatments required compounding. In turn, these providers developed the apothecary system of weights and measures, including the use of drams, scruples, and other terms that have since been largely replaced by the metric system. As their role evolved, most apothecaries entered the profession with a background in chemistry; hence they were sometimes called dispensing chemists.

To be legally recognized as a pharmacist in the United States today, an individual must have graduated from a recognized program and received a doctor of pharmacology (Pharm D) degree. Pharmacists increasingly work collaboratively in hospital settings and in some areas have received or are attempting to obtain a degree of prescriptive authority. Pharmacists fill prescriptions, **dispense** (or **furnish**) the drugs, and counsel the individuals obtaining the agent. Counseling is an important aspect of the pharmacist's role today; it includes advising individuals taking either prescription or nonprescription drugs or both, particularly regarding the way to safely take the agent(s), signs and symptoms of therapeutic as well as adverse effects, and the emerging body of evidence on drug–drug, drug–food, and/or drug–herb interactions.

The Cost of Drugs in Modern Society

The study of the costs and consequences of drug therapy for healthcare systems and society is called **pharmacoeconomics**. Development and marketing of a new drug is a complex and expensive process that generally requires years of research and development. Approximately 25 novel drugs are introduced each year, but not all are profitable. All manufacturers seek a blockbuster drug, or an agent that generates more than $1 billion in annual revenues. Pfizer had such an agent with its brand of atorvastatin (Lipitor): This pharmaceutical agent amassed more than $130 billion in revenues in the 14 years before its patent expired in 2011.[40]

Law described the use of pharmaceuticals in the modern world as part of the medicalization of society, or the belief that any condition, trivial or serious, can and should be treated with a drug instead of other interventions, especially nutrition and exercise.[41] In the United States, the cost of prescription and nonprescription drugs has increased substantially over the last 2 decades. Today, the United States is the largest market in the world for prescription drugs, accounting for as much as 75% of sales of the most popular agents and with 1 in 4 individuals using prescription agents.[42] The cost of drugs directly influences the fact that healthcare expenditures rise by more than 5% each year—a rate higher than inflation.[43]

The Role of Health Insurance Plans

Healthcare insurance also affects the marketing and use of pharmaceuticals. The first modern major U.S. commercial health plan was developed for teachers; it guaranteed hospital coverage and used a blue cross as its symbol—hence the Blue Cross plan for hospital-only insurance. Blue Shield plans emerged later to cover services delivered by physicians, and some of the hospital and physician coverage plans eventually merged to form combined Blue Cross Blue Shield plans.

Health insurance was primarily purchased by individuals until strict federal wage guidelines were put into place during World War II. At that time, it was determined that employers could use fringe benefits such as health insurance to attract employees (in lieu of offering higher wages), and such plans eventually became common elements in employee benefits packages. In the United States today, the majority of adults younger than 65 years have employer-sponsored health insurance, although that may change as healthcare exchanges become more widely available.[45]

Over the decades, healthcare coverage has expanded from catastrophic hospital care to include preventive care, ambulatory services, and, more recently, drug benefits. Drug benefits were added by commercial insurers in an attempt to curtail costs and add benefits for their subscribers. It has been estimated that in 1960, more than 95% of pharmaceuticals were paid for by individuals, whereas 30 years later, the majority were paid for by insurance plans; that share has increased with the expansion of Medicare coverage to include a drug benefit.[46]

Formularies

One popular method used by insurers to control pharmaceutical costs is a **formulary**. In the United States, each healthcare plan may have a different formulary, or list of drugs that it pays for. Often, pharmaceutical companies have negotiated favorable charges for drugs directly with the insurer in exchange for having their products listed on the formulary.

Some formularies are separated into cost-sharing tiers. When this arrangement is used, the top tier is usually composed of generic agents that are totally paid for by the insurer, without a consumer copayment being required. The other tiers contain more expensive agents and may require varying levels of copayments from the consumer. Some drugs may not be eligible for any reimbursement by the health insurance plan. A closed formulary allows only those drugs on the list to be prescribed and paid for by the insurer without an appeals process. In contrast, an open formulary places no limitations on which drugs the prescriber can chose to order.

Like traditional health insurance plans, Medicare and Medicaid as well as some large public or academic facilities attempt to control costs through the use of closed formularies. However, as an unintended consequence, it has been found that requiring copayments may decrease the use of medications, especially by individuals who have chronic conditions and who face high copayment charges for multiple medications.[47]

Medicare and Medicaid

Medicare and Medicaid are public insurance programs funded by either the federal government or a combination of the state and federal governments. Medicare primarily covers elderly individuals, while Medicaid is primarily geared toward insuring persons who demonstrate that they cannot pay for healthcare costs or obtain healthcare insurance. Medicare is completely a federal program; Medicaid is state managed.

A Medicare prescription drug plan (Medicare Part D) was enacted in 2003 and implemented in 2006. Private insurance companies, which in turn are reimbursed by the federal government, administer Medicare Part D. Approximately 2000 unique Part D plans exist, although numbers and types vary regionally. Concerns have been made about the complexity of this system, but early data suggest that Part D may decrease the numbers of individuals who forgo needed medications in an effort to save money.[48,49]

Under the Medicaid program, individuals usually are not assessed a copayment if the drug is Medicaid approved. Over-the-counter agents are not reimbursed for persons on Medicaid, although the generic equivalent written as a prescription may be covered.

Marketing Drugs

In recent years, the marketing of various pharmaceuticals to healthcare providers has provoked strong criticism. Some physicians have been given financial gifts in recognition of their willingness to prescribe specific drugs—a situation that creates a conflict of interest. In response to this phenomenon, a nonprofit group, No Free Lunch, was developed to encourage prescribers to be wary of marketing strategies from pharmaceutical groups that include free samples of drugs, drug-labeled paraphernalia, continuing education, and food.

In response to criticism of how brand-name drugs are marketed, the Pharmaceutical Research and Manufacturers of America (PhRMA) released a marketing guidance code.[50] For example, even pens and pads emblazoned with the names of the drugs are to be strictly limited or stopped; dinners or other activities for prescribers and family members are curtailed; and independent continuing education sponsored by pharmaceutical companies is supposed to be promoted separately from drug marketing. It remains to be seen how these changes will influence the prescribing habits of healthcare providers.

Drug Samples

Samples of pharmaceutical agents, usually prescription drugs, are commonly found in ambulatory facilities. Healthcare providers should be aware of whether they are legally allowed to dispense these samples. Although some professionals claim that sampling allows medically uninsured populations an alternative path to obtain access to necessary agents, studies have found that sampling is a method of marketing, encouraging individuals to continue on a specific pharmaceutical for the course of the condition or disease.[51]

Special Populations

Clinical Trials and Women

Until the 1990s, women of childbearing age frequently were excluded from clinical drug trials due to their potential for pregnancy and the related risk of inadvertent exposure of a fetus to the investigational drug. The disadvantage of this exclusion is that it means even commonly prescribed drugs may never have been evaluated for gender-related adverse effects or appropriate dosing for women. Yet, statistically, women have a higher incidence of adverse drug reactions than do men.[52-54]

Since the 1991 inception of the U.S. Office of Women's Health, researchers have been encouraged to include women as participants in clinical drug trials and to analyze trial data by gender. Inclusion of women as participants in clinical trials offers researchers the opportunity to evaluate gender-related differences that influence disease prevalence, presentation, and response to pharmacologic therapy. Analysis of these differences can provide insight into the biologic processes that contribute to these gender differences, and understanding these differences may lead to new directions in future research.

Pregnancy and the FDA

In 1980, the FDA published a description of five categories that ranked the risk of teratogenic effects of pharmaceutical agents to be used in drug labeling.[55] This list of five discrete **pregnancy categories**, A, B, C, D, and X, was unique to the United States. Other countries use a narrative approach to describe information available about use of drugs in pregnancy. Contrary to popular belief, the FDA did not assign specific drugs to these categories. Instead, the manufacturer reviewed the FDA categories and assigned a pregnancy category letter to the drugs marketed by that manufacturer.

The FDA Pregnancy Categories had several problems. Category C was the most problematic because it actually represented two separate concepts. An agent could be placed in Category C because there have been reports of teratogenicity in animals. For example, glucocorticosteroids were placed into this category because rabbits demonstrated embryotoxic and fetotoxic effects after exposure to these drugs, although no such findings have been reported in humans. However, a far more common reason than animal teratogenicity for classifying an agent into Category C is the second concept—namely, lack of information about the drug's effects. Most drugs were placed into Category C for this reason, and it is because of this vagueness that the categorization system was problematic.

The categories could also mislead healthcare providers because teratogenic risk does not necessarily increase as the categories move from A to X. Pregnancy Categories C, D, and X are based on risks weighed against benefits, which means a particular drug labeled Category C may carry the same risks as a drug labeled Category X, yet have a C classification because it has more benefits. Category X was reserved for the few agents that are known teratogens for which alternative nonteratogenic agents exist. Acne is an example of a condition that is not life threatening, but the retinoids used to treat acne can cause lifelong congenital effects to the intrauterine conceptus and so should never be taken by pregnant women.

In 2008, a new system for the pregnancy and lactation section of drug labeling was proposed and in 2014, the FDA released a final amendment to the regulations governing content and format of the "Pregnancy" and "Nursing Mothers" subsections of the "Use in Specific Populations" section of labeling prescription drugs.[56] This rule requires removal of the letter pregnancy categories. The package inserts will now include three separate sections that provide information in a narrative format: "Pregnancy," "Lactation," and "Females and Males of Reproductive Potential." Table 1-3 summarizes the new FDA labeling.

The goal of the new labeling is to provide information that will support counseling and the transfer of knowledge about the drug to the consumer.

Table 1-3 2014 Changes to FDA Drug Labeling for Pregnancy and Lactation

Category	Required Content
Pregnancy	***Pregnancy Registry subheading***: Existence of any pregnancy registries and contact information and instructions for how to enroll in pregnancy registries. ***Risk Summary subheading***: If the drug is absorbed systemically, content will include a summary of the risk for all developmental outcomes, using all available animal and human data. A statement that articulates the background risk will be included. ***Clinical Considerations subheading***: May also include dose adjustments for pregnancy, maternal adverse reactions, fetal adverse reactions, and the effect of the drug during labor and birth. ***Data subheading:*** Study type, exposure information (dose, duration, timing), fetal or neonatal adverse effects, number of subjects, and duration of study.
Lactation	***Risk Summary subheading:*** If the drug is absorbed systemically, the content will include data about the presence of the drug in human milk to the extent this information is available, effects of the drug on the breastfed child, and effects on breast milk production. ***Clinical Considerations subheading:*** Ways to minimize drug exposure in the breastfed child and information about monitoring or mitigating adverse reactions. The summary will include a risk and benefit statement. ***Data subheading:*** Study type, exposure information (dose, duration, timing), fetal or neonatal adverse effects, number of subjects and duration of study.
Females and Males of Reproductive Potential	This section is not required if none of the subheadings are applicable. When pregnancy testing or contraception are required or recommended before, during, or after drug therapy, or when there are human or animal data that suggest the drug has associated fertility effects, this information will be presented in subheadings "Pregnancy testing," "Contraception," and "Infertility."

Source: Modified from Food and Drug Administration. *Federal Regist.* 2014;79(233):72064-72103.[56]

Clinical Trials and the Elderly

Current rules regarding clinical drug trials necessitate that the published reports include the demographic characteristics of the subjects, including age, gender, and racial/ethnic backgrounds. Clearly, age is a major factor that must be involved in analysis because older individuals are more likely than younger persons to have a history of previous exposures to pharmaceuticals, multiple pathologic conditions, biologic variations in pharmacokinetics, and use of other agents (i.e., to be a polypharmacy user). Polypharmacy includes over-the-counter and herbal/botanical formulations. Use of multiple agents increases the risk of drug–drug, drug–herb, and drug–food interactions. Therefore, the elderly are not restricted from participation in clinical trials; indeed, they should be encouraged to enroll in such studies.

Rational Prescribing

Due to the complexity and seriousness involved in prescribing the appropriate agent for an individual, a rational approach has been advocated.[6,57] Several definitions exist for rational prescribing, as well as various examples. In general, rational prescribing includes four goals: (1) maximizing effectiveness of an agent; (2) minimizing side effects and risks; (3) customizing the agent for an individual; and (4) minimizing cost.[47,58]

Customization includes consideration of an individual's lifestyle, insurance drug benefits (if any), and desires. For example, use of an injectable pharmaceutical may be a problem for a woman with severe arthritis in her hands. When prescribing a statin for a mature woman, it would be wise to ask if her partner is also taking a statin. If so, the prescriber should consider prescribing the same drug for the woman under the assumption that the couple may share these medications, even though all individuals are warned not to do so. The two individuals also may share knowledge about the drug and be more likely to remember the name and dosing if they take the same agent.

In addition to seeking the most inexpensive sales outlet for the agent and using drug benefits if available, a few other practical options exist that clinicians may employ to help individuals save money. Often a tablet containing twice the dose does not cost twice as much; that is, the provider may be able to educate an individual on how to split a tablet. This action is not possible for capsules, extended-release agents, or some other formulations. For those individuals with chronic conditions, a prescription for 90 days generally is less costly than three 30-day refills, and it often carries a lower payment for persons with drug benefits. When drugs move from prescription to over-the-counter status, it may be less expensive for the individual to maintain a prescription for the first few years when the manufacturer has no OTC generic option available, even though ultimately there is evidence that OTC switching can save the public money.[43] Lastly, individuals should be counseled to continue medications such as antimicrobials until the prescription is finished, and to be aware of when therapies may no longer be warranted so that they do not have to pay for refills of unnecessary drugs.

The prescriber should keep in mind that rational prescribing is PERSON centered. The acronym PERSON denotes pragmatics, effectiveness, route/dose, safety, options, and needs/desires. *Pragmatics* applies, for example, when prescribing a statin that is already used in the home. Homeless individuals have no access to refrigerators, so prescribing a drug for such a person with diabetes that requires a low temperature for storage is irrational. *Effectiveness* is essential. If an agent is not effective, then it should not be prescribed at all. The effect desired should be considered as well: Is the drug meant to be curative, to be prophylactic, or simply to reduce symptoms or act palliatively? Likewise, *route* and *dose* need to be considered. Some individuals are unable to swallow, for example, so they need transdermal, topical, or parental formulations.

Safety, like effectiveness, is an essential consideration. The potential adverse effects and contraindications must be weighed against the disease condition, whether present or potential. Medications for women in special populations (e.g., pregnancy and lactation) should be carefully considered. Interactions between the agent and other drugs, herbs, or foods need to be addressed. *Options* include consideration of other pharmaceutical agents as well as nonpharmaceutical therapies such as exercise and nutrition. Less costly generics should be considered if possible. Knowledge of the marketplace enables a prescriber to know when it is less expensive to prescribe a generic drug than an OTC agent, or to appreciate when agents are covered by drug benefits. *Needs and desires* of the individual also should be considered. Some women will accept a prescription for a suppository but never fill it because of personal distaste for the application procedure. A woman may request a scopolamine patch in preparation for a planned cruise or prefer a certain kind of packaging for ease of use.

Monitoring is an important additional component in rational prescribing. The response of the individual helps determine future treatments. For example, optimally a drug should result in a positive therapeutic response. However, adverse effects may dictate a modification of the drug regimen, and toxic effects may require its complete discontinuation.

Irrational prescribing is never intended, yet it often occurs because the U.S. healthcare system is both complex and overburdened. Currently, interprofessional education is advocated as a method of promoting rational prescribing for all providers.[59] Intentional engagement of the goals and approaches to rational prescribing is of value to modern society as a whole.

How to Write a Prescription

A standard prescription contains several components. It should include the name, credentials, and contact information for the prescriber; the name and identifying information for the person for whom the prescription is written; the superscription or Rx insignia (derived from an abbreviation for the Latin words meaning "recipe" or "take"); the inscription or generic name of the drug with dose; the subscription or directions to the individual filling the prescription; the signature (from the Latin *signetur*, meaning "let it be labeled"), which details how the person for whom the drug is intended should use it; and the signed name of the authorized prescriber. Today, it is recommended that all prescriptions are written in English with no or minimal abbreviations. In particular, most Latin abbreviations should be avoided, as they often can be misinterpreted. For example, "qod" indicates every other day, but can be misread as "qid," resulting in eight administrations over a 48-hour period (as opposed to one administration over the same period). Some abbreviations exist in common usage and may continue to be seen, including in texts. These standard abbreviations include "po" (oral administration or by mouth); "bid," "tid," and "qid" (twice daily or three or four times daily, respectively); "prn" (as needed); as well as metric abbreviations such as "mg" and "mL" for milligrams and milliliters, respectively. Many facilities commonly maintain a list of acceptable abbreviations for charting as well as prescriptions. Box 1-2 lists recommendations to decrease medication errors when writing a prescription, and Figure 1-2 illustrates the components of a prescription.

Reduction of Medication Errors

In 1999, the U.S. Institute of Medicine released a study that estimated more than 90,000 individuals die in hospitals annually due to errors in the delivery of care.[7] Among these errors are many that are associated with pharmaceuticals, which are termed medication errors.

Although adverse effects have been estimated to occur with fewer than 0.5% of medication orders in hospitals, more than one-fourth of those that do occur are considered preventable.[7] Rates of adverse drug events in ambulatory facilities may even be higher. A suggested intervention to decrease medication errors is to use computerized ordering or electronic charting. Illegibility of a handwritten prescription increases the risk of a person receiving the wrong drug or dose. Electronic prescribing (e-prescribing) was recognized as a desirable goal in the 2003 Medicare Prescription Drug Improvement and Modernization Act, but rates of its implementation remain low.[60] The FDA has recognized that a myriad number of mobile apps exist, many of which provide information useful in avoiding medication errors, such as

Mary Breckinridge, CNM Certified Nurse-Midwife UCSF Women's Health UC # 54321 NPF: 1234-789	Kate Smith, MD Obstetrician/Gynecologist UCSF Women's Health BNDD No. AS345678 CA Lic. No. F28765

Name: Jenny Jones   Age: 24

Address: 326 Orange Vale Road, Fair Oaks, CA   Date: 8-24-15

℞ Metronidazole 500 mg tablets
sig: twice daily for 7 (seven) days
disp: 14 (fourteen)

Indication: Bacterial vaginosis

Refills: ⓪ 1 2 3 4 5

Allergies: None

Dispense as written ☐

Label: English ☒ Spanish ☐ Other ________

Mary Breckinridge
Signature

Figure 1-2 Sample prescription.

Box 1-2 Recommendations to Decrease Medication Errors When Writing a Prescription

Dos

Include numbers as both words and numerals (e.g., 60 [sixty] tablets).

Ensure clear writing, print in ink, or type the prescription.

Check for correct spelling (especially in an era of drugs with similar names).

Use English whenever possible instead of Latin.

State specific times (e.g., 8 A.M.) if possible.

Use a standard format, especially on preprinted blanks.

Use the most common formulation (e.g., 500 mg instead of 0.5 g).

Include a zero prefix with decimals less than 1 (e.g., 0.5 mg).

Use the abbreviation "mL" instead of "cc" because "mL" is less likely to be misread.

Don'ts

Do not use trailing zeros in decimals (e.g., 5.00).

Avoid unusual measurements such as teaspoons, tablespoons, pints, ounces, drams, grains, and minims.

Minimize vagueness (e.g., "prn"—at minimum, write "as needed for pain").

drug-to-drug interactions. To promote the development and use of quality apps for this purpose, the FDA issued nonbinding guidelines in 2013.[61]

Ethics and Prescribing Drugs

By definition, ethical dilemmas have no simple answers. Much of the discussion about ethical use of drugs concentrates on isolated topics such as pharmacotherapeutics, or use of a drug as a treatment for specific conditions. However, just as drugs have an important role in economics, they also have major ethical implications.[62] It is beyond the scope of this chapter to explore ethics and drug use in detail. However, the healthcare professional should consider how to personally approach a variety of issues, including prescribing for his or her own family; prescribing for oneself; selling nutritional supplements or other nonprescription items within the professional's office; use of placebos; support of selling agents overseas that are not marketed in the United States because of lack of effectiveness or risk of adverse effects; providing free samples of drugs; or acceptance of gifts from pharmaceutical companies, regardless of how minor the cost might be.[63]

Conclusion

Drugs are ubiquitous in modern society. Many medications have provided health, help, and hope for women. Unfortunately, some agents have also resulted in harm. Medicalization of conditions has often led women to seek pharmaceuticals as first-line treatments, even when other options may be equally effective or even safer. To promote the health of everyone in modern society, prescribing drugs should be conducted in a rational, legal, and ethical manner.

Resources

Organization	Description	Website
U.S. Food and Drug Administration (FDA)	The FDA is responsible for protecting public health by assuring the safety, effectiveness, quality, and security of human and veterinary drugs, vaccines, and other biological products, as well as medical devices. The FDA is also responsible for the safety and security of dietary supplements and products that give off radiation. In addition, the FDA regulates tobacco products.	www.fda.gov
U.S. Immigration and Customs (counterfeit drugs)	Investigative arm of the Department of Homeland Security. This agency works to identify and prevent sale of counterfeit pharmaceuticals.	www.ice.gov
U.S. Department of Justice, Drug Enforcement Administration (DEA)	The mission of DEA's Office of Diversion Control is to prevent, detect, and investigate the diversion of controlled pharmaceuticals and listed chemicals from legitimate sources while ensuring an adequate and uninterrupted supply for legitimate medical, commercial, and scientific need.	www.deadiversion.usdoj.gov

References

1. Roller ST, Pippins RR, Ngai JW. FDA's expanding postmarket authority to monitor and publicize food and consumer health product risks: the need for procedural safeguards to reduce "transparency" policy harms in the post-9/11 regulatory environment. *Food Drug Law J.* 2009;64(3):577-598.
2. Daemmrich A, Bowden ME. A rising drug industry. *Chem Eng News.* 2005;83(25):28-42.
3. Conrad P, Leiter V. From Lydia Pinkham to Queen Levitra: direct-to-consumer advertising and medicalization. *Sociol Health Illn.* 2008;30(6):825-838.
4. National Center for Health Statistics. *Health, US, 2013; with special feature on prescription drugs.* Hyattsville, MD: National Center for Health Statistics; 2014.
5. Greene JA, Podolsky SH. Reform, regulation, and pharmaceuticals: the Kefauver-Harris Amendments at 50. *N Engl J Med.* 2012;367(16):1481-1483.
6. Gupta SK, Nayak RP. Off-label use of medicine: perspective of physicians, patients, pharmaceutical companies, and regulatory authorities. *J Pharmacol Pharmacother.* 2014;5(2):88-92.
7. Kohn LT, Corrigan JM, Donaldson MS (Institute of Medicine). *To Err Is Human: Building a Safer Health System.* Washington, DC: National Academy Press; 2000.
8. Committee on the Assessment of the U.S. Drug Safety System, Baciu A, Stratton K, Burke SP, eds. *The Future of Drug Safety: Promoting and Protecting the Health of the Public.* Washington, DC: National Academies Press; 2007.
9. Brandt AM. FDA regulation of tobacco: pitfalls and possibilities. *N Engl J Med.* 2008;359(5):444-448.
10. Curfman GD, Morrissey S, Drazen JM. The FDA and tobacco regulation. *N Engl J Med.* 2008;359:1056-1057.
11. Hartung DM, Zarin DA, Guise JM, McDonagh M, Paynter R, Helfand M. Reporting discrepancies between the ClinicalTrials.gov results database and peer-reviewed publications. *Ann Intern Med.* 2014; 160(7):477-483.
12. Bongartz T, Sutton AJ, Sweeting MJ, Buchan I, Matteson EL, Montori V. Anti-TNP antibody therapy in rheumatoid arthritis and the risk of serious infections and malignancies. *JAMA.* 2006;295(19): 2275-2285.
13. Hanson GR, Venturelli PJ, Fleckenstein AE. *Drugs and Society.* 11th ed. Burlington, MA: Jones & Bartlett Learning; 2012.
14. Cohen JP, Paquette C, Cairns CP. Switching prescription drugs to over the counter. *BMJ.* 2005;330;39-41.
15. Consumer Healthcare Products Association. The value of OTC medicines to the United States. 2012. http://www.chpa.org/ValueofOTCMeds2012.aspx. Accessed June 10, 2014.
16. Fleming TR. Identifying and addressing safety signals in clinical trials. *N Engl J Med.* 2008;359(13):1400-1402.
17. Frank RG. The ongoing regulation of generic drugs. *N Engl J Med.* 2007;357(20):1993-1997.
18. Food and Drug Administration, Establishing a list of qualifying pathogens under the Food and Drug Administration Safety and Innovation Act. Final rule. HHS. *Fed Regist.* June 5, 20145;79(108):32464-32481. PMID: 24908687.
19. Pettit AC, Pugh ME. Index case for the fungal meningitis outbreak, United States. *N Engl J Med.* 2013; 368(10):970.
20. Centers for Disease Control and Prevention. Multistate outbreak of fungal infection associated with injection of methylprednisolone acetate solution from a single compounding pharmacy—United States, 2012. *MMWR.* 2012;61(41):839-842.
21. Rooks JP. Oxytocin as a "high-alert medication": a multilayered challenge to the status quo. *Birth.* 2009; 36(4):345-348.
22. Manias E, Williams A, Liew D, Rixon S, Braaf S, Finch S. Effects of patient-, environment- and medication-related factors on high-alert medication incidents. *Int J Qual Health Care.* 2014;26(3):308-320.
23. Pullirsch D, Bellemare J, Hackl A, et al. Microbiological contamination in counterfeit and unapproved drugs. *BMC Pharmacol Toxicol.* 2014;15(1):34.
24. Committee on Understanding the Global Public Health Implications of Substandard, Falsified, and Counterfeit Medical Products, Board on Global Health, Institute of Medicine; Buckley GJ, Gostin LO, eds. *Countering the Problem of Falsified and Substandard Drugs.* Washington, DC: National Academies Press; May 20, 2013.
25. United States Public Law, Title 21, Code of Federal Regulations (CFR) Part 1300 to 21 CFR §1308.
26. Ekins S, Andreyev S, Ryabov A, et al. A combined approach to drug metabolism and toxicity assessment. *Drug Metab Dispos.* 2006;34:495-503.
27. Ross NT, Wilson CJ. In vitro clinical trials: the future of cell-based profiling. *Front Pharmacol.* 2014;5:121.
28. Generic drugs versus brand names: switching could save money. Generic drugs have to go through the same

FDA approvals as brand names, so they have the same quality. *Harv Womens Health Watch.* 2013; 20(11):3.
29. 33 Fed. Reg. 9001 (1970) (codified at 21 C.F.R. §310.510).
30. Audet MC, Moreau M, Koltun WD, et al. Ortho Evra/Evra 004 study group. Evaluation of contraceptive efficacy and cycle control of a transdermal contraceptive patch vs. an oral contraceptive: a randomized controlled trial. *JAMA.* 2001;285(18):2347-2354.
31. Klein E, Bourdette D. Postmarketing adverse drug reactions: a duty to report? *Neurol Clin Pract.* 2013; 3(4):288-294.
32. Bresalier RS, Sandler RS, Quan H, et al. Adenomatous polyp prevention on Vioxx (APPROVe) trial investigators: cardiovascular events associated with rofecoxib in a colorectal adenoma chemoprevention trial. *N Engl J Med.* 2005;352(11):1092-1102.
33. Smith DA, Schmid EF. Drug withdrawals and the lessons within. *Curr Opin Drug Discov Devel.* 2006; 9(1):38-46.
34. Pirmohamed M. Personalized pharmacogenomics: predicting efficacy and adverse drug reactions. *Annu Rev Genomics Hum Genet.* 2014;15349-370.
35. Wilkes MS, Doblin BH, Shapiro MF. Pharmaceutical advertisements in leading medical journals: experts' assessments. *Ann Intern Med.* 1992;116(11): 912-919.
36. Donohue JM, Cevasco M, Rosenthal MB. A decade of direct-to-consumer advertising of prescription drugs. *N Engl J Med.* 2007;357:673-681.
37. U.S. House Committee on Energy and Commerce. Testimony. May 8, 2008. http://energycommerce.house.gov/cmte_mtgs/110-oi-hrg.050808.DTC.shtml. Accessed January 8, 2009.
38. Gerber DJ. Prescriptive authority: global markets as a challenge to national regulatory systems. *Houston J Int Law.* 2004;26:287.
39. U.S. Department of Justice, Drug Enforcement Administration, Office of Diversion Control. Pharmacist's manual. Section IX: valid prescription requirements. n.d. http://www.deadiversion.usdoj.gov/pubs/manuals/pharm2/pharm_content.htm. Accessed June 10, 2014.
40. Lessons from Lipitor and the broken blockbuster drug model. *Lancet.* 2011;378(9808):1976.
41. Law J. *Big pharma.* New York: Carroll & Graf; 2006.
42. The pharmaceutical and biotech industries in the United States. n.d. http://selectusa.commerce.gov/industry-snapshots/pharmaceutical-and-biotech-industries-united-states. Accessed June 10, 2014.
43. Schumock GT, Li EC, Suda KJ, et al. National trends in prescription drug expenditures and projections for 2014. *Am J Health Syst Pharm.* 2014;71(6): 482-499.
44. National health expenditures projections 2012-2022. n.d. http://www.cms.gov/Research-Statistics-Data-and-Systems/Statistics-Trends-and-Reports/NationalHealthExpendData/Downloads/Proj2012.pdf. Accessed June 10, 2014.
45. Buchmueller TC, Monheit AC. *Employer-sponsored health insurance and the promise of health insurance reform.* NBER Working Paper Number 14839. Cambridge, MA: National Bureau of Economic Research; 2009.
46. Lyles A, Palumbo FB. The effect of managed care of prescription drug costs and benefits. *Pharmacoeconomics.* 1999;15:129-140.
47. Wagner TH, Heisler M, Piette JD. Prescription drug co-payments and cost-related medication underuse. *Health Econ Policy Law.* 2008;3:51-67.
48. Madden JM, Graves AJ, Zhang F, et al. Cost-related medication nonadherence and spending on basic needs following implementation of Medicare Part D. *JAMA.* 2008;299(16):1922-1928.
49. Owens C, Baergen R, Puckett D. Online sources of herbal product information. *Am J Med.* 2014;127(2):109-115. [Epub October 7, 2013].
50. PhRMA. Code on interacting with healthcare professionals. 2008. http://www.phrma.org/sites/default/files/pdf/phrma_marketing_code_2008.pdf. Accessed June 10, 2014.
51. Hurley MP, Stafford RS, Lane AT. Characterizing the relationship between free drug samples and prescription patterns for acne vulgaris and rosacea. *JAMA Dermatol.* 2014;150(5):487-493.
52. Franconi F, Campesi I, Occhioni S, Antonini P, Murphy MF. Sex and gender in adverse drug events, addiction, and placebo. *Handb Exp Pharmacol.* 2012; 214:107-126.
53. Franconi F, Campesi I. Sex and gender influences on pharmacological response: an overview. *Expert Rev Clin Pharmacol.* May 24, 2014:1-17.
54. Heinrich J. *Drug Safety: Most Drugs Withdrawn in Recent Years Had Greater Risks for Women.* GAO 01-286R. Washington, DC: U.S. General Accounting Office; 2001.
55. Food and Drug Administration. *Federal Regist.* 1980; 44:37434-37467.
56. Food and Drug Administration. *Federal Regist.* 2014; 79(233):72064-72103.

57. Thomas CP, Kim M, Kelleher SJ, et al. Early experience with electronic prescribing of controlled substances in a community setting. *J Am Med Inform Assoc.* 2013; 20(e1):e44-e51.

58. Abood RR. *Pharmacy Practice and the Law.* 7th ed. Burlington, MA: Jones & Bartlett Learning; 2014.

59. Achike FI, Smith J, Leonard S, Williams J, Browning F, Gisson J. Advancing safe drug use through interprofessional learning (IPL): a pilot study. *J Clin Pharmacol.* 2014;54(7):832-839.

60. Thomas LJ, Coleman JJ. The medic's guide to prescribing: rational prescribing. *Student BMJ.* 2007;15: 133-168.

61. U.S. Department of Health and Human Services, Food and Drug Administration. Mobile medial applications: guidance for industry and Food and Drug Administration staff. 2013. http://www.fda.gov/downloads/MedicalDevices/DeviceRegulationandGuidance/GuidanceDocuments/UCM263366.pdf. Accessed July 9, 2014.

62. Sokol DK. "First do no harm" revisited. *BMJ.* 2013; 347:f6426.

63. Cutrona SL, Woolhandler S, Lasser KE, Bor DH, McCormick D, Himmelstein DU. Characteristics of recipients of free prescription drug samples: a nationally representative analysis. *Am J Public Health.* 2008;98(2):284-289.

2 Principles of Pharmacology

Laura W. Owens, Robin Webb Corbett, Tekoa L. King

Chapter Glossary

Absorption Movement of drug particles from the gastrointestinal tract to the systemic circulation by passive absorption, active transport, or pinocytosis.

Affinity Degree of attraction between a drug and a receptor. The greater the attraction, the greater the extent of binding.

Agonists Drugs that activate a receptor when bound to that receptor.

Agonist–antagonists Drugs that have agonist properties for one opioid receptor and antagonist properties for a different type of opioid receptor.

Alleles Alternative forms of a gene or DNA sequence that are located at a specific position on a specific chromosome. Each individual inherits two alleles for each gene. If the two alleles are the same, the person is homozygous. If they are different versions of the gene, the person is heterozygous. Genes can have several different forms or different alleles.

Antagonist Drug that prevents a receptor from being activated when bound to that receptor.

Bioavailability Percentage of an administered drug that is available to the target tissues.

Bioequivalence State in which a product's bioavailability falls within 80% to 125% of the bioavailability of the reference drug. If two products are bioequivalent, one can usually be substituted for the other.

Biotransformation Chemical changes a substance undergoes in the body.

Blood–brain barrier Characteristics of the capillaries surrounding the brain that create a natural barrier to the exchange of drugs between the systemic circulation and the circulation in the central nervous system.

Chronobiology (chronopharmacology) Use of knowledge of circadian rhythms to time administration of drugs for maximum benefit and minimal harm.

Clearance Measure of the body's ability to eliminate a drug.

Competitive antagonist Drug or ligand that reversibly binds to receptors at the same receptor site that agonists use (active site) without activating the receptor to initiate a reaction.

Cytochrome P-450 (CYP450) Generic name for the family of enzymes that are responsible for most drug metabolism reactions.

Dissolution Disintegration of solid drugs (tablets) into small particles in the gastrointestinal tract so that they can dissolve into a liquid.

Distribution Process by which a drug becomes available to body fluids and body tissues.

Dose–response relationship (dose–response curve) Change in the response to a drug caused by different doses of that drug. Dose–response curves help determine safe doses for drugs.

Drug–drug interactions Altered drug effects that occur when another drug is administered at the same time or in close proximity to the original drug's administration time.

Drug–herb interactions Altered drug effects that occur when certain herbs are taken at the same time or in close proximity to a drug's administration time.

Drug–nutrient interactions Altered drug effects that occur when certain foods or liquids are taken at the same time or in close proximity to a drug's administration time.

Efficacy Capacity to induce a therapeutic response. As opposed to effectiveness, which is the ability of a drug to produce a therapeutic response in real life conditions.

Elimination Removal of a drug or its metabolites whereby the drug or metabolites are changed to a water-soluble form, and thereby removed via the kidneys; less common elimination routes include liver, bile, feces, saliva, lungs, sweat, and breast milk.

Enteric coating Drug coating applied to slow the release and absorption of a drug in the stomach.

Excretion Elimination of a drug from the biologic system.

Extended release (sustained release, slow release) Drug designed to be released over an extended period of time.

First-pass metabolism (first-pass effect) Drug metabolism that occurs as a drug passes through the intestinal lumen, portal vein, and liver prior to entering the systemic circulation. Also known as hepatic first pass.

G-protein–coupled receptor Type of cell membrane receptor. The drug binds with this receptor, which then binds with guanosine triphosphate (GTP) and activates an effector (enzyme) in the cell.

Half-life Time it takes for half of the drug concentration to be eliminated from the body ($t½$).

Hydrophilic Drug that is water soluble. A drug or drug metabolite must be hydrophilic to be excreted in urine.

Inducers Drugs that stimulate production of one of the CYP450 enzymes, which in turn rapidly metabolizes the substrate drug. This can result in a decreased therapeutic effect of the substrate drug.

Inhibitors Drugs that prevent production of a CYP450 enzyme, which in turn decreases metabolism of the substrate drug. This results in an increased plasma level of the substrate drug and, therefore, an increased therapeutic effect, adverse drug reaction, and/or toxic effect.

Inverse agonists Drugs that bind to receptors that have an intrinsic or basal activity, which results in antagonism of this basal activity and downregulation of the receptor's effect. Antihistamines are inverse agonists.

Ligands Drugs or chemicals that bind to a specific receptor.

Lipophilic Drug that has a high affinity for fat. Lipophilic drugs transfer readily across the phospholipid cell membrane.

Loading dose Administration of a large initial drug dose.

Maximum effect Maximum drug effect; it varies by drug.

Metabolism Change of a drug, primarily in the liver by CYP450 enzymes, into metabolites that may be pharmacologically active or inactive. Drug metabolism alters a drug so that it may be eliminated.

Minimum effective concentration Minimum concentration of a drug in serum required to produce a desired pharmacologic effect.

Narrow therapeutic index As defined by the Food and Drug Administration, less than a twofold difference between the median effective dose and the median lethal dose.

Noncompetitive antagonists Drugs or ligands that reversibly bind to a receptor at a site different from the active site used by agonists; this binding causes a structural change that inhibits the agonist from binding to the active site. Noncompetitive antagonists do not compete for the active binding site but they do have an antagonist effect.

Partial agonist Drug molecule that elicits a partial pharmacologic response.

Peak levels Highest plasma drug concentrations.

P-glycoprotein Permeability glycoprotein (P-gp); a transmembrane protein that serves as a drug transporter and moves drugs out of cells. Also known as multidrug resistance protein 1 (MDR1) or ATP-binding cassette subfamily B member 1 (ABCB1).

Pharmacodynamics Study of drug concentration and the recipient's response; the study of a drug's effects, including the duration and the magnitude of the response in relationship to the drug dose.

Pharmacokinetics Process of drug absorption, distribution, metabolism, and elimination.

Phase I reactions First half of enzymatic metabolism, which makes a drug water soluble so it can be excreted; includes oxidation, hydrolysis, and/or reduction reactions.

Phase II conjugation reactions Second half of the drug metabolism process, which makes the drug polar and finalizes the changes that make it water soluble.

Polymorphism One of two or more naturally occurring variants of a particular DNA sequence on a chromosomal locus. The DNA variant is termed a polymorphism (as opposed to a mutation) when it appears in more than 1% of a population. Two types of polymorphisms are distinguished: insertions/deletions and single-nucleotide polymorphisms (SNP) wherein there is a change in the order of an amino acid base.

Polypharmacy Concurrent use of many different drugs and/or excessive use in excess of that which is clinically recommended.

Potency Concentration at which a drug elicits 50% of its maximal response.

Prodrugs Biologically inactive or partially active drugs that are changed as a result of the body's metabolism into active drugs.

Protein binding Fraction of total drug in the plasma that is bound to plasma proteins.

Receptor Protein or molecular complex that, when bound to a ligand (drug), either initiates a physiologic response or blocks the specific response that the receptor normally stimulates.

Steady state When drug elimination equals drug availability. Average concentration of the drug remains constant when it reaches a steady state.

Therapeutic effect Desired physiological or psychological response to a drug.

Therapeutic equivalence State in which two different drugs are pharmaceutically equivalent (contain the same active ingredient at the same dose) and have the same clinical effect with regard to both safety and efficacy when administered under specified conditions. The FDA has criteria for determining therapeutic equivalence.

Therapeutic index Guideline that estimates the margin of safety of a drug through the use of a ratio that measures the effective dose in 50% of the population and the lethal dose in 50% of the population.

Therapeutic range (therapeutic window) Plasma drug concentration between the minimum effective concentration in the plasma for obtaining the desired drug action and the mean toxic concentration.

Volume of distribution Relationship between the dose of the drug administered and the serum concentration after administration.

Xenobiotics Chemicals found in an organism that are not normally produced or expected to be present. Drugs can be xenobiotics, but the term is more frequently used to refer to toxins and poisons.

Introduction

During a typical lifespan, the average woman will take numerous medications, including prescription and nonprescription agents, and perhaps some natural medicinal substances such as herbs or other dietary supplements. These chemicals, via their action on physiologic processes, can be used to produce therapeutic benefit but can also cause toxic effects. This chapter reviews basic pharmacologic principles as applied to women's health.

The Nature of Drugs

Before a drug can elicit a physiologic response, it must be absorbed into the body and transported from a site of administration to the site of action. In most cases, the chemical (or drug) interacts with a specific target or **receptor** in the biologic system. There are several different types of receptors in the body. Many of them are located on the cell membrane (Figure 2-1). For a drug to possess the ability to produce medical benefits, it must have the appropriate size, electrical charge, shape, and composition to interact with a receptor and produce an effect. Interestingly, most receptors in the body exist naturally as targets for endogenous chemicals such as epinephrine, serotonin, or estrogen. Thus, drugs used for pharmacologic purposes often have some structural similarity to chemicals made naturally within the body. In addition, the drug should be able to leave the biologic system through elimination or inactivation in a reasonable amount of time so that the drug's actions are not inappropriately long or permanent.

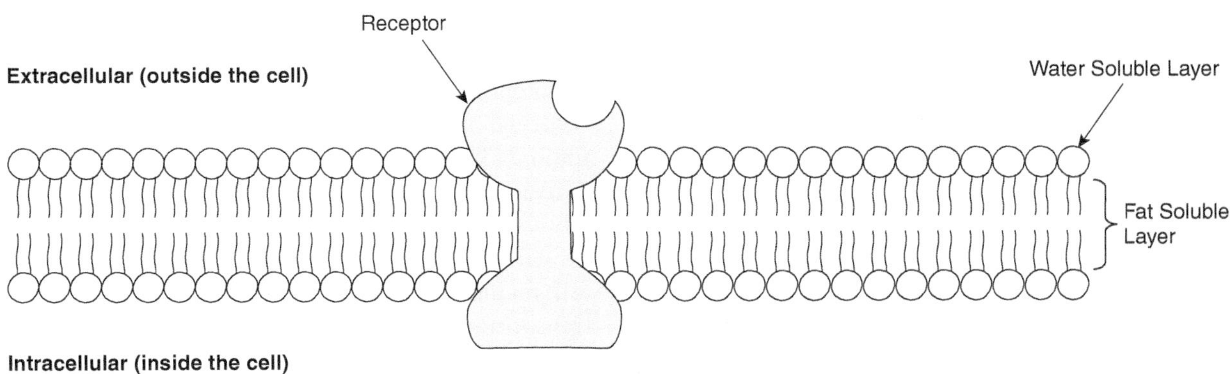

Figure 2-1 Cell membrane receptor.

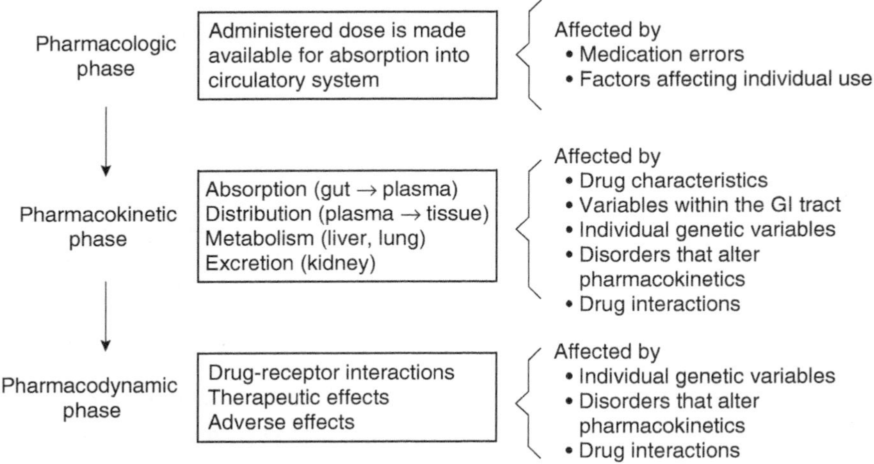

Figure 2-2 Factors that determine the intensity of drug responses.

Drugs can be solid, liquid, or gaseous at room temperature. This physical nature of the chemical often determines the best route through which the drug should be administered. Examples of routes of administration include intravenous (IV), intramuscular (IM), subcutaneous (SQ), inhalation, and transdermal (TTS), as well as enteral administration, such as oral (PO), rectal (PR), and sublingual (SL). Routes of administration vary depending on the physiochemical properties of the drug, including its molecular weight, fat or water solubility, and degree of ionization. Additionally, the route of administration affects the speed of absorption. Different routes may require various doses and dosage forms.

In considering all of the aforementioned factors, it is difficult to conceptualize how safe and effective drugs are developed and utilized for beneficial effects in the human body. The multitude of changes a drug undergoes between its administration and its stimulation of the intended response are divided into two major categories. **Pharmacokinetics** refers to the changes that a drug undergoes during its course through the body. **Pharmacodynamics** refers to the physiologic effects that the drug has on body function (Figure 2-2).

Pharmacokinetics

Pharmacokinetics specifically focuses on the kinetics of drug **absorption**, **distribution**, **metabolism**, and **excretion**. Clinical pharmacokinetics incorporates known pharmacokinetic principles of drug absorption, distribution, metabolism, and excretion but is based on the woman's disease state and takes into consideration individual-specific factors. A common example is when a laboratory measures a person's serum or plasma drug level. This numerical value is combined with knowledge of the disease state and conditions that influence the distribution of that particular drug. Kinetic principles can then be applied and used to modify the drug dose and subsequent drug serum levels to produce desirable changes in the individual's disease state. Examples of drugs for which serum plasma levels are drawn for clinical decision making include magnesium sulfate, vancomycin (Vanocin), theophylline (Theo-Dur), phenobarbital (Luminal), lithium (Lithobid), and digoxin (Lanoxin).

Absorption

After a drug is administered, it should be able to reach its intended site of action. This requires that the drug be absorbed into the circulation from its site of administration (Table 2-1).[1] Drugs can be absorbed via passive diffusion, active diffusion, or pinocytosis. Most drugs rely on passive diffusion. When a drug has a structure similar to a physiologic compound that moves across cell membranes via active transport, it is likely to be transported via active transport as well. Penicillin, for example, moves into the circulatory system via active transport. Macromolecules such as insulin and drugs made of large proteins access the circulatory system via pinocytosis.

Table 2-1 Absorption Speed of Various Drug Formulations

Type of Formulation	Absorption Rate
Oral Formulations	
Liquids, syrups, and elixirs	**Fastest**
Suspensions	↓
Powders	↓
Capsules	↓
Tablets	↓
Coated tablets	↓
Enteric-coated tablets	**Slowest**
Parenteral Formulations	
Intravenous (IV)	**Fastest**
Intramuscular (IM)	↓
Subcutaneous (SC)	↓
Intrathecal (IT)	↓
Epidural	**Slowest**

Source: Data from Guittierrez K. *Pharmacotherapeutics.* 2nd ed. St. Louis: Saunders Elsevier; 2008:44.[1]

Role of pH

Most drugs are weak organic acids or bases that exist in either an ionized or un-ionized form. Acidic drugs are in an un-ionized form that is lipid soluble or **lipophilic**; as a consequence, they diffuse easily across the phospholipid bilayer cell membrane. Basic drugs are in an ionized form and are water soluble or **hydrophilic**. These drugs cannot pass through the cell membrane into the intracellular compartment easily. The pH in the gastrointestinal tract also affects this process because the proportion of a drug that is un-ionized or lipophilic depends on the pH of the environment. The stomach is acidic with a low pH, and drugs that are weak acids are mostly in their un-ionized form in an acidic environment. Therefore, weak acids such as aspirin will readily be absorbed in the stomach. Conversely, the pH in the small intestine is more basic, and weak bases are more likely to be in their un-ionized form in this environment.

Oral Administration

Administering drugs orally is the preferred route of administration because it is safe, inexpensive, and convenient compared to other routes. Orally administered drugs (typically in tablet or capsule forms) must disintegrate into smaller particles, dissolve in the gastric fluid, and pass across the cell membranes within the gastrointestinal (GI) tract to be absorbed into the circulation. In addition, passage through the GI tract must alter the chemical characteristics of drugs that rely on passive diffusion so they become un-ionized and lipid soluble.

The oral route of administration does possess some disadvantages (Figure 2-3). Some drugs have limited absorption secondary to how their chemical characteristics respond to the environment of the GI tract, including the low pH of gastric acid, destruction by gastric enzymes, differences in gastric emptying rates, and

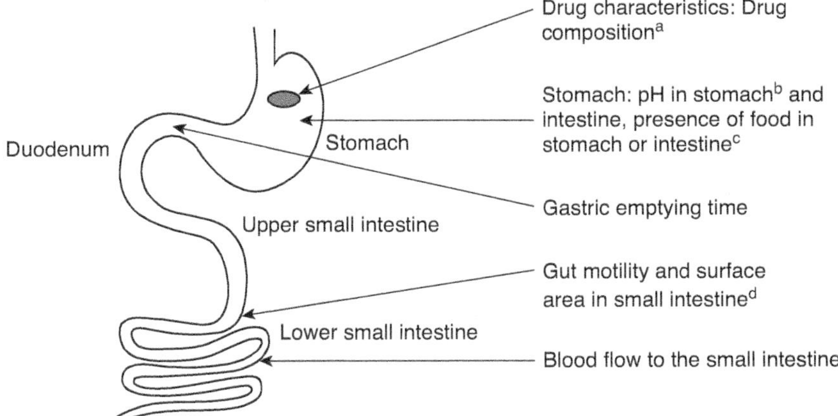

[a] Various aspects of the drug's chemical characteristics will affect absorption. For example, enteric coating will slow absorption, and drugs that are lipid-soluble will be absorbed more rapidly.

[b] Presence of antacid in the stomach will change the pH. This increases absorption of basic drugs and decreases absorption of acidic drugs.

[c] Food that is in the stomach or intestine can either facilitate or interfere with drug absorption.

[d] The small intestine has the greatest surface area, which is why most drugs are absorbed in the small intestine.

Figure 2-3 Factors that affect absorption of drugs.

adverse drug reactions such as vomiting due to gastric irritation. Infants and older individuals have less gastric acidity, which, in general, decreases drug absorption. The effect of food that is present in the GI tract also influences the absorption of drugs, albeit in a very drug-specific manner.[1] Some drugs are best taken with food to minimize gastrointestinal irritation, whereas other drugs' absorption may be impeded by food. Also, specific foods may enhance drug absorption.

Some drugs have an **enteric coating** that is intended to prevent the drug's disintegration and absorption in the stomach with subsequent absorption in the less acidic small intestine. In addition, **extended-release** (also known as **sustained-release** or **slow-release**) drugs may have multiple compressed coatings to allow release of the drug over time. These preparations are designed to produce slow, uniform absorption of the drug for 8 hours or more. The advantages of the coated preparations compared to their immediate-release counterparts include longer dosing intervals, maintenance of a therapeutic effect for a prolonged period of time, and decreased incidence and/or intensity of both undesired effects and nontherapeutic blood levels of the drug. Often, these drugs are designated by abbreviations such as *CR* (controlled release), *LA* (long acting), or *SR* (sustained release). To add to this confusion, "extended release" is the term recommended by the U.S. Pharmacopeia, but extended-release formulations can be labeled *XL*, *XR*, or *ER* depending on the choice of the pharmaceutical company that markets the drug.[3] These formulations should not be crushed, chewed, or scored (broken).

First-Pass Metabolism

After an orally administered drug enters the body, it passes through the intestine, intestinal wall, the portal blood system, and the liver before it enters the systemic circulation. Most drugs undergo metabolic changes during this trip via their interaction with (1) bacterial enzymes in the intestine; (2) permeability glycoprotein, usually referred to as **P-glycoprotein** (P-gp), which is a multidrug efflux pump present in the brush border membrane of gastrointestinal cells; (3) cytochrome 450 enzymes (CYP450 enzymes) present in gastrointestinal cells; and (4) CYP450 enzymes in the liver. Drug metabolism is called **biotransformation** because the structure of the drug is altered chemically. The biotransformation that occurs before the drug enters the systemic circulation is referred to as **first-pass metabolism** or the **first-pass effect**.[4,5]

As a result of first-pass metabolism, a proportion of the drug dose fails to enter the systemic circulation, thereby reducing the drug's bioavailability (Figure 2-4). Estrogen, for instance, is extensively metabolized in the liver via the first-pass effect. Alternative routes of administration for estrogen compounds such as patches and vaginal rings have been devised to decrease the amount of drug that must be administered to accommodate the first-pass effect.

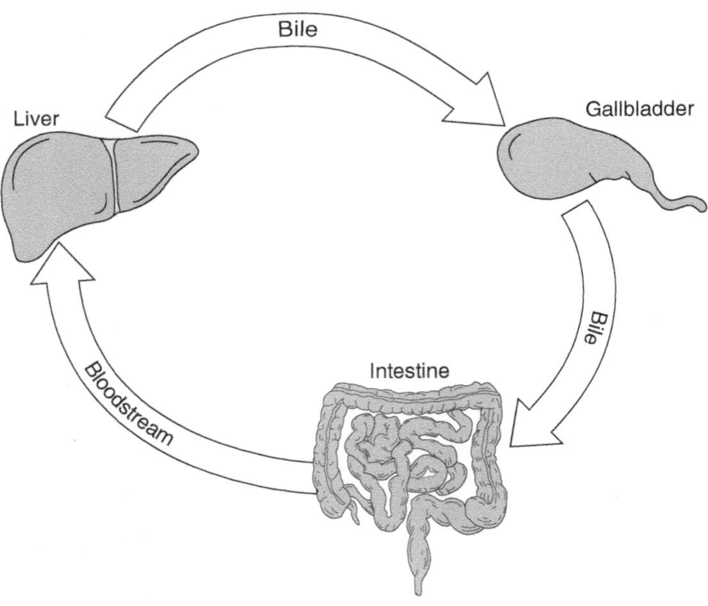

Figure 2-4 Hepatic first-pass metabolism.

Role of Enterohepatic Circulation

Some drugs are recycled through the enterohepatic circulation. When this occurs, there is an increased risk that their toxic effects will be manifested.[6] Once these drugs enter the liver and are taken up by hepatocytes, they are excreted into bile either unchanged or as metabolites. After the bile enters the gastrointestinal tract, the excreted drug is reabsorbed into the hepatic circulation, which can result in another peak in the plasma concentration of the drug or hepatotoxicity.

In summary, determinants of drug absorption following oral administration include properties that affect **dissolution** such as dosage forms, pH in the stomach and small intestine, and the size of the tablet. The next determinant is gastric emptying time, which is affected by the presence of food, antacids, or other drugs, as well as disease processes that might exist in the GI tract. Intestinal motility then affects the amount of time a drug is presented to the gastric lumen cells and, occasionally, the time available for drug degradation by microflora in the gut. Next, chemical properties of the drug such as water versus lipid solubility affect drug passage through the intestinal endothelial cells, and some drugs are metabolized by the intestinal endothelium or partially returned to the intestinal tract by P-gp. Finally, the extent to which a drug is metabolized via the first-pass effect will dictate the dose that must be used for oral administration.

Parenteral Administration

Drugs administered by parenteral routes (intravenous, subcutaneous, or intramuscular) bypass the GI tract, which allows for a more rapid, extensive, and predictable drug absorption as compared to other routes of administration. In the case of subcutaneous and intramuscular administration, the drug creates a depot under the skin and is absorbed into the systemic circulation by simple diffusion. The rate of absorption for these routes is limited by the area of the absorbing capillary membranes and by the solubility of the substance in the interstitial fluid. A subcutaneous injection can be used only for drugs that are not irritating to tissue; otherwise, severe pain, necrosis, and tissue sloughing may occur. The rate of absorption following subcutaneous injection of a drug often is sufficiently constant and slow to provide a sustained effect. This slow and constant rate is used and altered intentionally, as in the case of insulin: Altering the particle size, protein complex, and pH can provide for short (3–6 hours), intermediate (10–18 hours), and long-acting (18–24 hours) preparations of this hormone.

Drugs in aqueous solution are absorbed rapidly after intramuscular injection. This rate can be altered if the rate of blood flow surrounding the injected area is increased, as can happen during local heating (e.g., a hot bath), massage, or exercise. All of these measures increase vasodilatation, which in turn increases drug absorption into the systemic circulation. A slow, constant absorption from the intramuscular site can be achieved if the drug is injected in solution in oil vehicles; indeed, antibiotics are often administered in this manner.

Because intravenous administration injects the drug directly into the systemic circulation, 100% bioavailability is achieved. No first-pass effect occurs, and there are no barriers (e.g., skin) to drug absorption with this route. The drug delivery is controlled and achieved with an accuracy and immediacy not possible by the other routes. Drugs that cannot be administered intravenously include drugs in an oily vehicle, drugs that precipitate blood constituents or hemolyze erythrocytes, and drug combinations that result in the formation of precipitates.

Sublingual Administration

Sublingual administration occurs when a drug is placed under the tongue and absorbed into the blood. For some drugs, the sublingual route can be a convenient route of administration that bypasses the first-pass effect. The venous drainage from the mouth is to the superior vena cava, which protects the drug from rapid first-pass metabolism. Nitroglycerin is administered via sublingually because it is absorbed rapidly through this route; in contrast, if administered orally, it undergoes extensive metabolism by the liver until it reaches the point at which it essentially is removed from the circulation.

Transdermal Administration

Transdermal administration refers to the administration of a drug molecule through the skin for absorption into the circulation. Transdermal preparations are developed to deliver a consistent drug dose over a day or a period of days. Not all drug molecules can readily penetrate intact skin, but when they are able to do so, the amount absorbed depends on the surface area over which the drug is applied and on lipid solubility (the epidermis behaves as a lipid barrier). Transdermal administration can be convenient for some individuals, and this dosage form has become more popular in recent years. Controlled-release topical patches that have become increasingly available include nicotine for tobacco-smoking withdrawal, scopolamine (Transderm-Scop) for motion sickness, nitroglycerin for angina pectoris, estrogen (e.g., Vivelle, Climara, Estraderm) for menopausal therapy, and estrogens plus progestins for contraception. Systemic absorption of drugs occurs much more readily through abraded, burned, or denuded skin because the dermis is freely permeable. Also, when the skin is inflamed (causing an increase in cutaneous blood flow), drug molecules can more easily pass through the skin layer. Toxic effects can occur if highly lipid-soluble drug molecules are applied to skin that is not intact, so one must avoid transdermal administration in this situation. Conversely, lotion and ointments on the skin tend to impair drug transfer through transdermal administration.

Rectal Administration

When a drug is administered rectally, the drug molecule either is absorbed into the systemic circulation or placed to induce a localized effect, as in the case of hydrocortisone suppositories for hemorrhoids. This route of administration can be the preferred route when the individual is nauseated, vomiting, or unconscious. The potential for first-pass metabolism is less than that noted with the oral route of administration because approximately 50% of the drug that is absorbed from the rectum will bypass the portal system. However, rectal absorption often is irregular and incomplete, and many drugs can cause irritation of the rectal mucosa.

Pulmonary Administration

Some drugs are inhaled and subsequently absorbed through the pulmonary epithelium and mucous membranes of the respiratory tract. Systemic absorption of drug molecules through this route is typically rapid due to the lungs' large surface area. Advantages of this route of administration include rapid absorption of a drug molecule into the blood, avoidance of first-pass metabolism, and local application of the drug at the desired site of action in the case of pulmonary disease such as asthma. Inhaled drugs are often administered by nebulizer or a metered-dose inhaler that can create aerosols of small particles. For example, albuterol (Proventil HFA) may be administered by inhaler for individuals experiencing an acute asthma attack. More than one treatment may be required, depending on the severity of the attack and the person's response to the drug.

Topical Administration

When the drug is intended for local action (e.g., administration of eye drops for glaucoma), it is administered topically. Drug absorption through this route is continuous, although it has a slower onset of action. Systemic absorption is unlikely but does increase if the drug molecule is applied to mucous membranes. Drugs given via topical administration include ophthalmic drugs, which may take the form of drops or an ointment; erythromycin ointment (Ilotycin), for example, often is administered to newborns in the first few hours after birth to prevent ophthalmic neonatorum. Likewise, otic drugs (ear drops) may be given via topical administration to treat infections or to facilitate removal of cerumen. Both ophthalmic and otic drugs require diligence in identifying the correct eye/ear for administration, appropriate positioning of the individual for drug administration, and administration techniques specific to the drug medium.

In summary, factors that affect absorption are important considerations for the clinician because the drug must reach its intended site of action before it can begin to produce a change in the biologic system. However, in the end, the clinician is primarily concerned with bioavailability rather than the absorption of the drug. **Bioavailability** is a term used to indicate the proportion of a drug dose that reaches its intended site of action when administered by any route.

Distribution

Following a drug's administration and subsequent absorption into the systemic circulation, the drug becomes distributed into interstitial and intracellular fluids by passive mechanisms such as diffusion or by specific drug transport mechanisms. Distribution of the drug varies depending on multiple factors, including the size of the drug molecule, the drug's affinity for aqueous and lipid tissues, tissue permeability, systemic circulation, protein binding, and pH. These factors collectively determine the rate of delivery and potential amount of drug distributed into tissues.

There are two main phases of distribution. The first phase occurs when most of the well-perfused organs (e.g., liver, kidney, and brain) receive most of the drug. During the second phase of distribution, the less well-perfused organs receive concentrations of the drug. These less well-perfused organs include muscle, most viscera, skin, and fat. This second distribution phase may require minutes to several hours before the concentration of the drug in tissue is in equilibrium with the concentration in the circulation. Several clinically important pharmacokinetic processes occur as a drug is distributed.

Steady State

Steady state refers to the concentration of a drug in the systemic circulation that will eventually be achieved

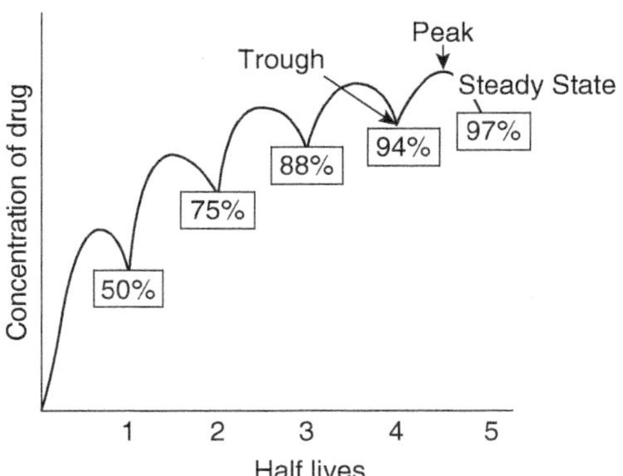

Figure 2-5 Steady state after repeated drug dosing.

when the rate of drug elimination equals the rate of drug availability.[7] This concept is often used in calculations of drug dose and interval between doses (Figure 2-5).

Half-Life

Half-life refers to the time it takes for the plasma concentration or the amount of drug in the body to be reduced by 50% or one half. Half-life is important because it determines the time required to reach steady state and the dosage interval. Steady state is usually reached after 4 to 5 half-lives. Complete **elimination** also takes approximately 4 to 5 half-lives once the drug is no longer administered; (Figure 2-6).

Another important concept when considering drug administration is loading dose. A **loading dose** is one or a series of doses that may be given at the onset of therapy with the aim of achieving the target plasma concentration rapidly. This dose, or series of doses, is used to rapidly attain a steady state when the treatment of the individual necessitates a quick therapeutic response.

Volume of distribution refers to the apparent volume (V_D) in which the drug is dissolved. In other words, V_D relates to the concentration of drug in plasma and the amount of drug in the body. The volume of distribution does not have a true physiologic meaning in terms of an anatomic space. However, it often is used to calculate the loading dose of a drug that will immediately achieve a desired steady-state drug level because it refers to the relationship between the dose of the drug administered and the serum concentration after administration.

Plasma Protein Binding

Protein binding is perhaps the most important factor when a drug is in the systemic circulation. Plasma protein

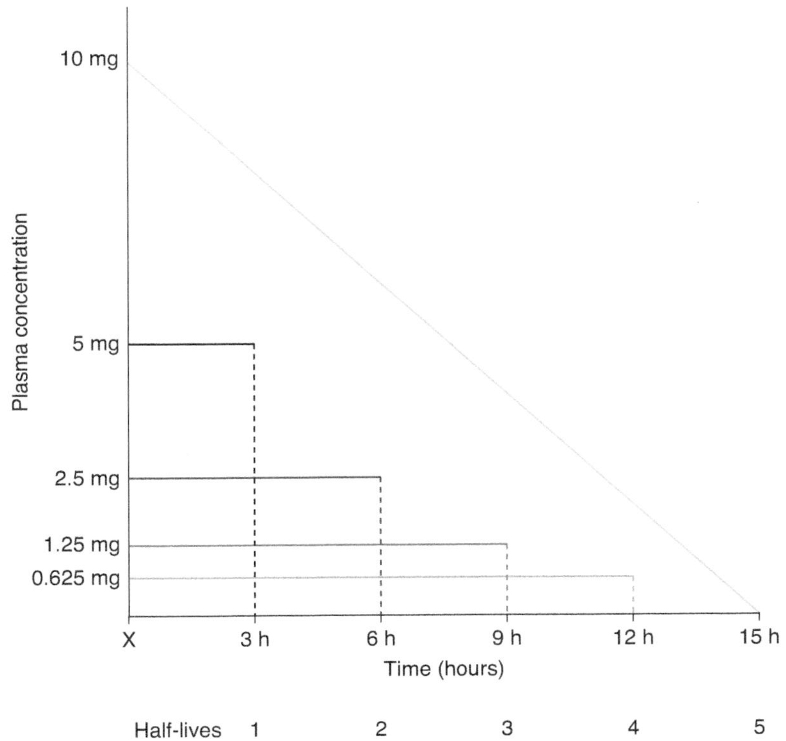

Figure 2-6 Elimination half-life determination.

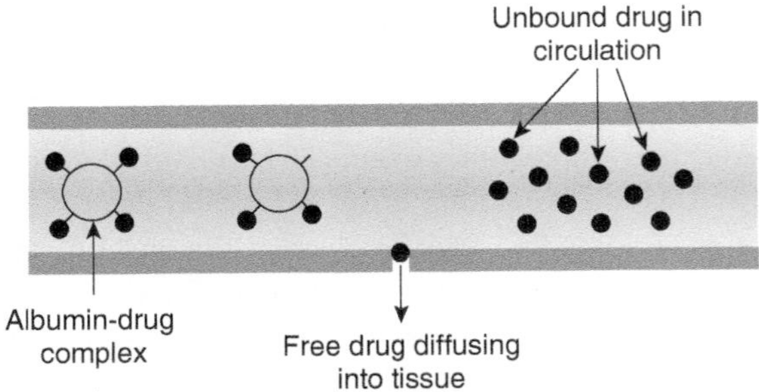

Figure 2-7 Protein binding of drugs.

binding refers to the fraction of total drug in the plasma that is bound to plasma proteins. Many drugs bind to proteins in plasma (Figure 2-7). More than 60 plasma proteins can bind to drugs, but albumin is the most common protein that does so. Albumin is a major carrier for acidic drugs, whereas the protein α_1-acid glycoprotein binds drugs that are basic in nature.

The amount of drug that is bound to plasma proteins is determined by the drug concentration in the systemic circulation, the affinity of the binding sites on the protein for the drug, and the number of binding sites. This concept is important because only the unbound (free) drug can distribute to its intended site of action in tissue; a drug's physiologic effect is related to the free concentration rather than the total circulating plasma drug concentration. The binding of drug to protein is readily reversible, lasting only a half of a millisecond, and the drug continually shifts from bound to unbound status.[6] Binding sites are limited, however, so they may eventually become saturated. When this phenomenon occurs, the risk for drug toxicity increases. For drugs that are normally highly protein bound, even small changes in the extent of binding can produce a large change in the amount of unbound drug and, in turn, a large change in drug effect. Factors that can increase or decrease the amount of protein available for protein-binding include myocardial infarction, surgery, neoplastic disease, rheumatoid arthritis, renal disorders, liver compromise, and burns.

In contrast to drugs that adhere to the protein-binding concept, many drugs accumulate in tissues at higher concentrations than in the extracellular fluids and blood. This pattern may be a result of active transport into the tissue, but more commonly it is a result of tissue binding. Tissue binding is often reversible. When a large fraction of drug is tissue bound, it may serve as a reservoir that prolongs drug action in that same tissue or at a distant site reached through the circulation. Caution must be exercised when prescribing drugs that are highly tissue bound. For example, the aminoglycoside antibiotic known as gentamicin (Garamycin) has a high affinity for kidney tissue, and it can cause local toxicity to the kidney if drug levels become too high.

Other examples of tissue binding include drugs that are lipophilic, which have a high affinity for fat and for bone.[8] Highly lipid-soluble drugs can be stored in fat tissues, which results in fat becoming a drug reservoir. Fat is a relatively stable reservoir because it has low blood flow. Bone is another tissue that is subject to tissue binding of lipophilic drugs. Such drugs can accumulate in bone by adsorption onto the bone crystal surface with eventual incorporation into the crystal lattice.

The Blood–Brain Barrier

The distribution of drugs into the central nervous system (CNS) from the blood is unique. The endothelial cells in the capillaries surrounding the brain are packed very tightly together, which disallows passive transport of materials in the blood out into the surrounding cerebral tissue. This **blood–brain barrier** creates a natural barrier to the exchange of drugs between the blood and the brain.[8,9] A drug must be able to travel *through* the endothelial cells to penetrate this barrier. In the rest of the body, the drug is often able to pass between endothelial cells because the cells are not joined as tightly. For a drug to be able to pass into the brain, it must be highly lipophilic; the more lipophilic a drug is, the more likely it is to pass through the blood–brain barrier.

Another natural drug barrier is the placenta. Fundamentally, the placenta is the organ of exchange between the mother and fetus. The placenta was once viewed as an absolute barrier to drugs and an agent of protection for the fetus, but today it is well known that this belief is flawed. The fetus is exposed to some extent to all drugs taken by the mother. Lipid solubility, the extent of plasma binding, and the degree of ionization of weak acids and bases are important general determinants of drug transfer across the placenta. Additionally, transmembrane proteins that function as efflux transporters are present in the placenta. The export transporters move drugs that diffuse into the placental cell back out into the maternal circulation and thereby limit fetal exposure to potentially toxic agents. Additional information about the use of drugs in pregnancy can be found in the *Pregnancy* chapter.

Drug Transporters: P-Glycoproteins

Some cells have transmembrane proteins that transport drugs and other chemicals out of the cell and into the

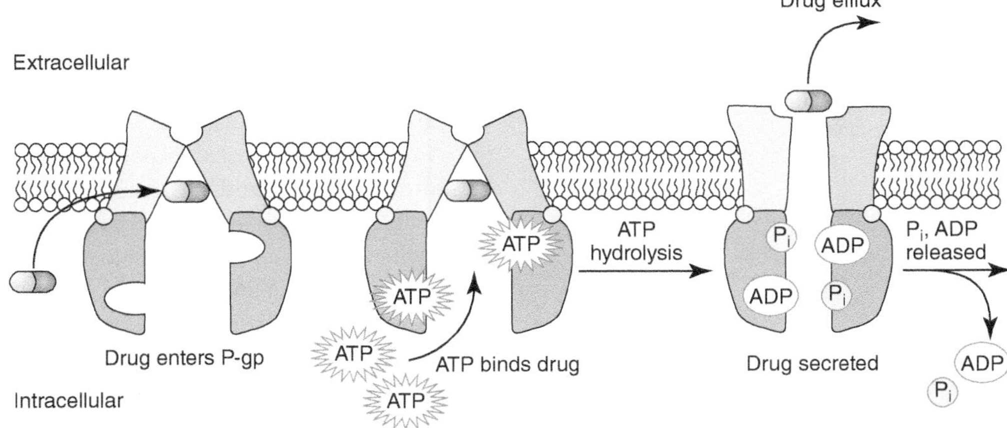

Figure 2-8 Drug transporters: P-glycoprotein in intestinal epithelial cell membranes.

circulation. One such drug transporter is permeability glycoprotein (P-gp), which is also known as multidrug resistance protein 1 (MDR1) or ATP-binding cassette subfamily B member 1 (ABCB1). P-gp, which is encoded by the *ABCB1* gene, functions as an efflux transporter. Fueled by ATP, this transmembrane protein transports drugs and other **xenobiotics** out of cells into the extracellular fluid (Figure 2-8).[10] P-gp is found in the plasma membranes of organs that affect drug absorption (epithelial cells in the intestinal tract), drug distribution (CNS, blood–brain barrier, and placenta), drug metabolism (liver), and drug elimination (kidney). The primary function of P-gp appears to be transporting harmful substances out of body tissues and preventing harmful agents from crossing the blood–brain barrier. P-gp substrates are generally large lipophilic compounds. Some drugs can inhibit or encourage expression of P-gp, thereby affecting the plasma concentration of the P-gp substrate.

Although the clinical implications and role of P-gp and other drug transporters have not been fully elucidated, it is clear they play important roles in drug response. Because these proteins are polymorphic, their role is reviewed further in the *Pharmacogenetics* chapter.

Metabolism

Termination of a drug's effects by the body is achieved via metabolism and elimination. Drug metabolism refers to the process by which a drug is chemically converted in the body to a metabolite. This transformation is usually enzymatic, and the enzymes responsible are mainly located in the liver. Other tissues, such as kidney, lung, small intestine, and skin, also contain enzymes that metabolize drugs. These reactions are classified as either **phase I reactions** or **phase II conjugation reactions.**[11]

The two-step process of phase I and phase II reactions make the drug molecule hydrophilic so the drug can be excreted via the kidney. Phase I reactions include oxidation, hydrolysis, and reduction reactions, which generally result in the loss of pharmacologic activity. Phase II conjugation reactions involve conjugation to form glucuronides, acetates, or sulfates. Both types of reactions play a major role in diminishing the biologic activity of a drug.

For most drugs, metabolism results in a pharmacologically inactive compound; however, a few drugs are transformed in the body to metabolites that have pharmacologic activity. These drugs are referred to as **prodrugs**. For example, valacyclovir (Valtrex) is not an effective antiviral drug, but its active metabolite, acyclovir, is active against herpes viruses.[12] Prodrugs are being developed intentionally to improve drug stability, increase systemic drug absorption, or prolong the duration of drug activity. When drugs are metabolized into inactive metabolites that are excreted, all is well. However, drug metabolism may also result in adverse health consequences. Therefore, a review of these mechanisms is in order.

The Cytochrome P-450 Enzymes

The **cytochrome P-450 (CYP450)** enzyme family is responsible for the majority of drug metabolism reactions.[13] The name P-450 was chosen because these enzymes are bound to membranes within mitochondria or endoplasmic reticulum within the cell (cyto) and because they contain a heme pigment that absorbs light at a wavelength of 450 nm when exposed to carbon monoxide. Each enzyme name

Table 2-2 Naming Convention for Cytochrome P-450 Enzymes

Nomenclature	Definition
CYP	Cytochrome P-450 enzyme
CYP1	Family designation
CYP1A	Subfamily A
CYPY1A1	Individual enzyme within subfamily
CYP1A1*1A	Allelic variant of the individual enzyme

reflects a family, subfamily, and then an individual number (Table 2-2). For example, CYP2D6 is number 6 in the subfamily "D" in the "2" family.[13] Currently, 57 different CYP450 enzyme genes have been identified, but only a few of these enzymes are responsible for the majority of drug metabolism in humans.[14] Three types of CYP450 isoforms (CYP1, CYP2, and CYP3) predominate in the metabolism of most commonly used pharmaceuticals.

The various ways these enzymes act represents perhaps the most interesting and most important set of processes that providers must know to prescribe drugs safely. Each CYP450 enzyme is encoded by a specific gene, and each human has two genes that determine expression of enzymatic activity—one inherited from the individual's mother and the other inherited from the individual's father. When a gene mutation occurs that results in an alternate version of the gene, the genes are referred to as **alleles**. Several alleles or variants of one gene may exist. When more than 1% of the population has naturally occurring variant alleles, the variations are collectively referred to as **polymorphism**. Some polymorphisms produce functional changes in the protein product of that gene. The genes that encode CYP450 enzyme activity, for example, are polymorphic. Thus, the clinical expression and functional ability of CYP450 enzymes to metabolize specific drugs ranges from absent to highly efficient depending on which alleles of the specific CYP450 gene an individual has inherited.[15]

The allele type is noted in the name following an asterisk. Thus, for example, CYP2C19*3 is a third allele variant of CYP2C19.

In addition, there are genetic, racial, and sex differences in CYP450 activity. These variations are reviewed in more detail in the *Pharmacogenetics* chapter.

Drug Interactions

Drugs can interact with many other substances, such as other drugs, herbs, and nutrients. These interactions can have important pharmacotherapeutic consequences.

Drug–Drug Interactions

The function of CYP450 enzymes can be significantly affected by the presence of drugs, food, herbs, and even vitamin supplements (Table 2-3). **Drug–drug interactions** refer to a modification of an expected drug response due to an exposure to another drug or substance at approximately the same time. Most commonly, drug–drug interactions occur when two drugs are coadministered and are metabolized by the same CYP450 enzyme.

Drugs are typically classified as **inhibitors** or **inducers** of CYP450 enzymatic activity. For example, Drug A might inhibit the activity of CYP3A4 and normally metabolizes Drug B. This results in an increase in the serum concentration of Drug B and subsequent risk of toxicity by Drug B. Conversely, administration of Drug A may induce more CYP3A4 activity and increase the metabolism of Drug B, thereby decreasing the serum concentration and the pharmacologic activity of Drug B. The effect of inducers occurs more slowly than the effect of inhibitors because it takes a while to produce more of the relevant CYP enzymes. Since most of these drug–drug interactions are due to CYP450 enzymes, it is important to determine the identity of the CYP450 enzyme that metabolizes a particular drug, to research the effects of the drug–drug interaction, and to educate individuals when coadministering drugs that are metabolized by the same enzyme.[12]

Coadministering drugs with known drug–drug interactions is sometimes done intentionally. An example of intentional coadministration can be found in the treatment of persons who are infected with the human immunodeficiency virus (HIV). Ritonavir (Norvir), a strong inhibitor of CYP3A4 and CYP2D6, is commonly coadministered with atazanavir (Reyataz), thereby increasing plasma levels and the anti-HIV activity of atazanavir. The ritonavir acts to boost the atazanavir concentration in the body.

Two different drugs can also be put together in one combination formulation to minimize drug interactions and facilitate patient adherence. Individuals with HIV and acquired immunodeficiency syndrome (AIDS) were prescribed a medication regimen that required taking 30 medications daily prior to the development of highly active antiretroviral therapy combination drugs; the combination drugs now allow them to take significantly fewer pills.

Drug–drug interactions can also occur when two drugs are given concomitantly and interact via their pharmacokinetic or pharmacodynamic processes. For example, additive effects of drugs that cause CNS sedation can, at the extreme, cause unconsciousness. When phenytoin (Dilantin) is given with salicylates (e.g., aspirin), the plasma

Table 2-3 Examples of CYP450 Enzymes That Frequently Metabolize Drugs and Their Pharmacologic Effects[a]

Inhibitors[b]: Generic (Brand)	Inducers[c]: Generic (Brand)	Substrates[d]: Generic (Brand)
CYP1A2		
Fluoroquinolones: ciprofloxacin (Cipro), clarithromycin (Biaxin) Combination oral contraceptives Other: amiodarone (Cordarone), cimetidine (Tagamet), erythromycin (E-Mycin), fluvoxamine (Luvox), isoniazid (INH)	Carbamazepine (Tegretol), insulin, phenobarbital (Luminal), phenytoin (Dilantin), primidone (Mysoline), rifampin (Rifadin), tobacco	Antidepressants: amitriptyline (Elavil), clomipramine (Anafranil), clozapine (Clozaril), desipramine (Norpramin), fluvoxamine (Luvox), imipramine (Tofranil) Antipsychotics: haloperidol (Haldol) Other: acetaminophen (Tylenol), caffeine, theophylline (Theo-Dur)
CYP2C9		
Anti-infectives: fluconazole (Diflucan), isoniazid (INH), metronidazole (Flagyl), ritonavir (Norvir), trimethoprim/sulfamethoxazole (Septra) Other: amiodarone (Cordarone), cimetidine (Tagamet), fluoxetine (Prozac), fluvoxamine (Luvox)	Carbamazepine (Tegretol), phenobarbital (Luminal), phenytoin (Dilantin), primidone (Mysoline), rifampin (Rifadin)	Carvedilol (Coreg), celecoxib (Celebrex), diazepam (Valium), glipizide (Glucotrol), glyburide (Micronase), ibuprofen (Advil, Motrin), irbesartan (Avapro), losartan (Cozaar)
CYP2C19		
Fluoxetine (Prozac), fluvoxamine (Luvox), isoniazid (INH), modafinil (Provigil) , omeprazole (Prilosec), ritonavir (Norvir), topiramate (Topamax)	Carbamazepine (Tegretol), phenobarbital (Luminal), phenytoin (Dilantin), rifampin (Rifadin)	Omeprazole (Prilosec), phenobarbital (Luminal), phenytoin (Dilantin)
CYP2D6		
Amiodarone (Cordarone), cimetidine (Tagamet), diphenhydramine (Benadryl), fluoxetine (Prozac), paroxetine (Paxil), quinidine, ritonavir (Norvir), sertraline (Zoloft)	No significant inducers	Antidepressants: amitriptyline (Elavil), clomipramine (Anafranil), desipramine (Norpramin), doxepin (Sinequan), fluoxetine (Prozac), imipramine (Tofranil), paroxetine (Paxil), venlafaxine (Effexor) Antipsychotics: haloperidol (Haldol), risperidone (Risperdal), thioridazine (Mellaril) Beta blockers: carvedilol (Coreg), metoprolol (Lopressor), propranolol (Inderal) Opiates: codeine, tramadol (Ultram) Other: donepezil (Aricept), ondansetron (Zofran)
CYP3A4		
Azole fungals: fluconazole (Diflucan), itraconazole (Sporanox), ketoconazole (Nizoral) Anti-infectives: clarithromycin (Biaxin), ciprofloxacin (Cipro), erythromycin (E-Mycin), isoniazid (INH), metronidazole (Flagyl), ritonavir (Norvir) Other: amiodarone (Cordarone), cimetidine (Tagamet), diltiazem (Cardizem), verapamil (Calan)	Carbamazepine (Tegretol), St. John's wort, dexamethasone, phenobarbital (Luminal), phenytoin (Dilantin), protease inhibitors, rifampin (Rifadin)	Alprazolam (Xanax), amlodipine (Norvasc), atorvastatin (Lipitor), cyclosporine (Sandimmune), diazepam (Valium), estradiol (Estrace), simvastatin (Zocor), sildenafil (Viagra), verapamil (Calan), zolpidem (Ambien)

[a] This table is not comprehensive as new information is being generated on a regular basis.
[b] These drugs inhibit the metabolism of substrates by these CYP450 enzymes.
[c] These drugs induce production of the CYP450 enzyme, which causes increased metabolism of the substrate.
[d] The plasma levels of these drugs are increased by inhibitors and decreased by inducers of the specific CYP450 enzyme responsible for their metabolism.
Source: Data from Lynch T, Pice M. The effect of cytochrome P450 metabolism on drug response, interactions, and adverse effects. *Am Fam Phys.* 2007; 76:391-396.[15]

levels of free phenytoin increase because the salicylates compete for plasma protein binding. Phenytoin has a very **narrow therapeutic index** and increased levels can reach toxic levels quickly, resulting in ataxia, nystagmus, or increased seizure activity.

P-Glycoprotein Drug Interactions

P-glycoprotein activity can also be increased or decreased by a number of endogenous and environmental stimuli. In a similar fashion to the CYP450 system, some drugs act as substrates (inducers) and others as inhibitors of P-glycoprotein expression. P-glycoprotein inhibition can result in increased plasma levels of a specific drug; conversely, P-glycoprotein induction can result in more rapid metabolism or elimination and decreased plasma levels of the drug in question. St. John's wort is a potent inducer of P-glycoprotein; when this herb is given concomitantly with digoxin (Lanoxin), the plasma levels of digoxin decrease because the augmented intestinal P-glycoprotein activity effectively keeps digoxin out of the systemic circulation.

Drug–Nutrient Interactions

Drug metabolism can also be influenced by diet. Previously these interactions were termed drug–food interactions, but they are more appropriately termed **drug–nutrient interactions**. Nutrients can affect drug bioavailability via two mechanisms: (1) decreased or delayed oral bioavailability via interference with absorption; and (2) increased bioavailability via inhibition of CYP3A in the cells of the intestinal wall.[16] This second mechanism increases plasma levels of the drug metabolized by CYP3A and can precipitate adverse drug reactions or toxicities.[17]

Components in grapefruits and grapefruit juices (naringin and furanocoumarins) are potent inhibitors of CYP3A (Box 2-1).[16,18,19] Persons who take a medication that has a narrow therapeutic index and is metabolized by CYP3A are more likely to have an adverse drug reaction if the medication is taken within 48 hours of ingesting grapefruit juice. Table 2-4 provides a list of drugs that have a clinically significant interaction with grapefruit juice.

Another clinically important drug–nutrient interaction is the hypertensive crisis that can occur among persons taking monamine oxidase (MAO) inhibitors while eating a diet of protein-rich foods that are high in tyramine (often foods that are aged, fermented, pickled, or smoked). Table 2-5 lists additional important drug–nutrient interactions.[20,21]

Table 2-4 Examples of Grapefruit Juice–Drug Interactions

Drug: Generic (Brand)	Clinical Effect of Increased Serum Concentration of Drug When Taken with Grapefruit Juice
Antiarrhythmics	
Amiodarone (Cordarone)	Thyroid, pulmonary, or liver injury; cardiac arrhythmias, prolonged QT syndrome, bradycardia
Quinidine	Torsades de pointes
Benzodiazepines	
Diazepam (Valium)	Increased CNS depression
Midazolam (Versed)	Increased CNS depression
Triazolam (Halcion)	Increased CNS depression
Calcium-Channel Blockers	
Felodipine (Plendil)	Flushing, peripheral edema, headaches, hypotension, tachycardia
Nicardipine (Cardene)	Flushing, peripheral edema, headaches, hypotension, tachycardia
Nimodipine (Nimotop)	Flushing, peripheral edema, headaches, hypotension, tachycardia
Verapamil (Covera-HS)	Flushing, peripheral edema, headaches, hypotension, tachycardia
CNS Depressants	
Buspirone (BuSpar)	Increased adverse effects of buspirone
Carbamazepine (Tegretol)	Increased adverse effects of carbamazepine
Clomipramine (Anafranil)	Increased effect of clomipramine
Sertraline (Zoloft)	Increased adverse effects of sertraline
Statins	
Atorvastatin (Lipitor)	Increased levels of atorvastatin can cause rhabdomyolysis
Lovastatin (Mevacor)	Increased levels of lovastatin can cause rhabdomyolysis
Pravastatin (Pravachol)	Increased levels of pravastatin can cause rhabdomyolysis
Simvastatin (Zocor)	Increased levels of simvastatin can cause rhabdomyolysis

Abbreviation: CNS = central nervous system.

Drug–Herb Interactions

Drug–herb interactions are particularly difficult to assess.[22] Most herbal products obtained over the counter are considered dietary supplements and, therefore, are not regulated as drugs.[23-25] Thus, there is wide variation in the pharmaceutically active compounds in different herbal preparations, and some may include components that are harmful. Nonetheless, adverse effects are known to occur when specific herbs and drugs are taken concomitantly with regulated medications. Individuals taking warfarin (Coumadin) can have increased bleeding if they take *Salvia miltiorrhiza* (Danshen) or garlic preparations.

Some of the most well-known herb–drug interactions are associated with use of St. John's wort.[27] This herb has

Table 2-5 Examples of Clinically Important Drug–Nutrient Interactions[a]

Drug: Generic (Brand)	Foods	Mechanism of Action	Clinical Implications
Angiotensin-converting enzyme (ACE) inhibitors	High-potassium foods such as bananas, oranges, legumes, meats, salt substitutes	ACE inhibitors spare potassium so the addition of food high in potassium can cause toxicity.	Bradycardia and potential cardiac arrest
Digoxin	High-fiber products such as bran, pectin, bulk laxatives	Decreases absorption of digoxin.	Insufficient digoxin effect
Monamine oxidase (MAO) inhibitors	Absolute: aged cheese, aged and cured meat, sausage, banana peel, fava bean pods, Marmite or yeast extracts, sauerkraut, soy sauce, tap beer Moderate: red and white wine, bottled or canned beer	Monoamine oxidase found in the GI tract inactivates tyramine. Tyramine can cause hypertension when absorbed into the systemic system.	Severe hypertensive reaction
Quinolones, antifungals, and tetracyclines	Dairy products, calcium supplements, calcium-fortified orange juice, antacids, iron-containing vitamins	Drugs bind to iron and calcium in the GI tract and form a compound that is excreted without entering the systemic system.	Decreased absorption of the antibiotic
Theophylline (Theo-Dur)	High-fat meal	High-fat meals increase absorption of theophylline.	Theophylline toxicity: nausea, vomiting, headache, irritability
Warfarin (Coumadin)[b]	Alcohol		More than three drinks/day increases effect of warfarin
	Foods with vitamin K must be used with consistency: broccoli, Brussels sprouts, turnip greens, kale, spinach	Large amounts of vitamin K interfere with the effect of warfarin.	Inadequate anticoagulation

[a] This table is not comprehensive as new information is being generated on a regular basis.

[b] Warfarin has multiple drug–drug, drug–nutrient, and drug–herb interactions.

Sources: Data from Chen J, Wilkinson J. The monoamine oxidase type B inhibitor rasagiline in the treatment of Parkinson disease: is tyramine a challenge? *J Clin Pharmacol.* 2012;52:620-628[19]; Gardner DM, Shulman KI, Walker SE, Tailor SA. The making of a user friendly MAOI diet. *J Clin Psychiatry.* 1996;57:99-104.[25]

Box 2-1 The Grapefruit Juice Story

In 1989, a group of researchers used grapefruit juice to mask the taste of alcohol in a study that was evaluating possible interactions between alcohol and felodipine (Plendil), a calcium-channel blocker used to treat hypertension. The study participants developed increases in plasma felodipine levels that were unrelated to alcohol or known felodipine pharmacokinetics. The culprit was the grapefruit juice!

Grapefruit has a number of constituents that inhibit the function of CYP3A4 enzymes in the cells of the intestinal lumen. Because CYP3A4 metabolizes many drugs before they enter the systemic system, inhibition of CYP3A4 can cause increased plasma levels of drugs, adverse drug reactions, and/or toxicity.

How much grapefruit juice does it take? Is it just the juice or does a grapefruit eaten for breakfast have the same effect? What about different types of grapefruit? Here is the story:

Grapefruit juice irreversibly inhibits CYP3A4, so new enzymes must be synthesized before normal function is restored. Thus, 30% of the inhibitory effect is still present 24 hours after ingestion of a single 8-oz glass of normal strength grapefruit juice. It is recommended that medications affected by grapefruit juice not be taken until 72 hours after the last glass of grapefruit juice. Unfortunately for grapefruit juice lovers, the effect is the same if they drink white, pink, or ruby red juice.

purported effectiveness for the treatment of individuals with depression. However, placebo trials of St. John's wort have been inconclusive and meta-analyses have concluded that it might be effective for mild depression only.[28] In addition, St. John's wort is an enzyme inducer and decreases the plasma levels of many drugs, including midazolam (Versed), digoxin (Lanoxin), warfarin (Coumadin), and oral oxycodone.[29,30] Women who are taking oral contraceptives can also experience breakthrough bleeding when St. John's wort is taken concomitantly with oral contraceptives, and this drug combination may interfere with the contraceptive effectiveness.[29]

Drug-Induced Toxicity

Finally, some metabolites of drugs and herbal dietary supplements are toxic to the liver or to the kidney.[31] In some instances, tests for liver function are required either before therapy with a specific drug is started or during therapy as a way to monitor liver function. The direct toxic effects of drugs or their metabolites on liver and/or kidney function are discussed in more detail in the *Drug Toxicity* chapter.

Excretion

Drug excretion refers to the elimination of a drug molecule or its metabolite from the biologic system. Drugs are primarily excreted via the kidneys, although some excretion does occur via saliva, feces, sweat, and mammary glands. Excretion of drugs in breast milk is important not because of the amounts eliminated, but because the excreted drugs are potential sources of unwanted pharmacologic effects in the nursing infant.

Excretion of drugs and metabolites into urine involves three distinct processes: glomerular filtration, passive tubular reabsorption, and active tubular secretion. All drugs that have a low molecular weight and are not bound to protein are filtered in the glomerulus into the glomerular filtrate. Lipid-soluble drugs move back into the blood via passive tubular reabsorption, but ionized hydrophilic drugs remain in the urine. Some drugs are actively secreted from the circulatory system into the proximal tubule. Penicillin-G is a good example of a drug that is eliminated via tubular secretion. Probenecid (Benemid), which is sometimes administered with Penicillin-G, blocks this mechanism and increases plasma levels of penicillin. Finally, the pH of the urine affects elimination.

Weak acids are excreted more easily in alkaline urine and more slowly when the urine is more acidic; the converse is true for drugs that are weak bases. Alterations in renal function will affect drug dose levels. When deciding on initial doses for drugs that are eliminated renally, the individual's renal function should be assessed. For example, gentamicin (Garamycin) is excreted via the kidney, and it can be toxic to proximal tubule cells. Therefore, when gentamicin is given in large doses or for a prolonged period of time, kidney failure can occur. As the kidney fails, less gentamicin is excreted, which predisposes the individual to additional kidney damage.

Clearance

Clearance is the measure of the body's ability to eliminate a drug.[32] This measure is often used in pharmacokinetic calculations, and it does not identify the mechanism or process of elimination (e.g., the clearance calculation does not consider whether the drug is eliminated by metabolic processes or excretion). This measure is the most important pharmacokinetic parameter because it determines the steady-state concentration for a given dosage route. The mechanisms of drug elimination are complex, but collectively, drug elimination from the body may be quantified using the concept of drug clearance.

Pharmacodynamics

Dose–Response Relationship

Pharmacodynamics is the study of the relationship between the concentration of a drug in the systemic circulation and the biologic response that occurs, often termed the **dose–response relationship**. A **dose–response curve** can be drawn by plotting the concentration of the drug on the x-axis and the response on the y-axis (Figure 2-9). The **minimum effective concentration** is the lowest dose at which a desired response is noted. A corollary concept, applied to the effect of antimicrobials, is minimum inhibitory concentration, meaning the lowest dose at which the antimicrobial inhibits visible growth of a microorganism overnight. The same dose of a drug often results in different plasma concentrations among individuals. This difference is secondary to individual differences in pharmacokinetic parameters. For example, the onset, intensity, and duration of response an individual experiences depend on both the dose of the drug administered and the pharmacokinetics of the drug in that individual.

Two important parameters can be calculated in drawing dose–response relationship curves for particular drugs. **Potency** is the concentration at which the drug elicits 50%

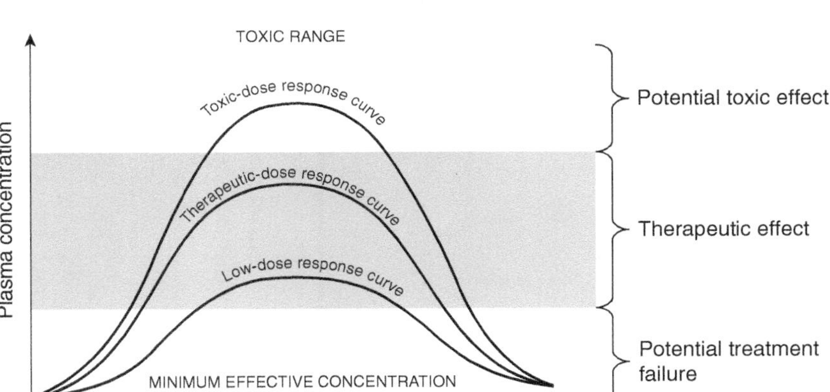

Figure 2-9 Dose–response curve.

of its maximal response. **Efficacy** is the maximal response produced by the drug. A clinical example of a study of pharmacodynamics is recording changes in blood pressure when a woman is being treated with antihypertensive medications. According to this concept, there is a drug receptor located within the target organ tissue. When a drug molecule finds and attaches to the receptor target, it forms a complex with that target that causes the biologic response, which is the specific mechanism of action of that drug.

Drug–Receptor Interactions: The Role of Cell Membrane Receptors

For a clinician to make rational therapeutic decisions, the prescriber must understand how drug–receptor interactions underlie the relationship between dose and response. A receptor is the cell component that interacts with a drug to produce a psychophysiologic effect. Drug receptors are often proteins, and common examples include receptors for hormones, growth factors, transcription factors, and neurotransmitters; the enzymes that play a role in crucial metabolic or regulatory pathways; proteins involved in transport; secreted glycoproteins; and structural proteins. Receptors are the governing agent in determining the dose for any drug. Specifically, the **affinity**, or propensity of a drug to bind with a specific receptor, determines the drug concentration necessary to achieve the desired effect. Drugs have a specific affinity for a particular cellular receptor. Drug binding to the receptor will either increase or decrease the rate of the biologic response controlled by that specific receptor. Note that drug–receptor binding does not change the physiologic activity, but simply either enhances or blocks it.

Four receptor systems are commonly cited: (1) embedded enzymes; (2) ligand-binding ion channels; (3) G-protein–coupled receptors; and (4) the nuclear receptors that are on the nuclear or mitochondrial membrane called transcription factors (Figure 2-10). The receptor of a cell membrane–embedded enzyme extends across the cell membrane, with the ligand-binding area located on the cell surface and the site for the enzyme activity located on the intracellular portion of the receptor. The response time of these receptors is usually within seconds. Insulin and atrial natriuretic factor are endogenous **ligands** that affect target cells via this signaling mechanism. Ligand-binding ion channels are similar to the embedded enzymes, in that the ion channels cross the cell membrane. These receptors control the flow of ions into and out of the cell. The ligand-binding domain is specific for a precise ion (e.g., calcium). With binding of the ligand to the receptor, the channel opens, allowing ions to flow into or out of the cell. Responses in this system commonly occur in milliseconds. The neurotransmitter acetylcholine and the amino acid glycine act through this receptor family.[33]

The **G-protein–coupled receptor** family is the largest group of cell-surface receptors, and approximately 30% of the drugs used today interact with these receptors (Box 2-2). Therefore, these receptors are of particular importance in pharmacology.[34] The G-protein–coupled receptor has three parts: the receptor, the G-protein, and the effector or second messenger. These receptors may be located on the cell surface or in a pocket accessible from the cell surface. Ligands bind to the receptors on the exterior portion of the cell membrane. Intracellularly, the bound receptors act as a catalytic enzyme. The second messenger then interacts

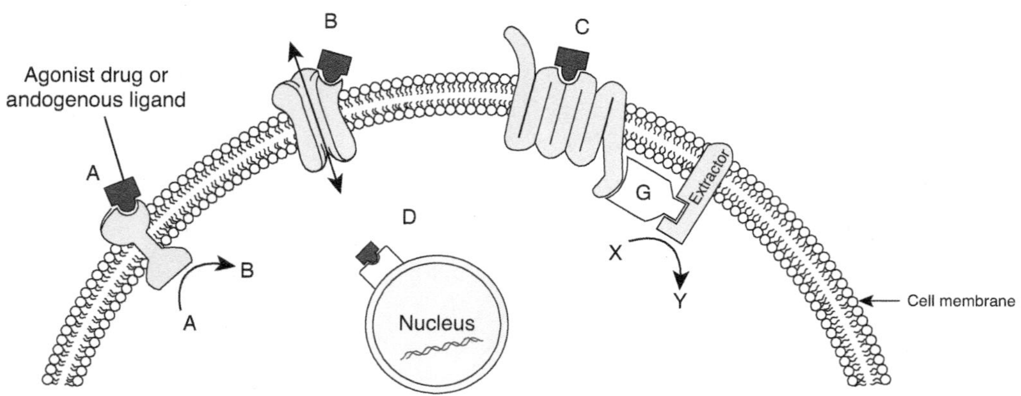

(A) Embedded enzyme: When a drug binds to the extracellular domain of this receptor, an enzymatic intracellular domain function is activated or inhibited. (B) Ligand-binding ion channel: The drug binds to the extracellular portion of this transmembrane protein complex, which causes it to change shape and alter conductance. (C) G-protein–coupled receptors are also known as seven transmembrane domain receptors. When a drug binds to the extracellular domain of this receptor, a G-protein in the intracellular space is activated to stimulate an effector mechanism. (D) Transcription factor: A lipid-soluble drug crosses the cell membrane and binds to an intracellular or nuclear receptor.

Figure 2-10 Four receptor types.

with intracellular components. The G-protein stimulates the enzyme adenyl cyclase to change ATP to cyclic AMP (cAMP) intracellularly, with subsequent activation of protein kinases and cellular reactions. Drugs acting via a G-protein–coupled receptor include beta blockers and antiasthma drugs.[35]

In contrast, transcription factors are intracellular receptors that have a longer response time. Lipid-soluble ligands cross the cell membrane to reach these receptors, which are located in the cell nucleus on DNA, where the transcription factors regulate protein synthesis. Activation of these receptors stimulate the transcription of messenger RNA templates for protein synthesis. With transcription factors there is a response time ranging from hours to days. Steroid hormones, such as estrogen and progesterone, act through these intracellular receptor sites.[36]

Agonists, Partial Agonists, and Antagonists

Agonists are drugs that elicit a pharmacologic response when interacting with the receptor. Such agents shift the equilibrium between the active and inactive forms

Box 2-2 Gone But Not Forgotten: Alfred Gilman

In 1941, two births occurred with significance for pharmacology—a book and a boy. In that year, two young researchers at Yale University, physician Louis Goodman and pharmacologist Alfred Gilman, published the first edition of their book, *The Pharmacological Basis of Therapeutics*. This internationally popular text has endured for more than 7 decades as the "bible" of pharmacology. As of 2011, a dozen editions had been published.

In the same year, Alfred Gilman and his wife had a son. In honor of their friend and the coauthor of the book, they named him Alfred Goodman Gilman. The younger Gilman went on to obtain both a degree as a physician and a PhD in pharmacology. He later was a contributing editor in the aforementioned prestigious text. But his major claim is his discovery regarding G-proteins. Martin Rodbell had found that guanosine-5′ triphosphate (GTP) was integral to actions within a cell. However, it was Alfred G. Gilman who discovered that the G-proteins actually are the molecular switches between activation of receptors on the cell and the actions within the cell. Knowledge of G-proteins and cellular activity is an invaluable asset in understanding drug actions and for drug design. For this work, Rodbell and Alfred G. Gilman shared the 1994 Nobel Prize in Physiology or Medicine.

Thus, two births in 1941 have added immeasurably to knowledge in pharmacology and health care.

of the receptor in the direction of the active form: By binding the active form more avidly (i.e., they induce a conformational change in the receptor that leads to a maximal effect), they drive the physiologic response in the direction of activation. Insulin and morphine are of examples of drugs that act as receptor agonists. Affinity refers to the degree of attraction between a drug and receptor. Drugs with high affinity bind more extensively to the receptor than a drug with less affinity. A **partial agonist** is a drug that elicits a partial pharmacologic response when bound to a specific receptor. Partial agonists have only a slightly higher affinity for the active receptor than for the inactive form, so they display some agonist activity and they interfere with the function of a full agonist. Buspirone (BuSpar), which is used to treat general anxiety disorder, is a partial agonist. **Agonist–antagonists** are similar to partial agonists in that they have an effect that is not as potent as full agonist stimulation. These drugs affect receptors that have different forms, and they act as an agonist at one form and as an antagonist at another. Butorphanol (Stadol), for example, blocks the effect of morphine at the mu opioid receptor but stimulates the kappa opioid receptor; the net result is analgesia that is not as potent as the effect obtained with morphine.

An **antagonist** is a drug that inhibits the action of an agonist when bound to the receptor and has no effect on the agonist itself. Antagonists may have a high affinity for the receptor, but they do not activate the receptor when bound to it. Although antagonists do not initiate a response, they prevent activation of the receptor by an agonist and, therefore, have a pharmacologic effect. The physiologic response to drugs acting as antagonists depends on the presence of an agonist. For example, antihistamines and naloxone (Narcan) are examples of antagonists.

Antagonists can be competitive or noncompetitive. A **competitive antagonist** occurs when the antagonist has equal affinity for both the active and inactive conformations of the receptor and competes with an agonist for binding to the active form of the receptor. Ligands with the highest affinity will bind with the receptor. If there is an equal affinity, then the ligand in the highest concentration will bind with the receptor. In contrast, **noncompetitive antagonists** bind with a part of the receptor away from the usual site to which an agonist binds. This causes a structural or functional change in the receptor that inactivates it, so agonist binding at the usual site fails to stimulate the expected physiologic response. The response to competitive antagonists is reversible, in that large enough amounts of the agonist may surmount the inhibitory effect, whereas the effect of noncompetitive antagonists is usually irreversible until the drug is inactivated.

The attractive feature of this model is that it explains **inverse agonists** rather well. If there is a basal tendency of the receptor to be in the active (agonist) state, then these active receptors will demonstrate a tonic, basal agonist effect even in the total absence of agonist ligands binding to them. If one adds an inverse agonist with a preference for the inactive receptor, the equilibrium shifts to the left, and the tonic agonist effect is lessened. Diphenhydramine (Benadryl) is an inverse agonist that binds to histamine receptors thereby suppressing the basal agonist activity.

Therapeutic Effect

All pharmacologic responses must have a maximum effect. The **maximum effect**, also referred to as the ceiling effect, is defined as the point at which no further response is achieved regardless of increasing drug concentration. If the clinician increases the dose of a drug but this does not lead to further clinical response, it is likely that the maximum effect has been reached. There is one other possible explanation: Some target organs may be more or less sensitive to the drug being administered. Therefore, it is important to note the drug dose required for the **therapeutic effect**. For some drugs, there is a narrow **therapeutic range** (or **therapeutic window**). The therapeutic range is the plasma concentration of the drug that produces the desired action without toxicity. Hence, a therapeutic range is between a minimal effective drug dose and the toxic concentration. Lithium (Eskalith), a drug frequently prescribed for women with bipolar disorder, has a narrow therapeutic range of 0.6–1.2 mEq/L with toxic concentrations at serum levels higher than 1.5 mEq/L.

Drugs also must be evaluated for the **therapeutic index** (Figure 2-11). The therapeutic index is the ratio of lethal doses in 50% of the population (LD_{50}) over the median minimum effective dose (ED_{50}) in 50% of subjects.[6] Thus, the therapeutic index is a quantitative measure of the safety of a drug. A drug has a narrow therapeutic index if the difference between the minimum effective concentration and the minimum toxic concentration is less than twofold. The FDA has named approximately 25 drugs as having a narrow therapeutic index (Table 2-6). A drug is safer when the value of the therapeutic index is higher. Lower therapeutic index numbers are associated with an increased risk of toxicity.

Identification of the therapeutic index sets the stage for considering **bioequivalence**. Bioequivalence is determined

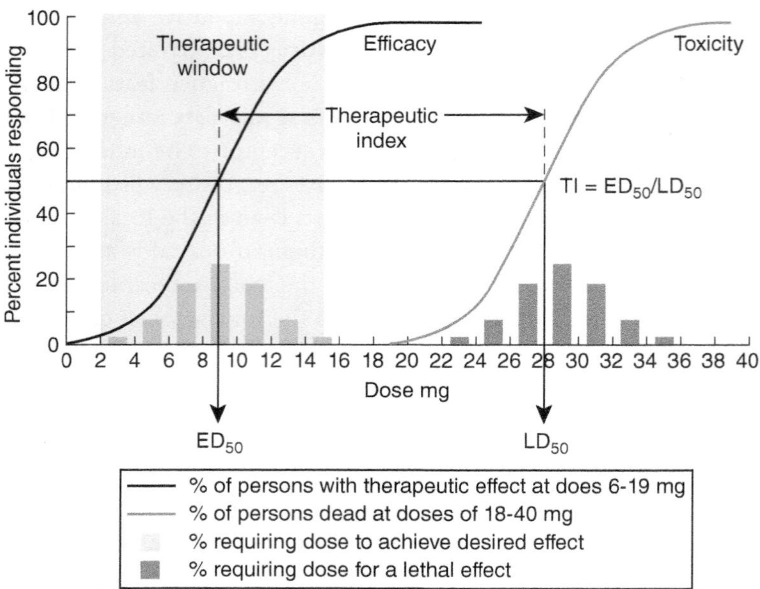

Figure 2-11 Therapeutic index.

by comparing the mean bioavailability of two drug products in multiple samples (individuals). If the mean bioavailability of one drug is within 80% to 125% of another drug, the two are determined to be bioequivalent and can usually be substituted for each other. However, bioequivalence does not guarantee **therapeutic equivalence**, because bioavailability depends on multiple individual factors. For example, an elderly woman with renal compromise may have a pharmacodynamic profile that allows her to metabolize one formulation of digoxin (Lanoxin) to obtain a therapeutic plasma level, but another formulation may result in subtherapeutic plasma levels. If the prescriber does not want the pharmacy to substitute one drug for another that has been determined to be bioequivalent, the words "no substitution" must be written on the prescription.

Table 2-6 Drugs with a Narrow Therapeutic Index

Drug: Generic (Brand)	Drug: Generic (Brand)
Amphotericin B (Amphotec)	Lithium (Eskalith)
Aminophylline	Metaproterenol sulfate (Alupent)
Carbamazepine (Tegretol)	Minoxidil (Rogaine)
Clindamycin (Cleocin)	Phenytoin sodium (Dilantin)
Clonidine (Catapres)	Prazosin hydrochloride (Minipress)
Digoxin (Lanoxin)	Primidone (Mysoline)
Dimercaprol	Procainamide hydrochloride (Procanbid)
Ethinyl estradiol/progestin oral contraceptives	Quinidine sulfate
Guanethidine sulfate	Theophylline (Theo-Dur)
Gentamicin (Garamycin)	Tricyclic antidepressants
Isoproterenol sulfate (Isuprel)	Warfarin (Coumadin)
Levothyroxine (Synthroid)	Valproic acid (Depakene)

Source: Data from Food and Drug Administration, Center for Drug Evaluation and Research.

When drugs with a narrow therapeutic index are being administered intravenously, the trough level should be drawn just before the next dose. In contrast, when gentamicin sulfate (Garamycin) is being administered, blood levels are obtained for **peak levels** 30 minutes after the intravenous infusion ends and trough levels are obtained just before the next dose. The drug dose may be adjusted according to the levels obtained. Peak and trough levels vary with the drug.

Pharmacotherapy

Pharmacotherapeutics refers to the clinician applying knowledge of the benefits and risks of drug therapy to individual care. In addition to pharmacokinetics and pharmacodynamics, other determinants of drug therapy include the age or gender of the person receiving the drugs, past and present health status, family history, lifestyle behaviors, and drug compliance. All of these factors must be considered when selecting and monitoring drug therapy. Understanding pharmacokinetics and pharmacodynamics is an important component of pharmacotherapy given the goal of achieving a desired beneficial effect with minimal adverse effects. The pharmacokinetic processes of absorption, distribution, metabolism, and excretion determine how rapidly, in which concentration, and for how long the drug will be present at the target organ. The pharmacodynamic concepts of maximum response, therapeutic index, and drug-receptor interactions determine the magnitude of the effect at a particular concentration. Knowing the relationship between drug concentrations and effects allows the clinician to take into account the various features of an individual that make this person different from the average individual in response to a drug.

Chronobiology/Chronopharmacology

Chronobiology or **chronopharmacology** is the study of pharmacokinetics as related to circadian rhythms or temporal changes. Variations in metabolism may differ by time of day, as well as by the age of the individual. In particular, elderly individuals may evidence changes in metabolism associated with time of day.[37] It has been suggested that use of drugs may be safer as well as more effective if timing of drug administration is considered.[38]

Timing of administration of antihypertensives at bedtime, for example, may result in better blood pressure control.[39] Intriguing chronopharmacology studies have also been conducted regarding the use of aspirin during pregnancy. One randomized controlled trial compared changes in blood pressure in women who took a placebo or low-dose aspirin at one of three times: in the morning, 8 hours after awakening, or at bedtime. Blood pressure was significantly reduced in the women who took aspirin compared to those who took the placebo only when the aspirin was taken 8 hours after awakening and at bedtime. Low-dose aspirin had no effect on blood pressure if taken in the morning.[40] These findings underscore the need for more studies in the area of chronopharmacology.

The Effects of Age

Clearly, a number of factors related to drugs influence drug dose, absorption, and efficacy; however, numerous factors related to the biologic system also influence drug therapy.[37] Newborns and children generally require lower drug doses secondary to their size and their immature hepatic and renal systems. Drugs cannot be metabolized or excreted as effectively due to the immature liver and kidneys, respectively. Likewise, older women may require a decreased dose and are at greater risk for toxicity due to the decreasing efficiency of hepatic metabolism and excretion associated with aging of the hepatic and renal systems. The lowered level of enzyme activity slows the rate of drug metabolism causing higher plasma drug levels per dose compared to young adults. Also, certain diseases that cause impaired renal and liver function mandate dosage adjustments.

Gender Differences in Drug Metabolism

Gender differences in drug metabolism may relate to several factors. Women are generally smaller in stature and weight than men; consequently, when women are prescribed the standard dose for men, they are often found to have higher plasma drug concentrations. In addition, individual differences in water and fat content can affect drug metabolism, as some drugs are more hydrophilic or lipophilic. Women have a slower gastrointestinal transit time during the luteal phase of the menstrual cycle and during pregnancy, which can also affect drug absorption. Women have a 50% to 75% higher risk for having an adverse drug event as men, in large part due to these many gender-related physiologic variations.[36]

Metabolic differences between the sexes have been noted for a number of drugs. This suggests that hormonal activity might affect the activity of certain CYP450 enzymes—a topic discussed in more detail in the *Pharmacogenetics* chapter. For example, women metabolize diazepam (Valium), prednisolone (Deltasone, Orapred), caffeine, and acetaminophen (Tylenol) slightly faster than their male counterparts. Conversely, men metabolize propranolol (Inderal), chlordiazepoxide (Librium), lidocaine, and some steroids faster than women.

Health Status

Both illness and some normal changes in health status can affect the pharmacokinetics and pharmacodynamics of a given drug. During pregnancy, a woman's reduced gastrointestinal motility and increased gastric pH affect drug absorption. Drug distribution may change because the maternal plasma volume increases by 50% in pregnancy. Serum albumin binding capacity is decreased during pregnancy, which results in an increase in unbound, active drug. Maternal hormones can affect drug metabolism by enhancing or inhibiting metabolism of various drugs. Drug excretion may also be affected due to the increase in renal blood flow. Pharmacokinetic and pharmacodynamic changes in pregnancy are discussed further in the *Pregnancy* chapter.

A woman with liver disease and tuberculosis will be unable to take some antitubercular drugs due to their hepatic toxicity. Congestive heart failure decreases hepatic blood flow by reducing cardiac output, which alters the extent of drug metabolism.

An alteration in production of the major drug-binding protein, albumin, can also alter the ratio of bound to unbound drug. Thus, a decrease in plasma albumin can increase the fraction of unbound (free) drug, which then becomes available to exert more of a pharmaceutical effect. The reverse is true when plasma albumin increases.

Genetic Factors

Drug action can vary as a result of genetic factors, a consideration discussed in more detail in the *Pharmacogenetics* chapter. Essentially, the metabolism rate for certain drugs can be slower or faster in some individuals based on genetic determinants. Some individuals are poor metabolizers of certain drugs because a specific CYP450 enzyme's activity is slower in those individuals compared to most persons in the general population.[41] Slower metabolism of drugs places these individuals at increased risk for adverse drug reactions and drug toxicity.

Lifestyle Behaviors

Lifestyle behaviors also are linked to pharmacodynamics and pharmacokinetics. For example, a woman who is prescribed a barbiturate—a drug that causes sedation and drowsiness—and who also ingests alcohol may have a drug–drug interaction that will enhance the sedative effect. Therefore, individuals need to be questioned frequently and directly with exacting questions such as "How much alcohol do you drink per day, and what do you drink?" rather than "Do you drink alcohol?" Women also need to be carefully questioned regarding self-medication with over-the-counter drugs, herbs, and dietary supplements. Any and all of these substances may interfere with a prescribed drug's effectiveness. For example, a pregnant woman with nausea and vomiting may self-medicate with the herb ginger. Generally in small and moderate doses, ginger may be helpful for some pregnant women; in pregnant women who are at high risk for hemorrhage, however, ginger inhibits platelet aggregation, thereby increasing their potential for bleeding.[42]

Individuals should also be questioned about their use of illegal substances. The use of illegal substances in addition to prescribed medications can result in acute toxicity. When a person who is taking heroin takes a barbiturate, for example, the combined sedative effect can result in a coma. Appropriate treatment is contingent upon the correct identification of the toxic substance. Illegal drug use is found in every age group, ethnicity, and socioeconomic status, so all individuals should be questioned about this practice.

The Role of Polypharmacy

Although there is no specific number of different drugs at which **polypharmacy** is universally defined, most studies have used five as the number of concurrently taken drugs that defines polypharmacy.[39] When a person is taking several medications due to multiple medical problems, the chance that a drug–drug interaction will occur increases. Because individuals may take several medications at a time and fail to report each one to their varied healthcare providers, the potential for drug–drug interactions can be high.[43]

Drug Adherence

Pharmacoadherence is the extent to which a person adheres to a medication regimen as mutually agreed upon with a healthcare professional.[44] Studies have found that 20% to 80% of individuals with chronic conditions requiring long-term pharmacologic regimens do not follow the prescribed regimen.[45] Measures of pharmacoadherence include direct, indirect, and subjective indexes. Direct measures may include biochemical assays as serum iron or total iron binding capacity levels for individuals with iron-deficiency anemia who are prescribed ferrous sulfate (Feosol). Indirect measures would include pill counts. Tailoring health education in accordance with the individual's culture, health literacy, and health numeracy may help improve pharmacoadherence. Health education is only one piece to this puzzle. Access to drugs and financial ability to pay for drugs can also adversely affect pharmacoadherance. Thus many factors need to be assessed when pharmacoadherance appears problematic.

Conclusion

According to the Institute of Medicine, in any 7-day period, 4 out of 5 adult individuals in the United States take prescription medications, over-the-counter medications, and supplements.[46] In this organization's report *Preventing*

Medication Error: Quality Chasm Series, medication errors were found to be a significant cause of morbidity and mortality. Providers of women's health care have a responsibility to understand the pharmacokinetics and pharmacodynamics of the drugs they order or administer. Multiple factors need to be considered, including age, gender, ethnicity, underlying health status, lifestyle behaviors that influence a drug's action, and effects. Routes and timing of drug administration vary depending on the drug and the woman's general health status. Monitoring for drug interactions with nutrients, herbs, and other drugs[46] and drug reactions is an important intervention. In addition, drug administration and responses vary across the lifespan, such that women who are pregnant, lactating, young, or elderly require special vigilance. Health education requires assessment of literacy, knowledge, and concerns, as well as the synergy of multidisciplinary healthcare members working together to provide the best care possible for women.

Resources

Organization	Description	Website
Indiana University School of Medicine	Drug interaction table of substrates, inhibitors, and inducers with links from the drug name to a PubMed list of citations that is continuously updated	http://medicine.iupui.edu/flockhart/table.htm
Concise Guide to Drug Interaction Principles for Medical Practice: Cytochrome P450s, UGTs, P-Glycoproteins	"Drugs" section in the Lexi-Complete PDA software package from Lexi-Comp; this PDA software includes a section on cytochrome P-450 enzyme activity for each drug narrative	
Merck Manual Online Medical Library	Overview of Pharmacokinetics and Overview of Pharmacodynamics: Articles that review the principles of pharmacokinetics with graphs and clinical correlates	www.merckmanuals.com/professional/clinical-pharmacology/pharmacokinetics/overview-of-pharmacokinetics
Interactive Clinical Pharmacology	Interactive colorful descriptions of many pharmacokinetic and pharmacodynamic concepts	www.icp.org.nz

References

1. Guittierrez K. *Pharmacotherapeutics.* 2nd ed. St. Louis: Saunders Elsevier; 2008:44.
2. Berman A. Reducing medication errors through naming, labeling, and packaging. *J Med Syst.* 2004; 28:9-29.
3. Gavhane YN, Yadav AV. Loss of orally administered drugs in GI tract. *Saudi Pharm J.* 2012;20(4): 331-344.
4. Soderberg Lofda K, Andersson M, Gustafsson L. Cytochrome P450-mediated changes in oxycodone pharmacokinetics/pharmacodynamics and their clinical implications. *Drugs.* 2013;73:533-543.
5. Gao Y, Shao J, Jiang Z, et al. Drug enterohepatic circulation and distribution: constituents of systems pharmacokinetics. *Drug Discovery Today.* 2014;19(3): 326-340.
6. Buxton ILO, Benet LZ. Pharmacokinetics: the dynamics of drug absorption, metabolism, and elimination. In: Brunton LL, Chabner B, Knollman B, eds. *Goodman & Gilman's the Pharmacological Basis of Therapeutics.* 12th ed. New York, NY: McGraw-Hill; 2011:17-40.
7. Meireles M, Martel F, Araújo J, et al. Characterization and modulation of glucose uptake in human blood–brain barrier model. *J Membr Biol.* 2013;246(9):669-677.
8. Smith B, Yogaratnam D, Levasseur-Franklin K, Forni A, Fong J. Introduction to drug pharmacokinetics in the critically ill patient. *Chest.* 2012;141(5):1327-1336.
9. Akhtar N, Ahad A, Khar RK, et al. The emerging role of P-glycoprotein inhibitors in drug delivery; a patent review. *Expert Opin Ther Pat.* 2011;21(4):561-576.
10. Corsini A, Bortolini M. Drug-induced liver injury: the role of drug metabolism and transport. *J Clin Pharmacol.* 2013;53(5):463-474.
11. Li F, Maag H, Alfredson T. Prodrugs of nucleoside analogues for improved oral absorption and tissue targeting. *J Pharm Sci.* 2008;97:1109-1134.
12. Krau SD. Cytochrome P450, part 1: what nurses really need to know. *Nurs Clin N Am.* 2013;48(4):671-680.
13. Wilkinson G. Drug metabolism and variability among patients in drug response. *N Engl J Med.* 2005;352(21):2211-2221.
14. Swen JJ, Nijenhuis M, de Boer A, et al. Pharmacogenetics: from bench to byte: an update of guidelines. *Clin Pharmacol Ther.* 2011;89(5):662-673.
15. Lynch T, Pice M. The effect of cytochrome P450 metabolism on drug response, interactions, and adverse effects. *Am Fam Phys* 2007;76:391-396.

16. Chan LN. Drug–nutrient interactions. *J Parenter Enteral Nutr.* 2013;37:450-459.
17. Pirmohamed M. Drug–grapefruit juice interactions. *BMJ.* 2013;346:f1.
18. Seden K, Dickinson L, Khoo S, Back D. Grapefruit–drug interactions. *Drugs.* 2010;70(18):2373-2407.
19. Chen J, Wilkinson J. The monoamine oxidase type B inhibitor rasagiline in the treatment of Parkinson disease: is tyramine a challenge? *J Clin Pharmacol.* 2012; 52:620-628.
20. Flockhart DA. Dietary restrictions and drug interactions with monoamine oxidase inhibitors: an update. *J Clin Psychiatry.* 2012;73(suppl 1):17-24.
21. Colalto C. Herbal interactions on absorption of drugs: mechanism of action and clinical risk assessment. *Pharmacol Res.* 2010;62:207-227.
22. Tsai H, Lin H, Simon Pickard A, Tsai H, Mahady G. Evaluation of documented drug interactions and contraindications associated with herbs and dietary supplements: a systematic literature review. *Int J Clin Pract.* 2012;66(11):1056-1078.
23. Kennedy DA, Seely D. Clinically based evidence of drug–herb interactions: a systematic review. *Expert Opin Drug Saf.* 2010;9(1):79-124.
24. Sahoo N, Manchikanti P, Dey S. Herbal drugs: standards and regulation. *Fitoterapia.* 2010;81:462-471.
25. Gardner DM, Shulman KI, Walker SE, Tailor SA. The making of a user friendly MAOI diet. *J Clin Psychiatry.* 1996;57:99-104.
26. Rahimi R, Abdollahi M. An update on the ability of St. John's wort to affect the metabolism of other drugs. *Expert Opin Drug Metab Toxicol.* 2012;8(6): 691-708.
27. Linde K, Berner MM, Kriston L. St John's wort for major depression. *Cochrane Database Syst Rev.* 2008; 4:CD000448. doi:10.1002/14651858.CD000448.pub3.
28. Russo E, Scicchitano F, Whalley B, et al. *Hypericum perforatum*: pharmacokinetic, mechanism of action, tolerability, and clinical drug–drug interactions. *Phytother Res.* 2014;28(5):643-655.
29. Nieminen T, Hagelberg N, Saari T, et al. St John's wort greatly reduces the concentrations of oral oxycodone. *Eur J Pain.* 2010:14:854-859.
30. Murphy PA, Kern SE, Stanczyk FZ, Westhoff CL. Interaction of St. John's wort with oral contraceptives: effects on the pharmacokinetics of norethindrone and ethinyl estradiol, ovarian activity and breakthrough bleeding. *Contraception.* 2005;71(6): 402-408.
31. Bunchorntavakul C, Reddy K. Review article: herbal and dietary supplement hepatotoxicity. *Aliment Pharmacol Ther.* 2013;37:3-17.
32. Li R, Barton HA, Varma MV. Prediction of pharmacokinetics and drug–drug interactions when hepatic transporters are involved. *Clin Pharmacokinet.* 2014; 53(8):659-678.
33. Hogg RC, Raggenbass M, Bertrand D. Nicotinic acetylcholine receptors: from structure to brain function. *Rev Physiol Biochem Pharmacol.* 2003;147:1-46.
34. Solinski HJ, Gudermann T, Breit A. Pharmacology and signalling of MAS-related G protein-coupled receptors. *Pharmacol Rev.* 2014;66(3):570-597.
35. Amezcua-Gutierrez MA, Cipres-Flores FJ, Trujillo-Ferrara JG, Soriano-Rusua MA. Clinical implications of recent insights into the structural biology of beta$_2$ adrenoreceptors. *Curr Drug Targets.* 2012; 13(10):1336-1346.
36. Witley H, Lindsey W. Sex-based differences in drug activity. *Am Fam Physician.* 2009;80(11):1254-1258.
37. Bruguerolle B. Clinical chronopharmacology in the elderly. *Chronobiol Int.* 2008;25(1):1-15.
38. Ohdo S, Koyanagi S, Matsunaga N, Hamdan A. Molecular basis of chronopharmaceutics. *J Pharm Sci.* 2011;100:3560-3576.
39. Zhao P, Xu P, Wan C, Wang Z. Evening versus morning dosing regimen drug therapy for hypertension. *Cochrane Database Syst Rev.* 2011;10:CD004184. doi:10.1002/14651858.CD004184.pub2.
40. Ayala DE, Ucieda R, Hermida RC. Chronotherapy with low-dose aspirin for prevention of complications in pregnancy. *Chronobiol Int.* 2013;30(1-2):260-279.
41. Samer CF, Lorenzini KI, Rollason V, Daali Y, Desmeules JA. Applications of CYP450 testing in the clinical setting. *Mol Diagn Ther.* 2013;17(3):165-184.
42. Liao YR, Leu YL, Chan YY, Kuo PC, Wu TS. Antiplatelet aggregation and vasorelaxing effects of the constituents of the rhizomes of *Zingiber officinale. Molecules.* 2012;17(8):8928-8937.
43. Hovstadius B, Petersson G. Factors leading to excessive polypharmacy. *Clin Geriatr Med.* 2012;28:159-172.
44. Chisholm-Burns MA, Spivey C. Pharmacoadherence: a new term for a significant problem. *Am J Health-Syst Pharm.* 2008;65:661-667.
45. Aronson J, Ferner RE. Clarification of terminology in drug safety. *Drug Safety.* 2005;28(10):851-870.
46. Institute of Medicine. *Preventing Medication Errors: Quality Chasm Series.* Washington, DC: Institute of Medicine; 2006.

3 Pharmacogenetics

Judith A. Lewis, Cindy L. Munro, Tekoa L. King

Chapter Glossary

Allele One of two or more versions of a gene. When genes are polymorphic and have alternate forms, these alternates are referred to as alleles.

Chromosomes Self-replicating genetic structures of cells containing the cellular DNA that bears the linear array of genes in its nucleotide sequence.

Extensive metabolizer Individual with two functional alleles, who therefore exhibits normal enzyme activity.

Gene Fundamental physical and functional unit of heredity; an ordered sequence of nucleotides located in a particular position on a particular chromosome that encodes a specific functional product.

Genetics Study of inheritance patterns of specific traits.

Genome Individual's complete set of DNA.

Genome-wide association studies (GWAS) Studies that compare the genome of a small group of individuals with a specific disease, drug response, or adverse drug reaction to a demographically similar group of individuals who do not have the disease or drug response. Detected differences in the genomes may allow identification of biomarkers, which can subsequently be tested for to personalize drug administration for maximum effectiveness and safety.

Genomics Study of all of the genes in an organism's makeup, including their interaction with the environment.

Genotype Genetic constitution of an organism, as distinguished from its physical appearance (its phenotype).

Intermediate metabolizer Individual with one functional allele and one nonfunctional allele, who therefore exhibits diminished enzyme activity.

Nucleotides Building blocks of DNA. A nucleotide has a base of adenine, thymine, guanine, or cytosine plus a sugar and phosphoric acid molecule. The order in which the nucleotide units appear (based on which of the four chemicals makes up the base) plays a role in storing and transferring genetic information.

Pharmacogenetics Study of inherited differences in drug metabolism and drug response. This information can be used to alter drug treatments for individuals with specific genetic variations.

Pharmacogenomics Study of how different genes in the full genome determine drug behavior. It uses information from the Human Genome Project, genomic approaches, and genome-wide association studies to identify genes involved in drug metabolism and drug response.

Phenotype Observable traits or characteristics of an organism. Examples include weight or the presence or absence of a disease. Phenotypic traits are not necessarily genetic, although they may result from an interaction between a genotype and the environment.

Polymorphism Difference in DNA sequence; one of two or more variants of a particular DNA sequence. The difference between a mutation and a polymorphism reflects the frequency of occurrence; polymorphisms occur in greater than 1% of the population.

Poor (slow) metabolizer Individual with two nonfunctional alleles of a gene, who therefore exhibits little or minimal enzyme activity.

Single-nucleotide polymorphism (SNP) DNA sequence variation that occurs when a single nucleotide (A, T, C, or G) in the genome sequence is altered. The abbreviation is pronounced "snip."

Slow acetylators Individuals with a polymorphism in one of the *N*-acetyltransferase enzymes that results in slow phase II drug metabolism. Such individuals have an increased risk for toxic reactions to drugs that are primarily metabolized via this phase II acetylation process.

Ultra-rapid metabolizer Individual with multiple copies of an allele, who therefore exhibits enhanced enzyme activity.

Introduction

Since the emergence of modern pharmacotherapeutics, it has been known that individuals respond to the same drug at a standard dose differently.[1-3] In fact, many of the drugs frequently prescribed by primary care providers exhibit wide interindividual variability in their effectiveness.[4] Variability in drug responses can be due to extrinsic factors such as smoking, diet, or drug–drug interactions, but may also be secondary to physiologic factors such as age, body mass index (BMI), or **genetics**. Genetic differences account for approximately 15% to 30% of interindividual differences in drug responses in general, but can be responsible for as much as 95% of interindividual variation for certain classes of drugs.[5] Genetic polymorphisms that affect the CYP450 enzyme family and other drug-metabolizing processes influence responses to as many as 30% of all drugs prescribed.[5] As knowledge of genetic determinants of drug response has grown, so has the field of **pharmacogenetics**—the branch of pharmacology that studies the variations in an individual's DNA sequence that affect drug metabolism and drug response.

In 2003, on the 50th anniversary of the publication of Watson and Crick's landmark article describing the molecular structure of DNA,[6] the National Institutes of Health held a conference to announce the completion of the sequencing of the human genome and the beginning of the study of **genomics**.[7] Along with the celebration of the completion of this massive undertaking, the conference laid the cornerstones of the postgenomic era in health care. **Pharmacogenomics** was acknowledged as one of the genomic applications that holds the greatest promise to transform the practice of health care in the twenty-first century. The goal of pharmacogenomics is to tailor drug dosing to an individual's unique genetic makeup. Pharmacogenomics applies knowledge of the whole genome to use of pharmaceuticals—in particular, knowledge about how certain genes within an individual's genotype affects therapeutic effects, side effects, adverse drug reactions, and toxic effects of drugs.

Pharmacogenomic studies are termed **genome-wide association studies (GWAS)**. These studies evaluate the genomes of many individuals who have a specific disorder or a specific response to a drug and compare them to the genomes of individuals without the disorder or drug response. Identification of genomic differences between the two groups then paves the way for developing drugs that will be effective for the affected individuals (Figure 3-1).[8,9] Although pharmacogenetics and

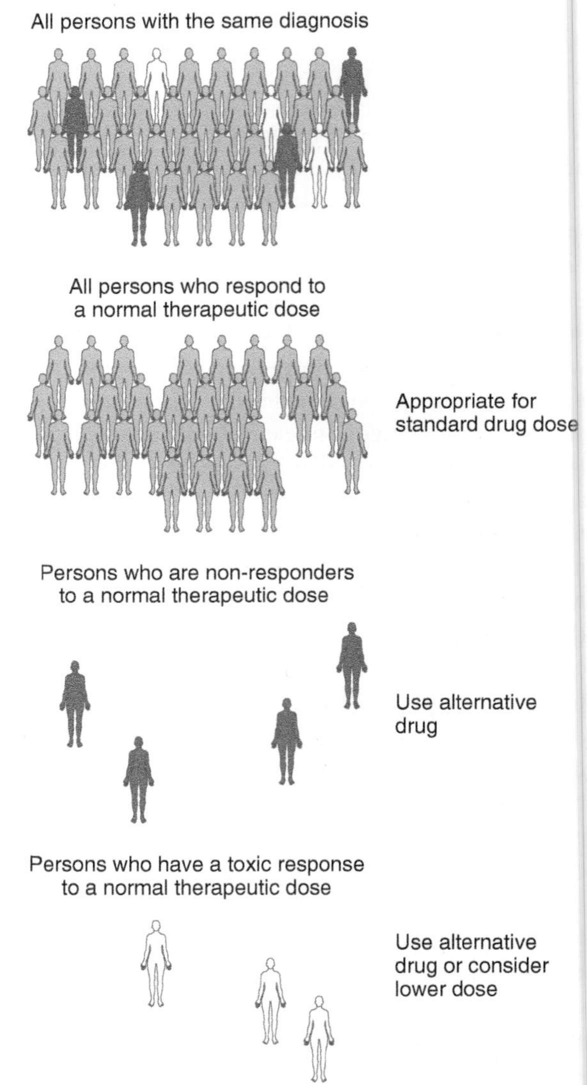

Figure 3-1 Potential of pharmacogenomics.

Box 3-1 A Quick Genetic Primer

Chromosomes are strands of DNA. All humans have 46 pairs of chromosomes, one in each pair inherited from the individual's mother and one inherited from the father. DNA is made up of building blocks (subunits) that are called **nucleotides**. Each nucleotide is made of a sugar, a phosphate molecule, and a chemical base, which is one of four chemicals: adenine (A), cytosine (C), guanine (G), or thymine (T). The order of A, C, G, and T makes the sequence of each person's DNA unique.

A **gene** is a segment of DNA located at a specific spot on the chromosome. Because each individual has two chromosomes, the pair of genes determines that individual's physical and physiologic function or **phenotype**. The genetic makeup of an organism is that organism's **genotype**. The term "genotype" is also used to refer to the two gene pairs inherited at a specific locus on the chromosome. A **genome** is an individual's complete set of DNA. Although the terms "genome" and "genotype" are often used interchangeably, there is a subtle distinction: Genome refers to all DNA, whereas genotype refers to all genes. Genes encode for the production of specific proteins or for the function of other genes.

When the ordering of A, C, G, or T is altered within a gene, an alteration that occurs in more than 1% of the population, it is referred to as a **polymorphism** and each different form of the gene is known as an **allele**. Some genes are highly polymorphic and have as many as 32 different alleles. The most common allele in a population is termed the "wild type" allele. When the polymorphism occurs within a single nucleotide, it is referred to as a **single-nucleotide polymorphism (SNP)**. The detection and elucidation of how different SNPs direct different functions are the basis of most pharmacogenetics research. When the polymorphism results in deletions or duplications, the result can be no enzyme activity or ultra-rapid metabolism secondary to an abundance of the metabolizing enzyme.

pharmacogenomics are technically different, in practice the two terms are often used interchangeably. In this text, the term "pharmacogenomics" refers to both single-gene and multigene data that are important for clinical practice. Box 3-1 provides a refresher of the genetics covered in this chapter.

Background

To date, the majority of pharmacogenomic research has been conducted in the area of drug metabolism, wherein genetic polymorphisms alter the function of the CYP450 enzymes.[10] Many polymorphisms of single gene nucleotides (SNPs) encode for the CYP450 enzymes (Figure 3-2). However, other findings from research are emerging. For example, polymorphisms that induce changes in cell membrane transport proteins (e.g., P-glycoproteins) can affect drug disposition within the body. Studies also are exploring genetic reasons why individuals fail to respond to common therapies, such as vaccines.[11] Pharmacogenomics encompasses five main areas of interest in how genetic differences affect drug response: (1) pharmacokinetics; (2) pharmacodynamics; (3) risk of adverse drug reactions; (4) racial and ethnic differences; and (5) gender differences. This chapter presents an overview of each of these categories.

Genomic Differences in Pharmacokinetics: Drug Metabolism and Drug Disposition

The primary pharmacokinetic processes affected by genetics occur during drug metabolism, because the genes that encode the CYP450 enzymes have many polymorphisms that affect the function of these enzymes. In general, CYP450 enzyme polymorphisms result in a person being either a **poor (slow) metabolizer**, an **intermediate metabolizer**, an **extensive metabolizer**, or an **ultra-rapid metabolizer** of a given medication.[12,13] Persons who are poor metabolizers will have significantly elevated plasma concentrations of a drug and a greater risk of toxicity than those who are extensive or ultra-rapid metabolizers when given the same dose. If a medication must be metabolized first so that the metabolite is the active drug,

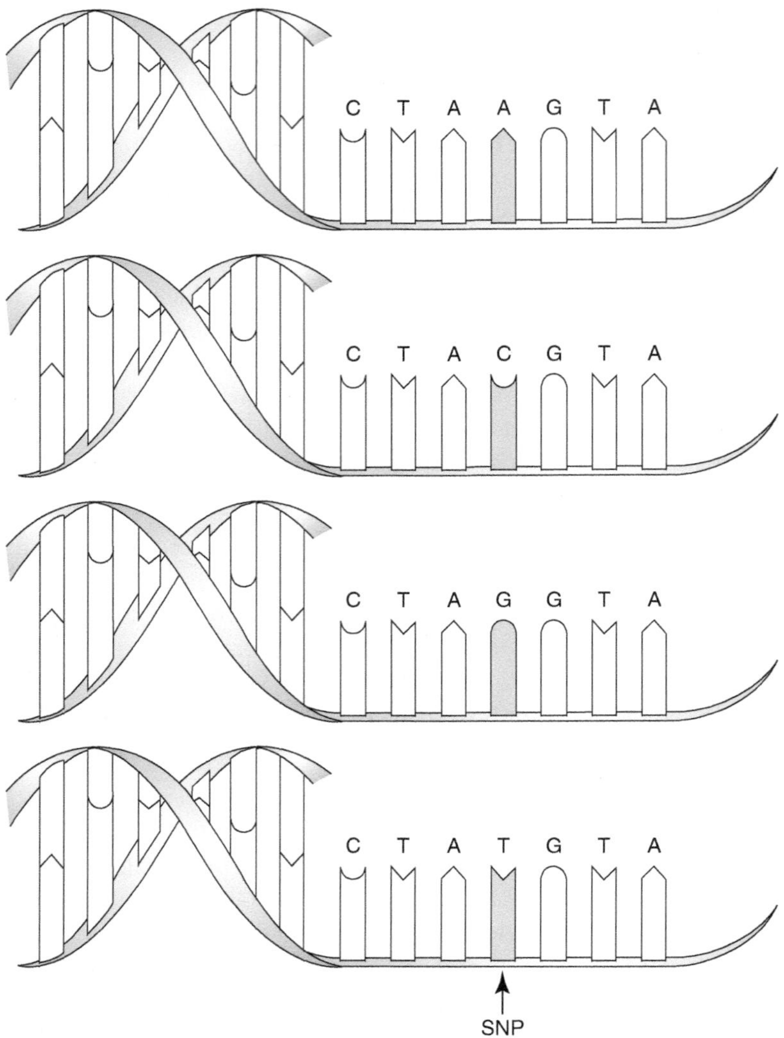

Figure 3-2 A single-nucleotide polymorphism is a change of a nucleotide at a single base-pair location on DNA.

a poor metabolizer may have a much weaker therapeutic response. In contrast, a polymorphism that involves duplication of CYP2D6 (which can result in as many as 13 copies of the gene) becomes an ultra-rapid metabolizer of drugs that are metabolized by CYP2D6. In this case, maintaining therapeutic drug levels may be difficult.

In 2006, a case report was published about a woman who was an ultra-rapid metabolizer for codeine but undiagnosed as such (Box 3-2). She took codeine for postpartum pain and the ultra-rapid metabolism of the drug resulted in an accumulation of active metabolites (i.e., morphine) that were passed through the breast milk to her infant, who later died of opiate poisoning.[14] Subsequently, the U.S. Food and Drug Administration (FDA) issued a warning about the use of codeine by breastfeeding women that notes the possibility of morphine toxicity in breastfeeding infants.[15] Although this is a rare and extreme example, the possibility of a genetic polymorphism should be considered for all persons who are either nonresponders or who develop toxic effects following administration of a medication. The various pharmacogenetic classes are listed in Table 3-1.

The ability to identify individuals who are poor or ultra-metabolizers will enable pharmacotherapeutic interventions to be identified that are both safer and more effective. In 2009, the Clinical Pharmacogenetics Implementation Consortium was formed. This organization develops peer-reviewed dosing guidelines for drugs that are substrates for clinically important CYP450 polymorphisms. In addition, the FDA now maintains a list of drugs that are mandated to include pharmacogenomic biomarker information on their

Table 3-1 Pharmacogenetic Classifications in Drug Metabolism

Classification	Genes	Impact on Active Drug	Impact on Prodrug
Ultra-rapid	Insertion of two or more copies in one gene	Active drug metabolized faster than usual, which leads to higher risk of inadequate effectiveness of the standard dose	Increased metabolism of prodrug leads to increased risk of toxicity from high levels of the active metabolites
Extensive	Each gene has normal function	Standard doses of the drug result in effectiveness without adverse effects	Prodrugs are converted to active metabolites that are effective without adverse effects
Intermediate	One gene of the pair has a variant that results in absent or reduced function	Decreased effectiveness in converting the active drug to the inactive metabolite results in increased risk of high blood levels and toxicity, but may also result in better than average effectiveness	Decreased conversion of the prodrug to the active metabolite results in decreased effectiveness of the standard dose
Poor	Both genes have a variant that results in absent or reduced function	Active drug conversion to the inactive metabolite is decreased, resulting in high blood levels of the active compound and increased risk for toxicity	When the prodrug is not able to be converted to the active metabolite, the result is nonresponse to therapy

drug labels. Websites for these organizations are listed at the end of this chapter. Polymorphisms of common CYP450 enzymes and some clinical examples are shown in Table 3-2.

Although much attention has been focused on the CYP family, other drug-metabolizing enzymes are also subject to genetic variations. For example, 10 common polymorphisms in the vitamin K epoxide reductase complex subunit 1 (*VKORC1*) gene account for as much as 25% of the dose response to warfarin (Coumadin).[16] People can be grouped as likely to need high, intermediate, or low doses of warfarin to achieve a therapeutic effect based on their

Box 3-2 Case Study: Caution with Codeine

A 20-year-old nulliparous woman immigrated to the United States from Saudi Arabia early in her pregnancy. At term, she had a prolonged labor and pushed for 3 hours in second-stage labor before becoming exhausted. A forceps delivery was performed and she had a midline episiotomy with a fourth-degree extension. Currently, she is 20 hours postpartum and has significant perineal edema. She has been requesting pain medication every 4 hours. Acetaminophen 325 mg/codeine 30 mg initially was ordered to be administered orally every 4 hours, but the woman stated that it was not adequately controlling her perineal pain. The dose was changed to acetaminophen 325 mg/codeine 60 mg orally every 4 hours; she states that her pain level is now acceptable. The woman planned to breastfeed but her nurse indicates she is having difficulty initiating breastfeeding because both mother and baby are very drowsy much of the time and the infant appears to have poor tone.

Treatment

This woman is a member of an ethnic group that has 16% to 28% incidence of a specific CYP2D6 genotype that causes conversion of codeine to its active metabolite, morphine, more quickly and more completely than in most individuals. Her drowsiness may be due to a lengthy and difficult labor and delivery, or it may be a sign that she is an ultra-rapid metabolizer of codeine, which leads to higher than expected maternal serum and breast milk morphine levels. All available alternative comfort measures should be utilized to minimize her need for opiate medication.

Her medication order should preferably be changed to a non-codeine-containing alternative. If this is not possible, she should be given the lowest possible dose of codeine to achieve acceptable pain relief for the shortest period of time possible. She must be counseled regarding the signs and symptoms of neonatal toxicity, such as drowsiness or sedation, difficulty breastfeeding, breathing difficulties, and decreased tone, especially if she needs to continue medication after discharge from the hospital. Her newborn's pediatric provider should be notified about the use of codeine during breastfeeding.

Table 3-2 Selected Polymorphisms[a] of CYP450 Enzymes and Their Clinical Implications

CYP450 Enzyme	Frequency of Poor Metabolizer Status	Example Drug Substrates	Clinical Example
CYP2C9	6–9% of Caucasians	Warfarin (Coumadin), phenytoin (Dilantin), NSAIDs	Warfarin has a very narrow therapeutic index; thus the dose must be finely calibrated to the response to avoid excessive bleeding or failure of therapeutic effect. The warfarin drug label provides dosing ranges based on CYP2C9 and *VKORC1* genotype.
CYP2C19	3–5% of Caucasians, 12–23% of Asians, 3.3% in Sweden, 14.6% in China, 18% in Japan	Metabolizes clopidogrel (Plavix), diazepam (Valium), phenytoin (Dilantin), propanolol (Inderal), proton-pump inhibitors, SSRIs, and clopidogrel (Plavix)	Citalopram (Celexa): The maximum recommended daily dose is usually 40 mg, but is 20 mg for persons who are CYP2C19 poor metabolizers. Omeprazole (Prilosec): Poor metabolizers have up to a fivefold higher blood level of omeprazole and better acid suppression and cure rates than the general population.
CYP2D6[b]	< 1% of Asians, 6–10% of Caucasians, 2–5% of African Americans; up to 29% of East Africans have multiple copies of this enzyme	Fluoxetine (Prozac), beta-adrenergic receptor blockers, antipsychotics, codeine, tamoxifen (Nolvadex) tricyclic antidepressants	Converts tamoxifen (Nolvadex) to the active metabolite. Ultra-rapid metabolizers have a better response to tamoxifen; poor metabolizers have shorter remission and worse disease prognosis.

Abbreviations: NSAIDs = nonsteroidal anti-inflammatory drugs; *VKORC1* = vitamin K epoxide reductase complex 1.
[a] Polymorphism of these enzymes results in ultra-rapid, intermediate, and poor metabolizing ability, thereby making these polymorphism responsible for blood levels of the substrate drug.
[b] Responsible for 20–23% of all drugs metabolized.
Sources: Data from Belle DJ, Singh H. Genetic factors in drug metabolism. *Am Fam Physician.* 2008;77(11):1553-1560[13]; Eichelbaum M, Ingelman-Sundberg M, Evans WE. Pharmacogenomics and individualized drug therapy. *Annu Rev Med.* 2006:27:119-137.[5]

VKORC1 type. As these issues with warfarin metabolism have become more widely recognized, alternative antiplatelet drugs have been developed; these agents are reviewed in more detail in the *Hematology* chapter. In 2007, the FDA changed the labeling on warfarin to reflect the need to evaluate genotype prior to drug dosing and administration.

Polymorphisms in Drug Transporters

Transport proteins are involved in the distribution of a number of therapeutic drugs. P-glycoprotein is an example of a transporter protein that has a role in excretion of metabolites into urine, bile, and the intestines. This protein also can decrease movement of various drugs such as digoxin (Lanoxin) across the blood–brain barrier, thereby limiting accumulation of those agents in the brain. Although polymorphisms in P-glycoprotein have been identified, the clinical relevance of polymorphisms of drug transporters has yet to be determined.

Rapid versus Slow Acetylators

As discussed in the *Principles of Pharmacology* chapter, drug metabolism occurs via phase I and phase II reactions that transform drugs from lipophilic to hydrophilic so they can be eliminated in urine. As part of this process, many drugs transfer an acetyl group from acetyl coenzyme A to an acceptor amine drug to form an amide. The enzyme *N*-acetyltransferase (NAT) catalyzes this process. At least three polymorphisms of NAT slow the process of NAT catalysis in the phase II reaction. Individuals who are **slow acetylators** have an increased risk for toxic reactions to drugs that are metabolized via this process, such as isoniazid (INH), sulfonamides, hydralazine (Apresoline), caffeine, and clonazepam (Klonopin). Slow acetylators who use isoniazid are at increased risk for isoniazid-induced neurotoxicity.[17] The incidence of slow acetylator status varies widely among ethnic groups, being present in 10% of Koreans, 25% of Thai, 20% of Chinese, 10% of Japanese, 60% of Indians, 50% of Germans, and 55% of Italians and Spanish individuals.[18]

Genomic Differences in Pharmacodynamics: Drug Response

A key molecule involved in drug response is the drug target or drug receptor. Dozens of receptors on cell membranes have been discovered. The genetic influence of polymorphisms in these receptors is independent of changes in drug metabolism, or even drug transport. One example of drug receptor concerns has emerged in connection with the beta-adrenergic receptor. Persons with asthma use $beta_2$ agonist drugs to relax smooth muscle surrounding the bronchial passages and thereby dilate those passages to improve air flow. Persons with genetic polymorphisms of the $beta_2$ adrenoreceptor have been found to have downregulation of the $beta_2$-adrenergic receptor rather than upregulation when they take these agents, which in turn worsens their disease and its accompanying symptoms. As many as 30% of persons with asthma have poor symptom control and recurrent exacerbations with treatment.[19] Specific sequelae include susceptibility to agonist-induced desensitization as well as various untoward cardiovascular effects.[20] Polymorphisms in several genes that encode for this receptor have been identified and the relationship between the polymorphic alleles and worsening clinical status has been identified in pharmacogenomic studies. Once knowledge of co-interactions has been elucidated, biomarkers that predict risk can be developed and genetic testing can be offered.

Drug receptors also provide the basis of some specifically developed drugs. These so-called designer drugs are usually thought of as prescription medications, but they may also be over-the-counter preparations or even botanicals. For example, studies of ginseng have identified a group of nuclear steroid hormone receptors in ginseng that may be manipulated to create a variation of ginseng that might be more effective as a pharmacologic agent.[21]

Role of Genetic Differences in the Risk of Adverse Drug Reactions

The risk of developing an adverse drug reaction can be increased secondary to poor metabolizer status or another genetic variation.[22] For example, CYP450 enzyme poor metabolizer status can result in toxic accumulation of a drug that then damages the liver. In contrast, some hypersensitivity drug reactions, such as Stevens-Johnson syndrome, occur secondary to polymorphisms of the human leucocyte antigen (HLA) genes that encode for the major histocompatibility complex (MHC) proteins. MHC proteins are present on the surface of cells, where they present small portions of antigen to T cells as part of the immune response. Polymorphisms in the MHC proteins allow some drugs to bind to them directly, thereby initiating a hypersensitivity reaction.[23] An example of this process is the association between carbamazepine (Tegretol) and Stevens-Johnson syndrome. Incidence of Stevens-Johnson syndrome is tenfold higher in persons of Southeast Asian descent compared to members of other racial/ethnic groups. Persons of Han Chinese ethnicity are most likely to have the polymorphic allele; thus, in this population, the FDA has recommended that genetic testing be completed before initiating carbamazepine therapy.[23] Similarly, genetic screening is recommended before starting abacavir therapy secondary to the risk of severe hypersensitivity reactions that occur in persons with the allele HLA-B*57:01.

Racial and Ethnic Differences in Drug Response

Polymorphisms of the genes encoding the CYP enzyme family are distributed differently among racial and ethnic groups. For example, the prevalence of CYP2D6 ultrarapid metabolizers is 1% to 10% in Caucasians, 3% to 5% in African Americans, 16% to 28% in North Africans, and 21% in Asians.[10] Likewise, the prevalence of poor metabolizer status varies across racial and ethnic groups. CYP2D6 is involved in metabolism of many commonly prescribed medications, including beta blockers, some tricyclic antidepressants, selective serotonin reuptake inhibitors, and codeine.[10] Both CYP2D6*17 (more common in African Americans than in other groups) and CYP2D6*10 (more common in Asians than in other groups) result in poor metabolism of drugs that are metabolized by these enzymes.

Polymorphic differences in drug receptors are also differentially distributed among racial and ethnic groups. It appears that persons of African American descent are more likely to respond with asthma exacerbation and increased morbidity when given long-acting beta-adrenergic agonists without concomitant therapy with an inhaled corticosteroid.[24] Although 49 polymorphisms have been identified in the gene that codes for the $beta_2$-adrengergic receptor, the knowledge of these relationships is not yet clear enough that clinical application of these findings is possible. Genome-wide association studies are pending.

Gender Differences in Drug Response

Genes encoding enzymes involved in drug metabolism are located on autosomes, rather than on sex chromosomes. Females and males in the same racial or ethnic group have similar distributions of particular polymorphisms. For this reason, the effects of gender on drug metabolism have often been assumed to result primarily from differences in average body size, renal excretion, and composition (body fat).[25] While these physiologic differences will differentially affect the pharmacokinetic properties of drugs, sex hormones can also influence the expression and activity of drug metabolism enzymes.[26,27] Activity of CYPs and other liver enzymes are modulated by sex hormones. Thus, even if a woman and a man have identical genes for CYP3A4, the amount and the activity of the CYP3A4 enzyme may differ in men versus women, resulting in different drug medication effects despite adjustment of the dose for body size. Research studies investigating the effects of sex hormones on drug metabolism are ongoing.

Women have a 50% to 75% higher risk than men of developing adverse drug reactions, including cardiac arrhythmias associated with medications that prolong the QT interval (an effect noted with some antihistamines, antibiotics, antiarrhythmics, and antipsychotics).[26] Two-thirds of reported drug-related arrhythmias occur in women. Long QT syndrome—the condition most commonly associated with adverse cardiac response to selected medications—is caused by polymorphisms in the potassium-channel genes *KCNQ1* and *KCNH2*. Although inheritance of the potassium-channel genes is generally considered autosomal dominant, for reasons not totally understood, there is a greater likelihood that women will transmit long QT syndrome to daughters than to sons.[28] Evidence also indicates that sex hormones modulate the response to medications that prolong the QT interval. Premenopausal women show greater QT prolongation during menses and ovulation than at other phases of the menstrual cycle.[29] A female with the *KCNQ1* or *KCNH2* polymorphism may have a lower threshold for developing an adverse reaction than a male who has identical potassium-channel mutations; in addition, her individual response to the medication may vary throughout her menstrual cycle.

Differences between women and men in response to pain medications have received a great deal of research attention. Sex differences in pain response are both complex and multifactorial in origin.[30,31] CYP450 enzyme polymorphisms can alter the effectiveness of pain medications, but differences in pain receptors may also be important. Some studies have reported that women respond with better analgesia and fewer side effects from kappa-receptor opiates than men do.[30,31] It has been hypothesized that estrogen affects opioid kappa-receptor density and binding. Other studies have reported that women respond better than men to mu-receptor agonists such as morphine.[32,33] A recent meta-analysis of sex differences in the response to opioids found that morphine is more potent in women than in men and that the onset/offset of morphine is slower in women.[34] Additional research is needed in this area before gender differences in the response to pain medications can be applied clinically.

The Future of Pharmacogenomics

To date, genome-wide association studies have identified some groups who will benefit from genome testing undertaken to direct pharmacotherapy, and the FDA has added pharmacogenomic information to the labels of several drugs, such as clopidogrel (Plavix), warfarin (Coumadin), and tramadol (Ultram).[35,36] For some drugs, this information includes actions to be taken in response to biomarker identification, such as genomic-specific dosing.[35,36] Table 3-3 lists the drugs for which genomics-based dosing guidelines are currently available.

The reliability of biomarkers used in pharmacogenomic testing is an area of active research. Although a variety of tests are available, there are also a plethora of unanswered questions about their use: How good is a particular test? Does it detect all etiologic polymorphisms of interest? Which group of individuals is most likely to benefit from this test? One example of how these issues are being handled involves a recent recommendation to categorize

Box 3-3 Polymorphisms and the Placenta: Effects on the Fetus

The placenta is a multifaceted organ. Despite its relatively short lifespan, the placenta can have long-term lasting effects on an individual's health. For example, the placenta expresses drug transporters that serve as efflux pumps. These transporters move drugs out of the placenta and back into the maternal compartment, thereby protecting the fetus from adverse drug effects. The placenta is of fetal origin and, therefore, the number and type of drug transporters expressed during gestation can be affected by polymorphism within the fetal genotype. A fetus with polymorphic drug transporters may not be as well protected against adverse effects of drugs, for example, and may be at more risk for developing a birth defect secondary to drug exposure. This scenario has been confirmed in mice that are at increased risk for cleft palate secondary to prenatal exposure to phenytoin (Dilantin).[38]

Fetal deletion of the *GSTT1(del)* gene results in deduced metabolism of nicotine metabolites. Fetuses with this genotype have been found to be at increased risk for low birth weight if their mother smokes during pregnancy.[39]

Table 3-3 Drugs with Dosing Guidelines Based on Genetic Polymorphisms[a]

Drug: Generic (Brand)	Indication	Polymorphism
Abacavir (Ziagen)	Antiretroviral to treat HIV infection	HLA-B
Allopurinol (Zyloprim)	Gout	HLA-B
Amitriptyline (Elavil)	Antidepressant	CYP2C19, CYP2D6
Azathioprine (Imuran)	Prevent transplant rejection	TPMT
Boceprevir (Victrelis)	Hepatitis C	IFNL3
Capecitabine (Xeloda)	Chemotherapy for cancer	DPYD
Carbamazepine (Tegretol)	Anticonvulsant used to treat epilepsy; also used to treat bipolar disorder and trigeminal neuralgia	HLA-B
Clomipramine (Anafranil)	Tricyclic antidepressant	CYP2C19, CYP2D6
Clopidogrel (Plavix)	Antiplatelet used to prevent intravascular clotting	CYP2C19
Codeine (usually found in combination products such as Tylenol 3)	Analgesic	CYP2D6
Desipramine (Norpramin)	Tricyclic antidepressant	CYP2D6
Doxepin (Deptran)	Tricyclic antidepressant	CYP2C19, CYP2D6
Fluorouracil (Adrucil)	Antimetabolite used to treat cancer	DPYD
Imipramine (Tofranil)	Tricyclic antidepressant	CYP2C19, CYP2D6
Ivacaftor (Kalydeco)	Cystic fibrosis	CFTR
Mercaptopurine (Purinethol)	Immunosuppressant	TPMT
Nortriptyline (Pamelor)	Tricyclic antidepressant	CYP2D6
Peginterferon alfa-2a (Pegasys)	Interferon used to treat chronic hepatitis C	IFNL3
Rasburicase (Elitek)	Contraindicated for persons who are G6PD deficient; treats the high levels of uric acid that occur when chemotherapy breaks down tumors	G6PD
Ribavirin (Rebetol)	Interferon used to treat hepatitis C	IFNL3
Simvastatin (Zocor)	Cholesterol-lowering drug	SLCO1B1
Tegafur (Uftoral)	Chemotherapy drug used to treat cancer	DPYD
Telaprevir (Incivek)	Hepatitis C	IFNL3
Thioguanine (Tabloid)	Acute myeloid leukemia	TPMT
Trimipramine (Surmontil)	Tricyclic antidepressant family	CYP2C19, CYP2D6
Warfarin (Coumadin)	Antithrombotic to prevent intravascular clotting	CYP2CP, VKORC1

[a] This table is not comprehensive as new information is being generated on a regular basis. Readers should refer to the Clinical Pharmacogenetics Implementation Consortium website for the current list.
Source: Data from Clinical Pharmacogenetics Implementation Consortium (CPIC), www.pharmgkb.org/page/cpic.

genetic tests into three tiers: (1) Tier 1/green genomic tests are based on evidence that supports implementation in practice; (2) Tier 2/yellow genomic tests are based on evidence that is insufficient to support their implementation in routine practice; and (3) Tier 3/red tests either have synthesized evidence that supports not using them or do not have relevant evidence available.[37] It is not yet clear if this classification system will be widely adopted.

Despite these unresolved issues, pharmacogenomics is likely to affect all healthcare fields in the future. Box 3-3 provides an example of how pharmacogenomic research may affect pregnant women and those who care for them.[38,39] As the knowledge base expands, several key areas within the field of pharmacogenomics bear watching.

Pharmacogenomics in Drug Development

Genome-wide association studies are a boon for drug development because they enable a drug researcher to identify a small homogenous group of individuals that would be most likely to benefit from a new drug. Once the etiologic SNP(s) or other genetic marker(s) are identified, biomarkers that reliably test for the polymorphism can be found and tested. There are multiple additional steps in this process as well as several scientific hurdles in study design and methodologies. However, once the trail from biomarker to genetic marker has been blazed, then regulatory agencies can look at population effects to determine which group of individuals will likely receive the greatest benefit from use of the test. All healthcare providers who prescribe drugs will want to pay close attention to this area of research.

Ethics and Pharmacogenomics

Most of the studies currently being conducted relate to genotypes and drug effectiveness and adverse effects. However, several topics germane to the overall field of genetics also have profound implications for pharmacogenomics. For example, informed decision making in an emerging area with multiple potential clinical implications obviously can be problematic.[40,41] Other ethical issues include the concept of patenting gene therapy and concerns related to access and privacy.

In the area of genetics as a whole, ethics is now recognized as a major thematic concern. Ethical dilemmas often occur when the needs of an individual differ from family beliefs or cultural mores.[42] These dilemmas may arise within the area of pharmacogenomics as well as within genetics as a whole. For example, to customize care, a person may need to have a personalized risk profile, and pharmacologic regimens based on individual genomic patterns. One major concern is that of access to these services. As pharmaceuticals become more individualized, it is expected that the already high cost of drugs in the United States will continue to increase. Health insurance—or, conversely, a lack of adequate prescription coverage—may increase disparities in adverse health outcomes and limit opportunities for some subgroups on the basis of their genetics. A full description of ethical considerations in pharmacogenomics is beyond the scope of this chapter, but should be acknowledged, and readers are encouraged to consider these factors when prescribing pharmaceuticals.

Resources for Pharmacogenomics

Healthcare providers who have an understanding of genomics and the application of genomic science to pharmacology can be more effective prescribers. Some excellent Internet resources are listed at the end of this chapter. In 2000, the National Coalition of Health Professions Education in Genetics (NCHPEG), an interdisciplinary group, published core competencies that serve as the framework for the education of health professionals in the area of genetics. These core competencies were reviewed, updated, and republished in late 2007.[43,44] One of the competencies specifically targets understanding of pharmacogenomics and the need to match prescribed drugs to individual genomic profiles. NCHPEG is working to ensure that resources are available so that all clinicians will have the tools necessary to "think genomically." As the era of personalized pharmacologic care emerges, genetic testing may be appropriate to determine the most effective pharmacologic regimen, the expected response to a medication, the appropriate dosage regimen, or the proper way of monitoring drug effectiveness. Current recommendations for drugs that may benefit from genetic testing can be found on the websites of the FDA and the Clinical Pharmacogenetics Implementation Consortium.

Conclusion

In the near future, the field of pharmacology undoubtedly will be deeply intertwined with expanding knowledge of pharmacogenomics. However, it would be premature to anticipate that widespread genotyping will be implemented within the next few years. More likely, such genotyping will occur sooner rather than later for persons with high-risk conditions and for drugs that are particularly difficult to manage with regard to adverse effects (e.g., meperidine [Demerol]) or achieving a therapeutic response (e.g., warfarin [Coumadin]).

As knowledge continues to grow about drug metabolism and genotypes, there also will be an explosion in research in other pharmacogenomic areas, including excretion, absorption, drug targets, and others. Clinical challenges include the probability that identification of genetic and pharmacogenomic risk factors will precede the development of new therapies or interventions for prevention.[45] Thus, healthcare professionals may be faced with the ability to identify drugs that are genetically contraindicated for a specific individual, but not have alternative options. In summary, clinicians need to be aware of the emerging information in pharmacogenomics. Eventually it will form one of the foundations of rational, genetically guided prescribing.

Resources

Organization	Description	Website
Clinical Pharmacogenetics Implementation Consortium (CPIC)	Shared project of PharmGKB and the Pharmacogenomics Research Institute, which is funded by the National Institutes of Health. The CPIC publishes peer-reviewed dosing guidelines for drugs (Table 3-3).	www.pharmgkb.org/view/dosing-guidelines.do?source=CPIC#
Food and Drug Administration, Table of Pharmacogenomic Biomarkers in Drug Labeling	List of drugs that have genomic information on the drug label. Some of these drugs require genomic testing prior to initiating therapy; others include genomic information in the precautions, warnings, or drug pharmacology.	www.fda.gov/drugs/scienceresearch/researchareas/pharmacogenetics/ucm083378.htm
GeneReviews	An expert-authored, peer-reviewed list of genetic diseases that addresses diagnosis, management, and genetic counseling for each disease	www.ncbi.nlm.nih.gov/books/NBK1116
Indiana University School of Medicine, Division of Clinical Pharmacology	Defines genetic influences on pharmacologic responses	www.drug-interactions.com
National Human Genome Research Institute	Includes many resources that address new knowledge based on the human genome	www.genome.gov
PharmGKB Pharmacogenetics Research Network	Nationwide collaboration of scientists studying the effects of genes on an individual's responses to a wide variety of medicines. The interactive website enables a clinician to explore the current state of knowledge about a specific drug or even a gene.	www.pharmgkb.org/index.jsp
University of California–San Diego Skaggs School of Pharmacy and Pharmaceutical Sciences	Pharmacogenomics education program	http://pharmacogenomics.ucsd.edu/home.aspx

References

1. Shin J, Kayser SR, Langaee TY. Pharmacogenetics: from discovery to patient care. *Am J Health Syst Pharm.* 2009;66(7):625-637.
2. Wolpert CM, Singer ML, Speer MC. Speaking the language of genetics: a primer. *J Midwifery Womens Health.* 2005;50(3):184-188.
3. Morse BL, Kim RB. Is personalized medicine a dream or a reality? *Crit Rev Clin Lab Sci.* 2014;2:1-11.
4. Evans WE, McLeod HL. Pharmacogenomics: drug disposition, drug targets, and side effects. *N Engl J Med.* 2003;348(6):538-539.
5. Eichelbaum M, Ingelman-Sundberg M, Evans WE. Pharmacogenomics and individualized drug therapy. *Annu Rev Med.* 2006;27:119-137.
6. Watson JD, Crick, FHC. Molecular structure of nucleic acids: a structure for deoxyribose nucleic acid. *Nature.* 1953;171:737.
7. National Institutes of Health. *From double helix to human sequence.* Scientific symposium; Bethesda, MD; April 14-15, 2003.
8. Wilkinson GR. Drug metabolism and variability among patients in drug response. *N Engl J Med.* 2006;21:2211-2221.
9. Service RF. Pharmacogenomics: going from genome to pill. *Science.* 2005;308:1858-1860.
10. Weinshilboum R. Inheritance and drug response. *N Engl J Med.* 2003;348(6):529-537.
11. Poland GA, Ovsyannikova IG, Jacobson RM. Application of pharmacogenomics to vaccines. *Pharmacogenomics.* 2009;10(5):837-852.
12. Samer CF, Lorenzini KI, Rollason V, Daali Y, Desmeules JA. Applications of CYP450 testing in the clinical setting. *Mol Diagn Ther.* 2013;17(3):165-184.
13. Belle DJ, Singh H. Genetic factors in drug metabolism. *Am Fam Physician.* 2008;77(11):1553-1560.
14. Koren G, Cairns J, Chitayat D, Gaedigk A, Leeder SJ. Pharmacogenetics of morphine poisoning in a breastfed neonate of a codeine-prescribed mother. *Lancet.* 2006;368(9536):704.
15. U.S. Food and Drug Administration. Public health advisory: use of codeine by some breastfeeding mothers may lead to life-threatening side effects in nursing babies. http://www.fda.gov/Safety/MedWatch/SafetyInformation/SafetyAlertsforHumanMedicalProducts/ucm152107.htm. Accessed July 30, 2014.
16. Ross S, Parer G. Pharmacogenetics of antiplatelets and anticoagulants: a report on clopidogrel,

warfarin, and dabigatran. *Pharmacogenomics.* 2013;14:1565-1572.

17. Sim E, Lack N, Wang CJ, et al. Arylamine *N*-acetyltranferases: structural and functional implications of polymorphisms. *Toxicology.* 2008;254(3): 170-183.
18. Walker K, Ginsberg G, Hattis D, Johns DO, Guyton KZ, Sonawane B. Genetic polymorphism in *N*-acetyltransferase (NAT): population distribution of NAT1 and NAT2 activity. *J Toxicol Environ Health B Crit Rev.* 2009;12(5-6):440-472.
19. Otega VE, Wechsler M. Asthma pharmacogenetics: responding to the call for a personalized approach. *Curr Opin Allergy Clin Immunol.* 2013;13:399-409.
20. Miller SM, Ortega VE. Pharmacogenetics and the development of personalized approaches for combination therapy in asthma. *Curr Allergy Asthma Rep.* 2013;13(5):443-452.
21. Yue PY, Mak NK, Cheng YK, et al. Pharmacogenomics and the yin/yang actions of ginseng: anti-tumor, angiomodulating and steroid-like activities of ginsenosides. *Chin Med.* 2007;15(2):6.
22. Ingelman-Sundberg M. Pharmacogenomic biomarkers for prediction of severe adverse drug reactions. *N Engl J Med.* 2008;358(6):637-639.
23. Karlin E, Phillips E. Genotyping for severe drug hypersensitivity. *Curr Allergy Asthma Rep.* 2014;14: 418-424.
24. Ortega VE, Meyers DA. Pharmacogenetics: implications of race and ethnicity on defining genetic profiles for personalized medicine: mechanisms of allergic diseases. *J Allergy Clin Immunol.* 2014;133:16-26.
25. Gandhi M, Aweeka F, Greenblatt RM, Blaschke TF. Sex differences in pharmacokinetics and pharmacodynamics. *Annu Rev Pharmacol Toxicol.* 2004;44: 499-523.
26. Anderson GD. Sex and racial differences in pharmacological response: where is the evidence? Pharmacogenetics, pharmacokinetics, and pharmacodynamics. *J Womens Health.* 2005;14:19-29.
27. Anderson GD. Gender differences in pharmacological response. *Int Rev Neurobiol.* 2008;83:1-10.
28. Imboden M, Swan H, Denjoy I, et al. Female predominance and transmission distortion in the long-QT syndrome. *N Engl J Med.* 2006;355(26):2744-2751.
29. Anthony M, Berg MJ. Biologic and molecular mechanisms for sex differences in pharmacokinetics, pharmacodynamics, and pharmacogenetics: part I. *J Womens Health Gend Based Med.* 2002;11:601-615.
30. Rasakham K, Liu-Chen LY. Sex differences in kappa opioid pharmacology. *Life Sci.* 2011;88(1-2):2-16.
31. Dahan A, Kest B, Waxman AR, Sarton E. Sex-specific responses to opiates: animal and human studies. *Anesth Analg.* 2008;107(1):83-95.
32. Fillingim RB, Gear RW. Sex differences in opioid analgesia: clinical and experimental findings. *Eur J Pain.* 2004;8:413-425.
33. Fillingim RB, Ness TJ, Glover TL, et al. Morphine responses and experimental pain: sex differences in side effects and cardiovascular responses but not analgesia. *J Pain.* 2005;6(2):116-124.
34. Niesters M, Dahan A, Kest B, et al. Do sex differences exist in opioid analgesia? A systematic review and meta-analysis of human experimental and clinical studies. *Pain.* 2010;151(1):61-68.
35. Pacanowski MA, Leptak C, Zineh I. Next-generation medicines: past regulatory experience and considerations for the future. *Clin Pharmacol Ther.* 2014; 95(3):247-249.
36. Wang L, McLeod HL, Weinshilboum RM. Genomics and drug response. *N Engl J Med.* 2011;364(12): 1144-1153.
37. Dotson WD, Douglas MP, Kolor K, et al. Prioritizing genomic applications for action by level of evidence: a horizon-scanning method. *Clin Pharmacol Ther.* 2014;95(4):394-402.
38. Daud A, Bergman J, Bakker M, et al. Pharmacogenetics of drug-induced birth defects: the role of polymorphisms on placental transporter proteins. *Pharmacogenomics.* 2014;15(7):1029-1041.
39. Hellden A, Madadi O. Pregnancy and pharmacogenomics in the context of drug metabolism and response. *Pharmacogenomics.* 2013;14(14):1779-1791.
40. Hampton T. Researchers draft guidelines for clinical use of pharmacogenomics. *JAMA.* 2006;296(12):1453-1454.
41. Rothstein MA. *Pharmacogenomics: Social, Ethical, and Clinical Dimensions.* Hoboken, NJ: Wiley-Liss; 2003.
42. Lea DH, Williams J, Donahue MP. Ethical issues in genetic testing. *J Midwifery Womens Health.* 2005; 50(3)234-240.
43. National Coalition for Health Professional Education in Genetics. Core competencies in genetics for health professionals. 2007. http://www.nchpeg.org/index.php?option=com_content&view=article&id=237&Itemid=84/. Accessed August 20, 2014.
44. Engstrom JL, Sefton MG, Mattheson JK, Healy KM. Genetic competencies essential for healthcare professionals in primary care. *J Midwifery Womens Health.* 2005;50:177-183.
45. Hunter DJ, Khoury MJ, Drazen JM. Letting the genome out of the bottle: will we get our wish? *N Engl J Med.* 2008;358(2):105-107.

4

Drug Toxicity

Nell L. Tharpe, Tekoa L. King

Chapter Glossary

Adverse drug events (ADEs) Any untoward medical occurrence that may present during treatment with a pharmaceutical product but that does not necessarily have a causal relationship with the pharmacologic treatment.

Adverse drug reactions (ADRs) Responses to a drug that are noxious and unintended and that occur at doses normally used for prophylaxis, diagnosis, or therapy of disease or for the modification of physiologic function.

Anaphylactoid reaction Severe systemic reaction with the same symptoms as anaphylaxis, which occurs after the first exposure to a substance. Anaphylactoid reactions occur as a reaction to the substance itself and are not allergic or dependent on immunoglobulin E.

Anaphylaxis Severe, potentially fatal, systemic allergic reaction that occurs suddenly after contact with an allergy-causing substance.

Antidotes Substances or agents that counteract or neutralize the effect of a poison or toxin by binding with it (chemical antidote) or preventing its intestinal absorption (mechanical antidote).

Antigen Substance that, when introduced into the body, is perceived as foreign and initiates an immune response.

Bioaccumulation Functional biologic process in which substances are taken up and stored faster than they are metabolized or excreted. This results in an increase in the concentration of a chemical within the organism over time.

Chelating agent Chemical compound that forms complexes with metals. The resultant chelate can then be excreted. Chelating agents are used to treat metal poisoning.

Drug allergy Hypersensitivity reaction to a medication.

Haptens Small molecules that elicit immune responses only when attached to larger carriers. A drug can be a hapten if it attaches to an intrinsic protein to form a complex that is then antigenic and can induce a hypersensitivity response.

Hypersensitivity reactions States of altered reactivity wherein the body reacts to a foreign substance with an exaggerated immune response.

Idiosyncratic reactions Unpredictable reactions that are uncommon and unexpected occurring after administration of the first dose of a medication, and are not within the known pharmacologic properties of the drug.

Pseudo-allergy Hypersensitivity reaction wherein a drug interacts directly with mast cells or complement to initiate a systemic anaphylactoid reaction; it is clinically similar to anaphylaxis. Also termed nonallergic anaphylaxis.

Red man syndrome Reaction appearing within 4–10 minutes after the commencement or soon after the completion of an infusion, characterized by flushing and/or an erythematous rash on the face, neck, and upper torso due to nonspecific mast cell degranulation rather than an IgE-mediated allergic reaction. Hypotension and angioedema may also occur. Treated with antihistamines.

Secondary side effects Adverse health conditions that occur secondary to a predictable drug effect. The development of thrush following treatment of antibiotics is a secondary side effect.

Side effects Drug effects that occur secondary to the intended therapeutic effect and are bothersome but not deleterious. Side effects may be unwanted or therapeutic for another indication.

Toxicants Toxic agents that are inorganic, such as heavy metals, chemicals, and industrial effluent.

Toxicity Consequence of a dose or exposure to an agent that is beyond the body's capability to metabolize under physiologic conditions; an adverse effect produced by a drug that is detrimental to the individual's health.

Toxicology Study of the adverse effects of chemical, physical, or biological agents on living organisms and the ecosystem, including the prevention and amelioration of such adverse effects.

Toxins Toxic agents produced by or occurring naturally in living organisms. *Environmental toxins* are toxins that are found in the environment due to chemical spills, waste, or pollution.

Type I hypersensitivity reactions True IgE-mediated allergic reactions.

Type II hypersensitivity reaction Cytotoxic reactions wherein IgG or IgM antibodies destroy cells containing antigens or haptens.

Type III hypersensitivity reaction Reactions in which soluble antigens not bound to cell surfaces (which occurs in Type II reactions) bind to antibodies and form complexes that are not easily cleared. These complexes are then deposited in organs where they induce an inflammatory response.

Type IV hypersensitivity reactions Delayed T-cell-mediated reactions.

Introduction

All drugs can be toxic if certain individual, environmental, dose, or genetic factors are present. Thus, knowledge of adverse effects of drugs is an integral component of the practice of pharmacotherapeutics. This chapter reviews adverse drug reactions, drug overdose, anaphylaxis, and poisoning.[1-3]

Toxicology is both the branch of pharmacology that studies the adverse health effects of drugs and a related science that studies the adverse effects of chemicals, physical agents, and radiation. Toxicology is usually subdivided into environmental, occupational, and medical branches. Toxicologists evaluate factors that modify the effects of **toxins** and **toxicants** on the biologic systems of individuals or populations and are instrumental in the development of preventive and safety practices to minimize exposures.

The concept of toxicology has existed throughout the ages. Out of necessity, humans learned which plants and animals were safe to eat and which were poisonous. The long-term effects of chemical warfare used during World War I and nerve agents used during World War II highlighted the potentially devastating effects of environmental toxins and stimulated the development of the modern science of toxicology.

In the 1930s, scientists pioneered the development of numerous synthetic chemicals with the goal of producing commercial products to enhance numerous aspects of daily life. The 1935 DuPont chemical company slogan, "Better Things for Better Living . . . Through Chemistry," summarized this approach. During the post–World War II years, significant advances in the prevention and treatment of disease were made possible due to the development of highly effective new pharmacologic agents. However, the extensive and often indiscriminate use of new chemicals, including drugs, revealed the toxic effects of many of these substances.

Rachel Carson's well-known book, *Silent Spring*,[4] published in 1962, clearly portrayed the alarming negative effects of widespread use of toxic compounds, such as dichloro-diphenyl-trichloroethane (DDT). Carson's work is considered the impetus behind the environmental movement and contributed to the development of the scientific discipline of environmental toxicology.

Adverse Drug Reactions

Adverse drug reactions (ADRs) were defined by the World Health Organization in 1972 as noxious and unintended human responses to pharmacologic agents occurring at doses normally considered therapeutic.[5] Adverse drug reactions can be related to the active component of the drug itself, or they can be a reaction to excipients, which are fillers in the medication, metabolites of the drug, or contaminants from the manufacturing process. ADRs are distinguished from **adverse drug events (ADEs)**, which are any untoward medical occurrence that may present during treatment with a pharmaceutical product. However, they may not be caused by the pharmacologic agent.

The primary resource for studying ADRs and ADEs is the U.S. Food and Drug Administration's (FDA) MedWatch Program, which has collected and analyzed drug-related adverse event data since 1998. The FDA Adverse Event Reporting System (FAERS) collects postmarketing reports on ADEs, ADRs, product quality problems, product use errors, and suspected therapeutic failures. The goal of FAERS is to improve public health through effective collection and analysis of safety reports. Federal regulations require drug manufacturers to submit all reports of adverse drug events they receive to FAERS. Healthcare providers and consumers may also voluntarily submit reports through the MedWatch website (its address is provided at the end of this chapter).

Clinical reviewers who work in the Center for Drug Evaluation and Research (CDER) and the Center for Biologics Evaluation and Research (CBER) review reports submitted to FAERS to monitor drug safety. The CDER and CBER evaluations form the basis for further epidemiologic studies when appropriate. As a result of these analyses, the FDA may take regulatory actions, such as updating a product's labeling information, reevaluating an approval decision, or recalling a drug from the market.

Incidence of Adverse Drug Reactions

Approximately 6.5% of all persons admitted to a hospital in the United States are admitted for treatment of a serious ADR.[6,7] The incidence of fatal ADRs is approximately 0.15% to 0.3%, or nearly 100,000 persons per year.[8] As use of prescription medications increases, so does the incidence of ADRs.

When Moore et al. conducted an analysis of all serious ADRs and ADEs reported to the FAERS database between 1998 and 2005, they found that 67% (n = 314,145) were manufacturer-submitted expedited reports addressing problems identified in the early postmarketing period.[9] In the interval from 2000 to 2009, the number of reports of serious ADEs submitted to FAERS increased at a mean annual rate of 11.3%.[10]

Thus, ADRs are an ongoing public health problem. Before they are marketed to the general public, most drugs are studied in fewer than 4000 individuals during preclinical trials.[11] Therefore, ADRs that occur at a rate of 1 per 1000 users (or less) are not likely to be detected during preclinical testing.[11] The relatively small numbers of ADRs are not the whole problem, however. Preclinical drug testing is usually conducted among a homogenous population to best determine the drug response for a specific indication. Once the drug receives FDA approval and is sold on the larger market, a larger heterogeneous population of individuals will use the drug; at that point, drug interactions not detected in preclinical testing are likely to appear. As reviewed in the *Pharmacogenetics* chapter, race, age, gender, and genetics are only some of the characteristics that can have significant effects on drug response. Postmarketing reports of ADRs, therefore, are an essential mechanism for identifying ADRs. Clinicians and consumers alike are strongly encouraged to report ADRs to the FAERS website.

Adverse drug events related to commercial dietary supplements is another area of concern, and one where the incidence of ADEs is not well known.[12] In contrast to prescription medications, supplements do not require FDA approval before being marketed to the public. Commercially available supplements can result in a wide array of serious ADRs, including cardiac arrhythmias, myocardial infarction, hepatoxicity, and mood alterations such as panic attacks and unprovoked aggression.

Factors That Increase the Risk of Adverse Drug Reactions

Multiple factors increase the risk that an ADR will occur, including characteristics of the drug, individual factors, and route of administration.[13] Drugs with a high molecular weight (e.g., insulin) and those that are CYP450 inducers or inhibitors can generate ADRs. Also, some drugs are more likely than others to form bonds with intrinsic proteins in which the resultant complex is antigenic. With regard to individual characteristics, persons who are young or older, women, and persons with serious illnesses have an increased risk for experiencing ADRs. Examples of conditions that increase the risk of ADRs include autoimmune disorders, concomitant viral infection, and liver dysfunction. In addition, certain genetic polymorphisms increase the risk for experiencing an ADR. Finally, medications that must be administered via the intravenous, intramuscular, or topical route are more likely to cause an ADR than are medications that are administered orally.

Adverse Drug Reactions in Women

While some ADRs affect both women and men, others are specific to women and their offspring. Historical examples include thalidomide, used in the 1960s, and diethylstilbestrol (DES), a drug commonly prescribed to pregnant women between the years 1938 to 1971.[14] Overall, women have a nearly twofold greater risk of experiencing an adverse reaction to drugs compared to men.[13,15] Of the 10 prescription drugs withdrawn from the market between 1997 and 2001, 8 had more health risks for women than for men.[16] Women may be physiologically more prone to develop ADRs, yet compared to men, women use more medications and report adverse reactions more often.[16] Further research is necessary to determine why the incidence of ADRs is higher in women than in men.

Classification of Adverse Drug Reactions

Several classification schemes for ADRs have been promoted based on putative etiology, time of onset, or predictability of drug response.[11,17–19] None are definitive, however, because the mechanism of action of ADRs is incompletely understood. In this chapter, the classification system used by the Joint Task Force on Practice Parameters, representing the American Academy of Allergy, Asthma, and Immunology, the American College of Allergy, Asthma, and Immunology, and the Joint Council of Allergy, Asthma, and Immunology, is used (Figure 4-1 and Table 4-1).[19]

ADRs are initially classified as Type A reactions that are due to the pharmacologic properties of the drug. Type A ADRs are predictable, non-immune, and often dose dependent. In contrast, Type B reactions are unpredictable and may have a mechanism of action that involves the immune system.[11] Type B hypersensitivity ADRs are further subclassified based on the immune or nonimmune mechanism of action (Figure 4-1).[11,17] Approximately 85% to 90% of ADRs are Type A, and 10% to 15% of ADRs are Type B.

Type A Adverse Drug Reactions

Type A ADRs occur as a result of drug side effects, drug–agent interactions, or drug toxicity. Known **side effects** and **secondary side effects** of drugs are predictable drug outcomes, and are addressed throughout this text in the sections on specific drugs. Drug interactions are reviewed in the *Principles of Pharmacology* chapter.

Drug Toxicity

Drug **toxicity** can occur as a result of toxic metabolites or drug overdose. If an active metabolite is generated following biotransformation, the metabolite may bind with the intended target receptors, enzymes, or proteins and cause an unintended toxic response. In other instances, especially in the presence of renal or hepatic dysfunction or in persons with genetic polymorphisms in the cytochrome P-450 enzyme system, metabolism may result in toxic metabolites or transform drugs or chemical agents to reactive species that cause cellular damage, toxicity, or both.[20]

A drug overdose occurs when the amount of a drug or a combination of drugs is cytotoxic to the individual. It may occur if an excessive dose is administered, during

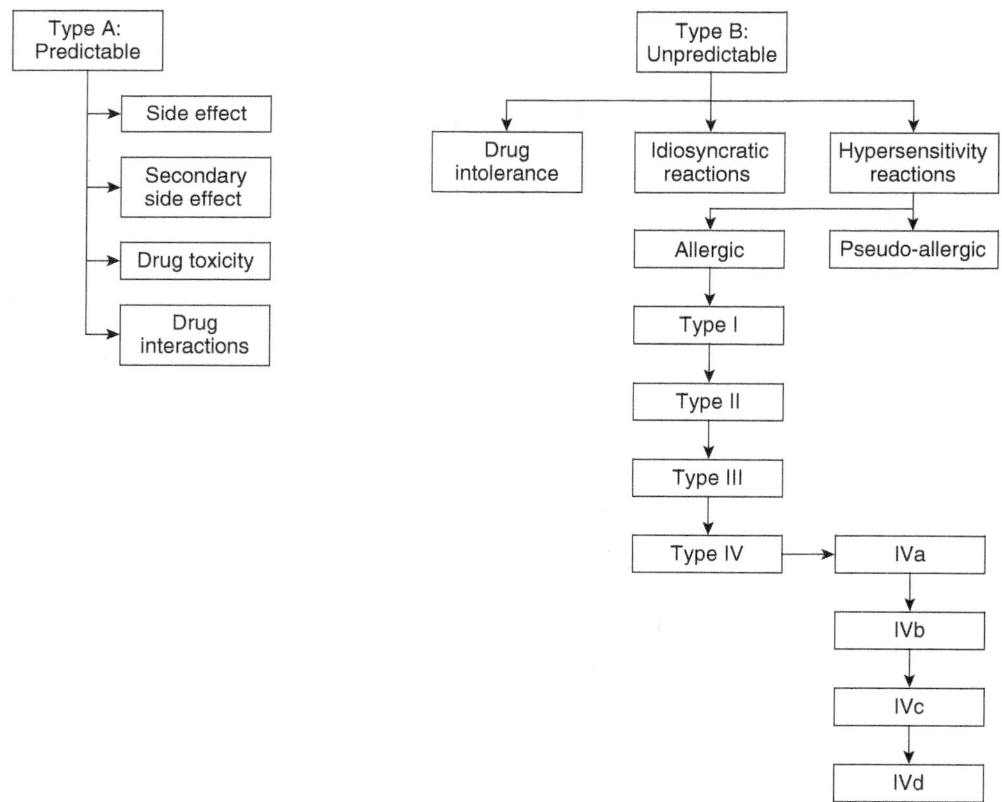

Figure 4-1 Classification of adverse drug reactions.

Table 4-1 Types of Adverse Drug Reactions

	Mechanism of Action	Chronology	Clinical Symptoms	Example
Type A: Predictable Based on Pharmacologic Mechanism of Action				
1. Side effect	Expected response of drug based on pharmacodynamics.	Variable	Variable	Dry mouth following use of anti-histamine
2. Secondary effect	Clinical condition that develops secondary to known effects of a drug.	Variable	Variable	Candidal vaginitis following course of antibiotics
3. Drug toxicity	Toxic effects of drug or drug metabolite.	Variable	Variable	Hepatotoxicity from acetaminophen overdose
4. Drug interaction	Generally involves inhibition or suppression of CYP450 enzymes, which results in diminished or enhanced drug response.	Variable	Variable	Seizure following concomitant use of theophylline and erythromycin
Type B: Drug Reaction Not Predicted from Pharmacologic Mechanism of Action				
1. Drug intolerance	An undesired drug effect produced at therapeutic or subtherapeutic doses. Presumed genetic polymorphism that may or may not be known. Immune mechanisms are not involved.	Variable but often soon after drug is absorbed	Variable	Aspirin-induced tinnitus at low dose of aspirin
2. Idiosyncratic reaction	Uncharacteristic reaction that is not explainable in terms of the known pharmacological actions of the drug but is reproducible on readministration. Presumed to occur secondary to an underlying abnormality of metabolism, excretion, or bioavailability.	Variable	Variable	Hemolytic anemia in person with G6PD deficiency after taking aspirin
3. Hypersensitivity reactions 3a. Allergic (Drug Allergy)				
Type I hypersensitivity (IgE-mediated)	IgE-mediated activation of mast cells and basophils releases histamine and leukotrienes.	Immediate: Minutes to few hours after drug exposure	Anaphylaxis, urticaria, angioedema, bronchospasm, pruritus, vomiting, diarrhea	Anaphylaxis following second exposure to β-lactam antibiotic
Type II hypersensitivity (cytotoxic)	IgG or IgM antibodies directed at drug-hapten coated cells.	Variable	Hemolytic anemia, neutropenia, thrombocytopenia	Thrombocytopenia following exposure to propylthiouracil (PTU)
Type III (immune complex)	IgM, IgG, and IgA. Tissue deposition of drug–antibody complexes.	1–3 weeks after drug exposure	Arthritis, nephritis, serum sickness, glomerulonephritis, vasculitis	Arthus reaction (local); serum sickness (systemic)
Type IV delayed drug hypersensitivity	MHC presentation of drug molecules to T cells and subsequent cytokine and inflammatory mediator release.	2–7 days after cutaneous drug exposure	Allergic contact dermatitis, maculopapular drug rash	Ampicillin rash
3b. Pseudo-allergic		Variable	Variable	Opioid-induced itching

Sources: Data from Aronson JK, Ferner RE. Clarification of terminology in drug safety. *Drug Saf.* 2005;28(10):851-870[18]; Doña I, Barrionuevo E, Blanca-Lopez N, et al. Trends in hypersensitivity drug reactions: more drugs, more response patterns, more heterogeneity. *J Investig Allergol Clin Immunol.* 2014;24(3):143-153[17]; Hausmann O, Schnyder B, Pichler WJ. Etiology and pathogenesis of adverse drug reactions. *Chem Immunol Allergy.* 2012;97:32-46[11]; Joint Task Force on Practice Parameters; American Academy of Allergy, Asthma, and Immunology; American College of Allergy, Asthma, and Immunology; Joint Council of Allergy, Asthma, and Immunology. Drug allergy: an updated practice parameter. *Ann Allergy Asthma Immunol.* 2010;105(4):259-273[19]; Reidl MA, Casillas AM. Adverse drug reactions: types and treatment options. *Am Fam Physician.* 2003;68:1781-1790.[13]

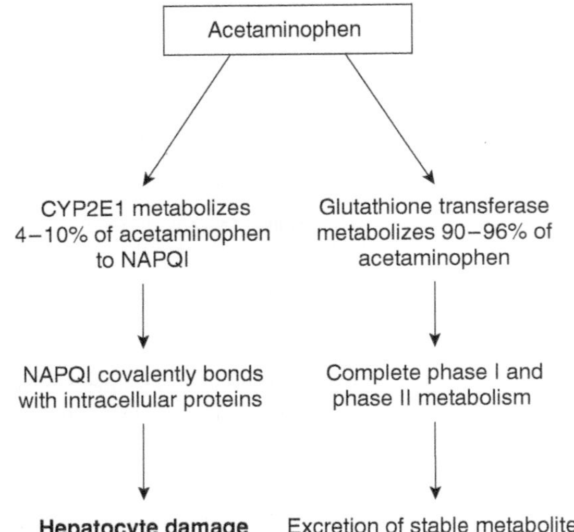

Figure 4-2 Drug toxicity: Mechanism of acetaminophen-induced hepatotoxicity.

administration of a therapeutic dose to a person who has renal or hepatic compromise, through a drug–agent interaction that decreases metabolism of the drug, or when metabolic or genetic variations result in decreased metabolism of the drug. For example, one of the most common causes of drug-induced liver disease is an overdose of acetaminophen (Tylenol).[21] In this case, the damage is caused by the metabolite *N*-acetyl-*p*-benzoquinone, which is normally detoxified during phase II metabolism. In the case of an overdose, the large amount of active metabolite generated overwhelms the ability of the liver to detoxify it, and liver damage ensues. Acetaminophen (Tylenol) is a common component in many over-the-counter cold products and, therefore, consumers can inadvertently self-administer an excessive dose (Figure 4-2).

Drug Interactions

Unexpected reactions can occur as a result of interactions between prescription drugs, over-the-counter medications, dietary supplements, or illicit agents. The accurate identification of drug interactions is challenging, particularly when more than two medications or supplements are involved. A number of "drug interaction checker" electronic tools are available to professionals and consumers as aids to help reduce preventable adverse effects.

Type B Adverse Drug Reactions

Type B ADRs are generally not dose dependent. These ADRs have traditionally been classified as unpredictable. Persons who experience Type B ADRs often have a genetic predisposition that increases the likelihood that a specific drug will elicit an ADR. New genetic tests can confer predictability for some ADRs such as carbamazepine (Tegretol)-induced cutaneous eruptions, so it is no longer correct to assume that all Type B ADRs are unpredictable. Similarly, not all hypersensitivity reactions are true drug allergies. For example, NSAID-induced respiratory symptoms occur secondary to an inhibition of the enzyme cyclooxygenase-1 (COX-1). The result is a diminution of prostaglandin production and an increase in leukotriene synthase, which causes bronchospasm.[11] As knowledge of drug response, genetic polymorphisms, and the immune mechanisms increases, our ability to identify individuals at risk for Type B ADRs and prevent ADRs will likely increase and classification of these ADRs may change.[4]

Drug Intolerance

Intolerance refers to a type of ADR in which the individual has an unusually low threshold for an expected side effect or an atypical ADR. The mechanism of action is presumed to be a combination of known pharmacologic effects and individual susceptibility. These ADRs are related to the pharmacologic effects and occur in persons who do not have known abnormalities of metabolism, excretion, or bioavailability. Thus, genetic predispositions that are as yet undiscovered are presumed to play a role in the development of drug intolerance.

Idiosyncratic Drug Reactions

Idiosyncratic drug reactions are uncharacteristic reactions that are presumed to be caused by an underlying abnormality in metabolism, excretion, or bioavailability.[19,22] These clinical reactions are unrelated to the pharmacologic properties of the drug (Box 4-1).[23]

Hypersensitivity Reactions

Hypersensitivity reactions are objectively reproducible symptoms or signs initiated by exposure to a defined stimulus at a dose tolerated by normal persons.[23] Hypersensitivity reactions can be immune mediated or non-immune mediated, although the end steps in the pathologic process and clinical symptoms are the same in both cases.[24] The term **drug allergy** is used to designate an immune-mediated or allergic hypersensitivity reaction; the term **pseudo-allergy** is used to refer to a nonimmune mediated reaction.[3]

Box 4-1 The Story of an Idiosyncratic Drug Reaction

CR, a 22-year-old college student, was given minocycline (Minocin) for treatment of new-onset pustular acne. Three weeks after CR started taking minocycline, she developed a fever, a generalized rash, and arthralgia. CR was examined at her college health center and noted to have some lymphadenopathy. She had no known exposure to any infectious diseases and no history of allergic reactions.

CR was admitted to the hospital for observation. Over the course of the next day, she developed angioedema and dyspnea. She had normal laboratory values, including a complete blood count (CBC) and tests of liver function and renal function. She also had a normal chest X ray and negative blood cultures. Tests for systemic lupus erythematosus, hepatitis, and other autoimmune disorders were all negative.

It was determined that CR had a serum sickness-like reaction, which is a well-known adverse effect of minocycline. CR was treated with steroids and the minocycline was discontinued. Her symptoms improved quickly and she was able to return to her normal activities 3 weeks after the initial onset of symptoms.

Allergic hypersensitivity reactions are further subdivided into categories based on the mechanism of action, although histamine is directly responsible for symptoms in each type. Individuals with hypersensitivity reactions frequently exhibit hives (urticaria) or rash, pruritus, wheezing, arthralgia, and localized edema. Hypotension, blistering of the skin, high fever, angioedema, or airway compromise signal the onset of a severe hypersensitivity reaction.

Substances with higher molecular weights and complex chemical structures, such as exogenous proteins (e.g., insulin), have a greater propensity for triggering immunogenic hypersensitivity or allergic reactions. Other drugs that have smaller molecular weights act as **haptens** by binding to endogenous proteins to form hapten–protein complexes that are antigenic.[25]

Type I Hypersensitivity Reactions

Type I hypersensitivity reactions are true IgE-mediated allergic reactions. As many as 70% of Type I reactions occur in females.[26] Immune sensitivity is enhanced by intermittent and repeated administration compared to continuous treatment. Immune sensitivity occurs most often following parenteral administration of a medication.

Following initial exposure to the drug, the drug-specific IgE antibody binds to surface receptors on mast cells and basophils throughout the body. When the drug enters the body and is detected a second time, the IgE-bound cells release histamine, prostaglandins, and leukotrienes, which cause the cascade of clinical manifestations within minutes to hours following exposure to the drug.[3,26] The amount and combination of pharmacologically active substances released contribute to the severity of the hypersensitivity reaction, which may consist of mild rhinorrhea, moderate urticaria and bronchial asthma, or severe anaphylaxis or **red man syndrome**. Anaphylaxis—the most severe form of the Type I hypersensitivity reaction—occurs within an hour after initial exposure.

Antibiotics are the most common etiology of mild and severe Type I hypersensitivity reactions and are particularly well known for their immunogenicity.[26,27] The drugs most often implicated are beta-lactam antibiotics such as amoxicillin (Amoxil), ampicillin (Principen), and penicillin.[28] Sulfonamides and cephalosporins have also been identified as triggers for these reactions.[29]

Anaphylaxis

In 2011, the World Allergy Organization published definitive diagnostic criteria for anaphylaxis (Table 4-2).[2,30] Acute anaphylaxis is characterized by respiratory difficulty and hypotension and requires rapid administration of epinephrine and prompt emergency treatment to secure the airway and provide fluid management.[31] Once the individual is stable, follow-up evaluation may include skin testing or radioallergosorbent testing to positively identify the allergen(s) (Figure 4-3). Drugs known to elicit anaphylaxis are listed in Table 4-3.[3,23,31] Treatment of anaphylactic reactions is discussed in Box 4-2.[31–33]

Type II Hypersensitivity Reactions

Type II and Type III hypersensitivity reactions both involve drug-specific IgG antibodies and the formation of immune complexes. In the case of **Type II hypersensitivity reactions**, the affected cells include erythrocytes, leukocytes, and platelets. Thus, the clinical syndromes associated with this type of ADR are hemolytic anemia, thrombocytopenia, or neutropenia. The immune complexes form when a drug acts as a hapten and binds to a protein, which makes the drug–protein complex antigenic. IgG or IgM antibodies tag

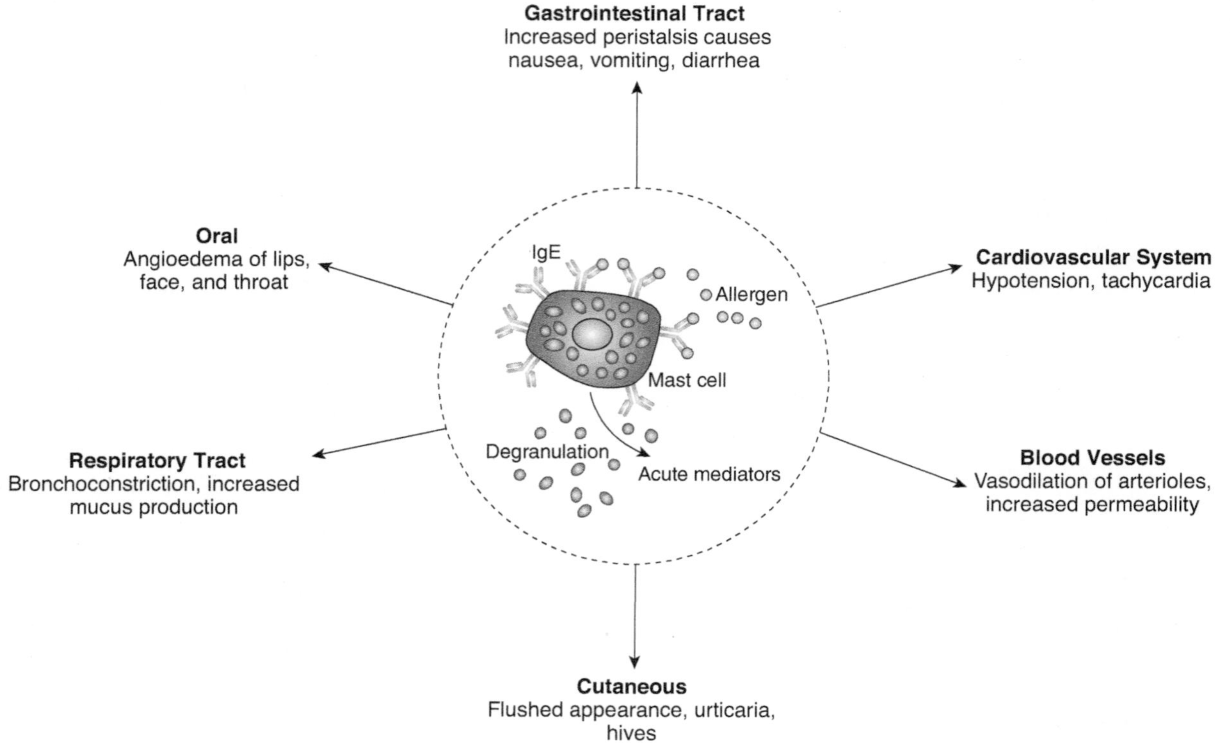

Figure 4-3 Mechanism of anaphylaxis.

Table 4-2 Criteria for Diagnosis of Anaphylaxis

Anaphylaxis is highly likely when any one of the following criteria are fulfilled:
1. Acute onset of an illness (minutes to several hours) with involvement of the skin, mucosal tissue, or both (e.g., generalized hives, pruritus or flushing, or swollen lips, tongue, or uvula) *and at least one of the following:* a. Respiratory compromise (e.g., dyspnea, wheeze–bronchospasm, stridor, reduced PEF, hypoxemia) b. Reduced blood pressure or associated symptoms of end-organ dysfunction (e.g., hypotonia [collapse], syncope, incontinence) *OR*
2. Two or more of the following that occur rapidly after exposure to a *likely allergen*[a] *for that patient* (minutes to several hours): a. Involvement of the skin–mucosal tissue (e.g., generalized hives, itch–flush, swollen lips, tongue, or uvula) b. Respiratory compromise (e.g., dyspnea, wheeze–bronchospasm, stridor, reduced PEF, hypoxemia) c. Reduced blood pressure or associated symptoms (e.g., hypotonia [collapse], syncope, incontinence) d. Persistent gastrointestinal symptoms (e.g., crampy abdominal pain, vomiting) *OR*
3. Reduced blood pressure after exposure to a *known allergen*[b] *for that patient* (minutes to several hours) a. Infants and children: low systolic blood pressure (age specific) or > 30% decrease in systolic blood pressure[c] b. Adults: systolic blood pressure < 90 mm Hg or > 30% decrease in systolic blood pressure from that person's baseline

Abbreviations: PEF = peak expiratory flow.

[a] Or other trigger—for example, immunologic but IgE-independent, or nonimmunologic (direct) mast cell activation.

[b] For example, after an insect sting, reduced blood pressure might be the only manifestation of anaphylaxis. In a similar example, during allergen immunotherapy, after injection of a known allergen in that patient, generalized urticaria (just one body organ system affected) might be the only initial manifestation of anaphylaxis.

[c] Low systolic blood pressure for children is defined as less than 70 mm Hg from 1 month to 1 year, less than 70 mm Hg from 1 to 10 years, and less than 90 mm Hg from 11 to 17 years. Normal heart rate ranges from 80 to 140 beats/min at age 1–2 years; from 80 to 120 beats/min at age 3 years; and from 70 to 115 beats/min after age 3 years. Infants are more likely to have respiratory compromise than hypotension or shock; and in this age group, shock is more likely to be manifest initially by tachycardia than by hypotension.

Source: Reproduced from Simons FER, Ardusso LRF, Bilò MB, et al. World Allergy Organization guidelines for the assessment and management of anaphylaxis. WAO position paper. *WAO J.* 2011;4:13-37.[2]

Table 4-3 Drugs Most Likely to Cause Anaphylaxis

Type I Hypersensitivity Anaphylaxis: Generic (Brand)	Pseudo-allergic Anaphylactoid Reaction: Generic (Brand)
Acetylsalicylic acid (aspirin)	Cephalosporins
Beta-lactam antibiotics	Codeine
Immunoglobulin preparations	Doxorubicin (Doxil)
Plasma expanders	Meperidine (Demerol)
Quinolones	Morphine
	Nonsteroidal anti-inflammatory drugs
	Penicillin
	Platinum-containing chemotherapy agents
	Quinolones
	Radio contrast media
	Taxanes

Sources: Data from Farnam K, Chang C, Teuber S, Gershwin ME. Nonallergic drug hypersensitivity reactions. *Int Arch Allergy Immunol.* 2012;159(4):327-345[23]; Pichler WJ, Adam J, Daubner B, Gentinetta T, Keller M, Yerly D. Drug hypersensitivity reactions: pathomechanism and clinical symptoms. *Med Clinic N Am.* 2010;94:645-66[43]; Wang H, Wang HS, Liu ZP. Agents that induce pseudo-allergic reaction. *Drug Discov Ther.* 2011;5(5):211-219.[30]

the hapten–protein complex and send signals leading to destruction of the cell.[34] Commonly implicated drugs are penicillins, cephalosporins, NSAIDs, propylthiouracil (PTU), sulfonamides, and vancomycin (Vanocin).

Type III Hypersensitivity Reactions

Type III hypersensitivity reactions are the rarest form of hypersensitivity reaction. In this case, the immune complexes precipitate in various tissues, resulting in complement activation and a local or systemic inflammatory response, such as serum sickness, vasculitis, arthus reaction, or drug-induced fever. The drug acts as a soluble **antigen**; it is not bound to cell surfaces (which occurs in Type II reactions) but rather binds to antibodies and forms complexes that are not easily cleared. These complexes become deposited in organs and induce an inflammatory response. Immune complex reactions generally occur 7–21 days following drug administration.[2,3,28,34]

Antitoxins for rabies or botulism, for example, can cause serum sickness. Penicillins, cephalosporins, neomycin, glucocorticoids, sulfonamide antibiotics, and sulfonamide diuretics can cause vasculitis. Diphtheria, tetanus, and hepatitis vaccines can cause arthus reactions. The drugs most often associated with drug fever are anticonvulsants, minocycline (Minocin), antibiotics, allopurinol (Zyloprim), and, rarely, heparin.[35] Type III reactions can also mimic disorders such as lupus and arthritis. For example, minocycline (Minocin) can induce a Type III reaction called "drug-induced lupus." Treatment includes discontinuation of the inciting medication supportive care and monitoring, as well as administration of anti-inflammatory agents.

Box 4-2 Treating Anaphylaxis and Anaphylactoid Reactions: Epinephrine

Epinephrine is an agonist for alpha- and beta-adrenergic receptors that, when stimulated, initiate vasoconstriction, increased peripheral vascular resistance, increased cardiac contractility, relaxation of respiratory smooth muscle, and decreased inflammatory response—all of which counter the histamine-initiated inflammatory responses.[3] There are no contraindications to use of epinephrine for a person experiencing a severe hypersensitivity reaction.

The dose of epinephrine for treatment of anaphylactoid reactions and anaphylaxis in adults is 0.3 to 0.5 mL in a concentration of 1:1000 given intramuscularly and repeated every 5 to 15 minutes as needed for 3 to 4 doses.[2,31] Individuals with a history of serious hypersensitivity reactions are frequently prescribed an epinephrine auto-injector (EpiPen). This device is designed to provide a unit dose of 0.3 mg epinephrine 1:1000 in 3 mL via an auto-injector syringe that can be injected through clothing; it allows the individual to rapidly self-administer the drug intramuscularly immediately following exposure to a known allergen.[2,31,32]

Additional treatments for hypersensitivity reactions include corticosteroids to limit inflammatory response, bronchodilators to maintain airway function, and NSAIDs for pain relief.[3] New preventive therapies under development and evaluation include immunotherapy with allergen extracts, administration of anti-IgE to individuals who have allergic asthma, and other immunomodulator treatments to preemptively modulate immune hypersensitivity reactions.[33]

Type IV Hypersensitivity Reactions

Type IV hypersensitivity reactions are delayed reactions. This type of reaction can occur following exposure to latex gloves, tuberculosis purified protein derivative (Mantoux) testing, and exposure to poison oak or poison ivy. In addition, many drugs can cause these reactions. In Type IV reactions, activation of T cells by molecules from the drug or substance results in cytokine and inflammatory mediator release approximately 2–7 days following exposure.[3,34]

Most Type IV hypersensitivity reactions are characterized by cutaneous involvement because the skin contains large quantities of T cells. The clinical picture includes contact dermatitis, drug-induced hypersensitivity syndrome (DRESS), maculopapular eruptions, Stevens-Johnson syndrome, and toxic epidermal necrolysis. Type IV reactions are divided into four subcategories based on the specific immune response generated.[3] Diagnosis is based on appearance, although patch testing may be performed following treatment to verify the allergen. Treatment consists of comfort measures and topical or systemic corticosteroid therapy as indicated, as the severity of these disorders ranges from mild to life threatening.

Pseudo-allergic Drug Reactions

Pseudo-allergic reactions can occur the first time an individual is exposed to the inciting drug without prior sensitization.[23] The **anaphylactoid reaction** to aspirin is a good example of pseudo-allergic reaction. This reaction is variously called "aspirin allergy," "aspirin-induced asthma," "aspirin-exacerbated respiratory disease (AERD)," and the "aspirin triad." Aspirin allergy can be mild or severe, and either respiratory or cutaneous reactions are possible. This anaphylactoid reaction occurs in 10% of adults with asthma and approximately 0.3% of the general population.[30] Symptoms of the respiratory version include profuse rhinorrhea, bronchospasm, periorbital edema, and flushing, which occur within a few hours of ingestion but not as immediately as allergic hypersensitivity **anaphylaxis**.[3]

Aspirin and some first-generation NSAIDs inhibit the enzyme COX-1, which produces prostaglandin E_2 (PGE_2). PGE_2 prevents the release of histamines and synthesis of leukotrienes that cause bronchoconstriction.[30] Thus, aspirin can facilitate the release of leukotrienes and cause bronchospasm in some individuals. Drugs known to elicit a pseudo-allergic reaction are listed in Table 4-3.[23] Treatment for a pseudo-allergic anaphylactoid reaction, which is the same as treatment for a Type I hypersensitivity anaphylaxis reaction, is listed in Box 4-2.[31–33]

Clinical Manifestations of Drug Reactions and Toxicity

Clinically, it can be helpful to categorize adverse drug reactions by the organ system affected or syndrome that is elicited rather than by the ADR classification. Clinical symptoms of drug hypersensitivity reactions are varied and can mimic many other clinical conditions or diseases, leading to delay in accurate diagnosis. While skin lesions are often an early presenting symptom, the ADR presentation may affect any major organ system—resulting in hepatitis, carditis, or pneumonitis, for example.[3] There are many different cutaneous drug reactions known best to dermatologists. This section reviews both these common cutaneous presentations of adverse drug reactions and exemplar rare disorders that are associated with significant morbidity.

Drug-Induced Cutaneous Conditions

Cutaneous manifestations are the most frequent type of drug reaction and often the cardinal sign of drug toxicity or hypersensitivity.[3,27] Drug-induced skin manifestations eruptions are usually Type IV hypersensitivity reactions that develop several days or a few weeks after the initial exposure to the inciting medication, or mild Type I hypersensitivity reactions such as the classic "ampicillin rash." Symptoms include rash, hives or urticaria, and sometimes angioedema that appears after the drug is discontinued.

The most common drug-induced eruptions are drug-induced exanthems or rashes, which account for approximately 75% of all cutaneous drug reactions.[27] While drug-induced rashes occur in response to many medications, their most frequent occurrence is secondary to the administration of antibiotics or sulfa drugs. Rash typically presents with intense pruritus and the formation of spreading macular, papular, or morbilliform (measles-like) eruptions that begin in dependent areas and then spread.[36] The morbilliform type is more frequently associated with Stevens-Johnson syndrome.

Urticaria is often the initial sign of a reaction to penicillins, cephalosporins, sulfa drugs, local anesthetics, or latex and is mediated by the release of histamine by cutaneous mast cells. If the rash is an IgE-mediated Type I hypersensitivity reaction, urticaria may occur as an isolated finding or as a precursor of acute anaphylactic reaction. Non-IgE-mediated hives also occur, most frequently in response to angiotensin-converting enzyme (ACE) inhibitors, opiates, and anesthetic agents. An idiopathic form of urticaria can worsen with exposure to aspirin, acetaminophen (Tylenol), or indomethacin (Indocin).

Maculopapular exanthems are the most common cutaneous delayed hypersensitivity reaction. Such a rash usually appears 7–20 days after drug exposure. The classic ampicillin rash is a maculopapular exanthem. Other drugs associated with this reaction are antiepileptic drugs, quinolones, and radiocontrast media.

Fixed drug eruptions can occur following exposure to NSAIDs (including aspirin), tetracyclines and sulfonamides, the phenolphthalein found in some laxatives, and barbiturates. These eruptions appear as either eczematous plaques or bullous lesions. When the individual is re-exposed to the same antigen, lesions recur in the same (fixed) locations where they appeared during the initial attack.

Vasculitis is a component of many cutaneous drug reactions and, therefore, the epidemiology of this reaction is difficult to determine. Vasculitis is the result of hapten–protein complexes that are deposited in small blood vessels. Arthralgia, myalgia, and a palpable purpura rash are the most common symptoms.[37] Propylthiouracil (PTU) and hydralazine (Apresoline) are highly associated with the development of vasculitis.

Photosensitivity reactions occur when persons using photosensitizing agents such as medications and personal care products are exposed to ultraviolet light. Photosensitivity drug reactions include phototoxic and photoallergic reactions. A phototoxic reaction presents as hypersensitivity to sun exposure, resulting in severe sunburn in exposed areas of the skin; it may or may not itch. Such reactions are a result of dose-related direct cellular damage caused by the photoactivated agent and usually develop within minutes or hours after exposure to the drug and light.[38] Phototoxic reactions can occur following use of tetracyclines (doxycycline, minocycline, and others), quinolones (ciprofloxacin), diuretics, and NSAIDs (naproxen, ibuprofen, and others). Likewise, photoallergic reactions are drug-related light sensitivities. These reactions take the form of unpredictable immune-mediated reactions that typically occur 24–72 hours after exposure to the agent and light. The rash is eczematous and itchy. Photoallergic reactions have a similar mechanism of action as contact dermatitis reactions, with the cutaneous effects appearing as eczematous patches in exposed areas, which can extend to unexposed skin.[38]

Angioedema, which is most frequently associated with ACE inhibitor administration, may occur independently or in association with urticaria. Angioedema involves the deep dermis and subcutaneous tissues and may cause laryngeal edema with resultant airway compromise.

Serum sickness is an immune-complex hypersensitivity disorder (Type III) that results from exposure to a foreign protein antigen or hapten, such as following tetanus antitoxin or antirabies serum administration.[34] The incidence of serum sickness is unknown.[39] This reaction was seen much more frequently in the mid-twentieth century when drug development was less precise and heterologous serum products were in use. Serum sickness is characterized by fever, followed by rash, and accompanied by general malaise that includes headache, nausea and vomiting, and prominent polyarthralgia or polyarthritis that occurs 8–14 days after the antigen exposure.[40] The majority of serum sickness cases occur secondary to use of cefaclor (Ceclor) or minocycline (Minocin).[39,42]

Drug reaction with eosinophilia and systemic symptoms (DRESS), formerly called drug-induced hypersensitivity syndrome, occurs in 1 per 1000 to 1 per 10,000 drug exposures.[43] DRESS is characterized by mucocutaneous rash, fever, centrofacial swelling, and internal organ involvement.[43] Anticonvulsants appear to have a toxic metabolite that induces this disorder; thus these drugs are responsible for 35% of the DRESS cases diagnosed today.[44] Similarly, sulfonamide antibiotics can cause drug-hypersensitivity syndrome via a metabolic pathway that produces toxic metabolites. Other drugs strongly associated with DRESS include allopurinol (Zyloprim) and dapsone, minocycline (Minocin), nevirapine (Viramune), and abacavir (Ziagen) (Table 4-4).

Stevens-Johnson syndrome (SJS) and *toxic epidermal necrolysis (TEN)* are acute idiosyncratic hypersensitivity reactions that occur rarely but are associated with significant morbidity and mortality. The overall incidence of SJS is 1–7 cases per 1 million individuals per year.[45] The drugs with the highest incidence of SJS/TEN are trimethoprim–sulfamethoxazole (Bactrim) (1–3 reactions per 100,000 users), sulfadoxine/pyrimethamine (Fansidar-R) (10 reactions per 100,000 users), and carbamazepine (Tegretol) (14 reactions per 100,000 users).[46] Other drugs associated with SJS/TEN are listed in Table 4-4. Overall, 1-year mortality rates from these reactions are 34%, with approximately 23% of deaths occurring in the first 6 weeks after diagnosis.[47]

Acute generalized exanthematous pustulosis (AGEP) is another rare type of drug reaction that occurs in 1–5 individuals per 1 million users.[37] The onset is acute and begins with erythema and edema in the facial area, then rapidly advances to include pustular rash, fever, and vasculitis.[48,49] The disorder is severe and generally lasts about a week, but long-term morbidity and mortality are rare. Approximately 60% of the individuals who develop AGEP have been exposed to aminopenicillins, quinolones, or macrolides.

Pemphigus is a rare form of skin drug eruption—that is, a blistering disease. The drugs most commonly involved are ACE inhibitors.[37]

Table 4-4 Selected Drugs That Can Cause Severe Cutaneous Hypersensitivity Reactions

Drugs Strongly Associated with AGEP	Drugs Strongly Associated with DRESS	Drugs Strongly Associated with SJS
Amoxicillin	Abacavir (Ziagen)[a]	Abacavir (Ziagen)[a]
Ampicillin (Amoxil)	Allopurinol (Zyloprim)[a]	Allopurinol (Zyloprim)[a]
Diltiazem	Amlodipine	Carbamazepine (Tegretol)[a]
(Hydroxy)chloroquine	Ampicillin (Amoxil)	Chlormezanone (Trancopal)
Macrolides	Bupropion (Wellbutrin)	Co-trimoxazole (Septra)
Pristinamycin	Captopril (Capoten)	Fosphenytoin (Cerebyx)
Quinolones	Carbamazepine (Tegretol)[a]	Lamotrigine (Lamictal)
Sulfonamides (anti-infective formulations)	Celecoxib (Celebrex)	Meloxicam (Mobic)
	Ethambutol (Myambutol)	Nevirapine (Viramune)[a]
	Ibuprofen (Advil)	Phenobarbitol (Luminal)
	Isoniazid (INH)	Phenytoin (Dilantin)[a]
	Ketoprofen (Orudis)	Piroxicam (Feldene)
	Phenobarbitol (Luminal)	Sulfadiazine (Diazin)
	Phenytoin (Dilantin)[a]	Sulfadoxine (Fansidar-R)
	Ranitidine (Zantac)	Sulfamethoxazole and trimethoprim (Bactrim)
	Rifampin (Rifadin)	Sulfasalazine (Azulfidine)
	Sulfamethoxazole and trimethoprim (Bactrim)	Tenoxicam (Tilcotil)

Abbreviations: AGEP = acute generalized exanthematous pustulosis; DRESS = drug reaction with eosinophilia and systemic symptoms; SJS = Stevens-Johnson syndrome.

[a] Individuals with HLA-A*A31:01, HLA-B*15:02, HLA-B*35:05, HLA-B*15:11, and CYP2B6 polymorphisms are at increased risk for developing SJS or DRESS when administered one of these medications. Genetic testing is recommended prior to administration for some of these medications.

Sources: Data from Ahronowitz I, Fox L. Severe drug-induced dermatoses. *Semin Cutan Med Surg.* 2014;33(1):49-58[37]; Dodiuk-Gad RP, Laws PM, Shear NH. Epidemiology of severe drug hypersensitivity. *Semin Cutan Med Surg.* 2014;33(1):2-9[39]; Papay J, Yuen N, Powell G, Mockenhaupt M, Bogenrieder T. Spontaneous adverse events of Stevens-Johnson syndrome/toxic epidermal necrolysis: detecting associations with medicines. *Pharmacoepidemol Drug Saf.* 2012;21:289-296.[46]

Hepatotoxicity

Drug-induced liver injury is the primary cause of the post-marketing withdrawal of prescribed drugs.[50,51] Although hepatotoxicity is a rare occurrence, acetaminophen (Tylenol) overdose was the leading cause of acute liver failure in the United States in 2008. More than 1000 drugs that cause hepatotoxicity have been identified.[51] Hepatotoxicity can result from toxicity of the drug itself or highly reactive toxic metabolites that are produced in excess or not reduced to nonreactive compounds. For example, isoniazid (INH) toxicity is secondary to the creation of toxic metabolites that directly harm hepatocytes (Figure 4-1). Clinically, two kinds of drug-related hepatotoxicity occur: (1) the hepatocellular type, which presents with a marked elevation in alanine aminotransferase; and (2) the cholestatic type, which is evidenced by an initial rise in serum alkaline phosphatase.[52] Drug-induced hepatitis can be acute or chronic in nature and can result in liver failure. Cirrhosis and hepatic cholestasis can also occur, with jaundice being prolonged in the presence of cholestasis. Extrahepatic symptoms, such as fever, rash, or serum-sickness syndrome, are not uncommon, particularly in individuals with immune-mediated hepatic injury. Treatment is based on symptoms and is largely supportive, although individuals with acute liver failure may require transplant.

Hepatotoxicity can also occur following use of dietary supplements. In May 2013, a cluster of individuals, after using a popular over-the-counter protein supplement marketed for weight loss, began to present with symptoms of severe hepatitis and liver failure.[53] By February 2014, 97 cases had been identified, which resulted in 47 hospitalizations, 3 liver transplants, and 1 death.[53] The product associated with these reactions, OxyElite, was removed from the market by the FDA.[54] This story highlights the importance of routine inquiry about use of dietary supplements and early reporting of ADRs to the FAERS.

An individual's risk of hepatotoxicity is affected by a multitude of factors. In particular, preexisting hepatic compromise, drug interactions, immune factors, and some genetic polymorphisms of the cytochrome P-450 system can increase the risk of hepatotoxicity.[55] Other associated factors include race, female gender, and chronic or acute alcohol intake.[55] Women develop hepatotoxicity more often than men do.[55,56] Concomitant use of some complementary and alternative therapies, such as kava-kava, germander, and others, can also contribute to hepatic injury.

Nephrotoxicity

The kidneys play a crucial role in drug excretion and detoxification. While only 7% of drugs fail to be approved due to nephrotoxicity, the percentage of individuals in the intensive care unit who develop nephrotoxicity ranges from 30% to 50%. This discrepancy demonstrates that the kidney is one of the major organs affected by drug-related toxic responses and an important focus of toxicological adverse event reporting.[57]

To form urine, the kidney receives approximately 25% of the cardiac output, which exposes renal glomerular, tubular, and interstitial cells to large concentrations of drugs and their metabolites. As urine is concentrated in the kidney's proximal tubule, nephrotoxins accumulate and may result in site-specific nephrotoxicity. Drug-related kidney damage may lead to vascular or direct tubular injury, allergic interstitial inflammation, glomerular basement membrane injury, chronic interstitial injury, papillary necrosis, direct tubular toxicity, free-radical injury, abnormal phospholipid metabolism, and intracellular calcium toxicity.[58] Four drug-induced toxic renal syndromes are distinguished: acute renal failure, chronic renal failure, nephritic syndrome, and renal tubular dysfunction.[58]

Acute kidney injury and nephrotoxicity are more common when one or more of the following factors are present: age older than 60 years, exposure to multiple nephrotoxic agents, diabetes, heart disease, and systemic infection. Risk of nephrotoxicity increases in the presence of multiple risk factors.[58]

A wide range of commonly administered prescription and over-the-counter drugs possess the potential for nephrotoxicity. Risk is elevated in the presence of preexisting renal compromise, low fluid volume, polypharmacy, bolus dosing, and drug interactions that increase circulating drug levels. Drugs that may contribute to nephrotoxicity include ACE inhibitors, acyclovir (Zovirax), cephalosporins, ciprofloxacin (Cipro), immunoglobulin, lithium (Lithobid), NSAIDs, penicillins, sulfonamides, rifampin (Rifadin), and valproic acid (Depakote).[59]

Drug Fever

Drug fever is a nonspecific sign of drug toxicity that mimics numerous medical conditions. While fever is a predictable side effect of some medications and vaccines, it can also be the primary indicator of an adverse drug reaction. Drug fever occurs more commonly in individuals who are taking multiple medications, the elderly, and persons who are infected with HIV.[60]

The physiologic mechanisms behind febrile reactions to pharmacologic agents are not well understood. Drug-related temperature elevations are associated with hypersensitivity (allergic) reactions, pharmacologic alterations in thermoregulatory mechanisms, alterations in skeletal muscle action and metabolism, idiosyncratic drug reactions, and as a direct result of drug pharmacokinetics.[60]

Febrile hypersensitivity reactions are most often associated with use of anticonvulsants, antibiotics, allopurinol (Zyloprim), and heparin. Antibiotics are associated with approximately one-third of all drug-related fevers, and they often confuse the clinical picture by simulating a relapse of the underlying condition that prompted use of antibiotics, thereby prolonging exposure to antibiotic treatment if drug-induced fever is not considered as the cause.

Some drugs, such as thyroid replacement hormone (Synthroid), agents with an anticholinergic effect (e.g., tricyclic antidepressants, antihistamines, and phenothiazines), and sympathomimetic agents (e.g., amphetamines, cocaine, and ecstasy), may disrupt physiologic thermoregulation of the body. Such dysregulation may result in temperature elevation that occurs secondary to increased heat production or diminished heat dissipation.[61]

Parenteral administration of medications may cause fever secondary to contamination of the medication or site, a localized inflammatory response, or a response to the drug, as is common following administration of some vaccines. Fever may also occur in response to the pharmacologic properties of the drug itself, most commonly following oncology-related chemotherapy and treatment of conditions such as secondary or tertiary syphilis or brucellosis.

Malignant Hyperthermia

Febrile **idiosyncratic reactions**, such as malignant hyperthermia, while highly unpredictable, may have a familial or genetic basis. Malignant hyperthermia is a potentially life-threatening pharmacogenetic disorder of skeletal calcium regulation that is primarily triggered by inhalation agents used during anesthesia induction and maintenance.[62] Malignant hyperthermia results in muscle rigidity and significant pyrexia. It requires prompt recognition and rapid initiation of treatment with dantrolene sodium (Dantrium) to prevent excess morbidity or mortality.[63]

Long QT Syndrome

Prolongation of the QT interval (*torsades de pointes*) is a side effect of a number of structurally unrelated drugs. The clinical presentation is usually syncope (hypotension) and palpitations (tachycardia) that are self-limited, but this syndrome can cause seizure-like activity and sudden cardiac arrest.[64] Drug-induced prolonged long QT syndrome is more prevalent in individuals with the following risk factors: female gender, hypokalemia, bradycardia, polymorphisms of the sodium ion channels, naturally occurring long QT syndrome, treatment of cardiac symptoms with QT-prolonging drugs, and profoundly low magnesium levels.[65] Approximately 10% to 15% of persons who develop drug-induced long QT interval have genetic polymorphisms that result in subclinical long QT intervals.[64]

Drugs most commonly associated with long QT syndrome include cardiac drugs such as disopyramide (Norpace), dofetilide (Tikosyn), ibutilide (Corvert), procainamide (Pronestyl), quinidine (Quinora and others), sotalol (Betapace), and bepridil (Vascor). Clarithromycin (Biaxin), erythromycin (E-mycin and others), droperidol (Inapsine), methadone (Dolophine), and antipsychotic agents, have a small, but documented risk of long QT syndrome, which may be exacerbated by concurrent administration of drugs that inhibit drug-elimination mechanisms.[65]

Evaluation of the QT interval is used as a marker during drug development for the prediction of serious adverse drug effects, syncope, and sudden cardiac arrest. However, the number of participants in drug trials needed to effectively quantify this risk remains unknown. When new drugs are administered to study participants with preexisting higher-than-average risk of sudden death, symptoms of long QT syndrome can be confounded by changes in the QT interval that occur secondary to disease states, or as physical manifestations of psychological conditions such as psychosis.

In addition, current evidence suggests that 5% to 10% of individuals with drug-induced long QT syndrome have common polymorphisms that affect normal action potentials, leading to subclinical long QT syndrome.[65] Cardiac evaluation with ECG is frequently recommended prior to initiating a medication associated with long QT syndrome. This is particularly appropriate for women who have specific factors that significantly elevate the risk of long QT syndrome, such as women older than 65 years, a family history of sudden death, use of medications that prolong the QT interval, and coadministration of pharmacologic agents that inhibit drug-elimination mechanisms (e.g., erythromycin [E-mycin and others], clarithromycin [Biaxin], ketoconazole [Nizoral], itraconazole [Sporanox], amiodarone [Cordarone], quinidine [Quinora and others], antidepressants, and antiretroviral agents).[65]

Drug-Induced Lupus

Drug-induced lupus is a drug-induced autoimmune disorder that is reversible following cessation of drug therapy.[66] This condition occurs in individuals on long-term therapy (> 1 month duration). It is more common in elderly individuals and in females.[66] Symptoms include malaise, fever, joint pain, and swelling. Although the mechanism responsible for this disorder is not definitively known, it is assumed that the offending drugs or a reactive metabolite blocks the innate process of tolerance, thereby facilitating production of autoantibodies, or that the drug (or metabolite) creates a hapten that functions as an autoantibody.[66]

While a wide array of medications may cause drug-induced lupus, the drugs most often associated with this disorder are procainamide (Pronestyl) and hydralazine (Apresoline). In addition, quinidine (Quinaglute), isoniazid (INH), methyldopa (Aldomet), minocycline (Minocin), and chlorpromazine (Thorazine) are known to induce lupus.[66] Other drugs that are considered probable causes of drug-induced lupus include anticonvulsants, statins, fluorouracil agents, terbinafine (Lamisil), antithyroid medications, and hydrochlorothiazide (HydroDIURIL).[66]

Thrombocytopenia

Bleeding and bruising following use of quinine for treatment of malaria were first reported in *The Lancet* in 1865.[67] Although quinine is not used to treat malaria today, it is still used for the treatment of nocturnal muscle cramps, and thrombocytopenia continues to be a complication of its use. The University of Oklahoma Health Sciences Center maintains an ongoing database of drugs that cause thrombocytopenia and at the time of this writing had identified 87 drugs with clear evidence for a causal association to thrombocytopenia, drawn from a total of 253 drugs associated with thrombocytopenia based on case reports.[68]

Drugs that induce thrombocytopenia do so by various mechanisms.[68] Ultimately, antibodies stimulated by the drug or drug–platelet complex destroy platelets. The overall incidence of drug-induced thrombocytopenia is 1–2 cases per 100,000 population per year, with some drugs being more likely to cause this complication than others.[68]

The drugs most often associated with drug-induced thrombocytopenia are quinine, platelet inhibitors such as abciximab (ReoPro), antirheumatic drugs such as gold salts, sulfonamide antibiotics such as trimethoprim–sulfamethoxazole (Bactrim), heparins, cimetidine (Tagamet), acetaminophen (Tylenol), diuretic agents such as chlorothiazide (Diuril), and some chemotherapeutic agents.[69,70] In the presence of polypharmacy, it can be challenging to isolate the potentially offending agent.

Treatment of drug-induced thrombocytopenia consists of discontinuing the medication and monitoring for platelet recovery. When pharmacologic treatment is necessary, an alternative medication must be substituted.

Preventing Adverse Drug Reactions

The Institute of Medicine has noted that hospitalized individuals experience an average of 1 medication error per day and that 380,000 preventable ADEs occur annually.[7] In a meta-analysis of 16 recent prospective studies on outpatient populations presenting for hospitalization or emergency department care (n = 48,797), Hakkarainen et al. found that 2% of adult outpatients were determined to have ADRs.[71] An evaluation of the ADRs revealed that 52% of these reactions were deemed preventable.[71] The same researchers performed an associated meta-analysis of 8 recent studies examining ADRs in the inpatient population (n = 24,128). They found that among inpatients, 1.6% had preventable ADRs, with 45% of the reactions identified being deemed preventable.[71]

Modifiable factors leading to ADRs and ADEs can be broadly classified as being related to either prescribing or adherence. These factors include inaccurate clinical diagnosis resulting in incorrect treatment; inaccuracy in the prescription process, such as incorrect spelling or dose, and errors in dispensing or administration. In addition, self-medication; misunderstanding regarding drug therapy; noncompliance with recommended drug therapy; and drug interactions secondary to polypharmacy or coadministration with certain foods, herbs, or other substances can result in ADRs. Finally, undiagnosed preexisting medical, genetic, or allergic conditions contribute to many ADRs; more of these reactions may be considered preventable in the future as we learn about genetic polymorphisms and develop genetic tests for these markers.

As a result of the national focus on medication errors, U.S. hospitals have set up internal systems designed to prevent errors. Practices such as unit-dose medications, limited-access medication carts, computer entry of medication orders, and integrated bedside documentation systems can reduce medication errors and prevent adverse drug events. With the advent of electronic health records and e-prescribing, more clinicians who practice in the community setting have put similar prevention strategies into place.

Prevention of ADRs and ADEs in the outpatient setting relies on accurate diagnosis, selection of an optimal and appropriate pharmacologic agent, assessment of potential for interactions with other agents, evaluation for genetic or physiologic variations or conditions that may affect drug metabolism, developmentally and culturally appropriate medication instruction, correct medication, dose, dispensing, and labeling, and compliance with recommended therapy by the individual.

Electronic prescribing in the outpatient setting is rapidly becoming routine. Electronic generation, transmission, and tracking of prescriptions is efficient and offers greater security than the paper-based prescription system. Additionally, e-prescribing can offer greater safety through cross-referencing for drug interactions, correct doses, and patient-specific factors including prior ADRs. In 2010, the Drug Enforcement Administration (DEA) created provisions that allow for e-prescribing of controlled substances, which represent an estimated 20% of all prescriptions.[72] Under the DEA's rules, electronic prescriptions for controlled substances are authorized only when each electronic prescription or electronic health record (EHR) application used by the practitioner and the pharmacy complies with the electronic application requirements in the DEA's interim final rule.[72] This compliance is determined by a qualified third party that audits the electronic prescription or EHR application or by review and certification of the application by an approved certification body.

Poisoning

Poisoning is the result of accidental or deliberate overdose of pharmacologic substances, or exposure to toxic levels of nonpharmacologic chemical, biologic, or physical agents that results in organ impairment or injury, or systemic effects.[73] Poisoning is now the leading cause of death by injury in the United States, and nearly 90% of poisoning deaths are drug related.[73] In 2008, the rate of poisoning deaths exceeded the rate of deaths from automobile accidents for the first time since 1980.[73] The Institute of Medicine's 2004 report on poisoning estimated that more than 4 million poison exposures occur annually in the United States, resulting in more than 30,000 fatalities in 2004.[74] By 2008, the number of fatalities attributed to drug-related poisoning had risen to 41,000.[74] Much of that increase is attributable to opioid-related deaths, which account for 40% of all drug-related deaths; this mortality includes preventable child deaths from ingestion of adult prescription medications.[73]

Poison control centers in the United States are now linked to a real-time poison control database and surveillance system that is continually updated and offers callers current research-based poison exposure management guidelines relevant to clinical and medical toxicology. In 2012, the 57 poison control centers in the United States served the nation's population of more than 318 million people.[75] There were 2,275,141 human exposure calls reported, resulting in 7.2 reported exposures per 1000 individuals.[75] Approximately 70% of these exposures were handled over the telephone by the poison control center and the exposed individual was not evaluated by a healthcare professional. Poisoning is not a reportable occurrence, so it is likely that individuals who were treated by healthcare professionals were not included in these numbers.

Poisoning occurs in children and adults from ingestion of household substances such as lead paint chips, solvents, or cleaners; inadvertent overdose of medication secondary to impaired renal or hepatic function; deliberate overdose of medications; poisoning from dietary supplements; foodborne toxins; or excessive exposure to environmental or occupational toxins.[74] Antidepressants are among the most common class of prescription drugs for which overdose is reported to poison control centers.

Although half of all poisonings occur in children younger than 6 years, according to 2013 data from the American Association of Poison Control Centers, the majority of adult poisoning victims (58.05%), whether intentional or unintentional, were women 20 years or older. Fatalities from poisoning are essentially evenly distributed between males and females, with the overwhelming majority (70%) occurring in individuals between the ages of 20 and 59 years.[75]

Reported poisonings occurring during pregnancy account for only a small number of the total number of human poisonings (0.3% [$n = 7671$]). Nearly 75% of poisonings during pregnancy were unintentional.[75] Hence, women's health clinicians must remain alert to the risk of poisoning in all women under their care, and should address the significant risk of accidental poisoning of children in the household.

Care of the Woman Who Is Poisoned

During evaluation of the suspected poisoning victim, the type of exposure, severity of symptoms, and level of toxicity should be determined. Physical toxins include energy, noise, cold, heat, and radiation. Chemical toxicants include many household products, chemicals used in industry, and most pharmacologics. Biologic toxins include vaccines and pharmacologic products from plant or animal sources, as well as occupational or environmental exposure to the same substances.

Criteria for consultation and hospitalization vary based on the agent, the age and health of the individual who has been poisoned, the type of poisoning, and other factors. Prompt access to emergency medical care by contacting 911 or a poison control center is indicated for signs of an acute allergic reaction, suspected overdose, fever, or dermatologic manifestations of SJS/TEN.

Care of an individual who has been poisoned begins with rapid assessment of the airway, breathing, and state of consciousness, while determining the offending agent(s) and time elapsed since exposure. Primary therapy consists of gastrointestinal decontamination via interruption of poison absorption and/or facilitation of poison excretion, and provision of appropriate antidotal therapy, if available. Cutaneous, mucous membrane, or ocular exposures are treated with irrigation using copious amounts of water or normal saline.

Gastrointestinal Decontamination

Gastrointestinal decontamination is appropriate if the poison was ingested within 1 to 2 hours and the poison is known to be amenable to reabsorption. A combination of adsorbing or binding agents, diluting agents, agents that enhance intestinal motility, and antidotal therapy, when applicable, should be accompanied by supportive and advanced medical care as indicated. Due to its hyperemetic effects, ipecac syrup is no longer recommended as first-line therapy.[76] Syrup of ipecac increases the risk of aspiration pneumonitis and interferes with the actions of activated charcoal. Gastric lavage is a time-consuming procedure that can delay administration of the more effective activated charcoal. Therefore, gastric lavage is no longer routinely recommended for treatment of poisoning.[77]

Activated Charcoal and Sorbitol

Activated charcoal is considered first-line therapy for ingested poisons. Activated charcoal is an inert fine carbon powder that is both insoluble and nonabsorbable, with an extensive network of interconnecting pores and large surface area. It acts by rapidly binding with (adsorbing) the chemical, thereby limiting systemic absorption and toxicity. Activated charcoal is most effective when it is administered within 1 hour following ingestion of the offending substance.[78] The recommended dose of activated charcoal for conscious adult poisoning victims is 50 g (25–100 mg range is acceptable).[78] Activated charcoal is mixed with water or sorbitol to form a slurry that is administered orally or via nasogastric tube. Sorbitol acts to enhance bowel motility, thereby facilitating elimination of the charcoal–poison complex and preventing constipation secondary to activated charcoal administration.[78]

Contraindications to use of activated charcoal include the following: unprotected airway, risk for gastrointestinal hemorrhage or perforation, recent surgery or medical condition that could be adversely affected by use, and ingestion of a poison that is not reabsorbable (e.g., heavy metal, lithium, alcohol).[78] In general, activated charcoal is administered as a single dose. Multidose regimens are used on occasion for life-threatening poisoning but the effectiveness is controversial and the decision to administer activated charcoal more than once is best made by poison control experts.

Cathartics and Whole-Bowel Irrigation

Cathartics and whole-bowel irrigation are forms of decontamination that rapidly empty the gastrointestinal tract of bulky or coated toxic materials and foreign bodies such as drug packets, sustained-release medications, and batteries. Polyethylene glycol solution (Colyte, GoLYTELY) may be administered to clear toxic substances not bound by activated charcoal. The adult dose is 1.5–2 liters per hour orally (or per nasogastric tube) until the rectal effluent is clear. Whole-bowel cleansing may reduce the binding capacity of activated charcoal; therefore, when indicated, polyethylene glycol solution is administered *after* the administration of activated charcoal.[79]

Specific Poison Antidotes

Antidotes are agents that are administered to counteract the effects of a poison or toxin. Antidotes act through inhibiting absorption, reversing the action of poisons, or neutralizing the poison. Pharmaceutical antidotes are agents that treat the toxic effects of specific drugs, such as naloxone (Narcan) for opioid overdose. Specific antidotes interact directly with the agent of overdose or poisoning, such as *N*-acetylcysteine (Acetadote, Mucomyst) for acetaminophen overdose, calcium gluconate for magnesium sulfate toxicity, or species-specific antivenin. The pharmacokinetics of the antidote must be known to use this treatment correctly. For example, the half-life of naloxone (Narcan) is 60–90 minutes, which is shorter than the half-life of many opioids, Therefore, this agent may need to be administered more than once.[80] Antidotes to common poisons are listed in Table 4-5.[81]

Poisoning Prevention

Many cases of inadvertent poisoning can be prevented through routine use of basic safeguards. All medications should be kept in their original containers, so that the name and recommended dose are clearly visible. Medication containers should be kept out of the reach of children, and child safety packaging should be used when there are children in the home or visiting the home. Alcohol and illicit or street drugs should be secured out of the reach of children. Household products should also be kept out of the reach of children, and agents with a high hazard for poisoning should be secured.

Appropriate prescribing and education about the risk of poisoning should be an integral part of prescriptive practice for health professionals. Multiple prescription or over-the-counter medications in the home and increased use of opioids and sedatives create opportunities for preventable poisoning to occur.

Toxicity from Heavy Metals

Heavy metals are naturally occurring substances that contribute, in trace amounts, to healthy physiologic functioning. Excess amounts of heavy metals can result in alterations in central nervous system function and organ damage, and can affect normal growth and development. Chronic exposure may result in progressive physical, muscular, and neurologic conditions that mimic numerous other health conditions.

Iron Toxicity

Iron is necessary for hematologic function and is commonly administered as replacement therapy to treat anemia. The vast majority of iron overdoses occur in children younger than 6 years. Prenatal vitamins and iron supplements have a high concentration of iron per tablet, so they pose an especially high risk for overdose. Toxicity is related to the dose of elemental iron ingested and results in free-radical formation and lipid peroxidation.

Iron toxicity initially presents with nausea, vomiting, and abdominal pain within the first 6 hours after ingestion. Vomiting may be severe and lead to hypovolemic shock.

Table 4-5 Antidotes to Common Poisons[a]

Poison: Generic (Brand)	Symptoms	Antidote
Acetaminophen (Tylenol)	Nausea, vomiting, malaise, right upper quadrant pain, confusion, jaundice, coma	*N*-acetylcysteine (NAC)
Alcohols	Drowsy, disinhibition, seizures, confusion, coma	Thiamine
Anticholinergics: antihistamines, atropine, tricyclic antidepressants, psychoactive drugs	Tachycardia, hyperthermia, mydriasis, urinary retention, delirium	Physostigmine
Anticoagulants	Bleeding	Vitamin K_1, protamine
Aspirin	Tinnitus, nausea and vomiting, fever, disorientation, lethargy, coma	Activated charcoal
Benzodiazepines	Drowsy, lethargic, ataxia, hypotension, coma, respiratory depression	Supportive care, flumazenil[b]
Beta blockers	Bradycardia, hypotension, arrhythmia	Glucagon
Calcium-channel blockers	Drowsy, confusion, chest pain, hypotension, chest pain, seizures, respiratory distress	Calcium, intravenous insulin in high dose with intravenous glucose
Cholinergics	Diarrhea, mitosis, emesis, lacrimation, lethargy, salivation	Atropine, pralidoxime (organophosphate overdose)
Clonidine withdrawal or hypertensive crisis from monoamine oxidase inhibitor (MAOI) interactions, or stimulant overdose	Hypertension, tachycardia	Phentolamine, beta blockers unless specifically contraindicated, benzodiazepine
Digoxin (Lanoxin)	Bradycardia, drowsiness, lethargy	Digoxin Fab antibodies
Heparin anticoagulation	Bleeding	Protamine
Iron	Stomach pain, nausea and vomiting, hypovolemic shock	Deferoxamine (Desferal)
Isoniazid (INH)	Nausea and vomiting, diarrhea, irritability, lethargy, light sensitivity, confusion, dizziness	Pyridoxine
Lead	Abdominal pain, cramping, anemia, constipation, headaches, reduced sensation	Chelation therapy: dimercaptosuccinic acid (DMSA), ethylenediaminetetraacetic acid (EDTA)
Levodopa withdrawal	Akinetic crisis, dystonic reaction	Bromocriptine
Methotrexate	Stomatitis, nausea and vomiting, diarrhea, pancytopenia, leukopenia, thrombocytopenia	Leucovorin (folinic acid)
Metoclopramide (Reglan) or narcoleptics	Dystonic reaction	Diphenhydramine (Benadryl)
Opioids	Nausea and vomiting, drowsy, cyanosis, coma	Naloxone[c]
Serotonin syndrome	Agitation, restlessness, confusion, tachycardia, headache, shivering, diarrhea, twitching muscles	Benzodiazepines such as diazepam (Valium)
Sulfonylurea-induced hypoglycemia	Confusion, hunger, dizziness, irritability, headaches, coma	Octreotide, glucose
Tricyclic antidepressants	Tachycardia, chest pain, drowsiness, seizure, dry mouth, dry skin, blurred vision, urinary retention	Sodium bicarbonate
Warfarin	Bleeding	Vitamin K_1

[a] This table provides a list of well-known antidotes. Use should be based on consultation with poison control experts, as the dosing, timing, and agent changes as new knowledge is incorporated into poison control protocols. This table may not represent the standard of care in a specific area. In case of emergency, a poison control center should be consulted.
[b] Use of flumazenil is contraindicated in the presence of tricyclic antidepressant overdose and in chronically habituated benzodiazepine users, as it may precipitate seizures in these cases.
[c] Use of naloxone is contraindicated in persons hypersensitive to it and in certain situations wherein the individual is tolerant to opioid agonists/ antagonists.

With continued deterioration, shock ensues, accompanied by metabolic acidosis. Hepatic necrosis may occur within 96 hours after ingestion of a toxic dose of iron salts and may lead to fatal liver failure. Serum iron levels aid in quantifying the severity of the overdose, with a level exceeding 500 mcg/dL considered serious toxicity, and a level greater than 1000 mcg/dL considered life threatening.[82] Treatment consists of volume replacement, airway protection, prompt intravenous administration of deferoxamine (Desferal) for serious toxicity, and supportive care.[82] Deferoxamine is a **chelating agent** that binds with circulating ferric iron to form a water-soluble solution that can be excreted via the kidneys.

Lead Poisoning

Lead is a naturally occurring elemental metal that was once used in many products such as paint, lead solder in food cans, and gasoline. Lead may be found in commercial products such as hair dye, batteries, and fishing weights. It is a waste product of the steel and iron industries and is released into the atmosphere as a result of coal-based power generation.[82,83] Lead cannot be destroyed, and it is transferred continuously between air, water, and soil. As a result, in areas with elevated environmental lead concentrations, exposure may occur secondary to atmospheric exposure, through ingestion of locally grown produce, or by contact with contaminated soil, dust, and water supplies.[83] For example, persons who reside in areas proximate to heavily trafficked roads are likely to be exposed to this metal from leaded gas.

The vast majority of adult lead poisoning cases are related to occupational exposures, although environmental exposures do occur secondary to exposure to lead paint (most commonly in houses built prior to 1970) and imported products such as health remedies, spices, foods, pottery, and cosmetics.[83]

Lead is absorbed through skin and mucous membranes, and it bioaccumulates in humans. Elevated blood lead levels as a result of **bioaccumulation** inhibit enzyme function in multiple biochemical pathways due to lead's affinity to bind to biologically active molecules in the body. Lead stored in bones may contribute to lead toxicity in women with hypothyroidism, during postmenopausal bone resorption, and during pregnancy when this metal passes to the fetus.[82] Lead toxicity in children can permanently affect neurocognitive development, and may also have immunological, cardiovascular, and endocrine effects.[83]

Elevated blood lead levels are most commonly diagnosed through screening because individuals with low levels of lead toxicity are typically asymptomatic. Screening is recommended for persons with occupational or environmental exposure who are pregnant or planning pregnancy, women who exhibit pica, and individuals with low intake of dietary calcium.[84] Elevated lead levels in pregnant women may cause low birth weight, smaller than usual head circumference, mental retardation, and impaired neurobehavioral development in their offspring.[82] Even low levels of lead poisoning have potential to affect the developing fetus, and women with elevated blood lead levels excrete lead in breast milk.

Blood lead levels should be less than 5 mcg/dL in children and less than 10 mcg/dL in adults. When lead levels exceed 5 mcg/dL, eliminating exposure to the source is frequently adequate to reduce these levels to the normal range.[84] Lead exposure can be diminished through covering of lead-painted walls, regular damp dusting of surfaces, hand washing before meals, washing of all fruits and vegetables before use, and allowing tap water to run for 30 seconds before drinking.[83] For those individuals with persistent elevated blood lead levels, significant symptoms, or nonpregnant women with fertility concerns, chelating agents may be administered under the direction of a medical toxicologist.

Primary prevention of elevated lead levels begins with home assessment for potential sources of lead exposure. Patterns of distribution of elevated blood lead levels often reflect racial and income disparities related to quality of housing, nutrition, and other environmental factors. Clinicians can be a reliable source of information about lead hazards, educate families about lead exposure, and know how to initiate an environmental assessment.[84]

Mercury Toxicity

Mercury toxicity causes anxiety, memory loss, fearfulness, excitability, and personality changes. The expression "mad as a hatter," refers to the mental disorder seen in persons who made hats in the eighteenth and nineteenth centuries in England and developed mercury toxicity; at that time, mercury was used in the production of the felt from which hats were constructed. The primary sources of exposure to mercury today are ingestion of fish containing significant bioaccumulations of methylmercury (e.g., tuna, swordfish, walleye, and pike), occupational exposures, and amalgam dental fillings.[85] Minute amounts of ethyl mercury are also used in the preservation of many pharmacologic products, most commonly ophthalmic and otic solutions, and some adult vaccines.

The preservative thimerosal is a mercury derivative (ethyl mercury) that was incorrectly postulated to contribute to autism and attention-deficit/hyperactivity disorder in young children through the administration of childhood vaccines that used thimerosal as a preservative. Thimerosal is no longer used in vaccines intended for children in the United States, but is present in some vaccines used for adults, such as the influenza vaccine, although thimerosal-free influenza vaccine is available and produced by one manufacturer. Thimerosal continues to be an important preservative of multidose vaccines in low- and middle-income nations.[86]

Mercury toxicity results in intention tremor of the hands, inflamed gums and excessive salivation, and mental and emotional changes. Mercury vapor is easily absorbed through the lungs, while only small amounts are absorbed through the GI tract. Mercury is excreted via the GI tract, respiratory system (mercury vapor), and kidneys. This metal accumulates in both the kidney and central nervous system, where it can cause nephrotoxicity and neurologic changes.[85]

While mercury toxicity in adults is now relatively uncommon, even small amounts of mercury can be harmful to the developing fetus. The bioaccumulation of mercury in fish is primarily in the methylmercury form, which is more toxic than elemental mercury, leading to recommendations that pregnant women avoid some specific types of fish (e.g., tilefish from the Gulf of Mexico, shark, swordfish, and king mackerel) and limit consumption of bluefin and albacore tuna.[87] Fetal exposure to methylmercury can cause impaired neurologic development, such as diminished ability related to cognition, memory, attention, language, and fine motor and visual spatial skills.[85]

Mercury toxicity is determined through evaluation of blood and urine concentrations. Normal adult serum mercury levels are less than 5 mcg/L, with symptoms of toxicity becoming apparent at a concentration of about 100 mcg/L. Thiol-based chelating agents are used to treat confirmed mercury toxicity.[85]

Endocrine Disruptors

Endocrine disruptors are synthetic chemicals that disrupt physiologic function through interference with normal hormone secretion or action. These chemicals mimic or block the action of hormones, resulting in developmental, neurologic, immune, and reproductive system aberrations.[88]

Exposure to endocrine disruptors may occur through the environment, such as drinking water contaminated with dioxin, polychlorinated biphenyls (PCBs), or dichloro- diphenyl-trichloroethane (DDT), or through the use of commercial products such as plastics, drugs, or cosmetics that contain preservatives such as paraben or ethylene oxide. Endocrine disruptors may be found in water, soil, and the atmosphere. These chemicals are lipophilic, so they can accumulate in the fatty tissues of plants and animals, and subsequently be ingested by humans through the diet.

Prominent among the endocrine-disrupting chemicals are the xenoestrogens or ecoestrogens, which are substances with significant estrogenic effects. Xenoestrogens bind to estrogen receptor sites. Genetic and environmental interactions associated with endocrine disruptors are postulated to contribute to the development of conditions such as breast cancer, infertility, endometriosis, immune disorders, childhood developmental and cognitive delay, and birth defects.[88] Due to their affinity to fatty tissues, effects of endocrine disruptors may be diminished in women with a lower body mass index.

Conclusion

Knowledge about adverse drug reactions, chemical toxicity, and poisoning relates to all aspects of pharmacotherapeutics and is integral to safe prescriptive practice. In spite of the best efforts of healthcare providers to prevent ADRs and ADEs, no agent is deemed 100% safe. Therefore, all practitioners must be prepared to evaluate individuals who present with signs or symptoms of drug-related reactions or potentially toxic exposures.

Regardless of whether an individual is treated on an outpatient basis or is hospitalized, it is essential that the clinician identify and record any toxicity- or drug-related adverse events in the woman's record. ADEs are reported to the FDA through MedWatch. Clinician reporting of ADEs helps build the database of information about drug reactions and provides invaluable data with which to determine drug safety, optimal doses, and identification of drug-related risk factors.

Over-the-counter and prescription pharmacologic agents offer a multitude of effective therapies for chronic and acute conditions. With thoughtful consideration about the balance between therapeutics' benefits and drug toxicity or adverse reactions, women's healthcare providers can help women live healthier lives.

Resources

Organization	Description	Website
Food and Drug Administration Adverse Event Reporting System (FAERS)	A computerized database that contains postmarketing reports of adverse events and medication errors submitted to the FDA. FAERS is part of the FDA's safety surveillance program for all approved drug and therapeutic biologic products. The goal of FAERS is to improve public health through effective collection and analysis of safety reports. Drug manufacturers are required by regulation to submit all reports of adverse drug events to FAERS. Healthcare providers and consumers may also voluntarily submit reports through the MedWatch website.	www.accessdata.fda.gov/scripts/medwatch
Food and Drug Administration, Drug Safety Communications	Information about drug alerts, drug safety communications, and drug recalls can be found on the FDA's website	www.fda.gov/Drugs/DrugSafety/default.htm
American Association of Poison Control Centers (AAPCC)	The AAPCC website includes a list of all U.S. poison control centers, updates and alerts about poisons, and information on prevention. U.S. data on poisonings are also available.	www.aapcc.org Poison Help Line: 1-800-2222-1222
Center for Research on Occupational and Environmental Toxicology	An organization composed of scientists, educators, and information specialists working at Oregon Health and Science University in Portland, Oregon, on occupational safety and health issues	www.croetweb.com
Centers for Disease Control and Prevention, Unintentional Poisoning	This website offers poisoning resources for families	www.cdc.gov/HomeandRecreationalSafety/Poisoning/index.html
Collaborative on Health and the Environment	This site offers a searchable database that summarizes links between chemical contaminants and approximately 180 human diseases or conditions	http://database.healthandenvironment.org
Extoxnet	This site provides toxicology information briefs on a number of topics	http://extoxnet.orst.edu/tibs/ghindex.html
Haz-Map	A clinical research tool for the evaluation of occupational toxicology based on disease categories and agents	www.haz-map.com/toxicology.htm
World Health Organization, Essential Medicines and Health Products Organization	*Safety of Medicines: A Guide to Detecting and Reporting Adverse Drug Reactions*—a guide to detecting and reporting adverse drug reactions	http://apps.who.int/medicinedocs/en/d/Jh2992e
Toxipedia	An online toxicology resource	www.toxipedia.org
Toxicology/occupational health resources	This site provides links to many online resources related to toxicology	www.lib.berkeley.edu/PUBL/tox.html

References

1. Edwards IR, Aronson JK. Adverse drug reactions: definitions, diagnosis, and management. *Lancet.* 2000;356(9237):1255-1259.
2. Simons FER, Ardusso LRF, Bilò MB, et al. World Allergy Organization guidelines for the assessment and management of anaphylaxis. WAO position paper. *WAO J.* 2011;4:13-37.
3. Pichler WJ, Adam J, Daubner B, Gentinetta T, Keller M, Yerly D. Drug hypersensitivity reactions: pathomechanism and clinical symptoms. *Med Clinic N Am.* 2010;94:645-664.
4. Carson R. *Silent Spring.* Boston, MA: Houghton Mifflin; 1962.

5. World Health Organization. International drug monitoring: the role of national centres. *WHO Tech Rep Ser.* 1972;498:1-25.
6. Davies EC, Green CF, Taylor S, Williamson PR, Mottram DR, Pirmohamed M. Adverse drug reactions in hospital in-patients: a prospective analysis of 3695 patient-episodes. *PLoS One.* 2009;4:e4439.
7. Aspden P, Wolcott JA, Bootman JL, Cronenwett LR, eds. *Preventing Medication Errors.* Washington, DC: National Academies Press; 2007:1-455.
8. Wilke RA, Lin DW, Roden DM, et al. Identifying genetic risk factors for serious adverse drug reactions: current progress and challenges [erratum, *Nat Rev Drug Discov.* 2008;7(2):185]. *Nat Rev Drug Discov.* 2007;6(11):904-916.
9. Moore TJ, Cohen MR, Furberg CD. Serious adverse drug events reported to the Food and Drug Administration 1998-2005. *Arch Internal Med.* 2007;167: 1752-1759.
10. Weiss-Smith S, Desgpande G, Chung S, Gogolak V. The FDA drug safety surveillance program: adverse event reporting trends. *Arch Intern Med.* 2011;171(6): 591-593.
11. Hausmann O, Schnyder B, Pichler WJ. Etiology and pathogenesis of adverse drug reactions. *Chem Immunol Allergy.* 2012;97:32-46.
12. Cohen P. Hazards of hindsight: monitoring the safety of nutritional supplements. *N Engl J Med.* 2014; 370(14):1277-1280.
13. Reidl MA, Casillas AM. Adverse drug reactions: types and treatment options. *Am Fam Physician.* 2003; 68:1781-1790.
14. Goodman A, Schorge J, Greene MF. The long-term effects of in utero exposures: the DES story. *N Engl J Med.* 2011;364(22):2083-2084.
15. Zopf Y, Rabe C, Neubert A, et al. Women encounter ADRs more often than do men. *Eur J Clin Pharmacol.* 2008;64:999-1004.
16. Heinrich J. *Drug safety: most drugs withdrawn in recent years had greater health risks for women.* GAO-01-286R. Washington, DC: U.S. General Accounting Office; 2001. http://www.gao.gov/assets/100/90642.pdf. Accessed September 29, 2014.
17. Doña I, Barrionuevo E, Blanca-Lopez N, et al. Trends in hypersensitivity drug reactions: more drugs, more response patterns, more heterogeneity. *J Investig Allergol Clin Immunol.* 2014;24(3):143-153.
18. Aronson JK, Ferner RE. Clarification of terminology in drug safety. *Drug Saf.* 2005;28(10):851-870.
19. Joint Task Force on Practice Parameters; American Academy of Allergy, Asthma, and Immunology; American College of Allergy, Asthma, and Immunology; Joint Council of Allergy, Asthma, and Immunology. Drug allergy: an updated practice parameter. *Ann Allergy Asthma Immunol.* 2010;105(4):259-273.
20. Zhou S, Chan E, Li X, Huang M. Clinical outcomes and management of mechanism-based inhibition of cytochrome P450 3A4. *Ther Clin Manage.* 2005;1: 3-13.
21. Larson AM, Polson J, Fontana RJ, Davern E. Acetaminophen-induced acute liver failure: results of a United States multicenter, prospective study. *Hepatology.* 2005;42:1364-1372.
22. Khan DA. Drug allergy. *J Allergy Clin Immunol.* 2010;125(2 suppl 2):S126-S137.
23. Farnam K, Chang C, Teuber S, Gershwin ME. Nonallergic drug hypersensitivity reactions. *Int Arch Allergy Immunol.* 2012;159(4):327-345.
24. Uetrecht J. Idiosyncratic drug reactions: past, present, and future. *Chem Res Toxicol.* 2008;21:84-92.
25. Faulkner L, Meng X, Park BK, Naisbitt DJ. The importance of hapten–protein complex formation in the development of drug allergy. *Curr Opin Allergy Clin Immunol.* 2014;14(4):293-300.
26. Gomes ER, Demoly P. Epidemiology of hypersensitivity drug reactions. *Curr Opin Allergy Clin Immunol.* 2005;5:309-316.
27. Gruchalla R. Understanding drug allergies. *J Allergy Clin Immunol.* 2000;105:S637-S644.
28. Torres MJ, Blank M. The complex clinical picture of β-lactam hypersensitivity: penicillins, cephalosporins, monobactams, carbapenems, and clavams. *Med Clin N Am.* 2010;94:805-820.
29. Ponka D. Approach to managing patients with sulfa allergy: use of antibiotic and nonantibiotic sulfonamides. *Can Fam Physician.* 2006;52(11):1434-1438.
30. Wang H, Wang HS, Liu ZP. Agents that induce pseudo-allergic reaction. *Drug Discov Ther.* 2011;5(5):211-219.
31. Liberman PL. Recognition and first-line treatment of anaphylaxis. 2013. *Am J Med.* 2014;127 (1 suppl):S6-S11.
32. Manivannan V, Hess EP, Bellamkonda VR, et al. A multifaceted intervention for patients with anaphylaxis increases epinephrine use in adult emergency department. *J Allergy Clin Immunol Pract.* 2014;2:294-299.
33. Babu KS, Polosa R, Morjaria JB. Anti-IgE: emerging opportunities for omalizumab. *Expert Opin Biol Ther.* 2013;13(5):765-777.

34. Uzzaman A, Cho SH. Classification of hypersensitivity reactions. *Allergy Asthma Proc.* 2012;33(suppl 1): S96-S99.
35. Patel RA. Drug fever. *Pharmacother.* 2010;30(1):57-69.
36. Stern RS. Utilization of hospital and outpatient care for adverse cutaneous reactions to medications. *Pharmacoepidem Drug Saf.* 2005;14:677-684.
37. Ahronowitz I, Fox L. Severe drug-induced dermatoses. *Semin Cutan Med Surg.* 2014;33(1):49-58.
38. Dubakiene R, Kupriene M. Scientific problems of photosensitivity. *Medicina.* 2006;42:619-624.
39. Dodiuk-Gad RP, Laws PM, Shear NH. Epidemiology of severe drug hypersensitivity. *Semin Cutan Med Surg.* 2014;33(1):2-9.
40. Katta R, Anusuri V. Serum sickness-like reaction to cefuroxime: a case report and review of the literature. *J Drug Dermatol.* 2007;6:747-748.
41. Kaplan RP, Potter TS, Fox JN. Drug-induced pemphigus related to angiotensin-converting enzyme inhibitors. *J Am Acad Dermatol.* 1992;26(2 Pt 2);364-366.
42. Wolf R, Orion E, Marcos B, Matz H. Life-threatening acute adverse cutaneous drug reactions. *Clin Dermatol.* 2005;23(2):171-181.
43. Criado PR, Criado RF, Avancini JM, Santi CG. Drug reaction with eosinophilia and systemic symptoms (DRESS)/drug-induced hypersensitivity syndrome (DIHS): a review of current concepts. *An Bras Dermatol.* 2012;87(3):435-449.
44. Kardaun SH, Sekula P, Valeyrie-Allanore L, et al. Drug reaction with eosinophilia and systemic symptoms (DRESS): an original multisystem adverse drug reaction: results from the prospective RegiSCAR study. *Br J Dermatol.* 2013;169(5):1071-1080.
45. Finkelstein Y, Macdonald EM, Li P, Hutson JR, Juurlink DN. Recurrence and mortality following severe cutaneous adverse reactions. *JAMA.* 2014;311(21):2231-2232.
46. Papay J, Yuen N, Powell G, Mockenhaupt M, Bogenrieder T. Spontaneous adverse events of Stevens-Johnson syndrome/toxic epidermal necrolysis: detecting associations with medicines. *Pharmacoepidemol Drug Saf.* 2012;21:289-296.
47. Knowles SR, Shear NH. Recognition and management of severe cutaneous drug reactions. *Dermatol Clin.* 2007;25:245-253.
48. Sidoroff A, Halevy S, Bavinck JN, Vaillant L, Roujeau JC. Acute generalized exanthematous pustulosis (AGEP): a clinical reaction pattern. *J Cutan Pathol.* 2001;28(3):113-119.
49. Schmid S, Kuechler PC, Britschgi M, et al. Acute generalized exanthematous pustulosis. *Am J Pathol.* 2002;161(6):2079-2082.
50. Lee WM. Drug-induced hepatotoxicity. *N Engl J Med.* 2003;349:474-485.
51. Makarova SI. Human *N*-acetyltransferases and drug-induced hepatotoxicity. *Curr Drug Metab.* 2008;9: 538-545.
52. Navarro VJ, Senior JR. Drug-related hepatotoxicity. *N Engl J Med.* 2006;354:731-739.
53. Cohen P. Hazards of hindsight: monitoring the safety of nutritional supplements. *N Engl J Med.* 2014;370:14:1277-1280.
54. U.S. Food and Drug Administration. OxyElite Pro supplements recalled. 2013. http://www.fda.gov/ForConsumers/ConsumerUpdates/ucm374742.htm. Accessed October 3, 2014.
55. Njoku DB. Drug-induced hepatotoxicity: metabolic, genetic and immunological basis. *Int J Mol Sci.* 2014;15:6990-7003.
56. Chalasani NP, Hayashi PH, Bonkovsky HL, et al. ACG clinical guideline: the diagnosis and management of idiosyncratic drug-induced liver injury. *Am J Gastroenterol.* 2014;109:950-966.
57. Fuchs TC, Hewitt P. Biomarkers for drug-induced renal damage and nephrotoxicity: an overview for applied toxicology. *AAPS J.* 2011;13(4):615-631. http://www.ncbi.nlm.nih.gov/pmc/articles/PMC3231866/#__ffn_sectitle. Accessed October 2, 1014.
58. Naughton CA. Drug-induced nephrotoxicity. *Am Fam Physician.* 2008;78(6):743-750.
59. Guo X, Nzerue C. How to prevent, recognize, and treat drug-induced nephrotoxicity. *Curr Drug Ther.* 2002;69:289-312.
60. Eyer F, Zilker T. Bench-to-bedside review: mechanisms and management of hyperthermia due to toxicity. *Crit Care.* 2007;11:236-238.
61. Rusyniak DE, Sprague JE. Toxin-induced hyperthermic syndromes. *Med Clin North Am.* 2005;89: 1277-1296.
62. Hopkins PM. Malignant hyperthermia: pharmacology of triggering. *Br J Anaesth.* 2011;107(1):48-56. http://bja.oxfordjournals.org/content/107/1/48.full.pdf+html. Accessed October 2, 1014.
63. Kim TW, Rosenberg H, Nami N. Current concepts in understanding malignant hyperthermia. *Anesthesiology News.* 2014. http://www.anesthesiologynews.com/download/MalignantHyperthermia_AN0214_WM.pdf. Accessed October 2, 1014.

64. Gupta A, Lawrence AT, Krishnan K, Kavinsky CJ, Trohman RG. Current concepts in the mechanisms and management of drug-induced QT prolongation and torsade de pointes. *Am Heart J.* 2007;153: 891-899.
65. Kannankeril P, Roden DM, Darbar D. Drug-induced long QT syndrome. *Pharmacol Rev.* 2010;62:760-781.
66. Vedove CD, Simon JC, Girolomoni G. Drug-induced lupus erythematosus with emphasis on skin manifestations and the role of anti-TNFα agents. *J Dtsch Dermatol Ges.* 2012;10:889-897.
67. Vipan W. Quinine as a cause of purpura. *Lancet* 1865;2:37.
68. Reese JA, Li X, Hauben M, et al. Identifying drugs that cause acute thrombocytopenia: an analysis using 3 distinct methods. *Blood.* 2010;116:2127-2133.
69. Priziola JL, Smythe MA, Dager WE. Drug-induced thrombocytopenia in critically ill patients. *Crit Care Med.* 2010;38:S145-S154.
70. Curtis BR. Drug-induced immune thrombocytopenia: incidence, clinical features, laboratory testing, and pathologic mechanisms. *Immunohematol.* 2014; 30(2):55-65.
71. Hakkarainen KM, Hedna K, Petzold M, Hägg S. Percentage of patients with preventable adverse drug reactions and preventability of adverse drug reactions: a meta-analysis. *PLoS One.* 2013;7(3):e33236.
72. Thomas CP, Kim M, Kelleher SJ, et al. Early experience with electronic prescripting of controlled substances in a community setting. *J Am Med Inform Assoc.* 2013;20(e1):e44-e51.
73. Warner M, Chen LH, Makuc DM, Anderson RN, Miniño AM. *Drug poisoning deaths in the United States, 1980-2008.* NCHS Data Brief, no 81. Hyattsville, MD: National Center for Health Statistics; 2011. http://www.cdc.gov/nchs/data/databriefs/db81.htm#poisoning. Accessed October 2, 1014.
74. Institute of Medicine, Committee on Poison Prevention and Control. *Forging a Poison Prevention and Control System.* Washington, DC: National Academies Press; 2004.
75. Mowry JB, Spyker DA, Cantilena LR Jr, Bailey JE, Ford M. 2012 annual report of the 98 American Association of Poison Control Centers' National Poison Data System (NPDS): 30th annual report. *Clin Toxicol.* 2013;51(10):949-1229. https://aapcc.s3.amazonaws.com/pdfs/annual_reports/2012_NPDS_Annual_Report.pdf. Accessed October 2, 1014.
76. Höjer J, Troutman WG, Hoppu K, et al. Position paper update: ipecac syrup for gastrointestinal decontamination. *Clin Toxicol.* 2013;51(3):134-139.
77. Benson BE, Hoppu K, Troutman WG, et al. Position paper update: gastric lavage for gastrointestinal decontamination. *Clin Toxicol.* 2013;51:140-146.
78. Chyka PA, Seger D, Krenzelok EP, et al. Position paper: Single-dose activated charcoal. *Clin Toxicol* 2005;43:61.
79. Position paper: whole bowel irrigation. *J Toxicol Clin Toxicol.* 2004;42:843.
80. Boyer EW. Management of opioid analgesic overdose. *N Engl J Med.* 2012;367:146-155.
81. Lam SW, Engebretsen KM, Bauer SR. Toxicology today: what you need to know now. *J Pharm Pract.* 2011;24(2):174-188.
82. Chang TP, Rangan C. Iron poisoning: a literature-based review of epidemiology, diagnosis, and management. *Pediatr Emerg Care.* 2011;27(10):978-985.
83. Agency for Toxic Substances and Disease Registry. Toxicological profile for lead 2007. http://www.atsdr.cdc.gov/toxprofiles/tp13.html. Accessed July 22, 2008.
84. Advisory Committee on Childhood Lead Poisoning Prevention. *Low level lead exposure harms children: a renewed call for primary prevention.* Atlanta, GA: Centers for Disease Control and Prevention; 2012. http://www.cdc.gov/nceh/lead/ACCLPP/Final_Document_030712.pdf. Accessed October 2, 1014.
85. Rice KM, Walker EM, Gillette WM, Blough ER. Environmental mercury and its toxic effects. *J Prev Med Public Health.* 2014;47(2):74-83.
86. Orenstein WA, Paulson JA, Brady MT, Cooper LZ, Seib K. Global vaccine recommendations and Thimerosal. *Pediatrics.* 2013;131:149-151. http://www.autismoava.org/archivos/Pediatrics-2012-Orenstein-peds.2012-1760.pdf. Accessed October 2, 1014.
87. U.S. Food and Drug Administration, Environmental Protection Agency. Fish: what pregnant women and parents should know. 2014. http://www.fda.gov/Food/FoodborneIllnessContaminants/Metals/ucm393070.htm. Accessed October 2, 1014.
88. Gore AC. Developmental programming and endocrine disruptor effects on reproductive neuroendocrine systems. *Front Neuroendocrinol.* 2008;29(3):358-374.

II Lifestyle and Preventive Healthcare Practices

Habits can be either healthy or unhealthy. However, even so-called healthy habits are not universally positive. In the chapter *Vitamins and Minerals,* nutritional supplements are discussed. Evidence about the benefits and risks of vitamins are described in this chapter. Other dietary supplements, although perhaps not harmful, are costly and of questionable effectiveness. Moreover, too much of a good thing may be bad: Megavitamins and minerals can be harmful and sometimes even teratogenic.

The iconic example of primary health prevention is the use of immunizations. For many years, only a relatively small number of vaccines were available, and they were intended primarily for children. Today, the number of vaccines, especially for adolescents and adults, has increased—and so has the controversy about their effectiveness and adverse effects. When individuals decide not to avail themselves of vaccines, the entire concept of herd immunity begins to unravel. The chapter *Immunizations* addresses these issues and provides national recommendations for regular vaccinations.

In two unhealthy situations, pharmacologic regimens have been developed that support efforts to regain health. The chapter *Drugs to Promote Optimum Weight* examines the myths and realities about drugs and weight loss. It addresses the use of pharmacologic agents used to augment diet and exercise in an attempt to attain a healthy body mass index. This topic is receiving increasing attention in a society in which obesity is an emerging epidemic. Although there is no single magic drug that can guarantee weight loss, at the end of this chapter, the reader will have an understanding of the agents available, their effectiveness, and their indications.

Nicotine replacement therapies (NRTs) have demonstrated value for individuals who find it difficult to discontinue smoking. The plethora of over-the-counter (OTC) gums, patches, and other options can be confusing for the woman who wishes to stop smoking. The chapter *Smoking Cessation* reviews available evidence on types of NRTs and the reported effectiveness of both OTC products and prescription-only therapies.

In addition to nicotine, drugs can be abused. The chapter *Drugs of Abuse* addresses licit agents such as alcohol, illicit drugs such as cocaine, and abuse of prescription drugs such as opiates. The last group of agents, often euphemistically termed "recreational drugs," are used by millions of Americans annually, but are associated with multiple long-term adverse effects and even death. Treatments with other agents may pose trading one habit for another. The delicate balances involved in selecting pharmacotherapeutic agents for individuals who abuse substances are examined in this chapter.

The last chapter in this section, *Complementary and Alternative Therapies*, presents an overview of herbs and botanical products that should be viewed as rigorously as prescription drugs. Randomized clinical trials have shown that some of these agents have therapeutic effects. Nevertheless, some herbs and botanical products have adverse drug–herb interactions that are clinically significant. Other widely used agents may be safe but are of questionable efficacy.

All of these chapters present information on agents that may not commonly be perceived as "drugs." However, information about these agents, both for good and for ill, can be important considerations for clinicians as they prescribe medications for women.

5 Vitamins and Minerals

Katie Ferraro

Based on the chapter by Jessica A. Grieger, Heather I. Katcher, Vijaya Juturu, and Penny M. Kris-Etherton in the first edition of Pharmacology for Women's Health

Chapter Glossary

Antioxidants Substances, including selected vitamins, that inhibit oxidation of other molecules, leading to cell death.

Dietary supplements Products intended to supplement the diet. Such products may contain vitamins and minerals, as well as herbs or other botanicals.

Functional foods Fortified, enriched, or enhanced foods that have potentially beneficial effects on health when consumed as part of a varied diet and marketed as such. Also known as nutraceuticals.

Megadose Exceptionally large amount of a vitamin or mineral. The exact dose has not been defined.

Minerals Inorganic micronutrients that are essential for life, maintain their chemical compositions, and usually are found in trace amounts in food.

Provitamin Compound that is converted to a vitamin within an organism; sometimes termed a vitamin precursor or previtamin. Not all vitamins have a provitamin/previtamin compound.

Vitamins Organic micronutrients that are essential for life, and can be changed by heat, air, or acids.

Introduction

As a formal area of research, the study of **vitamins** and **minerals**, commonly collectively referred to as micronutrients, is a relatively new one. Although vitamins were not identified until the early part of the twentieth century, researchers throughout history have sought to associate particular components of the diet with conditions and diseases of excess or deficiency. Even prior to the discovery of vitamin C, British sailors were nicknamed "Limeys," after the Royal Navy added lime juice to water to prevent scurvy. Ascorbic acid (vitamin C)—the *anti-scorbutic* (anti-scurvy) factor—was named long before the chemical structure of vitamin C was identified in 1933.[1]

Essential vitamins and minerals are those micronutrients that the body cannot make and, therefore, must be obtained through the diet. Despite the continually evolving body of evidence in the field, today, scientists are confident that all of essential vitamins and minerals have been discovered and isolated. For example, total parenteral nutrition (TPN) is now able to sustain human life in relatively good nutrient status even in the absence of food.

Historically, the focus of nutrition practice was on meeting nutrient needs and preventing vitamin and mineral deficiencies. More recently, the emphasis of nutrition policy and practice has shifted from solely treatment to the prevention and management of chronic diseases such as cardiovascular disease, diabetes, and cancer, even though there is no evidence to support these claims as yet.

Nutrition experts have long championed the message of *food first*—in other words, "food before supplementation"—because many of the nutrients found in food confer a wide range of remarkable health benefits. However, **dietary supplements** have become popular, and this trend has led to the emergence of nutraceuticals (also known as **functional foods**), which are products that have been fortified, enriched, or enhanced to provide a potentially beneficial effect on health when consumed as part of a varied diet.[2]

Unfortunately, many instances exist where the scientific evidence is insufficient to support the health benefits touted by marketers of dietary supplements and nutraceutical products. In addition, as scientific knowledge advances, questions about both benefits and potential risks associated with these agents are emerging. In some cases, evidence from clinical trials and documented cases of nutrient deficiencies indicates that the use of selected supplements should be recommended.[3] However, when the data are lacking or when adverse effects have been reported, recommendations for their use are not warranted. This chapter provides an overview of vitamins and minerals, reviews the current evidence for use of popular vitamin and mineral supplements, and provides guidance regarding appropriate recommendations for clinical practice, recognizing that when at all possible, food is preferentially favored as a primary source of essential vitamins and minerals.

Dietary Reference Intake Guidelines

The U.S. government has played a role in guiding food intake for more than a century. The first government dietary guide of a *Farmers' Bulletin* was published in 1894 and written by the first director of the U.S. Department of Agriculture's (USDA) Experiment Stations.[4] In 1916, nutritionist Caroline Hunt published the USDA's *Food for Young Children*. Hunt classified foods as belonging to one of five groups: milk and meat, cereals, vegetables and fruits, sugars and sugary foods, and fats and fatty foods.[5] These categories were used for decades. The 1940s ushered in the era of the Recommended Dietary Allowances (RDAs), a set of specific recommended intakes of calories and nine essential nutrients: protein, iron, calcium, vitamins A and D, thiamin, riboflavin, niacin, and vitamin C.[6] In 1997, the RDAs became part of an expanded system called the Dietary Reference Intakes (DRIs). Table 5-1 lists some commonly used and sometimes misused terms found in discussions of vitamins and minerals when consumed in diet or in supplements.

The DRIs are issued by the Food and Nutrition Board (FNB) of the Institute of Medicine, National Academy of Sciences, and are reviewed periodically. The most recent revision was of the calcium and vitamin D DRI recommendations, which were updated in 2010, whereas the remainder of the DRI values was established as part of the 1997–2004 DRIs. Several electronic dietary guidance resources for healthcare professionals are available and are listed in the Resources table at the end of this chapter.

Table 5-1 Lexicon of Dietary Intake Terms

Recommended Dietary Allowance (RDA)	Average daily level of intake sufficient to meet the nutrient requirements of nearly all (97–98%) of healthy persons in that age and gender group.
Adequate Intake (AI)	A value established when evidence is insufficient to develop an RDA and is set at a level assumed to ensure nutritional adequacy.
Tolerable Upper Intake Level (UL)	The maximum daily intake unlikely to cause adverse health effects. UL values have not been established for all vitamins and minerals, but for those that do exist, care should be taken not to exceed the UL.
Estimated Average Requirement (EAR)	The average daily nutrient intake level estimated to meet the requirement of half the healthy individuals in a particular life stage and gender group. The EAR is used in nutrition research and policymaking and provides the framework within which RDA values are set.

Sources: Data from National Institutes of Health, Office of Dietary Supplements. Nutrient recommendations: Dietary Reference Intakes (DRI). *Health Information.* http://ods.od.nih.gov/Health_Information/Dietary_Reference_Intakes.aspx. Accessed June 4, 2014[7]; U.S. Food and Drug Administration. Dietary Supplement Health and Education Act of 1994. *Regulatory Information.* October 25, 1994. http://www.fda.gov/RegulatoryInformation/Legislation/FederalFoodDrugandCosmeticActFDCAct/SignificantAmendmentstotheFDCAct/ucm148003.htm. Accessed June 4, 2014.[8]

Regulation of Dietary Supplements in the United States

The regulation of dietary supplements in the United States is under the auspices of the Food and Drug Administration (FDA), as stipulated by the Dietary Supplement Health and Education Act (DSHEA) of 1994. DSHEA defines a dietary supplement as a product (other than tobacco) that is intended to supplement the diet. Dietary supplements contain one or more of the following ingredients: a vitamin, a mineral, an herb or other botanical, an amino acid, a dietary substance used to increase the total dietary intake, or a concentrate, metabolite, constituent, extract, or combination of any of these ingredients.[8]

Although the FDA regulates foods, prescription drugs, medical devices, and supplements, the standards applied to regulation of supplements are substantially less stringent than those applied to foods, prescription drugs, and medical devices. Under DSHEA, dietary supplements that contain established ingredients—defined as those ingredients that were sold in the United States prior to 1994—can be marketed without the manufacturer having to provide any prior evidence regarding their effectiveness or safety. In general, manufacturers do not need to register their products with the FDA or obtain FDA approval before producing or selling dietary supplements. However, manufacturers must make certain that the product label information is truthful and not misleading, although some critics have questioned consistent FDA enforcement of the latter mandate.

Supplement Effectiveness

Whereas drug manufacturers can claim that their drug will diagnose, cure, mitigate, treat, or prevent a disease based on evidence provided to FDA, these claims cannot be made for dietary supplements. Claims about the advantages of a specific food dietary supplement as noted on the labels may be one of the three types listed in Table 5-2.

Safety of Supplements

Due to the natural and holistic attributes ascribed to dietary supplements, and because they are easily accessible, consumers may not recognize the inherent dangers associated with inappropriate use of these products. Dietary supplements may interact with other medications (or even other supplements), may cause side effects of their own, and may contain potentially harmful ingredients that are not disclosed on the supplement's label. Supplements have generally not been tested for safety when used by pregnant and nursing women or children. Dietary supplements sold in the United States are not required to contain standardized doses of active ingredients, and manufacturers often avoid having to disclose the actual supplement contents through the use of "proprietary blend" statements instead of transparent ingredient lists. Because federal law does not require that dietary supplements be tested for safety or efficacy prior to their sale, a consumer may be at risk for adverse health effects when using these products, especially when they take a **megadose**—a term without a specific definition, but one that is an exceptionally large dose. A list of credible groups that can be consulted by providers and consumers can be found in the Resources list at the end of this chapter.

Although some individuals may use dietary supplements without clear indications, for others these agents may be beneficial. Table 5-3 lists special populations who may benefit from dietary supplements.

Table 5-2 Types of Claims for Dietary Supplements

Nutrient content claim	Claim that characterizes the level of a nutrient in a food if it has been authorized by the FDA (e.g., "good source of vitamin A" or "twice the omega-3 fatty acids per capsule"). Nutrient content claims are generally considered to contain reliable information.
Health claim	Claim describing a relationship between a food substance and reduced risk of a disease or health-related condition (e.g., linking calcium and osteoporosis). Because the FDA allows health claims backed by both strong and weak evidence, health claims may represent either reliable or unreliable information.
Structure-function claim	Claim that may describe the role of a nutrient or dietary ingredient intended to impact the normal structure or function of the human body (e.g., "helps maintain normal cholesterol levels" or "antioxidants maintain cell integrity"). Structure-function claims are generally considered to be the least reliable of the claims.

Table 5-3 Examples of Special Populations Who May Benefit from Dietary Supplements

Cohort	Indications
Individuals on weight loss diets	Those on very low-calorie diets or restrictive diets can benefit from a multivitamin/mineral supplement.
Vegans and vegetarians	Animal products are the only appreciable sources of vitamin B_{12}; vegans should supplement with vitamin B_{12}. Individuals who do not consume dairy products may need calcium and vitamin D.
Infants, children, and adolescents	Those who live in areas where municipal water is not fluoridated may need a fluoride supplement. 400 IU of vitamin D is recommended per day for all infants beginning shortly after birth, as well for children and adolescents.
Reproductive-aged women (18–45 years)/ pregnant women	All women planning or capable of becoming pregnant should receive 400–800 mcg folic acid per day from fortified foods, supplements, or prenatal vitamins.
Older adults	Because of decreased gastric hydrochloric acid production and decreased intrinsic factor production (as well as reduced food intake), older adults may require supplemental vitamin B_{12}. Calcium and vitamin D may also need to be supplemented, depending upon intake, exercise level, and sunlight exposure.
Dark-skinned individuals	Darker-skinned persons receive a smaller effective dose of ultraviolet radiation than do lighter-skinned persons; depending upon sunlight exposure and intake levels, darker-skinned persons may benefit from vitamin D supplementation.
Cigarette smokers	Vitamin C may prevent cigarette smoke–induced oxidative damage. The DRI for vitamin C for smokers is 35 mg more per day compared to nonsmokers (female smokers ≥ 19 years: DRI is 100 mg vitamin D per day).
Chronic alcohol users	The metabolic effects of alcohol as a toxin coupled with poor dietary intake can result in deficiencies in vitamin status, particularly the B vitamins. Vitamin A supplements can be toxic when combined with alcohol.

Abbreviations: DRI = Dietary Reference Intake.

Vitamins

Vitamins are organic compounds that are essential in small quantities for normal growth, development, and metabolic processes. In general, vitamins are not endogenously produced and must be obtained from external sources. Thirteen specific vitamins have been identified. The vitamins are classified based on their solubility, with the B vitamins and vitamin C in the water-soluble vitamins class, and vitamins A, D, E, and K in the fat-soluble vitamins class. The B vitamins function as coenzymes in the conversion of macronutrients to energy and in the building and maintaining of body tissues and cell membranes. Some vitamins also have antioxidant properties, including vitamin A, vitamin E, and vitamin C and the mineral selenium. Box 5-1 discusses the history of naming of vitamins.

Box 5-1 Where Is Vitamin G? The Naming of Vitamins

The first third of the twentieth century was the age of discovery for vitamins. In the early 1900s, scientists conducted numerous research studies, especially with animals, in which they discovered nutritionally limited diets resulted in various disease conditions such as rickets, beriberi, pellagra, and scurvy. Casmir Funk, a European biochemist, suggested that the active factors in food that resolved these conditions were "vital amines" (vital amino acids). By the time it became apparent that these substances were not amino acids, vital or not, the name had become relatively common and eventually was shortened to *vitamin*.

Individuals may question why certain letters are missing in the names of vitamins. Some vitamins, such as vitamin G (riboflavin), vitamin H (biotin), and vitamin M (folic acid) were reclassified as part of the vitamin B complex. Others, such as vitamin F (essential fatty acids) and vitamin P (flavonoids), ultimately were found not to be vitamins at all. Vitamin J (catechol) and vitamin L_1 (anthranilic acid) were found to be protein metabolites. Vitamin K was named by German-speaking scientists who felt its association with coagulation (*koagulation*) warranted the specific letter.

Antioxidant Vitamins

Antioxidants are chemicals that are capable of slowing or preventing oxidation. Oxidation damages cells, and antioxidants serve to neutralize free radicals, thereby protecting against potential damage to cellular tissues. Antioxidant vitamins include vitamin E (α-tocopherol), vitamin C (ascorbic acid), and vitamin A (retinol, β-carotene). In 2012, a Cochrane systematic review of 78 randomized controlled trials with almost 300,000 participants found that taking supplements of the antioxidant vitamins did not decrease mortality rates, although in some studies vitamin A was associated with increased risk of death.[9] Despite increasing public interest, the U.S. Preventive Services Task Force (USPSTF) and the National Cancer Institute state that there is no clear evidence to support the use of antioxidant supplementation in cancer prevention.[10,11] The Academy of Nutrition and Dietetics encourages practitioners to promote food-based sources—as opposed to supplements—as the best nutrition-based strategy for achieving optimal health and reducing the risk of chronic disease.[3]

Fat-Soluble Vitamins

Fat-soluble vitamins are stored in body fat as well as the liver and other organs. Generally, fat-soluble vitamins pose a greater risk for toxicity than water-soluble vitamins when consumed in excess, because they can accumulate in the liver and fat tissue and are not excreted as rapidly as water-soluble vitamins. A summary table of all fat-soluble vitamins can be found at the end of this section (Table 5-5).

Vitamin A

Vitamin A is a fat-soluble vitamin that exists in four forms, each with a different biologic function: retinal, retinol, retinoic acid, and retinyl ester (the storage form). Retinal is required for vision, while retinoic acid is the principal hormonal metabolite required for growth and differentiation of epithelial cells. Vitamin A is involved with the maintenance of mucous membranes, skin, bone, and hair, and also acts as an antioxidant. When found in foods, two types of vitamin A are distinguished: (1) preformed vitamin A is found in animal foods, such as dairy products, fish, and meat (especially liver); and (2) **provitamin** A carotenoids are present in dark orange, yellow, and green plant foods like carrots, papayas, pumpkins, and squash. Both preformed vitamin A and provitamin A are metabolized in the cells to become the active forms of the vitamin—namely, retinal and retinoic acid.

The Tolerable Upper Intake Level (UL) for vitamin A is 3000 mcg per day for adults 19 years and older. The UL is for preformed vitamin A; there is no UL set for beta-carotene or other provitamin A carotenoids. Vitamin A deficiency is rare in the United States but may occur if the individual has a malabsorption syndrome that inhibits absorption of fats, cystic fibrosis, cholestasis, or cholestasis-related liver disease. On a global scale, however, vitamin A deficiency is the leading cause of preventable blindness in children, and vitamin A deficiency increases the risk of infection and death from diarrheal diseases and measles (rubeola). In pregnant women, vitamin A deficiency is linked to higher rates of maternal mortality.[12]

With regard to toxicity, the body, particularly in the liver, can store excessive amounts of all fat-soluble vitamins, including vitamin A. Levels of these vitamins can accumulate, and at high levels vitamin A can cause significant toxicity-related side effects known as hypervitaminosis A. Acute toxicity can occur following a dose of more than 660,000 IU. Symptoms include nausea and vomiting, blurry vision, vertigo, and malaise or drowsiness. Chronic toxicity can also occur if amounts higher than 10 times the RDA are consumed regularly. Symptoms include ataxia, alopecia, hepatotoxicity, bone and muscle pain, and visual impairments, in addition to other nonspecific symptoms.

High doses of preformed vitamin A in the drug isotretinoin (Accutane) are also known to be teratogenic if taken during pregnancy, and high-dose vitamin A supplements should be avoided by women of childbearing age. Overconsumption of beta-carotene can cause a temporary orange or yellowish hue of the skin (carotenodermia) that is neither teratogenic nor clinically dangerous, and can easily be relieved by discontinuation of beta-carotene intake.[13]

The RDAs for vitamin A for women are noted in Table 5-6 at the end of this section.[14] Vitamin A is listed on food and supplement labels in international units (IUs), although nutrition scientists preferentially use retinol activity equivalents (RAEs) to account for the different bioactivity levels of retinol and provitamin A carotenoids. Box 5-2 explains the conversion between units of mcg RAE and IU for vitamin A.

If treatment with vitamin A is needed, supplementation can be provided via oral capsules or intramuscular injection if malabsorption prevents oral use. Some weight reduction medications that decrease fat absorption, such as orlistat (Xenical), can also interfere with absorption of any of the fat-soluble vitamins, including vitamin A. Likewise, supplementation with this vitamin may be recommended for women after bariatric surgery. Because vitamin A can be teratogenic, women of a reproductive age should be counseled about the use of this drug. For example, many women take multiple vitamins containing iron during pregnancy and may need to increase their iron levels for therapeutic reasons. Under those circumstances, women should be educated not to double or triple the number of pills or capsules of a multivitamin because of the risk of toxicity and teratogenicity of vitamin A in particular. Similarly, women who are taking retinoids for dermatologic reasons should be advised not to add supplements containing vitamin A. Vitamin A supplementation was thought to be of value to prevent cardiovascular disease. However, after evaluation, it has not been shown to be effective for this purpose and is not recommended for prophylaxis or disease prevention.

Vitamin D

Vitamin D is a fat-soluble vitamin that promotes calcium absorption in the gut and normal bone mineralization and can be obtained from sun exposure, explaining why it is commonly known as the "sunshine vitamin." Vitamin D helps to maintain normal serum calcium and phosphate concentrations.[16] To be adequately activated, vitamin D must undergo two hydroxylations in the body. First, in the liver, vitamin D is converted to 25-hydroxyvitamin D [25(OH)D], also called calcidiol. Subsequently, calcidiol is hydroxylated in the kidneys to form 1,25-dihydroxyvitamin D [1,25$(OH)_2$D], also called calcitriol. Thus, a healthy liver and functional kidneys are required for optimal vitamin D activation; injury or damage to these organs can precipitate vitamin D deficiency.

Box 5-2 Converting Between mcg RAE and IU for Vitamin A

To convert vitamin A as retinol:
From IU to mcg: IU × 0.3 = mcg
From mcg to IU: mcg ÷ 0.3 = IU
Example: 5000 IU × 0.3 = 1500 mcg

To convert vitamin A as beta-carotene:
From IU to mcg: IU × 0.6 = mcg
From mcg to IU: mcg ÷ 0.6 = IU
Example: 5000 IU × 0.6 = 3000 mcg

Source: Modified from National Institutes of Health, Office of Dietary Supplements. Unit conversions. *Dietary Supplement Ingredient Database.* 2012. http://dietarysupplementdatabase.usda.nih.gov/ingredient_calculator/equation.php. Accessed June 4, 2014.[15]

Vitamin D is rare in most food sources. The flesh of fatty fish (such as salmon, tuna, sardines, and mackerel) and fish liver oils (such as cod liver oil) are the best sources, although smaller amounts of vitamin D are found in egg yolks, beef liver, and cheese. Mushrooms may contain vitamin D if they are exposed to ultraviolet light during the growing process. Fortified foods serve as the primary source of dietary vitamin D in the United States, where the majority of the fluid milk supply is voluntarily fortified with 100 IU vitamin D per 8 fluid ounce (1 cup) serving.[16]

Inadequate vitamin D status leads to rickets in children and osteomalacia and hyperparathyroidism in adults. Vitamin D deficiency can be caused by inadequate sunlight exposure, which leads to decreased synthesis of vitamin D in the skin; by inability of kidneys to convert 25(OH)D to its active form; or by impaired absorption of vitamin D from the digestive tract. Vitamin D insufficiency or deficiency is more likely among individuals with milk allergy, lactose intolerance, or malabsorption syndromes, and in adherents to certain types of restrictive vegetarianism or veganism. Other persons at increased risk for vitamin D insufficiency include exclusively breastfed infants, older adults, persons with limited sun exposure, persons with dark skin, persons who are taking a medication that accelerates metabolism of vitamin D such as phenytoin (Dilantin), and individuals who are obese or who have undergone gastric bypass surgery.[16,17]

At the other end of the intake spectrum, vitamin D toxicity is linked to nonspecific symptoms including anorexia, weight loss, excessive urination, and heart arrhythmias. Such toxicity can also cause elevated blood levels of calcium, leading to vascular and tissue calcification and damage to the heart, blood vessels, and kidneys. The toxicity threshold for vitamin D is suspected to be in the range of 10,000 to 40,000 IU per day, with serum 25(OH)D levels of 500–600 nmol/L (200–240 ng/mL).[16] The UL for vitamin D has been set at 4000 IU per day.[18]

Controversy Regarding Insufficiency versus Deficiency

There has been a resurgence of interest in vitamin D in the last several years. Supplementation has been suggested to be of value for heart, bone, and liver health as well as for prevention and treatment of diabetes mellitus, autism, multiple sclerosis, and cancer.[19] Multiple studies are currently exploring whether such relationships exist. However, many of these studies are limited by the fact that there is no general consensus on optimal serum concentrations of 25(OH)D for either bone health or general health. Although serum levels of 25(OH)D serve as a biomarker of exposure to vitamin D from sun, food, and supplemental sources, the degree to which levels predict health outcomes has not yet been determined.[18] Despite this lack of consensus, the information in Table 5-4 provides an overview of the correlation of 25(OH)D concentrations with potential health effects. Serum concentrations of 25 (OH)D are reported in both nanomoles per liter (nmol/L) and nanograms per milliliter (ng/mL), with 1 nmol/L equaling 0.4 ng/mL.[20]

Table 5-4 Serum 25-Hydroxyvitamin D [25(OH)D] Concentrations and Health

Concentration		Health Status
nmol/L	ng/mL	
< 30	< 12	Associated with vitamin D deficiency Increased risk for rickets in children and osteomalacia in adults—especially adults with 25(OH)D levels < 10 ng/mL
30–50	12–20	May be considered inadequate for bone and overall health in healthy individuals
≥ 50	≥ 20	Generally considered adequate for bone and overall health in healthy individuals
> 125	> 50	Emerging evidence suggests potential adverse effects at high levels, particularly at levels > 150 nmol/L (> 60 ng/mL)

Source: Modified from National Institutes of Health, Office of Dietary Supplements. Vitamin D fact sheet for health professionals. *Health Information*. June 24, 2011. http://ods.od.nih.gov/factsheets/VitaminD-HealthProfessional/. Accessed June 4, 2014.[16]

There has been a movement in the twenty-first century to treat persons with vitamin D levels between 12 and 20 ng/mL, or according to some sources, as high as 30 ng/mL. The theory is that these asymptomatic individuals may be at high risk of developing osteoporosis, especially because low vitamin D levels are associated with a decrease in serum calcium and increased activity of the parathyroid, which causes increased bone resorption. Other incidental findings suggest that vitamin D may be of value in preventing or treating memory loss, schizophrenia, or a myriad of cardiovascular conditions. However, the scientific studies in these areas have yielded inconsistent findings. At this time there is no consensus regarding vitamin D supplementation to treat women with insufficiency in an effort to decrease cardiovascular diseases, preeclampsia, preterm birth, or gestational diabetes, or to decrease mortality among older women. Studies are still being conducted to ascertain if some associations do exist. Until clear benefits are discovered, many providers neither screen for nor treat persons with vitamin D insufficiency, especially given estimates that 75% of the population of the United States may meet the current definition of having vitamin D insufficiency or deficiency.

Recommendations for Supplementation

In 2008, the American Academy of Pediatrics (AAP) doubled its vitamin D supplement recommendation; now the AAP recommends that exclusively and partially breastfed infants receive 400 IU per day supplemental vitamin D beginning shortly after birth until they are weaned to vitamin D–fortified whole milk or vitamin D–fortified formula and consuming at least 1000 mL per day. Nonbreastfed infants ingesting less than 1000 mL per day of vitamin D–fortified milk or formula are also recommended to receive 400 IU supplemental vitamin D per day.[21,22]

Data from the 2005–2006 National Health and Nutrition Examination Survey (NHANES) reveal that a large proportion of U.S. citizens who do not take vitamin D supplements do not consume the recommended DRI for this vitamin. However, when supplements were added into the calculation, the mean values of number of persons who consume adequate amounts were significantly increased.[23]

The DRI for vitamin D was revised in 2010; the current recommendation is 15 mcg (600 IU) vitamin D per day for persons 1–70 years and 20 mcg (800 IU) vitamin D per day for persons older than 70. The DRI for vitamin D is based on the presumption of minimal sunlight exposure.[15,18] Box 5-3 demonstrates how to convert vitamin D between IU and mcg units of measurement.

Vitamin D supplements in the form of capsules or tablets are available as vitamin D_3 (cholecalciferol) or vitamin D_2 (ergocalciferol). Vitamin D_3 increases 25(OH)D levels better than vitamin D_2. For individuals with normal intestinal absorption, every 100 IU of vitamin D_3 increases the 25(OH)D level by approximately 0.7–1.0 ng/mL (1.75–2.5 nmol/L).

The most commonly used dose for repletion is 50,000 IU orally once per week for 6 to 8 weeks. Once the 25(OH)D levels are stable, a maintenance dose of 600 to 800 IU per week is recommended. The dose for supplementation is also 600 to 800 IU per week. The once-weekly dosing regimen appears to improve vitamin D levels better than daily or monthly dosing, although some persons improve well with once-monthly dosing. Persons with malabsorption, such as those who have undergone bariatric surgery, are usually prescribed 10,000 to 50,000 IU per day.

Vitamin D metabolites such as calcitriol (Rocaltrol, Vectical) are also available in capsule form and can be used to treat vitamin D deficiency. These formulations are recommended for persons with liver or renal insufficiency, as they are more easily metabolized and have a more rapid onset of action compared to vitamin D_3 or vitamin D_2. Calcidiol is associated with a high incidence of hypercalcemia; if it is used, the woman's calcium levels must be monitored.

Box 5-3 Converting Between mcg and IU for Vitamin D

To convert vitamin D:

From IU to mcg: IU × 0.025 = mcg

From mcg to IU: mcg ÷ 0.025 = IU

Example: 400 IU × 0.025 = 10 mcg

Source: Modified from National Institutes of Health, Office of Dietary Supplements. Unit conversions. *Dietary Supplement Ingredient Database*. 2012. http://dietarysupplementdatabase.usda.nih.gov/ingredient_calculator/equation.php. Accessed June 4, 2014.[15]

Vitamin E

Vitamin E is a fat-soluble antioxidant vitamin that exists in any of eight chemical forms, including four tocopherols (α, β, γ, δ) and four tocotrienols (α, β, γ, δ); α-tocopherol is the form that is known to meet human requirements. In addition to its antioxidant properties, vitamin E protects cell membranes, enhances immune function, and may help prevent cataracts.[24] Nuts, seeds, and plant oils are the best dietary sources of vitamin E, although green leafy vegetables and fortified cereals also supply this fat-soluble vitamin.[24] A number of studies have indicated that current intake levels of vitamin E in the United States typically fall below the RDA levels, although some analyses indicate that these estimates may underrepresent fat and, therefore, vitamin E intake, because food preparation methods and the amount of fat added to foods is often unknown or underestimated.[25]

Despite what may be suboptimal intake levels, vitamin E–deficiency diseases in adults who reside in the United States are rare with the one exception of preterm infants of very low birth weight (less than 1500 g) who are at increased risk for deficiency.[26] The rare individuals with vitamin E deficiency may demonstrate ataxia, peripheral neuropathy, and an impaired immune response.

There are no adverse effects known from excessive consumption of dietary sources of vitamin E; however, due to the potential hemorrhagic effects associated with high supplemental vitamin E intake, a UL of 1000 mg per day has been determined by the Food and Nutrition Board.[25] The DRI for vitamin E is 15 mg per day for females 14 years and older, with needs increasing to 19 mg per day during lactation.[25]

The amount of vitamin E in foods and dietary supplements is listed in international units (IU). The naturally

Box 5-4 Relationships Between mg and IU Based on Form of Vitamin E

Vitamin E (Alpha-Tocopherol)	Natural Form (D-Alpha-Tocopherol)	Synthetic Form (DL-Alpha-Tocopherol)
1 mg	1.49 IU	2.22 IU
1 IU	0.67 mg	0.45 mg

Source: National Institutes of Health, Office of Dietary Supplements. Vitamin E fact sheet for professionals. *Health Information*. June 5, 2013. http://ods.od.nih.gov/factsheets/VitaminE-HealthProfessional/#en52. Accessed June 5, 2014.[27]

sourced vitamin E is called d-alpha-tocopherol, whereas the synthetically produced variety is dl-alpha-tocopherol.[27] Box 5-4 demonstrates how to convert between IU and mcg of vitamin E.

Two observational studies conducted in the early 1990s suggested that supplemental vitamin E might play a role in prevention of cardiovascular disease. However, further studies failed to confirm any cardiovascular protection. As a result, the American Heart Association maintains that there is no evidence to justify use of vitamin E or other oxidants to promote cardiovascular health and reduce the risk of disease.[28] Furthermore, the USPSTF recommends against the use of both beta-carotene and vitamin E supplements for the prevention of cardiovascular disease or cancer.[29]

Vitamin E is a component of a common drug composed of various vitamins and minerals, marketed as Preserve AREDS. This brand-name product is often prescribed to decrease development of visual conditions such as macular degeneration, although use of vitamin E alone has not been found to be therapeutic. Vitamin E is an antioxidant and an anticoagulant. Thus, the action of this drug can counter the action of vitamin K, even leading to a vitamin K deficiency.

A common myth exists that treatment of a scar with topical vitamin K will decrease the cosmetic appearance of the cicatrix. There is no evidence supporting this activity, and even some suggestion that vitamin E may actually enhance the scarring.

Vitamin K

Vitamin K is actually a group of different compounds. The phylloquinones (the vitamin K_1 series) are naturally occurring compounds that are found in dark green, leafy vegetables. The menaquinones (the vitamin K_2 series) are synthesized by bacteria. Like all fat-soluble vitamins, vitamin K requires some dietary fat and a supply of bile salts and pancreatic juices to promote its absorption.[30] This micronutrient assists with the production of prothrombin and is required for blood clotting, bone health, and the regulation of various enzyme systems.[30]

Vitamin K was discovered in the 1930s by a Danish biochemist, Henrik Dam. After the first clinical trials found a benefit from using vitamin K to treat persons with obstructive jaundice, it was then administered to newborns suffering from hemorrhagic disease. This use of vitamin K lowered the mortality from the disease from 4.6% to 1.8% and led to the Nobel Prize for Dam and the scientist who isolated the vitamin itself, Edward Doisy.[31] Use of vitamin K for preventing hemorrhagic disease of the newborn is discussed in more detail in the chapter *The Newborn*.

Vitamin K deficiency is rare among adults, because this vitamin is found in many foods and synthesized normally by gut bacteria in healthy individuals. Among older adults, suboptimal vitamin K intake levels have been linked with increased likelihood of hip fractures.[30] Persons at higher risk for vitamin K deficiency include individuals with kidney/liver damage or disease; those taking antibiotics for a long period of time; persons with malabsorption or cirrhosis; individuals with vitamin D deficiency; and persons who take antituberculosis drugs such as rifampin (Rifadin), anticoagulant drugs, or bile acid sequestrants such as cholestyramine (Questran).

The drug warfarin (Coumadin) blocks the enzyme that converts vitamin K to its active form in the liver. Thus, vitamin K supplementation is used therapeutically to correct the excess anticoagulation that can occur following use of warfarin when necessary, although concurrent use may also result in impairment of the activity of warfarin. Vitamin K's inhibition of anticoagulation is not observed with newer anticoagulants such as dabigatran (Pradaxa) and rivaroxaban (Xarelto). Because dark green, leafy vegetables contain vitamin K, individuals who are taking warfarin (Coumadin) should maintain a steady and regular intake of foods containing high levels of vitamin K. These individuals are advised to avoid any significant increase in consumption of dark green, leafy vegetables, but not to eliminate all vegetables entirely. Women with vitamin K deficiency may demonstrate easy bruising, bleeding from the gums, and heavy menstrual flow.

Evidence is lacking to support an RDA for vitamin K; rather, an Adequate Intake (AI) level of 90 mcg per day for adult women has been established. There is no UL for vitamin K.[14]

If treatment with vitamin K is necessary, doses of 1 to 25 mg can be administered orally as a tablet that contains 5 mg (Mephyton) or parenterally (Phytonadione). The onset of action is 6 to 10 hours following oral administration and 1 to 2 hours following intravenous administration. The peak effect occurs 24 to 48 hours following oral administration and 12 to 14 hours following intravenous injection. Anaphylaxis has been reported, albeit rarely, when vitamin K is administered via any of the parenteral routes.

Studies are ongoing to determine if a clear association exists among vitamin supplementation and promotion of bone health and prevention of a number of diseases or conditions. The latter include cardiovascular disease, Alzheimer's disease, cancer, and type 2 diabetes.

Summary of Fat-Soluble Vitamins

Although supplements containing fat-soluble vitamins are readily available, their use in preventing disease in healthy individuals has not been proven and they are not recommended for this purpose. Deficiencies are rare and limited to special populations. Fat-soluble vitamins can cause toxicity if taken in excess. Table 5-5 summarizes information related to the fat-soluble vitamins.

Table 5-5 Fat-Soluble Vitamins: A Summary

Fat-Soluble Vitamin	Function	Selected Food Sources	Recommended Intake Levels	Deficiency and Excessive Intake Considerations	Clinical and Supplementation Considerations
Vitamin A	Antioxidant Vision Growth and differentiation of epithelial cells Maintains mucous membranes, skin, bone, and hair	Preformed vitamin A from animal foods (dairy products, fish, meat, and liver) Provitamin A carotenoids in dark orange, yellow, and green plant foods	RDA: 700 mcg/day for females RDA during pregnancy is 770 mcg/day; during lactation, it is 1300 mcg/day if the woman ≥ 19 years RDA for women 14–18 years is 750 mcg/day during pregnancy and 1200 mcg/day during lactation	Deficiency: xerophthalmia (night blindness), increased mortality, risk of infections Excess: congenital birth defects, maternal mortality UL (for preformed vitamin A): 3000 mcg RAE (10,000 IU)	Supplements often are part of a combined multivitamin. Supplements can be teratogenic. Orlistat (Alli, Xenical) and cholestyramine can decrease vitamin A absorption. The retinoids acitretin (Soriatane) and bexarotene (Targretin) can increase the risk of hypervitaminosis A when taken with vitamin A supplements.
Vitamin D	Promotes calcium absorption and normal bone mineralization Maintains serum calcium and phosphate concentrations	Flesh of fatty fish (salmon, tuna, sardines, mackerel) Fish liver oils (cod liver oil) Egg yolks, beef liver, cheese Mushrooms if exposed to UV light Milk in United States is fortified with 100 IU per 8 fl oz (1 cup)	RDA: 15 mcg/day for females 9–70 years RDA: 20 mcg/day for females > 70 years	Deficiency: rickets in children and osteomalacia in adults Excess: nonspecific toxicity symptoms (anorexia, weight loss, excessive urination, heart arrhythmias) UL: 4000 IU/day	Corticosteroid medications such as prednisone can reduce calcium and impair vitamin D absorption. Orlistat (Alli, Xenical) and cholestyramine (Questran, LoCholest, Prevalite) can reduce vitamin D absorption. Phenobarbital and phenytoin (Dilantin) increase hepatic metabolism of vitamin D.
Vitamin E	Antioxidant Protects cell membranes Enhances immune function May help prevent cataracts	Nuts, seeds, and plant oils Green, leafy vegetables Fortified cereals	RDA: 15 mg/day for females and during pregnancy; 19 mg/day during lactation	Deficiency: rare but preterm infants are at increased risk Excess: rare but can cause hemorrhagic effects UL: 1000 mg/day for females ≥ 19 years	Vitamin E can inhibit platelet aggregation and antagonize vitamin K–dependent clotting factors; Cholestyramine (Questran, LoCholest, Prevalite) can reduce vitamin E absorption. Avoid large vitamin E doses when taking anticoagulant or antiplatelet medications such as warfarin (Coumadin). Vitamin E taken in conjunction with other antioxidants can suppress the rise in HDL and HDL2 that sometimes occurs in those individuals taking simvastatin (Zocor) and niacin. Advise against vitamin E and other antioxidant supplements during cancer chemotherapy or radiotherapy.
Vitamin K	Production of prothrombin, required for blood clotting Regulates bone health and other enzyme systems	Dark green, leafy vegetables	No RDA, AI: 90 mcg/day for females ≥ 19 years	Deficiency: premature and exclusively breastfed infants are at risk for hypoprothrombinemia Excess: can interfere with warfarin (Coumadin) therapy	Caution against significant changes in vitamin K–containing foods intake when taking warfarin (Coumadin), as the drug blocks the enzyme that converts vitamin K to its active form. Cholestyramine (Questran, LoCholest, Prevalite) can reduce vitamin K absorption.

Abbreviations: AI = adequate intake; HDL: high-density lipoprotein; RDA = recommended daily allowance; UL = tolerable upper intake level; UV = ultraviolet.

Water-Soluble Vitamins

The water-soluble vitamins consist of the B vitamins and vitamin C. Unlike the fat-soluble vitamins, the water-soluble vitamins are not stored in considerable amounts in the body and are excreted in the urine; in turn, they must be consumed on a more regular basis. In general, the B vitamin status of most healthy persons who reside in the United States is adequate, due in part to current grain intake levels that help meet B vitamin needs: Whole grains naturally contain B vitamins, and enriched grains have mandatory supplemental levels of the B vitamins thiamin, riboflavin, niacin, folic acid, and the mineral iron added to them. A summary table at the end of this section (Table 5-7) lists selected water-soluble vitamins and identifies the basic functions, selected food sources, recommended intake levels, deficiency and excessive intake considerations, and clinical and supplementation considerations of these agents.

B Vitamins

The eight B vitamins involved in cell metabolism function collectively as part of coenzymes. Coenzymes are small molecules that combine with an enzyme to activate it.[32] Despite a commonly held belief that B vitamins "give you energy," these vitamins do not directly supply the body with energy; rather, they indirectly assist the body's functioning by metabolizing energy from carbohydrates, lipids, and amino acids.

Thiamin (Vitamin B_1)

Thiamin is an essential coenzyme for several intracellular reactions. It is responsible for generating energy from carbohydrates and driving neural function. Thiamin was one of the first vitamins to be identified.[33] Thiamin was originally spelled with an "e"; the terminal "e" was dropped when it was discovered that the vitamin was not an amine, although it may still be spelled with an "e" depending on the text.[34]

Yeast and liver are high in thiamin, although in the United States, pork, whole grains, and enriched grain products are more commonly consumed sources of thiamin.[15] Thiamin deficiency can cause beriberi and Wernicke-Korsakoff syndrome, but widespread thiamin deficiencies are not a major American public health concern.[16]

However, women with a malabsorption condition may be at increased risk for the deficiency. Other conditions that have been reported to place a woman at risk for this deficiency include ulcerative colitis, cataracts, type 2 diabetes mellitus, nephropathy, and memory loss, although scientific evidence is not clear regarding the association. Women with hyperemesis of pregnancy who receive dextrose should also receive thiamin to reduce the risk of Wernicke-Korsakoff syndrome.

There are no known consequences of low-level thiamin excess, although very high doses—such as 1000 times the nutritional need of commercial thiamin hydrochloride—can suppress respiration and prove fatal. There is no UL for thiamin. The RDA is set at 1.2 mg per day for adult males and 1.1 mg per day for adult females.[35]

Riboflavin (Vitamin B_2)

Riboflavin plays a role in energy metabolism, nerve function, protection of biological membranes, and the synthesis of a number of vitamins. The word "riboflavin" is derived from the ribose component and the Latin word *flavus*, meaning "yellow"—which describes this compound's yellow color.[24] Meats and dairy foods are the primary sources of riboflavin in the American diet.

The riboflavin-deficiency disease is called ariboflavinosis; it is characterized by cheilosis, stomatitis, glossitis, and confusion. Riboflavin deficiency in the United States is rare, and a stand-alone riboflavin deficiency is even more rare, as B vitamin deficiencies tend to cluster. Persons with thyroid disease, which interferes with riboflavin utilization, and alcoholism are at highest risk for deficiency. Individuals with riboflavin deficiency may have normochromic, normocytic anemia.

No riboflavin-related toxicity disease has been reported; and as such, no UL has been set. The RDA for riboflavin is 1.1 mg per day for females. Because riboflavin is easily destroyed by light, milk is now stored in opaque containers to preserve its riboflavin content.

Newborns undergoing phototherapy often also are given riboflavin, because it promotes breakdown of bilirubin. Breastfeeding women should be cautioned about storing breast milk in glass containers, which may accelerate riboflavin losses of this valuable food.[36] Studies are being currently conducted to determine whether riboflavin may be effective for treatment of women with migraines or keratoconus.

Niacin (Vitamin B_3)

Niacin (nicotinic acid, nicotinamide, or vitamin B_3) is a water-soluble vitamin that plays a role in DNA synthesis and repair, cholesterol metabolism, and glucose homeostasis. The niacin-derived coenzymes NAD and NADP are involved in more than 200 enzymatic reactions that catalyze energy metabolism.[24] Niacin is synthesized endogenously through the conversion of tryptophan. The word "niacin" is the term that defines the direct vitamin precursors for NAD formation, whereas "niacin equivalents" refer to the non-vitamin NAD precursor tryptophan. One mg of niacin is equivalent to 60 mg tryptophan. The DRI for niacin (or niacin equivalents) is set at 14 mg per day for adult females.[16] Tryptophan represents approximately 1% of protein consumed in the diet, so eating 100 g dietary protein per day would yield 16 mg of niacin or roughly 100% of an adult's daily NAD needs without requiring the vitamin forms of niacin.[37] Dietary sources of niacin include whole-grain foods, enriched and fortified breakfast cereals, liver, poultry, fish, tomatoes, beef, and mushrooms.[15] Niacin is relatively stable, and is not readily destroyed by exposure to light or heat.[24]

The niacin deficiency disease is called pellagra, a term meaning "angry skin"; it is characterized by the "three D's"—diarrhea, dermatitis, and dementia.[37] Heavy reliance on refined foods led to widespread pellagra in the United States in the early parts of the twentieth century until an officer in the Public Health Service discovered that supplementing diets with eggs and milk alleviated the symptoms of pellagra.[15,24] The UL for niacin applies to synthetic forms obtained from supplements, fortified foods, or a combination of the two, and is set at 35 mg per day for adults.[16]

Prescription formulations of niacin are available as nicotinic acid or nicotinamide. Nicotinic acid (Niacin-50 [OTC], Niacor, Niaspan) is used to treat dyslipidemias. Nicotinic acid prevents hepatic production of very low-density lipoprotein (VLDL). Nicotinamide does not have therapeutic value for treating dyslipidemias. Additional information about use of this agent can be found in the *Cardiovascular Conditions* chapter.

Niacin is available in regular-release (Niacor) and extended-release (Niaspan) forms. Over-the-counter preparations of niacin are not FDA regulated and may contain variable amounts of the active vitamin. Sustained-release OTC formulations have been associated with hepatotoxicity and are not recommended. In contrast, immediate-release OTC formulations appear to be safe, as are prescription brands of sustained-release formulations (Niaspan). The dose is generally 300–500 mg per day, and higher doses are sometimes used.

The classic side effect of taking a high dose of niacin is a temporary facial and body flushing that lasts for 10 to 20 minutes. Flushing occurs in the majority of persons who take this supplement, but is less common with use of the sustained-release formulation and is further reduced with use of the coated caplets of Niaspan. Additional common side effects include nausea and paresthesias.

Adverse effects of niacin are also possible. Statin-induced myopathy is more likely in persons who also take niacin and especially in persons of Chinese ancestry. Therefore, the combination of statin and niacin should not be prescribed for this population. Nicotinic acid can also increase glucose levels, induce hyperuricemia, and exacerbate hypotension in persons treated with vasodilators. In addition, this agent increases the risk of developing infection or bleeding.

Studies are being conducted to explore whether supplementation with niacin may prevent or modify a number of different conditions. These conditions include migraines, vertigo, schizophrenia, Alzheimer's disease, diabetes, acne, hypertension, cataracts, and memory loss.

Pantothenic Acid (Vitamin B_5)

Pantothenic acid and its coenzyme form coenzyme A (CoA). This enzyme functions in a number of metabolic pathways and plays critical roles in ATP production and the synthesis of heme, cholesterol, bile salts, fatty acids, steroid hormones, and phospholipids. The name of this nitrogen-containing compound is derived from the Greek word *pantos*, meaning "everywhere." Pantothenic acid is found in almost every plant and animal tissue.[24] Pantothenic acid deficiency is extremely rare, and there is no known toxicity or UL set for this vitamin. Sufficient data are not available to set an RDA for pantothenic acid, although an AI level of 5 mg per day has been established.[16]

Some cosmetic companies add pantothenic acid to hair products with the intention of increasing hair health. However, no studies have confirmed such improvement occurs. Future studies may provide additional information regarding the merits of supplementation to decrease diabetic ulcerations/polyneuropathy, decrease high LDL cholesterol levels, and improve wound healing.

Pyridoxine (Vitamin B_6)

Vitamin B_6 is involved in more than 100 chemical reactions. Its three forms—pyridoxine, pyridoxal, and pyridoxamine—all have similar biologic responsibilities within the body.[24] Vitamin B_6 assists with the conversion of tryptophan to niacin, aids in glucose regulation, and promotes steroid hormone formation. Like other B vitamins, it is found in a variety of foods, including whole grains and fortified and enriched cereals, garbanzo beans, tuna, and liver.[15] The DRI for vitamin B_6 is 1.3 mg per day for adult women.[16]

Vitamin B_6 deficiency presents as microcytic hypochromic anemia, but deficiency is rarely seen in individuals who consume a well-balanced diet. Overconsumption and toxicity from vitamin B_6–containing foods is also unusual, although toxicity can occur with high-dose supplementation. The UL for vitamin B_6 is 100 mg per day. Some data support the practice of high-dose vitamin B_6 intake (more than 1000 mg per day) to alleviate premenstrual syndrome symptoms.[38,39]

Vitamin B_6 supplementation is commonly used in two additional medical conditions. First, isoniazid (INH) use can cause vitamin B_6 deficiency, which can result in INH-related neurotoxicity. Supplementation with 25–50 mg per day of pyridoxine (Neuro-K-250) is recommended to prevent INH-related neurotoxicity, and treatment with much higher doses can correct this neurotoxicity. Second, pyridoxine is often recommended for treatment of pregnancy-related nausea and vomiting.[40] This use is reviewed in more detail in the *Pregnancy* chapter. Studies are currently being conducted assessing supplementation for treatment of individuals with Parkinson's disease, autism, and attention-deficit disorders. Magnesium supplementation is used in the last case.

Biotin (Vitamin B_7)

Biotin can be obtained from dietary sources and is also produced by colonic bacteria, albeit in quantities insufficient to meet human needs. Biotin plays a role in gluconeogenesis and ATP production, as part of the citric acid cycle. The best food sources of biotin include peanuts, almonds, mushrooms, and cooked egg yolk.[15] Biotin's bioavailability is inhibited by the presence of avidin, a protein present in raw egg whites, so very high consumption of raw eggs (e.g., eating 12 raw eggs per day for a prolonged period of time) is ill advised.[24] Cooking heat denatures avidin, so large amounts of cooked egg intake are not linked to biotin deficiency.

Biotin deficiency is rare, although it can be an inborn error of metabolism. In that situation, clinical signs and symptoms may include conjunctivitis, neurologic symptoms, and various dermatologic conditions such as alopecia.

Data are insufficient to set an RDA for biotin, but the AI level is 30 mcg per day. There is no UL established for biotin and no known disease of excess.[16]

Folate (Vitamin B_9)

Folate (folic acid) is a water-soluble vitamin that assists in production and maintenance of cells (including red blood cells) and DNA synthesis and also functions in combination with vitamin B_{12} in amino acid metabolism. Folate is absorbed in the small intestine and then is stored in the liver. Unlike iron, folate is not heavily recycled, but instead needs daily replacement. The name "folate" comes from the Latin word *folium*, meaning "leaf"—an appropriate name considering that dark green, leafy vegetables are rich sources of food folate. Other folate-containing foods include organ meats, legumes, whole grains, and fortified and enriched cereal products.[15] Folic acid is the synthetic form of folate. Although folate is theorized to be more bioavailable from the supplement form compared to food-sourced folate, the degree and significance of this difference have not been determined.[41]

Folate deficiency during pregnancy increases the risk of neural tube defects (NTDs) such as spina bifida and anencephaly. In an effort to prevent NTDs, 53 countries, including the United States, now mandate fortification of wheat flour with folic acid.[42,43] Multiple studies have shown decreases of 19% to 32% in NTD prevalence in the United States since the implementation of folic acid fortification was finalized in 1998.[44] The DRI for folate is listed as dietary folate equivalents (DFE), and Box 5-5 provides more information about folate conversion.

Folic acid deficiency usually is linked to inadequate consumption, absorption, or storage. Severe folate deficiency manifests itself as megaloblastic macrocytic anemia, a condition that causes red blood cells to remain in their immature forms (megaloblasts). Vitamin B_{12} deficiency can also cause this type of anemia. High doses of folic acid are said to mask vitamin B_{12} deficiency; as such, the UL for folate has been set at 1000 mcg per day DFE from fortified foods or supplements. There is no known toxicity from high intake of food folate. Due to widespread enrichment and fortification efforts, folate deficiency in the United States

Box 5-5 Converting Between DFE and mcg for Folate and Folic Acid

1 DFE equals:
1 mcg food folate or
0.6 mcg folic acid from fortified food or
as a supplement consumed with food or
0.5 mcg of a supplement taken on an empty stomach

Source: Data from National Institutes of Health, Office of Dietary Supplements. Unit conversions. *Dietary Supplement Ingredient Database*. 2012. http://dietarysupplementdatabase.usda.nih.gov/ingredient_calculator/equation.php. Accessed June 4, 2014.[15]

Table 5-6 Selected Drug Interactions with Folic Acid[a]

Drug	Effects on Folic Acid	Effects on Drug
5-Fluorouracil (Adrucil)		Increases side effects
Alcohol (excessive intake)	Inhibits absorption	
Antacids	Inhibit absorption	
Bile acid sequestrants	Inhibit absorption	
Fosphenytoin (Cerebyx)		Decreases serum levels
Histamine-2 antagonists	Inhibit absorption	
Metformin (Glucophage)	Inhibits absorption	
Phenobarbitol (Luminal)		Decreases serum levels
Primidone (Mysoline)		Decreases serum levels
Proton pump inhibitors	Inhibit absorption	
Tetracyclines		Inhibit absorption

[a] This table is not comprehensive as new information is being generated on a regular basis.
Source: Data from Kaferle J, Strzoda CE. Evaluation of macrocytosis. *Am Fam Physician*. 2009;79(3):203-208.[45]

is rare, although it is still seen in individuals who abuse alcohol and with the use of certain medications such as anticonvulsant drugs. Table 5-6 lists selected medications that interact with folic acid.

In the late twentieth century, folic acid emerged as a potential "magic bullet" for a wide variety of conditions. However, much of the early information proved not to be statistically significant. There is some indication that the vitamin may decrease the risk of stroke and depression. In addition, when used in combination with other vitamins and minerals, folic acid may decrease the risk of macular degeneration. Conversely, evidence has failed to demonstrate a decrease in cardiovascular disease, in spite of the action of folic acid in decreasing homocysteine. This B vitamin has not been proven to decrease cancer in general, and it can interfere with chemotherapeutic agents such as methotrexate (Rheumatrex, Trexall), whose mechanism of action is as an antifolate drug.

Vitamin B_{12} (Cyanocobalamin)

Vitamin B_{12}, also known as cobalamin, was the last of the B vitamins to be discovered. It is used in ATP production, and functions with folate in amino acid metabolism. Vitamin B_{12} is unique in that it is found in appreciable amounts only in animal-derived foods.[15] As such, persons on strict vegetarian and vegan diets are advised to supplement with vitamin B_{12} to avoid deficiency. Good sources of vitamin B_{12} include clams, liver, oysters, crab, and eggs. Some debate exists about the addition of sea algae to the diet instead of animal products as a source of this B vitamin, but additional study is needed to ascertain whether it is beneficial.

Proper vitamin B_{12} absorption requires the presence of intrinsic factor, a protein produced by the stomach. The aging process is often associated with decreased hydrochloric acid production, which leads to a related reduction in intrinsic factor and subsequent inability to adequately absorb vitamin B_{12}. Vitamin B_{12} deficiency is thought to affect between 15% and 40% of the elderly population.[46] Women who have experienced bariatric surgery may require supplementation with vitamin B_{12} for life. However, because vitamin B_{12} is the only B vitamin that is stored in the body, it can take a period of 2 to 3 years before stores are depleted and deficiency occurs.

A secondary type of vitamin B_{12} deficiency is pernicious anemia, caused by an autoimmune disease wherein antibodies destroy the stomach cells that otherwise would produce intrinsic factor.[47] Pernicious anemia does not usually respond to increases in dietary or oral supplemental vitamin B_{12} intake, but instead is treated with this vitamin given by different routes of administration such as intramuscular and intranasal.

Vitamin B_{12} is also linked with mylenation of nerves and there are numerous neurologic symptoms associated with vitamin B_{12} deficiency. Interestingly, folic acid supplementation can mask vitamin B_{12} deficiency because the folic acid corrects the megaloblastic anemia but does not correct the neurologic damage. Permanent nerve damage can occur if vitamin B_{12} deficiency is not corrected. The DRI for vitamin B_{12} is 2.4 mcg per day for adults. An important point to note is that although the DRI recommendations do not increase with age, age is associated with atrophic gastritis that may reduce an individual's ability to digest food-bound vitamin B_{12}.[16] As such, providers are advised to encourage older adults to eat vitamin B_{12}–rich foods or to consume supplements when indicated.[47] There is no known toxicity from vitamin B_{12} and no UL has been set.

Anticonvulsants have been associated with decreased vitamin B_{12} absorption.[48] H_2-receptor antagonists including cimetidine (Tagamet), famotidine (Pepcid), nizatidine (Axid), and ranitidine (Zantac) cause a reduction in gastric acid that can reduce absorption of dietary sources of vitamin B_{12}. Metformin (Glucophage) inhibits vitamin B_{12} absorption and enhances the requirement of B_{12} among persons with diabetes.

Vitamin C

Unlike most animals, humans cannot synthesize vitamin C endogenously; thus, this micronutrient is an essential dietary constituent.[49] Vitamin C, which is also named ascorbic acid, has antioxidant properties, is involved in

Box 5-6 Can Vitamin C Cure the Common Cold?

- Vitamin C supplements do not reduce the incidence of common cold in the general population.
- Vitamin C supplements may shorten the duration and lessen the severity of the common cold.
- Vitamin C supplements can fill some nutritional gaps for persons with increased needs or decreased intake levels, such as older individuals and those who are heavy smokers.

Sources: Data from Douglas R, Hemila H, Chalker E, Treacy B. Vitamin C for preventing and treating the common cold. *Cochrane Database Syst Rev*. 2007;3:CD000980[53]; National Institutes of Health, Office of Dietary Supplements. Vitamin C fact sheet for health professionals. *Health Information*. June 5, 2013. http://ods.od.nih.gov/factsheets/VitaminC-HealthProfessional/#en4. Accessed June 7, 2014.[52]

collagen synthesis and protein metabolism, and increases the bioavailability and absorption of iron, copper, and chromium.[24] This vitamin is abundant in many fruits and vegetables, such as citrus fruits, peppers, strawberries, broccoli, Brussels sprouts, and papayas.[15]

The effects of scurvy—the disease caused by vitamin C deficiency—have been known for centuries. Although scurvy today is rare, overt deficiency symptoms may appear when intake falls below 10 mg per day for many weeks.[24] The RDA for vitamin C in adult women is 75 mg per day. Household survey data indicate that mean intakes in the United States generally exceed this amount.[50] Cigarette smokers need an additional 35 mg per day above the RDA, because cigarette smoke increases free-radical exposure.[25] Studies indicate that 70% to 90% of vitamin C can be absorbed when intake levels are moderate (30–180 mg per day), but that at doses exceeding 1 g per day, absorption drops to less than 50%.[51] Unused vitamin C, like all water-soluble vitamins, is excreted in the urine.

Vitamin C improves the absorption of nonheme iron, or the type of iron present in plant foods. Although this effect can be helpful in iron-deficient persons, it is a cause for concern in those with hereditary hemochromatosis, which is an iron overload disease, because iron toxicity can result in tissue damage.[25,51] Very high levels of vitamin C intake from supplements can cause gastrointestinal distress, including nausea, diarrhea, cramping, and kidney stones.[24] The UL for vitamin C is set at 2 g per day (2000 mg per day). The contents of many OTC cold remedies approach or exceed this amount of vitamin C, so it is wise to read the labels of such products carefully, and discontinue use if experiencing gastrointestinal symptoms.

Ever since Linus Pauling suggested that vitamin C could treat and/or prevent the common cold in the 1970s, much has been said about the effect of this vitamin on upper respiratory diseases. The results of studies have been inconsistent, but research currently supports the information found in Box 5-6.

Table 5-7 summarizes information on selected water-soluble vitamins.

Minerals

Minerals are inorganic compounds that support many cellular processes, act as electrolytes, or have a structural function. Forty minerals exist, of which approximately 16 are essential and need to be consumed in the diet. Unlike vitamins, which are classified based on solubility, minerals are classified based on human requirements for them. The major minerals—calcium, phosphorus, magnesium, potassium, sodium, and chloride—are required in amounts of more than 100 mg per day. Trace minerals are required in amounts less than 100 mg per day; they include iron, copper, selenium, iodine, chromium, manganese, molybdenum, and zinc. A summary table at the end of this section (Table 5-19) outlines the basic functions, selected food sources, recommended intake levels, deficiency and excessive intake considerations, and clinical and supplementation considerations of selected minerals.

Calcium

Calcium is the most abundant mineral in the human body. More than 99% of calcium in the body is found in the bones and teeth, where it plays an important structural function. The remaining 1% is found in the blood, muscle, and interstitial fluid, where it mediates vascular contraction and vasodilation, muscle contraction, nerve transmission, and secretion of hormones and enzymes.[54]

Calcium is found primarily in dairy foods and to some degree in collard greens, kale, broccoli, and salmon and sardines (with bones).[15] Increasingly, calcium-fortified foods are also available, including fruit juices, tofu, and cereals. Calcium absorption is affected by the calcium status of the body, the calcium content of a meal, age, pregnancy, vitamin D status, and plant components in the diet. Much as with many other vitamins or minerals, calcium absorption increases when calcium stores are low or when dietary calcium declines. Calcium absorption is highest in infancy and early puberty, and is also increased during the last two trimesters of pregnancy. The rate of absorption

Table 5-7 Water-Soluble Vitamins: A Summary

Water-Soluble Vitamin	Function	Selected Food Sources	Recommended Intake Levels	Deficiency and Excessive Intake Considerations	Clinical and Supplementation Considerations
Thiamin (Vitamin B_1)	Coenzyme, generates energy from carbohydrate Drives neural function	Widespread in food supply; pork; whole, enriched, and fortified grains	RDA: 1.1 mg/day for females ≥ 19 years RDA: 1.4 mg/day during pregnancy and lactation in females ≥ 14 years	Deficiency: beriberi and Wernicke-Korsakoff syndrome Excess: no known disease of excess No UL	No known major drug–drug interactions.
Riboflavin (Vitamin B_2)	Plays a role in energy metabolism, nerve function, protection of biological membranes, and synthesis of other vitamins	Meats and dairy foods	RDA: 1.1 mg/day for females ≥ 19 years RDA: 1.4 mg/day during pregnancy and 1.6 mg/day during lactation	Deficiency: rare but can cause ariboflavinosis Excess: no known disease of excess No UL	No known major drug–drug interactions. Large doses of tricyclic antidepressants may decrease amount of riboflavin in body.
Niacin (Vitamin B_3)	DNA synthesis and repair Cholesterol metabolism Glucose homeostasis	Whole, enriched, and fortified grains; liver, poultry, fish, beef; tomatoes and mushrooms	RDA: 14 mg/day for females ≥ 14 years RDA: 18 mg/day during pregnancy and 17 mg/day during lactation	Deficiency: pellagra Excess: niacin-related flushing UL: 35 mg/day for adults ≥ 19 years from synthetic supplements, fortified foods, or combination of both	Moderate concern for supplementation in combination with alcohol, allopurinol (Zyloprim), carbamazepine (Tegretol), clonidine (Catapres), antidiabetes drugs, bile acid sequestrants, statins, primidone (Mysoline), probenecid, and sulfinpyrazone (Anturane).
Pantothenic Acid (Vitamin B_5)	ATP production Synthesis of heme, cholesterol, bile salts, fatty acids, steroid hormones, and phospholipids	Widespread in foods	No RDA AI: 5 mg/day for females ≥ 14 years AI 6 mg/day during pregnancy and 7 mg/day during lactation	Deficiency: rare Excess: no known disease of excess No UL	No known major drug–drug interactions.
Pyridoxine (Vitamin B_6)	Converts tryptophan to niacin Glucose regulation Promotes steroid hormone formation	Widespread in foods Whole and fortified grains, garbanzo beans, tuna, liver	RDA: 1.0-1.7 mg/day RDA: 1.9 mg/day during pregnancy and 2.0 mg/day during lactation	Deficiency: rare but can cause microcytic hypochromic anemia Excess: no known disease of excess UL: 100 mg/day for females ≥ 19 years	Cycloserine (Seromycin) increases urinary excretion of vitamin B_6. Some antiepileptic drugs increase catabolism of vitamin B_6. Theophylline may lead to low vitamin B_6 levels and seizures.
Biotin (Vitamin B_7)	Gluconeogenesis ATP production	Peanuts, almonds, mushrooms, cooked egg yolks	No RDA AI: 30 mcg/day for females ≥ 19 years AI: 30 mcg/day during pregnancy and 35 mcg/day during lactation	Deficiency: only seen with very high raw egg white intake Excess: no known disease of excess No UL	No known major drug–drug interactions.
Folate (Vitamin B_9)	Cell production and maintenance Neural tube formation	Leafy green vegetables; whole, fortified, and enriched grains; organ meats; legumes	RDA: 400–800 mcg/day for ≥ 14 years RDA: 600 mcg/day during pregnancy and 500 mcg/day during lactation	Deficiency during pregnancy can cause neural tube defects; severe deficiency can cause megaloblastic macrocytic anemia Excess: high folic acid intake can mask vitamin B_{12} deficiency UL: 1000 mcg/day for females ≥ 19 years	Folic acid is the synthetic form of folate. Folic acid can interfere with methotrexate (Rheumatrex, Trexall). Antiepileptic medications can reduce serum folate levels. Consider additional folic acid with sulfasalazine (Azulfidine) when used to treat a person with ulcerative colitis.

(*continues*)

Table 5-7 Water-Soluble Vitamins: A Summary (*continued*)

Water-Soluble Vitamin	Function	Selected Food Sources	Recommended Intake Levels	Deficiency and Excessive Intake Considerations	Clinical and Supplementation Considerations
Cobalamin (Vitamin B_{12})	ATP production Functions with folate in amino acid metabolism	Found only in animal foods Clams, liver, oysters, crab Fortified breakfast cereals	RDA: 2.4 mcg/day for females ≥ 14 years RDA: 2.6 mcg/day during pregnancy and 2.8 mcg/day during lactation	Deficiency: seen in elderly and those with atrophic gastritis; megaloblastic anemia; secondary deficiency causes pernicious anemia Excess: no known disease of excess No UL	Vegans and strict vegetarians should supplement with vitamin B_{12}. Chloramphenicol (Chloromycetin) can interfere with red blood cell response to supplemental vitamin B_{12}. H_2 receptor antagonists can interfere with vitamin B_{12} absorption in persons with low intakes. Metformin (Glucophage) may reduce vitamin B_{12} absorption.
Ascorbic Acid (Vitamin C)	Antioxidant Collagen synthesis Protein metabolism	Citrus fruits Widespread in fruits and vegetables Peppers, strawberries, broccoli, Brussels sprouts, papayas	RDA: 75 mg/day for females ≥ 19 years RDA: 85 mg/day during pregnancy for females ≥ 19 years and 120 mg/day during lactation for females ≥ 19 years	Deficiency: scurvy Excess: can cause GI distress UL: 2,000 mg/day for persons ≥ 19 years	Vitamin C increases bioavailability and absorption of iron, copper, and chromium Smokers need an additional 35 mg/day above RDA. Vitamin C supplements do not prevent the common cold but may decrease duration and intensity of the common cold.

Abbreviations: AI = adequate intake; H_2 = histamine-2; RDA = recommended daily allowance; UL = tolerable upper intake level.

declines gradually with age in both men and women. Calcium absorption is enhanced by vitamin D, as the latter induces synthesis of intestinal proteins that promote calcium absorption. Conversely, phytic acid, which is found in fiber-containing whole-grain foods like wheat bran, beans, seeds, nuts, and soy isolates, and oxalic acid, which is found in spinach, collard greens, sweet potatoes, rhubarb, and beans, inhibit calcium absorption, although the degree to which calcium absorption is impacted varies.[55] Persons who eat a variety of foods do not necessarily need to be concerned about reduced absorption from phytic acid– and oxalic acid–containing foods.[54]

Bones increase most readily in size and mass during periods of growth such as childhood and adolescence. The National Osteoporosis Foundation estimates that 85% to 90% of adult bone mass has been established by 18 years in females, with peak bone mass occurring somewhere between the ages of 25 and 30 years; bone mass then declines at varying rates after that time.[56] Calcium DRIs reflect these age-related changes, with calcium needs being highest in children 9 to 18 years. DRI values for calcium for infants from birth to 12 months are Adequate Intake levels; the AI for life stage and gender group is believed to cover the needs of all healthy individuals in the groups, but lack of data or uncertainty about the data prevent experts from specifying with confidence the percentage of individuals covered by this intake. Table 5-8 lists the current DRI recommendations for calcium. There are no changes in calcium recommendations during pregnancy and lactation because the body becomes more efficient at absorbing calcium to meet the increased needs of the woman and fetus/newborn during pregnancy and lactation. The UL for calcium is set at 2500 mg per day for adults 19–50 years and in pregnant and lactating women, and at 2000 mg per day for those 50 years or older.[54]

Table 5-8 Dietary Reference Intakes: Recommended Dietary Allowances for Calcium

	Females	Pregnant or Lactating Females
9–13 years	1300 mg	
14–18 years	1300 mg	1300 mg
19–30 years	1000 mg	1000 mg
31–50 years	1000 mg	1000 mg
51–70 years	1200 mg	
> 70 years	1200 mg	

Source: Modified from National Institutes of Health, Office of Dietary Supplements. Calcium fact sheet for health professionals. *Health Information*. November 21, 2013. http://ods.od.nih.gov/factsheets/Calcium-HealthProfessional/#en1. Accessed June 7, 2014.[54]

Lactose-intolerant individuals should consume non-dairy sources of calcium. Other options to meet calcium needs include taking calcium supplements, lactase enzyme supplements, or pretreated dairy products (e.g., Lactaid). Other calcium-containing foods that are appropriate for lactose-intolerant individuals include hard cheeses because the majority of lactose has been removed during processing; yogurt that contains live active cultures, which aid in lactose digestion; and calcium-fortified lactose-free milk or milk alternatives like soymilk, almond milk, or rice milk.

In North America, calcium intake levels are generally less than recommended amounts, especially for females and older adults.[57] Increasing consumption of carbonated beverages, energy drinks and other sweetened refreshments, as well as high rates of lactose intolerance among certain ethnic and racial groups, are likely contributors to this substandard calcium intake.

Long-term calcium deficiency can result in osteoporosis. Hypocalcemia due to low dietary calcium is uncommon but can result from a medical condition or treatment such as renal failure, surgical removal of the stomach, or use of loop diuretics (e.g., furosemide). Hypocalcemia can cause numbness and tingling in the fingers, muscle cramps, convulsions, lethargy, poor appetite, and mental confusion, as well as abnormal heart rhythms and death.

Calcium toxicity from diet and supplements is rare because calcium absorption is limited by the gastrointestinal tract. Excessively high intake can have adverse effects including impaired kidney function and impaired absorption of minerals such as iron, zinc, magnesium, and phosphorus. Hypercalcemia can result from malignant cancer and from excess intake of vitamin D (supplement overuse at doses of 50,000 IU or higher). Symptoms of calcium toxicity include lax muscle tone, constipation, large urine volumes, nausea, and ultimately confusion, coma, and death.[54] Although it had been theorized that kidney stones resulted from high calcium intake, more recent studies have shown that a high dietary calcium intake decreases the risk of kidney stones.[58]

Calcium Supplements

Encouraging consumption of dietary sources of calcium is a recommended first-line approach to preventing calcium-deficiency–related disorders. Recommending calcium supplements should be considered only when adequate dietary intake of calcium is not possible. Often calcium supplements are combined with vitamin D supplements to promote absorption. Also, to maximize absorption of calcium, supplements may need to be divided over time because a dose should be less than 500–600 mg at one time.

Although calcium supplements may increase bone mineral density, this increase appears to be of modest value until the postmenopausal period. Older women—especially those at risk for or currently experiencing osteoporotic changes—appear to reduce their risk of fracture when their diet is augmented by calcium supplements.

Because of the importance of calcium to the cardiovascular system, studies have been conducted to evaluate the role of supplementation in reducing cardiac disease. To date, this research has failed to find a protective value of these supplements; in fact, in some cases the drugs may be associated with a small increase in cardiovascular risk. Alternatively, data have indicated that calcium supplements during pregnancy may decrease the risk of preeclampsia in women who are calcium deficient.

Several different forms of calcium exist, including calcium carbonate, citrate, phosphate, gluconate, and lactate. Two of the most common types of calcium supplements are calcium carbonate and calcium citrate. Calcium carbonate, which is the least expensive calcium supplement, should be taken with meals because it requires acid from the digestive process to make the calcium more soluble and readily absorbed. Calcium citrate supplements may be taken with or without food and have been suggested to be a better choice than carbonate for individuals with achlorhydria or those taking histamine-2 blockers or protein pump inhibitors. Calcium phosphate is available as a supplement, but there is debate on its effectiveness and it is less often used than carbonate and citrate. Calcium gluconate and lactate are rarely used as supplements because they contain less calcium than carbonate and citrate. Women should be advised to read labels carefully, as some supplements claiming to contain calcium are derived from dolomite or bone meal—these agents may also contain lead.

Table 5-9 provides additional information on calcium supplements. Persons taking calcium supplements who are also taking iron supplements should avoid taking these agents together, as these two minerals interfere with each other's absorption. Supplements can be obtained as dedicated products or as the active ingredient in an antacid promoted for the treatment of pyrosis (heartburn).

Multiple drug–drug and drug–food interactions are associated with calcium supplements. Calcium-containing antacids can interact with a large number of drugs, including iron, because they promote changes in gastric acidity. Owing to the many possible interactions, prescribers should

Table 5-9 Calcium Supplements

Calcium Supplements	Brands	Absorption Requires Hydrochloric Acid?	Meals or Not?	Calcium Content
Calcium carbonate	Caltrate Tums and other antacids Viactiv OsCal	Yes	Take with meals	Most supplements contain 500–600 mg calcium
Calcium citrate	Citracal Citracal Liquitab	No	Can be taken with or without meals	Most supplements contain 200–300 mg calcium

ask women if they are taking calcium before prescribing other agents. Table 5-10 lists the most important interactions that have clinical implications. In addition to drugs, consumption of caffeine and sodium increases urinary excretion of calcium, and foods with high levels of oxalates (e.g., spinach) form insoluble compounds with calcium, resulting in decreased absorption of this mineral.

Chromium

Chromium is a trace mineral that is not well understood. This mineral can be found in food as trivalent chromium or as hexavalent chromium, which is also an industrial pollutant. Some evidence suggests that chromium picolinate, when used as a nutritional supplement, may augment the actions of hypoglycemic medications such as insulin and metformin. The supplement also may have some utility in treating individuals with hypercholesterolemia, although additional research on both of these clinical indications is needed.[59] Table 5-11 lists some of the more common drug interactions associated with chromium.

Cobalt

Cobalt, a transition metal that exists in the oxidation states Co^{+2} and Co^{+3}, is an essential trace element. This mineral is an integral part of the chemical structure of vitamin B_{12}, which is required for folate and fatty acid metabolism. Cobalt is primarily absorbed from the pulmonary and gastrointestinal tracts, with smaller amounts absorbed through the skin. No RDI has been set for cobalt because cobalt deficiency is exceedingly rare.

Cobalt supplementation has been recommended by some scientists for treating anemia, nephritis, and infection in addition to the usual hemopoietic agents, but no treatment plan has been standardized. Conversely, excessive cobalt has been associated with risks including allergic dermatitis, rhinitis, and asthma. A rare form of cardiomyopathy was discovered when cobalt compounds were added to stabilize beer foam. At very high doses, cobalt toxicity can cause death. Although this mineral is available as a nutritional supplement, it is rarely used or recommended.[24]

Table 5-10 Selected Drug–Drug and Drug–Food Interactions with Calcium[a]

Drug	Effects on Calcium	Effects on Drug	Other Effects
Anti-infectives (e.g., quinolones, tetracyclines)		Decreases serum levels With tetracycline, insoluble compounds are made	
Bisphosphonates (e.g., alendronate risedronate)		Decreases serum levels	
Calcipotriene (Dovonex)		Decreases serum levels	
Calcium-channel blockers and other antihypertensives		Decreases serum levels	
Ceftriaxone (Rocephin)			If coadministered intravenously, major risk of precipitate that damages lungs and kidneys
Digoxin (Lanoxin)		Increases serum levels	Increased risk with potential arrhythmias
Levothyroxine (Synthroid)		Decreases serum levels	
Thiazide diuretics	Increases serum levels		Increased risk of kidney disorders

[a] This table is not comprehensive as new information is being generated on a regular basis.

Table 5-11 Selected Drug–Drug Interactions with Chromium[a]

Drug	Effects on Chromium	Effects on Drug	Other Effects
Antacids	Decreases serum levels		Inhibits gastric acidity
Corticosteroids	Decreases serum levels		Inhibits gastric acidity
H_2 blockers (such as cimetidine [Tagamet], famotidine [Pepcid], nizatidine [Axid], and ranitidine [Zantac])	Decreases serum levels		Inhibits gastric acidity
Insulin and other hypoglycemics		Increase hypoglycemic effects	
Nonsteroidal anti-inflammatory drugs (NSAIDs) and prostaglandin inhibitors (e.g., ibuprofen [Advil], indomethacin [Indocin], naproxen [Aleve], piroxicam [Feldene], and aspirin)	Increases serum levels		
Proton pump inhibitors (such as omeprazole [Prilosec], lansoprazole [Prevacid], rabeprazole [Aciphex], pantoprazole [Protonix], and esomeprazole [Nexium])	Decreases serum levels		Inhibits gastric acidity

[a] This table is not comprehensive as new information is being generated on a regular basis.
Source: Data from National Institutes of Health, Office of Dietary Supplements. Chromium dietary fact sheet for health professionals. *Health Information*. June 24, 2011. http://ods.od.nih.gov/factsheets/Chromium-HealthProfessional/#h9. Accessed January 28, 2015.[60]

Copper

Copper is an essential component of numerous copper metalloenzymes that are required for normal oxidative metabolism. The total amount of copper in the body is in the range of 75 to 100 mg, with copper being present in every tissue of the body. This mineral is stored primarily in the liver, with smaller amounts found in the brain, heart, kidney, and muscles. Copper is needed for synthesis of hemoglobin, proper iron metabolism, and maintenance of blood vessels. It also aids in overall healthy function of the blood vessels, nerves, immune system, melanin, and bones. Copper is involved in energy production, the conversion of dopamine to norepinephrine, and blood clotting. It is also important for the production of thyroxine and is necessary for the synthesis of phospholipids found in the myelin sheaths that cover and protect nerves.

Organ meats are the best dietary sources of copper, with oysters and other shellfish, whole grains, legumes, nuts, potatoes, and dark leafy greens also providing this mineral.[15] The RDA for copper is 900 mcg per day for adults.[14] The average daily Western diet contains adequate copper, approximately 40% of which is absorbed, with an equivalent amount returned to the gastrointestinal tract from the bile.[61]

Dietary copper is absorbed through the mucosa in the jejunum and transported via the portal blood to the liver. This mineral competes with zinc for absorption sites, so high levels of zinc can cause copper deficiency, and vice versa. There is no known disease of copper excess. Extra copper is not stored in the body; rather, the liver incorporates it into bile and removes it with fecal waste. However, some individuals may have an autosomal recessive genetic condition known as Wilson's disease or hepatolenticular degeneration, in which copper accumulates in tissues. Such persons may even need a liver transplant if the accumulation is severe. Clinical signs and symptoms of Wilson's disease include neurologic, psychiatric, and hepatic variations. For women with Wilson's disease, use of a copper intrauterine device is contraindicated. The UL for copper is set at 10,000 mcg per day for adults.[14]

Copper deficiency causes an extensive range of symptoms, including iron-deficiency anemia, ruptured blood vessels, osteoporosis, joint problems, brain disturbances, elevated low-density lipoprotein cholesterol (LDL-C) levels, reduced high-density lipoprotein cholesterol (HDL-C) levels, increased susceptibility to infections due to poor immune function, loss of pigments in the hair and skin, weakness, fatigue, breathing difficulties, skin sores, poor thyroid function, and irregular heartbeat. Persons at risk for copper deficiency include hospitalized adults and preterm infants receiving improper nutrition support.[24] Certain medications/drugs may interact with copper; Table 5-12 lists some of the most common of these interactions.

Iodine

Iodine is a nonmetallic trace mineral required for the synthesis of the thyroid hormones triiodothyronine (T_3) and thyroxine (T_4). Thyroid hormones regulate a number of physiologic processes, including growth, development, metabolism, and reproductive function. The pituitary gland secretes thyroid-stimulating hormone (TSH), which

Table 5-12 Selected Drug Interactions with Copper[a]

Drug	Effects
Antisecretory antihistamines such as famotidine (Pepcid, Pepcid AD), and nizatidine (Axid, Axid AR)	Drug decreases serum levels of copper by inhibiting absorption
AZT (Azidothymidine, Zidovudine, Retrovir)	Drug decreases serum levels of copper
Calcium and phosphorous	Drug decreases serum levels of copper by increasing excretion
Estrogen-containing agents (e.g., combined oral contraceptives)	Drug increases absorption of copper
Nonsteroidal anti-inflammatory drugs (NSAIDs), including etodolac (Lodine), ibuprofen, nabumetone (Relafen), naproxen (Aleve), and oxaprozin (Daypro)	Copper enhances anti-inflammatory effects
Vitamin C, iron, and manganese	Drug decreases serum levels of copper by inhibiting absorption

[a] This table is not comprehensive as new information is being generated on a regular basis.

stimulates iodine trapping, thyroid hormone synthesis, and release of T_3 and T_4. Thyroid function has a profound impact on overall health via modulation of carbohydrate, protein, and fat metabolism; vitamin utilization; the digestive process; hormone secretion; sexual and reproductive health; and many other physiologic parameters.

Iodine deficiency causes hypothyroidism. With this disorder, TSH levels become persistently elevated, which leads to hypertrophy of the thyroid gland, often expressed as a goiter.

Iodine deficiency during pregnancy can result in cretinism, which causes severe mental retardation, growth abnormalities, infertility, and increased mortality risk.[62] Excessive iodine intake can result in some of the same symptoms as iodine deficiency, including goiter, high TSH levels, and hypothyroidism. The UL for iodine does not apply to persons receiving iodine for medical treatment; moreover, with normal food and intake levels, iodine consumption is not likely to exceed the UL of 1100 mcg per day.[54,63] Drug interactions with iodine are relatively rare, although levels of iodine can interfere with effectiveness of lithium.

The amount of iodine found in most foods is typically quite small and varies depending on environmental factors such as the soil concentration of iodine and the use of fertilizers. Rich food sources of this nutrient include processed foods that contain iodized salt and dairy foods because iodine is used in milk processing. Other dietary sources of iodine include seaweed and peanuts.[15] Voluntary fortification of table salt with iodine was introduced in 1924 and resulted in a virtual elimination of endemic goiter from hypothyroidism in the United States. There is some concern that as various non-iodized salts are being promoted for cooking, the incidence of thyroid deficiency may increase. The DRI for iodine is 150 mcg per day for those 14 years and older, 220 mcg per day during pregnancy, and 290 mcg per day for women who are breastfeeding.[15]

Iron

Iron plays a key role in the synthesis of many enzymes and proteins and is involved in regulation of cell growth and cell differentiation.[14] This mineral serves as the site for oxygen binding in the hemoglobin molecule, which contains almost two-thirds of the total body iron. Twenty-five percent of total body iron is stored as ferritin and hemosiderin, primarily in the liver, spleen, and bone marrow. These stores are readily mobilized to meet daily needs when iron intake or absorption is inadequate. The RDA for iron is 18 mg per day for women 19–50 years, 27 mg per day during pregnancy, 9 mg per day during lactation for women 19 years or older, and 8 mg per day for postmenopausal women and those older than 50 years.[14] The Daily Value (DV) listed on food labels in the United States calls for 18 mg iron per day; therefore a food item that says one serving contains 50% DV for iron, contains 9 mg iron per serving. Table 5-13 outlines iron needs for infants, children, and women according to the DRIs.

Dietary iron is found in two forms: heme iron and nonheme iron. Heme iron is found exclusively in animal products, including meat, fish, and poultry. Nonheme iron refers to iron in all other forms; it is found in plant foods such as legumes, green leafy vegetables, strawberries, and some whole grains. Heme iron is more easily absorbed than is nonheme iron; however, the rate at which a person's body can absorb iron depends on a number of circumstances. For individuals with chronically low iron stores, such as those with vegetarian diets devoid of heme-based iron, iron absorption is greater. Well-nourished individuals with adequate iron stores can absorb 5% to 10% of dietary iron, whereas those who are iron deficient will absorb as much as 20% to 30% of dietary iron.[65]

Individuals who are at risk for iron-deficiency anemia should consider pairing the iron-rich foods in their diet with vitamin C–containing foods. For example, to maximize iron absorption from an iron-fortified cereal, the cereal should be consumed at the same time as the person eats a serving of vitamin C–rich citrus fruit or drinks

Table 5-13 Dietary Reference Intakes: Recommended Dietary Allowances for Iron

	Life Stage	Iron Needs (mg/day)
Infants	6–12 months	11
Children	1–3 years	7
	4–8 years	10
Females	9–13 years	8
	14–18 years	15
	19–30 years	18
	31–50 years	18
	51–70 years	8
	> 70 years	8
Pregnant women	14–18 years	27
	19–30 years	27
	31–50 years	27
Lactating women	14–18 years	10
	19–30 years	9
	31–51 years	9

Source: Data from Institute of Medicine, Food, and Nutrition Board. *Dietary Reference Intakes for Vitamin A, Vitamin K, Arsenic, Boron, Chromium, Copper, Iodine, Iron, Manganese, Molybdenum, Nickel, Silicon, Vanadium, and Zinc*. National Academies Press: Washington, DC; 2001.[14]

a small glass of orange juice. Traditionally iron supplements are suggested to be given at the same time as vitamin C supplements. However, some evidence indicates that this co-supplementation does not actually decrease or treat iron-deficiency anemia.[66] Iron absorption is diminished in the presence of substances that chelate iron—for example, oxalates, phytates, and tannins. Table 5-14 highlights these compounds and other factors, along with their dietary sources, that limit iron absorption. Box 5-7 explores the myth of spinach as a rich source of iron.

Iron-Deficiency Anemia

Iron deficiency is the most common micronutrient deficiency worldwide, affecting almost 2 billion persons globally.[67] Iron needs increase during periods of growth, and pregnant women and children are at increased risk for developing iron deficiency. Approximately 20% of perinatal mortality and 10% of maternal mortality in the developing world can be attributed to iron deficiency. Inadequate dietary iron intake is a primary cause of both iron deficiency and iron-deficiency anemia. Poor absorption, gastrointestinal problems, periods of growth, increased blood volume (e.g., during pregnancy), and other chronic conditions can also contribute to iron deficiency.

Table 5-14 Factors That Limit Iron Absorption

Factor	Sources
Oxalates	Chocolate, spinach, rhubarb, beet greens
Phytic acid, phytates	Whole grains, bran, unleavened bread, soybeans, and soy products
Tannins	Tea, coffee, some grains
Excessive dietary fiber	High-fiber foods such as bran cereals and fiber-fortified granola bars
Vegetarian diets	Low in or devoid of heme iron
Very low-calorie diets	Too low in energy and often low in iron

Box 5-7 The Myth of Spinach

For those of a certain age, Popeye the Sailor Man is a cartoon character well remembered for his abnormally large forearms and his strength in using those limbs in fights against evil enemies. Popeye was a victim of product placement, advertising his eponymous can of spinach as necessary for his strength. This connection was at least in part based on the concept that spinach was a rich source of iron, making the body stronger.

Popeye might have been amazed to learn that spinach, although a source of other healthy vitamins, is not a very good source of dietary iron. The basis of this myth began in the late nineteenth century when a German scientist misplaced a decimal point in publication of the iron content in the food, causing it to be listed as 10 times greater than was warranted by the evidence. Today, it is known that spinach is high in oxalates, binding to the iron that is present and potentially decreasing iron levels. Thus, perhaps Popeye experienced a potent placebo effect when consuming spinach.

Iron Supplements

Even conscientious individuals who strive to increase dietary iron intake may fall far short of meeting their actual iron needs. If an iron-deficient person is seeking to consume 50 to 60 mg of elemental iron per day, he or she would have to consume more than 3 pounds of meat per day to obtain the desired amount of iron from foods alone. Fortunately, iron supplements are among the most affordable and effective nutrient supplements available on the market. Approximately 14% to 18% of persons in the United States use a supplement that contains iron and as many as 60% of lactating women and 72% of pregnant women do so as well.[68–70]

Iron supplements can be found in several forms, and vary in regard to the amount of available elemental iron. Iron supplements include ferrous iron and ferric iron salts. These supplements include ferrous fumarate (33% elemental iron), ferrous sulfate (20% elemental iron), ferrous gluconate (12% elemental iron), and carbonyl iron (45% elemental iron). Thus, a typical 300-mg tablet of ferrous sulfate contains 50 to 60 mg oral elemental iron. Elemental iron doses should be in the range of 50 to 200 mg per day for adults and 6 mg per day per kilogram body weight in children. Ferrous iron has more bioavailability and is the most frequently used supplement. Carbonyl iron also is available in oral form and has been said to have fewer side effects than other iron supplements. Because it is released directly with gastric acid production, this formulation is claimed to result in a more gradual release.

Supplemental iron is usually administered to an iron-deficient person for 3 to 5 months, given 3 times daily. Iron supplements are best absorbed on an empty stomach; however, this practice can also cause irritation of the gastrointestinal tract. Gastrointestinal pain from iron supplements can be lessened by taking iron supplements with food, although this will decrease absorption rates. Iron is absorbed primarily in the duodenum, so enteric-coated or sustained-release formulations, even though they are generally more expensive, usually have less bioavailability and are less therapeutic. Most iron supplements are taken as oral tablets, caplets, or capsules, although parenteral formulations and even liquid preparations are available.

Iron supplements should be considered for individuals who are unable to obtain adequate iron from dietary sources alone. Some preparations also contain vitamin C, but it is suggested that adding ascorbic acid may simply increase absorption by 10% at most. Table 5-15 lists common oral iron preparations.

A woman who absorbs 10 to 20 mg of iron per day can expect to triple her red blood cell production rate and achieve a rise in hemoglobin concentration of 0.2 g/dL per day, with effects being seen somewhere between day 4 of treatment up to the second or third week of supplementation.[71] Common causes of persistently low hemoglobin levels in light of oral iron supplementation include a woman's inability to continue with supplementation due to the GI side effects, reduced iron absorption related to malabsorption from steatorrhea, hemodialysis, celiac sprue, or bleeding that may be taking place at a rate that is faster than blood cell replacement.

While inexpensive and rapidly effective, iron supplementation is not without risks. The FDA has decreed that all iron supplements must carry a warning regarding the finding that iron ingestion is a major cause of fatal poisoning in children younger than 6 years and indicating that the product should be kept out of reach of children. Individuals with the iron overload condition known as hemochromatosis should closely monitor their iron and vitamin C intakes, because vitamin C accelerates iron absorption. Hemochromatosis affects nearly 1 in 250 persons of northern European descent.[72] Those who receive frequent blood transfusions may also be at risk for iron overload and are advised to avoid iron supplementation. The UL for iron is 40 mg per day for persons aged 0–13 and 45 mg per day for those 14 and older.[14]

Drug–Iron Interactions

The most notable drug–drug interactions with oral preparations of iron affect drug absorption. Antacids, histamine-2 receptor antagonists, and proton pump inhibitors have all been shown to decrease iron absorption, while tetracycline and fluoroquinolone absorption may be inhibited if these antibiotics are co-administered with iron. These medications should be taken at least 2 hours before or after iron administration. Vitamin C (ascorbic acid) coadministration results in an increase in iron-associated side effects. Oral preparations should be administered between meals, as food can decrease iron absorption by 50%.

Magnesium

Magnesium is a major mineral and cofactor involved in more than 300 enzyme systems, regulating functions as diverse as protein synthesis, muscle and nerve action, blood glucose control, and blood pressure.[73] Accurately assessing magnesium status is challenging, as most magnesium is located inside of the cells or in bone. There is no universally agreed-upon or satisfactory method for assessing this status, and magnesium levels are not routinely evaluated in electrolyte testing in the hospital setting.[74]

Magnesium is widespread in plant and animal foods, with green leafy vegetables, legumes, nuts, seeds, and whole grains being good dietary sources. Refined-grain foods are lower in magnesium than their whole-grain

Table 5-15 Oral Iron Supplements

Drug: Generic (Brand)	Formulation and Elemental Iron Content	Dose and Indications	Contraindications/Precautions
Iron Salts			
Ferrous sulfate (FeoSol, Fer-Iron Drops, Fero-Grad, Mol-Iron, Slow Fe)	65 mg elemental iron in 325 mg tablet	3 tablets 3 times/day on an empty stomach for treatment of iron-deficiency anemia in adults Iron-deficiency anemia (*drug of choice*) Prevention of iron deficiency (e.g., during pregnancy or chronic blood loss)	Use with caution in persons with GI distress. May decrease dosing to 1 or 2 times daily or take with food if gastrointestinal side effects become problematic. Extended-release formulations are more expensive and may have less bioavailability. Discoloration of stool (dark green/black) should not be interpreted as a sign of bleeding. Fatal toxicity may occur in children from unintended overdose (lethal dose is 2–10 g in children).
Ferrous fumarate (Ferretts [OTC], Feostat, Feostat Drops, Hemocyte [OTC], Ircon, Nephro-Fer, Palafer, Span-FF)	33% elemental iron available in 63, 195, 200, 324, and 325 mg tablets; chewable 100 mg tablets; controlled-release 300 mg; oral suspension 100 mg/5 mL, 45 mg/0.6 mL 108 mg elemental iron in 325 mg tablet	PO 200 mg 3–4 times daily; no specific instructions available for iron-deficiency anemia in pregnancy Prevention of iron deficiency (e.g., during pregnancy or chronic blood loss)	Same as ferrous sulfate.
Ferrous gluconate (Fergon, Fertinic, Novoferrogluc)	12% elemental iron available in 300, 320, and 325 mg tablets; 86, 325, and 435 mg capsules, 300 mg film coated, and 300 mg/5 mL elixir 35 mg elemental iron in 325 mg tablet	PO 300–600 mg/day in divided doses Iron-deficiency anemia Prevention of iron deficiency (e.g., during pregnancy or chronic blood loss)	Same as ferrous sulfate.
Carbonyl iron (FeoSol caplets, FeoSol elixir, Icar-C, Icar C Plus SR Oral)	45 mg caplets (FeoSol), 65 mg tablets, 15 mg chewable tablets (Icar-C), 15 mg/1.25 mL suspension (Icar), 0.4 mg tablets (Icar C Plus SR Oral)	Feosol: 1 tablet or caplet once/day, or 5 mL daily Icar C Icar C Plus SR Oral: 0.4 mg Iron-deficiency anemia Prevention of iron deficiency (e.g., during pregnancy or chronic blood loss) Icar C Plus: folic acid–deficient megaloblastic anemia and prevention of neural tube defects	Carbonyl iron formulations contain pure (elemental) iron and thus are substantially more potent than iron salts. Hemochromatosis, hemosiderosis. Inhibits tetracycline absorption. Nausea, abdominal discomfort and pain, constipation, and diarrhea; may mask occult bleeding. Tooth discoloration (FeoSol elixir).

counterparts, as the bran portion of whole grains—which is removed during refining—is where most of the magnesium is located.[15] Tap water, mineral water, and bottled waters can also provide magnesium, albeit in varying amounts (ranging from 1 mg/L to more than 120 mg/L).[75] Household diet surveys indicate that magnesium intakes are generally lower than recommended amount.[76] The DRI for magnesium is 320 mg per day for females 31 years or older. Pregnancy needs are 400 mg per day for women 14–18 years, 350 mg per day for women 19–30 years, and 360 mg per day for women 31–50 years. During lactation, needs are 360 mg per day for women 14–18 years, 310 mg per day for women 19–30 years, and 320 mg per day for women 31–50 years.[78]

Magnesium deficiency and toxicity are both relatively rare. Deficiency may be seen in individuals who abuse alcohol and who have nutrient-poor diets or secondary malnutrition from impaired nutrient absorption.[24] Inadequate magnesium intake may also be seen in individuals with gastrointestinal diseases such as Crohn's, celiac disease, regional enteritis, and resection or bypass of the small intestine, especially the ileum.[73] High doses of magnesium from supplements often consumed in the form of magnesium-containing laxatives and antacids can cause diarrhea, nausea, and abdominal cramping, although this usually occurs at levels of more than 5000 mg per day.[79]

Magnesium can be found in several pharmaceutical agents. Magnesium sulfate is a long-standing treatment for women at risk of eclampsia, and the same agent has been found more recently to provide neuroprotection for the fetus/newborn. Additional information about these indications and treatments can be found in the *Pregnancy* chapter. Magnesium hydroxide is a common component of various laxatives and antacids. More than a century ago, Phillips, a pharmacist patented Milk of Magnesia for these indications.

Magnesium oxide is a commonly used supplement, although questions have arisen regarding the bioavailability of this agent. Intravenous magnesium is used to treat cardiac arrhythmias. Studies are being conducted to determine if magnesium supplementation can decrease the risk of various cardiac conditions, hypercholesterolemia, asthma, multiple sclerosis, and even attention-deficient disorders, although none have had definitive results to date.

Symptoms of magnesium toxicity appear when serum concentration levels exceed 1.74–2.61 mmol/L; such an excess can lead to hypotension, nausea, vomiting, facial flushing, urinary retention, ileus, depression, irregular heartbeat, and cardiac arrest. These symptoms may be exacerbated when kidney function is impaired and the body loses its ability to remove excess magnesium.[79] The UL for magnesium is 350 mg per day for all persons 9 years and older. Table 5-16 provides information on magnesium's interactions with medications.

Potassium

Potassium is an electrolyte that helps maintain kidney function and is involved in contractions of cardiac, skeletal, and smooth muscle cells. This mineral is of interest in the management of persons with hypertension because potassium has been shown to help lower blood pressure. Foods that contain large amounts of potassium include most fruits and vegetables—a fortunate occurrence, as fruits and vegetables are also naturally low in sodium, making them doubly important for individuals seeking to lower their blood pressure. Especially high-potassium foods include legumes, potatoes, seafood, dairy foods, potatoes, tomatoes, and bananas.[80]

As is the case with the other electrolytes, there is no RDA for potassium, although an AI of 4700 mg per day for adults has been established. The *Dietary Guidelines for Americans, 2010* also recommend a daily intake of 4.7 g of potassium per day, which is the amount of potassium in roughly five medium-sized baked potatoes, with their skins on, although only approximately 2% of adults in the United States adhere to this guideline.[81,82] The hypotensive effects of potassium have largely been based on studies that analyzed food-based potassium, not supplements.

Low dietary potassium intake culminating in potassium deficiency is uncommon, given that so many foods contain potassium. Prolonged periods of vomiting or diarrhea or abuse of diuretic drugs can lead to hypokalemia. Severe potassium deficiency causes blood pressure irregularities, irregular heart rhythms, muscular weakness, and dyspnea. Potassium toxicity is also rare, but can

Table 5-16 Selected Drug–Drug Interactions with Magnesium[a]

Drug	Effects on Magnesium	Effects on Drug	Comments
Antibiotics (e.g., quinolones, tetracyclines)		Decrease serum levels by forming insoluble compounds	Separate intake of magnesium-rich supplements or antibiotics by 4–6 hours
Bisphosphonates		Decrease serum levels by decreasing absorption	Separate intake of magnesium-rich supplements or medications and medications such as alendronate (Fosamax) by at least 2 hours
Diuretics (loop and thiazide)	Decrease serum levels (chronic use)		Chronic use leads to magnesium depletion
Diuretics (potassium sparing diuretics)	Increase serum levels by reducing magnesium excretion		
Proton pump inhibitors	Decrease serum levels (prolonged use more than 1 year)		

[a] This table is not comprehensive as new information is being generated on a regular basis.

Table 5-17 Selected Drugs That Increase Risks of Hypocalcemia or Hypercalcemia When Taken with Potassium Supplements[a]

Risk of Hypocalcemia	Risk of Hypercalcemia
Beta-adrenergic agonists	Angiotensin-converting enzyme (ACE) inhibitors
Bronchodilators	Angiotensin receptor blockers
Corticosteroids	Anticoagulant
Decongestants	Antihypertensive agents
Diuretics	Anti-infective agents
High-dose antibiotics (e.g., penicillin)	Cardiac glycosides
Mineralocorticoids	Nonsteroidal anti-inflammatory drugs
Substances with mineralocorticoid effects	Potassium-sparing agents/ diuretics

[a] This table is not comprehensive as new information is being generated on a regular basis.

result from IV potassium injections or very high doses of supplements, leading to life-threatening toxicity.[24] There is no UL set for potassium.[82] Multiple drug–drug interactions exist for potassium, and the major ones are associated with the risk of either hypocalcemia or hypercalcemia. Selected drugs that increase these risks are listed in Table 5-17.

Potassium Supplements

Potassium is available as a nutritional supplement, which are usually indicated for individuals taking loop diuretics or thiazides. The most common formulation is potassium gluconate, but this mineral can also be found as potassium iodide, nitrate, chloride, hydroxide bromide, oxide, cyanide, canrenoate, and citrate. However, some of these forms, such as potassium cyanide, are poisons and others are used for nonhealth purposes such as chemical fertilizers. Some brands of commercially available salt substitutes contain potassium chloride instead of sodium chloride. Potassium chloride may prove harmful for individuals with kidney problems or those who are taking medication for heart, kidney, or liver problems. Potassium supplements may be obtained as capsules, tables, elixirs, liquids, powders, or granules.

Selenium

Selenium was discovered in 1817 but was not recognized as an essential nutrient until the late 1950s. This essential trace mineral is involved in reproduction, thyroid hormone metabolism, and DNA synthesis, and has antioxidant properties that provide protection from oxidative damage.[83] Plant foods are the major dietary sources of selenium, although the content of selenium in food depends on the selenium content of the soil, which varies widely by geographic region. The primary sources of this mineral in the diet of persons who reside in the United States are breads, grains, meat, poultry, fish, and eggs.[84] The DRI for selenium is 55 mcg per day for persons 14 years and older.[25]

Blood and urine concentrations reflect recent selenium intake, whereas hair and nail samples can indicate longer-term intakes over months and years.[85] Selenium deficiency is rare in North America, although persons undergoing kidney dialysis and those living with HIV may be at increased risk for suboptimal selenium levels. Severe selenium deficiency causes Keshan disease, so named because it was first documented in the Keshan region of China, an area with very little selenium in its soil. Keshan disease disproportionately affects children, causing serious heart problems, and can be fatal. Very high selenium intake levels can cause selenosis, which is associated with symptoms such as a garlic-like odor of the breath, nausea, vomiting, diarrhea, and brittle teeth and fingernails.[25]

The UL for selenium is 400 mcg per day. Selenium may interact with cisplatin (Platinol-AQ), an inorganic platinum chemotherapy agent, potentially decreasing toxicity and/or levels of either drug.[85,86] Future studies are needed in this area to further elucidate these effects.

Zinc

Zinc is a trace mineral involved in more than 300 enzymatic reactions in the body, playing roles in immune function, protein and DNA synthesis, wound healing, cell division, and normal growth and development throughout the lifespan.[87] Zinc is also essential for the maintenance of proper taste and smell. The best dietary sources of zinc include shellfish, meat, organ foods, dairy foods, legumes, chocolate, and fortified cereal-grain products.[15] Zinc is best absorbed when consumed from animal versus plant foods. Much like iron, its absorption is increased in the presence of vitamin C.[24]

Zinc intake levels in the United States are generally considered to be adequate, although intake levels among older adults may be suboptimal. The RDA for zinc is 8 mg per day for females. The Institute of Medicine recommends 50% more zinc intake by vegetarians and vegans in particular compared to non-vegetarians due to differences in absorption levels from plant versus animal foods.[14]

Table 5-18 Selected Drug–Drug Interactions Associated with Zinc[a]

Drug	Effects on Zinc or the Drug	Comments
Amiloride (Midamor)	Increases serum levels of zinc by decreasing excretion	
Caffeine	Decreases serum levels of zinc	
Captopril (Capoten) and enalapril (Vasotec)	Increases serum levels of zinc by decreasing excretion	
Chlorthalidone (Thalitone)	Decreases serum levels of zinc	
Cholesterol-lowering drugs		Zinc interacts with LDL, HDL lipoproteins, and triglycerides, reducing HDL
Cholestyramine (Questran)	Increases serum levels of zinc by decreasing excretion	
Cisplatin (Platinol-AQ)	Increases cytotoxicity of cisplatin	
Deferoxamine (Desferal)	Decreases serum levels of zinc by increasing excretion	
Diuretics (loop and thiazide)	Decrease serum levels of zinc by inhibiting absorption	
Erythromycin (E-Mycin)	Decrease serum levels of zinc by inhibiting absorption	
Ethanol (alcohol)	Decreases serum levels of zinc	
Fluoroquinolone antibiotics	May decrease the effectiveness of fluoroquinolone antibiotics	
Interferon alfa-2B (Intron A)	May inhibit interferon release	
Insulin	Increase serum levels of insulin	Improves both insulin secretion and insulin sensitivity and exerts insulin-like effects
Pancreatic enzyme replacements	Increases serum levels of zinc by improving absorption	
Tetracycline anti-infectives	Decreases effectiveness of tetracyclines by binding with zinc	
Thyroid-active drugs		Zinc can alter thyroid hormone metabolism

Abbreviations: HDL = high-density lipoprotein; LDL = low-density lipoprotein.
[a] This table is not comprehensive as new information is being generated on a regular basis.

Zinc deficiencies can lead to growth restriction, delayed sexual maturity and hypogonadism in males, as well as eye and skin lesions, hair loss, and diarrhea.[87] Zinc toxicity is rare, but can be achieved with very high doses of supplemental zinc. The UL for zinc is 40 mg per day.

Zinc may affect other medications by inhibiting absorption, producing side effects, or enhancing actions. Insulin sensitivity is increased with zinc supplementation. Conversely, iron supplements may decrease zinc absorption. Table 5-18 highlights some drug interactions with zinc.

Table 5-19 summarizes information on micronutrient minerals.

Some vitamins and/or minerals interfere with the absorption or metabolism of other vitamins. For example, zinc inhibits copper absorption, vitamin E antagonizes the action of vitamin K, and iron inhibits zinc absorption.

Several studies have attempted to identify whether a single multivitamin/multimineral taken each day could prevent a number of diseases. There is no current evidence to support the effectiveness of this simple intervention.[88] Conversely, there has been a suggestion that use of multivitamin/multimineral supplements may be associated with a small risk of mortality, although those findings are subject to debate.[89,90]

Multivitamin/Multimineral Supplements

Approximately half of the adult population in the United States takes a multivitamin. Unfortunately, there is no standardization for the components of multivitamins/multiminerals and no database that summarizes the components found in the multitude of these products available. Evaluation of bioavailability is complicated because it depends on factors specific to the individual as well as the type of supplement, formulation, and combinations present in the overall vitamin pill.

Supplementation for Women After Bariatric Surgery

Obesity is a well-known problem of modern society. Bariatric surgery has emerged as a common treatment for individuals, especially those with morbid obesity or concomitant conditions. However, most of the surgical techniques interfere with absorption of food and nutrients so as to promote weight loss. No standard list of vitamins or minerals exists for women who undergo such procedures. However, most sources suggest supplementation with a daily multivitamin/mineral. Others recommend that the following vitamins

Table 5-19 Minerals: A Summary

Mineral	Function	Selected Food Sources	Recommended Intake Levels	Deficiency and Excessive Intake Considerations	Clinical and Supplementation Considerations
Calcium	Bone structure Vascular and muscle contraction Nerve transmission Secretion of hormones and enzymes	Dairy foods Salmon and sardines with bones Calcium-fortified foods	RDA: 1000 mg/day for females 19–50 years and 1200 mg/day for females ≥ 51 years	Deficiency: osteoporosis Excess: impaired kidney function and impaired absorption of iron, zinc, magnesium, and phosphorus UL: 2500 mg/day for persons 19–50 years; 2000 mg/day for persons > 50 years; 2500 mg/day during pregnancy and lactation for women ≥ 19 years	Calcium absorption enhanced by vitamin D. Calcium absorption inhibited by phytic acid (in whole-grain foods, beans, nuts, seeds, and soy isolates) and oxalic acid (in spinach, greens, sweet potatoes, rhubarb, and beans). Limit calcium supplement dose to 500 mg at one time. Calcium citrate supplements: take with or without food. Calcium carbonate supplements: take with food.
Copper	Synthesizes hemoglobin Assists in iron metabolism Helps produce thyroxine	Organ meats Oysters and shellfish Whole grains, legumes, nuts, potatoes, leafy greens	RDA: 900 mcg/day for females RDA: 1000 mcg/day during pregnancy and 1300 mcg/day during lactation	Deficiency: can be caused by high levels of zinc supplementation Excess: no known disease of excess but excess copper supplementation can cause zinc deficiency UL: 10,000 mcg/day for persons ≥ 19 years	None
Iodine	Synthesizes thyroid hormones	Iodized salt Seaweed, peanuts	RDA: 150 mcg/day for females ≥ 14 years RDA: 220 mcg/day during pregnancy and 290 mcg/day during lactation	Deficiency during pregnancy results in cretinism; deficiency can cause goiter Excess can also cause goiter, elevated TSH levels, hypothyroidism UL: 1100 mcg/day for persons ≥ 19 years	Taking high doses of iodine with antithyroid medication like methimazole (Tapazole) can have an additive effect, causing hypothyroidism. Taking potassium iodide with ACE inhibitors and/or potassium-sparing diuretics can increase risk of hyperkalemia.
Iron	Regulates cell growth and differentiation	Heme iron is in animal foods: meat, fish, and poultry Nonheme iron comes from plant foods: leafy greens; legumes; whole, fortified, and enriched grains	RDA: 18 mg/day for females ≥ 19–50 years and 8 mg/day for females ≥ 51 years RDA: 27 mg/day during pregnancy and 9 mg/day during lactation in women ≥ 19 years	Deficiency: iron deficiency and iron-deficiency anemia Excess: iron toxicity is a leading cause of childhood poisoning; use caution in the iron overload condition of hemochromatosis	Vitamin C enhances iron absorption. Oxalates, phytates, and tannins decrease iron absorption. Ferrous sulfate is most readily absorbable type of supplemental iron. Iron supplements are best absorbed on an empty stomach but may cause GI distress.
Magnesium	Cofactor in approximately 300 enzyme systems Regulates protein synthesis, muscle and nerve action, blood glucose control, and blood pressure	Widespread in plant and animal foods Green leafy vegetables, legumes, nuts, seeds, whole grains	RDA: 320 mg/day for females ≥ 31 years RDA: 310–400 mg/day during pregnancy and lactation, varies by age	Deficiency: rare Excess: no known disease of excess although can cause GI distress UL: 350 mg/day	Magnesium-containing supplements or medications can decrease absorption of oral bisphosphonates. Magnesium can form insoluble complexes with tetracyclines and quinolone antibiotics. Chronic use of loop diuretics can increase urinary magnesium losses. PPIs when taken for longer than 1 year can cause hypomagnesemia.

(*continues*)

Table 5-19 Minerals: A Summary (*continued*)

Mineral	Function	Selected Food Sources	Recommended Intake Levels	Deficiency and Excessive Intake Considerations	Clinical and Supplementation Considerations
Potassium	Maintains kidney function Muscle contractions Blood pressure management	Widespread in fruits and vegetables Legumes, potatoes, seafood, dairy foods, potatoes, tomatoes, and bananas	No RDA, AI: 4.7 g/day for females ≥ 14 years and during pregnancy RDA: 5.1 g/day during lactation	Deficiency: blood pressure irregularities, irregular heart rhythms, muscular weakness, hypotension, dyspnea Excess: use caution with supplements or salt substitutes containing potassium in persons with kidney problems or on medication for heart, kidney, or liver problems No UL	Use caution with ACE inhibitors. Avoid potassium with amiloride (Midamor), spironolactone (Aldactone), or triamterene (Dyrenium).
Selenium	Antioxidant Assists in reproduction, thyroid hormone metabolism, and DNA synthesis	Plant foods grown in areas with selenium-rich soil	RDA: 55 mcg/day for females ≥ 14 years RDA: 60 mcg/day during pregnancy and 70 mcg/day during lactation	Deficiency: Keshan disease Excess: selenosis UL: 400 mcg/day for persons ≥ 14 years	Cisplatin may reduce selenium levels. Advise against selenium and other antioxidant supplements during cancer chemotherapy or radiotherapy.
Zinc	Immune function, protein and DNA synthesis, wound healing, cell division, normal growth and development	Shellfish, meat, organ foods, dairy, legumes, chocolate, fortified grains	RDA: 8 mg/day for females ≥ 19 years RDA: 11 mg/day during pregnancy for females ≥ 19 years and 12 mg/day during lactation for females ≥ 19 years RDA for females 14–18 years: 9 mg, then 12 mg during pregnancy and 13 mg during lactation	Deficiency: growth retardation, delayed sexual maturity, hypogonadism, impotence, eye and skin lesions, hair loss, and diarrhea; can be caused by excess copper supplementation Excess: rare but can be achieved with high supplemental levels; excess zinc supplements can cause copper deficiency UL: 40 mg/day for persons ≥ 19 years	Quinolone antibiotics and tetracycline antibiotics interact with and inhibit absorption of zinc; take antibiotic 2 hours before or 4–6 hours after zinc supplement. Penicillamine absorption and action reduced by zinc; take zinc at least 2 hours before or after medication. Thiazide diuretics such as chlorthalidone (Hygroton) and hydrochlorothiazide (Esidrix and HydroDiuril) increase zinc excretion; zinc status should be monitored.

Abbreviations: ACE = angiotensin-converting enzyme; AI = Adequate Intake; GI = gastrointestinal; PPI = proton pump inhibitor; RDA = Recommended Daily Allowance; TSH = thyroid-stimulating hormone; UL = Tolerable Upper Intake Level.

and minerals be supplemented indefinitely or permanently, either in combination or separately: calcium, iron, vitamin A, vitamin B_1 (at least for the first 6 months), vitamin B_{12}, vitamin C, vitamin D, vitamin K, and zinc. More studies are needed for long-term analysis after bariatric surgery.

Special Populations: Pregnancy, Lactation, and the Elderly

Nutrients are important for brain development during fetal and early postnatal life. Certain nutrients, such as protein, certain fats, iron, zinc, copper, iodine, selenium, vitamin A, choline, and folate, have greater effects on brain development than others. Nutrient deficiency or nutrient excess can adversely affect brain development, depending on the timing, dose, and duration of exposure.

Many women in low-income countries consume inadequate levels of micronutrients due to limited intake of animal products, fruits, vegetables, and fortified foods. These diets can result in anemia, hypertension, complications of labor, and even death. Nevertheless, more evidence is required before multimicronutrient supplementation programs are implemented on a global scale. In the United States, women who are under-nourished and obese have a double nutritional burden, wherein individual nutritional needs present clinical challenges.[91]

Supplemental multivitamins, folic acid, calcium, and iron are commonly recommended for pregnant women. The evidence for taking folic acid supplements preconceptionally and in early pregnancy is strong, whereas the evidence for routine use of multivitamins with iron is controversial for otherwise healthy women. The benefits, risks, and pharmacotherapeutic considerations associated with vitamin use by pregnant women are reviewed in more detail in the *Pregnancy* chapter.

Both physiologic and lifestyle changes that affect mature women have an impact on absorption and metabolism of vitamins and minerals. For example, as individuals age, vitamin D is absorbed less efficiently. Older women who reside in nursing homes often do not get sufficient sunlight. This combination exacerbates the well-known risks related to falls and fractures.

Conclusion

Multiple studies have assessed the use of vitamins, minerals, or both as treatment of major clinical disease states. The use of supplements has not been universally recommended for prevention of cardiovascular disease or cancer, as few studies have provided strong evidence of reductions in these events when supplements are used. Therefore, diet remains the cornerstone in clinical management when vitamins and minerals are suggested as therapies.

The majority of observational studies evaluating the health effects of vitamins and minerals have found a lower risk of chronic disease among individuals with higher circulating levels or intakes of specific nutrients, vitamins, or minerals. However, these types of observational studies often do not report whether the subjects were taking other supplements before and during the study, and there is little information addressing other variables that might potentially affect the occurrence of the disease in question. In addition, dietary supplements have not been standardized, and trials have used different products with different bioavailabilities. For example, since food fortification has become popular, intakes of certain nutrients have often exceeded the RDI.

Despite the limitations of early epidemiologic evaluations, randomized trials have been conducted in this area and knowledge about the use of dietary supplements as specific pharmacotherapeutic agents is growing. For the most part, randomized trials that have compared use of a single vitamin supplement to no supplementation have found no effect on the disease of interest, and on occasion they have documented an increased risk for other disorders in the cohort using the vitamin. However, future studies may enhance the understanding of administration of a vitamin or mineral as a preventive or treatment agent, especially in the area of treatment of women with chronic diseases.

Resources

Organization	Description	Website
U.S. Pharmacopeial (USP) Convention	Scientific nonprofit organization that sets standards for the identify, strength, quality, and purity of medicines, food ingredients, and dietary supplements	www.usp.org
Consumer Lab	A privately held U.S. company that publishes test results on health, wellness, and nutrition products	www.consumerlab.com
NSF International	Organization that independently tests, audits, certifies, trains, and consults for the food, water, health science, sustainability, and consumer product sectors	www.nsf.org
Apps		
Myriad apps exist for devices in the area of vitamins and minerals. However, most are sponsored by companies that sell nutritional supplements and, therefore, they may be perceived to be biased. Websites such as those from federal agencies are increasingly including apps; the reader is advised to regularly consult the website of the U.S. Office of Dietary Supplements (http://ods.od.nih.gov/), among others, regarding introduction of new apps.		
Other Resources		
Interactive DRI for healthcare professionals	U.S. Department of Agriculture (and Institute of Medicine)	http://fnic.nal.usda.gov/fnic/interactiveDRI/
DRI tables	Institute of Medicine, Food and Nutrition Board	http://fnic.nal.usda.gov/dietary-guidance/dietary-reference-intakes/dri-tables
Dietary guidance interactive tools, calculators, and counters	U.S. Department of Agriculture	http://fnic.nal.usda.gov/dietary-guidance/interactive-tools/calculators-and-counters
ASA24 (Automated Self-Administered 24-Hour Recall) for consumers	National Cancer Institute	http://appliedresearch.cancer.gov/asa24/
NIH Office of Dietary Supplements (ODS)	Free dietary *Supplement Fact Sheets* are available from this source	http://ods.od.nih.gov/factsheets/list-all/

References

1. Carpenter K. The discovery of vitamin C. *Ann Nutr Metab*. 2012;61(3):259-264.
2. Crowe K, Francis C, Dietetics AoNa. Position of the Academy of Nutrition and Dietetics: functional foods. *J Acad Nutr Diet*. 2013;113(8):1096-103.
3. Marra M, Boyar A. Position of the American Dietic Association: Nutrient supplementation. *J Am Diet Assoc*. 2009;109(12):2073-2085.
4. Atwater W. Principles of nutrition and nutritive value of food. *U.S. Department of Agriculture, Farmers' Bulletin*. 1902;142.
5. Hunt C. Food for young children. *U.S. Department of Agriculture, Farmers' Bulletin*. 1917;808.
6. Davis C, Saltos E. Dietary recommendations and how they have changed over time. *America's Eating Habits: Changes and Consequences*. 1999:35.
7. National Institutes of Health, Office of Dietary Supplements. Nutrient recommendations: Dietary Reference Intakes (DRI). *Health Information*. http://ods.od.nih.gov/Health_Information/Dietary_Reference_Intakes.aspx. Accessed June 4, 2014.
8. U.S. Food and Drug Administration. Dietary Supplement Health and Education Act of 1994. *Regulatory Information*. October 25, 1994. http://www.fda.gov/RegulatoryInformation/Legislation/FederalFoodDrugandCosmeticActFDCAct/SignificantAmendmentstotheFDCAct/ucm148003.htm. Accessed June 4, 2014.
9. Bjelakovic G, Nikolova D, Gluud LL, Simonetti RG, Gluud C. Antioxidant supplements for prevention of mortality in healthy participants and patients with various diseases. *Cochrane Database Syst Rev*. 2012;3:CD007176.
10. Fortmann S, Burda B, Senger C, Lin J, Whitlock E. Vitamin and mineral supplements in the primary prevention of cardiovascular disease and cancer: an updated systematic evidence review for the U.S. Preventive Services Task Force. *Ann Intern Med*. 2013;159(12):824-834.
11. National Cancer Institute. Antixoidants and cancer prevention. *National Cancer Institute Fact Sheet*. January 16, 2014. http://www.cancer.gov/cancertopics/factsheet/prevention/antioxidants. Accessed June 4, 2014.
12. World Health Organization. Vitamin A deficiency. *Micronutrient Deficiencies*. http://www.who.int/nutrition/topics/vad/en/. Accessed June 4, 2014.
13. Johnson EJ, Russel RM. β-carotene. In: Coates PM, Betz JM, Blackman MR, et al., eds. *Encyclopedia of Dietary Supplements*. 2nd ed. London, UK. New York: Informa Healthcare; 2010:115-120
14. Institute of Medicine, Food, and Nutrition Board. *Dietary Reference Intakes for Vitamin A, Vitamin K, Arsenic, Boron, Chromium, Copper, Iodine, Iron, Manganese, Molybdenum, Nickel, Silicon, Vanadium, and Zinc*. National Academies Press: Washington, DC; 2001.
15. National Institutes of Health, Office of Dietary Supplements. Unit conversions. *Dietary Supplement Ingredient Database*. 2012. http://dietarysupplementdatabase.usda.nih.gov/ingredient_calculator/equation.php. Accessed June 4, 2014.
16. National Institutes of Health, Office of Dietary Supplements. Vitamin D fact sheet for health professionals. *Health Information*. June 24, 2011. http://ods.od.nih.gov/factsheets/VitaminD-HealthProfessional/. Accessed June 4, 2014.
17. Cranney C, Horsely T, O'Donnell S, Weiler H, Ooi D, Atkinson Sea. Effectiveness and safety of vitamin D. Evidence Report/Technology Assessment No. 158 prepared by the University of Ottawa Evidence-based Practice Center under Contract No. 290-02.0021. AHRQ Publication No. 07-E013. 2007.
18. Institute of Medicine, Food, and Nutrition Board. Dietary reference intakes for calcium and vitamin D. 2010. http://www.iom.edu/~/media/Files/Report%20Files/2010/Dietary-Reference-Intakes-for-Calcium-and-Vitamin-D/Vitamin%20D%20and%20Calcium%202010%20Report%20Brief.pdf. Accessed February 11, 2015.
19. Hoffmann MR, Senior PA, Mager DR. Vitamin D supplementation and health-related quality of life: a systematic review of the literature. *J Acad Nutr Diet*. 2015;115(3):406-418.
20. Felman D, Pike JW, Adams JS. Relevant lab values for adults and children. In: Felman D, Pike JW, Adams JS. *Vitamin D*. 3rd ed. Amsterdam: Elsevier; 2011: xxiv-xxx.
21. Wagner C, Greer F, Breastfeeding AAOPSO, Nutrition AAOPCO. Prevention of rickets and vitamin D deficiency. *Pediatrics*. 2008;122:1142-1152.
22. Perrine CG, Sharma AJ, Jefferds ME, Serdula MK, Scanlon KS. Adherence to vitamin D recommendations among US infants. *Pediatrics*. 2010;125(4):627-632.
23. Bailey RL, Dodd KW, Goldman JA, et al. Estimation of total usual calcium and vitamin D intakes in the United States. *J Nutr*. 2010;140(4):817-822.

24. McGuire M, Beerman K. *Nutritional Sciences from Fundamentals to Food.* 13th ed. Belmont, CA: Cengage; 2013.
25. Institute of Medicine, Food, and Nutrition Board. *Dietary Reference Intake for Vitamin C, Vitamin E, Selenium, and Carotenoids.* National Academies Press: Washington, DC; 2000.
26. Brion L, Bell E, Raghuveer T. Vitamin E supplementation for prevention of morbidity and mortality in preterm infants. *Cochrane Database Syst Rev.* 2003; 4:CD003665.
27. National Institutes of Health, Office of Dietary Supplements. Vitamin E fact sheet for professionals. *Health Information.* June 5, 2013. http://ods.od.nih.gov/factsheets/VitaminE-HealthProfessional/#en52. Accessed June 5, 2014.
28. Kris-Etherton PM LAHB, Steinberg D, Witztum J. Antioxidant vitamin supplements and cardiovascular disease. *Circulation.* 2004;110:637-641.
29. Fortmann S, Burda B, Senger C, Lin J, Whitlock E. Vitamin and mineral supplements in the primary prevention of cardiovascular disease and cancer: an updated systematic evidence review for the U.S. Preventive Services Task Force. *Ann Intern Med.* 2013;159(12):824-834.
30. Gallagher ML. Intake: the nutrients and their metabolism. In: Mahan LK, Escott-Stump S. Raymond JL, eds. *Krause's Food and the Nutrition Care Process.* 13th ed. St. Louis, MO: Elsevier Saunders; 2012:32-40.
31. Zetterstrom R, Dam C, Doisy E. The discovery of antihaemorrhagic vitamin and its impact on neonatal health. *Acta Paediatr.* 2006;95(6):642-644.
32. Sizer F, Whitney E. *Nutrition Concepts & Controversies.* 13th ed. Belmont, CA: Cengage; 2014.
33. Carpenter K. The discovery of thiamin. *Ann Nutr Metab.* 2012;61(3):219-223.
34. Lonsdale D. Thiamin(e): the spark of life. *Subcell Biochem.* 2012;56:199-227.
35. Institute of Medicine, Food, and Nutrition Board. *Dietary Reference Intakes for Thiamin, Riboflavin, Niacin, Vitamin B_6, Folate, Vitamin B_{12}, Pantothenic Acid, Biotin, and Choline.* National Academies Press: Washington, DC: 2000.
36. Schlenker E, Gilbert J. *Williams' Essentials of Nutrition and Diet Therapy.* 13th ed. Philadelphia, PA: Mosby; 2011.
37. Penberthy W, Kirkland J. Niacin. In: Erdman JW, MacDonald IA, eds. *Present Knowledge in Nutrition.* 10th ed. Ames, IA: Wiley-Blackwell; 2012:293-306.
38. Whelam A, Jurgens T, Naylor H. Herbs, vitamins and minerals in the treatment of premenstrual syndrome: a systematic review. *Can J Clin Pharmacol.* 2009; 16(3):e407-e429.
39. Bendich A. The potential for dietary supplements to reduce premenstrual syndrome (PMS) symptoms. *J Am Coll Nutr.* 2000;19(1):3-12.
40. Matthews A, Haas D, O'Mathuna D, Dowswell T, Doyle M. Interventions for nausea and vomiting in early pregnancy. *Cochrane Database Syst Rev.* 2014; 3:CD007575.
41. Gregory J. Case study: folate biovailability. *J Nutr.* 2001;131(4):13765-13825.
42. Centers for Disease Control and Prevention. CDC grand rounds: additional opportunities to prevent neural tube defects with folic acid fortification. *MMWR.* 2010:980-984.
43. Food and Drug Administration. *Food Standards: Amendment of Standards of Identity for Enriched Grain Products to Require Addition of Folic Acid. Final Rule. 21 CFR Parts 136, 137, and 139.* 1996.
44. Crider K, Bailey L, Berry R. Folic acid food fortification: its history, effect, concerns, and future directions. *Nutrients.* 2011;3(3):370-384.
45. Kaferle J, Strzoda CE. Evaluation of macrocytosis. *Am Fam Physician.* 2009;79(3):203-208.
46. Baik H, Russell R. Vitamin B_{12} deficiency in the elderly. *Annu Rev Nutr.* 1999;19:357-377.
47. Cattan D. Pernicious anemia: what are the actual diagnosis criteria? *World J Gastroenterol.* 2011; 17(4):543-544.
48. Aslan K, Bozdemir H, Unsal C, Guvenc B. The effect of antiepileptic drugs on vitamin B_{12} metabolism. *Int J Lab Hematol.* 2008;30(1):26-35.
49. Li Y, Schellhorn HE. New developments and novel therapeutic perspectives for vitamin C. *J Nutr.* 2007;137(10):2171-2184.
50. Moshfegh A, Goldman J, Cleveland L. *What We Eat in America, NHANES 2001–2002: Usual Nutrient Intakes from Food Compared to Dietary Reference Intakes.* National Academies Press: Washington, DC; 2005.
51. Jacob R, Sotoudeh G. Vitamin C function and status in chronic disease. *Nutr Clin Care.* 2002;5:66-74.
52. National Institutes of Health, Office of Dietary Supplements. Vitamin C fact sheet for health professionals. *Health Information.* June 5, 2013. http://ods.od.nih.gov/factsheets/VitaminC-HealthProfessional/#en4. Accessed June 7, 2014.

53. Douglas R, Hemila H, Chalker E, Treacy B. Vitamin C for preventing and treating the common cold. *Cochrane Database Syst Rev*. 2007;3:CD000980.
54. National Institutes of Health, Office of Dietary Supplements. Calcium fact sheet for health professionals. *Health Information*. November 21, 2013. http://ods.od.nih.gov/factsheets/Calcium-HealthProfessional/#en1. Accessed June 7, 2014.
55. National Institutes of Health, Office of Dietary Supplements. Vitamin D fact sheet for health professionals. *Health Information*. June 24, 2011. http://ods.od.nih.gov/factsheets/VitaminD-HealthProfessional/. Accessed June 4, 2014.
56. National Osteoporosis Foundation. Did you know? http://www.nof.org. Accessed June 7, 2014.
57. Mangano K, Walsh S, Insogna K, Kenny A, Kerstetter J. Calcium intake in the United States from dietary and supplemental sources across adult age groups: new estimates from the National Health and Nutrition Examination Survey 2003–2006. *J Am Diet Assoc*. 2011;111(5):687-695.
58. Curhan G, Willett W, Knight E, Stampfer M. Dietary factors and the risk of incident kidney stones in younger women: Nurses' Health Study II. *Arch Intern Med*. 2004;164(8):885-891.
59. Broadhurst CL, Domenico P. Clinical studies on chromium picolinate supplementation in diabetes mellitus: a review. *Diabetes Technol Ther*. 2006;8(6):677-687.
60. National Institutes of Health, Office of Dietary Supplements. Chromium dietary fact sheet for health professionals. *Health Information*. June 24, 2011. http://ods.od.nih.gov/factsheets/Chromium-Health Professional/#h9. Accessed January 28, 2015.
61. Milne D. Copper intake and assessment of copper status. *Am J Clin Nutr*. 1998;67(5 suppl):1041S-1045S.
62. Zimmermann M. Iodine deficiency. *Endocr Rev*. 2009;30(4):376-408.
63. Pennington J. A review of iodine toxicity reports. *J Am Diet Assoc*. 1990;90(11):1571-1581.
64. Fein SB, Labiner-Wolfe J, Scanlon KS, Grummer-Strawn LM. Selected complementary feeding practices and their association with maternal education. *Pediatrics*. 2008;122(suppl 2):S91-S97.
65. Academy of Nutrition and Dietetics. Anemia. In: *Nutrition Care Manual*. 2012. http://www.nutritioncaremanual.org. Accessed January 19, 2013.
66. Fishman SM, Christian P, West KP. The role of vitamins in the prevention and control of anaemia. *Public Health Nutr*. 2000;3(2):125-150.
67. World Health Organization. Quantifying selected major risks to health. In: *The World Health Report*. Geneva, Switzerland: World Health Organization; 2002:47-97.
68. United States Department of Agriculture, Agriculture Research Service. *What We Eat in America, 2009–2010*. http://www.ars.usda.gov/SP2UserFiles/Place/80400530/pdf/0910/Table_1_NIN_GEN_09.pdf. Accessed June 22, 2015.
69. Bailey R, Gahche J, Lentino C, Dwyer J, Engel J, Thomas P. Dietary supplement use in the United States, 2003–2006. *J Nutr*. 2011;141(2):261-266.
70. Cogswell M, Kettel-Khan L, Ramakrishnan U. Iron supplement use among women in the United States: science, policy and practice. *J Nutr*. 2003;133(6):1974S-1977S.
71. National Institutes of Health, Office of Dietary Supplements. Dietary supplement fact sheet: iron. *Health Information*. April 8, 2014. http://ods.od.nih.gov/factsheets/Iron-HealthProfessional/. Accessed June 10, 2014.
72. Burke W, Cogswell ME, McDonnell SM, Franks A. Public health strategies to prevent the complications of hemochromatosis. In: Khoury MJ, Burke W, Thomson EJ, eds. *Genetics and Public Health in the 21st Century: Using Genetic Information to Improve Health and Prevent Disease*. Oxford UK: Oxford University Press; 2000:447-462.
73. Rude R. Magnesium. *Modern Nutrition in Health and Disease*. 11th ed. Baltimore, MD: Lippincott Williams & Wilkins; 2012.
74. Witkowski M, Hubert J, Mazur A. Methods of assessment of magnesium status in humans: a systematic review. *Magnesium Res*. 2011;24:163-180.
75. Azoulay A, Garzon P, Eisenberg M. Comparison of the mineral content of tap water and bottled waters. *J Gen Intern Med*. 2001;16:168-175.
76. Moshfegh A, Goldman J, Ahuja J, Rhodes D, LaComb R. *What We Eat in America, NHANES 2005–2006: Usual Nutrient Intakes from Food and Water Compared to 1997 Dietary Reference Intakes for Vitamin D, Calcium, Phosphorus, and Magnesium*. National Academies Press: Washington DC; 2009.
77. Institute of Medicine, Food, and Nutrition Board. *Dietary Reference Intakes for Calcium, Phosphorus, Magnesium, Vitamin D, and Fluoride*. National Academies Press: Washington, DC; 1997.
78. National Institutes of Health, Office of Dietary Supplements. Magnesium fact sheet for health

professionals. *Health Information*. November 4, 2013. http://ods.od.nih.gov/factsheets/Magnesium-HealthProfessional/#en28. Accessed June 7, 2014.

79. Musso C. Magnesium metabolism in health and disease. *Int Urol Nephrol*. 2009;41:357-362.
80. U.S. Food and Drug Administration. Proton pump inhibitor drugs (PPIs): drug safety communication: low magnesium levels can be associated with long-term use. *MedWatch*. March 2, 2011. http://www.fda.gov/Safety/MedWatch/SafetyInformation/SafetyAlertsforHumanMedicalProducts/ucm245275.htm. Accessed June 7, 2014.
81. U.S. Department of Agriculture, U.S. Department of Health and Human Services. *Dietary Guidelines for Americans, 2010*. 7th ed. Washington, DC: U.S. Government Printing Office, December 2010. http://www.health.gov/dietaryguidelines/dga2010/dietaryguidelines2010.pdf. Accessed February 11, 2015.
82. Institute of Medicine, Food, and Nutrition Board. Dietary Reference Intakes for water, potassium, sodium, chloride, and sulfate. 2005. http://www.nal.usda.gov/fnic/DRI/DRI_Water/water_full_report.pdf. Accessed February 11, 2015.
83. Sunde RA. Selenium. In: Ross CA, Caballero B, Cousins RJ, Tucker KL, Ziegler TR, eds. *Modern Nutrition in Health and Disease*. 11th ed. Philadelphia, PA: Lippincott Williams & Wilkins; 2012:265-275.
84. Chun OK, Floegel A, Chung SJ, Chung CE, Song WO, Koo SI. Estimation of antioxidant intakes from diet and supplements in U.S. adults. *J Nutr*. 2010;140(3):317-324.
85. National Institutes of Health, Office of Dietary Supplements. Selenium fact sheet for health professionals. *Health Information*. July 2, 2013. http://ods.od.nih.gov/factsheets/Selenium-HealthProfessional/#en7. Accessed June 7, 2014.
86. Sieja K, Talerczyk M. Selenium as an element in the treatment of ovarian cancer in women receiving chemotherapy. *Gynecol Oncol*. 2004;93:320-327.
87. National Institutes of Health, Office of Dietary Supplements. Zinc fact sheet for health professionals. *Health Information*. June 5, 2013. http://ods.od.nih.gov/factsheets/Zinc-HealthProfessional/. Accessed June 7, 2014.
88. Singal M, Banh HL, Allan GM. Daily multivitamins to reduce mortality, cardiovascular disease, and cancer. *Can Fam Physician*. 2013;59(8):847.
89. Mursu J, Robien K, Harnack LJ, Park K, Jacobs DR Jr. Dietary supplements and mortality rate in older women: the Iowa Women's Health Study. *Arch Intern Med*. 2011;171:1625-1623.
90. Macpherson H, Pipingas A, Pase MP. Multivitamin–multimineral supplementation and mortality: a meta-analysis of randomized controlled trials. *Am J Clin Nutr*. 2013;97(2):437-444.
91. Dean SV, Lassi ZS, Imam AM, Bhutta ZA. Preconception care: nutritional risks and interventions. *Reprod Health*. 2014;11(suppl 3):S3.

6 Immunizations

Kathryn M. Osborne, Mary C. Brucker

Based on the chapter by Mary Beth Koslap-Petraco and Barbara Hackley in the first edition of Pharmacology for Women's Health

Chapter Glossary

Active immunity Immunity produced by an individual's own immune system. Also referred to as natural immunity and is usually permanent immunity.

Adaptive immunity Antigen-specific response. Ability of the body to create an immune response to an individual antigen and to remember to reproduce this response if the antigen reappears. Contrast with innate immunity.

Antibodies Protein immunoglobulins produced by B lymphocyte cells that aid in the elimination of antigens.

Antigens Live or inactivated substances capable of stimulating an immune response.

Cell-mediated immune response Immune response does not involve antibodies but does involve activated macrophages and cytotoxic T-cell lymphocytes. Also termed cellular immunity.

Cellular immunity Immune response that involves the following cellular components of the immune system: macrophages, T-cell lymphocytes, and natural killer cells. Also termed cell-mediated immune response.

Humoral immunity Immune response that relies on antibodies produced by B lymphocytes.

Immunization Process by which a person or animal becomes protected from a disease through use of a vaccine to provoke active immunity in the person's body.

Immunoglobulins Any of several preformed antibodies derived from human sera that can be administered to provide passive immunization.

Inactivated vaccines Vaccines that contain a bacterium or virus that is inactivated by heat or chemicals so it cannot replicate. The components of the organism that stimulate immunity are isolated and used for the vaccine. Inactivated vaccines cannot cause disease.

Infectious diseases Diseases caused by a pathogenic microorganism. It may or may not be communicable. For example, tetanus is an infectious disease but is not communicable.

Innate immunity Immune cells that respond nonspecifically to foreign material. For example, phagocytes will attack many different microbes. Contrast with adaptive immunity.

Live attenuated vaccines (LAVs) Vaccine made of bacteria or viruses that are alive but weakened so they are not likely to cause disease. A very small inoculum is used to stimulate active immunity. Live attenuated vaccines may, on rare occasions, cause disease in recipients with suppressed immune systems.

Passive immunity Nonpermanent immunity that results from the transfer of antibodies to an individual from another human or animal source.

Polysaccharide vaccines Inactivated vaccines that are composed of long chains of sugar molecules from the capsule of specific bacteria.

Recombinant vaccine Antigens used in vaccines that are produced by genetic engineering technology.

Toxoid Fractional vaccine made from an inactivated toxin.

Vaccination Process of administering an agent (vaccine) to produce immunity.

Vaccines Agents administered to produce immunity to a disease.

Historical Review

One of the greatest achievements in public health during the twentieth century was the decrease in the incidence of infectious diseases. Although much of this phenomenon can be attributed to improvements in sanitation and hygiene, the near-eradication of many diseases that have historically led to death and disability can be largely credited to successful **vaccination** campaigns.[1] For example, years ago it was common to find the abbreviation UCHD or "usual childhood diseases" on a woman's medical record, indicating that she had a history of rubella, varicella, and pertussis. These **infectious diseases** were communicable conditions that were highly contagious. Today, however, these diseases are rare due to widespread administration of **vaccines**.

A common misconception is that vaccinations are necessary only during childhood. In reality, multiple vaccine-preventable diseases have been recognized as prevalent among adults. Yet, despite strong recommendations for continued vaccination against several diseases throughout adulthood, surveys have revealed suboptimal levels of adult vaccination.[2] As a result, each year tens of thousands of adults continue to acquire diseases that could be prevented. Thus, the subject of **immunization** is important for healthcare providers who care for persons of any age. This chapter reviews the vaccines commonly recommended for adolescent girls and women throughout their lifespan.

Box 6-1 Gone But Not Forgotten: Examples of Vaccine-Preventable Diseases

In 1966, the World Health Organization (WHO) spearheaded a campaign to eradicate numerous infectious diseases, especially smallpox, which was once a global scourge. The goal for smallpox was achieved: The last naturally occurring case of smallpox occurred in 1977 in Somalia and the world was declared smallpox free in 1980.[4]

Currently WHO is working to eradicate poliomyelitis. Global efforts to eradicate this disease have resulted in a reduction in the incidence of polio from an estimated 350,000 cases in 1988 to 406 cases reported in 2013. Today, polio remains endemic in only three countries: Afghanistan, Nigeria, and Pakistan.[5]

Since the introduction of the first *Haemophilus influenzae* type b (Hib) vaccine in 1985, the annual incidence of this invasive disease in children younger than 5 years has dropped by 99%, to fewer than 1 case per 100,000 children in the United States. Although Hib has been virtually eliminated in the United States, the Centers for Disease Control and Prevention (CDC) recognizes that the risk for invasive Hib disease among under-immunized and unimmunized children persists and recommends continuing routine vaccination, with the first vaccines beginning at 2 months after birth.[6]

Public Health Impact of Vaccination Programs

Vaccines had a significant positive impact on public health in the twentieth century, as noted in Box 6-1. The 100% decrease in smallpox and diphtheria is an example of a great success story that occurred secondary to a widespread vaccination program. Other vaccine-preventable diseases such as tetanus, polio, measles (rubeola), mumps, rubella, and congenital rubella have virtually been eliminated in the United States since the introduction of effective vaccination programs. If these vaccination programs are not maintained, however, the incidence of many of these diseases is anticipated to rise to prevaccination levels.[3]

Disparities in Vaccination Rates

According to the National Health Interview Survey data from 2012, only 55.1% of persons 65 years or older received any tetanus toxoid–containing vaccine in the previous 10 years, and only 59.9% received a pneumococcal vaccine despite recommendations that all adults be vaccinated for pneumococcus.[7] Influenza vaccination rates for adults 65 years or older increased between 1980 and the early 1990s but have stabilized since 1997; fewer than 20% of persons in high-risk groups are vaccinated against influenza today.[3] Economic and racial disparities also exist. Although programs such as Vaccines for Children (authorized by the U.S. Congress in 1994) have dramatically reduced disparities in coverage, low-income persons as well as children and adults from minority racial and ethnic groups remain at greater risk for under-immunization across the United States.[7]

Healthy People 2020 Goals

The Centers for Disease Control and Prevention (CDC) published national targets related to vaccinations and infectious diseases as part of its *Healthy People 2020* goals. Among these goals, nine are specifically related to improving vaccination rates for all U.S. populations.[8] To date, none of the *Healthy People 2020* goals regarding vaccination and infectious disease has been met on any measure; indeed, substantial improvements in vaccination rates will be necessary to achieve those goals.[3] Providers in any setting, regardless of the age, gender, or socioeconomic level of the population served, can work to help reach the *Healthy People 2020* vaccination goals. Before reviewing vaccines, a brief review of immunity and the immune system is in order.

Basics of Immunity

Immunity is the ability of the human body to identify and eliminate foreign material. Immunity occurs as a result of a complex interaction between **antigens**, which are substances foreign to the human body; **antibodies**, which are immunoglobulins produced by lymphocytes; and other cells specific to the immune system. Effective responses to an infection vary based on an individual's genetics or health status at time of exposure as well as other characteristics, with some individuals being more susceptible to disease than others.[3]

The human body has a variety of physiologic defenses that act to repel microbes. For example, microbes must first penetrate physical barriers, such as the cornified epidermis of the skin or mucus produced by the respiratory tract, and chemical barriers, such as the exquisitely maintained pH of the vaginal mucosa. If these barriers are breached, then the immune system is triggered to respond in multiple ways to isolate invading microbes and render those microbes, now termed antigens, harmless.

Invading microbes first encounter the general defense mechanisms of the immune system, known as **innate immunity**, which includes circulating phagocytes, natural killer cells, nonspecific antibodies, and the complement system. The complement system is composed of small proteins that circulate as immune precursors. These proteins mark invading microbes as foreign and weaken their cell walls to allow antibodies, once activated, to penetrate and kill the microbes. This initial response can help contain the invading microbes until the cellular and humoral systems are activated and can respond to specific antigens.

The ability of the body to develop specific responses to specific antigens is known as **adaptive immunity** (Figure 6-1). The humoral system is composed chiefly of B lymphocyte cells that develop and secrete antibodies against specific antigens such as bacteria or viruses. Antibodies released by B lymphocytic cells generally attack free-floating extracellular antigens, a process referred to as **humoral immunity**.[9]

T cells—some of which help coordinate B lymphocytic cells and other immune responses, and some of which attack infected cells directly—dominate in the **cell-mediated immune response**. T cells also fight intracellular infections such as viruses and can function either offensively or defensively. The offensive T cells do not attack the virus directly, but use chemicals that eliminate the cells already

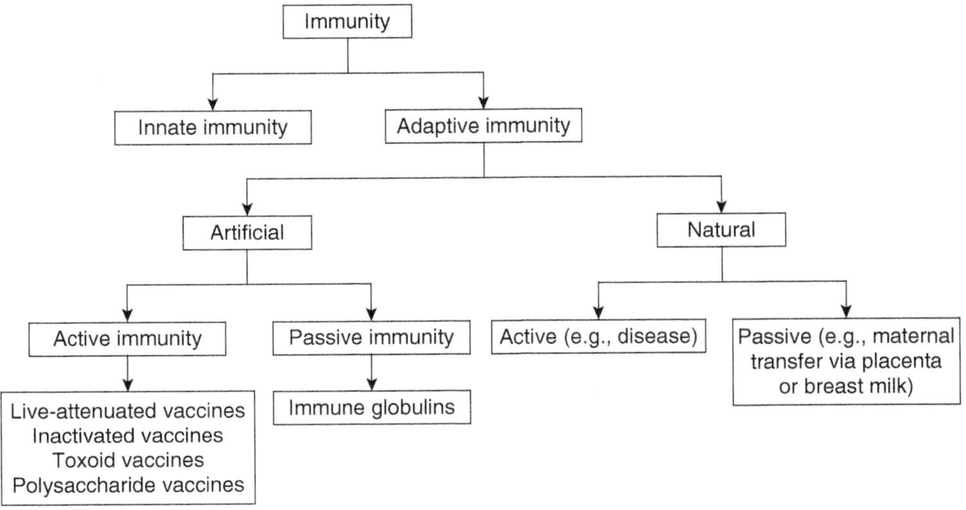

Figure 6-1 Types of immunity.

infected with the offending virus. Because they have been programmed by previous exposure to virus antigen, these cytotoxic T cells sense the presence of the virus in infected cells, latch onto the infected cell, and release chemicals to kill the cell and the virus inside. The defensive T cells also called helper T cells defend the body by secreting chemical signals that direct the activity of other immune system components. Helper T cells assist in activating cytotoxic T cells and also work closely with B lymphocytic cells. Any of the processes performed by T cells—that is, the cell-mediated immune response—can be affected by the general health or genetic makeup of an individual, which can either hinder or boost the immune response.

Two basic types of mechanisms help the body develop immunity against a disease-causing pathogen: active and passive. **Active immunity** is protection produced by the person's own immune system and usually is permanent. Stimulation of the immune system with antigens results in the production of antibodies and **cellular immunity** in response to antigens from naturally occurring infection or antigens introduced artificially through vaccination. Antibodies that are transferred to a human by another human or via vaccination result in **passive immunity**. An example of passive immunity is seen in infants who are being breastfed. These infants have immunity to certain diseases because maternal antibodies are present in breast milk and protect the infant. As is true of all passive immunity, this protection from antigens is temporary, as the passively received antibodies do not remain in the infant's system permanently.[3]

Some vaccines are antibodies and therefore provide passive immunity. Other vaccines initiate adaptive immunity primarily by creating memory B lymphocytic cells, which can release large numbers of antibodies directed against specific antigens once these antigens enter the human host, although some vaccines are T-cell mediated. However, because these immune mechanisms are just one part of a much more complex system, vaccinations may not produce the same level or durability of protection in all individuals.

Vaccine Products

Vaccines are substances or agents that are administered to deliberately provoke an immune response that is similar to the body's immune response to natural infection. These agents are administered through needle injection, oral ingestion, or intranasal aerosol. Development of a vaccine is a complicated process, as summarized in Box 6-2.

Box 6-2 Vaccine Production

Based on the stories found in multiple popular media, it might seem that once a pathogen is identified, development of a vaccine is a foregone conclusion. Moreover, it is assumed that the vaccine will always be rapidly available. Samples of antibodies are taken from survivors in these tales, and mysteriously the vaccine appears in the hands of the brilliant scientist from the nearby lab. In reality, vaccine production is far more complex and sophisticated.

For a virus, a cell medium composed of rapidly dividing cells, such as those derived from chicken embryos or human cells, provide the means to grow more viral proteins. In contrast, bacteria can be grown in bioreactors. In either case, the intention is to be able to harvest a large amount of the viral or bacterial antigen. The antigens are isolated and purified, including being subjected to ultrafiltration. Stabilizers and preservatives may be added to prolong shelf life. Ultimately, the vaccines are combined in a production vessel, placed into sterile containers, and labeled for use. Rigorous studies are also conducted to identify the effectiveness of vaccines.[3]

Vaccination is the process of administering the agent, whereas immunization denotes the body's process that results in active immunity.[9] Although such usage is not strictly correct, the terms "vaccination" and "immunization" often are used interchangeably. Several different types of vaccines are widely available in the United States. These agents have different pharmacologic effects and characteristics, as noted in Table 6-1. These variations determine the logistics of how the vaccine is used.

Live Attenuated Vaccines

Live attenuated vaccines (LAVs) are derived from live viruses or bacteria that have been weakened (attenuated) in a laboratory; most LAVs available in the United States are viral vaccines. When small doses of the weakened virus or bacteria are administered, they replicate and create an adequate amount of the organism to stimulate an immune response that is almost identical to the response triggered by a natural infection. In most instances, full immunity is achieved following a single dose, although a small number of recipients require a second dose because the immune

Table 6-1 Vaccine Products Available in the United States

Vaccine Type	Description	Examples
Live, Attenuated	Weakened version of the live microbe. These vaccines elicit a strong immune reaction. Rare possibility that this type of vaccine can cause disease.	Herpes zoster Influenza (nasal spray) Measles, mumps, rubella (MMR) Rotavirus Varicella (chickenpox)
Inactivated/Killed	Microbe killed via heat, chemical, or radiation. Immune response is not as robust, so these vaccines always require booster doses.	Hepatitis A (whole cell) Polio (IPV)
Toxoid (inactivated toxin)	Used to immunize against bacteria for which the bacterial toxin causes disease. The toxin is inactivated to make the vaccine.	Diphtheria, tetanus (also part of DTaP or Tdap combined immunization)
Subunit	Include only the antigen or several antigens from the microbe that best stimulate an immune reaction. The microbe is grown and then broken apart to harvest the relevant antigens.	Influenza (injection) Pertussis (part of DTaP combined immunization)
Recombinant subunit	The antigen is manufactured using recombinant DNA technology. The microbe genes are inserted into baker's yeast or another carrier nonpathogenic organism, which produces the desired antigen as it grows. The antigen is harvested from the yeast and used to produce the vaccine.	Hepatitis B Human papillomavirus (HPV)
Conjugate subunit	Used to immunize against microbes that have a polysaccharide coating that protects the antigenic material. The antigen is attached to the polysaccharide coat.	*Haemophilus influenzae* type b (Hib) Meningococcal Pneumococcal
DNA vaccine	Experimental but currently being tested in humans. The genes that encode for the antigen are injected into the body; they direct production of the antigen, which then initiates an immune response. Herpes and influenza are being tested with this type of vaccine.	

Source: Modified from Atkinson W, Wolfe S, Hambrosky J, eds. *Epidemiology and Prevention of Vaccine-Preventable Diseases*. 12th ed. Washington, DC: Centers for Disease Control and Prevention; 2012.[3]

system fails to respond with just one dose—a condition most commonly seen with vaccines against measles, mumps, and rubella (MMR) and against varicella. In rare instances, administration of an LAV results in a mild form of the disease. Severe or fatal reactions to LAVs, as a result of uncontrolled replication, occur only in individuals with compromised immune systems, such as those persons with HIV, with leukemia, or taking immunosuppressant drugs.[3,9]

Inactivated Vaccines

Inactivated vaccines are not alive and, therefore, do not replicate in the human body. These vaccines are produced by growing a virus or bacterium in culture media and then inactivating the organism with chemicals and/or heat. In contrast to LAVs, which result in immunity following a single dose, the first dose of an inactivated vaccine simply primes the immune system; subsequent doses are always required to achieve full immunity. Furthermore, antibody titers against inactivated antigens diminish over time, such that individuals require periodic "booster" doses to maintain full immunity. Inactivated vaccines never cause disease from infection, even in individuals with a compromised immune system. Table 6-2 summarizes the differences between live attenuated and inactivated vaccines.[4]

Some inactivated vaccines are derived from the killed pathogen itself. However, others are derived from inactivated toxins from bacteria and stimulate an immune response again toxoid-producing bacteria. This type of vaccine may be categorized as a **toxoid** vaccine.

Subunit vaccines are made from parts of a virus or bacterium instead of the whole organism (e.g., the pertussis component of the DTaP vaccine). Polysaccharides contain long chains of sugar molecules that make up the surface of some bacteria and cause an immune response by stimulating B lymphocytic cells without assistance from T-helper cells. However, pure **polysaccharide vaccines** are not highly immunogenic. Thus, some polysaccharide vaccines are conjugated to improve the response, especially within immature immune systems such as are found among infants and young children. Conjugation is a chemical process in which a polysaccharide from an antigen is attached to a carrier protein. Conjugation changes the response from T-cell independent to T-cell dependent, which makes the immune response more robust.

More recently, genetic engineering has enabled a gene for a vaccine protein to be inserted into another virus or into culture cells. The final vaccine protein is known as a **recombinant vaccine**. The hepatitis B vaccine currently

Table 6-2 Live Attenuated Vaccines versus Inactivated Vaccines

Effect	Live Attenuated Vaccines	Inactivated Vaccines
Ability to cause disease	Small dose of attenuated bacteria replicates and stimulates active immunity. Could rarely cause disease.	Killed bacteria or component of bacteria stimulates active immunity. Cannot cause disease.
Number of doses required	One dose required.	Subsequent doses required to stimulate B lymphocytic cells to make antibody that will remain in immunologic memory. Periodic booster doses may also be required.
Effect of circulating antibody	Circulating antibody can interfere with replication of the attenuated antigen and disrupt or obstruct the antibody response and subsequent development of active immunity.	Circulating antibody will not affect the antibody response and development of active immunity. Vaccines can be administered if antibody is present (e.g., in a newborn who might have transplacentally acquired the antibody).
Use in pregnancy	Contraindicated in pregnancy. Some may be contraindicated for persons with specific immunosuppressed states.	May be given during pregnancy.

Source: Modified from Atkinson W, Wolfe S, Hambrosky J, eds. *Epidemiology and Prevention of Vaccine-Preventable Diseases.* 12th ed. Washington, DC: Centers for Disease Control and Prevention; 2012.[3]

used in the United States is a recombinant vaccine, for example. Genetic engineering is also used to combine two types of human papillomavirus (HPV) vaccines. When virus-like particles are produced, they can stimulate an immune response, but because they do not contain HPV genetic material, they cannot cause the infection.

Factors Affecting Responses to Vaccines

Several factors influence the response of a given recipient to a vaccine, including the recipient's immune status, genetics, age, and the type of vaccine administered. The following factors are taken into consideration when making recommendations regarding the age at which each vaccine is given: (1) age-specific risks for disease; (2) age-specific risks for complications associated with the disease; (3) age-related response to vaccine; and (4) potential for passively transferred antibodies to interfere with the immune response of the vaccine.[1] For example, neonates will have received passively transferred antibodies during pregnancy and breastfeeding that could interfere with their independent immune response to a particular vaccine.

Another factor that affects whether receipt of a vaccine will induce durable immunity is the amount of time between the initial dose, subsequent doses in the series, and booster doses. Vaccines that require multiple boosters must not be administered earlier than recommended. Giving the booster dose too early will not increase the immune response because the immune system does not recognize the second vaccine as a separate event (Figure 6-2).[9]

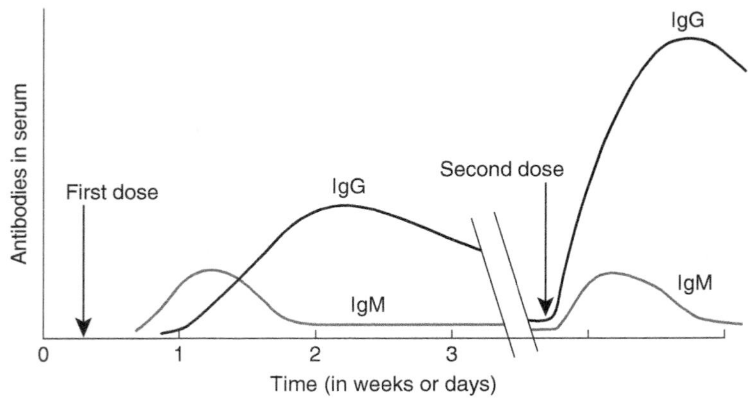

Figure 6-2 IgG and IgM following booster dose of vaccine.

Vaccine Schedules

The CDC Advisory Committee on Immunization Practices (ACIP) regularly issues recommendations about specific vaccines that should be offered to newborns, children, adolescents, and adults. Vaccination recommendations change frequently depending on the evolving epidemiology of vaccine-preventable diseases, the introduction of new vaccine products, and the supply of various agents, which can be adversely affected by production problems. Vaccine recommendations are released annually and are available for young children (0 to 6 years), older children and adolescents (ages 7 to 18 years), and adults.

Because of the rapidly changing nature of these recommendations, the recommended vaccine schedules/tables are likely to become outdated quickly and are not provided in this text. For example, in 2015, the CDC modified the adult schedule to change the suggestion that individuals 65 years or older might receive the 13 valent pneumococcal conjugate vaccine (PVC13) to a recommendation. Therefore, the major vaccines are reviewed in this chapter but providers are advised to check the CDC's website or vaccine app; both are listed in the resources provided at the end of this chapter.[10,11]

Age-Specific Vaccine Schedules

Each year an estimated 45,000 adults die from vaccine-preventable diseases.[12] One of the greatest challenges faced by healthcare providers is accessing a complete vaccination history for adolescents and adults. In general, if a full vaccination history is not available following every attempt to obtain such a history, healthcare providers should consider adolescent and adult women to be unvaccinated and administer the recommended age-appropriate vaccine—a process called catch-up vaccination. Box 6-3 describes a regular primary care visit with a focus on vaccination.

Box 6-3 A Primary Care Visit

JT is a 60-year-old, healthy woman who comes in today for a regular visit. She does not have any vaccination records and cannot remember receiving any vaccinations in several years. Her provider is faced with the challenge of what to do.

Based on the ACIP information obtained from the CDC website, the Tdap vaccine should be offered because she is overdue for her 10-year tetanus booster and because pertussis control is currently needed in the United States. At the time of this writing, ACIP recommends that Tdap replace the next Td booster dose for all adults. Subsequent booster doses should be given every 10 years with Td. Influenza vaccination is also recommended for this woman because it is indicated for all individuals 6 months or older.

The herpes zoster vaccine is of particular note because it is recommended for the prevention of shingles and should be offered as a one-time vaccine to all individuals 60 years or older.

Vaccines for measles, mumps, rubella, and varicella are unnecessary for this woman because she is old enough to have been born at a time when these diseases were epidemic. Adults who were born before 1957 should be considered immune to measles (rubeola), mumps, and rubella; adults born before 1980 should be considered immune to varicella.

Pneumococcal vaccines are recommended for use starting at age 65 for healthy adults. Thus, JT should be informed about their importance for the future, but it is too early to recommend this vaccine for JT today.

All the common inactivated vaccines can be given at the same time without decreasing the effectiveness of any individual vaccine. The response to live attenuated vaccines may be impaired if administered within 28 days of each other if given on different days but if given simultaneously, they do not interfere with the immune response. JT needs herpes zoster vaccine and influenza vaccine, both of which are live attenuated vaccines. She is counseled about vaccines and, after providing informed consent, she is given the influenza vaccine and Tdap today. She has chosen to delay the herpes zoster vaccine so she can check to make sure her insurance covers it and is told she should wait at least 30 days if she does not want the vaccine today. She makes an appointment to return for the herpes zoster vaccine in 2 months.

While many of the vaccines offered to adults and children are directed at the same vaccine-preventable illnesses, the specific vaccine products offered to newborns and children may need to be adapted for use in older individuals. For example, tetanus, pertussis, and diphtheria vaccines have long been offered to both adults and children. While all of the vaccine formulations provide protection against diphtheria and tetanus, and some provide protection against pertussis, there are major differences in each product in terms of the relative dose for each disease. A capitalized letter signifies a larger dose and a small letter signifies a smaller dose of the various components. Vaccines for adults and adolescents contain reduced amounts of diphtheria toxoid but similar levels of tetanus toxoid and inactivated pertussis antigen compared with pediatric formulations (Box 6-4). Formulations offered to infants and children include DTaP and DT; adolescent and adult formulations include Td and Tdap. While dosage levels of diphtheria toxoid are higher in vaccines for children than adults, dosages of other vaccine products such as hepatitis B are lower for pediatric individuals.[3]

Box 6-4 A Gynecologic Visit for an Adolescent

ML is a 17-year-old adolescent in the office today for a regular visit. She is using a ParaGard intrauterine device (IUD) and has been in a monogamous relationship for a year. You ask to see her vaccination record. It reveals she completed her five-dose DTaP series at age 6 years, four doses of inactivated polio vaccine, two measles, mumps and rubella (MMR), two varicella (VAR), and three hepatitis B (Hep B) vaccines. You must now consider which vaccines are indicated.

Because ML has not had any vaccinations since she was 6 years old, she needs catch-up vaccines. A Tdap booster is indicated for all adolescents at 11 years with catch-up if the booster was not previously administered.

Meningococcal vaccine is also indicated for all 11- to 12-year-olds with catch-up when indicated.

While the optimal time to give human papillomavirus (HPV) vaccine is before sexual debut, it is still useful to give this vaccine to older adolescents and young women. Even if ML is infected with one of the strains of HPV contained in the vaccine, the vaccine will protect her against the other strains for which it is indicated.

Another major difference between the various vaccine schedules is that more products using unique combinations of vaccines are available for use among children than are available for adults. While similar to each other, not all of them are approved for use in the exact same populations or may be used interchangeably, making the schedule very complex to administer in children. For example, two Tdap products are available: Boostrix and Adacel. Boostrix is available for use among individuals 10 years and older, including adults 65 or older, whereas Adacel is approved for use only in adolescents and adults 11–64 years.[4]

Prior to age 19 years, young women are considered to have complete vaccine coverage if they have received the full series of vaccines against hepatitis A and B; rotavirus; diphtheria, tetanus, and acellular pertussis; *Haemophilus influenzae* type B; pneumococcal vaccines; polio; influenza; measles, mumps and rubella; varicella; human papillomavirus; and meningococcal conjugate vaccine. The following vaccines are recommended for women 19 years and older: HPV; influenza; measles, mumps, and rubella; tetanus, diphtheria, and pertussis (Td/Tdap); varicella; and zoster. Under special circumstances, it may be suggested that a woman in this age group should have hepatitis A, hepatitis B, and pneumococcal vaccines (PCV13, PPSV23).[13] The herpes zoster vaccine is recommended for women 60 years or older. The pneumococcal product is indicated for individuals 65 years and older.

Common Vaccines for Women

Multiple vaccines exist for women of various ages in the United States. The following are among the most commonly administered. This discussion of vaccines is followed by a description of immunoglobulins, which, although they are not vaccines, are used in clinical practice essentially to provoke passive immunization among women in certain situations.

Hepatitis A

Hepatitis A virus (HAV) is acquired through fecal–oral transmission and replicates in the liver. The symptoms of acute HAV are indistinguishable from the symptoms of other types of acute viral hepatitis. The illness typically has an abrupt onset of fever, malaise, anorexia, nausea, abdominal pain, dark urine, and jaundice. Clinical illness usually does not last longer than 2 months, although 10% to 15% of persons have prolonged or relapsing signs and symptoms for up to 6 months. Virus may be excreted during a relapse. No carrier state exists for hepatitis A.[14]

The likelihood of symptomatic illness from HAV infection is directly related to age. In children younger than 6 years, most infections are asymptomatic. Children play an important role in HAV transmission, however. They may serve as a source of infection particularly for household or other close contacts. Historically, children 2–18 years have experienced the highest rates of hepatitis A. Since 2002, rates among children have declined due to immunization, and the incidence of hepatitis A is now similar in all age groups.

Other groups at increased risk for hepatitis A infection include international travelers, men who have sex with men, and persons who use illegal drugs. Food handlers are not at increased risk for hepatitis A because of their occupation, but are noteworthy because of their critical role in common-source food-borne HAV transmission if they are infected.[3]

Hepatitis A Vaccine

Vaccination against hepatitis A has been incorporated into the routine childhood vaccine schedule, but is generally offered only to adults who are at high-risk for contracting the infection. Two preparations of hepatitis A vaccine are currently available in the United States: Havrix, a combination vaccine developed in a preparation containing neomycin, and Vaqta, an inactivated whole virus. A single primary dose is followed in 6 months by the booster dose. Limited data indicate that the vaccines from different manufacturers are interchangeable.

The most commonly reported adverse reaction following vaccination is a local reaction at the site of injection. Injection-site pain, erythema, or swelling is reported by 20% to 50% of recipients. These symptoms are generally mild and self-limited. Mild systemic complaints (e.g., malaise, fatigue, low-grade fever) are reported by fewer than 10% of recipients. No serious adverse reactions have been reported.[3,14]

Hepatitis B

Hepatitis B is characterized by an insidious onset of malaise, anorexia, nausea, vomiting, right upper quadrant abdominal pain, fever, headache, myalgia, skin rashes, arthralgia and arthritis, and dark urine beginning 1–2 days before the onset of jaundice. Clinical signs and symptoms occur more often in adults than in infants or children, who usually have an asymptomatic acute course. However, 50% of adults who have acute infections are asymptomatic.

Box 6-5 A Case of a Chronic Carrier

Typhoid Mary was a cook who lived in New York during the turn of the last century. She was a carrier of typhoid: In other words, she was capable of infecting others but was herself asymptomatic. Because of her occupation, Mary transmitted the disease to a number of people, some who died of being infected with typhoid. Ultimately, Mary endured two decades of isolation until her death because no treatment for the chronic carrier state could be found. Although a number of diseases, such as tuberculosis, can have a chronic carrier state, hepatitis B is one of the few diseases with chronic carriers for which a vaccine exists.

Hepatitis B virus (HBV) is the most common known cause of chronic viremia, with more than 350 million persons estimated to be chronically infected worldwide. Box 6-5 describes a famous historical chronic carrier of another disease that like hepatitis can be present as a chronic condition in a person who is asymptomatic but infectious. HBV infection is an established cause of acute and chronic hepatitis and cirrhosis, and is the cause of as many as 80% of hepatocellular carcinomas.[15] Among known human carcinogens, it is second only to tobacco in causing actual cases of cancer.

The key route of transmission of hepatitis B is via contamination of mucosal surfaces with infective serum or plasma. Fecal–oral transmission does not appear to occur. In the United States, the most important route of transmission is via sexual contact, either heterosexual or homosexual, with an infected person. Direct percutaneous inoculation of HBV by needles during injection drug use is the second most common mode of transmission. Transmission of HBV may also occur by other percutaneous exposure, including tattooing, ear piercing, and acupuncture, as well as needlesticks or other injuries from sharp instruments sustained by medical personnel. These exposures account for only a small proportion of reported cases in the United States. Breaks in the skin without overt needle puncture, such as fresh cutaneous scratches, abrasions, burns, or other lesions, may serve as other routes for entry.

Transmission may also occur during mouth pipetting, eye splashes, or other direct contact with mucous membranes of the eyes or mouth. Transfer of infective material to skin lesions or mucous membranes via inanimate environmental surfaces may occur by touching surfaces of various types of hospital equipment. Contamination of mucosal surfaces with infective secretions other than serum or plasma could occur with contact involving semen. While most HBV infections in adults result in complete recovery, fulminant hepatitis occurs in about 1% to 2% of acutely infected persons.[15]

Because hepatitis B infection is common in certain subgroups in the United States and is epidemic in many parts of the world, it may be that an individual already has been infected and is not in need of vaccination. In this case, serologic testing can help distinguish whether an individual is acutely or chronically infected or is susceptible and could benefit from vaccination. Lab indices and their clinical interpretation are listed in Table 6-3.

Serologic Tests

Perinatal transmission of HBV from mother to infant at birth is very efficient. If the mother is positive for both HBsAg (hepatitis B surface antigen) and HBeAg (antigen contained in the core of HBV that indicates high infectivity), 70% to 90% of infants born to these women will become infected in the absence of postexposure prophylaxis. As many as 90% of infants who become infected will develop a chronic infection.[16] The risk of perinatal transmission is approximately 10% if the mother is positive only for HBsAg. Postexposure prophylaxis requires provision of hepatitis B immunoglobulin and initiation of the three-dose vaccine series immediately after birth. Infants who weigh less than 2000 g at birth and who are born to women who are HBsAg-positive have a decreased immune response to vaccine and a high risk of exposure during birth; these infants need an additional dose of vaccine (a total of four doses) starting at 1 month of age.[13]

Because not all women are tested for hepatitis B before the birth of the infant and some women may have become acutely infected after the last test result was obtained, a woman's status may not be known with accuracy when she gives birth. Therefore, hepatitis B vaccination for all infants soon after birth and before hospital discharge is the strategy recommended by the ACIP, even for those infants born to women who were tested and found to be HBsAg negative. Infants born to women whose status is unknown should receive hepatitis B vaccinations within 12 hours of birth and hepatitis B immunoglobulin (HBIG) no later than 7 days after birth if the mother tests positive. Because preterm infants' immune systems respond less robustly than term infants, infants weighing less than 2000 g who are born to women whose HBsAg status is unknown should also receive the hepatitis immunoglobulin, HBIG.[13]

Table 6-3 Interpretation of Hepatitis B Serologic Tests

Tests	Results	Interpretation
HBsAg Anti-HBc Anti-HBs	Negative Negative Negative	Susceptible
HBsAg Anti-HBc Anti-HBs	Negative Negative Positive with ≥ 10 mIU/mL[a]	Immune due to vaccination
HBsAg Anti-HBc Anti-HBs	Negative Positive Positive	Immune due to natural infection
HBsAg Anti-HBc IgM anti-HBc Anti-HBs	Positive Positive Positive Negative	Acutely infected
HBsAg Anti-HBc IgM anti-HBc Anti-HBs	Positive Positive Negative Negative	Chronically infected
HBsAg Anti-HBc Anti-HBs	Negative Positive Negative	Four interpretations possible[b]

[a] Postvaccination testing, when it is recommended, should be performed 1–2 months following dose number 3.

[b] (1) May be recovering from acute HBV infection; (2) may be distantly immune and the test is not sensitive enough to detect a very low level of anti-HBs in serum; (3) may be susceptible with a false positive anti-HBc; (4) may be chronically infected and have an undetectable level of HBsAg present in the serum.

Source: Data from Atkinson W, Wolfe S, Hambrosky J, eds. *Epidemiology and Prevention of Vaccine-Preventable Diseases.* 12th ed. Washington, DC: Centers for Disease Control and Prevention; 2012.[3]

Hepatitis B Vaccine

Hepatitis B vaccine is produced by two manufacturers, GlaxoSmithKline (Engerix-B) and Merck (Recombivax HB). The recommended dose of vaccine differs depending on the age of the recipient and type of vaccine; see Table 6-4 for the dosing schedule. Although the antigen content of the vaccines differ, vaccines made by different manufacturers are interchangeable with one exception: Only the Merck vaccine is approved for the alternate two-dose schedule for adolescents age 11–15 years. Providers must always follow the manufacturer's dosage recommendations. Both vaccines are now available as thimerosal-free preparations.[3]

Following three intramuscular doses of hepatitis B vaccine, more than 90% of healthy adults develop adequate antibody responses. Correct administration is also the key to durable immunity. The deltoid muscle is the recommended site for hepatitis B vaccination in adults; immunogenicity of the vaccine is lower when injections are given in the gluteus. However, there is an age-specific decline

Table 6-4 Recommended Doses of Currently Approved Formulations of Hepatitis B Vaccine by Age Group and Vaccine Type

	Single-Antigen Vaccine				Combination Vaccine					
	Recombivax HB		Engerix-B		Comvax		Pediatrix		Twinrix	
Age Group	**Dose (mcg)[a]**	**Volume (mL)**	**Dose (mcg)[a]**	**Volume (mL)**	**Dose (mcg)[a]**	**Volume (mL)**	**Dose (mcg)[a]**	**Volume (mL)**	**Dose (mcg)[a]**	**Volume (mL)**
Infants (< 1 year)	5	0.5	10	0.5	5	0.5	0	0.5	N/A	N/A
Children (1–10 years)	5	0.5	10	0.5	5	0.5	10	0.5	N/A	N/A
Adolescents										
11–15 years	10[b]	1.0	N/A	N/A	N/A	N/A	N/A	N/A	N/A	N/A
11–19 years	5	0.5	10	0.5	N/A	N/A	N/A	N/A	N/A	N/A
Adults (≥ 20 years)	10	1.0	20	1.0	N/A	N/A	N/A	N/A	20	1.0
Hemodialysis patients and other immuno-compromised persons	5	0.5	1.0	0.5	N/A	N/A	N/A	N/A	N/A	N/A
< 20 years[c]	5	0.5	10	0.5	N/A	N/A	N/A	N/A	N/A	N/A
≥ 20 years	40[d]	1.0	40[c]	2.0	N/A	N/A	N/A	N/A	N/A	N/A

Abbreviations: N/A = not applicable.
[a] Recombinant hepatitis B surface antigen protein dose.
[b] Adult formulation administered on a two-dose schedule.
[c] Higher doses might be more immunogenic, but no specific recommendations have been made.
[d] Dialysis formulation administered on a three-dose schedule at age 0, 1, and 6 months.
Source: Reproduced from Atkinson W, Wolfe S, Hambrosky J, eds. *Epidemiology and Prevention of Vaccine-Preventable Diseases.* 12th ed. Washington, DC: Centers for Disease Control and Prevention; 2012.[3]

in immunogenicity. After age 40 years, approximately 90% of recipients respond to a three-dose series; by 60 years, only 75% of persons vaccinated develop protective antibody titers.[3]

The HBV vaccine is 80% to 100% effective in preventing infection or clinical hepatitis in those who receive the complete course of vaccine. Larger vaccine doses (2 to 4 times the normal adult dose) or an increased number of doses may be required to induce protective antibodies in persons on hemodialysis and those who are immunocompromised.[15]

The most common adverse reaction following hepatitis B vaccine is pain at the site of injection. Mild systemic complaints such as fatigue, headache, and irritability have been reported. Fever has been reported in 1% of adults, but serious systemic adverse reactions and allergic reactions are rarely reported following administration of this vaccine. No evidence has been reported that administration of HBV vaccine at or shortly after birth increases the number of febrile episodes, sepsis evaluations, or allergic or neurologic events in the newborn period.

Hepatitis B vaccine has been suggested to cause or exacerbate multiple sclerosis (MS). A single study in a British population found a slight increase in risk of MS among hepatitis B vaccine recipients.[17] However, earlier large population-based studies have shown no association between receipt of hepatitis B vaccine and either the development of MS or exacerbation of the course of MS in persons already diagnosed with disease.[17,18]

Occupational Exposure to Hepatitis B

Occupational exposure to hepatitis B deserves special mention. Table 6-5 presents the recommended doses of hepatitis B vaccine for persons who are exposed to hepatitis B through occupational contact.

Combination Hepatitis A and Hepatitis B Vaccine

Combination hepatitis A and hepatitis B vaccine (Twinrix) contains approximately half the adult dose of hepatitis A vaccine and the usual adult dose of hepatitis B vaccine. By giving a reduced dose of hepatitis A vaccine, this formulation can be used in place of the three-dose single-agent hepatitis B vaccine schedule and provides good protection against both diseases. Twinrix is approved for persons 18 years and older.[19]

Table 6-5 Recommended Postexposure Prophylaxis for Occupational Exposure to Hepatitis B Virus

	Treatment		
Vaccination and Antibody Response of Exposed Workers[a]	**Source HBsAg**[b] **Positive**	**Source HBsAg**[b] **Negative**	**Source Unknown or Not Available for Testing**
Unvaccinated	HBIG[c] once and initiate HB vaccine series	Initiate HB vaccine series	Initiate HB vaccine series
Previously vaccinated			
Known responder[d]	No treatment	No treatment	No treatment
Known nonresponder[e]	HBIG once and initiate revaccination or HBIG twice[f]	No treatment	If known high-risk source, treat as if source were HBsAg positive
Antibody response unknown	Test exposed person for anti-HBs.[g] If adequate,[d] no treatment is necessary. If inadequate,[e] administer HBIG once and vaccine booster.	No treatment	Test exposed person for anti-HBs.[g] If adequate,[d] no treatment is necessary. If inadequate,[e] administer vaccine booster and recheck titer in 1–2 months.

[a] Persons who have previously been infected with HBV are immune to reinfection and do not require postexposure prophylaxis.
[b] Hepatitis B surface antigen.
[c] Hepatitis B immune globulin; dose is 0.06 mL/kg administered intramuscularly.
[d] A responder is a person with adequate levels of serum antibody to HBsAg (i.e., anti-HBs ≥ 10 mIU/mL).
[e] A nonresponder is a person with inadequate response to vaccination (i.e., serum anti-HBs < 10 mIU/mL).
[f] The option of giving one dose of HBIG and reinitiating the vaccine series is preferred for nonresponders who have not completed a second three-dose vaccine series. For persons who previously completed a second vaccine series but failed to respond, two doses of HBIG are preferred.
[g] Antibody to HBsAg.
Sources: Reproduced from Atkinson W, Wolfe S, Hambrosky J, eds. *Epidemiology and Prevention of Vaccine-Preventable Diseases.* 12th ed. Washington, DC: Centers for Disease Control and Prevention; 2012[3]; Centers for Disease Control and Prevention. Recommended adult vaccine schedule, by vaccine and age group: United States, 2015. http://www.cdc.gov/vaccines/schedules/downloads/adult/adult-schedule-easy-read-bw.pdf. Accessed February 5, 2015.[11]

Human Papillomavirus

Human papillomavirus (HPV) is the most common sexually transmitted infection in the United States. This infection is so prevalent that the CDC estimates that almost all sexually active adults will become infected at some point in their lives. An estimated 20 million people in the United States are currently infected with HPV, and at least half of those are adolescents and young adults age 15–24 years.

Although most HPV infections are asymptomatic and resolve spontaneously, certain types of the virus can cause cervical intraepithelial neoplasm (CIN) grade 2 or greater, adenocarcinoma in situ, and CIN grade 1. Oncogenic high-risk HPV types are detected in 99% of all cervical cancers. Less commonly, HPV can cause cancers of the anus, penis, oropharynx, vulva, and vagina. Of the more than 100 HPV types (Figure 6-3), types 16 and 18 account for approximately 70% of cervical cancers and 70% of anal/genital cancers, and types 6 and 11 account for 90% of genital warts. An estimated 17,000 women in the United States are diagnosed each year with cancer attributed to HPV. Non-oncogenic HPV types can cause genital warts and warts in the respiratory tract of children, a rare form of disease known as juvenile-onset recurrent respiratory papillomatosis (RRP).[20,21]

Human Papillomavirus Vaccine

The CDC recommends a three-dose HPV vaccine series for all adolescents age 11–12 years. Those young women age 13–18 years who have not been previously vaccinated should also receive the three-dose series. In addition, the CDC recommends that all women age 19–26 years who have not been previously immunized receive a three-dose series.[11]

Currently, three HPV vaccines are licensed by the Food and Drug Administration (FDA) for use in the United States. Human papillomavirus bivalent types 16 and 18 vaccine, recombinant (Cervarix, 2vHPV) prevents infection with HPV types 16 and 18, which cause of 70% of cervical cancers. Human papillomavirus quadrivalent types 6, 11, 16, and 18 vaccine, recombinant (Gardasil, 4vHPV) protects against HPV types 6, 11, 16, and 18. Types 6 and 11 cause approximately 90% of genital warts. The newest 9-valent vaccine (Gardasil-9, 9vHPV) protects against HPV types, 6, 11, 16, 18, 31, 33, 45, 52, and 58. This vaccine is effective against five additional cancer-causing types of HPV, which account for approximately 15% of cervical cancers. HPV vaccines are licensed for use in females, may be given with other age-appropriate vaccines, and are administered intramuscularly in a three-dose series over 6 months (the second dose is given 2 months after the first

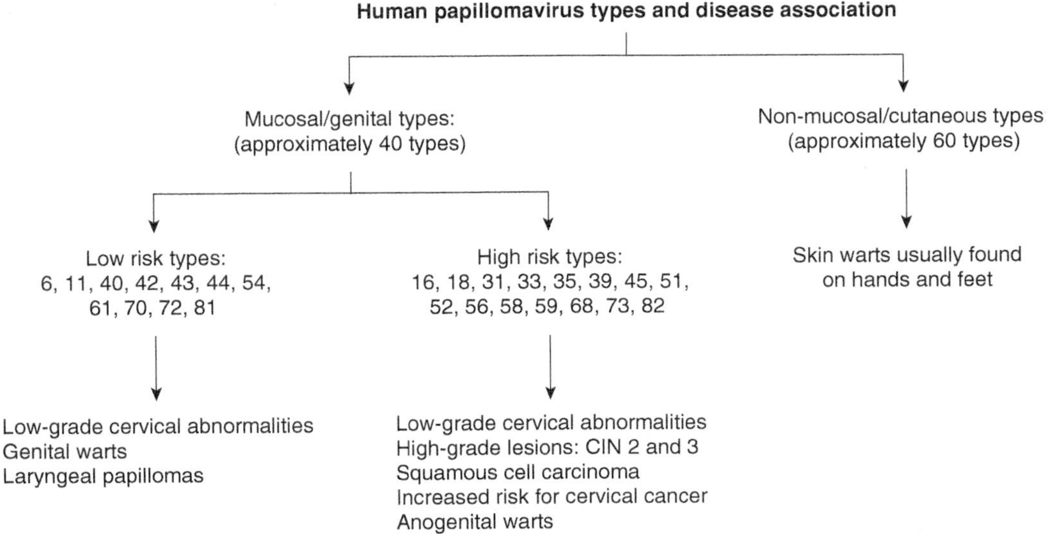

Figure 6-3 Human papillomavirus types and associated diseases.

dose and the third is given 6 months after the first dose).[21] Gardasil and Gardasil-9 have also been licensed for use in males. The efficacy of the 2vHPV and 3vHPV vaccines, after completion of the three-dose series, is identified in Table 6-6. The efficacy of the 9vHPV is approximately 96% for cervical cancer and vaginal epithelial neoplasia.

Close monitoring for adverse drug events associated with HPV vaccines has revealed that these vaccines have high levels of safety. The most commonly reported drug reactions are dizziness, fainting, nausea, headache, fever, hives, and injection-site pain, redness, and swelling.[22]

HPV vaccines are contraindicated for anyone with a history of hypersensitivity to any of the vaccine components, and women with moderate or severe acute illnesses should postpone vaccination until the illness subsides. The 4vHPV and 9vHPV vaccines are contraindicated for women with a history of hypersensitivity to yeast, and the 2vHPV prefilled syringes should not be given to women who have a latex sensitivity.

Table 6-6 Results of Selected Clinical Trials on HPV Vaccine Efficacy Against HPV Vaccine-Type Precancers and Anogenital Warts

Outcome	Vaccine	Sex	Vaccine Efficacy
Cervical precancer	2vHPV and 4vHPV	Females	> 93%
Vaginal/vulvar precancer	4vHPV	Females	100%
Anal precancer	4vHPV	Males	75%
Anogenital warts	4vHPV	Females Males	99% 89%

Source: Reproduced from Centers for Disease Control and Prevention. HPV vaccine information for clinicians: fact sheet. http://www.cdc.gov/std/HPV/STDFact-HPV-vaccine-hcp.htm. Accessed June 11, 2014.[22]

HPV vaccines should not be given to women who are pregnant. There are limited data on HPV vaccination in pregnancy, although the vaccines have not been causally associated with adverse pregnancy outcomes. Exposure to HPV vaccine during pregnancy should be reported to the manufacturer-supported pregnancy registry for this vaccine.

The HPV vaccination provides immunity only from new exposure to the virus; it does not treat existing infection or reduce the incidence of cervical cancer in women who were infected with HPV prior to vaccination. Furthermore, 30% of cervical cancers are caused by HPV types that are not covered by the vaccine. Therefore, it is important for healthcare providers to recommend that all women continue to seek cervical cancer screening according to evidence-based recommendations.[23]

Influenza

Influenza is a highly contagious disease of the respiratory system caused by a variety of influenza viruses. Spread by droplet, influenza is the most common vaccine-preventable disease in the United States. Symptoms include rapid onset of fever and chills, sore throat, muscle aches, fatigue, cough, headache, and runny nose. Influenza is considered a seasonal disease that usually occurs in the fall and winter, with peak occurrences in January. The risks for severe complications of influenza, most often associated with secondary bacterial pneumonia, are greatest for young children, persons 65 years and older, women who are pregnant,[25] and persons of any age with certain medical conditions.[24,26]

Influenza Vaccines

The CDC recommends that all persons older than 6 months receive an influenza vaccine each year during flu season.[11] Although the influenza vaccine usually becomes available in October, women may appropriately receive protection against the disease with vaccination any time during the flu season.[3]

Two types of influenza vaccines have been approved for use in adolescents: inactivated influenza vaccine (IIV) and live attenuated influenza vaccine (LAIV). Inactivated influenza vaccines are administered intramuscularly and are available in pediatric and adult doses. These vaccines are available in trivalent vaccines (which protect against three viruses) and quadrivalent vaccines (which protect against four viruses).[19] The efficacy of influenza vaccines varies and largely depends on the similarity of the vaccine strain to the strain of virus that is circulating in a given year.[3] Most influenza vaccines are inactive and grown in egg products, so women and girls who have an egg allergy should not receive standard IIVs.

Contraindications to use of any influenza vaccine are presented in Table 6-7. Precautions with use of influenza vaccines are necessary when individuals have moderate to severe illness or a history of Guillain-Barré syndrome within 6 months of receiving a previous influenza vaccine.[27] Side effects of IIVs are usually mild and short-lived and include soreness, redness or swelling at the injection site, low-grade fever, and aches.[28]

Live attenuated influenza vaccines, which are approved for use in persons 2–49 years, are available in quadrivalent formulas (LAIV4) and are delivered intranasally using a prepackaged sprayer. Because inactivated vaccines do not interfere with the immune response to live vaccines, LAIV4 may be administered on the same day or at any time prior to or following the administration of other IIVs (e.g., Tdap). It may also be administered on the same day as other live vaccines—although if they are not administered on the same day, other live vaccines should be given no less than 4 weeks apart. Side effects of LAIVs are mild and self-limiting and include cough, runny nose and nasal congestion, sore throat, and chills. Precautions with the use of LAIVs are the same as the precautions for IIVs.

In 2013, the FDA approved Flublok, a trivalent recombinant influenza vaccine (RIV3) that does not use egg products, for use in adults 18–49 years. Intranasally administered LAIV, marketed as Flumist, may be used only by healthy, nonpregnant women younger than 50 years; LAIV should not be administered to women who are pregnant or healthcare workers who care for severely immunocompromised individuals. The standard-dose IIV or high-dose IIV

Table 6-7 Contraindications and Precautions to the Use of Influenza Vaccines[a]

Vaccine	Contraindications	Precautions
IIV (includes IIV3, IIV4, and ccIIV)	History of severe allergic reaction to any component of the vaccine, including egg protein, or after previous dose of any influenza vaccine	Moderate to severe illness with or without fever History of Guillain-Barré syndrome within 6 weeks of receipt of influenza vaccine
RIV3	History of severe allergic reaction to any component of the vaccine Approved only for persons age 18–49 years	
LAIV[b]	History of severe allergic reaction to any component of the vaccine, including egg protein, or after a previous dose of any influenza vaccine Concomitant aspirin therapy in children and adolescents Age ≤ 2 years or ≥ 50 years Major comorbidities such as disorders of the respiratory system, cardiovascular system, and others; immunocompromise, pregnancy	Moderate to severe illness with or without fever History of Guillain-Barré syndrome within 6 weeks of receipt of influenza vaccine Asthma in persons 5 years or older Medical condition that might predispose to higher risk for complications attributable to influenza

Abbreviations: IIV = inactivated influenza vaccine; IIV3 = inactivated influenza vaccine, trivalent; IIV4 = inactivated influenza vaccine, quadrivalent; RIV3 = recombinant influenza vaccine; LAIV = live-attenuated influenza vaccine.

[a] Providers of vaccines should check FDA-approved prescribing information for influenza vaccines for the most complete and updated information, including, but not limited to, indications, contraindications, and precautions.

[b] A full list of precautions and contraindications can be found on the CDC website.

Source: Reproduced from Centers for Disease Control and Prevention. Prevention and control of seasonal influenza with vaccines: recommendations of the Advisory Committee on Immunization Practices—United States, 2013–2014.[29]

(Fluzone High-Dose) may be used for women 65 years or older.[30]

Measles, Mumps, and Rubella

Rubeola (measles), mumps, and rubella (German measles) are viral infections spread by airborne droplet transmission of respiratory secretions. Because these diseases were once thought to primarily affect children, early attempts at vaccine coverage focused on vaccinating all infants during the first year of life. Although dramatic reductions in the number of reported cases of disease occurred following introduction of these vaccines during the 1960s, during the past 20 years there has been a resurgence of reported cases, particularly among previously immunized adults.[3]

Measles, Mumps, and Rubella Vaccine

A single-dose vaccination with the live, attenuated combined vaccine against measles, mumps, and rubella (MMR) is recommended for all adults born after 1956 who do not have documentation of previous vaccination or laboratory-confirmed immunity to all three diseases.[11] Some individuals may think they are immunized, but actually received vaccines that are no longer recommended in regard to type or timing (Box 6-6). The CDC also recommends that certain groups of adults who are at increased risk for infection receive a second vaccine dose that is administered a minimum of 28 days after the first dose.[11] These groups include students in postsecondary educational institutions and individuals who work in a healthcare facility or plan to travel internationally. The CDC also recommends that healthcare facilities consider vaccinating personnel who were born before 1957 and lack laboratory-confirmed evidence of measles, mumps, and/or rubella immunity. The recommended vaccine schedule for these individuals is two doses of MMR vaccine (at least 28 days apart) for those who are not immune to measles or mumps and one dose of MMR vaccine for those who are not immune to rubella.[11]

Regardless of their year of birth, all women of childbearing age should have serologic confirmation of rubella immunity. Those women who lack evidence of immunity and are not pregnant should be vaccinated with a single dose of MMR vaccine. The MMR vaccine is contraindicated in pregnancy, so women who are pregnant and who are found to lack rubella immunity should be vaccinated with a single dose of MMR vaccine in the immediate postpartum period or after termination of a pregnancy.[11]

Adverse drug reactions associated with the MMR vaccine are uncommon, are usually self-limiting, and include fever, rash, and swelling of the lymph nodes in the cheeks or neck. Rarely, individuals may experience moderate to severe events that include seizures, temporary joint pain and stiffness, and temporary low platelet counts.

Concerns about administration of the vaccine to women who are pregnant stemmed from fears that the vaccine can cause congenital rubella syndrome. As a result, careful monitoring of inadvertent administration of the vaccine occurred from 1971 until 1989. During the monitoring period, there was no evidence of congenital rubella syndrome occurring in the offspring of any of the 321 women who were exposed to the vaccine during pregnancy and who carried their pregnancy to term.[31] Nonetheless, concern regarding the small theoretical risk of congenital rubella syndrome in the offspring of women exposed to the vaccine persists. Women who are pregnant or planning a pregnancy within 4 weeks should not be vaccinated. In the event of inadvertent exposure, women who are pregnant should be counseled about the potential risks. However, MMR exposure should not be considered a reason to recommend pregnancy termination.[32]

Box 6-6 Gone But Not Forgotten: Right Today, Wrong Tomorrow

A common mantra in health care is *Whatever is done today is likely to be found wrong in the future.* A good example of that epigram involves killed or unknown vaccines for measles that were administered between 1963 and 1967 and similar vaccines for mumps that were administered before 1979. Women who received these vaccines may not have maintained immunity and are at increased risk for infection. Thus, these individuals should be evaluated and receive a series of two doses of the vaccine in question.

Meningococcus

Meningococcus is an aerobic, gram-negative bacterium that is spread by droplet aerosol or secretions from the nasopharynx of infected persons or carriers. Most commonly, the invasive form of the disease manifests as meningococcal meningitis, a life-threatening disease with symptoms similar to other forms of meningitis, such as headache, stiff neck, and fever. Meningococcal disease may also present as meningococcal septicemia, pneumonia, arthritis, otitis media, and epiglottitis. Approximately 9% to 12% of cases of invasive meningococcal disease are fatal.[33]

Risk factors for meningococcal disease include age; this disease occurs most commonly in infants and children younger than 5 years, adolescents, young adults age 16–21 years, and adults older than 65 years. The other primary risk factor is crowded living conditions. The increased incidence of disease among first-year college students who live in residence halls led to a recommendation that all college freshmen who live in such settings consider vaccination. Since that time, many colleges and at least 35 states have mandated vaccination against meningococcal disease prior to college admission.[3] Individuals with certain diseases, such as functional or anatomic asplenia, and travelers to certain regions of the world are also at increased risk for infection.[33]

Meningococcal Vaccine

A single dose of meningococcal vaccine administered at age 11–12 years with a booster dose at age 16 years is recommended. Adolescents age 11–18 years who have HIV should receive two doses, at least 8 weeks apart. All adolescents age 13–18 years who have not been previously immunized should receive the vaccine. If the first dose is given at age 13–15 years, a booster dose should be administered at age 16–18 years but no sooner than 8 weeks following the first dose. A booster dose is not necessary for adolescents immunized at 16 years or older.[11]

Meningococcal conjugate vaccine products are occasionally referred to by the names that reflect their serotypes (e.g., A, C). These include MenACY-D, which is marketed under the brand name Menactra, and MenACWY-CRM, also known by the brand name Menveo. Both of these vaccines are quadrivalent meningococcal polysaccharide conjugate vaccines that are conjugated to diphtheria toxoid protein to improve immunogenicity. Both vaccines are available in single-dose vials, are administered intramuscularly, and may be given concomitantly with other vaccines.

A meningococcal polysaccharide vaccine (abbreviated as MPSV4 and marketed as Menomune) is also available and may be recommended if the other options are not available; this product is the only meningococcal vaccine licensed for persons older than 55 years. Adverse effects of these vaccines occur infrequently, but include fever, headache, erythema at the injection site, and dizziness with syncope following administration (most commonly in adolescents). Rare cases of Guillain-Barré syndrome have been reported following vaccination, although since 2010, ACIP has not included a history of Guillain-Barré syndrome as a precaution or a contraindication for meningococcal vaccination because the benefits of vaccination outweigh the potential risk for recurrent disease.[34]

Pneumococcal Disease

Pneumococcal disease is an acute bacterial infection caused by *Streptococcus pneumoniae* that usually presents as one of three clinical syndromes: pneumonia, bacteremia, and meningitis. The most common of these forms is pneumococcal pneumonia. Regardless of the syndrome that manifests, pneumococcal disease may cause severe debilitation; in many instances, it is fatal. Morbidity and mortality rates are higher among the elderly.[3]

Pneumococcal Vaccine

The CDC recommends vaccination against pneumococcal disease for all women 65 years and older, and for all women who smoke cigarettes, have asthma, or are residents of long-term care facilities.[11] For these women, the CDC recommendation calls for a single dose of pneumococcal polysaccharide (PPSV23).

Two vaccines are available for use in the United States: the pneumococcal conjugate vaccine (PCV13) and the pneumococcal polysaccharide vaccine 23—valent (PPSV23). While the PPSV23 vaccine covers more pneumococcal strains than the PCV13 vaccine (23 versus 13 respectively), it induces a weaker immune response in young children than in adults. Consequently, the PCV13 vaccine is the only product approved for use in children younger than 2 years, whereas the PPSV23 vaccine is the preferred product in older children and adults because of its broader coverage and stronger immunogenicity in this population. All women with certain high-risk conditions should be offered vaccination with PCV13 or PPSV23, and the current list of specific high-risk groups is available from the CDC. The PVC13 is also now available for women 65 years and older.[11,35]

Pneumococcal vaccines are administered by injection, either intramuscularly or subcutaneously. The most common adverse effect of pneumococcal vaccine is a local reaction that includes pain and swelling at the injection site, which generally resolves within 48 hours. Fewer than 1% of persons who receive the vaccine develop systemic reactions such as fever and myalgia.[35]

Polio

The response to polio infection is highly variable. As many as 95% of all persons with polio infections are asymptomatic. When they do appear, symptoms can vary from upper respiratory symptoms to gastrointestinal symptoms to nonparalytic aseptic meningitis. Fewer than 1% of all persons with polio infection develop flaccid paralysis. Many persons with paralytic poliomyelitis recover completely, and muscle function returns to some degree in most individuals who experience this condition.[36]

Polio Vaccine

Jonas Salk introduced the first inactivated polio vaccine (IPV) in 1955. Several years later, Albert Sabin introduced the live attenuated oral polio vaccine (OPV). Since 1980, the only indigenous polio cases in the United States have been vaccine acquired, with 8 to 9 such cases occurring annually. Since the Western Hemisphere was declared polio free in 1991, the risk of vaccine-acquired polio was no longer acceptable.[1] Thus, in 2000, the CDC and the ACIP changed the immunization schedule and opted for an IPV-only schedule; use of OPV was discontinued. The inactivated IPV in current use in the United States is an enhanced-potency IPV that was licensed in 1987.[36]

Routine vaccination of adults (18 years and older) who reside in the United States is not necessary or recommended because most adults already received a complete vaccine series in childhood and are immune. In addition, wild-type polio has been eliminated from the United States, so adults have a very small risk of exposure to wild-type poliovirus. Adults who are at increased risk of infection include travelers to epidemic areas (currently Afghanistan, Nigeria, and Pakistan), travelers to areas that have wild poliovirus circulation, some laboratory workers, and healthcare personnel in close contact with individuals who may be excreting wild-type polioviruses. For those at risk, a three-dose series is recommended if these individuals have not been previously immunized.[11,36]

Side effects of IPV may include minor local reactions (pain, redness). No serious adverse reactions to IPV have been documented.[3]

Tetanus, Diphtheria Toxoids, and Acellular Pertussis

Tetanus, an often fatal disease, is caused by an exotoxin that is produced when the bacterium *Clostridium tetani* enters the body through a wound and acts at several sites within the central nervous system to interfere with the release of neurotransmitters, resulting in symptoms that range from trismus (lockjaw), stiff neck, and difficulty swallowing to seizures. Alterations in temperature, blood pressure, and heart rate are also frequently seen.

Diphtheria is caused by the bacterium *Clostridium diphtheria* and is transmitted when the organism comes in contact with any mucous membrane, most commonly the mucous membranes of the nose and mouth. Symptoms of the disease are related to the site of infection, but usually involve the nose, throat, and pharynx.[3,37]

Pertussis is a highly communicable disease caused by the bacterium *Bordetella pertussis*, which is transmitted via the respiratory route through contact either with respiratory droplets or with airborne droplets of respiratory secretions.[38] The incidence of pertussis decreased dramatically following the introduction of the pertussis vaccine during the 1940s.[39] However, the incidence has gradually been increasing since the 1980s and the disease is currently considered endemic in the United States.[40] The increased incidence over the past 20 years most likely reflects waning population immunity.[39] There were 48,277 cases of pertussis reported in 2012, with evidence indicating that the disease is significantly underreported.[41]

Tetanus, Diphtheria Toxoids, and Acellular Pertussis Vaccine

Pertussis outbreak control efforts are aimed primarily at reducing morbidity and mortality from the disease among newborns and infants, with a secondary aim of decreasing morbidity among people of all ages. There is no vaccine for newborns. Vaccination of family members is a vaccine strategy, also known as cocooning, aimed at protecting this vulnerable population.[42] Thus the tetanus–diphtheria–pertussis (Tdap) vaccine is offered to all persons who have close contact with infants younger than 2 months, including parents, household contacts, childcare workers, and visitors such as grandparents.

Because of the increased incidence of pertussis in adolescent and adult populations, the pertussis vaccine has been added to the tetanus and diphtheria vaccine recommended for all individuals every 10 years. The CDC now recommends that all adolescents age 11–12 years receive one dose of Tdap vaccine. All women who have not received the Tdap vaccine, or whose vaccine status is unknown, should receive a single dose of Tdap followed by a booster with tetanus and diphtheria toxoids (Td) every 10 years.[11,42]

Two Tdap vaccines are currently licensed in the United States: Boostrix and Adacel. Both of these vaccines are supplied in single-dose vials or syringes. It is acceptable to administer Tdap regardless of the time since the last tetanus and diphtheria toxoid–containing vaccine was given. In fact, the CDC recommends that all women who are pregnant receive a single dose of Tdap, preferably between 27 and 36 weeks' gestation, during every pregnancy regardless of the interval between pregnancies.[11,42] The CDC recommendation for nonpregnant women calls for them to receive a tetanus and diphtheria toxoids (Td) booster dose 10 years following the initial Tdap dose and again every 10 years. Common side effects of Tdap administration include mild fever, redness or swelling at the injection site, and tenderness at the injection site.

Varicella

Varicella is an acute infection caused by the varicella zoster virus (VSV). Two forms of this infectious disease exist: primary varicella infection (also known as chickenpox) and herpes zoster, the recurrent varicella infection also known as shingles.

Primary varicella infections (chickenpox) are characterized by a generalized pruritic rash that progresses quickly from macules to papules to vesicular lesions. The clinical course of this disease is often more severe in adults, who also have a higher incidence of complications.[44] Herpes zoster (shingles), the recurrent form of this disease, is characterized by painful vesicles that usually erupt along a sensory nerve line. The vesicles are typically accompanied by moderate to severe pain and are seen most often on the trunk. Herpes zoster is caused by the activation of latent VZV. The reasons for this reactivation are poorly understood, although factors associated with herpes zoster include immunosuppression, aging, intrauterine exposure to VZV, and having had varicella prior to the age of 18 months.[3]

Although acute varicella is usually mild and self-limited, it may be associated with moderate to severe complications, including secondary bacterial infection of the lesions with *Staphylococcus* or *Streptococcus*, pneumonia, encephalitis, meningitis, and infection of other vital organs. Rarely, persons may develop Reye syndrome and Guillain-Barré syndrome. The most common complication of herpes zoster is postherpetic neuralgia, which may persist for a year or longer after the lesions resolve.[45]

Varicella Vaccine

The CDC recommends vaccination against herpes zoster for all women 60 years or older regardless of their history of prior infection.[11] This vaccine is administered by subcutaneous injection as a one-time dose, and it may be administered in conjunction with other age-appropriate vaccines.[2] The zoster vaccine (Zostavax) is a live attenuated virus vaccine and is contraindicated for women with a history of allergic reaction to any of the vaccine components, women who are immunosuppressed, and women who are pregnant.

The CDC also recommends vaccination against varicella (chickenpox) for all nonpregnant women who do not have evidence of immunity. Varicella vaccine (Varivax) is a live attenuated vaccine administered in a two-dose series by subcutaneous injection, with at least 4 weeks between doses. Varicella vaccine was first licensed for use in the United States in 1995,[1] so it is likely that care providers will see women who have not been previously immunized or who do not demonstrate evidence of immunity. Evidence of immunity can be demonstrated through documented receipt of two doses of vaccine administered at least 4 weeks apart, a history of healthcare provider–diagnosed varicella or herpes zoster, or serologic laboratory confirmation of immunity. Adults born in the United States before 1980 are also considered immune. The immune status of women who are pregnant and healthcare workers should be assessed with serologic confirmation of immunity. Women who are pregnant and who are not immune should receive the first dose of vaccine in the immediate period after giving birth or after termination of pregnancy. Varicella vaccine can also be administered post-exposure if the individual does not have contraindications to use of this vaccine to prevent or mitigate the severity of disease.

Varicella vaccine is contraindicated for persons with any of the following conditions: a history of allergic reaction to any of the vaccine components (gelatin, neomycin, or other components), immunosuppression, blood dyscrasia such as leukemia, receiving oral steroids, moderate or severe concurrent illness, receipt of blood products during the previous 3–11 months, and women who are pregnant.[43] As is true for many vaccines, the most common adverse effects after receipt of varicella vaccines are local; systematic reactions such as headache are less common.

Immunoglobulins

Immunoglobulins, also known as immune globulins or gamma globulins, are discussed in this chapter because they induce passive immunization. These preformed antibodies are not vaccines; indeed, such preparations are considered treatment rather than prophylaxis when they are administered following exposure to the diseases they are designed to prevent. Varicella zoster immunoglobulin (VariZIG) and hepatitis B immunoglobulin (HBIG) are examples of immunoglobulins commonly used to prevent development of the disease in individuals who have known exposure to that disease. Table 6-8 lists the immunoglobulins available for treatment in the United States today.

Varicella Immunoglobulin

In 2012, varicella zoster immunoglobulin (VariZIG), a purified human immunoglobulin preparation made from plasma containing high levels of anti-varicella IgG antibodies, was approved by the FDA for prophylaxis against varicella.[3] Box 6-7 lists the indications for use of VariZIG.[47] This agent has replaced the varicella zoster immunoglobulin

Table 6-8 Immunoglobulins Commonly Available in the United States

Immunoglobulin	Clinical Indication
Botulinum antitoxin (Botox)	Treatment of botulism. Also used to treat a variety of conditions including headaches, detrusor muscle dystrophy, limb spasticity, hyperhidrosis, and lateral canthal lines (crow's feet).
Cytomegalovirus intravenous immunoglobulin (CMV-IGIV)	Prophylaxis to prevent CMV infection for hematopoietic stem cell and kidney transplant recipients.
Hepatitis B immunoglobulin (HBIG)	Prophylaxis following exposure to hepatitis B.
Human rabies immunoglobulin (HRIG)	Treatment of rabies post exposure.
Immunoglobulin (IgG)	Prophylaxis following hepatitis A or measles exposure. Used to treat rubella during first trimester of pregnancy. Also used to treat varicella if varicella zoster immunoglobulin is unavailable.
Intravenous immunoglobulin (IVIG) and subcutaneous immunoglobulin (SCIG) replacement therapy	Prophylaxis and/or treatment for individuals with severe bacterial and viral infections and among potentially immunocompromised individuals (e.g., HIV infections in children, antibody-deficiency disorders, thrombocytopenic purpura, hypogammaglobinemia in chronic lymphocytic leukemia), persons with neurologic disorders such as myasthenia gravis, and persons with Guillain-Barré syndrome.
Respiratory syncytial virus (RSV-IGIV or RSV-mAb)	Prevention of RSV in infants < 35 weeks' gestation at birth or children with chronic lung disorders. RSV-IGIV is derived from human antibodies. RSV-mAb is a murine monoclonal antibody.
Rho(D) immunoglobulin (RhoGAM)	Prevention of maternal isoimmunization.
Tetanus immunoglobulin	Treatment of tetanus and postexposure prophylaxis.
Varicella zoster immunoglobulin (VariZIG)	Prophylaxis for postexposure in persons who are immunocompromised or pregnant and in perinatally exposed newborns.

Source: Data from Rubin FH. Passive immunization. *Merck manual professional online.* Last modification 2013. http://www.merckmanuals.com/professional/infectious_diseases/immunization/passive_immunization.html. Accessed October 7, 2014.[46]

Box 6-7 Persons for Whom Varicella Zoster Immunoglobulin (VariZIG) Is Indicated

Persons who have been exposed to varicella and are at high risk for complications of disease, but who are not candidates for the varicella vaccine

Immunocompromised persons

Neonates whose mothers have signs and symptoms of varicella perinatally (i.e., 5 days before to 2 days after giving birth)

Preterm infants born at 28 weeks' gestation or later who are exposed during the neonatal period and whose mothers do not have evidence of immunity

Preterm infants born earlier than 28 weeks' gestation or who weigh 1000 g or less at birth and were exposed during the neonatal period, regardless of maternal history of varicella disease or vaccination

Women who are pregnant without evidence of immunity

Source: Centers for Disease Control and Prevention. Updated recommendations for use of VariZIG—United States, 2013. 2013:62(28);574–576. http://www.cdc.gov/mmwr/preview/mmwrhtml/mm6228a4.htm. Accessed October 5, 2014.[47]

marketed as VZIG, which was removed from the market by its manufacturer a few years prior. VariZIG is lyophilized or freeze dried in a high vacuum; when reconstituted, it can be administered intramuscularly in a 5% solution of immunoglobulin-G (IgG) up to 10 days after exposure to the disease. Incubation periods may be prolonged after administration of the vaccine, so women should be monitored for 28 days after exposure. If a woman demonstrates any signs or symptoms of varicella within that time frame, antiviral therapy should be promptly initiated. The most common adverse drug reactions following administration of this vaccine are minor and include headaches and infection-site pain. Contraindications for VariZIG include a history of hypersensitivity/anaphylaxis with human immunoglobulins.

Hepatitis B Immunoglobulin

Hepatitis B immunoglobulin (HBIG) is a generic immunoglobulin that contains a high titer of anti-hepatitis B antibodies. This agent is used to treat individuals who have no evidence of immunity but are accidentally exposed to HBV. Many of these individuals are healthcare providers who become exposed during practice of their occupation. Others may be exposed through sexual contact with an infected individual or via perinatal exposure to a newborn.[3]

In addition to receiving HBIG, completion of the postexposure vaccine series is essential to prevent chronic infection, particularly among the children who may become chronic carriers. Newborns whose mothers are infected have the highest risk of becoming chronic carriers—a state that itself carries a high risk for developing hepatocellular carcinoma.

The efficacy of HBIG varies. Perinatally, HBIG and the first injection of the HepB vaccine series to the neonate has been found to be 85% to 95% effective in providing passive immunity in the newborn. For a healthcare worker, multiple doses of HBIG starting within 1 week after percutaneous exposure appears to be 75% effective, suggesting that perhaps HBIG and initiation of the vaccine series may be useful postexposure treatment for adults as well as newborns.[48]

Vaccine Safety

Vaccine products have been incredibly successful in reducing the incidence of many diseases in the United States and globally. However, the success of vaccine strategies in reducing the burden of disease is closely linked to the public's perception of vaccine safety. Vaccination rates in the United States remain suboptimal for most vaccine-preventable diseases among all age groups.[49] Individuals, including parents of minors, make decisions about vaccination based largely on perceived risks and benefits, and they may decide to stop vaccinating themselves and their family members when the perceived risks outweigh the benefits.

The pertussis epidemic of 1979 in Japan provides an example of how eroded public trust in a vaccine can impact a nation. In 1974, almost 80% of Japanese children had been vaccinated against pertussis. That same year, there were only 393 reported cases of pertussis and no deaths. By 1976, following widespread rumors that the vaccine was no longer necessary and not safe, the vaccination rate among infants had dropped to 10%. In 1979, there were more than 13,000 reported cases of pertussis and 41 deaths.[3]

To reduce the incidence of vaccine-preventable diseases, it is imperative that vaccines remain safe and that individuals receive accurate information about the risks and benefits of vaccine use. Several measures are in place to assure vaccine safety in the United States. First, all vaccines must be licensed by the FDA prior to use in the general public. That licensure is granted only after extensive safety and effectiveness studies conducted first in the laboratory, then in animals, and finally in three separate phases of human clinical trials which are conducted over several years and include thousands of volunteer participants. Following licensure, vaccine surveillance continues with the following initiatives: Phase 4 trials that are conducted to identify rare reactions that were not detected prior to licensure, monitoring for changes in the rate of known reactions, identification of risk factors for reactions, identification of vaccine lots that have higher rates of reactions or are associated with specific types of drug reactions, and monitoring for any signals that may indicate the need for further study or changes in vaccine recommendations.[3]

Monitoring vaccine benefit is relatively easy; assessing risk is much more difficult. Even if a condition or reaction appears to be triggered by a particular vaccine product, the exact cause of an adverse event can be difficult to determine. Vaccines include substances other than the active component, such as adjunctive elements and preservatives. In addition, they are often given as combination products, and several vaccines may be given at a single healthcare visit, making it difficult to discern which specific vaccine could have caused a reaction. Products could also become contaminated during their production or be reconstituted with inappropriate dilutants. Vaccination might also potentially trigger an adverse drug reaction only in susceptible individuals, rather than in the general population. Vulnerability may be clear in some cases (e.g., in individuals who have experienced prior episodes of Guillain-Barré syndrome), but may be hidden when unrecognized genetic or physiologic differences between individuals increase the risk of adverse drug events. While the relationship between an adverse drug event and vaccination could be causal, most such effects are thought to be coincidental. Determining which of these myriads of possibilities is the correct one is very challenging.

The CDC engages in three vaccine safety activities to help answer questions about vaccine safety. The Vaccine Adverse Event Reporting System (VAERS) is a national vaccine safety surveillance program cosponsored by the CDC and the FDA. VAERS accepts all reports of adverse effects from vaccine recipients and/or their guardians, healthcare providers, and vaccine manufacturers. Approximately 30,000 reports of adverse drug events are filed with VAERS each year; 10% to 15% of those are classified as serious (resulting in hospitalization, disability, life-threatening illness, or death).[50] Data are entered into a large database and analyzed each year. Findings are limited by the reporting process, which includes only those events that are actually reported, and the inability to draw causal relationships between the vaccine and any given adverse event. While case reports submitted to VAERS cannot determine the underlying relationship between an adverse event and a vaccine, potential problems can be identified and evaluated in future research on vaccine safety. Because large sample sizes are needed to identify rare events, reporting is essential. Therefore, healthcare providers need to be vigilant and report minor as well as major adverse events, and remote as well as recent adverse events associated with vaccine receipt.

The Vaccine Safety Datalink (VSD) was established in 1990 between the CDC's Immunization Office and nine large healthcare organizations. Using electronic health data, VSD conducts studies to examine, in greater detail, rare and serious adverse drug events that are reported in the literature or to surveillance systems such as VAERS.[51] The work of VSD has resulted in key contributions to the understanding of vaccine safety over the past 25 years. For example, VSD research has answered questions about the safety of additives in vaccine products and led to the removal of thimerosal from vaccines for children (except in some flu vaccines). In addition to studying reports of adverse drug events, VSD monitors adverse events associated with new vaccines. When new recommendations are made, it provides information to various organizations that establish national guidelines for vaccine use.

In 2001, the CDC's Immunization Safety Office, in conjunction with seven medical research centers and other partners, established the Clinical Immunization Safety Assessment Project (CISA). This project strengthens the ability to accurately monitor vaccine safety by conducting high-quality research and closely examining adverse drug events through individual case review.[52]

In addition to these measures taken by the CDC to assure vaccine safety, vaccine manufacturers often establish their own reporting registries for vaccine use following licensure of vaccine products by the FDA. For example, the manufacturer of Tdap vaccines continues to operate registries that gather data on the use of these vaccines in pregnant women. It is also important for individual healthcare providers to take steps that ensure the safest use of vaccine products, including the measures outlined in Box 6-8.

The National Childhood Vaccine Injury Prevention Act of 1986 requires that all healthcare providers report certain adverse events associated with vaccine administration to VAERS.[3] Furthermore, healthcare providers are encouraged to report all adverse drug events and side effects regardless of whether they are certain that the vaccine caused the reaction. Reporting guidelines for VAERS are available online at the CDC's website. The National Childhood Vaccine Injury Prevention Act also requires that all healthcare providers present the parents or guardians of children with vaccine information statements (VISs) on every vaccine that is administered in both private and public settings.[3]

Box 6-8 Steps Healthcare Providers Can Take to Promote Safe Use of Vaccines

Ensure that all vaccines are stored and administered as recommended by the manufacturer.

Follow recommendations for timing and spacing of vaccines.

Maintain currency regarding recommendations for vaccine scheduling.

In case of real or suspected adverse drug effects or adverse drug reactions, care for the woman and report the side effects.

Communicate the risks and benefits of vaccine products to individuals for whom care is provided.

Vaccine Controversies

Several years ago, the use of thimerosal in vaccine products came under intense scrutiny by national policymakers and the news media. The concern was raised because thimerosal (a preservative that was commonly used in the past) contains ethyl mercury. While methyl mercury is an environmental contaminant, ethyl mercury metabolizes to water (H_2O) once it enters the body. Methyl mercury, in contrast, persists in the tissues, leading to the danger of mercury poisoning. Attention by the news media has raised concerns among some parents and pregnant women that thimerosal contained in vaccines might harm their children. However, numerous studies to date have not found any association between thimerosal and adverse outcomes.[53–55]

One of the provisions of the FDA Modernization Act, which was signed into law in 1997, required that the FDA identify foods and drugs into which mercury was intentionally introduced and analyze the potential effects of each of the mercury compounds identified. Although to date no adverse effects of thimerosal used as a preservative in vaccines have been identified (other than irritation at the injection site), a decision was made in 1999 to reduce or eliminate thimerosal in vaccines as a precautionary measure. Thimerosal has not been used in routinely recommended childhood vaccines since 2001 (with the exception of some influenza vaccines), nor is it used in most commonly recommended vaccines for adults.[55]

Numerous other adverse events have been potentially linked to vaccine receipt, including a purported relationship between certain childhood vaccines and autism. Most of these associations either have not been found to be etiologically related (as noted in Box 6-9) or are currently under investigation. While it is beyond the scope of this chapter to cover these associations in detail, further information can be found on websites, particularly the Immunization Safety Review, sponsored by the Institute of Medicine and Global Advisory Committee on Vaccine Safety, which in turn is sponsored by the World Health Organization.

Box 6-9 To Treat or Not to Treat: Do Vaccines Cause Autism?

The number of children who have a diagnosis of autism has increased since the 1980s. At the same time, the number of vaccines recommended for children has increased. In 1998, Wakefield et al. authored an article that proposed the MMR vaccine causes autism via a series of physiologic reactions to the vaccine. Their study cited the cases of 12 children with developmental delays (8 had autism) who developed the condition within 1 month of receiving an MMR vaccination.[56] Since the publication of the Wakefield et al. article, several studies have evaluated the relationship between administration of these vaccines and subsequent development of autism. To date, none of the many well-designed studies done has found any association between vaccines and autism or other developmental delays. Moreover, the journal in which the original article was published, *The Lancet*, has published a retraction of the Wakefield et al. article secondary to the discovery of misconduct by the authors of the Wakefield study.[57]

What is the relationship between autism and vaccines? The MMR vaccine is given to children at age 2 years. This is also the age at which symptoms of autism usually first appear. Thus, there is a temporal association (but no causation) between the administration of vaccine and the development of this disorder. In addition, although it appears that the number of children with autism has increased in the last several years, the noted increase is likely secondary to a more inclusive case definition and improved awareness of the disorder.

For some individuals, the cell line source used to grow a virus in one of the first steps in development of a vaccine is concerning. Several antivaccine personal blogs and websites state or imply that vaccines are made from the fetal products from abortion. Although no vaccine contains fetal tissue, it is accurate to say that the two most common cell lines were derived from tissue obtained after two terminated pregnancies in the 1960s.[58] Neither of the pregnancies was aborted specifically to provide material for vaccines, but cell lines MRC-5 and WI-38 contain cells from those pregnancies.[59] The CDC provides a list of all ingredients used in vaccines in the United States, including the cell lines.[60] Several vaccines, but not all, incorporate material from these lines. For example, the vaccine for hepatitis A lists such a cell line as an ingredient, but a recombinant vaccine such as the one for hepatitis B does not. Most vaccines that contain the cell lines in question (e.g., MMR) do not have alternatives; thus the use of these cell lines may pose a dilemma for some women. Other women may express similar concerns about the use of embryo cell lines that involve animals.

Vaccine Storage and Administration

Improper administration of vaccine products can undermine the protection they provide against vaccine-preventable diseases. Strict adherence to vaccine handling and storage requirements and recommended techniques of administration (e.g., choice of site [deltoid versus gluteal muscle] and route [intramuscular versus subcutaneous]), spacing booster doses correctly, and using proper dosages (pediatric vs. adult) are essential. Failure to follow recommended guidelines can impede a complete and full immune response after vaccine receipt and can leave the recipient susceptible to infection.[11]

Although failure to comply with guidelines affects all vaccines, improper handling and administration are more likely to adversely affect live viral vaccines. Notably, storage of vaccines at improper temperatures can destroy components of the vaccine and render it ineffective. Given this risk, healthcare providers should inspect vaccines upon delivery to ensure they have been shipped and stored at proper temperatures, and should closely monitor the temperature of storage units. Expiration dates must also be carefully observed. These dates often change depending on the way the products are stored. For example, some vaccines expire more quickly when stored at room temperature than when they are refrigerated, and the expiration dates for vaccines that are packaged in multiple-dose vials that must be reconstituted often change following reconstitution. Expiration dates and lot numbers should be recorded when vaccines are received and placed into storage, and a new expiration date should be placed on the vial if or when the method of storage changes.[52]

Generally, vaccines are administered simultaneously with a healthcare visit. Doing so is more practical for both providers and women, and is highly recommended by the ACIP as an approach that improves the likelihood that an individual will receive all recommended vaccinations on time. Simultaneous receipt of multiple vaccines, whether they are live or inactivated ones, does not impair the immune response to any agent. However, if it is determined later that another live viral vaccine is needed, vaccination will need to be delayed. Unless they are given on the same day, live viral vaccines need to be spaced a minimum of 4 weeks apart.[2] Giving live viral vaccines too close together negatively affects the immune response of the second vaccine. This situation is most likely to occur when providing vaccine coverage to travelers. It is highly recommended that healthcare providers consult with an expert in travel vaccines before administering any vaccines so that a determination can be made concerning which vaccines are needed, and then a plan be made to administer them in a timely, convenient fashion that does not undermine their effectiveness.

Receipt of antibody-containing products such as immunoglobulins, whole blood, or other blood products can negatively affect the immune response to live vaccines but not inactivated ones. If a live vaccine is given first, 2 or more weeks should elapse before an antibody product is given. If an antibody-containing product is given first, then 3 or more months should elapse before vaccination.[11] The recommended time interval between the two varies by product. Providers should consult ACIP statements for guidance.

Live viral vaccines are generally more susceptible to damage if not handled properly; inactivated vaccines are also affected by such issues, albeit to a lesser degree. Storing the vaccine at the wrong temperature or exposing the vaccine to light, for example, can reduce the potency of some vaccines. Resources such as the Vaccine Storage and Handling Toolkit are very useful for practices needing detailed information on vaccine storage and administration issues.

Vaccines that require multiple doses also need to be spaced correctly. Each dose needs to be timed so that the body recognizes it as a separate event and will reboost the immune system to respond to the new vaccine. Vaccine schedules list the minimum interval between doses. Individuals who are late for the next dose in the series should receive that scheduled dose and continue on in the series; those who receive vaccinations later than recommended do not need to restart the series. However, if vaccines are administered earlier than recommended, even by a few days, that vaccine cannot be counted and the woman will need to return at the appropriate time for revaccination.[3]

Special Populations

Vaccines considered safe in healthy adults may not be appropriate for use in all populations. For example, vaccines administered to pregnant and lactating women may be unsafe for fetuses and newborns and individuals with chronic conditions may be more likely to experience vaccine-related adverse drug events. These concerns have led to close scrutiny of the safety of vaccine products in vulnerable populations, particularly individuals who are immunosuppressed, women who are pregnant or lactating and their newborns, and those individuals who are healthcare workers.

Adolescents

Although vaccine coverage for infants and young children has improved significantly over the past 30 years in the United States, vaccine coverage for adolescents is of importance, in large part because of the decreased frequency with which members of this age group visit a healthcare provider. Prior to age 11 years, girls are considered to have complete vaccine coverage if they have received the full series of vaccines against hepatitis A and B; rotavirus; diphtheria, tetanus, and acellular pertussis; *Haemophilus influenzae* type b (Hib); pneumococcal vaccines; polio; influenza; measles, mumps, and rubella; and varicella. All children younger than 11 years should also receive a full series of pneumococcal vaccines, and children at high risk for infection should receive meningococcal vaccine. The hepatitis B vaccine has been recommended in infancy for many years, so that it no longer appears on the vaccine schedules for adolescents and adults, aside from recommendations for catch-up. The following vaccines are recommended for girls 11–18 years who are considered fully vaccinated: tetanus, diphtheria, and acellular pertussis (Tdap); influenza

(IIV or LAIV); human papillomavirus (HPV2 or HPV4); and meningococcal conjugate vaccine.[13]

As more vaccines are added to the vaccine schedule, questions have begun to arise regarding the ability of adolescents to provide informed consent for vaccinations for themselves. Some health departments in the United States currently allow adolescents who are minors to sign for vaccines for themselves if the vaccine is part of the protocol for a visit for a sexually transmitted infection or disease. The Adolescent Working Group of the National Vaccine Advisory Committee is currently exploring the issue of how to ensure appropriate vaccination services for this population. Issues related to confidentiality during a visit for sexually transmitted infections or diseases are a prominent part of the discussion.

Women Who Are Pregnant

Table 6-9 summarizes the recommendations regarding vaccine use in pregnancy. Use of inactivated vaccines are safe to administer during pregnancy, whereas live viral vaccines are contraindicated for women who are pregnant.[32,43] Although there is very little evidence of a causal relationship between vaccines and teratogenic effects, there is a theoretical risk that live viral vaccines might cause infection and potentially harm the fetus. Smallpox is the only vaccine for which fetal injury has been identified following vaccination.[4] Rubella is also of concern, because fetuses born to women infected with the wild-type virus have a high risk a constellation of birth defects called congenital rubella syndrome. While no cases of congenital rubella syndrome have been reported in infants born to women inadvertently vaccinated with rubella vaccine in pregnancy, cases of subclinical infection with vaccine virus have been documented.[3]

Adverse fetal effects after exposure to measles, mumps, and varicella vaccines are much less likely to cause birth defects than after exposure to rubella vaccine. Eighteen years of close monitoring of the MMR vaccine, through a vaccine-in-pregnancy registry, and 17 years of monitoring of the varicella vaccine, have not revealed any increased risks for birth defects or congenitally acquired disease following administration of these vaccines.[3] Although the FDA approved closure of the vaccine-in-pregnancy registry for varicella, the manufacturer (Merck) continues to monitor inadvertent exposure.

Pregnant women who are exposed to MMR or varicella vaccines should be counseled about the theoretical risks associated with administration of live vaccines in pregnancy. Routine pregnancy testing of childbearing-age women prior to administering live attenuated vaccine is not recommended, and administration of live attenuated vaccine during pregnancy should not be an indication for elective pregnancy termination.[32,43] All nonpregnant women who are not immune should be vaccinated using the recommended dosage and administration and advised to avoid pregnancy for at least 4 weeks. Women who are pregnant who are not immune to rubella and/or varicella should be immunized in the immediate postpartum period or following pregnancy termination, and counseled to avoid pregnancy for at least 4 weeks.

In 2012, the Advisory Committee on Immunization Practices began recommending that all women who are pregnant (with each pregnancy) receive the Tdap vaccine, regardless of the interval since the last dose. This new recommendation was made in an attempt to prevent pertussis morbidity and mortality in infants.[42] Although the vaccine may be administered at any time during pregnancy, it is recommended during the third trimester, as this schedule facilitates a higher concentration of maternal antibodies that will be transferred to the fetus close to the time of birth. The monitoring of Tdap administration during pregnancy for adverse outcomes is ongoing through

Table 6-9 Vaccine Use in Pregnancy

Vaccine	Recommendation for Use During Pregnancy
Hepatitis A vaccine	Recommended if otherwise indicated
Hepatitis B vaccine	Recommended in some circumstances
Human papillomavirus (HPV) vaccine	Not recommended
Influenza inactivated (IIV) vaccine	Recommended
Influenza live attenuated (LAIV) vaccine	Contraindicated
Measles, mumps, and rubella (MMR)	Contraindicated
Meningococcal	May be used if otherwise indicated
Pneumococcal conjugate vaccine (PCV13)	Inadequate data for specific recommendation
Pneumococcal polysaccharide vaccine (PPSV23)	Inadequate data for specific recommendation
Polio vaccine	May be used if needed
Tetanus–diphtheria (Td)	Should be used if otherwise indicated
Tetanus–diphtheria–pertussis (Tdap)	Recommended
Varicella	Contraindicated
Zoster	Contraindicated

Source: Reproduced from Centers for Disease Control and Prevention. Guidelines for vaccinating pregnant women. http://www.cdc.gov/vaccines/pubs/preg-guide.htm. Accessed July 7, 2014.[43]

vaccine-in-pregnancy registries established by the manufacturers. Healthcare providers are encouraged to report administration of Adacel to women who are pregnant to Sanofi Pasteur (1-800-822-2463) and administration of Boostrix to women who are pregnant to GlaxoSmithKline Biologicals (1-888-825-5249).

All women who are or will be pregnant during the flu season should be offered the TIV influenza vaccine. Although the increased risks for hospitalization and other poor outcomes for women who are pregnant who contract influenza are greatest during the second and third trimesters, vaccination during any trimester is recommended because of the difficulty in predicting exactly when any given flu season will begin.

Women Who Are Lactating

Most live vaccines are not excreted in human milk. Therefore, both live and inactivated vaccines may be safely given to breastfeeding women. Rubella vaccine virus may be excreted in human milk. Although research data is limited, it appears that the virus rarely infects the infant and when infection does occur, it is usually a mild illness because the virus has been attenuated.[3,43] Women who are lactating should be counseled to receive age- and risk-appropriate vaccines and to have their infants vaccinated according to the recommended schedules.

Women 65 Years and Older

Women older than 65 years are more likely to have chronic diseases that place them at higher risk for infections or major complications of the chronic disease. In general, vaccines administered to these women are not different than those given to younger women, but there is a greater urgency for complete vaccinations. The vaccine for pneumococcal disease is indicated for women in this age group.[11]

Women Who Are Immunosuppressed

Individuals may be immunosuppressed from a multitude of causes, including cancer, chemotherapy, antirejection therapy following organ transplant, HIV infection, and high-dose corticosteroid use. Inactivated vaccines have been found to be well tolerated in immunosuppressed individuals.[3] However, use of live viral vaccines is problematic. Immunity occurs in response to live vaccine administration through replication of the vaccine virus; therefore, for persons who are immunosuppressed, this replication is uncontrolled (by a normally functioning immune system) and can lead to severe or fatal reactions. Given this risk, live vaccines should not be administered to individuals who are severely immunosuppressed, although inactivated vaccines may be given when indicated.[11]

Household members of immunosuppressed individuals should be vaccinated appropriately and may safely be given MMR, varicella, rotavirus, and LAIV vaccines. No special precautions need to be taken unless the vaccinated contact develops a rash after vaccination with varicella vaccine. In this case, contact should be avoided with immunosuppressed individuals until after the rash resolves.

Immunosuppressed individuals should receive vaccines against influenza (use the TIV vaccine), meningococcal and pneumococcal infections, Hib disease, and hepatitis B, although the response to these vaccines may be suboptimal.

Adults with HIV are at risk for complications after measles infection and varicella. For this reason, the ACIP recommends vaccinating asymptomatic or mildly immunosuppressed HIV-positive individuals for MMR or varicella. Because guidelines change frequently, women's healthcare providers should consult the latest recommendations before immunizing HIV-positive individuals with live viral vaccines.[3]

Healthcare Workers

Healthcare personnel are at a significant risk for acquiring and transmitting several diseases.[61] Based on documented nosocomial transmission rates, the ACIP recommends that all healthcare personnel have evidence of immunity against hepatitis B, influenza, measles, mumps, rubella, pertussis, and varicella. In the absence of evidence of immunity, such personnel should be immunized against these diseases according to the recommended schedules.

All healthcare personnel should receive an influenza vaccine annually during the flu season. Both LAIV and TIV are appropriate for use in healthcare personnel, although those who provide care for severely immunocompromised hospitalized women, women who are pregnant, or women who are older than 50, and those healthcare personnel who have their own contraindications for live vaccine, should not receive LAIV but instead should be administered a single dose of TIV.[12] Nonpregnant healthcare workers without evidence of immunity to measles or mumps should receive two doses of MMR vaccine that are administered at least 28 days apart. Healthcare workers without evidence of immunity to rubella should receive a single dose of MMR vaccine. As is true for most adults, healthcare personnel should receive a one-time dose of Tdap and boost with Td every 10 years. Nonpregnant workers without evidence of immunity to varicella should receive the two-dose series. All healthcare personnel also should have documented evidence of immunity to hepatitis B and varicella. Those who are not immune should receive the recommended doses of vaccines.[40]

Travelers

Travelers who plan to travel outside the United States should be current with their own vaccines. Vaccine recommendations vary by country and by regions within a country. Because the prevalence of vaccine-preventable diseases can change dramatically, with recommendations therefore changing accordingly, international travelers could benefit from referral to a travel clinic. For individuals who are unable to see a healthcare provider with expertise in travel recommendations, the CDC offers an interactive website that provides information for consumers and clinicians.[62] Readers are also advised to consult the CDC about vaccine use in women who are pregnant who anticipate travel outside the United States.

Conclusion

The advent of vaccination was a game changer in health care. Over the years, this practice has evolved from a focus on preventing childhood diseases to today's protection of girls and women from HPV-associated cancer. Expansion of this area of pharmacotherapeutics in the next decades is unpredictable; it is expected that new vaccines will emerge. Among the vaccines now being researched are several products to prevent a variety of cancers,[63] including breast cancer[64] and melanomas.[65] Infectious diseases also are targeted for new vaccines, including pneumonias caused by *Streptococcus*,[66] and viruses such as the Ebola virus[67] and the ever-elusive HIV vaccine.[68]

Research to genetically engineer plants so they manufacture proteins that elicit an immune response is under way. Imagine eating a banana or a mashed potato to become immunized against hepatitis B. Although this research has several challenges, it opens up possibilities that may in the future improve vaccine availability and lower the cost of vaccination. Delivery systems are likely to be intranasal, inhaled, or oral (including through food intake). Vaccines themselves may be modified to tolerate environmental temperature extremes and have longer shelf lives that facilitate global transport.[69] In conclusion, vaccinations are among the most cost-effective measures that have been developed for health maintenance and promotion. Great strides have been made to provide vaccines that are safe and effective. Providers who incorporate vaccines into their practice will extend the benefits of vaccination into traditionally under-immunized populations. Clinicians practicing in the area of women's health have been identified as common providers of many of the vaccinations given in the United States. Those who vigilantly screen for any potential adverse events and report these reactions to VAERS will help ensure that the products offered to the public are the safest ones possible.

Resources

Organization	Description	Website
General Information		
Centers for Disease Control and Prevention (CDC)	Influenza mobile application for clinicians; with this app, providers can find the CDC's latest recommendations about influenza, vaccination, and treatments	www.cdc.gov/flu/apps/cdc-influenza-hcp.html
Centers for Disease Control and Prevention (CDC), National Center for Immunizations and Respiratory Diseases Immunization	Federal website with multiple useful webpages for consumers and professionals; includes immunization schedules for children and adults, as well as an app of these tables (www.cdc.gov/vaccines/schedules/hcp/schedule-app.html)	www.cdc.gov/vaccines
Children's Hospital of Philadelphia, Vaccine Education Center	Website focused on pediatrics but with information about vaccines also used by adults; has a free downloadable mobile app for iPhone and Android devices called "Vaccines on the Go: What You Should Know"	www.chop.edu/service/vaccine-education-center/home.html

Clinical Immunization Safety Assessment (CISA)	Healthcare providers who have questions about vaccine safety relative to a specific person who resides in the United States may request a free case evaluation	www.cdc.gov/vaccinesafety/activities/cisa.html or email CISAeval@cdc.gov
Federal Drug Administration	Package inserts for U.S.-licensed vaccines	www.fda.gov/BiologicsBloodVaccines/Vaccines/ApprovedProducts/ucm093833.htm
National Network for Immunization Information (NNii)	Repository of information about vaccines, including those unusual in the United States, such as anthrax vaccine; affiliated with the American Academy of Pediatrics, the American Nurses Association, the American Academy of Family Physicians, and the American College of Obstetricians and Gynecologists, among others	www.immunizationinfo.org
Centers for Disease Control and Prevention (CDC), Vaccines for Women who are pregnant	Webpage within CDC website	www.cdc.gov/vaccines/adults/rec-vac/pregnant.html
Pregnancy Registry		
Boostrix	Registry for Boostrix	www.pregnancyregistry.gsk.com/boostrix.html
Adacel	Registry for Adacel	www.sanofipasteurpregnancyregistry.com/?fa=adacel
Gardasil	Registry for Gardasil	www.merckpregnancyregistries.com/gardisil.html
Varicella (pregnancy registry has formally closed)	New cases of exposure immediately before or during pregnancy or other adverse events after vaccination with Varivax, ProQuad, or Zostavax should continue to be reported	Report to Merck (1-877-888-4231) and to VAERS (https://vaers.hhs.gov/index)
Vaccine Safety		
Johns Hopkins University School of Public Health, Institute for Vaccine Safety	Designed to provide an independent assessment of vaccines and vaccine safety; the institute's goal is to work toward preventing disease using the safest vaccines possible	www.vaccinesafety.edu
Global Advisory Committee on Vaccine Safety (GACVS), World Health Organization	Manual on global perspective of adverse vaccine events and reactions	www.who.int/vaccine_safety/en
VAERS submission webpage	Online form to report adverse vaccine drug events	https://vaers.hhs.gov/esub/step1
Travelers' Vaccine Information		
Centers for Disease Control and Prevention (CDC), Travelers' Health	Requirements for vaccines listed by countries to be visited and other information	www.cdc.gov/travel/contentVaccinations.aspx

References

1. Centers for Disease Control and Prevention. Achievements in public health, 1990-1998: Control of infectious diseases. *MMWR.* 1999;48(29):621-629.
2. Centers for Disease Control and Prevention. Adult vaccination information for healthcare and public health professionals. http://www.cdc.gov/vaccines/hcp/patient-ed/adults/index.html. Accessed May 1, 2014.
3. Atkinson W, Wolfe S, Hambrosky J, eds. *Epidemiology and Prevention of Vaccine-Preventable Diseases.* 12th ed. Washington, DC: Centers for Disease Control and Prevention; 2012.
4. World Health Organization. Smallpox. http://www.who.int/csr/disease/smallpox/en/. Accessed May 1, 2014.
5. World Health Organization. Poliomyelitis. http://www.who.int/mediacentre/factsheets/fs114/en/. Accessed May 1, 2014.
6. Briere EC, Rubin L, Moro PL, Cohn A, Clark T, Messonnier N. Prevention and control of *Haemophilus influenzae* type b disease: recommendations of the Advisory Committee on Immunization Practices

(ACIP). *MMWR Recomm Rep.* 2014;63(RR-01):1-14. http://www.cdc.gov/mmwr/preview/mmwrhtml/rr6301a1.htm. Accessed May 1, 2014.

7. Walker AT, Smith PJ, Kolasa M. Reduction of racial/ethnic disparities in vaccination coverage, 1995-2011. *MMWR Surveill Summ.* 2014;63(suppl 1):7-12. http://www.cdc.gov/mmwr/preview/mmwrhtml/su6301a3.htm. Accessed June 6, 2014.
8. Centers for Disease Control and Prevention. Healthy People 2020: immunization and infectious diseases. http://www.healthypeople.gov/2020/topics-objectives/topic/immunization-and-infectious-diseases. Accessed May 2, 2014.
9. Centers for Disease Control and Prevention. Immunization: the basics. http://www.cdc.gov/vaccines/vac-gen/imz-basics.htm. Accessed June 4, 2014.
10. National Center for Immunization and Respiratory Diseases. General recommendations on immunizations: recommendations of the Advisory Committee on Immunization Practices (ACIP). *MMWR.* 2011; 60(RR02):1-60. http://www.cdc.gov/mmwr/preview/mmwrhtml/rr6002a1.htm. Accessed June 4, 2014.
11. Centers for Disease Control and Prevention. Recommended adult vaccine schedule, by vaccine and age group: United States, 2015. http://www.cdc.gov/vaccines/schedules/downloads/adult/adult-schedule-easy-read-bw.pdf. Accessed February 5, 2015.
12. Chiarella P, Massi E, De Robertis M, Fazio VM, Signori E. Strategies for effective naked DNA vaccination against infectious diseases. *Recent Pat Antiinfect Drug Discov.* 2008;32:93-101.
13. Centers for Disease Control and Prevention. Recommended vaccine schedule for persons age 0 through 18 years: United States, 2014. http://www.cdc.gov/vaccines/schedules/hcp/imz/child-adolescent.html. Accessed June 5, 2014.
14. Matheny SC, Kingery JE. Hepatitis A. *Am Fam Physician.* 2012;86(11):1027-1034.
15. Alavian SM, Miri SM, Jazayeri SM. Hepatitis B vaccine: prophylactic, therapeutic, and diagnostic dilemma. *Minerva Gastroenterol Dietol.* 2012;58(2): 167-178.
16. Geeta MG, Riyaz A. Prevention of mother to child transmission of hepatitis B infection. *Indian Pediatr.* 2013;50(2):189-192.
17. Martínez-Sernández V, Figueiras A. Central nervous system demyelinating diseases and recombinant hepatitis B vaccination: a critical systematic review of scientific production. *J Neurol.* 2013;260(8): 1951-1959.
18. Farez MF, Correale J. Immunizations and risk of multiple sclerosis: systematic review and meta-analysis. *J Neurol.* 2011;258(7):1197-1206.
19. Beran J. Bivalent inactivated hepatitis A and recombinant hepatitis B vaccine. *Expert Rev Vaccines.* 2007; 6(6):891-902.
20. Murphy J, Mark H. Cervical cancer screening in the era of human papillomavirus testing and vaccination. *J Midwifery Womens Health.* 2012;57(6):569-576.
21. Zonfrillo NJ, Hackley B. The quadrivalent human papillomavirus vaccine: potential factors in effectiveness. *J Midwifery Womens Health.* 2008;53(3):188-194.
22. Centers for Disease Control and Prevention. HPV vaccine information for clinicians: fact sheet. http://www.cdc.gov/std/HPV/STDFact-HPV-vaccine-hcp.htm. Accessed June 11, 2014.
23. Dunne EF, Markowitz LE, Saraiya M, et al. CDC grand rounds: reducing the burden of HPV-associated cancer and disease. *MMWR.* 2014;63(04): 69-72. http://www.cdc.gov/mmwr/preview/mmwrhtml/mm6304a1.htm. Accessed July 5, 2014.
24. Gabriel G, Arck PC. Sex, immunity and influenza. *J Infect Dis.* 2014;209(suppl 3):S93-S99.
25. Yudin MH. Risk management of seasonal influenza during pregnancy: current perspectives. *Int J Womens Health.* 2014;6:681-689.
26. Viasus D, Oteo Revuelta JA, Martínez-Montauti J, Carratalà J. Influenza A (H1N1) pdm09-related pneumonia and other complications. *Enferm Infec Microbiol Clin.* 2012;30(suppl 4):43-48.
27. Centers for Disease Control and Prevention. Key facts about influenza (flu) and flu vaccine. http://www.cdc.gov/flu/keyfacts.htm. Accessed June 8, 2014.
28. Centers for Disease Control and Prevention. Prevention and control of seasonal influenza with vaccines: recommendations of the Advisory Committee on Immunization Practices—United States, 2013-2014.
29. Centers for Disease Control and Prevention. Prevention and control of seasonal influenza with vaccines: recommendations of the Advisory Committee on Immunization Practices (ACIP), 2014-15 influenza season. http://www.cdc.gov/flu/professionals/acip/. Accessed October 21, 2014.
30. Centers for Disease Control and Prevention. Flublok seasonal influenza vaccination. http://www.cdc.gov/flu/

protect/vaccine/qa_flublok-vaccine.htm. Accessed June 5, 2014.

31. White SJ, Boldt KL, Holditch SJ, Poland GA, Jacobson RM. Measles, mumps, and rubella. *Clin Obstet Gynecol.* 2012;55(2):550-559.
32. Keller-Stanislawski B, Englund JA, Kang G, et al. Safety of immunization during pregnancy: a review of the evidence of selected inactivated and live attenuated vaccines. *Vaccine.* October 3, 2014. [Epub ahead of print].
33. American Academy of Pediatrics Committee on Infectious Diseases. Updated recommendations on the use of meningococcal vaccines. *Pediatrics.* 2014;134(2):400-403.
34. Cohn AC, MacNeil JR, Clark TA, et al. Prevention and control of meningococcal disease: recommendations of the Advisory Committee on Immunization Practices (ACIP). *MMWR Recomm Rep.* 2013;62(RR-2):1-28. http://www.cdc.gov/mmwr/preview/mmwrhtml/rr6202a1.htm. Accessed June 5, 2014.
35. Feldman C, Anderson R. Review: current and new generation pneumococcal vaccines. *J Infect.* 2014;69(4):309-325.
36. Goodrick S. Preventing polio. *Lancet Neurol.* 2014; 13(7):653.
37. Thwaites CL, Beeching NJ, Newton CR. Maternal and neonatal tetanus. *Lancet.* August 19, 2014. [Epub ahead of print].
38. Leschke TM, Blumin JH, Bock JM. Diagnosis and laryngeal complications of *Bordetella pertussis* infection in the ambulatory adult population. *Otolaryngol Head Neck Surg.* September 9, 2014. [Epub ahead of print].
39. Gabutti G, Azzari C, Bonanni P, et al. Pertussis: current perspectives on epidemiology and prevention. *Hum Vaccin Immunother.* 2014;11(1):108-117.
40. Jakinovich A, Sood SK. Pertussis: still a cause of death, seven decades into vaccination. *Curr Opin Pediatr.* 2014;26(5):597-604.
41. Centers for Disease Control and Prevention. Pertussis (whooping cough): about pertussis outbreaks. http://www.cdc.gov/pertussis/outbreaks/about.html. Accessed June 8, 2014.
42. Lloyd KL. Protecting pregnant women, newborns, and families from pertussis. *J Midwifery Womens Health.* 2013;58(3):288-296.
43. Centers for Disease Control and Prevention. Guidelines for vaccinating pregnant women. http://www.cdc.gov/vaccines/pubs/preg-guide.htm. Accessed July 7, 2014.
44. Papaloukas O, Giannouli G, Papaevangelou V. Successes and challenges in varicella vaccine. *Ther Adv Vaccines.* 2014;2(2):39-55.
45. Kawai K, Preaud E, Baron-Papillon F, Largeron N, Acosta CJ. Cost-effectiveness of vaccination against herpes zoster and postherpetic neuralgia: a critical review. *Vaccine.* 2014;32(15):1645-1653.
46. Rubin FH. Passive immunization. *Merck manual professional online.* Last modification 2013. http://www.merckmanuals.com/professional/infectious_diseases/immunization/passive_immunization.html. Accessed October 7, 2014.
47. Centers for Disease Control and Prevention. Updated recommendations for use of VariZIG—United States, 2013. 2013:62(28);574-576. http://www.cdc.gov/mmwr/preview/mmwrhtml/mm6228a4.htm. Accessed October 5, 2014.
48. Centers for Disease Control and Prevention. CDC guidance for evaluating health care personnel for hepatitis B virus protection and for administering postexposure management. *MMWR Recomm Rep.* 2013;62(RR10):1-19.
49. Centers for Disease Control and Prevention. Why immunize? http://www.cdc.gov/vaccines/vac-gen/why.htm. Accessed July 17, 2014.
50. Centers for Disease Control and Prevention. Vaccine Adverse Event Reporting System (VAERS). http://www.cdc.gov/vaccinesafety/Activities/vaers.html. Accessed July 17, 2014.
51. Centers for Disease Control and Prevention. Vaccine Safety Datalink (VSD). http://www.cdc.gov/vaccinesafety/Activities/vsd.html. Accessed July 17, 2014.
52. Centers for Disease Control and Prevention. Clinical Immunization Safety Assessment (CISA) project. http://www.cdc.gov/vaccinesafety/Activities/CISA.html. Accessed July 17, 2014.
53. Pichichero ME, Cernichiari E, Lopreiato J, Treanor J. Mercury concentrations and metabolism in infants receiving vaccines containing thimerosal: a descriptive study. *Lancet.* 2002;360(9347):1737-1741.
54. Heron J, Golding J, Team AS. Thimerosal exposure in infants and developmental disorders: a prospective cohort study in the United Kingdom does not show a causal association. *Pediatrics.* 2004;114(3): 577-583.
55. U.S. Food and Drug Administration. Thimerosal in vaccines. http://www.fda.gov/biologicsbloodvaccines/

safetyavailability/vaccinesafety/ucm096228.htm#t3. Accessed July 19, 2014.
56. Wakefield AJ, Murch SH, Anthony A, et al. Ileal-lymphoid-nodular hyperplasia, non-specific colitis, and pervasive developmental disorder in children. *Lancet.* 1998;351(9103):637-641.
57. Eggertson L. *Lancet* retracts 12-year-old article linking autism to MMR vaccines. *CMAJ.* 2010;182(4): E199–E200.
58. Plotkin SA, Cornfeld D, Ingalls TH. Studies of immunization with living rubella virus: trials in children with a strain coming from an aborted fetus. *Am J Dis Child.* 1965;110(4):381-389.
59. Jacobs JP, Jones CM, Bailie JP. Characteristics of a human diploid cell designated MRC-5. *Nature.* 1970;277:168-170.
60. Centers for Disease Control and Prevention. Vaccine excipient table. http://www.cdc.gov/vaccines/pubs/pinkbook/downloads/appendices/B/excipient-table-2.pdf. Accessed October 10, 2014.
61. Advisory Committee on Immunization Practices, Centers for Disease Control and Prevention (CDC). Immunization of health care personnel: recommendations of the Advisor Committee on Immunization Practices (ACIP). *MMWR.* 2011;60(RR07):1-45. http://www.cdc.gov/mmwr/preview/mmwrhtml/rr6007a1.htm?s_cid=rr6007a1_w. Accessed July 14, 2014.
62. Centers for Disease Control and Prevention. Travel health. http://wwwnc.cdc.gov/travel. Accessed October 5, 2014.
63. Smit MA, Jaffee EM, Lutz ER. Cancer immunoprevention: the next frontier. *Cancer Prev Res (Phila).* September 22, 2014. [Epub ahead of print].
64. Gross BP, Wongrakpanich A, Francis MB, Salem AK, Norian LA. A therapeutic microparticle-based tumor lysate vaccine reduces spontaneous metastases in murine breast cancer. *AAPS J.* September 16, 2014. [Epub ahead of print].
65. Ozao-Choy J, Lee DJ, Faries MB. Melanoma vaccines: mixed past, promising future *Surg Clin North Am.* 2014;94(5):1017-1030.
66. Tarahomjoo S. Recent approaches in vaccine development against *Streptococcus pneumoniae. J Mol Microbiol Biotechnol.* 2014;24(4):215-227.
67. Cohen J. Infectious disease. Ebola vaccine: little and late. *Science.* 2014;345(6203):1441-1442.
68. Hammer SM, Sobieszczyk ME, Janes H, et al. Efficacy trial of a DNA/rAd5 HIV-1 preventive vaccine. *N Engl J Med.* 2013;369(22):2083-2092.
69. Kumru OS, Joshi SB, Smith DE, Middaugh CR, Prusik T, Volkin DB. Vaccine instability in the cold chain: mechanisms, analysis and formulation strategies. *Biologicals.* 2014;42(5):237-259.

7 Drugs to Promote Optimum Weight

Cecilia M. Jevitt

Chapter Glossary

Anorexiants Drugs that decrease appetite. A synonym is anorectic.

Binge eating disorder Most common eating disorder, in which the individual suffering from the condition regularly eats excessive amounts of food.

Body mass index (BMI) Number calculated using a standard formula for weight and height that produces a reliable indication of body fatness. The formula has variations to reflect use of different measurement instruments (e.g., pounds versus kilograms).

Diet General foods eaten by an individual. The word often is used imprecisely to connote weight reduction. However, it may be configured to gain, lose, or maintain weight.

Obese Condition attributed to a person with a BMI of 30.0 or more. It may be subdivided further into three classes. Class 3 obesity (a BMI of 40 or more) is termed morbid obesity.

Obesigenic agents Pharmacologic medications whose side effects include weight gain.

Overweight Individual with a BMI between 25.0 and 29.9.

Yo-yo weight loss dieting Cycle of weight loss and weight gain.

Introduction

Maintaining an optimum weight is a health challenge. Before mechanization, humans spent hours each day on physical activities requiring energy, such as gathering or growing food. Physical expenditures of energy usually balanced intake. However, during the last half century, food intake has remained stable while activity levels have fallen. Mechanized farming, manufacturing, and information technology, along with individual car ownership and hours watching broadcast entertainment, minimize energy use. Few residents of postindustrial nations do daily heavy manual labor; thus, intake regularly exceeds energy expenditure. For weight loss to occur, regardless of medication use, energy expenditure must exceed intake. Theoretically, medications can support planned weight loss by suppressing appetite and signaling satiety. In clinical practice, medications that suppress appetite (**anorexiants**) or change metabolic pathways have risks and side effects that have, so far, generally outweighed their benefits.

Unlike the excessive intake of other illness-producing substances, such as tobacco or alcohol, food cannot be avoided entirely. Some food must be consumed several times a day for health, and food always remains an object of potential excessive intake. In the United States, eating has been integrated into family and work patterns as three meals a day. Meals are more than just necessary nutritional intake; that is, they also represent culturally influenced rest, relaxation, and communication times. Holidays have culturally specific celebratory foods, and religions have ceremonial meals and foods. Persistent willpower is necessary to avoid overeating in societies with an abundance of resources, regular relaxation times, and frequent celebrations.

Thirty percent of women in the United States are **overweight** and another 30% are **obese**, based on **body mass index (BMI)** calculations.[1] Optimum weight is not defined by clothing size or physical attractiveness; rather, it is

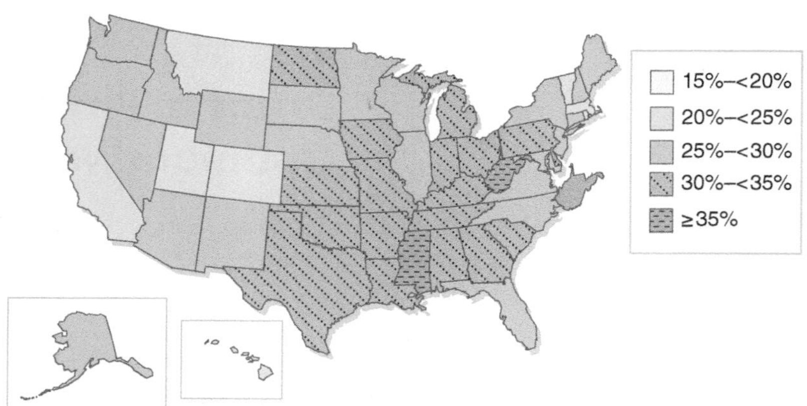

Figure 7-1 Obesity trends among U.S. adults: Prevalence[a] of self-reported obesity among U.S. adults by state and territory, 2013.

[a] Prevalence estimates reflect Behavioral Risk Factor Surveillance Systems methodologic changes started in 2011. These estimates should not be compared to prevalence estimates before 2011.

Source: Centers for Disease Control. National Center for Health Statistics. Prevalence of obesity: United States, 2013. 2013. http://www.cdc.gov/obesity/data/prevalence-maps.html Accessed September 21, 2014.[1]

weight that does not increase risk for disease. Obesity increases women's risks for abnormal menstrual patterns, infertility, early pregnancy loss, fetal malformations, surgical birth, postpartum hemorrhage, lactation difficulties, depression, diabetes, hypertension, heart disease, sleep apnea, joint pain, and a variety of cancers.[2] Being overweight is not as strongly linked with risk for disease as is being obese; however, uncontrolled weight gain is the first step toward obesity. The prevalence of overweight and obesity in postindustrial societies, as illustrated in Figure 7-1, mandates that clinicians of all specialties view BMI as a vital sign and be familiar with obesity prevention strategies and pharmacologic treatments.

Overweight and Obesity

BMI is a relative measure of weight and height using the formulas noted in Table 7-1, which are based on common measurements of body area.[3] Overweight is defined as a BMI between 26 and 29.9, whereas a BMI of 30 or more indicates obesity.[3,4] BMI is an imperfect measure of adiposity, however, because it can be inflated by extreme variations in bone and/or muscle mass.[3,4] Each BMI number represents approximately 5 pounds (2.27 kg). In general, women have a higher percentage of body fat per BMI level than men because men have more muscle mass.

Table 7-1 Weight Classifications by BMI and Body Fat Content

Classification	BMI[a]	Women: Percentage of Body Fat	Men: Percentage of Body Fat
Underweight	< 18.5	23–31	13–21
Normal	18.7–24.9	31–37	21–27
Overweight	25.0–29.9	37–42	27–31
Obesity class I	30.0–34.9	> 42	> 31
Obesity class II	35.0–39.9		
Obesity class III	≥ 40.0		

Abbreviations: BMI = body mass index.

[a] BMI is a relation between weight and height. It can be calculated in several ways, based on the choice of measurement instrument.

BMI = weight in kilograms divided by (height in meters)^2 *or*

BMI = weight in pounds × 703 divided by (height in inches)^2 *or*

BMI = weight in pounds × 4.88 divided by (height in feet)^2

Source: Data from National Institutes of Health, National Heart, Lung, and Blood Institute. Managing overweight and obesity in adults: systematic evidence review from the obesity expert panel: 2013. http://www.nhlbi.nih.gov/guidelines/obesity/ser/index.htm. Accessed March 23, 2014.[3]

Waist measurements in women (measured immediately above the iliac crest) more than 35 inches (88.8 cm) indicate excess abdominal fat and are correlated with the same health risks as if the woman were in the obese BMI category. Abdominal fat is metabolically active. It produces hormones, including leptin, and inflammatory cytokines, such as tumor necrosis factor alpha (TNFα) and interleukins including IL-6 and IL-1β.[5,6] Inflammatory changes in adipose tissue induce adipocytokine dysregulation, decreasing insulin sensitivity and release of anti-inflammatory adiponectin. Accumulating evidence supports chronic inflammation as the root of many of obesity's comorbid diseases—heart disease, hypertension, and diabetes, in particular.[7,8]

Women often strive for a weight they perceive as attractive instead of healthy. For example, if a woman is 5'6" tall (168 cm) and weighs 196 pounds (88.9 kg), she has a BMI of 32. Losing 5% of total body weight (10 pounds [4.54 kg], BMI = 30) reduces her risk for hypertension, diabetes, dyslipidemia, and heart disease.[3] Another 10% loss (20 pounds [8.94 kg], BMI = 27) further reduces risk and is achievable by most women with decreased intake and increased physical activity.[3] For each 1 kg (2.2 pounds) lost, the risk of metabolic syndrome is reduced by about 8% in a dose-dependent response.[3] To attain a normal or healthy BMI of 25, a 40-pound (18 kg) weight loss would be required. Losing and sustaining a loss of more than 10% body weight is difficult,[3] yet women often attempt even more unrealistic weight losses. For example, a loss of almost 80 pounds (36 kg) would be necessary for this woman to wear a size 8 dress.

Healthy intake reductions and exercise increases can produce a 1 pound per week weight loss.[3] Once weight is lost, intake limitations and activity increases must continue or weight will be regained. Controlling appetite and sustaining the motivation to exercise for years is a challenge that makes medications for weight loss and weight control attractive to many people.

Physiology of Weight Gain and Loss

Weight abnormalities can be caused by alterations in appetite and energy expenditure, physical or mental disease, eating disorders, and medications.

Mechanical and Neurohormonal Control of Energy Homeostasis

The body strives to balance energy intake with expenditure through central nervous system control. Hunger is stimulated before eating by afferent visual and olfactory sensory signals that prepare the body to eat and digest food. Peripheral distention and chemoreceptors in the gut and energy conversion in the liver signal the vagus nerve in the area postrema and the nucleus of the solitary tract.[9] Brain stem receptors detect circulating levels of nutrients and their metabolites.

Ingested neurotransmitter precursors alter central nervous system neuron–chemical activity, such as serotonin production, particularly in the hypothalamic nuclei and the limbic areas.[9] The serotonin, dopamine, norepinephrine, and endocannabinoid systems all modulate feelings of hunger and satiety. Food intake is decreased when serotonin (5-HT) or its precursors tryptophan and 5-HTP are increased. Therefore, several pharmaceutical agents may be given that address the various factors affecting weight, even though these drugs may not have specific U.S. Food and Drug Administration (FDA) indications for weight loss purposes. For example, selective serotonin receptor agonists are under investigation as appetite modulators.[10] Serotonin reuptake inhibitors, such as phentermine (Adipex-P), fenfluramine (Pondimin), and sibutramine (Meridia), are known to reduce hunger. Noradrenaline mechanisms, rather than 5-HT, may account for the appetite-reducing action of sibutramine (Meridia). Eating causes an increase in endogenous noradrenaline.[10] In turn, drugs such as amphetamines, phenylpropanolamine (Acutrim, Dexatrim), and sibutramine, which increase noradrenaline, reduce appetite and food intake. Dopamine activation decreases food intake. If selective dopamine agonists stimulate D1 or D2 receptors, food consumption decreases.[10] Bupropion (Wellbutrin) is both a noradrenaline and dopamine reuptake inhibitor. Bromocriptine (Parlodel), a D_2 receptor, is under investigation as an appetite suppressant.[10] Selective CB_1 receptor-blockers, such as rimonabant (Acomplia), decrease appetite with psychoactive effects.[10] Finally, endogenous cannabinoids interact with cannabinoid type 1 (CB_1) receptors in fat, liver, skeletal muscle, and other tissues to stimulate appetite. The hunger associated with smoking cannabis sativa, or marijuana, is an example of this effect.

In addition to the effects of neurotransmitters, a variety of hormones are involved in appetite and satiety, including insulin, leptin, ghrelin, neuropeptide Y, cholecystokinin, pancreatic polypeptide, peptide YY, and glucagon-like peptide. Many of these hormones are under investigation for use in weight control. Gut distention, adequate levels of nutrients, and neurotransmitters all combine to produce feelings of satiety. Medications to optimize weight could, therefore, work via several mechanisms including increasing and prolonging gastrointestinal distention, decreasing chemoreceptor signaling, or increasing the amount of neurotransmitters necessary for satiety.

Most body cells undergo periods of growth, programmed aging, and death (apoptosis). Adipose cells do not die, but rather expand or contract to accommodate excess energy stored as fat. Leptin, produced in abdominal fat stores, produces hunger signals that tell the body to increase eating and conserve fat stores. Leptin is produced even after weight loss, signaling the body to eat and regain lost weight.[5]

Age Variations in Energy Expenditure

Body size and composition, resting metabolic rate differences that are independent of body composition, and the thermal effect of food (the energy expenditure necessary to process food for use and storage above the basal metabolic rate) are influenced by genetic inheritance.[4] Studies attribute 25% to 50% of body composition to genetic factors, and the genetics of weight homeostasis is a current area of research interest.[4]

As women age, their caloric needs change. Growth to 18 years of age uses more calories than necessary for weight maintenance. Children's linear growth and ponderal growth occur at different times, preventing reliable use of BMI in persons younger than 18 years; instead, the World Health Organization's reference weights for children should be employed in this population.

Gender differences also exist. Women's thermal energy expenditures are approximately 16% lower than men's, so that women have lower daily caloric requirements than men. For reproductive-age women, basal metabolic rate and resting metabolic rate increase slightly during the luteal phase of the menstrual cycle. An adult woman with a BMI between 18.5 and 25 and a low activity level needs approximately 2000 calories per day to maintain body weight; by comparison, men in the same BMI and activity categories need 2500 calories per day. Institute of Medicine and U.S. Department of Agriculture nutrition guidelines are based on a 2000 calorie per day **diet**. Measuring intake against this standard may lead some women to unwittingly overeat, as some sedentary women need only 1500 to 1700 calories per day, particularly those with heights less than 63 inches (160 cm) and women who are older than 30 years.[4]

The decline in resting energy expenditure with age, coupled with a loss of fat-free body mass, lowers the basal metabolic rate. In men with stable weights, basal metabolic rate drops between 1% and 2% per decade. However, this decline accelerates for women after 50 years of age, and resting metabolic rate and fat-free mass further decrease postmenopausally in the absence of hormone therapy.[4]

Diseases Associated with Weight Alterations

Many physical diseases alter weight homeostasis. Physical causes of weight change, such as diabetes and thyroid abnormalities, must be investigated before weight maintenance therapies are initiated. Nicotine suppresses appetite, so tobacco cessation without lifestyle changes and behavioral therapy commonly is followed by weight gain. Some women recognize this association and unfortunately do not discontinue smoking for fear of weight gain, and women who stop tobacco use for pregnancy often restart in the postpartum period in an effort to control their weight.

The hormonal disturbances associated with obesity may cause anovulation, thereby reducing fertility. Weight loss of as little as 10% of body weight has been demonstrated to restore ovulation and fertility. Many published studies have shown that metformin (Glucophage) enhances insulin sensitivity and has been used preconceptionally to enhance weight loss and restore ovulation.[11,12]

Binge Eating Disorder

Most individuals occasionally overeat or binge on special occasions, but persons with **binge eating disorder** regularly eat excessive quantities of food.[13] Binge eating disorder is the most common eating disorder.[13] It is more common among women than among men, and it affects approximately 2% of the adult population living in the United States. Individuals with binge eating disorder are most often obese or go through cyclic bingeing and dieting (**yo-yo weight loss dieting**), alternating periods of overweight with periods of obesity. Table 7-2 lists the symptoms of binge eating disorder. Treatment plans using second-generation antidepressants such as fluvoxamine (Luvox) and fluoxetine (Prozac, Sarafem) along with weight-optimizing medications have been studied to reduce food binges; however, recent research indicates that psychological therapy in conjunction with topiramate (Topamax) is the most effective therapy.[14]

Bulimia Nervosa

Binge eating is a component of bulimia nervosa. Persons with bulimia nervosa eat excessively and then purge using induced vomiting, diuretics, or laxatives in an attempt to prevent weight gain. Binge eating alternates with purging, fasting, and excessive exercise.[15] Antianxiety agents along with weight-optimizing medications are being studied for treatment of this disorder.

Table 7-2 Signs of Eating Disorders

Binge Eating Disorder	Anorexia Nervosa
Consume an unusually large quantity of food Eat much more quickly than usual during binge episodes Continue eating until uncomfortably full Consume large amounts of food even when not hungry Eat alone because of embarrassment about the amount of food eaten Feel disgusted, depressed, or guilty after overeating Feel eating is out of control	Resistance to maintaining body weight at or above a minimally normal weight or age and height Intense fears of gaining weight or becoming fat, even though underweight Disturbances in the way in which body weight or shape is experienced, undue influence of body weight or shape on self-evaluation, or denial of the seriousness of the current low body weight Infrequent or absent menstrual periods in females who have reached puberty

Source: Reprinted from Heaner MK, Walsh BT. A history of the identification of the characteristic eating disturbances of bulimia nervosa, binge eating disorder and anorexia nervosa. *Appetite*. 2013;65:185-188, with permission from Elsevier.

Anorexia Nervosa

Anorexia nervosa is a serious mental illness. Individuals with this disease see themselves as overweight and starve and purge themselves in an attempt to attain an abnormally low body weight (Table 7-2). Anorexia nervosa is most common in female adolescents and young women, with an estimated 0.5% to 3.7% of women in the United States experiencing anorexia during their lives.[15] Challenges in treatment of anorexia are to overcome obsessions with eating and weight while stimulating appetite and changing self-image. Anorexia nervosa generally requires individual treatment with psychotropic medications within a program of biobehavioral support. Individuals with a history of anorexia should never be prescribed weight loss medications.

Obesigenic Medications

Several drug categories have weight gain as a possible or even common side effect. Table 7-3 lists some common drug categories whose side effects include weight gain. Prominent among these **obesigenic agents** are glucocorticoids and various psychiatric agents.

Glucocorticoids

Long-term use of glucocorticoids promotes weight gain. All glucocorticoids stimulate gluconeogenesis in the liver and inhibit peripheral glucose use. Glucocorticoids also cause protein breakdown in muscle, bone, and skin, which increases circulating amino acids. These amino acids stimulate hepatic enzyme activity, causing increased glycogen deposition and decreased glycolysis. High-dose exogenous steroid use promotes insulin resistance, with resulting carbohydrate intolerance and fasting hyperglycemia. Long-term steroid use mobilizes and remodels adipose deposits, resulting in characteristic fat deposits on the neck, supraclavicular area, and face.

Medications for Schizophrenia

Individuals with schizophrenia have a high prevalence of obesity and metabolic syndrome.[16–18] Olanzapine (Zyprexa), risperidone (Risperdal), quetiapine (Seroquel), and clozapine (Clozaril) are antipsychotic medications used in the treatment of schizophrenia that cause weight gain, which in turn often progresses to obesity.[16–18] Investigations using sibutramine (Meridia), topiramate (Topamax), naltrexone, or metformin (Glucophage) to counter this weight gain are ongoing.[16–21] Intake reduction and exercise programs have been shown to counteract antipsychotic medication related weight gain; however, illness can make adherence to these regimens particularly difficult.[22]

Hormonal Contraceptives

Excessive weight gain is a commonly reported side effect of hormonal contraceptives such as combined oral contraceptive pills and medroxyprogesterone acetate (DMPA);

Table 7-3 Drugs That May Cause Weight Gain

Drugs	Examples: Generic (Brand)
Classes of Drugs That Cause Weight Gain	
Antipsychotics	Olanzapine (Zyprexa), risperidone (Risperdal), quetiapine (Seroquel), clozapine (Clozaril)
Beta blockers	Atenolol (Tenormin), labetalol (Trandate), metoprolol (Lopressor)
Corticosteroids	Methylprednisolone (Solu-Medrol), prednisone (Deltasone)
Sulfonylureas	Chlorpropamide (Diabinese), glyburide (Micronase)
Thiazolidinedione (glitazones)	Rosiglitazone (Avandia), pioglitazone (Actos)
Tricyclic antidepressants	Amitriptyline (Elavil), nortriptyline (Aventyl), imipramine (Tofranil)
Individual Drugs That Cause Weight Gain	
Insulin	
Lithium (Eskalith)	
Valproate (Depakote)	

however, this side effect of contraceptives is not supported by FDA premarketing research.[23] Despite these data, many women continue to associate hormonal contraceptive use with weight gain.

One of the newer drugs on the market contains the progestin drospirenone; drospirenone is chemically related to spironolactone and has anti-mineralocorticoid properties that produce mild diuresis. This progestin is used in the oral contraceptives Yasmin (3 mg drospirenone and 30 mcg ethinyl estradiol) and YAZ (3 mg drospirenone and 20 mcg ethinyl estradiol). Drospirenone is favored by some endocrinologists for use by obese women with polycystic ovary syndrome because of its antiandrenergic properties. Early marketing of these products stressed their potential for inducing less bloating and fluid retention. Because of the marketing and the mild diuretic effect, some consumers viewed drospirenone as a weight loss medication, but no evidence has been found to support this claim.

Concerns have emerged regarding hormonal contraceptive failures among women who have BMIs higher than 35, particularly among those who use the contraceptive patch or combination pills. A Cochrane systematic review failed to find any such association, although the review also noted that well-controlled studies that included sufficient obese women were lacking.[23] Hormonal contraception is discussed in detail in the *Contraception* chapter.

Weight Loss Guidelines

Current guidelines support antiobesity drug use only as part of a comprehensive weight optimization plan that includes dietary modification, increased physical activity, lifestyle modification, and behavioral management, because integration of these components has an additive, synergistic effect.[2,3,24] Weight management through intake reduction, increased exercise, lifestyle modifications, and behavioral therapies lacks the potential physical and cognitive side effects associated with use of weight management medications alone. Therefore, nonmedicinal and nonsurgical weight loss interventions are recommended for overweight individuals (BMIs 26–29.9). A reduction of 500 to 1000 calories per day will provide for a sustainable weight loss of 1 pound per week. Total fats should account for 30% or less of dietary intake.[2,3,24]

Most weight loss is accomplished by decreased calorie intake; however, increased physical activity burns calories and stabilizes blood glucose through cellular use of noninsulin glucose. A walking program incrementally increased from 10 minutes to 30 to 60 minutes per day on 5 days each week can provide the physical activity necessary for weight stabilization and cardiac health.[2,3]

Lifestyle modifications are accomplished through behavioral changes. Consequently, individuals need insight into their eating behaviors to help them adopt and maintain healthier patterns. For example, through counseling, a woman might realize that she eats a quart of her favorite ice cream when she has an upsetting day at work. Substituting other stress-relieving tactics could lower consumption.

Weight loss medications are indicated for individuals with BMIs greater than 29 or individuals whose BMIs are greater than 26 and who have comorbidities such as hypertension or type 2 diabetes. Weight regain occurs with all weight loss medications once the medication is discontinued unless intake is kept low and physical activity is maintained.[2,24]

Weight loss surgery to correct obesity includes gastric banding and gastric bypass. The potentially serious side effects of these surgeries generally limit their use to individuals with a BMI of 40 or higher who have failed medical therapy, or those individuals with BMIs of 35 or greater who have comorbid conditions.[24] Following these surgeries, individuals will need vitamin and mineral supplementation for life. For example, calcium supplementation is essential to prevent postsurgical osteoporosis.

Pharmacokinetics and Pharmacodynamics of Weight Optimization Drugs

Medications to optimize weight fall into these three categories: (1) those that increase energy expenditure; (2) those that reduce appetite; and (3) those that decrease nutrient absorption (Figure 7-2 and Table 7-4). Single-drug weight loss therapies at best produce an 8% to 10% loss of initial body weight.[25] Because other weight loss treatments, such as reduction diets and exercise programs, have fewer side effects than weight loss medications and have equal weight loss success, the benefits and risks of these drugs must be carefully considered. Such medications are most effective when they are used to control appetite and signal satiety during a program of restricted intake and increased physical activity. Weight loss drugs may be of more value, when used in combination with dietary restriction, for obese individuals with mechanical arthritis or reduced cardiac function, which limits physical activity, than they would be

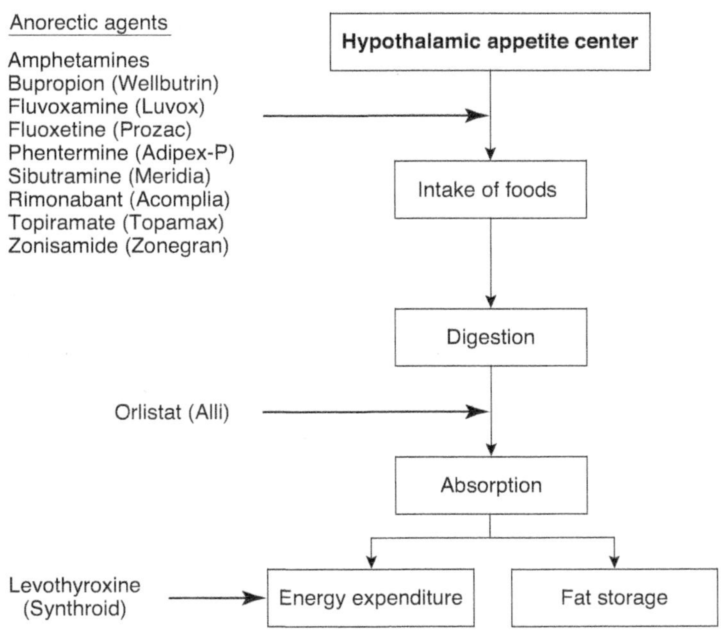

Figure 7-2 Weight loss drugs: site of action.

for other obese persons who could implement increased exercise programs with the dietary restrictions.

In general, weight loss drugs should not be used by individuals with hepatic or renal disease. Weight loss can precipitate or exacerbate gallstone formation; therefore, individuals with preexisting cholelithiasis should use these medications cautiously. Reproductive-age women with obesity or other conditions such as anorexia nervosa, as well as those taking many weight management medications, may experience menstrual irregularities and amenorrhea. Therefore, overweight or obese women seeking treatment for metrorrhagia or oligomenorrhea should be questioned routinely about use of antiobesity medications. A woman who has experienced infertility secondary to anovulation and amenorrhea may resume ovulation when she starts a weight loss activity and should consider using a reliable contraceptive method.

Drugs That Increase Energy Expenditure

Levothyroxine (T_4, Levo-T, Levoxyl, Synthroid) is the manufactured levo isomer of thyroxine. Indicated primarily for the treatment of hypothyroidism, it promotes protein and carbohydrate metabolism and increases gluconeogenesis. Exogenous levothyroxine has been administered since the 1950s for weight loss. Although this medication is not FDA approved for weight loss, weight loss clinics across the United States use high-dose levothyroxine to raise metabolism, thereby burning calories. The induced hyperthyroidism necessary for weight loss may produce serious and dangerous side effects.

Levothyroxine is a cardiostimulant and decreases cholesterol concentrations in the liver and bloodstream. Physiologic doses of the drug gradually reduce overweight or obesity that is secondary to hypothyroidism. Withdrawal of thyroid hormone may cause hypoglycemia, and long-term, high-dose levels have been associated with osteoporosis, especially in postmenopausal females.

Levothyroxine is contraindicated for individuals with uncontrolled adrenal insufficiency, untreated thyrotoxicosis, and myocardial infarction. It should be used cautiously by women with hypertension, angina, cardiac arrhythmias, previous myocardial infarction, or coronary artery disease. The cardiostimulatory effects of levothyroxine may precipitate cardiac arrhythmias and angina, and its use in individuals who are taking sympathomimetic agents for coronary artery disease treatment may result in coronary insufficiency. In addition, levothyroxine alters blood glucose levels and may alter the effectiveness of antidiabetes medications. Additional information regarding levothyroxine can be found in the chapter *Thyroid Disorders*.

Table 7-4 Medications Used in Weight Loss Therapy

Drug: Generic (Brand)	Mechanism of Action	Formulations	Dose	Clinical Considerations
Bupropion (Wellbutrin)	Induces anorexia	Tabs: 75 mg, 100 mg SR tabs: 100 mg, 150 mg, 200 mg XL tabs: 150 mg, 300 mg	150 mg PO in the morning; increase by 100 mg/day PO every 3 days to a maximum of 350 mg/day PO in divided doses	Do not break, crush, or chew SR or XL formulations. Should allow 8 hours between doses Bupropion has multiple adverse effects, drug–drug interactions, and contraindications. FDA black box warnings that bupropion may increase suicidal ideation in persons < 24 years and may cause neuropsychiatric symptoms.
Fluoxetine (Prozac, Sarafem)	Induces anorexia	Caps: 10 mg, 20 mg, 40 mg Tabs: 20 mg, 40 mg	60 mg/day PO	FDA approved for binge eating disorders.
Fluvoxamine (Luvox)	Induces anorexia	Tabs: 25 mg, 50 mg, 100 mg	50 mg/day PO at bedtime. May increase to maximum of 300 mg/day. If total dosage is more than 100 mg/day, give in divided doses.	Off-label use for binge eating disorders.
Lorcaserin HCl (Belviq)	Induces anorexia	10 mg orally 2 times/day		Evaluate response at 12 weeks and discontinue if weight loss is < 5% of baseline body weight. Multiple side effects and adverse effects. Many clinically significant drug–drug interactions.
Metformin (Glucophage)	Decreases intestinal glucose absorption	Tabs: 500 mg, 850 mg, 1000 mg ER tabs: 500 mg, 750 mg	850 mg PO 2 times/day	Do not break, crush, or chew ER formulations. Gastrointestinal side effects are common. Contraindicated for persons with cardiac, renal, or liver disease secondary to risk for lactic acidosis.
Naltrexone–Bupropion (Contrave)	Induces anorexia	Each tablet has naltrexone 8 mg/ bupropion 90 mg	1 tablet once/day for one week. Increase to 1 tablet 2 times/day during second week. Increase to 2 tablets in A.M. and 1 tablet at P.M. during third week. Increase to 2 tablets 2 times/day during week 4.	Evaluate response at 12 weeks and discontinue if weight loss is < 5% of baseline body weight. Allow 14 days to elapse before starting after discontinuing an MAO inhibitor. Bupropion has multiple adverse effects, drug–drug interactions, and contraindications. FDA black box warnings that bupropion may increase suicidal ideation in persons < 24 years and may cause neuropsychiatric symptoms.
Orlistat (Alli, Xenical)	Decreases nutrient absorption	Caps generic: 120 mg Caps trade: 60 mg	120 mg PO with each main meal containing fat. Maximum dose is 360 mg/ day PO.	For long-term use. Take with or up to 1 hour after a meal containing fat. Refrain from taking a multivitamin containing fat-soluble vitamins for at least 2 hours after taking orlistat.
Phentermine (Adipex-P)	Induces anorexia	Tabs: 5 mg, 18.75 mg, 30 mg, 37.5 mg ER: 8 mg, 30 mg	8 mg 3 times/day PO or 17–37.5 mg once/day PO taken 10–14 hours before bedtime	For short-term use. Take 30 minutes before meals.
Phentermine and topiramate (Qsymia)	Induces anorexia	Each tablet has phentermine 3.75 mg/topiramate 23 mg	1 tab PO daily for 14 days. Increase to 2 tabs daily for 12 weeks.	Evaluate response at 12 weeks and if weight loss is < 3% of baseline body weight, discontinue therapy or increase to 3 tablets/day. Allow 14 days to elapse before starting after discontinuing an MAO inhibitor. Has multiple drug–drug interactions.
Topiramate (Topamax)	Induces anorexia	Tablets: 25 mg, 50 mg, 100 mg, 200 mg Available as sprinkle capsules to place over food	27–600 mg once/day PO. Average dose is 50 mg/day.	Off-label use for binge eating disorders. Can be taken without regard to meals. Has multiple side effects, adverse effects, and drug–drug interactions. Gastrointestinal side effects are common. Must be withdrawn gradually. Contraindicated in persons with hepatic or renal disorders.
Zonisamide (Zonegran)	Induces anorexia	Caps: 25 mg, 50 mg, 100 mg	100 mg/day PO gradually increased to 400 mg/day. Can be increased to 600 mg/day for persons who < 5% of body weight at the end of 12 weeks.	Off-label use for binge eating disorders. Gastrointestinal side effects are common. Must be withdrawn gradually.

Drugs That Reduce Appetite

Amphetamine

Amphetamine, a Schedule C-II controlled substance, is a sympathomimetic adrenergic agonist that suppresses appetite. Amphetamine was widely used in the 1950s and 1960s for weight loss. Because of its addictive properties and psychiatric effects, this drug is no longer indicated for weight loss.

Fenfluramine and Dexfenfluramine

Fenfluramine (Pondimin) and dexfenfluramine (Redux) stimulate the release of serotonin and inhibit serotonin reuptake, thereby decreasing appetite. They also increase glucose uptake by skeletal muscles. Fenfluramine was prescribed with phentermine in a combination known as the fen-phen regimen. It is no longer marketed in the United States and is not FDA approved for use, although both fenfluramine and dexfenfluramine may still be available in Europe or via the Internet (Box 7-1).

> **Box 7-1** Gone But Not Forgotten: The Fen-Phen Fiasco
>
> The fen-phen (fenfluramine and phentermine) regimen was introduced in 1992. Weight loss using this drug regimen was highly successful, with losses of 15% of initial body weight being reported.[27] Associated cases of pulmonary hypertension and valvular heart disease were reported among 5% to 25% of women using this combination of drugs. The association was confounded by the fact that obesity alone is associated with cardiovascular disease. However, the FDA disapproved the combination in 1996, and the manufacturers voluntarily withdrew the drugs from the U.S. market in 1997, despite fenphen's widespread use and favorable safety record in Europe.
>
> Combined phentermine and fenfluramine is still available in Europe and over the Internet in the United States with a prescription. The severity of valvular disease decreases following the termination of fen-phen use; however, persons who have used fen-phen need to report dyspnea, decreasing exercise tolerance, syncope, angina, and edema immediately, as all of these are signs of cardiac disease.

Phentermine

Phentermine (Adipex-P, Atti-Plex-P, Fastin, Ionamin, Kraft-Obese, Pro-Fast SA, Pro-Fast SR, Tara-8), a noradrenergic drug that suppresses appetite by stimulating sympathetic activity, is chemically and pharmacologically related to the amphetamines. It is indicated for short-term (6 week) weight loss therapy. Phentermine can be purchased over the Internet without a prescription.

The most common side effects associated with phentermine include irritability, insomnia, and personality changes. Altered alertness places phentermine users at risk for accidents when driving or using heavy equipment. Use of this agent is contraindicated for persons with hypertension, heart disease, glaucoma, or depression. Because it is a sympathomimetic drug, it is also contraindicated for persons with hyperthyroidism. Long-term use of phentermine can cause dependence. Phentermine can aggravate anxiety, mania, agitation, and psychosis. Abrupt cessation of therapy is known to cause depression or extreme fatigue. Use should be gradually tapered before discontinuation. This agent should not be used for those with a history of anorexia nervosa, depression, or substance abuse. Phentermine interacts with monoamine oxidase (MAO) inhibitors, causing increased cardiac stimulation and hypotension. Insulin requirements and the actions of other hypoglycemic agents may be altered by phentermine use.

A phentermine–fluoxetine (phen-flu) combination is being investigated in Europe as a fen-phen replacement. In one study, phentermine–fluoxetine users had lower weight loss (9%) than phentermine–fenfluramine users (12.6%) but developed no cardiac valve lesions after 6 months of treatment.[27]

Sibutramine

Sibutramine (Meridia) is a serotonin and norepinephrine reuptake inhibitor that is theorized to suppress appetite by signaling early satiety. Sibutramine was indicated for weight loss for healthy individuals as part of a program of dietary management and increased physical activity. Some sources credit this drug with increasing resting energy expenditure. FDA approval of sibutramine was withdrawn in 2010 following accumulating reports of cardiovascular events, stroke, heart failure, and kidney failure. This agent has been removed from the U.S. market except for research studies.[19]

Topiramate and Zonisamide

The ability to induce anorexia and persistent weight loss in obese individuals was discovered during clinical trials of topiramate (Topamax) and zonisamide (Zonegran), two antiepileptic drugs with similar actions and indications. Topiramate and zonisamide have multiple indications, including the treatment of seizure disorders, alcoholism, bipolar disorder, diabetic neuropathy, mania, and migraine prophylaxis. The exact mechanisms of their weight loss action are unknown, although emerging research indicates that both of these agents inhibit the induction of carbonic anhydrases. Carbonic anhydrase enzymes are necessary for new lipogenesis in both the mitochondria and the cytosol of cells. Topiramate inhibits lipogenesis in adipocytes similarly to other sulfonamide carbonic anhydrase inhibitors.[26] It has been shown to produce significant weight loss and improve glucose homeostasis when used as an adjunct to diet and exercise therapy in persons with type 2 diabetes (Box 7-2).[26] Topiramate alone has been used to treat obesity associated with medications for bipolar disorder.

Topiramate and zonisamide have multiple adverse reactions, including agitation, anorexia, depression, dizziness, drowsiness, emotional lability, euphoria, hallucinations, hypoesthesia, decreased libido, erectile dysfunction, menstrual irregularities, psychosis, tinnitus, and xerostomia. Driving and operating heavy equipment should be undertaken with caution due to the central nervous system side effects. Gastrointestinal symptoms include abdominal pain, constipation, diarrhea, gastritis, flatulence, gastroesophageal reflux, nausea, vomiting, and pancreatitis. These agents may be such effective anorexiants because they cause hypoglycemia, anemia, osteopenia, and osteoporosis. Both topiramate and zonisamide are contraindicated for persons with biliary cirrhosis, hepatic or renal disease, chronic obstructive lung disease, emphysema, glaucoma, nephrolithiasis, and ocular disease.

Topiramate must be avoided during pregnancy. Use of this agent during pregnancy as an anticonvulsant revealed a significant increase in oral cleft deformities in newborns exposed to topiramate during the first trimester.[28]

Box 7-2 A Case of Chronic Obesity

MJ is a 37-year-old accountant who asked during her regular gynecologic visit, "Can you prescribe more of this weight loss medication for me?" MJ revealed that her primary care provider had prescribed phentermine for her a year ago but refuses to renew the prescription, partly due to concerns about her blood pressure. MJ lost 27 pounds (12 kg) while using phentermine, but since she discontinued the medication, she has regained 23 pounds (10 kg). MJ had four prior cycles of 25- to 30-pound (11.34–13.6 kg) weight loss and regain since age 20. Her highest weight was 212 pounds ([96.1 kg], BMI = 34.2). Prior weight loss medications included fen-phen, over-the-counter products containing ephedra, and two cycles of phentermine.

MJ is a nonsmoker who does little physical activity and dislikes exercise. At this visit, her weight was 198 pounds (90 kg), BMI was 32, and waist measurement was 45 inches (114 cm). Her blood pressure was 146/94 mm Hg. Her thyroid function was normal, total cholesterol was 295 mg/dL, triglycerides were 210 mg/dL, and high-density lipoprotein (HDL) was 34 mg/dL. Her fasting glucose was 112 mg/dL and her hemoglobin A_{1c} (HbA_{1c}) was 6.5 mg/dL. Because of her prior fen-phen use, an EKG had been done; the results were normal. MJ had four markers for metabolic syndrome: (1) obesity, (2) abdominal fat, (3) hypertension, and (4) elevated triglycerides, including elevated cholesterol and decreased high-density lipoprotein (HDL). The clinician reviewed her caloric needs, the effect of exercise on glycemic control and blood pressure, and metabolic syndrome. Weight optimization would be vital for preventing diabetes and heart disease. MJ would need a lifelong program of reduced intake and increased physical activity to prevent weight regain.

MJ hesitantly agreed to a referral to a local multidisciplinary weight loss program. During program participation, she walked at lunch hour, gradually increasing her walking to 45 minutes each day. The program provided low-fat, nutritious meal cooking classes. MJ initiated orlistat (Xenical) 120 mg with each meal. Ten weeks after initiation of this program, she was dissatisfied with her weight loss and found a new provider who prescribed topiramate (Topamax) to augment weight loss. Although she lost 8 pounds (3.5 kg) during 3 weeks of topiramate use, she felt confused and stopped using the topiramate.

At 30 weeks of program participation, MJ had lost 25 pounds (10 kg). This lowered her BMI to 27.9. Her total cholesterol was 170 mg/dL and her HDL was 72 mg/dL. Her HgA_{1c} was 4.8 mg/dL. Her blood pressure averaged 126/85 mm Hg. MJ hoped to double that loss and planned to initiate phentermine–topiramate (Qsymia).

Phentermine and Topiramate (Qsymia) Combination Therapy

A new combination of phentermine and topiramate (Qsymia) is available and received FDA approval in 2012. The dose of each medication within Qsymia is lower than when these drugs are used as monotherapy. Weight loss is more modest, but fewer side effects are observed.[27]

Fluoxetine and Fluvoxamine

Fluoxetine (Prozac) and fluvoxamine (Luvox) are SSRIs that have been studied as components of weight loss therapy for persons with binge eating disorder, bipolar disease–associated obesity, and obesity.[16,17] Fluoxetine (Prozac) has been approved by the FDA for the treatment of binge eating disorder. In studies, use of fluoxetine reduced food intake, improved insulin sensitivity, and decreased insulin requirements for individuals with type 2 diabetes.[17] Fluoxetine is not indicated for general treatment of obesity because of its frequent side effects, which include somnolence, agitation, alterations in libido and orgasmic dysfunction, diarrhea, and tremors.

Use of fluvoxamine (Prozac) to reduce binge eating disorders has been studied, and significant results in terms of decreasing binge episodes and lowering BMI over 9 weeks were found. Oral doses ranged from 50 to 300 mg per day. However, the majority of participants failed to complete the study due to nausea, somnolence, and dizziness.[14] Fluvoxamine is currently used off label for binge eating, but it is important to note that SSRIs have recently been associated with suicidal ideation among young adults (18–24 years), and a black box warning on the label urges caution with use of these drugs in persons younger than 24 years.

Bupropion

Bupropion (Wellbutrin) is a noradrenaline and dopamine reuptake inhibitor indicated for treatment of depression. Unintentional weight loss during bupropion use suggested its utility in weight loss therapy. This agent has also been used as an adjunctive therapy for the treatment of seasonal affective disorder, nicotine dependence, bipolar disorder, and obesity. Individuals with bulimia or anorexia nervosa who use bupropion are at increased risk for having seizures. Incremental initiation reduces the risk of seizures.

Bupropion may cause elevations in liver function tests. Central nervous system side effects include restlessness, agitation, anxiety, confusion, insomnia, paranoia, and hallucinations. Bupropion must be used cautiously by persons with cardiac disease, as it may cause hypertension. In addition, the FDA has two black box warnings on the label of bupropion cautioning use in persons younger than 24 years as it has been associated with suicidal ideation and neuropsychiatric symptoms.

Naltrexone–Bupropion (Contrave) Combination Therapy

Naltrexone (Revia, Depade) is an opioid antagonist used for the treatment of opioid and alcohol dependency. Bupropion (Wellbutrin) is a norepinephrine/dopamine reuptake inhibitor that has been used for many years to treat depression and smoking cessation. Combination therapy with naltrexone and bupropion produces weight loss and has a metabolic profile beneficial for the potential treatment of obesity. A fixed dose of sustained-released naltrexone–bupropion (Contrave) enhanced weight loss in four Phase 3 clinical trials.[29,30] Naltrexone–bupropion is more effective in promoting weight loss than orlistat (Xenical). Although the weight loss produced by the phentermine–topiramate (Qsymia) combination is superior to that observed with the naltrexone–bupropion (Contrave) combination, the latter therapy has fewer severe adverse effects. In addition, naltrexone–bupropion is well tolerated, with nausea being the most frequently reported adverse event. Unlike other centrally acting medications, including phentermine–topiramate, naltrexone–bupropion has no abuse potential. In 2014, naltrexone–bupropion received FDA approval as a weight loss drug using the brand name Contrave.

Drugs That Decrease Nutrient Absorption

Orlistat

Orlistat (Alli, Xenical) is a gastrointestinal lipase inhibitor that blocks the absorption of dietary fat by preventing gastric and pancreatic lipases from hydrolyzing dietary triglycerides into free fatty acids and monoglycerides. Numerous studies demonstrate reduced fasting insulin levels, reduced low-density lipoproteins (LDL), lowered HbA_{1c}, and improved glycemic control with orlistat use. This agent has minimal systemic absorption, with more than 80% being excreted unchanged in feces. The brand Alli became available over the counter in the United States in 60-mg dosing in 2007, although Xenical in 120-mg capsules continues to be available by prescription only.

One orlistat capsule is administered with each main meal containing fat or within 1 hour after the meal. The dose is omitted when meals are missed or contain no fat. Orlistat has a modest effect on weight loss. An individual can expect to lose approximately 6 pounds more per year than can be lost with diet alone.

The most common side effects of orlistat are steatorrhea, flatulence, abdominal bloating, increased defecation, oily spotting, and fecal urgency and incontinence. Side effects increase with the amount of dietary fat consumed, with adverse gastrointestinal events being most common when fat exceeds 30% of intake. Long-term use of orlistat is credited with improving the release of appetite-regulating gut hormones such as pancreatic lipase, thereby increasing feelings of satiety.[31] Poor lipid absorption decreases serum levels of β-carotene and vitamins A, D, and E, but vitamin deficiencies can be avoided by daily use of a fat-soluble vitamin-containing multivitamin that is taken at least 2 hours after orlistat use.

Rare cases of rash, urticaria, pruritus, and prolonged clotting times were reported during postmarketing surveillance. Orlistat is contraindicated for use by individuals with cholestasis, anorexia, or bulimia nervosa, and hyperoxaluria, and clotting times must be monitored in those persons using anticoagulant therapy. A related compound, cetilistat, is under investigation and shows promise as a weight loss agent, with fewer side effects than orlistat.[32]

Other Weight Loss Medications

Lorcaserin

Lorcaserin HCl (Belviq) was approved in 2012 by the U.S. Food and Drug Administration to augment lifestyle modification in obese (BMI ≥ 30) and overweight (BMI ≥ 27) persons who have one obesity-related comorbidity. This novel serotonin 5-HT_{2C} selective agonist has been shown in three Phase 3 studies to significantly reduce weight and cardiovascular risk factors such as diabetes. Therapeutic results should be evaluated by week 12. If at 12 weeks the woman has not lost 5% of body weight, lorcaserin should be discontinued, as she is then not likely to have lorcaserin-associated weight loss.

Lorcaserin is contraindicated for breastfeeding women, children younger than 18 years, and persons with renal or hepatic disease. Because individuals using lorcaserin reported feeling "high, sedated, or hallucinogenic" 2 to 6 times more than controls, this agent is classified as a Schedule IV controlled substance. In studies, 16% of lorcaserin users reported euphoria that lasted as long as 9 hours after the last dose. No data are available about lorcaserin overdoses.

Because it is a serotonergic drug, lorcaserin has the potential to cause serotonin syndrome or neuroleptic malignant syndrome–like reactions (NMS). Symptoms of these conditions include agitation, hallucinations, coma, seizures, autonomic instability, tachycardia, labile blood pressure, hyperthermia, and muscle rigidity. These reactions are most likely to occur when lorcaserin is accidentally used with other serotonergic agents such as bupropion (Wellbutrin), St. John's wort, or dextromethorphan. When they occur, emergency management is needed.

Other side effects of lorcaserin include regurgitant valvular heart disease, bradycardia, decreases in white blood cells, pulmonary hypertension, and prolactin level increases. Among men, priapism lasting longer than 6 hours has been reported. Among individuals with type 2 diabetes using oral hypoglycemic or insulin, lorcaserin-related weight loss may result in episodes of hypoglycemia.

Rimonabant

Rimonabant (Acomplia) is a novel appetite suppressant that blocks the cannabinoid-1 (CB-1) receptor subtype.[33] The use of cannabis sativa as an antiemetic and appetite stimulant in oncology established the role of endocannabinoids in appetite regulation.[34,35] Rimonabant was available in the United Kingdom and other European countries; however, the FDA denied its release in the United States in 2007, owing to safety concerns centered on increased anxiety, depression, aggression, psychosis, and suicidal thoughts in rimonabant users. After reports of severe psychological problems and suicide during rimonabant use accumulated in Europe, the European Medicines Agency withdrew its recommendation in January 2009. The manufacturer then suspended sales of the drug.

Metformin

Metformin (Glucophage) is a biguanide that decreases liver glucose production while increasing insulin sensitivity in the liver and peripheral tissues. This agent decreases intestinal glucose absorption and decreases triglyceride and LDL levels while increasing HDL levels. Among individuals who do not have diabetes, metformin does not affect pancreatic β-cell function or cause hypoglycemia. It induces weight loss in women with polycystic ovary disease. Metformin may be used as initial infertility treatment in anovulatory obese women with the aim of restoring ovulation following weight loss, although its efficacy in this indication has been called into question (Box 7-3).[36,37] Metformin 850 mg is taken orally twice a day with meals for weight loss. This dose produces weight loss comparable to daily sibutramine doses and prescription-strength orlistat.[36]

Adverse reactions to metformin use may include dizziness, headache, flushing, chills or sweating, myalgias, chest pressure, palpitations, and dyspnea. Metformin use

Box 7-3 A Case of Obesity and Infertility

SH is a 24-year-old primary schoolteacher who, after 3 years of marriage and 2 years of unsuccessful attempts to start a family, has asked for fertility help during her annual gynecologic exam. She is a nonsmoker with no chronic diseases. Her menstrual cycles are approximately 70- to 90-day intervals with 2–3 days of painless spotting during each menses.

SH's height is 64 inches (162.6 cm), weight is 207 pounds (93.9 kg), and BMI is 35.5. Her blood pressure is 131/84 mm Hg, pulse 80, and respirations 18. Her physical examination was essentially normal. SH has facial acne with mild facial and abdominal hirsutism.

The clinician explained the associations between excess adipose tissue, insulin resistance, excess estrogen storage, elevated androgens, and ovulatory irregularities. SH's menstrual irregularities, hirsutism, and acne suggested she may have polycystic ovary syndrome (PCOS). The clinician ordered a transvaginal ultrasound to visualize ovarian mass and rule out reproductive organ anomalies, fasting blood glucose, and tests of SH's thyroid-stimulating hormone level and serum androgen level so these results would be available when SH had her appointment with the reproductive endocrinologist. SH's transvaginal ultrasound was normal, as were the serum glucose and thyroid-stimulating hormone level. Her serum androgen was near the upper limits of normal.

The reproductive endocrinologist advised SH that she most likely had PCOS and that a 5% to 10% loss of body weight was the best initial treatment to restore ovulation. SH was prescribed metformin (Glucophage) 850 mg to be taken orally twice a day with meals. She was also prescribed spironolactone (Aldactone) 50 mg orally per day to minimize androgenic effects of PCOS. Obesity increases the risk of fetal deformities, and SH was advised to take folic acid 400 mcg orally daily. SH joined a weight loss program that focused on balanced, calorie-restricted nutrition, and she joined a women's gym.

At the end of 20 weeks, SH had lost 18 pounds (8.2 kg) and continued to take the metformin, spironolactone, and folic acid. She was losing patience with her planned meals and had stopped using the gym after 12 weeks. However, the 9% loss of body weight lowered her BMI to 32.4. Her blood pressure fell to an average of 124/70 mm Hg, and she had two menses that were a month apart. These successes encouraged SH to continue her planned eating and she returned to the gym. At the end of week 36, SH had maintained her weight at 189 pounds (85.7 kg, BMI = 32) for 5 months and was pregnant.

The 18-pound (8.2-kg) weight loss did not shift SH from an obese to an overweight BMI category; however, 20 pounds (9 kg) is the average annual loss associated with all weight management therapies. Women with BMIs of 30 or higher are at increased risk for many perinatal complications, including fetal malformations, gestational diabetes, hypertension, deep vein thrombosis, macrosomia, induction of labor, cesarean birth, and shoulder dystocia. The reproductive endocrinologist advised SH to discontinue the metformin and spironolactone during pregnancy but to continue the folic acid during the first trimester. Using Institute of Medicine guidelines, SH was advised not to diet during pregnancy, but to anticipate a 15-pound weight gain. A dietician reviewed carbohydrate counting and the American Diabetic Association Diet with SH, planning a 2000 calorie/day intake.

may cause many gastrointestinal symptoms, including cramping, diarrhea, nausea, vomiting, flatulence, indigestion, and abnormal stools. Some individuals experience an annoying metallic taste.

Over-the-Counter Medications

A variety of herbs, vitamin and mineral supplements, and fibers are available over the counter for weight loss. Questions about over-the-counter weight loss pills or preparations should be a part of every primary care exam. Women who use these compounds are motivated to optimize weight and may be receptive to trying prescription weight loss medications with proven efficacy. A major concern with weight loss supplements has become the discovery of product contamination with actual weight loss drugs such as sibutramine (Meridia). No over-the-counter weight loss supplement has been found to improve weight loss efforts better than intake restriction and increases in physical activity.[38,39]

Substances That Increase Energy Expenditure

Chromium Picolinate

An organic compound of trivalent chromium and picolinic acid, a derivative of tryptophan, is marketed as chromium picolinate. Chromium is an essential mineral that is an insulin cofactor. This ingredient has long been used as an adjunct for glucose control in diabetes management; indeed, most weight loss compounds contain chromium picolinate in 200 to 400 mcg per day doses. One meta-analysis indicates that use over 6–14 weeks in individuals with BMIs of 28–33 provides statistically significant weight loss compared to a placebo, but clinically this amounts to approximately 2.5 pounds (1.1–1.2 kg).[39] Restricting intake by 500 calories per day over the same time period could produce a loss of 3–7 pounds (1.4–3.2 kg). Chromium picolinate was well tolerated in the randomized controlled trials studying its use for this indication.[40]

In another study, chromium picolinate was associated with decreased fasting blood sugar and insulin levels, thereby increasing insulin sensitivity among women who had polycystic ovary syndrome that was resistant to treatment with clomiphene citrate (Clomid). These effects were comparable with metformin (Glucophage) treatment; however, metformin use was associated with decreased hyperandrogenism. Chromium picolinate had fewer side effects than metformin. Women using chromium picolinate and metformin had similar ovulation and pregnancy rates.[40]

In spite of the promising results cited, a Cochrane review found no evidence strong enough to guide clinicians in the use of chromium picolinate for weight loss.[41]

Garcinia Cambogia

Garcinia cambogia contains hydroxy-citric acid, which suppresses de novo fatty acid synthesis and is thought to reduce intake.[42,43] One randomized study demonstrated significantly greater weight loss with *Garcinia cambogia* use over 12 weeks' time compared to a placebo (8.14 ± 6.82 lb versus 5.28 ± 6.45 lb [0.7 ± 3.1 kg versus 2.4 ± 2.9 kg]).[42] Another randomized study showed no significant difference in weight loss between persons using *Garcinia cambogia* and individuals taking a placebo after 12 weeks.[43] One study of a nutraceutical containing *Garcinia cambogia, Ascophyllum nodosum* extract, and L-carnitine suggests that this product might be useful as an appetite modulator. Study participants using the combination as they desired reported decreased appetite and greater feelings of satiety.[43]

Ephedra

An alkaloid derived from the herb *Ephedra sinica* is available as ephedra. This pharmacologic agent increases metabolism, has anorexiant properties, and is a bronchodilator. Known as *ma huang* in Chinese medicine, it has been used for more than 5000 years to treat asthma, hay fever, and respiratory tract infections. In the past, ephedra was a component of many over-the-counter weight loss pills. Ephedra, however, can generate serious adverse reactions, including hypertension, dizziness, nausea, dysrhythmias, heart failure, and myocardial infarction. A series of sudden heart failure deaths in ephedra users with no prior heart disease prompted the FDA to ban ephedra sales in the United States in 2004; appeals courts upheld the ban in 2006. Ephedra is available outside the United States and is used extensively (both legally and illegally) by athletes for weight control. Strenuous exercise during ephedra use increases the risk of heat stroke, stroke, and sudden cardiac arrest; therefore, many sports organizations, including the International Olympics Committee, have banned its use.

Substances That Reduce Appetite

Yerba mate, an herbal product from the South American evergreen tree *Ilex paraguariensis*, contains large amounts of caffeine, which may delay gastric emptying time, thereby prolonging satiety. Adverse effects have not been reported, but studies of this product are limited. Side effects secondary to caffeine may be expected.

Another evergreen tree, *Pausinystalia yohimbe*, yields yohimbine, an α_2 receptor agonist that is intended to reduce appetite. Trials of the product marketed as yohimbe have produced conflicting results.[39] Yohimbine is a purported aphrodisiac; it is contraindicated for persons with renal disease. Extracts of black, green, and mulberry teas are under investigation as weight loss adjuvants.[39,44]

Other Botanical Products

Glucomannan

Many weight loss products contain fibers that increase the size of the intestinal food bolus, stimulating pressure receptors to signal satiety. *Amorphophallus konjac*, the konjac root, contains glucomannan, a dietary fiber composed of a polysaccharide chain and mannose. Glucomannan is hydrophilic and creates a larger food bolus, thereby signaling early satiety. This ingredient is used extensively in Japanese foods such as noodles and tofu. Weight loss using 2–4 g per day has been demonstrated with few side effects.[39,45]

In a double-blind study where the intervention participants used 1 g of glucomannan with 8 oz water before each of their three daily meals over 8 weeks, the glucomannan group averaged a 5.5 pound (2.5 kg) greater weight loss than control subjects with no prescribed change in intake or exercise. They also had significant reductions in serum cholesterol and LDL (21.7 and 15 mg/dL, respectively) compared to placebo users.[46] Glucomannan improved lipid parameters and glycemic status in one study of individuals with diabetes but no weight loss was associated with glucomannan.[47]

Guar gum, another dietary fiber, is derived from the Indian bean *Cyamopsis tetragonolobus.* It has not been shown to lower body weight.

Although the water-soluble fiber psyllium is well tolerated, it has not been shown to enhance weight loss, but it can improve lipid and glucose parameters.[39] All fiber products have the potential to cause diarrhea, flatulence, and gastrointestinal discomfort.

Fenugreek

Fenugreek has been found to reduce blood glucose through decreased insulin resistance. In a study of women with polycystic ovary syndrome where one group received fenugreek seed capsules plus metformin and a second group received only metformin, rates of insulin resistance after 8 weeks of treatment remained similar between the groups; however, women who received the fenugreek seed extract had improved ovary appearance by sonogram and improved menstrual cyclicity.[48]

Substances Intended to Decrease Nutrient Absorption

Chitosan is a polysaccharide produced from the chitin contained in the exoskeletons of marine crustaceans. Chitosan is marketed to decrease fat absorption but has not been shown to enhance weight loss. Its most frequent side effects are constipation and flatulence.[39] Over-the-counter orlistat (Alli) would be an effective substitute for chitosan.

Nonpharmacologic Weight Loss Methods

The National Physical Activity and Weight Loss survey was a nationwide telephone survey completed in 2002 that questioned 11,211 individuals about complementary and alternative medicine (CAM) therapy use for weight loss. Of those persons surveyed, 3% had used a CAM therapy in the preceding 12 months for weight loss. The most popular CAM modality used was yoga, including yoga breathing (57.4%). Other methods included meditation (8.2%), massage (7.5%), acupuncture (7.7%), and Eastern martial arts (5.9%). All other CAM therapies combined accounted for 13.3% of those used.[49] A meta-analysis of acupuncture and acupressure studies revealed no convincing research that either method reduces body weight.[39] Most studies investigating the effect of hypnosis on weight loss are at least a decade old and do not demonstrate significant weight loss with this modality.[50]

Special Populations

Children and Adolescents

Overweight and obesity are epidemic in children in the United States; however, weight loss medication use in children younger than 16 years is generally not recommended. The preferred interventions are to identify children at risk for overweight, then reduce their energy intake by trading calorie-dense, non-nutritious foods, such as cookies and soda, for more nutritious foods, such as fruits and complex carbohydrates, while increasing their physical activity. Play and sports participation will increase muscle mass while using stored fat for fuel. The high basal metabolic rate during children's growth augments weight loss when intake and activity are optimized.

The use of weight loss medications has been studied in children receiving second-generation antipsychotic medications with subsequent insulin resistance, obesity, and type 2 diabetes. In one study, children 10 to 17 years treated with atypical antipsychotics took metformin 500 mg with their evening meal for 1 week and then added another 500-mg dose with breakfast. In week 4, metformin was increased to 850 mg twice a day. Those individuals using metformin stabilized BMI, neither gaining nor losing weight, and developed increased insulin sensitivity over 16 weeks. Adolescents receiving the placebo continued to gain weight.[51]

Topiramate (Topamax) was used as an anorexiant in a small study of children 4 to 18 years with binge eating disorder or Prader-Willi syndrome. Doses were gradually increased until a dosage of 7.0 mg/kg per day was achieved. Topiramate was successful in reducing obsessive food cravings. However, at this dose, 71% of children complained of memory problems and almost 30% also complained of reduced psychomotor speed and language and attention problems. These effects disappeared after dosage reductions to 3.0 mg/kg per day or cessation of topiramate.[52]

Orlistat (Xenical, Alli) has been studied in obese adolescents and can be used safely with weight monitoring every 2–4 weeks. Forty percent of adolescents 12–16 years using orlistat plus mild caloric restriction, exercise, and behavioral therapy in one study had a 5% to 10% decrease in BMI compared to 20.2% of teens using a placebo. BMI reduction is a better measure of weight loss in adolescents because rapid adolescent height growth changes BMI. At the end of 1 year, weight had increased only 1 pound (0.53 kg) in the orlistat group, while the control group gained, on average, 6.9 pounds (3.14 kg).[53] Parents need to know that their offspring may purchase orlistat without a prescription and might use it during unsupervised weight loss attempts.

Adolescents may also purchase and use laxatives for weight loss without parental knowledge. This strategy, which is often used for purging by persons with eating disorders, provides a temporary 1- to 2-pound weight loss of fecal matter but no loss of stored fat. A study of 4292 adolescents using data from the 2001 National Household Survey on Drug Abuse found that approximately 10% of adolescent females used laxatives or vomited to lose weight during the preceding year.[54] Teens of both sexes may use laxatives and diuretics for small weight losses when trying to stay in a lower weight division for sports divided into weight categories, such as wrestling.

Pregnancy

Women should not adopt dietary restrictions to lose weight during pregnancy and most weight loss drugs are contraindicated for use during pregnancy. Recommended prenatal weight gain varies with prepregnant body mass index.[5] Physical activity can be increased to prevent excessive prenatal weight gain. Use of phentermine (Adipex-P) and sibutramine (Meridia) have not been determined to be appropriate for pregnant women however, no data link accidental phentermine and sibutramine use during pregnancy with teratogenic or fetotoxic effects. Orlistat (Xenical, Alli) will limit the absorption of essential fatty acid and vitamins needed for optimal fetal development, although animal studies have failed to demonstrate that this drug is linked to embryotoxicity or teratogenic effects. Both topiramate (Topamax) and zonisamide (Zonegran) are contraindicated during pregnancy, as topiramate use in the first trimester is associated with oral cleft defects.

Lactation

Milk production utilizes 500 calories of energy per day. As a result, lactation combined with restriction of calories to those needed to maintain ideal body weight will cause the loss of 1 pound per week. A 500 calorie per day restriction augments weight loss without decreasing the quantity or quality of milk production. Lactating women should not need drug therapy for gradual weight loss. The limited absorption of orlistat (Xenical, Alli) suggests that the drug is not excreted in breast milk, but no research is available to support this contention. Both topiramate (Topamax) and zonisamide (Zonegran) are contraindicated during breastfeeding. Although this topic has not been studied, potential excretion of these agents in breast milk would expose the infant to potent neuromodulators that might suppress appetite.

Elderly

Women's caloric needs decline when they reach a postmenopausal state. In turn, caloric intake must decrease or activity must increase to prevent weight gain. As estrogen levels drop, adipose depots are remodeled, and fat is moved from the breasts and hips to the abdomen. Waist measurements, therefore, may increase without weight gain. Whether estrogen therapy prevents or ameliorates this remodeling is being studied. Women's risk for hyperlipidemia, hypertension, heart disease, and type 2 diabetes increase postmenopausally, emphasizing the importance of weight optimization in this age group. Age-related decreases in liver and renal function must be considered when prescribing weight loss medications for postmenopausal women.

Conclusion

Intake and exercise adjustments can optimize body weight with few side effects or medication interactions and are the preferred methods of weight loss for individuals who are overweight. Multiple hormonal variations make weight loss more difficult for obese persons. Some medications, such as antipsychotics and glucocorticoids, actually can cause obesity. Prescription weight loss medications can augment diet, exercise, and biobehavioral therapy to initiate weight loss for obese individuals. Without dietary vigilance, however, weight will be regained once weight loss medications are stopped. Ongoing research into neuromodulators and hormones may provide new weight loss therapies over time.

Resources

Organization	Description	Website
National Institutes of Diabetes and Digestive and Kidney Diseases, Weight Control Information Network	Prescription medications for the treatment of obesity; drugs are compared for doses, side effects, and mechanism of action	www.win.niddk.nih.gov/publications/prescription.htm
Centers for Disease Control and Prevention	BMI calculator	www.cdc.gov/healthyweight/assessing/bmi/adult_bmi/english_bmi_calculator/bmi_calculator.html
WebMD, Drugs and Medications Search	Common drugs for treating anorexia nervosa	www.webmd.com/drugs/condition-1010-Anorexia+Nervosa.aspx?diseaseid=1010&diseasename=Anorexia+Nervosa&source=0

References

1. Centers for Disease Control. National Center for Health Statistics. Prevalence of obesity: United States, 2013. 2013. http://www.cdc.gov/obesity/data/prevalence-maps.html Accessed September 21, 2014.
2. American College Obstetricians and Gynecologists. *The Role of the Obstetrician–Gynecologist in the Assessment and Management of Obesity.* Committee Opinion No. 319. Washington, DC: American College Obstetricians and Gynecologists; 2005.
3. National Institutes of Health, National Heart, Lung, and Blood Institute. Managing overweight and obesity in adults: systematic evidence review from the obesity expert panel: 2013. http://www.nhlbi.nih.gov/guidelines/obesity/ser/index.htm. Accessed March 23, 2014.
4. National Research Council. *Dietary Reference Intakes: The Essential Guide to Nutrient Requirements.* Washington, DC: National Academies Press; 2006.
5. Ghigliotti G, Barisione C, Garibaldi S, et al. Adipose tissue immune response: novel triggers and consequences for chronic inflammatory conditions. *Inflammation.* May 14, 2014. [Epub ahead of print].
6. Jensen MD. Potential role of new therapies in modifying cardiovascular risk in overweight patients with metabolic risk factors. *Obesity.* 2006;14(3):143S-149S.
7. Ogden C, Carroll M, Kit B, Flegal K. Prevalence of childhood and adult obesity in the United States, 2011-2012. *JAMA.* 2014;311(8):806-814.
8. Phelan S, Wadden TA, Berkowitz RI, et al. Impact of weight loss on the metabolic syndrome. *Int J Obs.* 2007;31:1442-1448.
9. Hofbauer K, Nicholson J, Boss O. The obesity epidemic: current and future pharmacological treatments. *Annu Rev Pharmacol Toxicol.* 2007;47:565-592.
10. Pacher P, Batkai S, Kunos G. The endocannabinoid system as an emerging target of pharmacotherapy. *Pharmacol Rev.* 2006;58(3):389-462.
11. Ciaraldi TP, Aroda V, Mudaliar SR, Henry RR. Inflammatory cytokines and chemokines, skeletal muscle and polycystic ovary syndrome: effects of pioglitazone and metformin treatment. *Metabolism.* 2013;62(11):1587-1596.
12. Panidis D, Tziomalos K, Papadakis E, Katsikis I. Infertility treatment in polycystic ovary syndrome: lifestyle interventions, medications and surgery. *Front Horm Res.* 2013;40:128-141.
13. Faulconbridge LF, Bechtel CF. Depression and disordered eating in the obese person. *Curr Obes Rep.* 2014 1;3(1):127-136.
14. Reas DL, Grilo CM. Current and emerging drug treatments for binge eating disorder. *Expert Opin Emerg Drugs.* 2014;19(1):99-142.
15. Heaner MK, Walsh BT. A history of the identification of the characteristic eating disturbances of bulimia nervosa, binge eating disorder and anorexia nervosa. *Appetite.* 2013;65:185-188.
16. Gianfrancesco F, Pesa J, Ruey-Hua W, Nasrallah H. Assessment of antipsychotic-related risk of diabetes mellitus in a Medicaid psychosis population: sensitivity to study design. *Am J Health-Syst Pharm.* 2006;63:431-441.
17. Hasnain M, Vieweg WV. Weight considerations in psychotropic drug prescribing and switching. *Postgrad Med.* 2013;125(5):117-129.
18. Teff K, Rickels M, Grudziak J, et al. Antipsychotic-induced insulin resistance and postprandial hormonal dysregulation independent of weight gain or psychiatric disease. *Diabetes.* 2013;62(9):3232-3240.
19. Biedermann F, Fleischhacker WW, Kemmler G, et al. Sibutramine in the treatment of antipsychotic-induced weight gain: a pilot study in patients with schizophrenia. *Int Clin Psychopharmacol.* 2014;29(3):181-184.
20. Jarskog LF, Hamer RM, Catellier DJ, et al. Metformin for weight loss and metabolic control in overweight outpatients with schizophrenia and schizoaffective disorder. *Am J Psychiatry.* 2013;170(9):1032-1040.
21. Tek C, Guloksuz S, Reutenauer EL. Investigating the safety and efficacy of naltrexone for anti-psychotic

induced weight gain in severe mental illness: study protocol of a double-blind, randomized, placebo-controlled trial investigating the safety and efficacy of naltrexone for anti-psychotic induced weight gain in severe mental illness. *BMC Psychiatry.* 2013;13:176.
22. Giannopoulou I, Botonis P, Kostara C, Skouroliakou M. Diet and exercise effects on aerobic fitness and body composition in seriously mentally ill adults. *Eur J Sport. Sci.* 2014;14(6):620-627.
23. Lopez LM, Grimes DA, Chen M, et al. Hormonal contraceptives for contraception in overweight or obese women. *Cochrane Database Syst Rev.* 2013;4:CD008452.
24. Mechanick J, Youdim A, Jones D, et al. Clinical practice guidelines for the perioperative nutritional, metabolic, and nonsurgical support of the bariatric surgery patient: 2013 update cosponsored by American Association of Clinical Endocrinologists, the Obesity Society, and American Society for Metabolic & Bariatric Surgery. *Surg Obes Rel Dis.* 2013;9(2):159-191.
25. Whigman LD, Dhurandhar NV, Rahko PS, Atkinson RL. Comparison of combinations of drugs for treatment of obesity: body weight and echocardiographic status. *Int J Obesity.* 2007;31(5):850-857.
26. Scozzafava A, Supuran CT, Carta F. Antiobesity carbonic anhydrase inhibitors: a literature and patient review. *Expert Opin Ther Pat.* 2013;23(6):725-735.
27. Xiong GL, Gadde KM. Combination phentermine/topiramate for obesity treatment in primary care: a review. *Postgrad Med.* 2014;126(2):110-116.
28. Mines D, Tennis P, Curkendall SM, et al. Topiramate use in pregnancy and the birth prevalence of oral clefts. *Pharmacoepidemiol Drug Saf.* 2014;23(10):1017-1025.
29. Verpeut JL, Bello NT. Drug safety evaluation of naltrexone/bupropion for the treatment of obesity. *Expert Opin Drug Saf.* 2014;13(6):831-841.
30. Hurt RT, Edakkanambeth Varayil J, Ebbert JO. New pharmacologic management treatments for the management of obesity *Curr Gastroenterol Rep.* 2014; 16(6):394-398.
31. Olszanecka-Glinianowicz M, Dąbrowski P, Kocełak P, et al. Long-term inhibition of intestinal lipase by orlistat improves release of gut hormones increasing satiety in obese women. *Pharmacol Rep.* 2013;65(3):666-671.
32. Gras J. Cetilistat for the treatment of obesity. *Drugs Today (Barc).* 2013;49(12):755-759.
33. Manning S, Pucci A, Finer N. Pharmacotherapy for obesity: novel agents and paradigms. *Ther Adv Chronic Dis.* 2014;5(3):135-148.
34. Romero-Zerbo SY, Bermúdez-Silva FJ. Cannabinoids, eating behaviour, and energy homeostasis. *Drug Test Anal.* 2014;6(1-2):52-58.
35. Cristino L, Becker T, Di Marzo V. Endocannabinoids and energy homeostasis: an update. *Biofactors.* 2014; 40(4):389-397.
36. Spritzer PM. Polycystic ovary syndrome: reviewing diagnosis and management of metabolic disturbances. *Arq Bras Endocrinol Metabol.* 2014;58(2):182-187.
37. Ciaraldi TP, Aroda V, Mudaliar SR, Henry RR. Inflammatory cytokines and chemokines, skeletal muscle and polycystic ovary syndrome: effects of pioglitazone and metformin treatment. *Metabolism.* 2013;62(11): 1587-1596.
38. Kim HJ, Lee JH, Park HJ, Cho SH, Cho S, Kim WS. Monitoring of 29 weight loss compounds in foods and dietary supplements by LC-MS/MS. *Food Addit Contam Part A Chem Anal Control Expo Risk Assess.* 2014;31(5):777-783.
39. Pittler M, Ernst E. Dietary supplements for body-weight reduction: a systematic review. *Am J Clin Nutr.* 2004;79:529-536.
40. Sadoughi S. Metformin versus chromium picolinate in clomiphene citrate–resistant patients with PCOs: a double-blind randomized clinical trial. *Iran J Reprod Med.* 2013;11(8):611-618.
41. Tian H, Guo X, Wang X, et al. Chromium picolinate supplementation for overweight or obese adults. *Cochrane Database Syst Rev.* 2013;11:CD010063.
42. Heymsfield SB, Allison DB, Vasselli JR, Pietrobelli A, Greenfield D, Nunez C. *Garcinia cambogia* (hydroxycitric acid) as a potential anti-obesity agent: a randomized controlled trial. *JAMA.* 1998;280(18): 1596-1600.
43. Mayer MA, Finlayson G, Fischman D, et al. Evaluation of the satiating properties of a nutraceutical product containing *Garcinia cambogia* and *Ascophyllum nodosum* extracts in healthy volunteers. *Food Funct.* 2014;5(4):773-779.
44. Flanagan J, Bily A, Rolland Y, Roller M. Lipolytic activity of Svetol, a decaffeinated green coffee bean extract. *Phytother Res.* 2014;28(6):946-948.
45. Onakpoya I, Posadzki P, Ernst E. The efficacy of glucomannan supplementation in overweight and obesity: a systematic review and meta-analysis of randomized clinical trials. *J Am Coll Nutr.* 2014;33(1):70-78.
46. Walsh DE, Yaghoubian V, Behforooz A. Effect of glucomannan on obese patients: a clinical study. *Int J Obes.* 1984;8(4):289-293.

47. Chen HL, Sheu WH, Tai TS, Liaw YP, Chen YC. Konjac supplement alleviated hypercholesterolemia and hyperglycemia in type 2 diabetic subjects: a randomized double-blind trial. *J Am Coll Nutr.* 2003;22(1):36-42.
48. Hassanzadeh Bashtian M, Emami SA, Mousavifar N, Esmaily HA, Mahmoudi M, Mohammad Poor AH. Evaluation of fenugreek (*Trigonella foenum-graceum L.*): effects of seeds extract on insulin resistance in women with polycystic ovarian syndrome. *Iran J Pharm Res.* 2013;12(2):475-481.
49. Sharpe P, Blanck H, Williams J, Ainsworth B, Conway J. Use of complementary and alternative medicine for weight control in the United States. *J Altern Complement Med.* 2007;13(2):217-222.
50. Pittler MH, Ernst E. Complementary therapies for reducing body weight: a systematic review. *Int J Obesity.* 2005;29:1030-1038.
51. Klein D, Cottingham E, Sorter M, Barton B, Morrison J. A randomized, double blind, placebo-controlled trial of metformin treatment of weight gain associated with initiation of atypical antipsychotic therapy in children and adolescents. *Am J Psychiatry.* 2006;163:2072-2079.
52. Aarsen F, van den Akker E, Drop S, Catsman-Berrevoets C. Effect of topiramate on cognition in obese children. *Neurology.* 2006;67:1307-1308.
53. Chanoine JP, Hampl S, Jensen C, Boldrin M, Hauptman J. Effect of orlistat on weight and body composition in obese individuals. *JAMA.* 2005;293(23):2873-2883.
54. Cance J, Ashley O, Penne M. Unhealthy weight control behaviors and MDMA (ecstasy) use among adolescent females. *J Adolesc Health.* 2005;37:409.

8 Smoking Cessation

Donna D. Caruthers, Susan A. Albrecht

Chapter Glossary

Drug discrimination Psychobiologic cues that develop with drug use (e.g., nicotine) and can prompt additional drug-using behavior (e.g., smoking another cigarette).

Electronic cigarettes Battery-powered hand-held units that deliver vaporized nicotine for inhalation.

Lapses Momentary smoking events or slips by an abstinent tobacco user. The individual might take a puff of a cigarette or smoke a whole cigarette.

Passive smoking Another name for second-hand smoke.

Relapse Event when a tobacco user attempting cessation reinstitutes previous use of tobacco or more. This event often follows a lapse in smoking.

Second-hand smoke Smoke inhaled by someone other than the active smoker. Also called passive smoking or environmental tobacco smoking.

Third-hand smoke Particles and toxins found in smoke that linger in an environment on surfaces such as bedding, couches, and carpets and are exposed to individuals other than the active smoker.

Tolerance Condition that occurs when a tobacco user's response to the psychoactive drug of nicotine decreases and requires the individual to use large quantities or more frequent dosing of tobacco/nicotine-containing products. Tolerance to nicotine includes psychobiologic factors.

Vapes Battery-powered mobile vaporizers of liquid nicotine with the capability of delivering different doses of nicotine.

Introduction

Tobacco use is the foremost cause of death in women and men in the United States today, yet the number of women who smoke continues to increase.[1] The Centers for Disease Control and Prevention (CDC) in the United States estimates that 42.1 million adults (18.1%) smoke cigarettes.[1] The prevalence of smoking is higher among men (20.5%) than among women (15.8%), although reports indicate that women have nearly the same risk for death from smoking as do men.[2]

The landmark U.S. Surgeon General's report on smoking and implications for health was published in 1964, but the first report from that office on the adverse effects of smoking specific to women was not published until 1980.[3] In 2014, the Surgeon General released a report that addresses what has been learned about the health consequences of smoking in the 50 years since the original publication.[4] This report reviews mounting evidence documenting adverse effects of smoking on cardiovascular, pulmonary, gastrointestinal, reproductive, renal, dental, integumentary, neuro-cognitive, neurological, and ophthalmic systems. Women who smoke are at greater risk for multiple health complications as compared to women who do not smoke.[5] Lung cancer is the leading cause of cancer deaths in women; as smoking prevalence in women increases, the incidence of lung cancer deaths follows the direction of smoking prevalence.[6]

This chapter reviews smoking cessation therapies, with a focus on the pharmacologic treatment(s) for tobacco addiction in women.

Tobacco Use Among Women

Cigarette smoking was rare among women in the early part of the twentieth century. The number of women smokers gradually increased during that century, but then began to decline in the mid-1970s in an era of multiple antismoking campaigns. Nevertheless, today the rate of smoking among adolescent girls is approximately 20%.[1] Among adult women, smoking prevalence by ethnicity is highest among American Indian or Alaska Native women (26%), intermediate among White women (18.4%) and Black women (14.8%), and lowest among Hispanic women (7.8%) and Asian or Pacific Islander women (5.5%).[1] Approximately 11% of women report smoking during their pregnancy. Overall, 54% of women who attempt to quit smoking during pregnancy, are successful.[7]

Most women begin smoking during adolescence. The period of adolescence often involves risky behaviors, peer pressure, and changes in self-confidence. Notably, adolescents have an increased risk of developing an addiction to smoking.[8] Reasons for smoking initiation may include perceptions of peers, experimentation, and role models who smoke.[9] Adolescents may find that after they initiate tobacco use, continuing to smoke has perceived advantages with peers, elevates their mood, and helps control weight. Alcohol and tobacco reinforce the use of each substance in both adolescents and adults.[10]

Health Consequences of Smoking

Women are much more likely to suffer adverse health consequences from smoking than men. The continuum of the health consequences of tobacco use may begin within the womb and end with death, and those consequences are not limited to the leading lethal medical disorders, such as lung cancer and cardiovascular disease. Tobacco use has significant adverse effects on fertility, pregnancy, birth outcomes, and breastfeeding, and it increases the risk for sudden infant death syndrome (SIDS) in children who are exposed to smoke in the home. Pregnancy complications that are more likely to occur in women who smoke compared to women who do not smoke include ectopic pregnancy, spontaneous abortion, neural tube defects, preterm birth, preterm premature rupture of membranes (PPROM), placenta previa, hypertensive disorders, low birth weight, stillbirth, and perinatal mortality.[4] Women who quit smoking before or during pregnancy reduce the adverse effects of tobacco on reproductive outcomes.

Nonsmokers also have an increased incidence of adverse health effects secondary to environmental exposure to smoking. Adverse effects associated with **passive smoking**, also called **second-hand smoke** exposure, include lung dysfunction, acute respiratory infections, recurrent otitis media, bronchitis, pneumonia, and SIDS.[11] Research is now being conducted on the consequences of exposure to **third-hand smoke**, which refers to tobacco toxins that coat various environmental items (e.g., car cushions, beds, sofas). Third-hand smoke may potentially harm adults and children long after the active smoker has left the area.[12]

Effect of Gender on Smoking Cessation

Women also have a more difficult time ceasing smoking than do men. It is not known if this difference arises secondary to the physiologic effects of smoking or non-nicotine factors.[13] Premenopausal women may find quitting more difficult during the luteal phase of their menstrual cycle. Nicotine withdrawal symptoms may include depressive symptoms and irritability, as well as effects on the luteal phase of the menstrual cycle. Research suggests that women with severe premenstrual symptoms should start to quit smoking during the follicular phase of the menstrual cycle to minimize the experience of nicotine withdrawal symptoms, particularly those that are related to negative mood in the 2 weeks before menses.[13]

Women also are about half as likely to quit smoking through use of a nicotine patch when compared to men; it is not clear if the addition of counseling significantly improves these rates.[14] The nicotine inhaler appears to be more beneficial for women who are seeking to quit smoking than for men.[14] The effects of some of the non-nicotine pharmacologic therapies may be more beneficial for women, although this is an area in which more research is needed and clinical guidelines are not yet available.

Physiology of Tobacco Addiction

The primary addictive substance within tobacco is the plant alkaloid nicotine. Absorption and metabolism of nicotine are assisted by the nature of nicotine—that is, whether it is water soluble versus lipid soluble. Nicotine can be absorbed through the mucosa, through the skin, or across the pulmonary capillary–alveolar membranes when carried on tar droplets from cigarette smoke to the terminal airways and alveoli in the lung. Cigarette smoke is a very effective delivery method because the speed and dosing of nicotine via the lungs affect the brain faster than an intravenous injection. This is due to the large surface area of the pulmonary capillary–alveolar membrane and the subsequent acceleration of the spread of nicotine provided by the arterial side of the heart, which delivers blood to the brain without going through the venous system and liver.[15] An average cigarette contains approximately 10–14 mg of nicotine, of which approximately 1–1.5 mg is absorbed.

Nicotine is metabolized in the liver, and multiple active metabolites of this chemical have been identified. Cotinine appears to be the most important nicotine metabolite; it is metabolized more slowly than nicotine itself. Both cotinine and nicotine are metabolized via CYP450 enzymes. Genetic polymorphisms within the CYP450 enzymes responsible for nicotine metabolism may play a role in the ease or difficulty with which individuals achieve smoking cessation. For example, persons with the ultrarapid CYP2D6 polymorphism are more likely to be heavy smokers.[16]

Gender also affects the metabolism of nicotine. Premenopausal women metabolize nicotine more rapidly than do men, and nicotine metabolism is even faster in women who are pregnant or taking birth control pills.[17] The addition of menthol appears to be associated with a longer half-life for cotinine in women. In addition, women have a faster elimination rate of nicotine and its metabolites.

Nicotine is an agonist that stimulates presynaptic and postsynaptic nicotinic acetylcholine receptors (nAChRs), particularly the alpha$_4$ beta$_2$ subtype.[18,19] These receptors are located throughout the body but are found primarily in the brain. The beta$_2$ subunit influences self-administration of nicotine, whereas the alpha$_4$ subunit likely influences sensitivity to nicotine. The alpha$_4$ beta$_2$ subunit and alpha$_7$ likely reinforce the cardiovascular effects of nicotine use. The alpha$_7$ subunit may promote rapid synaptic transmission, which could influence learning, conditioning, and sensory gating.[18] Nicotine works as an agonist of nAChRs in the mesolimbic system, the frontal cortex, and the corpus striatum. Several different neurotransmitters are released from these nicotinic receptors (Figure 8-1).[18] In all, nicotine stimulates five different neurotransmitter classes: amino acids, monoamine catecholamines, monoamine indolamine, neuropeptides, and acetylcholine.

Of particular import is the dopamine release that occurs when nicotine binds to nAChRs in the ventral tegmental area located in the midbrain and the nucleus

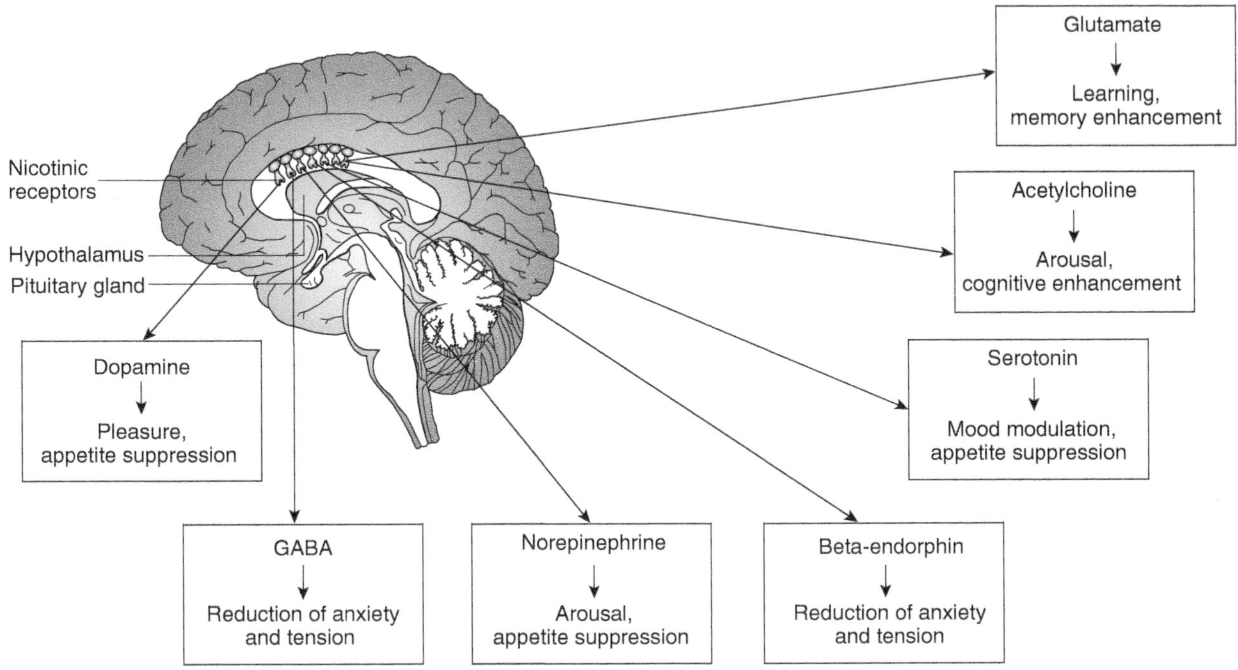

Figure 8-1 The effects of nicotine on nicotinic receptors in the brain.

accumbens, both of which are part of the reward pathway. Stimulation of the mesolimbic reward pathway via release of dopamine is an essential process in the development and maintenance of nicotine addiction, similar to what happens with other substances of abuse (e.g., heroin, alcohol, and cocaine).[18] Nicotine also stimulates the release of dopamine in the corpus striatum and frontal cortex. This pattern of spiked dopamine release in the brain is also similar to the function of other addictive substances in the brain.

The process of addiction is a biopsychological one. The biopsychological conceptual framework identifies an interaction between the biologic activity at the cellular level and psychological processes developed following sensory, mood, and environmental cues that contribute to conditioning to smoking.[18] With repeated use of nicotine, the central nervous system is remodeled through a psycho-pharmacologic process, which includes the development of **tolerance**, **drug discrimination**, withdrawal symptoms, and **relapse** potential during tobacco abstinence.[1,18] In addition, after some exposure to nicotine, the brain produces more acetylcholine nicotine receptors, which in turn provide more receptor sites for nicotine.[18] This part of the remodeling becomes important in the process of smoking cessation, **lapses**, and relapse. Positive psychoactive effects of nicotine, such as improved mood, arousal, and relaxation reinforce the use of nicotine. It has been noted that nicotine meets the U.S. Surgeon General's primary criteria for an addictive substance—that is, nicotine promotes compulsive self-administration, has psychoactive effects, and reinforces self-administration.

Nicotine Withdrawal

Nicotine addiction is associated with a withdrawal process when an individual attempts to quit or has a substantial delay in smoking. Symptoms of nicotine withdrawal include (1) depressed mood or dysphoria; (2) irritability/frustration/anger; (3) anxiety and restlessness; (4) increased appetite/hunger; (5) decreased heart rate; (6) difficulty concentrating/impaired cognitive function; (7) insomnia/sleep disturbance; (8) craving; and (9) somatic complaints of headaches, gastrointestinal disturbances, and dizziness.[20] Persons usually reach the peak of the physiologic withdrawal symptoms within 1–3 weeks of smoking cessation if nicotine replacements are not used.[20] The average woman who wishes to stop smoking will commonly make two or three attempts before succeeding in quitting. Although some resources qualify tobacco addiction as "high" or "low," there are no definitions for the term, and some women who smoke a few cigarettes daily may have as much difficulty stopping as women who smoke several packs per day.

Nicotine and Drug Interactions

Tobacco smoking has known interactions with several pharmaceutic agents secondary to both its pharmacokinetic and pharmacodynamic effects (Table 8-1). Some substances in tobacco induce CYP450 enzymes that are responsible for

Table 8-1 Nicotine–Drug Interactions[a]

Drug: Generic (Brand)	Interaction with Smoking	Clinical Considerations During Smoking Cessation
Benzodiazepines	Decreased sedation secondary to central nervous system stimulation	Dose may need to be lowered
Beta blockers	Less effective for blood pressure control secondary to decreased end-organ responsiveness from nicotine stimulation	Unclear
Caffeine	Increases clearance by approximately 50%	Assess total caffeine intake and monitor for caffeine toxicity
Clozapine (Clozaril)	Decreases plasma concentrations	Dose may need to be lowered
Fluvoxamine (Luzox)	Decreases plasma concentrations	Dose may need to be lowered but is not routine
Imipramine (Tofranil)	Decreases plasma concentrations	Dose may need to be lowered but is not routine
Insulin (subcutaneous)	Nicotine induces insulin resistance and vasoconstriction, which decreases absorption	Close monitoring of blood glucose levels and dose of insulin may need to be lowered
Oral contraceptives	Increased risk of adverse effects such as thromboembolism and myocardial infarction	Oral contraceptives are not recommended for women 35 years or older who smoke > 15 cigarettes/day
Propanolol (Inderal)	Increased clearance	Unclear clinical implications
Theophylline (Theo-Dur)	Increased clearance by approximately 50%	Dose may need to be lowered
Warfarin (Coumadin)	Prolonged International Normalized Ratio (INR)	Dose may need to be lowered

[a] This table is not comprehensive as new information is being generated on a regular basis.

metabolizing other drugs. Notably, warfarin (Coumadin), theophylline (Theo-Dur), insulin, beta blockers, corticosteroids, estrogens, and drugs for schizophrenia may require altered doses when an individual smokes cigarettes.[21] In addition, combined oral contraceptives and nicotine synergistically increase the risk for stroke and peripheral thrombus in women via a mechanism that has not been fully elucidated.[22]

Initiating Smoking Cessation

The 2008 publication *Smoking Cessation: Clinical Practice Guideline of the Agency for Health Care Policy and Research (AHCPR)* recommended that screening for tobacco use be undertaken at every healthcare visit for every individual.[23] The promotion and prescription of treatment for tobacco addiction start with the healthcare provider's knowledge and commitment to screening, provision of appropriate treatment, and adequate follow-up. Studies on smoking cessation suggest that lack of adherence by healthcare providers in assessing, monitoring, and following up on tobacco addiction and treatment contributes to the lack of initiation to quit smoking and/or relapse from cessation.[23,24]

Clinical guidelines for smoking cessation intervention suggest using the *Five A's* to initiate and monitor smoking cessation with individuals in any medical setting. The *Five A's* encourage the healthcare provider to ask, advise, assess, assist, and arrange follow-up.[23] In addition, assessment of smoking status, quantity, and cessation interest has been proposed as an addition to vital sign assessments.[23] Although this chapter does not focus on the behavioral components of an intervention program, various resources are available to assist healthcare providers as needed.[24]

Pharmacologic therapy should be considered for all individuals who smoke unless those therapies are contraindicated for that particular individual. However, rather than simply prescribing a drug, a dual treatment protocol is recommended, consisting of pharmacologic treatment and cognitive-behavioral therapy following a distinct healthcare message advocating cessation.[23]

Nonpharmacologic Therapies Used for Smoking Cessation

Nonpharmacologic therapy for smoking cessation includes group or individual therapy as well as alternative therapies such as hypnosis, acupuncture, acupressure, and meditation. Intensive person-to-person contact of more than 10 minutes per session is most effective when compared to no provider contact time (odds ratio [OR] 2.3; 95% confidence interval [CI], 2.0–2.7).[23] Group or individual therapy and alternative intervention delivery via the Internet and telephone are also effective. Intervention programs that combine three or more formats (e.g., telephone counseling, group counseling, individual therapy) are more effective than a single type of intervention (OR, 2.5; 95% CI, 2.1–3.0).[23]

Research has not substantiated support for hypnotherapy,[25] acupuncture, acupressure, laser therapy, or electrostimulation treatments for smoking abstinence.[26] Exercise has been used alone and in combination with other therapies to assist persons in their efforts to quit smoking. Although exercise may be more beneficial in women than in men,[23] evidence is limited regarding the support for exercise in achieving 12-month abstinence outcomes.[27]

Pharmacologic Therapies: Overview

There are currently seven pharmaceutical agents that are approved by the U.S. Food and Drug Administration (FDA) for treatment of smoking cessation. First-line therapy for tobacco dependence includes nicotine replacement therapies delivered via gum, patch, inhaler, spray, or lozenge as well as non-nicotine therapies (bupropion [Zyban]), and partial nicotine receptor agonists (varenicline [Chantix]).[29] Although considered experimental in the United States, a cannabinoid receptor antagonist (rimonabant) has been developed by Sanofi Aventis for smoking cessation purposes.[24] Table 8-2 identifies the effectiveness of the smoking cessation medications as compared to a placebo at 6 months after smoking cessation.[23,30]

Nicotine Replacement Therapy

Each year, approximately 3% of individuals who smoke successfully quit either by weaning or by abruptly stopping. Nicotine replacement therapies (NRTs) can increase the rate of quitting by 50% to 70%.[30] NRTs replace nicotine without the other toxic substances contained in cigarettes. Once NRTs are discontinued, abstinent individuals can experience nicotine withdrawal symptoms. Thus, these products are used to help persons withdraw from nicotine by mitigating withdrawal symptoms via exposure to less nicotine. NRTs can be very popular as an initial aid in smoking cessation because most of them are available on

Table 8-2 Odds of Abstinence After 6 Months of Smoking Cessation: Medication versus Placebo

Drug: Generic (Brand)	Odds of Abstinence 6 Months After Smoking Cessation: OR (95% CI)
Nicotine Replacement Medications	
Nicotine gum (2 mg) (≥14 weeks' use)	1.5 (1.2–1.7)
Nicotine inhaler	2.1 (1.5–2.9)
Nicotine lozenge	2.05 (1.62–2.59)
Nicotine nasal spray	2.3 (1.7–3.0)
Nicotine patch (6–14 weeks)	1.9 (1.7–2.2)
Nicotine patch (> 14 weeks)	1.9 (1.7–2.3)
Non-Nicotine Medications	
Bupropion SR (Zyban)	2.0 (1.8–2.2)
Varenicline (Chantix) 2 mg/day	3.1 (2.5–3.8)
Varenicline (Chantix) 1 mg/day	2.1 (1.5–3.0)
Combination Therapy	
Nicotine patch with bupropion SR	2.5 (1.9–3.4)
Nicotine patch with nortriptyline or nicotine inhaler	2.3 (1.3–4.6)
Nicotine patch with prn nicotine gum or nicotine spray	3.6 (2.5–5.2)
Medications That Are Not Effective	
Naltrexone (Vivitrol)	0.5 (0.2–1.2)
Selective serotonin reuptake inhibitors	1.0 (0.7–1.4)

Abbreviations: SR = sustained release.
Sources: Data from Fiore MC, Jaén CR, Baker TB, et al. *Treating tobacco use and dependence: 2008 update. Clinical practice guideline.* Rockville, MD: U.S. Department of Health and Human Services. Public Health Service; May 2008. http://www.ahrq.gov/professionals/clinicians-providers/guidelines-recommendations/tobacco/clinicians/update/index.html. Accessed October 23, 2014[23]; Nides M. Update on pharmacologic options for smoking cessation treatment. *Am J Med.* 2008;121(4 suppl 1):S20-S31.[28]

an over-the-counter basis and are less expensive than the non-nicotine drugs.

Nicotine gum was the first NRT product. Today, various dosing vehicles to deliver nicotine are available, such as gum, lozenge, patch, inhaler, and spray (Table 8-3). Each of the NRT delivery vehicles has demonstrated effectiveness in treating tobacco dependence with or without behavioral therapy; however, smoking cessation is most likely to be successful when any of the pharmacologic therapies is coupled with a cognitive-behavioral therapy.[23]

Mechanism of Action

NRT is designed to diminish the cravings for smoking and the withdrawal symptoms that often induce a person to lapse. One cigarette contains approximately 1–2 mg of nicotine. The amount of nicotine in each of the NRT products is listed in Table 8-3. Plasma levels of nicotine rarely exceed 15 ng/mL following use of the various NRT products. The NRT lozenge may provide a higher plasma level of nicotine compared to nicotine gum.[31] Patch therapy has the slowest absorption rate and produces the lowest plasma levels, which do not reach peak plasma levels until 8 hours following administration. Women who smoke may perceive the first day on an NRT to be easier than subsequent days on the same NRT dose secondary to the presence of to residual nicotine from the previous use of tobacco products.

Side Effects/Adverse Reactions

All of the NRT products have some uncomfortable side effects, as noted in Table 8-3. These side effects are generally related to the mode of delivery. For example, nicotine is an irritant when it comes in contact with skin and mucosa, which occurs in approximately 50% of users. Rotating patch sites and using hydrocortisone cream to treat irritated skin that is not directly under the patch are recommended. Side effects of nicotine gum and lozenges include irritation of the buccal cavity, mouth soreness, hiccups, dyspepsia, and an aching jaw. Individuals should be instructed to avoid operating motorized vehicles for 5 minutes after using the nasal spray because of the potential for coughing, watery eyes, and sneezing.

If individuals use an NRT prior to quitting smoking, nausea can occur due to nicotine overdose. NRTs should be used with caution within 2 weeks of a myocardial infarction, presence of serious arrhythmias, or escalating difficulty with angina pectoris, but has not been associated with increasing risk for cardiovascular events, even among persons with a history of such disease.[32]

Drug–Drug and Drug–Food Interactions

When administering the gum, lozenge, or the inhaler, individuals should be cautioned against ingestion of food and beverages such as coffee, juices, and soft drinks, and especially acidic beverages within 15 minutes of administering an NRT, because food and drinks may diminish the absorption of the NRT.[31] NRT is metabolized in the liver. Grapefruit juice can inhibit the metabolism of nicotine to cotinine, and it increases renal clearance of nicotine.[33]

Prescribing Information

Dosing with any of the NRT products should be individualized. The base smoking rate can assist in establishing the initial dose. For example, when daily smoking is no more than half of a pack per day, the 2-mg gum, 2-mg lozenge,

Table 8-3 Nicotine Replacement Therapies

Drug: Generic (Brand)	Amount of Nicotine in Formulation	Dose	Maximum Dose	Time to Peak Plasma Level	Side Effects	Contraindications
Gum (Nicorette)[a]	2 mg, 4 mg	< 25 cigs/day: 2 mg if smoking. > 25 cigs/day: 4 mg if smoking; 1 piece of gum every hour for 6 weeks, then 1 piece every 2–4 hours for 2–4 weeks, then 1 piece every 2–4 hours for 2–4 weeks, then 1 piece every 4–8 hours.	24 pieces per day if monotherapy and 15 pieces per day if used in combination with another NRT product	20–30 minutes	Irritation of buccal cavity, mouth soreness, hiccups, dyspepsia, aching jaw.	Myocardial infarction, heart disease, angina pectoris, serious arrhythmias, stroke, diabetes, hypertension, hyperthyroid, stomach ulcers, liver or kidney disease, pregnancy or breastfeeding
Inhaler (Nicotrol Inhaler)[b]	4-mg cartridge	6–16 cartridges/day for 12 weeks, then taper dose over 12 weeks.	16 cartridges/day	15 minutes	Inflammation of mouth and throat, coughing, rhinitis, stomach irritation.	Same as for gum
Lozenge (Commit)[a]	2 mg, 4 mg	Those who smoke first cig within 30 minutes of wakening: use 4 mg. Others use 2 mg first 6 weeks, every 1–2 hours; weeks 7–9, every 2–4 hours; weeks 10–12, every 4–8 hours.	24 per day	20–30 minutes	Irritation of teeth, gums, and throat; dyspepsia; diarrhea; constipation; flatulence; insomnia; hiccups; headache; coughing.	Same as for gum
Patch (Nicotrol, NicoDerm CQ)[a]	7–14 mg, light smoker; 21–22 mg, moderate smoker; 40+ mg, heavy smoker (two 21-mg patches)	> 10 cigs/day: 21 mg/24 hours for 6–8 weeks, then decrease to 14 mg/24 hours for 2–4 weeks, then decrease to 7 mg/24 hours for 2–4 weeks. ≤ 10 cigs/day: 14 mg/24 hours for 6 weeks, then decrease to 7 mg/24 hours for 2–4 weeks.	1 patch/24 hours	5–10 hours	Skin irritation, sleep disturbance, tachycardia, dizziness, headache, nausea, vomiting, muscle aches and stiffness; vivid dreams and nightmares; may take patch off after 16 hours if sleep disturbances occur.	Same as for gum
Spray (Nicotrol NS)[b]	0.5 mg per spray	1–2 sprays in each nostril every hour for 3–6 months, then taper dose over 4–6 weeks.	5 doses/hour or 40 doses/day	5–7 minutes	Throat irritation, sneezing, coughing, watery eyes, runny nose.	Same as for gum

Abbreviations: cigs = cigarettes; NRT = nicotine replacement therapy.
[a] Available over the counter.
[b] Available via prescription only.

and 7- or 14-mg patch may be considered for a starting dose of NRT. If a person smokes a pack of cigarettes per day, a typical starting dose for the patch would be a 21- or 22-mg patch. If the individual smokes two packs per day, the 40+-mg patch may need to be prescribed. Follow-up in 1- and 2-week intervals is recommended to monitor adherence, side effects, and self-reported smoking with NRT.

Directions for using nicotine replacement products are listed in Table 8-4. For example, the NRT gum should not be chewed like regular gum, and the NRT lozenge should not be used like candy. Both the gum and the lozenge require a slow alternating pace of stimulation of the product in the mouth and parking the lozenge or gum in the mouth. Stimulation of the drug, such as chewing, should occur with smoking urges. The patch, which provides long-acting nicotine to manage withdrawal, can be used in combination with the gum, which provides a short-acting dose to counteract acute withdrawal symptoms (Table 8-5).[32]

Most nicotine patches are applied and removed every 24 hours. The Nicotrol patch is unlike the other patches and is not used for 24 hours; instead, this patch should be worn for only 16 hours. Nicotine patches have been found to

Table 8-4 Consumer Directions for Using Nicotine Replacement Products

Type of NRT	Consumer Instructions
Nicotine gum or lozenge	Nicotine gum provides a steady supply of nicotine that is absorbed from the mucous membranes in your mouth. Any nicotine that you swallow will not have an effect. Chew slowly until you notice a peppery taste, then place the gum in the side of your mouth between your gum and your cheek. Leave each piece of gum in place for 30 minutes. Avoid consuming food, especially acidic foods, for 15 minutes before and after using this gum.
Nicotine inhaler	The inhaler comes with 42 cartridges and a mouthpiece. Place the cartridge in the inhaler and then place the inhaler in your mouth. Close your mouth around the inhaler. Suck on the inhaler with several short sucks to get the air saturated with nicotine into the back of your throat. Suck or puff on each cartridge for about 20 minutes. Use at least 6 cartridges a day and no more than 16 per day.
Nicotine nasal spray	Spray is a good form of NRT for persons who have had difficulty stopping smoking because the nicotine affects the brain faster than with other NRT products (approximately 10 minutes) and reduces cravings more quickly. Each spray is approximately 0.5 mg of nicotine. Blow your nose to clear it. Slightly tilt your head back and insert the bottle tip as far back as is easily done. Breathe in through your mouth and hold your breath. Press the bottom of the bottle to release the spray. Do not sniff through your nose or swallow while spraying. Breathe out through your mouth. Apply one spray to each nostril. Use the spray at least 8 times/day but no more than 40 times/day.
Nicotine patch	The nicotine patch provides a steady supply of nicotine that is absorbed from the skin and will continue to be absorbed several hours after the patch is removed. Place a new patch on your body every morning. Place the patch on a clean, dry, non-hairy area on your upper body or arm between your neck and your waist. Use a different site every day. It is safe to wear the patch in the shower, pool, or bath. If the skin becomes irritated, rub a small amount of 1% hydrocortisone cream over the irritated area once a day until healed. Do not put a patch on that area until it is healed.

be associated with sleep disturbances. For women who have sleep disturbances with the use of the 24-hour patches, the 16-hour patch may be more effective.

Nicotine patches are similar to a sandwich. The top layer, which is exposed to the air, is not permeable. The nicotine is placed between the outer layer and a permeable layer that is placed on the skin. This nicotine is slowly released over the course of the day through the skin to the capillaries.

Patches were originally all the same size and color. More recently, patches have been designed to be less obvious when worn on an area not covered by clothing (e.g., on an arm). The patch size has been scaled to reflect changes in dose for those products that provide a stepwise reduction in nicotine dosing as part of the treatment strategy.

Table 8-5 Dosing for Combined Use of Nicotine Replacement Patch and Gum

Number of Cigarettes Smoked per Day (cigs/day)	NRT Patch (mg)	NRT Gum
< 10[a]	7	2 mg every 1–2 hours with maximum of 15 pieces/day
10–20	14	
21–30	21	
31–40	28	
> 40	42	

Abbreviations: cigs = cigarettes; NRT = nicotine replacement therapy.
[a] Or if the individual weighs less than 45 kg.

Non-Nicotine Pharmacologic Therapies

Bupropion (Zyban, Wellbutrin) and varenicline (Chantix) may both aid in permanent smoking cessation.[34] Clonidine (Catapres) and nortriptyline (Aventyl) have also been found to be effective and are used as second-line therapies under a physician's guidance.

Table 8-6 Non-Nicotine–Containing Medications Used for Smoking Cessation

Drug: Generic (Brand)	Preparation	Mechanism of Action	Dose	Side Effects/Adverse Effects	Contraindications
Bupropion (Zyban, Wellbutrin)	150 mg; begin 7–14 days before scheduled quit date; available by prescription.	Nonsedating anxiolytic. Eliminates dysphoria by slowing metabolism of serotonin and increases firing of noradrenergic neurons. Dopamine reuptake inhibitor.	Start a week before the quit date and continue for 7–12 weeks after smoking cessation. Every day 150 mg for 3 days; then 150 mg 2 times/day.	Insomnia, dry mouth, dizziness, nausea, constipation, runny nose, jitters, tachycardia, trouble concentrating, skin rash, agitation, change in appetite, and serious neuropsychiatric events, including suicidal ideation and suicide attempts. Rarely, bupropion can cause seizures.	History of seizures, eating disorders, uncontrolled hypertension; use of MAO inhibitor in previous 14 days; use of Wellbutrin for depression.
Varenicline (Chantix)	0.5 mg, 1.0 mg, 2.0 mg; available by prescription.	Partial nicotine receptor agonist.	First 3 days 0.5 mg every day; days 4–7, 0.5 mg 2 times/day; days 8 and following, 1.0 mg 2 times/day until end of treatment.	Nausea, sleep disturbance and strange dreams, constipation, flatulence, vomiting, sensitivity to light, pancreatitis, hallucinations, and serious neuropsychiatric events, including suicidal ideation and suicide attempts.	18 years or older, alcohol and illicit drug use, use of insulin, anticoagulants, or theophylline. Use of bupropion at the same time for psychiatric disorder is not an absolute contraindication, but this drug should be used with caution during pregnancy or breastfeeding.

Abbreviations: MAO = monoamine oxidase; NRT = nicotine replacement therapy.

Both bupropion and varenicline are available by prescription in the United States. A Cochrane systematic review found varenicline to be more effective than bupropion (relative risk [RR], 0.68; 95% CI, 0.56–0.83) in maintaining smoking abstinence, but recommended that additional studies be conducted to verify this conclusion.[34] Table 8-6 provides information about non-nicotine medications currently approved by the FDA for smoking cessation therapy.

Bupropion Sustained Release (Zyban, Wellbutrin)

Bupropion (Zyban, Wellbutrin) was initially approved for the treatment of depression. The approval of bupropion for smoking cessation occurred in the mid-1990s following clinical drug trials that demonstrated its effectiveness for this indication. These trials were initiated after clinicians reported a decreased interest in smoking among persons treated with bupropion.

Bupropion is available for smoking cessation treatment under the trade name Zyban. The identical agent is also marketed as Wellbutrin, Wellbutrin SR (sustained release), and Wellbutrin XL (extended release) for treatment of depression. Zyban is the formulation that is specific for smoking cessation treatment. Zyban and Wellbutrin SR are bioidentical, and both contain 150 mg of bupropion. Zyban and Wellbutrin SR are available as 100-mg tablets; Wellbutrin SR is also available in 200-mg tablets. Differences in insurance coverage may exist for payment for these drugs. Wellbutrin may be covered for the treatment for depression, but Zyban may not be covered for smoking cessation. In contrast, some health insurance companies cover both formulations of bupropion for both treatment of depression and smoking cessation. This issue may be important for prescribing if smoking cessation drugs are not covered under a woman's insurance plan and a legitimate reason could be found for use of the agent as an antidepressant.

Mechanism of Action

Theoretically, bupropion mediates noradrenergic and dopaminergic mechanisms and acts as an antagonist at nicotinic receptors. Bupropion may also inhibit presynaptic reuptake of the noradrenergic and dopaminergic transporters, which can mimic the effects obtained from nicotine receptor stimulation and diminish nicotine withdrawal effects.[35] Bupropion is metabolized in the liver via CP450B6. Approximately 87% of bupropion and its metabolites are excreted in urine through the kidneys and another 10% via fecal elimination.[35,36] Depending on the woman's risk profile for comorbidities, laboratory values should be monitored for both liver and kidney function.

Side Effects/Adverse Reactions

The most common side effects of bupropion (Zyban) include insomnia and dry mouth. If insomnia becomes problematic, the evening dose can be moved to an earlier part of the evening, combined with observation to ascertain the woman's response in terms of insomnia.

In 2009, the FDA mandated that companies producing bupropion and varenicline add a black box warning to the label that warns the user of possible serious neuropsychiatric symptoms in persons who use these drugs. Postmarketing surveillance studies found a temporal relationship between both drugs and changes in behavior, hostility, agitation, suicidal ideation, and suicidal attempts. These symptoms tend to occur approximately 2 weeks after initiation of the drug. The actual incidence is unknown because the data come from the FDA's Adverse Events Reporting System (FAERS), which may reflect underreporting. Conversely, studies in the last decade have suggested that a reevaluation of the black box warning is warranted. Currently, a large study is underway exploring the relationship between neuropsychiatric changes and bupropion, varenicline, and NRTs.[37]

Drug–Drug Interactions

Bupropion, marketed as Wellbutrin, is also discussed in more detail in the *Mental Health* chapter. The active metabolite of bupropion, 4-hydroxybupropion, is metabolized by CYP2B6 and has inhibitory effects on CYP2D6.[38] Therefore, caution and observations for side effects are warranted if this medication is taken with other medications on the growing list of drugs that are known be metabolized by CYP2B6 or CYP2D6.[23] Hormones, including hormonal contraceptive methods, may inhibit CP450B6 activity, which is the enzyme responsible for metabolism of bupropion (Zyban). Thus, concomitant use of hormonal contraceptive methods and long-acting bupropion may increase plasma levels of bupropion SR, thereby increasing the risk of seizures and bupropion side effects. It has been suggested that women using combined oral contraceptives might need smaller doses of bupropion when starting on this drug and require adequate monitoring and follow-up.

Contraindications

Bupropion lowers the threshold for seizure activity. Contraindications for the use of bupropion include history of seizures, epilepsy, eating disorders, use of monoamine oxidase (MAO) inhibitors within 14 days of therapy, use of bupropion for treatment of depression, bipolar condition, severe hepatic cirrhosis, active brain tumor, discontinuation of alcohol or benzodiazepines, and severe hypertension.[36] Although bupropion (Zyban) and nicotine replacement may be used in combination, ongoing assessments are necessary if the woman has a history of cardiovascular disease.[39] The combination of these drugs has been safely used for individuals with a diagnosis of heart failure.

Clinical treatment studies have not identified gender differences in responses to use of bupropion (Zyban) to treat tobacco dependence. In addition, bupropion attenuates the weight gain associated with smoking cessation in both men and women. There is a positive correlation between increasing doses from 100 mg to 300 mg and cessation rates; however, the response to therapy diminishes by 45 weeks following the end of treatment. Therefore, women who smoke are more likely to achieve cessation when they use higher doses early in their treatment. There is no known difference over the lifespan of adults with respect to age and dosing with bupropion for tobacco dependence treatment.[23,40] Bupropion can be used during pregnancy.

Prescribing Information

Bupropion is started approximately 7 to 14 days before a scheduled quit date from tobacco use. If smoking continues beyond the seventh week of treatment, healthcare providers need to reevaluate the use of this drug. Initial assessment of kidney and liver function should be considered for persons with comorbid conditions.

Ongoing assessment of medication adherence is recommended. Although self-report is a typical method of assessing adherence, healthcare providers may consider reviewing medication refill rates as an additional indirect measure of adherence. Requesting that individuals maintain a medication log in the first 3 months of therapy may also provide information regarding adherence and side effects to medication.

Pharmacogenomics

Individuals with the specific variant gene of CYP2B6 have been found to be less likely to return to smoking 6 months following the initiation of smoking cessation with bupropion.[39] Genetic research regarding this drug suggests women with a particular genetic variation may be more susceptible to side effects with bupropion (Zyban), which in turn may eventually lead to poor adherence to the medication regimen and an increased risk for relapse to tobacco use.[40] This relationship has not been found in

Box 8-1 Varenicline and Neuropsychiatric Disorders

In 2007, an accomplished musician, who regularly played and recorded with such well-known groups as the Dallas Symphony and the band Edie Brickell and the New Bohemians, smoked but desired to quit. After a night during which he consumed large amounts of alcohol, he went to a friend's home, and both of them took their regular doses of varenicline. According to his friend, shortly thereafter the musician became incoherent and violent. Her neighbor, awakened by the noise, fired what he thought was a warning gun shot, but it hit and killed the musician.

This high-profile event was widely covered by national press. Later that same year, the FDA issued warnings regarding neuropsychiatric symptoms reported with the use of varenicline (Chantix) that included agitation, depression, suicidal ideation, and completed suicide. In 2009, these warnings were converted to a mandated black box warning.[44] At the same time, black box warnings were also issued for bupropion and other antidepressants.

However, studies in the decade after this tragic death have not found a clear causal relationship between the two smoking cessation drugs and neuropsychiatric disorders. Stapleton et al. reported the use of varenicline in a sample of individuals diagnosed with mental illness (i.e., depression, bipolar disorder, or psychosis) and found that varenicline did not affect the participants' mental illness.[45] A meta-analysis of 17 randomized placebo-controlled clinical trials involving more than 8000 participants found that varenicline improved tobacco abstinence rates and was not associated with increased rates of neuropsychiatric adverse events.[46] Thus, although a black box warning currently exists, this may not be the end of the story.

men. Although a history of discomfiting side effects and adherence difficulties is not indicative that a woman has this genetic variation, clinicians should consider that it is a possibility and reevaluate the treatment plan with the woman or consider alternative medications. Future studies are needed to examine pharmacogenomics with all of the first-line therapies and combinations of these medications.

Varenicline (Chantix)

Varenicline (Chantix) is the most recently approved pharmacologic agent for treatment of tobacco dependence. This drug is a partial agonist for neuronal nicotinic acetylcholine receptors. Smoking cessation rates in the clinical trials of this drug are reported to be as high as 44%.[41,42]

Mechanism of Action

Varenicline is theorized to influence the reward pathway response in the mesolimbic dopamine system of the brain and to decrease nicotine withdrawal symptoms. In the body, varenicline binds with $alpha_4$ $beta_2$ subtype neuronal nicotinic acetylcholine receptors and produces agonist activity at that receptor site while blocking the receptors from being stimulated by nicotine. Maximum plasma concentrations occur in 3 to 4 hours, and the drug's half-life is approximately 24 hours. Varenicline is minimally metabolized by the liver, with 92% of the drug being excreted by the kidneys.[43]

Side Effects/Adverse Reactions

The most common side effects associated with varenicline that are reported include nausea, abnormal or vivid strange dreams, constipation, flatulence, and vomiting. However, because both varenicline and bupropion act on nicotinic brain receptors, monitoring the response to these medications should include self-reported information from the person about known side effects and changes in behavior, along with laboratory monitoring of kidney and liver function. Similar to bupropion, changes in behavior with varenicline have been reported to include agitation/anxiety, depressive symptoms or mood, suicidal ideation, and suicide (Box 8-1).[23]

Drug–Drug Interactions

Clinically significant pharmacokinetic drug interactions with varenicline have not been reported. In addition, the safety of administering varenicline with bupropion SR (Zyban) has not been examined. Therefore, the concomitant use of these two drugs is not recommended at this time. Moreover, varenicline is not recommended for combination therapy with nicotine replacement therapy, due to the competing antagonist action of varenicline and nicotine at the same nicotinic receptor sites, as well as the partial stimulating agonist effect provided by varenicline, which is similar to that produced by nicotine.[47]

Contraindications

The initial studies of varenicline were predominantly completed with samples of healthy adults, and this drug is contraindicated for persons younger than 18 years. Caution should be exercised when considering varenicline for persons with comorbid disorders, including mental illness. Because most of this drug is excreted unchanged by the kidneys, varenicline should not be given to individuals with renal dysfunction (creatinine clearance < 30 mL), renal insufficiency, or renal failure.[23] The use of alcohol and illicit drugs should be avoided due to a lack of information about the effects of taking these agents, which act upon the same brain receptors concomitantly.

In 2009, the FDA issued a black box warning that varenicline may cause neuropsychiatric effects such as agitation, violence, suicide ideation, or suicide attempts.[44] Persons who take varenicline should be given a medication guide that reviews these adverse effects and are cautioned to stop using this medication if they experience any of these symptoms. There are no human studies to date regarding any effects of this agent on the fetus, on the neonate, or during nursing, but caution is advised regarding the use of varenicline in pregnant and nursing women.

Prescribing Information

Dosing of varenicline is increased according to a standard regimen during the first 8 days of treatment. Administration of varenicline is reported to be unaffected by food or time of day; however, directions for administration include (1) taking the varenicline after meals or food; (2) drinking 8 ounces of water with each dose for renal clearance; (3) starting varenicline 7 days before a selected quit day while still smoking; and (4) for support and motivation, use of the web-based GetQuit program, which is recommended by varenicline's manufacturer (Pfizer).

Data from clinical trials suggest there is no difference in dosing required for adults across the lifespan. Once individuals begin using varenicline, they may report that smoking after starting the medication is not as rewarding or satisfying as it was before using this drug. Treatment is recommended for a minimum of 12 weeks, but research findings suggest that treatment may need to be continued beyond the initial 12 weeks for one additional 12-week round.

Nortriptyline (Aventyl) and Clonidine (Catapres)

Second-line treatment options often used off-label because they do not have specific FDA approval for smoking cessation treatment include clonidine (Catapres) and nortriptyline (Aventyl).[48]

Evidence of the effectiveness of nortriptyline has not been consistent, however. The 2008 treatment guideline update indicates the odds ratio for abstinence using nortriptyline across studies was 1.8 (95% CI, 1.3–2.63) and the estimated abstinence rate was 23% when compared to a placebo at 6 months after smoking cessation was initiated.[23] However, nortriptyline has well-known adverse effects, including, but not limited to, abnormal heart rhythm, low blood pressure, hallucinations, Parkinson symptoms, and sexual problems. Most of the serious adverse effects are dose dependent, and it appears that the doses used for smoking cessation purposes do not usually engender these effects. Nevertheless, this drug is contraindicated for women with cardiovascular problems.[49]

Clonidine (Catapres) lacks adequate evidence to support its use as a first-line medication for the treatment of nicotine addiction.[23] In addition, the side effects experienced while taking this drug and discontinuing it have raised concerns because other medications with established efficacy are available.

In the event that an individual is not able to use first-line treatment medications, these second-line treatment medications can be considered, but only under careful monitoring by healthcare providers.

Combination Therapy

Within the last decade, studies have been conducted to assess the efficacy of combining different types of NRT or combining NRT with bupropion to increase the rate of successful tobacco cessation. In general, the results of these studies have been positive. The NRT patch provides the long-acting NRT while nicotine gum, an inhaler, or lozenge provides relief for breakthrough urges for nicotine.[50–52] Long-term use of a nicotine patch (more than 14 weeks) with as-needed use of NRT gum or spray has an odds ratio of effectiveness of 3.6 (95% CI, 2.5–5.2) compared to a placebo. According to the latest treatment guidelines, this combination of NRT medications has an estimated abstinence rate of 36%. Use of the NRT patch with bupropion had the next highest odds ratio (OR, 2.5; 95% CI, 1.9–3.4) and an abstinence rate of 29%. Use of the patch with nortriptyline or the NRT inhaler has also demonstrated abstinence rates of 27% and 26%, respectively.[23]

Box 8-2 A Smoking Cessation Plan

ML is 35 years old. Although she successfully quit smoking during her pregnancy, her daughter is now 18 months old, and ML has resumed smoking, going through one pack of cigarettes per day. During an annual visit to her healthcare provider, she mentioned that she wants to stop smoking permanently. Her clinician used the *Five A's*: ask, advise, assess, assist, and arrange. ML has asked for smoking cessation medication, and together she and her clinician chose a quit date.

ML's history is significant for depression, for which she takes amitriptyline (Elavil). She has no other medical problems, and her only other medications are the TriCyclen combination oral contraceptive (COC) and a multivitamin. She wishes to continue the COC. She is not breastfeeding her daughter.

As she left the office, ML had a plan to initiate the nicotine patch with as-needed use of other NRT programs. Combination therapies are more efficacious than monotherapies, so the nicotine patch alone is not the best choice. Varenicline is the most effective drug for smoking session but carries an FDA black box warning that it could increase suicidal ideation; thus NRT would be a better choice for ML as an initial therapy. Bupropion is not recommended for ML because both the antidepressant and the oral contraceptives have a potential drug–drug interaction that would increase the plasma levels of bupropion and increase her risk for seizure.

The nicotine patch comes in formulations of 7 mg, 14 mg, and 21 mg (NicoDerm) designed for 24-hour use or a 15-mg (Nicotrol) version that is used for 16 hours. Standard practice is to use a dose that corresponds to the number of cigarettes smoked per day. Thus, ML was given one 21-mg patch. Her provider gave her a prescription and education materials on how to use the patch, gum, and lozenges.

Smoking cessation is most effective if nonpharmacologic methods are combined with pharmacologic methods. ML's provider encouraged her to make an appointment with her therapist to discuss smoking cessation, advisability of future use of varenicline, and other nonpharmacologic therapies. She was given information about a smoking cessation group as well. ML made an appointment to return 1 week after her quit date to evaluate her progress.

Electronic Cigarettes and Mobile Vaporizer Units: Smoking Cessation Products or Just a Sales Smokescreen?

Electronic cigarettes (e-cigs) and handheld vaporizer units (**vapes**) are increasingly popular with both men and women—sometimes as part of an effort to quit smoking, but other times as a smokeless option when the use of tobacco indoors is prohibited.[53,54] Similar to smoking cigarettes, nicotine delivered by these units is absorbed through the pulmonary capillary system. This type of delivery provides nicotine to the brain in seconds, which is more rapid than the rate achievable with intravenous delivery. These nicotine-dispensing devices are not regulated by the FDA at this time. However, several cities have banned the use of these devices indoors, and other jurisdictions may follow.

E-cigs and vapes are battery-operated devices containing liquid nicotine. Like cigarettes and hookah/shisha water pipes, these units must heat the nicotine to produce some vapor to inhale. When a user inhales or puffs on the device, the inhalation triggers the battery and atomizer, which in turn leads to the release of vaporized nicotine. E-cig units are cylindrical in shape and often look like a cigarette. The cylinder of this device contains a light, battery, sensor, heater, cartridge, and a hole on the end that is opposite the light (Figure 8-2). The battery powers the unit, and the sensor microchip allows puffing or inhaling on the unit to be recognized. When the user inhales, the coil heats the nicotine liquid in the cartridge, which provides the vaporized nicotine to the user. Typically, these cartridges contain nicotine dissolved in propylene glycol and/or vegetable glycerin, with the addition of flavorings, including those of candy, fruit, and spices.[55]

The vape units are larger than the e-cig units. A cylindrical tube holds the battery, cartomizer, on/off button, and tip. The cartomizer includes a cartridge containing the atomizer (heating coil), sensor, and liquid nicotine. Unlike an e-cig, the vape unit has a tip through which the user inhales.

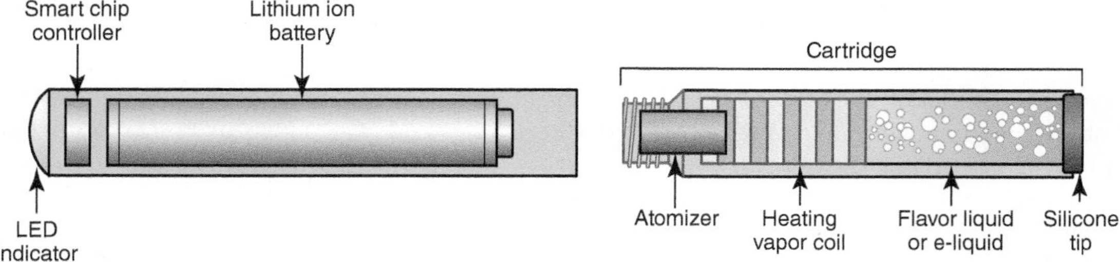

Figure 8-2 Components of a typical e-cigarette.

These units can be expensive, and they require users to refill the liquid. Moreover, unlike the e-cig, vape units can be loaded with different doses of nicotine, ranging from 0 to 24 mg in increments of 6 mg.

There are several purported reasons for using e-cigs and vape units. Some believe that they deliver less nicotine than regular cigarettes and are less toxic, and can be used to wean off use of cigarettes. However, there is no evidence at this time that these beliefs are valid.[56] Furthermore, some subpopulations among adults and adolescents prefer to use multiple modes of consuming nicotine, which may include smoked tobacco, oral tobacco products, and electronic nicotine devices.[57] The use of multiple devices raises concern about the total amount of nicotine intake and potentially harmful chemicals that these individuals are receiving.

Toxicity and safety continue to be concerns with regard to e-cigs and vapes. These devices should be kept out of the reach of children. The CDC has noted increased reports of poisoning related to the inhalation of the vapor, swallowing of the liquid, and/or contact of the liquid to the skin and/or eyes.[58]

Another concern pertains to the liquid used in the devices. To control costs, some users try to "home-brew" their own liquid. Low traces of chemicals emitted into the environment have also been reported.[59] Yet another controversy is the use of child-friendly flavors such as bubble gum, gummy bears, and cotton candy. Although there is a federal ban against selling regular cigarettes to minors, no such national law exists for e-cigarettes, and the concern is that the candy flavors available with these devices may cause youth to initiate smoking.

There is growing debate regarding the usefulness of e-cigs and vapes for smoking cessation. While some groups would like to see them regulated by the FDA, if not banned altogether, smoking cessation researchers note a potential need for new treatment options to assist with smoking cessation efforts.[60] Some studies have reported that regular cigarettes deliver 10 times the nicotine that e-cigs and vape units provide.[61] More studies are needed to fully understand these devices and their use for smoking cessation, particularly since legal and societal issues remain unclear.

Future Therapy

New therapies to treat tobacco dependence are under development and in testing. A nicotine conjugate vaccine (NicVAX), for example, is under investigation as a potential means of treating tobacco dependence as well as relapse. The vaccine stimulates the immune system to make antibodies that bind to nicotine, thereby preventing nicotine from crossing the blood-brain barrier. The result is that no pleasure is derived from the nicotine. Findings from Phase 2 trials indicate NicVAX is safe and influenced cessation efforts in 25% of persons with smoking histories of one pack per day or more.[62–64] Furthermore, these preliminary reports suggest the nicotine vaccine has minimal to no side effects.

Special Populations

Pregnancy and Lactation

A U.S. Public Health Service guideline suggests that women may be motivated to quit smoking while pregnant, during which time they are likely to be susceptible to messages and reinforcement for tobacco cessation. Furthermore, healthcare providers may promote relapse prevention by emphasizing the relationship between maternal smoking and poor health outcomes for both mother and child.[65] Women who are able to quit smoking by 16 weeks' gestation have no increased risk for low birth weight, stillbirth, or infant death compared to those who continue smoking into the second trimester.[66]

Bupropion has no known teratogenic effects, but the increased risk for seizures is a concern that has limited prescriptions of this agent as a smoking cessation drug for pregnant women. The safety of nicotine replacement during pregnancy has been evaluated in a few clinical trials that have shown some effectiveness and no adverse effects on women or their fetuses.[67] In the absence of conclusive data, it is currently believed that the benefits of smoking cessation outweigh the potential risks to the fetus from exposure to NRT products, and clinical practice guidelines in the United States recommend NRT products for pregnant women as long as the total dose of nicotine in the NRT is not larger than would have been received via the usual dose from that individual's daily smoking habit.[23]

Elderly

Efforts to help women who are perimenopausal or menopausal stop smoking deserve special mention. Smoking is associated with early onset of menopause, which in turn increases a woman's risk for many disorders, including cardiovascular events and osteoporosis. In the past, concern about weight gain has been a significant reason why women who smoke do not quit. Few studies have been conducted on specific NRT products used by women 65 years or older, but the nicotine patch is just as effective in this population as it is in other age groups. Because steroids inhibit CP450B6 activity, women on hormone therapy may need smaller doses of bupropion SR when starting this drug.[38,67]

Conclusion

Pharmacologic therapy is an important treatment option for women desiring to discontinue their use of tobacco. Varenicline is the most recent addition to the treatment options for tobacco addiction and is providing positive results. Bupropion provides women with a different option that also has the ability to attenuate weight gain and achieve a nearly 25% abstinence rate; it is as efficacious as NRT products when used as a monotherapy. The highest rates of abstinence occur with combination therapy consisting of the nicotine patch plus bupropion SR or varenicline, followed by the combination of the nicotine patch with as-needed use of NRT gum or spray.[23]

Research supports the need to treat women for longer than 12 weeks, particularly with individuals who are severely addicted.[23] Healthcare providers may need to consider menstrual cycles when initiating tobacco cessation in premenopausal women. Both younger and older women should not be ignored due to their age when it comes to providing tobacco addiction treatment. Members of both groups can obtain great health benefits by quitting smoking. Offering messages to promote cessation and prescribing medication is only the beginning when assisting women to abstain from tobacco. Follow-up is vital to assist women with support and monitoring of their progress, use of medications, side effects, and relapse prevention if needed.

Resources

Organization	Description	Website
Federal Government Sites		
Centers for Disease Control and Prevention: Quit Smoking Campaign	List of multiple credible resources for individuals interested in quitting smoking; includes a wide variety of web pages with information and tips	www.cdc.gov/tobacco/campaign/tips/quit-smoking/quitting-resources.html
National Institute on Drug Abuse	Multiple professional publications about tobacco addition/abuse (e.g., *NIDA Research Report: Tobacco Addiction; Drug Facts: Cigarettes and Other Tobacco Products*); information about adolescent smoking and use of e-cigarettes can be found here	www.drugabuse.gov/publications/research-reports/tobacco
National Institutes of Health/National Cancer Institute	Multiple web pages including information about smoking and suggestions on how to stop	www.smokefree.gov or http://betobaccofree.hhs.gov
Non-Federal Government Sites		
American Cancer Society	Information on tips to stop smoking; Spanish version available	www.cancer.org/%20healthy/stayawayfromtobacco/guidetoquittingsmoking/index
American College of Nurse-Midwives	Campaign with CDC that includes talking points for providers and women-focused information	www.midwife.org/Smoking-Cessation
American College of Obstetricians and Gynecologist	Several resources for providers of care of women and the women themselves; includes an e-module focused on smoking	www.acog.org/About-ACOG/ACOG-Districts/District-II/Smoking-Cessation-Tools-and-Resources

Organization	Description	Website
American Lung Association	Tips to stop smoking	www.lung.org/stop-smoking
Get Quit	Program specific to Chantix and sponsored by the drug's manufacturer	www.get-quit.com/sites/getquit/Pages/index.aspx
Apps and Other Resources		
Live Strong: My Quit Coach	App to personalize and track progress stopping smoking	www.livestrong.com/quit-smoking-app
National Institutes of Health/National Cancer Institute: Smoking Quitline	Telephone help in quitting and answers to smoking-related questions in English or Spanish for consumers	Toll-free call within the United States, Monday through Friday, 8:00 A.M. to 8:00 P.M. Eastern Time: 1-877-44U-QUIT (1-877-448-7848)
National Institutes of Health/National Cancer Institute: LiveHelp Online Chat	Consumer information and advice about quitting smoking through a confidential online text chat with an information specialist from NCI's Cancer Information Service	Monday through Friday, 8:00 A.M. to 11:00 P.M. Eastern Time: https://livehelp.cancer.gov/app/chat/chat_launch
National Institutes of Health/National Cancer Institute: Smoke Free site	Top-rated consumer-oriented free apps for smartphones, computers, and tablets sponsored by the federal government; includes *QuitStart*, *QuitGuide*, and *QuitPal*	www.smokefree.gov/apps-quitpal
National Institutes of Health/National Cancer Institute: Smoking Text	Mobile text messaging to help motivate people to continue not smoking	http://smokefree.gov/smokefreetxt; also available on Facebook (www.facebook.com/SmokefreeTXT)
Quit It Lite	Allows consumers to estimate how many cigarettes they have not smoked and how much money they have saved by not smoking	www.itunes.apple.com/us/app/quit-it-lite-stop-smoking-now/id468624531?mt=8

References

1. Agaku IT, King BA, Dube SR. Current cigarette smoking among adults—United States, 2005–2012. *MMWR.* 2014;63:29-34. http://www.cdc.gov/tobacco/data_statistics/mmwrs/byyear/2014/mm6302a2/intro.htm. Accessed October 16, 2014.
2. Thun MJ, Carter BD, Feskanich D, et al. 50-year trends in smoking-related mortality in the United States. *N Engl J Med.* 2013;368:351-364.
3. U.S. Department of Health and Human Services. *The health consequences of smoking for women: a report of the Surgeon General.* Washington, DC: U.S. Department of Health and Human Services, Public Health Service, Office of the Assistant Secretary for Health, Office on Smoking and Health; 1980.
4. U.S. Department of Health and Human Services. *The health consequences of smoking—50 years of progress: a report of the Surgeon General.* Atlanta, GA: U.S. Department of Health and Human Services, Centers for Disease Control and Prevention, National Center for Chronic Disease Prevention and Health Promotion, Office of Smoking and Health; 2014. Printed with corrections, January 2014.
5. U.S. Department of Health and Human Services. *Women and smoking: a report of the Surgeon General.* Rockville, MD: U.S. Department of Health and Human Services, Public Health Service, Office of the Surgeon General; 2001.
6. Healton CG, Gritz ER, Davis KC, et al. Women's knowledge of the leading causes of cancer death. *Nicotine Tob Res.* 2007;9(7):761-768.
7. Tong VT, Dietz PM, Morrow B, et al. Trends in smoking before, during, and after pregnancy: Pregnancy Risk Assessment Monitoring System, United States, 40 sites, 2000–2010. *MMWR Surveill Summ.* 2013;62:1-19. http://www.cdc.gov/mmwr/preview/mmwrhtml/ss6206a1.htm?utm_source=rss&utm_medium=rss&utm_campaign=trends-in-smoking-before-during-and-after-pregnancy-pregnancy-risk-assessment-monitoring-system-united-states-40-sites-20002010. Accessed October 16, 2014.
8. Hiemstra M, Otten R, de Leeuw RN, van Schayck OC, Engels RC. The changing role of self-efficacy in adolescent smoking initiation. *J Adolesc Health.* 2011;48:597-603.
9. Bricker JB, Peterson AV, Robyn Andersen M, Leroux BG, Bharat Rajan K, Sarason IG. Close friends', parents', and older siblings' smoking: reevaluating their influence on children's smoking. *Nicotine Tob Res.* 2006;8(2):217-226.
10. Hertling I, Ramskogler K, Dvorak A, et al. Craving and other characteristics of the comorbidity of alcohol and nicotine dependence. *Eur Psychiatry.* 2005;20(5-6):442-450.
11. Batscheider A, Zakrzewska S, Heinrich J, et al. Exposure to second-hand smoke and direct healthcare costs in children: results from two German birth cohorts, GINIplus and LISAplus. *BMC Health Serv Res.* 2012;12:344.
12. Matt GE, Quintana PJ, Destaillats H, et al. Thirdhand tobacco smoke: emerging evidence and arguments for a multidisciplinary research agenda. *Environ Health Perspect.* 2011;119(9):1218-1226.

13. Perkins KA. Smoking cessation in women: special considerations. *CNS Drugs.* 2001;15(5):391-411.
14. Perkins KA, Scott J. Sex differences in long-term smoking cessation rates due to nicotine patch. *Nicotine Tob Res.* 2008;10(7):1245-1250.
15. Benowitz NL. Nicotine pharmacology and addiction. In: Benowitz NL, ed. *Nicotine Safety and Toxicity.* New York: Oxford University Press; 1998:3-16.
16. Kukkanen J, Hukkanen J, Jacob P III, Benowitz NL. Metabolism and disposition kinetics of nicotine. *Pharmacol Rev.* 2005;57(1):79-115.
17. Benowitz NL, Sessov-Schlagger CN, Swan GE, Jacob P III. Female sex and oral contraceptive use accelerate nicotine metabolism. *Clin Pharmacol Ther.* 2006;79:480-488.
18. Benowitz NL. Neurobiology of nicotine addiction: implications for smoking cessation treatment. *Am J Med.* 2008;121(4 suppl 1):S3-S10.
19. Egleton RD, Abbruscato T. Drug abuse and the neurovascular unit. *Adv Pharmacol.* 2014;71:451-480.
20. Hughes JR, Gust SW, Skoog K, Keenan RM, Fenwick JW. Symptoms of tobacco withdrawal: a replication and extension. *Arch Gen Psychiatry.* 1991;48(1):52-59.
21. Kroon LA. Drug interactions with smoking. *Am J Health Sys Pharm.* 2007;64:1917-1921.
22. Ravel AP, Borges-Garcia R, Diaz F, Sick TJ, Bramlett H. Oral contraceptives and nicotine synergistically exacerbate cerebral ischemic injury in the female brain. *Transl Stroke Res.* 2013;4(4):402-412.
23. Fiore MC, Jaén CR, Baker TB, et al. *Treating tobacco use and dependence: 2008 update. Clinical practice guideline.* Rockville, MD: U.S. Department of Health and Human Services. Public Health Service; May 2008. http://www.ahrq.gov/professionals/clinicians-providers/guidelines-recommendations/tobacco/clinicians/update/index.html. Accessed October 23, 2014.
24. Perkins KA, Conklin CA, Levine MD. *Cognitive-behavioral Therapy for Smoking Cessation: A Practical Guidebook to the Most Effective Treatments.* London: Routledge Taylor & Francis Group; 2008.
25. Barnes J, Dong CY, McRobbie H, Walker N, Mehta M, Stead LF. Hypnotherapy for smoking cessation. *Cochrane Database Syst Rev.* 2010;20:CD001008. doi:10.1002/14651858.CD001008.pub2.
26. White AR, Rampes H, Liu JP, Stead LF, Campbell J. Acupuncture and related interventions for smoking cessation. *Cochrane Database Syst Rev.* 2014;1:CD000009. doi:10.1002/14651858.CD000009.pub4.
27. Ussher MH, Taylor AH, Faulkner GEJ. Exercise interventions for smoking cessation. *Cochrane Database Syst Rev.* 2014;8:CD002295. doi:10.1002/14651858.CD002295.pub5.
28. Nides M. Update on pharmacologic options for smoking cessation treatment. *Am J Med.* 2008;121(4 suppl 1):S20-S31.
29. Crooks PA, Bardo MT, Dwoskin LP. Nicotinic receptor antagonists as treatments for nicotine abuse. *Adv Pharmacol.* 2014;69:513-551.
30. Le Houezec J, Aubin HJ Pharmacotherapies and harm-reduction options for the treatment of tobacco dependence. *Expert Opin Pharmacother.* 2013;14(14):1959-1967.
31. Choi JH, Dresler CM, Norton MR, Strahs KR. Pharmacokinetics of a nicotine polacrilex lozenge. *Nicotine Tob Res.* 2003;5(5):635-644.
32. Stead LF, Perera R, Bullen C, et al. Nicotine replacement therapy for smoking cessation. *Cochrane Database Syst Rev.* 2012;11:CD000146. doi:10.1002/14651858.CD000146.pub4.
33. Hukkanen J, Jacob P III, Benowitz NL. Effect of grapefruit juice on cytochrome P450 2A6 and nicotine renal clearance. *Clin Pharmacol Ther.* 2006;80(5):522-530.
34. Hughes JR, Stead LF, Hartmann-Boyce J, Cahill K, Lancaster T. Antidepressants for smoking cessation. *Cochrane Database Syst Rev.* 2014;1:CD000031. doi:10.1002/14651858.CD000031.pub4.
35. Foley KF, DeSanty KP, Kast RE. Bupropion: pharmacology and therapeutic applications. *Expert Rev Neurother.* 2006;6(9):1249-1265.
36. Haustein KO. Bupropion: pharmacological and clinical profile in smoking cessation. *Int J Clin Pharmacol Ther.* 2003;41(2):56-66.
37. Kotz D, Simpson C, Viechtbauer W, van Schayck OC, West R, Sheikh A. Cardiovascular and neuropsychiatric safety of varenicline and bupropion compared with nicotine replacement therapy for smoking cessation: study protocol of a retrospective cohort study using the QResearch general practice database. *BMJ Open.* 2014;4(8):e005281. http://bmjopen.bmj.com/content/4/8/e005281.long. Accessed October 16, 2014.
38. Palovaara S, Pelkonen O, Uusitalo J, Lundgren S, Laine K. Inhibition of cytochrome P450 2B6 activity by hormone replacement therapy and oral contraceptive as measured by bupropion hydroxylation C. *Clin Pharmacol Ther.* 2003;74:326-333.

39. Lee AM, Jepson C, Hoffmann E, et al. CYP2B6 genotype alters abstinence rates in a bupropion smoking cessation trial. *Biol Psychiatry.* 2007;62(6):635-641.
40. Swan GE, Valdes AM, Ring HZ, et al. Dopamine receptor DRD2 genotype and smoking cessation outcome following treatment with bupropion SR. *Pharmacogenomics J.* 2005;5(1):21-29.
41. Obach RS, Reed-Hagen AE, Krueger SS, et al. Metabolism and disposition of varenicline, a selective alpha$_4$beta$_2$ acetylcholine receptor partial agonist, in vivo and in vitro. *Drug Metab Dispo.* 2006;34(1):121-130.
42. Gonzales D, Rennard SI, Nides M, et al. Varenicline, an alpha$_4$beta$_2$ nicotinic acetylcholine receptor partial agonist, vs sustained-release bupropion and placebo for smoking cessation: a randomized controlled trial. *JAMA.* 2006;296(1):47-55.
43. Zierler-Brown SL, Kyle JA. Oral varenicline for smoking cessation. *Ann Pharmacother.* 2007;41(1):95-99.
44. Food and Drug Administration. FDA: boxed warning on serious mental health events to be required for Chantix and Zyban. 2009. http://www.fda.gov/NewsEvents/Newsroom/PressAnnouncements/ucm170100.htm. Accessed October 16, 2014.
45. Stapleton JA, Watson L, Spirling LI, et al. Varenicline in the routine treatment of tobacco dependence: a pre-post comparison with nicotine replacement therapy and an evaluation in those with mental illness. *Addiction.* 2008;103(1):146-154.
46. Gibbons RD, Mann JJ. Varenicline, smoking cessation, and neuropsychiatric adverse events. *Am J Psychiat.* 2013;170:1460-1467.
47. Ramon JM, Morchon S, Baena A, Masuet-Aumatell C. Combining varenicline and nicotine patches: a randomized controlled trial study in smoking cessation. *BMC Med.* 2014;12(1):172.
48. Hall SM, Lightwood JM, Humfleet GL, Bostrom A, Reus VI, Muñoz R. Cost-effectiveness of bupropion, nortriptyline, and psychological intervention in smoking cessation. *J Behav Health Serv Res.* 2005; 32(4):381-392.
49. Dhippayom T, Chaiyakunapruk N, Jongchansittho T. Safety of nortriptyline at equivalent therapeutic doses for smoking cessation: a systematic review and meta-analysis. *Drug Saf.* 2011;34(3):199-210.
50. Croghan IT, Hurt RD, Dakhil SR, et al. Randomized comparison of a nicotine inhaler and bupropion for smoking cessation and relapse prevention. *Mayo Clin Proc.* 2007;82(2):186-195.
51. Hurt RD, Krook JE, Croghan IT, et al. Nicotine patch therapy based on smoking rate followed by bupropion for prevention of relapse to smoking. *J Clin Oncol.* 2003;21(5):914-920.
52. Jamerson BD, Nides M, Jorenby DE, et al. Late-term smoking cessation despite initial failure: an evaluation of bupropion sustained release, nicotine patch, combination therapy, and placebo. *Clin Ther.* 2001;23(5):744-752.
53. Elrashidi MY, Ebbert JO. Emerging drugs for the treatment of tobacco dependence: 2014 update. *Expert Opin Emerg Drugs.* 2014;19(2):243-260.
54. Cobb NK, Abrams DB. The FDA, e-cigarettes, and the demise of combusted tobacco. *N Engl J Med.* 2014;371(16):1469-1471.
55. Riker CA, Lee K, Darville A, Hahn EJ. E-cigarettes: promise or peril? *Nurs Clin North Am.* 2012;47:159-171.
56. Etter JF, Bullen C. Electronic cigarette: users profile, utilization, satisfaction, and perceived efficacy. *Addiction.* 2011;106:2017-2028.
57. Erickson DJ, Lenk KM, Forster JL. Latent classes of young adults based on use of multiple types of tobacco and nicotine products. *Nicotine Tob Res.* 2014;16:1056-1062.
58. Chatham-Stephens K, Law R, Taylor E, et al. Notes from the field: calls to poison centers for exposures to electronic cigarettes—United States, September 2010–February 2014. *MMWR.* 2014;63:292-293. http://www.cdc.gov/mmwr/preview/mmwrhtml/mm6313a4.htm. Accessed October 23, 2014.
59. Schober W, Szendrei K, Matzen W, et al. Use of electronic cigarettes (e-cigarettes) impairs indoor air quality and increases FeNO levels of e-cigarette consumers. *Int J Hyg Environ Health.* 2014;217:628-637.
60. Barbeau AM, Burda J, Siegel M. Perceived efficacy of e-cigarettes versus nicotine replacement therapy among successful e-cigarette users: a qualitative approach. *Addiction Sci Clin Pract.* 2013;8:5.
61. Wolters A, de Wert G, van Schayck OC, Horstman K. Vaccination against smoking: an annotated agenda

for debate. A review of scientific journals, 2001–13. *Addiction.* 2014;109(8):1268-1273.

62. Pentel PR, LeSage MG. New directions in nicotine vaccine design and use. *Adv Pharmacol.* 2014;69: 553-580.
63. Hatsukami DK, Rennard S, Jorenby D, et al. Safety and immunogenicity of a nicotine conjugate vaccine in current smokers. *Clin Pharmacol Ther.* 2005;78(5): 456-467.
64. Bloch M, Parascandola M. Tobacco use in pregnancy: a window of opportunity for prevention. *Lancet Glob Health.* 2014;2(9):e489-e490.
65. Rigotti NA, Park ER, Chang Y, Regan S. Smoking cessation medication use among pregnant and post-partum smokers. *Obstet Gynecol.* 2008;111(2 pt 1): 348-355.
66. Black MM, Nair P, Spanier AJ. Dose and timing of pre-natal tobacco exposure: threats to early child development. *Lancet Respir Med.* 2014;2(9):677-679.
67. Allen SS, Hatsukami DK, Bade T, Center B. Transdermal nicotine use in postmenopausal women: does the treatment efficacy differ in women using and not using hormone replacement therapy? *Nicotine Tob Res.* 2004;6(5):777-788.

9 Drugs of Abuse

Barbara Peterson Sinclair, Margaret S. Stemmler

With acknowledgment to Shirley A. Summers for her contribution to the first edition of Pharmacology for Women's Health

Chapter Glossary

Abuse Maladaptive pattern of drug or substance use that leads to significant impairment and manifests in tolerance, withdrawal, use of the substance in larger amounts or over a longer period time than intended, including use outside of social norms.

Addiction Recurring compulsion to use a substance (e.g., alcohol or drugs). In the past, "addiction" has been a nonspecific umbrella term, whereas today specific labels such as "abuse" and "dependence" are used to more precisely describe drug use and misuse.

Anxiolytic Agent used for the treatment of anxiety and related psychological and physical symptoms. Several chemically different drugs, such as benzodiazepines, selective serotonin reuptake inhibitors, and even alcohol, may be termed anxiolytics.

Cross-tolerance Tolerance to the effects of one drug when using another drug that has not been used before because both agents share a similar pharmacologic action.

Dependence Physiological need for a drug or substance, often, but not necessarily, involving abuse.

Drug misuse Inappropriate use of prescription or over-the-counter medications, such as using medications in ways not indicated, taking drugs when not prescribed or more than prescribed or for longer periods of time than indicated, sharing drugs with others, and discontinuing drugs early.

Hypnotics Agents that produce somnolence.

Illicit drugs Substances or drugs that are not permitted by law.

Licit drugs Substances or drugs that are permitted by law.

Narcotics Legal, not pharmacologic, term, usually associated with opioids.

Opioids Drugs that bind to opium receptors (e.g., endorphins or methadone), resulting in opium-like effects; often used interchangeably with "opiate," although some sources reserve the latter term for drugs derived from natural opium poppy and "opioid" for both natural and synthetic agents.

Relapse Return to drug use behavior after a period of abstinence; a recurring hallmark of addiction.

Sedatives Agents that decrease central nervous system arousal and/or anxiety. Some sedatives also may be labeled as anxiolytics.

Substance use disorders Conditions that reflect dependence by an individual, which can move through a continuum and are not simply the presence or absence of abuse or addiction.

Tolerance With continued drug/medication use, the need for a higher dose to achieve the same desired response. It can occur with any drug and is not exclusive to addiction.

Withdrawal Symptoms that occur when a person who is dependent on a psychoactive drug or substance discontinues use of the agent. Also known as abstinence syndrome.

Introduction

Substance use disorders carry great cultural stigma. Even today, many individuals (erroneously) perceive **addiction** to be the result of personal weakness and moral failing. In the arena of health care, several theories of drug or substance addiction have been suggested; the prevailing model of substance use disorder identifies a number of neurobiological, psychological, social, and environmental factors that influence substance use. These components are intertwined with one another and address many dimensions in life: genetics, gender, personal and family history, psychology, social networks, political factors, and community. Advances in science have established that these disorders reflect a maladaptive change within the brain that is manifested through drug effects, drug-seeking behaviors, and the physical symptom clusters associated with **withdrawal**. Box 9-1 lists the common symptoms generally associated with this condition.

Considerable attention has been given to the increasing prevalence of substance use disorders, but it is important to recognize that not everyone who is exposed to alcohol or other drugs will become addicted or even dependent. Adolescents tend to be at greater risk than adults for developing substance use disorders because psychoactive substances are more toxic to the immature brain.[2] Individuals with co-occurring mental health disorders tend to exhibit greater impulsivity and/or novelty-seeking behaviors, such that they may seek out psychoactive substances to feel better or to self-medicate.[3] Chronic pain affects approximately 10% of persons who reside in the United States, and frequent use of medication to relieve pain can sometimes result in dependency. However, undertreated chronic pain can result in a person's behaviors being mistaken for drug-seeking behavior.

Regardless of how initiation and escalation of substance use occurs, the course of substance **abuse** is progressive. Increased frequency of use and taking of larger doses, advancing routes of administration, and polypharmacy (also called polydrug use) are components of drug escalation that enhance the experiential effect; each increase adds to the addiction risk. Combinations of drugs may be used together to augment the overall effect of the combination or in the course of drug behavior. For example, alcohol is a common part of drug-taking behavior, whereas mixing heroin with methamphetamine or cocaine in a "speedball" represents a specific escalation to elicit a "roller-coaster" effect of using both a stimulant and a depressant.

This chapter focuses on pharmacologic substances that frequently are drugs of abuse. While behaviors such as gambling and use of agents such as caffeine may appropriately fall under the umbrella of substance use disorders, they are outside the scope of this chapter focused on pharmacology and are not discussed here.

Box 9-1 Symptoms Associated with Substance Use Disorders

- Tolerance
- Withdrawal
- Use of the substance for longer than intended
- Unsuccessful attempts to decrease or discontinue use of the substance
- Expending considerable time to obtain, use, and recover from the effects of the substance
- Missing social engagements because of substance use
- Craving to use the substance
- Continued use despite knowledge of adverse consequences
- Failure to fulfill major role obligations
- Use in physically hazardous situations
- Continued use despite social and interpersonal problems

Source: Data from American Psychiatric Association. *Diagnostic and Statistical Manual of Mental Disorders.* Arlington, VA: American Psychatric Publishing; 2013.[1]

Neurobiology of Addiction

The mesolimbic system reinforces positive feelings associated with activities needed for survival, such as eating to stave off hunger, drinking to quench thirst, feeling warmth on a frigid day, and libido and sexual behavior. Frequent alcohol and/or drug exposure modifies this region of the brain and influences the brain's neurotransmitter systems, which results in altered neuronal stimulation in the areas that affect reward, pleasure, memory, decision making, and perceptions of well-being.[4] Figure 9-1 depicts brain regions that play a role in addiction.

The mesolimbic system forms a ring or limbus around the brain stem. These structures are involved with internal homeostasis, memory, learning, motivation, and emotion. Structures in the mesolimbic system are also called

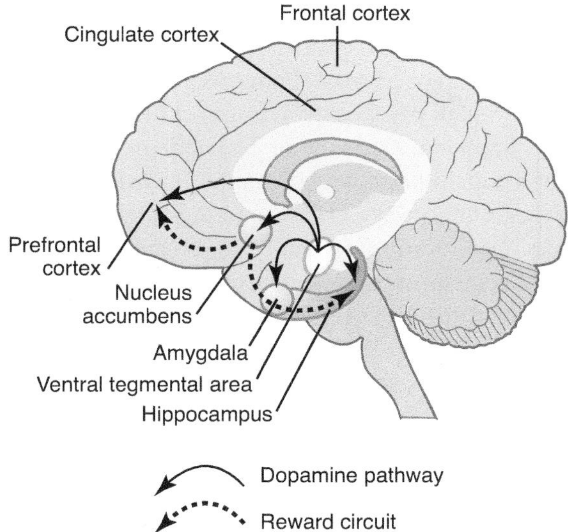

Figure 9-1 Structures in the mesolimbic system form the biological platform for addiction. Increased levels of dopamine in the neuronal synapses stimulate the reward pathway, which encourage the individual to continue taking drugs that keep dopamine levels high in the synapse.

the reward pathway. They are the biological platform for addiction starting with the neural pathways that connect the ventral tegmental area (VTA) to the nucleus accumbens (NAc), amygdala, and hippocampus. The neurons in the VTA release the neurotransmitter dopamine in response to a pleasurable experience. It is the dopamine that makes an individual feel pleasure. Sex, food, alcohol, barbiturates, benzodiazepines, and opioids stimulate neurons in the VTA. The NAc is a primary target of the dopamine released by the VTA. The NAc is also stimulated by amphetamines, opioids, cocaine, phencyclidine, ketamine, and nicotine. The result of drug use is increased levels of dopamine in the neuronal synapses in the reward pathway.

The reward pathway is connected to areas of the brain that control memory and behavior. This assures that the pleasure will be remembered and desired to be repeated. Dopamine released by neurons from the VTA also stimulates the amygdala and the hippocampus. The amygdala creates a conditioned response and the hippocampus lays down memories of the experience.[5]

When psychoactive drugs are used, they modulate the function of dopamine and other neurotransmitters that produce the sensations of pleasure and positive feelings. Synaptic neurotransmission is illustrated in Figure 9-2. With chronic use, the mesolimbic system becomes dysregulated, resulting in compulsion to continue drug use with greater amounts and/or more frequent dosing.[6,7]

Continued exposure to drugs of abuse interferes with the normal neural communication process. The prefrontal cortex is the brain region involved with rational thought and decision making. With ongoing drug use, synaptic remodeling in the prefrontal cortex leads to a smaller number of properly functioning dopamine receptors. The clinical result is **tolerance**, referring to the need for larger or more frequent doses of the drug to obtain the same pleasurable

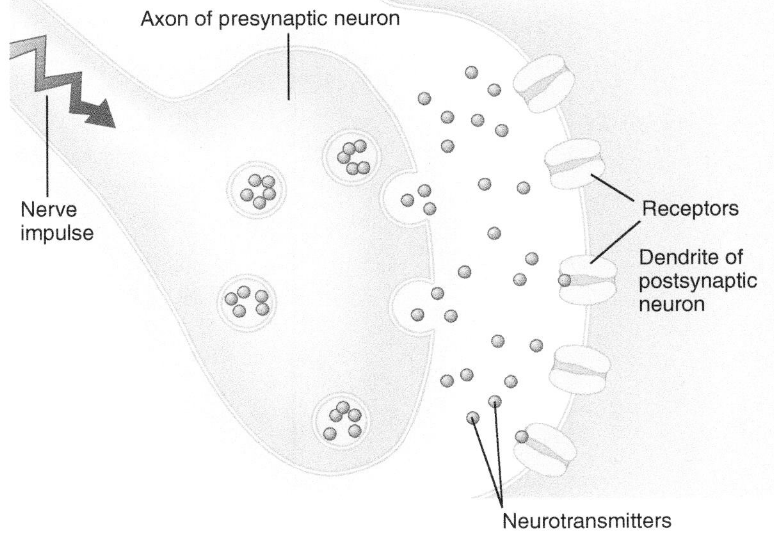

Figure 9-2 Synaptic neurotransmission.

effect. Individuals who develop tolerance to one drug may also demonstrate **cross-tolerance** to other drugs that work through a similar mechanism of action.

Individuals who abuse drugs often exhibit difficulty in making decisions or judging actions. The mesolimbic system responds to environmental stimuli with memory-associated cues of individuals, places, or objects linked to drug use behavior; thus, for example, seeing a place where drug use occurred can "trigger" a craving. When cue-induced reactions occur, they can lead to lapses into drug use, or they can instigate complete **relapse** and resumption of drug-using behaviors despite a long period of abstinence. It needs to be noted that this is a simplistic description of neural pathways that are complex and the subject of current research. A great deal remains to be learned about this process.

Even though psychoactive drugs act in a variety of ways on the brain, to a greater or lesser degree, their action involves dopamine activity (Figure 9-3). Drugs of addiction act in one of four ways: (1) by imitating natural neurotransmitters (e.g., morphine binds to opiate receptors and stimulates the postsynaptic neuron); (2) by stimulating the release of natural neurotransmitters (e.g., amphetamines stimulate the release of dopamine and directly mimic the effects of dopamine); (3) by blocking the release of

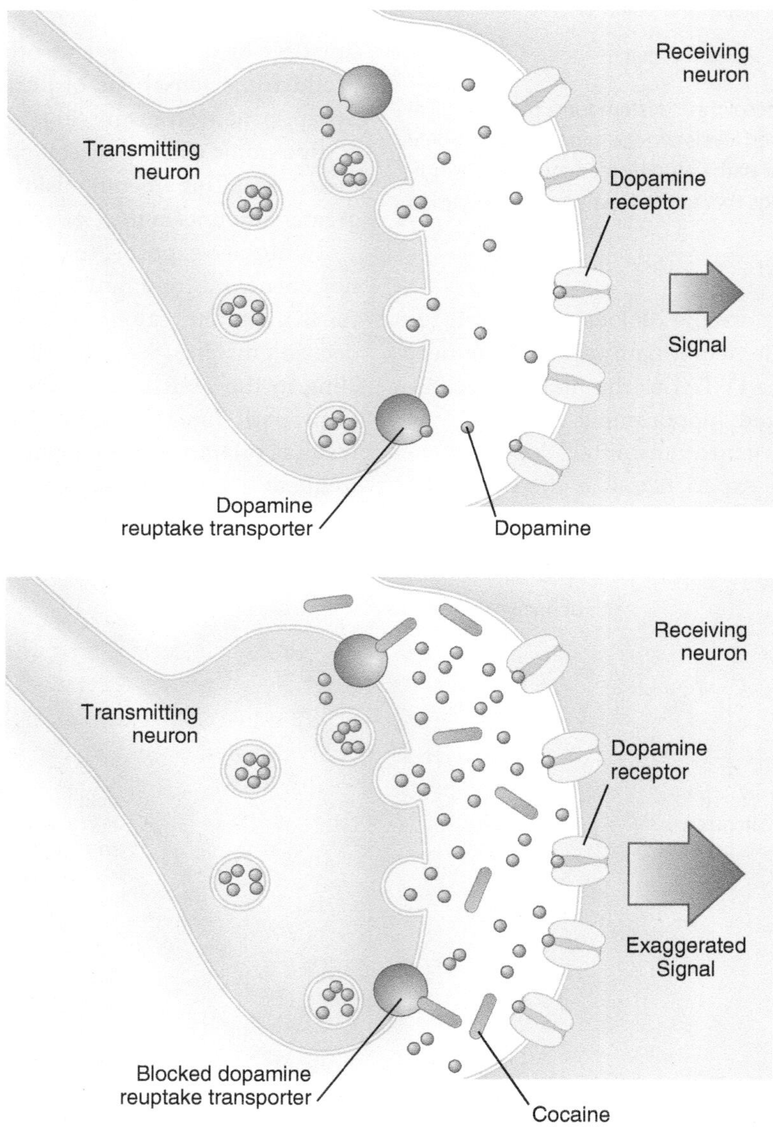

Figure 9-3 Effect of cocaine on dopamine reuptake.

a reuptake mechanism (e.g., cocaine blocks the reuptake of dopamine and 3,4-methylenedioxy-methamphetamine [MDMA; "ecstasy"] blocks the reuptake of serotonin); and (4) by binding to the gamma-aminobutyric acid (GABA) receptors (e.g., alcohol, barbiturates, and benzodiazepines work in this manner).

Treatment of Individuals with Substance Use Disorders

The most successful approach to substance use disorder treatment consists of comprehensive care, including both pharmacologic and counseling therapies. However, most individuals who abuse substances do not perceive that they need treatment.[8] In 2012, 23.1 million persons needed treatment, but only 11% received care. To some degree, treatment deficits survive as a result of the social stigma surrounding drug use. Limited access to services has been a problem not only for persons who abuse drugs, but also for healthcare professionals who want to refer a woman for treatment. The Patient Protection and Affordable Care Act (2012) and the Mental Health Parity and Addiction Equity Act (2008) both have proposed remedies for access to substance abuse treatment through the primary care setting. Time and evaluations will be needed to determine the outcome of these efforts.

Screening for Substance Use Disorders

Among the U.S. population, an estimated 20% to 25% use substances at risky levels that indicate a developing problem and 7% have substance use problems that require treatment.[8] Excessive alcohol intake, use of **illicit drugs**, and **drug misuse** of prescription medications are underdiagnosed by healthcare professionals. Nevertheless, concise, easy-to-administer screening tools are available that can be used in primary care settings. National studies reveal that nearly 70% of screenings are negative and require no intervention; only approximately 5% of the individuals will require extensive substance use evaluation and/or treatment.[9,10]

Behavioral Therapies for Individuals with Substance Use Disorders

Behavioral therapies, sometimes termed "talk therapies," are designed to help the individual bolster coping skills, learn to identify relapse triggers, and respond appropriately to a lapse in abstinence. Treatment options for women who abuse alcohol or other drugs individually or in groups include motivational interviewing, cognitive-behavioral therapies, and contingency management. The effectiveness of behavioral therapy has been reported to range between 25% and 40% as a means to achieve and sustain abstinence.[4]

The most commonly used adjunctive approaches are Alcoholics Anonymous (AA) and Narcotics Anonymous (NA). These 12-step support groups are intended to promote lifetime abstinence. The meetings are designed to provide no-cost, mutual support using a one-day-at-a-time approach. An alternative model is Smart Recovery, a no-cost program that addresses practical, supportive tools and cognitive therapies, accessible through the Internet and in-person meetings.

Women-only programs provide enhanced services, but they are not a requirement for treatment success.[11,12] Supplemental components in women-only programs address the needs of pregnant and parenting women with substance use disorders. Life management skills training, education completion, and job training constitute significant needs for many female participants. Women-only programs also have health agendas to provide prenatal education, child health, and parenting skills.

Women and Substance Use Disorders

Substance use disorders affect individuals across the full range of age, socioeconomic status, race, and ethnicity. Although trends in and preferences for illicit drugs vary around the country, the greatest percentage (21.3%) of substance users are found among young adults aged 18 to 25 years.[8] Initiation into drug use tends to occur during adolescence, and certain drugs (nicotine, alcohol, and marijuana) are often the first tried. During the early teen years, illicit drugs are used by similar percentages of young males and females—9.6% and 9.5%, respectively.[8] During high school, however, drug use by young men tends to surpass young women's use of all drugs with the exceptions of amphetamines, which young women use more than their male cohorts, and inhalants, which both genders use equally.[13]

Gender-related characteristics further influence substance use behaviors. For example, whereas men may try alcohol or other drugs independently, women tend to initiate substances upon their introduction by a trusted family member, intimate partner, or close friend; however, evidence of women playing an active role in their own initiation is emerging.[14] Women tend to escalate substance use more rapidly than men; they are less likely to seek and engage with treatment even though they demonstrate more severe addiction; and they experience higher levels of craving and relapse during abstinence.[8,15]

Drug use has an intense and overwhelming effect in women's lives. The female hormonal milieu, for example, influences women's drug-seeking and consumption patterns. Studies have shown that progesterone reduces the effects of some drugs (e.g., cocaine).[16] Substances have a greater reinforcing effect when taken before ovulation (follicular phase), a time when estrogen is the dominant hormone and the risk for pregnancy is highest. Consequently, drug intoxication puts women at higher risk for unintended pregnancy, sexually transmitted infections (STIs), and human immunodeficiency virus (HIV) exposure.[17,18]

Among women, substance use disorders are often socially rooted, revolving around intimate partner and family relationships. Besides harm to physical health, women experience a diminished sense of well-being through self-neglect and social isolation; their cultural roles are challenged, especially during pregnancy and in their roles as new mothers.[19,20] Current research is focused on discovering the nuances and differences in neurobehavioral effects of substance use disorders between women and men.[21,22]

Substance use influences women's lives differently across the lifespan. One's developmental stage in life may either encourage or discourage the possibility of substance abuse. Appropriately, much attention is given to prevention of substance abuse in youth and adolescence. For most individuals, initial exposures to drugs are not likely to occur until the middle and late adolescent years through experimentation that does not necessarily lead to addiction.

Substance Use During Pregnancy

The childbearing age range is considered from 15 to 45 years, the same age period when substance use is most prevalent. In national data and focused research, rates of substance abuse in pregnancy range from 4% (self-reported) to 19% (among pregnant women screened by urine toxicology at the time they give birth).[8,23] Women who abuse drugs are at great risk for pregnancy and sexually transmitted infections (STIs), including HIV, because psychoactive drugs tend to reduce inhibitions and interfere with women's decision making.

Poor attention to physical self-care and poor adherence to a contraceptive routine are common among women with substance use disorders.[18,24] Many women with substance use disorders tend to delay pregnancy recognition and avoid entry into prenatal care.[25] They continue to use their drug of choice because addiction overpowers their ability to stop.

Substance abuse increases the risk of harm to the woman, the pregnancy, and the family. Pregnancy outcomes hinge upon the type of substances abused, frequency of use, and gestational age at the time of exposure. A major challenge is that most illicit substances are not standardized in regard to ingredients, purity, or reporting of use. Substance abuse can alter the neurodevelopment of the fetus; however, to date, only alcohol exposure has been formally associated with a fetal or neonatal syndrome. Nevertheless, other drugs can influence fetal development. For example, methamphetamine and cocaine tend to reduce fetal growth, and exposure to anabolic steroids is associated with masculinization of a female fetus and interferes with growth of the long bones.[26]

Substance Use During Breastfeeding

In one study, more than 75% of women who were opioid dependent voiced a desire to breastfeed.[27] Unfortunately, the postpartum period is a vulnerable time when women may succumb to relapse, especially if they have been using the intrauterine fetus as a major reason for abstinence. The pharmacokinetics (e.g., molecular weight, lipid solubility) of the substances being abused determines advisability of establishing and/or continuing breastfeeding.

Substance Use and the Mature Women

Today, 22% of the U.S. population is older than 60 years, with women constituting approximately 55% of the senior cohort.[28] As they age, many women find themselves isolated with diminishing social supports. Notably, older women without such supports are more likely to use prescription medications and alcohol. Lack of treatment for depression also contributes to substance abuse, which can then lead to health consequences caused by over-sedation, injury due to falls, cognitive impairment, and drug interactions.[29]

Called a silent epidemic, alcohol abuse and misuse of prescription medications and over-the-counter (OTC) drugs by persons older than 60 years is a growing public health concern. Substance use disorders among elders are also undertreated.[29] However, women in the 50 to 59 year age group are more likely to seek substance abuse treatment than women in older age cohorts.

While alcohol is the primary substance of abuse among elder men, older women tend to abuse prescription drugs.[29] Categories of prescription drugs frequently abused by the elderly include tranquilizers, antidepressants, analgesics, sedatives, and stimulants. Prescription drug use is associated with a variety of medical conditions, hospital admissions, and psychological comorbidities.[30]

Polypharmacy—whether it involves prescription, OTC, or illicit drugs—raises the chance for drug–drug interactions. Alcohol is often used in conjunction with medications and illicit drugs, increasing the overall risk for harm. Aging metabolism, body composition, and general health status influence pharmacokinetics, such that the effects of the same drugs may differ for younger and older users. To date, there has been little study concerning substance use disorders and treatment effectiveness for older individuals.

Pharmacotherapy of Drugs of Abuse

For the purpose of this chapter, drugs of abuse are categorized as central nervous system (CNS) depressants, stimulants, sedative-hypnotics and anxiolytics, hallucinogens, and other drugs including anabolic steroids and OTC medications. Pharmacologic treatment as a stand-alone option is rarely sufficient to achieve long-term abstinence from alcohol or drugs. Unfortunately, there are no approved pharmacotherapies for most drugs of abuse; evidence-based pharmacotherapies are included in the discussion here when they exist. Medications used to treat substance use disorders are described on the basis of four functions: (1) to treat acute intoxication or overdose; (2) to treat acute withdrawal symptoms; (3) to maintain abstinence; or (4) to prevent relapse to the primary addictive substance. Empirical management for withdrawal and overdose conditions is addressed as well.

Alcohol

Approximately 7% of the U.S. population meets the diagnostic criteria for alcohol abuse or alcoholism.[8] Chronic alcohol use is responsible for liver cirrhosis, malnutrition, and esophageal and alimentary cancers.[31] Women who are heavy drinkers have higher risks for heart disease, liver damage, and physical disability than their male counterparts.[32] They are also at increased risk for anemia, osteoporosis, menstrual disorders, breast cancer, and infertility than non-alcohol users. Excess alcohol intake is associated with eating disorders, panic disorders, depression, and post-traumatic stress disorder.

Although the alcohol content of different drinks varies, the effects of alcohol are related to the amount imbibed and individual susceptibility, as described in Box 9-2. Alcohol is rapidly absorbed from the gastrointestinal tract and cleared from the blood in approximately one hour. Because alcohol has greater solubility in water than in fat, alcohol becomes distributed more quickly to tissues containing water. Women have proportionally more fat and less fluid than men, so when men and women ingest equal amounts of alcohol, women reach higher blood-alcohol concentrations faster.[33] Approximately 20% of alcohol consumed is absorbed from the stomach and 80% from the small intestine. The longer alcohol remains in the stomach, the more slowly it will be absorbed into the bloodstream. This factor explains why drinking and eating appears to have a sobering effect compared to drinking without eating at the same time. A small portion of consumed alcohol is excreted via the kidney, salivation, or exhalation (the basis of Breathalyzer tests), but 98% is metabolized in the liver. Alcohol pathways involve the enzymes alcohol dehydrogenase (DH) and aldehyde dehydrogenase (ALDH), which convert alcohol into acetaldehyde. This process is 60% more active in men—a difference that translates into higher alcohol absorption in women.

Box 9-2 Standard Measure of Alcohol Content

A standard drink is any drink that contains 0.6 ounce (14.0 grams or 1.2 tablespoons) of pure alcohol. This amount of pure alcohol can be found in combination drinks or in the following beverages:

- 12 ounces of beer (5% alcohol content)
- 8 ounces of malt liquor (7% alcohol content)
- 5 ounces of wine (12% alcohol content)
- 1.5 ounces of 80-proof (40% alcohol content) distilled spirits or liquor (e.g., gin, rum, vodka, whiskey)

Source: Reproduced from Alcohol and Public Health. Frequently Asked Questions Centers for Disease Control and Prevention, Division of Population Health, National Center for Chronic Disease Prevention and Health Promotion. http://www.cdc.gov/alcohol/faqs.htm. Accessed December 28, 2014.[35]

The neuropharmacology of alcohol is complex. Alcohol's rewarding effects result from the release of endogenous opioid peptides that activate dopamine. Chronic exposure overstimulates the mesolimbic system and causes neuroadaptations, such that withdrawal of alcohol prompts craving for alcohol.[34]

Treatment of a Woman with Acute Alcohol Intoxication

Treatment of alcohol intoxication is supportive until the effects of intoxication wear off. Fluid replacement, electrolytes, and B-complex vitamins are given to counteract the diuretic effect of alcohol and to protect against Wernicke's encephalopathy, a condition that occurs when the individual is thiamine deficient from chronic alcohol abuse.

Treatment of a Woman with Alcohol Withdrawal Syndrome

Alcohol is a CNS depressant. Abrupt discontinuation of chronic alcohol use sets off compensatory reactions in the sympathetic nervous system, leading to restlessness, irritability, poor concentration, emotional volatility, and elevated heart rate and blood pressure. In more severe withdrawal, hyperthermia, delusions, delirium tremens (DTs; i.e., disorientation, fluctuation of consciousness, and auditory, visual, or tactile hallucinations), and grand mal seizures may be experienced. Alcohol withdrawal is best treated in an inpatient setting that provides both pharmacologic and biopsychosocial therapies. The primary goal of medical treatment for alcohol withdrawal syndromes is to avoid seizures and delirium tremens. Benzodiazepines including diazepam (Valium) and chlordiazepoxide (Librium) are used to treat psychomotor agitation.

Treatment of a Woman with Alcohol Addiction

The objectives for treatment of alcohol addiction focus on treating withdrawal symptoms, maintaining abstinence, preventing relapse, and ensuring social and psychological rehabilitation. Although alcoholism is a chronic disease with high relapse potential, evaluations have found behavioral therapies to be essential in its treatment. Currently, there are three medications approved by the U.S. Food and Drug Administration (FDA) for the medically supervised treatment of alcohol addiction. Table 9-1 lists treatments for women with alcohol addiction.

Disulfiram (Antabuse)

Disulfiram (Antabuse) is an alcohol antagonist that has been available since the 1940s. It helps to maintain alcohol abstinence and prevent relapse. Disulfiram blocks the breakdown of alcohol's primary metabolite, acetaldehyde, causing unpleasant, averse symptoms when alcohol is ingested. The disulfiram–alcohol reaction causes increased heart rate and respiration, facial flushing, nausea, vomiting, and hypotension.[36] This reaction lasts as long as alcohol is being metabolized. Studies have shown that disulfiram reduces the number of days of alcohol use among treatment-adherent persons.[37] Individuals are encouraged to carry a safety card to notify healthcare providers or emergency personnel when they are using disulfiram.

Acamprosate (Campral)

Acamprosate (Campral) has been FDA approved since 2004 for maintaining abstinence in alcohol addiction. This drug decreases the severity of alcohol withdrawal and reduces alcohol intake among those person who relapse into alcohol use. Acamprosate balances glutamate and dopamine release in newly abstinent persons.[38] Anxiety, depression, and sleep disturbances associated with early abstinence are decreased. Use of this drug is recommended before abstinence, or as soon as possible in abstinence, or detoxification.[39]

Table 9-1 Pharmacotherapies for a Woman with Alcohol Addiction

Drug: Generic (Brand)	Formulations	Dose	Clinical Considerations	Side Effects/Adverse Reactions
Acamprosate (Campral)	333-mg delayed-release tablets	666 mg PO 3 times/day	Initiate as soon as possible after alcohol withdrawal. Do not use this drug to treat symptoms of withdrawal. Contraindicated for persons with renal impairment.	Sleep problems, headache, anxiety, depression, and weakness.
Disulfiram (Antabuse)	250- and 500-mg tablets	125–500 mg PO every day	Initiate no sooner than 12 hours after last ingestion of alcohol. Disulfiram reaction can occur up to 2 weeks after discontinuing the medication. Contraindications: cirrhosis, coronary artery disease, psychoses (past or current), renal impairment.	Minor: drowsiness, headache, impotence, headache, rash, acne, fatigue, and a metal or garlic aftertaste. Major: weakness, lack of energy, loss of appetite, nausea, and vomiting.
Naltrexone (ReVia)	50-mg tablets, 380-mg injectable kit	50 mg PO every day or 380 mg extended-release IM one time every 4 weeks	Contraindicated for persons using opioids and persons with liver impairment.	Nausea, headache, dizziness, fatigue, insomnia, anxiety, and nervousness.

The therapeutic effect of acamprosate is modest; it increases the chance of achieving abstinence after detoxification in 15% of individuals for 3 to 12 months after treatment. It increases cumulative duration of abstinence by 11%.[38] European studies indicate that this agent has greater effectiveness in women with anxiety, those with no family history of alcoholism, and women who have an older age at onset of alcoholism.[36,39] Although it is FDA approved, acamprosate is not used extensively in the United States. Taking acamprosate with food lowers its effectiveness, and the drug is contraindicated in persons with renal impairment.

Naltrexone (ReVia)

Naltrexone hydrochloride (ReVia) is a long-acting mu-opioid antagonist approved to reduce alcohol craving and extend time to relapse. This drug prevents a simple lapse from evolving into a relapse and then into heavy drinking behavior.[36,40] By binding to opioid receptors, naltrexone prevents development of the pleasurable effects associated with alcohol and other drugs. When taken orally, naltrexone is quickly absorbed and reaches peak levels within 1 to 2 hours; its effects persist for more than 72 hours.[36] Nausea affects adherence to this medication dosing plan.

Naltrexone is also available as an extended-release injectable (depot) suspension (Vivitrol, Vivitrex) that is administered monthly. The extended-release formulation is associated with less risk than the oral preparation because it does not undergo first-pass metabolism in the liver.[10] Extended-release administration also circumvents problems of adherence.

Although naltrexone can reduce craving, volume of alcohol consumed, and the number of heavy drinking days, it has minimal effects in maintaining abstinence.[40] Women are said to experience lower effectiveness with naltrexone, and a higher response to placebo.[41]

Naltrexone has a general favorable safety profile, but the FDA has issued a black box warning regarding its hepatoxicity. Naltrexone should be used with caution in individuals with acute hepatitis, liver failure, and active liver disease. Using opioids while taking naltrexone can produce life-threatening opioid intoxication and cause respiratory arrest, coma, and circulatory collapse. Health safety cards are recommended to notify healthcare providers of naltrexone use.

Opioids

Opioids are prescription drugs that are the most useful drug class for pain control via analgesia and anesthesia. Unfortunately, they are also one of the most highly abused drug classes.[42,43]

Frequently in the context of a substance use disorder, opioids are referred to as **narcotics**, although the latter term is a legal one (rather than a medical one). This label is codified in statutes associated with the U.S. Drug Enforcement Administration (DEA) and is not commonly used outside of the jurisprudence arena, although it may be heard in the popular media or among consumers.[44]

The body's opioid receptors are distributed throughout the central and peripheral nervous systems. Endogenous opioids (endorphins, enkephalins, and dynorphins) and opioids act in the same way on dopamine-containing neurons in the ventral tegmental area of the mesolimbic reward center. They block GABA's inhibitory receptors, causing even more dopamine to be released, resulting in euphoria. Dopamine floods the synapse; without it, craving then occurs.[45]

Street opioids present special challenges because the strength and purity of these drugs are unknown, making it easier for unintentional overdose to occur. Polypharmacy use combining opioids with alcohol, barbiturates, and other opioids can increase the sedative effects and respiratory depression.

Table 9-2 provides a list of opioids categorized according to schedule of controlled substances. Additional information about these schedules can be found in the chapter *Modern Pharmacology*.

Treatment of a Woman with Opioid Intoxication or Overdose

A person who has overdosed using an opioid may exhibit low blood pressure, slow respirations, pinpoint pupils, depressed sensorium, and coma. Treatment for acute overdose provides basic support of the essential body systems: airway, breathing, and circulation. If the woman is conscious, her stomach contents should be emptied by gastric lavage or initiation of vomiting. Persons who present with pinpoint pupils, slow respirations, and coma are assumed to have overdosed with an opioid. Expectant management consists of naloxone (Narcan) administered in titrated doses every 2 to 3 minutes until the symptoms are reversed.

Treatment of a Woman with Opioid Withdrawal

Withdrawal symptoms depend on the pharmacologic characteristics of the opioid drug involved. For instance, the short half-life of heroin results in more intense withdrawal symptoms compared to opioids with longer

Table 9-2 Opioids Listed by Schedule for Controlled Substances

Substance: Generic (Brand)	Street Name	Route of Administration	Medical Use
Schedule I			
Heroin	Big H, black tar, brown sugar, China white, junk, horse	Inhalation, intravenous, intramuscular	None
Schedule II			
Fentanyl (Duragesic)	China girl, Fat Albert	Oral, intravenous, intramuscular, transdermal	Postsurgical pain relief, management of acute or chronic pain, breakthrough cancer pain
Hydrocodone (Vicodin, Lortab, Lorcet)	Watson 387, vike	Oral	Moderate pain relief
Hydromorphone (Dilaudid)	Drug store heroin	Oral, intravenous, intramuscular, transdermal, suppositories	Postsurgical pain relief, management of acute or chronic pain, breakthrough cancer pain
Meperidine (Demerol)	Demmies	Oral, intravenous, intramuscular	Moderate to severe pain relief
Morphine (MS Contin, Kadian, and Avinza)	Morph, Miss Emma, M	Oral, intravenous, intramuscular, transdermal	Postsurgical pain relief, management of acute or chronic pain, breakthrough cancer pain
Oxycodone (OxyContin)	Hillbilly heroin, cotton	Oral, intravenous, intramuscular, transdermal	Postsurgical pain relief, management of acute or chronic pain, breakthrough cancer pain
Schedule III			
Codeine	Nods, lean, T-3, T-4	Oral	Pain relief, relief of cough and diarrhea

half-lives. Appearing as early as 4 to 6 hours after the last dose and peaking within 72 hours, most withdrawal symptoms subside after 7 to 10 days; however, postacute symptoms may last up to a month. Although healthcare providers suggest that symptoms are similar to the flu, most individuals with substance use disorders would not support that description.

The length of detoxification depends on the type of medication used, the treatment setting, the severity of the addiction, and the motivation of the individual. Typically, withdrawal in an inpatient facility can last for 10 to 14 days. Outpatient detoxification can last 14 to 21 days, and long-term withdrawal (often called tapering) can require up to 180 days. Controversial rapid (3 to 10 days) and ultrarapid (1 to 2 days) detoxification using an opioid antagonist such as naltrexone or naloxone in combination with other supportive medications like clonidine (Catapres) and benzodiazepines has been conducted in recent years. Individuals undergoing an ultrarapid detoxification are placed under anesthesia; the potential for adverse events as a result of ultrarapid detoxification is high, so women must be cautioned regarding all safety risks. Although more research is needed, ultrarapid detoxification does not appear to eliminate the withdrawal syndrome, nor does it sustain long-term abstinence.[46]

In 2001, the FDA transferred federal regulatory oversight of such programs to the Substance Abuse and Mental Health Services Administration (SAMHSA), which has developed an accreditation model for opioid treatment programs to allow providers more flexibility and greater clinical judgment in treating individuals dependent on opioids. The Drug Abuse Treatment Act of 2002 allows programs and physicians not affiliated with a certified opioid treatment clinic to provide services using Schedule III, IV, or V medications.

Drugs Used to Treat Opioid Addiction

The drugs used to treat opioid addiction affect the opioid receptors in various ways. Some interact with opiod receptors directly and others decrease or mitigate symptoms, such as agitation or gastrointestinal disorders.

Methadone (Dolophine)

Methadone (Dolophine), a long-acting, full mu-opioid agonist, is the medication most frequently used to treat opioid withdrawal or maintenance of abstinence. Administered daily, methadone suppresses withdrawal symptoms for 24 to 36 hours and blocks cravings. It does not produce a sensation of euphoria or sedation. Serious side effects of methadone can include respiratory depression, hypotension, sedation, or coma. Caution should be used when medicating a person on methadone who is concurrently using alcohol or taking CNS depressants or other opioid analgesics; the same is true for an individual scheduled for general anesthesia.

Methadone maintenance consists of a daily dose used as a substitute for illegal heroin with no attempt to reduce the dose. Methadone detoxification is intended to reduce the dose in a controlled manner with the ultimate goal of abstinence. Individuals can be maintained on a dose of methadone for any length of time, occasionally involving years.

Buprenorphine (Buprenex, Subutex)

Buprenorphine hydrochloride (Buprenex, Subutex) is a partial mu-opioid agonist. Suboxone, a partial mu-opioid agonist/mu-opioid antagonist, is a brand name for a combination of buprenorphine hydrochloride and naloxone hydrochloride. Buprenorphine is a potent drug that displaces morphine, methadone, and other full agonists. This agent reduces withdrawal symptoms, and unlike other treatment drugs, it has a lower potential for abuse and a reduced incidence of overdose or respiratory depression. Suboxone is the recommended form of maintenance treatment, as the addition of naltrexone prevents the individual from injecting the drug. Individuals are maintained on a daily schedule of sublingual tablets that must be placed under the tongue, allowed to fully dissolve, and not chewed or swallowed whole. These drugs should not be administered to persons who are hypersensitive to buprenorphine, and Suboxone should not be administered to those individuals who are hypersensitive to naloxone.

Clonidine (Catapres, Duraclon)

Clonidine (Catapres, Duraclon) is an antihypertensive medication that is used on an off-label basis to treat symptoms of opioid withdrawal, primarily by suppressing symptoms of restlessness, lacrimation, rhinorrhea, and sweating. Some providers and individuals prefer the use of clonidine instead of traditional medications such as methadone because no special dispensing license is required for this agent. Clonidine does not produce intoxication, and it does not reinforce drug-seeking behaviors. However, individuals with a history of drug abuse must be monitored closely, as clonidine can cause sedation and hypotension. Clonidine has additive drug–drug interactions with digitalis, calcium-channel blockers, and beta blockers that can cause bradycardia and atrioventricular (AV) block.

Naltrexone (ReVia)

Naltrexone (ReVia) is a mu-opioid antagonist that is approved for the treatment of opioid addiction. Naltrexone blocks the effects of heroin and other opioids. It has no positive reinforcing effects; consequently, there has been little acceptance of this drug for initial treatment. Rather, it is most effective for individuals who are already detoxified and want to prevent relapse. Treatment should not begin until the individual is opioid free, because administration of naltrexone can initiate opioid withdrawal syndrome in a person who is using any type of opioid. Contraindications to naltrexone include abuse of any opioids, use of legitimately prescribed opioid analgesics, opioid withdrawal symptoms, and failure of the naloxone challenge test (a screening test to determine the presence of any opioids in the body).[47]

Special Populations

Pregnancy

Approximately 13% of pregnant women report having a few drinks during pregnancy, 3% report binge drinking, and 0.7% report heavy drinking.[8] Prenatal exposure to alcohol is the leading cause of preventable birth defects and developmental disabilities. No amount of alcohol is known to be safe during pregnancy.

The adverse effects of alcohol are dose related or occur by threshold effect. Dose-related effects occur gradually; in contrast, threshold effects do not occur at low doses but do appear if the fetus is exposed to high doses. Since 1973, birth defects and developmental delays have been reported in children of women who were alcoholics themselves.[48] Fetal alcohol spectrum disorder (FASD) encompasses the range of fetal effects caused by maternal alcohol use: fetal alcohol syndrome (FAS), fetal alcohol effects (FAE), and alcohol-related neurodevelopmental disabilities (ARND). The most severe form, FAS, includes the classic craniofacial abnormalities, microcephaly, and delays in both prenatal and postnatal growth and development.[49] Although FAS is seen most often in children born to women who regularly drink large amounts of alcohol, studies suggest that FAS occurs in 0.2 to 2.0 infants per 1000 live births, and FASD occurs at least 4 times more often.

A decision to suddenly stop drinking during pregnancy can result in severe and dangerous withdrawal effects to both the woman and her fetus. To counteract these effects, most programs elect to treat the woman with short-acting barbiturates (e.g., chlordiazepoxide or diazepam). However, because barbiturates are potentially associated with cleft palates, a risk–benefit analysis should be undertaken before use. Other drugs effective in decreasing alcohol intake (i.e., naltrexone and acamprosate) are considered compatible in pregnancy. Although animal studies suggest adverse fetal effects from these agents, corresponding research in pregnant women has not been conducted.[50]

Women who abuse substances, especially depressants, may be ill prepared for the pain of labor. Their inability to cope with the intense stresses of labor heightens their experience of pain.[51] Methadone is not a pain reliever, however, so women who are on methadone should continue to take their regular dose.[52] The amount of analgesia that is needed during labor may be difficult to gauge, as the usual dose may need to be increased in women who abuse depressants. Butorphanol (Stadol) and nalbuphine (Nubain) are analgesics that should not be used during labor by women who are on methadone or who are abusing opioids because these medications are partial opioid antagonists.[52] Additionally, naloxone should not be administered at birth to newborns of opioid-dependent women, because it can cause an acute withdrawal reaction in the newborn.

Lactation

Contrary to some cultural myths, alcoholic beverages tend to inhibit the milk ejection reflex. Thus, alcohol should be consumed judiciously, if at all, by lactating women, especially given that its long-term effects on the nursling are unclear.[53,54]

Studies suggest that the woman who experiences opioid dependency may use methadone and buprenorphine during lactation because the amount of drugs found in breast milk has not been found to negatively influence neonatal abstinence syndrome (NAS).[55] The newborn with NAS presents a clinical challenge in terms of management of the withdrawal, and controversy exists regarding appropriate drug therapy. Although no universal treatment standard exists, the drugs most commonly used for treatment and weaning include methadone and buprenorphine as well as morphine, phenobarbital, and clonidine.

Elderly

The problem of addiction to **licit drugs** and illicit drugs is a growing concern among elderly populations. Among the most commonly abused agents in the category of depressants are alcohol and prescribed opioids.[56]

Stimulants

Stimulants are sympathomimetic drugs, a class with a long history of abuse that rivals the winding road followed by opioid addiction. Coffee, coca leaves, and khat (a plant-derived cathinone) are examples of stimulants that are used daily on a social basis to enhance life for persons around the world. Stimulants elevate mood, enhance physical and mental performance, increase vigilance, boost energy and alertness, and dampen appetite. They also elevate heart rate, blood pressure, cause vasoconstriction, and increase metabolism. As therapies, they are used for treating narcolepsy, producing weight loss, and improving concentration in attention-deficit disorder. Unfortunately, the rapid euphoria produced by stimulants attracts illicit recreational drug use. Stimulants of abuse are notably those with rapid absorption.[57,58] To date, there are no approved treatment medications for stimulant addiction. Table 9-3 lists stimulants in common use.

Nicotine

Nicotine is one of the most widely used legal stimulants and is considered one of the most treacherously addicting drugs. Despite its known health hazards, nearly 27% of the U.S. population are users of tobacco products, of whom 22.1% are cigarette smokers.[8] Nicotine and agents to

Table 9-3 Stimulants Associated with Drug Abuse by Schedule for Controlled Substances

Substance: Generic (Brand)	Street Name	Route of Administration	Medical Use
Schedule I			
MDMA	Adam, clarity, ecstasy, Eve, lover's speed, peace, STP, X, XTC	Oral	None
Schedule II			
Cocaine/crack	Coke, snow, flake, blow, crack, rock	Oral, inhalation, intravenous, intramuscular	Topical anesthetic
Dextroamphetamine (Dexedrine, Adderall)	Speed, upper, bennies, black beauties, dexies, LA turnaround, truck drivers, crosses	Oral	Obesity, narcolepsy, attention-deficit/hyperactivity disorder
Methamphetamine (Desoxyn)	Meth, speed, crystal, glass, ice, crank	Oral, inhalation, intravenous, intramuscular	None
Methylphenidate (Ritalin, Concerta)	JIF, MPH, R-ball, Skippy, smart drug, vitamin R	Oral	Attention-deficit/hyperactivity disorder

facilitate discontinuation of its use are discussed in detail in the chapter *Smoking Cessation*.

Cocaine

Cocaine is made from the leaf of the *Erythryoxylum coca* plant and is often mixed with other substances such as sugar, talcum powder, or cornstarch, and sometimes with other stimulant drugs. Crack is processed with ammonia or baking soda and water, heated, and then smoked. Cocaine effects last from 5 to 30 minutes depending on the route of administration (snorted, smoked, injected, or rubbed onto the gums). This pharmaceutical agent crosses the blood–brain barrier quickly and blocks the reuptake of dopamine, causing dopamine to accumulate in the synaptic cleft, which produces the euphoric effect.

When cocaine or crack is combined with heroin, the mixture is commonly known as a "speedball." This combination produces a "roller-coaster" of sensations in the user, and can lead to opioid overdose. When cocaine and alcohol are used at the same time, the metabolite cocaethylene is produced; this by-product is more toxic to liver cells than either drug used alone.

Amphetamines

Amphetamines are synthetic products that are chemically related to natural catecholamines (epinephrine and norepinephrine). These drugs act directly on the dopamine reward system, causing feelings of energy and exhilaration—effects similar to cocaine but with a prolonged duration. For example, the effects of amphetamine (Dexedrine, Obetrol) last from 2 to 4 hours, and those of methamphetamine (Desoxyn) last from 8 to 12 hours. Both of these products are oral prescription formulations (Schedule II) that are used as anorectics in obesity treatment. Illegally manufactured methamphetamine is inexpensive and available as "crystal" methamphetamine, a very pure form that is commonly snorted, injected, or smoked—like crack—in a glass pipe.

Amphetamines have short-term effects that increase wakefulness and sense of energy, and decrease appetite. Their physical effects include rapid or irregular heartbeat, elevation of core temperature, and hypertension. With chronic use, impulsivity, anxiety, irritability, paranoia, and aggressive or violent behavior are possible. Medical risks include hypertension, stroke, cardiovascular disease, and paranoid psychosis that is difficult to manage.

A combination medication of amphetamine and dextroamphetamine (Adderall) is a Schedule II drug prescribed for the treatment of attention-deficit/hyperactivity disorder (ADHD). Adderall increases the release of norepinephrine and dopamine. The drug is active for four to six hours. Its abuse potential is very high, as this medication is readily accessible and is misused for its value to increase productivity. This agent is also used in conjunction with binge alcohol drinking.[8]

Methylphenidate (Ritalin)

Methylphenidate (Ritalin, Concerta) is a medication indicated for reducing symptoms of ADHD and treating narcolepsy. It increases postsynaptic dopamine release and ultimately inhibits impulsiveness in persons with ADHD. Used orally, it is available in immediate-release and sustained-release formulations. Peak concentrations occur in 1 to 2 hours, and half-life is approximately 2 to 7 hours. When taken as prescribed, methylphenidate produces few serious side effects and can be quite effective. Minor side effects may include insomnia, stomachache, anorexia, and headache. Taken orally, snorted, or injected, methylphenidate is similar to amphetamines in terms of its toxicity and overdose potential.

3,4-Methylenedioxymethamphetamine (MDMA)

3,4-Methylenedioxymethamphetamine (MDMA) is also known as ecstasy. This illicit drug acts as both a stimulant and a psychedelic. It affects the brain by increasing three neurotransmitters—dopamine, norepinephrine, and serotonin—resulting in mood elevation, a sense of alertness, distortions in time, enhanced sensory perceptions, and decreased anxiety. MDMA is often used in combination with other drugs.[38,59] In frequent users, MDMA can cause side effects of anxiety, confusion, and insomnia that can last for days or weeks. Of special concern is the potential for overdose leading to hyperthermia, which can result in major organ failure.

Treatment for Stimulant-Related Substance Use Disorders

Treatment of a Woman with Stimulant Overdose

All stimulants elevate endogenous catecholamine and dopamine levels, resulting in movement disorders and hyperthermia. Acute toxicity can manifest as paranoia, psychosis, and movement disorders. No specific medications have been approved for treating stimulant overdose, but aggressive use of benzodiazepines or chlordiazepoxide (Librium) can provide treatment of psychomotor agitation and convulsions. Rapid cooling of hyperthermia is a critical first step after establishing an airway. Activated charcoal can be used if the agent was ingested orally. Vasodilators such as nitroglycerin are used to lower blood pressure.

Conversely, certain medications are contraindicated for stimulant overdose. Phenothiazines should not be given because they reduce the threshold for seizure activity and can worsen both hyperthermia and tachycardia. Beta blockers should be avoided because they have both alpha- and beta-adrenergic effects that could worsen the hypertension.

Treatment of a Woman with Stimulant Withdrawal

Withdrawal symptoms may begin within 1 to 2 hours after the last dose of a short-acting stimulant such as cocaine and within 14 hours after use of a long-acting stimulant such as methamphetamine. The acute phase of withdrawal is characterized by increased sleepiness, anxiety, dysphoria, inactivity, and craving, lasting from 7 to 10 days. The subacute phase then continues, with symptoms decreasing over approximately 14 to 21 days. Stimulant withdrawal is characterized by intense drug craving of long duration, hypersomnia, fatigue, headache, irritability, poor concentration, restlessness, and anhedonia (i.e., symptoms that manifest like depression). Persons withdrawing from stimulants should be monitored for suicide risk. Even after withdrawal of all such substances, the risk of relapse persists for years after detoxification.

Special Populations

Pregnancy

Cocaine has been associated with several poor outcomes as well as long-term problems such as abnormal neurodevelopment during childhood.[60] Amphetamines have been associated with preeclampsia, placental abruption, preterm birth, and fetal/newborn/infant death.[61] Identification of clear causality between use of these drugs and fetal/newborn effects is difficult to establish, however, especially because cocaine potency cannot be standardized and use of stimulants often is accompanied by use of other agents such as alcohol. The best information regarding cocaine in pregnancy indicates that the drug can be harmful to the developing fetus and child.

Lactation

None of the stimulants are considered safe for use during lactation. Long-term use of cocaine has been associated with lower prolactin levels, suggesting impairment of production of breast milk. Newborns are particularly vulnerable to cocaine and its metabolites, as neonates lack the enzyme that tends to inactivate these compounds.[62] The relationship between use of amphetamines and lactation appears similar to that associated with cocaine, but studies on this topic are scant.[63] In general, nonpharmacologic treatments such as breastfeeding, swaddling, and quiet environments are commonly used for newborns who appear to have neonatal abstinence syndrome or withdrawal from stimulants.

Elderly

Long-term cocaine use has been associated with conditions such as glaucoma and cardiac events—disorders that are more apparent in an older population. Amphetamine abuse is more common among individuals of reproductive age, so few data has been reported specific to this phenomenon in older adults.[56]

Sedatives, Hypnotics, and Anxiolytics

Hundreds of substances have been developed to affect CNS function by inducing sleep, relieving stress, and reducing anxiety. Barbiturates and benzodiazepines dominate the licit and illicit markets as the two major sedative-hypnotic **anxiolytic** classes. Unlike most other abused drug classes, sedative-hypnotics are rarely produced in clandestine laboratories; rather, legitimately manufactured pharmaceuticals are diverted to the illicit market. A notable exception is a relatively recent introduced drug, gamma-hydroxybutyric acid (GHB), which is discussed later in this chapter. This class of drugs is actually a mixed group chemically, yet all are CNS depressants. **Sedatives** decrease CNS arousal and anxiety, whereas **hypnotics** produce drowsiness or sleep.

Barbiturates

Since the early 1900s, barbiturates have been used therapeutically to treat anxiety, seizure disorders, and insomnia. They have a high potential for abuse, as they act by initially causing euphoria, loss of inhibition, and hypnotic effects, and depressing overall brain activity. Physical symptoms include drowsiness, slurred speech, loss of motor coordination, and impaired judgment.[64] Excessive use of barbiturates builds drug tolerance and physical **dependence** on the drug. Cumulative toxic effects can cause life-threatening cardiovascular and respiratory depression.

Barbiturates are grouped in three categories, based on the speed and duration of their effect. Ultra-short-acting barbiturates methohexital (Brevital) and thiopental (Pentothal) are highly lipophilic and produce anesthesia within approximately 1 minute after intravenous administration. Short-acting and intermediate-acting barbiturates are used primarily for insomnia and preoperative sedation, with their onset of action occurring from 15 to 40 minutes after administration and their effects lasting up to 6 hours. The intermediate-acting category is typically preferred by barbiturate abusers; it includes products such as amobarbital (Amytal), pentobarbital (Nembutal), secobarbital (Seconal), and an amobarbital/secobarbital combination (Tuinal). Finally, long-acting barbiturates are less lipophilic and accumulate more slowly in body tissues.

Barbiturates are used primarily for insomnia, anxiety, and seizure disorders; the most popular of these drugs include phenobarbital (Luminal) and mephobarbital (Mebaral). In general, barbiturates produce an unsatisfying sleep because they suppress the rapid eye movement (REM) component of sleep. As a consequence, users tend to wake feeling tired and irritable. Also, due the high risk of mortality in barbiturate overdose, fewer prescriptions of barbiturates have been written for insomnia in recent years. Barbiturates are contraindicated for persons with severe hepatic damage and porphyria. In addition, they should not be used concomitantly with alcohol, tranquilizers, or other CNS depressants.

Benzodiazepines

Of all the drugs that affect CNS functions, benzodiazepines are among those most widely prescribed. Therapeutically, these drugs are prescribed to produce sedation, induce sleep, relieve anxiety and muscle spasm, and prevent seizures. Benzodiazepines have a unique mechanism of action via a high affinity for the GABA-binding site on postsynaptic neurons in the VTA. Potentiating GABA binding results in CNS depression; prolonged use can lead to tolerance and physical dependence even at doses recommended for medical treatment.

The pharmacologic properties of the different benzodiazepines, such as rapidity of onset, half-life, and activity of metabolites, dictate their clinical use and are responsible for their abuse potential. As a rule, benzodiazepines act as sedatives in low doses; such is the case with flurazepam (Dalmane), temazepam (Restoril), midazolam (Versed), and triazolam (Halcion). As anxiolytics, mid-range doses of drugs such as alprazolam (Xanax), chlordiazepoxide (Librium), diazepam (Valium), lorazepam (Ativan), and oxazepam (Serax) are prescribed. Finally, hypnotics, such as clonazepam (Klonopin) and quazepam (Doral), are administered in high doses. Alprazolam and diazepam are the most frequently encountered benzodiazepines on the illicit market.

Flunitrazepam (Rohypnol) is a high-potency, short-acting benzodiazepine that is illegally marketed in the United States. It is known as a "date rape drug." When placed in the drink of an unsuspecting person, it incapacitates the individual and prevents resistance from sexual assault. Flunitrazepam produces anterograde amnesia, a condition in which events occurring while under the influence of the drug are forgotten.

Other Sedative-Hypnotics and Anxiolytics

Other sedative-hypnotics have abuse potential based on their tendency to induce psychological and physiologic dependence, although this risk is notably less remarkable than with benzodiazepines. For example, chloral hydrate has been given orally as a pill or syrup to induce sleep. Chloral hydrate mixed with alcohol is known as a Mickey Finn, a "knockout drink."

Buspirone (BuSpar) is an anxiolytic without sedative effects. It has an affinity for serotonin and D_2 dopamine receptors. Although it is promoted as a nonsedative, healthcare providers have noted increasing doses are required over time to achieve the original anxiolytic effect. In this case, withdrawal is associated with flu-like symptoms, insomnia, lethargy, muscle spasms, and, on occasion, suicidal thoughts; therefore, medical supervision is recommended for drug detoxification.

Treatment for Sedative-, Hypnotic-, and Anxiolytic-Related Conditions

Barbiturate or Benzodiazepine Overdose

Barbiturate toxicity presents as lethargy and somnolence that are accompanied by hypothermia, decreased pupillary light reflex, bradycardia, hypotension, and shock; when severe, it proceeds to coma. Treatment using pressor medications such as norepinephrine is used to correct hypotension. Activated charcoal is administered orally or by gastric lavage to bind and neutralize the offending drug. The use of ipecac syrup is contraindicated due to an increased risk for aspiration from the depressed neurologic responses. Barbiturates and benzodiazepines are excreted by the kidneys, so flushing with dextrose and sodium bicarbonate may be used as well.

Barbiturate or Benzodiazepine Withdrawal

Barbiturates and benzodiazepines require supervised withdrawal to prevent life-threatening events. Withdrawal symptoms begin within 20 hours after last use of short-acting compounds, and within 7 days after last use of long-acting forms. Common withdrawal symptoms include insomnia, irritability, mild tremor and muscle spasm, loss of appetite, sweating, and perceptual distortions. In more severe cases, weakness, vomiting, increased respirations, decreased blood pressure, seizures, and delirium with disorientation and hallucinations can occur. Outpatient detoxification can last as long as 3 to 4 months, during which time the sedatives are titrated at weekly intervals. Medically supervised inpatient withdrawal can last 15 to 30 days. Generally, a long-acting medication is substituted for a short-acting one to suppress withdrawal symptoms for a longer period of time. The rate of withdrawal depends on the severity of the symptoms.

Special Populations

Pregnancy

Barbiturates have not been proven to be teratogenic in pregnancy, although abuse close to the time of birth may result in a lethargic neonate owing to the drugs' long half-life.[65] Safety of benzodiazepines in pregnancy has been controversial: Some studies for both these types of drugs suggest a weak link with teratogenic effects such as cleft palate, whereas other research has failed to find any association.[65] Long-term use of these agents increases the risk associated with withdrawal effects for both the woman and the newborn.

Lactation

The sedative effects of both barbiturates and benzodiazepines suggest that women who are abusing these drugs should be counseled to discontinue them when breastfeeding. Both classes of drugs have long half-lives and metabolites that may contribute to neonatal sedation.[65]

Elderly

Barbiturates and benzodiazepines are among the more uncommon drugs of abuse for the mature woman; conversely, cannabis is among the most common.

Cannabis

Cannabis (also known as marijuana and weed, among many other names) is the most widely used psychoactive drug in the world; it is both an illicit drug and a medicinal drug in the United States. Cannabis does not readily fit within the traditional pharmacologic categories for drugs of abuse; however, it shares characteristics with most of the drug groups.

Historically, cannabis has been termed a gateway drug, although today that label is controversial. The gateway hypothesis is based on a concept that introduction to certain substances (e.g., marijuana, nicotine) promote later adoption of other drugs (e.g., heroin). Some authorities question whether this hypothesis implies an unproven causality, with use of these so-called gateway drugs actually being related to their accessibility and not predicting future drug use. Thus, although marijuana may be called a gateway drug in some resources, it may be more appropriate to avoid this term until a distinct link is made among use of various drugs.[66]

Today, it is generally believed that marijuana is safe for recreational use and that it is a medicinal agent, not a drug of abuse. Organic cannabis and hashish, a compressed resin form, have delta-9-tetrahydrocannabinol (THC) as the primary psychoactive ingredient. Synthetic cannabinoids ("spice" and "K2," dronabinol, and nabilone) are THC analogues that have the phytocannabinoid structure. Both natural and synthetic cannabinoids activate cannabinoid receptors, causing release of dopamine. Physical effects include euphoria, tachycardia, relaxed and enlarged bronchial passages, and redness in the eyes. Users may perceive hunger and thirst, grow cold, and feel sleepy or depressed. Because cannabinoid receptors are located throughout the brain (CB1 in presynaptic CNS) and other body systems (CB2 in peripheral nervous system), regular use is linked to nonspecific neurocognitive changes including short-term memory loss, decreased motor coordination, and in severe cases, psychosis or interpersonal violence.

Women experience more cannabinoid effects as compared to similar intoxication in men. Women recognize a shorter duration of effect, experience more dizziness, have greater spatial memory, slowed gastric emptying, and increased sexual arousal with low doses.[67] Frequent users are also at risk for respiratory cancers because marijuana smoke contains carcinogens—in fact, marijuana has 50% to 70% more carcinogenic hydrocarbons than does tobacco smoke.

Although marijuana is not regulated in terms of its purity or potency, a number of states have passed laws permitting the use of cannabis for medical purposes, such as controlling nausea and vomiting from cancer chemotherapy, stimulating appetite for individuals with acquired immunodeficiency syndrome (AIDS), and treating glaucoma and spasticity. Recreational use has also been legalized in a few states (Box 9-3). The only FDA-approved THC preparation

Box 9-3 Changes in Legal Status for Drugs

In the early twenty-first century, in addition to being recognized in a number of legal jurisdictions as a medicinal agent, cannabis has been approved for sale directly to consumers for private use in several states due to changing social mores. Private use can be for medicinal or recreational purposes.

Movement of a drug from illicit to licit status, or vice versa, is not unusual. Little more than a century ago, alcohol was removed from the legal marketplace when Prohibition was enacted through passage of the 18th Amendment to the U.S. Constitution. Despite this law, illicit alcohol continued to be available through the black market until the 20th Amendment was passed and repealed Prohibition, making alcohol a licit agent again. Laws making cannabis illegal, usually with the term "marijuana" or "marihuana" in the title of the act, have appeared in state statutes since the mid-nineteenth century; they were followed by a national law making cannabis illegal in the 1930s. Thus, the easing of restrictions by states in recent years reflects a change back to policies implemented decades ago.

Both restriction and liberalization of the marketing of agents such as alcohol and cannabis are fraught with potential problems. Prohibition did not cure alcoholism, but neither did repealing it. Proponents of legalizing these agents often argue that discontinuing penalties will increase the number of individuals who seek care, studies determining best practices will be more likely to be conducted, and standardization of purity and potency can be established. Opponents of state legalization of cannabis note that national laws remain in effect that make the agent illegal; in addition, concerns have been expressed about long-term and liberal use of cannabis in everyday life. It can be expected that legalization of cannabis will continue to be a point of discussion for several years to come.

for medical treatment is dronabinol (Marinol), a synthetic cannabinoid. Nonetheless, members of the public may often obtain and use other "street"-procured marijuana. Under controlled conditions, marijuana and dronabinol are found to decrease pain sensitivity, although dronabinol produces analgesia of longer duration.[68] Other clinical studies have confirmed that cannabinoids are effective for treating neuropathic pain but less beneficial in attenuating other types of pain.[69] Because of the anecdotal claim that medical marijuana reduces the opioid doses required for pain relief, it appears that cannabinoids and opioids have synergistic effects.[70] More research is needed regarding effectiveness of organic and synthetic cannabinoids for medical use.

Treatment of a Woman with Cannabis Withdrawal

Research has validated the existence of a cannabis withdrawal syndrome based on the symptoms experienced by nearly half of individuals in treatment.[71,72] Heavy users who experience withdrawal report anxiety, irritability, depressed mood, restlessness, disturbed sleep, and decreased appetite, though these symptoms resolve over a few weeks. No medication is currently approved for treatment of cannabis withdrawal. Successful suppression of withdrawal symptoms is reported with single-dose dronabinol administered daily or in a dose-dependent protocol.[73]

Special Populations

Pregnancy

Concern has been expressed that the potency of today's marijuana is more than 5 times greater than that of most marijuana encountered in the 1970s. Nevertheless, few studies have been conducted to rigorously explore the use of cannabis during pregnancy. Some suggestions of long-term cognitive changes among children exposed to cannabis while in utero have been made, but more research is needed.[74]

Lactation

Few studies have been conducted that have assessed the effects of marijuana among breastfeeding women, although the possibility of impaired judgment while caring for a newborn has been expressed as a concern. When cannabis is smoked, the infant may inhale the drug; thus women should be aware of and minimize these risks by not smoking around the newborn. As yet, no studies have addressed the potential long-term risks of cannabis use during breastfeeding.

Elderly

Medical marijuana is often prescribed for chemotherapy-induced nausea as well as for digestive conditions, chronic pain, and other disorders, and appears to be useful for most adult women with these conditions.[75]

Hallucinogens and Dissociative Anesthetics

Hallucinogens and psychedelics are substances that alter sensory processing in the brain, causing changes of perception, consciousness, and mood with particular distortions associated with thought, time, and space. Using hallucinogens is an ancient practice. The Maya used psilocybin mushrooms centuries ago. Since 1914, members of the Native American Church have formally used peyote and the mescal bean as sacramental plants for enhancing spiritual experiences.[76]

Dissociative anesthetics such as ketamine are characterized by analgesia and amnesia that have minimal effects on respiratory function. The woman appears to be awake with eyes open and ability to swallow, but without the ability to process information. Dissociative anesthesia is used for brief operative procedures or diagnostic procedures. Although abuse of dissociative anesthetics is rare, these medications can cause physical harm when taken illicitly.

Lysergic Acid Diethylamide

Developed in 1938, lysergic acid diethylamide (LSD) is a Schedule I drug. This drug was popular in the 1960s and 1970s.

The chemical structure of LSD—and those of psilocybin and peyote—are similar to that of serotonin. As agonists at the serotonin receptors, these agents disrupt the natural release of serotonin where perceptions are made and interpreted.[5] The individual's control of the behavioral, perceptual, and regulatory systems is then overrun. Hallucinogens and vivid dreaming occur while the individual remains conscious. Psychedelic experiences may be either pleasurable or quite terrifying and unpredictable. Due to its lipophilic nature, LSD can remain in fat stores and then be released back into circulation later, which can cause flashbacks. Physiologic symptoms can include rapid heart rate, increased blood pressure, tremors, dilated pupils, and hyperthermia.

Phencyclidine

Phencyclidine (PCP) is an illicit drug with notable hallucinogenic and dissociative properties. Although PCP's effects on the CNS vary, this agent is considered the most dangerous of the hallucinogens and is banned for human use. It affects numerous neurotransmitters, especially glutamate and dopamine. Low or moderate doses cause alterations in body image, distortions of space and time, feelings of invulnerability, and unpleasant delusions. In high doses, PCP can cause convulsions, coma, and death. Addiction can occur, and chronic users may have memory loss, speech difficulties, and depression persisting for as long as a year after the last use.[77]

Ketamine

A derivative of PCP, ketamine (Schedule III) was originally developed as an anesthetic. It is known for its profound anesthetic, amnestic, and sedative properties. Ketamine is frequently used in surgery for humans and animals. It is used on an off-label basis for treatment of neuropathic and cancer pain. In illicit use, ketamine is a club drug, is used as an antidepressant, and is used in drug-facilitated sexual assault. Its actions are similar to those of PCP, but less potent and of shorter duration. Adverse responses to ketamine include frightening sensory detachment similar to a bad trip on LSD. With high or frequent doses, ketamine can produce analgesia, amnesia, and coma.

Gamma-Hydroxybutyric Acid

Gamma-hydroxybutyric acid (GHB, Xyrem) is an FDA-approved (Schedule III) CNS depressant used for the treatment of cataplexy in narcolepsy. When manufactured illegally (Schedule I), it is sold in liquid form as "swigs." GHB and its analogues emerged in the 1990s as agents with alleged utility as anabolic agents for body building and as sleep aids.[78] GHB is also used to assist sexual assault or "date rape." As a club drug, it is used in conjunction with alcohol at nightclubs and "rave" parties. Overdose frequently requires emergency room care to reverse its severe depressant effects. A significant number of GHB-related fatalities have been reported due to respiratory depression and impaired judgment while operating vehicles.

Treatment for Hallucinogen and Dissociative Anesthetic–Related Conditions

Treatment of Hallucinogen or Dissociative Anesthetic Overdose

The most common adverse response to a large dose of a hallucinogenic agent is a bad experience that can can manifest as a temporary psychotic state. Although some reports of permanent psychosis have been published, it is not clear if these cases were due to the hallucinogen or to an underlying vulnerability. The pharmacologic treatment of choice is benzodiazepines to reduce anxiety. Treatment focuses on the presenting symptoms.

Treatment of Hallucinogen or Dissociative Anesthetic Withdrawal

PCP does not have specific symptoms of withdrawal. However, chronic use is associated with toxic psychosis that can take days or weeks to resolve. LSD and ecstasy do not produce physical dependence, although LSD may induce a hallucinogen-persisting perception disorder (HPPD), which includes flashbacks and persistent psychosis similar to those experienced following use of PCP. There are no specific pharmacologic treatments for PCP or LSD withdrawal.

Reports of GHB withdrawal symptoms are not common, because GHB has rapid absorption and elimination from the body. Onset of GHB effects begins within 10 to 15 minutes of ingestion, with peak levels occurring at 45 minutes. Withdrawal is characterized by anxiety, insomnia, and tremor; in severe cases, the syndrome can progress to severe delirium. Medications used to manage symptoms during withdrawal include diazepam (Valium), haloperidol (Haldol), and lorazepam (Ativan).

Special Populations

Pregnancy and Lactation

Hallucinogens have long been proposed as agents that can cause intrauterine chromosomal damage. However, research on this topic is scant, and most of these illicit drugs are adulterated with other agents, confounding any findings from studies. Nevertheless, little information suggests that hallucinogens are teratogenic, although they can result in impairment of the woman, thereby putting both her and her offspring in potential danger.[73]

Elderly

Few data exist regarding the use of hallucinogens among mature women. Wu et al. have reported that these agents are among the least used of illicit substances among older adults.[56]

Anabolic–Androgenic Steroids

Anabolic–androgenic steroids (AAS) were developed from the family of hormones that include testosterone and its related derivatives.[78,79] Although there has been an overall decline in the use of AAS since 2000, a recent, more drastic reduction is associated with media coverage of professional athletes who have abused "performance-enhancing drugs." These agents are classified as Schedule II drugs, and their therapeutic uses in women include the treatment of libido disorders and cachexia due to chronic disease such as HIV infection.

Use of anabolic–androgenic steroids is very infrequent among women. Certain groups of women (e.g., athletes, body builders, and some women with body dysmorphia) use anabolic–androgenic steroids to increase muscle size, reduce body fat, and improve body appearance.[26,80] In a small study, the initial onset of use by women occurred in early adulthood and was associated with lower doses than those used by men.[52] When combined with exercise, use of other performance-enhancing drugs, and a high-protein diet, anabolic steroids increase the size and strength of muscles, improve endurance, and decrease recovery time between workouts. Some steroids are taken orally, others are injected intramuscularly, and still others are creams or gels that are applied to the skin. More than 50% of users develop psychological dependence on anabolic–androgenic steroids.[81]

In women, anabolic–androgenic steroids have masculinizing effects, including acne, male-pattern hair growth on the face and body, development of angular facial features, voice changes, clitoral enlargement, and disrupted menstrual cycles.[26] Negative physical effects from use include alterations in serum lipids that can result in elevated blood pressure, thrombotic events, and cardiovascular disease. In addition, anabolic–androgenic steroids increases the risk for liver dysfunction and emotional liability that can lead to serious psychosis. Some of these effects are irreversible.

Treatment of a Woman with Steroid Withdrawal

Little research has been conducted on steroid withdrawal. Withdrawal symptoms include mood swings, reduced sex drive, fatigue, depression, restlessness, insomnia, aggression, headaches, and loss of appetite. Antidepressants can be utilized to combat depression, and analgesics can be used for body aches. Treatment includes education, psychological counseling, and ongoing medical surveillance.[81]

Special Populations

As noted, anabolic steroids are not a common drug of abuse among women regardless of age. The disruption of menses associated with anabolic–androgenic steroids use is likely to impair fertility. When they are taken during pregnancy, there is some evidence of masculinization of female fetuses and long bone impairment.[26] More research is needed in this area.

Inhalants

Inhalants are gases, solvents, or propellants whose vapors can produce a rapid euphoria when inhaled. These illicit substances are often used by young children and adolescents, with young teens from seventh to ninth grades being at greatest risk.[82] Older teens are known to initiate use of nitrous oxide "whippets."[13] Commercial solvents are inexpensive and easily accessible; they contain toxic ingredients including toluene, butane, heptane, hexane, benzene, and others. Many abused inhalants are everyday products—for instance, model airplane glue, paint thinners, degreasers, acrylic paints, gasoline, hair sprays, nail polish remover, shoe polish, butane lighters, nitrous oxide, video head cleaners, and whipped cream. In addition, amyl nitrate, a medication to treat angina, may be inhaled for sexual enhancement.

Substances can be sniffed or inhaled directly by bagging, huffing, or spraying. The response to inhalation is similar to CNS depressant effects, followed by dizziness, uncoordinated movement, and slurred speech. Intoxication lasts 5 to 15 minutes. With excessive inhalations, individuals may exhibit confusion, delirium, nausea, vomiting, and tremors. Long-term effects can include weight loss, irritability, and depression. In very severe situations, organ damage involving the liver, kidney, and brain is possible. Sudden sniffing death syndrome accounts for 50% of inhalant-related deaths, with 22% of these deaths occurring among first-time sniffers.[83]

Special Populations

Pregnancy and Lactation

Inhalants have a number of toxins that can be particularly harmful to a fetus or child. Some seemingly innocuous agents can be metabolized into ethanol, steroids, or other agents. Thus, inhalants are potentially problematic for the pregnant woman. In some cases, the newborn exposed to such agents may exhibit fetal solvent syndrome, a cluster of characteristics similar to fetal alcohol syndrome.[83] However, more data are needed to understand use of these agents during pregnancy and breastfeeding.

Elderly

Inhalants are not commonly abused by older women. Therefore, few data exist regarding use of these agents among mature adults of either gender.

Over-the-Counter Medication Abuse and Misuse

Self-administration of nonprescription medications offers the public both choices and opportunities for involvement in their own health care. As a result, and reflecting their publicly sanctioned sale, members of the public may believe all OTC drugs are safe.[50] In reality, as more pharmaceutical deregulation occurs, greater varieties of medications are becoming available, some of which are vulnerable to misuse or abuse. The categories of decongestants, antitussives, analgesics, antihistamines, and laxatives are most apt to be abused as reported by pharmacists, emergency department admissions, and national survey data.[84] Harm related to OTC misuse is primarily due to physiologic symptoms (e.g., tachycardia, hypertension, gastrointestinal irritation, and rebound symptoms).[84] Numerous studies have made an association between OTC medication abuse and use of illicit substances.[85]

Dextromethorphan

Dextromethorphan (Benylin, Delsym) is a dissociative agent that has been used for years as a cough suppressant. When taken in the designated dose, dextromethorphan is safe and effective. It is metabolized by cytochrome CYP2D6, a polymorphic enzyme that is present in approximately 85% of the population. Like ketamine and PCP, dextromethorphan's metabolite, dextrorphan, causes intense euphoria and "out of body" sensations.[86] The FDA has issued a warning about increased abuse of dextromethorphan, as overdoses of this agent are associated with cardiac arrhythmias, seizures, respiratory depression, and brain injury.

Special Populations

Pregnancy and Lactation

Dextromethorphan has not been found to be a major teratogen, although a few studies have suggested it has a weak association with some anomalies (no specific types have been identified). There is no evidence of untoward effects on the woman or the newborn during breastfeeding, although some cough remedies containing dextromethorphan may also have alcohol as an ingredient.[73]

Elderly

Abuse of dextromethorphan is not limited to adolescents. Middle-aged and older women also can experience what is termed "cough syrup psychosis" in a similar manner to younger women. One case study reported a woman who attempted suicide as well as tried to kill a relative. She survived and disclosed her ingestion of large amounts of dextromethorphan upon admission to a psychiatric unit.[87]

Future Pharmacotherapies for Substance Use Disorders

Drug actions within the brain can produce rewarding effects, craving responses, withdrawal reactions, and neuroadaptations. These neuropharmacologic actions have influenced our understanding of addiction, and they continue to guide researchers in the development of agents for treating such conditions.[5] Clinical trials for developing pharmacotherapies geared toward addiction are precise and complicated processes. Although many medications have demonstrated promise for treating some drugs of abuse, no highly efficacious agents have been approved for marketing in the United States in recent years. A few FDA-approved medications for nonrelated conditions have been identified as prospective treatments for alcohol and other drug addiction. For example, topiramate (Topamax) is an anticonvulsant for the treatment of epilepsy that interferes with alcohol reward, so it decreases the desire to drink. Varenicline (Chantix), a treatment for nicotine addiction, and ibudilast, a drug used in Japan for asthma treatment, are being evaluated as possible treatments for methamphetamine addiction.[88] Work continues on many fronts to find efficacious pharmacotherapies. Other supportive research has been reasonably successful, such as development of an implantable sustained-release delivery system for naltrexone intended to decrease alcohol craving or sustain abstinence for opioids.[89]

Conclusion

Substance use disorders are debilitating and foster a progressively adverse quality of life for individuals who live under their influence. Addiction is considered both a chronic and a relapsing disorder. It is characterized by compulsions to obtain and use alcohol or other drugs, loss of control in limiting their use, and negative body responses when drug intake is stopped.

Worldwide attention is focused on ways to impede addiction and to improve the lives of those who are harmed by it, although conflicting philosophies persist regarding the treatment of substance use disorder. Many providers believe that drug addiction should be treated by abstinence alone, whereas others support pharmacotherapy as an adjunct therapy. Still others suggest that all treatment for substance use disorder is ineffective. It is important for providers to evaluate, and then support, every possible means of effective and equitable treatment for all persons with substance use disorders. The best outcomes result from the combination of evidence-based counseling approaches with new pharmacotherapies that target neurologic mechanisms of the brain's reward system. However, further research is needed to expand the arsenal of medications used to treat substance use disorders and to promote greater effectiveness with application of traditional and new psychotherapeutic modalities.

Resources

Organization	Description	Website
National Institute on Alcohol Abuse and Alcoholism (NIAAA)	This site is the federal corollary to NIDA. Many of the programs and initiatives found at the site relate to alcohol use among young adults, a population that often mixes drugs with alcohol	www.niaaa.nih.gov/
National Institute on Drug Abuse (NIDA)	This site is the federal corollary to NIAAA. A wide variety of drugs that are abused, strategies for individuals to discontinue such use, and downloadable charts of agents can be found on this site	www.drugabuse.gov/
Centers for Disease Control and Prevention: Alcohol and Public Health	Single site with statistics from multiple sources about use of alcohol in the United States	www.cdc.gov/alcohol/onlinetools.htm
Drug Enforcement Administration: Drugs of Abuse	PDF article summarizes knowledge regarding agents that the federal government characterizes as drugs of abuse	www.dea.gov/docs/drugs_of_abuse_2011.pdf
Office of National Drug Control Policy	White House website specific to drug control policies and strategies of the federal executive branch	www.whitehouse.gov/ondcp

Consumer Self-Help Apps and Literature		
Multiple apps exist for consumers to track cravings and use of drugs. In addition, many provide motivational statements or advice to promote abstinence. Many apps are free or available for a modest fee. No single one has been found to be superior to others. It is likely that an individual woman may use several different apps based on her personal desires.		
Alcoholics Anonymous Big Book	Apps exist for iPhone and Android devices that include the "Big Book" with guidance for members of AA, as well as outlines of the 12-step program	www.aa.org
Narcotics Anonymous	Multiple products, including literature about how to initiate programs, purchase medallions to signify periods of abstinence, and obtain posters or educational materials	www.na.org

References

1. American Psychiatric Association. *Diagnostic and Statistical Manual of Mental Disorders.* Arlington, VA: American Psychatric Publishing; 2013.
2. Brown SA, McGue M, Maggs J, et al. A developmental perspective on alcohol and youths 16 to 20 years of age. *Pediatrics.* 2008;124(suppl 4):S290-S310.
3. Drapalski A, Bennett M, Bellack A. Gender differences in substance use, consequences, motivation to change, and treatment seeking in people with serious mental illness. *Substance Use Misuse.* 2011;46(6): 808-818.
4. Hanson GR, Venturelli PJ, Fleckenstein AE. *Drugs and Society.* 11th ed. Burlington, MA: Jones & Bartlett Learning; 2011.
5. Bear MF, Connors BW, Paradiso MA. *Neuroscience: Exploring the Brain.* 4th ed. Philadelphia, PA: Lippincott Williams & Wilkins; 2015.
6. Spanagel R, Heilig M. Addiction and its brain science. *Addiction.* 2005;100(12):1813-1822.
7. Gardner EL. Addiction and brain reward and anti-reward pathways. *Adv Psychosomatic Med.* 2011; 30:22-60.
8. Substance Abuse and Mental Health Services Administration. *Results from the 2012 National Survey on Drug Use and Health: Summary of National Findings.* Rockville, MD: Department of Health and Human Services; 2013.
9. Madras BK, Compton WM, Avula D, Stegbauer T, Stein JB, Clark HW. Screening, brief interventions, referral to treatment (SBIRT) for illicit drug and alcohol use at multiple healthcare sites: comparison at intake and 6 months later. *Drug Alcohol Depend.* 2009;99:280-295.
10. Substance Abuse and Mental Health Services Administration. *Treatment Improvement Protocols, No. 49.* Rockville, MD: Substance Abuse and Mental Health Service Administration; 2009.
11. Claus RE, Orwin RG, Kissin WB, Krupski A, Campbell K, Stark K. Does gender-specific substance abuse treatment for women promote continuity of care? *J Substance Abuse Treat.* 2007;32(1):27-39.
12. Grella C. *Substance abuse treatment services for women: a review of policy initiatives and recent research.* Los Angeles: UCLA Integrated Substance Abuse Programs; 2007.
13. Johnston LD, O'Malley PM, Miech RA, Bachman JG, Schulenberg JE. *Monitoring the future: national results on drug use. 1975–2013. Overview: key findings on adolescent drug use.* Ann Arbor, MI: Institute for Social Research, University of Michigan; 2014.
14. Bryant J, Treloar C. The gendered context of initiation to injecting drug use: evidence for women as active initiates. *Drug Alcohol Rev.* 2007;26:287-293.
15. Sartor CE, Lynskey MT, Heath AC, Jacob T, True W. The role of childhood risk factors in initiation of alcohol use and progression to alcohol dependence. *Addiction.* 2007;102(2):216-225.
16. Evans SM. The role of estradiol and progesterone in moduating the subjective effects of stimulants in humans. *Experim Clin Psychopharmacol.* 2007; 15(5):418-426.
17. Semple SJ, Strathdee SA, Zians J, Patterson TL. Life events and sexual risk among HIV-negative, heterosexual, methamphetamine users. *J Sex Res.* 2010;47(4):355-363.
18. Baskin-Sommers A, Sommer I. The co-occurrence of substance use and high-risk behaviors. *J Adolesc Health.* 2005;38:609-611.
19. Daley M, Shepard DS, Bury-Maynard D. Changes in quality of life for pregnant women in substance user treatment: developing a quality of life index for the addictions. *Substance Use Misuse.* 2005;40(3):375-394.
20. Arevalo S, Prado G, Amaro H. Spirituality, sense of coherence, and coping responses in women receiving treatment for alcohol and drug addiction. *Eval Program Plan.* 2008;31:113-123.
21. Lukas SE, Wetherington CL. Sex- and gender-related differences in the neurobiology of drug abuse. *Clin Neurosci Res.* 2005;5(2-4):75-87.

22. Bobzean S, DeNobrega AK, Perrotti LI. Sex differences in the neurobiology of drug addiction. *Experim Neurol.* 2014.
23. Azadi A, Dildy GA III. Universal screening for substance abuse at the time of parturition. *Am J Obstet Gynecol.* 2008;198(5):e30-e32.
24. Lee E, Maneno MK, Smith L, et al. National patterns of medication use during pregnancy. *Pharmacoepidemiol Drug Safety.* 2006;15(8):537-545.
25. Ayoola AB, Nettleman MD, Stommel M, Canady RB. Time of pregnancy recognition and prenatal care use: a population-based study in the United States. *Birth.* 2010;37(1):37-43.
26. American College of Obstetricians and Gynecologists. Performance enhancing anabolic steroid abuse in women. *Obstet Gynecol.* 2011;117(4):1016-1018.
27. O'Connor AB, Collett A, Alto WA, O'Brien LM. Breastfeeding rates and the relationship between breastfeeding and neonatal abstinence syndrome in women maintained on buprenorphine during pregnancy. *J Midwifery Womens Health.* 2013;58(4):383-388.
28. Vincent GK, Velkoff VA. *The next four decades: the older population in the United States: 2010–2050 population estimates and projections.* Washington, DC: Administration on Aging, Department of Commerce, U.S. Census Bureau; 2010.
29. Simoni-Wastila, Strickler G. Risk factors associated with problem use of prescription drugs. *Am J Public Health.* 2004;94(2):266-268.
30. Wang Y-P, Andrade LH. Epidemiology of alcohol and drug use in the elderly. *Curr Opin Psychiat.* 2013;26:343-348.
31. Centers for Disease Prevention and Control. Fact sheets: alcohol use and health. *Alcohol Public Health.* 2014. http://www.cdc.gov/alcohol/fact-sheet/alcohol-use. Accessed April 10, 2014.
32. Centers for Disease Prevention and Control. *Alcohol and Public Health Fact Sheets: Excessive Alcohol Use and Risks to Women's Health.* Atlanta, GA: Centers for Disease Control and Prevention; 2014.
33. National Institute on Alcohol Abuse and Alcoholism. Are women more vulnerable to alcohol's effects? *Alcohol Alert.* 1999;46. http://pubs.niaaa.nih.gov/publications/aa46.htm.
34. Koob GF. Neurobiological mechanisms of drug addiction: an introduction. In: Miller PM, ed. *Biological Research on Addiction.* Vol. 2. Salt Lake City, UT: Academic Press; 2013:1-3.
35. Alcohol and Public Health. Frequently Asked Questions Centers for Disease Control and Prevention, Division of Population Health, National Center for Chronic Disease Prevention and Health Promotion. http://www.cdc.gov/alcohol/faqs.htm. Accessed December 28, 2014.
36. Franck J, Jayaram-Lindstrom N. Pharmacotherapy for alcohol dependence: status of current treatments. *Curr Opin Neurobiol.* 2013;23:692-699.
37. Jorgensen C, Pedersen B, Tonnesen H. The efficacy of disulfiram for the treatment of alcohol use disorder. *Alcoholism Clin Experim Res.* 2011;35(10): 1749-1758.
38. Witkiewitz K, Saville K, Hamreus K. Acamprosate for treatment of alcohol dependence: mechanisms, efficacy, and clinical utility. *Therap Clin Risk Manage.* 2014;8:45-53.
39. Kalk NJ, Lingford-Hughes AR. The clinical pharmacology of acamprosate. *Br J Clin Pharmacol.* 2014; 77(2):315-323.
40. Garbutt JC. Efficacy and tolerability of naltrexone in the management of alcohol dependence. *Curr Pharm Des.* 2010;16:2091-2097.
41. Johnson B. Update on neuropharmacolgical treatments for alcoholism: scientific bais and clinical findings. *Biochem Pharmacol.* 2008;75(1):34-56.
42. Centers for Disease Control and Prevention. Web-based Injury Statistics Query and Reporting System (WISQARS). 2014. http://www.cdc.gov/injury/wisqars/fatal.html. Accessed December 28, 2014.
43. Centers for Disease Control and Prevention. National Vital Statistics System mortality data for 2012. http://www.cdc.gov/nchs/deaths.htm. Accessed December 28, 2014.
44. United States Department of Justice, Drug Enforcement Administration. Title 21 Code of Federal Regulations Part 1300 Definitions. http://www.deadiversion.usdoj.gov/21cfr/cfr/1300/1300_01.htm. Accessed December 9, 2014.
45. Nagi K, Pineyro G. Regulation of opioid receptor signalling: implications for the development of analgesic tolerance. *Mol Brain.* 2011:4.
46. Favrat B, Zimmerman G, Zullino D, et al. Opioid antagonist detoxification under anesthesia versus traditional clonidine detoxification combined with an additional week of psychosocial support: a randomized clinical trial. *Drug Alcohol Depend.* 2006;81: 109-116.
47. Jones ES, O'Connor PG. Diagnosis and pharmacologic management of opioid dependency. *Hosp Phys.* 2007;43:1015-1024.

48. Bowen SE. Two serious and challenging medical complications associated with volatile substance misuse: sudden sniffing death and fetal solvent syndrome. *Substance Use Misuse.* 2011;46:68-72.
49. Calhoun F, Warren K. Fetal alcohol syndrome: historical perspectives. *Neurosci Biobehav Rev.* 2007;31:1680171.
50. Substance Abuse and Mental Health Services Administration. *NSDUH Report: Misuse of Over-the-Counter Cough and Cold Medications Among Persons Aged 12 to 24.* Rockville, MD: Substance Abuse and Mental Health Services Administration; 2008.
51. Jones HE, Martin PR, Heil SH, et al. Treatment of opioid-dependent pregnant women: clinical and research issues. *J Substance Abuse Treat.* 2008; 35(3): 245-259.
52. Goff M, O'Connor M. Perinatal care of women maintained on methadone. *J Midwifery Womens Health.* 2007;52:236.
53. Haastrup MB, Pottegård A, Damkier P. Alcohol and breastfeeding. *Basic Clin Pharmacol Toxicol.* 2014; 114(2):168-173.
54. Schneider C, Thierauf A, Kempf J, Auwärter V. Ethanol concentration in breastmilk after the consumption of non-alcoholic beer. *Breastfeed Med.* 2013;8(3):291-293.
55. Gopman S. Prenatal and postpartum care of women with substance use disorders. *Obstet Gynecol Clin North Am.* 2014;41(2):213-228.
56. Wu LT, Blazer DG. Illicit and nonmedical drug use among older adults: a review. *J Aging Health.* 2011;23(3):481-504.
57. Wood S, Sage JR, Shuman T, Anagnostaras SG. Psychostimulants and cognition: a continuum of behavioral and cognitive activation. *Pharmacol Rev.* 2013;66:193-221.
58. Volkow ND. Stimulant medications: how to minimize their reinforcing effects? *Am J Psychiatry.* 2006; 163(3):359-361.
59. Maxwell JC. Psychoactive substances—some new, some old: a scan of the situation in the U.S. *Drug Alcohol Depend.* 2014;134:71-77.
60. Cressman AM, Natekar A, Kim E, Koren G, Bozzo P. Cocaine abuse during pregnancy. *J Obstet Gynaecol Can.* 2014;36(7):628-631.
61. Gorman MC, Orme KS, Nguyen NT, Kent EJ III, Caughey AB. Outcomes in pregnancies complicated by methamphetamine use. *Am J Obstet Gynecol.* 2014; 211(4):429,e1-e7.
62. Lactmed: A Toxnet Database. Drugs and lactation: cocaine.http://toxnet.nlm.nih.gov/cgi-bin/sis/search2/f?./temp/~zB8xZg:1. Accessed December 28, 2014.
63. Lactmed: A Toxnet Database. Drugs and lactation: amphetamines. http://toxnet.nlm.nih.gov/cgi-bin/sis/search2/f?./temp/~ZGq48u:1. Accessed December 28, 2014.
64. Katzung BG. Sedative-hypnotic drugs. In: Katzung BG, ed. *Basic and Clinical Pharmacology.* 13th ed. New York: McGraw-Hill; 2014:369-384.
65. Briggs G, Freeman R. *Drugs in Pregnancy and Lactation.* 10th ed. Philadelphia, PA: Lippincott Williams & Wilkins; 2014.
66. Vanyukov MM, Tarter RE, Kirillova GP, et al. Common liability to addiction and "gateway hypothesis": theoretical, empirical, and evolutionary perspective. *Drug Alcohol Depend.* 2012;123(suppl 1):S3-S17.
67. Craft RM, Marusich JA, Wiley JL. Sex differences in cannabinoid pharmacology: a reflection of differences in the endocannabinoid system. *Life Sci.* 2013;92(8-9):476-481.
68. Cooper Z, Comer SD, Haney M. Comparison of analgesic effects of dronabinol and smoked marijuana in daily marijuana smokers. *Neuropsychopharmacology.* 2013;38:1984-1992.
69. Kraft B, Frickey NA, Kaufmann RM, et al. Lack of analgesia by oral standardized cannabis extract on acute inflammatory pain and hyperalgesia in volunteers. *Anesthesiology.* 2008;109:101-110.
70. Ware MA. Clearing the smoke around medical marijuana. *Clin Pharmacol Therap.* 2011;90(6):769-771.
71. Budney AJ, Hughes JR. The cannabis withdrawal syndrome. *Curr Opin Psychiat.* 2006;19:233-238.
72. Levin KH, Copersino ML, Heishman SJ, et al. Cannabis withdrawal symptoms in non-treatment-seeking adult cannabis smokers. *Drug Alcohol Depend.* 2010;111:120-127.
73. Weinstein AM, Gorelick DA. Pharmacological treatment of cannabis dependence. *Curr Pharm Des.* 2011;17(14):1351-1358.
74. Warner TD, Roussos-Ross D, Behnke M. It's not your mother's marijuana: effects on maternal–fetal health and the developing child. *Clin Perinatol.* 2014;41(4):877-894.
75. Borgelt LM, Franson KL, Nussbaum AM, Wang GS. The pharmacologic and clinical effects of medical cannabis. *Pharmacotherapy.* 2013;33(2):195-209.
76. Gillespie NA, Neale MC, Prescott CA, Aggen SH, Kendler KS. Factor and item-response analysis

DSM-IV criteria for abuse of and dependence on cannabis, cocaine, hallucinogens, sedatives, stimulants and opioids. *Addiction.* 2007;102(6):920-930.

77. Gutierrez KJ. *Pharmacotherapeutics: Clinical Reasoning in Primary Care.* 2nd ed. Philadelphia, PA: W. B. Saunders; 2007.
78. Kanayama G, Hudson JI, Pope H. Illicit anabolic-androgenic steroid use. *Horm Behav.* 2010;58(1):111-121.
79. Drug Enforcement Administration. *Drugs of Abuse, 2011 Edition: A DEA Resource Guide.* Washington, DC: U.S. Department of Justice, Drug Enforcement Administration; 2011.
80. Ip EJ, Barnett MJ, Tenerowicz MJ, Kim JA, Wei H, Perry PJ. Women and anabolic steroids: an analysis of a dozen users. *Clin J Sport Med.* 2010;20(6):475-481.
81. Substance Abuse and Mental Health Services Administration. *Anabolic Steroids.* Vol. 5. Columbia, MD: Substance Abuse and Mental Health Services Administration; 2006.
82. Ahern NR, Falsafi N. Inhalant abuse: youth at risk. *J Psychosoc Nurs Ment Health Serv.* 2013;51(8):19-24.
83. Bowen SE. Two serious and challenging medical complications associated with volatile substance misuse: sudden sniffing death and fetal solvent syndrome. *Substance Use Misuse.* 2011;46:68-72.
84. Cooper RJ. Over-the-counter medicine abuse—a review of the literature. *J Substance Abuse.* 2013;18(2):82-107.
85. Reay G. *Physical dependence and addiction to prescription and over-the-counter medication. Report on an inquiry carried out by the All-Party Parliamentary Drugs Misuse Group, in the 2007-2008 Parliamentary session* [online]. 2009. http://www.drugscope.org.uk/Resources/Drugscope/Documents/PDF/Appgotcreport.pdf. Accessed March 8, 2015.
86. Burns JM, Boyer EW. Antitussives and substance abuse. *Subst Abuse Rehab.* 2013;4:75-82.
87. Modi D, Bhalavat R, Patterson JC II. Suicidal and homicidal behaviors related to dextromethorphan abuse in a middle-aged woman. *J Addict Med.* 2013;7(2):143-144.
88. Ray LA, Roche DJ, Heinzerling K, Shoptaw S. Opportunities for the development of neuroimmune therapies in addiction. *Int Rev Neurobiol.* 2014;118:381-401.
89. Goonoo N, Bhaw-Luximon A, Ujoodha R, Jhugroo A. Naltrexone: a review of existing sustained drug delivery systems and emerging nano-based systems. *J Controlled Release.* March 24, 2014:1-14.

© Sofimanning/Shutterstock

10 Complementary and Alternative Therapies

Wendell L. Combest, Austin J. Combest, Juliana van Olphen Fehr

Chapter Glossary

Botanical medicine Medicine that is derived from plant sources. Also known as phytotherapy.

Complementary and alternative medicine (CAM) Group of diverse medical and healthcare systems practices and products that are not presently considered to be part of conventional medicine.

Dietary supplements Products intended to supplement the diet that is not represented for use as a conventional food. They are not regulated by the FDA.

Homeopathy Type of alternative treatment or alternative medicine whose main tenet is that a person with a disease or condition can be treated by minute amounts of substances that in larger doses can cause the condition or symptoms of the condition.

Integrative medicine Use of traditional biomedical techniques and complementary and alternative medicine in a way that addresses the needs of the whole person.

Phytoestrogens Plant-derived agents that are nonsteroidal compounds that bind to estrogen receptors.

Phytotherapy Medicine that is derived from any part of a plant, including the root, leaves, fruit, flowers, or other parts of a plant. Also known as botanical medicine.

Probiotics Live organisms that, when administered in adequate amounts, confer health benefits to the host.

United States Pharmacopeia (USP) Nongovernmental, not-for-profit public health organization that serves as an official standards-setting authority for all prescription and over-the-counter medicines, including dietary supplements sold in the United States.

USP Verified Dietary Supplement Mark Label awarded to dietary supplements that have been approved by the United States Pharmacopeia.

Introduction

Complementary and alternative medicine (CAM) Is defined by the National Center for Complementary and Alternative Medicine (NCCAM) as "a group of diverse medical and healthcare systems practices and products that are not presently considered to be part of conventional medicine." Another widely used definition of CAM states that CAM is "a group of therapies not typically taught at U.S. medical schools or other schools of allied health or widely available at U.S. hospitals."[1] The National Health Interview Survey regularly queries about CAM use and has found approximately 38% of the adults use some CAM therapies.[2] CAM users are more likely to be women younger than 65 years.

The various CAM treatment modalities have been organized by NCCAM into four general domains, and a fifth called whole medical systems that combines aspects of the other four domains. The four domains are (1) mind-body medicine (e.g., meditation, prayer, art, music, dance therapies); (2) biologically based practices (e.g., herbal medicine, vitamins); (3) manipulative and body-based practices (e.g., chiropractic, osteopathic manipulation, massage); and (4) energy medicine involving energy fields (e.g., qi gong, Reiki, therapeutic touch) and bioelectromagnetic-based therapies (e.g., sound, magnet, and light therapies). The whole medical systems domain includes complete systems of practice and theory, such as the Western practices of **homeopathy** and non-Western systems such as traditional Chinese medicine (TCM) and Indian traditional medicine, called Ayurveda.

This chapter reviews botanical therapies used by women in the United States today, a field also referred to as **botanical medicine** or **phytotherapy**. The term "herbal" refers to the herbaceous parts of a plant, such as leaves and stems. The term "botanical" refers to foods or supplements that are derived from any part of the plant, including fruits, roots, and flowers. This chapter reviews the efficacy of specific botanical medicines where it is known and discusses the extent of knowledge about specific herbs that, to date, have not been proven to be efficacious. Other chapters mention specific CAM therapies as well.

History of Complementary and Alternative Medicine

Many of the therapies included under the mantle of CAM have been prominent components of healthcare systems in other countries, such as China and India, for centuries. Written references to medicinal herbs can be found in the earliest records from most cultures in the world. In fact, the use of herbs for medical treatment might be the oldest form of health care known, and it is the field of herbalism that is the direct precursor of pharmacology as it is practiced today. Many of the drugs used today are still derived from plant sources.

Although medical use of herbs and plants is an unbroken chain that reaches back into antiquity, other CAM therapies have followed a less clear path. Some therapies such as acupuncture and Ayurveda, which are labeled CAM in the United States, are part of mainstream medical care in India and China. As traditional allopathic medicine became more dominant during the late 1800s and early 1900s in the United States, alternative systems of health care used in this country became less popular. CAM therapies experienced a resurgence in the late twentieth century as part of the alternative health movement.[3]

Today, there is an emphasis on using both traditional biomedical techniques and CAM in a way that addresses the needs of the whole person. This approach is referred to as **integrative medicine**.

National Center for Complementary and Alternative Medicine

One of the major reasons for the rapid growth of CAM in the United States in the last part of the twentieth century was the formation of the Office of Alternative Medicine (OAM) in 1992. In 1999, the Office of Alternative Medicine was upgraded and became one of the 27 institutes and centers of the National Institutes of Health (NIH) that exists within the U.S. Department of Health and Human Services. Its name was ultimately changed to the National Center for Complementary and Alternative Medicine (NCCAM) to adequately reflect the complementary aspects of this group of therapies. According to its mission statement, NCCAM seeks to "explore complementary and alternative healing practices in the context of rigorous science, train CAM researchers, and disseminate authoritative information to the public and professionals."

Office of Dietary Supplements

Another key player in the advancement of knowledge of CAM in the United States is the Office of Dietary Supplements (ODS) at NIH, which was established in 1995 as a mandate of the Dietary Supplement Health and Education Act of 1994. Its mission is to "strengthen knowledge and understanding of dietary supplements by evaluating scientific information, stimulating and supporting research, disseminating research results, and educating the public to foster an enhanced quality of life and health for the U.S. population." The ODS, along with NCCAM, funds six dietary supplement research centers (mainly university based). Along with other governmental agencies, ODS also supports the International Bibliographic Information on Dietary Supplements, an extensive database of bibliographic citations and abstracts from the published research literature on dietary supplements.

German Commission E Monographs

Although no longer active, the German Commission E deserves mention. This commission, which was formed in Germany in 1978, produced 380 monographs on the safety and efficacy of drugs before the agency was disbanded in 1995. The monographs were imported, translated into English, and published by the American Botanical Council in 1998.[4] However, the English translations do not have citations, and thus, the information in these monographs is not dated.

Regulation of Dietary Supplements

In the United States, botanical medicines are sold and regulated as **dietary supplements**. The Dietary Supplement Health and Education Act (DSHEA) passed by the U.S. Congress in 1994 broadened the definition of dietary supplements to include vitamins, minerals, amino acids, and botanical and animal products.[3] The DSHEA defines a dietary supplement as "any product intended to supplement the diet which is not represented for use as a conventional food." Therefore, both botanical and non-botanical supplements can be sold in the United States without Food and Drug Administration (FDA) approval provided they do not make any claims that the dietary supplement diagnoses, treats, cures, or prevents any disease. Doing so makes the product subject to regulation as a drug.

The FDA regulates the marketing and sales of dietary supplements. The Federal Trade Commission (FTC) regulates the advertising of these products. The classification of a botanical product as a dietary supplement versus a medicine or drug has significant consequences for both consumers and providers. Table 10-1 summarizes these differences.

In 1998, the FDA redefined the word *disease* to help clarify permissible claims by dietary supplement manufacturers. Under this new definition, the following types of statements concerning the claims of dietary supplements are not permissible: "reduces the pain and stiffness of arthritis" or "lowers elevated cholesterol." So-called structure/function claims, however, are allowable. For example, manufacturers selling cranberry products can claim that the products support urinary health but they cannot claim that cranberry products prevent the occurrence of urinary tract infections. Following any allowable structure/function claim, the dietary supplement manufacturer must state on the product label, "This statement has not been evaluated by the FDA." Labels must also state, "This product is not intended to diagnose, treat, cure, or prevent any disease."

Labeling of dietary supplements requires that the product be labeled as such and all ingredients, including excipients, be listed in descending order of amount on the product's label. The identity of the plant parts present must be indicated as well as the name and location of the manufacturer or distributor.

Table 10-1 Comparison of Dietary Supplements and Drugs in the United States

	Dietary Supplement	Drug
Burden of proof of safety	Manufacturer	FDA
Label can denote use for treating disease	No	Yes
Must demonstrate safety before approval	No	Yes
Must demonstrate efficacy before approval	No	Yes
Requires investigational new drug (IND) application	No	Yes
Regulation of advertising	FDA	FTC

Abbreviations: FDA = Food and Drug Administration; FTC = Federal Trade Commission.

Other quality control measures for the dietary supplement industry include the work carried out by the **United States Pharmacopeia (USP)**, a nongovernmental, public health organization that is the official standards-setting authority for all prescription and over-the-counter (OTC) medicines, including dietary supplements, sold in the United States. The USP sets standards for the quality, strength, purity, and consistency of these products. The USP has a Dietary Supplement Verification program that tests many supplements for purity, potency, and overall quality. A manufacturer is allowed to use the **USP Verified Dietary Supplement Mark** on the label of its products if (1) all listed ingredients are the only ingredients in the container; (2) the supplement does not contain harmful levels of contaminants; (3) the supplement will not break down and release alternative ingredients into the body; and (4) the supplement has been made using Good Manufacturing Practices.

Safety of Botanical Medicines

Unlike food additives and drugs, dietary supplements do not require premarket approval for safety; therefore, the FDA must assume the burden of proving a product is unsafe if FDA personnel decide to investigate a particular marketed product. Thus both safety and efficacy—the two standards applied to pharmaceutical products—are not necessarily assessed for botanical products.

The medically active compound in a plant can come from the leaf, root, stem, or flower. In addition, the compound of interest may actually consist of several compounds that work synergistically. This combination may be active only if the plant is picked at a certain time of year or if it is dried or processed in a certain way. Given these factors, it is easy to see why the amount of active ingredient in the herbal supplements found on the over-the-counter shelves of a pharmacy vary widely.

Another concern is purity. For example, some botanical preparations have been discovered to be contaminated with heavy metals (e.g., iron in Ayurveda therapies imported from India). Products labeled as ginseng have been found to contain scopolamine.[5] Ginseng is very expensive to produce, which makes it an obvious target for replacement with non-ginseng substances.

Adverse Reactions to Botanical Medicines

Even when quality control is not a concern, adverse effects of botanical preparations that are truly pure can occur.

Adverse reactions associated with herbs may include idiosyncratic reactions, cardiotoxicity, renal toxicity, hepatotoxicity, convulsions, and drug–herb interactions.[6] In 2004, the FDA issued a rule banning ephedra from being included in dietary supplements after receiving reports of 34 deaths and more than 800 adverse medical events that were submitted between 1993 and 1997.

Hepatotoxicity is the adverse reaction most frequently reported in association with botanical medicines.[7,8] The well-known hepatotoxic effect of pyrrolizidine alkaloids is a good example of this problem. These compounds are present in many plants to varying degrees. Pyrrolizidine alkaloids are metabolized via CYP3A4 and CYP2B6 into pyrroles, which are capable of inducing hepatocellular injury. Comfrey, for example, contains pyrrolizidine alkaloids and large doses of comfrey tea have been the etiology of liver dysfunction in several of the case reports of herb-induced hepatoxicity. Table 10-2 lists the herbs that have been implicated in cases of hepatotoxicity. Because hepatotoxicity is rare, it can take large population exposures before a relationship between one herbal formulation and liver damage becomes evident. This may account for why some of the Chinese herbal medicines appear on this list. In addition, many Chinese herbal medicines contain species of *Senecio*, which is one of the three families of plants that contain large amounts of pyrrolizidine alkaloids.

Table 10-2 Selected Herbs That Have Been Implicated in Cases of Hepatotoxicity

Herb
Black cohosh (*Cimicifuga racemosa*)
Cascara sagrada (*Rhamnus purshiana*)[a]
Chaparral (*Larrea*)
Chinese herbal medicines:
Chaso
Jin Bu Huan (*Stephania sinica*)
Ma huang (ephedra)[b]
Sho (Do)-saiko-to
Shou-wa-pian
Comfrey (*Symphytum*)
Germander (*Teucrium chamaedrys*)
Kava (*Piper methysticum*)
Mistletoe (*Viscum album*)
Pennyroyal (*Mentha pulegium*)
Sassafras oil (*Sassafras*)
Senecio (*Senecio aconitifolius*)
Senna (*Cassia acutifolia*)
Skullcap (*Scutellaria*)
Valerian (*Valeriana officinalis*)

[a] Case report of cholestatic hepatitis.
[b] In 2004, the FDA issued a rule banning ephedra from all dietary supplements.
Sources: Data from Abdualmjid RJ, Sergi C. Hepatotoxic botanicals: an evidence-based systematic review. *J Pharm Pharm Sci*. 2013;16(3): 376-404[7]; Bunchorntavakul C, Reddy KR. Herbal and dietary supplement hepatotoxicity. *Aliment Pharmacol Ther*. 2013;37(1):3-17.[8]

Herb–Drug Interactions

Prescribers should be aware that 20% of persons in the United States use botanical products concomitantly with prescription drugs.[1] Herb–drug interactions are difficult to identify for several reasons. Herb–drug interactions are, in general, rare when both substances are taken in the prescribed manner for short periods of time. However, these interactions are undoubtedly underreported, so the true incidence is not known. In addition, most herbal preparations contain multiple compounds or a mixture of several different herbs; therefore when adverse effects are reported, it is not clear which compound is responsible for the reaction. The herbs that are most frequently associated with drug interactions include ginkgo, St. John's wort, ginseng, garlic, and kava.[9–12] Table 10-3 lists some of the well-known drug–herb interactions.

Efficacy of Botanical Medicines

The number of studies evaluating the efficacy of botanical medicines is beginning to increase. Because botanical medicines are complex compounds that are not easy to reproduce, determining the active ingredient(s) is a necessary first step that can take time and research. Many of the studies of medicinal use of herbs being published now are basic chemistry studies that either determine the active compound or test the in vivo effects of the active compound.

Randomized clinical trials (RCTs) of effectiveness of botanical medicines are often confounded by a large placebo effect in the control group. In addition, these trials may use different populations, different preparations, and different outcome measures. As a consequence, a botanical medicine might show effectiveness in some well-designed RCTs and no effectiveness in others. To date, most of the meta-analyses have reported negative results—but these negative findings should not be considered the final word. Until there is more standardization in the RCT methodologies, the meta-analysis technique will not be highly valuable in assessing the effectiveness of botanical therapies.

Finally, it is important to recognize that the doses of botanical medicines used in RCTs are not necessarily the

Table 10-3 Selected Drug–Herb Interactions[a]

Drug: Generic (Brand)	Effect
Asian ginseng root and	
Phenelzine (Nardil)	Case report of mania
Warfarin (Coumadin)	Decreased anticoagulant effect[b]
Echinacea and	
Acetaminophen (Tylenol)	Both acetaminophen and echinacea are potentially hepatotoxic; it is theorized that the combination could increase the risk of hepatotoxicity
Garlic and	
Antiretroviral drugs	Toxic gastrointestinal effects[c]
Chlorpropamide (Diabinese)	Enhanced hypoglycemic effect
Warfarin (Coumadin)	Increased anticoagulant effect[b]
Ginkgo and	
Aspirin and other NSAIDs	Increased bleeding
Digoxin (Lanoxin)	Increased blood levels of digoxin
Hypoglycemic agents	Ginkgo decreases blood sugar and may enhance the antihyperglycemic effect of oral medications used for diabetes
Omeprazole (Prilosec)	Increased metabolism of omeprazole and possible decreased effectiveness
Thiazide diuretics	Increased blood pressure
Trazodone (Desyrel)	Coma
Warfarin (Coumadin)	Increased anticoagulant effect[b]
Ginseng (Panax) and	
Opioids	Ginseng can inhibit analgesic effect of opioids
Warfarin (Coumadin)	Decreased serum concentrations of warfarin
Kava and	
Alprazolam (Xanax)	Semicomatose state
Levodopa (Sinemet)	Increased number of off periods
Opioids	Increased sedation
St. John's wort and	
Antiretroviral drugs	Decreased plasma levels of the antiretroviral drugs
Amitriptyline (Elavil)	Decreased plasma levels of amitriptyline
Benzodiazepines (midazolam [Versed], alprazolam [Xanax])	Decreased plasma levels of benzodiazepines
Cyclosporin (Neoral)	Decreased plasma levels of cyclosporine
Digoxin (Lanoxin)	Decreased plasma levels of digoxin
Loperamide (Imodium)	Acute delirium[b,c]
Methadone	Withdrawal syndrome[c]
Oral contraceptives	Decreased plasma levels of contraceptives; can cause contraceptive failure
Selective serotonin reuptake inhibitors	Serotonin syndrome
Simvastatin (Zocor)	Decreased plasma levels of simvastatin
Tacrolimus (Prototopic)	Decreased plasma levels of tacrolimus
Theophylline (Theo-Dur)	Decreased plasma levels of theophylline
Tolbutamide (Orinase)	Decreased plasma levels of tolbutamide
Warfarin (Coumadin)	Lowers INR

Abbreviations: INR = International Normalized Ratio; NSAID = nonsteroidal anti-inflammatory drug.
[a] This table is not comprehensive as new information is being generated on a regular basis.
[b] Causality uncertain.
[c] Case reports only.

same doses found on the shelf at the local drug store. Consumers and prescribers need to assess the value of the efficacy studies reported here with caution because until botanical medicines are standardized in the United States, their quality, purity, efficacy, and safety will not be guaranteed. Despite these caveats, there is growing evidence of the therapeutic usefulness of several botanical medicines commonly used in women's health.

Botanical Medicine in Women's Health

Women are much more likely to use botanical medicines than are men. Upchurch et al. conducted a secondary analysis of data from the 2002 National Health Interview survey and found that 40% of the women (n = 17,295) reported recent use of one or more CAM modalities.[13] The category of CAM most frequently used consisted of biologically based products (23.8%).[13] Musculoskeletal disorders and chronic pain were the conditions for which women most frequently used CAM therapies. Menopause was among the top 10 conditions for which herbal remedies were used. The remainder of this chapter provides selected examples of CAM products for which there is evidence about botanical therapies used predominately by women. It is important to note that this chapter does not provide a comprehensive review of the many different CAM therapies that could be used by women. Botanical medicines that play a predominant role in reproductive health are listed in Table 10-4 and botanical medicines commonly used for disease prevention are listed in Table 10-5.[14]

Depression

St. John's Wort (*Hypericum perforatum*)

Hypericum is a common ground cover with a pretty, five-petal yellow flower that blooms in the summer. The active agent, hypericin, contains many compounds, including naphthodianthrones that have several different versions of hypericin, flavonoids, hyperforin, amino acids, and tannins. The actual compound responsible for the therapeutic effects is unknown.[6] The mechanism for the apparent antidepressant effect of St. John's wort is unclear, but many studies indicate that this agent inhibits the reuptake of serotonin, dopamine, and norepinephrine in neuronal synapses in the brain.[9]

Table 10-4 Selected Botanical Medicines Used in Reproductive Health

Botanical Product	Clinical Indication	Evidence for Use
Black cohosh	Dysmenorrhea	No evidence of effectiveness
	Induction of labor	No evidence of effectiveness
	Menopausal symptoms	Conflicting studies; may have potential but more research needed
Blue cohosh	Induction of labor	Contraindicated
Castor oil	Induction of labor	No evidence of effectiveness
Chasteberry	Dysmenorrhea	No evidence of effectiveness
	Mastalgia	Effective
	Premenstrual syndrome	Effective for short-term use
Cramp bark	Dysmenorrhea	No evidence of effectiveness
Cranberry products	Prevention of urinary tract infection (UTI)	Probably effective for prevention of UTI but no evidence that cranberry is effective in treating UTIs
Dong quai (*Angelica sinensis*)	Menopausal symptoms	No evidence of effectiveness
Evening primrose	Premenstrual syndrome	No evidence of effectiveness
	Mastalgia	No evidence of effectiveness
	Menopausal symptoms	No evidence of effectiveness
Flax	Mastalgia	No evidence of effectiveness
Ginger	Nausea and vomiting in pregnancy	Effective
Ginseng	Menopausal symptoms	No evidence of effectiveness
Kava	Anxiety	Effective
Psidium guajava	Dysmenorrhea	Preliminary evidence of effectiveness
Red clover	Menopausal symptoms	No evidence of effectiveness
Rose tea	Dysmenorrhea	One study found that rose tea was effective; more studies needed
Sage	Menopausal symptoms	Preliminary evidence of effectiveness
Soy products	Menopausal symptoms	Effective for vasomotor symptoms; soy-based food products are more effective than tablets or capsules
St. John's wort	Depression	Good evidence for mild to moderate depression for short-term therapy
Wild yam	Menopausal symptoms	No evidence of effectiveness

Abundant evidence supports the benefit of this herbal supplement for treatment of mild to moderate depression. A meta-analysis of the RCTs on St. John's wort that were published in the late 1990s found that St. John's wort therapy is as effective as a placebo in improving symptoms of major depression (relative risk [RR], 2.47; 95% confidence interval [CI], 1.69–3.61; 29 trials, n = 5489) over a short period of treatment (mean = 6 weeks).[15] In many of these studies, the benefits of St. John's wort was shown to be equivalent to that of conventional antidepressant drugs. Fewer side effects were reported with use of St. John's wort compared to other antidepressant medications.

In general, the adverse effects of St. John's wort are minimal and lower in frequency than the side effects that occur after taking tricyclic antidepressants or selective serotonin reuptake inhibitors. That said, multiple side effects and a few adverse effects are associated with use of St. John's wort, including gastrointestinal distress, sexual dysfunction, dizziness, confusion, dry mouth, headache, and allergic skin reactions. Photosensitivity has been reported as well. Adverse effects include serotonin syndrome, which can occur when this herbal agent is taken concomitantly with selective serotonin reuptake inhibitors. In addition, case reports cite cardiovascular collapse during anesthesia, delayed emergence from anesthesia, and hypertensive crisis in persons taking St. John's wort.[6]

St. John's wort is a potent inducer of several CYP450 enzymes and has numerous clinically important interactions with drugs, such as anticoagulants, cyclosporine, digoxin (Lanoxin), protease inhibitors, and oral contraceptives (Table 10-3).[16] The FDA has issued a black box warning that advises against using St. John's wort in conjunction with protease inhibitors. Concomitant use of St. John's wort with drugs that have a narrow therapeutic index and are metabolized by a CYP450 enzyme induced by St. John's wort can lead to therapeutic failure. Examples include cyclosporine (Neoral), digoxin (Lanoxin), theophylline (Theo-Dur), tolbutamide (Orinase), and warfarin (Coumadin).

Table 10-5 Dietary Supplements Commonly Used for Disease Prevention

Conditions	Dietary Supplement	Common Dose	Effectiveness	Safety
Breast cancer prevention	Grapes (Contain resveratrol which is an antioxidant)	230 g/day	Inhibits growth in cancer cell lines and facilitated apoptotic effects of chemotherapy	+
Cancer (general)	Fish oil	No established dose	0	+
	Remifemin	20–40 mg 2 times/day	±	+
	Green tea	1–10 cups/day	±	+
Cardiovascular disease (general)	Red grape polyphenol extract	600 mg	±	+
	Green tea	1–10 cups/day	+	+
Cardiovascular disease (secondary prevention)	Fish oil	Capsule of EPA and DHA 850 to 1800 mg/day	+	+
Common cold	Echinacea	Capsule: 500–1000 mg 3 times/day for 5–7 days Tincture: 0.75–1.5 mL gargled and swallowed 2–5 times/day	±	+
Cognitive function dementia, Alzheimer's disease	Fish oil	No established dose	0	+
Memory enhancement (baseline healthy adult)	Gingko	Tablet: 120 mg 2 times/day	±	±
Memory enhancement (baseline mild impairment)	Gingko	Tablet: 120 mg 2 times/day	±	±
Osteoarthritis	Glucosamine	Capsule: 500 mg 3 times/day	+	+
	Chondroitin	Capsule: 400 mg 3 times/day	+	+
Travelers diarrhea	Probiotics	Tablets: 10–100 billion live organisms	+	+
Urinary tract infection	Cranberry	Juice: 90–480 mL cocktail or 15–30 mL unsweetened 100% juice/day Capsule: 1–6 of 300–400 mg 2 times/day Concentrate: 45 mL frozen concentrate 2 times/day	±	+
	Probiotics containing lactobacillus	Tablets: 5–10 billion CFUs/day	±	+

Abbreviations: 0 = evidence suggests not effective or safe; ± = evidence is equivocal but insufficient to prove effectiveness or safety; + = good evidence for effectiveness or safety; CFUs = colony forming units; DHA = docosahexaenoic acid; EPA = eicosapentaenoic acid.
Source: Adapted with permission from Najm W, Lie D. Dietary supplements commonly used for prevention. *Prim Care Clin Office Pract*. 2008;749-767.[14]

Urinary Tract Infections

Urinary tract infections (UTIs) are more common in women than in men. In fact, UTI is one of the most common bacterial infections in women.[17] Approximately 30% of all women will have a UTI before reaching the age of 24.[17]

Cranberry (*Vaccinium macrocarpon*)

Cranberry (*Vaccinium macrocarpon*) has been recommended for treating and preventing urinary tract infections, even though there is no evidence that cranberry is effective for this indication. Cranberry lacks direct antibacterial activity but appears to work via compounds in the berries that prevent microorganisms such as

Escherichia coli from adhering to epithelial cells lining the urinary tract. Cranberry also lowers urine pH enough to retard the breakdown of urine by *E. coli*, thus reducing the pungent ammonia-like odor associated with this infection.

Several meta-analyses and systematic reviews have evaluated the effectiveness of cranberry for prophylaxis of UTI and found it to be effective.[18–20] However, recent clinical trials not included in these meta-analyses failed to show a statistically significant effect on UTI prophylaxis.[21] The most recent Cochrane meta-analysis found cranberry-containing products are not associated with protective effects against UTIs (RR, 0.86; 95% CI, 0.71–1.04).[20] A subgroup analysis within the Cochrane review found that cranberry may be effective for women with recurrent UTIs. In contrast, the RCT carried out by Stapleton et al., which included 176 premenopausal women with a history of recent UTI,[21] found cranberry juice did not significantly reduce UTI risk. However, the researchers did find a reduction in urinary P-fimbriated *E. coli* strains, which supports the hypothesis that cranberry juice has advantageous biologic activity. In summary, cranberry products are not effective for treatment of a UTI. There are plausible biologic mechanisms for how cranberry might prevent recurrent UTI. RCTs that assessed cranberry products for prevention of recurrent UTI have conflicting results. Cranberry products are not recommended for prevention of UTI at this time.

Cranberry contains flavonoids that may interact with warfarin (Coumadin) in a way that causes an enhanced anticoagulant effect. For this reason, women on warfarin therapy should avoid using cranberry products in large amounts.

Probiotics

Probiotics are dietary supplements that contain "live organisms, which, when administered in adequate amounts, confer a health benefit on the host."[22] The use of probiotics to treat or prevent UTIs has been researched extensively.[23,24]

The mechanism by which *Lactobacillus* cultures may exhibit a protective effect is bacterial competition. In normal conditions, lactobacilli are the dominant bacteria in the vaginal flora. These bacteria are a known form of biofilm that has some antimicrobial activity in vitro and in animal models. Infection or incomplete cure of a genitourinary infection shifts the flora in the vagina such that coliform uropathogens predominate. Women who have recurrent UTIs are known to have vaginal microbacterial flora that does not include the usual amount of *Lactobacillus*. It has been theorized that *Lactobacillus*-containing probiotic products placed in the vagina will allow the *Lactobacillus* to compete with uropathogens, thereby preventing uropathogen colonization to the urethra and ascending infection into the bladder.

To date, none of the RCTs that have evaluated probiotics for prevention of UTIs have included adequate numbers of participants to show a significant change in the incidence of UTI.[23] Although one RCT did find a reduction in the occurrence of UTIs from 6 per year to 1.6 per year following weekly intravaginal use of *L. rhamnosus* and *L. fermentum*, use of a milk-based probiotic that stimulated growth of lactobacilli in the control group was equally effective.[25] More studies that utilize defined strains of *Lactobacillus* and larger numbers of participants are needed before the efficacy of probiotics in preventing UTIs can be determined.

Lactobacillus-containing products marketed for intravaginal use have very few adverse effects. The incidence of infection with lactobacilli is very low but can occur in persons who are immunocompromised or debilitated. None of the studies done to date have enrolled persons with these risk factors.[23]

Primary Dysmenorrhea

Dysmenorrhea is a type of pelvic pain occurring during menstruation that can be classified as either primary or secondary. Primary dysmenorrhea is very common, occurring in as many as 50% of all menstruating women; it usually presents within 3 years of menarche.[26] Uterine spasms are usually experienced as sharp intermittent pains that often radiate to the back of the legs or lower back. The etiology of this condition is not known but likely involves tissue ischemia and the release of prostaglandins, which mediate the pain and uterine contractions.[27] Several herbs have been widely used in treatments of dysmenorrhea, but evidence of effectiveness is generally weak.

Dong Quai (*Angelica sinensis*)

An extract from the root of a plant in the Apiaceae family *Angelica sinensis*, dong quai has been a popular remedy for dysmenorrhea in traditional Chinese, Japanese, and Korean medicine for centuries. The active constituent contains several different chemicals that have been tested in vitro, both individually and in combination, and found to have weak estrogenic activity. One presumed mechanism of action is an antagonistic effect on prostaglandin synthesis, which then inhibits uterine contractions. Constituents in dong quai are known to inhibit prostaglandin synthesis and have anticoagulant properties and antiplatelet action; however, no clinical trials have been conducted that demonstrate dong quai is effective for treating dysmenorrhea. Thus, there is insufficient evidence to support the use of dong quai for treatment of dysmenorrhea.

Adverse effects of dong quai include bloating and loss of appetite. Because dong quai has possible antithrombotic effects and progesterone effects, persons taking warfarin (Coumadin), hormone replacement therapy, oral contraceptives, or other herbs that cause blood thinning may consider this herb contraindicated. Individuals with a history of estrogen-dependent tumor should also use dong quai with caution.

Cramp Bark (*Viburnum opulus*) and Black Haw (*Viburnum prunifolium*)

A hot water infusion of the bark from cramp bark (*Viburnum opulus*) has been a traditional folk remedy for relieving menstrual cramps for centuries in the United States. The constituent vioudial extracted from the bark has been shown in animal studies to have smooth muscle-relaxing properties. Proanthocyanidins in the fruit have antioxidant, anti-inflammatory, and vasodilating activities.[28]

Black haw (*Viburnum prunifolium*) has long been used to treat menstrual cramps as well. In vitro studies in rabbits have shown it has smooth muscle-relaxing effects.[29] No clinical studies have been done in humans, however.

Rose Hips (*Rosa* spp.)

Rose hips have been used to treat dysmenorrhea in Eastern cultures. This botanical medicine has significant antioxidant potential due to its high content of both flavonoids and non-flavonoid polyphenols, as well as carotenoids.[30] One RCT attempted to determine the effectiveness of drinking rose tea for reducing pain associated with dysmenorrhea in Taiwanese adolescents (n = 130); the researchers found that the experimental group (n = 59) perceived less pain and had higher scores for psychological well-being over time (1, 3, and 6 months; $P > .001$).[31] The adolescents in the experimental group drank two teacups of rose tea for 12 days each month for 6 months. Limitations of this study included the subjective reporting of the participants and the fact that these findings cannot be generalized to all populations. Although the study contributes to current knowledge about rose tea and its use in the treatment of primary dysmenorrhea, it also emphasizes the need for further research.

Guava (*Psidium guajava* L.)

A popular Mexican phytomedicine prescribed for the treatment of dysmenorrhea is guava *Psidium guajava* L. (Myrtaceae) extract.[32] The primary action of the flavonols in *Psidium guajava* L. is antispasmodic, but this botanical product also has antioxidant and anti-inflammatory activity.[33] One RCT (n = 197) found that a dose of 6 mg per day of the extract significantly reduced menstrual pain as measured on a visual analogue scale ($P > .001$) when compared with nonsteroidal anti-inflammatory drugs (NSAIDs) and a placebo. However, all groups documented some reduction of pain associated with dysmenorrhea over the course of the trial.[34] A distinct advantage of using *Psidium guajava* L. to treat dysmenorrhea is that it does not have the adverse gastrointestinal side effects associated with NSAIDs, but more research is needed before this supplement can be recommended for routine use.

Other Herbs for Dysmenorrhea

Roots of the false unicorn (*Chamaelirium luteum*) were used by Native Americans and nineteenth-century eclectic physicians in North America to treat a variety of women's conditions, including dysmenorrhea. Black cohosh and chasteberry have also been used to treat dysmenorrhea, but there are no studies documenting the safety or effectiveness of these agents.[34]

Premenstrual Syndrome and Premenstrual Dysphoric Disorder

An estimated 85% to 90% of women experience regular premenstrual symptoms that include depression, irritability, mood swings, bloating, cyclic mastalgia, abdominal discomfort, emotional lability, headache, and constipation.[2] Premenstrual syndrome (PMS) is a disorder related to cyclical hormonal variation that causes disruption of emotional and physical well-being. PMS occurs during the luteal phase of the menstrual cycle and ceases after the start of menses. CAM therapies that show promise for treating PMS symptoms include calcium and vitamin B_6. Botanical medicines used for PMS include chasteberry and evening primrose oil.[35]

Chasteberry (*Vitex agnus-castus*)

Chasteberry (*Vitex agnus-castus*)—often referred to simply as *Vitex* by many herbalists—is a deciduous shrub native to the Mediterranean, Europe, and Central Asia. The dried ripe fruit of the chasteberry tree has been a popular botanical treatment for treatment of reproductive disorders for centuries. This fruit was used to decrease sexual desire in men in the Middle Ages, which is where it got its name. The dried fruit contains the iridoid glycosides aucubin and agnoside, plus flavonoids such as castican, orientin, isovitexin, and apigenin.[36] The essential oil fraction contains primarily limonene, cineole, and sabinene. The proposed mechanism of action for chasteberry is a decrease in prolactin, which reverses the normal luteal-phase suppression of luteinizing hormone (LH) and thereby allows full development of the corpus luteum and production of more progesterone, so the PMS symptoms are less severe.[37]

Several large, uncontrolled studies support the effectiveness and safety of chasteberry for treating PMS, and RCTs have shown chasteberry to be effective in reducing the symptoms of PMS as well.[37] A recent systematic review of eight RCTs found that in seven of the trials, chasteberry was superior to the placebo.[38]

The typical dose of chasteberry is 20–40 mg taken 1–3 times per day. Chasteberry is also sold as a liquid extract; with this formulation, the dose is 40 drops per day.[39]

Side effects of chasteberry appear to be mild, with reports citing gastrointestinal complaints, mild skin rash, nausea, headaches, acne, and increased menstrual flow.[40] Chasteberry may have estrogenic activity and should be avoided or used with caution by women with estrogen-sensitive disease. Chasteberry may also interfere with the efficacy of oral contraceptives and dopamine antagonists such as chlorpromazine (Thorazine) and prochlorperazine (Compazine).

One RCT has investigated the benefits of chasteberry for treatment of premenstrual dysphoric disorder (PMDD).[41] In this study, chasteberry was compared to drug treatment with fluoxetine (Prozac) for 2 months. Both treatments resulted in significant improvements in symptoms (64% with fluoxetine and 57.9% with chasteberry).

St. John's Wort (*Hypericum perforatum*)

Several studies have evaluated St. John's wort for treating symptoms associated with PMS. This herb appears to be effective in treating some of the PMS symptoms that women report, such as bloating and depression, although not all the studies have shown positive results.[42–44] For example, in an RCT conducted with 36 women who had regular menstrual cycles, St. John's wort was statistically superior to the placebo in improving physical and behavioral symptoms of PMS, but there was a lack of effect on mood and pain-related symptoms.[42] The most common dose is 900 mg per day.

Ginkgo Biloba

Ginkgo biloba, though better known for its well-documented clinical benefits in treating dementia, has also been shown to be effective for treating symptoms of PMS.[9] The dose used in the RCTs for this indication consisted of 80 mg of leaf extract taken twice daily starting on day 16 of the menstrual cycle and continuing until day 5 of the next cycle.[9]

Ginkgo biloba may inhibit CYP450 enzyme metabolism but clinically significant effects are not usually seen when standard doses are used.[45,46] Caution should be used by persons who are taking anticoagulants, as increased bleeding can occur. Persons who use anticonvulsants may have subtherapeutic plasma levels of the anticonvulsant if they also use Ginkgo biloba.

Evening Primrose (*Oenothera biennis*) Seeds

Evening primrose (*Oenothera biennis*) seeds are a rich source of the omega-6 fatty acid gamma-linoleic acid (GLA), which is a precursor to the synthesis of the important anti-inflammatory prostaglandin E_1.[34] Some women with PMS are deficient in GLA, particularly those who cannot convert the fatty acid linoleic acid to GLA.[47] Because of these properties, evening primrose oil (EPO) pressed from the seeds has become a popular remedy for PMS. However, little evidence supports use of this herb.[48]

Breast Pain (Mastalgia)

Mastalgia is a multifaceted condition that is poorly understood. An estimated 50% to 80% of women can expect to have some degree of mastalgia over the course of their lifetime. Mastalgia is classified as either being noncyclical or cyclical and associated with the menstrual cycle. In many women, cyclical mastalgia is associated with stress-induced hyperprolactinemia, which leads to hyperstimulation of the mammary gland, often resulting in pain.

Chasteberry (*Vitex agnus-castus*)

Since 1999, evidence has accumulated supporting the potential efficacy of chasteberry for the treatment of mastalgia.[34,49] Several formulations have been available in Germany since the 1950s (Femicur, Agnolyt, and Mastoynon) and are used for the treatment of mastalgia as well as menstrual cycle irregularities. The mechanism of action is presumed to be secondary to diterpenes such as the clerodadienols present in the dried fruit (berries), which are capable of binding to D_2 dopamine receptors, thereby causing suppression of prolactin release from the pituitary. It has also been postulated that as-yet-unidentified phytoestrogens in Vitex may competitively bind to estrogen receptors in the breast, thereby exerting antiestrogen effects. Some fruit extracts have constituents that competitively bind to both the alpha and beta isoforms of the estrogen receptor. Chasteberry was found to be effective in reducing both the intensity and the duration of breast pain in several RCTs and a systematic review.[49,50]

Evening Primrose (*Oenothera biennis*)

The oil from evening primrose seeds is a rich source of the omega-6 essential fatty acid gamma-linolenic. EPO is a popular treatment for mastalgia throughout Europe, especially in the United Kingdom. Nevertheless, there is insufficient evidence from the studies done to date to support use of EPO for treating mastalgia.[51]

Flax (*Linum usitatissimum*)

It has been hypothesized that the phytoestrogen lignin, which is present in the seeds of the flax plant (*Linum usitatissimum*), may offer benefit for treating mastalgia. A single RCT with 116 premenopausal women with severe breast pain found that flaxseed (25 g formulated into a muffin) given daily for 6 months resulted in decreased pain as measured by a visual analogue scale.[52] More research is needed to determine the potential clinical benefit of flaxseed in this condition.

Nausea and Vomiting During Pregnancy

Approximately 50% to 90% of women experience at least some level of nausea during the first trimester of pregnancy, while a somewhat lower percentage (25–55%) have episodes of vomiting.[53] Several CAM therapies, including acupressure and acupuncture, vitamin B_6, and ginger, are used to treat nausea and/or vomiting that occur during pregnancy. Vitamin B_6 is discussed in more detail in the *Pregnancy* chapter.

Ginger (*Zingiber officinale*)

Ginger (*Zingiber officinale*) has been used for centuries to treat many medical complaints, but particularly gastrointestinal disorders and nausea; it is also used as a digestive aid. The constituents in the ginger rhizome that are thought to be involved in its antiemetic activity are gingerols, shogoals, and galanolactone.[54] The mechanism of ginger's antiemetic effect is not completely understood but likely involves serotonin antagonism.[56]

A 2010 meta-analysis of 9 RCTs that enrolled 1081 women found that ginger resulted in a significant decrease in nausea when compared to a placebo treatment, but the relief was not always better than that obtained via use of vitamin B_6 or other drug therapies.[56] The dose of ginger (fresh or powdered) varies from 0.5 g to 2 g daily, with 1.0 g being the most typical dose. Ginger is available in a variety of forms, and an evaluation of products purchased in pharmacies and health food stores found a wide variation in the amount of active ingredients and suggested serving sizes.[57] Exact dosing relies on use of standardized extracts. Equivalent dosing is listed in Table 10-6.[58]

There is no clinical evidence to suggest that ginger has an adverse effect on fetal development and it has generally been considered safe for use during pregnancy in the Unites States. However, the German Commission E Monographs and other herbalist literature consider ginger a contraindicated treatment during pregnancy. This caution is based on the knowledge that ginger affects protein binding of testosterone and may have apoptotic effects in human lymphoma cells, both of which could have an adverse effect on an embryo. In traditional medical systems and herbalist literature, ginger is often contraindicated for use by pregnant women due to its reputation for inducing menstruation or promoting bleeding, but there is no clinical evidence that ginger acts as an abortifacient.[59]

Table 10-6 Equivalent Dosing of Ginger Products

The following equal 1000 mg standardized extract:
1 tsp fresh grated rhizome
2 oz drops liquid extract
2 tsp syrup (10 mL)
4 cups (8 oz each) ginger tea prepackaged
4 cups (8 oz each) ginger tea, steeping ½ tsp grated ginger for 5–10 minutes
8 oz ginger ale, made with real ginger
2 pieces crystallized ginger, each 1 inch square, ¼ inch thick
Chewable tablets contain 67.5 mg
Capsules come in various doses ranging from 100 mg to 1000 mg

Source: Adapted with permission from Bryer E. A literature review of the effectiveness of ginger in alleviating mild-to-moderate nausea and vomiting of pregnancy. *J Midwifery Womens Health*. 2005;50(1):e1-e3.[58]

Ginger is a potent thromboxane synthetase inhibitor and could have adverse effects on platelet aggregation. No such effects have been noted at normal doses or up to 15 g of raw ginger, but 10 g of dried ginger may decrease platelet aggregation times.[60] Ginger should not be taken concomitantly with warfarin (Coumadin) or nifedipine (Procardia). Ginger should be used with caution if taking other drugs that delay blood clotting such as aspirin.

Induction of Labor

A natural and safe form of inducing labor is often desired by both pregnant women and their caregivers. Acupuncture, castor oil, homeopathic compounds, and several herbs have all been used for this purpose. The American College of Nurse-Midwives distributed a questionnaire to 500 nurse-midwives to assess the frequency and type of labor inductions that these providers used. Five hundred questionnaires were mailed, and 172 were returned (a 34% response rate). Among the respondents, approximately 50% used herbal preparations to stimulate labor.[61] Of these, 93% used castor oil, 64% used blue cohosh, 45% used black cohosh, 63% used red raspberry leaf, and 60% used evening primrose oil.

Castor Oil (*Ricinus communis*)

Castor oil, obtained from the seeds of the castor bean plant (*Ricinus communis*), is classified as a stimulant laxative and is listed by the FDA as Generally Recognized as Safe (GRAS) as a stimulant laxative. The active compound in castor oil is likely ricinoleic acid. Its use in pregnant women is contraindicated because of the propensity to cause uterine contractions, which is also why it is used to induce labor at term. A dose of 15–60 mL will produce laxative effects.[62]

There are only a few studies that have evaluated the effectiveness of castor oil for labor induction. An RCT in 47 pregnant women found a significant increase in the probability of labor initiation during the first 24 hours after receiving 60 mL castor oil (54.2%) compared to the no-treatment control group (4.3%).[63] There was also a significant increase in the mean Bishop score in the castor oil group (2.50 ± 1.29 to 6.79 ± 3.20; $P < .001$).[63] A review of three RCTs conducted by the Cochrane Collaboration concluded that studies to date were of poor methodological quality and called for more research to determine the efficacy and safety of castor oil as a cervical priming and induction agent.[64]

Castor oil can cause nausea, vomiting, diarrhea, and gastrointestinal cramping. The ability of ricinoleic acid to cross the placenta seems plausible based on the small molecular weight, lipophilicity, and nonpolarity. Although the effects of castor oil on the fetus are unknown, an increase in meconium staining has been postulated. Given that the effectiveness has not been clearly demonstrated to date, side effects are distressing, and adverse fetal effects are possible, use of castor oil to induce labor is not recommended.

Blue Cohosh (*Caulophyllum thalictroides*)

Blue cohosh (*Caulophyllum thalictroides*) is a woodland perennial native to North America. Constituents in the root, including the glycosides caulosaponin and caulophyllosaponin as well as sparteine, have labor induction properties and have increased the rate and degree of uterine contractions both in vitro and in vivo. The medicinal compounds are derived from the root, which may also be called papoose root or squaw root.[65] Blue cohosh was used by Native American healers in a tea to relieve menstrual cramping and pains of labor. Interestingly, blue cohosh was listed in the U.S. Pharmacopeia as a labor inducer until 1905.

Blue cohosh is associated with case reports of perinatal stroke, myocardial infarction in a newborn, and hypoxic-ischemic encephalopathy following use to induce labor.[66] Given the potential for serious harm, blue cohosh should not be used by pregnant women.

Black Cohosh (*Cimicifuga racemosa*)

Black cohosh (*Cimicifuga racemosa*) is a perennial member of the buttercup family that, like blue cohosh, is native to North America. This plant is also called bugbane, snakeroot, and bugwort. Black cohosh belongs to a different family than blue cohosh, however, and the two should not be confused with each other. The roots and rhizomes of black cohosh contain a series of triterpene glycosides, mainly 27-deoxyactein and cimicifugoside, as well as the isoflavone formononetin, a phytoestrogen that functions as a weak partial agonist at the estrogen receptor. Black cohosh was extremely popular in 1800s and was a main ingredient in the famous Lydia Pinkham's Vegetable Compound used by many women for a variety of disorders, including menopause-associated hot flashes. Although black cohosh is effective for treating menopausal symptoms and has been used for induction of labor or correction of dysfunctional contractions, there are no studies of either the efficacy or the safety of its use by pregnant women.[67]

Menopause

Menopause is defined as occurring 12 months after cessation of menses. The average age of menopause is 51 years. The transitional phase prior to the onset of menopause is referred to as the climacteric or perimenopause. The menopausal symptoms most commonly reported are vasomotor symptoms such as hot flashes, headaches, and vaginal dryness. Because no pharmaceutical product, including hormone therapy, is without some adverse effects, women frequently seek out CAM options to ameliorate menopausal symptoms, as natural therapies are often thought to have less adverse effects. Women are also at increased risk for cardiovascular disorders as they age and the botanical medicines frequently used to treat menopausal symptoms have also been recommended as therapies for lowering hypercholesterolemia.

Phytoestrogens

Several plant-derived agents bind to estrogen receptors, and these compounds, called **phytoestrogens**, interact with estrogen receptors to function as estrogen agonists, antagonists, or partial agonists. The three main classes of phytoestrogens are isoflavones, lignans, and coumestrans.

Isoflavones are the most widely studied phytoestrogens. This class of organic chemicals has both phytoestrogen and antioxidant properties. Isoflavones are found in legumes, with soybeans having the highest concentration, followed by lentils, kidney beans, lima beans, broad beans, and chickpeas. Isoflavones have both estrogenic and antiestrogenic effects.[68] They have a stronger affinity for the estrogen receptor ER-β (found in kidney, brain, and heart tissue, as well as coronary arteries) than for the estrogen receptor ER-α (found in breast and uterine tissue).

Wild Soybean (Glycine max) *and Isoflavones for Indices of Cardiovascular Health*

Soybean products and isoflavones have also been extensively evaluated for positive effects on cardiovascular health and appear to have a modest effect in counteracting hypercholesteremia in some persons, particularly in lowering the levels of low-density lipids (LDL).[69] However, these products have not demonstrated a positive effect on high-density lipids (HDL), triglycerides, or blood pressure when the studies are evaluated as a whole. The Cochrane meta-analysis of RCTs that studied the effect of isoflavones on hypercholesterolemia did not find them to be clearly beneficial.[70] There is significant inter-individual variability in the effectiveness of these products, however, and they may be beneficial for some individuals.[71]

Soy (Glycine max) *and Isoflavones for Menopausal Symptoms*

Soy isoflavones from both soy products and red clover have been promoted for treatment of several menopausal vasomotor symptoms, but studies of their effectiveness for this indication have produced conflicting results.[72] It is difficult to conduct meta-analyses or systematic reviews of this body of work because the various studies have used different populations with variability in endogenous estrogen levels at baseline, different phytoestrogen compounds that have varying bioavailability, and different study measures. That said, some evidence supports the use of isoflavones for treating menopausal symptoms.

Soybeans are rich in the isoflavones genistein and daidzein, and they have been studied for their effects on multiple menopausal symptoms. High dietary intake of soy-based food products in Asia has been proposed as one explanation for the lower prevalence of menopausal symptoms in women from Japan, China, and Korea. A meta-analysis of 19 RCTs concluded that soy supplementation was effective in reducing the frequency of hot flashes in postmenopausal women but noted the high heterogeneity found in the studies.[73]

Approximately 30% to 50% of women metabolize daidzein into equol, a metabolite that has estrogenic effects. This individual variability in bioavailability of isoflavones may partly explain why some women have a more positive response to isoflavones than do others. It also appears that isoflavones from food products are more effective than dietary supplements that have higher concentrations of isoflavones.[74] In addition, soy-based isoflavones have the most benefit for women who have mild symptoms and who are in the perimenopausal period or early menopause.[68,72] The starting dose is 50 mg per day or greater, and therapy should continue for at least 12 weeks to determine effectiveness.[70]

Soy does not appear to have beneficial effects on bone. Isoflavones can stimulate growth of estrogen-sensitive breast tumors in vitro, but they do not appear to stimulate endometrial tissue or breast tissue in human studies at the doses that have been studied for short-term therapies. This outcome may reflect the fact that isoflavones have a higher affinity for the ER-β subtype. At the present time, it is recommended that women with breast cancer or other estrogen-dependent malignancies avoid isoflavone supplements.

Red Clover (Trifolium pratense)

The flower of the red clover plant (*Trifolium pratense*) contains the isoflavones coumestrol, genistein, and daidzein. Coumenstrol has anticoagulant and estrogenic properties.[75] Red clover has been studied for its potential to decrease hot flashes in menopause, decrease cholesterol, and increase arterial compliance and bone mineral density. Many studies testing red clover have used the product Promensil, a red clover dietary supplement containing 40 mg of total isoflavones per dose. A meta-analysis of RCTs that evaluated use of Promensil did not find it to be effective in reducing the incidence of vasomotor symptoms.[76] However, a subsequent RCT involving 109 postmenopausal women 40 years and older did show some effectiveness for this indication.[77] The treatment group received 2 daily capsules of 80 mg red clover isoflavones or a matched placebo. The red clover supplementation significantly reduced the frequency of hot flashes and the overall intensity of menopausal symptoms.

Wild Yam (Dioscorea villosa)

Because of the widespread belief that wild yam (*Dioscorea villosa*) roots contain dehydroepiandrosterone-like precursors of steroid hormones, wild yam has been used in a variety of treatments for dysmenorrhea and menopausal symptoms. Wild yam roots (particularly the Mexican wild yam) contain the saponin diosgenin, which was historically used to synthesize a variety of steroid hormones, including estrogen and progesterone. However, the conversion of diosgenin to steroid hormone cannot occur in the human body. To add further confusion to the matter, some manufacturers have adulterated wild yam preparations with synthetic steroid hormone, mainly progesterone, which might explain their observed effectiveness.

A double-blind, placebo-controlled, cross-over study tested the effectiveness of a topical wild yam cream in 23 menopausal women but statistically significant effects were seen following use of the wild yam cream compared to the placebo.[78]

Flaxseed (Linum usitatissimum)

The seeds of flax (*Linum usitatissimum*) are rich in secoisolariciresinol diglycoside, which can be converted by colonic bacteria to the active phytoestrogen lignans enterodiol and enterolactone. Flaxseed contains 25% protein, 3% to 6% soluble fiber, and 30% to 45% unsaturated fatty acids. Flaxseed oil is a good source of the omega-3 fatty acid alpha-linolenic acid. Like the isoflavone phytoestrogens, the lignans interact with the estrogen receptor as partial agonists. Flaxseed has been shown to lower total and LDL cholesterol levels. Part of this effect may be due to the lignans, which inhibit the activity of cholesterol-7 alpha-hydroxylase.

Similar to the case for other botanical medicines, studies of flaxseed for treating menopausal symptoms have yielded conflicting results, with some showing flax reduces the incidence of vasomotor symptoms and other reporting negative results.[79] For example, in one well-designed RCT (n = 188), postmenopausal women with or without breast cancer were given a flaxseed bar (410 mg of lignans) or a placebo bar for 6 weeks.[80] There were no statistical differences in the number of hot flashes (as assessed by self-reported diaries) between flaxseed and placebo bars. The largest and best-designed study was conducted by Dodin et al., who compared a flaxseed dietary supplement to a wheat germ placebo.[81] Results showed that total and LDL cholesterol were slightly reduced but no significant effects were seen on bone mineral density or menopausal symptoms. Flaxseed does not appear to have adverse effects or clinically significant drug–herb interactions.

Nonestrogenic Therapies for Menopausal Symptoms

It is recommended that women who have a history of or risk for estrogen-associated cancers avoid phytoestrogens. Thus, botanical medicines that mitigate menopausal symptoms but do not have estrogenic activity have been of interest. Black cohosh, ginseng, sage, evening primrose oil, and kava have been studied the most.

Black Cohosh (Cimicifuga racemosa)

The mechanism underlying the biologic effects of black cohosh (*Cimicifuga racemosa*) root may involve phytoestrogens, but more recent work suggests that black cohosh does not have estrogenic properties.[82] Therefore, it is likely that different preparations contain different compounds, which may account for the conflicting results in the studies conducted to date. Much of the early scientific work on black cohosh was done in Germany on a highly characterized alcoholic extract called Remifemin, standardized to contain 2.5% 27-deoxyactein. These studies found that black cohosh was more effective than the conventional treatment for relieving the depression and anxiety associated with menopause.[83] Subsequently, multiple RCTs have evaluated the effectiveness of black cohosh for relieving menopausal symptoms.[84] A meta-analysis of nine RCTs investigating the possible benefits of black cohosh found a significant reduction in the frequency of vasomotor symptoms compared to controls.[85] Only two of the nine trials in this meta-analysis tested black cohosh alone, whereas the other studies used combinations of black cohosh and other herbal products. In the two trials where black cohosh was used alone, there was only an 11% reduction in frequency of vasomotor symptoms. The Cochrane meta-analysis of black cohosh was inconclusive, but the authors indicated that this agent is promising and further research is needed.[85]

Black cohosh has been associated with case reports of hepatotoxicity.[7] Currently in the United States, it is not recommended for women who are pregnant, or for those with a history of estrogen-dependent cancers or liver dysfunction.

Ginseng (Panax ginseng)

The *Panax* genus includes several species of slow-growing perennials that have a long tradition in traditional Chinese medicine. The most commonly used species are Asian ginseng (*Panax ginseng*) and American ginseng (*Panax quinquefolius*). Siberian ginseng (*Eleutherococcus senticosus*) is sometimes promoted as an alternative to Asian ginseng, but it does not contain ginsenosides, which are the active constituents. *Panax quinquefolius* has a long history of use by North American Indians for treating multiple disorders. To date, research on the clinical effects of ginseng has been seriously confounded by use of the different forms in studies. *Panax ginseng* and *Panax quinquefolius* have different biologic properties.

Ginseng likely produces its beneficial effects via stimulation of the hypothalamus–pituitary–adrenal axis.[86] Ginseng is recommended as an "adaptogen," or tonic herb, used to stimulate the immune system and support the body under times of stress; it is widely used for many disorders in Chinese traditional medicine. Current studies of ginseng have yielded promising results with regard to this herb's ability to lower blood glucose levels and improve indices of immune function.[86] It has also been promoted for improving mood and cognition in menopause as well as for improving general menopausal symptoms, but has not shown positive effects in studies for the latter indication.[87]

In general, ginseng is a safe herb when taken in the usual doses. The most common side effects are headache, sleepiness, and gastrointestinal distress. Ginseng can induce hypoglycemia, so it should be used with caution by persons with diabetes. Ginseng is also associated with herb–drug interactions, as noted in Table 10-3. Combination products that include ginseng have been associated with case reports of severe adverse outcomes, but it is not clear if ginseng was the etiology of the reaction given that these products contain multiple biologically active ingredients.

Sage (Salvia officinalis)

Sage (*Salvia officinalis*) has been used as a culinary and medicinal herb for hundreds of years in Europe. Medicinally, it is most often used to treat mouth and throat inflammation, excessive sweating, and dyspepsia. In a recent open multicenter RCT ($n = 71$), a once-daily tablet of sage leaves taken for 8 weeks resulted in a significant decrease in both the intensity and the number of hot flashes, along with a 43% decrease in the Menopause Rating Scale (MRS).[88] Although these results are encouraging, sage requires further study in larger, better-designed trials before it can be recommended.

Large amounts and prolonged exposure to sage leaf and sage essential oil could result in restlessness, vomiting, tachycardia, and seizures. This toxicity is due to the presence of camphor and thujone. A dose consisting of 12 drops of the essential oil of sage, or 15 g of sage leaves, can engender toxic effects.[88]

Evening Primrose (Oenothera biennis)

The seeds of the popular medicinal plant evening primrose (*Oenothera biennis*) are a rich source (approximately 9% of the seed oil) of the essential omega-6 fatty acid GLA. Most of this botanical therapy's pharmacologic effects are due to the high GLA content. Evening primrose also contains linoleic acid, which is found in many other vegetable oils. Although some evidence suggests that evening primrose may be beneficial for a variety of diseases and conditions, only two clinical trials investigating the potential benefits for treatment of menopausal symptoms were found, and neither was able to show that evening primrose is therapeutically beneficial.[89]

Kava (Piper methysticum)

Kava (*Piper methysticum*) has a long history of both social and medicinal use as a tea and as a ground extract of its root. Several RCTs have been performed investigating the effects of kava on anxiety, producing good evidence that it is efficacious for this condition.[90] A recent comprehensive review of use of kava as a treatment for anxiety found that four out of six studies reviewed found significant improvement in symptoms of generalized anxiety disorder.[90] The mechanism of action appears to be secondary to the kavalactones present in the kava roots, which bind to GABA receptors, antagonize dopamine, inhibit norepinephrine uptake, inhibit monoamine oxidase B, and decrease glutamine release.

Kava dietary supplements are available as tablets, capsules, or powder that is mixed into a drink. Doses range from 50 mg to 240 mg of kavalactones, but the exact dose that is therapeutic is unknown.

Common side effects include headache and gastrointestinal distress. Chronic administration of large amounts can cause an unusual rash, which is reversible.[91] Kava is a potent inhibitor of CYP2E1, CYP1A2, and CYP2D6, so theoretically it may interact with drugs metabolized by these enzymes. There have been many case reports of liver damage following kava use, although it is not clear in how many cases kava was the causative agent. The FDA has issued a warning about possible liver failure associated with use of kava, and this herb should be used with caution.[92]

Conclusion

Most of the botanical compounds discussed in this chapter have been used for centuries, yet little is known about their safety or effectiveness. This issue is particularly important today, as more women are choosing to use dietary supplements and the number of products available in the marketplace is rapidly increasing. Because botanical medicines are classified as dietary supplements, they are largely unregulated. Large variations in the composition of ingredients make it difficult to determine therapeutic doses even when there is evidence of effectiveness. Drug–herb interactions are especially important, as they can potentially cause adverse effects.

There is good evidence that St. John's wort can improve depression, kava can improve symptoms of anxiety, and black cohosh can improve menopausal vasomotor symptoms when used for short periods of time. It also appears that soy from food products may have beneficial effects in treating menopausal symptoms.

Although this chapter focused on the botanical medicines used for specific reproductive health problems, CAM therapies are used for a wide diversity of health problems. The evidence for use of these therapies is conflicting for some products, yet many CAM therapies are effective and safe treatments for specific disorders. The practice of integrative medicine is increasingly important for all health-care providers.

Resources

Organization	Description	Website
National Center for Complementary and Alternative Medicine (NCCAM)	Website has multiple offerings to summarize the effectiveness of CAM therapies. The Herbs at a Glance page includes fact sheets on specific botanicals.	http://nccam.nih.gov
Office of Dietary Supplements, National Institutes of Health	Health information and summary of research on dietary supplements	http://ods.od.nih.gov
Natural Standard	Website was founded by research scientists and clinicians from more than 100 academic institutions throughout the world to provide quality, evidence-based information necessary for safer therapeutic decision making. The CAM information is presented in well-referenced, peer-reviewed, comprehensive monographs. Each monograph on a particular dietary supplement or CAM therapy provides rating scales to help evaluate the research evidence.	https://naturalmedicines.therapeuticresearch.com
Natural Medicine Comprehensive Database	Recognized by many as the gold standard in evidence-based information on natural products. More than 1000 natural products, including botanical products, are covered. This database provides current information on safety, efficacy, mechanism of action, adverse reactions, and interactions with food and drugs.	www.naturaldatabase.com
American Botanical Council (ABC)	Leading providers of science-based information on herbal medicine. ABC also offers the English translation of the Expanded German Commission E Monographs. The Commission E monographs produced by the German government in the 1970s evaluated the safety and efficacy of more than 300 herbal medicines.	www.herbalgram.org
Phytochemical and Ethnobotanical databases	These databases list chemical constituents and ethnobotanical uses of medicinal plants	www.ars-grin.gov/duke

References

1. Eisenberg DM, Davis RB, Ettner SL, et al. Trends in alternative medicine use in the United States, 1990–1997. *JAMA*. 1998;280:1569-1575.
2. Barnes PM, Bloom B, Nahin RL. *Complementary and alternative medicine use among adults and children: United States, 2007*. National Health Statistics Reports, no 12. Hyattsville, MD: National Center for Health Statistics; 2008. http://nccam.nih.gov/sites/nccam.nih.gov/files/news/nhsr12.pdf.
3. White House Commission on Complementary and Alternative Medicine Policy. *Final report*. March 2002. http://www.whccamp.hhs.gov/pdfs/fr2002_document.pdf. Accessed February 5, 2009.
4. Blumenthal M, Goldberg A, Brinkmann J. *Herbal Medicine: Expanded Commission E Monographs*. Austin, TX: American Botanical Council; 2000.
5. Draves AH, Walker SE. Analysis of the hypericin and pseudohypericin content of commercially available St. John's wort preparations. *Can J Clin Pharmacol*. 2003;10:114-118.
6. De Smet PA. Herbal remedies. *N Engl J Med*. 2002;347:2046-2056.
7. Abdualmjid RJ, Sergi C. Hepatotoxic botanicals: an evidence-based systematic review. *J Pharm Pharm Sci*. 2013;16(3):376-404.
8. Bunchorntavakul C, Reddy KR. Herbal and dietary supplement hepatotoxicity. *Aliment Pharmacol Ther*. 2013;37(1):3-17.
9. Tesch BJ. Herbs commonly used by women: an evidence-based review. *Am J Obstet Gynecol*. 2003;188:S44-S52.
10. Izzo AA, Ernst E. Interactions between herbal medicines and prescribed drugs. *Drugs*. 2001;61:2163-2175.
11. Hu Z, Yang X, Ho PC, et al. Herb–drug interactions: a literature review. *Drugs*. 2005;65:1239-1282.
12. Meng Q, Liu K. Pharmacokinetic interactions between herbal medicines and prescribed drugs: focus on drug metabolic enzymes and transporters. *Curr Drug Metab*. 2014;15(8):791-807.
13. Upchurch DM, Chyu L, Greendale GA, et al. Complementary and alternative medicine use among American women: findings from the National Health Interview Survey 2002. *J Womens Health*. 2007;16:102-113.
14. Najm W, Lie D. Dietary supplements commonly used for prevention. *Prim Care Clin Office Pract*. 2008;749-767.
15. Linde K, Berner MM, Kriston L. St. John's wort for major depression. *Cochrane Database Syst Rev*. 2008;4:CD000448. doi:10.1002/14651858.CD000448.pub3.
16. Zhou S, Chan E, Pan SQ, Huang M, Lee EJ. Pharmacokinetic interactions of drugs with St. John's wort. *J Psychopharmacol*. 2004;18:262-276.
17. Foxman B. Epidemiology of urinary tract infections: incidence, morbidity, and economic costs. *Dis Mon*. 2003;49(2):53-70.
18. Wang CH, Fang CC, Chen NC, et al. Cranberry-containing products for prevention of urinary tract infections in susceptible populations: a systematic review and meta-analysis of randomized controlled trials. *Arch Intern Med*. 2012;172(13):988-996.
19. Cravotto G, Boffa L, Genzin, Garella D. Phytotherapeutics: an evaluation of the potential of 1000 plants. *J Clin Pharm Ther*. 2010;35(1):11-48.
20. Jepson RG, Williams G, Craig JC. Cranberries for preventing urinary tract infections. *Cochrane Database Syst Rev*. 2012;10:CD001321. doi:10.1002/14651858.CD001321.pub5.
21. Stapleton AE, Dziura J, Hooton TM, et al. Recurrent urinary tract infection and urinary *Escherichia coli* in women ingesting cranberry juice daily: a randomized controlled trial. *Mayo Clin Proc*. 2012;87(2):143-150.
22. Food and Agriculture Organization (FAO), World Health Organization (WHO). *Health and nutritional properties of probiotics in food including powder milk with live lactic acid bacteria: report of a joint FAO/WHO expert consultation on evaluation of health and nutritional properties of probiotics in food including powder milk with live lactic acid bacteria*. Córdoba, Argentina: WHO; 2001.
23. Barrons R, Tassone D. Use of *Lactobacillus* probiotics for bacterial genitourinary infections in women: a review. *Clin Therapeutics*. 2008;30(3):453-468.
24. Grin PM, Kowalewska PM, Alhazzan W, Fox-Robichaud AE. *Lactobacillus* for preventing recurrent urinary tract infections in women: meta-analysis. *Can J Urol*. 2013;20(1):6607-6614.
25. Reid G, Bruce AW, Aylor M. Instillation of *Lactobacillus* and stimulation of indigenous organisms to prevent recurrence of urinary tract infections. *Microecol Ther*. 1995;23:32-45.
26. Proctor ML, Smith CA, Farquhar CM, Stones RW. Transcutaneous electrical nerve stimulation and acupuncture for primary dysmenorrhea. *Cochrane Database Syst Rev*. 2002;1:CD002123. doi:10.1002/14651858.

27. Sales KJ, Jabbour N. Cyclooxygenase and prostaglandins in pathology of the endometrium. *Reproduction.* 2003;126:559-567.
28. Fine AM. Oligomeric proanthocyanidin complexes: history, structure, and phytopharmaceutical applications. *Altern Med Rev.* 2000;5(2):144-151.
29. Cometa MF, Parisi L, Palmery M, Meneguz A, Tomassini L. In vitro relaxant and spasmolytic effects of constituents from Viburnum prunifolium and HPLC quantification of the bioactive isolated iridoids. *J Ethnopharmacol.* 2009;123(2):201-207.
30. Widén C, Ekholm A, Coleman MD, Renvert S, Rumpunen K. Erythrocyte antioxidant protection of rose hips. (*Rosa* spp.) *Oxid Med Cell Longev.* 2012;2021:621579.
31. Tseng Y, Chen C, Yang Y. Rose tea for relief of primary dysmenorrhea in adolescents: a randomized controlled trial in Taiwan. *J Midwifery Womens Health.* 2005;50(5):e51-e57.
32. Doubova S, Morales H, Hernández S, et al. Effect of a *Psidii guajavae folium* extract in the treatment of primary dysmenorrhea: a randomized clinical trial. *J Ethnopharmacol.* 2007:110;305-10.10.1016/j.jep.2006.09.033.
33. Sande KA, Grema YA, Geidam YM, Bukar-Kolo YM. Pharmacological aspects of *Psidium guajava*: an update. *Int J Pharmacol.* 2011;7:316-324.
34. Dennehy CE. Use of herbs and dietary supplements in gynecology: an evidence-based review. *J Midwifery Womens Health.* 2006;51:402-409.
35. Fugh-Berman A, Kronenberg F. Complementary and alternative medicine (CAM) in reproductive-age women: a review of randomized controlled trials. *Reprod Toxicol.* 2003;17:137-152.
36. Chen SN, Friesen JB, Webster D, et al. Phytoconstituents from *Vitex agnus-castus* fruits. *Fitoterpia.* 2011;82(4):528-533.
37. Wuttke W, Jarry H, Christoffel V, Spengler B, Seidlová-Wuttke D. Chaste tree (*Vitex agnus-castus*) pharmacology and clinical implications. *Phytomedicine.* 2003;10:348-357.
38. van Die MD, Burger HG, Teede HJ, Bone KM. *Vitex agnus-castus* extracts for female reproductive disorders: a systematic review of clinical trials. *Planta Med.* 2013;79(7):562-575.
39. Roemheld-Hamm B. Chasteberry. *Am Fam Phys.* 2005;72:821-824.
40. Daniele C, Kuhn JT, Pittler MH, Ernst E. *Vitex agnus castus*: a systematic review of adverse events. *Drug Saf.* 2005;28:319-332.
41. Atmaca M, Kumru S, Tezcan E. Fluoxetine versus *Vitex agnus castus* extract in the treatment of premenstrual dysphoric disorder. *Hum Psychopharmacol.* 2003;18(3):191-195.
42. Jang SH, Kim DI, Choi MS. Effects and treatment methods of acupuncture and herbal medicine for premenstrual syndrome/premenstrual dysphoric disorder: systematic review. *BMC Complement Altern Med.* 2014;14:11.
43. Canning S, Waterman M, Orsi N, Ayres J, Simpson N, Dye L. The efficacy of *Hypericum perforatum* (St John's wort) for the treatment of premenstrual syndrome: a randomized, double-blind, placebo-controlled trial. *CNS Drugs.* 2010;24(3):207-225.
44. Ghazanfarpour M, Kaviani M, Asadi N, et al. *Hypericum perforatum* for the treatment of premenstrual syndrome. *Int J Gynaecol Obstet.* 2011;113(1);84-85.
45. Di Lorenzo C, Ceschi A, Kupferschmidt H, et al. Adverse effects of plant food supplements and botanical preparations: a systematic review with critical evaluation of causality. *Br J Clin Pharmacol.* 2015;79(4);678-592.
46. Unger M. Pharmacokinetic drug interactions involving Ginkgo biloba. *Drug Metab Rev.* 2013;45(3):353-385.
47. Hardy ML. Herbs of special interest to women. *J Am Pharm.* 2000;40:234-242.
48. Bayles B, Usatine R. Evening primrose oil. *Am Fam Phys.* 2009;80(12):1405-1408.
49. Carmichael AR. Can *Vitex agnus castus* be used for the treatment of mastalgia? What is the current evidence? *Evid Based Complement Alternat Med.* 2008;5(3):247-250.
50. Srivastava A, Mansel RE, Arvind N, Prasad K, Dhar A, Chabra A. Evidence-based management of mastalgia: a meta-analysis of randomised trials. *Breast.* 2007; 16(5):503-512.
51. Basch E, Bent S, Collins J, et al. Flax and flaxseed oil: a review by the Natural Standard Research Collaboration. *Soc Integr Oncol.* 2007;5:92-105.
52. Goss PE, Li T, Theriault M, Pinto S, Thompson LU. Effects of dietary flaxseed in women with cyclical mastalgia. *Breast Cancer Res Treat.* 2000;64:49.
53. King TL, Murphy PA. Nausea and vomiting in pregnancy. *J Midwifery Womens Health.* 2009;54(6):430-444.

54. Abdel-Aziz H, Windeck T, Ploch M, Verspohl EJ. Mode of action of gingerols and shogaols on 5-HT_3 receptors: binding studies, cation uptake by the receptor channel and contraction of isolated guinea-pig ileum. *Euro J Pharmacol.* 2006;530:136-143.
55. Abdel-Aziz H, Nahrstedt A, Petereit F, Windeck T, Ploch M, Verspohl EJ. 5-HT_3 receptor blocking activity of arylalkanes isolated from the rhizome *Zingiber officinalis. Planta Med.* 2005;71(7):609-616.
56. Matthews A, Haas DM, O'Mathúna DP, Dowswell T, Doyle M. Interventions for nausea and vomiting in early pregnancy. *Cochrane Database Syst Rev.* 2014; 3:CD007575. doi:10.1002/14651858.CD007575.pub3.
57. Schwertner HA, Rios DC, Pascoe JE. Variation in concentration and labeling of ginger root dietary supplements. *Obstet Gynecol.* 2006;107(6):1337-1343.
58. Bryer E. A literature review of the effectiveness of ginger in alleviating mild-to-moderate nausea and vomiting of pregnancy. *J Midwifery Womens Health.* 2005;50(1):e1-e3.
59. Westfall RE. Use of anti-emetic herbs in pregnancy: women's choices and the question of safety and efficacy. *Complement Ther Nurs Midwifery.* 2004;10(1):30-36.
60. Bordia A, Verma SK, Srivastava KC. Effect of ginger (*Zingiber officinale Rosc.*) and fenugreek (*Trigonella foenumgraecum L.*) on blood lipids, blood sugar and platelet aggregation in patients with coronary artery disease. *Prostaglandins Leukot Essent Fatty Acids.* 1997;56(5):379-384.
61. McFarlin BL, Gibson MH, O'Rear J, Harman P. A national survey of herbal preparation use by nurse-midwives for labor stimulation: review of the literature and recommendations for practice. *J Nurse-Midwifery.* 1999;44(3):205-216.
62. Burdock GA, Carabin IG, Griffiths JC. Toxicology and pharmacology of sodium ricinoleate. *Food Chem Toxicol.* 2006;44:1689-1698.
63. Azhari S, Pirdadeh S, Lotfalizadeh M, Shakeri MT. Evaluation of the effect of castor oil on initiating labor in term pregnancy. *Saudi Med J.* 2006;27(7): 1011-1014.
64. Kelly AJ, Kavanagh J, Thomas J. Castor oil, bath and/or enema for cervical priming and induction of labour. *Cochrane Database Syst Rev.* 2013;7:CD003099. doi:10.1002/14651858.CD003099.pub2.
65. Dugoua JJ, Perri D, Seely D, Mills E, Koren G. Safety and efficacy of blue cohosh (*Caulophyllum thalictroides*) during pregnancy and lactation. *Can J Clin Pharmacol.* 2008;15:e66-e73.
66. Finkle RF, Zarlengo KM. Blue cohosh and perinatal stroke. *New Engl J Med.* 2004;351:302.
67. Dugoua JJ, Seely D, Perri D, Koren G, Mills E. Safety and efficacy of black cohosh (*Cimicifuga racemosa*) during pregnancy and lactation. *Can J Clin Pharmacol.* 2008;15:e257-e261.
68. Tempfer CB, Bentz EK, Leodolter S, et al. Phytoestrogens in clinical practice: a review of the literature. *Fertil Sterility.* 2007;87:1243-1249.
69. Sacks FM, Lichtenstein A, Van Horn L, et al. Soy protein, isoflavones, and cardiovascular health: an American Heart Association Science Advisory for professionals from the Nutrition Committee. *Circulation.* 2006;113(7):1034-1044.
70. Qin Y, Niu K, Zeng Y, et al. Isoflavones for hypercholesterolaemia in adults. *Cochrane Database Syst Rev.* 2013;6:CD009518. doi:10.1002/14651858.CD009518.pub2. Review. PubMed PMID: 23744562.
71. Dong JY, Tong X, Wu ZW, Xun PC, He K, Qin LQ. Effect of soy protein on blood pressure: a meta-analysis of randomized controlled trials. *Br J Nutr.* 2011;106:317-326.
72. North American Menopause Society. The role of soy isoflavones in menopausal health: report of the North American Menopause Society/Wulf H. Utian Translational Science Symposium in Chicago, IL (October 2010). *Menopause.* 2011;18(7):732-753.
73. Lethaby AE, Marjoribanks J, Kronenberg F, Roberts H, Eden J, Brown J. Phytoestrogens for vasomotor menopausal symptoms. *Cochrane Database Syst Rev.* 2007;4:CD001395. doi:10.1002/14651858.CD001395.pub3.
74. Belanos R, Del Castillo A, Francia J. Soy isoflavones versus placebo in the treatment of climacteric vasomotor symptoms: systemic review and meta-analysis. *Menopause.* 2010;17(3):660-666.
75. Kronenberg F, Fugh-Berman A. Complementary and alternative medicine for menopausal symptoms: a review of randomized controlled trials. *Ann Intern Med.* 2002;137:805-813.
76. Lethaby A, Marjoribanks J, Kronenberg F, Roberts H, Eden J, Brown J. Phytoestrogens for menopausal vasomotor symptoms. *Cochrane Database Syst Rev.* 2013;7:CD001395. doi:10.1002/14651858.CD001395.pub4.

77. Lipovac M, Chedraui P, Gruenhut C, et al. The effect of red clover isoflavone supplementation over vasomotor and menopausal symptoms in postmenopausal women. *Gynecol Endocrinol.* 2012;28(3):207-207.
78. Komesaroff PA, Black CV, Cable V, Sudhir K. Effects of wild yam extract on menopausal symptoms, lipids, and sex hormones in healthy menopausal women. *Climacteric.* 2001;4(2):144-150.
79. Dew TP, Williamson G. Controlled flax interventions for the improvement of menopausal symptoms and postmenopausal bone health: a systematic review. *Menopause.* 2013;20(11):1207-1215
80. Pruthi S, Qin R, Terstreip SA, et al. A Phase III, randomized, placebo-controlled, double-blind trial of flaxseed for the treatment of hot flashes: North Central Cancer Treatment Group No 807. *Menopause.* 2012;19(1):48-53.
81. Dodin S, Lemay A, Jacques H, Légaré F, Forest JC, Mâsse B. The effects of flaxseed dietary supplement on lipid profile, bone mineral density, and symptoms in menopausal women: a randomized, double-blind wheat germ placebo-controlled clinical trial. *J Clin Endocrinol Metab.* 2005;90(3):1390-1397.
82. Wuttke W, Jarry H, Haunschild J, Stecher G, Schuh M, Seidlova-Wuttke D. The non-estrogenic alternative for the treatment of climacteric complaints: black cohosh (*Cimicifuga* or *Actaea racemosa*). *J Steroid Biochem Mol Biol.* 2014;139:302-310.
83. Osmers R, Friede M, Liske E, Schnitker J, Freudenstein J, Henneicke-von Zepelin HH. Efficacy and safety of isopropanolic black cohosh extract for climacteric symptoms. *Obstet Gynecol.* 2005;105:1074-1083.
84. Shams T, Setia MS, Hemmings R, McCusker J, Sewitch M, Ciampi A. Efficacy of black cohosh–containing preparations on menopausal symptoms: a meta-analysis. *Altern Ther Health Med.* 2010;6(1):36-44.
85. Leach MJ, Moore V. Black cohosh (*Cimicifuga* spp.) for menopausal symptoms. *Cochrane Database Syst Rev.* 2012;9:CD007244. doi:10.1002/14651858.CD007244.pub2.
86. Kiefer D, Pantuso T. *Panax ginseng. Am Fam Physician.* 2003;68:1539-1542.
87. Shergis JL, Zhang AL, Zhou W, Xue CC. *Panax ginseng* in randomised controlled trials: a systematic review. *Phytother Res.* 2013;27(7):949-965.
88. Bommer S, Klein P, Suter A. First time proof of sage's tolerability and efficacy in menopausal women with hot flushes. *Adv Ther.* 2011;28(8):490-500.
89. Cancelo Hidalgo MJ, Castelo-Branco C, Blumel JE, Lanchares Pérez JL, Alvarez De Los Heros JI, Isona Study Group. Effect of a compound containing isoflavones, primrose oil, and vitamin E in two different doses on climacteric symptoms. *J Obstet Gynecol.* 2006;26(4):344-347.
90. Sarris J, LaPorte E, Schweitzer I. Kava: a comprehensive review of efficacy, safety, and psychopharmacology. *Aust NZ J Psychiatry.* 2011;45(1):27-35.
91. Couatre DL. Kava kava: examining reports of toxicity. *Toxicol Lett.* 2004;150:85.
92. Ulbricht C, Basch E, Boon H, et al. Safety review of kava (*Piper methysticum*) by the Natural Standard Research Collaboration. *Expert Opin Drug Saf.* 2005;4:779-794.

III Essential Drug Categories

During initial organization of this text, it became apparent that many drugs are specific for the treatment of a selected condition, whereas some drug categories include medications that are used for multiple conditions. Knowledge of the pharmacokinetics and pharmacodynamics of drugs used in many different settings enhances safe and rational prescribing. For example, understanding that a specific category of antibiotics acts by incapacitating bacterial cell wall synthesis enables the clinician not to choose a member of that category when the bacterium in question is *Chlamydia trachomatis*, an obligate intracellular parasite without cell walls. Knowledge that selected antihistamines cause profound sedation can support use of one such medication for mild insomnia and avoidance of the same agent for common allergies. Given that some drug categories are often used for many different indications, it appeared that the same material could be repeated in a number of chapters. Therefore, four chapters are clustered together into this section: *Antimicrobials*, *Analgesia and Anesthesia*, *Antihistamines*, and *Steroid Hormones*.

The *Antimicrobials* chapter includes a discussion of the most common anti-infective medications used and reviews the challenges of drug resistance, especially due to overuse and misuse of these drugs. *Analgesia and Anesthesia* examines drugs that are often used in the primary care arena. The analgesics can be over-the-counter drugs or medications made available by prescription only. Anesthesia may be used in an ambulatory setting as part of treatment for repair of a small laceration or for other procedures.

Antihistamines are an interesting drug family. Drugs in this category may be employed as treatments for such diverse conditions as gastrointestinal diseases, allergies, and sleeping difficulties. For each of these conditions, the basic pharmacologic principles underlying the drugs' mechanism of action remain the same.

Steroid hormones—specifically estrogens, progestins, and androgens—are a staple in a list of drugs used by women for multiple conditions. These compounds may be used as contraceptives, fertility drugs, menopause treatments, or remedies for menstrual irregularities.

11 Antimicrobials

Maureen T. Shannon, Tekoa L. King

Based on the chapter by Anne Marie Mitchell, Barbara J. Lannen, and Marie Daly in the first edition of Pharmacology for Women's Health

Chapter Glossary

Antibiotics (antibacterials) Natural or synthetic substances that destroy bacteria or inhibit their growth.

Antimicrobial stewardship Programs and interventions that monitor antimicrobial use in institutions in an effort to decrease misuse and overuse of antibiotics. These programs use many modalities, such as computer support decision analysis, review and feedback, and formulary restrictions.

Antifungals Agents that destroy or inhibit the growth of fungi.

Anti-infective Agent used to combat infection.

Antimicrobial Agent that destroys or prevents the development of microorganisms.

Antiparasitics Agents that destroy parasites.

Antipseudomonal penicillins Another term for extended-spectrum penicillins, which are primarily used to treat infections from *Pseudomonas aeruginosa*.

Antistaphylococcal penicillins Penicillins that have a bulky side chain, which prevents the bacterial beta-lactamase enzyme from binding to the drug and making it inactive. These penicillins are useful for treating staphylococcal species and streptococcal microorganisms. Also called penicillinase-resistant penicillins.

Antivirals Drugs used to treat viral infections.

Bactericidal Agent that is capable of killing bacteria.

Bacteriostatic Agent that is capable of inhibiting the growth of bacteria.

Beta-lactamase Enzyme that destroys the beta-lactam ring of penicillin-like antibiotics and makes them ineffective.

Broad-spectrum Referring to a penicillin that is effective against a variety of gram-positive and gram-negative organisms.

Concentration-dependent killing Action of a drug that is most effective when present at the site of infection or bacterial target in a concentration equal to or greater than 10 times the minimum inhibitory concentration.

Extended-spectrum Referring to a penicillin that has increased activity against gram-positive and gram-negative organisms.

Gram-negative Referring to bacteria that lose the color of the crystal violet stain and take the color of the red counterstain in Gram's method of staining.

Gram-positive Referring to bacteria that retain the color of the crystal violet stain in Gram's method of staining.

Methicillin-resistant *Staphylococcus aureus* (MRSA) *S. aureus* bacteria that produce altered penicillin-binding proteins to which the antistaphylococcal penicillins such as methicillin are unable to bind.

Minimum inhibitory concentration (MIC) Lowest concentration of an antimicrobial drug that will inhibit visible growth of a microorganism overnight during incubation.

Mycosis Infection caused by fungi.

Penicillin-binding proteins (PBPs) Bacterial enzymes such as transpeptidases to which the penicillins and cephalosporins bind and thereby act on bacterial microorganisms.

Penicillinase Bacterial enzyme that inactivates most penicillins.

Pseudomembranous colitis Colitis associated with antibiotic therapy, which is most often caused by *Clostridium difficile*, a normal part of the intestinal flora, because of disruption of the flora balance by broad-spectrum antibiotics. Symptoms include foul-smelling diarrhea with blood and mucus, cramps, fever, and leukocytosis. Treatment includes discontinuation of the antibiotic responsible and metronidazole therapy.

Selective toxicity Ability of an anti-infective agent to successfully target the cells of a microorganism without also destroying the human host cells.

Time-dependent killing Action of a drug that effectively kills a microorganism when exposed to the bacterial target for a period of time as long as the concentration exceeds the minimum inhibitory concentration for 50% of the dosing interval.

Introduction

In 1929, Sir Alexander Fleming, a Scottish bacteriologist, incubated his agar plates of staphylococci at room temperature and left them uncovered when he went on vacation, thinking they would grow more slowly than when placed at a higher temperature and, therefore, would be mature when he returned. However, when he returned, Fleming observed that the agar plates had a mold growing on them and that the bacteria did not grow near the mold. He named the mold *Penicillium*—and the discovery of modern antimicrobial drugs was launched.[1] Following World War II, penicillin was successfully mass produced by scientists in the United Kingdom and the United States. Streptomycin, chloramphenicol (Chloromycetin), and tetracycline were discovered in the 1940s through the 1950s, and new antibiotics are still being discovered today, albeit more infrequently than in earlier decades.

Antimicrobial drugs are among the most frequently prescribed pharmaceutical agents in the United States. Unfortunately, the development of antimicrobial resistance by pathogenic organisms is increasing rapidly and there is a documented causal relationship between overuse and misuse of anti-infectives and the emergence of antimicrobial-resistant organisms.[2] Many anti-infective agents are prescribed for conditions that do not actually require an anti-infective medication.[3] This chapter reviews the pharmacologic action of anti-infective drugs and presents guidelines for rational prescribing of this class of medication.

The terms **antimicrobial** and **anti-infective** describe all medications that are used for the treatment of infections caused by a variety of living organisms. The pathogen responsible for the infection could be a bacterium, fungus, virus, or protozoan. The antimicrobial drugs commonly called **antibiotics** are subcategorized as **antibacterials**, **antifungals**, **antivirals**, and **antiparasitics** based on the type of organism affected by the drug.

Classification of Bacteria and Other Pathogenic Organisms

The universe of microorganisms is quite diverse. The microbes that can be pathogenic in humans include bacteria, fungi, protozoa, complex organism parasites, and the nonliving obligate intracellular viruses. The primary mechanism of action of all antimicrobial agents is their ability to identify and target the biologic structure or function of a specific microbe that is different from normal cells in the human body, a function called **selective toxicity**.

Bacteria

Bacteria have three characteristics that are both essential for their survival and are different from humans: (1) the unique structure of their cell wall; (2) production of bacterial proteins; and (3) replication of bacterial chromosomes. Antibiotics (from the Latin *anti*, meaning "against," and the Greek *βιοτικός* or *biotikos*, meaning "fit for life") are antimicrobial agents that interfere with the bacterial peptidoglycan cell wall, inhibit protein synthesis, or interfere with bacterial DNA synthesis.

Bacteria are classified and named by their shape, reaction to staining with crystal violet dye, and oxygen requirements. In terms of shape, they are described as spherical (cocci), rod shaped (bacilli), or spiral (spirochetes). Cocci are further subdivided into (1) diplococci, such as those found in pairs like *Neisseria gonorrhoeae*; (2) streptococci, which are cocci found in a chain formation; and (3) staphylococci, which are cocci that exist in clusters.

All bacteria are classified as either gram-positive or gram-negative based on the structure of their cell walls. **Gram-positive** bacteria have a phospholipid bilayer cell membrane and a cell wall that is made of peptidoglycan. Peptidoglycan is composed of long sugar polymers with peptide side chains that form sturdy cross-links, which make the cell wall strong.[4] In contrast, **gram-negative** bacteria have a more complex cell wall structure. The cytoplasmic membrane of gram-negative bacteria is surrounded externally by a thin peptidoglycan wall, with the outermost layer then consisting of another phospholipid bilayer membrane (Figure 11-1). Gram-positive bacteria

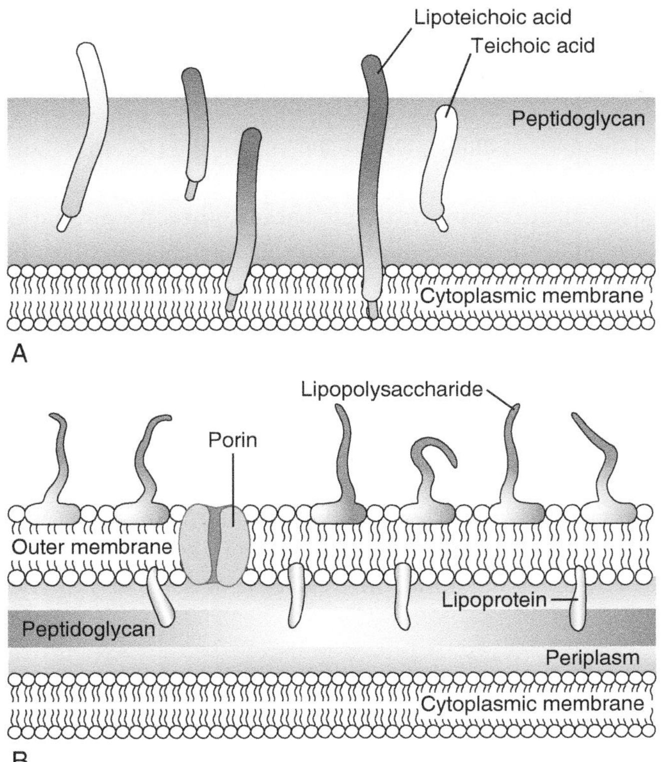

Figure 11-1 (A) Gram-positive cell wall. (B) Gram-negative cell wall.

are so named because the outermost thick cell wall retains dye, causing these bacteria to appear blue or violet when stained with crystal violet dye. Gram-negative bacteria, in contrast, do not retain the crystal violet dye and appear red or pink when stained with a counterstain.[5,6]

Finally, bacteria that use oxygen are called aerobes (e.g., *Mycobacterium tuberculosis*), and bacteria that do not require oxygen are called anaerobes (e.g., *Bacteroides*). Facultative anaerobic bacteria can survive and function with or without oxygen (e.g., group B streptococci).

Chlamydia is unique when compared to the bacteria just addressed because this organism lives within other cells. Originally, this microorganism was thought to be a virus since it is an obligate intracellular pathogen that cannot replicate outside of the host cell. However, scientists determined at the end of the twentieth century that it is more appropriately termed a bacterium. Genotyping within the last decade has revealed that evolution of this species is distinct from other bacteria. Therefore, it is assumed that this microorganism will continue to be termed a bacterium, but will remain in a separate category.

Biofilms are a group of bacteria that stick together, usually on a surface; nevertheless, they can be found in internal spaces as well. Such a community of adherent bacteria forms a matrix of extracellular polymeric substance (EPS) that encloses the community. When bacteria switch from the planktonic to biofilm form of growth, they exhibit different behaviors that reflect changes in genes that are upregulated or downregulated. These changes make the bacteria more resistant to antibiotics. It is estimated that biofilms are responsible for the majority of chronic infections, dental infections, chronic wounds, and catheter- or shunt-associated infections.

Fungi

Fungi include molds and yeasts that consist of filaments (hyphae), which create spores. The major difference between fungal cells and human cells is that the cell membrane of fungi is made of ergosterol instead of cholesterol. Antifungal agents interfere with the production or stability of ergosterol in different ways, thereby damaging fungi without harming adjacent human cells.

Viruses

Viruses (from the Latin *virus*, meaning "toxin or poison") are acellular obligate intracellular organisms made of either RNA or DNA. The viral RNA or DNA is covered by a protein coat called a capsid; the whole unit of viral genetic material and capsids is called a *virion*. Viruses cannot reproduce independenty. Instead, they have a typical life cycle that involves attachment to a host cell, release of the viral genes into the host cell, replication of viral components using host cell mechanisms, assembly of viral components, and then release of viral particles that will infect new host cells. Antiviral medications work by attacking a specific step in this life cycle. The best antivirals attack a viral protein that does not have a function in the human cell.

Parasites

Parasites are organisms that live on or in a host organism and can damage it. Parasites that infect humans range from single-celled organisms, such as protozoa (e.g., *Trichomonas*), to multicellular organisms, such as worms (i.e., helminths). Parasitic disease accounts for a large burden of human morbidity worldwide (e.g., malaria). Antiparasitic drugs are particularly difficult to develop because parasites—as multicellular organisms—share many similarities with human cells.[7]

Mechanism of Action of Antimicrobial Drugs

Antimicrobial drugs are compounds that were first derived from living organisms, specifically molds and plants, although many are now produced synthetically. Antimicrobial drugs work in one of two ways—those that inhibit bacterial growth are **bacteriostatic**, and those that kill bacteria are **bactericidal**. In practice, antimicrobial drugs are classified by their chemical structure and mechanism of action. Most antibiotics (1) attack the cell wall or cell membrane; (2) inhibit or alter protein synthesis; or (3) interfere with DNA replication. A few have other specific mechanisms of action, as shown in Figure 11-2.

Often, antimicrobial action is described on the basis of the **minimum inhibitory concentration (MIC)**, which is the lowest concentration of the antimicrobial drug that will inhibit visible growth of a microorganism overnight during incubation. The MIC is often used to determine bacterial resistance to an antimicrobial drug. Two other important concepts are **time-dependent killing** and **concentration-dependent killing** (Figure 11-3). Antibiotics that bind to their target bacteria for an extended period of time will kill the organism simply because they are present at the site of infection, in a concentration higher than the MIC, for more than 50% of the time within the dosing interval (time-dependent killing). In such a case, persistence of the antimicrobial action after the antimicrobial is removed is minimal. The beta-lactams, clindamycin (Cleocin), macrolides, and linezolid act in this manner. In contrast, aminoglycosides, quinolones, and vancomycin (Vanocin) rely on concentration-dependent killing. These agents work best when they are present in concentrations equal to or higher than 10 times the MIC at the site of their target organism. Interestingly, drugs that function

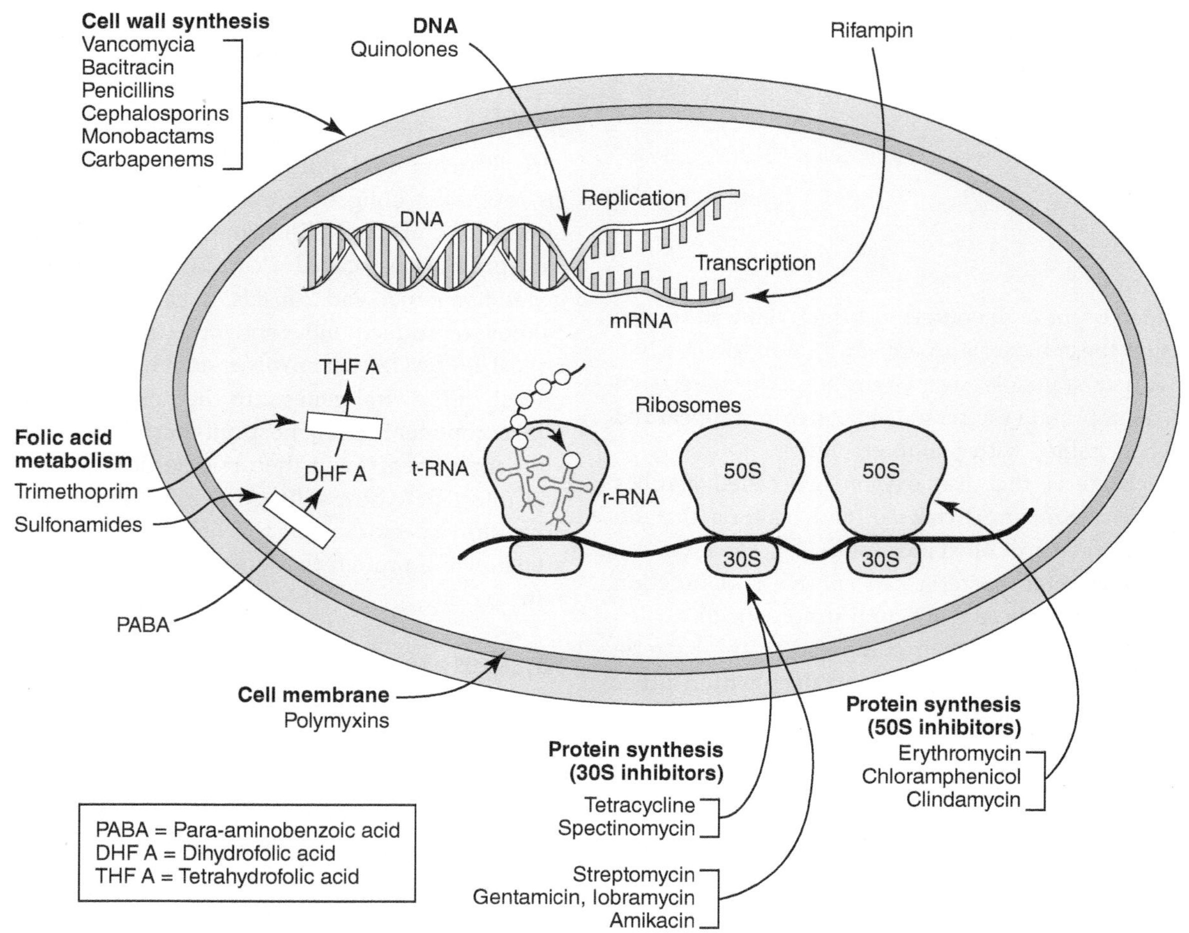

Figure 11-2 Mechanisms of action of common antimicrobial drugs.

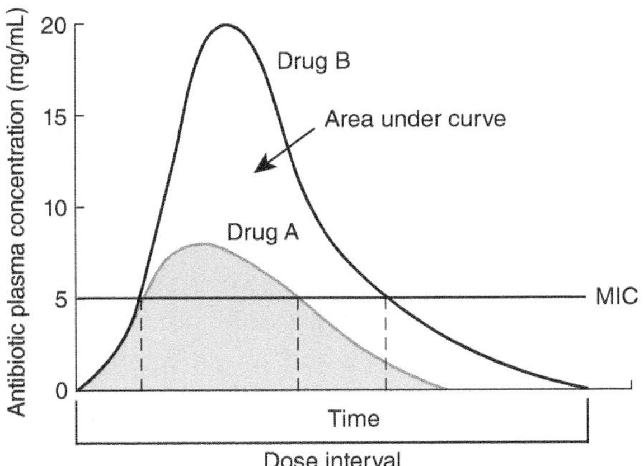

Figure 11-3 Drug A is present at a concentration of at least 5 mg/mL for 50% of the dosing interval which is necessary for time-dependent killing. Drug B reaches a concentration of 20 mg/mL which is 3 times the mean inhibitory concentration. This is needed for concentration-dependent killing.

via concentration-dependent killing often have a post-antibiotic effect, wherein bacteria are killed even though the drug concentration is less than the MIC.

Bacterial Resistance to Antimicrobial Drugs

The phenomenon of antimicrobial resistance is a global concern. Extreme care is necessary when prescribing antimicrobial therapy because overuse and inappropriate use of these agents are well-known causative factors contributing to the rising wave of microbial drug resistance.[8]

Antimicrobial resistance occurs as a result of changes in the genome of microbes that alter their function or structure. This can occur via spontaneous mutation, which generally results in the development of resistance to one drug, or conjugation or horizontal gene transfer, in which one extra-chromosomal DNA is transferred from one microbe to another microbe.[9,10] Conjugation frequently results in the development of multiple-drug resistance. Organisms that develop an alteration in their function or structure that confers resistance will survive exposure to an antimicrobial agent, and will pass this characteristic on to their offspring. In only a short time, a population of microbes that is resistant to antimicrobial agents will then develop. Table 11-1 summarizes the mechanisms of bacterial resistance and resultant effects for antibiotics. Clinical implications for each type of antimicrobial are discussed later in the chapter.

Principles of Rational Antimicrobial Therapy

In 2013, the World Economic Forum asserted that the greatest risk to human health today is antibiotic-resistant bacteria.[11] Antimicrobial resistance has led to increases in severity of disease, length of disease, complications, mortality, and healthcare costs of self-limiting infectious conditions. Incorrect antibiotic prescribing and overprescribing for disorders that do not require antimicrobial treatment are worldwide problems and two of the most important factors promoting antibiotic resistance.[12,13] The clinical development of new antimicrobials is a slow process, making it critical that the effectiveness of the antimicrobials currently in use be preserved.

Many reasons for misuse and overuse of antimicrobials have been identified, including lack of clinical guidelines,

Table 11-1 Mechanisms of Resistance to Antimicrobial Drugs

Action of Antimicrobial Drug	Mechanism of Bacterial Resistance	Example Bacteria That Use This Mechanism of Resistance	Examples of Drugs That Are Affected
Cell membrane alteration	Genetic alterations code for a different structure of the peptidoglycan cell wall to which penicillin cannot bind effectively.	Methicillin-resistant *Staphylococcus aureus, Neisseria gonorrhoeae, Streptococcus pneumoniae*	Penicillins, cephalosporins
Drug inactivation	Bacteria produce an enzyme that breaks down the antibiotic. The classic example is beta-lactamase, which breaks down penicillin and is produced by penicillin-resistant bacteria.	Methicillin-resistant *S. aureus, N. gonorrhoeae, Klebsiella, Bacteroides fragilis*	Penicillins, cephalosporins
Active efflux	Some drugs develop a method to actively pump antibiotic out of the cell before it reaches its internal target.	*Escherichia coli, Pseudomonas aeruginosa*	Tetracycline
Alteration of metabolic pathways	Bacteria develop alternative metabolic pathways that bypass the metabolic step with which the antibiotic interferes.	*E. coli, Klebsiella, Enterobacter, Proteus mirabilis, Proteus vulgaris*	Sulfonamides, trimethoprim

Box 11-1 Hand Hygiene: The Value of Soap

Hands are washed to prevent transmission of pathogenic organisms. But what is in soap? Which soap should be used? How long should one wash their hands? Does the temperature of the water mater? Do antiseptic gels, as an alternative to soap and water, work?

Soap is a cleansing agent made of an esterified fatty acid and sodium or potassium hydroxide; these components have the ability to surround oil particles so they can be dispersed in water. Soaps are also known as antiseptics, and are used to clean living tissue, in contrast to disinfectants that are used as cleansers for inanimate objects. Many soaps now are advertised as antibacterial and these usually contain triclosan. Triclosan is both an antibacterial and an antifungal agent and is present in approximately 75% of commercial soaps.[16] Hand sanitizers are also available; the active ingredient in these products may be isopropyl alcohol, benzalkonium chloride, triclosan, or povidone-iodine.

Although multiple studies have compared regular soap to antibacterial soap, there appears to be no difference between the two types of soaps in decreasing transmission of pathogens.[17] Both will reduce bacterial counts on the hands, but neither eradicates bacteria. Triclosan has been shown to alter hormonal regulation in animals. In addition, there is concern that widespread use of triclosan will foster the development of antibiotic resistance. The Food and Drug Administration (FDA) is currently reviewing the safety and effectiveness of this agent.

Isopropyl alcohol is an effective antibacterial agent that is superior to regular soap and water in eradicating bacteria. Alcohol in the presence of some water denatures proteins, and those hand-cleaning products that contain at least 60% alcohol are most effective.[18]

pressure from consumers, and prescriber ignorance about the best choice of antimicrobial, correct dose, and best duration of therapy.[14,15] Pharmaceutical companies' marketing of broader-spectrum antibiotics may also affect prescribing practices. In light of rapidly expanding bacterial resistance in the United States and globally, a systematic and rational approach to prescribing antimicrobial medications is essential.[11–13]

Rational prescribing maximizes effectiveness, minimizes risks, respects the individual's concerns, considers cost and convenience of administration, and evaluates the risk of antimicrobial resistance. Elements central to this approach that improve prescribing practices include prevention of infection[14–18] (Box 11-1) and slowing resistance via use of the narrowest-spectrum antibiotic that is effective for the shortest duration of treatment that is effective. The steps outlined in Box 11-2 are recommended for prescribers.[19,20]

Antimicrobial Stewardship

Multiple strategies have been instituted for the purpose of standardizing use of antimicrobial drugs. Programs designed to improve antimicrobial prescribing (right drug, dose, duration, and route of administration) to optimize health outcomes while minimizing adverse consequences fall under the umbrella of **antimicrobial stewardship**.[21] Examples include education and guidelines, formulary and restriction strategies, review and feedback, computer-assisted strategies, antimicrobial cycling, scheduled rotation of antimicrobials used in a hospital unit.[22–24] Resources for antimicrobial guidelines and professional association recommendations are listed in the Resources table at the end of this chapter.

Antibiotics That Inhibit Cell Wall Synthesis: Beta-Lactams and Vancomycin

Beta-lactams and vancomycin inhibit cell wall synthesis. The family of beta-lactams includes the penicillins, cephalosporins, carbapenems, and monobactams. Ethambutol also acts on the cell wall, but it is included under the category of antimycobacterial agents. Members of the beta-lactam family share a basic structure that includes a thiazolidine ring attached to a beta-lactam ring, which carries a secondary amino acid group. The beta-lactam ring is a critical element with respect to the antimicrobial activity of penicillin.

Box 11-2 Rational Antimicrobial Prescribing Practices

1. Confirm the presence of an infection through history and physical exam.
2. Identify the pathogen when possible.
3. Confirm the need for an antimicrobial agent.
4. Identify adjunct therapies, including infection control measures.
5. Recognize host factors that may impact pharmacodynamics and assess the individual's concerns and resources.
6. Select an appropriate antimicrobial agent using the dual principles of narrowest spectrum and shortest effective duration possible.
7. Know the pharmacokinetics, pharmacodynamics, and, in some instances, pharmacogenomics of the selected medications.
8. Educate the individual (and family) about appropriate use of antimicrobials, including finishing the full course of treatment and potential interactions with other drugs, food, and botanicals/herbals.
9. Monitor the therapeutic response and any adverse side effects.[1-3]

Sources: Data from Roe V. Antibiotic resistance: a guide for effective prescribing in women's health. *J Midwifery Womens Health*. 2008;53(3):216-226[19]; Waller DG. The science of prescribing. *Br J Clin Pharm*. 2012;74(4):559-560.[20]

Penicillins

Penicillins are bactericidal agents that are either natural (i.e., those developed from mold fermentation, such as penicillin G) or semisynthetic (i.e., those created by altering the structure of another chemical substance). Drugs in the penicillin family are classified on the basis of resistance and their spectrum of activity.

Mechanisms of Action and Spectrum of Activity

Penicillins interfere with the synthesis of the cell walls via the inhibition of **penicillin-binding proteins (PBPs)**[25]—that is, transpeptidases and autolysins. When penicillin binds to these proteins, the synthesis of the peptidoglycan wall is disrupted and cell lysis occurs. Penicillins are effective against gram-positive bacteria that have an exposed peptidoglycan cell wall. Because mammalian cells do not have a cell wall, penicillin has no direct effect on the cells of the human host.

Resistance to Penicillins

Figure 11-4 illustrates the mechanisms that bacteria have developed to incur resistance.[26] With regard to penicillins, these drugs poorly penetrate the intracellular space and, therefore, are ineffective against obligate intracellular organisms such as *Rickettsia* and *Chlamydia*. They are also ineffective against gram-negative bacteria because the peptidoglycan wall in gram-negative bacteria is not exposed to the antibiotic. Some gram-negative bacteria also have pores in the outer membrane that do not allow passage of beta-lactam antibiotics. Other bacteria have efflux pumps that remove the antibiotic from the periplasmic space. Some bacteria, such as *Mycoplasma*, do not make peptidoglycan and therefore, are impervious to the mechanism of action of beta-lactam antibiotics. Bacteria that do have peptidoglycan can alter the form of the peptidoglycan, thereby making the beta-lactam antibiotics ineffective. Finally, bacterial production of the enzymes **beta-lactamase** and **penicillinase** is a common mechanism of resistance. These enzymes break open the beta-lactam ring of the penicillin molecule and render it inactive.[9,27]

Classification of Penicillins

Penicillins are subdivided into four major groups: (1) narrow-spectrum penicillins that are penicillinase sensitive, such as penicillin G; (2) narrow-spectrum penicillins that are penicillinase resistant, such as the antistaphylococcal penicillins; (3) broad-spectrum penicillins, such as the aminopenicillins; and (4) extended-spectrum penicillins that include the antipseudomonal penicillins.

Narrow-Spectrum Penicillins Sensitive to Penicillinase

Table 11-2 lists the indications, doses, and adverse reactions to the most commonly used penicillins. The two natural, narrow-spectrum penicillinase-sensitive penicillin agents used today are benzylpenicillin, also known as penicillin G and penicillin V.

Penicillin G is unstable in an acid environment, and the majority of a dose given orally is destroyed by the strong acids in the stomach. Therefore, penicillin G is administered intravenously or intramuscularly. Procaine penicillin (Bicillin CR) is penicillin G in combination with a local anesthetic (procaine), making it useful for intramuscular injection. Benzathine benzyl penicillin (Bicillin LA) is a form of penicillin G that is slowly absorbed and

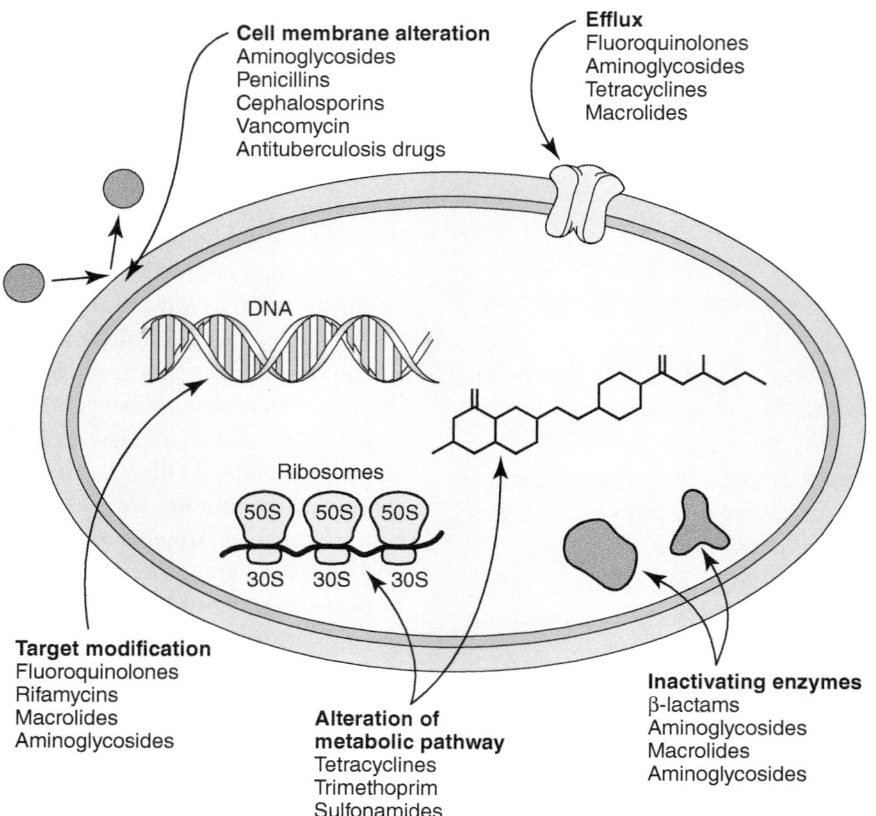

Figure 11-4 Major mechanisms of antimicrobial resistance.

hydrolyzed to penicillin G internally. It is used when prolonged concentrations are required. It is important not to confuse Bicillin CR and Bicillin LA. Bicillin CR contains both penicillin G and procaine. Bicillin LA contains penicillin G only and has a higher dose of the generic penicillin G per formulation. Both Bicillin CR and Bicillin LA are formulated as a total of 600,000 units per mL, 1.2 million units per 2 mL, or 2.4 million units per 4 mL. Both can be used to treat streptococcal infections but only Bicillin LA is approved for treatment of syphilis as the higher dose and longer duration of action is needed to treat the spirochete that causes syphilis. Bicillin CR is not as painful as Bicillin LA when given intramuscularly secondary to the procaine component.

Penicillin V potassium is stable in an acid environment, allowing it to be administered orally. Both injectable and oral formulations are available. This oral formulation may be taken 1 hour before or 2 hours after meals to enhance absorption.

The narrow-spectrum penicillinase-sensitive penicillins are indicated for infections caused by streptococci (e.g., pharyngitis), meningococci, enterococci, penicillin-susceptible pneumococci, and non-beta-lactamase-producing staphylococci. These drugs are also highly effective against spirochetes such as *Treponema pallidum*, *Clostridium* species, *Actinomyces*, group A *Streptococcus*,[28] and other gram-negative rods.

Clinical Indications for Penicillin G and Penicillin V

Penicillin G is used to treat infections such as endocarditis, meningitis (caused by *Neisseria meningitidis*), group B *Streptococcus* sepsis, Lyme disease, listeria, leptospirosis, and syphilis. It is used as prophylaxis to prevent group B *Streptococcus* sepsis in neonates born to women with this pathogen present in their genitourinary tract during labor and birth.

Penicillin V is used to treat tonsillitis, pharyngitis, and scarlet fever, as streptococcal pharyngitis has yet to demonstrate any resistance to penicillin. Penicillin V is also the first choice for prophylaxis against rheumatic fever.

Table 11-2 Penicillins

Penicillin: Generic (Brand)	Indications	Doses	Adverse Reactions	Clinical Considerations
Natural Penicillins				
Benzathine Penicillin G (Bicillin LA)	Syphilis, rheumatic fever, group A streptococcal pharyngitis	600,000–1.2 million U as single dose	Anaphylaxis, hypersensitivity reactions	Dose lasts 2–4 weeks. Do not give IV or SQ. Do not give concomitantly with tetracyclines.
Penicillin G Benzathine with procaine (Bicillin CR)	Moderate to severe upper respiratory infections, skin infection, soft-tissue infection, diphtheria	600,000–1.2 million U/day	Hypersensitivity occurs in 10–15% of individuals; risk of reaction is highest when combined with procaine and administered IM	Only parenteral PCN in use in outpatient settings. Reduce dose if renal impairment and hepatic disease occur. Do not give concomitantly with tetracyclines.
Penicillin G potassium (Pfizerpen)	Bacterial endocarditis, pneumococcal pneumonia, GBS, prophylaxis for laboring women	8–24 million units/day in divided doses	Anaphylaxis, hypersensitivity reactions	Do not give concomitantly with tetracyclines.
Penicillin V	Minor infections—drug of choice for group A beta-hemolytic *Streptococcus* Prophylaxis for rheumatic fever	2–4 g/day in divided doses—e.g., 500 mg every 4 hours	Low incidence of adverse reactions	May be taken with or without food. Do not give concomitantly with tetracyclines.
Penicillinase-Resistant Penicillins				
Cloxacillin (Cloxapen)	Treatment of soft-tissue infections caused by penicillinase-producing staphylococci that have demonstrated susceptibility to the drug	250–500 mg every 6 hours	High dose is associated with seizures and encephalopathy Thrombophlebitis has occurred with IV administration	Food interferes with absorption.
Dicloxacillin (Dynapen)		125–500 mg every 6 hours	Anaphylaxis, hypersensitivity reactions	Food interferes with absorption.
Nafcillin (Unipen)	Treatment of infections due to penicillinase-producing staphylococci	500 mg–1 g IV every 4–6 hours	Anaphylaxis, hypersensitivity reactions	Food interferes with absorption.
Oxacillin (Bactocill)		250–500 mg PO every 4–6 hours, 1–2 g IV every 4–6 hours; maximum of 9 g/day	Anaphylaxis, hypersensitivity reactions	Dose of oxacillin must be modified for persons with renal insufficiency.
Aminopenicillins				
Ampicillin[a]	Group B *Streptococcus faecalis*, *Proteus mirabilis*, *E. coli*, *Salmonella*, *Shigella*, *Haemophilus influenzae*	4–12 g/day IV, 250–500 mg every 6 hours PO	Rashes, diarrhea most common; also urticaria, nausea, vomiting	Assess for pseudomembranous colitis if diarrhea persists.
Amoxicillin (Amoxil)[a]	Not effective against *S. aureus*; used for acute otitis media, sinusitis	250–500 mg every 8 hours	Most common side effects are rash and diarrhea—less diarrhea than with ampicillin	Take on an empty stomach. Amoxicillin is more acid resistant than ampicillin and blood levels are greater; therefore, it is preferred when oral therapy is indicated.
Extended-Spectrum Penicillins				
Carbenicillin indanyl (Geocillin)	Same organisms susceptible to aminopenicillins plus *Pseudomonas aeruginosa*, *Enterobacter* species, *Proteus*, *Bacteroides fragilis*, and *Klebsiella*	1.5–3 g/day	Anaphylaxis, hypersensitivity reactions	Taken off the market in the United States.
Piperacillin/tazobactam (Zosyn)		12–24 g/day	Diarrhea, rashes, pain at IV site, confusion, dizziness, lethargy, constipation, nausea, vomiting, urticaria	Assess for pseudomembranous colitis (*C, difficile*) if diarrhea persists.
Ticarcillin (Ticar)		200–300 mg/kg/day; 12–24 g/day	Symptoms of sodium overload (CHF), interferes with platelet function and can promote bleeding	Should not be mixed with aminoglycosides in same IV solution.

Abbreviations: CHF = congestive heart failure; GBS = group B *Streptococcus*; PCN = penicillin.

[a] Epstein-Barr infection, acute lymphocytic leukemia, or cytomegalovirus infection increases the risk of developing ampicillin rash to approximately 60%.

Narrow-Spectrum Penicillins Resistant to Penicillinase

The second major category of penicillins, the narrow-spectrum penicillins resistant to penicillinase, also called **antistaphylococcal penicillins**, are characterized by a bulky attachment to the R side chain that prevents the bacterial beta-lactamase enzyme from binding to them. These semisynthetic penicillins are active against most staphylococcal species and streptococci microorganisms, but are not effective against the gram-positive enterococci, anaerobic bacteria, and gram-negative cocci and rods. Therefore, antistaphylococcal penicillin agents have a narrow spectrum of activity. Drugs in this category include cloxacillin (Cloxapen), dicloxacillin (Dynapen), nafcillin (Unipen), and oxacillin (Bactocill). Cloxacillin and dicloxacillin are administered orally and are appropriate for the treatment of mild to moderate localized staphylococcal infections.

Methicillin is an antistaphylococcal penicillin that is no longer commercially available. Approximately 30% of the population in the United States is colonized with *S. aureus*, and 1% are colonized with **methicillin-resistant *Staphylococcus aureus* (MRSA)**,[29] which is a growing clinical problem. Resistance to penicillin appears to result from production of altered PBPs to which the drugs are unable to bind. MRSA infections are categorized as community-associated or healthcare-associated diseases. Community-associated MRSA infections are predominately skin infections that manifest as abscesses, boils, or other pus-filled lesions. Currently, trimethoprim–sulfamethoxazole (Bactrim, Septra), clindamycin (Cleocin), tetracycline, and linezolid (Zyvox) are recommended for the treatment of dermatologic infections that are likely caused by MRSA (Box 11-3).[30,31] Healthcare-associated MRSA is an invasive infection most often seen

Box 11-3 Methicillin-Resistant *Staphylococcus Aureus*

MRSA is a strain of *S. aureus* that is resistant to all beta-lactam antibiotics, including those with beta-lactamase inhibitor combinations, such as ampicillin claviculate (Augmentin). Infections with this pathogen are categorized as either healthcare-associated MRSA (HA-MRSA) or community-associated MRSA (CA-MRSA).

Historically, HA-MRSA accounted for 90% of all MRSA infections. It is associated with a recent hospitalization and is more likely to occur in the elderly, African Americans, persons with open wounds or weakened immune systems, and men. Vancomycin has been the standard antibiotic used for treatment of HA-MRSA.

CA-MRSA is not associated with a recent hospitalization and is unfortunately becoming more common. In the United States, approximately 50% of all pigs and pig farmers carry MRSA. Consequently, there is concern that MRSA is becoming more prevalent and that animal sources may become an important reservoir for this pathogen. It is theorized that the large amounts of antibiotics used in pig farming (to keep the pigs healthy) may inadvertently create ideal incubators for breeding bacteria that are resistant to antibiotics. MRSA is a good example of this type of bacterium.

Approximately 75% of persons with CA-MRSA have a soft-tissue infection such as a furuncle (boil), cellulitis, impetigo, report of spider bite, or infected wound. Consequently, this condition should be part of the differential diagnosis for all soft-tissue infections seen in the outpatient setting. These soft-tissue infections form abscesses quite often. CA-MRSA strains are more virulent than HA-MRSA strains and can progress to toxic shock syndrome, sepsis, or necrotizing pneumonia.

The diagnosis of CA-MRSA can be made if the culture is positive for MRSA, and if the individual does not have a medical history of MRSA infection and does not have an indwelling catheter or other medical device that passes through the skin into the body. In addition, to warrant this diagnosis, the person in question will not have any of the following within the previous year: (1) hospitalization; (2) admission to a nursing home, skilled nursing facility, or hospice; (3) dialysis; or (4) surgery.[29]

The initial treatment is always incision, culture, and drainage. If incision and drainage are not possible or not considered sufficient treatment, the antibiotic recommendation for CA-MRSA is guided by the susceptibility of the cultured organism. If empiric therapy is started prior to knowledge of culture results, trimethoprim–sulfamethoxazole (Bactrim, Septra), 1–2 double-strength tablets every 8 to 12 hours, and clindamycin, 300 mg by mouth 4 times a day for 14 days, are the best first choices for women of childbearing age. Doxycycline (Vibramycin) can be used but is contraindicated for children and pregnant women. Linezolid (Zyvox) is the "big gun" that will eradicate CA-MRSA, but it has potential for antibiotic resistance, is expensive, and should not be used for outpatient empiric treatment.

in persons who have been hospitalized and have some degree of immunocompromise. Vancomycin (Vanocin) is the mainstay treatment of choice for hospital-associated MRSA infections, but current guidelines also suggest linezolid, daptomycin (Cubicin), and clindamycin can be used for this indication.[30,31]

Clinical Indications for Penicillinase-Resistant Penicillins (Antistaphylococcal Penicillins)

The primary use of antistaphylococcal penicillins is for treatment of cellulitis and soft-tissue infections caused by *S. aureus*. Dicloxacillin (Dynapen) has been and remains the first choice for treatment of lactational mastitis.[32] However, if any soft-tissue infection has signs that suggest MRSA is the etiologic agent, or if the individual is at risk for being infected with MRSA, then the first-choice treatment is an agent that is effective against MRSA.

Broad-Spectrum Penicillins

The two **broad-spectrum** penicillins in use today are the aminopenicillins known as ampicillin and amoxicillin (Amoxil). These agents are able to penetrate the porin channel in the outer cell membrane of gram-negative bacteria, but are susceptible to beta-lactamase. They are generally effective against the same bacterial strains as penicillin G, but have additional coverage against certain gram-negative bacteria, including *Haemophilus influenzae, Escherichia coli, Proteus mirabilis*, and enterococci.

Broad-spectrum penicillins can be administered either orally or intravenously. Amoxicillin (Amoxil) is the preferred oral agent because it is more acid resistant, resulting in greater absorption and higher plasma levels. It can be given 3 times per day rather than 4 times per day and is less likely to cause diarrhea when compared to ampicillin.

Combination aminopenicillins that consist of a beta-lactamase inhibitor and an aminopenicillin are also available. Such a combination allows the antimicrobial spectrum to be extended to include beta-lactamase-producing strains of bacteria. Amoxicillin in combination with clavulanic acid is an oral preparation that is effective against beta-lactamase-producing *S. aureus, N. gonorrhoeae, H. influenzae, E. coli, S. pneumoniae*, enterococci, and *Moraxella catarrhalis*. A combination of ampicillin and sulbactam (Unasyn) has similar benefits but is only used parenterally.[34]

Clinical Indications for Broad-Spectrum Penicillins

Ampicillin and amoxicillin are prescribed for the treatment of upper respiratory infections, pneumonia, sinusitis, uncomplicated urinary tract infections, orthopedic infections, gastrointestinal disorders, and many genital tract infections. They are the drugs of choice for meningococcal meningitis. Amoxicillin is also the drug of choice for infectious or subacute bacterial endocarditis prophylaxis. Box 11-4 provides the American Heart Association guidelines for this indication.[33]

Extended-Spectrum Penicillins

The three **extended-spectrum** penicillins available in the United States are ticarcillin (Ticar), carbenicillin indanyl (Geocillin), and piperacillin. The drugs in this category also are classified as **antipseudomonal penicillins** because they are primarily used, in combination with an aminoglycoside, to treat infections with *Pseudomonas aeruginosa*—infections that are particularly difficult to eradicate. Ticarcillin and piperacillin are limited to parenteral use only. Combination formulations that include beta-lactamase inhibitors—ticarcillin plus clavulanate (Timentin) and piperacillin plus tazobactam (Zosyn)—are also available. However, these drugs should not be mixed in the same intravenous solution, as inactivation may occur under those circumstances.

Metabolism

Metabolism of the penicillins varies greatly depending on the route of administration, stability, and protein binding capacity. Oral dicloxacillin (Dynapen), ampicillin, and amoxicillin (Amoxil) are well absorbed by the gastrointestinal tract. Intravenous administration results in rapid absorption and wide distribution to body tissues. Intramuscular administration is clinically effective; however, pain and local irritation at the injection site may prompt the provider to select an alternative route. Most of the penicillins are excreted as unchanged drugs through the kidneys. Elimination is rapid, so that the half-lives of penicillins are typically 30 to 90 minutes.

Side Effects and Adverse Reactions

Penicillins are generally nontoxic. The most common side effects of broad-spectrum penicillins are rash, nausea, vomiting, and diarrhea. These reactions occur more frequently with ampicillin than with any other penicillin. A nonpruritic maculopapular rash is quite common in children who take ampicillin or amoxicillin. It is frequently assumed to be a penicillin allergy, but, in fact, if the rash is nonpruritic, it is not a true hypersensitivity reaction. Persons who report ampicillin rash may be able to take penicillins subsequently without experiencing real allergic reactions.[35] Prolonged use has been implicated in the occurrence of secondary vaginal candidiasis infections due in large part to

Box 11-4 Infectious Endocarditis Prophylaxis Guidelines

The American Heart Association does not recommend routine prophylaxis for dental or other procedures. However, prophylaxis is recommended for individuals in the following circumstances:

- Presence of a prosthetic cardiac valve or prosthetic material used for cardiac valve repair
- History of previous infectious endocarditis
- Cyanotic congenital heart disease, completely repaired congenital heart disease with prosthetic material in first 6 months of life, or partially repaired congenital heart disease with residual defect
- Cardiac transplantation recipients developing cardiac valvulopathy

Subacute bacterial endocarditis (SBE) prophylaxis is recommended only for the following procedures:

- Invasive respiratory procedures (e.g., bronchoscopy)
- Dental procedures: Gingival or periapical region of teeth manipulated or oral mucosa perforated

When needed, the recommendation is amoxicillin 2 g given 30 to 60 minutes prior to the procedure if given intravenously and 1 hour prior to the procedure if given by mouth.

If the person receiving the drug is allergic to penicillin, the following alternatives may be used:

- Clindamycin (Cleocin) 600 mg by mouth 1 hour before the procedure or 600 mg intravenously 30 minutes before the procedure
- Cephalexin (Keflex) or cefadroxil (Duricef) 2 g by mouth 1 hour before the procedure
- Cefazolin (Ancef) or ceftriaxone (Rocephin) 1.0 g intramuscularly/intravenously 30 minutes before the procedure
- Azithromycin (Zithromax) or clarithromycin (Biaxin) 500 mg by mouth 1 hour before the procedure

Source: Data from Wilson W, Taubert KA, Gewitz M, et al. Prevention of infective endocarditis: guidelines from the American Heart Association: a guideline from the American Heart Association Rheumatic Fever, Endocarditis, and Kawasaki Disease Committee, Council on Cardiovascular Disease in the Young, and the Council on Clinical Cardiology, Council on Cardiovascular Surgery and Anesthesia, and the Quality of Care and Outcomes Research Interdisciplinary Working Group. *Circulation.* 2007;116(15):1736-1754.[33]

the failure to reestablish the normal lactobacilli-dominated vaginal flora following antimicrobial therapy.

Serious adverse effects of penicillins include allergic reactions, dermatologic reactions such as photosensitivity or morbilliform rash, and, more rarely, Stevens-Johnson syndrome or exfoliative dermatitis. Other adverse effects include encephalopathy, seizures, hepatitis, renal disorders such as interstitial nephritis, and hematologic disorders such as neutropenia or hemolytic anemia.

Ampicillin has been linked to development of pseudomembranous colitis. Thus, individuals presenting with a history of colitis or serious episodes of diarrhea associated with anti-infective therapy should be evaluated for **pseudomembranous colitis**—a condition often called *C. diff* because it is most frequently caused by an overgrowth of *Clostridium difficile.* Individuals with renal failure are vulnerable to seizures when penicillin is given in high doses; therefore, kidney function tests should be monitored in persons who have impaired renal function. Persons with hepatic impairment also require monitoring of liver function.

Allergic Reactions to Penicillins

Penicillin allergy is reported in approximately 8% of individuals who access healthcare services in the United States, yet only 10% of these persons have an actual immunopathologic allergy.[36] Although the World Allergy Organization's classification of immediate versus delayed reaction is generally used for classifying penicillin allergy reactions,[37] penicillins can actually cause any of the four types of allergic immunologic hypersensitivity reactions reviewed in the *Drug Toxicity* chapter. Type I hypersensitivity and Type IV delayed cutaneous reactions are the most common (Table 11-3). Immediate hypersensitivity reactions occur within 1 hour of administration and range from urticaria or angioedema to bronchospasm and anaphylaxis, which occurs in approximately 1 out of 10,000 administrations.[38] Accelerated reactions occur 1 to 72 hours after administration and include blood dyscrasias such as hemolytic anemia. Late reactions usually occur more than 72 hours after administration and can range from maculopapular rash to serum sickness or drug fever.[39]

Table 11-3 Penicillin Allergic Reactions: Mechanism of Action

Classification	Mechanism of Action	Time of Onset After Administration	Clinical Symptoms
Type I (immediate)	Penicillin-specific IgE antibodies bind to mast cells with release of histamine and inflammatory mediators	Within minutes to 1 hour	Urticaria, erythema or pruritus, hypotension, angioedema, bronchospasm, hypotension or shock, anaphylaxis
Type II (non-immediate; accelerated)	Cytotoxic response of IgG or IgM antibodies directed at drug–hapten-coated cells	Variable: 1 hour to 72 hours	Blood cell dyscrasias (hemolytic anemia, neutropenia, thrombocytopenia)
Type III (non-immediate)	Immune complex reaction: tissue deposition of drug–antibody complex with complement activation and inflammation	7–10 days	Serum sickness, fever, rash, arthralgias, lymphadenopathy, urticaria, glomerulonephritis, vasculitis
Type IV (delayed)	Cell-mediated response to T cells with cytokine and inflammatory mediator release	2–21 days	Allergic contact dermatitis, eczema, maculopapular, bullous, or pustular exanthema

Sources: Data from Demoly P, Romano A. Update on beta-lactam allergy diagnosis. Curr *Allergy Asthma Rep*. 2005;5(1):9-14.[39]; Napoli DC, Neeno TA. Anaphylaxis to benzathine penicillin G. *Pediatr Asthma Allergy Immunol*. 2000;14(4):329-332[38]; Solensky R, Khan DA. Drug allergy: an updated practice parameter. *Ann Aller Asthma Immunol*. 2010;105(4):259-273.[41]

Cross-Reactivity

Cross-reactivity is the term applied when a drug not previously given triggers a hypersensitivity reaction in an individual. Cross-reactivity can occur when two drugs have a common antigenic stimulus that elicits the hypersensitivity reaction. It is common between penicillins and cephalosporins, as both have the same beta-lactam core and R1 side chain.

The story of cephalosporin's cross-reactivity with penicillin allergy is interesting. The cephalosporin mold produces some penicillin-like compounds, so many early cephalosporin antibiotics actually contained traces of penicillin. In persons with a true immunoglobulin E (IgE)–type hypersensitivity reaction to penicillin, the incidence of cross-reactivity to first-generation cephalosporins ranges from 1% to 10.9% depending on the specific drug combinations.[40] When a cephalosporin is required for an individual who reports a penicillin allergy, penicillin skin testing is often undertaken to tailor the therapy. Persons who are skin-test negative can be safely given any cephalosporin. If the skin test is positive, an alternative drug can be used or desensitization to the cephalosporin can be performed. Table 11-4 reviews recommendations for administering cephalosporins to persons who report a penicillin allergy if penicillin skin testing is not available.[41,42]

It appears the R1 side chain is the primary determinant of cross-reactivity.[40-42] Ampicillin and amoxicillin (Amoxil) in particular have the same R1 side chain as some of the first- and second-generation cephalosporins (Table 11-5). Therefore, in addition to the clinical recommendations listed in Table 11-4, persons with an allergy to ampicillin or amoxicillin should avoid those first- and second-generation cephalosporins that have the same R1 side chains.[41,42]

Treatment of Persons Who Are Allergic to Penicillin

In persons with an established allergic response to penicillin, alternative options can often be found. However, the incidence of cross-allergenicity within the same drug class or among drugs that contain similar structural similarities, specifically first- and second-generation cephalosporins, occurs in approximately 1% to 20% of individuals with confirmed penicillin reactions.

Table 11-4 Use of Cephalosporins in Persons with a History of Penicillin Allergy

History	Clinical Recommendation
Penicillin reaction more than 10 years prior and/or reaction did not include symptoms of IgE-mediated hypersensitivity	Give cephalosporin as indicated. A reaction within 24 hours may occur in fewer than 1% of individuals.
Penicillin reaction occurred within 10 years and/or reaction included symptoms of IgE-mediated hypersensitivity	Give cephalosporin by graded challenge.[a] A reaction within 24 hours may occur in fewer than 1% of individuals.
History of anaphylaxis to penicillin	Desensitize to cephalosporin.

[a] Graded challenge: Tenfold increasing doses are given every 30–60 minutes until the recommended dose is administered. The starting dose is usually 1/100 or 1/10 of the full dose.

Sources: Data from Khan DA, Solensky R. Drug allergy. *J Allergy Clin Immunol*. 2010;125(2 suppl 2):S126-S137[42]; Solensky R, Khan DA. Drug allergy: an updated practice parameter. *Ann Aller Asthma Immunol*. 2010;105(4):259-273.[41]

Table 11-5 Penicillins and Cephalosporins with Identical R1 Side Chains

Penicillin: Generic (Brand)	Cephalosporin: Generic (Brand)
Amoxicillin (Amoxil)	Cefaclor (Ceclor)
Ampicillin	Cefadroxil (Duricef)
	Cefatrizine
	Cefprozil (Cefizil)
	Cephalexin (Keflex)
	Cephaloglycin (Kefglycin)
	Cephradine (Velosef)

Sources: Data from Campagna JD, Bond MC, Schabelman E, Hayes BD. The use of cephalosporins in penicillin-allergic patients: a literature review. *J Emerg Med.* 2012;42(5):612-620[40]; Khan DA, Solensky R. Drug allergy. *J Allergy Clin Immunol.* 2010;125(2 suppl 2):S126-S137[42]; Solensky R, Khan DA. Drug allergy: an updated practice parameter. *Ann Aller Asthma Immunol.* 2010;105(4):259-273.[41]

Approximately 90% of individuals who have experienced a severe allergic reaction to penicillin stop expressing penicillin-specific IgE over time. Skin testing with major and minor determinants of penicillin can determine which persons are currently at high risk for an allergic reaction. Major determinants are available commercially; they can identify 90% to 97% of currently allergic individuals, but caution must be exercised because 3% to 10% of such persons will still be missed without the full range of testing.[43]

When a woman is pregnant, there are no proven alternatives to penicillin for treating her if she has neurosyphilis or syphilis. When necessary, desensitization can be achieved in highly sensitive persons. The Centers for Disease Control and Prevention (CDC) has published guidelines for desensitizing individuals with a history of penicillin allergy.[44] This procedure is performed by administering small, gradually increasing amounts of penicillin V, orally or intravenously. After desensitization, the individual is maintained on penicillin for the course of therapy.

Drug–Drug Interactions

In general, drug–drug interactions with penicillin are uncommon. Probenecid (Benemid) slows tubular excretion of penicillin, thereby increasing plasma levels. Historically, probenecid was used when penicillin was indicated to treat persons with gonorrhea to prolong blood levels of penicillin and thereby augment therapy. Methotrexate (Rheumatrex), aspirin, and indomethacin (Indocin) can also potentially slow tubular secretion, although the clinical implications of such interactions are not clear. The combined use of bactericidal and bacteriostatic antibiotics can result in antagonism; thus, if taken concomitantly with penicillin, tetracycline (Achromycin), chloramphenicol (Chloromycetin), and other bacteriostatic drugs may decrease the bactericidal action of penicillin. Penicillin and ampicillin can increase bleeding when coadministered with warfarin (Coumadin).[45] Penicillin can decrease clearance of methotrexate (Rheumatrex), causing a risk for toxicity of this antifolate drug. Cholestyramine (Questran) decreases absorption and, therefore, the effects of oral penicillins. Neomycin can decrease absorption of penicillin V.

Evidence regarding penicillin and its effect on combination oral contraceptives is contradictory. Oral estrogens undergo hepatic metabolism to form conjugates that gastrointestinal flora then hydrolyze. This process allows for reabsorption of estrogens and maintenance of their pharmacologic effect. The alteration of gastrointestinal flora that occurs with the use of antibiotics can result in breakthrough bleeding and pregnancies. The estimated likelihood of this interaction is rare (approximately 1%), so the recommendation to counsel women about the potential for oral contraceptive failure remains controversial. In addition, it is difficult to link contraceptive failure directly to penicillin use because no oral contraceptive is 100% efficacious.[45] To date, the only antibiotics that have been shown to definitively decrease the effectiveness of oral contraceptives are rifampin (Rifadin) and griseofulvin (Grifulvin V). A number of other antibiotics, including penicillins, have been linked to unintended pregnancy anecdotally or in retrospective surveys, but prospective, randomized controlled trials have not been undertaken to confirm this connection. A true drug interaction may occur in a small subset of women, so most experts agree that the conservative approach is to advise use of an additional nonhormonal contraceptive method while taking any antibiotic.

Special Populations: Pregnancy, Lactation, and the Elderly

Animal studies have not revealed any fetal risks associated with use of penicillin during pregnancy. Penicillin crosses the placenta and can be found in amniotic fluid soon after administration. It is the drug of choice for treating penicillin-susceptible infections during pregnancy. Penicillin in general penetrates breast milk, with peak levels occurring about 6 hours after the drug is taken. Breastfeeding infants should subsequently be observed for any gastrointestinal upset, candidiasis, or allergic response, although major adverse effects have not been noted.

Some parenteral penicillins have higher sodium content and may need to be monitored in elderly persons if those individuals have or are at risk for cardiac and renal conditions. Evidence suggests that infections in general may be linked to atherosclerosis and thrombosis, which are more common as we age. Assuming this phenomenon truly exists, it is theorized that use of antibiotics may have a prophylactic effect. One study found that recent use of penicillin decreased stroke by 19% in elderly subjects on antihypertensive therapy (relative risk [RR] = 0.81; 95% confidence interval [CI], 0.70–0.94).[46]

Cephalosporins

Cephalosporins are semisynthetic beta-lactam antibiotics that are structurally similar to penicillins in many respects. These compounds contain a beta-lactam ring that is primarily responsible for their antimicrobial activity. However, the cephalosporins are less susceptible to cleavage by beta-lactamases than are the penicillins, and they have two sites that can be modified, which accounts for the larger number of agents in this class that have been developed for clinical use.

Cephalosporins, which were isolated from the fungus *Cephalosporium* shortly after penicillins were discovered, are categorized into five generations (Table 11-6). Progression from the first through the fourth generation reveals increased activity against gram-negative bacteria and anaerobes, better resistance to the destructive effects of beta-lactamase, and improved ability to penetrate the central nervous system. The cephalosporins' toxicity is low, and these drugs are among the most widely prescribed antibiotics. They are often used to treat respiratory tract infections, skin infections, endocarditis prevention, meningitis, gonorrhea, and some gastrointestinal illnesses.

Mechanism of Action and Spectrum of Activity

The cephalosporins are bactericidal and inhibit cell wall synthesis of microorganisms. As with penicillins, this action involves cephalosporins binding with the PCPs, impairing construction of the bacterial cell wall and lysis of the cell wall through activation of autolysin.

Unique properties of individual cephalosporins are determined by changes made to the structure of the cephalosporin formula. These agents are active against most gram-positive bacteria. The first-generation cephalosporins have the strongest activity against those gram-positive bacteria susceptible to this class of antibiotic—an important concept to remember when choosing one for specific infections. Each generation of cephalosporins has a broader spectrum of activity against aerobic gram-negative bacteria, but each generation also has less activity against gram-positive bacteria. Collectively, these agents have limited activity against anaerobes. In general, older first-generation formulations are less expensive but have a narrower antimicrobial spectrum of activity than the more recently developed agents.

Cephalosporins of any generation do not have appreciable activity against a number of common organisms, including penicillin-resistant *Pneumococcus*, MRSA, *Staphylococcus epidermidis*, *Enterococcus*, *Listeria*, *Mycoplasma*, *Campylobacter*, and intracellular organisms such as *Chlamydia pneumoniae* and *Chlamydia trachomatis*.

Mechanism of Resistance

Resistance to cephalosporins occurs via the same mechanisms that confer resistance to penicillins.

First-Generation Cephalosporins

The primary employment of first-generation cephalosporins is to treat skin and soft-tissue infections. Cefazolin (Ancef, Kefzol), a first-generation parenteral antibiotic, is often given prophylactically for surgical procedures such as a planned cesarean birth. These drugs should not be used for the treatment of respiratory infections because they are not active against *H. influenzae*. First-generation cephalosporins should not be prescribed for serious systemic infections because of their limited spectrum of activity.[47]

Second-Generation Cephalosporins

Second-generation cephalosporins are active against the organisms that are affected by first-generation drugs but interestingly, in the case of cefotetan (Cefotan) and cefoxitin (Mefoxin), less so because these two agents have an additional methoxy group that results in diminished activity against staphylococci and streptococci. Second-generation cephalosporins can be used to treat some aerobic and facultative gram-negative bacteria such as *E. coli*, *K. pneumoniae*, and *P. mirabilis*. These agents are also active against beta-lactamase-producing strains of *H. influenzae* and *M. catarrhalis* as well as *Streptococcus pneumoniae*. Second-generation cephalosporins are indicated for the treatment of sinusitis, otitis, and lower respiratory tract infections. In addition, they may be useful in treating peritonitis, diverticulitis, and pelvic infections.

Table 11-6 Cephalosporins[a]

Cephalosporin: Generic (Brand)	Indications	Dose	Route	Adverse Reactions	Clinical Considerations
First Generation					
Cefadroxil (Duricef)	Gram-positive cocci causing skin and soft-tissue infections such as *S. aureus* and streptococci	500 mg: 1 g 1–2 times/day	PO	Adverse reactions seen in all generations[b]	Most active against gram-positive organisms and the least expensive
Cefazolin sodium (Ancef, Kefzol)		250 mg: 2–3 times/day	IM/IV	Adverse reactions seen in all generations[a,b]	The drug of choice for prophylaxis in most surgical procedures
Cephalexin (Keflex)		250–500 mg every 6 hours	PO	Adverse reactions seen in all generations[b]	
Second Generation					
Cefotetan (Cefotan)	More active against gram-negative organisms and anaerobic organisms—used to treat serious upper and lower respiratory infections, genitourinary infections, gonococcus *Haemophilus influenzae*, *E. coli*, group A beta-hemolytic streptococci, staphylococci	1–2 g every 12 hours	IV/IM	Adverse reactions seen in all generations[b] Disulfiram-like reaction if taken with alcohol	Less effective than first generation against gram-positive organisms
Cefaclor (Ceclor)		250–500 mg every 8 hours	PO	Adverse reactions seen in all generations[b]	
Cefprozil (Cefzil)		250–500 mg every 12–24 hours	PO	Adverse reactions seen in all generations[b]	
Cefuroxime (Ceftin)		125–500 mg every 12 hours	PO/IV	Adverse reactions seen in all generations[b,c]	
Cefmetazole (Zefazone)		2 g every 6–12 hours	IV		
Third Generation					
Cefoperazone (Cefobid)	Serious infections resistant to first and second generations; drugs of choice for meningitis caused by gram-negative bacilli; nosocomial infections caused by gram-negative bacilli	2–4 g/day divided every 12 hours	IV/IM	Adverse reactions seen in all generations[b,c] Disulfiram-like reaction if taken with alcohol	Good alternative to aminoglycosides due to their lack of toxicity even at high doses
Ceftriaxone (Rocephin)		250 mg: 2 g once/day	IM/IV	Adverse reactions seen in all generations[b,c]	
Cefotaxime sodium (Claforan)		1–2 g 2 times/day	IM	Adverse reactions seen in all generations[b,c]	
Cefdinir (Omnicef)		300 mg 2 times/day	PO	Adverse reactions seen in all generations[b,c]	
Cefditoren (Spectracef)		200–400 mg 2 times/day	PO	Adverse reactions seen in all generations[b,c]	
Cefixime (Suprax)		200 mg 2 times/day or 400 mg/day	PO	Adverse reactions seen in all generations[b,c]	
Ceftibuten (Cedax)		400 mg/day	PO	Adverse reactions seen in all generations[b,c]	Oral suspension contains 1 g sucrose/tsp
Cefopodoxime (Vantin)		100–200 mg every 12 hours; 200 mg/day	PO	Adverse reactions seen in all generations[b,c]	
Ceftazidime (Fortaz, Tazicef)		1–2 g every 8–12 hours	IV	Adverse reactions seen in all generations[b,c]	
Fourth Generation					
Cefepime (Maxipime)	Very broad antibacterial spectrum	500 mg: 1 g 2 times/day	IM/IV	Adverse reactions seen in all generations[b,c] Encephalopathy, headache, bleeding, anemia	Good penetration in cerebrospinal fluid
Fifth Generation					
Ceftaroline (Teflaro)	Effective against MRSA	600 mg every 12 hours IV for 5–14 days	IV	Adverse reactions seen in all generations[b,c] Hemolytic anemia, superinfection with *C. difficile* if used for an extended period of time	

[a] This is not a complete list of the cephalosporins available in the United States today. Although the agents in the table are the most commonly prescribed, there are several other agents in each of the first four generations.
[b] Common adverse reactions and side effects for all generations of cephalosporins include diarrhea, nausea, dyspepsia, pain and inflammation at the IV site, rashes, urticaria, and pruritus. If diarrhea persists, assess for pseudomembranous colitis.
[c] Uncommon adverse reactions and side effects for all generations of cephalosporins include vomiting, oral or vaginal candidiasis, pseudomembranous colitis, fever, and allergic reaction.

Third-Generation Cephalosporins

Third-generation cephalosporins provide even greater gram-negative bacteria coverage in addition to being effective against the bacteria that are affected by second-generation cephalosporins, and select forms cross the blood–brain barrier, making them an effective treatment for meningitis. They are very useful for treating infections caused by *Enterobacteriacea* such as *E. coli*, *P. mirabilis*, *Klebsiella*, *Enterobacter*, and *Serratia*. These agents are usually reserved for treatment of serious infections caused by organisms that are resistant to other medications, and they are the current recommended treatment for several sexually transmitted diseases. Cefixime (Suprax) is the only recommended oral antimicrobial to which *N. gonorrhoeae* has not developed resistance; it is currently available as a single 400-mg dose. Ceftriaxone (Rocephin) is notable for a few special characteristics. It has a very long half-life and, therefore, can be dosed once per day. It is commonly used intramuscularly to treat endometritis, gonorrhea, and other mixed microbial infections.

Fourth-Generation Cephalosporins

A newer agent, cefepime (Maxipime), is a fourth-generation cephalosporin that is highly resistant to hydrolysis by beta-lactamases. This drug has been found to be very active against penicillin-resistant strains of streptococci and is able to penetrate the central nervous system.

Fifth-Generation Cephalosporins

Ceftaroline (Teflaro) is the sole cephalosporin in the fifth-generation category. This drug has a spectrum of activity similar to ceftriaxone (third generation), but improved activity against gram-positive organisms. Ceftaroline can be used to treat MRSA and may be equivalent to vancomycin for treatment of severe respiratory infections.

Metabolism

Most cephalosporins have relatively short half-lives, in the range of 1 to 2 hours.[48] They are excreted renally as unchanged drugs; thus their concentration in the urine remains high, and these agents need to be used with caution if the individual has any renal compromise. Tissue concentrations vary, but tend to be lower than serum concentrations.[49] Second-generation cephalosporins have significant individual differences in activity and toxicity. Excretion of third-generation cephalosporins administered via intravenous infusion is managed through the biliary tract; thus adjustment of dosing is not necessary in patients with renal insufficiency. Cefepime (Maxipime) is excreted by the kidneys.

Side Effects and Adverse Reactions

Cephalosporins are generally well tolerated and are one of the safest groups of antimicrobial drugs. Serious adverse effects are rare. Serum sickness-like reactions consisting of erythema multiforme, skin rashes with polyarthritis, arthralgia, and fever have been reported in children but not in adults. Anaphylaxis is rare. Local irritation may occur at the injection site, or thrombophlebitis may occur after intravenous administration. Maculopapular rashes and/or pruritus also occur in approximately 1% to 3% of persons who take these antibiotics. Gastrointestinal irritation from oral formulations may result in nausea and generalized intestinal upset. Fungal overgrowth such as vaginal candidiasis may occur with extended use. Some cephalosporins, such as cefmetazole (Zefazone), cefoperazone, and cefotetan (Cefotetan), contain an *N*-methylthiotetrazole group, which can cause hypothrombinemia and a disulfiram-like reaction.[48] The mechanism is reduction of prothrombin levels through the drugs' interference with vitamin K metabolism and blocking of aldehyde dehydrogenase, causing alcohol intolerance. Thus, caution is required when treating individuals with a history of bleeding disorders or excessive alcohol intake. In addition, persons receiving these drugs should be informed about these potential reactions so they can monitor for any signs of abnormal bleeding and avoid alcohol intake. Another adverse reaction, pseudomembranous colitis, may occur following the administration of a cephalosporin, requiring discontinuation of the drug and treatment for *C. difficile* overgrowth. Individuals with a history of gastrointestinal disease, especially colitis, should avoid cephalosporins.

Allergic Reactions to Cephalosporins

Hypersensitivity reactions to cephalosporins are the same as the reactions that occur after taking penicillin. Anaphylaxis and urticaria can occur immediately, but, as with penicillin, the most common reaction is a maculopapular pruritic rash.[50] Cross-reactivity between cephalosporins and penicillins occurs in approximately 2% of individuals who have a history of an immediate hypersensitivity reaction to penicillin and a positive skin test for penicillin allergy.[50] However, the degradation of cephalosporins and the resultant antigenic material is quite different from the process observed with penicillin; therefore, individuals who do not tolerate penicillin may be able to take cephalosporins without developing an allergic response, while individuals who are allergic to a specific cephalosporin may be able to take other cephalosporins or some penicillins. Similarly, some cephalosporins exhibit cross-reactivity with other cephalosporins.[50] Therefore, if an individual reports an allergy to a cephalosporin, skin testing may be indicated before administering another agent in this general class. Because the antigenic components of the cephalosporin molecule are not well characterized, if the skin test is negative, the individual can be given the cephalosporin as a graded challenge. If the skin test is positive, a drug from a different class should be used.

Drug–Drug Interactions

The use of alcohol when taking cefotetan (Cefotan), cefoperazone (Cefobid), or cefmetazole (Zefazone) may lead to an acute disulfiram-like reaction characterized by headache, flushing, dizziness, nausea, vomiting, or abdominal cramps within 30 minutes of alcohol use and lasting up to 3 days. This reaction may occasionally be termed an Antabuse effect, after a common brand name for disulfiram. Persons taking these cephalosporins should be cautioned to not drink alcohol while on the antibiotic therapy. A uricosuric agent such as probenecid may reduce renal excretion of some cephalosporins, allowing plasma levels of the drug to be maintained for a longer time and providing for an extended therapeutic effect.

Special Populations: Pregnancy, Lactation, and the Elderly

Cephalosporins are in general safe for use during pregnancy and do not appear to have any teratogenic effects.[41] Ceftaroline (Teflaro) has not been evaluated for use during pregnancy and should be avoided until data are available. The pharmacokinetic properties of cephalosporins are altered in pregnant women, resulting in shorter half-lives, lower serum levels, and increased clearance in these patients, although generally no change in dosing is necessary. Cephalosporins are excreted in breast milk in small quantities, but no untoward effects have been found. Cefdinir (Omnicef) has not been detected in breast milk, suggesting it might be an excellent choice when alternatives are considered.

Cephalosporins generally are safe and effective drugs for the elderly. Because these drugs are excreted renally, dose adjustments may be needed if an elderly individual has decreased renal function.

Carbapenems and Monobactams

Carbapenems and monobactams are two classes of penicillins used by hospitals. The medications in these classes are the most broad-spectrum antibiotics in use today and, therefore, are used to treat infections that are resistant to all other agents. Their mechanism of action is the same as the mechanism utilized by all penicillins. Carbapenems and monobactams interfere with the construction of the bacterial cell wall, leading to their bactericidal effects.

The carbapenems include imipenem (Primaxin), meropenem (Merrem IV), and ertapenem (Invanz). All of these drugs are available in parenteral form only. These medications have three special characteristics. First, they are very small, which allows them to enter porins in the outer membrane of gram-negative organisms. Second, they are resistant to beta-lactamases. Third, they are able to attack a broad range of PBPs. That said, carbapenems are not effective against MRSA, which has an altered form of PBP the carbapenems cannot bind to, and they are not effective against intracellular bacteria such as Chlamydiae.

Aztreonam (Azactam) is a bactericidal monobactam. It has a limited spectrum of activity, as it is effective only against gram-negative aerobic bacteria—for example, *Haemophilus influenzae*, *Pseudomonas aeruginosa*, *Enterobacteriaceae* (e.g., *Escherichia coli*, *Klebsiella pneumoniae*, *Salmonella*, *Shigella*), *Neisseria meningitidis*, and *Neisseria gonorrhoeae.* Similar to third-generation cephalosporins, aztreonam is able to penetrate cerebrospinal fluid. It is not absorbed through the gastrointestinal tract, however, so it must be given by the parenteral route of administration. Aztreonam is excreted renally. Because this agent's structure differs from the structures of penicillin and the cephalosporins, it is regarded as being safe to use in persons with allergies to these drugs.

Vancomycin

Vancomycin (Vanocin) was first isolated from a soil sample collected in the interior jungles of Borneo by a scientist at Eli Lilly.[52] This agent has traditionally been considered the drug of last resort because of its toxic side effects. The primary use of vancomycin has been to treat infections caused by MRSA and antibiotic-induced pseudomembranous colitis.

Mechanism of Action and Spectrum of Activity

Vancomycin does not contain a beta-lactam ring. Rather, its mechanism of action is the inhibition of the synthesis of the bacterial cell wall via binding with cell wall precursors (not PBPs), which makes it bactericidal for dividing microbes. Vancomycin is a very large molecule, which prevents it from passing through the porins in gram-negative cell membranes; thus it is effective against only gram-positive organisms and is primarily used to treat gram-positive bacteria that have resistance to penicillins and cephalosporins.[53]

Mechanism of Resistance

The primary mechanism of resistance to vancomycin is via genetic alteration of the cell wall, so it is resistant to binding by vancomycin. Vancomycin-resistant enterococci emerged in 1987. Vancomycin-intermediate *S. aureus* (VISA), vancomycin-resistant *S. aureus* (VRSA), and vancomycin-resistant *C. difficile* strains were identified in the 1990s.[54]

Clinical Indications

The CDC has established guidelines that restrict the use of vancomycin to specific life-threatening, gram-positive infections.[55] It is almost exclusively used intravenously in hospital settings. This drug has several common adverse side effects, such as red man syndrome, and can rarely be the cause of nephrotoxicity and ototoxicity. It is commonly associated with thrombophlebitis, requiring frequent changing of the intravenous site.[56]

Antibiotics That Inhibit or Alter Protein Synthesis

This section reviews the antibiotics that work by either inhibiting or altering protein synthesis in bacteria. The actions of these antibiotics have either a bacteriostatic or bactericidal effect based on their dosing and the sensitivity of the bacteria to the medication. Antibiotics whose mechanism of action inhibits or alters bacterial protein synthesis include the macrolides, clindamycin (Cleocin), the tetracyclines, the oxazolidinone linezolid (Zyvox), the ketolides (telethromycin [Ketek]), chloramphenicol (Chloromycetin), and the aminoglycosides.

Macrolides

Macrolides and lincosamides are a group of anti-infective agents that have a high molecular weight—hence their name (Table 11-7). Macrolides and lincosamides have a large macrocyclic ring containing 14 to 16 atoms with deoxy sugars attached to the ring. Erythromycin (E-mycin), the prototypical drug in this group, was developed in 1952 from *Streptomyces erythreus.* Clarithromycin (Biaxin) and azithromycin (Zithromax) are derivatives of erythromycin that are categorized as macrolides. The lincosamide clindamycin (Cleocin) is slightly different chemically from the macrolides but functions similarly and is discussed separately. Ketolides are a newer generation of drugs similar to macrolides that are used for multidrug-resistant respiratory infections. Telithromycin (Ketek) is the only ketolide available for clinical use at this time; it has significant activity against *S. pneumoniae* strains that are resistant to penicillin and macrolides. All of these agents are considered broad-spectrum antimicrobials.

Mechanism of Action and Spectrum of Activity

Macrolides and lincosamides bind to the P site of the 50s subunit of the bacterial ribosome, which inhibits RNA-dependent protein synthesis. The ketolides have a similar mechanism of action to macrolides and lincosamides; however, the difference in the structure of a ketolide allows it to be less susceptible to removal by bacteria's export pumps and, therefore, it can more effectively bind to the ribosome in targeted bacteria.[57] These drugs may be bacteriostatic or bactericidal depending on the drug concentration, species of bacteria, and growth phase of the bacteria.

Macrolides concentrate in macrophages, polymorphonuclear cells, and other leukocytes that migrate to the site of infection. Thus, their tissue concentration is higher than their plasma concentration. Via their leukocyte host, these drugs are active against intracellular microbes such as *Chlamydia*, *Legionella*, *Mycoplasma pneumoniae*, and *Rickettsia* species.

Macrolides and lincosamides have an antibacterial spectrum similar to that of penicillin; however, because they do not have a beta-lactam ring, they are effective against beta-lactamase-producing bacteria. Erythromycin is often used instead of penicillin for persons who are allergic to the latter. Nevertheless, it is not effective against gram-negative bacteria such as *H. influenzae*, so it is not a substitute for broad-spectrum penicillins such as ampicillin, nor is it a replacement for cephalosporins.

Succeeding generations of macrolides have a broader spectrum of activity. Clarithromycin (Biaxin) is effective against *Bordetella pertussis*, *Campylobacter*, *Chlamydia*, *Helicobacter*, *Legionella* species, *H. influenzae*, and *Mycobacterium tuberculosis*. Azithromycin (Zithromax) is less effective than erythromycin or clarithromycin against gram-positive bacteria, but is more effective against *H. influenzae* and *M. catarrhalis*, which is why it is one of the

Table 11-7 Macrolides, Clindamycin, and Ketolides

Macrolide: Generic (Brand)	Indications	Doses	Route	Adverse Reactions	Clinical Considerations
Azithromycin (Zithromax)	Gram-negative organisms, particularly GU pathogens: *Chlamydia trachomatis, Neisseria gonorrhoeae, Treponema palladium*	500 mg for 1 day, then 250 mg for 4 days	PO	Serious allergic reactions have occurred but are more common with erythromycin. Is not metabolized via CYP450 enzymes and has fewer drug–drug interactions.	Absorbed faster when taken with food. Need to take a loading dose to obtain effective plasma concentrations.
Clarithromycin (Biaxin, Biaxin XL)	*Haemophilus influenzae*, non-tuberculosis mycobacteria, *Helicobacter pylori* (part of triple therapy for *H. pylori*)	250–500 mg every 12 hours for 7–14 days	PO	Multiple drug–drug interactions.	Food delays the onset of action. Suspension should not be refrigerated.
Clindamycin (Cleocin)	Serious infections caused by anaerobes or *Staphylococcus*; used in combination therapy for polymicrobial infections; bacterial vaginosis, acne vulgaris	PO: 150–450 mg every 6 hours; IV/IM: 300–600 mg every 6–8 hours	PO, IM/IV, intravaginal	Diarrhea most common; dizziness, headache, vertigo, hypotension, nausea, vomiting, rashes.	Persistence of diarrhea indicates the need to assess for pseudomembranous colitis. A single IM injection that is > 600 mg is not indicated; nor is a single IV dose >1200 mg.
Erythromycin (E-mycin, Ery-Tab)	Mild to moderate upper and lower respiratory tract infections, skin infections, *Bordetella pertussis, Corynebacterium diphtheriae*; HIV-related infections and atypical organisms—Chlamydiae, Rickettsiae, Legionellae	250–500 mg 4 times/day	PO/IV	Ototoxicity following IV administration. Prolonged QT interval. Cholestatic hepatitis can aggravate myasthenia gravis symptoms. Multiple drug–drug interactions.	Due to GI upset, compliance can be difficult. Most erythromycins need to be taken with food. Erythromycin has multiple drug interactions.
Telithromycin (Ketek)	Multidrug-resistant community-acquired pneumonia, acute bacterial sinusitis due to *S. pneumoniae, H. influenzae, M. catarrhalis, C. pneumoniae, Mycoplasma pneumoniae*	800 mg every day for 7–10 days	PO	Hepatotoxicity; visual changes; prolonged QT interval.	Contraindicated for women with myasthenia gravis, as it may worsen this condition.

Abbreviations: GI = gastrointestinal; GU = genitourinary.

current drugs of choice for treating community-acquired pneumonia. Telithromycin (Ketek) is prescribed when multidrug-resistant community-acquired or acute bacterial sinusitis is diagnosed.

Mechanism of Resistance

The primary mechanism of resistance to macrolides and lincosamides is via mutation or methylation of the bacterial ribosome, i.e., a target-site modification and, less often, efflux pump.[58,59] Today, significant resistance to macrolides is observed in many common pathogens. Because there is regional variation in the incidence of pathogenic bacteria resistant to macrolides, clinicians need to be aware of changing recommendations for treatment of common conditions such as community-acquired upper respiratory tract infections, which are often caused by *S. pneumoniae*. In general, higher rates of resistance to penicillin will parallel higher rates of resistance to macrolides and lincosamides.

Clinical Indications

Erythromycin

Erythromycin (E-Mycin) is FDA approved to treat upper and lower respiratory tract infections, especially in individuals who have a penicillin allergy. This agent is effective against *Streptococcus pyogenes, S. pneumoniae, M. pneumoniae,* and *Legionella,* with the caveat that resistance to *S. pyogenes* and *S. pneumoniae* can be significant in some areas. In addition, erythromycin is the agent of choice in treating corynebacterial sepsis and neonatal and ocular infections. *C. trachomatis, Helicobacter, Listeria,* and other mycobacteria also are susceptible to erythromycin, but because azithromycin (Zithromax) has a more tolerable side-effect profile, it is more often recommended as first-line treatment for disorders caused by these microbes. Erythromycin, along with the other macrolides, is a drug of choice for individuals infected with *B. pertussis*, as it eliminates this pathogen from the nasopharynx and lowers infectivity.[60]

Clarithromycin

Clarithromycin (Biaxin) is derived from erythromycin and is almost identical with respect to its antibacterial activity. Clarithromycin has a half-life of 6 hours, compared to 1.5 hours for erythromycin; thus less frequent dosing is possible. Clarithromycin also is used for the treatment of *H. pylori* infection, a common cause of gastrointestinal reflux disease.

Azithromycin

Azithromycin (Zithromax) has unique properties that allow for once-a-day dosing. The slow release of the drug from tissues gives this medication a tissue half-life of 2 to 4 days, with an elimination half-life of almost 3 days. It is rapidly absorbed, and the oral preparation is well tolerated. The benefit of prescribing azithromycin is that it has fewer gastrointestinal side effects than the other macrolides, and its effects continue for several days after the last dose is given due to the drug's long half-life. The 15-member lactone ring results in far fewer drug–drug interactions than occur with erythromycin or clarithromycin. Azithromycin is the drug of choice for treating *C. trachomatis* infection.

Metabolism

Macrolides are weak bases, and their action is enhanced in an alkaline pH.[57] The erythromycin base is inactivated by stomach acid; thus this drug is made available as either enteric or film-coated formulations. Erythromycin estolate (Eryc, EryTab) is an acid-stable salt, and erythromycin ethyl succinate (EES) is an acid-stable ester that is converted to erythromycin base in vivo. Macrolides are absorbed from the gastrointestinal tract, metabolized in the liver via the cytochrome P450 system, and primarily excreted in bile, with 5% of excretion occurring through urine. Erythromycin estolate and azithromycin are better absorbed when taken with food, whereas erythromycin ethylsuccinate is better absorbed in the absence of food.

Side Effects and Adverse Reactions

Nausea, vomiting, diarrhea, and anorexia are the most common side effects associated with use of erythromycin (E-Mycin) and, to a lesser extent, clarithromycin (Zithromax) and azithromycin. These gastrointestinal effects are frequent and significant enough that they prompt some individuals to discontinue taking erythromycin. Erythromycin is a prokinetic agent, and the stimulation of motilin may potentially be one of the etiologic mechanisms by which this drug induces gastrointestinal symptoms.[58] The longer half-lives associated with clarithromycin and azithromycin as compared to erythromycin result in reduced incidence of gastrointestinal side effects with these two drugs. The selection of one agent over the other, therefore, may be determined by tolerability and cost. Telithromycin is usually well tolerated, but produces gastrointestinal side effects similar to those associated with other macrolides.

Erythromycin estolate (Eryc, EryTab) has the potential to produce acute cholestatic hepatitis. Given this risk, it is not an appropriate antibiotic for pregnant women or persons of any age who have compromised hepatic function. In high concentrations, erythromycin has the potential to prolong the cardiac QT interval, causing the fatal dysrhythmia of torsades de pointes.[58] To minimize this risk, erythromycin should be avoided by persons with congenital QT prolongation. Telithromycin (Ketek) has been associated with hepatotoxicity and can worsen myasthenia gravis.

Drug–Drug Interactions

Erythromycin (E-Mycin) and clarithromycin (Biaxin) are strong inhibitors of CYP3A4 and, in turn, are associated with many clinically important drug–drug interactions.[57,58,61,62] Selected common and significant drug–drug interactions associated with use of macrolides are listed in Table 11-8. Grapefruit juice is an inhibitor of the CYP3A4 enzyme system, which is responsible for the first-pass metabolism of erythromycin and clarithromycin. This effect causes increased bioavailability of these drugs and results in increased serum levels. Individuals should be counseled to avoid grapefruit juice during macrolide therapy.[61]

Erythromycin is a potent inhibitor of CYP3A4 and therefore has multiple drug interactions. Erythromycin should not be given concomitantly with cisapride (Propulsid), ergotamine (Cafregot), astemiazole (Hismanal), lovastatin (Mevacor), or simvastatin (Zocor). Erythromycin prolongs cardiac repolarization and is associated with case reports of torsades de pointes. Erythromycin is metabolized by CYP34A and therefore, other drugs that are strong inhibitors of CYP3A4 should not be used concomitantly with erythromycin as this combination increases the risk

Table 11-8 Macrolides: Selected Drug–Drug Interactions[a]

Drug: Generic (Brand)	Clinical or Pharmacokinetic Effect If Taken with Macrolides
Erythromycin and Clarithromycin	
Amitriptyline (Elavil)	Increased concentration, risk of torsades de pointes
Antiarrhythmics	Increased concentration, prolonged QT interval, torsades de pointes, death
Antipsychotics	Increased concentration, risk of torsades de pointes, disorientation with clozapine (Clozaril)
Azole antibiotics	Increased concentration, prolonged QT interval, torsades de pointes, death
Benzodiazepines (Triazolam)[b]	Amnesia, psychomotor impairment, unconsciousness, increased sedation
Buspirone (BuSpar)	Increased plasma levels of buspirone and increased sedation
Calcium-channel blockers	Increased plasma levels of calcium-channel blockers causing hypotension, tachycardia, edema, dizziness
Carbamazepine (Tegretol)	Toxic serum levels
Cisapride (Propulsid)	Increased plasma level of cisapride
Clozapine (Clozaril)	Disorientation
Corticosteroids	Increased plasma levels of corticosteroids
Cyclosporine (Neoral)	Nephrotoxic serum levels
Digoxin (Lanoxin)	Increased levels of digoxin, mild to moderate gastrointestinal symptoms
Diltiazem (Cardizem, Tiazac)	Fivefold increased risk of sudden cardiac death
Ergot alkaloids (e.g., Cafergot)	Increased risk for ergotism (peripheral vasoconstriction)
Felodipine (Plendil)	Increased plasma levels of felodipine
Fexofenadine (Allegra)	Increased plasma levels of fexofenadine
Fluoxetine (Prozac)	Delirium
HMG-CoA reductase inhibitors: simvastatin (Zocor), lovastatin (Mevacor), atorvastatin (Lipitor)	Increased plasma levels of simvastatin, lovastatin, and atorvastatin, resulting in severe toxicity
Itraconazole (Sporanox)	Fivefold increased risk of sudden cardiac death
Methylprednisolone (Medrol)	Decreased clearance of methylprednisolone; effect unknown
Midazolam (Versed)	Increased plasma levels of midazolam
Pimozide (Orap)	Prolonged QT interval
Rifabutin (Mycobutin)	Uveitis
Sildenafil (Viagra)	Priapism
Theophylline (Theo-Dur)	Increased plasma levels of theophylline that may lead to toxicity
Valproate (Depakote)	Increased plasma levels of valproate
Verapamil (Calan)	Fivefold increased risk of sudden cardiac death
Warfarin (Coumadin)	Hemorrhage
Azithromycin	
Aluminum and magnesium antacids	Decreased plasma levels of azithromycin
Digitoxin (Crystodigin)	Increased plasma levels of digitoxin
Telithromycin	
Cisapride (Propulsid), pimozide (Orap)	Increased plasma levels of cisapride and pimozide, resulting in severe toxicity
Digoxin (Lanoxin)	Increased plasma levels of digoxin
Ergot alkaloids	Increased plasma levels of ergotamine and dihydroergotamine
HMG-CoA reductase inhibitors: simvastatin (Zocor), lovastatin (Mevacor), atorvastatin (Lipitor)[c]	Increased plasma levels of simvastatin, lovastatin, and atorvastatin, resulting in severe toxicity
Itraconazole (Sporanox), ketoconazole (Nizoral)	Increased plasma levels of telithromycin
Metoprolol (Lopressor)	Increased plasma levels of metoprolol
Midazolam	Increased levels of midazolam
Theophylline (Theo-Dur)	Increased plasma levels of theophylline

[a] This table is not comprehensive. Healthcare providers who recommend a macrolide should evaluate all drugs taken concomitantly for macrolide associated drug–drug interactions.
[b] The benzodiazepines lorazepam (Ativan) and oxazepam (Alepam) are not metabolized by CYP450 enzymes and have no adverse interactions with macrolides.
[c] The HMG-CoA reductase inhibitors pravastatin (Pravachol) and lovastatin (Mevacor) are not metabolized by CYP2C9 and do not have adverse interactions with macrolides.
Sources: Data from Abu-Gharbieh E, Vasina V, Poluzzi E, De Ponti F. Antibacterial macrolides: a drug class with a complex pharmacological profile. *Pharmacol Res*. 2004;50(3):211-220[58]; Rubenstein E. Comparative safety of the different macrolides. *Int J Antimicrob Agents*. 2001;18:S71-S76[62]; Zuckerman JM. Macrolides and ketolides: azithromycin, clarithromycin, telithromycin. *Infect Dis Clin North Am*. 2004;18(3):621-649.[57]

of sudden cardiac death. Drugs in this category include the azoles ketoconazole (Nizoral) and itraconazole (Sporanox). Persons taking antiarrhythmic drugs such as amiodarone (Cordarone) should use erythromycin with caution, as it has been assocatied with prolonged QT syndrome and ventricular arrhythmias.

Telithromycin (Ketek) has the potential for numerous drug interactions because it is an inhibitor of and a substrate for CYP34A. Other drugs that inhibit the CYP34A enzyme can increase plasma levels of telithromycin (e.g., ketoconazole [Nizoral]). Conversely, drugs that are CYP34A enzyme inducers can decrease telithromycin levels, resulting in treatment failure, including phenobarbital (Luminal), rifampin (Rifadin), and phenytoin (Dilantin). However, due to its inhibition of the CYP34A enzyme, telithromycin can increase the plasma levels of several drugs, in some cases to toxic levels. For example, cisapride (Propulsid) and pimozide (Orap) are contraindicated for use with telithromycin, and certain statins, such as simvastatin (Zocor), lovastatin (Mevacor), and atorvastatin (Lipitor), should not be used with telithromycin.

Special Populations: Pregnancy, Lactation, and the Elderly

Macrolides do not appear to be associated with teratogenic effects.[63] Erythromycin does cross the placenta, but because plasma levels vary widely in pregnancy, it does not consistently treat the fetus for infection. However, erythromycin in combination with ampicillin is the drug regimen of choice for treating women with preterm premature rupture of membranes[64] and erythromycin is an approved alternative drug for chlamydial infections if needed.[65] Azithromycin (Zithromax) is also the drug of choice for treatment of *C. trachomatis* infections among pregnant women.[65] Clarithromycin (Biaxin) and azithromycin (Zithromax) have demonstrated adverse effects on the fetus in animal studies, but comparative human studies are lacking and no adverse effects have been reported as case studies. Nevertheless, these drugs are not recommended as first-line agents except in situations where no reasonable alternative therapy exists.

Some studies have shown a correlation between use of erythromycin in breastfeeding women and infantile hypertrophic pyloric stenosis in the early newborn.[66] Therefore, macrolides should be used with caution in women who are breastfeeding neonates.

Erythromycin is safe to use among elderly individuals who do not have severe cardiac, renal, or hepatic impairment or are not on any of several other medications that could interact with this drug.

Clindamycin

Clindamycin (Cleocin) is a synthetic derivative of lincomycin. Because it is very similar to the macrolides, it is often classified with them. Clindamycin has broad coverage against gram-positive bacteria, many anaerobes and intracellular bacteria such as *Mycoplasma*. It is more active than the macrolides against several anaerobic bacteria, such as *Bacteroides fragilis*. It is not effective for the treatment of disorders caused by gram-negative aerobic bacteria. The mechanism of action and the mechanism of resistance to clindamycin are the same as those for the macrolides. Consequently, bacteria that are resistant to erythromycin are frequently resistant to clindamycin.

Clinical Indications

Clindamycin (Cleocin) primarily is used to treat serious infections caused by anaerobes or *Staphylococcus*. It is useful against polymicrobial infections such as pelvic inflammatory disease and bacterial vaginosis, and is often administered as part of combination therapy for polymicrobial infections. This agent is used in combination with chloroquine to treat malaria. Clindamycin is effective against acnes vulgaris, which is caused by *Propionibacterium acnes*. Although this agent is effective against many gram-positive cocci as well, it is associated with a high incidence of diarrhea and a risk for developing pseudomembranous colitis. Given these risks, it is not considered a first-line treatment (over penicillins or cephalosporins) for disorders caused by gram-positive cocci. Clindamycin can be used to treat soft-tissue infections caused by MRSA, as many strains of MRSA remain susceptible to this agent.

Metabolism

Clindamycin is easily absorbed orally, and food does not affect its absorption. It is also absorbed topically enough to reach therapeutic systemic levels; for this route of administration, it is formulated as a gel, cream, or lotion. Clindamycin is 90% protein bound and metabolized via the liver but not via the cytochrome P450 system.

Side Effects and Adverse Reactions

Diarrhea occurs in 2% to 20% of persons who take clindamycin. Pseudomembranous colitis secondary to overgrowth of *C. difficile* is rare but accounts for approximately 3 million cases of diarrhea and colitis per year in the United States and the possibility of developing *C. diff* is listed in a black box warning on the product label. Hypersensitivity reactions occur in approximately 10% of persons who use clindamycin.

Drug–Drug Interactions

Clindamycin enhances the action of muscle relaxants such as pancuronium (Pavulon). It should not be given concurrently with erythromycin (E-Mycin) because the two antimicrobials have antagonistic effects.

Special Populations: Pregnancy, Lactation, and the Elderly

There are no reports linking clindamycin with teratogenic effects. This drug is secreted into breast milk, but no adverse effects on nursing infants have been confirmed. Studies have shown no clinically important differences between young and elderly subjects with normal hepatic function and normal renal function. Antibiotic-associated colitis and diarrhea occur more frequently in the elderly and may be more severe in this population. These individuals should be carefully monitored for the development of diarrhea.

Aminoglycosides

The aminoglycosides are important secondary to their effectiveness against gram-negative bacilli and relative lack of antimicrobial resistance.[67] The first aminoglycoside, streptomycin, was formulated in 1944 by Selman A Waksman, who won the 1952 Nobel Prize for this discovery.[68] Gentamicin (Garamycin) was formulated in 1963 and offered better coverage of gram-negative bacterial infections. Other aminoglycosides were subsequently developed, including amikacin (Amikin), netilmicin (Netromycin), and tobramycin (Nebcin). Currently, seven aminoglycosides are available for therapeutic use in the United States. Kanamycin has the most severe adverse effects and is periodically not available in the United States secondary to an inability to manufacture the drug. Kanamycin is rarely used anyway given the adverse effects. Paromomycin is an oral but poorly absorbed aminoglycoside that is primary used to treat intraintestinal amebic infection. The five aminoglycosides primarily in use are presented here. The most commonly used aminoglycosides are gentamicin (Garamycin), tobramycin (Nebcin), and amikacin (Amikin) (Table 11-9).

Mechanism of Action and Spectrum of Activity

Aminoglycosides are potent bactericidal antibiotics that work through irreversible inhibition of bacterial protein synthesis.[67] Energy is needed for aminoglycoside uptake into the bacterial cell, and this step can be inhibited or reduced in a low-pH environment such as lung or bronchial secretions. Aminoglycosides may act synergistically with other drugs that disrupt the bacterial cell walls, and this combination is used to treat some infections. Aminoglycosides work via concentration-dependent killing and have a post-antibiotic effect.[69]

These agents are active against aerobic gram-negative bacteria such as *E. coli, Klebsiella, P. mirabilis, Enterobacter, Acinetobacter, P. aeruginosa,* and some mycobacteria. Despite being active against gram-negative organisms, they are not used to treat *N. gonorrhoea* because drugs that produce fewer adverse reactions are available for use against this organism. Amikacin (Amikin) has the broadest spectrum of activity and is useful for the treatment of gentamicin- or tobramycin-resistant bacteria and in the treatment of infections caused by *Nocardia* and nontuberculous mycobacteria. Gentamicin and generic tobramycin are the drugs of choice against sensitive bacteria because of their lower cost and the extensive clinical experience with these drugs. Streptomycin is used primarily in the treatment of multidrug-resistant tuberculosis. It is both ototoxic and nephrotoxic and, therefore, is not used if other efficacious drugs are available.

Metabolism

Because aminoglycosides are poorly absorbed from the gastrointestinal tract, they are administered through the parenteral route to treat systemic infections. Excretion occurs rapidly by glomerular filtration, resulting in a half-life varying from 2 to 3 hours in a person with normal renal

Table 11-9 Aminoglycosides

Aminoglycoside: Generic (Brand)	Indications	Doses	Adverse Reactions	Clinical Considerations
Amikacin (Amikin)	Bacteremia, peritonitis, meningitis	5 mg/kg every 8 hours		Inactivated by penicillin; should not be mixed in the same IV fluid. Kidney levels and electrolyte levels should be monitored with all aminoglycosides.
Gentamicin (Garamycin)	Systemic infections, gram-negative bacteremia, peritonitis, meningitis, pneumonia, urosepsis *Pseudomonas aeruginosa, Escherichia coli, Klebsiella, Serratia, Proteus mirabilis*	1.7 mg/kg every 8 hours	Ototoxic, nephrotoxic; hypersensitivity reactions; hypomagnesemia common	Same as for amikacin.
Neomycin (Neo-Fradin Cortisporin, Neosporin)	Infectious diarrhea; gastrointestinal sterilization prior to surgery; topical infections of ear, eye, and skin	1 g × 3 doses preoperatively; topical 1–3 times/day	Most ototoxic and nephrotoxic; oral has caused intestinal malabsorption; topical can cause dermatitis	Not used parenterally.
Streptomycin	Meningitis, pneumonia, urosepsis, tuberculosis, endocarditis, plague, tularemia, glanders, brucellosis	0.5–2 g every 24 hours	Has been associated with neurologic disorders	First aminoglycoside discovered. Used in combinations with other drugs to treat tuberculosis.
Tobramycin (Nebcin, TobraDex)	Same as gentamicin; more active against *P. aeruginosa* compared to gentamicin	1.7 mg/kg every 8 hours	Same as gentamicin	Inhaled drug used for cystic fibrosis.

function. Aminoglycosides have good tissue penetration but reach only a low concentration in cerebrospinal fluid, lungs, alveoli, and bile.

Mechanism of Resistance

Bacteria can become resistant to aminoglycosides in one of three ways: via changes in the cell wall active transport system that facilitates entry into the intracellular compartment, by alteration of the 30S ribosome to prevent binding, or via enzymatic deactivation of the drug. Many enterococci that cause urinary tract infections are resistant to aminoglycosides and *P. aeruginosa* resistance is increasing. With these exceptions, resistance to aminoglycosides is currently very low.

Clinical Indications

Aminoglycosides are mostly used intravenously to treat serious gram-negative infections such as *P. aeruginosa.* These agents have been frequently used in combination with beta-lactam antibiotics to treat polymicrobial infections, because joint effects on gram-positive and gram-negative bacteria are synergistic. The beta-lactam effect on the cell wall facilitates uptake of the aminoglycoside into the cell cytoplasm, where it can reach the ribosomes. Readers may recognize the classic "amp and gent" (ampicillin and gentamycin) combination that is often used in hospital settings to treat infections presumed to be caused by streptococci. That said, aminoglycoside resistance is increasing and a fluoroquinolone is more often substituted for the gentamycin today. Alternatively, aminoglycosides may be used in combination with clindamycin (Cleocin) to extend coverage to anaerobic organisms. Gentamicin/tobramycin and neomycin/bacitracin (Neosporin ointment) combinations are used topically to treat eye infections.

Side Effects and Adverse Reactions

Common minor side effects of aminoglycosides include nausea, vomiting, diarrhea, headache, dizziness, tinnitus, vertigo, and roaring in the ears, all of which are mild and transient. The more serious adverse reactions are important considerations that limit use of these drugs; they include nephrotoxicity, ototoxicity, neuromuscular blockade, drug fever, and electrolyte imbalance. The rate of nephrotoxicity has been reported to be as high as 10% to 20% in some settings and is, in most cases, reversible.[70] In contrast, aminoglycoside-associated ototoxicity is irreversible. Gentamicin (Garamycin) can cause severe vestibular loss. Both ototoxic and nephrotoxic effects are directly related to the length of treatment and serum levels experienced by an individual. Management during treatment should include monitoring of blood serum levels and limited short-term therapy. A single daily dosage of an aminoglycoside is generally safe, efficacious, and cost-effective.

Drug–Drug Interactions

Drugs that are potentially nephrotoxic should not be taken concomitantly with aminoglycosides so as to avoid the additive risk of nephrotoxicity. Penicillins, cephalosporins, vancomycin (Vanocin), nonsteroidal anti-inflammatory drugs, salicylates, and loop diuretics all have potential to increase the risk of nephrotoxicity when taken with aminoglycosides. When penicillins and aminoglycosides are present together in high concentrations, the penicillins can inactivate the aminoglycosides.

Special Populations: Pregnancy, Lactation, and the Elderly

The parenteral aminoglycosides have been associated with teratogenic effects in animal studies, but limited human data on these risks are available. Animal studies have revealed changes in size and weight among rat pups, and nephrotoxicity in fetal rats. Streptomycin is associated with hearing loss in children exposed in utero to this medication and, therefore, is contraindicated during pregnancy. Aminoglycosides are poorly excreted into breast milk, so they are considered safe for use by women who are breastfeeding.

Aminoglycosides should be used with caution among the elderly because of potential for diminished renal function related to aging—a condition that may prolong the half-life of the drug and increase the risk of toxicity.

Tetracyclines

Tetracyclines were extracted from *Streptomyces* soil microorganisms found in Missouri mud in 1948 and became the first class of antimicrobials to be labeled *broad spectrum*[71] (Table 11-10). However, due to their widespread use in the 1950s and 1960s, a large number of resistant bacterial strains exist today, which limits their therapeutic use. Doxycycline (Vibramycin) and minocycline (Dynacin, Minocin) are the most commonly used formulations of tetracycline.

Mechanism of Action and Spectrum of Activity

Tetracyclines are primarily bacteriostatic, acting by binding to the 30S subunits of the ribosomes in susceptible microorganisms, and thereby inhibiting protein synthesis. These pharmaceuticals enter organisms through a combination

Table 11-10 Tetracyclines

Tetracycline: Generic (Brand)	Indications	Doses	Adverse Reactions	Clinical Considerations
Demeclocycline	Rickettsial fevers, various infections caused by *M. pneumoniae*, *C. trachomatis*, *C. psittaci*, *H. ducreyi*, *V. cholerae*, *E. coli*	600 mg/day in divided doses 2–3 times/day	Same as for tetracycline	Take medication 1 hour before or 2 hours after a meal.
Doxycycline (Vibramycin, Doxy Caps)	Mild to moderate infections, *Chlamydia trachomatis*, more severe gonorrhea, lymphogranuloma venereum, early syphilis, acne, acute exacerbation of bronchitis; prophylaxis of rat, bat, and raccoon bites; anthrax; malaria; and *Borrelia burgdorferi* (Lyme disease)	100 mg 1–2 times/day	Photosensitivity, gastrointestinal upset, rash, blood dyscrasias, hepatotoxicity	Associated with less nephrotoxicity. Can be taken with food.
Minocycline (Dynacin, Minocin)	Urethritis, gonorrhea; has been used to reduce symptoms of arthritis	100 mg 2 times/day	Can cause damage to the vestibular system, causing dizziness and vertigo and blue–black hyperpigmentation of skin and mucous membranes	More expensive.
Tigecycline (Tygacil)	Broad spectrum including MRSA, vancomycin-resistant enterococci, most aerobic gram-positive and gram-negative bacteria, except *Pseudomonas aeruginosa* and *Proteus*	100 mg IV followed by 50 mg IV every 12 hours for 5–14 days	Diarrhea, nausea, and vomiting during first few days of therapy; photosensitivity	Has a structure that makes it difficult for bacteria to develop resistance.
Tetracycline	Mild to moderate infections, gonorrhea, severe acne	1–2 g/day 2–4 times/day	Photosensitivity, will accumulate in kidneys, may increase blood urea nitrogen, can cause liver toxicities	Do not take with products containing calcium, magnesium, zinc, or iron; antacids; and milk products. Food affects absorption.

of passive diffusion and active transport, ultimately preventing the addition of amino acids to growing peptides.

Tetracyclines are broad-spectrum antibiotics that are effective against both gram-positive and gram-negative aerobes, thereby providing a good alternative for individuals who have a penicillin allergy. However, due to increasing bacterial resistance, they are now more often prescribed for the treatment of susceptible atypical organisms such as *Mycoplasma*, *Chlamydia*, and *Rickettsia* species; *Borrelia* species (especially *Borrelia burgdorferi*, the cause of Lyme disease); and *P. acnes*.

This class of antibiotic should not be used for common infections unless the organism has been shown to be sensitive through a culture and sensitivity test. Tetracyclines—specifically, doxycycline—are considered a first-line drug of choice for *C. trachomatis*, *Ureaplasma urealyticum*, and *B. burgdorferi*. This class is also used to prevent and treat malaria and may be used in different combination regimens for therapeutic treatment of duodenal ulcers caused by *H. pylori*. Tetracyclines are active against *Bacillus anthracis* and *Vibrio cholerae*.

Tigecycline (Tygacil) is similar to tetracycline, but is a glycylcycline. Tigecycline first became available in the United States in 2005. It is very effective against organisms that are resistant to other forms of tetracyclines and penicillins, as well as against many resistant strains of staphylococci and *S. aureus*.

Mechanism of Resistance

Prevalence of resistance varies among different regions of the United States and globally. Resistance to one agent does not imply resistance to other tetracyclines. The primary mechanism of resistance is efflux pumping of the drug out of the intracellular compartment; to a lesser extent, genetic mutation of the ribosome may prevent binding of the drug to the ribosome.[72]

Clinical Indications

One of the most common uses of tetracyclines is the treatment of acne vulgaris. These agents are the drugs of choice for treating infections caused by *Chlamydia*, *Rickettsia*, and spirochetal infections such as syphilis or Lyme disease. They are used to treat syphilis in persons who are penicillin-allergic, and may also be used to treat pneumonia, sinusitis, or urinary tract infections.

Metabolism

Differences among the tetracyclines include variety in absorption after oral administration and elimination.

Absorption occurs primarily in the upper intestinal tract and the small intestine: 60% to 70% for tetracycline and 95% to 100% for doxycycline (Vibramycin) and minocycline (Dynacin, Minocin). Both doxycycline and minocycline have longer half-lives than tetracycline itself, enabling the former agents to be given on a less frequent dosing schedule. The tetracyclines become widely distributed to tissues throughout the body, with the exception of cerebrospinal fluid. The shorter-acting tetracyclines are eliminated unchanged without being metabolized in the liver. The longer-acting tetracyclines have some metabolism in the liver and are unaffected by kidney dysfunction; as a consequence, they are safer for use in those individuals with renal impairment.

The short-acting tetracyclines—that is, tetracycline and oxytetracycline (Terramycin)—have a serum half-life of 6 to 8 hours. Intermediate-acting formulations—that is, demeclocycline (Declomycin) and methacycline (Rhodomycin)—have a longer serum half-life of 12 hours and are not commonly used. The longest-acting agents are doxycycline (Vibramycin) and minocycline (Minocin), with a half-life of 16 to 18 hours, enabling them to be given via a once-a-day dosing regimen.

Tigecycline has excellent tissue penetration and is excreted via the biliary tract; thus it is the preferred agent for individuals with renal compromise. This agent has a very long half-life of 36 hours. It is FDA approved for treatment of complicated skin and soft-tissue infections.

Side Effects and Adverse Reactions

Tetracyclines have many side effects and some adverse effects. These drugs can cause photosensitivity, especially among individuals with fair skin. Gastrointestinal disturbances are not unusual following both oral and intravenous administration. Nausea, vomiting, and diarrhea result from direct irritation to the intestinal tract. Anorexia has also been reported. Vertigo and dizziness have occurred with both doxycycline and minocycline.

Tetracyclines, like other antibiotics, are associated with pseudomembranous colitis caused by *C. difficile*, a superinfection of the bowel. For individuals who have preexisting renal or liver impairment, the risk for hepatotoxicity and nephrotoxicity needs to be considered. Tetracyclines are potent chelators of metal ions and can cause tooth discoloration of permanent teeth. These drugs are contraindicated for pregnant women and children 8 years and younger.

Drug–Drug and Drug–Food Interactions

The many drug–drug interactions associated with use of tetracyclines, and with doxycycline (Vibramycin) in particular, are listed in Table 11-11. Concomitant use of tetracyclines with oral contraceptives have been suggested to be problematic, although as previously noted, only rifampin (Rifadin) has been definitively shown to decrease

Table 11-11 Tetracyclines: Selected Drug–Drug Interactions[a]

Drug: Generic (Brand)	Effect If Taken with Tetracyclines
Drug–Drug Interactions	
Atovaquone (Mepron)	Decreased plasma levels of atovaquone, by as much as 40%; this combination is contraindicated for persons who need to take atovaquone for malarial prevention or treatment
Barbiturates[b]	Decreased doxycycline plasma levels
Carbamazepine (Tegretol)	Decreased plasma levels of tetracyclines
Colestipol (Colestid)	Decreased plasma levels of tetracyclines
Digoxin (Lanoxin)	Decreased plasma levels of tetracyclines
Ergotamine (Cafergot)	Increased risk for ergotism; bilateral upper limb ischemia
Isotretinoin (Accutane)	Increased risk for idiopathic intracranial hypertension
Lithium (Eskalith, Lithobid)	Increased lithium levels and possible toxicity
Methotrexate (Trexall, Rheumatrex)	Increased methotrexate plasma levels and possible toxicity
Molindone (Moban)	Decreased absorption of tetracyclines
Phenytoin (Dilantin)	Decreased plasma levels of tetracyclines
Quinapril (Accupril)	Decreased absorption of tetracyclines
Quinine	Increased quinine plasma levels and possible toxicity
Rifampin (RIF, Rifadin)[b]	Decreased doxycycline levels
Sucralfate (Carafate)	Decreased absorption of tetracyclines
Theophylline (Theo-Dur)	Increased theophylline levels
Warfarin (Coumadin)	Increased risk of bleeding
Drug–OTC Preparations Interactions	
Antacids	Decreased absorption of tetracyclines
Bismuth (Pepto-Bismol, Kaopectate)	Decreased absorption of tetracyclines
Iron-containing vitamins	Decreased absorption of tetracyclines
Laxatives	Decreased absorption of tetracyclines
Sodium bicarbonate (baking soda)	Decreased absorption of tetracyclines
Zinc	Decreased absorption of tetracyclines
Drug–Food Interactions	
Cheese	Decreased absorption of tetracyclines
Ethanol[b]	Decreased doxycycline plasma levels if chronic ethanol consumption
Iron-fortified cereals	Decreased absorption of tetracyclines
Milk, yogurt, and dairy products	Decreased absorption of tetracyclines

[a] This table is not comprehensive as new information is being generated on a regular basis.
[b] These interactions are specific for doxycycline as opposed to all tetracyclines.

the effectiveness of oral contraceptives. Tetracyclines form chelate complexes with many drugs that contain metal ions such as antacids, calcium, zinc, and iron. These chelate complexes are not absorbed, leading to reduced bioavailability of the tetracycline.[73] Milk products also contain ions and, therefore, may decrease absorption of tetracycline. The presence of food in the stomach may reduce absorption of tetracycline by as much as 50%. However, food taken with doxycycline (Vibramycin) or minocycline (Minocin) decreases absorption by only 20%, a level that is not considered clinically significant. Doxycycline is the only tetracycline extensively metabolized in the liver and subject to drug–drug interactions via inhibition or induction of CYP450 enzymes. Tetracyclines should not be used concomitantly with penicillins because the tetracycline diminishes the bactericidal activity of the penicillin.

The combination of diuretics and tetracyclines can result in decreased renal function and elevations in blood urea nitrogen and serum creatinine. Rifampin (Rifadin), phenobarbital (Luminal), phenytoin (Dilantin), and carbamazepine (Tegretol) induce CYP450 enzymes, thereby increasing doxycycline's metabolism and shortening its half-life.

Special Populations: Pregnancy, Lactation, and the Elderly

Tetracyclines should not be used by women during pregnancy or children 8 years and younger. Tetracycline becomes deposited in the teeth of the fetus, leading to discoloration and enamel dysplasia. It may also be deposited in the bones of the developing fetus, causing bone deformities and growth restriction. Tetracyclines are not contraindicated for breastfeeding women, most likely because the drug binds to milk calcium in the breast, which reduces transfer of the drug to the infant and results in low neonatal absorption.

Tetracyclines should be used with caution by anyone with renal impairment, as these drugs are eliminated renally. Reduction of kidney function is common among the elderly, so dose adjustments may be necessary in this population.

Oxazolidinones

The first oxazolidinone was formulated in the 1970s for control of bacterial and fungal diseases of certain foliage such as tomatoes and other plants. Due to initial adverse effects they were not marketed for human use. Further chemical modifications resulted in safer agents with superior properties and this class of drug became available in the United States in 2000.[74]

Mechanism of Action and Spectrum of Activity

Oxazolidinone, a monoamine oxidase (MAO) inhibitor, inhibits protein synthesis by interfering with the complex formation. Because of the unique binding site of oxazolidinone, it has no known cross-resistance with other drugs. The most commonly used oxazolidinone is linezolid (Zyvox), an antimicrobial that is bactericidal against streptococci and bacteriostatic against staphylococci and enterococci. Linezolid is primarily used to treat multidrug-resistant bacterial infections. It is active against gram-positive anaerobic cocci and gram-positive rods as well as against *Legionella*, *C. pneumoniae*, *S. pneumoniae*, and *H. influenzae*. Linezolid is approved for the treatment of community-acquired pneumonia, healthcare-associated pneumonia, complicated and uncomplicated skin infections, and vancomycin- and methicillin-resistant infections caused by multiresistant microbes.

Metabolism

Linezolid (Zyvox) is rapidly and extensively absorbed after oral administration, and peak serum levels are achieved within 1 to 2 hours. The time to peak concentration is delayed when linezolid is administered with a high-fat meal. This drug is well distributed in the tissues and is metabolized in the liver; approximately 65% of the dose is eliminated via nonrenal clearance. Linezolid may be administered intravenously or orally, with 600 mg given twice a day.

Side Effects and Adverse Reactions

The most common reactions reported—affecting 2% or more of individuals receiving linezolid—include diarrhea, headache, nausea, vomiting, insomnia, constipation, rash, and dizziness. More serious adverse reactions include peripheral and optic neuropathy, sometimes progressing to loss of vision in individuals who take the drug for longer than 28 days. An individual who experiences any visual impairment during linezolid therapy should stop taking the drug and have an ophthalmic evaluation performed. Seizures have been reported in some individuals, so persons at risk for seizures should not be administered linezolid. Myelosuppression occurs in approximately 3% of individuals who take linezolid for longer than a 2-week period and is more common among persons with renal impairment. The effects are reversible over time. Linezolid has also been associated with lactic acidosis, serotonin syndrome, and peripheral and optic neuropathy.[75]

Drug–Drug Interactions

Linezolid is a weak MAO inhibitor, and, therefore, this agent is associated with many clinically important drug–drug interactions. The *Mental Health* chapter reviews drug–drug interactions associated with MAO inhibitors in more detail. Persons taking linezolid should be counseled to avoid over-the-counter formulations that contain sympathomimetics such as phenylpropanolamine (Dexatrim) or pseudoephedrine (Sudafed). Likewise, they should not consume foods high in tyramine to avoid the potentially serious adverse effect of a hypertensive crisis. A small percentage of persons (fewer than 5%) will develop serotonin syndrome when linezolid is administered concomitantly with selective serotonin reuptake inhibitors.

Special Populations: Pregnancy, Lactation, and the Elderly

There is a paucity of data regarding the use of linezolid by women who are pregnant or breastfeeding. Nevertheless, it is likely that this agent may transfer through breast milk to the infant. Because myelosuppression has been observed in animal studies and reversible thrombocytopenia has been reported in adults, linezolid may not be the best choice of an anti-infective agent during pregnancy or breastfeeding.

No differences have been found in safety or effectiveness when linezolid is administered to elderly individuals. However, as is true for most antibiotics, this drug should be used with caution by persons with renal and hepatic impairment regardless of age.

Chloramphenicol

Chloramphenicol (Chloromycetin) was first isolated in 1947 from *Streptomyces venezuelae*, an organism found in a soil sample in Venezuela. It is not a first-line antibiotic because of its potential for causing aplastic anemia. Indeed, this agent is indicated only for treatment of life-threatening infections such as bacterial meningitis or rickettsial infections in individuals for whom the benefits outweigh the risks of potential toxicity.

Mechanism of Action and Spectrum of Activity

Choramphenicol is a protein synthesis inhibitor that readily penetrates bacterial cells. It binds to the 50S subunit of the bacterial ribosome. Chloramphenicol can also inhibit mitochondrial protein synthesis in mammalian cells; erythropoietic cells seem to be particularly sensitive to the drug. This antimicrobial agent has a wide range of activity against gram-positive, gram-negative, aerobic, and anaerobic bacteria, including typhoid fever, bacterial meningitis, rickettsial diseases, and brucellosis.

Metabolism

Chloramphenicol (Chloromycetin) is well absorbed orally or intravenously. The half-life of the active drug is 4 hours. The major route of elimination is hepatic metabolism to an inactive metabolite, which is then excreted in the urine. For this reason, any renal insufficiency can result in increased plasma concentrations.

Side Effects and Adverse Reactions

Nausea, vomiting, unpleasant taste, diarrhea, and perineal irritation may occur following the oral administration of chloramphenicol. Cases of contact dermatitis have been reported. Hypersensitivity is uncommon, but may appear as a macular or vesicular rash; fever may appear simultaneously or be the sole manifestation.

Adverse reactions include optic neuritis and gray syndrome. Gray syndrome is characterized by circulatory collapse, cyanosis, myocardial depression, and death. It is associated with high serum levels of chloramphenicol and is most likely to occur in persons who have hepatic or renal impairment; it is also a risk for newborns. The most important adverse effect, however, is on the bone marrow: Chloramphenicol is associated with a dose-related blood dyscrasia toxicity presenting as anemia, leukopenia, or thrombocytopenia or aplastic anemia. The product label carries a black box warning about the possibility of blood dyscrasias. In particular, chloramphenicol-associated aplastic anemia caused fatal cases of pancytopenia.

Drug–Drug Interactions

Chloramphenicol is a potent inhibitor of CYP2C619 and CYP3A4 and a weaker inhibitor of CYP2D6; consequently, it is associated with several clinically important drug–drug interactions. Chloramphenicol prolongs the half-lives of drugs that have a narrow therapeutic window, such as cyclosporine (Neoral), chlorpropamide (Diabinese), phenytoin (Dilantin), tacrolimus (Prototropic), tolbutamide (Orinase), and warfarin (Coumadin). Drugs that induce these enzymes, such as phenobarbital (Luminal) and rifampin (Rifadin), may shorten the half-life of chloramphenicol and result in subtherapeutic concentrations. All medications taken by a person who is started on chloramphenicol should be checked for drug–drug interactions given these risks.

Special Populations: Pregnancy, Lactation, and the Elderly

Although chloramphenicol (Chloromycetin) is lipid soluble and easily crosses the placenta, there are no reports linking this agent with birth defects. The drug can cause gray baby syndrome in neonates of women who were treated during pregnancy near the time of birth and in neonates given the drug directly. Fatal chloramphenicol toxicity is due to failure of the drug to be metabolized in the liver and inadequate renal excretion. Neonates should never be given this drug without close monitoring of serum levels. Chloramphenicol is secreted in breast milk but not in sufficiently large concentrations to produce gray baby syndrome, and no infant toxicity has been reported in the literature from use by lactating women. Nevertheless, this antibiotic is not recommended for use during pregnancy or by breastfeeding women due to its potential toxic effects.

There are no data about increased risk in the elderly following use of chloramphenicol. Caution should be exercised, however. When other antimicrobial drugs that are equally effective and potentially less toxic than chloramphenicol are available, they should be used instead.

Antibiotics That Affect DNA

Several antibiotics may potentially alter the DNA in bacteria. Included in this section are the fluoroquinolones and antiprotozoans. Rifampin (Rifadin) and possibly isoniazid (INH) may also alter bacterial DNA, but these drugs are included under the "Antimycobacterial Agents" section in this chapter.

Fluoroquinolones

Quinolones originally were used for eradication of gram-negative organisms found in urinary tract infections. The fluoroquinolones were formulated by adding a fluorine molecule to the quinolone structure, thereby increasing the drug's therapeutic use. This drug family, which is more commonly called the fluoroquinolones today, has bactericidal effects.

Like cephalosporins, fluoroquinolones are categorized by generations (Table 11-12). The first-generation formulations are rarely used today. Nalidixic acid was found to be a carcinogen and removed from use. Several of the second- and third-generation fluoroquinolones have also been removed from clinical practice secondary to toxicities or removed from the market as the manufacturer discontinued production. The fluoroquinolones most frequently used in clinical practice today are the second-generation ciprofloxacin (Cipro), the third-generation levofloxacin (Levaquin), and the fourth-generation moxifloxacin (Avelox). The third generation offers improved coverage against gram-positive organisms and a notably longer half-life. A number of broader-spectrum fluoroquinolones have been developed (e.g., sparfloxacin, trovafloxacin) but have been withdrawn from the U.S. market due to problems with toxicity.

Mechanism of Action and Spectrum of Activity

Fluoroquinolones block bacterial DNA synthesis by interfering with the function of two enzymes, topoisomerase II (gyrase) and topoisomerase IV.[76] Humans lack these enzymes, but they are required for the bacterial transcription process. Thus, fluoroquinolones prevent replication of bacteria or render them infertile. These drugs have a concentration-dependent bactericidal effect as well as a postantibiotic effect. They are given at high doses once or twice a day, rather than being administered as more frequent, albeit lower doses.[76]

Fluoroquinolones are broad-spectrum antibiotics. Notably, they are used for various respiratory infections caused by aerobic gram-negative bacteria such as *H. influenzae*. These drugs are also effective against *Shigella*, *Salmonella*, toxigenic *E. coli*, *Campylobacter*, and mycobacteria. They are used for the treatment of atypical pneumonias caused by *Chlamydiophila pneumoniae*, *Legionella pneumonophilia*, and *Mycoplasma pneumoniae*. In addition, fluoroquinolones can be used to treat infections causes by *Chlamydia trachomatis*, and some are effective against methicillin-susceptible strains of *Staphylococcus*, a gram-positive organism.

Mechanism of Resistance

Bacteria can develop resistance to fluoroquinolones via mutations in chromosomal genes or acquisition of resistance genes from plasmids. The likelihood of resistance is thought to increase with the duration of therapy, which is why shorter-duration regimens are used when possible. Fluoroquinolone resistance is increasing and is currently found in MRSA, some *Pseudomonas aeruginosa*, and *Neisseria gonorrhoeae*.

Clinical Indications

Fluoroquinolones are FDA approved for treatment of a wide range of infections. Except for the second-generation agents (which are increasingly resistant to *S. pneumoniae*), they are excellent drugs for respiratory infections. With the exception of moxifloxacin (Avelox), all fluoroquinolones

Table 11-12 Selected Fluoroquinolones[a]

Fluoroquinolone: Generic (Brand)	Indications	Doses	Adverse Reactions[b]	Clinical Considerations
Second-Generation Quinolones				
Ciprofloxacin (Cipro)	Mild to moderate UTI, lower respiratory tract infections, sinusitis, GI and skin infections, prostate infections, typhoid fever, bone and joint infections, anthrax prevention, gonorrhea, meningococcal carrier; effective against gram-negative organisms; weak activity against *S. pneumoniae* and no activity against anaerobes	PO: 250–750 mg 1–2 times/day IV: 200–400 mg every 12 hours	Mild GI/CNS symptoms, blood glucose abnormalities; can cause rupture of the Achilles tendon (contraindicated for children 18 years and younger)	Avoid when administering compounds with cations. Need proper hydration. Will cause precipitates to form if given in the same IV line with ampicillin or aminophylline.
Norfloxacin (Noroxin)		400 mg PO 2 times/day for 3 days	Mild GI/CNS symptoms; risk for tendon rupture (do not use in children 18 years and younger)	
Ofloxacin (Floxin)		200–400 mg 2 times/day	Dizziness, drowsiness, headache, GI symptoms, tendon rupture (do not use in children 18 years and younger)	
Third-Generation Quinolones				
Levofloxacin (Levaquin)	Same as second-generation, plus many gram-positive bacteria; less active than ciprofloxacin against *Pseudomonas* species	PO: 250–500 mg once daily IV: 500 mg	Mild GI/CNS symptoms, prolonged QT interval, rarely peripheral neuropathy	Improved pharmacokinetics allow once daily administration.
Fourth-Generation Quinolones				
Gemifloxacin (Factive)	Same as second-generation; increased activity against *S. pneumoniae* and anaerobes	320 mg PO once daily for 5 days	Mild GI/CNS symptoms, prolonged QT interval, hypersensitivity reaction	Used for community-acquired pneumonia and acute exacerbation of chronic bronchitis.
Moxifloxacin (Avelox)		PO: 400 mg once daily IV: 400 mg	Altered sense of taste, prolonged QT interval Hyperglycemia or hypoglycemia	Use with caution in persons with diabetes.

Abbreviations: CNS = central nervous system; GI = gastrointestinal; UTI = urinary tract infection.

[a] This is not a complete list of the quinolones available in the United States today. There are several other agents in each of the generations.

[b] Pseudomembranous colitis may occur with all quinolones; monitor for persistence of diarrhea.

Sources: Data from King DE, Malone R, Lilley S. New classification and update on the quinolone antibiotics. *Am Fam Phys.* 2000;61(9):2741-2748[79]; Liu HH. Safety profile of the fluoroquinolones. *Drug Saf.* 2010;33(5):353-369;[78] O'Donnell JA, Gelone SP. The newer fluoroquinolones. *Infect Dis Clin North Am.* 2004;18(3):691-716[76]; Sousa J, Alves G, Fortuna A, Falcao A. Third and fourth generation fluoroquinolone antibacterials: a systematic review of safety and toxicity profiles. *Curr Drug Saf.* 2014;9(2):89-105.[77]

may be used for the treatment of urinary tract infections caused by multidrug-resistant bacteria. Norfloxacin (Noroxin) is approved in the United States only for treatment of urinary tract infections. A 7-day course of ofloxacin (Floxin) is an alternative to doxycycline (Vibramycin) or azithromycin (Zithromax) for *C. trachomatis* infections. A single oral dose of ofloxacin or ciprofloxacin (Cipro) is effective against some strains of *N. gonorrhoeae* but is not the first-line therapy due to increasing resistance. A 14-day course of ofloxacin has been effective in treatment of pelvic inflammatory disease, when combined with an antibiotic with anaerobic activity. A 3-day course of ciprofloxacin is effective against chancroid.

Fluoroquinolones are also used for the treatment of bone, joint, and soft-tissue infections. Norfloxacin, ciprofloxacin, and a 5-day course of ofloxacin are effective against shigellosis and traveler's diarrhea. Newer fluoroquinolones such as moxifloxacin (Avelox) and gatifloxacin (Tequin) are indicated for treating community-acquired pneumonia (*S. pneumoniae*) and may be comparable to the beta-lactams as a therapy for this infection.

Gemifloxacin (Factive) and moxifloxacin (Avelox) are often referred to as the *respiratory fluoroquinolones* because of their enhanced gram-positive activity against the atypical chlamydial *Mycoplasma* and *Legionella* pneumonia infections. Ciprofloxacin (Cipro) and levofloxacin (Levaquin), along with azithromycin (Zithromax), are the antibiotics of choice for *Legionella pneumophila*. Ciprofloxacin is the preferred agent for prophylaxis and treatment of anthrax.

Metabolism

Fluoroquinolones are absorbed well and 80% to 95% bioavailable when taken orally. They have a wide distribution to tissues and body fluids.[76] Peak concentrations in serum are usually attained within 3 hours of administration. Taking the medication with food does not seem to affect the extent of quinolone absorption, but it may delay the time to reach peak drug concentrations in serum. Serum half-life ranges from 3 to 5 hours for norfloxacin (Noroxin) and ciprofloxacin (Cipro) to 20 hours for sparfloxacin (Zagam). Elimination for the majority of preparations is renal; consequently, doses must be adjusted for persons with renal impairment. Pefloxacin (Pelflacine) and moxifloxacin (Avelox) are metabolized predominantly in the liver, whereas norfloxacin (Noroxin), gemifloxacin (Factive), and ciprofloxacin (Cipro) are eliminated via both the hepatic and renal routes.

Side Effects and Adverse Reactions

Fluoroquinolones are, in general, well tolerated. The most common side effects associated with all these agents are nausea, vomiting, diarrhea (5–10% incidence), headache (5% incidence), dizziness, and insomnia.[77] Rashes occur in approximately 1% of all individuals who take these drugs. Interestingly, approximately 14% of women 40 years or younger who take gemifloxacin (Factive) for more than 7 days develop a rash; thus this drug is given for a maximum of 5 days of continuous therapy if possible. The rash is even more likely to occur if the woman is taking estrogen-containing products in addition to the fluoroquinolone. Photosensitivity may also occur. These drugs have been found to induce both hyperglycemia and hypoglycemia, particularly in persons with diabetes. Moxifloxacin appears to carry the highest risk for dysglycemia.

Box 11-5 Don't Forget *C. diff*

NC is a 42-year-old woman who completed a course of ciprofloxacin (Cipro) for presumed *Mycoplasma* pneumonia 2 weeks ago. NC reported diarrhea and abdominal cramping for 4 days that did not resolve following a day of bowel rest and use of loperamide (Imodium). She is having three or four episodes of foul-smelling diarrhea per day and feels very ill but is afebrile.

There is a suspicion that NC may have a pseudomembranous colitis caused by *Clostridium difficile* (called *C. diff*, pronounced "see-diff"). This gram-positive, spore-forming rod is a normal inhabitant of the intestine, but it has become resistant to fluoroquinolones. Thus, when ciprofloxacin eradicates most of the gut flora, the *C. difficile* colony blossoms. Infection with *C. difficile* is an identified risk associated with several antimicrobial drugs. There is some evidence that *C. difficile* may also be acquired via oral ingestion of the heat-resistant spores, which then convert to the vegetative forms in the intestine.

C. difficile releases toxins that cause the symptoms of pseudomembranous colitis. If untreated, *C. diff* overgrowth can cause sepsis, bowel perforation, or toxic megacolon, although these complications are more common in persons at higher risk for infection—namely, the elderly and persons who were recently hospitalized with a serious medical condition or need for a surgical procedure.

The antibiotics that effectively treat *C. difficile* are metronidazole (Flagyl) 500 mg 3 times a day for 10–14 days and vancomycin (Vanocin) 500 mg 4 times a day for 10–14 days. Metronidazole can cause a metallic taste in the mouth, nausea, and occasionally vomiting. Vancomycin should be used by persons who do not tolerate metronidazole or by women who are pregnant. Some evidence indicates that probiotics are also effective in helping restore the normal gut flora in persons with *C. diff*.

Follow-up is very important, because approximately 25% of persons with *C. difficile* overgrowth will become reinfected following treatment. It is not clear if these reinfections represent a relapse or a true reinfection from ingesting *C. difficile* spores. Treatment of reinfection consists of a second course of the same antibiotic used the first time, and most relapses respond to such retreatment if needed. NC had a resolution of symptoms 5 days after she started treatment with metronidazole (Flagyl).

Some serious adverse effects can occur following use of these antibiotics. Fluoroquinolones may exacerbate muscle weakness in persons who have myasthenia gravis and are contraindicated for these individuals. In 2008, the FDA issued a black box warning noting that fluoroquinolones increase the risk for developing tendinitis and tendon rupture in persons of all ages.[78] Levofloxacin, gemifloxacin, and moxifloxacin may cause a prolonged QT interval and are contraindicated for individuals with a known prolonged QT interval or hypokalemia.

In 2013, the FDA added a black box warning to the label of these drugs, warning about the possibility of peripheral neuropathy. When peripheral neuropathy occurs, it may either resolve or be permanent.

Fluoroquinolones occasionally can cause interstitial nephritis. The clinical presentation of antibiotic-induced interstitial nephritis varies, but it should be suspected in any individual on a fluoroquinolone who develops an acute renal dysfunction.[78] Fluoroquinolone use has also been associated with central nervous system effects including hallucinations, slurred speech, confusion, and even seizures in 1% to 2% of recipients. These symptoms usually resolve once the medication is discontinued, but the presence of a neurologic disorder might predispose users to these symptoms and, therefore, needs to be assessed.[78]

In addition, the development of pseudomembranous colitis secondary to overgrowth of *C. difficile* is particularly notable risk associated with fluoroquinolone treatment.[78] *C. difficile* overgrowth is resistant to fluoroquinolones; thus, as use of these drugs has increased, so has the incidence of pseudomembranous colitis (Box 11-5). Finally, fluoroquinolones cause hypersensitivity reactions including anaphylaxis, albeit very rarely.

Drug–Drug Interactions

Fluoroquinolones have multiple drug–drug interactions of clinical import.[79] Ciprofloxacin (Cipro), for example, is a strong inhibitor of CYP1A2. Well known drug–drug interactions associated with fluoroquinolones are listed in Table 11-13. Clinicians who prescribe fluoroquinolones should check all medications taken by their patients for clinically significant drug–drug interactions, as some combinations are contraindicated. Absorption of fluoroquinolones is impaired in the presence of magnesium, calcium, aluminum, and zinc. Therefore, any form of antacid, vitamin, or dairy product containing these cations must be avoided prior to taking the medication and within several hours after administration.

When fluoroquinolones are taken with caffeine, warfarin (Coumadin), cyclosporine (Neoral), or theophylline (Theo-Dur), they cause increased serum concentrations of these drugs. There is an increased risk of seizures when ciprofloxacin is used concurrently with foscarnet (Foscavir).[19]

Table 11-13 Fluoroquinolones: Selected Drug–Drug Interactions[a]

Drug: Generic (Brand)	Effect If Taken with Fluoroquinolone
All Quinolone Interactions	
Aluminum- or magnesium-containing antacids	Reduced bioavailability of fluoroquinolone
Antiarrhythmics: Class Ia and III (quinidine, ibutilide [Covert], Sotalol [Betapace], dofetilide [Tikosyn], amiodarone [Cordarone], verapamil [Calan])	Increased concentration of antiarrhythmic, prolonged QT interval, torsades de pointes, death; fluoroquinolones should not be used by persons who are taking antiarrhythmic drugs
Antipsychotics (e.g., haloperidol [Haldol], risperidone [Risperdal], clozapine [Clozaril])	Increased concentration of antipsychotic medication, risk of torsades de pointes, disorientation with clozapine
Multivitamins containing calcium, iron, or zinc	Reduced bioavailability of fluoroquinolones
Nonsteroidal anti-inflammatory drugs (NSAIDs)	CNS stimulation and convulsive seizures
Sucralfate (Carafate)	Decreased absorption of fluoroquinolones
Ciprofloxacin, Enoxacin, and Norfloxacin Interactions in Addition to Those Listed for All Fluoroquinolones	
Carbamazepine (Tegretol)	Increased levels of carbamazepine
Clozapine (Clozaril)	Increased levels of clozapine
Cyclosporine (Neoral)	Increased serum concentration of cyclosporine and risk for nephrotoxicity
Duloxetine (Cymbalta)	Increased plasma levels of duloxetine
Foscarnet (Foscavir)	Increased risk of seizures
Glyburide (Micronase)	Hypoglycemia requiring urgent treatment
Nitrofurantoin (Macrobid)	Nitrofurantoin antagonizes the antibiotic effect of norfloxacin in the urinary tract
Phenytoin (Dilantin)	Increased plasma levels of phenytoin and possible phenytoin toxicity
Tacrine (Cognex)	Increased plasma levels of tacrine
Theophylline (Theo-Dur)	Increased theophylline levels and potential theophylline toxicity
Tizanidine (Zanaflex)	Increased plasma levels of tizanidine
Warfarin (Coumadin)	Increased plasma levels of warfarin
Drug–Food Interactions	
Caffeine	Increased plasma levels of caffeine
Milk, yogurt, and dairy products	Decreased bioavailability of fluoroquinolones

[a] This table is not comprehensive as new information is being generated on a regular basis.

Table 11-14 Nitroimidazoles

Nitroimidazole: Generic (Brand)	Indication	Dose	Adverse Reactions	Clinical Considerations
Metronidazole (Flagyl)	*Trichomonas vaginalis* (TV), bacterial vaginosis (BV), amebiasis, pseudomembranous colitis, component of treatment of polymicrobial infections	TV: 2 g single dose BV: 250 mg 3 times/day or 375–500 mg 2 times/day Amebiasis: 500–750 mg 3 times/day Pseudomembranous colitis: 250–500 mg 3-4 times/day for 10–14 days	Dizziness, headache, abdominal pain, anorexia, nausea, vomiting, unpleasant taste, leucopenia, peripheral neuropathy, disulfiram-like reaction with alcohol	Avoid alcohol due to pronounced gastrointestinal upset, flushing, and palpitations. Use with caution in persons with hepatic insufficiency.
Tinidazole (Tindamax)	Bacterial vaginosis, *T. vaginalis*, giardiasis, amebiasis	BV: 1 g once daily for 5 days or 2 g once daily for 2 days TV and giardiasis: 2 g single dose Amebiasis: 2 g/day for 3 days	Dizziness, headache, constipation, dyspepsia, metallic or bitter taste, vomiting, vaginal candidiasis	Take with food to minimize gastrointestinal discomforts. Avoid alcohol while taking.

Special Populations: Pregnancy and Lactation

Fluoroquinolones are generally contraindicated for pregnant women and children 8 years or younger unless there are no safer alternatives, because these drugs cause cartilage abnormalities in animals. Studies evaluating outcomes of infants born to women exposed to norfloxacin or ciprofloxacin during the first trimester have identified no increase in teratogenic risks.[31] Nevertheless, because other, equally effective drugs are better studied and known to be safe in pregnancy, fluoroquinolines are not generally used in pregnant women.

Current studies suggest that the amount of fluoroquinolones present in breast milk is quite low. However, if ciprofloxacin (Cipro) is used by a lactating mother, the infant needs to be observed closely for diarrhea. Ciprofloxacin is considered compatible with breastfeeding by the American Academy of Pediatrics. Levofloxacin (Levaquin), ofloxacin (Floxin), and norfloxacin (Noroxin) have milk/plasma ratios even lower in breast milk than does ciprofloxacin, and these agents often are the first-line choices for breastfeeding mothers when this class of drugs is indicated.

Antiprotozoans: Nitromidazoles

A wide variety of protozoal parasites affect humans and are transmitted by insects, other mammals, or other humans. There are no effective vaccines for contact with these protozoa, so chemotherapy is the only practical treatment, and maintaining the integrity of the immune system is crucial. Protozoal infections include malaria, amebiasis, giardiasis, trichomoniasis, toxoplasmosis, giardiasis, cryptosporidiosis, and trypanosomiasis (sleeping sickness).[80] Toxoplasmosis is primarily treated with drugs discussed elsewhere, such as pyrimethamine (Daraprim), sulfadiazine, and clindamycin (Cleocin). Many of the other infective protozoans are found primarily in developing countries; the discussion here concentrates on the antiprotozoal drugs most commonly used in the United States—namely, the nitroimidazoles, metronidazole (Flagyl), and tinidazole (Tindamax). The drugs used to treat lice, scabies (1% permethrin [Nix]), and pinworms (mebendazole [Vermox]) are also reviewed (Table 11-14).

Metronidazole

Metronidazole (Flagyl) is a nitroimidazole drug that was introduced in 1959 for its antiprotozoal activity in treating *Trichomonas vaginalis*. This drug penetrates well into tissue and has been found to be bactericidal and effective for treatment of infections caused by both anaerobic bacteria and protozoa.

Mechanism of Action and Spectrum of Activity

Metronidazole is a prodrug that works in a unique way. Susceptible anaerobic organisms are able to donate electrons to the metronidazole molecule. This changes metronidazole into a highly reactive nitro anion radical that kills the host organism via alteration of the DNA and perhaps alterations of other significant biologic proteins within that organism. Thus, metronidazole enters the cell by diffusion and has a cytotoxic effect via the transformation into destructive free radicals.[80] Because aerobic bacteria are unable to activate metronidazole, they are not susceptible to its effects.

Metronidazole is effective against the anaerobes *B. fragilis*, *C. difficile* (and other *Clostridium* species), *Fusobacterium* species, *Gardnerella vaginalis*, and *H. pylori*. The drug is used for treatment of anaerobic intra-abdominal and pelvic infections. Because it penetrates well into the cerebrospinal fluid, it is useful for the treatment of meningitis or brain abscess caused by *B. fragilis*. Metronidazole is effective against pseudomembranous colitis caused by *C. difficile*.[81] It has also been used in combination with a proton pump inhibitor and clarithromycin or tetracycline for the treatment of *H. pylori* infection.[82] Resistance to metronidazole is being seen increasingly in all organisms that have traditionally been susceptible to this agent, so treatment failures do occur.

Clinical Indications

Metronidazole is effective against *T. vaginalis* and is the standard treatment for bacterial vaginosis. It has also demonstrated clinical effectiveness for the treatment of amebiasis, giardiasis, and some bacterial infections (e.g., *Bacteriodes*, *Clostridium*, *Helicobacter*, and *Campylobacter* species). Owing to these characteristics, it is a component of prophylaxis against postoperative mixed aerobic and anaerobic infections. Two of its most important indications today are treatment of *H. pylori* and *C. difficile* infections.

Metabolism

Metronidazole (Flagyl) is readily absorbed throughout the body, appearing in spinal fluid, breast milk, and saliva, and with peak plasma concentrations occurring 1 to 2 hours after oral administration. Its bioavailability is approximately 90% following oral absorption, with a half-life of approximately 8 hours.[83] When this agent is administered intravaginally, serum levels are lower—approximately 2% of the serum level found following administration of a 500-mg oral dose.

Metronidazole (Flagyl) is metabolized in the liver via hydroxylation. Approximately 60% to 80% of the drug is excreted through the urine, with the remaining 15% being excreted through feces. Metronidazole is metabolized in the liver and excreted renally.

Side Effects and Adverse Reactions

Gastrointestinal problems such as nausea, metallic taste, and diarrhea are the most commonly reported side effects. Individuals with hepatic insufficiency may have difficulty metabolizing metronidazole. More serious, but rare adverse effects include peripheral neuropathy, seizures, and pancreatitis. Seizures have been reported with high doses, and peripheral neuropathy with prolonged use of metronidazole.[80] Because metronidazole has been shown to be carcinogenic in mice and rats, its label carries a black box warning that states unnecessary use of the drug should be avoided.

Drug–Drug Interactions

Metronidazole (Flagyl) inhibits CYP2C9 and CYP3A4, which results in many drug–drug interactions (Table 11-15). This agent is structurally similar to disulfiram, and if the two are taken together, acute psychosis can occur.[83,84] Some individuals who drink alcohol while taking metronidazole will develop a disulfiram-like (Antabuse-like) effect of pronounced GI upset, flushing, and palpitations. Therefore, individuals should be counseled to avoid alcohol while taking metronidazole and for at least 24 hours after the last dose. This restriction includes alcoholic drinks, alcohol-based cough syrups, flavorings, or other products.[80]

Metronidazole (Flagyl) increases the plasma levels of several drugs, including cyclosporine (Neoral), carbamazepine (Tegretol), lithium (Eskalith, Lithane), phenytoin (Dilantin), tacrolimus (Prototropic), and warfarin (Coumadin). The drugs that are CYP34A inducers—such as phenobarbital (Luminal), phenytoin (Dilantin), and rifampin (Rifadin)—increase the metabolism of metronidazole, thereby decreasing its effectiveness.[80]

Special Populations: Pregnancy, Lactation, and the Elderly

The use of metronidazole (Flagyl) has been controversial in pregnancy. Early animal studies showed the drug to be mutagenic and potentially carcinogenic. Although it has not been shown to act this way in humans, some have advised against the use of metronidazole by pregnant women, especially during the first trimester of pregnancy. However, most sources now advocate use during any trimester of pregnancy if the drug is needed to treat a symptomatic condition.[85]

No reports of untoward effects in breastfed infants with any of the dosage regimens have been published, but metronidazole is excreted into breast milk in larger than usual amounts (approximately 20%). If a breastfeeding woman takes this medication, the American Academy of Pediatrics recommends discontinuing breastfeeding for 12 to 24 hours to allow excretion of the dose, or the mother can pump her breast milk and discard it ("pump and dump") in order not to suppress lactation.

Metronidazole should be used with caution by older adults who have renal impairment or hepatic or biliary disease.

Tinidazole

Tinidazole (Tindamax) is a nitroimidazole, approved in 2004, that is similar to metronidazole in its effect against amebiasis, giardiasis, and trichomoniasis. It has a better toxicity profile than metronidazole, however.

Table 11-15 Drug–Drug Interactions Associated with Metronidazole[a]

Drug: Generic (Brand)	Reaction and Clinical Considerations
Alcohol, including over-the-counter cough syrups, ethanol-containing medications, and licit consumption	Possible disulfiram-like reaction including significant nausea, vomiting, tachycardia, diarrhea, chills, and sweating
Antiarrhythmics: Class Ia and III (quinidine, ibutilide [Covert], Sotalol [Betapace], dofetilide [Tikosyn], amiodarone [Cordarone], verapamil [Calan])	Increased risk of prolonged QT interval
Aripiprazole (Abilify)	Increased serum concentrations of aripiprazole
Busulfan (Myleran)	Increased serum concentration of busulfan and possible toxic effects; avoid this combination
Disulfiram (Antabuse)	Enhanced adverse or toxic effects of metronidazole; avoid this combination
Ergot derivatives (drugs used to treat migraine and Parkinson disease)	Decreased elimination of ergot derivatives
Fluorouracil (Efudex)	Increased concentration of fluorouracil
Lithium (Lithobid)	Promotion of renal retention of lithium, increasing lithium levels and possible toxicity
Mebendazole (Vermox)	Enhanced risk of toxic effects of metronidazole, particularly risks of Stevens-Johnson syndrome and toxic epidermal necrolysis
Mifepristone	Enhanced risk of toxic effects of metronidazole, particularly risks of Stevens-Johnson syndrome and toxic epidermal necrolysis
Phenytoin (Dilantin)	Decreased clearance of phenytoin, resulting in increased serum concentration of phenytoin and possible ineffectiveness of metronidazole
Phenobarbital	Decreased serum concentration of metronidazole
Rifampin (Rifadin)	Decreased clearance of rifampin, resulting in increased serum concentration of rifampin and possible ineffectiveness of metronidazole
Warfarin (Coumadin) and other anticoagulants	Increased anticoagulant effects, leading to prolongation of prothrombin time

[a] This table is not comprehensive as new information is being generated on a regular basis.
Source: Data from Miljkovic V, Arsic B, Bojanic Z, et al. Interactions of metronidazole with other medicines: a brief review. *Pharmazie.* 2014;69(8):571-577.[84]

Mechanism of Action and Spectrum of Activity

Tinidazole (Tindamax) has a mechanism of action similar to that of metronidazole. Free nitro anion radicals are generated as a result of reduction of the nitro group of tinidazole by *T. vaginalis*, which is responsible for the antiprotozoal activity. The mechanism by which tinidazole acts against *Giardia* and *Entamoeba* species is unknown. Approximately 38% of *T. vaginalis* isolates exhibiting reduced susceptibility to metronidazole also show reduced susceptibility to tinidazole in vitro, but this appears much less common in practice. To reduce development of resistance, it is recommended that tinidazole be used only in cases where metronidazole is shown to be ineffective.

Clinical Indications

Tinidazole (Tindamax) is indicated for the treatment of *T. vaginalis* infections, bacterial vaginosis, and infections caused by *E. histolytica* and *G. lamblia*. It has been documented to have in vitro activity against *Bacteriodes*, *Fusobacterium*, and *Clostridium* species. It is also used in the treatment of amebiasis and giardiasis.[80,86,87]

Metabolism

Oral tinidazole (Tindamax) is readily absorbed by simple diffusion. The drug becomes widely distributed among all tissues, and it crosses the placental and blood–brain barriers. Peak plasma concentrations are reached in 2 to 3 hours, and the half-life is 12.7 hours. Tinidazole is excreted mainly in the urine; plasma clearance is reduced in the presence of hepatic impairment.[80,86]

Side Effects and Adverse Reactions

The most common side effects associated with tinidazole (Tindamax) include dizziness and headache, gastrointestinal effects such as constipation or diarrhea, vomiting, dyspepsia, and a metallic or bitter taste. Rarely, hypersensitivity reactions have occurred.[86] Like metronidazole, tinidazole is carcinogenic in mice and rats; thus, its label carries a black box warning that states unnecessary use of the drug should be avoided.

Drug–Drug Interactions

Although tinidazole (Tindamax) is a CYP3A4 and CYP2B6 inhibitor, there have been few reports of drug interactions. However, alcohol should be avoided when this medication is used, as with metronidazole.[80,86]

Special Populations: Pregnancy, Lactation, and the Elderly

There is some evidence of teratogenic potential in animal studies of tinidazole (Tindamax), and the manufacturer recommends this agent be avoided in the first trimester of pregnancy.[86] Current recommendations suggest interruption of breastfeeding for up to 3 days following administration of tinidazole due to lack of safety studies.[86] This span is longer than is recommended for use of metronidazole (Flagyl) and reflects both the lack of knowledge and a cautious approach by the professional organizations that issue such guidelines.

There are not enough studies of use of tinidazole (Tindamax) in the elderly to assess any changes in the response with aging. Caution should be exercised in the presence of hepatic or renal insufficiency due to decreased clearance.

Sulfonamides

Sulfonamides were the first agents formulated for the treatment of bacterial infections in the 1930s. They were actually discovered in 1936 by Gerhard Domagk, who found that an industrial dye named Prontosil was able to cure infections in mice. He subsequently used the drug to treat his daughter, who was very ill with a streptococcal infection that failed to respond to standard treatments. Domagk won the Nobel Prize in 1938 for his discovery. Because Adolf Hitler prohibited German scientists like Domagk from accepting this prize, he declined it. Domagk was eventually given the award in 1947.[88]

The term "sulfa drug" generally refers to antimicrobial drugs that contain a sulfonamide. Because many drugs used for different purposes have a sulfonamide moiety (SO_2NH_2) in the formulation, the term "sulfa drug" is imprecise and not recommended for use. Drugs that contain a sulfonamide moiety are initially divided into antimicrobial sulfonamides such as sulfisoxazole (Gantrisin) and nonantimicrobial sulfonamides such as the sulfonylureas used to treat diabetes. Allergies to sulfonamides are common, so any drug that has a sulfonamide group moiety may elicit an allergic reaction in a sensitive person.

Antimicrobial sulfonamides are broad-spectrum bacteriostatic drugs (Table 11-16). They are categorized as short-acting, intermediate-acting, long-acting, or ultra-long-acting agents. Long-acting sulfonamides have been associated with fatal hypersensitivity reactions, especially in children, which severely limits their use. In addition, these drugs can be divided into three major groups:

- Oral absorbable agents that are absorbed from the stomach and small intestine, metabolized in the liver, distributed widely throughout the body tissues, and cross the placenta.
- Oral, nonabsorbent agents, which includes sulfasalazine (Azulfidine). These drugs are relatively poorly absorbed from the gastrointestinal tract and, because of this effect, have been used to treat inflammatory bowel disorders and to suppress susceptible bowel flora before surgery.
- Topical preparations, such as sulfacetamide (Bleph 10) is a topical treatment for ophthalmic infections.

Mechanism of Action and Spectrum of Activity

Although a wide variety of chemical modifications of the sulfonamides have been synthesized, all share essentially the same mechanism of action. These agents are structurally similar to *para*-aminobenzoic acid (PABA), which is required for bacterial folic acid synthesis. The sulfonamides compete with PABA for incorporation into folic acid. Once the sulfonamide is incorporated, the synthesis of folic acid stops. Thus, sulfonamides are bacteriostatic in that they inhibit bacterial growth by interfering with microbial folic acid synthesis. Sulfonamides are rapidly absorbed and metabolized in the liver via acetylation and glucuronidation.

Sulfonamides are active against gram-positive bacteria, gram-negative bacteria, and protozoal infections. Acute toxoplasmosis can be treated with sulfadiazine in combination with pyrimethamine. Sulfasalazine (Azulfidine) is used to treat inflammatory bowel disease including ulcerative colitis and enteritis.

Mechanism of Resistance

Most bacterial species have developed some resistance to sulfonamides. For example, some bacteria have developed decreased permeability to the drug. Others have gene

Table 11-16 Sulfonamides

Sulfonamide: Generic (Brand)	Indications	Dose	Side Effects and Adverse Effects	Clinical Considerations[a,b]
Mafenide (Sulfamylon)	Topical antibiotic used to treat second- and third-degree burns	Apply to burned area 1–2 times/day	Hypersensitivity reaction, blood dyscrasias, Stevens-Johnson syndrome	Adverse effects are possible regardless of the route of administration. Prolonged use may result in fungal or bacterial superinfection. Use with caution in persons with renal impairment.
Silver sulfadiazine (Silvadene)	Topical antibiotic used to treat second- and third-degree burns	Aerosol, cleanser or cream; apply to a thickness of 1/16 inch; burned area should be covered with cream at all times		
Sodium sulfacetamide (Bleph-10)	Conjunctivitis or superficial ocular infection Trachoma	1–2 drops every 2–3 hours for 7–10 days; used with systemic therapy for trachoma		
Sulfur and sulfacetamide (AVAR)	Acne vulgaris, acne rosacea, seborrheic dermatitis	Apply in thin film 1–3 times/day	Contact dermatitis, blood dyscrasias, Stevens-Johnson syndrome, drug-induced lupus, hepatic necrosis, hypersensitivity reaction	
Sulfacetamide (Klaron, Ovace Wash)	Acne vulgaris (Klaron lotion), bacterial infections (Ovace Plus lotion), scaling dermatoses (Cream, shampoo, or Ovace Plus lotion)	Apply to infected area 2 times/day	Contact dermatitis Blood dyscrasias Stevens-Johnson syndrome Drug-induced lupus Hepatic necrosis Hypersensitivity reaction	Avoid contact with eyes or mucous membranes.
Sulfisoxazole (Gantrisin)	Urinary tract infections, otitis media, sinusitis, bronchitis, pneumonia, traveler's diarrhea, diverticulitis, rheumatic fever prophylaxis	1–2 g every 6 hours (dose varies depending on the indication)		Primarily used as a pediatric drug. Short acting. Maximum adult daily dose is 8 g. Fluid intake should be sufficient with all sulfonamides.
Sulfadiazine	Same as sulfisoxazole; when combined with pyrimethamine, is used to treat toxoplasmosis.	1 g every 4–6 hours	Nausea, rash, hypersensitivity reaction, confusion, dizziness, diarrhea, blood dyscrasias, Stevens-Johnson syndrome, kernicterus, renal damage	Short acting.
Trimethoprim and sulfamethoxazole (TMP/SMX) (Bactrim DS, Septra DS)	Same as sulfisoxazole plus *Shigella flexneri*, MRSA, *Listeria*	Oral single-strength is 80 TMP/400 SMK; usual dose is 1–4 times/day Oral double strength is 160 TMP/800 SMX; usual dose is 2 times/day Suppression of: UTI varies Dosing based on trimethoprim component as mg/kg/day for IV dosing	Nausea, vomiting, and rash; hypersensitivity reaction; hyperkalemia and blood dyscrasias; many drug–drug interactions	Intermediate-acting; adverse effects are much more likely in persons infected with HIV.

[a] These drugs are not teratogenic but should not be given in the third trimester of pregnancy due to risk of hyperbilirubinemia, severe jaundice, hemolytic anemia, and theoretically kernicterus in the newborn.

[b] All sulfonamides are contraindicated for persons with glucose-6-phosphate dehydrogenase deficiency (G6PD), as they can precipitate hemolysis in this population.

mutations in the PABA binding site that disallows the sulfonamide to attach to the target. Still others have developed active efflux mechanisms that eliminate the drug from the intracellular space.

Trimethoprim/Sulfamethoxazole

The combination of trimethoprim/sulfamethoxazole (TMP/SMX; Bactrim, Septra) has a unique mechanism of action whereby both drugs independently affect one part of the pathway that results in synthesis of tetrahydrofolic acid, which is essential for the production of bacterial folic acid. Both drugs are bacteriostatic when used alone, but bactericidal when used in this combination formulation. TMP/SMX is effective against many urinary, respiratory, and gastrointestinal pathogens in addition to MRSA and protozoan pathogens. This combination formulation is especially therapeutic for urinary tract infections caused by *E. coli*, *Klebsiella*, *Enterobacter*, *P. mirabilis*, and *Proteus vulgaris* and, therefore, is well known to women's health-care providers. However, resistance is widespread and geographically specific, so providers need to know their local patterns of resistance before prescribing this drug.

Side Effects and Adverse Reactions

Sulfonamides are associated with multiple side effects, including nausea, vomiting, diarrhea, rash, fever, headache, and depression. Most concerning, however, are allergic reactions to sulfonamides. Allergic reactions to these agents are the second most frequent cause of allergic drug reactions, after those caused by beta-lactam antibiotics.[89]

Sulfa Allergy

Hypersensitivity reactions to sulfonamides are caused by a reactive metabolite resulting from the CYP450 enzyme-facilitated metabolism of the parent drug. Persons who have the slow-acetylator phenotype may be at increased risk for developing sulfonamide allergic reactions.[90] Immediate Type I hypersensitivity reactions are rare. Rash, which usually appears within 3 days of initiation of therapy and resolves as soon as the drug is discontinued, is the most common allergic reaction. More seriously, the sulfonamides are among the most common causes of Stevens-Johnson syndrome, a rare condition that can evolve into toxic epidermal necrolysis with a mortality rate of 30%. Therefore, Stevens-Johnson syndrome should be considered if a woman presents with a history of sulfonamide use and inflammation of the mucous membranes and/or a painful, blistering rash.

Less common reactions to sulfonamides include drug-induced lupus, serum sickness-like syndrome, hemolytic anemia, and aseptic meningitis. These drugs can crystalize in the renal tubules, causing acute renal failure, and they can block secretion of creatinine. Acute pancreatitis has been associated with sulfonamide use. Individuals with glucose-6-phosphate dehydrogenase (G6PD) deficiency are at risk for a sulfonamide-induced hemolytic anemia. Sulfonamides may also cause neutropenia, agranulocytosis, or induction of thrombocytopenia.

Cross-Reactivity of Sulfonamide Allergic Reaction

The sulfonamide allergy is important because other frequently used classes of drugs, such as sulfonylureas, diuretics, celecoxib (Celebrex), dapsone, and sumatriptan (Imitrex), have a sulfonamide moiety, and the existence of cross-reactivity has been controversial.[90,91] Cutaneous rashes develop in 3% to 4% of persons who take drugs that have a sulfonamide component. This rash usually presents 72 hours to 2 weeks after administration. Approximately 0.4% of persons who take a sulfonamide develop a severe hypersensitivity reaction such as anaphylaxis or Stevens-Johnson syndrome.[91] The exception is persons who are HIV positive: These individuals have a greater incidence of developing rashes to sulfonamide antibiotics for reasons that have not been fully elucidated.

Cross-reactivity of the allergic reaction between sulfonamide antibiotics and sulfonamide nonantibiotics does not occur because the reactive metabolite responsible for the reaction is not generated in the metabolism of sulfonamide nonantibiotics. However, approximately 10% of persons who report a reaction to sulfonamide antibiotics will also have a reaction to sulfonamide nonantibiotics. It is theorized that these persons have an innate tendency to develop drug reactions, which in this case occur secondary to an underlying mechanism that is not related to the sulfonamide moiety.[91]

Manufacturers of sulfonamide-containing drugs vary in how they label their products with regard to sulfonamide allergy. Moreover, there are no clear clinical guidelines for practitioners. Consequently, decisions about prescribing sulfonamide nonantibiotics to persons who have reported a sulfa allergy following a course of a sulfonamide antibiotic must be individualized.

Drug–Drug Interactions

Sulfonamides cause drug–drug interactions via several mechanisms. Table 11-17 presents a sample of these interactions. Agents that increase the risk of sulfonamide toxicity include phenylbutazone (Butazolidin), salicylates, and probenecid (Benemid). Agents that decrease the plasma levels of sulfonamides include procaine, rifampin (RIF, Rifadin), and dapsone (Aczone).

Trimethoprim is a potent inhibitor of renal tubular secretion, which can result in increased plasma levels of many drugs. Dapsone (Aczone), digoxin (Lanoxin), dofetilide (Tikosyn), methotrexate (Trexall), phenytoin (Dilantin), repaglinide (Prandin), rifampin (RIF, Rifadin), rosiglitazone (Avandia), and warfarin (Coumadin) plasma levels can be increased when these drugs are administered concomitantly with trimethoprim/sulfamethoxazole.

Special Populations: Pregnancy, Lactation, and the Elderly

Sulfonamides are not teratogenic, but they should not be administered during the last month of pregnancy because they compete for bilirubin-binding sites on plasma albumin

Table 11-17 Selected Drug–Drug Interactions Associated with Sulfonamides[a]

Drug: Generic (Brand)	Mechanism of Action	Clinical Effect
Angiotensin-converting enzyme (ACE) inhibitors	Trimethoprim reduces potassium excretion and is synergistic with the same effect produced by ACE inhibitors	Hyperkalemia
Amantadine (Symmetrel)	CYP2C9 inhibition increases serum concentration of amantadine	Mental confusion, myoclonus
Angiotensin II receptor blockers	Trimethoprim reduces potassium excretion and is synergistic with the same effect produced by ACE inhibitors	Hyperkalemia
Azithropine (Imuran)	Trimethoprim enhances the myelosuppressive effect of azithropine	Myelosuppression
Digoxin (Lanoxin)	CYP2C9 inhibition increases serum concentration of digoxin	Digoxin toxicity
Fluvastatin (Lescol)	CYP2C9 inhibition	Myalgia, myositis, rhabdomyolysis
Methenamine (Hiprex)	Formation of insoluble precipitate in urine	Bladder impairment; combination is contraindicated
Methotrexate (Rheumatrex)	Inhibition of anion transporter in renal tubule; displaces methotrexate from binding sites so plasma levels of free methotrexate are increased	Methotrexate toxicity; combination is generally contraindicated
Nonsteroidal anti-inflammatory drugs (NSAIDs)	CYP2C9 inhibition; trimethoprim reduces potassium excretion synergy—the same effect produced by NSAIDs	Hypertension, hyperkalemia
Oral hypoglycemic drugs such as glyburide, gliclazide, and repaglinide	CYP2C9 inhibition and displacement of the sulfonylurea hypoglycemic drug from plasma protein-binding sites	Hypoglycemia
Phenytoin (Dilantin)	CYP2C9 inhibition increases serum concentration of phenytoin	Phenytoin toxicity
Potassium-sparing diuretics and thiazide diuretics	Trimethoprim reduces potassium excretion and is synergistic with the same effect produced by diuretics	Hyperkalemia
Rifampin (RIF, Rifadin)	CYP2C9 inhibition increases serum concentration of rifampin	
Warfarin (Coumadin)	CYP2C9 inhibition	Hemorrhage

[a] This table is not comprehensive as new information is being generated on a regular basis.
Source: Data from Ho JMW, Juurlink DN. Considerations when prescribing trimethoprim–sulfamethoxazole. *CMAJ.* 2011;183(16):1851-1858.[92]

and may increase neonatal blood levels of unconjugated bilirubin, increasing the risk of neonatal kernicterus. Trimethoprim has a small association with an increased risk for cardiovascular defects and oral clefts in fetuses. The risk of megaloblastic anemia in a folate-deficient woman is more commonly realized during pregnancy with the use of sulfonamides.

Sulfonamides should be used with caution by breastfeeding women with fragile newborns, premature infants, infants with G6PD deficiency, or infants younger than 2 months with hyperbilirubinemia.[93] Sulfisoxazole is considered the preferred sulfonamide for breastfeeding women due to its reduced transfer to the nursing infant.

A major concern for elderly individuals is renal impairment; because of this risk, fluid intake of 2 liters daily is advised to reduce the formation of renal crystals and stones when taking sulfonamides. With the combination of trimethoprim/sulfamethoxazole (Bactrim, Septra), older adults are more susceptible to the adverse effects of skin reactions and bone marrow depression. Folic acid deficiency may occur in debilitated individuals and alcoholics because of the interference of folic acid metabolism with this drug; therefore these individuals should be advised to supplement with folic acid.

Nitrofurantoin

Nitrofurantoin (Macrodantin) is a urinary tract antimicrobial that is available as macrocrystals as well as a combination of monohydrate/macrocrystals (Macrobid). It is bacteriostatic in low concentrations and bactericidal in high concentrations. Nitrofurantoin is used as a urinary antiseptic, being prescribed exclusively for treatment or prophylaxis of urinary tract infections because of its pharmacologic and chemical properties.

Mechanism of Action, Spectrum of Activity, and Metabolism

The mechanism of action of nitrofurantoin is not well understood; however, this compound is involved with bacterial metabolism and may work by disrupting bacterial cell formation. Nitrofurantoin achieves high concentrations only in kidney tissue and urine, where it is active against most organisms responsible for urinary tract infections. It is not effective against *Pseudomonas, Enterobacter, Klebsiella*, and *Proteus* microbes.

Nitrofurantoin is absorbed and metabolized efficiently, minimizing its side effects in most individuals. Excretion is through the kidneys. The drug does not reach therapeutic levels in most body tissues and, therefore, should not be used in upper tract and complicated infections. It has minimal side effects on bowel and vaginal flora, but has been used effectively in prophylaxis of urinary tract infections for more than 40 years. There is low bacterial resistance to this drug, but the cure rate for acute cystitis is approximately 80% to 85% when it is given twice daily for 7 days, which is lower than the cure rate seen following treatment with TMP/SMX.

Side Effects and Adverse Reactions

Nitrofurantoin can cause gastrointestinal distress. This drug can trigger peripheral polyneuropathy, especially in individuals with impaired renal function, anemia, diabetes, electrolyte imbalance, or vitamin B deficiency, and in those who are debilitated. This drug should be used with caution among individuals with peripheral neuropathy. It can also cause hematologic reactions, such as agranulocytosis, leukopenia, and thrombocytopenia, and hemolytic anemia in infants and individuals with G6PD deficiency. A hypersensitive reaction to the drug manifests as an acute pulmonary reaction characterized by cough, dyspnea, chest pain, chills, and fever that resolves in 2 to 4 days after the drug is discontinued. Persons with this reaction should not be prescribed nitrofurantoin again.

Drug–Drug Interactions

Probenecid (Benemid), an antigout agent, should be avoided by persons taking nitrofurantoin; when taken simultaneously with nitrofurantoin, probenecid inhibits renal excretion of the antimicrobial agent. Concomitant use of magnesium or quinolones should be avoided due to their antagonistic action with nitrofurantoin.

Special Populations: Pregnancy, Lactation, and the Elderly

Nitrofurantoin is safe for use in pregnancy and often is used for the treatment of asymptomatic bacteruria and cystitis in pregnant women. Because it is not a sulfa-containing drug, there are no limitations on its use in the third trimester. No concerns have been reported among healthy breastfeeding mothers and their infants. As previously noted, nitrofurantoin should be avoided or used with caution in a lactating woman whose infant has G6PD deficiency.

Nitrofurantoin is not contraindicated for healthy, mature individuals. However, the elderly woman who has severe renal disease should avoid use of this drug because such disease could reduce nitrofurantoin excretion, leading to systemic toxicity. Elderly individuals are also more susceptible to the acute pulmonary reaction associated with this drug.

Antimycobacterial Agents

Mycobacterium tuberculosis, the bacterium responsible for tuberculosis infection, was first isolated in 1882 by Robert Koch, a German physician who eventually received the Nobel Prize for his discovery.[94] Thirty percent of the world's population is infected with *M. tuberculosis*, making it the most common infection globally.[95] Both multiple-drug-resistant tuberculosis (MDR-TB) and extensively drug-resistant tuberculosis (XDR-TB) are increasing. In 2012, surveillance reports from drug resistance surveys indicated that 3.6% of persons with newly diagnosed *M. tuberculosis* cases and 20% of persons previously treated for the disease have MDR-TB.[96]

M. tuberculosis is an intracellular pathogen that resides within macrophages. To be successful in eradicating this bacterium, pharmacologic agents must confront and overcome three characteristics: (1) a lipid-rich cell wall membrane; (2) efflux pumps in the cell membrane that remove potentially harmful chemicals; and (3) the bacterium's ability to hide inside the host's cells, thereby creating an additional layer of protection. Given these obstacles, *M. tuberculosis* can prove inaccessible to many pharmacologic agents. Additionally, this pathogen has the ability to develop resistance that requires combination therapies to be continued for months, or in some cases years, to successfully eradicate it. Management of mycobacterial infections requires long-term persistence with the treatment regimen.[95]

Tuberculosis (TB) can affect any organ in the body, but it most often affects lung tissue. Once the infection has been acquired, it may or may not become active depending on the individual's age, immunity status, and the presence of other medical conditions. Once exposed and infected, a healthy individual will develop a cell-mediated immunity 2 to 12 weeks after the initial infection, but remains asymptomatic because the macrophages and T cells surround and isolate the small amounts of bacteria remaining in nodules. These bacteria, however, may become activated at a later point in time. Thus, latent tuberculosis infection (LTBI) is an inactive form of TB that is detected through an abnormal skin test. The individual with latent TB does not yet have any lung damage, is not contagious, and is asymptomatic. Nevertheless, this individual has approximately a 10% risk of developing the active form of TB and requires treatment.[96,97]

The FDA has approved several drugs for treatment of TB, which are classified as first-, second-, or third-line drugs and are prescribed based on factors such as type of tuberculosis and presence of comorbidities. Table 11-18 lists the first-line drugs, and Figure 11-5 illustrates their mechanism of action. Currently, there are four approved regimens for treating LTBI.[98] The first-line agents that form the four-drug regimen for treatment of active TB are isoniazid (INH), rifampin (RIF, Rifadin), ethambutol (EMB, Myambutol), and pyrazinamide (PZA). Streptomycin is added in situations that meet certain specifications. In addition, two newer forms of rifampin—rifabutin (Mycobutin) and rifapentine (Priftin)—can be used for persons who have shown intolerance to rifampin.[97] The specific drug regimens recommended for treatment of LTBI are reviewed in the *Respiratory Conditions* chapter.

Isoniazid

Isoniazid (INH, Nydrazid, Lionized) is an antibacterial medication that has been used to both prevent and treat TB since 1952. Isoniazid should be a part of treatment for

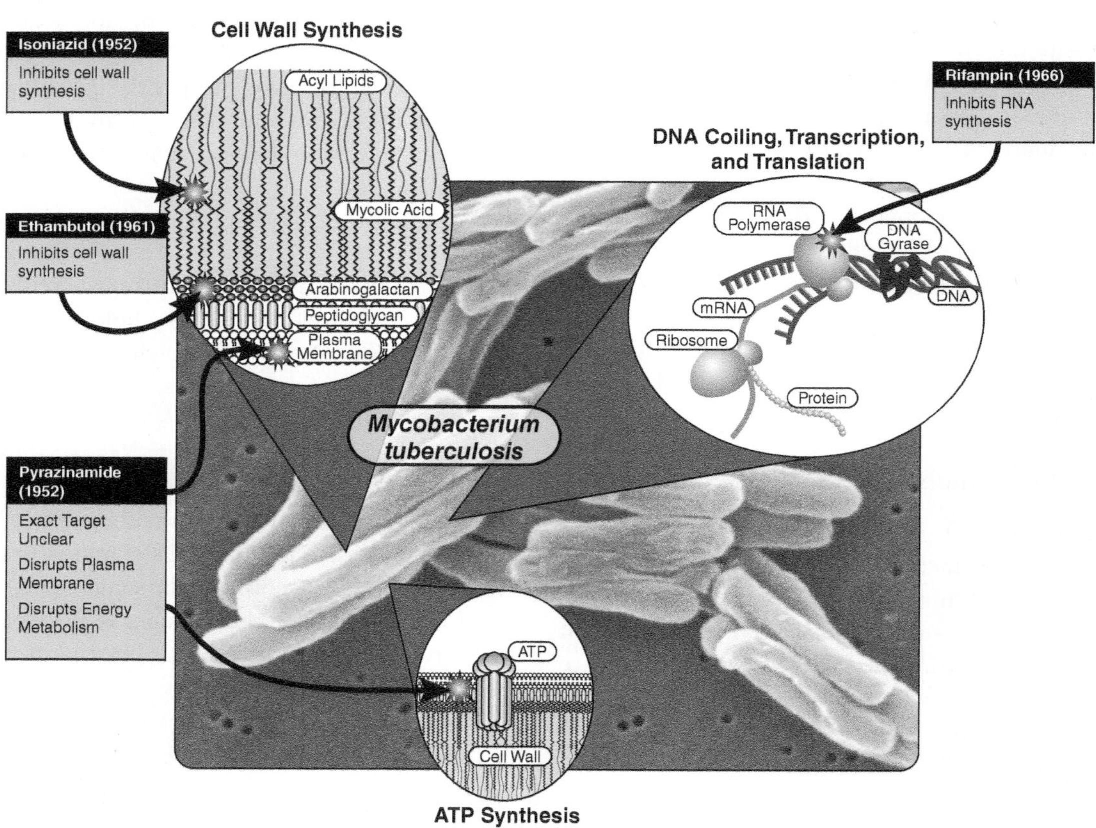

Figure 11-5 The mechanism of action of antituberculosis drugs used in the first-line treatment protocols. Tuberculosis, which results from an infection with *Mycobacterium tuberculosis*, can usually be cured with a combination of first-line drugs taken for several months. Shown here are the four drugs in the standard regimen of first-line drugs and their modes of action. Also shown are the dates these four drugs were discovered—all more than 40 years ago.

Source: National Institute of Allergy and Infectious Diseases; National Institutes of Health; Centers for Disease Control and Prevention.

Table 11-18 Antimycobacterial Agents

Drug: Generic (Brand)	Indications	Doses	Adverse Reaction	Clinical Considerations
Ethambutol (Myambutol)	First-line TB; used in pregnancy	5–25 mg/kg; maximum 2.5 g/dose	Red–green color blindness, blurred vision, GI disturbance, rash	Use extreme caution in women with renal failure or optic neuritis.
Isoniazid (INH, Lionized)	First-line TB; used in pregnancy	5 mg/kg; maximum 300 mg/dose	Peripheral neuropathies, hepatitis, nausea, vomiting, mild CNS effects	Contraindicated in acute hepatic disease. Vitamin B_6 may prevent peripheral neuropathy and CNS effects. Multiple drug–drug interactions.
Pyrazinamide (PZA)	First-line TB; not used in pregnancy	15–30 mg/kg; maximum 2 g/dose	Mild elevation of serum aminotransferases and uric acid, rashes, arthralgia, GI disturbances	Contraindicated in acute hepatic disease and acute gout. May make glucose control more difficult in persons with diabetes.
Rifabutin (Mycobutin)	For MAC prophylaxis in persons with HIV or for persons intolerant to rifampin	300 mg/day	GI upset, skin rashes, hepatotoxicity, neutropenia, thrombocytopenia, uveitis, arthralgias, and neutropenia seen with high doses	Causes orange discoloration in urine, tears, and sweat. Has the most drug–drug interactions of all the first-line TB agents. NNRTIs and PIs are contraindicated if the woman is on rifabutin. Multiple drug–drug interactions.
Rifampin (Rifadin)	First-line TB; used in pregnancy	10 mg/kg; maximum 600 mg/dose	GI upset, hepatitis, skin rashes, blood dyscrasia, headaches, fatigue, dizziness	Causes orange discoloration in urine, tears, and sweat. Contraindicated in acute hepatic disease. Interferes with oral contraceptives; use an alternative method. NNRTIs and PIs are contraindicated if the woman is on rifampin. Multiple drug–drug interactions.
Rifapentine (Priftin)	For MAC prophylaxis in persons with HIV or for persons intolerant to rifampin	600 mg/week taken as 300 mg twice weekly, supplied as 150-mg tablets	GI upset, skin rashes, uveitis seen with high doses; hepatotoxicity, neutropenia, and thrombocytopenia are rare reactions	Causes orange discoloration in urine, tears, and sweat. Take on an empty stomach. Multiple drug–drug interactions.

Abbreviations: MAC = *Mycobacterium avium* complex; NNRTI = nonnucleoside reverse transcriptase inhibitor; PI = protease inhibitor.

all persons with TB unless there is a compelling reason to omit it, such as allergy to the pharmacologic agent.[99]

Mechanism of Action

Isoniazid is a prodrug with a primary mechanism of action that involves disruption of mycolic acid, an essential component in the bacterium's lipid cell wall synthesis, resulting in death of the bacterium.[99] Alternative mechanisms that have been proposed include DNA impairment of the bacterium, decrease in cellular respiration, and lipid peroxidation of the bacterial wall.

Metabolism

Isoniazid is readily absorbed by the gastrointestinal tract and diffuses well to all body tissues, although absorption can be reduced by concomitant use of aluminum-containing antacids. The medication reaches a peak plasma concentration within 2 hours of dosing. It is metabolized by the liver and excreted in the urine.

Side Effects and Adverse Reactions

Isoniazid is metabolized in the liver to inactive metabolites, principally by acetylation, the rate of which is genetically determined. The rate of acetylation does not alter the treatment course but does change the half-life, and persons with the poor acetylator phenotype have an increased incidence of drug–drug interactions. Side effects include rash, fever, and neuritis, all of which occur in fewer than 2% of persons taking this drug.[98]

Isoniazid increases secretion of pyridoxine (vitamin B_6) in urine and can cause vitamin B_6 deficiency, which manifests as peripheral neuritis, although this is rare at the 5 mg/kg dose level. Peripheral neuropathy is more common in pregnant women and in persons with seizure disorders, diabetes, anemia, alcoholism, malnutrition, or HIV infection. To prevent or treat peripheral neuropathies, supplementation with 25 mg of pyridoxine per day is recommended. Other less common neurologic side effects include muscle twitching, ataxia, convulsions in those persons who have seizure disorders, paresthesias, and optic neuritis and atrophy. The coadministration of pyridoxine prevents the development of these effects in the majority of individuals who take isoniazid.

Isoniazid can stimulate true hypersensitivity reactions, of which hepatotoxicity is the most serious. Hepatotoxicity occurs in 5% to 20% of persons on a regular multidrug regimen primarily due to the coadministration of rifampin (Rifadin); however, the incidence of hepatotoxicity changes in different populations (e.g., it increases with increasing age).[100] Fatal hepatitis is a rare occurrence. Adults started on isoniazid should have baseline values of liver enzymes recorded, with monitoring during therapy then being individualized.

Hematologic side effects can occur in some persons, including vasculitis and the development of antinuclear antibodies. Fewer than 1% of persons using this drug will develop a lupus-like syndrome. Rarely, persons taking isoniazid will develop psychosis.

Rifampin

Rifampin (RIF, Rifadin) is one of the three drugs in the family of rifamycins, which include rifampin, rifabutin (Mycobutin), and rifapentine (Priftin). All three rifamycins can be used to treat tuberculosis, but rifampin is included in the first-line regimens that are recommended by the CDC.[101] Rifampin is a bactericidal antibiotic first introduced in the late 1960s. This agent is one of the four drugs used in the standard regimen for treating active tuberculosis.[97]

Mechanism of Action and Spectrum of Activity

Rifampin binds to the enzyme DNA-dependent RNA polymerase, thereby blocking RNA transcription. This pharmacologic agent is most active against bacteria undergoing cell division and those that are semidormant. In addition to *M. tuberculosis*, rifampin inhibits the growth of several gram-positive and some gram-negative bacteria, including *S. aureus, E. coli, Proteus, Klebsiella, H. influenzae, N. meningitides, M. kansasii*, and *M. leprae*. Rifampin often is used in combination with isoniazid for the treatment of active TB, although it may be given alone as an alternative to isoniazid for the treatment of latent TB.[98] It also has an inhibitory effect against other mycobacteria, including *M. avium, M. intracellulare*, and *M. scrofulaceum*. Rifampin is very effective in the treatment of mycobacterial infection because it has the ability to penetrate phagocytic cells, killing organisms that are not well accessed by other therapeutic agents.

Rifampin, in combination with a second therapeutic agent, is a good choice for the treatment of microbes that are harbored within abscesses and lung cavities. Further uses have been in the treatment of osteomyelitis, prosthetic valve endocarditis, and Hansen's disease (leprosy). Finally, rifampin has been used in the treatment of methicillin-resistant *S. aureus* infection in combination with other antibiotics.

Metabolism

Rifampin is well absorbed after oral administration, with a half-life of 2 to 5 hours. Food decreases the peak plasma concentrations by 30%; therefore, rifampin should be taken on an empty stomach. It is metabolized in the liver and excreted through bile, primarily in the stool, with less than 30% being excreted in the urine. It is widely distributed to tissues; however, levels in the central nervous system reach only approximately 5% of those in plasma.

Side Effects and Adverse Reactions

In general, rifampin is well tolerated; however, side effects include rash, fever, nausea, and vomiting. The medication stains tears, sweat, and urine orange, and all persons taking this drug will experience this effect. This phenomenon does not pose any serious risk and spontaneously resolves after the medication has been discontinued. High doses of rifampin can rarely cause a flu-like symptom that is not dangerous.

More serious adverse reactions include hepatotoxicity, which is more common when rifampin is given with isoniazid (approximately 3% incidence) than when rifampin is administered alone (1% incidence, but this regimen is not recommended).[100] Rifampin can rarely stimulate a Type II hypersensitivity reaction that is manifested as thrombocytopenia, hemolytic anemia, acute renal failure, or thrombocytopenic purpura.

Pyrazinamide

Pyrazinamide (PZA) is a derivative of niacinamide and is active against mycobacteria and tubercle bacilli.[95] This agent is used in combination with isoniazid and rifampin for the 6-month therapy course when treating active TB.

Pyrazinamide is not used as monotherapy. The addition of pyrazinamide to the initial 2 months of treatment allows the regimen used to treat active TB to be reduced from 9 months to 6 months.[95]

Mechanism of Action

Pyrazinamide, a prodrug, is metabolized to the active metabolite pyrazinoic acid. This conversion requires acidic conditions, and it has been suggested that the necrotic TB cavities' inflammatory cells provide this environment through their production of lactic acid. The pyrazinoic acid that results inhibits fatty acid synthesis in the microbe. In addition, pyrazinoic acid lowers the pH below that necessary for growth of *M. tuberculosis*. Pyrazinamide is bacteriostatic and works best against dormant or semidormant mycobacterial populations. Thus, when it is used with isoniazid and rifampin, it helps eliminate all forms of the organism faster and can allow for a shorter period of therapy.[97]

Metabolism

Pyrazinamide is well absorbed, with a bioavailability of greater than 90%. However, its half-life varies depending on the user's weight and gender. Pyrazinamide crosses the blood–brain barrier when the meninges are inflamed. It is metabolized in the liver, and approximately 70% of the drug is excreted in the urine.

Side Effects and Adverse Reactions

Arthralgia, mild nausea, and vomiting are common but not severe side effects of pyrazinamide unless higher doses are used. Transient rashes can occur, and it is important to counsel individuals that photosensitivity can occur when taking this drug. Hyperuricemia often occurs as result of the inhibition of the excretion of uric acid by pyrazinamide metabolites. However, this condition generally remains asymptomatic, with only rare instances of acute gout reported in association with pyrazinamide use. Nevertheless, the use of pyrazinamide by persons with gout should be avoided whenever possible.

The most serious side effect of pyrazinamide is hepatotoxicity. Rare instances of death associated with hepatic failure have been reported. However, these instances primarily occurred when the drug was prescribed for more than 2 months. Baseline plasma alanine/aspartate aminotransferase levels should be obtained prior to the initiation of therapy and repeated during the course of pyrazinamide use. Use of this medication by persons with preexisting hepatic disease should be avoided.

Ethambutol

Ethambutol (Myambutol) is bacteriostatic against actively growing *M. tuberculosis*. This agent is used in combination with isoniazid, rifampin, and pyrazinamide, primarily to add extra coverage in case the organism is resistant to isoniazid.

Mechanism of Action

Ethambutol works by inhibiting the cell wall formation of the TB bacilli.[95] Ultimately, the cell wall is rendered more permeable, improving drug access to the intracellular space within the microbe.[95]

Metabolism

Ethambutol is well absorbed from the gastrointestinal tract and becomes widely distributed in the body tissues. It is metabolized in the liver and excreted renally. This drug accumulates in individuals with renal insufficiency, and the dose requires downward adjustment for these persons.

Side Effects and Adverse Reactions

In general, adverse reactions to ethambutol occur in 2% of those using the drug. Arthralgia is the most common side effect, but it is rarely cause for discontinuation of the medication. A decrease in the renal secretion of uric acid may result in hyperuricemia.[95] Cutaneous reactions and peripheral neuritis are rare adverse effects.

The most important side effect with ethambutol use is optic neuritis, which results in a loss of visual acuity and the development of red–green color blindness. The risk of this effect is dose dependent, with approximately 15% of persons who take a dose of 50 mg/kg per day developing this condition compared to fewer than 1% of those who take 15 mg/kg per day. The optic neuritis is reversible once the drug is discontinued, but the time for resolution to occur reflects the degree of visual impairment experienced. Consequently, it is recommended that visual acuity and color discrimination testing be done prior to and at regular intervals during ethambutol therapy.

Mechanism of Resistance to Antituberculosis Agents

The tubercular bacilli are able to mutate into drug-resistant strains quite effectively, and thus drug resistance is an increasingly difficult problem. For example, several mutations in DNA-dependent RNA polymerase confer resistance to rifampin. In addition, some strains have duplicated the target enzyme, modified cell permeability, or denatured rifampin via covalent bonding once it is in the intracellular space.[102] Drug-resistant strains to each of the primary agents used to exist, but cross-resistance is not common, so combination therapies are generally effective. However, strains that are resistant to isoniazid and rifampin, called multiple-drug-resistant (MDR) strains, are becoming more prevalent and require a complicated therapeutic approach best managed by specialists in this field.

Drug–Drug Interactions

Drug–drug interactions are among the most important considerations for persons prescribing and taking isoniazid or rifampin. Isoniazid is an inhibitor of several CYP450 enzymes, and as one would expect, it has multiple drug–drug interactions because the inhibition is permanent until new CYP450 enzyme is synthesized. Rifampin is a potent inducer of several CYP450 enzymes and, therefore, decreases the therapeutic effects of more than 100 other medications. This can lead to adverse health consequences when rifampin is given to persons taking some commonly used drugs such as oral contraceptives, warfarin (Coumadin), or sulfonylureas. Some of the common drug–drug interactions of these two drugs are listed in Table 11-19 and Table 11-20.[95]

Table 11-19 Isoniazid: Selected Drug–Drug Interactions[a]

Drug: Generic (Brand)	Effect If Taken with Isoniazid
Acetaminophen (Tylenol)	Increased plasma levels of acetaminophen and increased risk of hepatotoxicity. Risk is greatest 24 hours after the last dose of isoniazid is taken. Contraindicated combination.
Carbamazepine (Tegretol)	Increased plasma levels of carbamazepine and increased risk for hepatotoxicity.
Chlorzoxazone (Paraflex)	Increased plasma levels of chlorzoxazone.
Diazepam (Valium)	Increased plasma levels of diazepam.
Levodopa (Sinemet)	Hypertension, flushing, tachycardia. Isoniazid acts as an MAO inhibitor, causing excess catecholamine when given with levodopa, which is a dopamine precursor.
Phenytoin (Dilantin)	Increased plasma levels of phenytoin.
Rifampin (Rifadin)	Increased risk for hepatotoxicity.
Theophylline (Theo-Dur)	Increased plasma levels of theophylline.
Triazolam (Halcion)[b]	Increased plasma levels of triazolam.
Valproic acid (Depakote)	Increased plasma levels of valproic acid and increased risk of hepatotoxicity.
Warfarin (Coumadin)	Increased plasma levels of warfarin.

[a] This table is not comprehensive as new information is being generated on a regular basis.
[b] This interaction is documented; there are case reports of increased plasma levels of other benzodiazepines when taken with isoniazid, but studies are needed to elucidate the relationships.

Table 11-20 Rifampin, Rifabutin, and Rifapentine: Selected Drug–Drug Interactions[a]

Drug: Generic (Brand)	Effect If Taken with Rifampin, Rifabutin, or Rifapentine
Antiarrhythmics	
Amiodarone (Cora)	Increased amiodarone metabolism; avoid concomitant use.
Digoxin (Lanoxin)	Digoxin dosage may need to be increased.
Quinidine	Quinidine dosage may need to be increased.
Anticoagulants	
Warfarin (Coumadin)	Increased renal clearance of warfarin and decreased effectiveness.
Antimicrobials	
Chloramphenicol (Chloromycetin)	Increased risk of aplastic anemia; avoid concomitant use.
Clarithromycin	Increased serum concentrations of the active metabolite of clarithromycin.
Doxycycline (Vibramycin)	50% increase in the doxycycline dosage may be necessary.
Erythromycin (E-mycin)	Erythromycin metabolism is increased and plasma levels lowered; efficacy can be decreased.
Anticonvulsants	
	Increased clearance noted; monitor clinical condition. May require an increased dosage. Measurement of phenytoin and valproic acid concentrations is suggested.
Angiotensin II Receptor Blockers	
Irbesartan (Avapro), losartan (Cozaar)	Increased metabolism, which decreases the effect of the angiotensin II receptor blocker.
Antifungals	
Fluconazole (Diflucan)	Fluconazole dosage may need to be increased.
Itraconazole (Sporanox)	Substantial reduction in plasma level noted; concomitant use not recommended.
Ketoconazole (Nizoral)	Substantial reduction in plasma level noted; concomitant use not recommended.
Benzodiazepines	
Buspirone (BuSpar)	Increased metabolism, which decreases effect of buspirone.
Diazepam (Valium)	Increased metabolism, which decreases effect of diazepam.
Triazolam (Halcion)	Increased metabolism, which decreases effect of triazolam.
Zolpidem (Ambien)	Increased metabolism, which decreases effect of zolpidem.
Beta Blockers[b]	
Labetalol (Trandate), metoprolol (Lopressor), acebutolol (Sectral)	Increased clearance, resulting in reduced effects. Monitor and increase dosage as necessary.
Calcium-Channel Blockers	
Diltiazem (Cardizem), verapamil (Calan), nifedipine (PO only) (Procardia)	Substantial reduction in diltiazem, verapamil, and nifedipine concentrations; avoid concomitant use with rifampin.

Glucocorticoids	
Methyl prednisolone (Medrol)	Decreased plasma levels of glucocorticoids; dose must be adjusted.
Hormonal Therapy and Oral Contraceptives	
Contraceptives, oral	Documented clinical failures; use nonpharmacologic contraceptive agent.
Levothyroxine (Synthroid)	Decreased plasma levels of levothyroxine.
Opioids	
Methadone, morphine, codeine	Decreased plasma levels of methadone are significant and dose of methadone might need to be doubled. Morphine dose may need to be increased to have efficacy.
Protease Inhibitors	
	Concomitant use with protease inhibitors is contraindicated. Rifabutin should be used if rifamycin is necessary, with appropriate manufacturer-recommended dosage adjustment.
Psychotropic Drugs	
Haloperidol (Haldol)	Decreased plasma levels of haloperidol.
Nortriptyline (Aventyl)	Decreased plasma levels of nortriptyline.
Quetiapine (Seroquel)	Decreased plasma levels of quetiapine.
Selective Serotonin Reuptake Inhibitors	
Citalopram (Celexa), escitalopram (Lexapro), fluvoxamine (Luvox)	Serotonin syndrome.
Statins	
Fluvastatin (Lescol), lovastatin (Mevacor, Altocor), simvastatin (Zocor)	Increased statin metabolism and reduced efficacy; substantially increasing the dose may be necessary.
Sulfonylureas	
Chlorpropamide (Diabinese), glyburide (Micronase, Diabeta), tolbutamide (Orinase)	Increased hypoglycemic effect.
Theophylline (Theo-Dur)	Theophylline is more extensively metabolized and plasma levels fall.

[a] This table is not comprehensive as new information is being generated on a regular basis.
[b] Except the following beta blockers: atenolol (Tenormin), levobunolol (Betagan), and nadolol (Corgard).

All food can impair absorption of isoniazid and rifampin. Isoniazid is a weak MAO inhibitor, and there are case reports of reactions occurring when this agent is taken with cheese or wine. Antacids inhibit oral absorption of isoniazid and ethambutol.

Special Populations: Pregnancy, Lactaction, and the Elderly

Animal studies have reported teratogenic effects for all four of the antituberculosis drugs, but all are still recommended for use by pregnant women who have active TB given the adverse effects of the disease.[101] If isoniazid is used by a woman during pregnancy, 25 mg per day of pyridoxine (vitamin B_6) should be prescribed as well.

All four medications are secreted in breast milk in minute quantities, ranging from 0.75% to 2.3% of the maternal dose at most. Careful monitoring of the breast-feeding infant for hepatotoxicity and neuritis is required. Breastfeeding women taking isoniazid should also take supplemental pyridoxine, but there are no contraindications to use of these drugs by lactating women and no reports of adverse effects on nursing infants.

Similarly, all four drugs are recommended for use in the treatment elderly individuals for TB if needed. Because elderly persons are more likely to have kidney or liver dysfunction, monitoring for liver toxicity is important.

Antifungal Agents

There are approximately 200,000 identified fungi species; however, only a small percentage of these are known to cause significant disease in humans. Fungi species include molds, yeasts, smuts, mushrooms, and the pathogens *Aspergillus fumigatus, Candida albicans, Cryptococcus, Histoplasma, Pneumocystis jirovecii.* The source of penicillin, *Penicillium chrysogenum,* is also a fungi. There has been a dramatic increase in the incidence of fungal infections over the last 20 years related to the emergence of broad-spectrum antibiotics; advances in critical care, surgery, and cancer treatment; and HIV. Antifungal agents have gone through revolutionary changes and have become much less toxic; however, the emergence of azole-resistant organisms, as well as the increased incidence of mycotic infections, has generated new challenges.[103]

The fungi that cause infections in humans are eukaryotic organisms that grow as either multicellular filaments called hyphae (molds) or single-cell organisms (yeasts), which often branch into pseudohyphae. They usually reproduce by making spores. Fungi possess a chitinous cell wall, which is the major focus of most antifungal medications.

Fungal infections are called **mycoses** and are categorized as superficial (localized to skin, hair, or nails), subcutaneous (confined to the dermis or subcutaneous tissue), systemic (infection in internal organs), or opportunistic (infection secondary to immunocompromise in the host). One interesting property of these infections is that they are not transmissible. Dermatophytes are fungi that live only on dead tissue such as nails or skin.

Chemically, the five classes of antifungal agents are azoles, polyenes, allylamines, echinocandins, and a class that includes two agents (flucytosine [Ancobon, 5-FC] and griseofulvin [Grifulvin V]) that disrupt bacterial DNA or RNA. Clinically, antifungal agents are categorized as either systemic or topical. Topical and vaginal preparations are reviewed in more detail in the *Dermatology* and *Vaginal Conditions* chapters, respectively. Antifungal agents administered systemically can be given either orally or parenterally. Parenteral agents such as amphotercin B are reserved for treatment of invasive disease. Because they are also associated with many toxicities, they are best used by specialists who care for persons with life-threatening illness. Table 11-21 reviews the orally administered antifungal agents.

Azoles

Azoles are classified as imidazoles or triazoles, according to the number of nitrogen atoms they have in the azole ring.[103,104] The imidazoles include ketoconazole (Nizoral), miconazole (Monistat), and clotrimazole (Lotrimin). The triazoles include itraconazole (Sporanox), fluconazole (Diflucan), posaconazole (Noxafil), isavuconazole (Cresemba), and voriconazole (Vfend). In general, the imidazoles are used to treat the superficial mycoses, which are discussed in more detail in the *Dermatology* and *Vaginal Conditions* chapters, and triazoles are used to treat systemic mycoses. However, both imidazoles and triazoles can be used either orally or topically; thus these categorizations are not always precise or clinically useful.

Mechanism of Action and Spectrum of Activity

The azoles are primarily fungistatic, rather than fungicidal. They act by inhibiting one of the fungal CYP450 enzymes, thereby decreasing production of ergosterol, which is an essential component of the fungal cell wall. Specificity is conferred via this mechanism because human cell membranes are made with cholesterol, whereas fungi cell membranes are made with ergosterol.

Overall, the spectrum of activity of azoles is broad, in that they are generally effective against endemic **mycosis**, *Candida* species, *Cryptococcus neoformans*, the dermatophytes, and even *Aspergillus* infections. However, the spectrum of activity of individual azoles varies considerably, and resistance to specific azoles is increasing. These two factors significantly affect the choice of drug for specific indications. For example, fluconazole is effective against yeasts but not effective for treating molds. Fungal resistance has developed to all the azoles via several different mechanisms, including efflux pumps, gene mutations that affect the structure of the fungal cell wall, and overexpression of the target enzyme.[105]

Chlortriamzole

Chlortriamzole (Lotrimin) is available as a cream, lotion, powder, solution, or tablets for intravaginal application. Topical application of this agent is effective for treatment of most Candida species. Fungicidal concentrations remain in the vagina for about 3 days after the last application of the drug. Approximately 1% of persons who used this drug report stinging, burning, or skin rash.

Fluconazole

Fluconazole (Diflucan) is the most widely used antifungal despite its high cost. It is most often prescribed for the treatment of mucocutaneous candidiasis. Fluconazole is also active against tinea corporis, tinea cruris, and tinea pedis. It has also been used to treat mammary candidiasis in breastfeeding women.[103]

This agent has almost 100% bioavailability and excellent cerebrospinal fluid penetration, providing a therapeutic advantage for the treatment of cryptococcal meningitis. Fluconazole has a high degree of water solubility, and gastric absorption is not affected by pH or the presence of food. The serum half-life is long, which allows once daily dosing. It is widely distributed in the tissues, and it is eliminated unchanged in the urine.

Fluconazole is the systemically used azole with the fewest side effects or adverse effects. Minor gastrointestinal upset has been reported with use of this agent. The issues that limit its use are that resistance in *Candida* species appears to develop quickly and drug–drug interactions must be assessed before prescribing fluconazole.

Itraconazole

Itraconazole (Sporanox) has largely replaced ketoconazole (Nizoral) in the treatment of systemic infections and is available in oral and intravenous formulations. Itraconazole is indicated for the treatment of dimorphic fungi—*Histoplasma*, *Blastomyces*, and *Sporothrix*. This agent also is active against *Aspergillus*.[103]

The antifungal activity of itraconazole is potent but can be limited by bioavailability. Absorption is improved when this agent is taken with food, but inhibited by an alkaline gastric environment. In addition, itraconazole has poor cerebrospinal fluid penetration. The half-life of itraconazole is 24 to 42 hours. This drug undergoes extensive

Table 11-21 Antifungals Administered Orally

Drug: Generic (Brand)	Indications	Dose	Side Effects and Adverse Effects	Clinical Considerations
Triazoles				
Fluconazole (Diflucan)	Candidiasis, cryptococcal meningitis	Vaginally: 150 mg as single dose Oral: 200 mg for 1 day, then 100 mg once daily	SE: Minimal gastrointestinal side effects AE: Hepatic dysfunction, alopecia following long course of therapy	Multiple drug–drug interactions. Perform active medication review prior to use.
Itraconazole (Sporanox)	Candidiasis, blastomycosis, histoplasmosis, severe tinea, onychomycosis, aspergillosis	Dose varies: 100–200 mg once daily	SE: Gastrointestinal, diarrhea AE: Hepatic dysfunction, triad of hypertension, hypokalemia and peripheral edema; cardiac dysrhythmias, bronchospasm when taken with other drugs	Administer with food or acidic carbonated beverage. FDA black box warning about risk of congestive heart failure and drug interactions. Multiple drug–drug interactions, with several that are contraindicated for coadministration.
Ketoconazole (Nizoral)	Candidiasis, blastomycosis, histoplasmosis, severe tinea, onychomycosis	200–400 mg once daily	SE: Headaches, dizziness, nausea AE: Hepatic dysfunction	FDA black box warning about possible hepatotoxicity and prolonged QT interval. Multiple drug–drug interactions. Perform active medication review prior to use.
Posaconazole (Noxafil)	Invasive *Aspergillus*, cryptococcal disease, and *Candida* infections	100–400 mg PO 2–3 times/day	SE: Gastrointestinal, rash, headache AE: Hepatic dysfunction	Administer with high-fat food or acidic carbonated beverage. Multiple drug–drug interactions. Perform active medication review prior to use.
Voriconazole (Vfend)	Aspergillosis not responsive to other drugs, invasive candidiasis	200–300 mg 2 times/day	SE: Gastrointestinal, rash, photosensitivity AE: Hepatic dysfunction, transient visual disturbances, photophobia, neurologic toxicity, prolonged QT interval, alopecia and nail changes, Stevens-Johnson syndrome, skin cancers, perostitis	Persons taking this drug should avoid sun exposure. Discontinue drug if skeletal pain occurs. Multiple drug–drug interactions. Perform active medication review prior to use.
Allylamines and Benzylamines				
Terbinafine (Lamisil)	Onychomycosis	250 mg/day for 6–12 weeks	Ophthalmic changes	Oral dose associated with some drug–drug interactions common to all azoles. Topical preparations generally considered safe.
Polyenes				
Amphotericin B (Fungizone, Amphotec, Abelcet, AmBisome)	Systemic mycoses, cutaneous candidiasis	IV: Up to 5 mg/kg/day depending on product Topical: 3% cream/lotion Ointment: Applied 2–4 times/day	Azotemia, anemia, chills, fever, myalgias, abdominal pain, weight loss and vomiting; burning, itching, and erythema with topical application	Ineffective against dermatophytic infections.
Echinocandins				
Caspofungin (Cancidas)	Aspergillosis not responsive to other drugs, invasive candidiasis	50–70 mg daily	Phlebitis, histamine effect with rapid infusion	No change in dose needed for persons with renal impairment.
Other				
Flucytosine (Ancobon, 5-FC)	Cryptococcal meningitis, chromoblastomycosis	100–150 mg/kg/day; used only in combination with amphotericin B or itraconazole	Leukopenia, thrombocytopenia, rash, nausea, vomiting, diarrhea	Toxicity is increased in persons with HIV. Modify dose in persons with renal impairment.
Griseofulvin (Grifulvin V)	Dermatophytosis of skin, hair, and nails: tinea corporis, tinea cruris, tinea capitis, tinea pedis, tinea unguium	500 mg to 1 g daily	Headache, nausea, vomiting, diarrhea, photosensitivity, fatigue, vertigo, syncope, mental confusion	Monitor renal, hepatic, and hematologic functions with prolonged therapy. Absorbed better with a fatty meal. Can lower effectiveness of oral contraceptives.

hepatic metabolism and, therefore, is associated with many drug–drug interactions. Itraconazole's label carries an FDA black box warning that recommends it not be prescribed to persons who have ventricular dysfunction or congestive heart failure and notes that itraconazole is associated with hepatotoxicity. Hair loss is the other rare adverse effect associated with use of this drug.[103]

Isavuconazole

Isavuconazole (Cresemba) was approved in 2015. Isavuconazole has an expanded spectrum of activity in that it is effective for treatment of Mucorales in addition to yeasts and molds. The drug is available as an oral or intravenous solution and is generally used to treat invasive infections.

Ketoconazole

Ketoconazole (Nizoral) is one of the oldest azoles and the most studied of this class. It is available as a shampoo, cream, foam, or gel for treatment of superficial fungal and yeast infections. Topical agents are used to treat dermatophytosis and candidiasis, and shampoos are employed for treatment of seborrheic dermatitis. Interestingly, the topical formulations of ketoconazole have anti-inflammatory effects that are equal to those produced by 1% hydrocortisone cream. Infections of the hair and nails may require a longer period of treatment. Ketoconazole is lipophilic and is easily stored in tissue. The cream contains sulfites, so it should not be used by persons who are allergic to those compounds.

Ketoconazole is also available as an oral preparation for systemic use; however, it is less selective against fungal enzymes than the newer azoles that have been developed for use against systemic infections. In this indication, it has largely been replaced by itraconazole, because ketoconazole has more adverse effects and drug–drug interactions.

Approximately 3% of persons using ketoconazole (Nizoral) report nausea, vomiting, or anorexia.[103] Ketoconazole can cause mild elevations in liver enzymes or fatal hepatotoxicity. The overall rate of hepatic dysfunction is 1% to 2%.[106] The label for oral ketoconazole carries a black box warning that addresses severe adverse reactions including (1) an association with hepatotoxicity that includes some fatalities and (2) an association with adrenal insufficiency due to its inhibition of CYP 17-alpha-hydroxylase and CYP11A1, which can, at high doses, block steroidogenesis. In addition, its ability to inhibit CYP450 enzymes and cause drug–drug interactions is probably the most clinically significant aspect of oral ketoconazole. Its coadministration with cisapride, pimozide, quinidine, or dofetilide is contraindicated secondary to the risk of increased plasma levels that can cause prolonged QT interval.[103] Finally, more rarely, anaphylaxis, suicidal ideation, severe depression, and other hypersensitivity reactions such as hemolytic anemia have been reported. Currently, the FDA has restricted the use of oral ketoconazole to only life-threatening systemic mycotic infections (e.g., blastomycosis, coccidioidomycosis, histoplasmosis, chromomycosis, paracoccidioidomycosis) when other antifungal agents are not available or cannot be tolerated.[103]

Miconazole

Miconazole (Monistat, Miconazole, Vagistat) is used externally for treatment of athlete's foot and fungal infections on skin, candidal intertrigo, and orally or intravaginally to treat candidiasis infections. Miconazole is available in many different forms including an aerosol powder, cream, lotion, ointment, suppository, and a combination product with zinc oxide that is used to treat diaper rash. Miconazole can diminish the therapeutic effects of progesterone. This can occur if both are used intravaginally during pregnancy. Adverse reactions are rare for any of the topical formulations but drug–drug interactions and adverse effects can occur when administered orally. Hypersensitivity reactions are rare but have been reported.

Posaconazole

Posaconazole (Noxafil) is the newest azole that the FDA has approved for treatment of invasive *Aspergillus* and *Candida* infections. The drug can be administered orally or intravenously. Absorption is better if it is taken with food. Like the other azoles, posaconazole is contraindicated for coadministration with several drugs secondary to its strong CYP3A4 inhibitory effect.

Voriconazole

Voriconazole (Vfend) has poor oral bioavailability and the oral tablets must be taken 2 to 3 hours either before or after a meal. It is indicated for systemic *Candida* species infections, including those known to be resistant to other forms of therapy, and is the current agent of choice for treatment of *Aspergillus* infections, fungal infections refractory to other agents, and severe corneal infections of the eye.[103] Voriconazole is used most frequently for individuals who are immunocompromised, such as those with organ transplants and hematologic cancers.

Voriconazole penetrates into the CNS and is metabolized in the liver, so the dose should be reduced for individuals with hepatic impairment or this agent avoided altogether. Persons with polymorphisms for the CYP2C19 enzyme have altered responses to this drug. Slow metabolizers, often persons of Asian decent, are at increased risk for toxicity including hepatotoxicity. Voriconazole exhibits nonlinear pharmacokinetics in that a 50% increase in dose could result in a 100% increase in serum levels. Thus it is common to monitor serum levels when this drug is used to treat invasive infections. Rashes (7%) and elevated hepatic enzymes have been observed with the use of voriconazole.[103] Visual disturbances occur in 30% of individuals who are given this medication, including blurring and alterations in color vision that may resolve without intervention. Visual and auditory hallucinations after the first dose have been reported.

Metabolism

The imidazoles are poorly absorbed in the gastrointestinal tract and are primarily formulated as topical creams and lotions for treating dermatologic or vaginal mycoses. The triazoles are absorbed in the gastrointestinal tract, but there are individual differences with regard to their oral bioavailability and their effectiveness with food intake.[104] Some of the azoles achieve good tissue penetration, including in the central nervous system, whereas others do not access all sites of mycotic infections. The azoles are metabolized in the liver via interaction with the CYP450 enzyme system; they are eliminated by the kidneys, except fluconazole (Diflucan), which is excreted renally as the unchanged drug.[103]

Side Effects and Adverse Reactions

Over-the-counter azole creams and lotions have very low toxicity and few side effects. The most common side effects associated with the oral agents are gastrointestinal symptoms. Itraconazole, in particular, may induce diarrhea, which actually occurs secondary to the cyclodextrin added to this agent to enhance its solubility.

Each of the triazoles has a different adverse-reaction profile, just as they have different spectra of activity (as noted in Table 11-21). All can induce hepatotoxicity, albeit to varying degrees. Although the hepatotoxicity is usually reversible after discontinuation of the drug, a few of these drugs have labels with black box warnings about the risk of hepatotoxicity. All individuals taking azoles orally or parenterally need to be aware of the signs and symptoms of hepatitis, including fatigue, anorexia, nausea, fever, and jaundice. In some situations, liver enzymes should to be monitored in persons taking prescription oral antifungal agents.

Drug–Drug Interactions

All of the triazoles are inhibitors of CYP3A4 and, therefore, can cause increased plasma levels of drugs metabolized by this enzyme, some of which are serious and potentially fatal. Thus, the azoles are another category of drugs for which knowledge of drug–drug interactions is critical for both the prescriber and the person taking the medication. A complete medication review is necessary before prescribing these drugs.

Common drug–drug interactions are listed in Table 11-22.[103] Fluconazole (Diflucan) and voriconazole (Vfend) inhibit CYP2C9 and CYP2C19 as well as CYP3A4. Because these drugs are also substrates for some of the CYP450 enzymes, coadministration with inducers such as phenytoin (Dilantin) can result in subtherapeutic levels of the azole.[104] Ketoconazole (Nizoral) is the most potent inhibitor of CYP3A4, followed by itraconazole (Sporanox), miconazole (Monistat), and, to a lesser degree, fluconazole (Diflucan).

Drug–Food Interactions

Ketoconazole and itraconazole require an acidic environment of absorption. Antacids, proton pump inhibitors, and H_2 antagonists should not be coadministered with these drugs. Conversely, absorption of fluconazole is independent of the presence or absence of food. Grapefruit juice can delay absorption of itraconazole and, therefore, should be avoided during therapy.[103]

Special Populations: Pregnancy, Lactation, and the Elderly

All the triazoles are associated with teratogenic effects in animals; thus the general recommendation is to use them only if the benefit outweighs the risk to the fetus. Voriconazole (Vfend) should not be administered to pregnant women. Ketoconazole (Nizoral) is classified as safe for breastfeeding women by the American Academy of Pediatrics if safer alternatives are not available. In contrast, the lack of data about these agents' effects on a nursing infant suggest breastfeeding women should not use the other orally administered triazoles.

Lower dosages may be required for elderly individuals with renal impairment. Itraconazole (Sporanox) can cause a dose-dependent inotropic effect leading to congestive

Table 11-22 Azoles: Select Examples of Drug–Drug Interactions[a]

Drug: Generic (Brand)	Azole	Effect
Severe Effects: Contraindicated Combinations[a]		
Carbamazepine (Tegretol)	Voriconazole	Increased plasma level of carbamazepine
Cisapride (Propulsid)	All	Prolonged QT interval; avoid coadministration
Cyclosporine (Neoral)	All	Nephrotoxicity
Digoxin (Lanoxin)	Itraconazole, ketoconazole	Digoxin toxicity
Disopyramide (Norpace)	Itraconazole, ketoconazole	Prolonged QT interval
Dofetilide (Tikosyn)	Itraconazole, ketoconazole	Increased plasma levels of dofetilide and cardiac failure
Ergotamine (Cafergot)	All	Ergotism; avoid coadministration
Felodipine (Plendil)	Itraconazole, ketoconazole	Hypotension
Lovastatin (Mevacor, Altocor)[b]	All	Increased plasma levels of lovastatin and hypotension, case report of rhabdomyolysis; avoid coadministration
Quinidine	All	Increased plasma levels of quinidine and cardiac failure; avoid coadministration
Pimozide (Orap)	All	Increased plasma levels of pimozide and cardiac failure; avoid coadministration
Simvastatin	Ketoconazole, posaconazole	Increased plasma levels of simvastatin and hypotension; avoid coadministration
Moderately Severe Effects		
Carbamazepine (Tegretol)	Fluconazole	Increased carbamazepine levels
Methyl prednisolone (Medrol)	Ketoconazole	Adrenal suppression
Midazolam (Versed)	Fluconazole, ketoconazole, itraconazole	Increased sedation
Phenytoin (Dilantin)	Fluconazole, miconazole	Nystagmus and ataxia
Rifabutin (Mycobutin)	Fluconazole	Ocular toxicity (uveitis)
Rifampin (RIF, Rifadin)	Ketoconazole	Increased clearance of the azole and reduced concentrations of rifampin
Sulfonylureas	Fluconazole, miconazole	Hypoglycemic reactions
Tacrolimus (Prototropic)	Ketoconazole, miconazole	Decreased plasma levels of tacrolimus
Theophylline (Theo-Dur)	All	Increased plasma levels of theophylline
Triazolam (Halcion)	Ketoconazole, itraconazole	Increased plasma levels of triazolam and increased sedation
Warfarin (Coumadin)	All	Increased plasma levels of warfarin
Drugs That Alter Azole Metabolism		
Antacids	Ketoconazole, itraconazole	Decreased absorption of the azole
Barbiturates	All	Decreased plasma levels of the azole
Carbamazepine (Tegretol)	All	Decreased plasma levels of the azole
Cimetidine (Tagamet)	Terbinafine	Increased plasma levels of terbinafine
H_2 receptor antagonists	Ketoconazole, itraconazole	Decreased absorption of the azole
Isoniazid (INH)	Itraconazole	Decreased plasma levels of the azole
Phenobarbital (Luminal)	Itraconazole	Decreased plasma levels of the azole
Phenytoin (Dilantin)	All	Decreased plasma levels of the azole
Proton pump inhibitors	Ketoconazole, itraconazole	Decreased absorption of the azole
Rifampin (RIF, Rifadin)	All	Decreased plasma levels of the azole

[a] This table is not comprehensive as new information is being generated on a regular basis.
[b] This interaction is expected to occur with other statin drugs as well as with lovastatin.

heart failure in individuals with impaired ventricular function. It may also cause hypokalemia with high doses, so it should be used with caution.

Allylamines and Benzylamines

The allylamines include naftifine hydrochloride (Naftin) and terbinafine (Lamisil); the single benzylamine available is butenafine (Lotrimin Ultra [OTC], Mentax). These agents work well for infections caused by dermatophytes but are not quite as effective against *Candida* infections. Naftifine hydrochloride and butenafine are topical treatments for fungal species, and terbinafine is approved for oral and topical treatment. Topical formulations are 1% creams applied twice daily to the affected area. Butenafine is more effective than the other two options in treating *C. albicans* infection. Systemic oral terbinafine (250-mg tablet once daily) is effective for nail onychomycosis.

Mechanism of Action

These drugs prevent ergosterol synthesis via binding to the enzyme squalene epoxidase. The allylamines and benzylamines are both fungistatic and fungicidal.[64]

Metabolism

Absorption of naftifine and butenafine is low; consequently, no systemic effects have been reported with these drugs.[103] Oral terbinafine undergoes some hepatic metabolism via the CYP450 enzyme system, and approximately 80% of the drug is excreted in the urine. Terbinafine accumulates in skin, nails, and fatty tissue and has a very long half-life (300 hours); its slow elimination from these tissues may account in part for its effectiveness in treating nail infections.

Side Effects and Adverse Reactions

The most common side effects that have been reported for naftifine and butenafine are burning and stinging of the affected area. Rare incidents of liver failure have occurred with the use of terbinafine, along with ophthalmic changes, neutropenia, and renal dysfunction. The label for oral terbinafine carries a black box warning stating it is associated with hepatic toxicity.

Drug–Drug Interactions

Terbinafine is a potent inhibitor of CYP2D6 and has multiple drug–drug interactions, which include increased plasma levels of tricyclic antidepressants, beta blockers, selective serotonin reuptake inhibitors, MAO inhibitors, and caffeine.[103] Alcohol can cause increased liver damage if taken with terbinafine. Cimetidine (Tagamet) decreases the clearance of terbinafine and increases its plasma levels. Conversely, rifampin (RIF, Rifadin) increases metabolism of terbinafine and decreases its plasma levels.

Special Populations: Pregnancy, Lactation, and the Elderly

Naftifine hydrochloride, butenafine, and topical formulations of terbinafine are safe for use during pregnancy. No fetal harm has been noted in animal studies, but lack of human studies does not allow a full assessment of fetal risk. Naftifine is absorbed systemically, so the manufacturer recommends that it be used with caution by breastfeeding women. The effects of butenafine on a breastfeeding infant are unknown, but are thought to be clinically insignificant. Systemic use of terbinafine should be avoided during pregnancy, and this agent is not recommended for use by women who are breastfeeding secondary to high milk/plasma ratios.

Elderly individuals tend to be on more medications that may interact with these drugs. If an elderly individual has renal or hepatic impairment, the dosage of terbinafine should be reduced.

Polyenes

The polyenes include amphotericin B and nystatin (Mycostatin). Amphotericin B was the only antifungal agent available for treating systemic fungal infections for many years. This broad-spectrum antifungal drug is available for both topical and intravenous use. Therapy with this agent is limited due to its nephrotoxicity and other adverse effects, but amphotericin B does remain the drug of choice for many systemic mycoses, usually during life-threatening situations.[103]

Nystatin is limited to topical use and is effective against *Candida* but not other dermatophytes. It is available as a cream, ointment, powder, liquid, and suspension; a pastille is used to treat oral candidiasis (thrush). It is well tolerated; however, the imidazoles or triazoles are more effective for the treatment of vaginal candidiasis.

Mechanism of Action and Spectrum of Activity

Amphotericin B and nystatin bind to ergosterol in the fungal cell membrane, resulting in leakage of the cell contents and reduced viability, which makes these agents both fungistatic and fungicidal. Amphotericin B is effective against *C. albicans*, *C. neoformans*, *Histoplasma capsulatum*, *Blastomyces dermatitidis*, *Coccidioides immitis*, and *Aspergillus fumigatus*. Topical amphotericin B is limited to treatment of candidiasis of the skin.

Metabolism

Gastrointestinal absorption of amphotericin B is negligible, and this drug is available only in a parenteral formulation. With parenteral administration, it becomes distributed throughout the body and is excreted renally; because of its extensive binding to tissues, however, its half-life is 15 days. Nystatin is not absorbed by the gastrointestinal tract, skin, or vagina.

Side Effects and Adverse Reactions

Nystatin has very few side effects or adverse effects.[103] Renal damage is the most significant dose-dependent adverse reaction associated with amphotericin B and can be irreversible. Newer formulations in which the drug is surrounded by lipid envelopes are beginning to be used in the hope that they will decrease the incidence of renal damage. Hematologic effects have occurred with administration of this medication. Individuals taking nystatin should be regularly monitored for anemia. Almost all persons receiving amphotericin B intravenously experience chills, fever, myalgias, joint pain, abdominal pain, weight loss, and vomiting. Other side effects include burning, itching, and erythema from topical application.[103]

Drug–Drug Interactions

If amphotericin B and azole antifungals are given at the same time, the antifungal effect of amphotericin B is antagonized. Coadministration of amphotericin B with any medication in a long list of individual agents can cause nephrotoxicity, hypokalemia, or prolonged QT interval. This drug is best used only by specialists who treat life-threatening systemic fungal infections.

Special Populations: Pregnancy, Lactation, and the Elderly

Amphotericin B and nystatin are safe for use during pregnancy. There are no reports linking these drugs with fetal congenital defects. They may be used during pregnancy if the woman would clearly benefit from them. They are not absorbed through the gastrointestinal tract and, therefore, the amount in breast milk should not cause any untoward effects in the nursing infant. Nevertheless, because amphotericin has significant toxicity, it is not recommended for women who are breastfeeding.[107]

Amphotericin B should not be administered to an elderly person who might have renal impairment.

Echinocandins

Caspofungin acetate (Cancidas), micafungin (Mycamine), and anidulafungin (Eraxis) belong to the echinocandin class of antifungals. In susceptible fungi, they cause lysis of the cell wall. These agents are approved for treatment of esophageal candidiasis, disseminated and mucocutaneous *Candida* infections, and invasive aspergillosis intolerant of other drugs, and in febrile persons with neutropenia in whom a fungal infection is suspected.[103]

Caspofungin acetate, micafungin, and anidulafungin are available only in intravenous form because they are not absorbed when administered orally. These agents are not metabolized via the CYP459 enzymes and, therefore, do not have the drug–drug interactions associated with the azoles and allylamines.

Other Antifungals

Griseofulvin

Griseofulvin (Fulvicin, Grifulvin V) is an older antifungal medication that has not been as widely used due to the enhanced safety panel of some of the newer antifungal agents. Griseofulvin is used to treat superficial mycoses such as ringworm of the skin and nails and is available as a suspension or in tablets for oral administration.

Griseofulvin interferes with cell division of the fungal cells by inhibiting mitosis. It also acts at the cellular level to bind to keratin and, therefore, acts to protect new skin and nail growth from becoming infected. It is effective in the treatment of mycotic infections of the hair, skin, and nails due to *Microsporum*, *Trichophyton*, and *Epidermophyton* species. It is not effective against *Candida* species, but for years has been the agent of choice for treating tinea capitis, especially in children. *M. canis* is a dermatophyte that causes tineacapitis.[103] Although now largely replaced by other agents, griseofulvin is more effective in treating *Microsporum canis* infections than is terbinafine (Lamisil).

Serious reactions to griseofulvin are uncommon. Gastrointestinal discomfort such as nausea, vomiting, flatulence, diarrhea, dry mouth, and angular stomatitis may occur in association with use of this agent. Headaches have been observed in as many as 15% of individuals taking griseofulvin, but they usually disappear spontaneously with continued therapy. Additionally, some individuals experience photosensitivity, fatigue, vertigo, syncope, and mental confusion. Hematologic effects can include leukopenia, neutropenia, monocytosis, and punctate basophilia. In addition, hepatotoxicity has been reported. Therefore, it is recommended that weekly laboratory tests be obtained during the first month of treatment with griseofulvin to monitor for hepatotoxicity and hematologic changes. Subsequent periodic monitoring should continue thereafter based on the results of the laboratory testing.[103]

Griseofulvin is an inducer of CYP1A2, which facilitates metabolism of oral contraceptives and warfarin (Coumadin). Thus, concomitant use of griseofulvin may interfere with oral contraceptive or warfarin effectiveness. This agent can also increase sensitivity to alcohol, causing a serious reaction. Griseofulvin can decrease the effects of warfarin and decrease levels of barbiturates and cyclosporine (Sandimmune).

Griseofulvin is contraindicated for use during pregnancy secondary to older reports of teratogenic effects in humans. Its effects on a nursing infant are unknown, so it is generally not recommended for use by breastfeeding women. No special considerations have been noted for use of griseofulvin by elderly patients.

Flucytosine

Flucytosine (5-fluorocystocine, Ancobon) is a water-soluble pyrimidine analogue that is effective against *C. neoformans*, some *Candida* species, and chromoblastomycosis. Resistance to flucystosine develops when it is used as a single agent to treat these infections. Therefore, it is used in combination with other antifungal agents. Its clinical therapeutic use is limited to treatment of cryptococcal meningitis in conjunction with amphotericin B and to treatment of chromoblastomycosis in conjunction with itraconazole (Sporanox).

Flucytosine is well absorbed from the gastrointestinal tract and becomes widely distributed in the body tissues, with peak plasma concentrations occurring in 1 to 2 hours. Approximately 80% of the drug is excreted unchanged in the urine. Its normal half-life is 3 to 6 hours, but in the presence of renal impairment is much more prolonged; consequently, persons with renal failure or HIV must have plasma levels monitored frequently.

Side effects associated with use of flucytosine include rash, nausea, vomiting, diarrhea, and enterocolitis. Flucytosine may also depress the bone marrow, causing leucopenia and thrombocytopenia.

This drug should not be used if a woman is pregnant or breastfeeding, as it is an antimetabolite and noted to have teratogenic effects.

Antiviral Agents (Nonretroviral)

Virus comes from the Latin word meaning "toxin or poison." Viruses consist of single- or double-stranded RNA or DNA genetic material enclosed within a protein coat called a capsid, which protects the genetic material. In addition, some viruses have a fat envelope that is derived from the infected host's cells and surrounds the protein coat, thereby providing another layer of protection. All viruses are obligatory intracellular pathogens with the unique ability to cause infections in humans by hijacking the normal functions of human cells.

Antiviral therapy was the focus of much pharmacologic research in the 1950s, when the effort to find a cure for cancer viruses was directed toward finding compounds that could inhibit DNA synthesis. However, many of the antiviral agents that are now in use were developed in the past three decades. Currently, research is focused on finding new antiviral agents that have greater specificity with fewer toxic effects on the host cell.

Viral replication consists of several generic steps (Figure 11-6), which include the following:

1. Binding and fusion or attachment to the host cell
2. Penetration into the host cell
3. Reverse transcription or uncoating of the virus to reveal the genetic material
4. Integration into the cell nucleus and replication of the genetic material

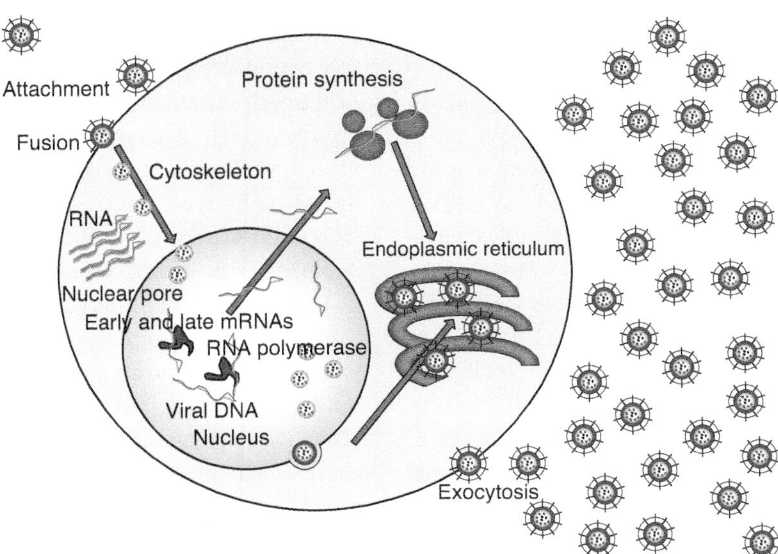

Figure 11-6 Viral life cycle.

5. Assembly of virus particles
6. Lysis of the host cell to release the newly made viruses

A key point regarding viral invasion is that the replication of the virus actually peaks before the individual has any manifestations of clinical symptomatology. This situation provides the virus with a distinct advantage and poses additional challenges to the host and the clinician in providing remedial curative and finally preventive efforts.[108]

Antiviral agents can target any one of the viral replications steps.[108] Uncoating inhibitors amantadine (Symmetrel, Symadine) and rimantadine (Flumadine) prevent the viral genetic material from being released from the protein coat once the virus is inside the host cell. Nucleic acid synthesis inhibitors are phosphorylated by the virus within the host cell into a metabolite that accumulates and inhibits replication of DNA or RNA. Acyclovir (Zovirax) is an example of a nucleic acid synthesis inhibitor. Nucleoside reverse transcriptase inhibitors also prevent DNA or RNA replication after the drug is phosphorylated, but in this case cellular kinases do the job instead of viral kinases. These drugs are approved for treatment of HIV. Non-nucleoside reverse transcriptase inhibitors bind to HIV reverse transcriptase and block viral reproduction; they are also part of the regimen used to treat HIV. Protease inhibitors block the activity of proteolytic enzymes that are needed for production of new viruses. Entry inhibitors work by either binding to the host cell's CCR5 receptor to prevent attachment to an essential HIV viral protein or preventing the fusion of the host cell's and the virus's membranes. The integrase inhibitor blocks the integration of HIV DNA into the host cell's chromosome by inhibiting HIV-encoded integrase. These drugs work in various combinations that are part of the individual's HIV antiretroviral regimen.[109]

Many viruses are pathogenic in humans. They include the viruses that cause cold sores, cytomegalovirus (CMV), Epstein-Barr virus (EBV), hepatitis, herpes simplex virus (HSV), HIV, influenza, and varicella-zoster virus (VZV), to name just a few. In fact, eight herpes viruses within the family Herpesviridae are pathogenic in humans. This is not a comprehensive list; rather, it is a selective one including the viruses most often encountered in generally healthy adults who seek treatment in primary care practice. Women's healthcare providers are most often called upon to provide an antiviral therapy for herpes simplex virus, influenza, varicella-zoster virus infection, or hepatitis. The antiretroviral drugs used to treat HIV/AIDS and hepatitis are reviewed in the *Sexually Transmitted Infections* chapter. The anti-influenza antiviral drugs are reviewed in the *Respiratory Conditions* chapter.

Drugs for Herpes: Acyclovir, Famciclovir, Penciclovir, and Valacyclovir

Acyclovir (Zovirax) is the first agent introduced of the four nucleoside analogue formulations known to be effective for treatment of intracellular viral parasites. Famciclovir (Famvir) and valacyclovir (Valtrex) are the other systemic agents available. Penciclovir (Denavir) is a topical agent. All four of these drugs are similar in their method of action; however, the indications for the use of penciclovir are restricted to oral or skin HSV infections, whereas the other agents can be used systemically to treat HSV and VZV infections[108]; see Table 11-23. Other antiviral drugs such as ganciclovir (Cytovene) and valganciclovir (Valcyte) are used to treat CMV, often in persons who are hospitalized. These antivirals have multiple adverse effects and are not reviewed in this text.

Mechanism of Action and Spectrum of Activity

All four of these drugs have the same mechanism of action. They require viral kinase or a trigger for initial phosphorylation. The active metabolite accumulates only in the infected host cells and then inhibits replicative function of the viral DNA polymerase.[108,110] Valacyclovir is a prodrug of acyclovir and is converted rapidly and completely to acyclovir after oral administration. Penciclovir is a prodrug of famciclovir.[110]

Acyclovir is indicated for treatment of HSV infection, prevention of recurrent HSV flares, and treatment of VZV infection. When used for treatment of genital herpes, oral acyclovir shortens the symptoms of the infection by approximately 2 days and also reduces the incidence of viral shedding by approximately 7 days. Famciclovir and valacyclovir are preferred for the treatment and prevention of HSV because both have been found to have a slight superiority in effectiveness when compared to acyclovir, in that they reduce the pain and shorten the duration of the outbreak more than does acyclovir.[108,111] Epstein-Barr virus, CMV, and human herpesvirus-6 (HHV-6) infections have been treated with acyclovir; however, this drug's in vitro activity has been found to be weak and thus, ganciclovir (Cytovene) or valganciclovir (Valcyte) are preferred. Penciclovir has very poor bioavailability, and its use is recommended only for the treatment of HSV infections of the lips and face. It is not recommended for use in mucous membrane infections.[108,110]

Table 11-23 Antiviral Drugs Used to Treat Herpes Virus

Drug: Generic (Brand)	Indications	Dose	Adverse Reactions	Clinical Considerations
Acyclovir (Zovirax)	Herpes simplex, genital herpes, herpes zoster, varicella-zoster	Initial: 200 mg 5 times/day for 10 days Recurrent: 200 mg 5 times/day for 5 days Chronic suppressive therapy: 400 mg 2 times/day for 12 months Herpes zoster: 800 mg 5 times/day for 7–10 days	Nausea, vomiting, headache, CNS reactions, rash, malaise; use with caution in persons with renal impairment	Do not exceed maximum dosage; start all antiherpes drugs as soon as symptoms begin
Famciclovir (Famvir)	Herpes simplex, genital herpes	Initial: 250 mg 3 times/day for 7–10 days Recurrent: 1000 mg 2 times/day for 1 day Suppressive: 250 mg 2 times/day for up to a year	Headache, GI side effects, numbness	Can decrease duration of postherpetic neuralgia
	Herpes zoster	500 mg 3 times/day for 7 days		
Penciclovir (Denavir)	Herpes simplex of lips and face	10 mg/g in cream base; apply every 2 hours while awake for 4 days	Headache, local edema, pruritus, urticarial, parosmia	Use restricted to HSV infection of lips and face; safety and effectiveness in children ≤ 12 years not established
Valacyclovir (Valtrex)	Herpes simplex, genital herpes	Initial: 1 g 2 times/day 10 days Recurrent: 500 mg 2 times/day for 3 days Suppressive: 1 g once daily	GI side effects, dizziness, headache, abdominal pain	Not approved for immunocompromised individuals; not affected by food
	Herpes zoster	1 g 3 times/day for 7 day		

Metabolism

The bioavailability of acyclovir is only approximately 15% to 30%. It is poorly absorbed from the gastrointestinal tract. Acyclovir diffuses into most tissues and penetrates into cerebrospinal fluid. It is excreted through the renal system as an unchanged drug; the liver metabolizes only 10%, and the half-life is approximately 3 hours for individuals with normal renal function. Famciclovir and valacyclovir are both more bioavailable than acyclovir. The bioavailability of famciclovir is 70% to 80%, whereas the bioavailability of valacyclovir is approximately 50%. Penciclovir has poor bioavailability and in healthy adults has not demonstrated measurable levels in plasma or urine.[108,110]

Side Effects and Adverse Reactions

Acyclovir (Zovirax), famciclovir (Famvir), and valacyclovir (Valtrex) are all generally tolerated with minimal discomfort. The primary concerns are headache, nausea, and diarrhea. Intravenous infusion has been associated with renal complications. Adequate hydration and avoidance of rapid infusion rates can prevent adverse effects. More serious side effects have been noted with long-term use of the drugs.

Acyclovir should be used cautiously by persons who have neurologic disorders. Approximately 1% of all individuals receive parenteral acyclovir report neurologic reactions. The primary concerns associated with penciclovir use, which occur in fewer than 1% of persons who use the drug, include headache and local reactions, such as erythema, hyperesthesia, or skin discoloration, to the site of the topical agent's application.[108]

Drug–Drug Interactions

All four of these antiviral drugs may diminish the therapeutic effect of vaccines. Probenecid (Benemid), cimetidine (Tagamet), and theophylline (Theo-Dur) all increase plasma levels of acyclovir and valacyclovir. Acyclovir and valacyclovir can decrease excretion of tenofovir (Viread) and enhance the CNS depressant effect of zidovudine (Retovir). Famciclovir potentiates digoxin (Lanoxin); when these two drugs are coadministered, the levels of digoxin need to be monitored.[108,110]

Special Populations: Pregnancy, Lactation, and the Elderly

All four of the antiviral drugs are considered safe for use during pregnancy and recommended for use in the third trimester of pregnancy for the prevention of recurrent outbreaks.[112] Analysis of data collected by a pregnancy registry between 1984 and 1999 did not find any teratogenic effects in humans secondary to acyclovir use. However, animal studies have reported teratogenic effects, and a pregnancy registry has been established for famciclovir (1-888-669-6682).

No concerns have been reported for the infants of breastfeeding women who take one of these drugs. However, fewer data are available regarding famciclovir; therefore, acyclovir would be the preferred drug in breastfeeding women. Intravenous administration of acyclovir is the method of treatment for the newborn with neonatal HSV infection or herpes simplex encephalitis, and few adverse reactions have been noted with this usage.

Because renal dysfunction is more likely among elderly persons, close monitoring should be undertaken when these antiviral drugs are used in the older adult population. The dose of acyclovir may need to be reduced if the individual, regardless of age, has renal impairment.

Conclusion: Appropriate Prescribing Practices

Antimicrobial drugs are an essential tool used in the primary health care of women. It is incumbent upon clinicians to use this resource wisely and well; anti-infective agents can be of great benefit to the women. These drugs can also have unintended consequences if used carelessly or without a systematic approach. The principles presented in this chapter will assist the clinician in maximizing the effectiveness of this resource.

Resources

Organization	Description	Website
Centers for Disease Control and Prevention	Healthcare providers' TB program materials	www.cdc.gov/tb/education/provider_edmaterials.htm
Food and Drug Administration	Drug Safety and Availability website lists FDA drug safety communications, drug recalls, and the index to drug-specific information, which lists any FDA black box warnings	www.fda.gov/Drugs/DrugSafety/default.htm
Infectious Disease Society of America	A comprehensive list of guidelines for infectious diseases that can be sorted by disease or organism	www.idsociety.org/IDSA_Practice_Guidelines/
United States National Library of Medicine Toxicology data network (TOXNET)	Lactmed is a TOXNET database that summarizes the safety of drugs used during lactation	http://toxnet.nlm.nih.gov/cgi-bin/sis/search2

Apps		
Centers for Disease Control and Prevention	Latent tuberculosis infection (LTBI) mobile application for healthcare providers; CDC-developed app for healthcare providers	Download from Apple app store

References

1. Ligon BL. Penicillin: its discovery and early development. *Semin Pedatr Infect Dis.* 2004;15(1):52-57.
2. Kallen AJ, Mu Y, Bulens S et al. Health care-associated invasive MRSA infections, 2005-2008. *JAMA.* 2010; 304(6):641-648.
3. Brooks BD, Brooks AE. Therapeutic strategies to combat antibiotic resistance. *Adv Drug Deliv Rev.* 2014;30(78C):14-27.
4. Chapot-Chartier MP, Kulakauskas S. Cell wall structure and function in lactic acid bacteria. *Microb Cell Fact.* 2014;13(suppl 1):S9.
5. Cabeen MT, Jacobs-Wagner C. Bacterial cell shape. *Nat Rev Microbiol.* 2005;3(8):602.
6. Reynolds J, Moyes RB, Breakwell DP. Differential staining of bacteria: acid-fast stain. *Curr Protoc Microbiol.* November 2009; Appendix 3H.
7. Phillips MA, Stanley SL Jr. Chemotherapy of protozoal infections: amebiasis, giardiasis, trichomoniasis, leishmaniasis, and other protozoal infections. In: Bruton LL, Chabner BA, Knollmann BC, eds. *Goodman and Gillman's the Pharmacological Basis of Therapeutics.* 12th ed. New York: McGraw-Hill Medical; 2011:1419-1443.
8. Hughes D. Selection and evolution of resistance to antimicrobial drugs. *IUBMB Life.* 2014;66(8): 521-529.
9. Martinez JL. General principles of antibiotic resistance in bacteria. *Drug Disc Today: Technol.* 2014;11: 33-39.
10. Aminov RI. The role of antibiotics and antibiotic resistance in nature. *Environ Microbiol.* 2009;11(12): 2970-2988.
11. Spellberg B, Bartlett JG, Gilbert DN. The future of antibiotics and resistance. *N Engl J Med.* 2014;368(4): 299-302.
12. Llor C, Bjerrum L. Antimicrobial resistance: risk associated with antibiotic overuse and initiatives to reduce the problem. *Ther Adv Drug Saf.* 2014;5(6): 229-241.

13. Slama TG, Amin A, Brunton SA, et al.; Council for Appropriate and Rational Antibiotic Therapy. A clinician's guide to the appropriate and accurate use of antibiotics: the Council for Appropriate and Rational Antibiotic Therapy (CARAT) criteria. *Am J Med.* 2005;118(suppl 7A):1S-6S.
14. Davey P, Brown E, Charani E, et al. Interventions to improve antibiotic prescribing practices for hospital inpatients. *Cochrane Database Syst Rev.* 2013;4:CD003543. doi:10.1002/14651858.CD003543.pub3.
15. Arnold SR, Straus SE. Interventions to improve antibiotic prescribing practices in ambulatory care. *Cochrane Database Syst Rev.* 2005;4:CD003539. doi:10.1002/14651858.CD003539.pub2.
16. Perencevich EN, Wong MT, Harris AD. National and regional assessment of the antibacterial soap market: a step toward determining the impact of prevalent antibacterial soaps. *Am J Infect Control.* 2001;29(5):281-283.
17. Food and Drug Administration. Triclosan: what consumers should know. http://www.fda.gov/ForConsumers/ConsumerUpdates/ucm205999.htm. Accessed December 11, 2014.
18. Boyce JM, Pittet D; Healthcare Infection Control Practices Advisory Committee; HICPAC/SHEA/APIC/IDSA Hand Hygiene Task Force. Guideline for hand hygiene in health-care settings. Recommendations of the Healthcare Infection Control Practices Advisory Committee and the HICPAC/SHEA/APIC/IDSA Hand Hygiene Task Force. Society for Healthcare Epidemiology of America/Association for Professionals in Infection Control/Infectious Diseases Society of America. *MMWR Recomm Rep.* 2002;51(RR–16):1-45, quiz CE1-4.
19. Roe V. Antibiotic resistance: a guide for effective prescribing in women's health. *J Midwifery Womens Health.* 2008;53(3):216-226.
20. Waller DG. The science of prescribing. *Br J Clin Pharm.* 2012;74(4):559-560.
21. Dodds Ashley ES, Kaye KS, DePestel DD, Hermsen ED. Antimicrobial stewardship: philosophy versus practice. *Clin Infect Dis.* 2014;59(S3):S112-S121.
22. MacDougal C, Polk RE. Antimicrobial stewardship programs in health care systems. *Clin Microbiol Rev.* 2005;18(4):638-656.
23. Dellit TH, Owens RC, McGowan JE Jr, et al.; Infectious Diseases Society of America; Society for Healthcare Epidemiology of America. Infectious Diseases Society of America and the Society for Healthcare Epidemiology of America guidelines for developing an institutional program to enhance antimicrobial stewardship. *Clin Infect Dis.* 2007;44(2):159-177.
24. Society for Healthcare Epidemiology of America; Infectious Diseases Society of America; Pediatric Infectious Diseases Society. Policy statement on antimicrobial stewardship by the Society for Healthcare Epidemiology of America (SHEA), the Infectious Diseases Society of America (IDSA), and the Pediatric Infectious Diseases Society (PIDS). *Infect Control Hosp Epidemiol.* 2012;33(4):322-327.
25. Frere JM, Page MG. Penicillin-binding proteins: evergreen drug targets. *Curr Opin Pharmacol.* 2014;18C:112-119.
26. Tang SS, Apisarnthanarak A, Hsu LY. Mechanisms of β-lactam antimicrobial resistance and epidemiology of major community and healthcare-associated multidrug resistant bacteria. *Adv Drug Deliv Rev.* 2014;78C:3.
27. Jacoby GA, Munoz-Price LS. The new beta lactamases. *N Engl J Med.* 2005;352(4):380-391.
28. Shulman ST, Bisno AL, Clegg HW, et al. Clinical practice guideline for the diagnosis and management of group A streptococcal pharyngitis: 2012 update by the Infectious Disease Society of America. *Clin Infect Dis.* 2012;55(10):1279-1282.
29. Kriebs J. Methicillin-resistant *Staphylococcus aureus* infection in the obstetric settings. *J Midwifery Womens Health.* 2008;53(3):247-250.
30. Liu C, Bayer A, Cosgrove SE, et al. Clinical practice guidelines by the Infectious Diseases Society of America for the treatment of methicillin-resistant *Staphylococcus aureus* infections in adults and children. *Clin Infect Dis.* 2011;52:e18-e55.
31. Holland TL, Arnold C, Fowler VG Jr. Clinical management of *Staphylococcus aureus* bacteremia: a review. *JAMA.* 2014;312(13):1330-1341.
32. Betzold CM. An update on the recognition and management of lactational breast inflammation. *J Midwifery Womens Health.* 2007;52(6):595-605.
33. Wilson W, Taubert KA, Gewitz M, et al. Prevention of infective endocarditis: guidelines from the American Heart Association: a guideline from the American Heart Association Rheumatic Fever, Endocarditis, and Kawasaki Disease Committee, Council on Cardiovascular Disease in the Young, and the Council on Clinical Cardiology, Council on Cardiovascular Surgery and Anesthesia, and the Quality of Care

and Outcomes Research Interdisciplinary Working Group. *Circulation.* 2007;116(15):1736-1754.

34. Lode HM. Rational antibiotic therapy and the position of ampicillin/sulbactam. *Int J Antibrob Agents.* 2008;32(1):10-28.
35. Salkind AR, Cuddy PG, Foxworth JW. Is this patient really allergic to penicillin? An evidence-based analysis of the likelihood of penicillin allergy. *JAMA.* 2001;285(19):2498-2505.
36. Macy E. Penicillin and beta-lactam allergy: epidemiology and diagnosis. *Curr Allergy Asthma Rep.* 2014; 14(11):476.
37. Johansson SG, Bieber T, Dahl R, et al. Revised nomenclature for allergy for global use: report of the Nomenclature Review Committee of the World Allergy Organization, October 2003. *J Allergy Clin Immunol.* 2004;113(5):832-836.
38. Napoli DC, Neeno TA. Anaphylaxis to benzathine penicillin G. *Pediatr Asthma Allergy Immunol.* 2000;14(4):329-332.
39. Demoly P, Romano A. Update on beta-lactam allergy diagnosis. *Curr Allergy Asthma Rep.* 2005;5(1):9-14.
40. Campagna JD, Bond MC, Schabelman E, Hayes BD. The use of cephalosporins in penicillin-allergic patients: a literature review. *J Emerg Med.* 2012; 42(5):612-620.
41. Solensky R, Khan DA. Drug allergy: an updated practice parameter. *Ann Aller Asthma Immunol.* 2010;105(4):259-273.
42. Khan DA, Solensky R. Drug allergy. *J Allergy Clin Immunol.* 2010;125(2 suppl 2):S126-S137.
43. Gruchalla RS, Pirmohamed M. Antibiotic allergy. *N Engl J Med.* 2006;354(6):601–609.
44. Centers for Disease Control and Prevention. Management of patients who have a history of penicillin allergy: sexually transmitted diseases treatment guidelines. 2010. http://www.cdc.gov/STD/treatment/2006/penicillin-allergy.htm.
45. Pai MP, Momary KM, Rodvold KA. Antibiotic drug interactions. *Med Clin North Am.* 2006;90(6): 1223-1255.
46. Brassard P, Bourgault C, Brophy J, Kezouh A, Suissa S. Antibiotics in primary prevention of stroke in the elderly. *Stroke.* 2003;34(9):163-166.
47. Stevens DL, Bisno AL, Chambers HF, et al. Practice guidelines for the diagnosis and management of skin and soft tissue infections: 2014 update by the Infectious Diseases Society of America. *Clin Infect Dis.* 2014;59(2):e10-e52.
48. Christian SS, Christian JS. The cephalosporin antibiotics. *Prim Care Update Ob/Gyn.* 1997;4: 168-174.
49. Sader HS, Jacobs MR, Fritsche TR. Review of the spectrum and potency of orally administered cephalosporins and amoxicillin/clavulanate. *Diag Microb Infect Dis.* 2007;57(3 suppl):S5-S12.
50. Kim MH, Lee JM. Diagnosis and management of immediate hypersensitivity reactions to cephalosporins. *Allergy Asthma Immunol Res.* 2014;6(6): 485-495.
51. Czeizel AE. Use of cephalosporins during pregnancy and in the presence of congenital abnormalities: a population-based case control study. *Am J Obstet Gynecol.* 2001;184(6):1289-1296.
52. Levine DP. Vancomycin: a history. *Clin Infect Dis.* 2006;42(suppl 1):S5-S12.
53. Levine DP. Vancomycin: understanding its past and preserving its future. *South Med J.* 2008;101(3): 284-291.
54. McDonald LC, Killgore GE, Thompson A, et al. Emergence of an epidemic, toxin gene variant strain of *Clostridium difficile* responsible for outbreaks in the United States between 2000 and 2004. *N Engl J Med.* 2005;353(23):2433-2441.
55. CDC. Recommendations for preventing the spread of vancomycin resistance: recommendations of the Hospital Infection Control Practices Advisory Committee (HICPAC). *MMWR.* 1995;44(RR12);1-13. http://wonder.cdc.gov/wonder/prevguid/m0039349/m0039349.asp. Accessed August 17, 2014.
56. Moellering RC Jr. Vancomycin: a 50-year reassessment. *Clin Infect Dis.* 2006;42(suppl 1):S3-S4.
57. Zuckerman JM. Macrolides and ketolides: azithromycin, clarithromycin, telithromycin. *Infect Dis Clin North Am.* 2004;18(3):621-649.
58. Abu-Gharbieh E, Vasina V, Poluzzi E, De Ponti F. Antibacterial macrolides: a drug class with a complex pharmacological profile. *Pharmacol Res.* 2004;50(3): 211-220.
59. Woeczprel K, Osek J. Antimicrobial resistance mechanisms among *Campylobacter. Biomed Res Int.* 2013;2013:340605.
60. Tiwari T, Murphy TV, Moran J. Recommended antimicrobial agents for the treatment and postexposure prophylaxis of pertussis: 2005 CDC guidelines. *MMWR.* 2005;54(RR14):1-16. http://www.cdc.gov/mmwr/preview/mmwrhtml/rr5414a1.htm. Accessed December 11, 2014.

61. Kanazawa S, Ohkubo T, Sugawara K. The effects of grapefruit juice on the pharmacokinetics of erythromycin. *Eur J Clin Pharmacol.* 2001;56(11): 799-803.
62. Rubenstein E. Comparative safety of the different macrolides. *Int J Antimicrob Agents.* 2001;18:S71-S76.
63. Lin KJ, Mitchell AA, Yau WP, Louik C, Hernández-Díaz S. Safety of macrolides in pregnancy. *Am J Obstet Gynecol.* 2013;208(3):e1-e8.
64. American College of Obstetricians and Gynecologists (ACOG). Practice bulletin no. 139: premature rupture of membranes. *Obstet Gynecol.* 2013;122(4): 918-930.
65. Centers for Disease Control and Prevention. Sexually transmitted diseases treatment guidelines, 2010. *MMWR Recomm Rep.* 2010;59(RR–12):1-110.
66. Sørensen HT, Skriver MV, Pedersen L, Larsen H, Ebbesen F, Schønheyder HC. Risk of infantile hypertrophic pyloric stenosis after maternal postnatal use of macrolides. *Scand J Infect Dis.* 2003;35(2): 104-106.
67. Bennett CC. The aminoglycosides. *Prim Care Update Ob/Gyn.* 1996;3(6):186-191.
68. Woodruff HB, Selman A. Waksman, winner of the 1952 Nobel Prize for physiology or medicine. *Appl Environ Microbiol.* 2014;80(1):2-8.
69. Pagkalis S, Mantadakis E, Mavros MN, Ammari C, Falagas ME. Pharmacological considerations for the proper clinical use of aminoglycosides. *Drugs.* 2011;71(17):2277-2294.
70. Xie J, Talaska AE, Schacht J. New developments in aminoglycoside therapy and ototoxicity. *Hear Res.* 2011;281(1–2):28-37.
71. Nelson ML, Levy SB. The history of the tetracyclines. *Ann NY Acad Sci.* 2011;124(1):17-32.
72. Nguyen F, Starosta AL, Arenz S, Sohmen D, Dönhöfer A, Wilson DN. Tetracycline antibiotics and resistance mechanisms. *Biol Chem.* 2014;395(5): 559-575.
73. Mazzei T. The difficulties of polytherapy: examples from antimicrobial chemotherapy. *Intern Emerg Med.* 2011;6(suppl 1):S103-S109.
74. Shaw KJ, Barbachyn MR. The oxazolidinones: past, present, and future. *Ann NY Acad Sci.* 2011;1241: 48-70.
75. Narita M, Tsuji BT, Yu VL. Linezolid-associated peripheral and optic neuropathy, lactic acidosis, and serotonin syndrome. *Pharmacotherapy.* 2007;27(8): 1189-1197.
76. O'Donnell JA, Gelone SP. The newer fluoroquinolones. *Infect Dis Clin North Am.* 2004;18(3): 691-716.
77. Sousa J, Alves G, Fortuna A, Falcao A. Third and fourth generation fluoroquinolone antibacterials: a systematic review of safety and toxicity profiles. *Curr Drug Saf.* 2014;9(2):89-105.
78. Liu HH. Safety profile of the fluoroquinolones. *Drug Saf.* 2010;33(5):353-369.
79. King DE, Malone R, Lilley S. New classification and update on the quinolone antibiotics. *Am Fam Phys.* 2000;61(9):2741-2748.
80. Phillips MA, Stanley SL. Chemotherapy of protozoal infections: amebiasis, giardiasis, trichomoniasis, trypanosomiasis, leishmaniasis, and other protozoal infections. In: Brunton LL, Lazo JS, Parker KL, eds. *Goodman & Gillman's the Pharmacological Basis of Therapeutics.* 12th ed. New York: McGraw-Hill Medical; 2011:1419-1442.
81. Winslow BT, Onysko M, Thompson KA, Caldwell K, Ehlers GH. Common questions about *Clostridium difficile* infection. *Am Fam Phys.* 2014;89(6): 437-442.
82. Alahdab YO, Kalayci C. *Helicobacter pylori*: management in 2013. *World J Gastroenterol.* 2014;20(18): 5302-5307.
83. Lau AH, Lam NP, Piscitelli SC, Wilkes L, Danziger LH. Clinical pharmacokinetics of metronidazole and other nitroimidazole anti-infectives. *Clin Pharmacokinet.* 1992;23(5):328-364.
84. Miljkovic V, Arsic B, Bojanic Z, et al. Interactions of metronidazole with other medicines: a brief review. *Pharmazie.* 2014;69(8):571-577.
85. Koss CA, Baras DC, Lane SD, et al. Investigation of metronidazole use during pregnancy and adverse birth outcomes. *Antimicrob Agents Chemother.* 2012; 56(9):4800-4805.
86. Armstrong NR, Wilson JD. Tinidazole in the treatment of bacterial vaginosis. *Int J Womens Health.* 2009;1:59-65.
87. Stover KR, Riche DM, Gandy CL, Henderson H. What would we do without metronidazole? *Am J Med Sci.* 2012;343(4):316-319.
88. Raju TN. The Nobel chronicles. *Lancet.* 1999; 353(9153):681.
89. Schnyder B, Pichler WJ. Allergy to sulfonamides. *J Allergy Clin Immunol.* 2013;31(1):256-257.
90. Wulf NR, Matuszewski KA. Sulfonamide cross-reactivity: is there evidence to support broad

cross-allergenicity? *Am J Health-Syst Pharm.* 2013; 70(17):1483-1494.

91. Strom BL, Schinnar R, Apter AJ, et al. Absence of cross-reactivity between sulfonamide antibiotics and sulfonamide nonantibiotics. *N Engl J Med.* 2003; 349(17):1628-1635.
92. Ho JMW, Juurlink DN. Considerations when prescribing trimethoprim–sulfamethoxazole. *CMAJ.* 2011;183(16):1851-1858.
93. Chin KG, McPherson CE III, Hoffman M, Kuchta A, Mactal-Haaf C. Use of anti-infective agents during lactation. Part 2: aminoglycosides, macrolides, quinolones, sulfonamides, trimethoprim, tetracyclines, chloramphenicol, clindamycin, and metronidazole. *J Hum Lact.* 2001;17(1):54-65.
94. Kaufmann SH, Baumann S, Nasser EA. Exploiting immunology and molecular genetics for rational vaccine design against tuberculosis. *Int J Tuberc Lung Dis.* 2006;10(10):1068-1079.
95. Shi R, Itagaki N, Sugawara I. Overview of anti-tuberculosis (TB) drugs and their resistance mechanisms. *Mini Rev Med Chem.* 2007;7(11):1177-1185.
96. World Health Organization. *Global tuberculosis report.* Geneva, Switzerland: World Health Organization; 2013.
97. Ahmad S, Mokaddas E. Current status and future trends in the diagnosis and treatment of drug-susceptible and multidrug-resistant tuberculosis. *J Infect Pub Health.* 2014;7(2):75-91.
98. Centers for Disease Control and Prevention. Treatment options for latent tuberculosis infection. January 20, 2012. http://www.cdc.gov/tb/publications/factsheets/treatment/LTBItreatmentoptions.htm. Accessed December 14, 2014.
99. Timmins GS, Deretic V. Mechanism of action of isoniazid. *Mol Microbiol.* 2006;62(5):1220-1227.
100. Tostmann A, Boeree MJ, Aarnoutse RE, et al. Antituberculosis drug-induced hepatotoxicity. *J Gastroenterol Hepatol.* 2008;23(2):192-202.
101. Centers for Disease Control and Prevention. Treatment of tuberculosis. *MMWR Recomm Rep.* 2003:52(RR–11):1-77.
102. Tupin A, Gualtieri M, Roquet-Banères F, Morichaud Z, Brodolin K, Leonetti JP. Resistance to rifampicin: at the crossroads between ecological, genomic, and medical concerns. *Int J Antimicrob Agents.* 2010;35(6):519-523.
103. Zhang AY, Camp WL, Elewski BE. Advances in topical and systemic antifungals. *Dermatol Clin.* 2007;25(2):165-183.
104. Lewis RE. Current concepts in antifungal pharmacology. *Mayo Clin Proc.* 2011;86(8):805-817.
105. Pfaller MA. Antifungal drug resistance: mechanisms, epidemiology, and consequences for treatment. *Am J Med.* 2012;125(1 suppl):S3-S13.
106. Food and Drug Administration. FDA drug safety communication: FDA limits use of Nizoril (ketoconazole) oral tablets due to potentially fatal liver injury and risk of drug reactions and adrenal gland problems. http://www.fda.gov/drugs/drugsafety/ucm362415.htm. Accessed August 28, 2014.
107. Mactal-Haaf C, Hoffman M, Kuchta A. Use of anti-infective agents during lactation. Part 3: antivirals, antifungals, and urinary antiseptics. *J Hum Lact.* 2001;17(2):160-166.
108. Acosta EP, Flexner C. Antiviral agents (nonretroviral). In: Bruton LL, Chabner BA, Knollmann BC, eds. *Goodman and Gillman's the Pharmacological Basis of Therapeutics.* 12th ed. New York: McGraw-Hill Medical; 2011:1593-1623.
109. Flexner C. Antiretroviral agents and treatment of HIV infection: antiviral agents (nonretroviral). In: Bruton LL, Chabner BA, Knollmann BC, eds. *Goodman and Gillman's the Pharmacological Basis of Therapeutics.* 12th ed. New York: McGraw-Hill Medical; 2011: 1632-1665.
110. James SH, Prichard MN. Current and future therapies for herpes simplex virus infections: mechanism of action and drug resistance. *Curr Opin Virol.* 2014; 8:54-61.
111. Brantley JS, Hicks L, Sra K, Tyring SK. Valacyclovir for the treatment of genital herpes. *Expert Rev Anti Infect Ther.* 2006;4(3):367-376.
112. Hollier LM, Wendel GD. Third trimester antiviral prophylaxis for preventing maternal genital herpes simplex virus (HSV) recurrences and neonatal infection. *Cochrane Database Syst Rev.* 2008;1:CD004946. doi:10.1002/14651858.CD004946.pub2.

© Sofmanning/Shutterstock

12 Analgesia and Anesthesia

James R. Walker, Tekoa L. King

Based on the chapter by Elissa Lane Miller in the first edition of Pharmacology for Women's Health

With acknowledgment to Nell Tharpe

Chapter Glossary

Analgesia Absence of pain in response to stimulation that would normally be painful.

Anesthesia Total or partial loss of sensation.

Atypical analgesics Antiseizure, antidepressant, or other medications that are not classic analgesics but have analgesic properties and are used as adjunct analgesics

Breakthrough pain Transitory flare of moderate to severe pain that occurs unexpectedly despite otherwise controlled pain.

Ceiling effect Dose beyond which no additional therapeutic effect is gained.

Equianalgesic Different doses of two analgesics that provide an approximately equal analgesic effect; 30 mg of morphine is a common standard for calculating equianalgesic doses.

Multimodal analgesia Use of more than one medicine or class of medication or the use of more than one analgesic technique to produce analgesia through multiple mechanisms.

Nociception Ability to sense pain. Nociceptors are pain-sensing nerve endings.

Opiate Opioid that contains the compounds found in opium.

Opioid Any natural or synthetic drug that has actions similar to morphine.

Patient-controlled analgesia (PCA) Method of allowing a person in pain to self-administer pain medication.

Preemptive analgesia Use of analgesia before the onset of noxious stimuli or a painful procedure.

Tolerance State of adaptation in which exposure to a drug induces changes that result in a diminution of one or more of the drug's effects over time. Also, the need for an increased dosage of a drug to produce the same level of analgesia that previously existed.

Introduction

Pain is probably the most common reason individuals seek medical attention. It is estimated that as many as 43% of all adults have chronic pain,[1] and virtually everyone will have acute pain at some point in their lives. **Nociception** is the ability to sense pain. Pain is a subjective experience, and no tests exist to measure the specific qualitative or quantitative nature of a person's pain. This chapter reviews the pharmacology of drugs used to treat pain and common drugs used for analgesia and anesthesia.

Accurate assessment, diagnosis, and management of pain can be challenging for even the most experienced practitioner because many factors affect a person's perception, experience, and expression of pain. A comprehensive assessment of pain is mandated by The Joint Commission–approved pain assessment and management standards that were established in 1999. Thus, a formal assessment and documentation of that assessment are now mandated for all persons cared for by institutions accredited by The Joint Commission. Pain assessment, in essence, has become the fifth vital sign. Standardized pain assessment tools can be found in the list of resources at the end of this chapter.

The Physiology and Pathophysiology of Pain

Pain is defined by the International Association for the Study of Pain as "an unpleasant sensory and emotional experience associated with actual and potential tissue damage or described in terms of such damage."[3] The phenomenon of pain is complex. It includes sensory and emotional components and is initiated from both peripheral and central mechanisms that employ a host of receptors and substances that are involved in transmission and modulation of pain. The pain threshold is the amount of stimulation required before the sensation of pain is experienced by an individual.[3] Pain tolerance is the greatest intensity of painful stimulation that an individual is able to tolerate in a given situation.[3]

Pain can be classified according to its duration, etiology, and intensity. Acute pain is the "normal, predictable physiological response to a noxious chemical, thermal, or mechanical stimulus and typically is associated with invasive procedures, trauma, and disease. Acute pain generally is time-limited, lasting six weeks or less."[4] Chronic pain persists "beyond the usual course of an acute disease or healing of an injury (e.g., more than three months)."[4] Referred pain occurs when an individual experiences pain at a site adjacent to or at a distance from the site of injury. A classic example of referred pain is the pain that a woman feels in her shoulder when an ectopic pregnancy ruptures; this pain is referred to the shoulder from bleeding that irritates the peritoneum. **Breakthrough pain** is a transitory flare of moderate to severe pain that occurs unexpectedly despite otherwise controlled pain. Breakthrough pain typically lasts 30 minutes or less; however, it may occur several times daily.[5] Each of these types of pain requires a different pharmacologic approach.

Pain may also be differentiated by etiology; that is, it is either nociceptive or neuropathic. Nociceptive pain occurs in the presence of local tissue damage. With this type of pain, activation of nociceptive receptors located in the skin and other tissues activate a variety of chemical mediators such as bradykinin, prostaglandin, potassium, leukotrienes, or histamine that initiate transmission of impulses to the somatosensory cerebral cortex where the perception of pain occurs (Figure 12-1).

Nociceptive pain may be further subdivided into somatic pain and visceral pain. Visceral pain originates from receptors located in the internal organs, which are activated by compression, infiltration, stretching, or ischemia. Visceral pain is often diffused and poorly localized, and may be referred to other regions of the body. Examples of visceral pain include the pain associated with myocardial infarction, cholelithiasis, and appendicitis. Somatic pain is caused by stimulation of nociceptive receptors located in the skin and other superficial structures. Somatic pain tends to be easily localized, and may be described as dull or aching. Examples of somatic pain include musculoskeletal injuries, tendinitis and bursitis, and postsurgical pain. Nociceptive pain is typically well managed by drugs from the nonsteroidal anti-inflammatory drug (NSAID) and opioid classes.

Neuropathic pain results from an injury or malfunction in the peripheral or central nervous system. Although the pain in such a case may initially be the result of an injury, neuropathic pain persists long after the original injury has resolved. The resulting compression or injury to a peripheral nerve or to the central nervous system (CNS) may persist for months to years. While acute pain may be useful as a warning signal of injury, neuropathic pain

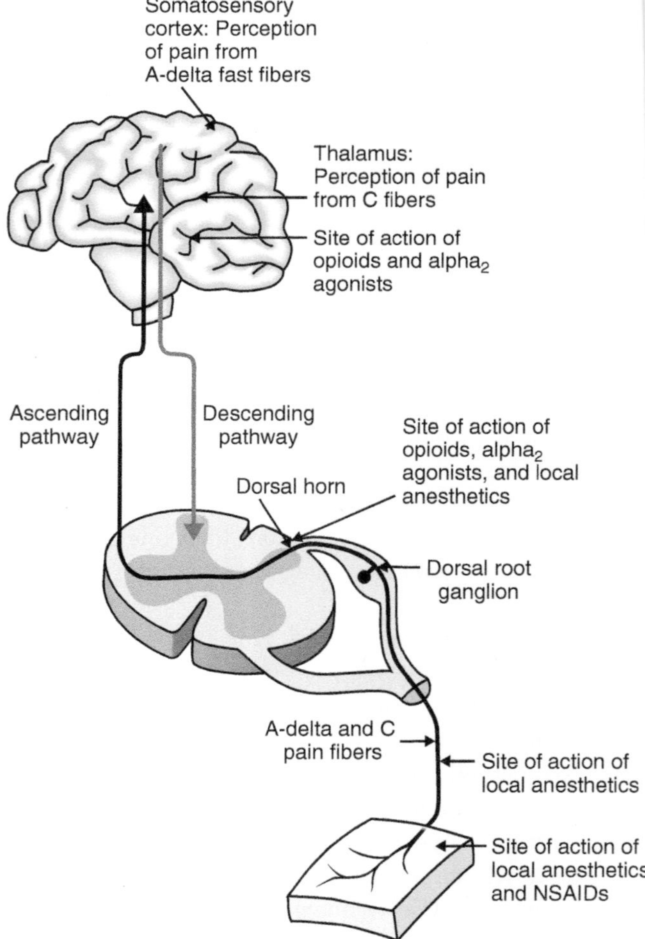

Figure 12-1 Pain pathway and primary sites of action of common analgesics and anesthetics.

serves no useful purpose and may be classified as a disease state in and of itself. Examples of neuropathic pain include postherpetic neuralgias, nerve entrapment syndromes, diabetic neuropathies, and phantom limb pain.

Neuropathic pain is frequently described as burning, lancinating, tingling, or like an electrical shock. Typically, this type of pain does not respond well to opioids or NSAIDs. Complete resolution of neuropathic pain may not always be possible, but it can often be improved by use of antidepressants, anticonvulsants, or local anesthetics.

An individual may also experience a mixture of nociceptive and neuropathic pain that requires a combination of therapies, both pharmacologic and nonpharmacologic. Cancer pain is often mixed, for example, and requires a multimodal treatment approach.

Transmission of Pain Impulses

The perception of pain depends on the cascade of physiologic events that begins with detection of a noxious stimulant, which is followed by conduction of pain impulses to the brain where the insult is interpreted as pain. Most pain medications affect the neurotransmitters that facilitate conduction of the pain signal within the synapse between nerve cells along the nerve pathway from the site of injury to the brain (Figure 12-1). Several neurotransmitters, such as endorphins, cannabinoids, serotonin, norepinephrine, and substance P, serve as physiologic agonists or antagonists to the pain signal.[6] Although a detailed review of the pathophysiology and neurobiology of pain is beyond the scope of this chapter, the interested reader is referred to seminal reviews of this phenomenon.[7–10]

Transduction, the first step of the cascade, begins with a noxious stimulus that causes the release of neurotransmitters—such as prostaglandins, histamine, leukotrienes, bradykinin, and substance P—that stimulate nociceptors and initiate nerve conduction or signal transduction. NSAIDs inhibit the release of prostaglandins at the site of injury.

When tissue is damaged, a local inflammatory response is also initiated. Several of the inflammatory mediators act on the nociceptor nerve endings to sensitize them. This results in a lower threshold for impulse conduction and a higher excitability of the nerve ending. This process, which is referred to as peripheral sensitization or primary hyperalgesia, is generally reversible once the tissue heals.[8]

The nerve signal is then transmitted via the afferent C fibers and A-delta fibers to the substantia gelatinosa, located in the dorsal horn of the spinal cord.[7] These fibers release neurotransmitters that facilitate signal transmission across the dorsal horn and to the thalamus or midbrain, and eventually to the somatosensory cerebral cortex via the ascending spinothalamic tract. If the pain stimulus is intense, central sensitization may occur in the dorsal horn whereby the nerve endings develop a lower threshold to pain stimuli. For example, central sensitization occurs after surgery and is one factor responsible for severe postoperative pain.

Opioids bind to presynaptic and postsynaptic opioid receptors in the central nervous system. When they bind to presynaptic opioid receptors, neurotransmitter release (e.g., substance P, glutamate, norepinephrine, serotonin) is inhibited, thereby preventing signal transmission. When opioids bind to postsynaptic opioid receptors, the neuron becomes hyperpolarized, thereby preventing signal transmission up the spinal cord to the brain.

Descending nerves from the CNS modulate the transmission of the pain signal in the dorsal horn. The primary neurotransmitters involved are norepinephrine and serotonin.[8] Tricyclic antidepressants inhibit the reuptake of serotonin, prolonging its effect and thereby enhancing the inhibition of afferent fibers in the spinal cord.

Pain perception occurs in the cortex. Fibers from the thalamus send the message to several centers in the cortex that identify the type of pain, its location, and other pain-related characteristics. Several different neurotransmitter receptors in the CNS cause a mild euphoria and decrease in pain perception when stimulated or antagonized by specific opioids.

Genetics of Pain

There is significant interindividual variation in pain sensitivity and vulnerability to chronic pain conditions. To date, studies of the genetic contributions to pain sensitivity have found several genes that control nociception. Migraine was the first painful disorder to be associated with a specific genetic polymorphism. Variants in the gene that encodes for the mu-opioid receptor affect pain perception and influence how an individual responds to morphine and other mu-opioid agonist drugs.

Gender Differences in Pain

Gender differences in the pain response have been studied extensively in the last few decades.[12,13] Women have a higher prevalence of several painful conditions, including arthritis, fibromyalgia, irritable bowel syndrome, and pain from other autoimmune diseases.[12] Sex hormones such as estrogen and progesterone are known to play a role in the function of several pain-related neurotransmitters. For example, low estrogen levels result in suppression of endogenous neurotransmissions affecting the mu receptors, thereby resulting in higher levels of pain.[14]

Sex differences also exist in the response to opioid analgesia. Some evidence indicates that estrogen reduces the efficacy of mu-opioid agonists; as a consequence, these drugs may be less effective in the treatment of visceral pain in women than in men.[15] Women also experience more side effects of mu-opioids than do men.[16] However, studies on sex differences in pain perception have yielded conflicting results and the neurobiologic causes of variability in pain responses between men and women have yet to be adequately explored, especially in humans.

Analgesia: An Introduction

Analgesia is the absence of pain in response to stimulation that would normally be painful. This word comes from the Greek *an-* ("without") and *algesia* ("to feel pain"). **Anesthesia** is the loss of all sensation, including pain. Anesthetic and analgesic drugs can be given through many different delivery systems to provide regional analgesia or anesthesia, local anesthesia, or systemic analgesia, including via oral, parenteral, and transdermal techniques.

Atypical analgesics is the term used for drugs that can mitigate pain but are not members of the opioid or nonsteroidal anti-inflammatory drug families. Drugs used for treating seizures, for example, have some efficacy in mitigating neuropathic pain.

Multimodal analgesia refers to the use of two or more medications from different drug classes to produce analgesia through multiple mechanisms.[17,18] Because multimodal techniques capitalize on different physiologic mechanisms to block pain, the result is a synergistic or potentiating effect that allows for use of lower doses of the individual agents. Multimodal analgesia has excellent results and has become commonplace in treating postoperative pain.

Preemptive analgesia refers to the administration of analgesic medication prior to a painful procedure or surgery for the purpose of decreasing peripheral and central sensitization to painful stimuli, thereby decreasing postoperative pain.[17,19,20] While animal studies have been promising, the clinical studies of preemptive analgesia have yielded equivocal results.

Finally, analgesic techniques can be defined by the protocols for administration. **Patient-controlled analgesia (PCA)** is being used increasingly for acute and postoperative pain. When individuals are able to control the timing of the administration of pain medications, they have better health outcomes, higher consumer satisfaction scores, and no increase in the incidence of adverse reactions.[21]

Approach to Pain Management

In 1990, the World Health Organization (WHO) introduced the analgesic ladder for the treatment of pain.[22] Although originally intended as a standard for the management of cancer-associated pain, the analgesic ladder serves as a useful guideline for the management of both acute and chronic pain from any cause. The WHO ladder provides a stepwise approach to pain management. Step 1 recommends treatment of mild pain with non-opioid analgesics such as acetaminophen, aspirin, or NSAIDs. Step 2 adds a moderate opioid agonist in combination with non-opioids for moderate pain or pain of shorter duration, such as postoperative pain. Step 3 recommends use of stronger opioids on a round-the-clock rather than as-needed (prn) schedule for persistent pain. Figure 12-2 illustrates WHO's stepped approach to pain management.

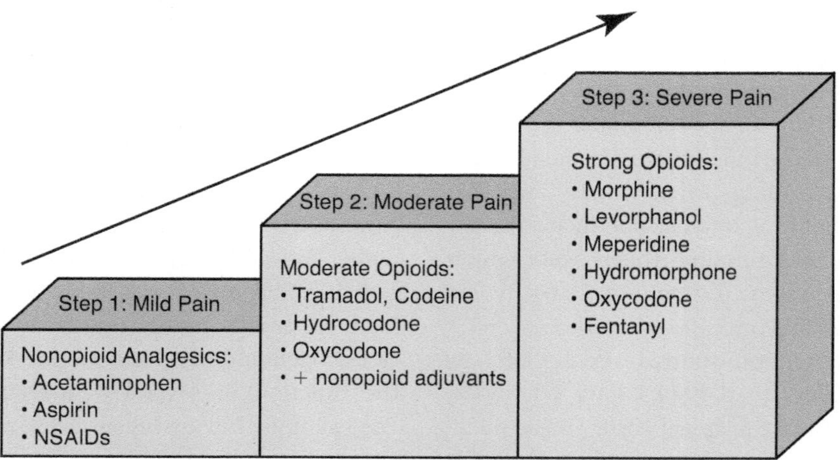

Figure 12-2 World Health Organization analgesic scale.

Pain management begins with the selection of the appropriate analgesic at the appropriate dosage and administration regimen. Management of chronic pain is best achieved when medications are administered on a regular, rather than as-needed, schedule.[23] Breakthrough pain is best managed with rapid-onset medications that have short half-lives. Pain that consistently recurs before the onset of regularly scheduled medication may indicate opioid **tolerance** or disease progression and, therefore, signals the need for dose escalation and reevaluation.[24]

Non-opioid Analgesics

Non-opioid analgesics include two major classes: NSAIDs and acetaminophen. Six classes of NSAIDs are distinguished based on chemical structure. Although salicylates such as aspirin are included in the NSAID class, in clinical practice the term "NSAID" is not used to refer to salicylates. The primary difference between non-opioid analgesics and opioid analgesics include the following: (1) NSAIDs have a **ceiling effect**—that is, after a certain plasma level is achieved, increasing the dose will increase the side effects, but not the analgesic effect; (2) NSAIDs have antipyretic effects, but opioids do not; and (3) NSAIDs do not produce physical dependence or psychological dependence.[25] The NSAIDs that are frequently used are categorized as selective or nonselective based on their mechanism of action. Commonly used nonprescription and prescription NSAIDs are reviewed in Table 12-1 and Table 12-2.[26]

Mechanism of Action of Non-opioid Analgesics

A summary of the pharmacokinetics of non-opioid analgesics is provided in Table 12-3. The mechanism of action of acetaminophen has not been fully elucidated, although it is believed that this drug inhibits prostaglandin synthesis in the CNS and blocks pain impulse generation peripherally. The antipyretic effect occurs secondary to inhibition of the heat-regulating center in the hypothalamus. Acetominophen is not an anti-inflammatory agent and, therefore, is not considered an NSAID.

All drugs in the NSAID family mitigate pain via inhibition of cyclooxygenase (COX), the enzyme responsible for synthesis of prostaglandins, prostacyclin, and thromboxane. Prostaglandins cause pain through promotion of inflammatory responses such as edema and local vasodilation, and by stimulating nociceptors to transmit pain impulses.

COX converts arachidonic acid from the cell membrane into prostaglandin H_2, the precursor of a variety of prostaglandins (Figure 12-3). COX has three forms: COX-1, COX-2, and COX-3.

- COX-1 is constitutive and found in virtually all tissues. It is involved in the production of prostaglandins

Table 12-1 Over-the-Counter Non-opioid Analgesics for Treating Mild Pain

Drug: Generic (Brand)	Formulations	Usual Adult Dose	Maximum Daily Dose	Clinical Considerations
Acetaminophen (Tylenol)	Regular strength 325 mg; extra strength 500 mg; extended release 650 mg	650–1000 mg PO every 4–6 hours	4000 mg/24 hours[a]	Acetaminophen has antipyretic and analgesic properties but is not anti-inflammatory. Should be avoided by persons with liver impairment or those who regularly consume more than 3 alcoholic drinks/day. Use during pregnancy is associated with higher risk for hyperkinetic disorder and autism-like behaviors in children.
Nonsteroidal Anti-inflammatory Drugs (NSAIDs)				
Aspirin (ASA)[b]	Low-dose ("Baby") ASA 81 mg Adult tablets come as 325 or 500 mg	325–1000 mg PO every 4 hours	4000 mg	Aspirin is associated with Reye's syndrome in children. Antiplatelet effect is irreversible for the life of the platelets. Gastritis and bleeding are common with chronic use. Persons with asthma may be intolerant to ASA. Discontinue 1 week prior to elective surgery.
Ibuprofen (Motrin, Advil, Nuprin, Rufen)[b]	200 mg	400–800 mg PO every 4–6 hours	3200 mg	Analgesic and antipyretic effects are relatively immediate. Anti-inflammatory effects require longer therapy and higher doses. Contraindicated in third trimester of pregnancy.
Naproxen (Aleve)[b]	250, 375, 500 mg	200–800 mg PO every 4 hours	1500 mg	Analgesic and antipyretic effects are relatively immediate. Anti-inflammatory effects may require longer therapy.

[a] The recommended maximum dose per day is currently 4000 mg. Because there is a narrow margin between this dose and the risk for hepatotoxicity, some authors suggest that 3000–3250 mg should be the maximum dose per day that is recommended for healthy individuals and that the maximum recommended dose be lower for persons at risk for hepatic injury.
[b] NSAIDs are contraindicated during pregnancy.
Source: Modified from Miller E. World Health Organization pain ladder. *J Midwifery Womens Health.* 2004;49(6):542-546.[26]

Table 12-2 Prescription Non-opioids for Treating Mild Pain

Drug: Generic (Brand)	Formulations	Usual Adult Dose	Maximum Daily Dose	Clinical Considerations
Salicylic Acid Derivatives				
Choline magnesium trisalicylate	500, 750, 1000 mg	1000–2000 mg every 12–24 hours	4500 mg	Does not inhibit platelet aggregation. Less effective analgesia than aspirin or ibuprofen.
Choline salicylate (Arthropan)	870 mg/ 5 mL	325–500 mg every 3–4 hours	3600-5400 mg/day	Same basic side effects as aspirin.
Nonselective Nonsteroidal Anti-inflammatory Drugs				
Diflunisal[a,b] (Dolobid)	250, 500 mg	1000 mg initially, followed by 500 mg every 8–12 hours	1500 mg	Slower onset than aspirin but 500 mg of diflunisal is superior to 650 mg of aspirin. May take up to 14 days for full therapeutic effects to be reached.
Etodolac[a,b] (Lodine)	400, 500 mg	200–800 mg 2 times/daily	1200 mg	Relatively minor gastrointestinal side effects in comparison with other NSAIDs. Also available in extended-release formulations for once-daily dosing.
Fenoprofen[a,b] (Nalfon)	200, 400 mg	200–600 mg every 6–8 hours	3200 mg	Fenoprofen is the most nephrotoxic of all NSAIDs. Drug-induced nephritic syndrome has been reported.
Ketoprofen[a,b] (Orudis)	25-, 50-, 75-mg capsules; 100-, 150-, and 200-mg ER	25–50 mg every 6–8 hours	300 mg (or 200 mg ER)	Severe gastric toxicity associated with ketoprofen may require discontinuation. Also available in extended-release formulation for once-daily dosing.
Ketorolac[a,b] tromethamine (Toradol)	10-mg tablets, 15 mg/mL, 30 mg/mL	Oral: 10 mg every 4–6 hours; IV/IM: 30 mg every 6 hours	Oral: 40 mg IV: 120 mg	Therapy should be limited to 5 days. Step down to ibuprofen after 5 days.
Meclofenamate sodium[a,b] (Meclomen)	50 mg, 100 mg	50–100 mg every 4–6 hours	400 mg	Relatively severe gastric toxicity may require coadministration of a cytoprotective agent. May cause photosensitivity. Sunscreen recommended.
Mefenamic acid[a,b] (Ponstel)	250 mg	500 initially, then 250 mg every 6 hours	1000 mg	FDA approved for treatment of primary dysmenorrhea, but no clinical evidence that it is more effective than other NSAIDs. Treatment of mild to moderate pain should be limited to less than 7 days.
Selective Nonsteroidal Anti-inflammatory Drugs				
Celecoxib[a,b] (Celebrex)	50, 100, 200, 400 mg	50–100 mg 2 times/daily	400 mg	COX-2 specific: Persons with sulfonamide allergy or sensitivity should avoid celecoxib. Use cautiously in the elderly, and in persons with asthma, renal or hepatic disease, or on anticoagulants or antihypertensives.

Abbreviations: COX = cyclooxygenase; ER = extended release; NSAIDs = nonselective anti-inflammatory drugs.
[a] The labels of all NSAIDs carry an FDA black box warning indicating that these drugs increase the risk for serious cardiovascular thrombotic events, myocardial infarction, stroke, gastrointestinal bleeding, ulceration, and perforation of the stomach or intestines.
[b] All NSAIDs are contraindicated for treatment of individuals with perioperative pain in the setting of coronary artery bypass graft.
Source: Modified from Miller E. World Health Organization pain ladder. *J Midwifery Womens Health.* 2004;49(6):542-546.[26]

that have many important "housekeeping" functions, including (1) protection of gastric mucosa; (2) inhibition of gastric secretions; (3) stimulation of platelet aggregation; (4) renal vasodilation; and (5) stimulation of uterine contractions.

- COX-2 is inducible in macrophages and at tissue injury sites. At the site of tissue injury, COX-2 is released and subsequently converts arachidonic acid to prostaglandins that mediate local inflammatory responses and sensitize receptors to painful stimuli. COX-2 is constitutive in some tissues. In the brain, COX-2 facilitates synthesis of prostaglandins that mediate fever and pain perception. In the kidney, constitutive COX-2 facilitates production of prostaglandins that support renal function.
- COX-3 is a variant of COX-1, so some scientists prefer the term *COX-1b* or *COX-1 variant* (COX 1v). COX-3 acts centrally within the blood–brain barrier to regulate fever and pain sensitivity.[27]

NSAIDs are generally classified according to the specific COX enzyme that is inhibited. Aspirin and other

Table 12-3 Pharmacokinetics of Non-opioid Analgesics

Drug: Generic (Brand)	**Time to Peak Concentration (Hours)**	**Half-Life (Hours)**	**Protein Binding**	**Metabolism**
Acetaminophen (Tylenol)	0.7	1–4	> 50%	CYP2E1 and CYP1A2
Salicylates				
Aspirin	Variable	0.3	75–90%	Liver
Choline salicylate (Arthropan, Trilisate)	0.5	2–3	80–90%	Liver
Magnesium salicylate (Magan, Doan's caplets)	0.5	2–3	80–90%	Liver
Sodium salicylate (generic)	0.5–0.75	2–3	80–90%	Liver
First-Generation NSAIDs (Nonselective COX Inhibitors)				
Diclofenac (Voltaren, Cataflam)	2	2	99%	CYP2C9
Diflunisal (Dolobid)	2–3	8–12	99%	Liver
Etodolac (Lodine)	1.5	7.3	99%	CYP2C9
Fenoprofen (Nalfon)	2	3	99%	Liver
Flurbiprofen (Ansaid)	2.5	5.7	99%	CYP3C9
Ibuprofen (Motrin, Advil, others)	1–2	1.8–2	99%	CYP2C9 and CYP2C19
Indomethacin (Indocin)	21.5	4.5	90%	CYP2C9
Ketoprofen (Orudis, Oruvail)	0.5–2	2	99%	CYP2C9
Ketorolac (Toradol)	2–3	5–6	99%	CYP2C9
Meclofenamate (generic)	0.5–2	1.3	99%	Liver
Mefenamic acid (Postel)	2–4	2	90%	CYP2C9
Meloxicam (Mobic)	4–5	20	99%	CYP2C9
Nabumetone (Relafen)	9–12	22	99%	CYP2C9 and CYP1A2
Naproxen (Aleve, Anaprox, Naprosyn)	2–4	12–17	99%	CYP2C9
Piroxicam (Feldene)	3–5	50	99%	CYP2C9
Sulindac (Clinoril)	2–4	7.8	93%	Liver
Tolmetin (Tolectin)	0.5–1	2–7	99%	Liver
Second-Generation NSAIDs (COX-2 Inhibitors)				
Celecoxib (Celebrex)	3	11	97%	CYP2C9 and CYP3A4

Abbreviations: COX = cyclooxygenase; NSAIDs = nonsteroidal anti-inflammatory drugs.

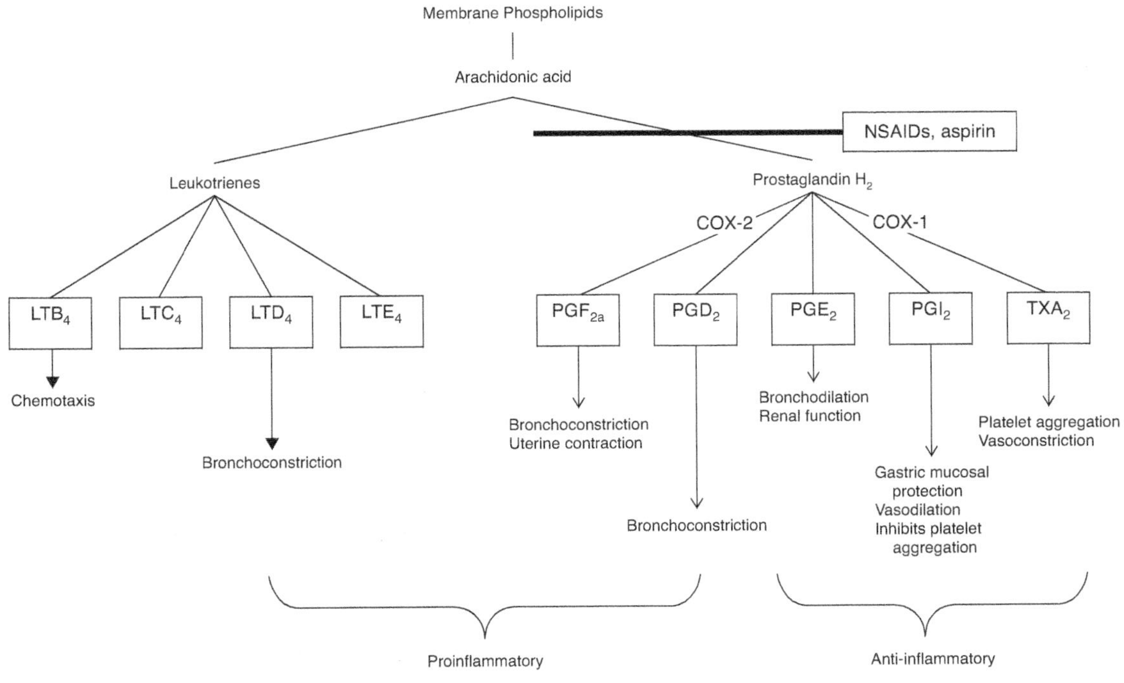

Figure 12-3 COX pathways.

first-generation NSAIDs inhibit all three COX enzymes and, therefore, are called nonselective COX inhibitors. Second-generation NSAIDs inhibit both COX-2 and COX-3. Acetaminophen is hypothesized to affect only COX-3, which may explain its lack of anti-inflammatory effect.[28] Although all NSAIDs prevent production of prostaglandins via inhibition of the COX enzymes, there are clinically important differences in the pharmacokinetics and pharmacodynamics of individual drugs.

Aspirin

Aspirin, or acetylsalicylic acid (ASA), is the prototype for nonsteroidal anti-inflammatory drugs. Aspirin-containing compounds have been used to treat pain since the beginning of recorded history. Medicine made from willow bark, which contains salicin, was recommended for treatment of fever, pain, and inflammation by the ancient Greeks.[29] Introduced as a patented pill by Bayer in 1899, aspirin's mechanism of action remained unclear until 1971, when its COX-inhibiting abilities were demonstrated.[30] Newer NSAIDs have been developed, but aspirin continues to be one of the most valuable and widely used agents. It remains the standard against which all other NSAIDs are compared.

Pharmacokinetics

Aspirin, a weak acid, is rapidly absorbed from the stomach and small intestine. Absorption following oral administration is rapid and complete. Following absorption, aspirin is rapidly converted to salicylic acid, the active metabolite. The half-life of salicylic acid ranges from 3.5 to 4.5 hours.

Salicylic acid is distributed to all body tissues via plasma albumin, to which it is extensively bound. Once the plasma proteins are saturated, the unbound fraction increases disproportionately, which can lead to aspirin toxicity. Aspirin inhibits COX-1 and COX-2 irreversibly, so its duration of action is secondary to the rate at which the COX system replaces itself in the affected target organ. This results in a duration of action of 6 to 12 hours in general, although the antiplatelet effects last 8 to 10 days. The antiplatelet effect is not reversible until new platelets are available. Excretion of salicylic acid and its metabolites occurs renally and is dependent upon urinary pH. Excretion is facilitated by alkalinization of the urine and inhibited by acidic urine.

Pharmacodynamics

Aspirin has four major therapeutic indications: (1) reduction of fever; (2) relief of mild to moderate pain; (3) reduction of inflammation; and (4) suppression of platelet aggregation. Aspirin's antipyretic effect is achieved by lowering the set point of the hypothalamus through inhibition of COX-2. By inhibiting prostaglandin synthesis in the hypothalamus, aspirin reduces fever, but does not lower normal body temperature.

The analgesic effects of aspirin are achieved both peripherally and centrally. Through aspirin's action of suppressing prostaglandin synthesis at the site of local tissue injury, local pain receptors are rendered less sensitive. Central prostaglandin inhibition results in decreased transmission of pain impulses through the spinal column. Aspirin suppresses inflammation through nonselective inhibition of the COX system, which results in an overall reduction of prostaglandins.

Aspirin is an initial drug of choice for inflammatory conditions such as rheumatoid arthritis, tendinitis, and bursitis. However, it must be given in doses to produce plasma drug levels of 150 mcg/mL to 300 mcg/mL to achieve sufficient anti-inflammatory effects. Because signs of salicylate toxicity can begin to emerge at levels as low as 200 mcg/mL, becoming severe at levels greater than 400 mcg/mL, the usefulness of aspirin for relief of chronic inflammatory conditions can be limited by adverse effects. Aspirin and other NSAIDs have a ceiling effect; that is, increasing the dose beyond a certain amount will not increase analgesia but will increase toxicity.[31]

Platelet aggregation is facilitated by the action of thromboxane A_2 (TXA_2), a prostaglandin-related compound induced by COX-1. By irreversibly acetylating COX-1, aspirin inhibits the formation of thromboxane A_2, thereby reducing platelet stickiness and inhibiting platelet aggregation. Because platelets do not have the ability to synthesize new COX-1, platelet aggregation is inhibited for the life of the platelet, which is approximately 8 to 10 days.

Clinical Indications for Aspirin

Aspirin is indicated for relief of mild to moderate pain, including arthritis, fever reduction, and suppression of inflammation. It is also useful for treatment of dysmenorrhea, although it may increase menstrual bleeding when used for this purpose. Aspirin is not effective for visceral pain.

The antiplatelet effect of aspirin promotes bleeding. A daily dose of low-dose aspirin is recommended to inhibit platelet aggregation for persons with or at risk for ischemic stroke, transient ischemia attacks, acute myocardial infarction, and chronic stable angina. Low-dose aspirin has been colloquially called "baby aspirin" in the past, but that terminology has fallen into disfavor because of potential confusion with pediatric use. Approximately 50 million persons in the United States (36% of the adult population) take aspirin daily for cardiovascular protection.[32]

In the past, persons who took aspirin daily to prevent clotting were counseled to stop taking the aspirin several days before having a surgical procedure. Studies comparing the benefits and risks of aspirin therapy, however, have concluded that stopping aspirin before surgery is not always necessary and depends on the individual risk and the procedure being performed.[33,34] Although regular use of high-dose aspirin has been found to decrease the risk of colorectal cancer (these cancers overexpress COX-2), the United States Preventive Services Task Force does not recommend the use of aspirin or NSAIDs for this purpose given the significant risk of gastrointestinal (GI) bleeding associated with the use of aspirin.[35]

Side Effects/Adverse Effects

The most common side effects of aspirin therapy are gastrointestinal in nature. The incidence of gastrointestinal complications varies depending on specific population characteristics, use of additional medications, duration of therapy, and dose. Overall, approximately 50% of persons who take aspirin report some gastric upset. Nausea, heartburn, and gastric distress may be seen with low or intermittent dosing secondary to suppression of the prostaglandins that facilitate production of gastric mucosa. Long-term use may result in gastric ulceration and bleeding. Aspirin-induced ulcers are often asymptomatic, and perforation and hemorrhage can occur without premonitory signs. In the Women's Health Study, approximately 50% of the participants reported some gastric upset, whereas the incidence of any gastrointestinal bleeding was 5% and the incidence of a GI hemorrhage that required a blood transfusion was 0.6%.[36] To date, no evidence has been published showing that enteric-coated or buffered tablets decrease the risk of GI bleeding.[37]

The FDA publishes regulations requiring all products that contain aspirin to (1) display the names *aspirin* and *NSAID* prominently on the principal display panel of the label; (2) include a warning about severe gastrointestinal bleeding on the outside of the container or wrapper of the package; and (3) include a warning that severe liver damage can result if large doses are used or if the individual consumes three or more alcoholic drinks per day.

Factors that increase the risk of gastric ulceration include advanced age, previous history of peptic ulcer disease, infection with *Helicobacter pylori*, history of intolerance of ASA or other NSAIDs, cigarette smoking, and alcohol use. The incidence of gastrointestinal complications increases in persons taking larger doses; however, even the lowest 81-mg dose doubles the incidence of gastrointestinal complications when compared to placebo.[31] Concomitant use of a proton pump inhibitor or histamine-2 antagonist to reduce gastric acid production can be useful for those persons on long-term aspirin therapy. Misoprostol (Cytotec), a synthetic prostaglandin, promotes gastric mucus production and is the only agent proven to be effective for the prevention and treatment of clinically significant ASA-associated ulcers.[38]

Although short-term use of aspirin at low therapeutic levels rarely causes serious adverse effects, toxicity is associated with long-term use at high-dose anti-inflammatory levels. Prostaglandins promote renal vasodilation and other normal renal functions. High-dose or long-term use of ASA by persons with renal impairment can result in acute renal function impairment by inhibition of prostaglandin through the COX-1 pathway. Sodium retention, edema, decreased urine output, and increased blood urea nitrogen and serum creatinine all are signs of renal impairment that must be monitored for those individuals taking high-dose, long-term ASA therapy. Interruption of ASA therapy typically reverses these effects. Renal papillary necrosis also may be associated with long-term ASA use.

Aspirin can cause hepatic injury and various blood dyscrasias, although these complications are rare. Hepatotoxicity from aspirin is most likely to occur in children who have a concomitant viral illness that results in the clinical presentation called *Reye's syndrome*.[39] Reye's syndrome is not common today, secondary to the recommendation that children not be given aspirin.

Finally, daily aspirin therapy is associated with a small increased risk for hemorrhagic stroke; in all trials conducted to date, however, this risk was offset by a much larger reduction in myocardial infarction and stroke from clots.[36] Thus, when considering daily aspirin therapy for cardiovascular protection, the risk of gastrointestinal hemorrhage and hemorrhagic stroke must be compared to the risk for a cardiovascular event, and the recommendation for taking aspirin needs to be individualized when considering prophylactic use of aspirin. (See the *Cardiovascular Conditions* chapter for more detailed information on use of aspirin for cardiovascular protection.)

Aspirin Hypersensitivity

Aspirin is associated with three types of hypersensitivity reactions: aspirin-exacerbated respiratory disease (AERD), aspirin-intolerant urticaria/angioedema, and (rarely) anaphylaxis.[40,41] AERD has a prevalence of 0.3% to 0.9% in the general population, but this prevalence is increased to 10% to 20% in persons with asthma.[42] However, AERD occurs in 30% to 40% of persons who have asthma and nasal polyps.[43] AERD is also more common in women than in men and generally develops in adulthood.

In 1922, Widal first described the clinical syndrome of aspirin allergy, asthma, and nasal polyps—a syndrome later named Samter's triad.[41] The mechanism of action of Samter's triad is related to aspirin inhibition of the COX pathways, which shifts arachidonic acid metabolism to the leukotriene pathway, which then results in increased production of leukotrienes that cause bronchoconstriction. This disorder also appears to have a genetic component.[43] The symptoms usually appear 30 to 120 minutes after the individual ingests aspirin.

Aspirin-intolerant urticaria is the least understood of the three types of hypersensitivity reactions, but appears to occur secondary to aspirin-stimulating histamine release of cutaneous mast cells. True anaphylaxis from aspirin use is probably extremely rare.

Persons with aspirin hypersensitivity can be treated with leukotriene receptor antagonists such as zileuton (Zyflo) or montelukast (Singular). Aspirin desensitization can be performed if aspirin therapy is necessary, but this should be done in a hospital under close monitoring. Finally, avoiding aspirin and aspirin-containing products is the best way to prevent these symptoms. Approximately 20% of persons with aspirin allergy will also exhibit allergic reactions to nonselective NSAIDs because they cross-react with aspirin; thus, these individuals should not use nonselective NSAIDs. Selective COX-2 inhibiting NSAIDs and nonacetylated salicylates are recommended for treatment of pain in persons who have an aspirin hypersensitivity.

Salicylism: Aspirin Toxicity

Salicylism, or aspirin toxicity, occurs when serum plasma levels of aspirin rise above 300 mcg/mL, which is just slightly higher than therapeutic levels. Signs of salicylism include tinnitus, dizziness, headache, sweating, and tachypnea. Acid–base imbalances may result in respiratory alkalosis. In most cases, salicylism is easily reversed by discontinuing the drug. Some experts suggest that tinnitus can be used as a marker for high therapeutic levels of ASA.[44] The dose at which tinnitus occurs is considered the individual's maximal therapeutic dose. However, this method for determining maximal dosing is not safe for the elderly, who may not develop tinnitus until toxic levels are present. Many over-the-counter drugs contain aspirin and, therefore, aspirin overdose can occur unintentionally.

Drug–Drug Interactions

Aspirin can be involved in drug–drug interactions via several mechanisms. The ability of aspirin to compete for plasma protein sites can result in increased plasma levels of other drugs that bind to the same plasma proteins. This is the etiology of the well-known drug–drug interaction that occurs when valproic acid (Depakote) and aspirin are taken concomitantly. When aspirin is used in combination with another NSAID, the two medications have an additive effect on the risk for developing gastrointestinal side effects. In addition, NSAIDs compete for the sites where aspirin and NSAIDs block COX-1, thereby preventing aspirin from having the irreversible anticoagulation effect that can be one of the desired therapeutic outcomes.[45] Significant drug interactions associated with aspirin are summarized in Table 12-4.

Contraindications

Absolute contraindications to ASA use include previously demonstrated hypersensitivity, recent history of gastrointestinal bleeding, and bleeding disorders. Aspirin should not be used by children and adolescents suspected of having influenza or varicella because there is a reported association between use of aspirin to treat viral syndromes and the development of Reye's syndrome. The etiologic relationship is controversial, but the recommendation that children not be given aspirin stands nonetheless. Aspirin should be used cautiously by persons with renal impairment, cigarette or alcohol use, *H. pylori* infection, gout, mild diabetes, uncontrolled hypertension, or heart failure.

Special Populations: Pregnancy, Lactation, and the Elderly

Aspirin is not recommended for use by women during pregnancy primarily because other drugs that are known to be safe are available for mild to moderate pain or fever. ASA suppression of COX-2 has a theoretical risk of interfering with implantation of the embryo, but this has not been proven in human studies. Known risks of chronic ASA use during normal pregnancy include anemia from occult gastrointestinal blood loss. Inhibition of prostaglandin production may also suppress spontaneous uterine contractions and delay or prolong labor.[46]

Suppression of prostaglandins is necessary for the maintenance of pregnancy, so there is a theoretical benefit to use of aspirin later in pregnancy.[47] Very-low-dose aspirin (60 to 80 mg per day), started in the late first trimester, is recommended for women with a previous history of preeclampsia in more than one pregnancy and for

Table 12-4 Selected Drug–Drug Interactions Associated with Aspirin/Salicylates and NSAIDs[a]

Drug: Generic (Brand)	Drug–Drug Interactions If Taken Concomitantly with Aspirin or NSAIDs
Alcohol	Increases gastrointestinal bleeding
Aminoglycosides	NSAIDs inhibit aminoglycoside renal clearance
Antacids	Increased pH of gastric contents may affect enteric-coated acetylsalicylic acid (ASA); aluminum hydroxide decreases naproxen absorption
Anticoagulants	ASA and NSAIDs prolong bleeding time
Antihypertensive agents	NSAIDs antagonize antihypertensive effects of beta blockers, ACE inhibitors, vasodilators, and diuretics Hyperkalemia may occur when NSAIDs are used with ACE inhibitors or potassium-sparing diuretics
Cephalosporins	Increase bleeding risk with ASA
Corticosteroids	Increase risk of gastrointestinal ulceration and reduction of serum salicylate levels
Digoxin (Lanoxin)	NSAIDs inhibit renal clearance of digoxin
Fluconazole (Diflucan)	Increases plasma concentration levels of celecoxib
H_2 receptor antagonists	Increase potential salicylate toxicity; reduce effectiveness of naproxen sodium
Hypoglycemic agents	Large doses of ASA may increase the hypoglycemic effect of these drugs
Lithium (Eskalith, Lithobid)	NSAIDs increase the steady-state concentration of lithium and can lead to lithium toxicity
Methotrexate (Rheumatrex, Trexall)	All NSAIDs except celecoxib result in reduced clearance of methotrexate, with resulting increased plasma methotrexate levels
NSAIDs	Routine but not intermittent use of ibuprofen reduces the antiplatelet effects of ASA
Phenobarbital (Luminal)	ASA levels may be reduced via enzyme induction
Phenytoin (Dilantin)	ASA and ibuprofen increase serum phenytoin levels by competition for protein-binding sites
Propranolol (Inderal)	Competition for receptors may reduce anti-inflammatory effectiveness of ASA
Pyrazolone derivatives (phenylbutazone, oxyphenbutazone, and possibly dipyrone)	Concomitant use with ASA increases the risk of gastric ulceration
Selective serotonin reuptake inhibitors	NSAIDs increase risk of gastrointestinal bleeding
Spironolactone (Aldactone)	ASA may decrease sodium excretion
Uricosuric agents (probenecid, sulfinpyrazone, and phenylbutazone)	ASA decreases effectiveness
Urinary alkalinizers	Reduction of ASA effectiveness by increasing renal elimination of salicylic acid
Valproate (Depakote)	ASA inhibits oxidation of valproate and reduces clearance with resulting potential increase in valproate toxicity

Abbreviations: ACE = angiotensin-converting-enzyme; ASA = aspirin; NSAIDs = nonsteroidal anti-inflammatory drugs.

[a] This table is not comprehensive as new information is being generated on a regular basis.

women who have had a preterm delivery associated with preeclampsia.[48] Evidence supports the administration of very-low-dose aspirin during the second and third trimesters for prevention of fetal growth restriction, premature birth, preeclampsia, and stillbirth in women at risk for these complications.[49,50]

Low-dose aspirin is also sometimes recommended for women at risk for thrombotic events (e.g., antiphospholipid antibody syndrome [APS]). Among women with APS who have experienced previous stillbirth, recurrent fetal loss, or thrombotic events, consideration should be given to aspirin and anticoagulant therapy during pregnancy and in the first six weeks postpartum.[50]

Aspirin freely crosses the placenta. Some evidence suggests that use of high-dose ASA at or near term is associated with restriction or premature closure of the ductus arteriosus in the fetus.[51] Routine high-dose aspirin use in pregnancy has also been associated with stillbirth, renal toxicity, and intracranial hemorrhage in preterm infants.[52] The American Academy of Pediatrics (AAP) lists ASA as a drug that has been associated with serious neonatal side effects and should be avoided during lactation.[53]

Elderly women are more susceptible to the adverse effects of aspirin as compared to younger women. Gastrointestinal, renal, and central nervous system effects are found more frequently in the elderly. Additionally, increased risk for drug interactions exist. Increase in serum potassium for those persons with chronic renal insufficiency or those on potassium-sparing antibiotics is a rare but serious adverse effect.

Other Salicylates

Nonacetylated salicylates include choline salicylate (Arthropan), magnesium salicylate (Doan's pills), sodium salicylate, and diflunisal (Dolobid). Like aspirin, these drugs inhibit both COX-1 and COX-2; thus they have similar indications for their use, including treatment of mild to moderate pain. However, these agents do not have the same antiplatelet effect as aspirin, and they are not recommended for protection against stroke or myocardial infarction. The most common side effects associated with these other salicylates are gastrointestinal in nature, although the incidence of gastric ulceration is much reduced compared to the frequency of side effects associated with use of ASA.

Nonsteroidal Anti-inflammatory Drugs

Nonselective NSAIDs were developed to achieve the benefits of aspirin with fewer side effects. In 1969, ibuprofen (e.g., Advil, Motrin), the prototype drug, was introduced in the United Kingdom.[28] Numerous NSAIDs have since been developed, and collectively they are the most frequently used drugs in the United States. Nonselective NSAIDs such as ibuprofen inhibit COX-1 and COX-2. The newer selective NSAIDs inhibit COX-2 only, so they have a potential lower risk for gastrointestinal side effects. As the population ages, we can assume more persons will take NSAIDs, and more adverse effects will occur. Therefore, an in-depth knowledge of the pharmacologic effects of this class of drugs is essential for all primary care providers.

Nonselective NSAIDs

NSAIDs are weak organic acids that are well absorbed in the stomach and have negligible first-pass metabolism.[25] They achieve peak concentrations within 1 to 4 hours and are clinically divided into short-acting (less than 6 hours) or long-acting (more than 6 hours) options depending on the specific drug's half-life. Food does not interfere with absorption of the NSAIDs. All NSAIDs are highly protein bound and undergo hepatic metabolism via the CYP450 enzymes and excretion via the kidney. Like aspirin, ibuprofen (Advil) and other first-generation NSAIDs nonselectively inhibit COX-1 and COX-2 and have antipyretic, anti-inflammatory, and analgesic properties. Unlike aspirin, NSAIDs' effects on platelet inhibition are reversible.

Probably the most important clinical aspect of NSAID pharmacokinetics and pharmacodynamics is that there is considerable individual variability in response, the mechanism of which is not well known. Regardless, if one NSAID does not produce a therapeutic response, trying a different one may elicit the desired response.

Clinical Indications

Clinical indications for NSAIDs are the same as for use of aspirin, with a few exceptions. Because NSAIDs do not have a permanent effect on platelet aggregation, they are not used for clotting prophylaxis or heart health.

Dosing

Doses and clinical considerations of commonly prescribed NSAIDS are listed in Table 12-2. For those persons taking ibuprofen (Advil), 2400 mg per day is therapeutically equivalent to 4 g of aspirin per day. It is important to remember that lower doses can be used for treatment of pain, but higher doses are needed to treat inflammation. In addition, it takes 2 to 4 weeks of regular use to realize the full anti-inflammatory benefit. NSAIDs are more effective than a daily 4-g dose of acetaminophen for treatment of osteoarthritis and rheumatoid arthritis.[53,54]

Side Effects/Adverse Effects

NSAIDs are associated with multiple adverse/side effects (Table 12-5).[55] The most common NSAID-related toxicities are gastrointestinal ulceration and nephrotoxicity.

Table 12-5 Adverse Effects of Nonsteroidal Anti-inflammatory Drugs

System	Nonselective NSAIDs	Selective NSAIDs	Adverse Effects	Clinical Considerations
Cardiovascular	Yes	Yes	Selective NSAIDs increase the risk for myocardial infarction and cardiovascular events. NSAIDs may exacerbate existing heart failure and hypertension.	Contraindicated for persons recovering from coronary bypass surgery. Ibuprofen (Advil) and celecoxib (Celebrex) at high doses are proposed to have the highest risk for myocardial infarction among the common NSAIDs.
Central nervous system	Yes	Yes	Aseptic meningitis, psychosis, cognitive dysfunction. ASA can cause tinnitus.	Psychosis and cognitive dysfunction are most prevalent in the elderly. These effects are associated most closely with use of indomethacin.

Gastrointestinal	Yes	Less than nonselective NSAIDs	Nonselective NSAIDs increase the risk for peptic ulcer and GI hemorrhage.	Risk increases with age, dose, and duration of therapy.
Hepatic	Yes	Yes	Hepatotoxicity is rare but increases if the individual is using other medications concomitantly with NSAIDs. Diclofenac (Voltaren) is reported to cause hepatitis.	Acute liver injury occurs in 3.7/100,000 NSAID users. Sulindac (Clinoril) increases this risk to 27/100,000 NSAID users. Some authors recommend checking liver function tests 8 weeks after starting chronic therapy.
Hematologic	Yes	No	Nonselective NSAIDS have a reversible effect on platelet aggregation. Chronic aspirin therapy slightly increases the risk for hemorrhagic stroke.	Concomitant use of NSAIDs and aspirin negates the effect of aspirin on platelet aggregation.
Renal	Yes	Yes	Nonselective and COX-2 selective NSAIDs can cause acute renal failure, but the risk is higher with use of COX-2 selective NSAIDs. Interstitial nephritis and nephrotic syndrome are more likely with nonselective NSAIDs.	Risk is highest in first 30 days of therapy. COX-2 selective NSAIDs should be avoided in persons with renal compromise.
Pulmonary	Yes	No	Bronchospasm in persons with aspirin hypersensitivity.	ASA and NSAIDs have some cross-reactivity.
Skin reactions	Yes	Yes	Stevens-Johnson syndrome and toxic epidermal necrolysis.	Rare: reported in approximately 1/100,000 persons using NSAIDs.
Allergic reaction	Yes	Yes	Selective NSAIDs have a sulfa group and may induce allergic reactions in persons who are allergic to sulfa drugs. Case reports exist but it does not appear to be common.	Use selective NSAIDs cautiously in persons who are allergic to sulfa drugs.

Abbreviations: ASA = aspirin; COX = cyclooxygenase; GI = gastrointestinal; NSAIDs = nonsteroidal anti-inflammatory drugs.

Gastrointestinal Complications

Although most NSAIDs have minimal side effects following the short-term recommended use, the most common side effect by far is gastrointestinal distress. Approximately 10% of persons using one of these drugs will discontinue the drug secondary to these symptoms.[55] In addition, asymptomatic ulcers and gastrointestinal mucosal erosion will occur in 5% to 20% of users, and 1% to 2% will experience peptic ulcer, gastrointestinal hemorrhage, or perforation. The mortality of these serious gastrointestinal disorders is 10% to 15%.[55] Although most persons who develop a serious GI adverse event while taking a nonselective NSAID are asymptomatic prior to the event, five specific risk factors have been identified (Table 12-6).[56,57]

Ibuprofen (Advil) and celecoxib (Celebrex) are associated with the lowest relative risk of gastrointestinal events when compared to other NSAIDs. Aspirin, naproxen (Naprosyn), ketoprofen (Orudis), meloxicam (Mobic), and indomethacin (Indocin) are associated with intermediate risk. The NSAIDs with the highest relative risk include piroxicam (Arantil, Feldene) and ketorolac (Toradol).[58]

Prevention and Treatment of Gastrointestinal Ulcers

Primary and secondary prevention and/or treatment of NSAID-induced ulcers is an important component of therapy. Choices include use of COX-2 selective NSAIDs instead of a nonselective NSAID as well as the addition of medications that affect the acid levels in the gastrointestinal tract, which include mucosal barrier agents

Table 12-6 Risk Factors for Upper Gastrointestinal Complications Following NSAID Use

Known Risk Factors
Anticoagulation medications
Corticosteroids
NSAID use: • High doses of NSAIDs (≥ 2 times normal dose) • Use of multiple NSAIDs • Low doses of aspirin and concomitant NSAID use
Older age (≥ 65 years)
Prior clinical event (ulcer, hemorrhage)
Serious systemic disorder
Possible Risk Factors
Alcohol consumption
Cigarette smoking
Infection with *Helicobacter pylori*

Sources: Data from Agency for Health Care Research and Quality. Choosing non-opioid analgesics for osteoarthritis: clinicians guide. http://www.effectivehealthcare.ahrq.gov/repFiles/Osteoarthritis_Clinician_Guide.pdf[57]; Laine L. GI risk and risk factors of NSAIDs. *J Cardiovasc Pharmacol.* 2006;47(suppl 1):S60-S66[56]; Vonkeman HE, van de Laar MAFJ. Nonsteroidal anti-inflammatory drugs: adverse effects and their prevention. *Semin Arthritis Rheum.* 2010;39(4):294-312.[55]

(e.g., sucralfate), proton pump inhibitors (PPIs; e.g., omeprazole [Prilosec]), histamine receptor antagonists (H_2RAs; famotidine [Pepcid]), and misoprostol (Cytotec).

Mucosal barrier agents and histamine receptor antagonists are not sufficiently effective and are not recommended for prevention or treatment of GI ulcers induced by NSAIDs.[59] Misoprostol reduces the incidence of ulcers by approximately 40%, but must be taken several times per day and has unpleasant side effects such as diarrhea.[59,60] Therefore, proton pump inhibitors are the drugs of choice for both primary prevention and secondary prevention in persons who have experienced a previous NSAID-induced ulcer.[59,60] Proton pump inhibitors are not effective in preventing the less common lower GI events.

PPIs are preferred for persons who have additional risk factors for ulcers. Persons at high risk for gastrointestinal hemorrhage (e.g., individuals with a history of NSAID-induced ulcer) should be offered either a COX-2 selective NSAID if they are not at risk for myocardial infarction or a nonselective NSAID and PPI. When nonselective NSAIDs are combined with daily, low-dose aspirin for cardiovascular protection, the NSAID can diminish the antiplatelet effect of aspirin by competitively occupying the COX-2 binding site on the platelet, thereby negating the therapeutic effect of aspirin.

Nephrotoxicity

Nephrotoxicity may occur secondary to the vasoconstrictive action of NSAIDs. Constriction of renal arterioles leads to reversible renal ischemia and a diminished glomerular filtration rate. These effects are exacerbated in individuals with fluid deficits or preexisting renal compromise, particularly in persons older than 65 years.

Acute tubulointerstitial nephritis secondary to NSAID therapy is twice as likely to occur in women as in men. Concomitant use of other nephrotoxic substances increases this risk. Nephritis presents with hematuria, pyuria, proteinuria, and elevated serum creatinine levels. Nephritis and renal ischemia typically resolve spontaneously following discontinuation of the drug; however, infrequently persistent changes occur, leading to renal failure.

Cardiotoxic Effects

Cardiotoxic effects associated with NSAIDs—in particular with COX-2 inhibitors—include mild elevations in blood pressure, increased risk of acute myocardial infarction, and stroke. Women who take NSAIDs on a regular basis have an increased risk of hypertension. An analysis of the Nurses' Health Study found a relative risk of 1.78 (95% confidence interval [CI], 1.21–2.61) among older women and 1.60 (95% CI, 1.1–2.32) among younger women for developing incident hypertension if taking NSAIDs daily for pain other than headache.[61,62] Research indicates that the cardiac risk appears to increase when the recommended NSAID dose is exceeded or the drug is used for long-term therapy. Based on the individual's age and cardiac risk profile, the risk of acute myocardial infarction or stroke may offset the GI benefit of COX-2 inhibitors.

Drug–Drug Interactions

Because most NSAIDs are tightly bound to plasma proteins, they have a potential to interact with many drugs. Coadministration of aspirin and some NSAIDs may reduce the cardioprotective effects of aspirin because of competition for binding sites on the COX enzyme.[62,63] Significant drug interactions associated with nonselective NSAIDs are summarized in Table 12-4.

Special Populations: Pregnancy, Lactation, and the Elderly

NSAIDs are not generally recommended for use in pregnancy. Naproxen (e.g., Naprosyn, Aleve) and ibuprofen (Advil) should not be used after 36 weeks' gestation to avoid increased blood loss during parturition and to avoid premature closure of the ductus arteriosus in the fetus.[52] Some research suggests that NSAIDs may also decrease the amount of amniotic fluid. NSAIDs are excreted in breast milk; however, because they are highly protein bound, very little actually transfers into breast milk.[64] Although the American Academy of Pediatrics considers use of nonselective NSAIDs to be compatible with lactation,[53] some authors recommend caution when exposing NSAIDs to newborns because they competitively displace bilirubin from plasma proteins and can increase the incidence of newborn jaundice.[64]

Elderly women are more susceptible to the adverse effects of gastrointestinal bleeding, hypertension, and renal function compromise if taking NSAIDs.[58] Persons older than 65 years who are considering long-term NSAID therapy should be evaluated for *H. pylori* infection, and that infection should be treated prior to initiation of NSAIDs if it is present. In general, if NSAIDs are needed, COX-2 selective NSAIDs are recommended secondary to older women's decreased risk of GI complications. Because the elderly often experience persistent pain and practice polypharmacy, the potential for significant drug–drug or drug–herb interactions should be carefully evaluated when considering routine NSAID therapy for them.

Selective NSAIDs

Celecoxib (Celebrex) is the only selective COX-2 inhibitor currently available in the United States. Rofecoxib (Vioxx) was voluntarily withdrawn from the market following research studies that demonstrated an increased risk of myocardial infarction among individuals using this drug (Box 12-1). Valdecoxib (Bextra) was also voluntarily withdrawn from the market for similar concerns.[65,66]

Mechanism of Action

Celecoxib selectively inhibits COX-2, thereby mitigating inflammation and pain. Because it has minimal action on COX-1, celecoxib does not have significant effects on gastric irritation, renal function, or platelet aggregation. COX-2 selective NSAIDs are rapidly absorbed from the gastrointestinal tract. Taking NSAIDs with food delays this absorption but does not affect peak concentration. Like the nonselective NSAIDs, selective NSAIDs are extensively protein bound and are metabolized in the liver and excreted through the kidneys.

Clinical Indications

Celecoxib is indicated for relief of signs and symptoms of osteoarthritis, rheumatoid arthritis in adults, and juvenile rheumatoid arthritis in children 2 years or older, and for treatment of ankylosing spondylitis, primary dysmenorrhea, and acute pain.

Adverse Effects

Adverse effects of COX-2 selective NSAIDs are listed in Table 12-5. Despite early hopes that celecoxib might have all the advantages of COX-2 inhibition without increased gastrointestinal toxicity, such promises have not been clearly demonstrated. The Celecoxib Arthritis Safety Study (CLASS) identified a reduced incidence of gastric ulceration with short-term use (less than 6 months).[67] However, the same study did not show any statistically significant reduction of gastric ulceration when celecoxib was compared with long-term use of traditional NSAIDs (more than 12 months).[67] Subsequent studies have yielded mixed results. At this time, then, the benefits of celecoxib in preventing gastrointestinal adverse effects remain unclear, especially with long-term use.

The most serious adverse effects of COX-2 inhibitors are cardiovascular in nature. In randomized clinical trials (RCTs), persons taking high doses of celecoxib (400–800 mg per day) have demonstrated an increased risk of both fatal and nonfatal myocardial infarctions (0.52% in persons taking a placebo versus 0.8% in persons taking

Box 12-1 The Story of Vioxx

The FDA approved rofecoxib (Vioxx) for relief of arthritis symptoms in 1999 based on data from trials of 3 to 6 months' duration. In 2000, the Vioxx Gastrointestinal Outcomes Research (VIGOR) study, which compared rofecoxib with naproxen (Aleve), indicated an increased risk for myocardial infarction in individuals taking 50 mg of rofecoxib.[65] Merck & Co. voluntarily withdrew rofecoxib, which had been marketed as an arthritis medication, from the market on September 30, 2004.

The largest prescription drug withdrawal in history, this move precipitated a public outcry against the FDA's drug approval and monitoring process. Merck claimed that the data were flawed. Although the FDA reviewed the data, it chose not to act but to await further investigation.

The Adenomatous Polyp Prevention on Vioxx (APPROVe) trial was the final blow for rofecoxib.[66] Even after excluding those individuals with a history of cardiovascular disease from the trial, the risk of myocardial infarction among persons taking rofecoxib was almost twice that among those persons taking a placebo. The study was halted early, and at that point, Merck voluntarily withdrew rofecoxib from the market.

The proposed mechanism by which rofecoxib increases the risk of myocardial infarction is through inhibition of COX-2, which mediates prostaglandin I_2 production. Prostaglandin I_2 inhibits platelet aggregation, causes vasodilation, and prevents vascular smooth muscle cell proliferation.

Although this mechanism is thought to be a class action, celecoxib (Celebrex) is less COX-2 specific than either rofecoxib or valdecoxib (Bextra) and may drive the mechanism less toward thrombosis. In April 2005, the FDA requested Pfizer to withdraw valdecoxib from the market. Currently, celecoxib is the only selective COX-2 inhibitor marketed in the United States.

celecoxib).[68] However, recent epidemiologic studies have not found any increased risk of cardiovascular complications in persons who take celecoxib.[69] Although a few studies have not found that celecoxib induces adverse cardiovascular effects, the overall body of evidence published to date suggests this drug is associated with an increased risk; thus it is recommended that celecoxib be given at the lowest therapeutic dose and used cautiously in those persons with increased risks for cardiovascular or renal disease.

Drug–Drug Interactions

Like first-generation NSAIDs, celecoxib may displace other protein-bound drugs, leading to adverse reactions. Unlike nonselective COX inhibitors, it does not interfere with the antiplatelet effect of aspirin, because mature human platelets lack COX-2.[70] Drug–drug interactions associated with celecoxib are listed in Table 12-4.

Contraindications

Celecoxib is contraindicated for those persons with known hypersensitivity to this medication. It should not be given to individuals who are allergic to sulfonamides or those who have experienced asthma or urticarial or allergic reactions to aspirin or other NSAIDs. In addition, celecoxib should not be used for analgesia by persons undergoing coronary artery bypass surgery, or in those with gastrointestinal bleeding.

Special Populations: Pregnancy, Lactation, and the Elderly

Celecoxib can be used by women during pregnancy prior to 30 weeks' gestation, but is contraindicated for the reminder of the pregnancy. Like other NSAIDs, this agent is contraindicated in the third trimester of pregnancy because it may promote premature closure of the ductus arteriosus.

Celecoxib is transferred into human milk, but its levels are so low that harm to the nursing child is unlikely.[71] The American Academy of Pediatrics does not make any recommendations regarding the use of celecoxib during lactation.

Celecoxib peak plasma concentrations are approximately 40% higher in the elderly than in younger individuals. For this reason, and because of the increased incidence of underlying comorbidities, the risk of significant cardiovascular and gastrointestinal events and acute renal failure is increased when celecoxib is used by persons older than 65 years.

Acetaminophen

Acetaminophen (Tylenol) is similar to aspirin and other NSAIDs in that it has both antipyretic and analgesic properties. However, acetaminophen has no clinically significant anti-inflammatory properties, nor does it suppress platelet aggregation, reduce renal blood flow, or increase gastric irritation.

Mechanism of Action

Acetaminophen is a selective inhibitor of prostaglandin synthesis. Unlike aspirin and other NSAIDs that inhibit prostaglandin both in the central nervous system and the periphery, acetaminophen's effects primarily are found in the central nervous system, with only limited effects occurring at peripheral sites.

Pharmacokinetics

Acetaminophen is readily absorbed following oral dosing and is widely distributed. Metabolism takes place in the liver by two different pathways. At therapeutic doses, most acetaminophen is conjugated with glucuronic acid and other liver enzymes into nontoxic metabolites and excreted through the kidney. Small amounts are converted into toxic metabolites by a secondary pathway, involving the CYP450 system. Relatively small amounts of this toxic metabolite can be further converted by glutathione into nontoxic forms for excretion.

When liver function is impaired or overdose occurs, the primary metabolic pathway is overwhelmed and acetaminophen must be metabolized via the secondary system. (For more detailed explanation of acetaminophen hepatotoxicity, see the *Drug Toxicity* chapter.) Alcohol or large amounts of the drug deplete glutathione, preventing the further metabolism of the toxic metabolites, and liver damage results.

Clinical Indications

Acetaminophen is indicated for relief of mild to moderate pain and reduction of fever. It is safe for use in children and adolescents suspected of having influenza or varicella because it has never been linked to Reye's syndrome. Acetaminophen is the preferred analgesic for persons with gastric ulceration or aspirin hypersensitivity.

Side Effects/Adverse Effects

Adverse effects of acetaminophen are rare at therapeutic doses. In contrast, routine use of acetaminophen at doses of 5 g or more per day has been associated with an increased risk for hypertension in women. A causal relationship between acetaminophen and hypertension has not been clearly established, nor is the mechanism of action whereby acetaminophen might cause elevations in blood pressure known.

Acetaminophen and Hepatotoxicity

Acetaminophen overdose can cause severe and sometimes fatal hepatotoxicity. This drug is the leading cause of liver injury in the United States because it is relatively easy to take an overdose of acetaminophen (Box 12-2). The minimum toxic single dose for healthy adults is between 7.5 g and 10 g, but liver toxicity can occur at normal therapeutic doses in persons who consume alcohol in large amounts or regularly.

Over the last few decades, the FDA has issued several recommendations regarding the hepatotoxicity risk associated with acetaminophen. Any products containing acetaminophen must carry an alcohol warning on their label that cautions users that they are high risk for liver disease if they are using acetaminophen and if they drink more than three alcoholic drinks per day.

Many over-the-counter (OTC) combination products contain acetaminophen; however, the consumer may not be aware that acetaminophen is in the medication, so overdose can occur inadvertently. The FDA has recommended that OTC combination products stop using the abbreviation APAP to designate the presence of acetaminophen on the product label because most consumers do not know that "APAP" is an acronym for "acetaminophen." This step remains voluntary, however, and has not been widely implemented.

In 2009, the FDA urged that all OTC analgesic preparations prominently display the names of the ingredients. Also in 2009, an FDA advisory committee recommended the following changes for acetaminophen preparations: (1) decrease the maximum total daily dosage from 4 g to 3250 mg; (2) decrease the maximum single dose to 650 mg or less (currently, OTC formulations of 500 mg per tablet allow a single dose to be 1000 mg if the person takes two tablets); and (3) eliminate some combination products, such as TheraFlu. Commercial labeling of acetaminophen-containing products now reflects these recommendations, although formulations that have more than 325 mg per tablet are still available because some pharmaceutical companies have resisted changing their formulations.

In 2014, the FDA recommended that combination analgesics that contain acetaminophen reduce the acetaminophen dose to no more than 325 mg per tablet. This change was largely designed to prevent acetaminophen overdose in persons taking pain medications that combine acetaminophen with an opioid such as hydrocodone. Manufacturers of several popular pain medications such as Vicodin have decreased the acetaminophen

Box 12-2 Don't Underestimate That Tablet of Tylenol: A Therapeutic Misadventure

JT, a frequent social drinker, spent an afternoon on the beach partying with friends. The next morning she had a headache, which she thought came from being in the sun too long. JT took four extra-strength tablets (2 g) of acetaminophen (Tylenol), forgot to eat breakfast, and went to work. About 72 hours later, she developed acute liver failure. How did this happen?

Approximately 90% of acetaminophen is metabolized into sulfate and glucuronide metabolites that are nontoxic and eliminated via the kidney. However, approximately 4% to 6% of acetaminophen is metabolized via CYP2E1 into a toxic metabolite NAPQI, which, under normal circumstances, is rapidly altered by glutathione into the same nontoxic water-soluble metabolite produced via the primary metabolic system.

Alcohol is a substrate for CYPE1 and increases the amount of CYPE1 twofold in persons who drink heavily. Alcohol also inhibits the production of glutathione. Thus, the drinks JT had the day before on the beach created more CYP2E1 and depleted the enzyme responsible for converting acetaminophen to a nontoxic metabolite. The acetaminophen she ingested was metabolized preferentially by CYPE1, which created sufficient NAPQI to produce liver failure, even though her total dose was below the usual toxic dose.

This relationship between chronic alcohol use and liver toxicity at high therapeutic doses is controversial. However, in 1998, the FDA issued a warning that persons who drink more than three glasses of alcohol per day should consult their healthcare provider before using acetaminophen.

Box 12-3 Information About Acetaminophen for Healthcare Providers

The maximum amount of acetaminophen in a prescription tablet, capsule, or other dosage unit is now reduced to 325 mg, although some individuals may still have acetaminophen products in their medicine cabinets that contain 500 mg/tablet. This reduction does not apply to over-the-counter products, although some manufacturers have voluntarily reduced the acetaminophen dose in some products. The total number of tablets or capsules that may be prescribed and the time intervals at which they may be prescribed will not change as a result of the smaller amount of acetaminophen. For example, suppose a product previously contained 500 mg of acetaminophen with an opioid and was prescribed as 1 to 2 tablets every 4 to 6 hours; once reformulated to contain 325 mg of acetaminophen, this product may continue to use the same dosing instructions as before the change.

Instructions for consumers should include the following:

- Do not exceed the acetaminophen maximum total daily dose (4 g/day).
- Read all labels of prescription and over-the-counter products to identify acetaminophen-containing products. The label may describe acetaminophen as APAP, AC, Acetam, Acetaminoph, or Acetamin.
- Do not take more than one product containing acetaminophen at a time.
- Do not to drink alcohol while taking acetaminophen-containing medications, as concomitant use of alcohol increases the risk of liver toxicity.
- Stop any acetaminophen-containing product immediately if any of the following symptoms appear: rash, swelling of the face, mouth, or throat, difficulty breathing, or itching.

dose per tablet in response to this recommendation. A summary of steps that healthcare providers can take to determine the total dose of acetaminophen is presented in Box 12-3.

The mechanism of action of acetaminophen toxicity is well known. As the normal pathway for acetaminophen metabolism becomes saturated, excess acetaminophen is metabolized through CYP450 enzymatic reactions that result in the formation of toxic metabolites. The clinical presentation occurs in three distinct stages that develop rapidly from the presenting gastroenteritis (24 hours), to subclinical hepatotoxicity (24 to 72 hours), to fulminant hepatic failure (72 to 96 hours).

Suspected or confirmed acetaminophen overdose is treated with acetylcysteine (Acetadote, Mucomyst), which is most effective when administered within 8 hours of overdose. Acetylcysteine prevents the toxic metabolite *N*-acetyl-*p*-benzoquinoneimine from binding to hepatocytes, thereby preventing the development of hepatotoxicity. Acetylcysteine may be administered orally or intravenously and has been shown to transfer across the placenta to the fetus.

Drug–Drug Interactions

Alcohol is the source of the most significant drug interaction associated with acetaminophen (Table 12-7). In turn,

Table 12-7 Selected Drug–Drug Interactions Associated with Acetaminophen[a]

Elevated Risk of Hepatotoxicity	**Decreased Analgesic Effect of Acetaminophen**	**Decreased Absorption of Acetaminophen**
Alcohol	Barbiturates	Cholestyramine (Questran)[b]
Barbiturates	Carbamazepine (Tegretol)	Food intake
Carbamazepine (Tegretol)	Hydantoins (Dilantin)	St. John's wort
Cholestyramine (Questran)	Isoniazid (INH)	
Hydantoins (Dilantin)	Rifampin (Rifadin)	
Isoniazid (INH)	Sulfinpyrazone (Anturane)	
Elevated Risk of Nephrotoxicity	**Increased Serum Acetaminophen Levels**	**Elevated International Normalized Ratio**
Rifampin (Rifadin)	Diflunisal (Dolobid)	Oral anticoagulants
Sulfinpyrazone (Anturane)		

[a] This table is not comprehensive as new information is being generated on a regular basis.
[b] Separate dosing by more than 1 hour.

the FDA now requires alcohol warnings on the labels of all acetaminophen products.[72] Concurrent use of acetaminophen and drugs that induce CYP450 enzymes such as rifampin (Rimactane), barbiturates, carbamazepine (Tegretol), and sulfinpyrazone (Anturane) also increases the risk of hepatotoxicity and may decrease the effectiveness of acetaminophen.

Routine use of acetaminophen can increase the risk of bleeding in those persons taking warfarin (Coumadin). Although the mechanism underlying this interaction is unknown, it has been suggested that acetaminophen may be related to genetic polymorphism or alterations in the metabolism of warfarin's *R*- or *S*-enantiomers.[73] Episodic use of acetaminophen by individuals taking warfarin does not increase the International Normalized Ratio, a test used to monitor the anticoagulant effects of warfarin. However, persons taking warfarin who also use acetaminophen 2 g per day for 3 consecutive days should have their anticoagulant status monitored.[74] Acetaminophen remains the drug of choice for analgesic and antipyretic control for these persons.

Contraindications

Acetaminophen should be avoided by persons with impaired liver function or acetaminophen hypersensitivity. This drug can theoretically cause hemolytic anemia in persons with known glucose-6-phosphate dehydrogenase (G6PD) deficiency. Although some case reports have linked acetaminophen to hemolytic anemia in persons with G6PD deficiency, other studies suggest acetaminophen is safe in this population provided these individuals do not exceed recommended therapeutic doses.[75]

Special Populations: Pregnancy, Lactation, and the Elderly

Acetaminophen crosses the placenta. Epidemiologic studies have found use of this drug during pregnancy is associated with cryptorchidism and an increased risk for asthma in offspring.[76–79] Additionally, acetaminophen use during pregnancy has been linked with increased frequency of the child being diagnosed with hyperkinetic disorder, being prescribed medication for attention-deficit/hyperactivity disorder (ADHD), or exhibiting ADHD-like behaviors.[80] However, other studies have not found acetaminophen to be linked to any congenital anomalies. Because all studies conducted to date have been retrospective analyses, causation has not yet been proven. Thus, at this time, acetaminophen is considered safe for short-term use by pregnant women.

Acetaminophen is excreted in breast milk, but no adverse effects among nursing infants have been reported. The American Academy of Pediatrics considers acetaminophen compatible with breastfeeding.[53]

Elderly women may be at increased risk for acetaminophen toxicity because of frequently undiagnosed subclinical hepatic insufficiency. When used at low doses with increased dosing frequencies, however, acetaminophen is safer than other drugs typically used for persistent pain.

Opioid Analgesics

Opioid refers to any natural or synthetic drug with actions similar to that of morphine. **Opiate** refers only to those opioids that contain compounds found in opium. *Narcotic* is a less precise term that has been used to refer to any drug that causes central nervous system depression or has a potential for causing physical dependency, and generally is a term associated with illegal use rather than pharmacologic use.

The Controlled Substances Act of 1970 created five schedule classifications for drugs or other substances that have significant potential for addiction and abuse. Opioids are assigned to a particular schedule based on their potential for abuse, their accepted medical use, and the potential for development of physical and/or psychological dependence on the drug. Prescriptive authority to prescribe opioids is regulated by the states and discussed in more detail in the *Modern Pharmacology* chapter.

Mechanism of Action of Opioids

The three main opioid receptors are labeled as mu, kappa, and delta.[81] All are G-protein–coupled receptors embedded in the plasma membrane of neurons.

- Mu receptors are found primarily in the central nervous system's pain-modulating areas, the dorsal horn of the spinal cord, and the intestinal tract. Activation of mu receptors results in analgesia, euphoria, and respiratory depression. Morphine is the prototypical mu receptor agonist.
- Kappa receptors are concentrated in the cerebral cortex of the brain, the substantia gelatinosa of the dorsal horn of the spinal cord, and the uterus. Activation of kappa receptors results in analgesia and sedation.
- Delta receptors are located in the limbic area of the brain and in the spinal cord. Delta receptors are thought to play a part in euphoria and may have a role in analgesia at the level of the spinal cord.

Table 12-8 Stimulation of Opioid Receptors

Drug: Generic (Brand)	Mu (μ)	Kappa (κ)	Delta (δ)
Effect	Analgesia, sedation, vomiting, respiratory depression, pruritus, constipation, anorexia, urinary retention, euphoria, physical dependence	Analgesia, sedation, dyspnea, respiratory depression, miosis, euphoria, dysphoria, psychomimetic effects	Analgesia, sedation, release of growth hormone
Pure Agonists			
Codeine	+		+
Fentanyl (Duragesic, Sublimaze)	+++		
Hydrocodone (Vicodin, Vicoprofen, Lortab, Lorcet, Zohydro ER)	+		
Hydromorphone (Dilaudid)	+++		
Levorphanol (Levo-Dromoran)	+++		
Meperidine (Demerol)	+++		
Methadone (Dolophine)	+++		
Morphine	+++	+	
Oxycodone (Percocet, OxyContin, Roxicodone)	+	++	
Oxymorphone (Opana, Numorphan)	+++		
Sufentanil (Sufenta)	+++	+	+
Agonist–Antagonists			
Butorphanol (Stadol)	±	+++	
Nalbuphine (Nubain)	– –	++	
Partial Agonists			
Buprenorphine (Buprenex, Suboxone)	±	– –	– –
Antagonists			
Nalmefene (Revex)	– – –	– –	–
Naltrexone (ReVia)	– – –	– –	–
Naloxone (Narcan)	– – –	– –	–

Abbreviations: +++ = strong agonist; ++ = moderate agonist; + = weak agonist; ± = partial agonist; – = antagonist.

The responses occurring with opioid receptor activation are summarized in Table 12-8.

All drugs have intrinsic affinity, a measure of the strength of the interaction between the drug and receptor, and effectiveness, the effect the drug has on the receptor. In the case of opioids, agonists have both strong affinity and effectiveness, partial agonists have affinity but elicit weak effectiveness, and antagonists have affinity but do not elicit any effectiveness. The pharmacologic effects of opioids relate to their differing degrees of affinity and effectiveness at the mu, kappa, and delta opioid receptors.

Gender Differences in Opioid Response

The response to opioids varies by gender. When the drugs are administered via patient-controlled analgesia (PCA) device, women use less opioid medications compared to men. When the drugs are administered by a healthcare provider, men use less opioid medications compared to women. Experimental models examining the gender differences in opioid response have not found any difference, however. Thus, the observed differences may be related to psychosocial, hormone, and neurobiologic variations between the genders.[12,13,82]

Classification of Opioids

Opioids are either hydrophilic or lipophilic. They can also be classified by their chemical origin (natural, semisynthetic, or synthetic), by their potency (strong, moderate, weak), or by their action on different types of receptors (agonist, partial agonist, agonist–antagonist, pure antagonist) (Table 12-9).

Opioid Agonists

Opioid agonists produce analgesia by binding to opioid receptors in the central nervous system, spinal cord, and gastrointestinal tract. Pure mu agonists are generally

Table 12-9 Classification of Opioids

	Drug: Generic (Brand)	Drug: Generic (Brand)	Drug: Generic (Brand)	Drug: Generic (Brand)
Effect on receptor	***Agonists*** Alfentanil (Alfenta), fentanyl (Duragesic, Sublimaze), morphine, sufentanil (Sufenta)	***Partial Agonists*** Buprenorphine (Buprenex, Suboxone)	***Agonist–Antagonists*** Butorphanol (Stadol), nalbuphine (Nubain), pentazocine (Talwin)	***Antagonists*** Naloxone (Narcan), nalmefene (Revex), naltrexone (ReVia, Vivitrol)
Chemical origin	***Natural*** Codeine, morphine	***Semisynthetic*** Buprenorphine (Buprenex), hydromorphone (Dilaudid), hydrocodone (Vicodin), oxycodone (OxyContin, Percocet), oxymorphone (Numorphan)	***Synthetic: Phenylpiperidines*** Fentanyl (Duragesic, Sublimaze), meperidine (Demerol), sufentanil (Sufenta)	***Synthetic: Pseudopiperidines*** Methadone (Dolophine)
Potency	***Strong*** Alfentanil (Alfenta), fentanyl (Duragesic, Sublimaze), morphine, sufentanil (Sufenta)	***Intermediate*** Butorphanol (Stadol), nalbuphine (Nubain), pentazocine (Talwin)	***Weak*** Codeine	

preferred for the management of moderate to severe pain. Not only are they available in a variety of formulations, but pure mu opioid agonists also have no analgesic ceiling. This characteristic makes them particularly useful for treatment of chronic pain, because doses may be increased indefinitely as long as adverse effects are avoided. An opioid with high intrinsic ability, such as morphine, achieves its maximal pharmacologic effects with relatively low receptor occupancy. By comparison, codeine, a weak mu agonist, has less analgesic potency.

Pharmacokinetics of Opioid Agonists

Most opioids are easily absorbed from the gastrointestinal tract, undergoing variable but significant hepatic first-pass effects. Thus, opioids administered orally typically require significantly larger doses than other forms for **equianalgesic** effects. Opioids are poorly protein bound. Most of these agents are metabolized by the CYP2D6 and CYP34A enzymes and excreted renally. Genetic variations and impaired hepatic or renal function affect metabolism; consequently, appropriate dosing must be individualized. For example, some persons genetically have a duplication of CYP2D6, which makes them ultra-metabolizers of codeine. Because codeine is a prodrug and its metabolite is the active drug morphine, ultra-rapid metabolism can result in plasma levels of morphine that are 50% higher than expected, causing an exaggerated analgesic and potentially toxic effect.[83]

Lipid solubility varies widely among opioids and accounts for the variations in these drugs' onset and duration of action. Morphine has relatively low lipid solubility, so it has a slow onset and prolonged duration of action relative to more lipid-soluble drugs such as fentanyl. Lipophilic opioids are more easily administered through transdermal and buccal routes.

Many opioids have active metabolites that affect the pharmacodynamic response with regard to both analgesic effects and adverse effects. Table 12-10 summarizes the pharmacokinetics of commonly used opioids.

Table 12-10 Pharmacokinetics of Opioids

Drug: Generic (Brand)	Bioavailability	Time to Peak Effect	Onset of Action	Half-Life	Duration of Action	Clinical Considerations
Pure Agonists						
Codeine	80%	0.5–1 hour	10–30 minutes	2–4 hours	4–6 hours	Approximately 10% is metabolized to morphine; slow metabolizers will have poor pain control
Fentanyl (Duragesic)	NA	IV/SQ: < 10 minutes	7–12 minutes	3–12 hours	1–2 hours	Fentanyl is highly lipid soluble; risk of delayed respiratory depression is less than that of morphine

(continues)

Table 12-10 Pharmacokinetics of Opioids (*continued*)

Drug: Generic (Brand)	Bioavailability	Time to Peak Effect	Onset of Action	Half-Life	Duration of Action	Clinical Considerations
Fentanyl (Duragesic) transdermal	92%	12–24 hours	NA	3–12 hours	72 hours	
Fentanyl (Duragesic) transmucosal	50%	15–30 minutes	7–12 hours	3–12 hours	1–2 hours	
Hydrocodone (Vicodin)	Unknown	0.5–1 hour	10–30 minutes	2–4 hours	3–6 hours	Available only in combination with acetylsalicylic acid or acetaminophen
Hydromorphone (Dilaudid)	24%	Oral: 1–2 hours IM/IV: 0.5–1 hour	30–45 minutes	2–3 hours	Oral: 3–6 hours IM/IV: 3–4 hours	Preferred for individuals with renal impairment
Levorphanol (Levo-Dromoran)	20–40%	Oral: 1–2 hours IM/IV: 0.5–1 hour	10–60 minutes	12–15 hours	3–6 hours	Half-life can be as long as 30 hours with repeated dosing, which suggests drug accumulation occurs
Meperidine (Demerol)	50–60%	0.5–1 hour	10–45 minutes	3–4 hours	2–4 hours	Not preferred for long-term use because of increased risk of toxicity from active metabolites
Methadone (Dolophine)	80%	1–2 hours	30–60 minutes	8–59 hours	4–7 hours	May prolong QT interval; use cautiously in persons with heart disease or those on medications that affect QT interval; sedation lasts 24–48 hours
Morphine	20–40%	Oral: 1–2 hours IV: 0.5–1 hour	IV: 3–5 minutes IM: 10–20 minutes	2–3 hours	3–6 hours	Active metabolite (morphine-6 glucuronide) is more potent than the parent drug
Morphine (CR) (Kadian)	20–40%	6–8 hours	120 minutes	2–3 hours	8–12 hours	Administered once or twice daily
Morphine (SR) (MS-Contin)	20–40%	6–8 hours	120 minutes	2–3 hours	12–24 hours	Administered once or twice daily
Oxycodone (various)	60–87%	1–2 hours	15–30 minutes	2–3 hours	3–6 hours	Available as a single entity or in combination with acetaminophen or aspirin
Oxymorphone (Numorphan)	10%	Oral: 1.5–3 hours IM/IV: 0.5–1 hour	3–6 minutes	3–4 hours	Oral: 4–6 hours IM/IV: 3–6 hours	Useful for individuals subject to multiple drug interactions because it does not affect CYP2D6 or CYP34A enzymes

Table 12-11 Equianalgesic Doses of Opioids

Drug: Generic (Brand)	Intravenous (mg)	Oral (mg)
Buprenorphine (Buprenex)	0.3	—
Butorphanol (Stadol)	2	—
Codeine	120	200[a]
Fentanyl (Sublimaze)	0.1	—
Hydrocodone[b] (Vicodin, Vicoprofen, Lortab, Lorcet)	—	20–30[b]
Hydromorphone (Dilaudid)	1.5	7.5
Meperidine (Demerol)	75	300[c]
Methadone (Dolophine)	10	3–5
Morphine	10	30
Nalbuphine (Nubain)	10	—
Oxycodone (Percocet)	—	20
Sufentanil (Sufenta)	0.002	—

Abbreviations: — = not available.

[a] Equianalgesic doses of codeine are not well defined because of the variability in codeine metabolism.

[b] These products contain 5, 7.5, or 10 mg of hydrocodone per tablet with either acetaminophen or aspirin. The equianalgesic doses of hydrocodone are not calculated for combination products because the analgesic efficacy is potentiated by the other drugs present in the combination.

[c] Contraindicated in persons receiving monoamine oxidase inhibitors. The maximum dose is 600 mg/24 hours because toxic metabolites can accumulate and cause seizures.

Dosing Considerations

Opioids are commonly prescribed for moderate to severe pain. These drugs may be administered in a variety of ways, including via the oral, rectal, parenteral, transdermal, buccal, intranasal, and epidural routes. Each route has specific advantages and disadvantages. For instance, most opioids have a high hepatic first-pass effect, requiring larger oral doses to attain equianalgesic effects. Rectal routes tend to have erratic absorption. Parenteral routes produce a more rapid onset of action but may be problematic for persons needing long-term use.

Morphine is the prototype mu opioid agonist and is the standard against which all other opioids are compared for equianalgesic dosing, also referred to as a *morphine equivalent dose* (Table 12-11). When persons are switched from one opioid to another, a conversion table such as Table 12-11 is used to determine the morphine equivalent dose of the new drug. These tables are available in pharmacies and online. The Resources section at the end of this chapter lists online sources and apps that provide opioid conversion tables.

Table 12-12 and Table 12-13 list doses of opioid agonists and opioid agonist–antagonists used to treat moderate to severe pain.[26]

Table 12-12 Opioids for Treating Moderate to Severe Acute or Chronic Pain

Drug: Generic (Brand)	Usual Adult Dose		Clinical Considerations
	Oral	IV or IM	
Codeine	30–60 mg	130 mg	60 mg PO is equivalent to 650 mg of aspirin. Some persons have no analgesic effect from codeine. FDA black box warning states that ultra-rapid metabolism of codeine to morphine may result in respiratory depression in children.
Fentanyl[a] (Duragesic, Sublimaze)	NA	50–100 mcg every 1–2 hours	Not recommended for acute pain except as a component of regional anesthesia. Can be given transdermally every 72 hours for chronic, malignant pain. Also available as intranasal or buccal formulations. Use only in opioid-tolerant individuals.
Hydrocodone[a] (Vicodin)	5–10 mg	NA	10 mg PO is equivalent to 60–80 mg of codeine. Available in combination formulations only with aspirin, ibuprofen, or acetaminophen. FDA black box warning includes CYP3A4 interactions. Concomitant use of hydrocodone and CYP3A4 inhibitors could increase hydrocodone concentrations. Sudden discontinuation of a drug that is a CYP3A4 inducer could also cause increase hydrocodone concentrations and hydrocodone toxicity.
Hydrocodone[a] (Zohydro ER)	10 mg		Extended-release opioid agonist indicated for managing severe chronic pain. FDA black box warning covers CYP3A4 interactions. Concomitant use of hydrocodone and CYP3A4 inhibitors may increase hydrocodone concentrations. Sudden discontinuation of a drug that is a CYP3A4 inducer could increase hydrocodone concentrations and hydrocodone toxicity.
Hydromorphone[a] (Dilaudid)	2–4 mg every 3–4 hours	1.5–4 mg every 3–4 hours	Hydromorphone has the same efficacy as morphine, but is 5 times more potent in oral form. Causes less nausea, vomiting, constipation, and euphoria than morphine. Should be reserved for persons with severe, chronic pain.
Levorphanol[a] (Levo-Dromoran)	2–4 mg	2 mg	Long half-life and risk of accumulation and CNS depression with repeated dosing.
Meperidine[a] (Demerol)	300 mg every 2–3 hours; maximum dose, 600 mg/24 hours	75–100 mg every 3 hours; maximum dose, 600 mg/24 hours	American Pain Society recommends this drug not be used as an analgesic. Although it remains available, its use is becoming rare. Treatment should be limited to 48 hours or less. Accumulation of the active metabolite can cause dysphoria and seizures, especially at amounts totaling more than 600 mg/24 hours.
Morphine[a]	10–30 mg every 3–4 hours[a]	IM: 5–10 mg every 3–4 hours IV: 2.4–5 mg every 3–4 hours	For relief of moderate to severe pain. The 10 mg dose of morphine is the standard against which all opioids are measured for equianalgesic dosing.
Morphine (MS Contin)	15 mg every 8–12 hours	NA	Extended-release formulation of morphine for opioid-tolerant persons. Should not be discontinued abruptly.
Oxycodone[a] (Percocet, OxyContin)	5–15 mg every 4–6 hours	NA	10 mg is equivalent to 90 mg of codeine PO or 10 mg of morphine SQ. Available in combination formulations and in sustained-release tablets. Has a high potential for abuse. Titrate the dose when discontinuing therapy to prevent withdrawal symptoms.
Tramadol (Ultram)	50–100 mg every 4–6 hours		50 mg is equivalent to 60 mg of codeine; 100 mg is equivalent to 60 mg of codeine with 650 mg of aspirin. Tramadol has both opioid and non-opioid properties. It also inhibits reuptake of serotonin and norepinephrine, but does not have the anticholinergic side effects of tricyclic antidepressants. Most useful for moderate pain. Unlike other opioids, it has a limited dose of 400 mg/24 hours.

[a] The warning labels of all opioid agonists carry an FDA black box warning that reviews the risk for life-threatening respiratory depression, addiction and abuse, neonatal withdrawal syndrome, and medication errors.

Source: Data from Miller E. World Health Organization pain ladder. *J Midwifery Womens Health*. 2004;49(6):542-546.[26]

Table 12-13 Opioid Agonist–Antagonists for Treating Moderate Pain of Limited Duration[a]

Drug: Generic (Brand)	Formulations	Usual Initial Adult Dose	Clinical Considerations
Buprenorphine (Buprenex)[a]	Oral formulations combined with naloxone and used to treat opiate addiction	0.3 mg/mL: Initial dose = 1 mL 2 mg sublingual tablet: Initial dose = 2 mg Butrans transdermal patch: 5–20 mcg/hour applied once per week	Approved for management of moderate to severe pain and treatment of opioid dependence. Associated with respiratory depression, which may not be fully reversible with naloxone. FDA black box warning describes life-threatening respiratory depression, addiction, abuse and misuse of transdermal patch, and neonatal opioid withdrawal syndrome for transdermal patch.
Butorphanol (Stadol)[a]	1–2 mg/mL	IV: 0.5–2 mg every 3–4 hours IM: 1–4 mg every 3–4 hours	Also available as a nasal spray.
Nalbuphine (Nubain)[a]	10 or 20 mg/mL	IM: 10 mg every 3–4 hours	Dysphoria is less common than with pentazocine, but more common than with morphine.
Pentazocine (Talwin)[a]	30 mg/mL	30 mg every 3–4 hours	Confusion and dysphoria are frequent side effects, especially in the elderly. Overdose is treatable with naloxone (Narcan) but not by other narcotic antagonists.

[a] Unlike pure opioid agonists, agonist–antagonists have a ceiling effect. Thus, their usefulness for persons with severe or chronic pain is limited. Use of agonist–antagonists may cause opioid withdrawal.

Source: Data from Miller E. World Health Organization pain ladder. *J Midwifery Womens Health*. 2004;49(6):542-546.[26]

The opioid dose required to achieve analgesia varies widely among individuals. Each woman's response to prior exposure to the drug, hepatic and renal function, and route of administration should be considered when determining the specific dose to be prescribed. Conversion to a different route or different drug requires careful consideration of the pharmacodynamics and pharmacokinetics of the preparation.

Side Effects/Adverse Effects

Opioids produce excellent analgesia but have significant adverse effects, including life-threatening respiratory depression, orthostatic hypotension, nausea, constipation, urinary retention, and dysphoria. Most of these adverse effects can be minimized by titrating slowly up to the lowest effective dose. Nevertheless, because these drugs also have a risk for addiction and abuse, they are best prescribed by a practitioner who is well versed in their use.

Nausea and vomiting are the most common side effects in the early stages of therapy and may require coadministration of a phenothiazine for control. Tolerance to these effects develops quickly, however, and routine use of phenothiazines to treat opioid-induced nausea is controversial. Although these medications are commonly used for this purpose, some sources suggest that phenothiazines may have additive sedating and dysphoric side effects without significantly improving pain control. Tolerance for constipation does not develop, and individuals on long-term narcotic therapy may need to be started on a bowel regimen to minimize this effect.

Respiratory depression is the most serious adverse effect of opioids, but it does not frequently occur with therapeutic doses. However, respiratory rate should be monitored for all individuals receiving intravenous opioids, and the drug should be withheld from those persons with respiratory rates less than 12 breaths per minute. Tolerance to respiratory depression develops with long-term use of opiates such as in individuals taking these drugs for chronic pain.

Opioid overdose is characterized by the classic symptom triad of coma, respiratory depression, and pinpoint pupils. Treatment is aimed at ventilatory support and reversal of opioid toxicity by administration of opioid antagonists such as naloxone (Narcan). Because naloxone has a shorter half-life than many opioids, repeat dosing may be necessary. A newer antagonist, nalmefene (Revex), has a longer half-life and may be preferred in some settings.

Table 12-14 summarizes the adverse effects of opioids and treatment/prevention strategies for these effects.[84]

Contraindications

All pure opioid agonists should be used cautiously by persons with impaired pulmonary function, such as those with asthma, emphysema, or other respiratory compromise. Caution should also be exercised when using these drugs to treat persons with head injuries, liver impairment, inflammatory bowel disease, prostatic hypertrophy, preexisting hypotension, or reduced blood volume.

Table 12-14 Adverse/Side Effects of Opioids

Adverse Effect	Clinical Considerations
Biliary colic	Avoid use of morphine for persons with biliary dysfunction. May substitute meperidine.
Constipation	Increase fluids, fiber, and physical activity. Regular use of stimulant laxatives and/or stool softeners may be warranted.
Cough suppression	Codeine and hydrocodone are sometimes administered for this purpose. When cough suppression is undesirable, auscultate lungs for the presence of rales (crackles). Instruct in deep breathing and coughing at regular intervals.
Euphoria/ dysphoria	Euphoria may enhance pain relief but contributes to addiction potential. Dysphoria is most likely to occur when opioids are taken in the absence of pain.
Hormonal	Decreased estrogen and testosterone leads to decreased libido, osteoporosis, and reduced bone mineral density. Can also cause amenorrhea or hypomenorrhea.
Increased intracranial pressure (ICP)	ICP corresponds to respiratory depression. At a normal respiratory rate, ICP remains normal.
Miosis	Keep room lights bright during waking hours to avoid impaired vision.
Neurotoxicity	Maintain hydration and reduce dose.
Nausea and vomiting	Pretreat with an antiemetic when necessary. Having the person lie still may reduce incidence. Although opioids directly stimulate the vomiting center in the brain, some nausea and bloating may be indicative of delayed gastric emptying. Use of a prokinetic drug such as metoclopramide may be helpful.
Orthostatic hypotension	Change positions slowly. Assist with ambulation as necessary.
Pruritus	Opioids cause histamine release.
Respiratory depression	Monitor respiratory rate. Titrate slowly. Avoid simultaneous use of other respiratory depressants. Agonist–antagonists produce less respiratory depression than pure agonists.
Sedation	Administer smaller doses more often. Use drugs with shorter half-lives. Administer small doses of a CNS stimulant in the morning and early afternoon.
Urinary retention	Encourage voiding every 4 hours. Palpate for bladder distention. Catheterization may be required.

Drug–Drug Interactions

The sedation and respiratory depression caused by opioids can be intensified by any drug that causes central nervous system depression. Barbiturates, benzodiazepines, and alcohol are especially problematic, and providers should caution those individuals for whom they prescribe opioids about the dangers of mixing any of these medications.

Morphine and other opioids may exacerbate hypotension in individuals taking antihypertensive drugs or other medications that lower blood pressure. Constipation and urinary retention may also be exacerbated by anticholinergic drugs. Meperidine, dextromethorphan, and tramadol are weak serotonin reuptake inhibitors (SRIs), and are best avoided by persons taking monamine oxidase (MAO) inhibitors. Case reports have described the development of serotonin toxicity in persons concurrently taking MAO inhibitors and SRIs.[85]

Table 12-15 summarizes the major drug–drug interactions associated with opioids.[85,86]

Table 12-15 Significant Drug–Drug Interactions of Opioids

Opioid: Generic (Brand)	Drug: Generic (Brand)	Effect
All	Antihistamines, CNS depressants (barbiturates, alcohol), chlorpromazine (Thorazine)	Potentiates sedation and respiratory depression
All	Warfarin (Coumadin)	Increased warfarin levels
All	Cimetidine (Tagamet)	Inhibits opioid metabolism, resulting in increased CNS toxicity
All	MAO inhibitors	Increased risk of hypertensive crisis
All	Erythromycin	Increased opioid effects
Codeine	Quinidine, bupropion, celecoxib (Celebrex), cimetidine (Tagamet)	Inhibits CYP2D6, thereby inhibiting codeine conversion to morphine, decreasing analgesic effect
Fentanyl (Duragesic)	Ketoconazole (Nizoral)	Increased levels of fentanyl through inhibition of CYP3A4
Meperidine (Demerol)	MAO inhibitors	Hyperpyrexia, serotonin toxicity
	Phenytoin (Dilantin), phenobarbital	Decreased meperidine levels
Methadone (Dolophine)	CYP3A4 inducers: carbamazepine (Tegretol), erythromycin, phenytoin (Dilantin), antiretroviral medications, rifampin (Rifadin)	Increased methadone metabolism; may induce withdrawal
	CYP3A4 inhibitors: fluconazole (Diflucan), SSRIs, TCAs	Increased methadone levels; methadone can also increase TCA levels
	CYP3A4 inhibitors: grapefruit and ciprofloxacin (Cipro)	Prolonged QT syndrome and torsades de pointes
Morphine	Antihypertensives	Increased orthostatic hypotension
	Dexamethasone, rifampin	Induced CYP2D6, thereby increasing plasma levels of morphine

(continues)

Table 12-15 Significant Drug–Drug Interactions of Opioids (*continued*)

Opioid: Generic (Brand)	Drug: Generic (Brand)	Effect
Morphine (*continued*)	Tricyclic antidepressants	Inhibit morphine glucuronidation, which causes increased blood levels of morphine Morphine also causes decreased metabolism of TCAs, which causes toxicity of TCAs
Tramadol (Ultram)	SSRIs and MAO inhibitors	Use with SSRIs causes a decreased analgesic effect and increased risk for serotonin syndrome
	CYP2D6 inhibitors such as quinidine	Tramadol is a CYP2D6 substrate; decreased or abolished analgesic effect of tramadol

Abbreviations: CNS = central nervous system; MAO = monoamine oxidase; SSRIs = selective serotonin reuptake inhibitors; TCA = tricyclic antidepressant.

Morphine

Morphine is primarily metabolized by demethylation and glucuronidation. Because only a very small portion is metabolized via the CYP450 enzymes, drug–drug interactions are extremely rare, and there are no genetic differences in response to this drug.[86]

Codeine

Codeine, a prodrug metabolized to morphine by CYP2D6, is a natural mu opioid agonist. This agent has an analgesic potency of about 50% that of morphine. Because codeine is metabolized by CYP2D6, it is subject to multiple drug–drug interactions; there are a large number of polymorphisms of the CYP2D6 enzyme. As stated previously, persons who are ultra-rapid metabolizers of codeine experience minimal analgesia when using this medication.

The FDA recently released a public health advisory about codeine secondary to a rare effect. A nursing mother who is an ultra-rapid metabolizer took codeine for postpartum pain, and the high levels of morphine in her breast milk resulted in a fatal neonatal respiratory depression. Lactating women, therefore, should use the lowest effective dose of codeine.

Codeine has an unusual emetic response, in that low doses are more emetic than higher doses. The mechanism underlying this response is not clear. At doses greater than 60 mg, the incidence of side effects and adverse effects increases without a concomitant increase in analgesia.

Fentanyl

Fentanyl (Duragesic, Sublimaze) is a strong synthetic mu opioid agonist approximately 80 times more potent than morphine. It has a short duration of action and is primarily metabolized by CYP3A4 to inactive metabolites. CYP3A4 inhibitors can cause increased fentanyl levels.

Hydrocodone

Hydrocodone (Vicodin) is the most commonly used oral opioid. It is recommended for the treatment of moderate or moderately severe pain and is also used to treat persistent cough. Hydrocodone, a prodrug, is metabolized via CYP2D6 to hydromorphone, the active metabolite. Similar to the situation with codeine, persons who are CYP2D6 deficient secondary to a polymorphism or those who take CYP2D6 inhibitors may have a decreased analgesic effect. An extended-release formulation (Zohydro ER) has been approved by the FDA for managing chronic pain.

Hydromorphone

Hydromorphone (Dilaudid) is a semisynthetic potent mu opioid agonist that, like morphine, is minimally metabolized via the CYP450 enzyme system. The metabolites of hydromorphone are not active.

Meperidine

Meperidine (Demerol) is a semisynthetic weak mu opioid with approximately 10% of the effectiveness of morphine.[81] It has an active metabolite, normeperidine, which has a longer half-life (15–30 hours) than the parent drug (3 hours). Normeperidine has some analgesic effect, but more importantly, it can cause CNS hyperexcitability—manifested as anxiety, mood changes, myoclonus, and seizures.[87] Normeperidine, when given to women in labor, can cause respiratory depression in newborns.

Although meperidine was the drug of choice for treating moderate to severe pain for much of the twentieth century, its toxic effects are significant, and meperidine is no longer recommended for treatment of postsurgical pain, labor pain, or pain among the elderly.[88] This agent is also contraindicated for individuals who take MAO inhibitors.

Methadone

Methadone is a synthetic full mu agonist that is used to treat heroin addicts, but also has benefits in the treatment of chronic and neuropathic pain states. This agent is metabolized by CYP3A4 and CYP2D6 and excreted via feces, so it can be used by persons with renal impairment. Methadone is associated with multiple drug–drug interactions, however. It has no active metabolites, but the analgesic effect lasts approximately 4 to 8 hours, and the plasma half-life is 8 to 59 hours, which is longer than its duration of analgesic action. Thus, repeated dosing can result in accumulation of the drug, resulting in sedation and confusion. Changing doses must be done with caution.

Oxycodone

Oxycodone (OxyContin, Percocet) is a semisynthetic opioid that is an agonist for the mu, kappa, and delta receptors. Oxycodone is an analgesic by itself, but oxymorphone, its metabolite, also has analgesic effects. Oxycodone is metabolized by CYP3A4 to noroxycodone and noroxymorphone, and by CYP2D6 to oxymorphone. Oxymorphone undergoes hepatic conjugation and renal excretion. Because oxycodone is metabolized by CYP3A4 and CYP2D6, it is subject to multiple drug–drug interactions. Tablets must not be crushed, broken, or chewed. There are no food–drug interactions. Adverse effects and efficacy for oxycodone are similar to those of morphine.

Oxymorphone

Oxymorphone (Opana, Numorphan) is a semisynthetic mu agonist that is approximately 6 to 8 times more potent than morphine.[89] It is slightly more toxic than morphine, but less toxic than the full synthetic preparations. Oxymorphone is used to treat acute and chronic pain and has a safety and efficacy profile similar to that of morphine and oxycodone. It undergoes hepatic conjugation and renal excretion.

Partial Agonists

Opioids with low intrinsic activity, such as buprenorphine (Buprenex), achieve relatively minimal pharmacologic effects even when drug receptor occupancy is high. These opioids are termed partial agonists.

Agonist–Antagonists

Agonist–antagonists, such as butorphanol (Stadol) and nalbuphine (Nubain), elicit agonist effects at one receptor while producing antagonist effects at another. These agents produce analgesia but typically result in less respiratory depression than pure agonists. Unlike pure agonists, agonist–antagonists do exhibit a ceiling effect. Increasing dosage beyond the maximal dose does not increase pain relief, but does increase toxicity. Concurrent use with pure agonists may cause a reduction of analgesia and narcotic withdrawal symptoms if the agonist–antagonist occupies a receptor that normally binds the pure agonist.

Antagonists

Opioid antagonists, such as naloxone (Narcan), competitively antagonize activity of opioids at the mu, kappa, and delta opioid receptors, having the greatest affinity for the mu receptors. Naloxone (Narcan), naltrexone (ReVia, Vivitrol), and nalmefene (Revex) are competitive antagonists used to counter opiate overdose. An intravenous dose of naloxone works in about 2 minutes, with effects lasting approximately 45 minutes. Naloxone should be used with extreme caution in persons who are opioid dependent, as abrupt reversal of opioid effects can precipitate acute withdrawal symptoms. Naltrexone is a competitive antagonist used to treat alcohol and opioid dependence. The clinical uses of naltrexone are discussed in more detail in the *Drugs of Abuse* chapter.

Miscellaneous Analgesic Agents

Tramadol

Tramadol (Ultram) is a unique opioid that does not fit in the usual classifications, although it is a controlled drug. This synthetic weak mu opioid agonist inhibits the reuptake of serotonin and norepinephrine. Its mechanism of action is not completely understood. Tramadol is used for management of moderate to severe pain and as a treatment for both acute and chronic pain. It is metabolized by CYP2D6 and CYP3A4 and has the usual drug–drug interactions associated with inducers and inhibitors of these enzymes. Tramadol can decrease the threshold for seizures when combined with serotonin reuptake inhibitors or tricyclic antidepressants or in persons with epilepsy. However, drug–drug interactions are not common when tramadol is used in therapeutic doses.

Dextromethorphan

Dextromethorphan (Benylin, Triaminic Cold and Cough, Robitussin) is a common constituent of cold and cough preparations. Although it is a synthetic opioid derivative, its activity does not rely on binding with opioid receptors. The antitussive effects of dextromethorphan are poorly understood. When taken in doses exceeding the maximum recommended dosage, this drug acts as a dissociative hallucinogen, similar to ketamine and phencyclidine (PCP), due to its antagonism of the *N*-methyl-D-aspartate (NMDA) receptors. Dextromethorphan is metabolized in the liver to form dextrorphan, an active metabolite, and by CYP2D6 to inactive metabolites. It should not be taken concomitantly with selective serotonin reuptake inhibitors, tricyclic antidepressants, or MAO inhibitors.

Whereas the antitussive effects of codeine can be reversed by opioid antagonists such as naloxone, the antitussive effects of dextromethorphan cannot. This suggests that dextromethorphan works through a non-opioid antitussive mechanism.

Special Populations

Treatment of Persons with Chronic Pain

Treatment of nonmalignant chronic pain is an increasingly frequent problem as the population ages, and long-term treatment with opioids is increasing as concern about addiction becomes less important than treating pain in the medical community. In general, pharmacologic treatment of chronic pain is directed at two fronts: the underlying disease process and the treatment of pain. NSAIDs, aspirin, acetaminophen, opioids, and adjunctive analgesics all have a role depending on the specific situation.[90] In practice, balancing pain relief and unacceptable side effects is an ongoing clinical challenge.

When increasing doses are needed to treat chronic pain, the underlying problem could be a progressive disease process or a therapeutic paradox called opioid tolerance and/or opioid hyperalgesia. The interaction between these two phenomena reduces analgesic efficacy, and it is important that prescribers recognize these syndromes.[91]

- Opioid tolerance is increasingly being treated with an opioid rotation technique. Development of tolerance to one opioid does not confer cross-tolerance to another, so rotating opioids toward equianalgesic dosing is sometimes effective in treating opioid tolerance.
- Opioid hyperalgesia is a state of nociceptive sensitization caused by exposure to opioids that occurs secondary to neuroplastic changes in the CNS.[92] NMDA receptor agonism appears to play a role in the development of hyperalgesia. NMDA antagonists such as ketamine can prevent or reverse opioid hyperalgesia, and research on newer agents that inhibit NMDA receptors is ongoing.[93]

Pseudo-addiction is a third behavior that affects use of opioids. Addiction is a primary, chronic, neurobiologic disease, for which genetic, psychosocial, and environmental factors influence its development and manifestations. It is characterized by behaviors that include impaired control over drug use, compulsive use, continued use despite harm, and craving. Pseudo-addiction occurs when pain is not sufficiently relieved with a standard opioid dose and the individual then exhibits some of the signs of addiction, such as tolerance and frequent requests to obtain analgesic drugs. Distinguishing between opioid addiction and pseudo-addiction can be difficult to make, as there are no specific distinctions between the two. Rather, pseudo-addiction behaviors are somewhat dependent upon staff responses to requests. In short, undertreatment of pain causes the sufferer to adopt more exaggerated expressions of pain, which in turn causes additional miscommunication. Careful history and a willingness to treat with larger doses as needed are important clinical strategies when caring for a person with acute or chronic pain.

Pregnancy and Lactation

All opioids cross the placental barrier and are excreted in breast milk. Maternal opioid use, especially use of codeine or hydrocodone, during the first trimester slightly increases the risk for congenital heart defects.[94] Opioids commonly used to treat labor pain are reviewed in the *Labor* chapter. The American Academy of Pediatrics considers opioids to be compatible with breastfeeding, although excessive use may result in increased sedation of the newborn.[53]

Elderly

Chronic pain of multiple etiologies is a common problem among the elderly population, and one that is often undertreated. Treatment of pain in older individuals is complicated by the greater frequency of comorbidities in this population, such as renal or hepatic impairment and cardiovascular disease, which increases the risks associated with opioid use, and by polypharmacy among the elderly, which increases the risk of drug interactions. Notably, age-related decreases in hepatic blood flow and renal function decrease metabolism and excretion of drugs, thereby increasing the potential for drug toxicities.

Older persons may be more sensitive to both the analgesic and adverse effects of opioids. Opioid use must be carefully monitored to achieve maximum analgesia with minimum adverse effects. Individualization of dosage, method of delivery, and careful attention to the person's response to any medication is necessary for individualized therapy to achieve maximum analgesia while minimizing adverse effects. The use of meperidine should be avoided in elderly women.[94,95] The active metabolite of meperidine, normeperidine, accumulates in elderly individuals because of their typically slowed renal clearance; this buildup can result in serious CNS side effects including tremors, seizures, confusion, and hyperexcitability.[96]

Combination Analgesics

Because multiple pain pathways and receptors are involved in the pain response, a wide variety of fixed-dose formulations that combine agents with different physiologic targets have been developed. Several rationales are applied when selecting fixed-dose combination analgesics. Combining analgesics with different mechanisms of action can have several different effects, including (1) increasing the analgesic effectiveness beyond what the individual agents are capable of via a synergistic effect; (2) increasing the analgesic duration; (3) diminishing or minimizing side effects and adverse effects; and (4) reducing opioid tolerance or hyperalgesia.[98] Most of the combination products on the market today include acetaminophen, aspirin, or ibuprofen in combination with an opioid, and the majority of studies on the effectiveness of pain relief supports the theory that these combination products relieve pain better than single agents.[98] Combination therapy is recommended by both the World Health Organization and the American Pain Society.

When using combination products, the dose-limiting factor is the dose of the non-opioid agent rather than the dose of the opioid component. Because acetaminophen toxicity can occur following use of these combination products, in 2011, the FDA recommended that manufacturers of combination opioids limit the dose of acetaminophen to 325 mg per tablet (from the previous standard of 500 mg/tablet). Despite the change in acetaminophen dose, individuals taking combination products should be cautioned to pay close attention to the total daily dosage of acetaminophen, ibuprofen, or aspirin from any source. Table 12-16 lists commonly used combination products and the doses recommended for treatment of mild, moderate, and severe pain.

Table 12-16 Combination Opioids for Treating Moderate Pain or Pain of Limited Duration

Dose per Tablet	Usual Initial Adult Dose	Clinical Considerations
Oxycodone/Acetaminophen[a]		
Percocet (2.5/325; 5/325; 7.5/325; 10/325)	5–10 mg PO oxycodone every 3–4 hours	Dose is typically prescribed by opiate strength, but maximum dosage may be limited by acetaminophen content. FDA black box warnings describe abuse potential, respiratory depression, neonatal opioid withdrawal syndrome, and acetaminophen-induced hepatotoxicity.
Tylox (5/325) mg	5–10 mg PO oxycodone every 3–4 hours	
Oxycodone/Aspirin		
Percodan (5/325)	5–10 mg PO oxycodone every 3–4 hours	Dose is typically prescribed by opiate strength, but maximum dosage may be limited by aspirin content. FDA black box warning describes acetaminophen-induced hepatoxicity.
Hydrocodone/Acetaminophen[a]		
Lorcet (5/325; 7/325; 10/325)	5–10 mg PO hydrocodone every 4–6 hours	Dose is typically prescribed by opiate strength, but maximum dosage may be limited by acetaminophen. FDA black box warning describes acetaminophen-induced hepatoxicity. Moved from Schedule II to Schedule III in 2014.
Lortab (2.5/325; 5/325; 7.5/325; 10/325)	5–10 mg PO hydrocodone every 4–6 hours	
Norco (2.5/325; 5/325; 7.5/325; 10/325)	5–10 mg PO hydrocodone every 4–6 hours	
Vicodin (5/325)	5–10 mg PO hydrocodone every 4–6 hours	
Vicodin ES (7.5/325)	5–10 mg PO hydrocodone every 4–6 hours	
Codeine/Acetaminophen[a]		
Tylenol No. 1 (7.5/300)	30–60 mg PO codeine every 4–6 hours	Codeine is a weak analgesic. Doses greater than 65 mg have increased side effects without increased pain relief. Dose is typically prescribed by opiate strength, but maximum dosage may be limited by acetaminophen. FDA black box warnings describe acetaminophen-induced hepatoxicity and ultra-rapid metabolism leading to respiratory depression and death in children. Nausea and vomiting are common side effects.
Tylenol No. 2 (15/300)	30–60 mg PO codeine every 4–6 hours	
Tylenol No. 3 (30/300)	30–60 mg PO codeine every 4–6 hours	
Tylenol No. 4 (60/300)	30–60 mg PO codeine every 4–6 hours	

[a] Maximum daily dose for a particular combination product should not exceed the maximum dose of acetaminophen (4 g/day).

Adjunctive Analgesics

Adjunctive analgesics are medications that enhance the analgesic effect of other agents. These analgesics allow for lower doses of the primary analgesic to be administered when used in combination primary/secondary therapy and are particularly useful for the management of neuropathic pain (Box 12-4). Commonly used adjunctive analgesics include tricyclic antidepressants, antiepileptics, local anesthetics, central nervous system stimulants, antihistamines, muscle relaxers, glucocorticoids, and bisphosphonates. Table 12-17 provides examples of the use of adjunctive agents with summaries of their risks and benefits.[99]

Inhalents

Most inhalants are also anesthetics, although not all. Anesthetics are drugs that produce a loss of sensitivity to stimuli. General anesthetics produce unconsciousness. Local and regional anesthetics block pain without loss of consciousness. General anesthetics may be delivered by inhalation or intravenous administration. With few exceptions, general and regional anesthetics are administered by specialists in anesthesia and are outside the scope of this discussion.

One inhalent of note is the analgesic nitrous oxide (Nitronox), a tasteless, odorless gas. It is sometimes used for analgesia during labor or dental procedures and is

Box 12-4 Neuropathic Pain

Ms. J is a 67-year-old woman who comes to the clinic with concerns of sharp, burning pain, and increased skin sensitivity in her scapular area. She states that her skin is so sensitive that she has trouble wearing a bra. On inspection, there are no lesions, redness, or edema. Light touch with a cotton ball produces concerns of stabbing pain. A careful health history reveals that Ms. J experienced an outbreak of shingles 6 weeks ago that spontaneously resolved without treatment. The healthcare provider diagnoses her present condition as postherpetic neuralgia (PHN).

Postherpetic neuralgia is generally a self-limiting condition, but it can last indefinitely. It is defined as pain that lasts beyond 1 month after the vesicular rash associated with shingles subsides. Age is the greatest risk factor for PHN. At age 60 years, approximately 60% of persons with shingles develop PHN, and the incidence increases with age. Treatment is aimed at pain control while waiting for the process to subside.

Because the pain associated with PHN is neuropathic in nature, treatment rarely requires the use of opioids, although they may be indicated in some cases. A variety of treatments have proven useful in treating this condition. Although acetaminophen may be adequate to treat mild cases of PHN, more troublesome cases usually require more definitive treatment with tricyclic antidepressants (TCAs), antiepileptic drugs (AEDs), or topical analgesics.

Amitriptyline (Elavil), imipramine (Tofranil), and nortriptyline (Pamelor) are suitable first-line TCAs. TCAs are best tolerated when started at small doses and given at bedtime. The dose can be titrated upward slowly every 2 to 4 weeks to achieve effective pain relief. TCAs may require as long as 3 months to achieve therapeutic results.

Gabapentin (Neurontin) and carbamazepine (Tegretol) are suitable first-line AEDs. Pregabalin (Lyrica) is a newer AED that is FDA approved for the PHN indication, but its high cost may render it unavailable to persons on fixed incomes. AEDs may have significant side effects such as memory impairment, sedation, liver toxicity, or electrolyte disturbances, which can make them problematic for some elderly persons. However, analgesic effects are typically achieved at relatively low doses, which helps to reduce the incidence of these problems.

Topical analgesics such as capsaicin have proven efficacious of PHN but must be used 5 to 7 times daily to achieve effective relief. Lidocaine patches have also shown effectiveness in this indication, but the pain relief typically lasts only 4 to 12 hours.

After reviewing her treatment options, Ms. J chooses to try lidocaine patches for immediate pain relief and start amitriptyline at 25 mg to be taken nightly. If pain relief is not adequate, her amitriptyline may be titrated upward by 25 mg every 2 to 4 weeks until adequate analgesia or a maximum dose of 150 mg per day is achieved.

Table 12-17 Adjuvant Analgesics

Drug Category	Beneficial Effects	Adverse Effects/Side Effects	Clinical Considerations
Alpha agonists: clonidine (Catapres)	Reduces sympathetically mediated pain	Anticholinergic effects (dry mouth, urinary retention, constipation), headache, nausea, allergic reaction	Act synergistically with opioids to produce antinociceptive effects.
Antiepileptics: carbamazepine (Tegretol), gabapentin (Neurontin), pregabalin (Lyrica)	Reduce neuropathic pain; pregabalin is also indicated for fibromyalgia; carbamazepine is effective for treating pain associated with trigeminal neuralgia	Carbamazepine is myelosuppressive; persons with bone marrow suppression should use with caution; though rare, pregabalin may cause angioedema	Gabapentin is currently the first choice for neuropathic pain secondary to proven efficacy, a low side-effect profile, and minimal drug–drug interactions.
Antihistamines: hydroxyzine (Vistaril)	Enhance analgesia, reduce anxiety, promote sleep, reduce nausea	Increased risk of respiratory depression	Use with caution in the elderly secondary to increased risk for tardive dyskinesia.
Bisphosphonates: etidronate (Didronel), pamidronate (Aredia)	Reduce cancer-related bone pain	Osteonecrosis of the jaw	Mechanism of action not understood.
Cannabinoids	Decrease hyperalgesia effect from opioids and act synergistically with the analgesic effect of opioids	CNS depression	Analgesic effect is mild. Studies comparing cannabinoids to placebo reveal efficacy, but studies comparing cannabinoids to other drugs are lacking.
CNS stimulants: dextroamphetamine (Concerta, Ritalin)	Potentiate analgesia and reduce opioid-induced sedation	Nausea, loss of appetite, diarrhea, constipation, nervousness, insomnia, irritability in first days of therapy, hypertension	Can be habit forming. Contraindicated for persons with glaucoma, hypertension, cardiovascular disease, substance abuse, or hyperthyroidism.
Corticosteroids: dexamethasone (Decadron)	Reduce edema, reduce inflammation, enhance appetite	Long-term therapy may cause gastric ulceration, osteoporosis, hyperglycemia, immunosuppression, adrenal insufficiency, or psychosis	Risk of adverse effects increases with increases in dose and longer duration of therapy.
GABA agonists: baclofen (Lioresal)	Potentiate antineuralgic effect of carbamazepine	Drowsiness, weakness, hypotension, confusion	Require slow tapering to avoid possible seizures.
Local anesthetics: lidocaine	Reduce neuropathic pain	Minimal adverse effects with transdermal formulations	Available in transdermal patches; has good efficacy for postherpetic pain.
NMDA antagonists: ketamine	Inhibit hyperalgesia effect from opioids and act synergistically with the analgesic effect of opioids	Hallucinations, memory impairment	Ketamine has a narrow therapeutic window.
SNRIs: duloxetine (Cymbalta)	Duloxetine is FDA approved for treatment of pain from diabetic neuropathy but is not as effective as TCAs	No anticholinergic or antihistamine effects, but minimal analgesic effects	The SNRIs have minimal analgesic effect, but are helpful in reducing the anxiety, depression, and insomnia that accompany chronic pain. Bioavailability of duloxetine is reduced by about one-third in smokers, but dosage adjustment is not recommended.
Topical: capsaicin	Used in topical creams to relieve pain of peripheral neuropathy	Burning at site of application	Analgesic effect is dose dependent and can last for weeks following one dose.
Tricyclic antidepressants: amitriptyline (Elavil)	Reduce neuropathic pain, elevate mood, promote sleep, enhance appetite	Increase anticholinergic effects of opioids (dry mouth, urinary retention, constipation), nightmares, confusion, cardiotoxicity	Inhibit serotonin and norepinephrine uptake. Effective for diabetic neuropathy and postherpetic neuralgia. Weight gain may limit usefulness. Use in elderly is controversial.

Abbreviations: CNS = central nervous system; GABA = gamma-aminobutyric acid; NMDA = *N*-methyl-D-aspartic acid; SNRIs = selective serotonin–norepinephrine reuptake inhibitors; TCAs = tricyclic antidepressants.

administered by advanced practice nurses, midwives, or nurses without direct specialist supervision. Nitronox is a blend of 50% oxygen and 50% nitrous oxide, which is self-administered by the laboring woman through a mask or mouthpiece. Nitrous oxide's onset of effect is rapid (1 minute or less) and is equally rapidly reversed upon discontinuation, making it especially useful during the second stage of labor, since it has few effects on the newborn.[100]

Local Anesthetics

The first local anesthetic used in clinical practice was cocaine. Sigmund Freud first noticed the anesthetic properties of this agent, and his friend Karl Koller performed the first operation using cocaine as a topical ocular anesthetic.[101]

Two major groups of local anesthetics are used: esters and amides. Esters (cocaine, procaine [Novocaine], tetracaine [Pontocaine], and benzocaine) have a shorter duration of action than amides, because their half-life in plasma ranges between less than 1 minute and 6 minutes. Esters are rapidly hydrolyzed in the blood by plasma cholinesterases. Hypersensitivity is more common with the ester-type local anesthetics. Individuals who experience an allergic response to one such local anesthetic should be considered allergic to all ester-type local anesthetics.

The amide local anesthetics are used more often in clinical practice. They include lidocaine (Xylocaine), mepivacaine (Carbocaine), bupivacaine (Marcaine), prilocaine (Citanest), and ropivacaine (Naropin). These agents have a low molecular weight and are highly lipophilic, which facilitate their wide distribution throughout the body tissues, especially in highly perfused organs. The amides are metabolized in the liver via the cytochrome P450 enzyme system. Allergic reactions to the amides are uncommon, but some products contain preservatives that may provoke an allergic reaction.

Mechanism of Action

Local anesthetics control pain by blocking sodium channels in the axonal membranes, thereby preventing the conduction of sensory impulses. Sodium channel blockade makes it impossible for an action potential to be propagated along a neuron. The onset of the sensory block follows an orderly progression. Sympathetic and pain sensory information is carried by small unmyelinated C fibers, which are the first to be blocked. The sensory block then progresses to the larger, myelinated A-delta fibers, which transmit temperature and pain sensory information. The largest fibers are the A-alpha fibers, which transmit proprioception information. Onset and duration of local anesthetic action depend on the agent's molecular size, lipid solubility, and degree of ionization, all of which vary among the local anesthetics in use (Table 12-18).

Duration of action is also influenced by regional blood flow. For this reason, local anesthetics are often combined with a vasoconstrictive drug such as epinephrine. With this combination therapy, epinephrine decreases local blood flow, thereby delaying systemic absorption and reducing the risk of toxicity by prolonging the achieving maximum duration of the local anesthesia while requiring less anesthetic. However, use of epinephrine may result in systemic effects such as palpitations, tachycardia, hypertension, and nervousness. In most cases, these effects are negligible and treatment is symptomatic.

Side Effects/Adverse Effects

The two major mechanisms of local anesthetic toxicity occur secondary to accidental injection into the bloodstream and subsequent systemic effects or direct toxicity from inadvertent intrathecal injection. The first symptoms of systemic toxicity are tongue numbness and a metallic taste. Dizziness, tinnitus, seizures, and then cardiac arrest

Table 12-18 Characteristics of Local Anesthetics

Classification	Drug: Generic (Brand)	Maximum Adult Dose (Plain)	Maximum Adult Dose with Epinephrine	Onset of Action	Duration of Action
Amides	Bupivacaine (Marcaine)	175 mg	250 mg	5 minutes	4–8 hours
	Lidocaine (Xylocaine)	300 mg[a]	500 mg[b]	2 minutes or less	30–120 minutes
	Ropivacaine (Naropin)	200 mg	NA	10 minutes	2–3 hours
Esters	Procaine (Novocain)	500 mg	600 mg	2–5 minutes	30–45 minutes
	Tetracaine (Pontocaine)	20 mg	20 mg	15 minutes or less	2–3 hours

[a] 4 mg/kg, which is 30 cc of 1% lidocaine.
[b] 7 mg/kg, which is 50 cc of 1% lidocaine with epinephrine solution.

can follow. Coadministration of epinephrine can reduce toxicity by reducing local blood flow and slowing systemic absorption to allow for a more even balance of drug distribution and metabolism. Direct toxicity following an intrathecal injection results in a very rapid onset of the regional block, hypotension, respiratory depression, and loss of consciousness.

Lidocaine

Lidocaine is the local anesthetic most commonly used in primary care. It works by blocking sodium channels at the axonal membrane, thereby reversibly stopping impulse conduction along the nerve. Lidocaine is completely absorbed following parenteral administration. This agent is rapidly metabolized by the liver and excreted through the kidneys. Its peak anesthetic effect occurs within 2 to 5 minutes and lasts from 15 to 45 minutes. Combination with a vasoconstrictor such as epinephrine delays systemic absorption of lidocaine, thereby prolonging the anesthetic effect.

Lidocaine suppresses myocardial excitability and conduction and may be given intravenously for its antidysrhythmic properties. If given in excess, it can cause bradycardia, heart block, reduced myocardial contractility, and cardiac arrest. Lidocaine also causes peripheral vasodilation that can result in hypotension. Allergic reactions to lidocaine are rare, but do occur. Cutaneous lesions, urticaria, edema, and anaphylactoid reactions are characteristic of lidocaine allergy.

Lidocaine is also used topically to treat neuropathic pain and is formulated as a 10 by 14 inch stretchy adhesive patch that contains 700 mg of lidocaine in an aqueous base.[102] The patch must be applied to intact skin and can be left on for 12 hours. A maximum of 3 patches can be worn at one time. Lidocaine delivered topically has minimal to no systemic effects.[103] Additional topical uses of local anesthetics are discussed in the *Dermatology* chapter. Local anesthetics for the woman giving birth also are discussed in the *Labor* chapter.

Complementary and Alternative Medicines

Relief of pain is the most common reason why individuals seek out complementary and alternative medicine (CAM). Individuals may use CAM for a variety of reasons, including the widely held perception that such therapies are safer than prescription medications. Women may also choose CAM therapies because previous medically supervised treatments have proved unsuccessful. CAM therapies may be combined with conventional therapies as well. Unfortunately, many CAM therapies have been inadequately studied, and little evidence is available about their safety or efficacy or possible interactions with conventional medications. This section presents CAM therapies commonly used for pain within the context of the available scientific evidence.

Herbals

Arnica (*Arnica montana*, leopard's bane) is used topically as a counterirritant, anti-inflammatory, and pain reliever. Studies have shown this herb to be as effective as ibuprofen (Advil) for treatment of osteoarthritis of the hand,[104] as well as safe and effective for treatment of mild to moderate osteoarthritis of the knee.[105] Arnica interacts with antihypertensive drugs and is considered poisonous when taken internally.

Capsaicin (*Capsicum frutescens*, African chilies, Mexican chilies, grains of paradise) has been used topically to treat postherpetic neuralgia, diabetic neuropathy, osteoarthritis, and rheumatoid arthritis. It works by binding to nociceptors in the skin. Initial excitation of the neurons is perceived as a sensation of itching or burning and is accompanied by local vasodilation. Following this initial excitation, there is a period of reduced sensitivity, which, with repeated applications, may cause degeneration of epidermal nerve fibers, resulting in persistent hypoanalgesia.[106] Studies of capsaicin for the treatment of chronic low back pain, knee pain, and soft-tissue pain have yielded conflicting results, with some showing a significant reduction in pain, and others showing no real clinical benefit from this therapy.[106,107] Capsaicin is generally well tolerated and appears to have no significant adverse effects.

Devil's claw (*Harpagophytum procumbens*) has been found to be effective in controlling pain associated with osteoarthritis of the knee and hip and with nonspecific low back pain. This herbal product is most efficacious when taken as an aqueous extract of 50 to 100 mg.[108] It has been used in the treatment of menstrual cramps, but there are no studies of its effectiveness for this use. Devil's claw interacts with warfarin, causing an increase in anticoagulation.[109] It may also have hypoglycemic effects and should be used cautiously by persons with diabetes who are using hypoglycemic agents.

Ginger (*Zingiber officinale*) has been used for the treatment of inflammation associated with rheumatoid arthritis. It is believed to inhibit prostaglandin and leukotriene synthesis.[110] Randomized studies have not demonstrated any increased efficacy of ginger over placebo or ibuprofen. However, no side effects or drug interactions have been reported.[111]

Willow bark (*Salix alba*) has moderate evidence supporting its effectiveness in the treatment of nonspecific low back pain. Daily doses standardized to 120 mg or 240 mg salicin (the active ingredient in willow bark) have been shown to be better than placebo in producing short-term improvements in pain and rescue medication.[112] However, willow bark has not been found to be effective for treatment of osteoarthritis.[113] Although there is little research on safety and drug interactions of willow bark, salicin is a salicylate, and individuals should be advised to take the same precautions when taking this herbal product as they would with aspirin.[114]

Butterbur (*Petasites hybridus*) has been found to reduce the frequency, intensity, and duration of migraine attacks in persons who experience three to seven attacks per month.[115] Butterbur is a member of the same plant family as ragweed, marigolds, and chrysanthemums and may cause allergic reactions in some individuals. Some butterbur preparations contain pyrrolizidine alkaloids, which may cause liver toxicity.[116]

Conclusion

As knowledge of molecular mechanisms of action and technology advance, new pain medications and new modalities for administering pain medications are emerging from the research pipeline and entering clinical practice. Researchers looking for new analgesics are exploring molecular receptor targets for new drugs and genetic variability in both pain perception and response to pain medications. The role of the immune system in pain pathways is just beginning to become clear. The latest modality for delivering systemic drugs is transdermal iontophoresis, a process that facilitates delivery of a charged molecule across intact skin using a small electrical current. Fentanyl is being used in this manner in palliative hospice settings, and it appears that iontophoresis may be superior to patient-controlled analgesia in certain settings.

Unrelieved pain causes needless suffering, and healthcare providers have an obligation to assess, believe, and document a woman's report of pain and to intervene to relieve or avert that pain. Because pain is a highly subjective and variable experience, treatment must be individualized, taking into account the type of pain, comorbid conditions, gender, age, and other individual characteristics.

Resources

Organization	Description	Website
Partners Against Pain	Offers and reviews multiple pain assessment tools as well as pain treatment forms and drug abuse assessment tools	www.partnersagainstpain.com/hcp/
American Pain Society (APS)	Clinical practice guidelines for use of pain medications and treatment of painful conditions are available at this website; APS also provides several monographs, books, and online continuing medical education (CME) courses for primary care providers, including the book *Pain: Current Understanding of Assessment, Management, and Treatments*	www.americanpainsociety.org/resources/content/apsclinicalpracticeguidelines.html www.americanpainsociety.org/education/content/enduringmaterials.html
Medscape Pain Learning Center	Online CME courses for healthcare providers that address pain medications	www.medscape.org/resource/pain/cme
Apps		
American Chronic Pain Association	2014 edition of *Resource Guide to Chronic Pain Medication and Treatment*	http://theacpa.org/uploads/documents/ACPA_Resource_Guide_2014_FINAL%20(2).pdf
Opioid Dosage Conversion Apps	Several apps can be downloaded that convert the dose of opioids from one medication to another to maintain equianalgesic dosing	www.itunes.apple.com http://play.google.com/store/apps
Drug Monographs	Medscape, Epocrates, and LactMed are apps that provide drug monographs; Micromedix, Lexicomp, UpToDate, and Pepid are subscription drug databases	

References

1. Institute of Medicine. *Relieving Pain in America: A Blueprint for Transforming Prevention, Care, Education, and Research.* Washington, DC: National Academies Press; 2011.
2. Rollason V, Samer C, Piguet V, Dayer P, Desmeules J. Pharmacogenetics of analgesics: toward the individualization of prescription. *Pharmacogenomics.* 2008;9(7):905-933.
3. International Association for the Study of Pain. Part III: pain terms, a current list with definitions and notes on usage. 1994. In: Mersekey H, Bogduk N, eds. *Classification of Chronic Pain.* 2nd ed. Seattle, WA: IASP Press; March 2012:209-214. http://www.iasp-pain.org/Taxonomy. Accessed December 31, 2014.
4. Federation of State Medical Boards. *Model Guidelines for the Use of Controlled Substances for the Treatment of Pain.* Washington, DC: Federation of State Medical Boards; 2013.
5. Portenoy RK, Bennett DS, Rauck R, et al. Prevalence and characteristics of breakthrough pain in opioid-treated patients with chronic noncancer pain. *J Pain.* 2006;7(8):583-591.
6. Rao PN, Mohamed T. Current and emerging "at-site" pain medications: a review. *J Pain Res.* 2011;4:279-286.
7. Moffat R, Rae CP. Anatomy, physiology, and pharmacology of pain. *Anesth Inesn Care Med.* 2010; 12(1):12-18.
8. Fong A, Schug SA. Pathophysiology of pain: a practical primer. *Plast Reconstructive Surg.* 2014;134 (4 suppl 2):8S-14S.
9. Melzack R, Coderre TJ, Katz J, Vaccarino AL. Central neuroplasticity and pathological pain. *Ann NY Acad Sci.* 2001;933:157-174.
10. Melzack R. From the gate to the neuromatrix. *Pain.* 1999;82(S):S121-S126.
11. Tremblay J, Hamet P. Genetics of pain, opioids, and opioid responsiveness. *Metabol Clin Experiment.* 2010;59(suppl 1):S5-S8.
12. Craft RM. Sex differences in opioid analgesia: "from mouse to man." *Clin J Pain.* 2003;19(3):175-186.
13. Bartley EJ, Fillingrim RB. Sex differences in pain: a brief review of clinical and experimental findings. *Br J Anaesth.* 2013;111(1):52-58.
14. Smith YR, Stohler CS, Nichols TE, Bueller JA, Koeppe RA, Zubieta JK. Pronociceptive and antinociceptive effects of estradiol through endogenous opioid neurotransmission in women. *J Neurosci.* 2006;26(21):5777-5785.
15. Sandner-Kiesling A, Eisenach JC. Estrogen reduces efficacy of mu but not kappa-opioid agonist inhibition in response to uterine cervical distention. *Anesthesiology.* 2002;96(2):375-380.
16. Fillingim RB, Ness TJ, Glover TL, et al. Morphine responses and experimental pain: sex differences in side effects and cardiovascular responses but not analgesia. *J Pain.* 2005;6(2):116-124.
17. Rosero EB, Joshi GP. Preemptive, preventive, multimodal analgesia: what do they really mean. *Plast Reconstr Surg.* 2014;134(4 suppl 2):85S.
18. Żukowski M, Kotfis K. The use of opioid adjuvants in perioperative multimodal analgesia. *Anaesthesiol Intens Ther.* 2012;44:42-46.
19. Katz J, Clarke H, Seltzer, Z. Preventive analgesia: quo vadimus? *Anesth Anal.* 2011;113(5):1242-1253.
20. Polomano RC, Rathmell JP, Krenzischek D, Dunwoody CJ. Emerging trends and new approaches to acute pain management. *J Peri Anesthes.* 2008;1(suppl 1): S43-S53.
21. Hudcova J, McNicol ED, Quah CS, Lau J, Carr DB. Patient controlled opioid analgesia versus conventional opioid analgesia for postoperative pain. *Cochrane Database Syst Rev.* 2006;4:CD003348. doi: 10.1002/14651858.CD003348.pub2.
22. World Health Organization. *Cancer Pain Relief and Palliative Care: Report of a WHO Expert Committee.* World Health Organization Technical Report Series 804. Geneva, Switzerland: World Health Organization; 1990.
23. Miaskowski C, Cleary J, Burney R, et al. *Guideline for the Management of Cancer Pain in Adults and Children.* Glenview, IL: American Pain Society; 2005.
24. Fine PG, Portenoy RK. *A Clinical Guide to Opioid Analgesics.* Minneapolis, MN: McGraw-Hill; 2004.
25. Munir M, Enany N, Zhang JM. Nonopioid analgesics. *Med Clin North Am.* 2007;91(1):97-111.
26. Miller E. World Health Organization pain ladder. *J Midwifery Womens Health.* 2004;49(6):542-546.
27. Kis B, Snipes J, Busija, D. Acetaminophen and the cyclooxygenase-3 puzzle: sorting out facts, fictions, and uncertainties. *J Pharmacol Exper Ther.* 2005;315(1):1-7.
28. Chandrasekharan NV, Dai H, Roos LT, et al. COX-3, a cyclooxygenase-1 variant inhibited by acetaminophen and other analgesic/antipyretic drugs: cloning, structure, and expression. *PNAS.* 2002;99(21):13926-13931.

29. Brune K, Hinz B. The discovery and development of anti-inflammatory drugs. *Arthritis Rheum.* 2004; 50(8):2391-2399.
30. Vane JR. Inhibition of prostaglandin synthesis as a mechanism of action for aspirin-like drugs. *Nat New Biol.* 1971;231(25):232-235.
31. Brown C. Effective use of nonsteroidal anti-inflammatory drugs. *Female Patient.* 2002;27:20-30.
32. Campbell CL, Smyth S, Monalescot G, Steinhubl SR. Aspirin dose of the prevention of cardiovascular disease: a systematic review. *JAMA.* 2007;297(18): 2018-2024.
33. Gerstein NS, Schulman PM, Gerstein WH, Petersen TR, Tawil I. Should more patients continue aspirin therapy perioperatively? Clinical impact of aspirin withdrawal syndrome. *Ann Surg.* 2012;255(5): 811-819.
34. Douketis JD, Spyropoulos AD, Spencer FA, et al. The perioperative management of antithrombotic therapy: antithrombotic therapy and prevention of thrombosis, 9th ed.: American College of Chest Physicians evidence-based clinical practice guidelines. *Chest.* 2012;141(2 suppl):e326S-e350S.
35. Rostom A, Dube C, Lewin G, et al. *Use of Aspirin and NSAIDs to Prevent Colorectal Cancer.* AHRQ Publication No. 07-0596-EF-1.Rockville, MD: Agency for Healthcare Research Quality; 2007.
36. Ridker PM, Cook NR, Lee IM, et al. A randomized trial of low-dose aspirin in the primary prevention of cardiovascular disease in women. *N Engl J Med.* 2005;352(13):1293-1304.
37. Takada M, Fujimoto M, Hosomi K. Difference in risk of gastrointestinal complications between users of enteric-coated and buffered low-dose aspirin. *Int J Clin Pharmacol Ther.* 2014;52(3):181-191.
38. Ho CW, Tse YK, Wu B, Mulder CJ, Chan FK. The use of prophylactic gastroprotective therapy in patients with nonsteroidal anti-inflammatory drug- and aspirin-associated ulcer bleeding: a cross-sectional study. *Aliment Pharmacol Ther.* 2013;37(8):819-824.
39. Aithal GP, Day CP. Nonsteroidal anti-inflammatory drug-induced hepatotoxicity. *Clin Liver Dis.* 2007; 11(3):563-575.
40. Palikhe NS, Kim SH, Park HS. What do we know about the genetics of aspirin intolerance? *J Clin Pharm Ther.* 2008;33(5):465-472.
41. Kong JS, Teuber SS, Gershwin ME. Aspirin and nonsteroidal anti-inflammatory drug hypersensitivity. *Clin Rev Allergy Immunol.* 2007;32(1):97-110.
42. Lee RU, Stevenson DD. Aspirin-exacerbated respiratory disease: evaluation and management. *Allergy Asthma Immunol Res.* 2011;3(1):3-10.
43. Kim SH, Sanak M, Park HS. Genetics of hypersensitivity to aspirin and nonsteroidal anti-inflammatory drugs. *Immunol Allergy Clin North Am.* 2013; 33(2): 177-194.
44. Grosser T, Smyth E, FitzGerald GA. Anti-inflammatory, antipyretic, and analgesic agents: pharmacotherapy of gout. In: Brunton LL, Chabner BA, Knollmann BC, eds. *Goodman & Gilman's the Pharmacological Basis of Therapeutics.* 12th ed. New York: McGraw-Hill; 2011:959-1004.
45. Lau WC, Gurbel PA. Antiplatelet drug resistance and drug–drug interactions: role of cytochrome 450 3A4. *Pharm Res.* 2006;23(12):2691-2707.
46. Risser A, Donovan D, Heintzman J, Page T. NSAID prescribing precautions. *Am Fam Phys.* 2009;80(12): 1371-1378.
47. James AH, Braneazio LR, Price T. Aspirin and reproductive outcomes. *Obstet Gynecol Surv.* 2008;63(1):49-57.
48. American College of Obstetricians and Gynecologists Task Force on Hypertension in Pregnancy. Hypertension in pregnancy. *Obstet Gyencol.* 2013;122(5): 1122-1131.
49. Bujold E, Roberge S, Lacasse Y, et al. Prevention of preeclampsia and intrauterine growth restriction with aspirin started in early pregnancy: a meta-analysis. *Obstet Gynecol.* 2010;116:402-414.
50. Committee on Practice Bulletins—Obstetrics, American College of Obstetricians and Gynecologists. Practice Bulletin No. 132: antiphospholipid syndrome. *Obstet Gynecol.* 2012;120(6):1514-1521.
51. Henderson JT, Whitlock EP, O'Connor E, Senger CA, Thompson JH, Rowland MG. Low-dose aspirin for prevention of morbidity and mortality from preeclampsia: a systematic evidence review for the U.S. Preventive Services Task Force. *Ann Intern Med.* 2014;160:695-703.
52. Yurdakok M. Fetal and neonatal effects of anticoagulants used in pregnancy: a review. *Turkish J Pediatr.* 2012;54(3):207-215.
53. American Academy of Pediatrics. The transfer of drugs and other chemicals into human milk. *Pediatrics.* 2001;108(3):776-789.
54. Geba GP, Weaver AL, Polis AB, Dixon ME, Schnitzer TJ; VACT Group. Efficacy of rofecoxib, celecoxib, and acetaminophen in osteoarthritis of the knee: a randomized trial. *JAMA.* 2002;287(1):64-71.

55. Vonkeman HE, van de Laar MAFJ. Nonsteroidal anti-inflammatory drugs: adverse effects and their prevention. *Semin Arthritis Rheum.* 2010;39(4):294-312.

56. Laine L. GI risk and risk factors of NSAIDs. *J Cardiovasc Pharmacol.* 2006;47(suppl 1):S60-S66.

57. Agency for Health Care Research and Quality. Choosing non-opioid analgesics for osteoarthritis: clinicians guide. http://www.effectivehealthcare.ahrq.gov/repFiles/Osteoarthritis_Clinician_Guide.pdf.

58. Castellsague J, Riera-Guardia N, Calingaert B, et al. Individual NSAIDs and upper gastrointestinal complications: a systematic review and meta-analysis of observational studies (the SOS Project). *Drug Saf.* 2012;35(12):1127-1146.

59. Wilcox CM, Allison J, Benzuly K, et al. Consensus development conference on the use of nonsteroidal anti-inflammatory agents, including cyclooxygenase-2 enzyme inhibitors and aspirin. *Clin Gastroenterol Hepatol.* 2006;4(9):1082-9.

60. Schlansky B, Hwang JH. Prevention of nonsteroidal anti-inflammatory drug-induced gastropathy. *J Gastroenterol.* 2009;44(suppl 19):44-52.

61. Forman JP, Stampfer MJ, Curhan GC. Non-narcotic analgesic dose and risk of incident hypertension in U.S. women. *Hypertension.* 2005;46(3):500-507.

62. Meek IL, van de Laar MAFJ, Vonkeman HE. Nonsteroidal anti-inflammatory drugs: an overview of cardiovascular risks. *Pharmaceuticals.* 2010;3:2146-2162.

63. Gladding PA, Webster MWI, Farrell HB, Zeng ISL, Park R, Ruijne N. The antiplatelet effect of six nonsteroidal anti-inflammatory drugs and their pharmacodynamics interactions with aspirin in healthy volunteers. *Am J Cardiol.* 2008;101(7):1060-1063.

64. Sammaritano LR, Bermas BL. Rheumatoid arthritis medications and lactation. *Curr Opin Rheumatol.* 2014;265(3):354-360.

65. Bombardier C, Laine L, Reicin A, et al. Comparison of upper gastrointestinal toxicity of rofecoxib and naproxen in patients with rheumatoid arthritis. VIGOR Study Group. *N Engl J Med.* 2000;343(21):1520-1528.

66. Bresalier RS, Sandler RS, Quan H, et al. Cardiovascular events associated with rofecoxib in a colorectal adenoma chemoprevention trial. *N Engl J Med.* 2005;352(11):1092-1102.

67. Silverstein FE, Faich G, Goldstein JL, et al.; Celecoxib Long-Term Arthritis Safety Study. Gastrointestinal toxicity with celecoxib vs nonsteroidal anti-inflammatory drugs for osteoarthritis and rheumatoid arthritis: the CLASS Study: a randomized controlled trial. *JAMA.* 2000;284(10):1247-1255.

68. Mukherjee D, Nissen SE, Topol EJ. Risk of cardiovascular events associated with selective COX-2 inhibitors. *JAMA.* 2001;286(8):954-958.

69. Hirayama A, Tanashashi N, Daida H, et al. Assessing the cardiovascular risk between celecoxib and nonselective nonsteroidal anti-inflammatory drugs in patients with rheumatoid arthritis and osteoarthritis. *Cric J.* 2014;78(1):194-201.

70. Li XC, Fries S, Li R, et al. Differential impairment of aspirin-dependent platelet cyclooxygenase acetylation by nonsteroidal anti-inflammatory drugs. *Proc Natl Acad Sci USA.* 2014;111(47):16830-16835.

71. Hale TW, McDonald R, Boger J. Transfer of celecoxib into human milk. *J Hum Lact.* 2004;20(4):397-403.

72. Food and Drug Administration. Over-the-counter drug products containing analgesic/antipyretic active ingredients for internal use: required alcohol warning; final rule; compliance date. 77N-094W; 21CFR-Part201 Food and Drug Administration HHS. *Fed Regist.* 1999;64(51):13066-13067.

73. Hughes GJ, Patel PN, Saxena N. Effect of acetaminophen on International Normalized Ratio in patients receiving warfarin therapy. *Pharmacotherapy.* 2011;31(6):591-597.

74. Lopes RD, Horowitz JD, Garcia DA, Crowther MA, Hylek EM. Warfarin and acetaminophen interaction: a summary of the evidence and biologic plausibility. *Blood.* 2011;118(24):6269-6273.

75. Sklar GE. Hemolysis as a potential complication of acetaminophen overdose in a patient with glucose-6-phosphate dehydrogenase deficiency. *Pharmacotherapy.* 2001;22(5):656-658.

76. Henderson AJ, Shaheen SO. Acetaminophen and asthma. *Pediatr Respir Rev.* 2013;14:9-16.

77. Jensen MS, Rebordosa C, Thulstrup AM, et al. Maternal use of acetaminophen, ibuprofen, and acetylsalicylic acid during pregnancy and risk of cryptorchidism. *Epidemiology.* 2010;21(6):779-785.

78. Mazaud-Guittot S, Nicolaz CN, Desdoits-Lethimonier C, et al. Paracetamol, aspirin, and indomethacin induce endocrine disturbances in the human fetal testis capable of interfering with testicular descent. *J Clin Endocrinol Metab.* 2013;98(11):E1757-E1767.

79. Thiele K, Kessler T, Arck P, Erhardt A, Tiegs G. Acetaminophen and pregnancy: short- and long-term

consequences for mother and child. *J Reprod Immunol.* 2013;97:128-139.

80. Liew Z, Ritz B, Rebordosa C, Lee PC, Olsen J. Acetaminophen use during pregnancy, behavioral problems, and hyperkinetic disorders. *JAMA Pediatr.* 2014;168(4):313-320.
81. Dietis N, Rowbotham DJ, Lambert DG. Opioid receptor subtypes: fact or artifact? *Br J Anaesth.* 2011;107(1):8-18.
82. Niesters M, Dahan A, Kest B, et al. Do sex differences exist in opioid analgesia? A systematic review and meta-analysis of human experimental and clinical studies. *Pain.* 2010;151(1):61-68.
83. Kirchheiner J, Schmidt H, Tzvetkov M, et al. Pharmacokinetics of codeine and its metabolite morphine in ultra-rapid metabolizers due to CYP2D6 duplication. *Pharmacogenomics J.* 2007;7:257-265.
84. Benyamin R, Trescot AM, Datta S, et al. Opioid complications and side effects. *Pain Physician.* 2008;11 (2 suppl):S105-S120.
85. Gillman PK. Monoamine oxidase inhibitors, opioid analgesics and serotonin toxicity. *Br J Anaesth.* 2005; 95(4):434-441.
86. Trescott AM, Datta S, Lee M, Hansen H. Opioid pharmacology. *Pain Physician.* 2008;11(2 suppl): S133-S153.
87. Latta K, Bingsberg B, Barkin R. Meperidine: a critical review. *Am J Ther.* 2002;9(1):53-68.
88. Thorson D, Biewen P, Bonte B, et al. *Acute Pain Assessment, and Opioid Prescribing Protocol: Health Care Protocol.* Bloomington, MN: Institute for Clinical Systems Improvement; January 2014.
89. Chamberlin KW, Cottle M, Neville R, Tan J. Oral oxymorphone for pain management. *Ann Pharmacother.* 2007;41(7):1144-1152. Epub June 26, 2007.
90. Manchikanti L, Abdi S, Atluri S, et al. American Society of Interventional Pain Physicians (ASIPP) guidelines for responsible opioid prescribing in chronic non-cancer pain: part 2 guidance. *Pain Physician.* 2012;15(3 suppl):S67-S116.
91. Chang G, Chen L, Mao J. Opioid tolerance and hyperalgesia. *Med Clin North Am.* 2007;91(2):199-211.
92. Lee M, Silverman SM, Hansen H, Patel VB, Manchikanti L. A comprehensive review of opioid-induced hyperalgesia. *Pain Physician.* 2011;14(2):145-161.
93. Silverman SN. Opioid induced hyperalgesia: clinical implications for the pain practitioner. *Pain Physician.* 2009;12(3):679-684.
94. Broussard CS, Rasmussen SA, Reefhuis J, et al. Maternal treatment with opioid analgesics and risk for birth defects. *Am J Obstet Gynecol.* 2011;204(4):314. e1-e11.
95. Fick DM, Cooper JW, Wade WE, Waller JL, Maclean JR, Beers MH. Updating the Beers criteria for potentially inappropriate medication use in older adults. *Arch Intern Med.* 2003;163(22):2716-2724.
96. Hanlon JT, Aspinall SL, Semla TP, et al. Consensus guidelines for oral dosing of primarily renally cleared medications in older adults. *J Am Geriatr Soc.* 2009; 57(2):335-340.
97. Chutka DS, Takahashi PY, Hoel RW. Inappropriate medications for elderly patients. *Mayo Clin Proc.* 2004;79:122-139.
98. Smith HS. Combination opioid analgesics. *Pain Physician.* 2008;11(2):201-214.
99. Khan MIA, Walsh D, Brito-Dellan N. Opioid and adjuvant analgesics: compared and contrasted. *Am J Hospice Palliative Med.* 2011;28(5):378-383.
100. Likis FE, Andrews JC, Collins MR, et al. Nitrous oxide for the management of labor pain: a systematic review. *Anesth Analg.* 2014;118(1):153-167.
101. Ruetsch YA, Boni T, Borgeat A. From cocaine to ropivacaine: the history of local anesthetic drugs. *Curr Top Med Chem.* 2001;1(3):175-182.
102. Mick G, Correa-Llanes G. Topical pain management with the 5% lidocaine medicated plaster: a review. *Curr Med Res Opin.* 2012;28(6):937-951.
103. Pasero C. Pain control: lidocaine patch 5%. *Am J Nurs.* 2003;103(9):77-78.
104. Widrig R, Suter A, Saller R, Melzer J. Choosing between NSAID and arnica for topical treatment of hand osteoarthritis in a randomised, double-blind study. *Rheumatol Int.* 2007;6:585-591.
105. Cameron M, Chrubasik S. Topical herbal therapies for treating osteoarthritis. *Cochrane Database Syst Rev.* 2013;5:CD010538. doi:10.1002/14651858. CD010538.
106. Sharma SK, Vij AS, Sharma M. Mechanisms and clinical uses of capsaicin. *Eur J Pharmacol.* 2013;720(1-3):55-62.
107. Mason L, Moore RA, Derry S, Edwards JE, McQuay HJ. Systematic review of topical capsaicin for the treatment of chronic pain. *BMJ.* 2004;328(7446): 991-999.
108. Brien S, Lewith GT, McGregor G. Devil's claw (*Harpagophytum procumbens*) as a treatment for

osteoarthritis: a review of efficacy and safety. *J Altern Complement Med.* 2006;12(10):981-993.

109. Izzo AA, Di Carlo G, Borrelli F, Ernst E. Cardiovascular pharmacotherapy and herbal medicines: the risk of drug interaction. *Int J Cardiol.* 2005;98(1):1-14.

110. Srivastava KC, Mustafa T. Ginger (*Zingiber officinale*) in rheumatism and musculoskeletal disorders. *Med Hypotheses.* 1992;39(4):342-348.

111. Bliddal H, Rosetzsky A, Schlichting P, et al. A randomized, placebo-controlled, cross-over study of ginger extracts and ibuprofen in osteoarthritis. *Osteoarthritis Cartilage.* 2000;8(1):9-12.

112. Oltean H, Robbins C, van Tulder MW, Berman BM, Bombardier C, Gagnier JJ. Herbal medicine for low-back pain. *Cochrane Database Syst Rev.* 2014;12: CD004504. doi:10.1002/14651858.CD004504.pub4.

113. Biegert C, Wagner I, Ludtke R, et al. Efficacy and safety of willow bark extract in the treatment of osteoarthritis and rheumatoid arthritis: results of 2 randomized double-blind controlled trials. *J Rheumatol.* 2004;31(11):2121-2130.

114. Clauson KA, Santamarina ML, Buettner CM, Cauffield JS. Evaluation of presence of aspirin-related warnings with willow bark. *Ann Pharmacother.* 2005; 39(7-8):1234-1237.

115. Lipton RB, Göbel H, Einhäupl KM, Wilks K, Mauskop A. *Petasites hybridus* root (butterbur) is an effective preventive treatment for migraine. *Neurology.* 2004; 63(12):2240-2244.

116. Danesch U, Rittinghausen R. Safety of a patented special butterbur root extract for migraine prevention. *Headache.* 2003;43(1):76-78.

© Sofimanning/Shutterstock

13 Antihistamines

Rebekah Jackowski McKinley

Based on the chapter by Lillie Rizack and Lawrence Carey in the first edition of Pharmacology for Women's Health

Chapter Glossary

Anticholinergic Drug that blocks the effect of the neurotransmitter acetylcholine peripherally and centrally, which results in multiple symptoms such as dry mouth, urinary retention, and mydriasis.

Antihistamines Class of drugs that blocks the effect of endogenously released histamines.

Histamine Amine with multiple biologic functions; an immune mediator that is synthesized and released by mast cells, basophils, and eosinophils. Histamine acts as a neurotransmitter in the brain and regulates gastric acid secretion.

Paradoxical reactions When a drug has the opposite effect of the one expected. Also called paradoxical effects.

Introduction

Antihistamines are a class of drugs that block the effects of histamine. Like analgesics and anti-infective agents, antihistamines are used in the treatment of many different disorders. This chapter reviews the general class of antihistamines, including both first- and second-generation formulations, with a focus on their pharmacologic effects, side effects, adverse effects, and drug–drug interactions.

Histamine

Histamine is a naturally occurring chemical messenger that has many different biologic roles. Histamine receptors can be found in most organs of the body. The function of histamine that is most well known is its role in mediating the body's inflammatory response. Mast cells and basophils release histamine after exposure to an antigen or trauma. Histamine, in turn, induces vasodilation and increases the permeability of local capillaries as part of the inflammatory response. Pruritus, hypotension, and bronchoconstriction are additional histamine effects noted during an inflammatory response.

Histamine is also present in neurons in the central nervous system, where it acts as a neurotransmitter and is involved in multiple functions, including wakefulness, memory, pain perception, and appetite. Histamine is also released from the enterochromaffin-like cells found in the gastric mucosa; such release increases the production of gastric acid secretions.[1] Table 13-1 provides an overview of the effects of histamine on various organ systems.

Histamine Receptors

Currently, four subtypes of histamine receptors have been identified: H_1, H_2, H_3, and H_4 (Table 13-1). Histamine receptors have constitutive activity in that they are able to initiate downstream events without ligand binding. This capability arises because the active and inactive states are in equilibrium with some being active and others being inactive at any one moment in time. H_1 receptors are found in vascular, smooth muscle, and nervous tissue and are primarily involved in inflammation, immediate hypersensitivity, and allergic reactions. H_1 receptors in the brain are concentrated in the cerebellum and forebrain, where histaminergic neurons are thought to play a role in excitation of the neuronal circuit and arousal when stimulated.[4] Agonist stimulation of H_2 receptors, which are located

Table 13-1 Histamine's Effects on Various Organ Systems

System	Histamine Effect	Physical Manifestation	Receptor
Cardiovascular			
Cardiac	Increased heart rate Increased contractility	Not usually clinically evident	H_2
Vascular	Dilation of arterioles and capillaries Constriction of veins and vascular endothelial cells Increased permeability of endothelial cells	Erythema Edema	H_1, H_2
Nervous			
CNS	Neurotransmission	Circadian rhythms Wakefulness	H_1, H_2, H_3
Afferent	Sensitization of nerve endings due to depolarization	Pruritus Pain	H_1, H_3
Gastrointestinal	Potentiates gastrin-induced acid secretion	Increased gastric acid	H_2, H_3, H_4
Skin	Combined vascular and afferent nerve effects	Urticaria	H_1
Respiratory			
Lungs[a]	Bronchoconstriction Prostanoid secretions	Wheezing Inflammation	H_1, H_2, H_3
Nose	Triggers goblet cells to decrease mucus viscosity Afferent nerve effects Vascular effects	Rhinorrhea Rhinitis Congestion secondary to edema	H_1, H_2, H_3
Immune system	Initiates inflammatory response Vasodilation	Inflammation, urticaria, anaphylaxis	H_1, H_2, H_3, H_4

[a] Individuals with asthma may have increased sensitivity to histamines.

Sources: Data from Bielory L, Ghafoor S. Histamine receptors and the conjunctiva. *Curr Opin Allergy Clin Immunol.* 2005;5(5):437-440[2]; Chambers C, Kvedar JC, Armstrong AW. Histamine pharmacology. In: Golan D, ed. *Principles of Pharmacology: The Pathophysiologic Basis of Drug Therapy.* Philadelphia, PA: Lippincott Williams & Wilkins; 2012:765-773[1]; Holgate Canonica GW, Simons FE, et al. Consensus Group on New-Generation Antihistamines (CONGA): present status and recommendations. *Clin Exp Allergy.* 2003;33(9):1305-1324.[3]

primarily in the gastric mucosa, induces secretion of gastric acid.

Research currently is being conducted to assess the location and function of H_3 and H_4 receptors. H_3 receptors appear to be found primarily in the brain, but have also been identified in eye, heart, and breast tissue. These receptors appear to be involved in circadian rhythms, alertness, allergic reactions, and possibly carcinomas.[5–9] H_4 receptors have been found in immune cells, hematopoietic cells, and breast tissue, and play a role in inflammation and allergic reactions.[5,7,10–16] Histamine receptors are G-protein–coupled receptors (Figure 13-1).

Antihistamines

The vast diversity of histamine functions is one reason why antihistamine drugs have many biologic effects and different therapeutic uses. Antihistamines traditionally are called histamine receptor antagonists or competitive antagonists. However, newer research classifies them as inverse agonists, in that they stabilize inactive forms of the histamine receptor and inhibit the spontaneous receptor activity that occurs naturally without the presence of an agonist, thereby shifting the balance toward inactive receptor status.[10–12,14–17]

Traditionally, new drugs have been created based on their ability to stimulate or inhibit a receptor. However, as knowledge about G-protein signaling activities has emerged, new options for drugs have presented themselves. For example, agents that target the signaling pathways or change the G-protein itself rather than the receptor may emerge as new therapies in the future.[18] It has been suggested that the term H_1 (or H_2) antihistamines, rather than H_1 (or H_2) blockers or antagonists, be used to reflect current understanding of histamine receptors and antihistamines. This terminology is used in this chapter.

Drugs targeting H_1 receptors are generally used to treat allergies and allergic reactions, nausea and vomiting, and motion sickness. First-generation H_1 antihistamines are subdivided into five categories based on their chemical structures: alkylamines, ethanolamines, ethylenediamines, phenothiazines, and piperazines (Table 13-2). Although

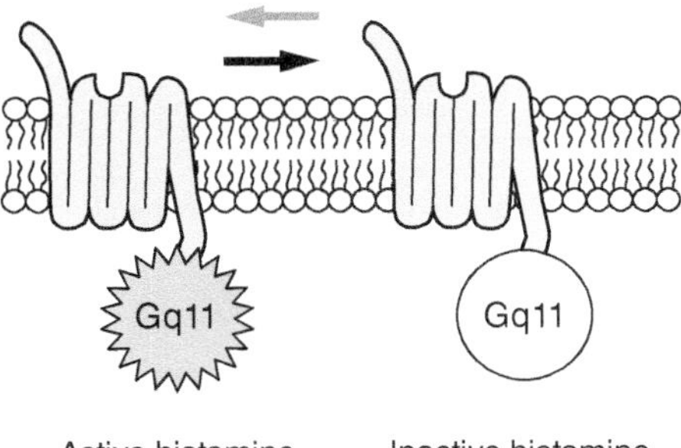

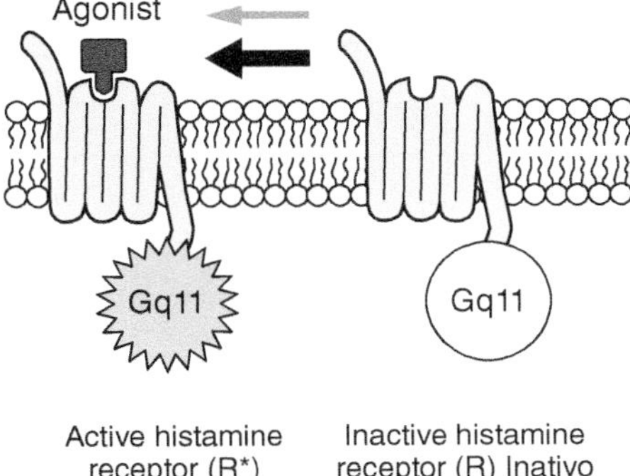

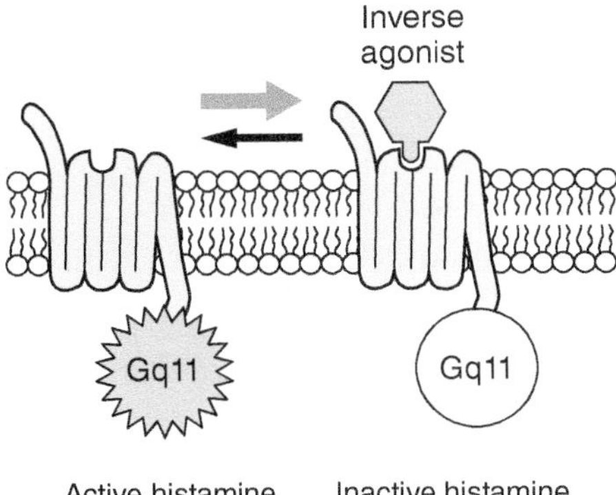

Figure 13-1 Stimulation of histamine receptors.

these chemical classes are well delineated, there is no distinct pharmacologic quality that separates one from the other. Some agents, however, are used for specific therapeutic reasons; for example, piperazines such as hydroxyzine (Vistaril) are used mainly for treatment of allergic reactions and for synergistic use with opiates, whereas the activity of meclizine (Antivert) is limited to prevention of motion sickness and nausea and vomiting. On a clinical basis, these subgroups are rarely discussed; rather, specific agents within the first-generation antihistamines are chosen based on their side-effect profile and distinct indication.

Drugs that inhibit stimulation of H_2 receptors are used to treat a variety of gastrointestinal disorders, such as peptic ulcer disease, erosive esophagitis, and gastroesophageal reflux disease. They are also prescribed to treat hypersecretory conditions such as Zollinger-Ellison syndrome, wherein increased levels of the hormone gastrin are produced.

As more is revealed about the role of H_3 and H_4 receptors, new drugs targeting these receptors are expected to emerge. For example, studies are beginning to demonstrate that H_3 and H_4 receptors may control cell proliferation, inflammation, and regulation of neurotransmitters. These findings may result in the future development of novel oncologic, neurologic, and anti-inflammatory agents.[7,22,23]

Antihistamines have anticholinergic effects that range from mild to severe depending on how well the drugs cross the blood–brain barrier and the strength of their affinity for cholinergic receptors. The ability of antihistamines to block the neurotransmitter acetylcholine can adversely affect many functions, including, but not limited to, memory, ability to concentrate, visual acuity, conduction through the sinoatrial and atrioventricular nodes in the heart, salivary secretion, and peristalsis in the intestinal tract. In contrast, antihistamines are sometimes used therapeutically specifically for their anticholinergic effects.

H_1 Antihistamines

Clinically, H_1 antihistamines are classified into two generations (or categories). The older first-generation agents have a short duration of activity—approximately 4 to 6 hours. They are lipophilic and cross the blood–brain barrier easily. In addition, the first-generation drugs are less specific for the H_1 receptor and, therefore, can cause a plethora

Table 13-2 Uses and Side Effects of Antihistamines

Antihistamine: Generic (Brand)	Uses	Side Effects: CNS Sedation	Gastrointestinal	Anticholinergic	Cardiovascular
H_1: First Generation					
Alkylamines					
Brompheniramine (Dimetane)	Allergies, pruritus, conjunctivitis	Low		Moderate	High
Ethylenediamines					
Chlorpheniramine (Chlor-Trimeton)	Allergies, rhinitis, conjunctivitis, pruritus, urticaria	Moderate		High	Moderate
Ethanolamines					
Clemastine (Tavist)	Allergies, rhinitis, pruritus, angioedema	High	Low	High	
Dimenhydrinate (Dramamine)	Antiemetic	High		High	High
Diphenhydramine (Benadryl, Unisom SleepGels)	Insomnia, upper respiratory allergies	High	Low	High	Low[a]
Doxylamine (Unisom SleepTabs)	Insomnia, nausea	High			
Piperazines					
Hydroxyzine (Atarax)	Allergies, pruritus, nausea and vomiting, insomnia	Moderate		Low	Low[a]
Meclizine (Antivert, Bonine)	Antiemetic	Low			
Phenothiazines					
Chlorpromazine (Thorazine)	Psychotic disorders, nausea, hiccups	Moderate		Moderate	Moderate
Prochlorperazine (Compazine)	Psychotic disorders, nausea	Low		Moderate	Low
Promethazine (Phenergan)	Allergies, nausea and vomiting	High		High	
H_1: Second Generation					
Cetirizine (Zyrtec)	Allergies	Low[a]	Low	Low	Low
Desloratadine (Clarinex)	Allergies	Low	Low	Low	Low
Fexofenadine (Allegra)	Allergies	Low[a]		Low	Low
Loratadine (Claritin, Alavert)	Allergies	Low[a]	Low	Low	Low[a]
H_2					
Cimetidine (Tagamet)	PUD, GERD, HS		Low		
Famotidine (Pepcid)	PUD, GERD, HS, E		Low		
Nizatidine (Axid)	PUD, GERD, HS, E		Low		
Ranitidine (Zantac)	PUD, GERD, HS		Low		

Abbreviations: CNS = central nervous system; E = esophagitis; GERD = gastroesophageal reflux disease; HS = hypersecretion; PUD = peptic ulcer disease.
[a] May be seen in higher doses.
Sources: Brock TP, Williams DM. Acute and chronic rhinitis. In: Alldredge BK, Corelli RL, Ernst ME, et al., eds. *Koda-Kimble and Young's Applied Therapeutics: The Clinical Use of Drugs.* 10th ed. Philadelphia, PA: Lippincott Williams & Wilkins; 2013;619-643[19]; Chambers C, Kvedar JC, Armstrong AW. Histamine pharmacology. In: Golan D, ed. *Principles of Pharmacology: The Pathophysiologic Basis of Drug Therapy.* Philadelphia, PA: Lippincott Williams & Wilkins; 2012:765-773[1]; Ergun T, Kus S. Adverse systemic reactions of antihistamines: highlights in sedating effects, cardio-toxicity, and drug interactions. *Curr Med Chem-Anti-inflammatory Anti-Allergy Agents.* 2005;4(5):507-515[4]; Fugit RV, Berardi RR. Upper gastrointestinal disorders. In: Alldredge BK, Corelli RL, Ernst ME, et al., eds. *Koda-Kimble and Young's Applied Therapeutics: The Clinical Use of Drugs.* 10th ed. Philadelphia, PA: Lippincott Williams & Wilkins; 2013;660-698[20]; Leurs R, Church MK, Taglialatela M. H_1-antihistamines: inverse agonism, anti-inflammatory actions, and cardiac effects. *Clin Exp Allergy.* 2002;32(4):489-498[17]; Nagel DS, Shields HM. Integrative inflammation pharmacology: peptic ulcer disease. In: Golan D, ed. *Principles of Pharmacology: The Pathophysiologic Basis of Drug Therapy.* Philadelphia, PA: Lippincott Williams & Wilkins; 2012;807-817.[21]

of central nervous system effects. The second-generation H_1 antihistamines have a longer duration—approximately 24 hours. They are more specific for the H_1 receptor and have fewer side effects. However, the second-generation drugs have more drug–drug interactions (Table 13-3).

All H_1 antihistamines, regardless of type, are metabolized in the liver.[24] These drugs are usually well absorbed after oral administration and are highly lipophilic. They are used primarily for treating allergic reactions, motion sickness, and, on occasion, nausea and vomiting.

Table 13-3 Common Doses and Drug–Drug Interactions Associated with Antihistamines

Antihistamine: Generic (Brand)	Usual Adult Dose	Known Drug–Drug Interactions and Adverse Effects
H_1: First Generation		
Alkylamines		
Brompheniramine (Dimetane)	4 mg PO every 4–6 hours or 8–12 mg of sustained-release form 2–3 times daily; max dose 12 mg/24 hours	MAO inhibitors can prolong and intensify the effects of the antihistamines.
Chlorpheniramine (Chlor-Trimeton)	4 mg PO every 4–6 hours; max dose 24 mg/24 hours Extended-release forms: 8–12 mg 2–3 times daily; max dose 24 mg/24 hours	MAO inhibitors, tricyclic antidepressants, phenothiazines, and benztropine can cause additive anticholinergic effects. CNS depressants can cause additive CNS depressant effects.
Ethanolamines		
Clemastine (Tavist)	1–2 PO mg 2 times daily; max dose 2 mg/24 hours	MAO inhibitors, clozapine, tricyclic antidepressants, phenothiazines, and other H_1 antagonists can cause additive anticholinergic effects. Alcohol, antipsychotics, barbiturates, chloral hydrate, opiate agonists, and hypnotics can cause enhanced CNS depressant effects.
Dimenhydrinate (Dramamine)	50–100 mg PO, IV, IM every 4–6 hours Max PO dose = 400 mg/24 hours Max IM dose = 100 mg/4 hours	
Diphenhydramine (Benadryl, Unisom SleepGels)	25–50 mg PO, IM, IV every 4–6 hours; max dose 300 mg/24 hours	
Doxylamine (Unisom SleepTabs)	Sleep: 25 mg PO at bedtime Antihistamine: 7.5-12.5 mg PO every 4–6 hours; max dose 75 mg/24 hours	MAO inhibitors, clozapine, tricyclic antidepressants, phenothiazines, and other H_1 antagonists can cause additive anticholinergic effects. Increased sedation if used in combination with other CNS depressant drugs. May enhance effects of epinephrine. May partially counteract the effects of heparin or warfarin.
Piperazines		
Hydroxyzine (Atarax)	25 mg PO 2–4 times daily for allergies 25–100 mg IM 3 times daily for nausea and vomiting 50–100 mg PO before bedtime for insomnia	MAO inhibitors, tricyclic antidepressants, phenothiazines, and benztropine can cause additive anticholinergic effects. Alcohol, antipsychotics, barbiturates, chloral hydrate, opiate agonists, and hypnotics can cause enhanced CNS depressant effects.
Meclizine (Antivert, Bonine)	25–50 mg PO 1 hour before travel, 25–50 mg PO once/daily	
Phenothiazines		
Chlorpromazine (Thorazine)	10–50 mg PO 2–4 times/day; 25–50 mg IM, which can be repeated in 1 hour Max dose is 2000 mg/24 hours	Chlorpromazine is an alpha-adrenergic antagonist, so increased pulse and hypotension can occur. Use with caution if the individual has heart disease, has a history of alcohol abuse, or is elderly. Can lower the seizure threshold, so do not use if taking anticonvulsants. Antihistamines may lead to prolonged QT interval. Can exacerbate psychotic symptoms in persons on amphetamines, SSRIs, St. John's wort, or barbiturates.
Prochlorperazine (Compazine)	5–10 mg PO, IM, IV 3–4 times daily max dose 40 mg/24 hours Sustained-release formulations available 25 mg PR every 12 hours for nausea	Can cause sedation, extrapyramidal symptoms, and anticholinergic effects. May be potentiated if given concomitantly with metoclopramide (Reglan). MAO inhibitors, tricyclic antidepressants, phenothiazines, and benztropine (Cogentin) can cause additive anticholinergic effects. Antacids that contain aluminum or magnesium, warfarin, or antiseizure drugs potentiate sedation of opioids and sedatives. Can reverse the vasopressor effect of epinephrine.

(*continues*)

Table 13-3 Common Doses and Drug–Drug Interactions Associated with Antihistamines (*continued*)

Antihistamine: Generic (Brand)	Usual Adult Dose	Known Drug–Drug Interactions and Adverse Effects
Promethazine (Phenergan)	12.5–25 mg PO, PR, IM, IV every 4–6 hours	FDA black box warning that intra-arterial and SQ administration can cause gangrene and other serious tissue injury. Sedation, extrapyramidal symptoms, and anticholinergic effects are known side effects. May be potentiated if given concomitantly with metoclopramide (Reglan). MAO inhibitors, tricyclic antidepressants, phenothiazines, and benztropine can cause additive anticholinergic effects. Can reverse the vasopressor effect of epinephrine.
***H_1*: Second Generation**		
Cetirizine (Zyrtec)	5–10 mg PO once daily	Alcohol,[a] barbiturates, tricyclic antidepressants, and opiate agonists can increase CNS depressant effects.
Desloratadine (Clarinex)	5 mg PO once daily	Erythromycin (E-mycin), azithromycin (Zithromax), ketoconazole (Nizoral), cimetidine (Tagamet), and fluoxetine (Prozac) interfere with metabolism of desloratadine, resulting in increased concentrations of desloratadine. Alcohol, opiate agonists, and other CNS depressants can cause enhanced CNS depressant effects.
Fexofenadine (Allegra)	60 mg PO once daily	Most fruit juices, erythromycin (E-mycin), ketoconazole (Nizoral), rifampin (Rifadin), antacids, and verapamil (Calan).
Loratadine (Claritin, Alavert)	10 mg PO once daily or 5 mg PO 2 times daily	Macrolide antibiotics, ketoconazole (Nizoral), cimetidine (Tagamet), amiodarone (Cordarone), and nefazodone (Serzone) interfere with metabolism of loratadine, resulting in increased concentrations of loratadine. Alcohol, antipsychotics, barbiturates, chloral hydrate, opiate agonists, and hypnotics can cause enhanced CNS depressant effects.
H_2		
Cimetidine (Tagamet)	800 mg PO at night or 300 mg PO 4 times/day with meals and once at night, or 400 mg PO 2 times daily for treatment of ulcer 400 mg PO at night for prevention of ulcer 200 mg PO prn with max dose 400 mg/day × 14 days for OTC treatment of heartburn	Decreases absorption of ketoconazole (Nizoral), itraconazole (Sporanox). Increased levels of alcohol, amiodarone (Cordarone), benzodiazepines, calcium-channel blockers, carbamazepine (Tegretol), cyclosporine (Neoral), diazepam (Valium), labetalol (Trandate), lidocaine, loratadine, phenytoin (Dilantin), procainamide, propranolol (Inderal), quinidine (Quinatime), theophylline (Theo-Dur), tricyclic antidepressants, valproic acid (Depakote), verapamil (Calan), and warfarin (Coumadin).
Famotidine (Pepcid)	40 mg PO at bedtime or 20 mg PO 2 times/day for treatment of ulcer 20 mg PO at bedtime for maintenance 20 mg PO 2 times/day for 6 weeks for treatment of GERD 10–20 mg PO prn for OTC treatment of heartburn	Alcohol. Decreases absorption of ketoconazole (Nizoral) and itraconazole (Sporanox).
Nizatidine (Axid)	300 mg PO at bedtime or 150 mg PO 2 times/day for treatment of ulcer 150 mg 2 times/day for treatment of GERD 75 mg PO prn for OTC treatment of heartburn with max dose 150 mg/day	
Ranitidine (Zantac)	150 mg PO 2 times/day or 300 mg at bedtime for treatment of ulcer 150 mg PO 2 times daily for treatment of gastric ulcer or GERD 75–150 mg PO prn for OTC treatment of heartburn with max dose 300 mg/day	

Abbreviations: CNS = central nervous system; GERD = gastroesophageal reflux disease; MAO = monoamine oxidase; max = maximum; OTC = over the counter; prn = as needed.

[a] Increased sedation seen primarily in women.

H_1 antihistamines cross the blood–brain barrier readily, where their actions within the central nervous system result in sedation—their best-known side effect. In some cases, H_1 antihistamines are used therapeutically to enhance sedation. However, tolerance to this effect appears to develop quickly, generally within 3 to 4 days.[25,26] Risk of tolerance explains why over-the-counter antihistamines such as diphenhydramine hydrochloride (Benadryl and Unisom SleepGels) and doxylamine succinate (Unisom SleepTabs), which are used as sleep aids, are recommended for short-term, intermittent use only.

H_1 antihistamines also have **anticholinergic** side effects, which can aid in the treatment of allergy-related rhinorrhea or the prevention of nausea, but can occasionally cause urinary retention and blurred vision. The anticholinergic effect can help mitigate or prevent some of the extrapyramidal effects of antipsychotics. Diphenhydramine, in particular, is given intravenously for the treatment of acute dystonic reactions.[27] H_1 antihistamines are frequently formulated in over-the-counter combination products (Box 13-1).

Box 13-1 Beware of Brand Names

Much has been written about the confusion caused by sound-alike brand names. However, little has been written about the variations of drugs made available under the *same* brand name. For example, most consumers and providers assume that the same brand name in different packaging indicates the same agent with different formulations or perhaps just marketed by different companies. Unfortunately, this assumption is not always correct.

On occasion, a brand name is so well recognized that the manufacturer chooses to use it as part of its overall market strategy. For example, Tylenol is a major drug brand, with more than $100 million in annual sales. The average person might think that Tylenol is synonymous with the generic drug acetaminophen, and that this agent is found in the remedy for allergy symptoms called Tylenol Allergy Multi-Symptom, albeit accompanied with the antihistamine chlorpheniramine maleate in this combination. However, Tylenol Simply Sleep, another of the manufacturer's products, has no acetaminophen and is composed solely of diphenhydramine hydrochloride, an antihistamine used as a sleep aid.

Another well-recognized brand name used for sleep is Unisom. Currently, when a Unisom product is used, the active ingredient will be an antihistamine—but not necessarily the same one. Tablets (Unisom SleepTabs) contain doxylamine succinate, whereas liquid/gelatin preparations (Unisom SleepGels) contain diphenhydramine hydrochloride.

In spite of the variations seen with branding, there is one constant: Reading labels continues to be a wise recommendation for all.

Contraindications to Use of H_1 Antihistamines

Contraindications to the H_1 antihistamines include any condition in which anticholinergic effects could have an adverse health effect, such as angle-closure glaucoma, hyperthyroidism, prostatic hypertrophy, and bladder neck obstructions, as well as conditions in which drowsiness poses a problem, such as driving, operating machinery, or consumption of alcohol. Because antihistamines are excreted via urine, individuals with renal impairment may need reductions in the antihistamine dose. **Paradoxical reactions** have occasionally been noted with this class of medications and appear with a higher frequency in children. Paradoxical reactions can include dermal reactions and hyperactivity.[28] An example of a paradoxical effect would be increased pruritus or hyperactivity instead of sedation following administration of diphenhydramine.

Side Effects/Adverse Effects of H_1 Antihistamines

Table 13-4 summarizes the side effects seen with the different classes of antihistamines.[1,2,17,29–31] H_1 antihistamines are associated with many side effects and adverse effects. Gastrointestinal side effects include nausea, vomiting, and epigastric distress. However, antihistamines are unique in that they are often used because their side effects have therapeutic effects. For example, the most common side effect of H_1 antihistamines is sedation; consequently, they are widely marketed in over-the-counter formulations as sleep aids. In contrast, H_1 antihistamines have an additive sedative effect when combined with other sedating drugs or alcohol; in this scenario, the sedation side effect can be considered an adverse effect.

Because H_1 antihistamines cross the blood-brain barrier, multiple adverse effects secondary to antagonist action on H_1 receptors in the central nervous system are common. These adverse effects include altered cognition, somnolence, psychomotor incoordination, or memory impairment, which are most likely in older individuals.[29] Occupation of serotonin receptors can result in increased

Table 13-4 Examples of Side Effects Seen Within Antihistamine Classes

Side Effect	H_1 Antihistamines (First Generation)	H_1 Antihistamines (Second Generation)	H_2 Antihistamines
Neurologic	Drowsiness, dizziness, sedation, somnolence, dystonic reaction	Same as first generation, but with less frequency	Headache, dizziness, insomnia
Gastrointestinal	Anorexia, constipation, epigastric distress	Abdominal pain, diarrhea, vomiting (especially in children)	Diarrhea
Anticholinergic	Urinary retention, blurred vision, constipation, dry mouth, dry mucous membranes	Rare	N/A
Cardiovascular	Changes in heart rate, changes in blood pressure	Rare	Rare changes in heart rate or rhythm

Sources: Chambers C, Kvedar JC, Armstrong AW. Histamine pharmacology. In: Golan D, ed. *Principles of Pharmacology: The Pathophysiologic Basis of Drug Therapy.* Philadelphia, PA: Lippincott Williams & Wilkins; 2012:765-773[1]; Ergun T, Kus S. Adverse systemic reactions of antihistamines: highlights in sedating effects, cardio-toxicity and drug interactions. *Curr Med Chem-Anti-inflammatory Anti-Allergy Agents.* 2005;4(5):507-515[4]; Golightly LK, Greos LS. Second-generation antihistamines: actions and efficacy in the management of allergic disorders. *Drugs.* 2005;65(3):341-384[31]; Leurs R, Church MK, Taglialatela M. H_1-antihistamines: inverse agonism, anti-inflammatory actions and cardiac effects. *Clin Exp Allergy.* 2002;32(4):489-498[17]; Mahdy AM, Webster NR. Histamines and antihistamines. *Anesthes Intensive Care Med.* 2011;12(7):324-327[30]; Simons FE, Simons KJ. Histamine and H_1-antihistamines: celebrating a century of progress. *J Allergy Clin Immunol.* 2011;128(6):1139-1150.[29]

appetite and weight gain. Other central nervous system effects include dystonic reactions, dyskinesia, and hallucinations.[30] The anticholinergic effects such as dry mouth or dry eyes become treatments for allergic conjunctivitis, but blurred vision and urinary retention—classic adverse anticholinergic effects—can also occur.

Drug–Drug Interactions Associated with H_1 Antihistamines

The primary drug–drug interactions of importance with the H_1 antihistamines are the additive sedative effect these drugs have when taken with other medications that cause sedation, such as sedatives, narcotics, antipsychotics, anxiolytics, alcohol, barbiturates, and hypnotics (Table 13-3). These sedating antihistamines also have an additive antimuscarinic action with drugs such as atropine and tricyclic antidepressants.

Second-Generation H_1 Antihistamines

Second-generation H_1 antihistamines are more highly selective for peripheral H_1 receptors than H_1 receptors in the central nervous system.[33] Generally, second-generation H_1 antihistamines are less sedating and have fewer anticholinergic side effects than the traditional H_1 antihistamines. However, because allergic reactions can themselves be sedating, it can be difficult to differentiate an antihistamine sedation side effect from sedation caused by the allergic condition alone.[22,23,32,34] Studies on sedative effects of antihistamines have been conducted with healthy volunteers who are not experiencing the fatigue of an allergic response; thus they have not clarified this question. The longer half-life of second-generation H_1 antihistamines allows once-a-day dosing. This factor, along with their favorable side-effect profile, often makes second-generation antihistamines preferable to their first-generation counterparts.

Two drugs in this class, astemizole (Hismanal) and terfenadine (Seldane-D), were removed from the market secondary to the occurrence of arrhythmias, which were the result of overdose or drug–drug interactions with such agents as erythromycin (E-mycin) and ketoconazole (Nizoral) that increased plasma levels of the drug[26,34,35] (Box 13-2). Some second-generation antihistamines—azelastine (Optivar), emedastine (Emadine), epinastine hydrochloride (Elestat), olopatadine (Patanol), and the newer agents alcaftadine (Lastacaft) and bepotastine (Bepreve)—are used primarily in ophthalmic or topical solutions.[4, 36–38]

Contraindications to Use of Second-Generation H_1 Antihistamines

The contraindications to use of second-generation H_1 antihistamines are essentially the same as the contraindications to use of first-generation H_1 antihistamines, especially for persons with conditions where anticholinergic effects would be undesirable. Although the sedation effect of second-generation H_1 antihistamines is much less than the sedation experienced by persons who take first-generation H_1 antihistamines, persons who drive a car or who work with heavy machinery should take the first few doses when not operating vehicles or equipment.[39]

Box 13-2 The Terfenadine (Seldane-D) Story

Terfenadine (Seldane-D) is an antihistamine that was developed, approved, and marketed for the treatment of allergies. Terfenadine is a prodrug, which is metabolized to the active drug fexofenadine by intestinal CYP3A4. However, when taken in high doses, terfenadine acts somewhat like quinidine in blocking sodium ion channels, thereby prolonging the cardiac action potential, which can cause prolonged QT interval and cardiac arrhythmias. This toxicity became apparent approximately 10 years after terfenadine was first introduced in clinical practice. Why did it take so long for the adverse effects of this drug to become apparent?

Most cases of terfenadine toxicity occurred in persons with preexisting cardiac disease or in persons who took an overdose of the drug. The active agent fexofenadine is not toxic, but when too much terfenadine was taken, less was metabolized, and the toxic effects of the prodrug terfenadine became evident. In addition, two oral antifungal agents, ketoconazole (Nizoral) and itraconazole (Sporanox), were first introduced in the 1980s. Both of these drugs block the metabolism of terfenadine.

The first report of cardiotoxicity secondary to use of terfenadine was published in 1989. In early 1997, the FDA recommended that terfenadine-containing drugs be replaced by fexofenadine. Seldane-D was removed from the U.S. market in late 1997 after the manufacturer of Seldane-D received approval for fexofenadine (Allegra).

Drug–Drug Interactions with Second-Generation H_1 Antihistamines

Few drug–drug interactions have been reported involving second-generation H_1 antihistamines (Table 13-3). Drug–drug interactions can theoretically occur among compounds that interact with or affect cytochrome P450 (CYP) activity. Notably, loratadine (Claritin) and fexofenadine (Allegra) are metabolized via the liver and the CYP450 enzyme system. Other drugs and substances that can affect CYP450 activity include antifungals, macrolides, and grapefruit juice; thus it is prudent to exercise caution when combining loratadine and fexofenadine with other substances that are metabolized by one of the CYP450 enzymes.[32] Drug interactions can also be additive. For example, cetirizine hydrochloride (Zyrtec) was found in one study to cause additional sedation when taken with alcohol.[33] Subsequent studies did not initially replicate this finding, but upon reexamination of the first study, these effects were found to be more common among women even when controlling for weight and body mass.[33,39]

Topical antihistamines are used for the treatment of allergic rhinitis and allergic conjunctivitis, atopic dermatitis, and chronic urticaria. The onset of action is rapid, and the duration of the effect is similar to that experienced with oral administration.[33,40,41] Antihistamines also have a role in the control of inflammatory responses, such as the flare and wheal noted in skin reactions. Additionally, they are used as adjunctive therapy when attempting to control pruritus of the eyes and skin. Diphenhydramine (Benadryl) and promethazine (Phenergan) occasionally are used as local anesthetics for individuals allergic to the standard agents. These agents work in the same way as procaine and lidocaine—namely, by blocking sodium channels.[27]

H_2 Antihistamines

H_2 antihistamines are used to treat gastric disorders wherein hyperacidity is a factor. These drugs competitively and reversibly inhibit the action of histamine at H_2 receptors, without the troublesome side effects encountered when using anticholinergic drugs for similar gastrointestinal problems.[27] Several of these agents are available over the counter (Box 13-3).

H_2 receptors are also present in other tissues throughout the body; however, the therapeutic dose needed for decreasing gastric acid usually has little effect on other systems. Of the four currently available agents, cimetidine (Tagamet) is administered most frequently (up to 4 times daily), whereas the other three agents—ranitidine (Zantac), famotidine (Pepcid), and nizatidine (Axid)—are dosed once or twice daily. All of the H_2 antihistamines have an extended half-life that may result in increased effects or toxicity in persons with renal impairment; thus it is wise to monitor renal function if long-term use is indicated.[42]

Contraindications

These drugs are rather benign from a contraindication standpoint. Indeed, they are generally considered safe to use except in those cases where a hypersensitivity or drug–drug interactions specific to an individual drug has been identified.

Box 13-3 A Case of Heartburn

LN is a 40-year-old female who reports a 3-month history of heartburn. She says her problem started after she was diagnosed with tension headaches, for which she takes nonsteroidal anti-inflammatory agents (NSAIDs), such as naproxen. Upon further questioning, it becomes evident that LN has been taking the NSAIDs frequently and often without food. There is a strong suspicion that she has developed a gastric complication secondary to the NSAID use, such as peptic ulcer disease.

Treatment

In addition to reviewing nonpharmacologic methods of treating tension headaches, the first step is to switch LN's pain reliever to acetaminophen (Tylenol), which does not cause gastric ulceration. Second, consider starting an H_2 antagonist, such as ranitidine (Zantac), at a dose of either 150 mg administered orally twice daily or 300 mg administered orally once a day for up to 8 weeks (in conjunction with treatment of *Helicobacter pylori* as appropriate). LN may need longer maintenance treatment of 150–300 mg taken orally each day at bedtime. Other H_2 antihistamines may be used; however, famotidine (Pepcid) should not be a consideration for LN because approximately 4% to 5% of individuals who use famotidine develop headaches associated with the drug itself.

Side Effects

Because H_2 antihistamines do not cross the blood–brain barrier readily, side effects are usually benign and infrequent. H_2 antihistamines' side effects are primarily gastrointestinal in nature, with an occasional mild central nervous system or dermatologic reaction being noted. Table 13-4 summarizes the side effects seen with the different classes of antihistamines. Individuals at higher risk for experiencing these side effects include older individuals, persons taking high doses, and persons with impaired renal function.

Drug–Drug Interactions

Cimetidine (Tagamet) affects CYP450-mediated drug metabolism, which results in decreased clearance of coadministered medications, especially those whose mechanism of action involves the same pathway. This is most significant if cimetidine is taken concomitantly with medications that have a limited therapeutic range. However, because cimetidine has many drug–drug interactions, it is not considered the first-line drug for inhibiting gastric secretions. Ranitidine (Zantac) also has some drug–drug interactions, but to a lesser extent (Table 13-3). All of the H_2 antihistamines can be involved in drug–drug interactions indirectly as a result of altered gastric pH if the other drug requires a specific pH for its absorption.[1]

Cimetidine (Tagamet) can cause gynecomastia in men. Although this is a well-known side effect, its mechanism of action is not clear. Moreover, cimetidine has been implicated as having the beneficial effect of increasing HDL and lowering LDL in both men and women. The clinical significance of this effect remains unclear.

Special Populations

Pregnancy

Antihistamines are widely used drugs both for the treatment of women with nausea and vomiting and for those with allergies. These drugs—particularly doxylamine succinate (Unisom) and most first-generation H_1 antihistamines—are effective for relieving nausea and vomiting during the first trimester of pregnancy.[43–47] It is generally believed that first-generation H_1 antihistamines do not have teratogenic or fetotoxic effects, given that they have been used for many years without noticeable problems. Nevertheless, recent studies have noted some case reports linking antihistamines to birth defects, suggesting they should be used with caution during pregnancy.[48] There are limited data on the use of H_2 antihistamines in pregnancy, but two studies have confirmed the generally held belief that there are no known teratogenic associations with these drugs.[49,50]

Lactation

The use of first-generation H_1 antihistamines during lactation is not considered safe, because these drugs are secreted in breast milk and can cause neonatal sedation.[2] If an antihistamine is necessary, cetirizine and loratadine are preferable, as they have been found in low levels in breast milk.[2] Cimetidine is considered by the American Academy of Pediatrics to be most compatible with breastfeeding.[51] Growth depression has been seen in rats following administration of both famotidine and nizatidine. Ranitidine has been shown to be excreted in breast milk, more so than with nizatidine and famotidine; it would appear that nizatidine and famotidine may be the preferred H_2 antihistamines for lactating women.[52] In addition, some sources suggest that the sedating antihistamines may decrease milk supply due to their anticholinergic effects.[53]

Elderly

First-generation H_1 antihistamines can be problematic for older individuals. These drugs can cause sedation and have adverse effects on cognition and balance—morbidities an older person may be less able to tolerate. Polypharmacy can also be a problem, as the first-generation drugs have multiple drug–drug reactions.[54] Second-generation H_1 antihistamines are generally better tolerated by older individuals. Adjustments in doses may need to be considered for all antihistamines for persons with renal or liver dysfunction.[55]

Antihistamines in the Future: H_3 and H_4 Receptor Antagonists

Drugs that are specific antagonists to the H_3 and H_4 receptors are not yet available for clinical use, although they are the subject of current research. H_3 receptors are found primarily in the central nervous system, and drugs that affect this receptor are being evaluated for use in treating cognitive disorders, sleep/wake disorders, epilepsy, and neuropathic pain.[56] H_4 modulators are being evaluated for use in treating inflammatory diseases, cancer, neuropathic pain, vestibular disorders, and type 2 diabetes.[57] Several novel drugs are in Phase 2 trials and may be expected to be approved for clinical use in the near future.

Conclusion

Antihistamines are a large class of drugs with several subdivisions. H_1 antihistamines generally are employed for the treatment of allergic reactions, but are also used for sedation and as antiemetics. Two generations of H_1 antihistamines exist; the second generation generally is more specific with fewer side effects but more drug interactions. H_2 antihistamines are used specifically for gastrointestinal disorders related to increased gastric acid. All of the antihistamines are generally safe, albeit with caution advised in case of polypharmacy or specific conditions.

Resources

Organization	Description	Website
University of Utah College of Pharmacy	Oral Antihistamines Drug Class Review (2nd Generation). This report reviews the clinical application of second-generation H_1 antihistamines. Updated May 2014.	https://medicaid.utah.gov/pharmacy/ptcommittee/files/Criteria%20Review%20Documents/Antihistamines%202nd%20Generation%20Agents%20May%202014.pdf
Oregon Health & Science University	Drug Class Review: Newer Antihistamines Final Report Update 2. Comparative clinical effectiveness and harms of different antihistamines.	www.ncbi.nlm.nih.gov/books/NBK50558/
U.S. National Library of Medicine	Liver Tox. This site summarizes potential hepatotoxicity for a list of first- and second-generation individual antihistamines.	http://livertox.nih.gov/Antihistamines.htm

References

1. Chambers C, Kvedar JC, Armstrong AW. Histamine pharmacology. In: Golan D, ed. *Principles of Pharmacology: The Pathophysiologic Basis of Drug Therapy.* Philadelphia, PA: Lippincott Williams & Wilkins; 2012:765-773.
2. Bielory L, Ghafoor S. Histamine receptors and the conjunctiva. *Curr Opin Allergy Clin Immunol.* 2005;5(5):437-440.
3. Holgate ST, Canonica GW, Simons FE, et al. Consensus Group on New-Generation Antihistamines (CONGA): present status and recommendations. *Clin Exp Allergy.* 2003;33(9):1305-1324.
4. Ergun T, Kus S. Adverse systemic reactions of antihistamines: highlights in sedating effects, cardio-toxicity and drug interactions. *Curr Med Chem-Anti-inflammatory Anti-Allergy Agents.* 2005;4(5):507-515.
5. Bakker RA. Histamine H_3-receptor isoforms. *Inflamm Res.* 2004;53(10):509-516.
6. Smolinska S, Jutel M, Caremeri R. Histamine and gut mucosal immune regulation. *Eur J Allergy Clin Immun.* 2014;69:273-281.
7. Medina V, Cricco G, Nuñez M, et al. Histamine-mediated signaling processes in human malignant mammary cells. *Cancer Biol Ther.* 2006;5(11):1462-1471.

8. Müller T, Myrtek D, Bayer H, et al. Functional characterization of histamine receptor subtypes in a human bronchial epithelial cell line. *Int J Mol Med.* 2006;18(5):925-931.
9. Rosa AC, Fantozzi R. The role of histamine in neurogenic inflammation. *Br J Pharmacol.* 2013; 170(1): 38-45.
10. de Esch IJ, Thurmond RL, Jongejan A, Leurs R. The histamine H_4 receptor as a new therapeutic target for inflammation. *Trends Pharmacol Sci.* 2005;26(9): 462-469.
11. Salcedo C, Pontes C, Merlos M. Is the H_4 receptor a new drug target for allergies and asthma? *Front Biosci (Elite Ed).* 2013;5:178-187.
12. Dunford PJ, Williams KN, Desai PJ, Karalsson L, McQueen D, Thurmond RL. Histamine H_4 receptor antagonists are superior to traditional antihistamines in the attenuation of experimental pruritus. *J Allergy Clin Immunol.* 2007;119(1):176-183.
13. Fogel WA, Lewinski A, Jochem J. Histamine in idiopathic inflammatory bowel diseases: not a standby player. *Folia Med Cracov.* 2005;46(3-4):107-118.
14. Fung-Leung WP, Thurmond RL, Ling P, Karlsson L. Histamine H_4 receptor antagonists: the new antihistamines? *Curr Opin Investig Drugs.* 2004;5(11): 1174-1183.
15. Monczor F, Fernandez N, Fitzsimons CP, Shayo C, Davio C. Antihistaminergics and inverse agonism: potential therapeutic applications. *Eur J Pharmacol.* 2013;715:26-32.
16. Zhang M, Venable JD, Thurmond RL. The histamine H_4 receptor in autoimmune disease. *Expert Opin Investig Drugs.* 2006;15(11):1443-1452.
17. Leurs R, Church MK, Taglialatela M. H_1-antihistamines: inverse agonism, anti-inflammatory actions, and cardiac effects. *Clin Exp Allergy.* 2002;32(4): 489-498.
18. Sjogren B, Blazer LL, Neubig RR. Regulators of G-protein signaling proteins as targets for drug discovery. *Prog Mol Biol Transl Sci.* 2010;91:81-119.
19. Brock TP, Williams DM. Acute and chronic rhinitis. In: Alldredge BK, Corelli RL, Ernst ME, et al., eds. *Koda-Kimble and Young's Applied Therapeutics: The Clinical Use of Drugs.* 10th ed. Philadelphia, PA: Lippincott Williams & Wilkins; 2013;619-643.
20. Fugit RV, Berardi RR. Upper gastrointestinal disorders. In: Alldredge BK, Corelli RL, Ernst ME, et al., eds. *Koda-Kimble and Young's Applied Therapeutics: The Clinical Use of Drugs.* 10th ed. Philadelphia, PA: Lippincott Williams & Wilkins; 2013;660-698.
21. Nagel DS, Shields HM. Integrative inflammation pharmacology: peptic ulcer disease. In: Golan D, ed. *Principles of Pharmacology: The Pathophysiologic Basis of Drug Therapy.* Philadelphia, PA: Lippincott Williams & Wilkins; 2012;807-817.
22. Lebois EP, Jones CK, Lindsley CW. The evolution of histamine H_3 antagonists/inverse agonists. *Curr Top Med Chem.* 2011;11(6):648-660.
23. Kollmeier A, Francke K, Chen B, et al. The histamine H_4 receptor antagonist, JNJ 39758979, is effective in reducing histamine-induced pruritus in a randomized clinical study in healthy subjects. *J Pharmacol Exp Ther.* 2014;350(1):181-187.
24. Histamine and antihistamines. In: Brody TM, Crespo LM, Wecker L, eds. *Brody's Human Pharmacology: Molecular to Clinical* [e-book]. 5th ed. Philadelphia, PA: Elsevier-Mosby; 2010;154-161. Accessed May 1, 2014.
25. Richardson GS, Roehrs TA, Rosenthal L, Koshorek G, Roth T. Tolerance to daytime sedative effects of H_1 antihistamines. *J Clin Psychopharmacol.* 2002;22(5):511-515.
26. Verster JC, Volkerts ER. Antihistamines and driving ability: evidence from on-the-road driving studies during normal traffic. *Ann Allergy Asthma Immunol.* 2004;92(3):294-303; quiz 303-305, 355.
27. Katzung BG. Histamine, serotonin, and the ergot alkaloids. In: Katzung BG, Masters SB, Trevor AJ, eds. *Basic and Clinical Pharmacology.* 12th ed. New York: McGraw-Hill; 2012;273-281.
28. Demoly P, Messaad D, Benahmed S, Benahmed S, Sahla H, Bousquet J. Hypersensitivity to H_1-antihistamines. *Allergy.* 2000;55(7):681.
29. Simons FE, Simons KJ. Histamine and H_1-antihistamines: celebrating a century of progress. *J Allergy Clin Immunol.* 2011;128(6):1139-1150.
30. Mahdy AM, Webster NR. Histamines and antihistamines. *Anesthes Intensive Care Med.* 2011;12(7): 324-327.
31. Golightly LK, Greos LS. Second-generation antihistamines: actions and efficacy in the management of allergic disorders. *Drugs.* 2005;65(3):341-384.
32. Church DS, Church MK. Pharmacology of antihistamines. *World Allergy Organ.* J 2011;4(3 suppl): S22-S27.
33. Walsh GM, Annunziato L, Frossard N, et al. New insights into the second-generation antihistamines. *Drugs.* 2001;61(2):207-236.
34. Paakkari I. Cardiotoxicity of new antihistamines and cisapride. *Toxicol Lett.* 2002;127(1-3):279-284.

35. Woolsey RL, Chen Y, Freiman JP, Gillis RA. Mechanism of the cardiotoxic effects of terfenadine. *JAMA.* 1993;269(12):1532-1536.
36. Bielory L. Role of antihistamines in ocular allergy. *Am J Med.* 2002;113(suppl 9A):34S-37S.
37. Gallois-Bernos AC, Thurmond RL. Alcaftadine, a new antihistamine with combined antagonist activity at histamine H_1, H_2, and H_4 receptors. *J Receptor Ligand Channel Res.* 2012;5:9-20.
38. McLaurin EB, Marsico NP, Ackerman SL, et al. Ocular itch relief with alcaftadine 0.25% versus olopatadine 0.2% in allergic conjunctivitis: pooled analysis of two multicenter randomized clinical trials. *Adv Ther.* 2014;31(10):1059-1071.
39. Verster JC, Volkerts ER. Antihistamines and driving ability: evidence from on-the-road driving studies during normal traffic. *Ann Allergy Asthma Immunol.* 2004;92(3):294-303.
40. Korsgren M, Andersson M, Larsson L, Aldén-Roboisson M, Greiff L. Onset of action of topical antihistamine as assessed by histamine challenge-induced plasma exudation responses. *Ann Allergy Asthma Immunol.* 2006;96(2):345-348.
41. Abelson M, Gomes P, Pasquine T, et al. Efficacy of olopatadine ophthalmic solution 0.2% in reducing signs and symptoms of allergic conjunctivitis. *Allergy Asthma Proc.* 2007;28(4):427-433.
42. Bonat J, Dragon C, Arcangelo V. Gastroesophageal reflux disease and peptic ulcer disease. In: Arcangelo V, Peterson A, eds. *Pharmacotherapeutics for Advanced Practice: A Practical Approach.* 2nd ed. Philadelphia, PA: Lippincott Williams and Wilkins; 2006;372-385.
43. Clark SM, Dutta E, Hankins GD. The outpatient management and special considerations of nausea and vomiting in pregnancy. *Semin Perinatol.* 2014; 38(8):496-502.
44. Koren G. Treating morning sickness in the United States: changes in prescribing are needed. *Am J Obstet Gynecol.* 2014;211(6):602-6.
45. Magee LA, Mazzotta P, Koren G. Evidence-based view of safety and effectiveness of pharmacologic therapy for nausea and vomiting of pregnancy. *Am J Obstet Gynecol.* 2002;186(5):S256-S261.
46. Mazzotta P, Magee LA. A risk–benefit assessment of pharmacological treatments for nausea and vomiting of pregnancy. *Drugs.* 2000;59(4):781-800.
47. Kallen B. Use of antihistamine drugs in early pregnancy and delivery outcomes. *J Matern Fetal Neonatal Med.* 2002;11:146-152.
48. Gilboa SM, Strickland MJ, Olshan AF, et al. Use of antihistamine medications during early pregnancy and isolated major malformations. *Birth Defects Res Part A Clin Mol Teratol.* 2009;85(2):137-150.
49. Garbis H, Elefant E, Diav-Citrin O, et al. Pregnancy outcome after exposure to ranitidine and other H_2-blockers: a collaborative study of the European Network of Teratology Information Services. *Reprod Toxicol.* 2005;19(4):453-458.
50. Mazzotta P, Koren G. Nonsedating antihistamines in pregnancy. *Can Fam Physician.* 1997;43: 1509-1511.
51. American Academy of Pediatrics Committee on Drugs. The transfer of drugs and other chemicals into human milk. *Pediatrics.* 2001;108(3):776-789.
52. Hagemann TM. Gastrointestinal medications and breastfeeding. *J Hum Lact.* 1998;14(3):259-262.
53. Hale T. *Medications and Mother's Milk.* 15th ed. Amarillo, TX: Hale; 2012.
54. Hansen J, Klimek L, Hörmann K. Pharmacological management of allergic rhinitis in the elderly: safety issues with oral antihistamines. *Drugs Aging.* 2005; 22(4):289-296.
55. Tawadrous D, Dixon S, Shariff SZ, et al. Altered mental status in older adults with histamine$_2$-receptor antagonists: a population-based study. *Eur J Intern Med.* 2014;25(8):701-709.
56. Kiss R, Keserű GM. Histamine H_4 receptor ligands and their potential therapeutic applications: an update. *Expert Opin Ther Pat.* 2012;22(3):205-221.
57. Tiligada E, Zampeli E, Sander K, Stark H. Histamine H_3 and H_4 receptors as novel drug targets. *Expert Opin Investig Drugs.* 2009;18(10):1519-1531.

14 Steroid Hormones

Mary C. Brucker, Frances E. Likis

Chapter Glossary

Androgens Original anabolic steroid and one of the major sex steroids.

Androstane derivatives Sex steroids that possess 19 carbons; this category includes androgens.

Androstenedione Androgen that is converted, along with testosterone, to estrone (E_1).

Antiestrogens Agents that block the actions of estrogens.

Antiprogestin Agent that blocks the action of progestins.

Aromatization Chemical reaction needed for production of stable endogenous estrogen.

Conjugation Chemical process that attaches a molecule to an existing drug or chemical. The resultant conjugated drug is water soluble and therefore able to be excreted renally.

Esterification Chemical process that converts an acid into an ester. When estrogens are esterified, they become more lipid-soluble and oral bioavailiablity is improved.

Estradiol (E_2) Main endogenous estrogen of the reproductive years.

Estrane derivatives Sex steroids that possess 18 carbons; this category includes estrogens.

Estriol (E_3) Weak estrogen that is produced primarily by the placenta.

Estrogens One of the major sex steroids for women.

Estrogen receptors Receptors found throughout the body that bind with estrogens through the cell membrane.

Estrone (E_1) The major estrogen in the postmenopausal period.

Micronization Chemical process that reduces the diameter/size of a chemical. The process can improve absorption.

Phytoestrogens Nonsteroidal botanicals that possess estrogenic activity themselves or are metabolized into compounds with estrogen activity.

Pregnane derivatives Sex steroids that possess 21 carbons; this category includes progestins and corticoids.

Progesterone One of the major endogenous sex steroids for women.

Progestins Umbrella term for naturally occurring agents (progesterone) and synthetic (progestogens).

Progestogen Synthetic progesterone.

Relative binding affinity (RBA) Method that attempts to characterize the potency of progestins by addressing their binding affinity with progesterone receptors.

Steroidogenesis Process by which steroid hormones are derived. In humans, the process is initiated from cholesterol, and through a series of steps, estrogen, progesterone, androgens, testosterone, cortisol, corticoids, and aldosterone are produced.

Testosterone Endogenously derived from the androgen group; important sex hormone for men and women.

Introduction

Endogenous hormones play essential roles in physiologic functions within the human body. The steroid hormones that were traditionally thought to affect reproduction only, actually have global effects on a woman's body.[1] However, it was not until the twentieth century that these agents were isolated and ultimately synthesized. From a modern perspective, sophisticated chemical analysis is done every day. Thus, it might seem amazing that it took U.S. chemist Edward Doisy 4 tons of sows' ovaries, or approximately 8000 individual ovaries, to obtain a mere 12 milligrams of **estradiol (E_2)** in the late 1920s.[2] A few months later, the German scientist Adolf Butenandt reported that he had independently isolated 20 milligrams of estradiol from the urine of more than 2000 pregnant women. Butenandt also is credited with isolating **testosterone** through an experiment in which he obtained 15 milligrams of androsterone from approximately 17,000 liters of male urine.[3] Eventually, both Doisy and Butenandt received Nobel Prizes in chemistry.

Isolation of **progesterone** followed within a decade. In 1937, Russell Marker, an American chemist, was the first to isolate pregnanediol and then convert it to progesterone. Marker had been intrigued with botanicals and imported Mexican yams, purportedly illegally, into his laboratory for study. Some reports state it took between 9 and 10 tons of Mexican yams to ultimately produce approximately 3 kilograms of progesterone. At the time, these few kilograms were highly valuable, with an estimated worth of approximately $250,000. They provided Marker with the ability to cofound a new pharmaceutical company. Named *Syntex*, a word derived from combining "synthetic" and "Mexican," it flourished for years, even after Marker left, primarily producing oral contraceptives and cortisol until it was acquired and subsumed by Roche Group, the pharmaceutical division of the Swiss company Hoffmann-La Roche AG, in 1990.[4,5]

Today, **estrogens**, **progestins**, and **androgens** are popular pharmaceuticals. These sex steroids are used for numerous indications, especially in the area of women's health care, and synthetic agents are widely available. However, the future of hormone therapies is likely to involve the development of agents that are more than simple replicates of endogenous hormones. New designer hormones attempt to maximize therapeutic effects while minimizing adverse effects and have opened a new realm of possibilities for treatment.

The classic definition of a hormone is an agent produced in one gland that travels through the bloodstream to stimulate, via chemical action, a function in another part of the body, from the Greek *horman*, meaning "to urge on". Hormones are responsible for paracrine communication, which is intercellular communication via local diffusion of regulating substances that affect nearby tissue, as well as autocrine communication, which is intracellular communication whereby a single cell produces regulating substances that act upon receptors on or within the same cell.

Based on their chemical composition, hormones are subdivided into the following classes: amines, peptides, prostaglandins, and steroids. All steroid hormones are derived from cholesterol, yet small changes in the molecules produce the three different types of steroids: (1) mineralocorticoids, such as aldosterone, that affect salt (mineral) balance; (2) glucocorticoids, such as cortisol, that affect glucose metabolism; and (3) gonadocorticoids, or sex steroids.[6] The gonadocorticoids include estrogen, progesterone, and androgen. The gonadocorticoids are grouped together as a family because of their shared ability to affect reproductive function.

This chapter provides an overview of the pharmacology of the sex steroid hormones. Pharmacotherapeutics of sex steroids are discussed in depth in additional chapters including *Contraception, Sexual Dysfunction,* and *The Mature Woman.*

Physiologic Functions of Sex Steroids

Steroidogenesis

Steroidogenesis is the process by which steroids are biosynthesized or produced endogenously. All steroids are formed from cholesterol, a 27-carbon steroid. Sex steroids are formed when cholesterol is further broken down into one of three groups. These groups are classified by their number of carbon atoms: **pregnane derivatives** have 21 carbons, **androstane derivatives** have 19 carbons, and **estrane derivatives** have 18 carbons. These groups—which are the precursors of progesterone, androgens, and estrogens, respectively—are summarized in Table 14-1 and depicted in Figure 14-1.[2,7]

Estrogen and Progesterone

Estrogen and progesterone are the primary sex steroids in females. Estrogen, a term derived from the Greek for "mad desire," is the sex steroid responsible for the majority of the development and maintenance of the female reproductive system and secondary sex characteristics. Estrogen

Table 14-1 Cholesterol Derivations and Products

Derivation from Cholesterol	Number of Carbons	Products
Pregnane	21	Progestogens and corticoids
Androstane	19	Androgens
Estrane	18	Estrogens

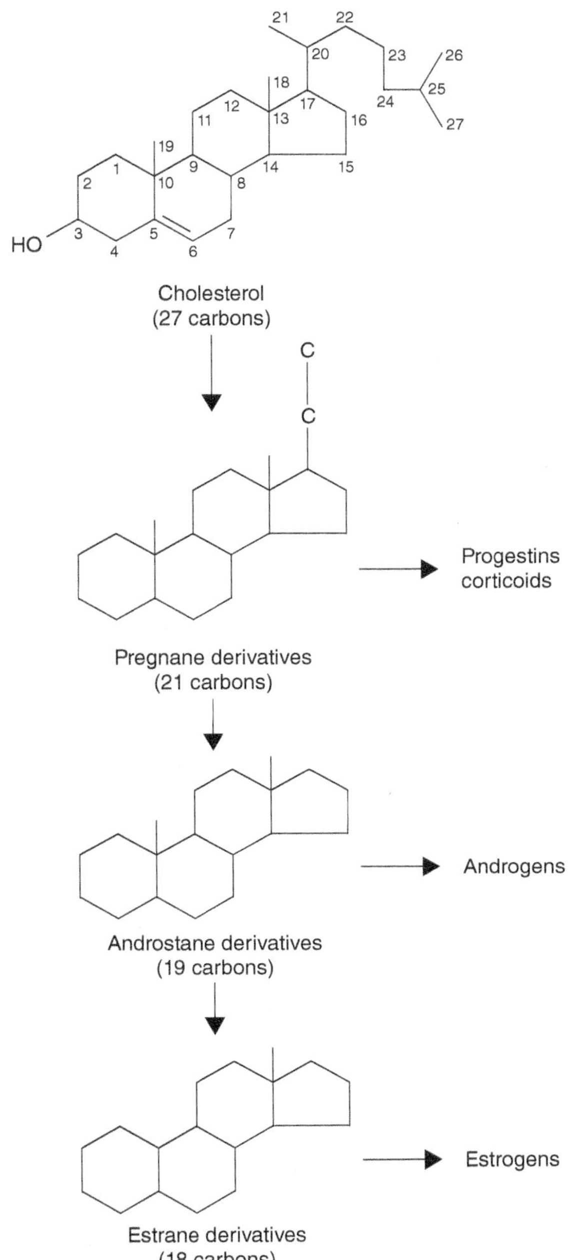

Figure 14-1 Biosynthesis of sex steroids.

also makes contributions to skeletal shape, urogenital tone and elasticity, and bone changes that allow for the growth spurt that occurs during puberty.[8]

Progesterone acts on the reproductive tract, where it causes the endometrium to change from proliferative to secretory during the second half of the menstrual cycle. Progesterone is a potent mitogen or promoter of cell division in the development of normal breast tissue[9] and it also induces thickening of the cervical mucus. Progesterone also has critical effects on other systems, including the central nervous system, the immune response, coagulation, gallbladder activity, and core temperature to name a few. Both estrogen and progesterone have essential roles in the menstrual cycle and during pregnancy/lactation. Progesterone, in particular, has an important role in female contraception.

Combined Estrogen and Progestins

Although both estrogen and progestins have been used as medications for decades, much remains to be discovered about these hormones. In particular, many of the studies exploring outcomes of women using estrogen-containing contraceptives or perimenopausal hormone therapy involve combination agents. Few data exist regarding the potential synergy or interactions of these agents, especially when both hormones are used simultaneously. At best, some studies have explored differences between women using a single hormone versus outcomes in women using both, such as in investigations that have compared progestin-only contraception with combined hormonal contraceptives. The following discussions of these hormones, particularly regarding their benefits and risks, should be viewed within this context.

Overview of the Menstrual Cycle

Knowledge of menstrual physiology is needed to understand the pharmacologic applications of sex steroid hormones. Details of the complexity involved in this natural phenomenon have continued to emerge in the last few decades as researchers have studied primates and humans, instead of earlier knowledge obtained from murine models. This body of research has revealed that prior assumptions

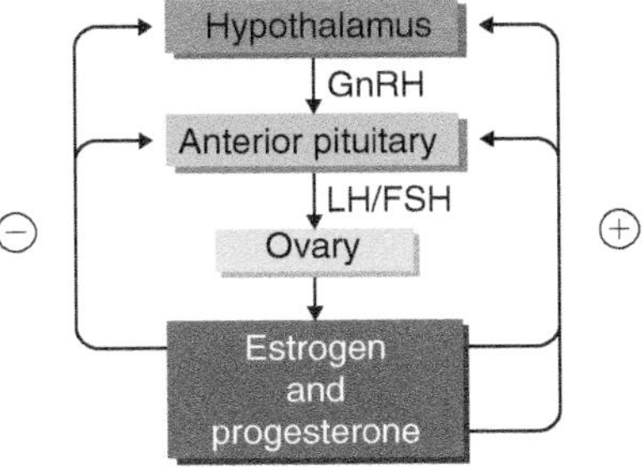

The hypothalmus–pituitary–ovarian axis operates under a negative feedback loop except during the immediate preovulatory period of days 12–14, when it becomes a positive feedback loop.

Figure 14-2 Hormonal regulation of the menstrual cycle.

based on rat models were false. This subsection provides a brief overview of this sophisticated process; however, the interested reader is directed to reproductive physiology texts, such as that by Speroff and Fritz, for more detailed information.[2]

The menstrual cycle is the result of intricate interactions among a number of hormones in the hypothalamic–pituitary–ovarian axis, as illustrated in Figure 14-2. During the first half, or follicular ovarian phase of the menstrual cycle, release of gonadotropin-releasing hormone (GnRH) from the hypothalamus stimulates secretion of follicle-stimulating hormone (FSH) and luteinizing hormone (LH) from the pituitary. FSH promotes maturation of follicles in the ovaries, which begin to secrete estrogen as they mature. Simultaneously, during this first half of the menstrual cycle, the endometrium proliferates under the influence of estrogen. Table 14-2 summarizes the hormonal fluctuations that occur during the normal menstrual cycle. Once critical blood levels of estrogen are attained, feedback to the pituitary signals a release of LH and more FSH. The surge of LH results in ovulation, the release of an egg from the dominant follicle.

Table 14-2 Overview of Endogenous Estrogen and Progesterone During the Menstrual Cycle

Days	Ovarian Cycle	Endometrial Cycle	Estrogen and Progesterone	Actions
1–5	Follicular	Menstrual	Low estrogen and progesterone	Inhibin falls. LH and FSH begin to slowly rise, starting on approximately day 27.
6–14	Follicular	Proliferative	Building estrogen and (to lesser extent) progesterone	LH initiates luteinization and progesterone production in the granulosa layer. The rise of progesterone facilitates positive feedback action of estrogen and may be necessary for the midcycle FSH peak, although the complete reason for midcycle FSH peak remains unclear. Estrogen production becomes sufficient to achieve and maintain the threshold concentration of estradiol that is required to induce the LH surge. A midcycle increase in local and peripheral androgens occurs, derived from the thecal tissue of unsuccessful follicles. A few hours after the LH surge, changes in hormone-level release suppression of oocyte maturation.
14	Ovulation	Proliferative	High estrogen and building progesterone	High levels of estrogen induce the LH surge at midcycle, and high levels of estrogen lead to sustained, elevated LH secretion. Suppression of inhibition of oocyte maturation allows final maturation of the oocyte. LH surge occurs and is responsible for luteinization of the granulosa, and synthesis of progesterones and prostaglandins in the follicle. Progesterone and prostaglandins work together to digest, weaken, and eventually rupture the follicular wall. The midcycle FSH peak frees the oocyte from follicular attachments and ensures sufficient LH receptors to allow an adequate normal luteal phase.
15–26	Luteal	Secretory (implantation phase)	Progesterone most dominant, but estrogen present	Progesterone from the corpus luteum acts both centrally and within the ovary to suppress new follicular growth. High levels of progesterone inhibit pituitary secretion of gonadotropins by inhibiting GnRH pulses at the level of the hypothalamus. High levels of progesterone antagonize the pituitary response to GnRH by interfering with estrogen action. Regression of the corpus luteum may involve luteolytic action of its own estrogen production, mediated by an alteration in local prostaglandin concentration. In early pregnancy, hCG maintains luteal function until placental steroidogenesis is established.
27–28	Luteal	Late secretory (ischemic)	Dropping estrogen and progesterone	The degeneration of corpus luteum results in low levels of estrogen, progesterone, and inhibin. The low level of inhibin removes the suppression of FSH on the pituitary. The low level of estrogen and progesterone allows an increase in GnRH pulsatile secretion and the removal of the pituitary from the negative feedback suppression. The removal of inhibin and estradiol and increased GnRH pulses allow an increase in FSH (and, to a lesser extent, LH). The increasing FSH is instrumental in the maturation of a dominant follicle.

Abbreviations: FSH = follicle stimulating hormone; GnRH = gonadotropin-releasing hormone; hCG = human chorionic gonadotropin; LH = luteinizing hormone.

In the second half, or luteal ovarian phase of the menstrual cycle, the follicle becomes the site of the corpus luteum, which primarily secretes large amounts of progesterone. Under the influence of progesterone, the endometrium height stabilizes while the glands become tortuous, layers of the endometrium develop, and a glycogen-rich fluid is secreted from the endometrium. These endometrial changes are in preparation for implantation should fertilization occur.

If the egg is not fertilized, progesterone produced by the corpus luteum suppresses secretion of LH and FSH and the corpus luteum degenerates in about 14 days. When the corpus luteum degenerates, progesterone levels fall and this change in hormone levels results in ischemia of the endometrium and initiation of menstruation.

In addition to their association with the ovaries and endometrium, estrogen and progesterone influence cyclic changes in other reproductive organs. As estrogen levels increase immediately prior to ovulation, the cervical mucus becomes clear, thin, abundant, and stretchy. During the second half of the menstrual cycle, when progesterone predominates, the cervical mucus decreases in amount and becomes opaque, thick, and viscous. Estrogen stimulates movement in the fallopian tubes to facilitate ovum transport, whereas progesterone reverses this effect.[2,10] Understanding the physiologic functions of estrogen and progesterone is essential for rational prescribing of the pharmacologic preparations of both hormones.

Estrogen

Estrogen is the generic term for a chemically similar family of endogenous hormones and exogenous compounds with an affinity for **estrogen receptors**.[6,8] Estrogen receptors are intracellular receptors present on the membrane of the cell nucleus. Two types of estrogen receptors (ER-α and ER-β) have been identified throughout the body in both males and females. These receptors have different tissue distributions. Specifically, a woman's body has more ER-α receptors than men, with many of them found in the female reproductive organs and liver and more ER-β receptors found in other tissues.[8] Strong receptor activity has been suggested to enhance the innate immunocompetency of an individual.[11,12] More receptor activity is likely to appear in cells with alpha receptors, although major research into ER-β is under way and may result in a deeper understanding of estrogen receptors in general.[13]

ER-α is expressed in the tissue of the uterus, ovary (theca cells), bone, breast, brain, liver, and adipose tissue. ER-β is expressed in the colon, ovary (granulosa cells), bone marrow, salivary gland, vascular endothelium, and brain.[14] The complexity of this distribution becomes important when designing new drugs. One type of drug, an estrogen agonist/antagonist (EAA), is an agent that can bind to either ER-α or ER-β and can cause either agonist or antagonist properties at the receptor site.[6] The EAAs, which are also known as selective estrogen receptor modulators (SERMs), are discussed later in this chapter.

Receptors remain under intensive study, and there is discussion of potential cloning of receptors as well as investigation of the relationships between specific receptors and risks of cancer. Estrogen receptors also are important factors when a woman is being treated for an estrogen-sensitive cancer. Chemotherapeutic agents that interfere with estrogens are addressed in the *Cancer* chapter.

As cholesterol undergoes steroidogenesis, estrogens are derived from androgens via **aromatization**, or development of a benzene ring. Three estrogens are produced naturally in the female body: **estrone (E_1)**, estradiol (E_2), and **estriol (E_3)**. These three estrogens vary in quantity and in potency. In this context, potency is defined as the hormone's affinity for estrogen receptors. Among reproductive-aged women, 17 β-estradiol (estradiol) is produced in the largest quantity through biosynthesis in the ovary. More than 95% of endogenous estradiol is produced in the ovaries, with the remainder produced via peripheral aromatization of estrone.[8] Of the three types of estrogens produced endogenously, estradiol is the most potent because it has the highest binding affinity for estrogen receptors, and it binds to both ER-α and ER-β receptors. Following menopause, estradiol levels drop to 10% or less of premenopausal levels.

Estrone is a metabolite of estradiol and is less potent than estradiol. It is primarily produced via the conversion of **androstenedione** in adipose tissue. In postmenopausal women, the ovary ceases producing estradiol, but the adrenal gland continues making androstenedione, the immediate precursor to estrone; additionally, estrone continues to be produced in the tissues of the body, particularly in adiposity or fat, so the levels of estrone remain unchanged while the plasma levels of estradiol fall markedly. As a result, estrone begins to be the estrogen present in largest quantity in postmenopausal women.[8]

The third endogenous estrogen, estriol, is a metabolite of estradiol and estrone in the periphery and is not secreted by the ovaries. Instead, estriol is the principal estrogen produced by the placenta during pregnancy, although it can be found in very small quantities among women who are not pregnant.[2,8]

Pharmacologic Uses of Estrogen

The pharmacotherapeutic uses of estrogen are discussed in depth in other chapters of this text. In brief, exogenous estrogens primarily are used by women for contraception and menopausal hormone therapy. In the 1960s and 1970s, one type of oral contraceptives, called sequentials, contained estrogen only for three weeks before progesterone was added for the final week of a monthly cycle. These contraceptives were removed from the market in the mid-1970s. Today, all of the estrogen-containing oral contraceptives are tablets that contain both estrogen and a progestin of some dose; thus they are referred to as combined hormonal contraceptives.

Three major combined hormonal contraceptive methods contain estrogen: combined oral contraceptives, the contraceptive vaginal ring (NuvaRing), and the transdermal contraceptive patch (Evra). The estrogenic component of combined hormonal contraceptives exerts its major effect via suppression of FSH, which prevents the selection and emergence of a dominant follicle. Estrogen also stabilizes the endometrium to minimize breakthrough bleeding. In addition, estrogen potentiates the action of the progestin component, which allows for lower doses of progestin.[6] Additional information about hormonal contraception can be found in the *Contraception* chapter.

Hormone therapy for treatment of menopausal symptoms is usually divided into two categories: (1) estrogen therapy provided to women who have had a hysterectomy and no longer have a uterus; and (2) estrogen plus progestin therapy, sometimes called hormone therapy. A progestin is added to estrogen for women who have an intact uterus to protect against estrogen-induced endometrial cancer. More information on these therapies can be found in the chapter *The Mature Woman*. Note that the word *replacement* in the previously used term, *hormone replacement therapy*, is no longer recommended when referring to these therapies because these formulations do not contain dosages sufficient to reach or replace premenopausal hormone levels.[15] Estrogen is prescribed for perimenopausal and postmenopausal women to alleviate menopausal symptoms that are troublesome for some individual women.

Pharmacologic Properties of Estrogen

Estrogens, like all steroids, are highly lipid soluble. Therefore, they diffuse easily through cell membranes. When estrogen reaches one of the many different tissues that contain cells with estrogen receptors, it passes into the cell and through the nuclear membrane. Inside the nucleus, it attaches to an estrogen receptor. The hormone/receptor unit then binds to co-factors and the resultant compound attaches to DNA binding sites and initiates gene transcription. Such transcription provides a virtual script that directs the production of specific proteins that will affect physiologic action.[16]

In the bloodstream, the vast majority of estrogen (69%) is bound to a protein called sex hormone-binding globulin (SHBG). Another 30% of estrogen is loosely bound to albumin, which leaves only 1% of the free estrogen available to diffuse into cells within tissues.[2] SHBG levels are increased in hyperthyroidism and pregnancy and when exogenous estrogens are present; conversely, levels of this globulin are decreased when androgens, progestins, insulin, and corticoids are administered or when central obesity exists.[13] Thus, the amount of circulating free estrogens is also influenced by these factors.

The effect of estrogen, whether produced endogenously or administered exogenously, depends on several factors. The first consideration is the relative potency of the estrogen type. Potency depends on the amount of free hormone available to diffuse across cell membranes and bind to a receptor, the hormone's affinity for estrogen receptors, and how long the estrogen remains bound to the receptor. The amount of free hormone available depends on the amount of SHBG present; SHBG is produced in the liver. Ultimately, the effect(s) estrogen has on physiologic function depends on the agonist or antagonist response that occurs following binding to the estrogen receptor within the target cell.[16]

After potency and receptor agonist/antagonist properties, the metabolism of endogenous estrogen is the next important factor to be considered in evaluation of pharmacologic products. Estrogens are well absorbed from the gastrointestinal tract as well as through the skin or mucous membranes.[15] Estrogen is metabolized into biologically less active or inactive forms via two mechanisms: (1) **conjugation** into water-soluble and nonbiologically active metabolites, which can then be excreted via the kidney; or (2) conversion into estrone or estriol, which are biologically active, but approximately 10 times less potent than estradiol.[16]

Estrogens are conjugated naturally in the liver, where they are altered to become structurally similar to bile acids. These metabolites are then excreted into the gastrointestinal tract via the bile ducts. In the intestine, normal bacterial flora unconjugate the estrogens, making them once again lipid soluble. This lipid-soluble, biologically active form is reabsorbed via the entero-hepatic circulation and thereby recycled into the circulation as an active metabolite.[16]

Orally ingested exogenous estrogen is metabolized rapidly into estrone in both the intestine and liver before it reaches the general circulation. This first-pass effect markedly decreases the amount of estrogen available for circulation. Non-oral estrogen formulations circumvent this first-pass effect and can reach therapeutic plasma levels at lower doses than oral formulations, although often it takes a longer time to achieve peak levels when non-oral formulations are used. For example, an oral contraceptive reaches peak plasma levels at 2 hours, whereas the estrogen patch (Evra) takes 48 hours to do so.

Estrogen Preparations

Pharmacologic estrogen preparations can be divided into six main groups: (1) human natural estrogens; (2) nonhuman natural estrogens; (3) synthetic estrogen mixtures; (4) synthetic estrogen analogues with a steroid molecular structure; (5) synthetic estrogen analogues without a steroid skeleton; and (6) plant-based estrogens without a steroid skeleton (Table 14-3).[15] The plant-based estrogens are also known as **phytoestrogens**; these naturally occurring products are available without a prescription. Estrogen formulations can be composed of one estrogen only or they can be combination products with varying amounts of chemically distinct estrogens. All formulations have a high affinity for estrogen receptors and stimulate estrogen function.[14]

The only human estrogen that is available as an FDA-approved drug is 17 β-estradiol, which is used for treatment of menopausal symptoms. Oral estradiol is micronized to enhance absorption. Estradiol also is absorbed rapidly through the skin, so it is commonly used in non-oral formulations such as transdermal and topical estrogen products.[1,4]

The nonhuman conjugated equine estrogens (CEEs) are derived from the urine of pregnant mares and primarily used for treatment of menopausal symptoms. Conjugated formulations of estrogen are made water soluble to promote oral absorption. The conjugated equine hormone marketed as the brand name Premarin contains at least 10 active estrogens—primarily sodium estrone sulfate (approximately 45%) and sodium equilin sulfate (approximately 25%). CEEs are the most frequently used estrogen products worldwide, and also the estrogen formulations that have been used in the majority of published clinical trials.[15,16] At this time, a generic version of CEE (Premarin) is not available in the United States.

Table 14-3 Pharmacologic Formulations of Estrogen

Category	Examples of Available Formulations and Clinical Use
Human natural estrogens, including estrone (E_1), 17 β-estradiol (E_2), and estriol	17 β-estradiol used for treatment for menopausal symptoms. Alkyl group often modified to facilitate different methods of administration.
Nonhuman estrogens	Conjugated equine estrogens (Premarin): a combination of several different estrogens isolated from the urine of pregnant mares. Used for treatment of menopausal symptoms.
Phytoestrogens	Plant derived xenoestrogens. Naturally occurring nonsteroidal plant compounds that are structurally similar to estradiol. Phytoestrogens are weakly estrogenic. Found in a wide variety of foods and botanicals, although doses are not standardized.
Synthetic estrogen mixtures	Synthetic conjugated estrogens (Cenestin, Enjuvia) are derived from yam or soy plants. Esterified estrogens (Menest) are derived from conjugated equine estrogens. Both synthetic estrogens are used to treat menopausal symptoms.
Synthetic estrogen analogs with a steroid molecular structure	Ethinyl estradiol is a synthetic compound that has ethinyl added to estradiol in order to make the formulation active when taken orally. Used in contraceptive agents and some formulations that treat menopausal symptoms. Estropipate (Ortho-Est) is a synthetic salt of estrone sulfate and piperazine. Used for treating menopausal symptoms.

Source: Data from North American Menopause Society. *Menopause Practice: A Clinician's Guide.* 5th ed. Cleveland, OH: North American Menopause Society; 2010.[15]

Two types of synthetic estrogen mixtures exist that are primarily used for menopausal hormone therapy: synthetic conjugated estrogens and esterified estrogens. The synthetic conjugated estrogen mixtures are derived from yam or soy plants and contain several types of estrogen. Both synthetic conjugated estrogen products available in the United States (Cenestin with 9 estrogens and Enjuvia with 10 estrogens) contain the primary estrogens in CEE, but the products are not considered equivalent to Premarin. **Esterification** is the process whereby estrogen is bound to a sulfate in order to alter the pharmcokinetics. Esterified estrogens are more lipophilic and have an extended half-life. The esterified estrogens (Menest) are derived from CEE, and their principal component is sodium estrone sulfate.[15,16]

Ethinyl estradiol and estropipate are the two synthetic estrogens with a steroid molecular structure. Prior to development of **micronization**, estradiol medications could not be well absorbed by the gastrointestinal tract. Ethinyl estradiol was a breakthrough drug—the result of researchers' realization that adding ethinyl to estradiol creates an estrogen that is active after oral administration.[2] Ethinyl estradiol is the form of estrogen found in the contraceptive vaginal ring (NuvaRing), the transdermal contraceptive patch (Evra), some menopausal treatments (e.g., Femhrt), and almost all of the combined oral contraceptives.

A few older combined oral contraceptives containing mestranol instead of ethinyl remain on the market, but most have been replaced by products that contain ethinyl estradiol. Estropipate (Ortho-Est) is used by postmenopausal women as hormone therapy and is an oral form of estrone sulfate with piperazine added for solubility and stability.[15]

Nonsteroidal synthetic estrogen analogues include diethylstilbestrol (DES), dienestrol, benzestrol, hexestrol, methestrol, methallenestril, and chlorotrianisene.[9] None of these compounds is currently available in the United States.[10,17] DES has an important role in the history of prescribing sex steroids. Phytoestrogens are plant-derived compounds that have estrogenic activity. They are nonsteroidal and have weak estrogen effects. Phytoestrogens are discussed in more detail later in this chapter.

Routes of Administration

Estrogen may be administered by the oral, vaginal, topical, transdermal, and injection routes. Vaginal formulations of estrogens include creams, rings, and tablets. Transdermal and topical estrogen products include patches, gels, and emulsions. An estradiol transdermal spray for women with postmenopausal vasomotor symptoms is marketed with the brand name Evamist.[18]

Benefits

The effectiveness of estrogen as a contraceptive (with added progestin), for treatment of women with vasomotor symptoms and vulvovaginal atrophy, and for prevention of osteoporosis among women is well established. Contraceptive formulations containing estrogen and progestins are highly effective for preventing pregnancy and also provide several major noncontraceptive benefits, as discussed in the chapter *Contraception*. As women age and endogenous estrogen levels decline, exogenous estrogens are an effective treatment for women who experience vasomotor symptoms such as hot flashes and night sweats. Decreased estrogen levels can also lead to vulvar and vaginal atrophy. Estrogen therapy improves vaginal atrophy and associated symptoms, such as vaginal dryness, urinary symptoms (for some women), and dyspareunia. In addition, estrogen therapy decreases bone resorption, which prevents bone loss and reduces the risk of osteoporotic fracture. Estrogen use by older women is discussed in detail in the chapter *The Mature Woman*.

Several other potential benefits of estrogen have been investigated. Toward the end of the twentieth century, a large body of observational data suggested that estrogen might be cardioprotective, especially for mature women. The vast majority of these studies were conducted among women using conjugated equine estrogens and for varying periods of time in relationship to natural menopause as well as varying durations of use. However, other findings regarding estrogen's ability to reduce the risk of heart disease were conflicting. A large randomized controlled trial in the early twenty-first century, known as the Women's Health Initiative, was designed to clarify questions about estrogen's cardioprotective effects. The study failed to find cardiac benefits, although some authorities questioned those results.[19] Points that were debated included the unknown influence of length of time between menopause and hormone initiation, the ages of the participants, the effect of preexisting coronary conditions, and the type of hormone and dose used. Many of the questions remain unanswered even today. For example, an observational study of almost 500,000 women using estradiol with or without a progestin was published in 2015. This research suggested that use of estradiol was associated with fewer cardiac events and deaths than otherwise would have been expected in the study population and reignited the debate about the type of estrogen that should be used.[20]

The preponderance of evidence, however, has not found clear cardiac benefits associated with estrogen therapy. Therefore, the North American Menopause Society (NAMS) does not recommend estrogen for protection against development of heart disease in women of any age.[14] Additional benefits of perimenopausal and postmenopausal estrogen use that have been reported in a number of studies include improved sleep, improved mood, increased sexual desire, and maintained or improved cognition, but the evidence for these effects is inconclusive to date.[14,15]

Side Effects/Adverse Effects

Estrogen has unintended effects that range from simply bothersome to serious complications. The most common side effects of estrogen are of the bothersome type, including nausea, breast tenderness, headache, and dizziness. Non-oral formulations can have side effects specific to the route of delivery. For example, women using estrogen patches may experience skin irritation, while women using the vaginal ring may experience vaginal discharge. Some major adverse effects also exist.

Thromboembolic Disease

Perhaps the most serious adverse effects associated with the use of estrogen are deep vein thrombosis (DVT) and other associated thromboembolic events such as pulmonary emboli. Early studies of oral contraceptives noted that the incidence of DVT decreased as the dosage of estrogen was lowered.[21,22] In 2007, it was suggested that use of transdermal contraceptive patches might also increase the risk of DVT and other associated conditions such as stroke and myocardial infarction. This finding was somewhat surprising because transdermal patches avoid the first-pass effect; consequently, it was thought women were exposed to lower doses of estrogen through this route of administration. However, this area of research remains under investigation.[22]

The risk of DVT is increased when estrogen is used by postmenopausal women. In addition to estrogen, some progestins used in contraceptives appear to be associated with a risk for developing DVT either independently or synergistically with estrogen.

Endometrial Cancer

Estrogen dosing, when administered alone, often is termed *unopposed.* Unopposed estrogen therapy increases the risk of endometrial cancer. In turn, women who take estrogen and who have an intact uterus also should receive a progestin regularly for the express purpose of decreasing their risk of developing endometrial cancer. Progestins can be administered orally daily or sequentially, via an intrauterine contraceptive device, or using another set pattern. Women who have experienced a hysterectomy may take unopposed estrogen with such a risk.

Breast and Ovarian Cancer

Estrogen is theorized to be associated, at least to some degree, with the development of breast cancer, albeit not necessarily as the single etiologic agent. Most breast tumors have estrogen receptors and some have progesterone receptors. The risk for breast cancer appears to be increased in women who also have obesity, infertility, delayed pregnancy, early menarche, and late menopause—all factors that are associated with periods of added estrogen exposure without the protection of progesterone.[2] Progesterone's role is less clear in breast cancer, even though it is known that progesterone plays a role in mitotic activity, as demonstrated during both the thelarche and luteal phases of the menstrual cycle.

In the Women's Health Initiative study, researchers found that women taking both estrogen and progestin had a small but significant increase in breast cancer (hazard ratio [HR], 1.26; 95% confidence interval [CI], 1.00–1.59; $N = 290$ cases), while women taking only estrogen had no significant increase in risk.[23,24] A later review of women and breast cancer investigated risks for women 5 years after the initial Women's Health Initiative report. In this study, scientists found that taking combined hormone therapy for 5 years doubled the risk for breast cancer, although the risk declined rapidly after discontinuation of this therapy.[25] Such a difference between estrogen-only regimens and combination estrogen/progestin regimens underscored the lack of knowledge about the combination therapy. These findings also emphasize the importance of shared decision making. As part of the informed consent (or refusal) process, women should be told that all risks—and even benefits—of estrogen therapy are probably not known at this time. If a woman chooses to use hormone therapy, she should always receive the lowest dose that relieves her symptoms, and use of estrogen therapy should be reviewed at each healthcare visit.

Ovarian cancer has been believed to be less influenced by estrogen and progestins than either endometrial or breast cancer, and many studies have failed to find clear evidence of an increased risk for women taking estrogen or any association with increasing duration of use.[2] However, approximately half of all studies are unpublished. In 2015, a review of 52 studies that were both published and unpublished, which collectively involved more than 12,000 women in the United States and Europe, found a significant association between estrogen use and ovarian cancer. Among women using estrogen-only therapy or estrogen/progestin combinations for 5 years or less, there was an increase in ovarian cancer incidence of more than 40% (risk ratio [RR], 1.43; 95% CI, 1.31–1.56; $P < 0.0001$).[26] The increased risk based on these epidemiologic findings decreased over time, but was still apparent 10 years after discontinuation of the estrogen product. Moreover, women with the *BRCA1* gene have a 60% lifetime risk of ovarian cancer. Women with the *BRCA2* gene have a 30% lifetime risk of developing ovarian cancer.[27] In conclusion, the risk of ovarian cancer may be negatively influenced by estrogen and/or estrogen and progestins, but additional studies are needed to clarify these relationships.

Phytoestrogens

Phytoestrogens are weak plant-derived substances that are structurally similar to estrogens and bind to estrogen receptors.[8,28] Some scientists advocate that phytoestrogens should be termed "estrogen agonists" and/or "estrogen antagonists" because these foods and supplements can bind to estrogen receptors and be viewed similarly to the so-called designer drugs that are discussed later in this chapter.

Phytoestrogens can be classified into three groups: isoflavones, lignans, and coumestans. The most common pharmacologic use of phytoestrogens is for the treatment of women with menopausal symptoms, and isoflavones are the most widely used and studied for this purpose. The isoflavones include genistein, daidzein, glycitein, biochanin A, and formononetin. Isoflavones appear to have a higher binding affinity for ER-β receptors than ER-α receptors.[15,16] Soy and red clover are commonly used sources of isoflavones. Soy supplementation appears to have a positive impact on serum lipids, but the clinical implication of this effect is not fully known.[29,30] Food sources of soy include soybeans, soy flour, soy protein isolate, miso soup, tempeh, tofu, and soy milk. Soy supplements are available as over-the-counter products (e.g., Health Woman, Soy Care, GeniSoy), as are supplements containing red clover (e.g., Promensil). These soy and red clover products are considered dietary supplements and, as such, are subject to less regulation than prescription drugs with regard to safety and effectiveness.[15] In general, the effectiveness of most phytoestrogen supplements remains unproven, although most data suggest that dietary supplements are less useful than foods containing the agents.

Xenoestrogens (Ecoestrogens, Estrogen Look-Alikes)

Nonpharmacologic agents such as pesticides may also be metabolized into estrogen components or activate estrogen receptors. These agents have been known by several names, including estrogen look-alikes, xenoestrogens (from the Greek word for "stranger"), and ecoestrogens; the last name recognizes their association with environmental pesticides. Estrogen look-alikes were discovered several years ago when animal reproduction plummeted in areas where the water was polluted with chemicals called endocrine disruptors. Subsequent investigation revealed feminization of and decreased fecundity among alligators in those polluted waters.

Many ecoestrogens appear to have long half-lives. Questions have emerged concerning whether ecoestrogens might play a role in the decreasing sperm counts among men in modern society, especially considering the food chain wherein animals may be exposed to xenoestrogens in their environments and then eaten as part of a regular diet. Few studies have been conducted in this area. Some suggestions have been made that organochlorines may be associated with shortened menstrual cycles in women who eat fatty fish from polluted waters more than once a month. Thus, environmental pollutants may have negative effects via steroidal pathways and endocrine disruption.[31] Xenoestrogens theoretically may have estrogenic, antiestrogenic, or mixed antagonist/agonist effects.

Estrogen Antagonists/Agonists

Antiestrogens are medications that are estrogen antagonists. Pure antiestrogens, such as fulvestrant (Faslodex), which is used to treat women with resistant breast cancer, have no agonist effects, but few of these hormones are available for clinical use. Medications that have estrogenic effects on some tissues while blocking the effects of estrogen on other tissues are increasingly being called estrogen agonist/antagonists (EAAs). EAAs include selective estrogen receptor modulators (SERMs)[32] as well as selective estrogen enzyme modulators (SEEMs).

Although the terms may be relatively new, some drugs that fit into this category have existed for decades. Clomiphene citrate (Clomid) and tamoxifen citrate (Nolvadex) are mixed antagonist/agonist compounds derived from triphenylethylene. Raloxifene hydrochloride (Evista) is an SERM derived from benzothiphene.[2] These medications differ in their indications and properties, so each is described separately here. SEEMs do not target estrogen receptors, but rather interfere with enzymatic pathways that result in synthesis of the estrogen itself. These drugs are used for the treatment of cancer, particularly breast cancer. Among the pharmaceuticals that may be characterized as SEEMs are various progestins as well as tibolone (Livial) and its metabolites, some of which inhibit enzymatic activities. Other EEAs can stimulate the local production of estrogen sulfates or block the aromatase action. The area of EEAs is likely to expand with additional designer formulations.

Clomiphene Citrate

The SERM clomiphene citrate (Clomid, Serophene, Milophene) is an estrogen antagonist/agonist that is commonly used as an ovulatory stimulant. This agent acts as an estrogen antagonist unless endogenous estrogen levels are extremely low, in which case it acts as an estrogen agonist. Clomiphene works by binding to estrogen receptors in the pituitary gland, thereby blocking those receptors from detecting circulating estrogen. As a result, the hypothalamus increases its secretion of gonadotropin-releasing hormone, which stimulates the pituitary to secrete follicle-stimulating hormone and luteinizing hormone. These hormones stimulate and initiate an ovulatory menstrual cycle.

Side effects of clomiphene include hot flashes, mood swings, ovarian enlargement, and multiple gestation, as well as some less frequently encountered symptoms—visual disturbances, breast tenderness, pelvic discomfort, and nausea. In pregnancies that occur among women taking clomiphene, 8% are multiple gestations and the vast majority of these are twins. There is no evidence that clomiphene increases the risk of congenital anomalies, nor is there evidence for a causal relationship between clomiphene and ovarian cancer.[33] Clomiphene is contraindicated for women who are pregnant, those who have ovarian enlargement, and those who have abnormal vaginal bleeding.[33]

Tamoxifen Citrate

Tamoxifen citrate (Nolvadex, Soltamox) is a nonsteroidal antiestrogen/agonist used to treat breast cancer, to reduce the incidence of breast cancer recurrence, and to prolong survival in women who have been treated for breast cancer, as well as to prevent breast cancer in women who are at high risk for this disease. Tamoxifen is actually a prodrug metabolized by CYP2D6 to endoxifen, which is the active metabolite. Ednoxifin is an estrogen receptor antagonist at selected sites such as the breasts, but acts as an estrogen agonist at other sites such as the endometrium, bones, and lipids. Thus, tamoxifen offers positive benefits in the form of protection from breast cancer and promotion of bone density, but also carries potentially serious risks such as endometrial cancer and thromboembolic events.[34]

The most common side effects associated with tamoxifen are hot flashes, nausea, vomiting, and irregular menses, including amenorrhea and oligomenorrhea. Persons who have genetic polymorphisms that result in reduced amounts of CYP2D6 may get benefit from taking tamoxifen, and this is one of the drugs for which genetic tests to determine the status of the CYP2D6-related genes prior to prescribing the drug are being discussed. Tamoxifen contraindications include concomitant use of warfarin-type (Coumadin-type) anticoagulant therapy, history of thromboembolic events, or pregnancy.[2,34,35] Toremifene citrate (Fareston) is a SERM that is similar in structure to tamoxifen; it is used to treat women with metastatic cancer.[9]

Raloxifene

Raloxifene HCl (Evista) is an estrogen antagonist/agonist that is FDA approved for the prevention and treatment of osteoporosis in postmenopausal women. This agent also is as effective as tamoxifen in reducing the risk of invasive breast cancer (RR = 1.02; 95% CI, 0.82–1.28).[35] Raloxifene acts as an estrogen agonist in bone but, unlike tamoxifen, does not cause endometrial proliferation. It is associated with an increased risk for thromboembolic events, but the risk is lower than that with tamoxifen. Almost 30% of women taking raloxifene report hot flashes, and approximately 10% report leg cramps. Contraindications to raloxifene use include lactation, pregnancy, and active or past history of thromboembolic events.[35]

Tibolone

Tibolone (Livial, Tibofem), an SEEM, is a synthetic steroid that is structurally related to the 19-nortestosterone commonly used in contraceptives. This drug is not available in the United States, although it is widely used in Europe for treatment of endometriosis and for postmenopausal hormone therapy. It has weak estrogenic, androgenic, and even progestin properties. It is effective in relieving hot flashes, improving mood, and possibly increasing libido and sexual response, although a systematic review found it to be less effective for women with perimenopausal symptoms.[36] Tibolone does not cause endometrial proliferation, so it is not associated with irregular vaginal bleeding and does not require a periodic use of progestin. In clinical practice, some premenopausal women continue to experience intermittent and occasional breakthrough bleeding when taking tibolone. This clinical sign does warrant further investigation to rule out endometrial abnormalities. Such bleeding is more likely to stem from polyps, fibroids, or elevated endogenous estrogen levels and not from endometrial proliferation. Ultrasound, hysteroscopy, or serum estrogen levels might be considered to determine its source. Tibolone is associated with a decrease of HDL—a cause for potential concern for some individuals. Tibolone also serves to prevent bone loss and may decrease fracture risk; however, its effects on breast cancer remain unknown.[37] While it is available in 90 countries, tibolone has not received FDA approval because of its association with an increased risk of stroke and the 12% incidence of uterine bleeding that results in the need for investigation.

Progestins

Progesterone is the precursor to androgens and estrogens. The primary source of endogenous progesterone production is the corpus luteum of the ovary, and levels of this hormone are highest during the second half of the menstrual cycle. If pregnancy occurs, progesterone also is produced by the placenta. The term *progesterone* is derived from the Latin word that means "for pregnancy." Small amounts of progesterone are secreted by the adrenal glands in women of all ages.

Endogenous progesterone binds to the progesterone receptor, resulting in dissociation of selected proteins, phosphorylation of the receptor itself, and activation of transcription factors. Progesterone inhibits estrogens by decreasing the number of estrogen receptors and increasing metabolism of estrogen to inactive metabolites. This hormone induces secretory changes in the endometrium, thereby decreasing the risk of endometrial hyperplasia; decreases uterine contractility during pregnancy; and maintains pregnancy.

Two forms of progesterone receptors exist, designated as PRA and PRB.[38] The two forms are structurally identical except that PRB contains 164 additional amino acids. The latter has yet to be associated with any events of clinical significance, although this is an area of ongoing research.

The Controversial Lexicon

In the literature, as well as in common use, there is a lack of standardization regarding the use of terms *progesterone, progestin, progestogen, progestagen,* and *gestogens.*[39] In general, the endogenous product is commonly known as *progesterone.*[40] For clarity, in this text the term *progestin* will be an umbrella term that includes both naturally occurring progesterone and other synthetic agents. The term **progestogen** will be reserved to describe the synthetic bioactive agents that are similar to progesterone.

Pharmacologic Uses of Progestins

Progestins are primarily used for contraception and for menopausal hormonal therapy, especially to oppose estrogenic-related endometrial hypertrophy, a known precursor of endometrial cancer. These agents can be used for contraception either alone or in combination with estrogen. Progestin-only contraceptive formulations include pills (so-called *minipills,* which is a misnomer because it implies low dose), injections (such as depot medroxyprogesterone acetate [Depo-Provera MPA]), implants (Nexplanon), the levonorgestrel-releasing intrauterine systems (Liletta, Mirena, Skyla), and emergency contraceptive pills (Plan B). Combination contraceptive formulations that contain estrogen and progestin include combined oral contraceptives, the contraceptive vaginal rings, and the transdermal contraceptive patch. The contraceptive mechanisms of action of progestins include suppression of the LH surge, which prevents ovulation, and thickening of the cervical mucus, which inhibits sperm penetration and transport.

A progestin-releasing intrauterine contraceptive device frequently is advocated for treatment of women with heavy menses. Although it is not a panacea, this therapy has been linked with decreases in bleeding and increased satisfaction by women compared to other oral medications and is less invasive than surgery.[41]

Although not as effective as single-agent estrogen for vasomotor therapy, progestins can be used to treat these menopausal symptoms. For this purpose, progestins usually are administered in conjunction with estrogen in the form of estrogen-plus-progestin therapy for women who have a uterus.

A progesterone challenge test continues to be used occasionally for specific situations in the care of women. This progestin withdrawal regimen is often used to induce bleeding in women who are amenorrheic or to regulate menses when a woman is experiencing abnormal uterine bleeding. If a woman is not pregnant and her hypothalamus–pituitary–ovarian axis is intact, vaginal bleeding should occur within a few days after cessation of the progestin therapy. Bleeding indicates that the woman is producing endogenous estrogen. The test is described in more detail in the *Pelvic and Menstrual Disorders* chapter.

Progestins also have been advocated for use during infertility treatments, especially in the form of vaginal suppositories administered in early pregnancy to support the endometrium for women who have experienced past spontaneous abortions, based on evidence that the drugs may decrease miscarriage (RR, 0.53; 95% CI, 0.35–0.79).[42] Progesterone in the form of 17-hydroxy-progesterone has been found to be an effective method to reduce preterm labor for selected groups of women at risk of preterm birth. A systematic review found that progesterone significantly reduced the risk of repeat preterm birth for women with a history of one preterm birth (five studies; 602 women; average RR, 0.31; 95% CI, 0.14–0.69). The same review found that women with a short cervix had a significant reduction in preterm birth when they received progesterone (two studies; 438 women; RR, 0.64; 95% CI, 0.45–0.90).[43] In these situations, progesterone was administered prophylactically.[44] There are insufficient data to suggest that this agent can be used as a tocolytic.[45] These pregnancy-related uses of progestins are discussed in more detail in the *Pregnancy* chapter.

Use of progestin for treatment of premenstrual symptomatology has a long history. However, studies have failed to demonstrate a clear benefit from the administration of this agent.[46]

A nonreproductive indication for progestins may be treatment of individuals who have experienced traumatic brain injury (TBI). Progestins have been proposed as potential neuroprotective agents. Conflicting data have been collected on this effect, and large studies are needed to clarify progestins' role in TBI treatment.[47,48]

Pharmacologic Properties of Progestins

Half-Life

Progesterone is rapidly absorbed and has a half-life of 5 minutes.[9] Early oral progesterones had rapid inactivation and poor bioavailability—limitations that served as the impetus for the development of synthetic drugs. More recently, techniques to micronize crystals have been developed. Oral absorption is improved when oral progesterone, like oral estrogen, is micronized.[4]

Relative Binding Affinity and Progesterone Potency

In the 1970s, it was common for providers to attempt to customize an oral contraceptive to a specific individual. Clinical symptoms such as nausea, acne, and weight gain were characterized as excessive estrogen or androgen effects, and progestins were divided into different categories, such as estrogenic, to determine the exact combined oral contraceptive (COC) that would be appropriate for the woman. To a large degree, these decisions were made based on studies about **relative binding affinity (RBA)** or progesterone potency. Relative binding affinity has limited clinical importance, particularly since most data are derived from studies of other species. Nor is potency of clinical significance, as agents have been formulated to accommodate the dose of a specific type of progestin needed for contraceptive effect. Potency occasionally continues to be mentioned in connection with these agents, as some COCs are advertised as having the lowest steroidal content—a marketing technique of questionable veracity. The concept of the quest for the perfect COC for an individual woman has been addressed by Speroff and Darney, who characterized the use of potency as an artificial exercise and further stated it had not withstood the test of time.[49]

Progestin Pharmacologic Preparations

Two types of progestins exist: natural progesterone and synthetic progestogens. The primary distinction between the two is whether they are identical to endogenous progesterone.[15] Classification of the progestins is depicted in Figure 14-3.

Natural Progesterone

Natural progesterone pharmacologic agents are chemically identical to endogenous progesterone.[4] Progesterone products approved by the FDA include oral capsules (Prometrium), vaginal gels (Crinone and Prochieve), a vaginal insert (Endometrin), and an intramuscular injection (Progesterone).[10] These agents have fewer undesirable side effects than medroxyprogesterone acetate (MPA), the most commonly prescribed progestin.

Synthetic Progestogens

Synthetic progestogens are similar, but not identical, to endogenous progesterone. Most progestogens are derived from progesterone or testosterone. The one exception is drospirenone, which is derived from spironolactone.[51] Drospirenone is a novel progestin that possesses antimineralocorticoid activity with a potassium-sparing diuretic effect similar to that in spironolactone; this agent is found in some combined oral contraceptives (Yasmin, Yaz). Because of the antimineralocorticoid activity, measurements of potassium levels are often obtained to establish a baseline or for continued monitoring while drospirenone is being used. This pharmacologic activity is evident clinically as effects on physiologic parameters, body weight, general well-being, and fluid-related symptoms, and drospirenone is generally not recommended for women who have hypertension. Drospirenone-containing pills were initially characterized as a weight loss contraceptive, but the average woman neither gains nor loses weight while taking this medication; however, some reports indicate that users experience less breast tenderness, abdominal bloating, fatigue, and depressed mood than are associated with other combined oral contraceptivess.[52]

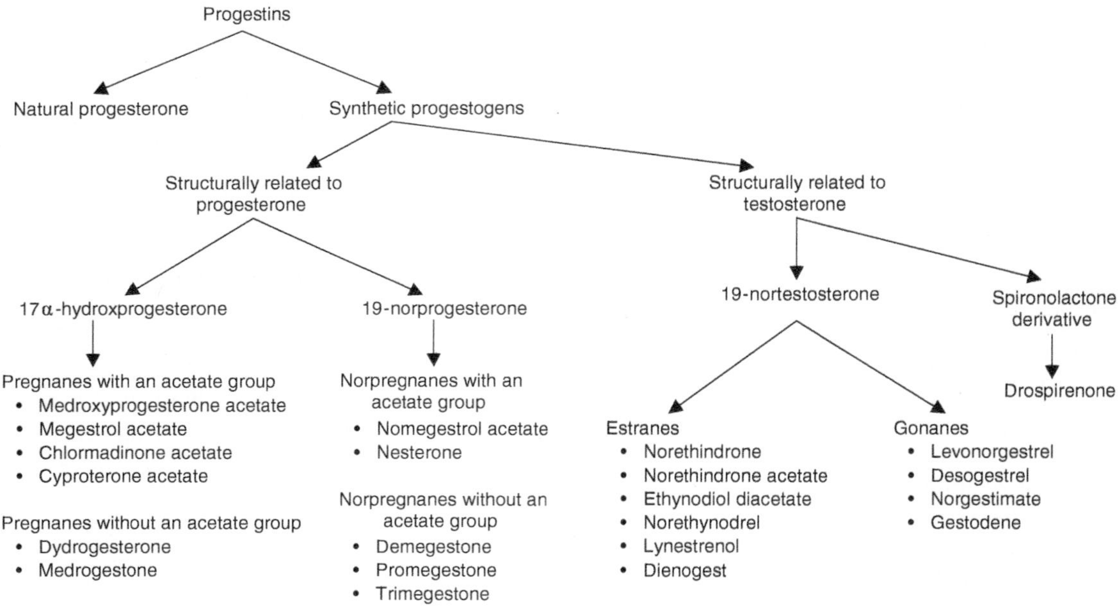

Figure 14-3 Classification of progestins.

Sources: Data from Simon JA. Exogenous progestogens through the life cycle: with a focus on their role in secondary amenorrhea and menopause. *Women's Health Care: Pract J Nurse Pract.* 2007;6(4):7-12[50]; Stanczyk FZ. All progestins are not created equal. *Steroids.* 2003;68(10-13):879-890.[51]

The progestogens that are structurally related to progesterone are divided into the pregnanes, which possess a methyl group at carbon 10, and the norpregnanes, which lack this methyl group. Pregnanes are derived from 17 α-hydroxyprogesterone, and the norpregnanes are derived from 19-norprogesterone. The pregnanes and norpregnanes can be further subdivided according to whether they contain an acetate group (Figure 14-3).[51] Pregnanes used in current clinical practice are medroxyprogesterone acetate and megestrol acetate (Megace). Medroxyprogesterone acetate—which is commonly called by its abbreviation, MPA—is available in oral and injectable formulations. The oral formulation (Provera) is primarily used as the progestin component of estrogen and progestin therapy and may be prescribed separately or combined with estrogen in one dedicated product (Premphase, Prempro). Intramuscular and subcutaneous formulations are used for contraception. The intramuscular formulation depot medroxyprogesterone acetate (DMPA) is marketed under the brand name Depo-Provera. Megestrol acetate (Megace) is used for breast and endometrial cancer treatment and is also given as an appetite stimulant for women with anorexia or cachexia.

Progestogens that are derived from testosterone are classified as estranes or gonanes. The estranes and gonanes are primarily used in oral contraceptives, although some menopausal hormone therapy formulations contain these progestins. The estranes include norethindrone and other progestins that are metabolized to norethindrone, including norethindrone acetate, ethynodiol diacetate, norethynodrel, lynestrenol, and dienogest. The gonanes include levonorgestrel and related progestins, such as desogestrel, norgestimate, and gestodene.[51] Some non-oral progestogen formulations contain active metabolites of these progestins. For example, the transdermal contraceptive patch (Evra) contains norelgestromin, which is the active metabolite of norgestimate. The contraceptive vaginal ring (NuvaRing) and single-rod implant (Nexplanon) contain etonogestrel, which is the active metabolite of desogestrel.

Routes of Administration

Routes for progesterone administration include oral, vaginal, transdermal, injection, implant, and intrauterine. Oral formulations include progestogens and micronized progesterone. A vaginal progesterone gel (Prochieve) and a contraceptive vaginal ring containing progestin and ethinyl estradiol (NuvaRing) are currently available. Transdermal patches with estrogen and progestin are available for contraception (Evra), and estrogen-plus-progestogen therapy (CombiPatch, Climara Pro) is used for women with menopausal symptoms. Transdermal progestin delivery options via a gel and a spray are under investigation.[53,54]

Benefits

Progestins have several well-recognized benefits. Contraceptives containing progestins either exclusively or in combination with estrogen are highly effective agents in preventing pregnancy. They have a powerful influence on the endometrium, including transformation of the endometrium to a secretory type, thereby decreasing the risk of endometrial hyperplasia and ultimately endometrial cancer. These agents also can help stabilize the endometrium as part of treatment of abnormal uterine bleeding. In addition, some evidence suggests that progestins may have a neuroprotective ability.

Side Effects/Adverse Effects

Side effects of progestins may include a wide variety of symptoms, including abnormalities of menstruation (breakthrough bleeding, amenorrhea), weight gain or loss, breast tenderness, and somnolence, among others. The cluster of symptoms of edema, breast tenderness, mild depression, and somnolence often is described as "premenstrual-like" and may contribute to women self-discontinuing therapy. There are many anecdotal reports of women who are prescribed both estrogens and progestins for vasomotor symptoms of menopause, but who choose to take estrogen only.

Certain progestins contain oils that may provoke allergies in women. These include vaginal gels (Crinone, Prochieve) that contain palm oil, capsules (Prometrium) that contain peanut oil, and progestin injectables that contain sesame oil.

Thromboembolic Events

Initially it was theorized that the estrogen in combination oral contraceptives accounted for the increased risk of deep vein thrombosis and other thromboembolic events observed among women using these products. This theory was further supported when DVT rates directly decreased as estrogen dose. However, with the advent of new progestins in COCs in the 1990s, there appeared to be a disparity in risk of DVT regardless of the stable dose and type of estrogen between women using older and newer types of progestins, especially among those individuals with an increased inheritable risk. It has been proposed that progesterone tends to inhibit the thrombotic activity of estrogen; however, the third-generation progestins do so less efficiently, especially for women with factor V Leiden.[55] Women taking estrogen-progestin therapy for contraception, abnormal uterine bleeding, menopausal symptoms, or other reasons should be counseled about this potential adverse effect. Reproductive-aged women using progestin formulations for contraception should be reassured that these risks are still lower than the risk of DVT during pregnancy. These risks are not limited to oral contraceptives: The FDA required changes in labeling for the contraceptive patch when it became apparent that an increase in thromboembolic activity was associated with the product.[56]

Cardiovascular Risks

Several progestins, including the gonanes, estranes, and MPA, have been reported to increase LDL levels and may slightly decrease HDL levels, although micronized progesterone has not been found to affect lipid levels to any significant degree.[40] The relationship of estrogen and progestin with the heart health of mature women and risk of subsequent cardiac events continues to be explored and is discussed in the chapter *The Mature Woman.*

Breast Cancer

Among the sex steroids, estrogen was first associated with breast cancer, and this association persists even today in the minds of most women. However, additional studies have called into question the role of progestins in relationship with the disease.[57] As is true of estrogen, progestins clearly are not a simple etiologic agent for inducing breast cancer. Nevertheless, progesterone has major effects on the normal breast. The Women's Health Initiative study reported that women taking both estrogen and progestin experienced a small but significant increase in breast cancer incidence. In addition, postmenopausal mammograms have been reported to be more difficult to read for women taking progestins.[58] At present, the role of progestins in breast cancer remains an enigma; given that breast cancer is an area of intense scrutiny today, however, answers may become available in the near future.

Bone Disorders

As with many other areas involving progestins, controversy exists concerning the relationship between progestins and bone development. In the late 1990s, studies were published that raised concerns about long-term use of the contraceptive injection medroxyprogesterone acetate in oil

(Depo Provera, DMPA) by adolescents owing to the risk of decreased bone density. In 2005, the FDA mandated that this agent's label carry a black box warning indicating that use of the agent should be time limited unless other options were not available.[59] However, studies of postmenopausal women using estrogen alone or estrogen/progesterone combination therapy tended to demonstrate that these therapies provided bone protection. Studies have since indicated that progestins appear to be extensively metabolized in osteoblasts and involved with progesterone receptors in bone.[60] Research involving adolescents has found that these young women appear to regain their bone density after discontinuation of the drug.[61] Therefore, many scientists have advocated removal of the black box warning.[62]

Until more information is available, it is generally advised that progestins never be considered for bone protection, and long-term use of DMPA be prescribed cautiously, in combination with health education to enable a woman to make a good decision for herself. Larger studies regarding bone fractures, not simply using bone density as a surrogate, also are needed.[63]

Phytoprogesterones: Myth or Reality?

In contrast to phytoestrogens, there are no phytoprogesterones. Although some consumers may think that consumption of certain foods, such as Mexican yams, will increase progesterone levels, that belief is a myth. This misconception may have stemmed from Russell Marker's work with yams. However, to isolate progesterone in food, certain laboratory manipulations are necessary, and the food itself cannot provide progesterone naturally.

Antiprogesterones and Progesterone Receptor Modulators

Mifepristone (Mifeprex, formerly RU486), a derivative of norethindrone, is a progesterone and glucocorticoid antagonist, indicating that it competes for binding to these receptors. Mifepristone usually is an **antiprogestin** but has agonist activity in some situations; thus it is identified as a progestin receptor modulator (SPRM) or a progestin agonist/antagonist.[40] Mifepristone currently is approved in the United States for use in conjunction with the prostaglandin analogue misoprostol (Cytotec) to terminate pregnancies with a gestation duration of less than 50 days. The vast majority of women will have a complete medical abortion following administration of mifepristone and misoprostol; the remainder will require surgical intervention to complete the abortion. Mifepristone also is effective as an emergency contraceptive agent. This pharmacologic agent has potential as a long-term contraceptive and as a treatment for uterine fibroids, endometriosis, steroid-receptive cancers, Cushing's disease, psychotic major depression, and Alzheimer's disease.[54] However, the politics of abortion continue to influence funding for research and the conduct of studies in this area.

Onapristone, asoprisnil, ulipristal, and proellex are antiprogestins that are structurally similar to mifepristone, and numerous other selective progesterone receptor modulators are under investigation.[54,64] Ulipristal (ella) also has been used for treatment of women with fibroids and as an option for emergency contraception.[65,66]

Androgens

Although androgens typically are viewed as male hormones, they are also important for women's health. Androgens are primarily produced in the corpus luteum and the adrenal cortex. Androstenedione and dehydroepiandrosterone are weak androgens that are the precursors to testosterone, which is itself a precursor for estrogen biosynthesis. For the normal woman, testosterone levels decline gradually from a high in the 20s, to a nadir during menopause. For women who experience a surgical menopause, levels drop dramatically. Androgens have high binding affinity, so it is estimated that almost 40% of endogenous testosterone is bound to SHBG and approximately 60% is bound to albumin, leaving 2% or less in the female circulation.[67]

Androgens are reported to affect women's sexual desire, muscle mass and strength, hair, bone mineral density, adipose tissue distribution, energy, and psychological well-being.[15] Exogenous androgenic agents are available, but are less commonly used in clinical practice than the estrogens and progestins. As with estrogens and progestins, receptor-mediated activity appears to be the major mechanism of action for androgens. Androgens penetrate cell membranes of the target cell and bind to androgen receptors located in the cytoplasm.

Pharmacologic Uses of Androgens

The primary indication for prescribing androgens is in the area of sexual well-being of the mature woman. After menopause, some women report that they not only have a lower libido, but also are less responsive sexually.

In addition, some women experience fatigue and general lack of muscle strength in addition to lack of sex drive. The agents that are suggested for women with these symptoms include estrogen with testosterone. Several brand-name preparations exist, including Estratest, Estratest HS, and Premarin with methyltestosterone. Methylation of testosterone enables this hormone to be orally ingested and allows it to be changed to estrogen more slowly than testosterone alone.[68–70] Use of testosterone for the mature woman is controversial and is discussed in more detail in the chapter *The Mature Woman*.

A weak androgen, danazol (Danocrine), may be used for the treatment of endometriosis. These endometrial implants have been found to have androgen receptors. The use of danazol is discussed in more detail in the chapter *Pelvic and Menstrual Disorders*.

Dehydroepiandrosterone (DHEA) is a precursor to androgens and estrogens. Some companies advertise this agent as an option for perimenopausal women to increase estrogenic activity. However, little evidence exists to support the value of oral supplements of this drug.[71]

Antiandrogens are used in combination with GnRH analogues to suppress androgen production, especially among transgendered individuals who are transitioning from male to female. Estrogens are also administered for this purpose, although the heightened risk of DVT remains a concern.[72]

Benefits

Some studies have suggested that androgens may effectively treat women with hot flashes of menopause, but adverse effects may cause early discontinuation and questions remain about long-term use.[70] Although not FDA indicated for bone protection, estrogen and testosterone have been found to increase bone density, even when compared to estrogen alone.[73,74]

Side Effects/Adverse Effects

Side effects of testosterone include acne, alopecia, edema, deepened voice, enlarged clitoris, irregular menses, and hirsutism. Serious adverse effects for women in some studies have included increased LDL levels and decreased HDL cholesterol levels. High doses of testosterone have been associated with liver cancer. The relationship between breast cancer and androgenic therapy is unknown, although most breast cancer tumors have androgen receptors. Testosterone is the prototype drug for anabolic steroids, a category of drugs of potential abuse, especially in the area of weight training and bodybuilding.[75]

Bioidentical Compounds

Bioidentical hormones are compounds with the same chemical and structure as hormones produced in the body. Although it is possible to formulate a bioidentical version of any hormone, this discussion is limited to bioidentical estrogen, progestins, and testosterone. Advocates for bioidentical hormones suggest that these products are natural, safer, and more effective than synthesized hormones, despite the lack of evidence to support this assertion.[76]

Some FDA-approved bioidentical agents exist, including 17 β-estradiol products (Table 14-3) and natural progesterone formulations, including oral capsules (Prometrium), vaginal gels (Crinone and Prochieve), a vaginal insert (Endometrin), and an intramuscular injection (Progesterone).[10,77] However, when the term *bioidentical hormone* is used in relation to a sex steroid hormone agent, it most often indicates products formulated by compounding pharmacies. Such products may be customized based on saliva or blood tests that measure endogenous hormone levels. However, evidence of effectiveness for these formulations is lacking. Compounded bioidentical hormones are not monitored by the FDA for dosage and purity, and inconsistencies have been found on both fronts.

The market for bioidentical hormones is growing as women seek natural remedies.[78] Lack of evidence should not limit study in this area, as rigorous research with standardized formulations may reveal effective treatment modalities.

Conclusion

Although estrogens, progesterones, and androgens first were isolated less than a century ago, their use in women's health care today is ubiquitous. Moreover, use of hormone therapy in the future will likely continue to expand as new agents are developed or designed because of increased understanding of receptors and enzymes. Ideally, these new designer drugs will promote therapeutic effects while decreasing the risks associated with endogenous hormones. Simultaneously, additional studies are likely to bolster our knowledge about other naturally occurring hormones such as phytoestrogens and xenoestrogens as well as the burgeoning field of bioidentical hormones.

Resources

Organization	Description	Website
North American Menopause Society (NAMS)	Professional organization dedicated to issues surrounding menopause. Major source of information about hormone therapy for mature women. Some materials are free; others are limited to members of NAMS. The free consumer app "MenoPro" features information for consumers as well as the ability to keep notes regarding bothersome symptoms to discuss with the provider. The NAMS professional journal, *Menopause*, is also available as an app.	www.menopause.org
Videos		
Multiple videos can be found online via a variety of sources. YouTube (www.youtube.com) has several free videos discussing steroidogenesis as well as videos animating cellular actions with receptors. These videos provide a visual interpretation of important concepts. As with much of the information on the Internet, the reader is advised to seek out credible sources.		

References

1. Kreeger KY. The rhythms that bind women. *Scientist* 2001;15(15):20.
2. Fritz MA. Speroff L. *Clinical Gynecologic Endocrinology and Infertility*. 8th ed. Philadelphia, PA: Lippincott Williams & Wilkins; 2011.
3. Sneader W. *Drug Discovery: A History*. New York: John Wiley and Sons; 2005.
4. Lehmann PA. Early history of steroid chemistry in Mexico: the story of three remarkable men. *Steroids.* 1992;57(8):403-408.
5. O'Dowd MJ. *The History of Medications for Women: Materia Medica Woman*. New York: Parthenon; 2001.
6. Likis FE. Contraceptive applications of estrogen. *J Midwifery Womens Health.* 2002;47(3):139-156.
7. Dahlman-Wright K, Cavailles V, Fuqua SA, et al. International Union of Pharmacology. LXIV. Estrogen receptors. *Pharmacol Rev.* 2006;58(4):773-781.
8. Food and Drug Administration, Center for Drug Evaluation and Research. FDA statement ongeneric Premarin. 1997. http://www.fda.gov/Drugs/DrugSafety/PostmarketDrugSafetyInformationforPatientsandProviders/ucm169045.htm. Accessed March 30, 2015.
9. Chrousos GP. The gonadal hormones and inhibitors. In Katzung BG, Trevor AJ, eds. *Basic & Clinical Pharmacology.* 13th ed. New York: McGraw-Hill; 2015:696-722.
10. U.S. Food and Drug Administration, Center for Drug Evaluation and Research. Electronic orange book: approved drug products with therapeutic equivalence evaluations, 2007. http://www.fda.gov/Drugs/InformationOnDrugs/ucm129662.htm. Accessed March 30, 2015.
11. Cunningham M, Gilkeson G. Estrogen receptors in immunity and autoimmunity. *Clin Rev Allergy Immunol.* 2011;40(1):66-73.
12. Kovats S. Estrogen receptors regulate innate immune cells and signaling pathways. *Cell Immunol.* 294(2):63-69.
13. Morani A, Warner M, Gustafsson JA. Biological functions and clinical implications of oestrogen receptors alfa and beta in epithelial tissues. *J Intern Med.* 2008;264(2):128-142.
14. North American Menopause Society. The 2012 hormone therapy position statement of the North American Menopause Society. *Menopause.* 2012;19(3):257-271.
15. North American Menopause Society. *Menopause Practice: A Clinician's Guide.* 5th ed. Cleveland, OH: North American Menopause Society; 2010.
16. Ruggiero RJ, Likis FE. Estrogen: physiology, pharmacology, and formulations for replacement therapy. *J Midwifery Womens Health.* 2002;47(3):130-138.
17. Reed CE, Fenton SE. Exposure to diethylstilbestrol during sensitive life stages: a legacy of heritable health effects. *Birth Defects Res C Embryo Today.* 2013;99(2):134-146.
18. Buster JE, Koltun WD, Pascual ML, Day WW, Peterson C. Low-dose estradiol spray to treat vasomotor symptoms: a randomized controlled trial. *Obstet Gynecol.* 2008;111(6):1343-1351.
19. Harman SM, Vittinghoff E, Brinton EA, et al. Timing and duration of menopausal hormone treatment may affect cardiovascular outcomes. *Am J Med.* 2011;124:199-205.
20. Mikkola TS, Tuomikoski P, Lyytinen H, et al. Estradiol-based postmenopausal hormone therapy and risk of cardiovascular and all-cause mortality. *Menopause.* March 23, 2015. [Epub ahead of print.]
21. Westhoff CL. Oral contraceptives and thrombosis. *Am J Obstet Gyncol.* 1998;179(3 pt 2):S38.

22. Cole JA, Norman H, Doherty M, Walker AM. Venous thromboembolism, myocardial infarction and stroke among transdermal contraceptive system users. *Obstet Gynecol.* 2007;109(2 pt 1):333-346.
23. Rossouw JE, Anderson GL, Prentice RL, et al.; Writing Group for the Women's Health Initiative Investigators. Risks and benefits of estrogen plus progestin in healthy postmenopausal women: principal results from the Women's Health Initiative randomized controlled trial. *JAMA.* 2002;288(3):321-333.
24. Stefanick ML, Anderson GL, Margolis KL, et al.; WHI Investigators. Effects of conjugated equine estrogens on breast cancer and mammography screening in postmenopausal women with hysterectomy. *JAMA.* 2006;295:1647-1657.
25. Chlebowski RT, Kuller L, Anderson G, et al. *Breast Cancer After Stopping Estrogen Plus Progestin in Postmenopausal Women.* Presented at the Women's Health Initiative 31st Annual San Antonio Breast Cancer Symposium (SABCS); December 12, 2008. Abstract 64.
26. Collaborative Group on Epidemiological Studies of Ovarian Cancer. Menopausal hormone use and ovarian cancer risk: individual participant meta-analysis of 52 epidemiological studies. *Lancet.* 2015; 385(9980):1835-1842.
27. Neves-E-Castro M. Association of ovarian cancers with postmenopausal hormonal treatments. *Clin Obstet Gynecol.* 2008;51(3):607-617.
28. Krebs EE, Ensrud KE, MacDonald R, Wilt TJ. Phytoestrogens for treatment of menopausal symptoms: a systematic review. *Obstet Gynecol.* 2004; 104(4): 824-836.
29. Reynolds K, Chin A, Lees KA, Nguyen A, Bujnowski D, He J. A meta-analysis of the effect of soy protein supplementation on serum lipids. *Am J Cardiol.* 2006; 98(5):633-640.
30. Dewell A, Hollenbeck PL, Hollenbeck CB. Clinical review: a critical evaluation of the role of soy protein and isoflavone supplementation in the control of plasma cholesterol concentrations. *J Clin Endocrinol Metab.* 2006;91(3):772-780.
31. Singleton DW, Khan SA. Xenoestrogen exposure and mechanisms of endocrine disruption. *Front Biosci.* 2003;8:s110-s118.
32. Mirkin S, Pickar JH. Selective estrogen receptor modulators (SERMs): a review of clinical data. *Maturitas.* 2015;80(1):52-57.
33. Practice Committee of the American Society for Reproductive Medicine. Use of clomiphene citrate in women. *Fertil Steril.* 2013;100(2):341-348.
34. Hu R, Hilakivi-Clarke L, Clarke R. Molecular mechanisms of tamoxifen-associated endometrial cancer. *Oncol Lett.* 2015;9(4):1495-1501.
35. Vogel VG, Costantino JP, Wickerham DL, et al.; National Surgical Adjuvant Breast and Bowel Project. Effects of tamoxifen vs raloxifene on the risk of developing invasive breast cancer and other disease outcomes: the NSABP Study of Tamoxifen and Raloxifene (STAR) P-2 trial. *JAMA.* 2006;295(23):2727-2741.
36. Formoso G, Perrone E, Maltoni S, et al. Short and long term effects of tibolone in postmenopausal women. *Cochrane Database Syst Rev.* 2012;2:CD008536.
37. Cummings SR, Ettinger B, Delmas PD, et al., LIFT Trial Investigators. The effects of tibolone in older postmenopausal women. *N Engl J Med.* 2008;359(7): 697-708.
38. Jacobsen BM, Horwitz KB. Progesterone receptors, their isoforms and progesterone regulated transcription. *Mol Cell Endocrinol.* 2012;357(1-2): 18-29.
39. Spark MJ. Progest-erone, ogen, in? Which is it? *BMJ.* 2009;339:b5142.
40. Levin ER, Hammes SR. Estrogens and progestins. In Brunton LL, Chabner B, eds. *Goodman & Gilman's The Pharmacological Basis of Therapeutics.* 12th ed. New York: McGraw-Hill; 2011:1163-1194.
41. Lethaby A, Cooke I, Rees MC. Progesterone or progestogen-releasing intrauterine systems for heavy menstrual bleeding. *Cochrane Database Syst Rev.* 2005;4:CD002126.
42. Wahabi HA, Fayed AA, Esmaeil SA, Al Zeidan RA. Progestogen for treating threatened miscarriage. *Cochrane Database Syst Rev.* 2011;12:CD005943.
43. Dodd JM, Jones L, Flenady V, Cincotta R, Crowther CA. Prenatal administration of progesterone for preventing preterm birth in women considered to be at risk of preterm birth. *Cochrane Database Syst Rev.* 2013;7:CD004947.
44. Meis PJ, Kebanoff M, Thom E, et al., for the National Institute of Child Health and Human Development Maternal-Fetal Medicine Units Network. Prevention of recurrent preterm delivery by 17 alpha-hydroxyprogesterone caproate. *New Engl J Med.* 2003; 348:2379-2385.
45. Su LL, Samuel M, Chong YS. Progestational agents for treating threatened or established preterm labour. *Cochrane Database Syst Rev.* 2014;1:CD006770.
46. Ford O, Lethaby A, Roberts H, Mol BWJ. Progesterone for premenstrual syndrome. *Cochrane Database Syst Rev.* 2012;3:CD003415.

47. Ma J, Huang S, Qin S, You C. Progesterone for acute traumatic brain injury. *Cochrane Database Syst Rev.* 2012;10:CD008409.
48. Skolnick BE, Maas AI, Narayan RK, et al.; SYNAPSE Trial Investigators. A clinical trial of progesterone for severe traumatic brain injury. *N Engl J Med.* 2014;371(26):2467-2476.
49. Speroff L, Darney PD. *A Clinical Guide for Contraception.* 5th ed. Philadelphia, PA: Lippincott Williams & Wilkins; 2011.
50. Simon JA. Exogenous progestogens through the life cycle: with a focus on their role in secondary amenorrhea and menopause. *Women's Health Care: Pract J Nurse Pract.* 2007;6(4):7-12.
51. Stanczyk FZ. All progestins are not created equal. *Steroids.* 2003;68(10-13):879-890.
52. Foidart J. Added benefits of drospirenone for compliance. *Climacteric.* 2005;8(3):28-34.
53. Sitruk-Ware R. Routes of delivery for progesterone and progestins. *Maturitas.* 2007;57(1):77-80.
54. Chabbert-Buffet N, Meduri G, Bouchard P, Spitz IM. Selective progesterone receptor modulators and progesterone antagonists: mechanisms of action and clinical applications. *Hum Reprod Update.* 2005;11(3): 293-307.
55. Kemmeren JM, Algra A, Meijers JC, Bouma BN, Grobbee DE. Effects of second and third generation oral contraceptives and their respective progestogens on the coagulation system in the absence or presence of the factor V Leiden mutation. *Thromb Haemost.* 2002;87(2):199-205.
56. U.S. Food and Drug Administration. Ortho Evra (norelgestromin/ethinyl estradiol) information. http://www.fda.gov/Drugs/DrugSafety/PostmarketDrugSafetyInformationforPatientsandProviders/ucm110402.htm. Accessed March 30, 2015.
57. Lange CA, Yee D. Progesterone and breast cancer. *Womens Health (London).* 2008;4(2):151-162.
58. Warren R. Hormones and mammographic breast density. *Maturitas.* 2004;49(1):67-78.
59. U.S. Food and Drug Administration. "Black box" warning added to contraceptive injection. *FDA Consum.* 2005;39(2):3.
60. Quinkler M, Kaur K, Hewison M, Stewart PM, Cooper MS. Progesterone is extensively metabolized in osteoblasts: implications for progesterone action on bone. *Horm Metab Res.* 2008;40(10):679-684.
61. Committee Opinion No. 602: Depot medroxyprogesterone acetate and bone effects. *Obstet Gynecol.* 2014; 123(6):1398-402.
62. Kaunitz AM, Grimes DA. Removing the black box warning for depot medroxyprogesterone acetate. *Contraception.* 2011;84(3):212-213.
63. Lopez LM, Grimes DA, Schulz KF, Curtis KM, Chen M. Steroidal contraceptives: effect on bone fractures in women. *Cochrane Database Syst Rev.* 2014;6:CD006033.
64. Sarkar NN. The state-of-the-art of emergency contraception with the cutting edge drug. *Ger Med Sci.* 2011; 9:Doc16 doi:10.3205/000139. Epub July 11, 2011.
65. Donnez J, Hudecek R, Donnez O, et al. Efficacy and safety of repeated use of ulipristal acetate in uterine fibroids. *Fertil Steril.* 2015;103(2):519-527.
66. Corbelli J, Bimla Schwarz E. Emergency contraception: a review. *Minerva Ginecol.* 2014;66(6):551-564.
67. Snyder PJ. Androgens. In Brunton LL, Chabner B. eds. *Goodman & Gilman's The Pharmacological Basis of Therapeutics.* 12th ed. New York: McGraw-Hill; 2011: 1195-1208.
68. Shulman LP. Androgens and menopause: more fuel for the fire. *Menopause.* 2006;13(2):168-170.
69. Penteado SR, Fonseca AM, Bagnoli VR, Abdo CH, Junior JM, Baracat EC. Effects of the addition of methyltestosterone to combined hormone therapy with estrogens and progestogens on sexual energy and on orgasm in postmenopausal women. *Climacteric.* 2008;11(1):17-25.
70. Somboonporn W, Bell RJ, Davis SR. Testosterone for peri and postmenopausal women. *Cochrane Database Syst Rev.* 2005;4:CD004509.
71. Eden JA. DHEA replacement for postmenopausal women: placebo or panacea? *Climacteric.* March 3, 2015:1-2.
72. Meriggiola MC, Gava G. Endocrine care of transpeople. Part II. A review of cross-sex hormonal treatments, outcomes and adverse effects in transwomen. *Clin Endocrinol (Oxford).* February 18, 2015. doi:10.1111/cen.12754.[Epub ahead of print.]
73. Watts NB, Notelovitz M, Timmons MC, Addison WA, Wiita B, Downey LJ. Comparison of oral estrogens

and estrogens plus androgen on bone mineral density, menopausal symptoms, and lipid-lipoprotein profiles in surgical menopause. *Obstet Gynecol.* 1995;85: 529-537.

74. Davis SR, McCloud PI, Strauss BJG, Burger HG. Testosterone enhances estradiol's effects on post-menopausal bone density and sexuality. *Maturitas.* 1995;21:227-236.
75. Rahnema CD, Crosnoe LE, Kim ED. Designer steroids: over-the-counter supplements and their androgenic component: review of an increasing problem. *Andrology.* February 13, 2015. doi:10.1111/andr.307. [Epub ahead of print.]
76. Cirigliano M. Bioidentical hormone therapy: a review of the evidence. *J Womens Health.* 2007;16(5):600-631.
77. ESHRE Capri Workshop Group. Hormones and cardiovascular health in women. *Hum Reprod Update.* 2006;12(5):483-497.
78. Fishman JR, Flatt MA, Settersten RA Jr. Bioidentical hormones, menopausal women, and the lure of the "natural" in U.S. anti-aging medicine. *Soc Sci Med.* 2015;132:79-87.

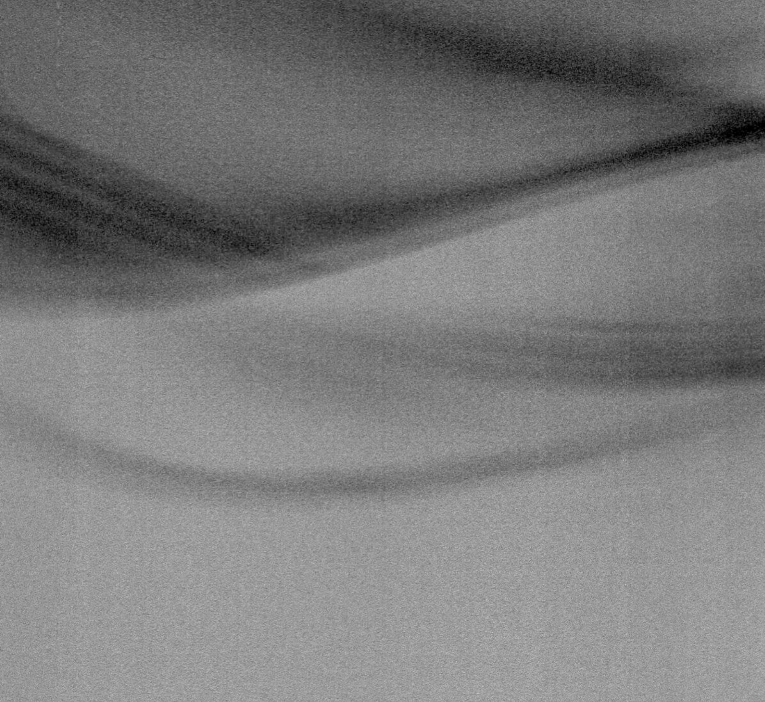

IV
Pharmacotherapeutics for Common Conditions

Pharmacotherapeutics is the study of effects of drugs in clinical practice; therefore, this section includes more chapters than the other sections, and here can be found specifics of pharmacologic management for common health conditions. This section starts with *Cardiovascular Conditions*, which are the number one killer of women today. *Hematology* discusses treatment of women with conditions such as anemia and venous thromboemboli. Multiple sclerosis, lupus, and other conditions often occur more frequently among women than among men, and these disorders and treatments are addressed in the *Autoimmune Conditions* chapter. The next chapter, *Diabetes*, discusses the disease of the same name, whose incidence is increasing and whose pharmacologic repertoire for treatment similarly is growing.

The *Thyroid Disorders* chapter examines another condition that is more common among women than men, and one that requires close monitoring for appropriate drug treatment. *Respiratory Conditions* includes treatments for women with mild allergic responses to those with potentially severe pneumonias. *Gastrointestinal Conditions* encompasses treatments for women who experience difficulty with the alimentary tract, from heartburn to constipation. *Lower Urinary Tract Disorders* includes infections as well as incontinence, both conditions of concern for women. Professionals who care for women are often presented with challenges addressed in the next chapter, *Sexually Transmitted Infections*.

The central nervous system plays an important role in health and disease. The chapter *The Central Nervous System* begins with a basic review of the anatomy and function of the central nervous system, followed by a review of pharmacologic management of epilepsy, Parkinson's disease, and Alzheimer's disease, among others. Psychotropic drugs, antianxiety drugs, and other drugs common in the twenty-first century are included in the *Mental Health* chapter.

Dermatology includes a discussion of the expected topical agents for acne and other skin blemishes. This chapter also includes a discussion of a new area of dermatology—cosmeceuticals. *Ophthalmic and Otic Disorders* reviews agents used for specific conditions in this highly specialized area. The last chapter in this section, *Cancer*, acknowledges the importance of chemotherapeutics today.

Many of the chapters in this section include drugs that are not commonly initiated by primary care providers. For example, chemotherapeutics are the purview of the oncology team. However, it is common that women who have complex medical conditions continue to seek care with their trusted healthcare professional and may seek help for some of the side effects of drugs used to treat their disorders. Thus, an individual scope of practice may be broader or more limited, yet basic information necessary for the primary care provider can be found in these chapters.

15
Cardiovascular Conditions

Laura V. Tsu

Based on the chapter by Angela R. Mitchell and Tekoa L. King in the first edition of Pharmacology for Women's Health

Chapter Glossary

Alpha-receptor antagonists Class of drugs that act as antagonists when bound to the alpha-adrenergic receptors located on vascular smooth muscle.

Adrenergic receptors Class of G protein–coupled receptors that are the targets for the catecholamines norepinephrine and epinephrine. Alpha-adrenergic and beta-adrenergic receptors are two subtypes of adrenergic receptors.

Angiotensin I Molecule formed by the action of renin on angiotensinogen, which is constittively present in plasma. It has no biologic activity, but is the precursor of angiotensin II, which is biologically active.

Angiotensin II Peptide hormone that causes increased blood pressure via vasoconstriction, release of aldosterone, increased heart muscle contractility, and sympathetic discharge. It is formed from angiotensin I, which is formed from angiotensinogen.

Angiotensin II receptor blockers (ARBs) Class of pharmaceuticals used to treat hypertension. These drugs block the binding of angiotensin II to AT_1 receptors, thereby preventing the agonist effect of angiotensin II.

Angiotensin-converting enzyme (ACE) inhibitors Class of pharmaceuticals used to treat hypertension. These drugs prevent the conversion of angiotensin I to angiotensin II.

Anticoagulant drugs Drugs that interfere in any of the coagulation cascade steps.

Antiplatelet drugs Drugs that prevent platelet aggregation.

Beta-adrenergic receptor antagonists (beta blockers) Class of pharmaceuticals used to treat hypertension. These drugs bind to beta-adrenergic receptors, thereby blocking the binding of norepinephrine and epinephrine.

Calcium-channel blockers (CCBs) Class of pharmaceuticals used to treat persons with hypertension by preventing calcium from entering muscle cells, which results in muscle relaxation and widening of blood vessels. Also known as calcium-channel antagonists and calcium-channel receptor antagonists.

Catecholamines Hormones derived from tyrosine; they include norepinephrine, epinephrine, and dopamine.

Central $alpha_2$-agonists Agents that suppress stimulation of sympathetic discharge in the central nervous system. Also called selective $alpha_2$-receptor agonists.

Chronotropic Having the effect of making the heart rate faster or changing the heart rate rhythm.

Dihydropyridines Class of calcium-channel blockers that have a selective effect in relaxing the smooth muscle that surrounds arterial vessels; they are used to treat individuals with hypertension.

Direct renin inhibitors Class of pharmaceuticals used to treat hypertension; they inhibit the action of renin.

Diuretics Any drugs that increase the amount of urine and cause diuresis.

Epinephrine Agent that is both a hormone and a neurotransmitter in the sympathetic nervous system as well as a nonselective agonist for alpha- and beta-adrenergic receptors. Also called adrenaline.

Inotropic Having the effect of altering muscular contractions, either weakening them (negative inotropic effect) or strengthening them (positive inotropic effect).

Non-selective alpha-adrenergic antagonists Drugs that have an antagonist effect on both $alpha_1$ and $alpha_2$ receptors. These drugs are generally reserved for treatment of hypertensive emergencies.

Norepinephrine Similar to epinephrine, a hormone and neurotransmitter that initiates the physiologic actions that appear during the flight-or-fight stress response. Like epinephrine, it has an agonist effect on alpha- and beta-adrenergic receptors.

Renin–angiotensin–aldosterone system (RAAS) Hormone system that functions as a negative feedback loop to control blood pressure and fluid balance.

Selective alpha-adrenergic antagonists Class of drugs that block the $alpha_1$ receptors peripherally, causing decreased peripheral vascular resistance and lowering of blood pressure.

Sodium chloride symporter Ion pump that removes sodium and chloride ions from the distal convoluted tubule of the kidney.

Statins Class of drugs that inhibit 3-hydroxy-3-methylglutaryl coenzyme A (HMG-CoA) reductase, an enzyme that is part of an essential early step in the biosynthesis of cholesterol.

Introduction

Cardiovascular disease (CVD) is the most common cause of death in women in the United States.[1,2] For the purposes of this chapter, the term *CVD* refers to several diseases, including hypertension, hyperlipidemia, coronary heart disease, angina, heart failure, and peripheral arterial disease. More than one in three female adults has some form of CVD, and females represent 51% of deaths from CVD.[3] Approximately 6.6 million women in the United States have coronary heart disease, with 2.6 million of those having a history of a myocardial infarction. Because women tend to experience myocardial infarctions at a later age compared to men, they are also more likely to die when they experience a heart attack (26% of women compared to 19% of men age 45 years or older).[3]

Today women are living longer lives, but often with multiple comorbid cardiovascular conditions. Diabetes and hypertension are more detrimental to women than to men, and these diseases are more strongly associated with cardiovascular disease among African Americans than among Caucasians.[4] Thus, it is imperative that practitioners treat and educate women about these conditions. This chapter reviews treatments for CVD disorders.

Various degrees of illness are associated with this constellation of disorders. The American Heart Association (AHA) has outlined the varying levels of risk for CVD with recommended treatments based on the degree of risk, as summarized in Table 15-1.[1] At the time of this writing, AHA has not issued new guidelines, although the recommendations regarding indications for specific cholesterol targets have been questioned in light of more recent information from the American College of Cardiology (ACA) and AHA and they may be modified in the future.[5]

Table 15-1 Recommendations for Prevention of Cardiovascular Disease in Women

Risk Factors	Recommendations
High risk (one or more high-risk states)	
Established coronary heart disease Cerebrovascular disease Peripheral artery disease Abdominal aortic aneurysm End-stage or chronic renal disease Diabetes mellitus 10-year Framingham global risk > 10%[a]	Class 1 recommendations (Intervention is useful and effective): Blood pressure control LDL-lowering therapy (goal < 100 mg/dL) Beta blocker ACE inhibitor/ARB Class II recommendations (Weight of evidence/opinion is in favor of usefulness/efficacy): LDL-lowering therapy (goal < 70 mg/dL for high-risk women) Non-HDL-lowering therapy (goal < 130 mg/dL for high-risk women) Glycemic control for women with diabetes Aspirin/antiplatelet Omega-3 fatty acids
At risk (one or more major risk factors)	
Cigarette smoking SBP ≥ 120 mm Hg, DBP ≥ 80 mm Hg, or treated hypertension Total cholesterol ≥ 200 mg/dL, HDL-C < 50 mg/dL, or treated for dyslipidemia Obesity Poor diet Physical inactivity Family history of premature CVD occurring in first-degree relatives in men < 55 years or in women < 65 years Metabolic syndrome Evidence of subclinical atherosclerosis Poor exercise capacity on treadmill test Systemic autoimmune collagen-vascular disease History of preeclampsia, gestational diabetes, or pregnancy-induced hypertension	Class 1 recommendations (Intervention is useful and effective): Blood pressure control LDL lowering therapy if ≥190 mg/dL Class II recommendations (Weight of evidence/opinion is in favor of usefulness/efficacy): Therapy for high LDL, non-HDL and triglycerides, and/or HDL in select women Aspirin

Ideal cardiovascular health (all of these)
Total cholesterol < 200 mg/dL (untreated)
BP < 120/< 80 mm Hg (untreated)
Body mass index < 25 kg/m^2
Abstinence from smoking
Physical activity at goal for adults > 20 years: ≥ 150 min/week moderate intensity, ≥ 75 min/week of vigorous intensity, or combination
Healthy (DASH-like) diet

Abbreviations: ACE = angiotensin-converting enzyme; ARB = angiotensin receptor blocker; BP = blood pressure; DASH = Dietary Approaches to Stop Hypertension; DBP = diastolic blood pressure; HDL = high-density lipoprotein; LDL = low-density lipoprotein; SBP = systolic blood pressure.
[a] Data from the Framingham Heart Study have been used to develop a risk assessment tool that estimates an individual's 10-year risk for having a myocardial infarction or coronary death.
Source: Mosca L, Benjamin EJ, Berra K, et al. Effectiveness-based guidelines for the prevention of cardiovascular disease in women—2011 update: a guideline from the American heart association. *Circulation.* 2011;123:1243-1262.

Prevention of Cardiovascular Disease

Primary prevention of CVD is an important component of healthcare services that should regularly be offered to women. However, evidence-based strategies for primary prevention of CVD in women have not conclusively been determined because of the lack of research in this area. Since 1997, numerous national campaigns to raise awareness of CVD as leading killer of women in the United States have been undertaken; nevertheless, public attention to this issue remains suboptimal, especially among racial and ethnic minorities.[6]

Prevention strategies are based on varying levels of risk for developing CVD. Lifestyle modification is the cornerstone of any CVD risk-reduction strategy. This approach includes recommendations for smoking cessation, physical activity, dietary intake, weight management, and use of omega-3 fatty acids.

Smoking, obesity, and physical inactivity are primary risk factors that are modifiable. Additional information concerning smoking cessation can be found in the *Smoking Cessation* chapter. There is a known relationship between body mass index (BMI) and development of CVD and other metabolic disorders.[7] The Dietary Approaches to Stop Hypertension (DASH) diet and the Mediterranean diet have been shown to lower blood pressure (BP) and cholesterol by focusing on a diet rich in fruits and vegetables.[7,8] These diets may also support weight loss if combined with increased physical activity. Sodium intake should be limited to no more than 2.4 grams daily and no more than 1 ounce of alcohol consumption per day.[9] Recommendations for women for prevention of CVD include at least 150 minutes of moderate exercise each week, 75 minutes of vigorous exercise each week, or an equivalent combination of both.[1]

The AHA recommends that women who have a high risk for developing CVD should add omega-3 fatty acid supplementation to their diets, especially if the woman has hypercholesterolemia or hypertriglyceridemia. Previous trials have shown benefit among participants who have had a previous myocardial infarction or heart failure. However, a randomized clinical trial of more than 12,000 participants assigned to omega-3 fatty acid supplementation versus placebo found no difference in cumulative rates of death, nonfatal myocardial infarction (MI), and nonfatal stroke at the end of five years.[10] Therefore, it is unclear if such supplementation provides a significant benefit in terms of cardioprotection. If omega-3 supplementation is used, the recommended dose is 1800 mg per day of eicosapentaenoic acid (EPA), which can be from a combination of fish and capsule supplementation.[1] Fish oil supplementation products can contain a varying amount of EPA and docosahexaenoic acid (DHA), so women should check the ingredients on the bottle to ensure they are consuming an adequate amount of EPA.

Controversy persists regarding the use of low-dose aspirin for primary prevention of CVD in women. An early review of five randomized trials of women who received aspirin therapy found a 32% reduction in the risk of the first myocardial infarction and a 15% reduction in the risk of all vascular events.[11] However, subsequent observational studies from the Women's Health Initiative found that there was no risk reduction from daily aspirin therapy for women who are at low risk for CVD.[12] The 2011 guideline states that for high-risk women with diabetes, aspirin 75–325 mg daily is reasonable.[1] Aspirin therapy can also be useful for women 65 years or older if their blood pressure is controlled and the benefit in preventing ischemic stroke and myocardial infarction outweighs the risk of gastrointestinal bleeding and hemorrhagic stroke. For women younger than 65 years, routine aspirin is not recommended for prevention of a myocardial infarction.[1]

Other approaches to lifestyle modification are holistic in nature. Reductions in elevated glucose and low-density lipoprotein (LDL) have also been achieved through activities such as relaxation, meditation, yoga, breathing exercises, and stress management. These activities can decrease the sympathetic responses that cause elevations in glucose and cholesterol levels.

In summary, programs that include counseling, smoking cessation, education, increased physical activity, and dietary modification are most likely to achieve successful lifestyle modification.[13] Even when successful, maintaining lifestyle modifications remains a challenge for most individuals. When rigorous lifestyle modifications are insufficient to achieve therapeutic goals within 3 to 6 months, pharmacotherapy is recommended. Drug therapy is utilized to control hypertension, to treat dyslipidemia, and to reduce morbidity and mortality among women with CVD. When selecting therapy, all of these goals should be considered.

Hypertension

One in three adults in the United States has hypertension, and this disease is often known as a "silent killer" because it affects many individuals without their knowledge. More men have hypertension than women until age 45 years; then the balance is equal during ages 45–64 years, but subsequently more women have hypertension than men after age 65 years.[3] The risk of hypertension increases in persons with the following risk factors: African American race, CVD risk factors, BMI greater than 27.3, physical inactivity, excess alcohol intake, and history of hyperlipidemia or diabetes. Currently, approximately 80% of persons who have hypertension are aware they have it and approximately 75% are being treated, but only approximately 50% have controlled blood pressure.[14] The medications used to control hypertension among women each affect one or more steps in several blood pressure regulatory systems. Thus a brief review of those systems is in order.

Physiology of Blood Pressure Control

Arterial blood pressure is the pressure that is exerted on the artery wall by blood flowing through these vessels. The systolic blood pressure is the pressure during cardiac contraction, and the diastolic pressure is the pressure during the filling of the cardiac chambers. The difference between these two measurements is referred to as the pulse pressure. The mean arterial pressure is the average pressure maintained in the arteries through the entire cardiac cycle. Factors that influence the mean arterial pressure include heart rate, stroke volume, and peripheral resistance. Several factors are involved in regulating arterial blood pressure, including the renin–angiotensin–aldosterone system, the sympathetic response of the autonomic nervous system, and peripheral autoregulation.

The Renin–Angiotensin–Aldosterone System

The **renin–angiotensin–aldosterone system (RAAS)** is the target of many antihypertensive agents, as illustrated in Figure 15-1. The juxtaglomerular cells in the kidneys produce renin in response to several factors, including a drop in perfusion, a decrease in sodium in the kidney, and beta-adrenergic stimulation. Once renin is produced and enters the circulation, it converts angiotensinogen into angiotensin I. **Angiotensin I**, although active, is converted into **angiotensin II** by angiotensin-converting enzyme (ACE). Angiotensin II can bind to two receptors—AT_1 and AT_2. AT_1 receptors are located throughout the body, including the brain, kidney, myocardium, peripheral vasculature, and adrenal glands. AT_2 receptors are located in the adrenal medullary, uterus, and brain and have no impact on blood pressure. Angiotensin II causes blood pressure elevation through potent vasoconstriction via stimulation of **catecholamines** and activation of the central sympathetic nervous system. Angiotensin-converting enzyme also stimulates the production of aldosterone, which in turn stimulates more sodium reabsorption in the kidney. The increased sodium reabsorption leads to decreased production of renin, which becomes the final link in the negative feedback loop that controls blood pressure in the glomerulus. Angiotensin II is converted to angiotensin III within the adrenal gland, and both angiotensin II and angiotensin III stimulate aldosterone production. This cascade of events is a sophisticated hormonal system that affects peripheral vascular resistance and blood pressure.

The RAAS has a dual function. Stimulation of the RAAS cascade increases blood pressure, which can cause damage to the endothelial, cells that line blood vessels. Thus stimulation of the RAAS also initiates a local inflammatory response that repairs damage to the endothelial cells. The long-term effects of this cycle of damage and repair are microvascular injury and endothelial cell dysfunction. The end-organ damage that ultimately results includes myocardial infarction, stroke, kidney disease, and peripheral artery disease.

It appears that chronic activation of the RAAS may have an etiologic role in the pathophysiology of diabetes as well as hypertension although the exact mechanism underlying this process has not been fully elucidated. It is well known that persons with hypertension are more likely to develop diabetes than are persons without hypertension. In addition, inhibition of the RAAS cascade by some antihypertensive medications has a positive effect on prevention of diabetes and diabetes complications.

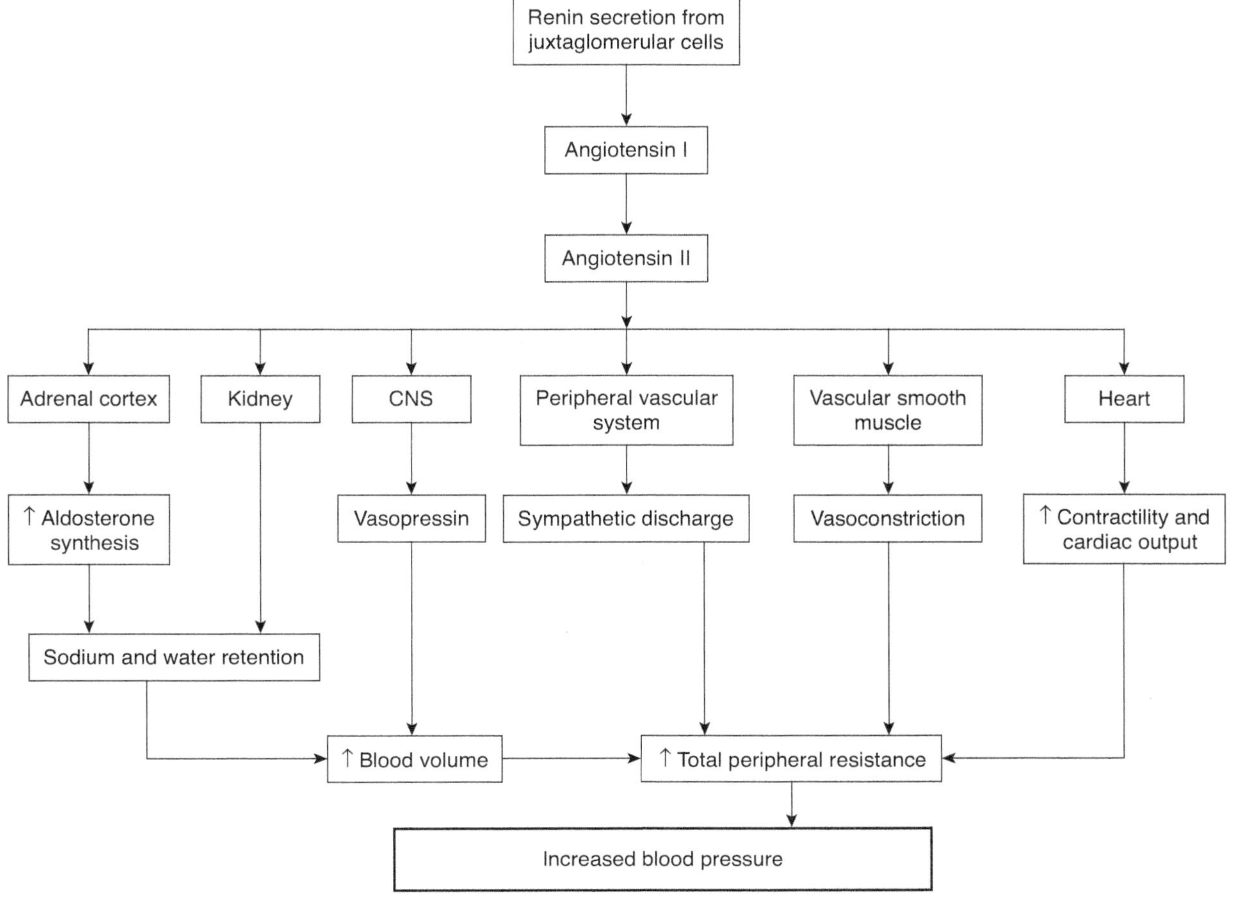

Figure 15-1 Renin–angiotensin–aldosterone system.

The Adrenergic Receptors

Arterial blood pressure is also controlled by the central and autonomic nervous systems. **Norepinephrine** and **epinephrine** are the primary neurotransmitters in the sympathetic nervous system, and the receptors for these hormones, called **adrenergic receptors**, are located in most organs. Adrenergic receptor stimulation in the smooth muscle that encases arteries and veins causes vasoconstriction or vasodilation. Two subtypes of adrenergic receptors exist, alpha and beta. These receptors are further subdivided into alpha$_1$, alpha$_2$, and two beta subtypes. The endothelial cells that line arterial and venous blood vessels have all the subtypes of adrenergic receptors.

The alpha$_1$ receptors cause vasoconstriction of peripheral arteries and veins when activated. The alpha$_2$ receptors suppress the release of norepinephrine presynaptically, thereby suppressing sympathetic output from the central nervous system. These receptors also increase vagal tone and suppress insulin secretion.

The two major subtypes of beta receptors are labeled beta$_1$ and beta$_2$. Cardiovascular structures typically have more beta than alpha receptors. The beta$_1$ receptors are concentrated in the cardiac muscle, conduction nodes, and kidney, whereas the beta$_2$ receptors are located in the lungs, liver, pancreas, and coronary arterioles. Stimulation of beta$_2$ receptors in the arterioles and venules causes vasodilation. Stimulation of beta$_1$ receptors in the heart causes increased heart rate and increased contractility.

Many of the drugs used to treat various cardiovascular conditions are selective or nonselective antagonists to the alpha or beta receptors. Drugs that block both subtypes of the alpha receptor are called **non-selective alpha-adrenergic antagonists**. Drugs that are selective for the alpha$_1$ or alpha$_2$ receptors are called **selective alpha-adrenergic antagonists**.

Drugs that are selective for the $alpha_1$ receptor are used to treat hypertension. Similarly some drugs are non-selective for the beta receptor subtypes and others are selective. Finally some drugs such as labetalol (Trandate) have a combined effect on both alpha and beta receptors.

The Baroreceptor Reflex

Another major factor in blood pressure regulation is the baroreceptor reflex, which originates in the aortic arch and carotid arteries. Baroreceptors are nerve endings in the wall of the artery that sense changes in blood pressure. When the blood pressure drops, the baroreceptors transmit signals that cause a reflex increase in heart rate and contractility and vasoconstriction in blood vessels, leading to increased blood pressure.

Diagnosis of Hypertension

Hypertension is diagnosed when systolic arterial blood pressure (SBP) is 140 mm Hg or higher or the diastolic blood pressure (DBP) is 90 mm Hg or higher on two or more separate occasions.[15,16] Hypertension can be described as primary or secondary. Primary hypertension is also known as essential or idiopathic, because there is no clear etiology. Secondary hypertension is caused by a primary disease of the kidney, adrenal gland, thyroid gland, coarctation of the aorta, or use of drugs such as combined oral contraceptives, estrogen, corticosteroids, sympathetic stimulants, appetite suppressants, antihistamines, and monoamine oxidase inhibitors. The majority of individuals with the diagnosis of hypertension have primary hypertension.

Several subclassifications are made for hypertension: prehypertension, stage 1 hypertension, and stage 2 hypertension. Normal blood pressure is SBP less than 120 mm Hg and DBP less than 80 mm Hg, and prehypertension is SBP 120–139 mm Hg or DBP 80–89 mm Hg. Stage 1 hypertension is SBP 140–159 mm Hg or DBP 90–99 mm Hg, and stage 2 hypertension is SBP 160 mm Hg or higher or DBP 100 mm Hg or higher.[15,17] Pharmacologic treatment should be offered if blood pressure values are consistently elevated and lifestyle modification has had no impact. Lifestyle and pharmacologic treatment should be initiated immediately if a person has end-organ damage secondary to elevated blood pressure.

Treatment of Women with Hypertension

The treatment goal for persons with hypertension is to decrease the risk of cardiovascular events, strokes, and kidney disease.[17] With every increase of 20/10 mm Hg increments, the risk for developing cardiovascular events and strokes doubles.[15] In 2014, the Eighth Joint National Committee (JNC 8) guideline for management of high blood pressure in adults was released.[18] The guideline incorporates data from recent randomized clinical trials to determine the evidence-based recommendations for blood pressure goals and initial medication recommendations, which are summarized in Table 15-2.

Table 15-2 Management of Blood Pressure in Adults

Criteria	Goal Blood Pressure	Initial Medications Recommended
< 60 years	Systolic < 140 mm Hg[a] Diastolic < 90 mm Hg[b]	Non-African American[c]: thiazide-type diuretic, calcium-channel blocker, ACE inhibitor or ARB African American[b]: thiazide-type diuretic or calcium-channel blocker
> 60 years	Systolic < 150 mm Hg[a] Diastolic < 90 mm Hg[a]	
> 18 years with diabetes	Systolic < 140 mm Hg[b] Diastolic < 90 mm Hg[b]	
> 18 years with chronic kidney disease	Systolic < 140 mm Hg[a] Diastolic < 90 mm Hg[a]	ACE inhibitor or ARB to improve kidney outcomes regardless of race or diabetes status[c]

Abbreviations: ACE = angiotensin-converting enzyme; ARB = angiotensin receptor blocker.

[a] This recommendation is based on expert opinion.

[b] This is a strong recommendation based on high quality evidence from well-designed randomized controlled trials or meta-analyses of such studies

[c] This is a moderate recommendation based on randomized controlled trials that have some limitations, well-designed non-randomized controlled trials, well designed observational studies, or meta-analyses of such studies

Source: James PA, Oparil S, Carter BL, et al. 2014 evidence-based guideline for the management of high blood pressure in adults: report from the panel members appointed to the Eighth Joint National Committee (JNC 8). *JAMA*. 2014;311:507-520.[18]

In addition to JNC 8, several guidelines for blood pressure management from other organizations are available.[16,17] These other guidelines differ slightly from JNC 8 in terms of BP goals for special populations, such as individuals with diabetes or chronic kidney disease and the elderly.

Pharmacologic Treatments for Women with Hypertension

The major categories of antihypertensive drugs include **diuretics, angiotensin-converting enzyme (ACE) inhibitors, angiotensin II receptor blockers (ARBs)**, and **calcium-channel blockers (CCBs)**. Other classes of medications for hypertension include **beta-adrenergic receptor antagonists (beta blockers)**, alpha$_1$ blockers, **central alpha$_2$-agonists**, direct vasodilators, and **direct renin inhibitors**.

Drugs commonly used for women with primary hypertension are those that reduce blood volume so as to reduce central venous pressure and cardiac output, those that reduce systemic vascular resistance, and those that reduce cardiac output through the mechanism of decreasing heart rate and stroke volume. Women with secondary hypertension usually are treated by focusing on the underlying disease, although they, too, may be prescribed antihypertensive drugs.

Historically, pharmacologic management of hypertension used a stepwise progression, starting with a specific medication if there was a compelling indication, or beginning with a thiazide diuretic if no compelling indication existed.[15] Based on updated studies incorporated into JNC 8, the first-line treatment for most individuals now consists of a drug from one of the following classes: thiazide diuretic, ACE inhibitor, ARB, or calcium-channel blocker.[18] If the goal BP is not reached within a month of treatment, the dose of the initial mediation can be increased or another major medication class can be added. If the goal BP still cannot be reached with two medications, a third antihypertensive can be added. Box 15-1 presents a common clinical scenario in which a woman may need additional medication for blood pressure control.

As most persons with hypertension will require at least two medications to achieve their BP goal, practitioners can consider starting a two-medication regimen initially if the woman has stage 2 hypertension.[16–18] The combination of an ACE inhibitor and ARB is not recommended due to the increased risk of renal injury and hyperkalemia when agents from these two classes are taken concomitantly.[19] The most common reason for discontinuing antihypertensive therapy is the development of side effects that adversely affect quality of life. Thus, when initially prescribing antihypertensive medications, frequent follow-up is necessary.

Box 15-1 A Regular Follow-up Visit for a Woman with Diabetes and Hypertension

SW is a 53-year-old white female presenting for regular follow-up care for her diabetes, hyperlipidemia, hypertension, coronary artery disease, and depression. SW had a myocardial infarction 2 years ago. She is able to manage her medications; however, she struggles with her diet and exercise regimens. She successfully quit smoking 6 months ago. She has been checking her glucose and blood pressure routinely and brings her logbook with her to the visit. Her glucose has been controlled well, as evidenced by a hemoglobin A_{1c} of 6.8 mg/dL at her last visit, as well as her LDL of 75 mg/dL, HDL of 46 mg/dL, and triglycerides of 110 mg/dL. Her blood pressure recordings from her logbook are 142/89, 138/92, 145/88, and 135/83 mm Hg. Over the past few visits, her blood pressure readings have been elevating.

Today her vital signs are height, 5 feet 5 inches (161.1 cm); weight, 220 pounds (99.8 kg); blood pressure, 140/90 mm Hg; heart rate, 82 bpm; respirations, 17 breaths/min; and pulse oximetry, 98%. Current medications include metformin (Glucophage) 1000 mg 2 times daily, ASA (aspirin) 81 mg once daily, exenatide (Byetta) 5 mcg SQ 2 times daily, metoprolol succinate (Toprol XL) 50 mg once daily, sertraline (Zoloft) 100 mg once daily, atorvastatin (Lipitor) 20 mg once daily, and hydrochlorothiazide (HydroDIURIL) 25 mg once daily. SW has no problems to report. Her physical exam is unremarkable.

SW is considered at high risk given her history of coronary artery disease and diabetes. She has taken some steps to reduce her risk, including quitting smoking and controlling her diabetes and lipid values. When initially diagnosed, she would have been counseled about her diet and need for exercise. Her blood pressure goal should be less than 140/90 mm Hg.

Previously her blood pressure was controlled well on the agents she is currently taking. She has a compelling indication for metoprolol succinate (Toprol XL) because of her previous myocardial infarction. However, she is not at her goal, and ACE inhibitors are preferred for persons with type 2 diabetes. She would benefit from the addition of an ACE inhibitor, and it can be given in combination with hydrochlorothiazide. A reduction in the hydrochlorothiazide may need to be done in the initialization of the ACE inhibitor because of the synergistic effect of the medications. If SW develops a troublesome cough that is interfering with her daily activities, a change from an ACE inhibitor to an ARB would be recommended.

Drug–Drug Interactions with Any Antihypertensive

A few drug interactions exist that affect all classes of antihypertensives. Nonsteroidal anti-inflammatory drugs (NSAIDs) inhibit vasodilation, and they also promote salt and water retention. Thus, NSAIDs can interfere with or reverse the antihypertensive effect of these drugs and should be used cautiously. Vasoconstricting agents such as decongestants in over-the-counter (OTC) cold remedies and the nasal vasodilators also found in OTC preparations can also increase blood pressure. Counseling about OTC drugs that increase blood pressure should occur when an antihypertensive agent is initially prescribed. Tricyclic antidepressants can lower blood pressure, for example; when they are taken concomitantly with antihypertensives, nocturnal or orthostatic hypotension can occur. Table 15-3 lists some examples of drugs that have an independent effect on blood pressure.

Diuretics

The mechanism of action for all diuretics is increased salt concentration in urine, which causes increased water excretion. The general mechanism of action is via a reduction in reabsorption of sodium ions, as these ions move through the renal tubule cells. The three classes of diuretics are distinguished one the basis of where they inhibit sodium reabsorption: Thiazide-type diuretics act in the distal tubule and connecting segment, loop diuretics act in the ascending limb of the loop of Henle, and potassium-sparing diuretics affect the aldosterone-sensitive principal cells in the cortical collecting tubule. Figure 15-2 illustrates the action of these agents.

The thiazide and loop diuretics are derived from sulfanilamide, which is in the family of sulfa drugs; thus individuals who are allergic to sulfonamides may be allergic to these diuretics. The clinical relevance of this potential cross-reactivity is unclear and controversial. Although the Food and Drug Administration (FDA) has approved labeling that states sulfanilamide diuretics may be contraindicated for persons who are allergic to sulfa drugs, this cross-reactivity remains rare. A review of the literature did not find strong evidence to support avoiding therapy in these individuals.[20] Prescribers should be aware of the potential problem, and individuals with a sulfa allergy should be monitored carefully if diuretics are initiated.

Table 15-3 Drugs That Affect Blood Pressure[a]

Agents with Hypotensive Effects	Agents with Hypertensive Effects
Anesthetics	Bromocriptine (Parlodel)
Atypical antidepressants (e.g., trazodone [Desyrel])	Corticosteroids
Antipsychotics (e.g., Clozapine [Clozaril])	Cyclosporine (Sandimmune)
Benzodiazepines (e.g., lorazepam [Ativan], alprazolam [Xanax])	Estrogens (combination oral contraceptives)
Digoxin (Lanoxin)	Herbs: feverfew, ginseng, goldenseal, St. John's wort
Dopamine agonists (e.g., levodopa-carbidopa [Sinemet])	Immunosuppressants (e.g., cyclosporine [Sandimmune], tacrolimus [Prograf])
Nitrates (e.g., nitroglycerin [Nitrostat])	Monoamine oxidase (MAO) inhibitors (e.g., phenelzine [Nardil])
Opiates	Nonsteroidal anti-inflammatory drugs (e.g., ibuprofen [Motrin], celecoxib [Celebrex])
Tricyclic antidepressants (e.g., amitriptyline [Elavil])	Stimulants (e.g., nicotine, amphetamines)
	Sympathomimetics (e.g., pseudoephedrine [Sudafed])
	Weight loss agents (e.g., sibutramine [Meridia], phentermine [Adipex])

[a] This table is not comprehensive as new information is being identified on a regular basis.

Thiazides

Thiazides (Table 15-4) can be used as monotherapy or in combination with other medications. These agents lower blood pressure further than other antihypertensive agents when used as monotherapy.[21] Thiazides have a synergistic relationship with other antihypertensive drugs and can be used in combination with other antihypertensive medications.

Thiazide diuretics inhibit the **sodium chloride symporter** in the distal convoluted tubule. Inhibition of the sodium-channel transport mechanism results in increased sodium excretion and, therefore, increased water excretion. With chronic therapy, thiazide diuretics also lower BP due to a decrease in peripheral vascular resistance. Because most of the filtered plasma is reabsorbed in the loop of Henle, thiazides are less potent than other diuretics. Overall, approximately 3% to 5% of the filtered sodium is inhibited from reabsorption if thiazides are used at maximal doses.

Hydrochlorothiazide (Esidrix, HydroDIURIL, Microzide) and chlorthalidone (Hygroton) are the two most commonly used thiazide diuretics in clinical practice. The antihypertensive effect of hydrochlorothiazide is optimal at 12.5–50 mg per day. Doses of more than 50 mg do not offer much benefit and result in a higher incidence of electrolyte abnormalities. There is significant inter-individual variability in the clinical response to a specific

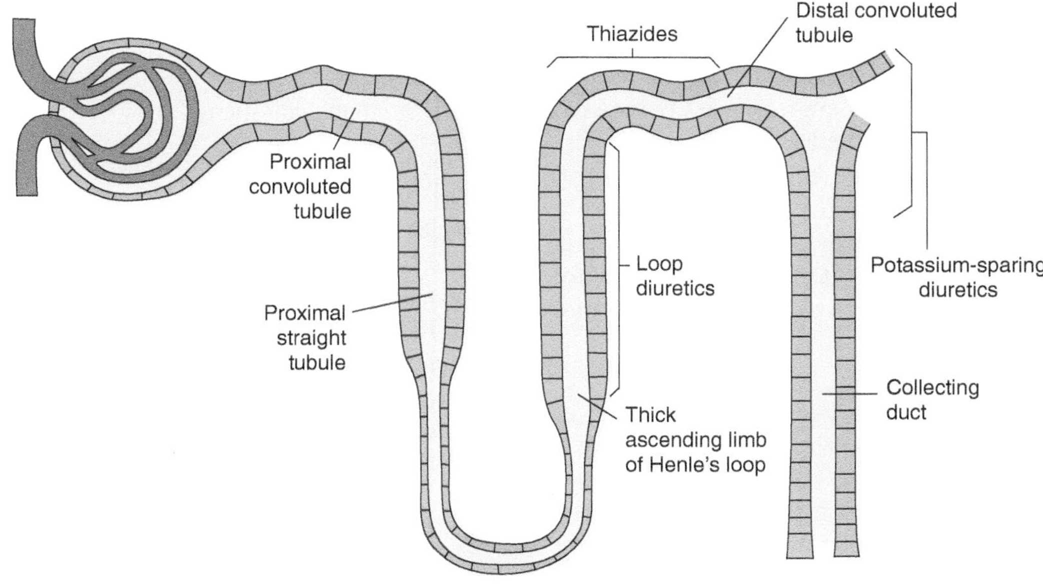

Figure 15-2 Site of action of diuretics.

dose of hydrochlorothiazide and, thus, dosing must be individualized.

The antihypertensive effect of chlorthalidone is optimal at 12.5–25 mg per day. Chlorthalidone (Hygroton) has a longer half-life than does hydrochlorothiazide and more potent. Chlorthalidone has been shown to be more effective than hydrochlorothiazide in some studies but not others and thus, neither drug is clearly more effective than the other in the studies conducted to date.

Side Effects/Contraindications

As a class of drugs, thiazides generally are well tolerated. Most of the side effects involve metabolic effects secondary to fluid and electrolyte imbalance such as hypokalemia, hyperuricemia, hypercalcemia, hyponatremia, impaired carbohydrate tolerance, and hyperlipidemia, with the most common being hypercalcemia. These side effects can be minimized with lower doses of hydrochlorothiazide (HydroDIURIL) or chlorthalidone (Hygroton), such as 6.25–12.5 mg per day. Few central nervous system or gastrointestinal effects are associated with thiazide use. Thiazides can also cause photosensitivity and rarely leukopenia or pancreatitis.

Drug–Drug Interactions

Cross-sensitivity is known to exist between thiazides and sulfa drugs; thus, an allergic reaction is possible if an individual has a sulfa allergy and takes a thiazide-type drug. Caution should be exercised when an individual combines thiazides with NSAIDs or steroids, because the

Table 15-4 Thiazide Diuretics[a]

Drug: Generic (Brand)	Formulation	Dose per Day	Frequency per Day	Duration of Action
Chlorothiazide (Diuril)	250-mg, 500-mg tablets	500 mg–2 g PO	2 divided doses	6–12 hours
Chlorthalidone (Hygroton)	25-mg, 50-mg, 100-mg tablets	50–100 mg PO	Single dose	24–72 hours
Hydrochlorothiazide (Esidrix, HydroDIURIL, Microzide)	25-mg, 50-mg tablets 12.5-mg capsules	12.5–50 mg PO	Single dose	6–12 hours
Indapamide (Lozol)	1.25-mg, 2.5-mg tablets	1.25–5 mg PO	Single dose	14–25 hours
Metolazone (Zaroxolyn)	2.5-mg, 5-mg, 10-mg tablets	2.5–5 mg PO	Single dose	> 24 hours

[a] Use cautiously among individuals who have renal impairment, hepatic impairment, gout, diabetes, and dehydration. These drugs are often formulated in combination with other antihypertensive drugs.

antihypertensive effect of the thiazide can be diminished while the risk of acute renal failure is increased. Thiazides can increase lithium levels and should not be administered in combination with quinidine, as a prolonged QT interval may result in polymorphic ventricular tachycardia.

Corticosteroids can enhance the adverse effect of hypokalemia. If hypokalemia occurs for any reason with thiazides, digitalis (Lanoxin) toxicity can become more likely. When beta blockers are taken concurrently with thiazides, there is an increased risk of hyperglycemia and hyperlipidemia.

Loop Diuretics

Loop diuretics (Table 15-5) act as a membrane transporter that is made up of sodium, potassium, and chloride in the thick ascending limb of the loop of Henle and competes for the chloride-binding site. Loop diuretics will be effective even in persons with significant renal failure. Because calcium and magnesium reabsorption depends on the concentrations of sodium and chloride, these diuretics enhance urinary loss of calcium—thus, they act in a different manner than thiazide diuretics, which promote calcium retention. This effect can be clinically useful when treating persons with hypercalcemia. Loop diuretics also have direct vascular effects such as increasing systemic venous capacitance, which decreases left ventricular filling pressure and subsequently lowers blood pressure. In short, the effects of decreased blood volume and vasodilation result in lowered blood pressure and decreased edema. Loop diuretics are excreted by the renal system. Loop diuretics are not as effective as thiazides in lowering blood pressure, but they are the most effective for persons who have edema secondary to heart failure.

Table 15-5 Loop Diuretics[a]

Drug: Generic (Brand)	Formulations	Dose per Day[a]	Duration of Action
Bumetanide (Bumex)	0.5-mg, 1-mg, 2-mg tablets	0.5–2 mg PO	4–6 hours
Ethacrynic acid (Edecrin)	25-mg tablets	50–200 mg PO, maximum of 400 mg/day	12 hours
Furosemide (Lasix)	20-mg, 40-mg, 80-mg tablets	20–80 mg PO is usual starting dose for woman with hypertension; maximum of 600 mg/day	6–8 hours
Torsemide (Demadex)	5-mg, 10-mg, 20-mg, 100-mg tablets	5–20 mg PO, maximum of 200 mg as single dose	6–8 hours

[a] All of these drugs can be prescribed in a single daily dose or as a divided dose taken twice daily.

Side Effects/Contraindications

The majority of loop diuretics' side effects are related to intense diuresis leading to electrolyte disturbances such as hyponatremia, hypokalemia, hypomagnesemia, and hypocalcemia. The same sodium/potassium/chloride membrane transporters exist in the inner ear, so loop diuretics can—albeit rarely—cause ototoxicity if given in high doses intravenously. The major precautions to consider prior to starting loop diuretics include sodium depletion, volume depletion, and allergic reaction due to potential cross-sensitivity among persons with a sulfa allergy.

Drug–Drug Interactions

Loop diuretics can have several drug–drug interactions. When taken with aminoglycosides or cisplatin (Platinol), a synergism can occur that increases the risk of ototoxicity. Similar to the case with thiazides, NSAIDs or probenecid (Benemid) can blunt the effect of loop diuretics if taken concurrently. The risk of hypokalemia increases if other drugs that cause hypokalemia are taken with loop diuretics. If hypokalemia occurs, digitalis toxicity becomes more likely in persons taking digoxin (Lanoxin).

Potassium-Sparing Diuretics

Potassium-sparing diuretics (Table 15-6) are rarely used as first-line agents for treatment of hypertension. These diuretics do have some antihypertensive effects, although their primary function is in the treatment of heart failure. Potassium-sparing diuretics act by blocking the effects of aldosterone on the collecting and late distal tubules, thereby preventing reabsorption of sodium back into the cells that line the nephron. When sodium is reabsorbed into the luminal cells, potassium is secreted. Thus when sodium reabsorption is prevented, potassium is conserved. Two types of potassium-sparing diuretics are available: the ENaC-channel blockers, triamterene (Dyrenium) and amiloride (Midamor); and the aldosterone antagonists, spironolactone (Aldactone) and eplerenone (Inspra). Triamterene and amiloride block sodium channels in cells in the late distal tubule. The aldosterone antagonists competitively block the intracellular receptor for aldosterone. When the aldosterone receptor is bound to aldosterone, proteins are synthesized that activate sodium channels and increase the synthesis of new potassium

Table 15-6 Potassium-Sparing Diuretics[a]

Drug: Generic (Brand)	Formulations	Dose per Day	Duration of Action
Amiloride (Midamor)	5-mg tablets	5–10 mg PO daily or in 2 divided doses; maximum 20 mg per day	24 hours
Eplerenone (Inspra)	25-mg, 50-mg tablets	50–100 mg PO daily or in 2 divided doses	4–6 hours
Spironolactone (Aldactone)	25-mg, 50-mg, 100-mg tablets	25–100 mg PO daily or in 2 divided doses	48–72 hours
Triamterene (Dyrenium)	50-mg, 100-mg tablets	100–300 mg PO daily or in 2 divided doses; maximum 300 mg per day	7–9 hours

[a] Caution should be used in persons with renal impairment, electrolyte disturbances, or serum or potassium higher than 5.5 mEq/L.

channels. Thus, the aldosterone antagonists reduce sodium reabsorption and reduce potassium secretion. Potassium-sparing diuretics are eliminated by renal excretion, with the exception of triamterene, which is metabolized into an active metabolite that is then eliminated via urinary excretion.

Side Effects/Contraindications

The most common side effect of potassium-sparing diuretics is hyperkalemia, especially when a potassium-sparing diuretic is administered in combination with other agents that have some potassium-sparing properties, such as ACE inhibitors or ARBs. Potassium levels need to be determined prior to initiation of treatment and monitored if potassium-sparing diuretics are to be used in addition to other agents that increase the risk of hyperkalemia. Aldosterone antagonists have a steroidal chemical structure and can therefore have endocrine side effects such as gynecomastia and menstrual irregularities.

Drug–Drug Interactions

Concomitant use of lithium (Lithobid) or NSAIDs should be undertaken with caution, as use of either with triamterene (Dyrenium) can cause lithium toxicity. NSAIDs can increase the risk of renal toxicity when taken with these diuretics. ARBs and other potassium-sparing agents increase the risk for hyperkalemia and are generally contraindicated if a person is taking potassium-sparing diuretics. Close monitoring is recommended for any individual who is taking a potassium-sparing diuretic and any other medication that has the potential to increase potassium levels, such as combined hormonal contraception that contains drospirenone (Yasmin, Yaz).

Diuretics and Special Populations: Pregnancy, Lactation, and the Elderly

Conflicting thoughts have been voiced about the use of diuretics during pregnancy, as these agents may increase the risk of impaired placental blood flow. Diuretics can cause decreased amniotic fluid volume and decreased placental perfusion, and there have been case reports of neonatal hypoglycemia, hypokalemia, and hyponatremia when these medications were taken close to birth. However, the most popular diuretic, hydrochlorothiazide (HydroDIURIL), is considered safe for use by women during pregnancy. Thiazides have been used for treatment of chronic or gestational hypertension, but they should not be used for the treatment of preeclampsia.

Diuretics also are generally considered safe for women who are breastfeeding. Higher doses have been associated with intense diuresis that results in decreased milk production. For example, it is suggested that hydrochlorothiazide be limited to 50 mg daily. Chlorothiazide (Diuril) and hydrochlorothiazide have the shortest half-lives of the thiazides and may be preferred for a breastfeeding woman because of that factor.[22] No information is available about lactation and use of triamterene (Dyrenium) and eplerenone (Inspra), so alternatives to these medications is suggested when a woman is breastfeeding.

Providers need to be cautious when prescribing thiazides for elderly women and should start with a lower-than-recommended daily dose in this population, such as hydrochlorothiazide 6.25–12.5 mg daily. One benefit of hydrochlorothiazide is that over several years of treatment, small improvements in total body bone density have been noted.[23]

Angiotensin-Converting Enzyme Inhibitors

ACE inhibitors (Table 15-7) are a widely used class of antihypertensive drugs and the fourth most common medication prescribed in the United. States. ACE inhibitors are effective for many women. The antihypertensive medications that do not have the adverse lipid and glucose metabolic effects associated with beta blockers and thiazides include ACE inhibitors, ARBs, and direct renin inhibitors. In addition, because ACE inhibitors block the RAAS cascade, they protect against end-organ disease such as renal failure.

Table 15-7 Angiotensin-Converting Enzyme Inhibitors

Drug: Generic (Brand)	Formulations	Dose	Duration of Action
Benazepril (Lotensin)	5-mg, 10-mg, 20-mg, 40-mg tablets	Initially 10 mg PO, maintenance 20–40 mg daily; maximum of 80 mg daily	24 hours
Captopril (Capoten)	12.5-mg, 25-mg, 50-mg, 100-mg tablets	Initially 25 mg 2–3 PO times/day; maximum of 450 mg daily. Take 1 hour before meals.	2 hours
Enalapril (Vasotec)	2.5-mg, 5-mg, 10-mg, 20-mg tablets	Initially 2.5 mg PO daily, maintenance 10–20 mg daily	12–24 hours
Fosinopril (Monopril)	10-mg, 20-mg, 40-mg tablets	Initially 10 mg PO daily, maintenance 20–40 mg daily; maximum of 80 mg daily	24 hours
Lisinopril (Prinivil, Zestril)	2.5-mg, 5-mg, 10-mg, 20-mg, 30-mg, 40-mg tablets	Initially 10 mg PO daily, maintenance 20–40 mg daily; maximum of 40 mg daily	24 hours
Moexipril (Univasc)	7.5-mg, 15-mg tablets	Initially 7.5 mg PO daily, maintenance 15–30 mg daily; maximum of 30 mg daily. Take 1 hour before meals PO.	> 24 hours
Perindopril (Aceon)	2-mg, 4-mg, 8-mg tablets	Initially 4 mg PO daily, maintenance 4–8 mg daily; maximum of 16 mg daily	25–120 hours
Quinapril (Accupril)	5-mg, 10-mg, 20-mg, 40-mg tablets	Initially 10 mg PO daily, maintenance 20–40 mg daily	24 hours
Ramipril (Altace)	1.25-mg, 2.5-mg, 5-mg, 10-mg tablets	Initially 2.5 mg PO daily, maintenance 2.5–20 mg daily; maximum of 20 mg daily. May sprinkle over 4 ounces of applesauce or with water if difficult to swallow.	24 hours
Trandolapril (Mavik)	1-mg, 2-mg, 4-mg tablets	Initially 1 mg PO daily, maintenance 2–4 mg daily; maximum of 8 mg daily. Initially 2 mg if person is African American.	72 hours

ACE inhibitors are approved for the treatment of hypertension, left ventricular systolic dysfunction, myocardial infarction, chronic kidney disease, renal protection in persons with diabetes, and for individuals who are at high risk for cardiovascular events. The majority of ACE inhibitors are available in generic formulations. Despite the different formulations, there is no significant reason to choose one ACE inhibitor rather than another, other than pragmatic reasons such as local cost or coverage on a formulary.

Some pharmacogenomic variations appear to exist with these drugs, and there is significant individual variability in response to them. African Americans often do not have the same benefit in blood pressure reduction with ACE inhibitors when compared to the response to calcium-channel blockers or thiazide diuretics[18,24]; consequently, these drugs are not recommended as the first-line treatment for African Americans.[18]

Most ACE inhibitors are actually prodrugs metabolized in the liver to an active metabolite. These agents prevent the conversion of angiotensin I into angiotensin II—hence the name *ACE inhibitor*. The ACE enzyme that catalyzes the alteration of angiotensin I into angiotensin II exists primarily in endothelial tissue in the pulmonary vasculature, and angiotensin II is therefore primarily produced in the blood vessels as blood passes through the lungs. ACE, in addition to its effects on angiotensin, blocks the degradation of plasma bradykinin and stimulates the synthesis of vasodilating prostaglandins. Bradykinin is a vasodilator; thus the excess bradykinin levels that result following use of ACE inhibitors results in vasodilation, decreased peripheral vascular resistance, and a lowered blood pressure through this independent pathway.

ACE inhibitors work well in combination with thiazides. The thiazides induce sodium depletion, which activates the renin–angiotensin–aldosterone system and shifts blood pressure control to angiotensin, which is then blocked by the ACE inhibitor. The mechanism of action whereby the ACE inhibitor suppresses the renin–angiotensin–aldosterone system may also explain why ACE inhibitors prevent the development of diabetes in persons with hypertension. Angiotension II increased hepatic glucose production and decreases insulin sensitivity. When the production of angiotensin II is blocked, these effects of glucose metabolism are inhibited.

Side Effects/Contraindications

One obvious side effect of the initial dose of ACE inhibitors is hypotension with symptoms of weakness, dizziness, or syncope. This effect is more common in persons who are volume depleted or those who have heart failure. Common side effects of ACE inhibitors include a dry cough that is secondary to elevated levels of bradykinin and substance P. The excess bradykinin is responsible for the dry cough that occurs in as many as 20% of persons who take these drugs. This dry cough is more common in women and among individuals of Asian and African backgrounds.[16] If an ACE inhibitor cough develops, the drug is discontinued, and an ARB is most often used as a substitute. Angioedema is a rare but serious complication, and individuals should seek urgent medical attention if they experience swelling of their tongue or face.

The major adverse effects associated with ACE inhibitors are hyperkalemia and deterioration of renal function. A baseline serum creatinine and potassium level should be obtained prior to initiating these drugs and again after the first week of therapy. Small rises in both creatinine and potassium are expected due to reduced pressure within the renal glomerulus and decreased filtration. An increase of more than 30% in the serum creatinine level is considered significant and warrants further investigation and possible referral. If the potassium level rises to more than 5.6–6.0 mEq/L, the ACE inhibitor should be stopped and renal function monitored carefully. Angioedema is a rare but serious complication that is secondary to the increase in bradykinins. It usually develops in the first week of therapy. Angioedema is life-threatening and individuals should seek urgent medical attention if they experience swelling of the tongue or face.

Contraindications to ACE Inhibitors

Contraindications to use of ACE inhibitors include any history of angioedema, regardless of the cause, pregnancy, renal artery stenosis, and previous allergy to ACE inhibitors.

Drug–Drug Interactions

Since ACE inhibitors can cause hyperkalemia, this class of antihypertensive medication should be used with caution by individuals taking potassium supplements, potassium-sparing diuretics, or any other medications that can increase potassium levels. The combined use of ACE inhibitors, diuretics, and NSAIDs can lead to a significant risk for acute renal failure, especially among the elderly. Both ACE inhibitors and NSAIDs can cause functional renal insufficiency, so this drug combination is considered potentially nephrotoxic. Major drug–drug interactions associated with ACE inhibitors are listed in Table 15-8.[25,26]

Table 15-8 Major Drug Interactions Associated with ACE Inhibitors and Angiotensin Receptor Blockers[a]

Drug: Generic (Brand)	Second Agent	Effect
Aliskiren	ACE inhibitor	Hyperkalemia and nephrotoxicity
Allopurinol (Zyloprim)	ACE inhibitor	Increases risk of Stevens-Johnson syndrome
Alpha blockers	ACE inhibitor	Augmentation of first-dose syncope associated with alpha blockers
Antacids	Fosinopril (Monopril)	Reduces bioavailability of fosinopril
Aspirin	ACE inhibitor or ARB	Possible antagonism of ACE inhibitor effects; not usually clinically significant at low doses of aspirin
Azathioprine (Imuran)	ACE inhibitor	Leukopenia
Clonidine (Catapres)	ACE inhibitor	Potentiate antihypertensive effects of clonidine
Co-trimoxazole (Septra)	ACE inhibitor	Hyperkalemia and sudden death
Cyclosporine (Neoral)	ACE inhibitor	Hyperkalemia and nephrotoxicity
Digoxin (Lanoxin)	ACE inhibitor	Hyperkalemia
	Captopril (Capoten)	Decreased clearance of captopril
Fluconazole (Diflucan)	Losartan (Cozaar)	Prevents conversion of losartan to its active metabolite, thereby decreasing hypotensive effect of losartan
Indomethacin (Indocin)	ACE inhibitor	Hyperkalemia
Immunosuppressants	Captopril (Capoten)	
Interferon alpha$_2$	ACE inhibitor	Granulocytopenia
Heparin and low-molecular weight heparins	ACE inhibitor	Hyperkalemia
Ketoconazole (Nizoral)	Losartan (Cozaar)	Inhibits CYP enzyme responsible for metabolizing losartan and thereby decreases effectiveness
Lithium (Lithobid)	ACE inhibitor or ARB	Lithium toxicity
Nonsteroidal anti-inflammatory drugs (NSAIDs)	ACE inhibitor or ARB	NSAIDs decrease the efficacy of ACE inhibitors and ARBs; their combination may increase the nephrotoxic effect
Phenobarbital (Luminal)	Losartan (Cozaar)	Phenobarbital induces CYP3A4 and decreases serum levels of losartan
Potassium-sparing diuretics	ACE inhibitor or ARB	Enhanced hyperkalemic effect

(continues)

Table 15-8 Major Drug Interactions Associated with ACE Inhibitors and Angiotensin Receptor Blockers[a] *(continued)*

Drug: Generic (Brand)	Second Agent	Effect
Rifampin (Rifadin)	Losartan (Cozaar)	Decreased effectiveness of losartan
Sirolimus (Rapamune)	ACE inhibitor	Angioedema in persons who have not had this response with the specific ACE inhibitor previously
Tacrolimus (Protopic)	ACE inhibitor	Hyperkalemia and nephrotoxicity
Tetracyclines	Quinapril (Accupro)	Magnesium carbonate in quinapril reduces absorption of tetracycline
Trimethoprim	ACE inhibitor	Hyperkalemia

Abbreviations: ACE = angiotensin-converting enzyme; ARB = angiotensin receptor blocker.
[a] This table is not comprehensive as new information is being identified on a regular basis.
Sources: Data from Regulski M, Regulska K, Stanisz B et al. Chemistry and pharmacology of angiotension-converting enzyme inhibitors. *Curr Pharmaceut Des*. 2015;21(13):1764-1775[26]; Unger T, Kaschina E. Drug interactions with angiotensin receptor blockers: a comparison with other antihypertensives. *Drug Safety*. 2003;26(10):707-720.[25]

ACE Inhibitors and Special Populations: Pregnancy, Lactation, and the Elderly

ACE inhibitors should not be used by women during pregnancy. These drugs have been linked to an increase in the risk of birth defects in the last 6 months of pregnancy.[26] They also should not be used by childbearing-age women who are considering pregnancy unless there is a compelling indication that outweighs the risk.

Most ACE inhibitors—but especially benzepril (Lotensin), captopril (Capoten), and quinapril (Accupril)—are found in low amounts in breast milk and are considered compatible with breastfeeding. Lisinopril (Zestril) has insufficient information regarding its use during lactation, and alternative therapy is suggested in breastfeeding women.[22]

Age is not a contraindication to the use of ACE inhibitors. Multiple benefits for the elderly using ACE inhibitors have been reported, including reduced decline of muscle strength.[27] The exact mechanism of action leading to this effect is not known.[27]

Angiotensin Receptor Blockers

Angiotensin II receptor blockers (ARBs) are also known as angiotensin II receptor antagonists (Table 15-9). This class of drugs is effective for the treatment of hypertension and heart failure. Although many of the ARBs are not currently available in a generic formulations, others can be found in formulations combined with other antihypertensive drugs, most commonly hydrochlorothiazide.

Two types of receptors can be found for angiotensin II—namely, the AT_2 and AT_1 receptors. ARBs possess a high affinity for the AT_1 receptor and bind specifically to it, thereby blocking the effects of angiotensin II on these receptors. These drugs have a slow dissociation from the

Table 15-9 Angiotensin Receptor Blockers

Drug: Generic (Brand)	Formulations	Dose	Duration of Action
Candesartan (Atacand, Atacand HCT)	4-mg, 8-mg, 16-mg, 32-mg tablets	Initially 16 mg PO, maintenance dose 8–32 mg daily; maximum dose 32 mg. Take daily or as divided dose.	> 24 hours
Eprosartan (Teveten, Teveten HCT)	400-mg, 600-mg tablets	Initially 600 mg PO daily, maintenance dose 400–600 mg; maximum dose 800 mg daily	5–9 hours
Irbesartan (Avapro, Avalide)	75-mg, 150-mg, 300-mg tablets	Initially 150 mg PO daily, maintenance dose 300 mg, maximum dose 300 mg daily.	> 24 hours
Losartan (Cozaar, Hyzaar)	25-mg, 50-mg, 100-mg tablets	Initially 50 mg PO daily, maintenance dose 25–100 mg daily; maximum of dose 100 mg daily	6–9 hours
Olmesartan (Benicar, Benicar HCT)	5-mg, 20-mg, 40-mg tablets	Initially 20 mg PO daily, maintenance dose 20–40 mg; maximum dose 40 mg daily	13 hours
Telmisartan (Micardis, Micardis HCT)	20-mg, 40-mg, 80-mg tablets	Initially 40 mg PO daily, maintenance dose 20–80 mg; maximum dose 80 mg daily	24 hours
Valsartan (Diovan, Diovan HCT, Exforge)	40-mg, 80-mg, 160-mg, 320-mg tablets	Initially 80–160 mg PO daily, maintenance dose 80–320 mg; maximum dose 320 mg daily	24 hours

AT_1 receptor that results in a long half-life, which has some clinical benefits. For example, the effects continue even if a dose is missed. It is hypothesized that these drugs are more effective in inhibiting the effects of angiotensin II than are ACE inhibitors because multiple physiologic pathways create angiotensin II—not just conversion from angiotensin I. ARBs in combination with a thiazide work well, and this is a common combination when two agents are needed to meet blood pressure goals.

Side Effects/Contraindications

The rate of discontinuation of ARBs due to side effects is similar to the discontinuation rate of placebo tablets, making them a generally well-tolerated category of drug.[28] Because these agents do not increase levels of bradykinin, ARBs are not associated with a dry cough. Hyperkalemia and a rise in serum creatinine are frequent concerns for persons using ARBs. If serum values of potassium or creatinine increase, the provider should review the individual's drug list, recommend the initiation of a low-potassium diet, and consider prescribing a diuretic (e.g., a loop or thiazide diuretic) to increase potassium excretion. When a person with chronic kidney disease is started on these drugs, serum potassium levels should be evaluated within 1 to 2 weeks.

Angiotensin II normally effects a constriction of the efferent arterioles of the glomeruli in the kidney; thus, when an ARB is used, the sudden lack of angiotensin results in vasodilation and lower intraglomerular pressure that allows an initial decrease in the glomerular filtration rate, which in turn leads to a rise in serum creatinine levels and does not reflect actual worsening of renal function. A 20% to 30% rise in creatinine is an expected outcome, and the individual should continue on the drug. If the level continues to rise, the drug should be discontinued.

Drug–Drug Interactions

Interactions between ARBs and other drugs are similar to those associated with ACE inhibitors, as listed in Table 15-8. Hypotension can occur in volume- or salt-depleted individuals, so these agents should be used cautiously in combination with potassium-sparing diuretics and potassium supplements. Losartan (Cozaar) is the one exception to the benign profile enjoyed by most ARBs. Losartan is metabolized by CYP2C9 into an active metabolite that accounts for the therapeutic effect; in turn, agents that inhibit CYP2C9 such as ketoconazole (Nizoral) may decrease the effectiveness of losartan. Conversely, rifampin (Rifadin) induces CYP2C9 and shortens the half-life of losartan, again decreasing effectiveness. Valsartan must be taken 1 to 2 hours before a meal in order to preserve the desired bioavailability as its absorption is decreased in the presence of food.[25]

ARBs and Special Populations: Pregnancy, Lactation, and the Elderly

ARBs should be avoided by all women of childbearing age as they are associated with teratogenic and fetotoxic effects. Insufficient information exists regarding the use of ARBs among women who are breastfeeding. Therefore, alternative drugs are recommended, especially if the nursling is a newborn or preterm infant.[22]

Aging is associated with loss of arterial elasticity and an increased risk of hypertension. As previously noted, older women also are at increased risk of comorbidities, any of which may require different treatments and which often involve the renal system. ARBs are not contraindicated for postmenopausal woman, but these women should be screened and monitored carefully because of the possibility of chronic diseases.

Direct Renin Inhibitors

Direct renin inhibitors suppress plasma renin activity, thereby preventing the conversion of angiotensinogen into angiotensin I at a different point in the RAAS cascade compared to ACE inhibitors and ARBs. Aliskiren (Tekturna) is the only drug in this category approved for use by the FDA at this time. The release of renin in the kidney is controlled by three major pathways: The macula densa pathway and intrarenal baroreceptor pathway are within the kidney, and the beta-adrenergic receptor pathway is in the central nervous system. Blocking the conversion of angiotensinogen into angiotensin I effectively inhibits all three pathways that stimulate the RAAS reflex cascade, which leads to a reduction in the overall production of angiotensin I and angiotensin II.

The recommended initial dose of aliskiren is 150 mg daily; however, if the goal blood pressure is not obtained, the dose can be increased to 300 mg daily. This agent can be used as monotherapy or in combination with all other antihypertensive agents. Aliskiren added to amlodipine (Norvasc), ramipril (Altace), and hydrochlorothiazide has been found to produce significantly greater reductions in blood pressure when compared to monotherapy.[29] However, due to a lack of evidence regarding its benefit in cardiovascular outcomes and increased cost, the role of aliskiren compared to other agents with better outcomes is currently unclear.

Side Effects/Contraindications

Aliskiren (Tekturna) should not be prescribed for persons who are taking an ACE inhibitor or ARB. Many of the same side effects seen with use of ACE inhibitors and ARBs are observed with use of direct renin inhibitors, such as angioedema, hypotension, and hyperkalemia. Similarly, the same concerns about possible impaired renal function and hyperkalemia apply with the use of direct renin inhibitors, and the same precautions should be taken in monitoring individuals who use direct renin inhibitors as are applied in individuals who take ACE inhibitors or ARBs.

Direct Renal Inhibitors and Special Populations: Pregnancy, Lactation, and the Elderly

Aliskiren (Tekturna) is contraindicated in pregnancy for same reasons that ACE inhibitors and ARBs are contraindicated in this population. When pregnancy is detected, the medication should be discontinued as soon as possible, as there is a risk of teratogenic and fetotoxic effects such as neonatal skull hypoplasia, anuria, reversible or irreversible renal function, and fetal death.[29] Little is known about the use of aliskiren by women during breastfeeding, but alternative therapy should probably be used if possible.

Conversely aliskiren is potentially a good choice as an antihypertensive agent for older individuals. Research published in 2014 suggested that it was superior to ramipril (Altace) for individuals in this subgroup. As is true for any drug used for older women, aliskiren must be evaluated in light of the health of the woman and her use of other medications.[30]

Beta-Adrenergic Receptor Antagonists (Beta Blockers)

Drugs categorized as beta-adrenergic receptor antagonists are generally referred to as beta blockers (Table 15-10). These drugs are effective and generally well tolerated antihypertensive agents. Prior to the introduction of ACE inhibitors and ARBs, beta blockers and diuretics were the first-line drugs used to treat hypertension. Since that time, clinical trials have found that ACE inhibitors and ARBs are of more benefit than are beta blockers for individuals who do not have a compelling indication for beta blockers, such as coronary artery disease.[18,31] Beta blockers are the first choice for management of hypertension if the person has a history of a prior myocardial infarction.[17,32] In this clinical scenario, a beta blocker has been found to reduce mortality and morbidity.

In general, all beta blockers inhibit or block the effects of norepinephrine and epinephrine outside of the central nervous system, thereby disallowing the natural effect of these neurotransmitters. Beta blockers are subdivided into two different categories: nonselective and selective. Drugs that are more selective for beta1 receptors in the heart versus beta$_2$ receptors in the bronchi and peripheral blood vessels are classified as cardioselective beta blockers. Medications such as atenolol (Tenormin), betaxolol (Kerlone), bisoprolol (Zebeta), and metoprolol (Lopressor, Toprol XL) are cardioselective. Because these drugs are less likely to cause bronchoconstriction or vasoconstriction than nonselective beta blockers, they generally are preferred for use by individuals who have chronic obstructive pulmonary disease or peripheral arterial disease. The cardioselective nature of these drugs is lost at higher doses, though this level varies from individual to individual.

Beta blockers' inhibition of the beta-adrenergic receptors in the cardiac muscle results in negative **inotropic** and **chronotropic** effects, thereby decreasing cardiac conduction velocity and automaticity. Currently it is theorized that the antihypertensive mechanism is primarily related to reduction of cardiac output, decreased renin release from the kidneys, and a central nervous system effect to reduce general sympathetic activity. Such effects should be carefully considered. For example, slowing of the atrioventricular conduction could be a desired therapeutic effect for one person, whereas it could be potentially life threatening for another.

The beta blockers are well absorbed after oral administration; peak concentrations occur in approximately 1 to 3 hours, and sustained-released formulations are available. Many beta blockers are available in an immediate-release dose or a sustained- or extended-release formulation.

Side Effects/Contraindications

Common side effects of beta blockers include bradycardia, hypotension, fatigue, dizziness, and dyspnea. Other side effects that need to be considered prior to use include second- or third-degree atrioventricular block, cold extremities, diarrhea, nausea, depression, and impotence. Negative effects on blood glucose levels and lipid levels can also develop when beta blockers are taken. The Glycemic Effects in Diabetes Mellitus Carvedilol–Metoprolol

Table 15-10 Characteristics of Beta Blockers

Drug: Generic (Brand)	Category	Formulations	Dose	Cardioselective	Duration of Action
Acebutolol (Sectral)	Second generation selective $beta_2$ blocker	200-mg, 400-mg capsules	Initially 400 mg PO daily in 1–2 divided doses, maintenance dose 200–800 mg; maximum dose 1.2 g/day	No	12–24 hours
Atenolol (Tenormin)	Second generation selective $beta_2$ blocker	25-mg, 50-mg, 100-mg tablets	Initially 25–50 mg PO daily, increase after 1–2 weeks; maximum dose 100 mg daily	Yes	12–24 hours
Betaxolol (Kerlone)	Third generation selective $beta_2$ blocker with additional actions	10-mg, 20-mg tablets	Initially 10 mg PO daily; maximum dose 20 mg daily	Yes	14–22 hours
Bisoprolol (Zebeta)	Second generation selective $beta_2$ blocker	5-mg, 10-mg tablets	2.5–5 mg PO daily; maximum dose 20 mg daily	Yes	9–12 hours
Carvedilol (Coreg, Coreg CR)	Third generation non-selective $beta_2$ blocker with additional actions	3.125-mg, 6.25-mg, 12.5-mg, 25-mg tablets 10-mg, 20-mg, 40-mg, 80-mg capsules	Initially 6.25 mg PO twice daily, increase over 1- to 2-week periods; maximum dose 25 mg 2 times/day. Coreg CR: initially 20 mg daily, increase over 1–2 weeks to a maximum dose of 80 mg daily.	No, mixed alpha and beta blocker	8–10 hours
Labetalol (Trandate)	Third generation non-selective $beta_2$ blocker with additional actions	100-mg, 200-mg, 300-mg tablets	Initially 100 mg PO 2 times/day, maintenance dose 200–400 mg daily; maximum dose 2.4 g daily	No, mixed alpha and beta blocker	8–12 hours
Metoprolol (Lopressor, Toprol-XL)	Second generation selective $beta_2$ blocker	25-mg, 50-mg, 100-mg tablets XL: 25-mg, 50-mg, 100-mg, 200-mg tablets	Metoprolol: initially 50 mg PO 2 times/day, maintenance dose 100–450 mg daily in 2–3 divided doses. Metoprolol XL: initially 25–100 mg PO daily; maximum dose 400 mg daily.	Yes	Immediate release: variable, dose related XL: 24 hours
Nadolol (Corgard)	First generation non-selective beta blocker	20-mg, 40-mg, 80-mg tablets	Initially 40 mg PO daily, maintenance dose 40–80 mg daily; maximum dose 320 mg daily	No	17–24 hours
Nebivolol (Bystolic)	Third generation selective $beta_2$ blocker with additional actions	2.5-mg, 5-mg, 10-mg, 20-mg tablets	5 mg PO daily, can increase every 2 weeks to maximum dose 40 mg daily	Cardioselective and vasodilatory	12–19 hours
Penbutolol (Levatol)	First generation non-selective beta blocker	20-mg tablets	20 mg PO daily	No	> 20 hours
Pindolol (Visken)	First generation non-selective beta blocker	5-mg, 10-mg tablets	Initially 5 mg PO twice daily, may increase dose after 3–4 weeks in 10-mg increments; maximum dose 60 mg	No	7–15 hours
Propranolol (Inderal, Inderal LA)	First generation non-selective beta blocker	10-mg, 20-mg, 40-mg, 60-mg, 80-mg tablets Oral sustained-release: 60-mg, 80-mg, 120-mg, 160-mg capsules	Propranolol: initially 40 mg PO 2 times/day, maintenance dose 120–240 mg in 2–3 divided doses; maximum dose 640 mg daily in divided doses. Propranolol LA: initially 80 mg PO daily; maximum dose 640 mg daily.	No	Immediate release: 6–12 hours Extended release: 24–27 hours
Timolol (Blocadren)	First generation non-selective beta blocker	5-mg, 10-mg, 20-mg capsules	Initially 10 mg PO 2 times/day, usual maintenance dose 20–40 mg/day; maximum dose 60 mg/day in 2 divided doses	No	4 hours

Comparison in Hypertensives (GEMINI) trial demonstrated that newer generations of beta blockers do not have the same negative effect on glycemic control.[33]

Beta blockers with shorter half-lives have more negative effects following abrupt withdrawal than beta blockers with longer half-lives. Abrupt withdrawal of these drugs can cause exacerbation of ischemic heart disease because of the sudden increase in sympathetic response. There is no specific method for tapering a person off of a beta blocker; however, decreasing the dose slowly and over an extended period of time has been found to diminish the clinical negative adrenergic effects.

Drug–drug interactions associated with use of beta blockers generally take the form of either additive effects, which cause hypotension or bradycardia, or inhibition, which negates the therapeutic effect of the beta blocker.

Table 15-11 Major Drug–Drug Interactions Associated with Beta Blockers[a]

Drug: Generic (Brand)	Effects with Concomitant Use of Beta Blockers
Aminophylline	Inhibits bronchodilation effect of aminophylline
Amiodarone (Cordarone)	Bradycardia or arrhythmia
Antidiabetic agents	Enhanced hypoglycemia
Calcium-channel blockers	Potentiation of bradycardia, myocardial depression, hypotension
Cimetidine (Tagamet)	Prolongs half-life of propranolol (Inderal)
Clonidine (Catapres)	Rebound hypertension during clonidine withdrawal
Diltiazem (Cardizem)	Bradycardia
Fluoxetine (Prozac)	Potentiates the beta blocker's effects
Isoproterenol (Isuprel)	Isoproterenol and beta blockers inhibit the effects of each other, resulting in hypertension and inhibition of bronchodilation
Methyldopa (Aldomet)	Rebound hypertension
Nonsteroidal anti-inflammatory drugs (NSAIDs)	Attenuation of the beta blocker's effect if NSAIDs are used for a prolonged period of time
Prazosin (Minipress)	Augmentation of first-dose syncope, hypotension
Rifampin (RIF, Rifadin)	Increased metabolism of beta blockers
Theophylline (Theo-Dur)	Attenuation of the bronchodilation effect of theophylline; can be minimized by using cardioselective beta blockers
Verapamil (Calan)	Bradycardia, heart block

[a] This table is not comprehensive as new information is being identified on a regular basis.

Drug–drug interactions associated with beta blockers are listed in Table 15-11.

Beta Blockers and Special Populations: Pregnancy, Lactation, and the Elderly

Some of the beta blockers are used during pregnancy to control hypertension, thyrotoxicosis, and arrhythmias. Labetalol (Trandate) is an alternative to methyldopa (Aldomet), which is an alpha$_2$-adrenergic antagonist, for the management of chronic hypertension during pregnancy if needed.[34] Atenolol (Tenormin) is associated with adverse fetal outcomes and reduced placental function and should be avoided.[35]

Propranolol (Inderal), labetalol, atenolol, nadolol (Corgard), and metoprolol (Lopressor) are excreted into breast milk in varying amounts. Only small amounts of propranolol have been found in breast milk, making it a safe choice in breastfeeding, whereas larger amounts of atenolol pass into the milk, suggesting that an alternative drug should be chosen.[22]

Beta blockers are not used as first-line antihypertensive agents in elderly women unless they have a compelling indication such as heart failure, postmyocardial infarction, or high coronary disease risk.[17,18] The major consideration for older women using beta blockers is that of comorbidities such as peripheral arterial disease (peripheral arterial occlusive disease), chronic obstructive pulmonary disease, or asthma. Diuretics, ARBs, and calcium-channel blockers are more effective for preventing cardiovascular outcomes and stroke and are associated with decreased morbidity in the elderly.[18,36]

Calcium-Channel Antagonists

Calcium-channel antagonists are most often referred to as calcium-channel blockers (CCBs) (Table 15-12). One of the key factors leading to elevated blood pressure is peripheral resistance. Calcium-channel antagonists reduce this resistance via dilation of the peripheral arteries. In addition to being useful as antihypertensive agents, the calcium-channel blockers, which are subcategorized as non-dihydropyridines, are effective for the treatment of cardiac arrhythmias.

Calcium-channel blockers bind to L-type calcium channels located on the cell membranes of vascular smooth muscle, cardiac muscle, and cardiac nodal tissue cells, thereby preventing the influx of calcium into these cells. The contraction of vascular smooth muscle is highly dependent on the influx of calcium. These drugs inhibit the influx of calcium into the arterial smooth muscle but have little effect on venous vasculature. Ultimately, calcium-channel blockers cause dilation of the peripheral arteries, with an ensuing reduction in blood pressure. The net effect is that the cell cannot contract as strongly because less calcium is available to drive the intracellular contraction mechanism—a phenomenon known as a negative inotropic effect. The heart rate also slows because the calcium-channel blocker inhibits the influx of calcium into the nerves that direct contraction; as a consequence, the action potential along the nerves is slowed—a phenomenon called a negative chronotropic effect. The clinical effects of calcium-channel blockers are peripheral vasodilation, decreased heart rate, increased cardiac contractility, and decreased cardiac conduction. The effect of calcium-channel blockers is slightly different within the cardiac cell. The depolarization of the sinoatrial and atrioventricular nodes is controlled primarily by the recovery of the slow calcium channels.

Table 15-12 Calcium-Channel Blockers

Drug: Generic (Brand)	Formulations	Dose	Duration of Action
Dihydropyridines			
Amlodipine (Norvasc)	2.5-mg, 5-mg, 10-mg tablets	Initially 5 mg PO daily, maintenance 5–10 mg; maximum dose 10 mg daily	24 hours
Felodipine (Plendil)	2.5-mg, 5-mg, 10-mg capsules	Initially 2.5–10 mg PO daily; maximum dose 20 mg daily	24 hours
Nicardipine (Cardene, Cardene SR)	Cardene: 20 mg, 30 mg Cardene SR: 30 mg, 60 mg	Cardene: start 20 mg PO 3 times/day, maintenance dose 20–40 mg PO 3 times/day; maximum dose 120 mg/day Cardene SR: start 30 mg PO 2 times/day, maintenance dose 30–60 mg PO 2 times/day; maximum dose 120 mg/day	Cardene: < 8 hours Cardene SR: 8–12 hours
Nifedipine (Adalat CC, Procardia XL)	Adalat CC: 30-mg, 60-mg, 90-mg extended-release tablets Procardia XL: 30-mg, 60-mg, 90-mg extended-release tablets	30–60 mg PO daily, maintenance dose 30–90 mg daily; maximum dose 90–120 mg daily	2–5 hours
Non-dihydropyridines			
Diltiazem (Cardizem CD, Cardizem LA, Tiazac, Dilacor XR, Dilacor XT)	Cardizem CD: 120-mg, 180-mg, 240-mg, 300-mg, 360-mg tablets Cardizem LA: 120-mg, 180-mg, 240-mg, 300-mg, 360-mg, 420-mg extended-release tablets Tiazac: 120-mg, 180-mg, 240-mg, 300-mg, 360-mg, 420-mg extended-release tablets Dilacor XR, Dilacor XT: 120-mg, 180-mg, 240-mg extended-release capsules	Cardizem CD: initially 180–240 mg PO daily; maximum dose 480 mg daily Cardizem LA: initially 180–240 mg PO daily; maximum dose 540 mg daily Tiazac: initially 120–240 mg PO daily; maximum dose 540 mg daily Dilacor XR/XL: initially 180 mg PO daily, maintenance dose 180–480 mg; maximum dose 540 mg daily	Immediate release: 5–10 hours
Verapamil (Calan, Calan SR, Isoptin SR, Verelan, Verelan PM)	Calan: 40-mg, 80-mg, 120-mg tablets Calan SR: 120-mg, 180-mg, 240-mg extended-release capsules Isoptin SR: 120-mg, 180-mg, 240-mg extended-release capsules Verelan: 120-mg, 180-mg, 240-mg, 360-mg extended-release capsules Verelan PM: 100-mg, 200-mg, 300-mg extended-release capsules	Calan: initially 80 mg PO 3 times/day; maximum dose 360 mg daily Calan SR: initially 180 mg PO daily; maximum dose 480 mg daily Isoptin SR: initially 120–180 mg PO daily Verelan: initially 120 mg PO daily, maintenance dose120–240 mg; maximum dose 480 mg daily Verelan PM: initially 200 mg PO daily, maintenance dose 200–400 mg; maximum dose 400 mg daily	Immediate release: 6–8 hours

There are three different subclasses of calcium-channel blockers, each of which has a different basic chemical structure and mechanism of action. The **dihydropyridines** reduce systemic vascular resistance and arterial pressure, and are primarily used to treat hypertension. The phenylalkylamine class, which includes verapamil (Calan), is selective for suppressing myocardium and has minimal vasodilation effects. Finally, the benzothiazepine class, which includes diltiazem (Cardizem), is an intermediate class that has both cardiac suppression and vasodilation effects. The non-dihydropyridine calcium-channel blockers, verapamil (Calan) and diltiazem (Cardizem), depress the rate at which the sinus node fires by slowing the recovery of these channels. This phenomenon can be extremely helpful in treating a person with supraventricular tachycardia, but could be detrimental in someone who has a preexisting heart block.

Although persons with uncomplicated hypertension tend to respond well to calcium-channel blockers, such drugs should be avoided in individuals with atrioventricular or sinoatrial nodal abnormalities or overt heart failure. These drugs are effective in reducing high blood pressure not caused by elevated renin levels, which is why this class of medications has been shown to be effective in the African American population.[25] Calcium-channel blockers are also effective for treatment of hypertension in persons who have concomitant asthma, hyperlipidemia, diabetes, or renal dysfunction.[37]

Many other antihypertensive agents work synergistically with calcium-channel blockers, such as ACE inhibitors, selective beta blockers, and diuretics. Several combination formulations of antihypertensive agents are now on the market, and their greater convenience tends to increase adherence to hypertensive medications. Many of the calcium-channel blockers are also available in generic preparations.

Side Effects/Contraindications

In the mid-1990s, observational studies indicated that short-acting, immediate-release calcium-channel blockers might cause an increase in myocardial infarction, gastrointestinal bleeding, and cancer, which led to a decrease in use. Subsequent randomized trials have shown that long-acting calcium-channel blockers decrease the frequency and number of cardiovascular events and that there is no association between these drugs and gastrointestinal bleeding or cancer.

Most of the side effects of calcium-channel blockers stem from the very mechanism that helps reduce blood pressure. As peripheral resistance is lowered, stimulation of the baroreceptor-mediated sympathetic response occurs, which causes tachycardia and increased stroke volume. Approximately 22% of persons who take dihydropyridine calcium-channel blockers will also develop peripheral edema; diuretics are not helpful in alleviating this side effect. Headache, palpitations, and flushing are other common side effects. Non-dihydropyridine calcium-channel blockers are more commonly associated with bradycardia, hypotension, and constipation.

Drug–Drug Interactions

Many of the calcium-channel blockers are both substrates and inhibitors of CYP3A4. Thus, they can inhibit their own metabolism, which in turn increases plasma levels and can result in toxicity. If cardiotoxicity occurs, the pharmacologic effects of these agents result in profound hypotension, bradycardia, and conduction disturbances leading to cardiovascular collapse.[38]

Most of the drug–drug interactions result in increased levels of either the calcium-channel blocker or the interacting drug and enhanced therapeutic responses that can have toxic effects. For example, the use of verapamil (Calan) by persons also taking digoxin (Lanoxin) will require monitoring the digoxin level on a regular basis to avoid digoxin toxicity. The combination of a calcium-channel blocker and quinidine may lead to severe hypotension. Hyperglycemia also may occur secondary to calcium-channel blockers' inhibition of insulin release from the pancreas. Lactic acidosis can occur as well. Overdose of calcium-channel blockers requires active cardiovascular support in an inpatient setting.

Table 15-13 Major Drug–Drug Interactions Associated with Calcium-Channel Blockers[a]

Drug: Generic (Brand)	Effects with Concomitant Use of Calcium-Channel Blockers
Amiodarone (Cordarone)	Additive reduction in heart rate and myocardial contractility
Anesthetics	Additive effect of increasing hypotensive effect
Atorvastatin (Lipitor)	Increased serum levels of atorvastatin
Azole antifungals	Increased hypotensive effect
Beta blockers	Generally well tolerated and can be used therapeutically, but there is an additive effect that can cause bradycardia and heart block
Carbamazepine (Tegretol)	Increased serum levels of carbamazepine via reduced elimination
Cimetidine (Tagamet)	Potentiation of the calcium-channel blocker's effects
Cyclosporine (Sandimmune)	Increases effect of cyclosporine
Digoxin (Lanoxin)	Increased levels of digoxin and possible digoxin toxicity. This effect is especially potent with verapamil, and combining digoxin with verapamil is contraindicated.
Grapefruit juice	Increases serum levels of calcium-channel blockers
Lithium (Eskalith, Lithobid)	Increased risk of neurotoxicity
Lovastatin (Mevacor)	Increased serum levels of lovastatin
Nafcillin	Reduced effect of the calcium-channel blocker
Phenobarbital (Luminal)	Increases clearance of verapamil
Phenytoin (Dilantin)	Reduced effect of the calcium-channel blocker
Quinidine	Excessive hypotension
Rifampin (Rifadin)	Decreased effect of the calcium-channel blocker, hypertension
Simvastatin (Zocor)	Increased serum levels of simvastatin
Theophylline (Theo-Dur)	Decreased clearance of theophylline and increased serum levels

[a] This table is not comprehensive as new information is being identified on a regular basis. In addition, individual calcium-channel antagonists may have a specific drug–drug interaction that other members of the same class do not have.

Drug–drug interactions associated with calcium-channel blockers are summarized in Table 15-13.

Calcium-Channel Blockers and Special Populations: Pregnancy, Lactation, and the Elderly

Calcium-channel blockers are used in pregnancy when the benefit of blood pressure reduction outweighs the risk. Long-acting formulations of nifedipine (Procardia) doses of 30 to 90 mg daily have been used without major adverse reactions. Nifedipine has been regularly used as a tocolytic to stop preterm labor because the calcium-channel blocker decreases the amount of intracellular calcium present in myometrial cells thereby preventing uterine contraction.

Calcium-channel blockers appear to cross into breast milk, but the levels are low; thus these agents are considered compatible for breastfeeding dyads.[22] Nifedipine is used by lactating women who experience nipple vasospasm (Raynaud disease).

Calcium-channel blockers are not contraindicated in otherwise healthy older women. Studies have indicated that they are as effective for cardiac and cerebral protection and treatment as other antihypertensives.[39]

Selective and Nonselective Alpha-Adrenergic Antagonists

Alpha-receptor antagonists are not commonly used as first-line monotherapy. However, they are complementary to the other groups of antihypertensives and they can be added when monotherapy is not sufficient to meet BP goals. These agents include drugs that are nonselective as well as newer agents that are relatively selective for the alpha$_1$ receptor, which are the agents in most common use. Selective alpha-adrenergic antagonists block the alpha$_1$ receptors in the peripheral vasculature, thereby inhibiting the effect of catecholamines, which results in vasodilation and decreased peripheral resistance. These agents, which are listed in Table 15-14, have largely replaced nonselective agents.

Side Effects/Contraindications

The primary side effects of selective alpha-adrenergic antagonists are postural hypotension and tachycardia that occur 1 to 3 hours after the initial doses. These effects can be reduced with a lower initial dose, the avoidance of concurrent use of diuretics, and ingestion at bedtime. Other common side effects are fatigue, nasal congestion, and headache. Women who are taking an alpha-adrenergic antagonist are also at increased risk of floppy iris syndrome if undergoing cataract surgery.

Table 15-14 Selective Alpha-Adrenergic Antagonists

Drug: Generic (Brand)	Formulations	Dose	Duration of Action
Doxazosin (Cardura)	1-mg, 2-mg, 4-mg, 8-mg tablets	Initially 1 mg PO daily; maximum dose 16 mg daily	> 24 hours
Prazosin (Minipress)	1-mg, 2-mg, 5-mg capsules	First dose at bedtime, 1 mg PO 2–3 times daily; maintenance dose 6–15 mg daily; maximum dose 20 mg daily	10–24 hours
Terazosin (Hytrin)	1-mg, 2-mg, 5-mg, 10-mg capsules	1 mg PO at bedtime; may increase dose slowly, maintenance dose 1–5 mg daily; maximum dose 20 mg/day. May be given in single or divided doses.	12 hours

Drug–Drug Interactions

The drug–drug interactions associated with use of alpha-adrenergic antagonists are primarily secondary to additive effects or inhibitory effects from concomitant use of drugs that have an independent effect on blood pressure. In particular, the combination of verapamil with any alpha-adrenergic antagonist can result in profound hypotension.

Alpha-Adrenergic Antagonists and Special Populations: Pregnancy, Lactation, and the Elderly

Alpha$_1$ receptor antagonists are rarely used in pregnancy because the beta blockers and calcium-channel blockers are effective and have few or no effects on the fetus. Little information exists regarding alpha-adrenergic antagonists when used by women during pregnancy and lactation. It is unknown if these drugs are excreted in breast milk.

There are no alterations in dosing for elderly women; however, consideration for increased dizziness and syncopal episodes should be considered. Alpha-adrenergic antagonists are not recommended as routine hypertensive treatment by the Beers criteria.[40] In addition, because these drugs cross the blood–brain barrier, they can cause depression, vivid dreams, and lethargy, all of which can be more troublesome to the elderly.

Central Alpha$_2$-Receptor Agonists (Selective Alpha$_2$-Receptor Agonists)

Central alpha$_2$-receptor agonists (Table 15-15) are not first-line antihypertensive drugs due to their negative side-effect profile and the limited data showing they can result in improved outcomes. These drugs exert their effects primarily by stimulating the alpha$_2$ receptors within the central nervous system, which reduces the sympathetic outflow from the vasomotor center and increases vagal tone. The result is a slower heart rate and decreased cardiac output. All of the central alpha$_2$-receptor agonists can cause severe hypertension if abruptly withdrawn.

Table 15-15 Central Alpha$_2$-Receptor Agonists

Drug: Generic (Brand)	Formulations	Dose	Duration of Action
Clonidine (Catapres, Catapres TTS)	0.1-mg, 0.2-mg, 0.3-mg tablets 0.1-mg, 0.2-mg, 0.3-mg weekly patches	Initially 0.1 mg PO 2 times/day, maintenance dose 0.1–0.2 mg PO 2 times/day; maximum dose 2.4 mg total daily	Tablets: 6–10 hours Patch: > 24 hours
Guanfacine (Tenex)	1-mg, 2-mg tablets	Initially 1 mg PO daily at bedtime, maintenance dose 1–2 mg daily; maximum dose 2 mg daily	24 hours
Methyldopa (Aldomet)	250-mg, 500-mg tablets	Initially 250 mg PO 2–3 times/day maintenance dose 250–500 mg 2 times/day; maximum dose 3000 mg daily	Single dose: 12–24 hours Multiple doses: 24–48 hours

Side Effects/Contraindications

Side effects of centrally acting alpha$_2$-receptor agonists include sedation, dizziness, and dry mouth. The last effect occurs in as many as 50% of persons who take clonidine (Catapres). Central nervous system effects also include parkinsonian symptoms and decreased libido, which can result in sexual dysfunction and impotence. The incidence of these symptoms is lower among persons who use the transdermal patch, yet this route of administration can cause contact dermatitis in approximately 15% to 20% of persons who use it. Abrupt discontinuation of these drugs may cause withdrawal symptoms such as headache, tachycardia, tremors, or sweating secondary to the sudden increase in sympathetic discharge. In addition, the arterial pressure can rebound and rise higher than it was previously. Rarely, a symptomatic bradycardia or sinus arrest can occur in persons with sinoatrial node dysfunction or persons who are taking other medications that affect the atrioventricular node.

Methyldopa (Aldomet) is a prodrug that has active metabolites that have adverse effects. Methyldopa can induce a transient sedation and depression, and in rare cases it may cause hemolytic anemia or liver disease. Hyperprolactinemia can become significant enough to cause gynecomastia and galactorrhea. Hepatotoxicity is a rare but serious adverse effect associated with the initiation of methyldopa. It is recommended that clinicians obtain a baseline complete blood count and perform liver function tests prior to starting this drug. Methyldopa is contraindicated for persons with hepatic disease, hypersensitivity to methyldopa, and those taking MAO inhibitors because the combination of methyldopa and MAO inhibitors can cause hallucinations and severe hypertension.

Drug–Drug Interactions

Alpha$_2$-receptor agonists are antagonized by tricyclic antidepressants, and they can potentiate the effects of central nervous system depressants such as alcohol, phenothiazines, and barbiturates. Methyldopa can increase the risk for lithium toxicity and heighten the effects of levodopa (Sinemet). Conversely, iron tablets can decrease the extent of methyldopa absorption. The use of clonidine (Catapres) with beta blockers may potentiate bradycardia and worsen rebound hypertension when the beta blockers are discontinued.

Central Alpha$_2$-Receptor Agonists and Special Populations: Pregnancy, Lactation, and the Elderly

Methyldopa (Aldomet) has been extensively used during pregnancy to manage moderate to severe chronic hypertension and is considered safe in pregnancy and compatible with breastfeeding.[34,41] This agent is not used to treat preeclampsia. Guanfacine (Tenex) is also considered safe in pregnancy, although no information is available regarding its use during lactation. Clonidine (Catapres) crosses the placenta, so caution is necessary secondary to the rebound hypertension that can occur if it is stopped abruptly. Clonidine does enter and may concentrate in breast milk, but its effects on the newborn are not clear.[22,42]

Methyldopa can cause drug-induced immune-mediated hemolysis, leading to a positive antibody (Coombs) test, but little drug passes into breast milk, suggesting it is the best option for the lactating woman.[22]

Alpha$_2$-receptor agonists are not recommended as routine hypertensive treatment for the elderly according to the Beers criteria.[40] No dosing changes are recommended based on a person's age; however, these medications should be used cautiously in the elderly because they can cause increased central nervous system depression.

Vasodilators

Vasodilators (Table 15-16) were among the first antihypertensive drugs available in the U.S. market. Today, hydralazine (Apresoline) and minoxidil (Loniten) are not commonly used as monotherapy in the treatment of hypertension, but they are effective in combination with other agents.

Table 15-16 Vasodilators

Drug: Generic (Brand)	Formulations	Dose	Duration of Action
Hydralazine (Apresoline)	10-mg, 25-mg, 50-mg, 100-mg tablets 20 mg/mL for intravenous use	Initial 10 mg PO 4 times/day, increase by 10–25 mg/dose gradually; maximum dose 300 mg daily	Up to 8 hours
Minoxidil (Loniten)	2.5-mg, 10-mg tablets	Initial 5 mg PO daily, maintenance dose 5–10 mg daily; maximum dose 100 mg daily	48–120 hours

Vasodilators relax the arteriolar smooth muscles, which results in dilation of blood vessels and a subsequent reduction in blood pressure. This drop in perfusion pressure can trigger the baroreceptor reflex, which will cause an increase in heart rate and cardiac output. The baroreceptor reflex can be blunted with the use of a concomitant beta blocker, which is especially important in order to avoid precipitation of angina in individuals with a previous myocardial infarction.

Side Effects/Adverse Effects

Common side effects of vasodilators include headache, nausea, diarrhea, palpitations, and nasal congestion. Less common side effects are blood dyscrasias, a lupus-like drug syndrome, and a positive direct antibody (Coombs) test. Individuals who have mitral valve rheumatic heart disease should not take vasodilators.

Drug–Drug Interactions

Among the important drug reactions with hydralazine (Apresoline) are hypotension that may be profound when the agent is taken concomitantly with diazoxide (Proglycem) or tizanidine (Zanaflex). Concomitant use of NSAIDs may diminish the hypotensive effect of hydralazine. Conversely, hydralazine can potentiate the orthostatic hypotensive effects of drugs such as MAO inhibitors.

Vasodilators and Special Populations: Pregnancy, Lactation, and the Elderly

Hydralazine (Apresoline) has long been used in pregnancy to correct acute severe hypertension associated with preeclampsia or eclampsia as needed. It is not used as a maintenance drug. There is no evidence of teratogenic or fetotoxic effects. Animal studies of minoxidil (Loniten) have revealed some birth defects and miscarriages among some species. Although the drug is not listed as a human teratogen, it is not commonly used for pregnant women.

Hydralazine is considered compatible with breastfeeding. It is generally preferred to minoxidil in this population because there is minimal information about the use of the latter among lactating women.

Today the majority of individuals hospitalized tend to be older. A study in 2011 revealed that use of hydralazine for hypertensive emergencies among older individuals often was associated with a misdiagnosis and caused a number of adverse effects, primarily hypotension.[43]

Complementary Treatments for Hypertension

Many studies have been completed over the past several years investigating alternative treatments for hypertension. However, the data in most of these studies are conflicting and often fail to provide a clear answer. There are no proven effective herbal products for treatment of hypertension, although a few have some promise as diuretics.[44]

Hyperlipidemia

Hyperlipidemia increases the risk for poor outcomes from atherosclerotic disease states, such as coronary heart disease, cerebrovascular disease, and peripheral vascular disease. The guidelines for treatment of blood cholesterol to reduce atherosclerotic cardiovascular risk in adults were updated in 2013 to provide guidance on the pharmacologic treatment of hyperlipidemia.[45] To better understand the pharmacologic interventions for dyslipidemia, a brief review of the physiologic mechanisms of cholesterol and lipid metabolism is in order.

Physiology of Lipid Metabolism

Cholesterol, a fat-like substance produced in the liver, is an essential element in bile salts, the precursor of steroid hormones, and a major component of cell membranes. Approximately 15% of cholesterol comes from diet; the rest is made endogenously in the liver and intestinal cells. Cholesterol, which is one of the most important lipids in the body, is insoluble; consequently, in the circulation, it is transported bound in lipid protein complexes called lipoproteins. Figure 15-3 provides an illustration of cholesterol metabolism.

All lipoproteins contain triglyceride, cholesterol, proteins, and other lipids besides cholesterol, although

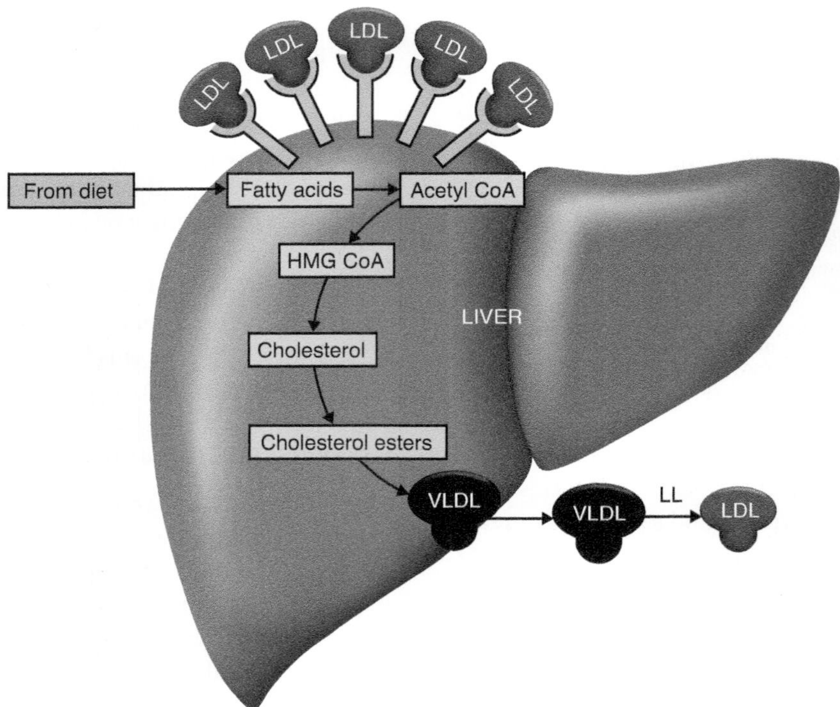

HMG CoA = 3-hydroxy-3-methyl-glutaryl-CoA reductase; LDL = low density lipoprotein; LL = lipoprotein lipase; VLDL = very low density lipoprotein.

Figure 15-3 Cholesterol metabolism.

they vary with regard to the ratio of lipid to protein. The lipoproteins that have more lipids are less dense, and those that have a greater proportion of protein are more dense. The three most commonly discussed lipoproteins that transport cholesterol are low-density lipoprotein (LDL), which transports cholesterol to peripheral tissues and is absorbed by the liver when cholesterol is needed for liver function; high-density lipoprotein (HDL), which transports cholesterol from the tissues to the liver, where it is broken down to become bile; and very-low-density lipoprotein (VLDL), which transports triglycerides from the liver to peripheral tissues. Once VLDLs give up triglycerides, they are converted to LDLs.

Atherosclerosis is a chronic inflammatory process that occurs within the walls of arteries—that is, it is not a phenomenon that develops overnight. Atherogenesis begins with entrapment of LDLs in the blood vessel wall. The LDLs are digested by macrophages, which become filled with lipid and evolve into foam cells that also get trapped in the endothelial wall. These foam cells eventually coalesce into a fatty streak, which is a smooth, raised plaque just beneath the endothelium. Fatty streaks form early in life and can progress to become rough, calcified atherosclerotic lesions that cause arterial stenosis or infarctions. LDL accounts for 60% to 70% of the body's total supply of cholesterol and is a major atherogenic lipoprotein. Lowering LDL reduces an individual's overall risk for CVD.[45]

Some medications used for other indications have an independent effect on lipids. For example, glucocorticoids, thiazide diuretics, cyclosporins, and tacrolimus (Prograf) raise the blood levels of triglycerides, LDL cholesterol, and HDL cholesterol. Estrogens increase blood levels of triglycerides and HDL cholesterol, but lower levels of LDL cholesterol. Androgens have the opposite effect: They increase triglyceride and LDL cholesterol levels and lower HDL cholesterol levels. Progestins raise blood levels of LDL cholesterol but lower levels of triglycerides and HDL cholesterol.

Pharmacologic Treatments for Hyperlipidemia

Decreasing the plasma levels of atherogenic lipoproteins such as LDL, non-HDL, VLDL, and triglycerides reduces the risk of developing CVD.[15] Treatment may be accomplished via several nonpharmacologic and pharmacologic treatments, either alone or in combination. Initial treatment should target the underlying cause of the hyperlipidemia. For most individuals, lifestyle modification is a necessary first step in treatment and risk reduction. When lifestyle modifications are not sufficient, drugs are required to obtain optimal goals.

HMG CoA reductase inhibitors (commonly called **statins**, bile acid–sequestering agents, nicotinic acid, fibric acid derivatives, cholesterol absorption inhibitors, and combinations of these agents are available to help individuals reach lipid goals. Each pharmacologic approach has a different effect on LDLs, HDLs, and triglycerides, as summarized in Table 15-17.

In contrast to the previous guidelines, which recommended treatment with pharmacologic therapy to target specific LDL goals,[46] the 2013 guidelines for treatment of blood cholesterol to reduce atherosclerotic cardiovascular risk in adults primarily recommend statin treatment for four populations:[45] (1) individuals with atherosclerotic cardiovascular disease; (2) individuals with primary elevation of LDL to 190 mg/dL or higher; (3) persons with diabetes who are between 40 and 75 years of age, with LDL in the range of 70–189 mg/dL and without atherosclerotic cardiovascular disease; and (4) persons without atherosclerotic cardiovascular disease or diabetes, with LDL in the range of 70–189 mg/dL and an estimated 10-year atherosclerotic cardiovascular disease risk of 7.5% or higher. A 10-year risk calculator can be found at the AHA website and it is listed in the Resources table at the end of this chapter.[47] This risk calculator incorporates gender, age, cholesterol levels, diabetes status, race, smoking status, blood pressure, and treatment; it advocates statin use instead of non-statin pharmacotherapy due to a lack of clinical trials demonstrating improved clinical outcomes with non-statin therapy.[45]

Table 15-17 Effects of Pharmacologic Treatments for Dyslipidemia

Drug	LDL	HDL	Triglycerides
Bile acid sequestrants	Modest effect	No effect	Minimal effect or increase
Ezetimibe (Zetia)	Effective	Modest effect	No effect
Fibrates	Minimal to no effect or increase	Modest effect	Effective
HMG CoA reductase inhibitors (statins)	Effective	Modest effect	Modest effect
Niacin	Modest effect	Effective	Effective

Abbreviations: HDL = high-density lipoprotein; LDL = low-density lipoprotein.

Because the new guidelines differ substantially from the previous hyperlipidemia guidelines, there has been much discussion regarding the increased number of persons who would be treated with statins under the current recommendations as compared to the previous guidelines. A population-based sample study estimated that an additional 12.8 million persons (10.4 million of whom did not have cardiovascular disease) would have been treated with statins from 2005 to 2010 if the new guidelines were used.[48] Both professionals and consumers have been somewhat confused about the new guidelines and the shift to statins instead of the emphasis on cholesterol levels (i.e., the "Know your numbers" approach) associated with earlier guidelines. It will likely take time before the recommendations are widely understood and adopted by all professionals.[49]

HMG CoA Reductase Inhibitors (Statins)

HMG CoA reductase inhibitors (statins) are the first-line treatment in reducing LDL. These agents are the most effective class of drugs available to reduce cholesterol levels. Statins have demonstrated the ability to reduce a woman's risk for developing CVD. Specifically, an aggressive reduction of LDL in a woman who has stable coronary artery disease decreases her risk of major cardiovascular events.[45]

Statins reduce cholesterol production by the liver through inhibition of 3-hydroxy-3-methyl-glutaryl-CoA reductase (HMG CoA), an enzyme involved in cholesterol production. These agents stimulate the upregulation of LDL receptors in the liver, which bind to LDL and thereby increase the extraction of LDL from the plasma pool. Some statins will cause a reduction in triglycerides and elevation of HDL, which occur secondary to the primary mechanism of reducing LDL. In addition to LDL reduction, statins have cardioprotective effects by improving endothelial function, improving plaque stability, and reducing endothelial inflammation.[50]

Statins all demonstrate the same basic mechanism of action, but there are significant differences in their potency and pharmacokinetic profiles that are of clinical import. Not all statins are equally aggressive in lowering LDL. High-intensity formulations lower LDL by approximately 50% or more, moderate-intensity statins lower LDL by approximately 30% to 50% and low-intensity statins lower LDL by 30% or less. Table 15-18 reviews the statins and doses that are considered high, moderate, or low intensity. Rosuvastatin (Crestor), Atorvastatin (Lipitor), and simvastatin (Zocor) cause the greatest drop in LDL levels. For persons who require statin therapy, high-intensity statin

Table 15-18 HMG CoA Reductase Inhibitors (Statins)

Drug: Generic (Brand)	Formulations	High-, Moderate-, and Low-Intensity Doses[a]	Half-Life	Metabolism
Atorvastatin (Lipitor)	10-mg, 20-mg, 40-mg, 80-mg tablets	High intensity: 40–80 mg PO/day Moderate intensity: 10–20 mg/day	9–32 hours	CYP3A4 (major), P-glycoprotein
Fluvastatin (Lescol)	20-mg, 40-mg tablets	Moderate intensity: 40 mg PO 2 times/day Low intensity: 20–40 mg/day	< 3 hours	CYP2C9 (minor)
Fluvastatin ER (Lescol XL)	80-mg extended-release tablet	Moderate intensity: 80 mg PO/day	9 hours	CYP2C9 (minor)
Lovastatin (Mevacor)	10-mg, 20-mg, 40-mg tablets	Moderate intensity: 40 mg PO/day Low intensity : 20 mg/day	2–4 hours	CYP3A4 (major), P-glycoprotein
Lovastatin ER (Altoprev)	20-mg, 40-mg, 60-mg extended-release tablets	Moderate intensity: 40 mg PO/day	12–14 hours	CYP3A4 (major), P-glycoprotein
Pitavastatin (Livalo)	1-mg, 2-mg, 4-mg tablets	Moderate intensity: 2–4 mg PO/day Low intensity: 1 mg/day	Approximately 12 hours	Minimal metabolism
Pravastatin (Pravachol)	10-mg, 20-mg, 40-mg, 80-mg tablets	Moderate intensity: 40–80 mg PO/day Low intensity: 10–20 mg/day	Approximately 3 hours	Minimal metabolism
Rosuvastatin (Crestor)	5-mg, 10-mg, 20-mg, 40-mg tablets	High intensity: 20–40 mg PO/day Moderate intensity: 5–10 mg/day	20 hours	Minimal metabolism
Simvastatin (Zocor)	5-mg, 10-mg, 20-mg, 40-mg, 80-mg tablets	Moderate intensity: 20–40 mg PO/day[b] Low intensity: 10 mg/day	Approximately 3 hours	CYP3A4 (major)

[a] All statins, except for atorvastatin, rosuvastatin, and pitavastatin, should be taken in the evening or at bedtime.
[b] Simvastatin 80 mg can be used only by women taking that dose more than 12 consecutive months without evidence of myopathy.[54]

therapy is recommended, except when there are increased risk factors for adverse effects. Such scenarios include in persons 75 years or older, when drug–drug interactions are a concern, and if the person is unable to tolerate a high-intensity statin.[45] Considerable individual variability in response to statins has been noted, which may be secondary to genomic polymorphisms that direct the activity of the metabolizing enzymes.[51]

Individuals are encouraged to take their statin at night because HMG CoA is more active in the evening.[52] Timing the dose this way allows for the highest plasma levels of statins when there are the highest levels of HMG CoA that the statin will inhibit. The three statins that can be taken at any time of the day—atorvastatin (Lipitor), rosuvastatin (Crestor), and pitavastatin (Livalo)—all have long durations of action and can inhibit HMG CoA sufficiently when taken at any time during the day. Simvastatin (Zocor) 80 mg is limited to women taking that dose more than 12 consecutive months without evidence of myopathy.[53]

Side Effects/Adverse Effects

There are several combination products in which a statin is combined with niacin, an antihypertensive agent, and/or another lipid-lowering drug. For example, The FDA has approved lovastatin/extended release niacin (Advicor) and simvastatin/ezetimibe (Vytorin). The fixed-dose combination formulations are called "polypills." The effectiveness of these combination products in comparison to individual agents has not been fully determined for primary prevention of cardiovascular disease whereas adverse effects may limit their use.

The polypill has been studied for secondary prevention of cardiovascular disease in persons who are at very high risk for cardiovascular disease. Although there are several theoretical advantages for the polypill, studies conducted to date have not demonstrated convincing evidence for their use. For example, the simvastatin/ezetimibe combination is approved for treatment of homozygous familial hypercholesterolemia as an adjunct to diet. Studies have not shown significant improvement in cardiovascular indices with use of Vytorin versus monotherapy with either simvastatin or ezetimibe. There are significant adverse effects and drug–drug interactions associated with the use of Vytorin. The FDA has several warnings and contraindications listed in the safety information about this product. The combination of lovastatin and niacin (Advicor) is associated with an increased risk for myopathy and rhabdomyolysis.

Side Effects/Adverse Effects

The most common side effects of statins are muscle pain and soreness or muscle cramps, which occurred in an estimated 10% to 20% of participants in observational studies.[54] (Box 15-2) Other side effects may include abdominal pain, constipation, diarrhea, and nausea. Many persons cannot tolerate higher doses of statins, especially simvastatin, because of myalgia.[54] For individuals who cannot tolerate the high-intensity dose of a statin due to these adverse effects, the dose of statin can be decreased to the moderate-intensity level. Myopathy is more likely if statins are given concomitantly with other drugs that elevate the plasma levels of statins. Adverse effects are rare at effective doses of the statin. Statins are contraindicated for women who are pregnant or who have active liver disease with persistent elevation of liver enzymes. However, persons with stable chronic liver disease can use statins if indicated.

Several uncommon side effects are associated with statins. First, asymptomatic elevations in hepatic aminotransferase activity can occur, which is more likely in persons with underlying liver disease. Elevations that are less than three times higher than the baseline value are considered normal and do not require intervention.

While serious liver injury can occur with statins, it is rare and, therefore, routine monitoring of liver function is not recommended by the FDA.[55] Baseline liver enzyme tests should be performed prior to initiation of statin therapy, but only as clinically indicated thereafter. Women should be counseled to report any of the following symptoms for further follow-up: unusual fatigue or weakness, loss of appetite, upper abdominal pain, dark-colored urine, and yellowing of the skin or whites of the eyes.

Another adverse reaction associated with statins is skeletal muscle abnormalities, which can range from simple myalgia to rare development of rhabdomyolysis. Creatinine kinase levels should be obtained if an individual reports significant muscle pain or weakness. The statin should be discontinued if the creatinine kinase level is elevated more than 10 times the upper limit of normal or the individual has intolerable symptoms. Individuals taking statins should be educated regarding the warning signs of rhabdomyolysis (muscle weakness, muscle aching, and/or dark-colored urine).

Lastly, a meta-analysis revealed that use of statins is associated with a small increase (9%) in the risk of developing diabetes.[56] However, the absolute risk of diabetes development is low and is small when compared to the benefit of cardiovascular event reduction with use of statins.

Drug–Drug Interactions

Drug–drug interactions associated with use of statins are listed in Table 15-19. Pravastatin (Pravachol), fluvastatin (Lescol), rosuvastatin (Crestor), and pitavastatin (Livalo) are the least likely statins to have drug interactions because they are not metabolized by the CYP450 enzyme system. Lovastatin (Mevacor, extended-release Altoprev), simvastatin (Zocor), and atorvastatin (Lipitor)

Box 15-2 Case Study: Statin Failure

PC is a 76-year-old woman who is being evaluated for side effects from statin therapy. She reports that she originally started on atorvastatin (Lipitor) 20 mg daily after having a stroke. She subsequently developed leg pain and fatigue, so she discontinued use of the drug. She then started on ezetimibe (Zetia) 10 mg daily. She denies any problems at this time. Her vital signs are height, 5 feet 8 inches (172.7 cm); weight, 150 pounds (68 kg); blood pressure, 115/72 mm Hg; heart rate, 72 bpm; and respirations, 16 breaths/min. When PC had her fasting lipid panel done, the results were total cholesterol, 302 mg/dL; LDL, 181 mg/dL; HDL, 60 mg/dL; and triglycerides, 307 mg/dL. Her other fasting lab results were all within normal ranges.

PC is similar to many individuals who experience fatigue and muscle aches without any increase in their blood levels of creatine phosphokinase (CPK) when starting statins. It is often difficult to convince a person who has no symptoms of disease of the benefit of a medication when side effects from the treatment appear. The provider discussed diet and exercise habits with PC. She agreed to attempt another statin, rosuvastatin (Crestor) 10 mg daily at bedtime and to continue on the ezetimibe (Zetia). Rosuvastatin is a moderate-intensity statin that is acceptable for PC because she is postmenopausal and has a history of statin intolerance; if she were younger than 75 years, it would have been acceptable to initiate therapy with a high-intensity statin, such as atorvastatin (Lipitor) 40–80 mg or rosuvastatin 20–40 mg.

The other item of concern is PC's hypertriglyceridemia. If she tolerates the statin, other agents such as omega-3 fatty acids and fibrates (excluding gemfibrozil [Lopid]) may need to be added to lower her triglycerides. It would also be reasonable to try any other statin at a low dose.

Table 15-19 Major Drug–Drug Associations with Statins[a]

Drug: Generic (Brand)	Agent Affected	Effect
Calcium-channel blockers	All statins	Increased serum levels of statins and increased risk for myopathy and rhabdomyolysis
Cimetidine (Tagamet)	All statins	Increased oral bioavailability of statins, thereby increasing serum levels
Cyclosporine (Neoral)	All statins, but increased significantly with pravastatin (Pravachol)	Increased serum levels of statins and increased risk for myopathy and rhabdomyolysis
Diltiazem (Cardizem)	Simvastatin (Zocor)	Increased serum levels of simvastatin
Fibrates	All statins	Additive increased risk for myopathy and rhabdomyolysis
Grapefruit juice[b]	All statins except pravastatin (Pravachol)	Increased oral bioavailability of statins, thereby increasing serum levels
Itraconazole (Sporanox)	All statins, especially simvastatin (Zocor)	Increased serum levels of statins and increased risk for myopathy and rhabdomyolysis
Ketoconazole (Nizoral)	All statins	Increased serum levels of statins and increased risk for myopathy and rhabdomyolysis
Macrolide antibiotics (e.g., erythromycin [E-Mycin])	All statins	Increased serum levels of statins and increased risk for myopathy and rhabdomyolysis
Niacin	Lovastatin (Mevacor), pravastatin (Pravachol), simvastatin (Zocor)	Increased serum levels of statins and increased risk for myopathy and rhabdomyolysis
Phenytoin (Dilantin)	Atorvastatin (Lipitor), simvastatin (Zocor)	Decreased serum levels of statin with subsequent subtherapeutic effect
Phenytoin (Dilantin)	Fluvastatin (Lescol)	Increased serum levels of phenytoin
Protease inhibitors	All statins	Increased serum levels of statins and increased risk for myopathy and rhabdomyolysis
Rifampin (Rifadin)	All statins	Decreased serum levels of statin with subsequent subtherapeutic effect
Selective serotonin reuptake inhibitors	Atorvastatin (Lipitor), Lovastatin (Mevacor), simvastatin (Zocor)	Increased serum levels of statins and increased risk for myopathy and rhabdomyolysis
Sildenafil	All statins	Increased serum levels of statins and increased risk for myopathy and rhabdomyolysis
Tacrolimus (Prograf)	Atorvastatin (Lipitor), Lovastatin (Mevacor) simvastatin (Zocor)	Increased serum levels of statins and increased risk for myopathy and rhabdomyolysis
Verapamil (Calan)	Atorvastatin (Lipitor), Lovastatin (Mevacor), simvastatin (Zocor)	Increased serum levels of statins and increased risk for myopathy and rhabdomyolysis
Warfarin (Coumadin)	Fluvastatin (Lescol), Lovastatin (Mevacor), simvastatin (Zocor)	Increased anticoagulant effect of the warfarin

[a] This table is not comprehensive as new information is being identified on a regular basis.
[b] Significant interaction only if large quantities of grapefruit juice are ingested. A single glass of grapefruit juice per day does not result in clinically significant increases in serum levels of the statin.

are CYP3A4 substrates and, therefore, their metabolism can be inhibited by CP3A4 inhibitors such as macrolide antibiotics, selective serotonin receptor inhibitors, cyclosporine (Neoral), ketoconazole (Nizoral), verapamil (Calan), ritonavir (Norvir), tacrolimus (Protropic), and grapefruit juice. Statins are contraindicated for persons taking gemfibrozil (Lopid) because gemfibrozil increases plasma levels of the statins via an effect that blocks biliary excretion and is associated with a significant risk for rhabdomyolysis. Polymorphisms or genetic differences may increase the risk for drug–drug interactions in certain individuals as well.[51]

Statins and Special Populations: Pregnancy, Lactation, and the Elderly

Statins are contraindicated for use during pregnancy because they can cause adverse fetal outcomes; notably, central nervous system and limb abnormalities were found in animal studies. Statins enter breast milk, so they are also contraindicated for women who are breastfeeding.[22] Providers should use caution when prescribing statins to women of childbearing age and should consider nonpharmacologic treatments if possible. Nevertheless, the updated guidelines identify statins as the initial medication of choice for treatment of children and adolescents with high LDL.[57] Statins can and are commonly recommended for older individuals, although monitoring may be more rigorous because of potential or real comorbidities.[58]

Fibric Acid Derivatives

Fibric acid derivatives (fibrates) are drugs of choice for persons with hypertriglyceridemia and are often used in combination with statins for the treatment of dyslipidemia (Table 15-20). These drugs are not generally used as monotherapy for hyperlipidemia.[59]

Fibrates typically decrease serum triglycerides by 30% to 50% and increase HDL by 5% to 15%. Their effect on LDL varies. These agents' primary mode of action is via activation of nuclear transcription factors called peroxisome proliferator-activated receptors. These factors, which are primarily located in the liver and brown adipose tissue, effect several changes in lipid metabolism once bound to the fibrate. Specifically, they reduce triglyceride production by stimulating triglyceride oxidation in the liver and increasing the activity of lipoprotein lipase, an enzyme that hydrolyzes the lipids in VLDL into free fatty acids, which then increases the clearance of triglyceride-rich VLDL. However, for those persons with extremely high triglyceride levels, an increased LDL level may occur when gemfibrozil (Lopid) is used.[60]

Table 15-20 Fibric Acid Derivatives

Drug: Generic (Brand)	Formulations	Dose	Effect on Lipids
Fenofibrate (Antara)	30-mg, 43-mg, 90-mg, 130-mg tablets	Initially 43–130 mg PO/day	Decreases LDL 20–30%; increases HDL 10–20%; decreases triglycerides 23–54%. Avoid statins.
Fenofibrate (Lofibra)	54-mg, 160-mg tablets	Initially 54–160 mg PO/day. Adjust dose for renal impairment.	Decreases LDL 20–30%; increases HDL 10–20%; decreases triglycerides 23–54%. Avoid statins.
Fenofibrate (Tricor)	48-mg, 145-mg tablets	Initially 48–145 mg PO/day; maximum dose 145 mg daily	Decreases LDL 20–30%; increases HDL 10–20%; decreases triglycerides 23–54%
Fenofibrate (Triglide)	160 mg	160 mg PO/day	Decreases LDL 20–30%; increases HDL 10–20%; decreases triglycerides 23–54%
Gemfibrozil (Lopid)	600 mg	600 mg PO 2 times/day 30 minutes prior to meals	Decreases LDL 0–10%; increases HDL 10–20%; decreases triglycerides 20–60%. Avoid statins.

Side Effects/Contraindications

Side effects of fibric acid derivatives include skin rashes, nausea, diarrhea, myopathy, arrhythmias, hypokalemia, and elevation in liver transaminase values. Liver transaminase levels should be monitored and the drug discontinued if these levels increase to more than three times the upper limit of normal. Fibric acid derivatives also should be discontinued in persons who develop an elevation of plasma creatinine phosphokinase. Fibrates appear to slightly increase the risk that an individual will develop pulmonary embolism or pancreatitis (1.1% with fibrates versus 0.7% with placebo and 0.8% with fibrates versus 0.5% with placebo, respectively).[61] Fibrates should be avoided by persons who have hepatic or renal dysfunction, including hepatic disease and biliary cirrhosis.

Drug–Drug Interactions

Interactions between fibric acid derivatives and warfarin (Coumadin) may occur in which the fibrate is displaced from albumin-binding sites, such that the dose of warfarin may need to be decreased. Because bile acid resins may bind fibrates, the fibrate should be administered 1 hour before or 4 hours after the woman takes a bile acid resin. Concomitant use of fibrates and statins should be avoided, as using both drugs increases the incidence of myopathies. Cyclosporine's effectiveness may be decreased when it is given with fibrates, and the risk of nephrotoxicity is increased with this combination. Fibrates also may potentiate the effect of antiglycemic drugs.

Fibrates and Special Populations: Pregnancy, Lactation, and the Elderly

No studies have been published regarding the use of fibrates during pregnancy in humans, but in animal studies these drugs have shown embryocidal and teratogenic effects. Therefore, fibrates are not recommended for use by pregnant women. Fibrates are also secreted in breast milk and in animal studies have been shown to cause tumor formation. Fibrates have a lower molecular weight that suggests they transfer into breast milk easily. Consequently, they should not be used by breastfeeding women secondary to the potential for newborn toxicity. There are no specific dosing considerations for the elderly.

Bile Acid Sequestrants

Bile acid sequestrants (resins) are among the oldest treatments for hyperlipidemia (Table 15-21). These drugs can be

Table 15-21 Bile Acid Sequestrants

Drug: Generic (Brand)	Formulations	Dose	Effect on Lipids
Cholestyramine (Questran)	4-g packet	Initially 1 packet mixed with fluid 1–2 times/day, maintenance 2–4 packets/day; maximum of 6 packets/day	Decreases LDL 15–30%; increases HDL 0–5%; increases triglycerides 0–10%
Colesevelam (Welchol)	625-mg tablet 3.75-g packet	3 tablets PO 2 times/day or 6 tablets/day 3.75 g once daily	Decreases LDL 15–18%; increases HDL 3–5%; increases triglycerides 0–10%
Colestipol (Colestid)	5-g packet	5–30 g daily or in divided doses	Decreases LDL 15–30%; increases HDL 0–5%; increases triglycerides 0–10%
	1-g tablet	Initially 2 g PO daily or 2 times/day, maintenance dose 2–16 g/day; maximum dose 16 g/day	

used as monotherapy or in combination with other hyperlipidemia pharmacotherapy. Resins are useful for persons with renal or hepatic disease because these drugs are not absorbed by the intestines. Gastrointestinal side effects are the primary reason for their discontinuation, and it is often difficult for an individual to reach treatment goals using these agents. A majority of persons with hyperlipidemia, like those with hypertension, need multiple drugs to get them to their treatment goals and reduce their risk of CVD.

Bile acids are metabolites of cholesterol and are normally absorbed in the intestinal lumen. Bile acid sequestrants are resins that bind to bile acids in the intestine, thereby preventing them from being reabsorbed.[62] The bile acid sequestrant is not absorbed either. This phenomenon results in an increase in conversion of cholesterol into bile acids in the liver. When bile acid sequestrants are used to treat primary hypercholesterolemia, a reduction of 9% to 18% ($P = 0.001$) can be expected in serum cholesterol levels.[63] The mean reduction in LDL is 20% with a dose of 4.5 g per day of colesevelam (Welchol). Another use of these drugs is to reduce pruritus caused by the accumulation of bile acids in persons with cholestasis.

Side Effects/Contraindications

Side effects of bile acid sequestrants are primarily gastrointestinal: bloating, dyspepsia, constipation, nausea, and flatulence. Severe hypertriglyceridemia is a contraindication because these drugs can increase triglyceride levels. Bile acid sequestrant resins can interfere with the intestinal absorption of other medications such as thiazides, propranolol (Inderol), cardiac glycosides, warfarin (Coumadin), other anticoagulants, some vitamins, and statins. Other medications should be given 1 hour prior to taking bile acid sequestrants or 4–6 hours after the bile acid sequestrant dose. The use of these medications is contraindicated for persons with biliary and bowel obstruction.

Bile Acid Sequestrants and Special Populations: Pregnancy, Lactation, and the Elderly

Bile acid sequestrants are not absorbed systemically, but they can interfere with intestinal absorption of vitamins A, D, E, and K as well as folic acid and iron. When used by pregnant women to treat intrahepatic cholestasis of pregnancy, the addition of a vitamin K supplement is recommended because vitamin K is not absorbed if bile salts are not present. The value of supplementing other fat-soluble vitamins is not clear. Bile acid sequestrants are not found in appreciable amounts in breast milk, but if they are taken for long periods of time so that the mother becomes deficient in fat-soluble vitamins, this deficiency could have an adverse effect on an infant.

There are no specific dosing considerations for the elderly. While previously the only treatment option for approved for children and adolescents, bile acid sequestrants are no longer first-line agents in this population due to their limited effectiveness when compared to statins, as well as their gastrointestinal side effects.[57]

Niacin (Nicotinic Acid)

Niacin (nicotinic acid) reduces LDL and effectively increases HDL. Available formulations are listed in Table 15-22. Niacin is one of the oldest drugs used to treat dyslipidemia. It is also the one drug used to treat dyslipidemia that can be obtained over the counter without a prescription.

In the AIM-HIGH trial, extended-release niacin combined with statin therapy was compared to statin monotherapy in persons with low HDL levels.[64] This trial was stopped early because of futility. The drug failed to reduce the risk of cardiovascular events, including heart attacks and strokes.

Niacin is a water-soluble B vitamin, also known as vitamin B_3, which inhibits the breakdown of fat in adipose tissue. Niacin has two forms-niacinamide and nicotinic acid. Both have different physiologic effects. Nicotinic acid

Table 15-22 Nicotinic Acid

Drug: Generic (Brand)	Formulations	Dose	Clinical Considerations
Niacin (Niacor)	Immediate-release 500-mg tablets	Initially 250 mg PO daily (1/2 tablet), maintenance 1–2 g daily in 2–3 divided doses; maximum of 6 g daily in 3 divided doses	Take in divided doses with food to minimize GI irritation. Take ASA or NSAID 30 min prior to the niacin.
Niacin ER (Niaspan)	500-mg, 750-mg, 1000-mg tablets	Initially 500 mg PO once daily, maintenance 1–2 g daily; maximum of 2 g daily	Needs to be taken at bedtime with a low-fat snack. Take ASA or NSAID 30 min prior to the niacin.
Niacin SR (Slo-Niacin)	250-mg, 500-mg, 750-mg tablets	250–750 mg PO once daily	Risk of hepatotoxicity

Abbreviations: ASA = acetylsalicylic acid; NSAID = nonsteroidal anti-inflammatory drug.

is an effective dyslipidemic agent whereas niacinamide does not have this effect. Additional information about this vitamin as well as other B vitamins is found in the chapter *Vitamins and Minerals.* The reduced plasma levels of free fatty acids result in a decrease in the secretion of VLDL and cholesterol from the liver, which in turn leads to a reduction in LDL. When the production of LDL decreases, the liver increases absorption of LDL from plasma. The overall breakdown rate of HDL in the liver then decreases, and HDL plasma levels increase. Niacin also decreases the amount of circulating fibrinogen and increases tissue plasminogen, which slows the rate of atherogenesis or thrombosis.

In studies using this agent, nicotinic acid has slowed the progression of arteriosclerosis of the carotid arteries.[65] Niacin is more effective at increasing HDL (30–40%) than are other agents such as statins (5–11%).[65] It has also been found to be as effective in reducing triglycerides as are fibrates.

Niacin is available as immediate-release, sustained-release, and extended-release formulations. The immediate-release formulations are likely to cause flushing and a feeling of warmth secondary to a prostaglandin-stimulated vasodilation. The sustained-release formulation is less likely to cause flushing, but can also increase the risk of hepatotoxicity. The extended-release formulation does not cause flushing and can be more attractive because it does not engender uncomfortable side effects. However, the extended-release formulations are also less effective than the immediate-release formulations, have a rare association with hepatotoxicity when taken in doses more than 2 g per day, and are not currently available without a prescription.

Niacin can be used in combination with statins, but this combination increases the risk of myopathy. Given this risk, serum creatine kinase levels should be monitored if this combination is prescribed.

Side Effects/Contraindications

Facial flushing is the most common side effect associated with taking niacin. The flushing and pruritus can be quite intense for 15–30 minutes and are dose dependent. However, 325 mg of aspirin or 200 mg of ibuprofen taken 30 minutes prior to taking the dose of niacin can decrease the flushing. Gradually titrating the dose over several days will allow the individual to develop a tolerance so that the flushing does not occur. In addition, taking niacin in combination with a low-fat snack and avoiding hot beverages and alcohol can substantially decrease flushing.

Three additional important side effects are associated with niacin: hyperuricemia, myopathy, and impaired insulin sensitivity. Myopathy is the underlying reason that the combination of niacin and statins (niacin/lovastatin [Advicor]) is associated with an increased risk for rhabdomyolysis. Niacin should be used with caution by persons with diabetes and by individuals with a history of gout. This drug should be avoided by women with peptic ulcer disease because it can cause release of histamine, which results in increased gastric motility and acid production. Liver function should be monitored secondary to the increased risk of hepatotoxicity.

Drug–Drug Interactions

The combination of any statin and niacin should be closely monitored, as there is an increased risk for rhabdomyolysis when these two drugs are taken in combination. If the individual is also taking bile acid sequestrants, the dose of niacin should be taken 1 hour before or 4–6 hours after the bile acid sequestrant to ensure absorption. The risk of rhabdomyolysis is also increased if the woman ingests red yeast rice concomitantly with niacin.

Niacin and Special Populations: Pregnancy, Lactation, and the Elderly

Although niacin is a B vitamin, which is necessary in fetal development, the doses used to lower cholesterol are quite high. Because it is not known if the higher doses used to treat hyperlipidemia might have an adverse effect on the fetus, it is generally recommended that these doses not be used by pregnant women. Niacin enters breast milk but is can be used by women who are breastfeeding.[22] No evidence exists that dosing or adverse effects differ for older women.

Cholesterol Absorption Inhibitors

Ezetimibe (Zetia) is the only drug in the cholesterol absorption inhibitors class. This drug is used alone and is also marketed in a fixed-combination formulation with simvastatin (Vytorin). The combination therapy of ezetimibe and simvastatin was found to reduce LDL more than monotherapy with either drug.[60] However, the combination product did not appear to improve intima-media thickness within arteries, which was used as a surrogate marker for atherosclerosis.[66] Another trial comparing statins with niacin or ezetimibe found that the decreased LDL observed with ezetimibe therapy actually worsened intima-media thickness.[67] Currently, the benefit of ezetimibe in management of hyperlipidemia remains unclear, as there are no studies that demonstrate its benefits in reducing cardiovascular outcomes. The mechanism of action of ezetimibe involves inhibition of intestinal absorption of cholesterol, which occurs primarily in the duodenum and proximal jejunum. The only formulation of ezetimibe available is a 10-mg tablet. This agent has a half-life of 22 hours.

Side Effects/Contraindications

The major side effects of ezetimibe are abdominal pain and diarrhea. Use of this agent in women with liver damage is contraindicated because the drug is metabolized hepatically.

Drug–Drug Interactions

Ezetimibe should be given at least 2 hours before or 4 hours after bile acid sequestrants. Use by women who also are receiving cyclosporine (Sandimmune) may result in increased levels of ezetimibe. Although the drug may be combined with a statin, the risk of rhabdomyolysis is increased if the woman takes statins concomitantly with ezetimibe.

Cholesterol Absorption Inhibitors and Special Populations: Pregnancy, Lactation, and the Elderly

No research has been conducted in pregnant women using ezetimibe, and this drug should be used only if the benefits outweigh the risks. It is unknown if the medication is excreted in breast milk, and its use during lactation should be avoided for fear of disrupting the neonatal lipid metabolism.[22] Ezetimibe may be used by older women in a similar manner that it is used by younger females.

Complementary Therapies for Women with Hyperlipidemia

The two dietary supplements known to be effective treatments for hyperlipidemia are niacin and omega-3 fatty acids. Other products such as oat bran, plant sterols, and blond psyllium may potentially have benefits in this indication, but no solid evidence supports their use at this time.

Omega-3 Fatty Acids and Omega-3 Acid Ethyl Ester

Omega-3 acid ethyl ester (Lovaza) is the only FDA-approved prescription omega-3 fatty acid available on the market. Each tablet contains 900 g of EPA and DHA. The FDA has approved using Lovaza for the treatment of severe hypertriglyceridemia (triglycerides ≥ 500 mg/dL), and the American Heart Association recommends use of this drug as an adjunct to other therapies by persons who have hypertriglyceridemia that has not responded to lifestyle changes for secondary prevention of myocardial infarction. A wide variety of OTC preparations of fish oils are available, but they might not contain the same concentration of pharmacologic-grade omega-3 fatty acids.

The exact mechanism of action of omega-3 fatty acids is unknown at this time. It has been hypothesized that they reduce triglyceride levels via the inhibition of acyl CoA:1,2 diacylglycerol acyltransferase, increased hepatic beta-oxidation, or a reduction in the hepatic synthesis of triglycerides.

Side Effects/Contraindications

The most common side effects of omega-3 fatty acids include gastrointestinal symptoms such as taste aversion and dyspepsia.

Drug–Drug Interactions

Omega-3 acid ethyl ester may increase bleeding time. Consequently, it needs to be used with caution by women who are also taking anticoagulants and/or NSAIDs.

Omega-3 Fatty Acids and Special Populations: Pregnancy, Lactation, and the Elderly

It has been established that women in the United States tend to have low intake of foods with a high content of omega 3 fatty acids. Supplements are considered to be free of mercury and can be taken safely by pregnant women. Nevertheless, there is no indication that pregnant women should take these nutritional supplements for treatment of hypercholesterolemia. Omega-3 fatty acids are compatible with breastfeeding.

Controversy exists about whether omega-3 fatty acids can decrease rates of cardiovascular disease among the elderly. In addition, conflicting data have been published about the use of these agents to increase cognitive function and improve mood among older adults. However, there are no studies suggesting a change in dosing is warranted for the older woman.

Cerebral Vascular Disease

A cerebral vascular event, or stroke, is defined as a sudden neurologic deficit in the brain caused by either ischemia or hemorrhage. Approximately 6.8 million persons in the United States have had a stroke, including 3.8 million women.[68] Cerebral vascular accident is the third leading cause of death in women. Women tend to live longer than men, so they also tend to be more adversely affected by the residual deficits of stroke, as they are more likely to be living alone and widowed, are more often institutionalized, and have poorer recovery from stroke than men.[68] While age-specific mortality is higher for men than women, this trend reverses at 85 years and older ages, so at that point more women die each year from stroke than men.[68]

The risk factors for stroke are different between genders, with sex-specific risk factors for women including pregnancy, preeclampsia, gestational diabetes, use of combination hormonal contraceptives, and postmenopausal hormone use.[68] Other risk factors that are stronger or more prevalent in women than in men include incidence of atrial fibrillation (AF), diabetes, and hypertension.[68] Management of these risk factors should be considered in both primary and secondary prevention of stroke in women.

Use of hormonal contraceptives may increase the risk of stroke in women with a priori risk factors for stroke, including cigarette smoking and prior thromboembolic event. If hormonal contraceptives are used, aggressive reduction of other stroke risk factors should be implemented.[68] Hormone therapy should not be used for primary or secondary prevention of stroke in postmenopausal women.

The majority of strokes are ischemic in origin (87%), and the remaining are hemorrhagic. The discussion in this section focuses on medications used for secondary prevention of ischemic stroke. First, however, a short review of platelet activation and aggregation is in order.

The Life Cycle of a Platelet

Technically, platelets are not cells because they do not have a nucleus. Rather, platelets are fragments of cytoplasm from a large cell called a megakaryoblast. Platelets form when the cell membrane of the megakaryoblast sends tendrils of membrane into the cytoplasm, which divides it into many compartments. These compartments are sealed off and extruded from the megakaryocyte as a platelet. Each platelet has cytoplasm and numerous granules that contain the chemicals involved in clotting.

The platelet must be activated before it engages in clotting activity. Endothelial damage triggers this activation, whereby the platelet changes from smooth and round to swollen with extruded, sticky, spiky processes. The change in shape exposes a phospholipid surface that is used by various coagulation factors. Once attached to the endothelial wall at the site of injury, degranulation of the platelet occurs, with the chemicals that initiate the clotting process being released. Adenosine diphosphate (ADP) attracts more platelets to the area; thromboxane A_2 attracts more platelets and triggers more degranulation. Pharmacologic therapies for prevention of stroke are targeted at inhibiting platelet coagulation. Further description of the clotting process can be found in the *Hematology* chapter.

Pharmacologic Treatment for Cerebrovascular Disease

Initial therapy for acute cerebral vascular accident includes agents used to assure medical stability, and assessment for eligibility for use of thrombolytic drugs. Several of the drug classes discussed previously in this chapter have beneficial effects for secondary prevention of a stroke or transient ischemic attack (TIA). Blood pressure medications should be initiated or restarted in women who have a blood pressure of 140/90 mm Hg or higher a few days after a stroke.[69] The optimal drug is not clearly defined, but available data support the use of diuretics and ACE inhibitors. Statin therapy with intensive lipid-lowering effects should also be started if the stroke has an atherosclerotic origin. The management of women with stroke or transient ischemic attack and other comorbid atherosclerotic cardiovascular disease should follow the 2013 ACC/AHA cholesterol guidelines, which include lifestyle, dietary, and medication recommendations.[69]

Pharmacologic therapy that specifically targets platelet aggregation is classified into three categories of antithrombotic agents: (1) **antiplatelet drugs** that prevent platelets from clumping to form a clot, such as aspirin and clopidogrel (Plavix); (2) **anticoagulant drugs** that slow the clotting process, thereby reducing fibrin formation and preventing new clots from forming, such as heparin or warfarin (Coumadin); and (3) fibrinolytic drugs that break apart fibrin molecules. The fibrinolytic drugs are used in the acute management of ischemia that might be fatal, such as myocardial infarction, pulmonary embolism, and the initial stage of ischemic stroke. Because they are not used in primary care, these drugs are not covered in this text. Instead, this section reviews antiplatelet agents used for secondary prevention of ischemic stroke. The anticoagulant drugs are discussed in more detail in the *Hematology* chapter, as they are also used in the treatment of venous thrombi. Both antiplatelet and anticoagulant drugs have a role in managing stroke, and evidence-based recommendations for their use were released by the AHA and American Stroke Association in 2014.[69]

Acetylsalicylic Acid (Aspirin)

Aspirin is the drug most widely used to prevent stroke. For women who had a non-cardioembolic stroke, aspirin 50–325 mg daily is recommended for prevention of a future stroke. Previously, the combination of aspirin and clopidogrel (Plavix) after a stroke or transient ischemic attack was not recommended due to an increased risk of major hemorrhage without any increase in clinical benefit. However, more recent data demonstrate the benefit of aspirin and clopidogrel combination therapy initiated 24 hours after a minor stroke or transient ischemic attack, and continuing for 90 days.[69–71]

In brief, aspirin irreversibly inhibits platelet cyclooxygenase (COX) by forming a covalent bond at the active site of the COX enzyme inside the platelet cell. When aspirin is not present, the COX enzyme facilitates the conversion of arachidonic acid into thromboxane A_2. Thromboxane A_2 then diffuses across the platelet membrane and binds to a receptor on another platelet, which results in platelet aggregation. Aspirin's effect lasts for the life of the platelet, which is 5 to 7 days.

The recommended dose of aspirin for secondary prevention after a stroke is 50–325 mg daily.[69] However, separate guidelines cite multiple studies that have found low-dose aspirin, 81 mg, is effective and associated with fewer bleeding events than higher doses.[72] The antiplatelet effect of aspirin has an onset of less than 60 minutes, and doses of 100 mg or less can have an inhibitory effect on COX.

Side Effects/Contraindications and Drug–Drug Interactions

Aspirin has multiple drug–drug interactions and side effects, as discussed in more detail in the *Analgesia and Anesthesia* chapter. The most concerning adverse effect is bleeding and gastrointestinal irritation, which can evolve into perforated ulcers. In addition, it is clear that higher doses do not enhance the anticlotting therapeutic effect, but they do increase the incidence of bleeding.

Aspirin and Special Populations: Pregnancy, Lactation, and the Elderly

Aspirin is specifically contraindicated in the third trimester of pregnancy because use of aspirin close to birth may prolong gestation or potentially cause premature closure of the ductus arteriosus in the fetus. Aspirin does cross into breast milk, and although low-dose aspirin used as a antiplatelet therapy may be safe for breastfeeding women, high doses should be avoided by the breastfeeding woman.[22] If a woman does take low-dose aspirin, she should time its administration so that it occurs approximately 2 hours after feeding to minimize risk to the infant of disruption of the child's platelets. There are no specific dosing considerations for the elderly.

Aspirin and Extended-Release Dipyridamole

The fixed-dose formulation of aspirin and extended-release (ER) dipyridamole (Aggrenox) was the first combination agent to show more benefit than had been obtained by the use of aspirin as monotherapy. Today, it is a recommended first-line treatment for secondary prevention of stroke in addition to aspirin alone.[69,72]

Dipyridamole inhibits the function of an intracellular enzyme that normally breaks down cyclic adenosine monophosphate. The cyclic adenosine monophosphate remains active, increasing the reuptake of intracellular calcium into the storage tubules, which prevents platelet activation and excretion of the granules that contain clotting factors.

Aggrenox is a combination of dipyridamole ER and aspirin (200 mg and 25 mg, respectively) that is taken twice daily. Slow titration can be instituted by taking the medication at bedtime for 2 to 3 days, then increasing to twice-daily dosing.

Side Effects/Contraindications

Headache is a common side effect with this combination therapy and is more common among women than among men. Abdominal pain, dyspepsia, nausea, and diarrhea also are commonly reported. Because Aggrenox contains aspirin, the side effects, adverse effects, and contraindications that exist for aspirin are also applicable to this combination therapy. These side effects are common and are the reason individuals stop therapy more often with Aggrenox than with low-dose aspirin alone.

Clopidogrel

Clopidogrel (Plavix) is an inhibitor of adenosine diphosphate (ADP), which exerts its antiplatelet effect on the membrane's G-protein–coupled receptors that lead to platelet shape change, and blocks the glycoprotein IIb/IIIa receptor. Clopidogrel is a prodrug that needs to be primarily metabolized by the CYP2C19 enzyme, and requires 3 to 7 days to achieve its maximum antiplatelet effect. It is available as a 75-mg tablet that is taken daily.

In studies comparing clopidogrel monotherapy to aspirin monotherapy and aspirin/dipyridamole combination therapy, researchers did not observe any difference in outcomes among the groups.[69] Therefore, while clopidogrel monotherapy is not recommended as an initial option for prevention of recurrent stroke, it is a reasonable alternative to aspirin monotherapy or the aspirin/dipyridamole combination, especially if the woman is intolerant to other therapies.[69]

Side Effects/Contraindications

The side effects of clopidogrel are less toxic than the side effects associated with another ADP receptor antagonist, ticlopidine (Ticlid). Although the incidence of gastrointestinal bleeding is less than is seen among persons taking aspirin, it is a well-known risk associated with use of clopidogrel. Clopidogrel is contraindicated for women who have active bleeding, peptic ulcer disease, and coagulation disorders.

Drug–Drug Interactions

Clopidogrel should be used cautiously with other antiplatelet agents, as their effects may be potentiated. It also has been associated with interactions with phenytoin (Dilantin), tamoxifen (Nolvadex), tolbutamide, streptokinase, and the proton pump inhibitors omeprazole (Prilosec) and esomeprazole (Nexium).

Clopidogrel and Special Populations: Pregnancy, Lactation, and the Elderly

Clopidogrel appears to be safe in pregnancy, and no teratogenic effects have been observed with its use in animal studies. It is theorized that clopidogrel is excreted in breast milk, but there is no evidence as to the clinical significance; consequently, use of this drug during lactation is not recommended. There are no specific dosing considerations for the elderly.

Peripheral Arterial Occlusive Disease

Approximately 5 million people in the United States suffer from peripheral arterial occlusive disease,[2] also known as peripheral vascular disease. In 2013, the ACC/AHA established clinical practice guidelines for the screening, evaluation, risk reduction, and treatment of persons with such disease.[73] For the purpose of this chapter, peripheral arterial occlusive disease is defined as a pathological condition of noncoronary arterial circulation secondary to occlusion or dilation. Atherosclerosis is the most common pathophysiology contributing to peripheral arterial occlusive disease. Individuals with peripheral arterial occlusive disease have a 20% to 60% increased risk of cardiovascular events such as myocardial infarction or stroke. Many women older than 65 years are asymptomatic, yet have a high risk of mortality secondary to this disorder, and it is recommended that they be treated even if they do not exhibit symptoms.

Common symptoms of peripheral arterial occlusive disease are pain in the legs at rest, intermittent claudication, and poor healing in wounds that affect the extremities. The risk factors for peripheral arterial disease are the same as the risk factors for most other CVD. Smoking is a powerful predictor of peripheral arterial occlusive disease, with more than 80% of those persons with peripheral arterial occlusive disease being current or past smokers. Diabetes, a cardiovascular risk equivalent, is also a major risk factor, and improved glycemic control can reduce the risk. Hyperlipidemia, elevated LDL, and reduced HDL also have a strong relationship with the progression of peripheral arterial occlusive disease. Hypertension has a weaker relationship with peripheral arterial occlusive disease, but use of ACE inhibitors has shown some benefit in treatment of peripheral arterial occlusive disease. Peripheral arterial occlusive disease is a major risk factor for the development of chronic disease, decreased functional capacity, amputation, and death.[73]

The diagnosis of peripheral arterial occlusive disease is based on symptoms, physical exam, and the ankle-brachial index. The ankle-brachial index is a noninvasive test that is highly sensitive and specific for diagnosing peripheral arterial occlusive disease.

The foundation of peripheral arterial occlusive disease treatment is lifestyle modification, which includes time-intensive interventions that can have long-reaching impact on a woman's quality of life. Smoking cessation is essential in treating any person with symptoms of peripheral arterial occlusive disease. Treatment of hyperlipidemia, diabetes, and hypertension according to recommendations from national guidelines should also be implemented.[73]

Pharmacologic Treatment of a Woman with Peripheral Arterial Occlusive Disease

Antiplatelet therapy is a cornerstone of treatment of a woman with peripheral arterial occlusive disease, and is highly recommended if the woman has intermittent claudication, has critical limb ischemia, or is asymptomatic with an ankle-brachial index 0.9 or less.[73] Antiplatelet therapy is not recommended if the ankle-brachial index is in the range of 0.91 to 0.99, and warfarin (Coumadin) is not recommended unless the woman has another indication for anticoagulation therapy.[73] Aspirin, 75–325 mg daily, is the recommended first-line antiplatelet drug. Clopidogrel (Plavix) is as effective as aspirin, and can be used if the woman is allergic or intolerant to aspirin.

For women who have intermittent claudication, cilostazol (Pletal) 100 mg twice daily can help improve symptoms and increase walking distance among individuals with lower-extremity peripheral arterial occlusive disease.[73] Cilostazol (Pletal) is a phosphodiesterase III inhibitor that inhibits platelet aggregation, causes vasodilation, and inhibits vascular smooth muscle cell proliferation. It is contraindicated for women with heart failure. Pentoxifylline (Trental) is also another option for intermittent claudication, but is not as effective as cilostazol. The prescription for pentoxifylline is 400 mg three times daily.

In addition, the ACC/AHA recommends that persons who are at risk for or who have peripheral arterial occlusive disease be treated for risk factors that cause this disease.[73] If a woman has an elevated blood pressure, she should be treated with an ACE inhibitor or a beta blocker. Individuals with concomitant peripheral arterial occlusive disease and diabetes will benefit from tight glycemic control with antiglycemic agents, either oral or parenteral. Optimal control of these comorbidities will help delay and prevent critical limb ischemia and the need for surgical intervention.

Heart Failure

Heart failure is a growing concern as the nation ages. Among individual in the United States who are 40 years or older, there is a 20% lifetime risk of developing a form of heart failure.[74] Currently, more than 5 million adults in the United States have diagnosed heart failure, and the prevalence is anticipated to rise due to the aging population. Despite improved and earlier detection and treatment, the mortality rate for this condition remains high, at approximately 50% within 5 years of diagnosis of heart failure. Women account for the majority of heart failure deaths (approximately 60%) in the United States annually.[3] The two leading causes of heart failure are coronary artery disease and hypertension.

The most common clinical signs of heart failure are fluid retention, fatigue, and dyspnea. Heart failure is commonly categorized as diastolic or systolic, and is now also referred to as heart failure with preserved ejection fraction (HFpEF) and heart failure with reduced ejection fraction (HFrEF), respectively.[74] HFpEF is diagnosed when the ejection fraction is higher than 40%, and HFrEF is diagnosed when the ejection fraction is 40% or less. Diastolic heart failure (or HFpEF) occurs when the ventricle fails to properly fill, and systolic dysfunction (or HFrEF) occurs when reduced contractility is present. The incidence of diastolic heart failure increases with age, and this condition is more common in women than in men.[75]

Heart failure is classified by the ACCF/AHA into four stages. Stage A refers to women who are at high risk for heart failure, but who do not have structural heart disease or symptoms. Stage B refers to persons with structural heart disease who do not have signs or symptoms of heart

Table 15-23 ACCF/AHA Stages and NYHA Functional Classification of Heart Failure

Stage	ACCF/AHA Stages
A	At high risk for heart failure but without structural heart disease or symptoms of heart failure.
B	Structural heart disease but without signs or symptoms of heart failure.
C	Structural heart disease with prior or current symptoms of heart failure.
D	Refractory heart failure requiring specialized interventions.

Source: Reprinted from Yancy CW, Jessup M, Bozkurt B, et al. American College of Cardiology Foundation; American Heart Association Task Force on Practice Guidelines. 2013 ACCF/AHA guideline for the management of heart failure: a report of the American College of Cardiology Foundation/American Heart Association Task Force on Practice Guidelines. *J Am Coll Cardiol.* 2013;62:e147-e239, with permission of Elsevier.

failure. Stage C is used to denote persons with structural heart disease with prior or current symptoms of heart failure. Stage D is the term for individuals with refractory heart failure requiring specialized interventions.[74] These are defined in Table 15-23.

Diastolic Heart Failure

Diastolic heart failure accounts for approximately 50% of women with clinical heart failure.[74] However, estimates of its prevalence vary based on the differing ejection fraction cut-off criteria. Measurement of diastolic dysfunction is limited in clinical practice because there is significant overlap between diastolic and systolic heart failure in terms of signs and symptoms that are detected on physical exam, ECG, and radiograph studies.

Pathophysiology of Diastolic Heart Failure

Diastolic heart failure occurs when there is impaired or incomplete myocardial relaxation and ventricle filling, which results in the clinical symptoms of heart failure. Diastolic dysfunction is technically abnormal function of the ventricle. There are two leading causes of diastolic dysfunction: cardiac ischemia and left ventricular hypertrophy. In addition, there are two types of ischemia, one related to supply and one related to demand. Demand ischemia is present when an increased oxygen demand is associated with increased physical activity. In this scenario, there is a relative insufficient supply of blood. Supply ischemia, in contrast, is seen when coronary blood flow is insufficient.

Pharmacologic Treatment of Women with Diastolic Heart Failure

The treatment for a woman with diastolic heart failure should be based on several national cardiology guidelines.[74,76] Many of the drugs recommended as treatments for women with systolic heart failure are also used for as treatments for women with diastolic heart failure. To date, however, few large clinical trials have been conducted that demonstrated improved clinical outcomes with these medications for women with diastolic heart failure.

Addressing the etiology of the diastolic dysfunction is key.[74,76] Left ventricular hypertrophy related to hypertension is a primary cause of diastolic dysfunction. Therefore, systolic and diastolic BP should be controlled according to clinical practice guidelines. Beta blockers, ACE inhibitors, ARBs, and calcium-channel blockers can all be utilized for this purpose. Diuretics can also be used for relief of symptoms, but women with diastolic heart failure will generally not require as high of a dose of a diuretic as do women with systolic heart failure.

Addressing other cardiac problems such as atrial fibrillation that stress the heart is vital in the management of diastolic heart failure. Medications that improve coronary ischemia need to be considered. Beta blockers have beneficial effects in slowing the heart rate and improving ventricular filling. Many calcium-channel blockers are not considered for use in systolic heart failure, but verapamil (Calan) is especially helpful in relaxing the myocardium, improving ventricular filling, and decreasing ischemic episodes in diastolic heart failure.

The RAAS is also activated in the pathophysiology of individuals with diastolic heart failure. ACE inhibitors and ARBs have demonstrated significant improvements in clinical outcomes among individuals with systolic heart failure. In contrast, several studies of ACE inhibitors or ARBs in treatment of persons with diastolic heart failure have yielded inconclusive results.[77–80] Therefore, there are no clear recommendations for specific drug classes to be used for women with diastolic heart failure because of the lack of evidence from clinical trials. Nevertheless, it remains important to use these medications to control BP so as to prevent progression of the disease state.

Systolic Heart Failure

Pathophysiology of Systolic Heart Failure

Systolic heart failure is a progressive syndrome that starts with an insult or injury to the myocardium. Over time, the accumulated injury leads to structural changes the size of heart chambers. These changes cause hemodynamic stresses to the wall of the heart that eventually result in decreasing cardiac performance, such as poor filling or weak ejection. The poor performance continues to cause further cardiac remodeling.

When a person has poor cardiac output, the RAAS is activated secondary to reduced renal blood flow. The result of this process is production of angiotensin II, which increases peripheral vascular resistance via vasoconstriction. Angiotensin II also directly stimulates the release of catecholamines from noradrenergic receptors, which increases heart rate and contractility. Ultimately, it stimulates the adrenal cortex to release aldosterone, which stimulates reabsorption of sodium and water. These effects initially maintain cardiac output, but over time in the presence of a damaged myocardium, these effects become maladaptive. Drugs that block or inhibit angiotensin II have demonstrated positive effects on long-term outcomes.

Ultimately, many neurohormonal peptides are involved in the development and progression of systolic heart failure, such as increased levels of norepinephrine, endothelin, vasopressin, and cytokines. Norepinephrine is known to increase heart rate and vasoconstriction. Individuals with heart failure who also have higher levels of norepinephrine have a poorer prognosis than those persons with lower norepinephrine levels, because the constant activation of the sympathetic nervous system downregulates the beta receptors. Therefore, drugs that cause suppression of the sympathetic nervous system are beneficial for persons with systolic heart failure.

Aldosterone increases retention of sodium, and new findings indicate that it is also involved in the development of cardiac fibrosis. Major reductions in mortality have been found with the use of drugs that reduce aldosterone levels. Angiotensin II is known to be a potent vasoconstrictor, which leads to increased vascular resistance.

Treatment of Women with Systolic Heart Failure

Treatment for a woman with heart failure is based on the stage of the disease. Table 15-24 lists doses of beta blockers for women with systolic heart failure.

Stage A Systolic Heart Failure

The purpose of identifying a person at stage A is to recognize risk factors for heart failure early and aggressively reduce those risks. If an individual smokes, smoking cessation should be discussed and positive reinforcement should be offered to nonsmokers and especially ex-smokers.

ACE inhibitors continue to have benefit for the treatment and prevention of heart failure, even beyond BP reduction. ACE inhibitors reduce risk by blocking—but not completely halting—the effects of the RAAS.[81] ACE inhibitors also improve survival and decrease mortality in women as well as in men.[82] Overall, the dose of an ACE inhibitor should be titrated to target doses, but the benefit of an ACE inhibitor at a lower dose is superior to no use at all.[83] The same precautions that apply when prescribing ACE inhibitors to treat hypertension need to be taken into consideration when using these agents to manage heart failure. Adverse effects and drug interactions of ACE inhibitors were discussed in conjunction with the treatment of women with hypertension earlier in this chapter.

Table 15-24 Initial and Target Doses of Beta Blockers for the Treatment of Women with Heart Failure

Drug: Generic (Brand)	Initial Dose	Target Dose
Bisoprolol (Ziac)	1.25 mg PO/day	10 mg/day
Carvedilol (Coreg, Coreg CR)	3.125 mg PO 2 times/day	25–50 mg 2 times/day
Metoprolol XL (Toprol XL)	12.5–25 mg PO/day	200 mg/day

Stage B Systolic Heart Failure

If structural changes are present but no symptoms of heart failure are found, the woman meets the criteria for stage B heart failure. The provider should continue to recommend all treatments used for persons with stage A heart failure. An individual with stage B heart failure may have a history of myocardial infarction or may have a left ventricular ejection fraction of 40% or less. This woman will benefit from use of both a beta blocker and an ACE inhibitor.[74,76] Beta blockers—specifically, bisoprolol (Ziac), carvedilol (Coreg, Coreg CR), and extended-release metoprolol succinate (Toprol XL)—have been shown to reduce the morbidity and mortality associated with stage B heart failure. Not all beta blockers are indicated in the treatment of heart failure, however, and some, such as propranolol (Inderal), atenolol (Tenormin), and metoprolol (Lopressor), may exacerbate symptoms of heart failure. Table 15-24 outlines the initial and target doses of these three drugs.

Women with stage B heart failure should continue to be optimized on an ACE inhibitor in addition to a beta blocker. Use of an ARB instead of an ACE inhibitor is recommended if the woman is intolerant to the ACE inhibitor. The addition of an ARB to an ACE inhibitor and beta blocker can be considered if the woman is titrated to the target doses of the ACE inhibitor and beta blocker, yet is still persistently symptomatic.[74,76] Note that this is not common practice, however, owing to the increased risk of renal injury and hyperkalemia when ACE inhibitors and ARBs are used concomitantly.

Digoxin (Lanoxin) is a medication that was once extremely popular as a treatment for heart failure. Currently, it is reserved for individuals in later stages of heart failure due to its adverse-effect profile and limited effectiveness. Non-dihydropyridine calcium-channel blockers such as verapamil (Calan) are not recommended for persons with any stage of systolic heart failure because they have negative inotropic effects.

Stage C Systolic Heart Failure

Individuals who have symptoms of heart failure with structural changes in the myocardium have progressed to stage C heart failure. Several medications can be added to help with symptom management in such persons and to reduce hospitalizations, morbidity, and mortality—namely, ARBs, aldosterone antagonists, nitrates, and hydralazine (Apresoline).

When a person has fluid overload, diuretics can provide symptomatic relief. Such individuals optimally should be titrated with a beta blocker and ACE inhibitor or ARB. The addition of diuretics such as thiazides or loop diuretics along with sodium restriction will help control fluid overload. The diuretics may be used as needed, or they may need to be a part of ongoing therapy. Initially, loop diuretics are recommended to manage edema. Often furosemide (Lasix) is the drug of choice; however, the pharmacokinetics of furosemide are not as predictable as those of other loop diuretics such as torsemide (Demadex) and bumetanide (Bumex). Failure to respond to one loop diuretic suggests that another may be tried and benefit may be gained. Individuals with normal renal function are expected to benefit from the normal maximum dosing. However, those women who develop diuretic resistance may require higher doses of loop diuretic or addition of another type of diuretic to provide sequential nephron blockade.[74,76]

Aldosterone Antagonists

Aldosterone antagonists have a role in management of a woman with heart failure beyond their diuretic effect. Aldosterone is a key component in the development of hypertension and heart failure secondary to its role in stimulating sodium and water retention. The RALES trial (Randomized Aldactone Evaluation Study), which included 1663 individuals with HFrEF and ejection fraction less than 35%, showed an approximately 30% reduction in mortality with the use of spironolactone compared to placebo.[84] More recently, the EMPHASIS heart failure trial compared eplerenone to placebo among 2737 participants with HFrEF and ejection fraction less than 35%. This trial also demonstrated that eplerenone reduced the rate of death and hospitalization, although an increased risk of hyperkalemia was observed.[85]

Spironolactone (Aldactone) blocks the aldosterone receptors when prescribed at doses of 12.5–25 mg per day. Eplerenone (Inspra) is a more selective aldosterone antagonist, which is dosed at 25–50 mg per day. Due to its selectivity, eplerenone has fewer side effects than does spironolactone; however, spironolactone is more commonly used because it is available in a generic formulation.

Because many of the drugs (e.g., ACE inhibitors, ARBs) used to treat heart failure can cause potassium retention, electrolyte levels should be monitored carefully when these drugs are used in combination.[74] Triple therapy consisting of an ACE inhibitor, an aldosterone antagonist, and an ARB should be avoided, as the incidence of adverse effects with this combination usually outweighs the benefits.[74]

Vasodilators

The combination of isosorbide dinitrate (Isordil, Sorbitrate) and hydralazine (Apresoline) also reduces mortality among persons with stage C heart failure. These drugs cause vasodilation of both arteries and veins and can be added to a well-established therapy of ACE inhibitors and beta blockers. In addition, there is benefit seen among African Americans with use of these drugs and in combination with other standard treatments.[86] The isosorbide dinitrate/hydralazine combination can be used in place of an ACE inhibitor or ARB if the woman has drug intolerance, hypotension, or renal insufficiency.[74,76] The standard dose of hydralazine is 25 mg three times daily, which is commonly titrated up; a dose of 100 mg three times daily may be indicated. This standard dosing is combined with isosorbide dinitrate at a dose of 40 mg four times daily.

Calcium-Channel Blockers

In general, non-dihydropyridine calcium-channel blockers are not recommended for individuals with systolic heart failure because they have a negative inotropic effect, which can lead to worsening of heart failure symptoms and mortality. However, the dihydropyridine calcium-channel blockers amlodipine (Norvasc) and felodipine (Plendil) do not have negative effects on heart failure. Both of these agents are able to provide benefits through improvements in blood pressure control and decreased angina symptoms. Caution needs to be exercised when prescribing these drugs, as they are associated with a high incidence of peripheral edema.

Digoxin

Digoxin (Lanoxin) has been used as a medicine for more than two centuries. Until recently, it was the mainstay of therapy for heart failure. Digoxin is extracted from the leaves of the plant *Digitalis lanata*, a common garden flower in the United States. Digoxin can be beneficial for persons with current or prior symptoms of heart failure and reduced left ventricular ejection fractions, decreasing their hospitalizations for heart failure.[74] The use of this drug is also well established for treating arrhythmias such as atrial fibrillation. Digoxin is approved for use in combination with ACE inhibitors, beta blockers, and diuretics, with the caveat that the individual must be assessed and monitored for digoxin therapeutic levels, renal function, and signs and symptoms of toxicity.

Digoxin has an inotropic effect on the heart, making the force of the myocardial muscle stronger during contraction. This effect is caused by inhibition of the sodium/potassium ATPase pump on cell membranes, which increases the intracellular calcium and results in increased contractility. Digoxin also slows electrical conduction between the atria and ventricles, so it can be used to treat some arrhythmias. The half-life of digoxin is 36 hours, with its onset of action occurring in 1.5 to 6 hours.

One important point to remember about the use of digoxin in women with heart failure and normal sinus rhythm is that this drug decreases hospital admissions but does not improve mortality rates.[87] Lower doses of digoxin should be used in women compared to doses recommended for men, especially if the woman is older than 70 years, has impaired renal function, or has a low body mass. A worrisome finding is that there appears to be an increase in total mortality and secondary outcomes of death from CVD or worsening heart failure with the use of digoxin in women when compared to the outcomes in men.[87] Several theories have been offered to explain this finding. Perhaps women have higher serum levels of digoxin, or perhaps hormonal therapy interferes with the metabolism of digoxin, leading to higher levels of digoxin.[88] A recent observational trial of more than 17,000 men and 19,000 women found no difference in risk of mortality based on gender.[89] Overall, women may continue to benefit from digoxin therapy; when taking this drug, they should be monitored closely and their medication levels maintained at a lower end of the therapeutic window.

Side Effects/Adverse Effects of Digoxin

Two of the ways primary care providers may interact with women who are taking digoxin is in monitoring for side effects, adverse effects, and drug–drug interactions. Digoxin has a very narrow therapeutic index, so persons taking this medication must be educated about the signs and symptoms of toxicity, which include nausea, vomiting, palpitations, confusion, blurred vision, disturbances of color vision with a tendency to see yellow-green coloring, photophobia, abdominal pain, and seizures. Laryngeal edema is a rare adverse effect of digoxin. Digoxin has been designated by the Institute for Safe Medicine Practices as a high-alert medication because there is a heightened risk of significant harm if it is used in error. For those women with normal renal function, 60% to 80% of the drug is excreted in the urine unchanged. Therefore, impaired renal function is an increased risk for toxicity.

Although digoxin toxicity usually appears at a serum level of higher than 2 mcg/mL, the recommended drug level for heart failure is 0.5–0.9 mcg/mL.[74] Clinical symptoms of digoxin toxicity may be seen in some individuals before toxic levels are reached. When toxicity is present, the medication should be withheld until the symptoms resolve and the digoxin level returns to normal. For life-threatening situations, digoxin immune fab (Digibind) can be used to bind digoxin in the blood. This agent, which is used as an antidote to digoxin toxicity, is derived from sheep immunoglobulin fragments taken from animals that were immunized with a derivative of digoxin.

Drug–Drug Interactions Associated with Digoxin

Because digoxin has a narrow therapeutic index, it is associated with many significant drug interactions, some of which are listed in Table 15-25.

Digoxin and Special Populations: Pregnancy, Lactation, and the Elderly

Digoxin can be used during pregnancy and is occasionally used to treat fetal tachycardia. Digoxin appears in breast milk in concentrations similar to the concentration in

Table 15-25 Major Drug Interactions Associated with Digoxin[a]

Drug: Generic (Brand)	Effects
Amiodarone (Cordarone), itraconazole (Sporanox), ketoconazole (Neoral), nicardipine (Cardene), nifedipine (Procardia), ritonavir (Norvir), verapamil (Calan)	Reduces clearance of digoxin, which raises serum levels and causes possible digoxin toxicity
Beta blockers, calcium-channel blockers, methyldopa (Aldomet)	Slows heart rate, leading to an additive effect of hypotension
Cholestyramine (Questran), sucralfate (Carafate)	Interferes with intestinal absorption, which lowers serum levels and decreases the therapeutic effect
Potassium-depleting diuretics	Uncorrected potassium depletion makes the heart more sensitive to digoxin; this combination can cause digoxin toxicity and/or arrhythmias
Rifampin (Rifadin)	Increases nonrenal clearance and decreases the therapeutic effect

[a] This table is not comprehensive as new information is being identified on a regular basis.

maternal plasma, so it should be used with extreme caution by women who are breastfeeding infants.

Digoxin is also a Beers criteria drug. Although it is most commonly used by elderly individuals, these are also the persons at highest risk of side effects or toxicity from the narrow therapeutic window.

Stage D Heart Failure

Stage D is the final stage of heart failure, in which women have symptoms refractory to optimal therapy. End-of-life care should be discussed with persons with this diagnosis. At this point, all pharmacologic options have been maximized. Often these individuals benefit from routine, continuous infusions of positive inotropic drugs for palliation. Control of fluid status is a key to providing comfort to decrease hospitalizations related to pulmonary edema.

Cardiac Arrhythmias

Abnormal electrical conduction in the heart causes irregular rate and/or rhythm. The term *cardiac arrhythmia* refers to several different conditions, some of which are asymptomatic, whereas others are life threatening. The most common symptomatic arrhythmia, atrial fibrillation, is reviewed in this chapter. Although treatment of other arrhythmias differs somewhat, the management of atrial fibrillation can be used as an example to illustrate the general principles used in the management of all arrhythmias.

Physiology of Cardiac Rhythms

Normally, electrical conduction controls the rhythm of the heartbeat. Each beat originates in the sinoatrial node in the right atrium. The electrical impulse spreads through the bundle of His in the atrioventricular node and then down the Purkinje fibers in both ventricles, which initiates ventricular contraction. The ability of the sinoatrial node to automatically stimulate a contraction is called *automaticity*. The cells in the sinoatrial node and atrioventricular node differ from other heart muscle cells in another way as well: These cells depend on calcium for the initial depolarization phase of the action potential, whereas other cells in the heart depend on sodium for the depolarization phase.

The atria and the ventricles are electrically separate entities, except for the anteroseptal region in the atrioventricular node in the bundle of His. In addition to the specialized cells that generate the coordinated electrical impulses, all heart muscle cells have the capacity to contract without electrical stimulation. The cells that make up the atrioventricular node, bundle of His, and Purkinje fibers can initiate an action potential strong enough to stimulate a contraction.

Usually, the sinoatrial node works more quickly than other cells and, therefore, controls the usual rate and rhythm, resulting in a heart rate of 60 to 100 beats per minute. However, when the heart muscle contracts secondary to stimulation by a cell other than the cells in the sinoatrial node, an ectopic beat occurs. Because every cell in the heart can transmit an action potential, abnormal electrical conduction circuits can develop. These abnormal circuits can cause fibrillation when one chamber of the heart responds to an abnormal circuit, which is a manifestation of a reentry circuit. Arrhythmias are classically divided into two types—those that alter the automaticity of the sinoatrial node and those that occur secondary to abnormal impulse conduction.

Persons at risk for developing arrhythmias include those who have hypertension, coronary artery disease, heart failure, congenital heart abnormality, hyperthyroidism, diabetes, sleep apnea, alcohol consumption, use of stimulant drugs, and advanced age. With greater age, the heart muscle becomes weaker and more susceptible to abnormal conduction and abnormal firing.

The risks associated with arrhythmias include fainting, falling, and fractures secondary to syncope. Even more importantly, thromboembolic events that may lead to stroke can occur when the blood in the heart is in stasis.

Pharmacologic Treatment of Arrhythmias

The drugs used to treat arrhythmias are organized into four categories based on their mechanisms of action (Table 15-26). The class I drugs are sodium-channel blockers, which decrease the automaticity of the sinoatrial node and slow the heart rate. The class II drugs are beta blockers, which inhibit the tonic sympathetic influence on the sinoatrial node, thereby slowing the heart rate so the myocardium does not have to work as hard. The class III drugs inhibit repolarization by blocking potassium channels, which both slows the heart and prevents reentry circuits. The class IV drugs comprise the non-dihydropyridine calcium-channel blockers, which act on the sinoatrial and atrioventricular nodes—the cells in these nodes are more calcium dependent than sodium dependent for the depolarization phase of the action potential.

Table 15-26 Classes of Drugs Used to Treat Women with Arrhythmias

Class I[a]	Class II[b]	Class III[c]	Class IV[d]
Class Ia	Acebutolol (Sectral)	Amiodarone (Cordarone)	Diltiazem (Cardizem)
Disopyramide (Norpace)	Atenolol (Tenormin)	Dofetilide (Tikosyn)	Verapamil (Calan, Covera-HS)
Procainamide (Procan, Procan)	Betaxolol (Kerlone)	Dronedarone (Multaq)	
Quinidine (Cardioquin, Quinora)	Bisoprolol (Zebeta)	Ibutilide (Corvert)	
Class Ib	Carvedilol (Coreg)	Sotalol (Betapace)	
Lidocaine (Xylocaine)	Esmolol (Brevibloc)		
Mexiletine (Mexitil)	Metoprolol (Toprol-XL, Lopressor)		
Class Ic	Nadolol (Corgard)		
Flecainide (Tambocor)	Propranolol (Inderal)		
Propafenone (Rythmol)	Sotalol (Betapace)		
	Timolol (Blocadren)		

[a] Class I drugs are sodium-channel blockers
[b] Class II drugs are beta blockers
[c] Class III drugs inhibit repolarization by blocking potassium channels, which both slows the heart and prevents reentry circuits
[d] Class IV drugs are non-dihydropyridine calcium-channel blockers

Atrial Fibrillation

Atrial fibrillation is the most common cardiac dysrhythmia among adults, affecting 2.7 to 6.1 million adults in the United States. This incidence is expected to double over the next 25 years due to the aging of the population.[90] The incidence of atrial fibrillation varies with ethnicity, gender, and age. Although the total incidence of men and women with this condition is similar, approximately 60% of persons with atrial fibrillation who are older than 75 years are women.[68] Advancing age is the highest predictor of atrial fibrillation development, with only 1% of those individuals with this arrhythmia being younger than 60 years.[90]

Atrial fibrillation can be asymptomatic or can cause palpitations, the most common symptom. Other symptoms include weakness, chest pain, or fatigue. Atrial fibrillation increases the risk of ischemic stroke four- to five-fold, and the absolute risk ranges from 1.5% for those 50–59 years old to almost 25% for those 80 years or older.[68] Female gender is an additional risk factor for development of stroke; it is included in the CHA_2DS_2-VAS_c score, an updated scoring system to estimate stroke risk among individuals with atrial fibrillation.[91]

The drug used to treat atrial fibrillation are directed at three targets: (1) controlling the heart rate; (2) preventing thrombus formation and stroke; and (3) correcting the rhythm disturbance if controlling the rate is unsuccessful. Beta blockers and calcium-channel blockers (described earlier in this chapter) are used to stabilize the heart rate. The anticoagulant drugs used to prevent thrombus are discussed in more detail in the *Hematology* chapter.

This section provides a brief description of the class I and class III antiarrhythmic drugs used to correct rhythm disturbances in individuals who are hemodynamically stable, who require additional medication, and whose care generally is provided in the outpatient setting with careful monitoring and frequent supervision. Initiation of therapy and management of women who need antiarrhythmic drugs is usually outside the scope of primary care, although primary care providers may care for persons using these agents for other healthcare concerns. The interested reader is referred to the 2014 guidelines for the management of individuals with atrial fibrillation for a full description of currently recommended management of arrhythmias.[90]

Antiarrhythmic Drugs

Class Ia, Ic, and III antiarrhythmic drugs are used to convert atrial fibrillation into a regular rhythm if standard pharmacologic therapies or electrical conversion has been unsuccessful. Efforts to convert atrial fibrillation into a sinus rhythm are not always successful and may produce an independent increased risk for thromboembolism. Therefore, either electrical conversion or pharmacologic conversion generally is offered only to persons already on anticoagulants. These same medications can then be utilized to maintain normal sinus rhythm after conversion.

Because antiarrhythmic drugs affect the electrical conduction within the heart, they have the potential to create arrhythmias and must be used with caution. The side effect of greatest concern is development of a prolonged QTc interval, which can turn into torsades de pointes (a French term meaning "twisting of the points"), which can then evolve into ventricular fibrillation and sudden death. Risk factors for developing torsades de pointes include female gender, bradycardia, advanced age, electrolyte imbalances, baseline prolonged QT interval, and concomitant use of other QT-prolonging medications.[90,92] Routine monitoring of the QTc interval and avoiding other medications that can increase the QTc interval will decrease the risk that the woman might develop torsades de pointes.

Amiodarone (Cordarone) is the class III drug most often recommended for management of women in the outpatient setting. The dose of amiodarone is based on the severity of the arrhythmia. Side effects include pulmonary fibrosis, optic nerve neuropathy, hypotension, hyperthyroidism or hypothyroidism, hepatotoxicity, peripheral neuropathy, headache, ataxia, and skin discoloration. This drug also has multiple drug–drug interactions. Amiodarone is contraindicated for individuals with severe sinoatrial node dysfunction, second- or third-degree atrioventricular heart block, sinus bradycardia, or hypotension.

In summary, cardiac arrhythmias are common in the elderly and a frequent comorbidity in persons with hypertension or other cardiovascular disease processes. The management of cardiac arrhythmias is complex and requires specific knowledge and training in cardiac physiology and the pharmacology of a class of drugs that have multiple adverse effects.

Conclusion

Women need to appreciate the importance of their cardiovascular health. Primary prevention can lead to significant reduction in their lifetime risk of developing CVD. Screening and recognizing risks early is the key to reducing CVD events. Many cardiac events occur in combination and require multiple pharmacologic interventions. Often one drug is insufficient to reach the clinical goals, so multiple drugs may be needed. The healthcare provider needs to be aware of the risk factors for an individual woman and her existing CVD conditions to provide optimal treatment. Continued monitoring of risk factors is necessary, and maintenance treatment goals need to be evaluated frequently. In the area of CVD pharmacology, recommendations and guidelines continue to change as more is revealed about this amazing physiologic system.

Resources

Organization	Description	Website
National Heart, Lung, and Blood Institute	Federal government site that contains professional and consumer information about cardiovascular conditions, among others. General topics include heart information for women, and for women of color. Systematic reviews are included on the page for professionals.	www.nhlbi.nih.gov/
American Heart Association	Organization that focuses on cardiovascular health. Its site includes web pages for professionals, including pocket guidelines for a variety of conditions (e.g., atrial fibrillation).	www.heart.org/HEARTORG/
American College of Cardiology	National organization for cardiologists. Although most of the material requires membership, some information regarding cardiovascular health can be found on this site.	www.acc.org/
Apps		
A myriad of apps exist for devices in the area of consumer-oriented information about cardiovascular disorders. Many are free and can be suggested to women. Some general apps can help women track drug administration.		
National Heart, Lung, and Blood Institute	The 10-year risk calculator for heart attacks can be found at this site. A BMI calculator, including iOS app, is included on this site.	www.nhlbi.nih.gov
American Heart Association	Mobile apps for the iOS and Android platforms offer pocket guidelines for a variety of conditions (e.g., atrial fibrillation).	www.heart.org/HEARTORG
	Cardiovascular Risk Calculator. This calculator can be used on the website or downloaded to a mobile device as an app.	https://my.americanheart.org/professional/StatementsGuidelines/Prevention-Guidelines_UCM_457698_SubHomePage.jsp
American College of Cardiology	A number of free apps, including guidelines and tips for prevention of cardiac disease, are available for professionals at the webpage for mobile resources.	www.acc.org/tools-and-practice-support/mobile-resources

References

1. Mosca L, Benjamin EJ, Berra K, et al. Effectiveness-based guidelines for the prevention of cardiovascular disease in women—2011 update: a guideline from the American Heart Association. *Circulation.* 2011;123: 1243-1262.
2. Roger VL, Go AS, Lloyd-Jones DM, et al., for the American Heart Association Statistics Committee and Stroke Statistics Subcommittee. Heart disease and stroke statistics—2012 update: a report from the American Heart Association. *Circulation.* 2012; 125:e2-e220.
3. Go AS, Mozaffarian D, Roger VL, et al., on behalf of the American Heart Association Statistics Committee and Stroke Statistics Subcommittee. Heart disease and stroke statistics—2013 update: a report from the American Heart Association. *Circulation* 2013; 127:e6-e245.
4. Cheng S, Claggett B, Correia AW. Temporal trends in the population attributable risk for cardiovascular disease: the Atherosclerosis Risk in Communities Study. *Circulation.* 2014;130(10):820-828.
5. Keaney, JF Jr, Curfman GD, Jarcho JA. A pragmatic view of the new cholesterol treatment guidelines. *N Engl J Med.* 2014;370(3):275-278.
6. Mosca L, Hammond G, Mochari-Greenberger H; American Heart Association Cardiovascular Disease and Stroke in Women and Special Populations Committee of the Council on Clinical Cardiology, Council on Epidemiology and Prevention, Council on Cardiovascular Nursing, Council on High Blood. Fifteen-year trends in awareness of heart disease in women: results of a 2012 American Heart Association national survey. *Circulation.* 2013;127:1254-1263.
7. Dahlof B, Sever PS, Poulter NR, et al. Prevention of cardiovascular events with an antihypertensive regimen of amlodipine adding perindopril as required versus atenolol adding bendroflumethiazide as required, in the Anglo-Scandinavian Cardiac Outcomes Trial—Blood Pressure Lowering Arm (ASCOT-BPLA). *Lancet* 2005;366(9489):895-906.
8. Stradling C, Hamid M, Taheri S, Thomas GN. A review of dietary influences on cardiovascular health: part 2: dietary patterns. *Cardiovasc Hematol Disord Drug Targets.* 2014;14(1):50-63.
9. Weinstein AR, Sesso HD, Lee IM, et al. Relationship of physical activity vs. body mass index with type 2 diabetes in women. *JAMA.* 2004;292:1188-1194.
10. Risk and Prevention Study Collaborative Group, Roncaglioni MC, Tombesi M, Avanzini F, et al. *n*-3 fatty acids in patients with multiple cardiovascular risk factors. *N Engl J Med.* 2013;368(19):1800-1808.
11. Eidelman RS, Hebert PR, Weisman SM, Hennekens CH. An update on aspirin in the primary prevention of cardiovascular disease. *Arch Intern Med.* 2003; 163:2006-2010.
12. Ridker PM, Cook NR, Lee IM, et al. A randomized trial of low-dose aspirin in the primary prevention of cardiovascular disease in women. *N Engl J Med.* 2005; 352(13):1293-1304.
13. Pritchett AM, Forest JP, Mann DL. Treatment of the metabolic syndrome: the impact of lifestyle modification. *Curr Artheroscler Rep.* 2005;7:95-102.
14. Nwankwo T, Yoon SS, Burt V, Gu Q. Hypertension among adults in the United States: National Health and Nutrition Examination Survey, 2011–2012. *NCHS Data Brief.* 2013;1-8.
15. National High Blood Pressure Education Program. *The Seventh Report of the Joint National Committee on Prevention, Detection, Evaluation, and Treatment of High Blood Pressure.* Bethesda MD: National Heart, Lung, and Blood Institute; 2004.
16. Weber MA, Schiffrin EL, White WB, et al. Clinical practice guidelines for the management of hypertension in the community: a statement by the American Society of Hypertension and the International Society of Hypertension. *J Clin Hypertens.* 2014;16:14-26.
17. Go AS, Bauman MA, Coleman King SM, et al. An effective approach to high blood pressure control: a science advisory from the American Heart Association, the American College of Cardiology, and the Centers for Disease Control and Prevention. *Hypertension.* 2014; 63:878-885.
18. James PA, Oparil S, Carter BL, et al. 2014 evidence-based guideline for the management of high blood pressure in adults: report from the panel members appointed to the Eighth Joint National Committee (JNC 8). *JAMA.* 2014;311:507-520.
19. Gradman AH, Parisé H, Lefebvre P, Falvey H, Lafeuille MH, Duh MS. Initial combination therapy reduces the risk of cardiovascular events in hypertensive patients: a matched cohort study. *Hypertension.* 2013; 61:309-318.
20. Wulf NR, Matuszewski KA. Sulfonamide cross-reactivity: is there evidence to support broad cross-allergenicity? *Am J Health Syst Pharm.* 2013;70: 1483-1494.

21. Musini VM, Nazer M, Bassett K, Wright JM. Blood pressure-lowering efficacy of monotherapy with thiazide diuretics for primary hypertension. *Cochrane Database Syst Rev*. 2014;5:CD003824.
22. National Institutes of Health, U.S. National Library of Medicine, Toxnet Toxicology Data Network, Lactmed. Drugs and lactation database (Lactmed). http://toxnet.nlm.nih.gov/newtoxnet/lactmed.htm. Accessed April 7, 2015.
23. Bolland MJ, Ames RW, Horne AM, Orr-Wa BJ, Gamble GD, Reid IR. The effect of treatment with thiazide diuretics for 4 years on bone density in normal postmenopausal women. *Osteoporos Int*. 2007;4:479-486.
24. Peck RN, Smart LR, Beier R et al. Difference in blood pressure response to ace-inhibitor monotherapy between black and white adults with arterial hypertension: a meta-analysis of 13 clinical trials. *BMC Nephrol*. 2013;14:201.
25. Unger T, Kaschina E. Drug interactions with angiotensin receptor blockers: a comparison with other antihypertensives. *Drug Safety*. 2003;26(10):707-720.
26. Regulski M, Regulska K, Stanisz B et al. Chemistry and pharmacology of angiotension-converting enzyme inhibitors. *Curr Pharmaceut Des*. 2015; 21(13):1764-1775.
27. Onder G, Penninx BW, Balkrishan R, et al. Relation between use of angiotensin-converting enzyme inhibitors and muscle strength and physical function in older women: an observational study. *Lancet*. 2002; 359(9310):926-930.
28. Law MR, Wald NJ, Morris JK, Jordan RE. Value of low dose combination treatment with blood pressure lowering drugs: analysis of 354 randomised trials. *BMJ*. 2003;326:1427.
29. Müller DN, Derer W, Dechend R. Aliskiren: mode of action and preclinical data. *J Mol Med*. 2008;86: 659-662.
30. Baschiera F, Chang W, Brunel P; AGELESS Study Group. Effects of aliskiren- and ramipril-based treatment on central aortic blood pressure in elderly with systolic hypertension: a substudy of AGELESS. *Vasc Health Risk Manag*. 2014;10:389-397.
31. Wiysonge CS, Bradley HA, Volmink J, Mayosi BM, Mbewu A, Opie LH. Beta-blockers for hypertension. *Cochrane Database Syst Rev*. 2012;11:CD002003.
32. O'Gara PT, Kushner FG, Ascheim DD, et al., for the American College of Cardiology Foundation/American Heart Association Task Force on Practice Guidelines. 2013 ACCF/AHA guideline for the management of ST-elevation myocardial infarction: a report of the American College of Cardiology Foundation/American Heart Association Task Force on Practice Guidelines. *Circulation*. 2013;127:e362-e425.
33. Bakris GL, Fonseca V, Katholi RE, et al. Metabolic effects of carvedilol vs metoprolol in patients with type 2 diabetes mellitus and hypertension: a randomized controlled trial. *JAMA*. 2004;292:2227-2236.
34. Firoz T, Magee L, MacDonell K, et al., for the Community Level Interventions for Pre-eclampsia (CLIP) Working Group. Oral antihypertensive therapy for severe hypertension in pregnancy and postpartum: a systematic review. *BJOG*. 2014;121(10):1210-1208.
35. Al Khaja KA, Sequeira RP, Alkhaja AK, Damanhori AH. Drug treatment of hypertension in pregnancy: a critical review of adult guideline recommendations. *J Hypertens*. 2014;32:454-463.
36. Aronow WS, Fleg JL, Pepine CJ, et al. ACCF/AHA 2011 expert consensus document on hypertension in the elderly: a report of the American College of Cardiology Foundation Task Force on Clinical Expert Consensus Documents developed in collaboration with the American Academy of Neurology, American Geriatrics Society, American Society for Preventive Cardiology, American Society of Hypertension, American Society of Nephrology, Association of Black Cardiologists, and European Society of Hypertension. *J Am Coll Cardiol*. 2011;57:2037-2114.
37. Wright JT Jr, ALLHAT Collaborative Research Group. Outcomes in hypertensive black and nonblack patients treated with chlorthalidone, amlodipine, and lisinopril. *JAMA*. 2005;293:1595-1608.
38. Thakra R, Shulman R, Bellingam G, Singer M. Management of a mixed overdose of calcium channel blockers, β-blockers and statins. *BMJ Case Rep*. 2014; pii: bcr2014204732. doi:10.1136/bcr-2014-204732.
39. Caballero-Gonzalez FJ. Calcium channel blockers in the management of hypertension in the elderly. *Cardiovasc Hematol Agents Med Chem*. 2015;12(3):160-165.
40. American Geriatrics Society 2012 Beers Criteria Update Expert Panel. American Geriatrics Society updated Beers criteria for potentially inappropriate medication use in older adults. *J Am Geriatr Soc*. 2012;60:616-631.
41. Umans JG. Medications during pregnancy: antihypertensives and immunosuppressives. *Adv Chronic Kidney Dis*. 2007;14:191-198.
42. Podymow T, August P. Hypertension in pregnancy. *Adv Chronic Kidney Dis*. 2007;14:178-190.

43. Campbell P, Baker WL, Bendel SD, White WB. Intravenous hydralazine for blood pressure management in the hospitalized patient: its use is often unjustified. *Am Soc Hypertens*. 2011;5(6):473-477.
44. Wright CI, Van-Buren L, Kroner CI, Koning MM. Herbal medicines as diuretics: a review of the scientific evidence. *J Ethnopharmacol*. 2007;114:1-31.
45. Stone NJ, Robinson J, Lichtenstein AH, et al. 2013 ACC/AHA guideline on the treatment of blood cholesterol to reduce atherosclerotic cardiovascular risk in adults: a report of the American College of Cardiology/American Heart Association Task Force on Practice Guidelines. *J Am Coll Cardiol*. 2013;pii: S0735-S1097.
46. National Cholesterol Education Program (NCEP) Expert Panel on Detection, Evaluation, and Treatment of High Blood Cholesterol in Adults (Adult Treatment Panel III). Third Report of the National Cholesterol Education Program (NCEP) Expert Panel on Detection, Evaluation, and Treatment of High Blood Cholesterol in Adults (Adult Treatment Panel III) final report. *Circulation*. 2002;106:3143-3421.
47. American Heart Association. 2013 prevention guideline tools CV risk calculator. http://my.americanheart.org/professional/StatementsGuidelines/PreventionGuidelines/Prevention-Guidelines_UCM_457698_SubHomePage.jsp. Accessed April 7, 2015.
48. Pencina MJ, Navar-Boggan AM, D'Agostino RB Sr, et al. Application of new cholesterol guidelines to a population-based sample. *N Engl J Med*. 2014;370(15):1422-1431.
49. D'Agostino RB Sr, Ansell BJ, Mora S, Krumholz HM. Clinical decisions: the guidelines battle on starting statins. *N Engl J Med*. 2014;370(17):1652-1658.
50. Colhoun HM, Betteridge DJ, Durrington PN, et al. Primary prevention of cardiovascular disease with atorvastatin in type 2 diabetes in the Collaborative Atorvastatin Diabetes Study (CARDS): multicentre randomized placebo-controlled trial. *Lancet*. 2004;364(9435):685-696.
51. Bottorff MB. Statin safety and drug interactions: clinical implications. *Am J Cardiol*. 2006;97(suppl):27C-31C.
52. Kajinami K, Akao H, Polisecki E, Schaefer EJ. Pharmacogenomics of statin responsiveness. *Am J Cardiol*. 2005; 96(9A):65K-70K, discussion 34K-35K.
53. Food and Drug Administration. New restrictions, contraindications, and dose limitations for Zocor (simvastatin) to reduce the risk of muscle injury. http://www.fda.gov/drugs/drugsafety/ucm256581.htm. Accessed April 7, 2015.
54. Fernandez G, Spatz ES, Jablecki C, Phillips PS. Statin myopathy: a common dilemma not reflected in clinical trials. *Cleve Clin J Med*. 2011;78:393-403.
55. Food and Drug Administration. FDA announces safety changes in labeling for some cholesterol-lowering drugs. http://www.fda.gov/NewsEvents/Newsroom/PressAnnouncements/ucm293623.htm/ Accessed April 7, 2015.
56. Sattar N, Preiss D, Murray HM, et al. Statins and risk of incident diabetes: a collaborative meta-analysis of randomised statin trials. *Lancet*. 2010;375(9716):735-742.
57. Expert Panel on Integrated Guidelines for Cardiovascular Health and Risk Reduction in Children and Adolescents; National Heart, Lung, and Blood Institute. Expert Panel on Integrated Guidelines for Cardiovascular Health and Risk Reduction in Children and Adolescents: summary report. *Pediatrics*. 2011;128:S213-S256.
58. Mahvan TD, Hilaire ML, Vigil A, Mlodinow S. Cholesterol management in geriatric patients: new guidelines. *Consult Pharm*. 2015;30(2):68-76.
59. Grundy SM, Vega GL, Yuan Z, Battisti WP, Brady WE, Palmisano J. Effectiveness and tolerability of simvastatin plus fenofibrate for combined hyperlipidemia: the SAFARI Trial. *Am J Cardiol*. 2005;95:462-468.
60. Bottorff MB. Statin safety and drug interactions: clinical implications. *Am J Cardiol*. 2006;97(suppl):27C-31C.
61. Keech A, Simes RJ, Barter P, et al. Effect of long-term fenofibrate therapy on cardiovascular events in 9795 people with type 2 diabetes mellitus (the FIELD study): randomised controlled trial. *Lancet*. 2005;366(9500):1849-1861.
62. Jacobson TA, Armani A, McKenney JM, Guyton JR. Safety considerations with gastrointestinally active lipid-lowering drugs. *Am J Cardiol*. 2007;99:47C-55C.
63. Insull W, Toth P, Mullican W, et al. Effectiveness of colesevelam hydrochloride in decreasing LDL cholesterol in patients with primary hypercholesterolemia: a 24-week randomized controlled trial. *Mayo Clin Proc*. 2001;76:971-982.
64. AIM-HIGH Investigators, Boden WE, Probstfield JL, et al. Niacin in patients with low HDL cholesterol levels receiving intensive statin therapy. *N Engl J Med*. 2011;365(24):2255-2267.

65. Taylor AJ. Arterial biology for the investigation of the treatment effects of reducing cholesterol (ARBITER) 2: a double-blind, placebo-controlled study of extended-release niacin on atherosclerosis progression in secondary prevention patients treated with statins. *Circulation.* 2004;110:3512-3517.
66. Kastelein JJ, Akdim F, Stroes ES, et al. for ENHANCE Investigators. Simvastatin with or without ezetimibe in familial hypercholesterolemia. *N Engl J Med.* 2008; 358(14):1431-1443.
67. Villines TC, Stanek EJ, Devine PJ, et al. The ARBITER 6-HALTS Trial (Arterial Biology for the Investigation of the Treatment Effects of Reducing Cholesterol 6-HDL and LDL Treatment Strategies in Atherosclerosis): final results and the impact of medication adherence, dose, and treatment duration. *J Am Coll Cardiol.* 2010;55:2721-2726.
68. Bushnell C, McCullough LD, Awad IA, et al., for the American Heart Association Stroke Council, Council on Cardiovascular and Stroke Nursing, Council on Clinical Cardiology, Council on Epidemiology and Prevention, and Council for High Blood Pressure Research. Guidelines for the prevention of stroke in women: a statement for healthcare professionals from the American Heart Association/American Stroke Association. *Stroke.* 2014;45:1545-1588.
69. Kernan WN, Ovbiagele B, Black HR, et al., on behalf of the American Heart Association Stroke Council, Council on Cardiovascular and Stroke Nursing, Council on Clinical Cardiology, and Council on Peripheral Vascular Disease. Guidelines for the prevention of stroke in patients with stroke and transient ischemic attack: a guideline for healthcare professionals from the American Heart Association/American Stroke Association. *Stroke.* 2014;45(7):2160-2236.
70. Diener HC, Bogousslavsky J, Brass LM, et al., for the MATCH Investigators. Aspirin and clopidogrel compared with clopidogrel alone after ischemic stroke or transient ischaemic attack in high-risk patients (MATCH): randomized, double-blind, placebo-controlled trial. *Lancet.* 2004;364(9431):331-337.
71. Wang Y, Wang Y, Zhao X, et al., for the CHANCE Investigators. Clopidogrel with aspirin in acute minor stroke or transient ischemic attack. *N Engl J Med.* 2013;369(1):11-19.
72. Lansberg MG, O'Donnell MJ, Khatri P, et al., for the American College of Chest Physicians. Antithrombotic and thrombolytic therapy for ischemic stroke: *Antithrombotic Therapy and Prevention of Thrombosis*, 9th ed: American College of Chest Physicians evidence-based clinical practice guidelines. *Chest.* 2012;141(2 suppl):e601S-e636S.
73. Anderson JL, Halperin JL, Albert NM, et al. A report of the American College of Cardiology Foundation/American Heart Association Task Force on Practice Guidelines. *Circulation.* 2013;127:1425-1443.
74. Yancy CW, Jessup M, Bozkurt B, et al. American College of Cardiology Foundation; American Heart Association Task Force on Practice Guidelines. 2013 ACCF/AHA guideline for the management of heart failure: a report of the American College of Cardiology Foundation/American Heart Association Task Force on Practice Guidelines. *J Am Coll Cardiol.* 2013;62: e147-e239.
75. Masoudi FA, Havranek EP, Smith G, et al. Gender, age, and heart failure with preserved left ventricular systolic function. *J Am Coll Cardiol.* 2003;41: 217-223.
76. Heart Failure Society of America; Lindenfeld J, Albert NM, Boehmer JP, et al. HFSA 2010 comprehensive heart failure practice guideline. *J Card Fail.* 2010; 16:e1-e194.
77. Cleland JG, Tendera M, Adamus J, Freemantle N, Polonski L, Taylor J, for the PEP-CHF Investigators. The perindopril in elderly people with chronic heart failure (PEP-CHF) study. *Eur Heart J.* 2006;27:2338-2345.
78. Massie BM, Carson PE, McMurray JJ, et al., for the I-PRESERVE Investigators. Irbesartan in patients with heart failure and preserved ejection fraction. *N Engl J Med.* 2008;359(23):2456-2467.
79. Yusuf S, Pfeffer MA, Swedberg K, et al., for the CHARM Investigators and Committees. Effects of candesartan in patients with chronic heart failure and preserved left-ventricular ejection fraction: the CHARM-Preserved Trial. *Lancet.* 2003;362(9386):777-781.
80. Pitt B, Pfeffer MA, Assmann SF, et al., for the TOPCAT Investigators. Spironolactone for heart failure with preserved ejection fraction. *N Engl J Med.* 2014; 370(15):1383-1392.
81. Meurin P. The ASCOT trial: clarifying the role of ACE inhibition in the reduction of cardiovascular events in patients with hypertension. *Am J Cardiovasc Drugs.* 2006;6:327-334.
82. Keyhan G, Chen SF, Pilote L. Angiotensin-converting enzyme inhibitors and survival in women and men with heart failure. *Eur J Heart Fail.* 2007;9:594-601.

83. Rochon PA, Sykora K, Bronskill SE, et al. Use of angiotensin-converting enzyme inhibitor therapy and dose-related outcomes in older adults with new heart failure in the community. *J Gen Intern Med.* 2004;19:676-683.
84. Pitt B, Zannad F, Remme WJ, et al. The effect of spironolactone on morbidity and mortality in patients with severe heart failure: Randomized Aldactone Evaluation Study. *N Engl J Med.* 1999;341(10):709-717.
85. Zannad F, McMurray JJ, Krum H, et al. for the EMPHASIS-Heart Failure Study Group. Eplerenone in patients with systolic heart failure and mild symptoms. *N Engl J Med.* 2011;364(1):11-21.
86. Taylor AL, Ziesche S, Yancy C, et al. Combination of isosorbide dinitrate and hydralazine in blacks with heart failure. *N Engl J Med.* 2004;351(20):2049-2057.
87. Digitalis Investigation Group. The effects of digoxin on mortality and morbidity in patients with heart failure. *N Engl J Med.* 1997;336(8):525-533.
88. Rathore SS, Wang Y, Krumholz H. Sex based differences in the effect of digoxin for the treatment of heart failure. *N Engl J Med.* 2002;347(18):1403-1411.
89. Flory JH, Ky B, Haynes K, et al. Observational cohort study of the safety of digoxin use in women with heart failure. *BMJ Open.* 2012;2:e000888.
90. January CT, Wann LS, Alpert JS, et al. 2014 AHA/ACC/HRS guideline for the management of patients with atrial fibrillation: a report of the American College of Cardiology/American Heart Association Task Force on Practice Guidelines and the Heart Rhythm Society. *J Am Coll Cardiol.* 2014;pii:S0735-S1097.
91. Lip GY, Nieuwlaat R, Pisters R, Lane DA, Crijns HJ. Refining clinical risk stratification for predicting stroke and thromboembolism in atrial fibrillation using a novel risk factor-based approach: the euro heart survey on atrial fibrillation. *Chest.* 2010;137:263-272.
92. Trinkley KE, Page RL 2nd, Lien H, Yamanouye K, Tisdale JE. QT interval prolongation and the risk of torsades de pointes: essentials for clinicians. *Curr Med Res Opin.* 2013;29:1719-1726.

16 Hematology

Samantha A. Karr, Kristi Watson Kelley

Based on the chapter by Patrick J. M. Murphy, Brian Meadors, and Tekoa L. King in the first edition of Pharmacology for Women's Health

Chapter Glossary

Antiplatelet drugs Drugs that decrease platelet aggregation.

Anticoagulant drugs Drugs that interfere in any of the coagulation cascade steps.

Contact activation pathway See *intrinsic pathway.*

Direct factor X_a inhibitors Drugs that prevent factor X_a from cleaving prothrombin into thrombin.

Direct thrombin inhibitors Drugs that prevent thrombin from activating platelets to release enzymes that accentuate the coagulation process.

Extrinsic pathway (tissue factor pathway) Series of reactions within the coagulation process that begin when coagulation factor VII comes in contact with tissue factor expressed on the surface of cells. When factor VII binds to tissue factor, the resulting complex initiates a series of reactions that lead to the formation of thrombin. This pathway, more commonly referred to as the *tissue factor pathway,* initiates the coagulation process.

Hypochromic anemia Anemia characterized by red blood cells in which the central area is enlarged and pale. It occurs secondary to a deficiency of hemoglobin, which contains the pigment that imparts the red color to the cell.

Intrinsic factor Glycoprotein produced by the parietal cells of the stomach. Vitamin B_{12} binds to intrinsic factor in the ileum, and the vitamin B_{12}/intrinsic factor complex is then able to enter the portal circulation.

Intrinsic pathway Series of transformations that coagulation factors undergo that are initiated by factors present in blood. The intrinsic cascade begins when coagulation factors present in blood come in contact with collagen in subendothelial connective tissue that becomes exposed after endothelial cells are injured. Also referred to as the *contact activation pathway.*

Macrocytic anemia Anemia characterized by red blood cells that are larger than usual.

Megaloblastic anemia Macrocytic anemia characterized by deficient DNA synthesis. This anemia frequently occurs secondary to a deficiency of vitamin B_{12} or folic acid.

Microcytic anemia Anemia characterized by red blood cells that are smaller than usual.

Pernicious anemia Anemia that occurs secondary to vitamin B_{12} deficiency.

Racemic mixture Mixture that contains equal amounts of left- and right-handed enantiomers of a molecule. These molecules have the same chemical composition, but the structures of the left-handed and right-handed versions are different.

Thrombolytic drugs Drugs that dissolve blood clots via thrombolysis.

Thrombosis Disorder that occurs when a thrombus blocks the blood vessel and causes ischemia in tissues nourished by that vessel.

Vitamin K antagonists Drugs that block the absorption or function of vitamin K, thereby decreasing the concentration of several coagulation factors. Warfarin (Coumadin) is a vitamin K antagonist.

Introduction

Common non-neoplastic hematologic disorders include anemias and coagulopathies that can cause a thrombus or embolus. Drugs used to treat anemias and coagulopathies act by activating, inhibiting, or supplementing biomolecules normally present in the vasculature. This chapter reviews the physiologic and pathophysiologic states associated with decreased red blood cell concentrations and then addresses treatments for the most common forms of anemia. An overview of coagulopathies and drugs—parenteral and oral anticoagulants, direct thrombin inhibitors, **antiplatelet drugs**, and **thrombolytic drugs**—used to treat coagulation disorders is presented. Because many of the drugs that are used for persons with hematologic disorders affect red blood cell production, a brief review of the physiology is in order.

Erythropoiesis and Iron Metabolism

Erythropoiesis, the process encompassing the development and maturation of erythrocytes (also called red blood cells [RBCs]), begins in red bone marrow. It starts with differentiation of a pluripotent stem cell and concludes in the blood with the formation of the mature erythrocyte. Erythropoietin and cytokines stimulate differentiation of a pluripotent stem cell into a proerythroblast, which upon subsequent cell divisions incorporates hemoglobin (Hgb) to form an erythroblast. This erythroblast collects increasing amounts of hemoglobin while undergoing additional rounds of cell division and gradually extrudes its nucleus, resulting in the development of a reticulocyte. The reticulocyte enters the systemic circulation. Over the course of the first 7 days in the circulation, this reticulocyte loses its remaining nuclear components, thereby forming a mature erythrocyte. Approximately 40% to 50% of total blood volume is made of erythrocytes, which circulate for approximately 120 days before being catabolized in the spleen and reticuloendothelial system.

Role of Erythropoietin, Hemoglobin, and Iron in Erythropoiesis

Erythropoietin and hemoglobin are essential for erythrocyte maturation. Erythropoietin is a glycoprotein produced by the kidneys in response to decreased oxygen levels in the blood. Once released, erythropoietin stimulates production of erythrocytes via interactions with growth factors involved in the transformation of erythrocyte precursor cells. Erythropoietin also protects erythrocytes from apoptosis. Under normal physiologic conditions, this glycoprotein maintains a constant rate of new erythrocyte production that balances natural erythrocyte loss. When erythropoietin production or release is impaired, such as occurs in chronic kidney disease, erythrocyte production decreases.

Hemoglobin is composed of an iron–porphyrin ring and four globin chains (two alpha-globin chains and two beta-globin chains). Hemoglobin reversibly binds to oxygen; the body capitalizes on this mechanism to transport oxygen from the lungs and release it to tissues. Hemoglobin accounts for more than 90% of the protein content in the mature RBC and provides the characteristic red (normochromic) appearance of these cells. Approximately 75% (2.5 g) of the iron in the body is present in hemoglobin. Following destruction of erythrocytes by the reticuloendothelial system, iron and other cellular components are recycled for the production of future erythrocytes.

Role of Folate and Vitamin B_{12} in Erythropoiesis

Folate (also known as folic acid, B_9) and vitamin B_{12} (also known as cobalamin) are dietary nutrients and are discussed in more detail in the *Vitamins and Minerals* chapter. Both folate and vitamin B_{12} required for DNA synthesis. Blood cell lineage development, and erythropoiesis in particular, are acutely sensitive to folate and vitamin B_{12} concentrations in the body because a relatively high fraction of erythrocytes is undergoing cellular division at any one time. Within the cell, vitamin B_{12} demethylates the inactive dietary form of folate (5-methyl tetrahydrofolate) into folinic acid (5-formyl tetrahydrofolate), which is the active metabolite. Folinic acid is an enzyme that facilitates DNA synthesis.

Absorption of vitamin B_{12} occurs in the ileum. Absorption of vitamin B_{12} is dependent on **intrinsic factor**, a glycoprotein secreted from parietal cells in the gastric mucosa that complexes with vitamin B_{12} to facilitate absorption. When super-physiologic levels of inactive folate are present within cells, an alternative pathway can facilitate the conversion of inactive folate to its active metabolite folinic acid, even in the absence of vitamin B_{12}.

The Role of Iron

The total body store of iron in a premenopausal woman is approximately 250 to 300 mg.[1] While the recommended daily iron intake is 10 mg to 30 mg, only 5% to 10% of the ingested iron is usually absorbed, although the percentage of ingested iron that is absorbed can increase to approximately 30% in states of iron deficiency. The body loses approximately 1 to 2 mg of iron every day through the skin, minor blood loss, and enteric desquamation; in turn, approximately 1 to 2 mg of iron is absorbed daily.[1] Thus, internal iron recycling accounts for the majority of iron hemostasis within the body. This mineral is also discussed in the *Vitamins and Minerals* chapter.

Intestinal absorption is affected by the charged state of the iron atom. Heme or ferrous (Fe^{2+}) iron is more readily absorbed than non-heme oxidized or ferric (Fe^{3+}) iron. The latter form is not soluble in its charged state, but rather must be reduced to Fe^{2+} before it can be transported into the duodenal enterocyte. Non-heme iron is absorbed better in an acidic environment because the acidic environment promotes the change from ferrous to ferric iron. Orally administered iron is absorbed into mucosal cells within the duodenum and proximal jejunum. Once absorbed into the duodenal enterocytes, an export protein, ferroportin, moves the iron out of the enterocyte and into the circulation; there, the iron becomes bound to a transport protein, transferrin, and is carried to the red bone marrow.[1,2] The iron is then incorporated into hemoglobin in the bone marrow, and subsequently into the developing erythroblast. Most iron in the body is present in the hemoglobin. The remainder is found in the muscle protein myoglobin, an iron-containing enzyme; iron storage proteins such as ferritin; and iron transporter proteins such as transferrin.

Following catabolism of an erythrocyte by the spleen, iron is recycled. During this process, it is again bound to transferrin and returned to the bone marrow for a successive round of erythropoiesis.

Ferritin is a globular protein that serves as the intracellular iron storage repository. Free iron is toxic to cells because it can catalyze the formation of free radicals; therefore, iron is bound to proteins in various ways so that it can be released for use as needed. Because blood levels of ferritin reflect the total body store of iron, the ferritin level will reflect the degree of severity of iron-deficiency anemia.

Drugs That Cause Hematologic Disorders

Drug-induced hematologic disorders are generally a rare adverse side effect of drug therapy. Nevertheless, several drugs have a clinically significant association with a hematologic disorder. Many drugs are reported to cause hemolytic anemia or agranulocytosis—the list is too long to review in detail in this chapter. The interested reader is referred to reviews on the subject.[3–7] Table 16-1 presents examples of drugs that are commonly used in primary care and are associated with specific hematologic disorders.

Table 16-1 Examples of Drugs That Induce Hematologic Disorders

Disorder and Description	Exemplars of Drugs That Induce Disorder: Generic (Brand)
Aplastic anemia: Pancytopenia secondary to bone marrow suppression.	Anticonvulsants Antithyroid drugs Antituberculosis drugs Carbamazepine (Tegretol) Chloramphenicol (Chloromycetin) Felbamate (Felbatol) Nonsteroidal anti-inflammatory drugs (NSAIDs) Phenytoin (Dilantin) Sulfonamides Ticlopidine (Ticlid) Trimethoprim–sulfamethoxazole (Bactrim) Valproic acid (Depakote)
Agranulocytosis/neutropenia[a]: Decrease in peripheral neutrophil count.	Analgesics Anticonvulsants Cefotaxime (Claforan) Cefuroxime Chlorpromazine (Thorazine) Cimetidine (Tagamet) Clozapine (Clozaril) Diclofenac (Voltaren) Fluoxetine (Prozac) Ibuprofen (Advil) Iron-chelating agents Methyldopa (Aldomet) Metoclopramide (Reglan) Penicillins, including ampicillin, nafcillin, penicillin, oxacillin (Bactocil) Phenytoin (Dilantin) Procainamide (Pronestyl) Propylthiouracil (Propyl-Thyracil)
G6PD deficiency: Glucose-6-phosphate dehydrogenase is an enzyme that protects red blood cells (RBCs) from oxidative destruction. The genetic mutation that causes G6PD deficiency results in RBCs that are at increased risk for drug-induced destruction.	Acetaminophen (Tylenol) Antimalarial drugs Aspirin Dapsone Nitrofurantoin (Macrobid) NSAIDs Primaquine
Hemolytic anemia[b]: Destruction of RBCs by autoantibodies directed toward an antigen on the RBC. The autoantibody can be formed when the drug becomes part of the antigen (haptene reaction) or the drug alters the antigen to make it more antigenic.	Acetaminophen (Tylenol) Cephalosporins Cimetadine (Tagamet) Ciprofloxacin (Cipro) Dapsone (Dapsone) Diclofenac (Cambia) Insulin Levodopa (Sinemet) Lorazepam (Ativan) Methyldopa (Aldomet) Nonsteroidal antiinflammatory drugs (NSAIDs) Penicillins (Large doses) Phenazopyridine (Pyridium) Piperacillin (Zosyn) Rifampin (Rifadin) Tetracyclines Tolbutamide (Orinase) Trimethoprim/sulfamethoxazole (Bactrim)

(*continues*)

Table 16-1 Examples of Drugs That Induce Hematologic Disorders (*continued*)

Disorder and Description	Exemplars of Drugs That Induce Disorder: Generic (Brand)
Thrombocytopenia: Low platelet count caused by drug-induced formation of antibodies that destroy platelets. Antibodies are directed toward an antigen on the platelet. The antibody can be formed when the drug becomes part of the antigen (haptene reaction) or the drug alters the platelet antigenic material on the platelet to make it more antigenic. Can also be secondary to decreased platelet production following use of drugs the suppress bone marrow.	Acetaminophen (Tylenol) Aspirin Beta-lactam antibiotics Carbamazepine (Tegretol) Cimetidine (Tagamet) Heparin Measles/mumps/rubella (MMR) vaccine Naproxen (Naprosyn) Phenytoin (Dilantin) Platelet inhibitors Ranitidine (Zantac) Rifampin (Rifadin) Sulfonamides Tirofiban (Aggrastat) Trimethoprim/sulfamethoxazole (Bactrim) Valproic acid (Depakene) Vancomycin (Vanocin)
Thrombotic microangiopathy: Microangiopathic hemolytic anemia, thrombocytopenia, and organ injury.	Immunosuppressive agents such as cyclosporine Quinine

[a] The systematic review by Andersohn et al. found 36 drugs with level 1 evidence for causality, 89 drugs with level 2 evidence for causality, and 55 drugs with level 3 evidence for causality.

[b] More than 100 drugs are known to cause hemolytic anemia. This list gives examples of those commonly used in primary care.

Sources: Data from Andersohn F, Konze C, Garbe E. Systematic review: agranulocytosis induced by nonchemotherapy drugs. *Ann Intern Med.* 2007;146(9):657-665[5]; Arndt PA, Garratty G. The changing spectrum of drug-induced immune hemolytic anemia. *Semin Hematol.* 2005;42:137[4]; Aster RH. Adverse drug reactions affecting blood cells. *Handb Exp Pharmacol.* 2010;196:57-76[6]; Garratty G. Immune hemolytic anemia associated with drug therapy. *Blood Rev.* 2010;24:143[3]; Youngster I, Arcavi L, Schechmaster R, et al. Medication and glucose-6-phosphate-dehydrogenase: an evidence-based review. *Drug Saf.* 2010;107(3):737-741.[7]

Anemias

Anemias are a collection of conditions characterized by (1) a loss of hemoglobin (e.g., hemorrhage or increased hemolysis of red blood cells); (2) a decrease in production of hemoglobin (e.g., aplastic anemia); and/or (3) production of variant forms of hemoglobin (e.g., thalassemia, sickle cell anemia). Anemias occur secondary to one of several factors, including deficiency of a nutrient essential for the development and maturation of erythrocytes, such as occurs in folate or vitamin B_{12} deficiency, and impaired bone marrow production of erythrocytes, which can occur during chronic infection. Acute or chronic blood loss can also be a source of anemia. Anemia can also arise secondary to genetic alterations in the type of hemoglobin made, which is the underlying pathophysiology that occurs in sickle cell anemia and the thalassemias.

The most common anemias are nutritional deficiency–associated anemias, which appear after a period of inadequate consumption or inadequate absorption of iron, vitamin B_{12}, and/or folic acid. Treatment in primary care is directed at replacing the individual's absent nutrient with vitamin supplementation. Successful therapeutic intervention requires identification of the type of anemia as well as the underlying cause of the disease. The treatment goals for the individual who is anemic are to ameliorate the symptoms, rectify the underlying cause, and prevent recurrence.

Anemia in Women

Women are more likely than men to become anemic secondary to their increased needs for iron and obligate blood loss during menses and childbirth.[8] An estimated 10% to 20% of menstruating women and 16% to 29% of pregnant women are classified as anemic based on the presence of low hemoglobin concentrations (< 11 g/dL during the first and third trimesters, < 10.5 g/dL during the second trimester).[8] Anemia occurs less frequently among women who are taking estrogen–progestin oral contraceptives and more often in women who are using copper-containing intrauterine devices. Even healthy women develop a characteristic physiologic anemia during pregnancy secondary to an increase in plasma volume that is proportionately more than the increase in RBCs. Low birth weight, preterm birth, and newborn mortality are all associated with maternal anemia during pregnancy.[9]

Anemia-Induced Morphologic Changes in Red Blood Cells

Several types of anemia are distinguished, although all are characterized by adverse effects on RBCs at some point in the life cycle of the erythrocyte. For example, aplastic anemia occurs when the bone marrow does not make enough erythrocytes.

Aberrant erythrocyte maturation manifests as changes in erythrocyte size and color, along with measures of hematocrit and/or hemoglobin content. Assessment of these changes can assist the healthcare provider in making a specific diagnosis. Anemias caused by deficiencies of either folic acid or vitamin B_{12} may be identified as **macrocytic anemia** and **megaloblastic anemia**, whereas anemias caused by iron deficiencies result in decreased production of hemoglobin and subsequent smaller red cells and are classically identified as **microcytic anemia** and **hypochromic anemia**.[8] A typical mature RBC is the same diameter as the nucleus of a white blood cell. When the measured RBC diameter is greater than the nucleus of surrounding white blood cells, the RBCs are termed macrocytic. Conversely, when the RBC diameter is less than the nucleus of white blood cells, they are microcytic.

Megaloblasts are oversized erythroblasts present in the bone marrow, whereas macrocytes are oversized erythrocytes present in the circulation. Both megaloblasts and macrocytes are found in substantially increased concentrations when insufficient stores of either folic acid or vitamin B_{12} are available to the bone marrow. Microcytes are abnormally small circulating erythrocytes, and their pale (hypochromic) coloration may result from severely decreased hemoglobin content. Anemias that are either mild or in their initial stages may not display the classical morphologic changes in red blood cell size and color.

Microcytic Anemia: Iron Deficiency

Common etiologies of iron-deficiency anemias involve states where the body requires increased RBC synthesis, such as blood volume expansion during pregnancy, occult blood loss from a gastrointestinal ulcer or tumor, or overt blood loss from excessive menstruation. Less common etiologies of iron-deficiency anemia include decreased iron availability secondary to dietary insufficiency or impaired intestinal absorption.

Classic signs of iron-deficiency anemia include the presence of microcytic and hypochromic RBCs that have a mean corpuscular volume (MCV) that is less than 80 fL; however, these cells may not be observed in all instances. Plasma ferritin concentrations can be particularly useful for identifying a reduction of iron stores. Aggregated ferritin stores in bone marrow are depleted or absent when iron-deficiency anemia becomes clinically evident. The treatment of an individual with iron-deficiency anemia is iron replacement.

Oral Iron Formulations

Iron is available in both oral and parenteral preparations. The three orally administered iron salts are ferrous sulfate, ferrous gluconate, and ferrous fumarate. Ferrous sulfate is available as an elixir that contains 44 mg of elemental iron per 5 mL. Additional information about the oral formulations of iron can be found in the *Vitamins and Minerals* chapter. Parenteral iron preparations—iron dextran, ferric gluconate, and iron sucrose—are available for use by individuals who are unable to absorb sufficient quantities of orally administered iron or who cannot tolerate the gastrointestinal-associated side effects of oral iron therapy.

The recommended dose of oral iron for treating iron-deficiency anemia in adults is approximately 150 to 200 mg of elemental iron daily, given in 2 to 3 divided doses. This is roughly equivalent to a 325-mg tablet of ferrous sulfate taken 3 times per day. However, due to the relatively limited intestinal absorption of orally administered iron, divided dosing is required. The amount of elemental iron present in oral iron preparations varies from approximately 10% to 33% and must be taken into account when calculating the dose. It can take as long as 6 to 8 weeks before iron therapy corrects anemia and as long as 6 months before iron stores are fully replenished.

Food decreases intestinal iron absorption by approximately 50%, and iron is best absorbed in an acidic environment. Therefore, iron tablets should be taken between meals; taking ascorbic acid (vitamin C) with iron may enhance the mineral's absorption. Because iron is absorbed in the proximal portion of the small intestine, enteric-coated formulations do not readily supply the iron needed and should be avoided. Failure to respond to oral iron therapy may be due to malabsorption or continued blood loss, both of which are indicative of the need for further clinical evaluation. Coadministration of drugs such as tetracycline (Theo-Dur), proton pump inhibitors, calcium, and antacids decrease absorption.[1] If antacids are required for other conditions, their administration should be separated by at least 2 to 3 hours from oral iron supplement administration. Additional information and drug–drug interactions associated with oral iron products can be found in the *Vitamins and Minerals* chapter.

Side Effects/Adverse Effects

Gastrointestinal disorders including nausea, epigastric distress, and constipation are quite common following oral administration of iron salts. The reported side effects of oral iron therapy correlate to the concentration of elemental iron ingested. Because all three iron salts can produce these effects, equipotent doses of oral iron therapy should have the same degree of side effects. For persons who have difficulty with these symptoms, using the ferrous sulfate elixir in a dose as tolerated can be an effective solution.

Parenteral Preparations of Iron

Parenteral iron preparations are generally prescribed for individuals who are unable to absorb sufficient quantities of orally administered iron or who cannot tolerate the gastrointestinal side effects of oral iron therapy. For example, persons with celiac disease have limited oral iron absorption and may not receive therapeutic levels with oral therapy. Persons being treated for peptic ulcers, inflammatory bowel disease, enteritis, or ulcerative colitis may also benefit from parenteral iron therapy, as this route of administration will not exacerbate their preexisting condition or cause additional gastrointestinal side effects. Additionally, parenteral therapy is commonly used for individuals undergoing cancer chemotherapy or hemodialysis.

The parenteral preparations of iron include iron dextran (DexFerrum), which comes in high-molecular-weight (DexFerrum) and low-molecular-weight (INFeD) formulations; ferric carboxymaltose (Injectafer)[9,10]; sodium ferric gluconate complex (Ferrlecit); iron sucrose (Venofer); and ferumoxytol (Feraheme) (Table 16-2).

Side Effects and Adverse Effects

Pain and localized discoloration at the injection site are the most commonly reported side effects for both iron dextran and ferric carboxymaltose. Headache, fever, arthralgia, pruritus, and rash can also occur.

The primary disadvantage of all parenteral iron preparations is infusion reactions,[8] which—though rare—are most likely to occur following administration of high-molecular-weight iron dextran.[9] The low-molecular-weight dextran formulations have demonstrated a threefold lower incidence of serious toxicity compared to the high-molecular-weight formulations (11.3 versus 3.3 life-threatening adverse drug events per million doses, respectively).[11] For ferric gluconate, ferric sucrose, and dextran, the incidence of adverse effects is 0.9, 0.6, and 3.3 per million doses, respectively. Although these are very low rates, a test dose

Table 16-2 Parenteral Iron Formulations for Iron-Deficiency Anemia

Drug: Generic (Brand)	Elemental Iron Concentration (mg/mL)	Dose	Clinical Considerations
Ferric carboxymaltose (Ferinject)	50 in 750 mg/ 15 mL vial	IV: 750–1000 mg over 15–30 minutes Maximum dose per session: 500 mg elemental iron over 4 hours Total maximum dose: 1000 mg elemental iron	Low risk of hypersensitivity reaction. Nausea, headaches, dizziness, and hypertension are mild but common side effects. Better tolerated than oral ferrous sulfate.
Ferric gluconate complex (Ferrlecit)	12.5	125 mg elemental iron infused over 1 hour Maximum dose per session: 250 mg elemental iron Total maximum dose: 1000 mg elemental iron	Administered in conjunction with erythropoietin to maximize RBC production in persons undergoing hemodialysis. Contraindications: Hypersensitivity to ferric gluconate; any anemia not associated with iron deficiency; iron overload. Adverse effects: Flushing/hypotension; may augment hemodialysis-induced hypotension.
Ferumoxytol (Feraheme)	30	IV Maximum dose per session: 510 mg elemental iron Total maximum dose: 1020 mg elemental iron	Can cause severe hypotension in approximately 2% of recipients. Also used as an MRI contrast agent. Persons receiving ferumoxytol will need to notify the radiologist if MRI is needed within 3 months of the iron injection.
Iron dextran, high molecular weight (DexFerrum)	50	IM (Z-track technique) or slow IV bolus Test dose: 25 mg over 5 minutes Maximum dose: 100 mg elemental iron	Contraindications: Hypersensitivity to iron dextran; any anemia not associated with iron deficiency. IV route is preferred because of the decreased risk of anaphylaxis. When given intramuscularly, iron dextran must be given via the Z-track method to prevent leakage of the medication into surrounding tissues at the injection site.
Iron dextran, low molecular weight (INFeD)	50	IV: Test dose required—25 mg over 30 seconds; wait 1 hour, then 925 mg over 4–6 hours (100 mg/2 minutes) Maximum dose: 1000 mg elemental iron	Fewer serious adverse drug events than high-molecular-weight formulation. Allows for highest dose of iron to be administered at one time compared to other parenteral agents.
Iron sucrose (Venofer)	20	IV: 100–400 mg infused over 15–60 minutes Maximum dose per session: 200–250 mg elemental iron Total maximum dose: 1000 mg elemental iron	Administered in conjunction with erythropoietin to maximize RBC production in persons undergoing hemodialysis. Contraindications: Hypersensitivity to iron sucrose; any anemia not associated with iron deficiency.

Abbreviations: LBW = lean body weight in kg; MRI, magnetic resonance imaging.

Sources: Data from Camaschella C. Iron-deficiency anemia. *N Engl J Med.* 2015; 372:1832-1843[9]; DeLoughery TG. Microcytic anemia. *N Engl J Med.* 2014; 371:1324[8]; Keating GM. Ferric carboxymaltose: a review of its use in iron deficiency. *Drugs.* 2015;75(1):101-127.[10]

Table 16-3 Folic Acid and Vitamin B_{12} Formulations

Drug: Generic (Brand)	Formulations	Indication/Dose	Clinical Considerations
Cyanocobalamin (Cobolin-M, Nascobal, CaloMist)	Tablet/lozenge: Multiple formulations Injection: 1000 mcg/mL Nasal spray: 500 mcg/actuation (Nascobal) 25 mcg/actuation (CaloMist)	For vitamin B_{12} deficiency: PO: 250 mcg/day Intranasal: 500 mcg in one nostril once weekly Maintenance: 25 mcg in each nostril daily to twice daily (following correction of deficiency) IM/SQ: 100 mcg/day for 6–7 days Maintenance: 100 mcg/month Pernicious anemia: PO: 1000–2000 mcg/day IM/deep SQ: 1 mg/day for 1 week, then 1 mg/week for 4 weeks, then 1 mg/month Intranasal: 500 mcg in one nostril weekly	Contraindications: Hypersensitivity to cyanocobalamin or any component of formulation. Avoid IV administration: anaphylaxis can occur. Test dose is recommended for persons suspected of cyanocobalamin sensitivity prior to administration. IM/SQ/PO routes are used for treatment; oral and intranasal administration routes are used after hematologic remission and no signs of nervous system involvement. Administer nasal sprays at least 1 hour before or after ingestion of hot foods or liquids.
Folic acid (Folacin-800, FA-8)	Capsule: 0.8 mg, 5 mg Tablet: 0.4, 0.8, 1 mg Injection: 5 mg/mL (10 mL)	Usual: 0.4 mg/day for prophylaxis during pregnancy[a] 1 mg/day for 1–4 months for deficiency and replacement	Contraindications: Hypersensitivity to folic acid. Not appropriate for anemias other than megaloblastic/macrocytic anemia, vitamin B_{12} deficiency, and uncorrected pernicious anemia.
Leucovorin calcium	Tablet: 5, 10, 15, 25 mg Injection: 50, 100, 200, 350, 500 mg	For folate-deficient megaloblastic anemia IV/IM: Up to 1 mg/day	Contraindications: Hypersensitivity to folic acid. Only for use if not responsive to folate or when oral therapy is not an option; much more expensive than folate.

[a] Recommended dose for women with a history of neural tube defects is 4 mg per day for 4 or more weeks prior to conception and during the first 12 weeks of pregnancy.

is still recommended. Epinephrine and respiratory support should be readily available during test dose administration.

Erythropoiesis-Stimulating Agents

In individuals undergoing hemodialysis, sufficient quantities of intravenously administered iron are required to maximize RBC synthesis. Similarly, persons undergoing chemotherapy may need an agent that stimulates erythropoiesis in the bone marrow to prevent severe anemia. For these situations, an erythropoiesis-stimulating agent, erythropoietin (Procrit, Epogen), is available. Although erythropoietin improves hemoglobin levels, it is also associated with an increased risk of thrombosis and possible tumor growth. Erythropoietin is reviewed in more detail in the *Cancer* chapter.

Macrocytic Anemia

Macrocytic anemia usually occurs secondary to either folate or vitamin B_{12} deficiency, or both. When one or both of these vitamins are deficient, defective RNA and DNA are made within the red blood cells, which causes a macrocytic, megaloblastic anemia. Macrocytic anemia can also be caused by hypothyroidism, liver disease, hemolysis, blood dyscrasias, or drug therapy.[12] Treatments for macrocytic anemia are listed in Table 16-3.

Folate Deficiency

Folate-deficiency anemia primarily involves inadequate ingestion, absorption, or storage of dietary folic acid. Folate deficiency can arise during pregnancy, in the elderly, among individuals who abuse alcohol, or as an adverse drug reaction. Many drugs, some of which are commonly used in primary care of women, are known to cause folate deficiency and may require folate replacement if prescribed (Table 16-4).[12]

Folate is absorbed in the small intestine and stored in the liver, where it undergoes enterohepatic recirculation. In contrast to iron, which is heavily recycled, the body requires daily replacement of folate. Folate deficiency develops within weeks if this nutrient is not replaced. Deficiencies of either folate or vitamin B_{12} can result in the production of

Table 16-4 Drugs That Cause Folate Deficiency

Drugs
Anticonvulsants such as carbamazepine (Tegretol), phenytoin (Dilantin), and valproic acid (Depakote)
Methotrexate (Rheumatrex)
Phenytoin (Dilantin)
Pyrimethamine (Daraprim)
Sulfasalazine (Azulfidine)
Trimethoprim–sulfamethoxazole (Bactrim)

Source: Data from Kaferle J, Strzoda CE. Evaluation of macrocytosis. *Am Fam Physician.* 2009;79(3):203-208.[12]

significant quantities of macrocytes (RBC mean corpuscular volume > 100 fL). Therefore, it is important to distinguish which nutrient deficit is present to provide the appropriate treatment approach. Excessive folic acid ingestion can correct the macrocytic anemia but does not correct the underlying pathology of vitamin B_{12} deficiency.

Folic acid is used prophylactically to prevent folate–deficient megaloblastic anemias and used therapeutically to treat folate deficiency and the initial stages of severe vitamin B_{12}–deficient megaloblastic anemias. Folic acid is very well tolerated by the body and has minimal adverse effects, even if taken at super-therapeutic doses.

The most common indications for prophylactic treatment with folic acid are pregnancy and lactation. In early pregnancy, folate deficiency increases the risk of neural tube defects in a developing fetus. In the United States, the practice of folic acid supplementation has decreased this risk by approximately 66% in women who do not have an a priori increased risk for neural tube defects (e.g., women with a prior infant with a neural tube defect or women taking anticonvulsants).[13] In 1992, the Centers for Disease Control and Prevention (CDC) recommended that all women of childbearing age take a folic acid supplement of 400 mcg per day via ingestion of fortified foods or supplements and that a 400 mcg per day supplement be continued during the first trimester of pregnancy.[13] In addition to the CDC recommendation, United States Task Force for Preventive Care has designated daily 400 to 800 mcg per day as a Grade A recommendation.

Pharmacotherapeutic doses of folic acid are most commonly administered orally and are readily absorbed (Table 16-3). For individuals who have diagnosed folate-deficiency anemia or impaired folate absorption, a dose of 1 to 2 mg per day of an oral supplement is sufficient to force absorption and stimulate erythropoiesis. Replacement therapy should continue for 4 months, as this is the length of time that folate stores in the body last.

Side Effects/Adverse Effects

Although folic acid is generally well tolerated, common adverse effects reported include gastrointestinal symptoms—a bad taste in the mouth with large doses, nausea, and loss of appetite—and neurologic symptoms—confusion, irritability, and even sleep disturbances. The incidence of these adverse events has not been defined, however, and it can be difficult to determine whether the adverse events are due to the administration of folic acid or the deficiency it is trying to correct. The only serious adverse effect reported is allergy to folic acid.

In the case of severe folate–deficiency anemia, treatment may include intramuscular injections of both folic acid and vitamin B_{12}, followed by subsequent doses of oral folic acid alone (1–2 mg/day for 1–2 weeks, followed by 400 mcg/day maintenance doses). Megaloblasts will dissipate from the bone marrow after 48 hours of treatment, reticulocyte levels will increase after 2 to 3 days, and RBCs and hemoglobin concentrations will increase to normal levels within 2 to 6 weeks.

Leucovorin can be administered in instances where persons are not able to tolerate or do not respond to oral folic acid. Leucovorin is reduced folic acid. This agent is most often used to combat the harmful effects methotrexate (Rheumatrex) during chemotherapy but may be used to treat severe megaloblastic anemia that is secondary to folate and vitamin B_{12} deficiency.

Vitamin B_{12} Deficiency

Vitamin B_{12} is also known as cobalamin, a name referencing its molecular structure, which is coordinated by an atom of cobalt. Vitamin B_{12} deficiency causes neurologic, hematologic, and psychiatric symptoms as well as macrocytic anemia.[14,15] Deficiency of this essential nutrient can occur secondary to pernicious anemia, impaired gastrointestinal absorption of the vitamin from regional enteritis, celiac disease, bariatric surgery, pancreatitis, a vegetarian or vegan diet, or some drugs.[14] Drugs known to cause vitamin B_{12} deficiency are listed in Table 16-5.

Vitamin B_{12} is displaced from food in the stomach by intrinsic factor, which is produced by the parietal cells of the stomach. Thus, insufficient intrinsic factor is the most common cause of vitamin B_{12} deficiency.[15] Individuals with atrophic or autoimmune gastritis, for example, have decreased intrinsic factor secretion. **Pernicious anemia** is the term for anemia resulting from impaired vitamin B_{12} absorption secondary to a lack of intrinsic factor.

The anemia associated with vitamin B_{12} deficiency occurs because vitamin B_{12} is an essential step in activating folic acid, which is required for RBC production. This vitamin is also involved in myelination of nerves. Thus, in addition to causing anemia, vitamin B_{12} deficiency can lead to neurologic damage (e.g., paresthesias, cognitive impairment, and even "megaloblastic madness"— a constellation of psychiatric symptoms, possibly due to myelin synthesis).[14]

Table 16-5 Drugs That Cause Vitamin B_{12} Deficiency

Cimetidine (Tagamet)
Metformin (Glucophage)
Neomycin (No-Fradin)
Nitrous oxide anesthesia
Proton pump inhibitors

Box 16-1 Why Is JL So Tired?

JL is a 22-year-old female college student who comes into the school healthcare clinic because she is always tired and has been unable to keep current with her schoolwork. In taking JL's history, the clinician learns that JL has been a vegetarian for several years and is now following a vegan diet. She does not eat any dairy products. Her menses are regular, and she has very light bleeding.

JL's physical examination is normal. She does not have any symptoms of viral or infectious disease. She does not have any neurologic symptoms of vitamin B_{12} deficiency. The clinician suspects JL may be anemic and queries her further about her diet. JL is juggling working and going to school. She has relied on cooked beans/burritos and pasta because they are quick and easy to prepare, and she says she has not been hungry recently. The clinician orders a complete blood count (CBC) with differential, ferritin level, homocysteine, and methylmalonic acid level. She arranges for JL to return in a week to review the results.

JL's CBC reveals a macrocytic anemia with a normal folate level and a high homocysteine level, which results in a presumptive diagnosis of vitamin B_{12} and/or folate deficiency. Because folate is fortified in grains in the United States and would be present naturally in pasta and beans, the clinician suspects the source of JL's anemia is vitamin B_{12} deficiency. The clinician reviews dietary sources of these vitamins. She tells JL how to obtain folate in green, leafy vegetables and fruits. Because vitamin B_{12} is highly bioavailable in dairy products, she explores the idea of eating dairy products and JL agrees to consider it. In addition, the clinician encourages JL to review the food labels of food products, especially breakfast cereals, to see if the products are fortified with vitamin B_{12}. The clinician prescribes JL a vitamin supplement that is vegan friendly and contains a combination of folic acid 2.5 mg, cyanocobalamin 1000 mcg, and pyridoxine 25 mg. She tells JL that it can take a few months for the anemia to resolve and arranges for a follow-up visit in 1 month to see if JL is feeling less tired and to determine how the changes in her diet are working.

In contrast to folate deficiency, it can take months to years of impaired vitamin B_{12} absorption before the deficiency is detected clinically because the body contains robust stores of vitamin B_{12}. Vitamin B_{12}–associated neurologic damage may take longer to correct than vitamin B_{12}–deficiency anemia, however, and may be irreversible if not treated within 2 to 6 months of developing symptoms. High doses of folate can successfully treat the hematologic consequences of vitamin B_{12} deficiency, but folate will not resolve the neurologic effects (Box 16-1).

Cyanocobalamin, a crystalline form of vitamin B_{12}, is available in oral, intramuscular, and intranasal formulations. This agent is most commonly administered intramuscularly for acute treatment and then given orally or intranasally for maintenance. Some individuals with pernicious anemia, such as those who have had bariatric surgery, will need vitamin B_{12} replacement for life.[15] The oral formulation contains an extremely high dose of vitamin B_{12}, of which a small portion is absorbed via a route that does not rely on intrinsic factor. The higher dose is well tolerated, nontoxic, and beneficial for addressing the neurologic effects of vitamin B_{12} deficiency.[15] In particular, oral dosing appears to be as beneficial as intramuscular dosing in resolving hematologic and neurologic symptoms, with no difference in adverse effects.[16] As a result, some clinicians may recommend high-dose oral administration instead of the intramuscular injections that were standard therapy in years past. The intranasal preparation has not been tested for improvement of the severe vitamin B_{12} deficiency neurologic symptoms. Although vitamin B_{12} is available as sublingual tablets and oral solution, there is no evidence to support these formulations' efficacy in treating vitamin B_{12} deficiency, although they may have benefit in prophylaxis or maintenance therapy.

The hematologic response to vitamin B_{12} drug therapy is typically rapid, occurring in less than 48 hours. Neurologic impairments may improve, and ultimately resolve, more gradually over 6 months of treatment.[15]

Side Effects/Adverse Effects

In general, cyanocobalamin is well tolerated. Persons receiving subcutaneous or intramuscular injections of this agent may experience injection-site reactions. Arthralgias, headaches, dizziness, and nasopharyngitis have all been reported, but serious adverse effects such as anaphylaxis and angioedema are rare. All persons receiving cyanocobalamin should be monitored periodically while on therapy for both effectiveness in replenishing vitamin B_{12} and tolerability of the replacement therapy selected.

Aplastic Anemia

Aplastic anemia occurs when the bone marrow does not produce enough new cells to replace red blood cells in the circulation. This type of anemia can develop secondary to an autoimmune process in the case of inherited aplastic anemia or acquired aplastic anemia resulting from exposure to radiation or chemotherapy; more rarely, it may be caused by drugs as noted in Table 16-1. Interestingly, the scientist Marie Curie died of aplastic anemia that probably developed following her exposure to radiation. A detailed discussion of the management of aplastic anemia is beyond the scope of this chapter. Persons with aplastic anemia may need transfusions or immunosuppressive therapy and possibly a hematopoietic stem cell transplant.[17,18]

Special Populations: Pregnancy, Lactation, and the Elderly

The treatment of anemia during pregnancy is the same as the treatment for nonpregnant women. Anemia that first occurs during pregnancy is almost always a dilutional physiologic anemia that resolves following supplementation with iron. Because some women may first have their blood indices observed during pregnancy, folate deficiency and vitamin B_{12} deficiency may also be diagnosed during pregnancy and correspondingly treated with the appropriate supplement. There are no adverse effects of iron, folate, or vitamin B_{12} when used by pregnant or lactating women. Erythropoietin (Procrit) is not used during pregnancy.

Anemia is more common among the elderly and may occur secondary to nutritional deficiencies or comorbidities. In addition to treatment of the underlying vitamin deficiency, erythropoietin may be used by elderly women if the cause of anemia is a renal disorder or other condition in which erythropoietin is approved for use so as to avoid blood transfusion.[19]

Hemoglobinopathies: Sickle Cell Anemia and Thalassemias

Hemoglobinopathies comprise a diverse set of disorders that result from mutations in the genes that encode for the globin chains within the hemoglobin molecule. Two categories of hemoglobinopathies are distinguished: sickle cell disorders and thalassemias. Both cause hemolytic anemia. Persons who are heterozygous for one gene that codes for an abnormal globin chain are usually asymptomatic and not anemic. Conversely, persons who have homozygous genes for the aberrant globin chain have profound anemia and are primarily cared for by hematology specialists.

Sickle cell disease encompasses a group of conditions that arise due to mutations of the beta-globin. In homozygous sickle cell anemia, both beta-globins are abnormal, and the result is a type of hemoglobin called HbS. This abnormal hemoglobin forms long polymer chains when deoxygenated; the chains cause the red blood cell to be rigid and shaped like a sickle. The rigid elongated cells may occlude the vasculature, which causes a vaso-occlusive crisis typified by ischemia, hemolysis, severe pain, and, ultimately, organ damage. These sickle red blood cells are more easily destroyed than are regular red blood cells, which is why sickle cell disease causes a hemolytic anemia.

Historically, the primary treatment for sickle cell vaso-occlusive crises has been liberal use of opioids to decrease pain. As the molecular mechanisms that underlie the functions of sickle red blood cells have been elucidated, however, new and novel pharmacotherapeutic treatments have emerged. To date, the FDA has approved use of hydroxyurea (Hydrea), which increases the production of another type of hemoglobin, fetal hemoglobin (Hbf). Fetal hemoglobin has two alpha-globin chains and two gamma-globin chains; this type of hemoglobin does not form polymer chains.[20] Hydroxyurea significantly decreases the incidence of vaso-occlusive crises and need for blood transfusions in persons with sickle cell disease. Due to an associated risk of congenital malformations, hydroxyurea should be discontinued 3 months before conception and avoided during pregnancy. Other disease-modifying agents for sickle cell disease are currently under study, although no other agents have been FDA approved as yet due to lack of sufficient efficacy or insufficient data regarding their safety.

Thalassemias are conditions that result from reduced or no production of one of the globin chains. Reduction of the alpha chains causes alpha thalassemia, and reduction in the beta chains causes beta thalassemia. Persons with beta thalassemia (Cooley's anemia) are dependent on transfusions for survival. Alpha thalassemia is usually a milder form of thalassemia.

Four genes encode for the alpha-globin chain. No alpha globin is made in the most serious form of alpha thalassemia wherein all four genes are inactive, and the resulting hemoglobin is called Bart's hemoglobin. This fatal condition causes hydrops fetalis and intrauterine demise. When three of the four genes are inactive, the individual will have moderate anemia that is periodically severe and treated with transfusions. Iron overload is the expected complication and is treated with iron chelation.

Iron Chelation Therapy

For individuals with either alpha and beta thalassemia, frequent hypertransfusion therapy results in iron overload; thus iron chelation to correct iron overload is the mainstay of therapy. Currently, three iron chelator drugs are available for treating chronic iron overload: deferoxamine (Desferal), deferiprone (Exjade), and deferasirox (Ferriprox).[21,22]

Deferoxamine is administered either intravenously or subcutaneously, usually for 8 to 12 hours during the night for 5 to 7 days per week. Deferiprone can be given orally 3 times per day, and deferasirox is given orally 2 times per day. The most common adverse effect of deferoxamine is irritation at the site of administration, but it can (rarely) cause high-frequency hearing loss, allergic reactions, or decreased night vision. Nightly infusions of deferoxamine can result in 20 to 50 mg of iron loss, excreted in urine and stool. All of the oral chelating agents have an FDA black box warning on their labels indicating that they may cause agranulocytosis and should not be used in combination with other drugs that induce neutropenia.

Special Populations: Pregnancy, Lactation, and the Elderly

Women who have sickle cell disease, sickle cell trait, beta thalassemia, or beta thalassemia trait will present with anemia during pregnancy. In general, treatment of women with anemia is based on an evaluation that determines how much of their anemia is microcytic and secondary to low iron stores versus how much is macrocytic and secondary to the hemoglobinopathy.

Coagulation Disorders

Coagulation disorders include disorders that predispose the individual to hemorrhage or to **thrombosis** and include some conditions that predispose persons to both hemorrhage and thrombosis. Blood clots or thrombi are composed of platelets, fibrin, and captured red cells. Thus, drugs used to promote coagulation or prevent it are directed toward one of the following physiologic targets:

- **Anticoagulant drugs** interfere with fibrin formation and are primarily used to treat or prevent venous thrombi, as these thrombi are formed under low shear conditions and have more fibrin than platelets in the complex. The three types of anticoagulants are **vitamin K antagonists**, **direct thrombin inhibitors**, and **direct factor Xa inhibitors**.
- Antiplatelet drugs interfere with platelet adhesion or platelet function. They are used primarily to treat arterial thrombi, as these thrombi are formed under high shear conditions and contain more platelets than fibrin. Arterial thrombi develop on top of an atherosclerotic plaque and manifests as a myocardial infarction, ischaemic stroke, or peripheral artery disease. Examples of antithrombotic agents include aspirin and clopidogrel (Plavix).
- Fibrinolytic agents degrade fibrin.

This section reviews von Willebrand disease and the unique drug desmopressin (DDAVP, Stimate), as well as anticoagulants used in the management of venous thrombi. Antiplatelet drugs used for secondary prevention of ischemic stroke or myocardial infarction are reviewed in the *Cardiovascular Conditions* chapter. Evidence-based practice guidelines for use of antiplatelet and anticoagulant drugs for prevention of various types of ischemic stroke are listed in the Resources table at the end of this chapter. The fibrinolytic agents are used in the hospital as part of initial treatment for thrombotic disorders and are not reviewed in this text. First, a brief review of coagulation is in order.

Hemostasis

Hemostasis is achieved through the formation of a platelet plug that is subsequently strengthened by the recruitment and activation of fibrin to form a thrombus. Historically, this coagulation process was described as a cascade of events that occurred in two pathways. Coagulation initiated via the **intrinsic pathway (contact activation pathway)** used coagulation factors present in blood, whereas coagulation initiated via the **extrinsic pathway (tissue factor pathway)** started after exposure to tissue factor, which is constitutively present on the cell membranes of cells outside the vasculature. These two "waterfall" cascades converge into a common pathway that results in the generation of a fibrin clot.

Today, it is clear that the intrinsic and extrinsic pathways are linked from the outset; thus, rather than focusing on two cascade-type pathways, coagulation has been reframed as a process with four distinct phases.[23] First is the initiation phase, which has two steps. In the first step, two pathways are initiated: the tissue factor pathways and the contact activation or intrinsic pathway. Tissue factor is not usually exposed to plasma. When tissue factor is exposed to plasma via injury or damage to the endothelial cell lining of the vasculature, it binds to factor VII_a (the subscript a means this factor is activated, and there is always a small amount of activated factor VII in plasma). Other coagulation factors are then activated, with the result being the production of factor X_a, which cleaves prothrombin into thrombin. This process is referred to as the tissue factor pathway. Thrombin—the final enzyme in the clotting cascade—directly produces fibrin. Four of the coagulation factors involved in the production of thrombin—factors VII, IX, X, and prothrombin—require vitamin K for their biosynthesis. A lack of vitamin K results in decreases of serum concentration of these factors, which inhibits coagulation. Vitamin K antagonists interrupt the coagulation cascade at this juncture.

Thrombin is also the final enzyme produced by the contact activation/intrinsic pathway. In this set of steps, several coagulation factors enzymatically react after coming in contact with exposed collagen from the subendothelial tissue. The two pathways merge with the production of factor X_a. Direct factor X_a inhibitors interrupt the process at this point. The contact activation/intrinsic pathway is slower than the tissue-factor pathway; the latter is the primary pathway that initiates coagulation and the formation of blood clots. Direct thrombin inhibitors bind to thrombin and inactivate it.

The second step of the initiation phase involves platelets. When endothelial cells are damaged, platelets aggregate in response to the presence of exposed collagen from the endothelial cells. Glycoprotein II_b/III_a (GP II_b/III_a), a receptor on the cell membrane of the platelet, is activated. Once activated, GP II_b/III_a undergoes a conformational change and joins with other GP II_b/III_a receptors on other platelets to form a heterodimer (Figure 16-1). This heterodimer binds to fibrinogen, which is present in plasma and forms cross-links with other platelets in the area that have activated GP II_b/III_a receptors on their extracellular surface. At this point, von Willebrand factor (VWF), a large glycoprotein that is constitutively produced in endothelial cells, joins the process and further strengthens the bonds by forming links between the GP II_b/III_a receptors and collagen from the endothelial cell.

Polymorphisms in the GP II_b/III_a receptor can occur. In addition, it appears that estrogen may have more of a platelet aggregation effect in women with certain polymorphisms of this receptor. This phenomenon might explain why hormone therapy increased the incidence of cardiovascular events in women who took nonphysiologic doses of estrogen in randomized trials of estrogen therapy for postmenopausal symptoms.[24]

The second phase of coagulation is the amplification phase and formation of the loose platelet plug. In this phase, thrombin sets the stage for phase 3 by activating the platelets that are present. Direct thrombin inhibitors prevent thrombin from amplifying the process at this point. The activated platelets expose receptors and binding sites, and they release granules that contain additional clotting factors, thereby triggering additional platelet activation and increased clotting. This positive feedback mechanism propagates the process. The platelets change shape to accommodate the formation of the plug. Interestingly, thrombin also initiates the processes (phase 4 of the coagulation process) that create the chemicals that slow and stop the clot process—specifically, activation of protein C and protein S.

Phase 3 of the coagulation process is the propagation phase, in which a large burst of thrombin that alters fibrinogen into fibrin stabilizes and creates the actual blood clot.[25]

Finally, the fibrinolytic system, which thrombin originally activated in phase 2, matures, and the fourth phase of fibrinolysis can occur. Three types of natural anticoagulants come into play during this final phase of the coagulation process: antithrombin, plasmin, and proteins C and S.

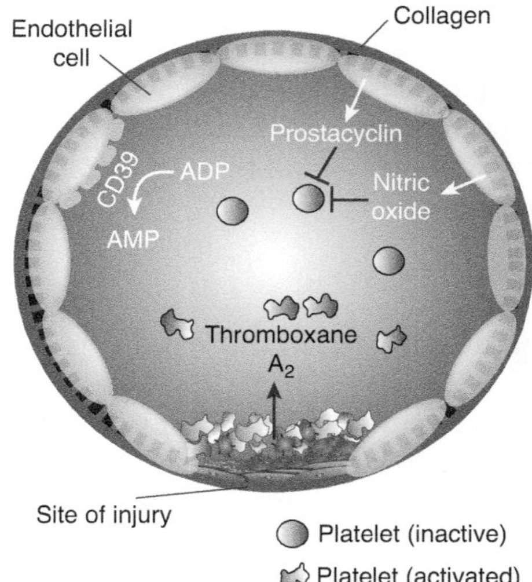

Figure 16-1 Formation of a platelet plug.

- Antithrombin inhibits five of the activated clotting factors: IX_a, X_a, XI_a, XII_a, and thrombin. Inhibition of factor X_a and thrombin is especially important because it stops the acceleration of clotting that is initiated from either the tissue factor pathway or the contact platelet process. As a consequence of the antithrombin activity, fibrinogen is prevented from being converted into fibrin and, therefore, is unable to extenuate clotting. Antithrombin is unable to disrupt fibrin that has already polymerized, however, so it is ineffective at removing a clot that has already formed.
- Plasmin is an enzyme that is normally present in the blood in the inactive precursor form of plasminogen. Once converted from plasminogen, plasmin is able to digest fibrin polymers and dissolve fully formed blood clots once tissue repair has concluded.
- Protein C and protein S, which inhibit two of the coagulation factors, are both dependent on vitamin K for their synthesis.

Figure 16-2 shows the coagulation cascade and mechanisms of action of commonly used anticoagulant drugs.

Thrombosis and Thrombocytic Structures

A thrombus is a pathogenic blood clot that adheres to the wall of a blood vessel or the heart and prevents blood flow. Venous thrombosis and arterial thrombosis differ in etiology and clinical presentation. While an arterial thrombus most commonly causes localized tissue injury at the site of formation, a venous thrombus typically causes harm at a remote location in the vasculature.

During the formation of an arterial thrombosis, an atherosclerotic plaque or other damage to the arterial wall leads to platelet recruitment and platelet adhesion at the site of injury. Platelet adhesion causes the cellular release of ADP and thromboxane A_2 into the blood and activation of additional platelets. As the number of thrombocytes increases, the size of the platelet plug expands and the blockage of the artery increases. Impaired blood transport activates the coagulation process and reinforcement of the platelet plug with a fibrin meshwork. The thrombus prevents blood flow and downstream tissue perfusion, resulting in localized tissue injury.

The classic factors to which venous thrombus formation is attributed are referred to as Virchow's triad, which includes venous stasis, endothelial injury, and hypercoagulation. An arterial thrombosis most commonly develops secondary to formation of an atherosclerotic plaque or other damage to an arterial wall. A venous thrombosis originates as a result of slow-moving or stagnant blood flow, which leads to the activation of the coagulation cascade and formation of fibrin. The morphology of a venous thrombus consequently differs from that of its arterial

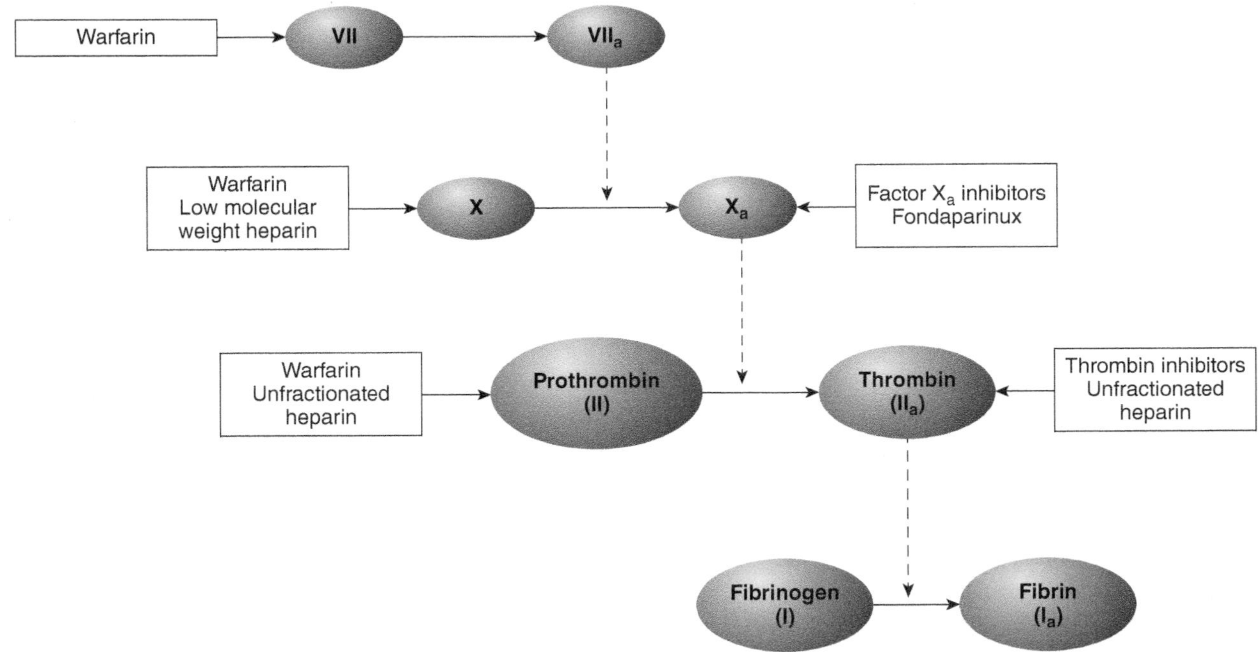

Figure 16-2 Coagulation cascade and mechanisms of action of anticoagulant drugs.

counterpart. Venous thrombi typically possess long tails of accumulated platelets and RBCs. The tail of the venous clot may detach and travel through the vasculature to a distant site, resulting in an embolism, which is referred to as thromboembolism.

Bleeding Disorders: von Willebrand Disease

The primary indications for antifibrinolytic drugs in primary care are bleeding disorders such as the hemophilias, factor deficiencies, and von Willebrand disease (VWD). Hemophilias are a group of genetic disorders that are primarily evident in males; thus they are not covered in this chapter. Inherited factor deficiencies do affect women but as a group they are rare and treatment usually consists of replacement of the deficient factor. The most common disorder that causes bleeding in women is von Willebrand disease.[26]

Von Willebrand disease is caused by impairment in the synthesis or action of von Willebrand factor (VWF). It can occur secondary to a genetic mutation or be acquired. Approximately 50% of adolescents with severe menstrual bleeding at menarche have an inherited coagulopathy, of which von Willebrand disease is the most common form.[27] Treatments specifically for menorrhagia are reviewed in the *Pelvic and Menstrual Disorders* chapter.

Desmopressin

The primary pharmacologic therapy for von Willebrand disease itself is desmopressin (DDAVP, Stimate), which stimulates release of endogenous VWF from endothelial cells.[26–30] The two additional therapies used for this indication are replacement of VWF with human plasma–derived VWF concentrate as prophylaxis to prevent bleeding episodes and use of agents that promote hemostasis.[26]

Desmopressin is a synthetic derivative of vasopressin, the antidiuretic hormone that increases VWF concentrations two- to five-fold following each intravenous, subcutaneous, or intranasal spray dose.[26] This agent can be used therapeutically to treat a bleeding episode or prophylactically to prevent one.

Desmopressin can cause tachyphylaxis after repeated doses, so its administration is limited to once per day. Common side effects include vasodilation and facial flushing, headache, nausea, and tingling. Hyponatremia can occur if excess fluids are taken, which in turn can cause seizures and death if not treated. Rare anaphylactic hypersensitivity reactions have been reported. NSAIDs will aggravate the hyponatremia effect and should not be used by persons with VWD.

Antifibrolytic Therapy, Estrogen, and Recombinant Factor VII_a

Although desmopressin is the primary therapy for VWD, antifibrinolytic agents such as aminocaproic acid or tranexamic acid have been used to prevent dissolution of clots, particularly in women with menorrhagia or following dental procedures.[29,30] Estrogen increases the synthesis of VWF and may be helpful for some women. Because of the controversy surrounding the side effects of long-term therapy with estrogen, this option is best discussed with a specialist.

Recombinant factor VII_a bypasses the need for factor VIII in the contact activation pathway and allows the coagulation cascade to proceed without VWF. Recombinant factor VII_a carries a risk of thrombosis, so it should be used with caution and by specialists in treating women with this disorder.

Special Populations: Pregnancy, Lactation, and the Elderly

Pregnancy shifts the coagulation system to a pro-coagulable state, and VWF levels rise secondary to stimulation from pregnancy-related hormones. Thus, women who have VWD rarely need treatment during pregnancy.[31] Desmopressin is safe for use during pregnancy. Use of tranexamic acid (Cyklokapron) is controversial secondary to limited data in humans, although some experts recommend it. The manufacturer recommends using tranexamic acid with caution during breastfeeding. Women with VWD may be at increased risk for postpartum hemorrhage and are usually managed with replacement therapy around the time of birth by maternal–fetal medicine specialists and hematologists.

Anticoagulant Drugs

Pathologic blood clotting can occur through multiple mechanisms, including infection, cancer, injury, or thrombophilia. Thrombophilias can be inherited or acquired. Approximately 5% to 8% of the population in the United States has a genetic thrombophilia, yet most persons never have any problems with clotting until an additional risk factor is present. Common thrombophilias in women include deep vein thrombosis (DVT), stroke, and pulmonary embolism. Less common etiologies include inherited disorders such as factor V Leiden, protein C deficiency, and protein S deficiency, and acquired disorders such as antiphospholipid antibody syndrome. Overall, the incidence of thromboembolism increases with age.[32]

Venous thromboembolism is of particular concern for women.[33] Early treatment is critical to avoid life-threatening complications. In addition, prophylactic therapy to prevent pulmonary embolism has been shown to substantially improve clinical outcomes of individuals with symptomatic DVT.[34,35] Long-term hormone therapy, pregnancy, and combined oral contraceptive use are all correlated with increased incidence of thrombosis and subsequent pathologies. Combination oral contraceptives are the most common cause of thrombosis in young adult women, and this risk is even higher for women who smoke and use combined oral contraceptives.[36] The increased risk of thrombosis during pregnancy may be attributed to impaired venous return by the uterus or the presence of the hypercoagulable state associated with pregnancy.[37] The randomized controlled trials of hormone therapy (HT) for postmenopausal women found HT to be associated with a twofold increase in venous thromboembolism.[38]

Parenteral Anticoagulants

Parenteral anticoagulants are used for prophylaxis and acute treatment of individuals with thrombosis, particularly venous thrombosis. A general comparison of these agents is presented in Table 16-6, and dosing information is given in Table 16-7.[39,40] Antithrombin inhibitors include unfractionated heparin, multiple formulations of low-molecular-weight heparin, and fondaparinux (Arixtra). These drugs significantly increase the activity of antithrombin by forming a drug–antithrombin protein complex. As a result of this complex formation and the increased antithrombin activity, factor X_a is inhibited, thus preventing coagulation signaling and fibrin production from either the tissue factor or the contact pathway (Figure 16-3). Uncontrolled bleeding is the major side effect of all these medications and should be carefully monitored.

Table 16-6 Comparison of Parenteral Anticoagulants

Feature	Heparin	Low Molecular Weight Heparin	Fondaparinux
Source	Porcine intestine	Porcine intestine	Synthetic
Molecular weight	15,000 Da	Mean: 5000 Da (range 4000–8000 Da)	1500 Da
Biologic target	X_a, II_a, thrombin	X_a, II_a	X_a
Pharmacokinetics			
Half-life	1 hour	14 hours	17 hours
Bioavailability	30%	90%	100%
Onset of action	Immediate	1–2 hours	1–2 hours
Dosing	Continuous IV or SQ 2 times/day titrated to response	1–2 times/day SQ titrated to response	Once daily SQ, fixed dose of 2.5 mg/day
Effect on platelets	High dose can interfere with platelet aggregation and cause bleeding	No effect	No effect
Crosses placenta/use in pregnancy	No; safe for use in pregnancy	No; safe for use in pregnancy	No; insufficient data so it is not recommended for use in pregnancy
Requires coagulation monitoring	Yes	No	No
Adverse Effects			
Major bleeding	3.2%	0.9%	
HIT	1–5%	< 1%	< 1%
Immediate hypersensitivity reaction	Yes	Yes	No
Osteoporosis and spontaneous vertebral fracture	Yes	Yes, but less than with heparin	Less than with heparin or LMWH

Abbreviations: HIT = heparin-induced thrombocytopenia; LMWH = low-molecular-weight heparin.
Sources: Data from Garcia DA, Baglin TP, Weitz JI, Samama MM. Parenteral anticoagulants: antithrombotic therapy and prevention of thrombosis, 9th ed.: American College of Chest Physicians evidence-based clinical practice guidelines. *Chest.* 2012;141(2 suppl):e24S-e43S[40]; Wells PS, Anderson DR, Rodger MA, et al. A randomized trial comparing 2 low-molecular-weight heparins for the outpatient treatment of deep vein thrombosis and pulmonary embolism. *Arch Intern Med.* 2005;165:733.[41]

Table 16-7 Parenteral Anticoagulants

Drug: Generic (Brand)	Formulations	Indication/Dose	Clinical Considerations
Unfractionated Heparin			
Heparin (UFH)	Multiple injection and solution formulations, ranging from 1 unit/mL to 20,000 unit/mL	DVT prevention: SQ: 5000 units every 8–12 hours DVT/PE treatment: IV: 80 unit/kg IVP followed by infusion of 18 unit/kg/hours to maintain antifactor X_a levels at 0.3–0.7 unit/mL SQ: 17,500 units or 250 unit/kg, then 250 unit/kg every 12 hours to maintain antifactor X_a levels at 0.3–0.7 unit/mL	Contraindications: Hypersensitivity to heparin or any component of the formulation; thrombocytopenia; uncontrolled active bleeding except when due to DIC; suspected intracranial hemorrhage. Heparin is supplied in a wide range of strengths. Fatal medication errors related to overdose have occurred. Initial bolus is weight based, followed by infusion titrated based on aPTT or antifactor X_a determinations.
Low-Molecular-Weight Heparin			
Dalteparin (Fragmin)	Injection: 2500–18,000 IU available	DVT prophylaxis: 2500–5000 units daily Extended DVT or PE treatment: SQ: 200 units/kg daily for 1 month, then 150 unit/kg/dose in months 2–6	FDA approved for DVT prophylaxis in persons who require surgery and are at risk for thromboembolism, and for prophylaxis against recurrence of DVT or PE. Dose for DVT prophylaxis depends on the type of surgery/procedure the person will undergo. Extended treatment of individuals with DVT or PE is only for persons with cancer.
Enoxaparin (Lovenox)	30 mg/0.3 mL to 100 mg/1 mL	DVT prophylaxis: SQ: Dosing ranges from 30 mg every 12 hours to every 24 hours to 40 mg every 24 hours, depending on the type of surgery Duration is usually for approximately 10 days post surgery or until the risk of DVT has diminished or the individual is anticoagulated on warfarin DVT treatment: SQ: 1 mg/kg/dose every 12 hours or 1.5 mg/kg/dose every 24 hours	FDA approved for treatment of individuals with DVT and for prophylaxis for DVT and acute coronary syndromes. Contraindications: Hypersensitivity to heparin or any component of the formulation, hypersensitivity to pork products, thrombocytopenia, major bleeding. FDA black box warning: Persons with recent or anticipated epidural or spinal anesthesia are at risk of spinal or epidural hematoma and subsequent paralysis. Multiple dosing regimens are used for prophylaxis and treatment for each LMWH. They depend on variables such as weight, age, type of surgery, overall risk, condition (i.e., pregnancy, cancer), renal function, and others.
Tinzaparin (Innohep)	Injection: 20,000 IU/mL (2 mL)	DVT prophylaxis: SQ: 75 antifactor X_a units/kg generally given 7–10 days postoperatively DVT treatment: SQ: 175 antifactor X_a IU/kg every 24 hours for 6 days or longer, until adequate anticoagulation with warfarin	FDA approved for treatment of individuals with DVT and PE and prevention of VTE following surgery. Duration of therapy is determined by the type of surgery as well as other risk factors.
Factor X_a Inhibitor			
Fondaparinux (Arixtra)	Injection: 2.5–10 mg options are available	DVT prophylaxis: SQ: 2.5 mg every 24 hours; initial dose is given 6–8 hours after surgery; usual duration is 5–9 days DVT treatment: SQ: body weight 50–100 kg: 7.5 mg every 24 hours; body weight > 100 kg: 10 mg every 24 hours Usual duration: 5–10 days	FDA approved for prophylaxis of DVT in persons undergoing surgery, and for treatment of persons with VTE or PE. Contraindications: Not recommended for use for DVT prophylaxis in persons weighing less than 50 kg. Hypersensitivity to fondaparinux, hemophilia, leukemia with bleeding, peptic ulcer disease, hemorrhagic stroke, surgery, thrombocytopenic purpura, severe renal disease. FDA black box warning: Persons with recent or anticipated epidural or spinal anesthesia are at risk of spinal or epidural hematoma and subsequent paralysis.

Abbreviations: aPTT = activated partial thromboplastin time; DIC = disseminated intravascular coagulation; DVT = deep vein thrombosis; IVP = intravenous push; LMWH = low-molecular-weight heparin; PE = pulmonary embolism; VTE = venous thromboembolism.

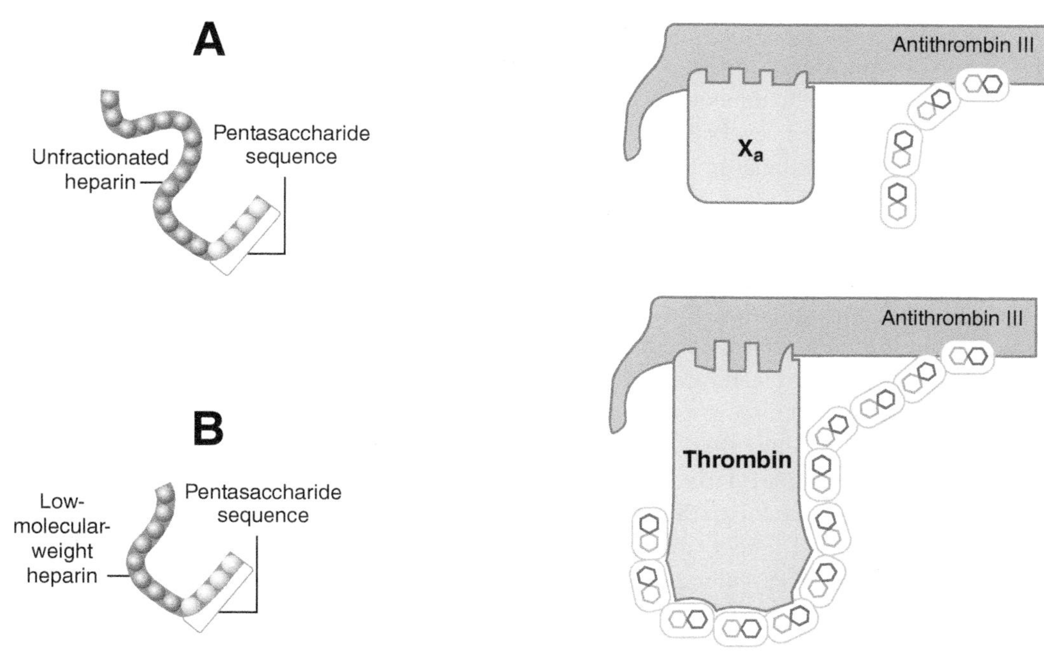

Figure 16-3 Parenteral anticoagulants: mechanism of action.

Unfractionated Heparin

Unfractionated heparin was first isolated from an extract of liver in 1916, but it was not available for clinical use until the 1930s. The process of synthesizing a pure form of heparin suitable for use in humans was devised by Best, who applied the same techniques he used in his discovery of insulin. The first formulations of clinically usable insulin and heparin were both produced by a Canadian team from the University of Toronto.

Heparin is a polysaccharide mixture consisting of molecules with molecular weights ranging from 3 to 30 kDa.[39] Heparin is obtained from animal sources including swine and cattle. A five-sugar (pentasaccharide) sequence that forms the site of interaction between heparin and antithrombin is intermittently dispersed along the molecule. Its multiple negatively charged sugar moieties makes heparin a large, highly polar molecule that must be administered intravenously or subcutaneously. The size and polarity of the molecule prevent heparin from transferring across cellular membranes, including the placenta, and heparin is not detected in breast milk.

Heparin has no effect on existing clots; rather, it prevents formation of new thrombi. Under normal conditions, the plasma protein antithrombin forms complexes with thrombin (factor II_a), factor IX, and factor X. The complexes effectively block the ability of these factors to propagate the coagulation process. Unfractionated heparin forms a complex with antithrombin that vastly accelerates the rate at which these reactions take place.

Heparin is metabolized in the liver and excreted through the kidneys. The drug has a half-life of 1.5 hours in individuals with normal liver and kidney function. The duration may increase several-fold if hepatotoxicity or nephrotoxicity is present. Heparin is associated with extensive plasma protein binding and individual variations in response to its use. Pharmacologic use requires ongoing monitoring. Activated partial thromboplastin time (aPTT) values are typically measured before and after therapy to verify the preferred anticoagulant effect of heparin and to ensure proper dosing. The therapeutically desired aPTT ratio (i.e., the ratio of normal aPTT to heparin-treated aPTT) is 1.5:2.5.[39] Another approach to monitoring heparin levels is to ensure antifactor X_a levels stay within the therapeutic range of 0.3–0.7 unit/mL. A standard low-dose unfractionated heparin regimen administered for prophylaxis of VTE is 5000 units administered subcutaneously 2 hours prior to surgery, followed by 5000 units every 8 to 12 hours postoperatively until the person is ambulatory.[39]

Side Effects and Adverse Effects

Heparin-associated side effects commonly relate to the drug's action and potential for initiating the immune response. The most common side effects (occurring in more than 10% of users) are excessive bleeding and thrombocytopenia. Heparin-induced thrombocytopenia is an immunogenic reaction observed in fewer than 3% of individuals receiving extended (more than 4 days) heparin therapy; it occurs when antibodies develop to the heparin–platelet complex. The paradoxical effect of heparin-induced thrombocytopenia results in vascular damage and activation of the clotting cascade, potentially leading to thrombosis and DVT, pulmonary embolism, and myocardial infarction. Hypersensitivity reactions to heparin may also occur due to the animal source of the drug. A test dose prior to fully commencing therapy can be used to verify the lack of a hypersensitivity reaction for an individual.

Reversal of Bleeding

Protamine sulfate (Protamine) may be administered to treat a heparin overdose. This agent is a positively charged protein that binds and sequesters the negatively charged molecules of heparin. The drug dose is calculated based on a concentration of 1–1.5 mg protamine sulfate per 100 units of unfractionated heparin if given within 30 minutes of the last dose of heparin. Typical administration of protamine sulfate is via a slow intravenous infusion of 50 mg for at least 10 minutes.

Low-Molecular-Weight Heparins

The class of drugs known as low-molecular-weight heparins (LMWHs) includes molecules that are smaller (2–9 kDa) and more uniform than unfractionated heparin. The pharmacokinetic properties of LMWHs provide several advantages over unfractionated heparin. Distribution and bioavailability of LMWHs are greater than that of unfractionated heparin. These agents are associated with fewer adverse drug events, require only one to two doses per day, and do not require aPTT monitoring, all of which make them more amenable for ambulatory and in-home care settings.

LMWHs form a complex with antithrombin, like unfractionated heparin; however, LMWHs are smaller than the unfractionated versions, and the resulting heparin–antithrombin complex blocks factor X_a very well but does not block the action of thrombin (Figure 16-3). Despite slightly different mechanisms of action, both types of heparin are equally efficacious for most disorders that require anticoagulation. A standard treatment regimen for postoperative DVT prophylaxis is 7 to 10 days of the LMWH.

Currently, three LMWH preparations are available in the United States: enoxaparin (Lovenox), dalteparin (Fragmin), and tinzaparin (Innohep). Each differs slightly in terms of its physical and chemical properties and, although all three are suitable for DVT prophylaxis, each has slightly different FDA-approved indications. If used for treatment of persons with DVT or PE, LMWH therapy will be supplemented and then replaced by warfarin (Coumadin) for outpatient continuation of therapy for nonpregnant individuals. Note that standard dosing for enoxaparin is given in milligrams, whereas dosing for dalteparin and tinzaparin is given in antifactor X_a international units (IU).

Side Effects and Adverse Effects

Hemorrhage is the most common adverse effect of LMWHs, although the associated risk is less with LMWHs than with unfractionated heparin. Thrombocytopenia is more than 300% less likely to occur with LMWH therapy compared to unfractionated heparin therapy; however, it remains a serious concern.

Reversal of Bleeding

Protamine sulfate may be used in the treatment of an individual with an LMWH overdose, although it is an unlabeled indication. The dose of protamine sulfate varies with the specific formulation (e.g., 1 mg protamine per 1 mg enoxaparin; 1 mg protamine per 100 IU of dalteparin or tinzaparin) and the amount of time since LMWH was administered.

Fondaparinux

Fondaparinux (Arixtra) is a synthetic preparation of the active pentasaccharide present in both unfractionated heparin and LMWH. Like LMWH, fondaparinux selectively interacts with antithrombin to form an inhibitory complex that prevents factor X_a from converting prothrombin to thrombin. Fondaparinux reversibly binds to antithrombin and has a higher affinity than unfractionated heparin or LMWH. Routine laboratory evaluation of bleeding times (e.g., aPTT) is not necessary for persons on fondaparinux. Most treatment regimens consisting of this drug are prescribed for 5 to 10 days.

Side Effects/Adverse Effects

As with the other parenteral anticoagulants, hemorrhage is the most common adverse effect of fondaparinux, although the associated risk is less than with LMWH or unfractionated heparin. Thrombocytopenia does not seem to occur to the same extent as with unfractionated heparin or LMWH, and fondaparinux has been successfully used to treat persons with a history of heparin-induced thrombocytopenia (HIT).[41]

Reversal of Bleeding

Unlike with the other parenteral anticoagulants, protamine is not an effective antidote for hemorrhage in persons taking fondaparinux because it does not bind to protamine. The package insert for Fondaparinux clearly states that no reversal agent is available for use in cases of overdose. However, some reports indicate that recombinant factor VII_a may be effective in persons taking fondaparinux who need reversal.

Oral Anticoagulants

Oral anticoagulants include: (1) the vitamin K antagonist warfarin (Coumadin); (2) the direct thrombin inhibitor dabigatran etexilate (Pradaxa); and (3) the direct factor X_a inhibitors rivaroxaban (Xarelto), Edoxaban (Savaysa), and apixaban (Eliquis). Table 16-8 presents an overview of the oral anticoagulant drugs.[42–46]

Warfarin

Warfarin (Coumadin) is a vitamin K antagonist that indirectly inhibits the coagulation cascade. This drug was initially produced as a pesticide for rats and mice and is still

Table 16-8 Comparison of Oral Anticoagulants for Treatment of Persons with Venous Thromboembolism

Feature	**Warfarin (Coumadin)**	**Target-Specific Anticoagulants**			
		Dabigatran (Pradaxa)	**Rivaroxaban (Xarelto)**	**Apixaban (Eliquis)**	**Edoxaban (Savaysa)**
Mechanism of action	Inhibits the production of vitamin K–dependent clotting factors (II, VII, IX, X) and proteins C and S	Inhibits thrombin	Inhibits factor X_a	Inhibits factor X_a	Inhibits factor X_a
Half-life	40 hours	12–72 hours, significantly prolonged in persons with renal impairment	5–9 hours, slightly prolonged in persons with renal impairment	8–15 hours, slightly prolonged in persons with renal impairment	8–10 hours
Onset of action	36–72 hours	2–3 hours	2 hours	3 hours	1–3 hours
Indications	Prophylaxis and treatment of persons with venous thromboembolism (both DVT and PE) and to reduce risk of recurrence	Treatment of individuals with venous thromboembolism (both DVT and PE) and to reduce risk of recurrence	Prophylaxis and treatment of persons with venous thromboembolism (both DVT and PE) and to reduce risk of recurrence	Prophylaxis of DVT following hip or knee replacement surgery	FDA approved in January 2015 for treatment of persons with DVT, PE, and nonvalvular atrial fibrillation
Dose	Individual-dependent dose administered once daily	150 mg 2 times/day	Treatment of individuals with DVT/PE: 15 mg 2 times/day with food for the first 21 days, then 20 mg once daily with food for the duration of treatment Prophylaxis: 10 mg once daily	Prophylaxis: 2.5 mg twice daily, with the first dose taken 12–24 hours after surgery	30–60 mg once daily
Contraindications	Numerous	Pathological bleeding; hypersensitivity reaction; mechanical heart valves	Pathological bleeding; hypersensitivity reaction	Pathological bleeding; hypersensitivity reaction	Pathological bleeding
Pregnancy and breastfeeding	Avoid use in pregnancy; may be used during breastfeeding	Safe for use during pregnancy; avoid during breastfeeding (no adequate studies)	Safe for use during pregnancy; avoid during breastfeeding (no adequate studies)	Safe for use during pregnancy; avoid during breastfeeding (no adequate studies)	

(*continues*)

Table 16-8 Comparison of Oral Anticoagulants for Treatment of Persons with Venous Thromboembolism (*continued*)

Feature	Warfarin (Coumadin)	Target-Specific Anticoagulants			
		Dabigatran (Pradaxa)	Rivaroxaban (Xarelto)	Apixaban (Eliquis)	Edoxaban (Savaysa)
Drug interactions	Numerous—CYP3A4, CYP2C9, CYP1A2 inhibitors	Avoid with strong P-glycoprotein inducers or inhibitors	Avoid with drugs that are P-glycoprotein and strong CYP3A4 inhibitors, HIV protease drugs, antimycotics Use caution with rifampin, phenytoin, carbamazepine, and phenobarbital	Avoid with drugs that are P-glycoprotein and strong CYP3A4 inhibitors, HIV protease drugs, antimycotics Use caution with cimetidine, SSRIs, and diltiazem	Strong P-glycoprotein inhibitors
Adverse drug reactions	Bleeding, hemorrhage Rare: skin necrosis, purple toe syndrome	Bleeding; gastrointestinal—dyspepsia, gastritis	Bleeding, musculoskeletal events	Bleeding	Bleeding and anemia
Major bleeding	1.8%	0.3–0.9%	0.7%	0.1–0.3%	
Monitoring	INR	Nothing specific; may consider periodic monitoring of CBC	Nothing specific; may consider periodic monitoring of CBC	Nothing specific; may consider periodic monitoring of CBC	
Reversal	Vitamin K, fresh frozen plasma, recombinant factor VII_a	No reversal agent	No reversal agent	No reversal agent	No reversal agent

Abbreviations: CBC = complete blood count; DVT = deep vein thrombosis; HIV = human immunodeficiency virus; INR = International Normalized Ratio; PE = pulmonary embolism; SSRI = selective serotonin reuptake inhibitor.

Sources: Data from Ageno W, Gallus AS, Wittkowsky A, Crowther M, Hylek EM, Palareti G. Oral anticoagulant therapy: antithrombotic therapy and prevention of thrombosis, 9th ed.: American College of Chest Physicians evidence-based clinical practice guidelines. *Chest*. 2012;141(2 suppl): e44S-e88S[44]; Di Nisio M, Middeldorp S, Buller HR. Direct thrombin inhibitors. *N Engl J Med*. 2005;353:1028-1040[43]; Dobesh PP, Fanikos J. New oral anticoagulants for the treatment of venous thromboembolism: understanding differences and similarities. *Drugs*. 2014;74:2015-2032[46]; Mahan CE. Practical aspects of treatment with target specific anticoagulants: initiation, payment and current market, transitions, and venous thromboembolism treatment. *J Thromb Thrombolysis*. 2015;39(3):295-303[45]; Devabhakthuni S, Yoon C, Pincus KJ. Review of the target-specific oral anticoagulants in development for treatment and prevention of venous thromboembolism. *J Pharm Pract*. 2015;1:1-15.[47]

used for this purpose. As is the case for many of the drugs used today, the origins of its use as a human therapy begin with observations of animal diseases. In the early 1920s, cattle in the United States and Canada began to hemorrhage following ingestion of moldy sweet clover hay. The etiology of the agent in the moldy hay that caused the cattle to become deficient in prothrombin remained a mystery until the 1940s, when chemists at the University of Wisconsin were able to isolate the active chemical. A few years after it was on the market as a pesticide, warfarin was found to be effective in preventing thrombosis and embolism.

Warfarin is the only oral vitamin K antagonist anticoagulant available in the United States and is used extensively for treatment of persons with VTE or PE, and long-term prevention of venous thrombi formation. Warfarin disrupts the biosynthesis of four vitamin K–dependent coagulation factors (factors II, VII, IX, and X), which blocks activation of the tissue factor pathway, contact pathway, and common coagulation pathway. It also inhibits the synthesis of the vitamin K–dependent protein S and protein C.

Warfarin prevents the synthesis of new vitamin K–dependent clotting factors but has no effect on the factors currently in circulation, which accounts for the delay in its anticoagulant effect. This drug requires 4 to 5 days for the peak antithrombotic effects to develop. The vitamin K–dependent clotting factors inhibited by warfarin have varying half-lives, with factor II having the longest half-life, up to 72 hours. To ensure that the anticoagulant effect of warfarin has reached its full extent, overlap with a parenteral anticoagulant is required for the first 5 days of treatment. If the parenteral anticoagulant is discontinued prematurely, adequate protection of warfarin against recurrent VTE may not be realized, even if the therapeutic range is reached in the first few days of therapy.

Warfarin is continued for at least 3 to 6 months to prevent recurrence of a thrombosis that is secondary to a nonrecurring event (e.g., surgery). Individuals who are receiving treatment for idiopathic (i.e., no precipitating cause identified) DVT or pulmonary embolism and those who have an irreversible risk factor (e.g., an inherited thrombophilia) are usually prescribed warfarin for at least 6 to 12 months and then evaluated for the need for ongoing treatment. Individuals who have experienced two or more venous thromboembolisms are typically candidates for chronic warfarin treatment.

Box 16-2 Why Is SM's INR High?

SM is a 34-year-old female (5′ 7″, 170 lb [77.3 kg], BMI 26.6 kg/m^2) who presented to the emergency room with warmth, redness, and swelling in her left lower extremity. SM has no significant past medical history or family history. Her only current medication is ethinyl estradiol 30 mcg/drospirenone 3 mg combined oral contraceptive (COC), 1 pill daily.

SM is diagnosed with DVT. Her baseline screening for coagulopathies reveals that she is heterozygous for factor V Leiden. SM is started on enoxaparin 120 mg daily (1.5 mg/kg/day treatment dose for DVT) for immediate treatment and warfarin 7.5 mg daily. She continues on this regimen for 5 days, at which point her INR is 2.1. At this time, enoxaparin is discontinued and warfarin is continued at 7.5 mg daily. SM is followed up in the anticoagulation clinic and her INR values are monitored for 2 to 4 months.

Two months after the DVT diagnosis, SM develops a urinary tract infection and is given trimethoprim–sulfamethoxazole 160/800 mg (Bactrim) to be taken 2 times per day for 3 days. On the last day of therapy for the urinary tract infection, her INR is in the supratherapeutic range (e.g., 4.1). SM is counseled to withhold one dose of warfarin. One week later, her INR is in the therapeutic range.

SM was appropriately started on parenteral and oral anticoagulation therapy for the diagnosis of DVT. She will no longer be able to take a combined oral contraceptive due to the presence of mutations in her factor V Leiden, which cause a hypercoagulable state that could be exacerbated by combination oral contraceptives. Since SM is of childbearing age, she and her clinician reviewed options for contraception during the period of anticoagulation. She is aware that warfarin is teratogenic and understands the duration of action of the drug. She chose a copper intrauterine device for her contraceptive. The culprit for increasing SM's INR in August was with trimethoprim–sulfamethoxazole, which has a known drug–drug interaction with warfarin.

Management of persons taking warfarin can be complex (as noted in Box 16-2) and may be handled by special anticoagulation clinics. Computer-based dosing algorithms are often used. Although primary care providers may care for persons using warfarin, specialists usually initiate and oversee warfarin dosing and monitoring. The text in this chapter presents an overview of this complicated drug.

Pharmacokinetics

Warfarin is able to pass through cell membranes with relative ease and is readily absorbed from the intestines. Once in the blood, this agent becomes extensively (99%) bound to plasma albumin. The drug has a half-life of 36 to 48 hours and is metabolized in the liver via CYP450 enzymes. Anticoagulant effects will continue up to 5 days after discontinuation of the drug due to its long half-life.

Warfarin has a narrow therapeutic range. In addition, the activity and metabolism of this drug are highly variable from one person to another, which makes achieving a therapeutic level often difficult in clinical practice.[47,48] The etiology of this variability in action is partially genetic. Warfarin is actually a **racemic mixture** of *R*- and *S*-warfarin. *S*-warfarin has more anticoagulant activity than does *R*-warfarin, and the two are metabolized by different CYP450 enzymes within the liver. *S*-warfarin is metabolized by CYP2C9, and polymorphisms in CYP2C9 (specifically CYP2C9*2 and CYP2C9*3) explain many of the differences in clinical response to warfarin. These CYP2C9 variants are found in approximately 10% to 20% of Caucasians and African Americans. Polymorphisms in the gene *VKORC1*, which encodes for vitamin K function, also affect warfarin activity, and differences in this gene also contribute to genetic variation. The frequency of the variant *VKORC1* gene is approximately 80% in Asians.

In 2007, the FDA approved a label change for warfarin that provides information about how the drug's pharmacokinetics are altered in persons with specific genetic polymorphisms. Healthcare providers are not required to perform genetic testing prior to initiating warfarin therapy, but these tests are available and are increasingly being used in instances where attaining a therapeutic INR has proved elusive. Genetic testing may help offer guidance on initial dosing as well; however, these tests can be expensive and the information that they provide is not always timely.[48]

Side Effects/Adverse Effects

The most common and significant adverse drug reaction with warfarin is both minor and major bleeding. Indeed, warfarin's label carries an FDA black box warning that the drug can cause major or fatal bleeding. If uncontrolled bleeding develops, warfarin should be immediately discontinued. Although bleeding can be a complication of anticoagulation therapy, severe bleeding is infrequent. Possible signs of bleeding other than bright red bleeding include dark, tarry stool and minor bleeding at the gums during oral hygiene.

Warfarin can cause an immediate hypersensitivity reaction, including anaphylaxis. Adverse effects other than hemorrhage and drug–drug interactions are relatively infrequent, however. A small dose (2.5 mg orally) of vitamin K can compete with warfarin and reverse the warfarin-induced inhibition of clotting factor biosynthesis, thus making it a useful treatment for warfarin overdose; however, unless clinically significant bleeding occurs or urgent reversal is needed, one or more doses of warfarin be initially withheld, depending on the degree of INR elevation.

Contraindications

Warfarin is contraindicated in individuals with impaired liver activity secondary to alcoholism, because the vitamin K deficiency common in persons with impaired liver function increases this drug's anticoagulant effect. Other contraindications include history of hemorrhagic stroke, known hypersensitivity to warfarin, pregnancy (except for women with a mechanical heart valve), threatened abortion, history of blood dyscrasias, planned optic or central nervous system surgery, malignant hypertension, active bleeding, history of falls, and inability to adhere to therapy.

Dosing

Initial dosing for warfarin is typically between 5 and 10 mg daily; however, starting doses of less than 5 mg might be warranted in elderly individuals; in persons with impaired nutrition/albumin status, chronic liver disease, or congestive heart failure; when high risk of bleeding exists; and when interacting drugs are present. Because initial dosing requirements can be difficult to predict, several published dosing algorithms, computer programs, and other resources can help offer guidance, as noted in the Resources table at the end of this chapter.

Clinical Management

The two most common methods for monitoring therapeutic actions of warfarin are calculation of prothrombin time (PT; normal value = 12 seconds) and the International Normalized Ratio (INR). The therapeutic range for INR is between 2.0 and 3.0, with a target INR of 2.5. If an individual taking warfarin has an INR value greater than or less than the desired value, the dose of warfarin can be altered to bring the INR into the therapeutic range.

It is usually recommended that individuals not change between brands of warfarin because different formulations may have differing bioavailability, despite their generic equivalency. If a change in brand of warfarin becomes necessary due to availability or for formulary purposes, increased monitoring during the first several days to weeks after the switch can help detect a subsequent change in INR due to the new formulation.

Drug–Drug Interactions

Warfarin has an extensive collection of drug–drug, drug–food, and drug–herb interactions. Some of the more common interactions are listed in Table 16-9. Certain

Table 16-9 Drug–Drug Interactions Associated with Warfarin[a]

Drugs That Increase Anticoagulation Effect: Generic (Brand)	Drugs That Decrease Anticoagulation Effect: Generic (Brand)
Acetaminophen (Tylenol) in quantities > 2 g daily	Alcohol
Allopurinol (Zyloprim)	Antacids (if administered close to warfarin; separate administration by several hours)
Amiodarone (Cordarone)	Antihistamines
Androgens	Azathioprine (Imuran)
Aspirin	Barbiturates
Cephalosporins, second and third generation	Carbamazepine (Tegretol)
Cimetidine (Tagamet)	Cholestyramine (Questran)
Ciprofloxacin (Cipro), Levofloxacin (Levaquin)	Clozapine (Clozaril)
Disulfiram (Antabuse)	Dicloxacillin (Dynapen)
Dong Quai	Diuretics
Erythromycin (E-Mycin)	Estrogens
Fish oil	Griseofulvin (Grifulvin V)
Fluconazole (Diflucan)	Nafcillin (Unipen)
Fluorouracil (Efudex, Fluoroplex)	Oral contraceptives
Fluoxetine (Prozac)	Phenobarbital (Luminal)
Gingko	Phenytoin (Dilantin)
Ginseng	Rifampin (Rifadin)
Glucagon	Secobarbital (Seconal)
Isoniazid (INH)	Spironolactone (Aldactone)
Metronidazole (Flagyl)	St. John's wort
Omeprazole (Prilosec)	Sucralfate (Carafate)
Sertraline (Zoloft)	Trazodone
St. John's wort	Vitamin C, high doses
Sulfonamides	Vitamin K
Tamoxifen (Nolvadex)	
Tetracycline	
Trimethoprim–sulfamethoxazole (Bactrim)	

[a] This table is not comprehensive as new information is being generated on a regular basis. More common examples are included for reference.

drugs may increase or decrease the anticoagulant effects of warfarin, thereby increasing the potential for hemorrhage or thrombosis, respectively. Some drugs may increase warfarin effects by displacing warfarin from albumin or inhibiting hepatic warfarin metabolism, whereas other drugs may decrease warfarin effects by reversing the inhibition of clotting factor biosynthesis or increasing hepatic warfarin metabolism. In addition, warfarin can affect the metabolism of other drugs. For example, the metabolism of hypoglycemic agents and anticonvulsants is decreased when these agents are taken with warfarin, which can lead to toxic effects. Awareness of these interactions are important for primary care providers.

Approximately 17% to 26% of persons who take warfarin use herbal supplements,[49] and in one study of 17,861 persons on warfarin, 68% were prescribed at least one agent that interacts with warfarin.[50] Unfortunately, drug information references are not always consistent with the information discussed regarding drug–drug interactions with warfarin. In one review, some of the major drug information databases were compared to the information provided in the product labeling by the manufacturer; 648 drug–drug interactions with warfarin were listed in total across four sources, but only 50 were common to all sources. When in doubt, it is recommended that providers check more than one drug information reference.[50]

Drug–Food Interactions

In addition to use of other drugs, diet, smoking, and alcohol affect the metabolism and biologic activity of warfarin. Avoidance of alcohol is recommended while using any anticoagulant, but especially warfarin. Cigarette smoking has been shown to increase warfarin requirements via modification of cytochrome P450 CYP1A2 metabolism. Similarly, smoking cessation typically results in decreased warfarin dosing requirements.[52] In addition to cigarette smoking, marijuana is a commonly used substance that may alter warfarin dosing requirements.[53]

The amount of vitamin K in one's diet can significantly impact the effect of warfarin. Individuals are counseled to stay on a regular diet without changing the proportions or types of food ingested. Table 16-10 identifies the vitamin K content in some common foods. Vitamin K content of foods is also available from the U.S. Department of Agriculture (USDA), which provides food composition lists, and in charts noted in the Resources listed at the end of this chapter. Green, leafy vegetables (e.g., spinach, broccoli, kale, collard greens) tend to contain the largest amounts of vitamin K. However, even high amounts of vitamin K are acceptable and can be accounted for in the treatment plan for persons taking warfarin.

Table 16-10 Vitamin K Content of Selected Foods[a]

High Vitamin K Content (≥ 25 mcg per serving size of ½ cup to 1 cup)	Moderate Vitamin K Content (10–24 mcg per serving size of ½ cup to 1 cup)	Low Vitamin K Content (0–9 mcg per serving size of ½ cup to 1 cup)
Apple peel, green	Alfalfa seeds	Alcoholic beverages
Asparagus: canned, cooked, frozen	Apple peel, red	Apple juice
Avocado, peeled	Apple pie	Apple sauce
Beans: snap, raw	Artichokes	Apples: gala, golden delicious, red delicious
Blueberries	Beans: kidney	Bacon
Broccoli	Beans: snap	Bagel
Brussels sprouts[b]	Blackberries	Banana
Cabbage	Bread stuffing	Barley
Cabbage: Chinese	Carrots	Beans: baked, pinto, white
Coleslaw	Cauliflower	Beef
Collard greens[b]	Celery	Biscuits
Cow peas	Chicken	Burrito
Cucumber skin, raw	Grapes	Butter
Endive, raw[b]	Leeks	Cake
Fish: tuna in oil	Lentils	Candy
Kale[b]	Margarine	Cereals
Lettuce: red leaf[b]	Miso	Cheese
Mayonnaise	Orange	Chicken
Nuts: pine, pistachio	Peppers: green, boiled	Cookies
Okra	Pies	Corn
Parsley[b]	Plums	Dairy products
Peas	Raspberries	Eggs
Prunes	Potatoes	Fish
Spinach	Salad dressing	Fruit: melons, peaches, pears
Swiss chard[b]	Tomatoes	Ham
Tea		Melons
Turnip greens		Milk
		Pasta
		Potatoes
		Rice

[a] This list is not comprehensive. The vitamin K content of most foods, including most brand packaged foods, can be found in charts that are available from the USDA food composition lists.

[b] These foods have very high amounts of vitamin K (≥ 200 mcg).

The Role of Vitamin K

Vitamin K is essential for the formation of several clotting factors and anticoagulant proteins. Two forms of vitamin K, phylloquinone (vitamin K_1) and menaquinone (vitamin K_2), are normally absorbed in the intestine in the presence of bile salts. These precursors of vitamin K are ubiquitous in most diets (Table 16-10) and are also produced by the bacteria that inhabit the intestines. Deficiency is extremely rare, except in the case of newborns, who do not have intestinal flora at the time of birth. The chapter *The Newborn* reviews the use of vitamin K therapy for newborns. Vitamin K deficiency can also occur if the bile is obstructed or if its action is blocked by warfarin (Coumadin), other drugs that are vitamin K antagonists (e.g., anticonvulsants, antibiotics, isoniazid [INH]), parenchymal liver diseases such as cirrhosis, or malabsorption syndromes.

Vitamin K can be administered intravenously, intramuscularly, or orally. The intravenous formulation AquaMephyton is used for newborns to prevent hemorrhagic disease of the newborn. The American College of Chest Physicians publishes recommendations for vitamin K therapy if persons on anticoagulant therapy have an INR that is higher than therapeutic values.[54] After one oral dose of vitamin K, concentrations of blood coagulation factors increase in approximately 6 to 12 hours. Oral formulations of vitamin K are recommended for pregnant women who need to take an anticonvulsant agent (e.g., phenytoin [Dilantin]) and for individuals on long-term isoniazid therapy.

Target-Specific Oral Anticoagulants: Direct Thrombin Inhibitors

Direct thrombin inhibitors (DTIs) are a new class of oral anticoagulants that bind to thrombin. Dabigatran (Pradaxa) is currently the only DTI on the market in the United States, although additional agents are under study. Direct thrombin inhibitors offer greater convenience relative to warfarin for anticoagulation, as no regularly required monitoring or dosage adjustment is required with these agents. However, there are also no currently available reversal agents for DTIs in the case of overdose or bleeding.

The FDA has approved dabigatran for prophylaxis and treatment of individuals with DVT and PE. Clinical trials data indicate that it has similar efficacy and safety to warfarin for these indications.[55,56]

Target-Specific Oral Anticoagulants: Factor X_a Inhibitors

Rivaroxaban (Xarelto), apixaban (Eliquis), and edoxaban (Savaysa) are newer oral anticoagulant agents that work by inhibiting factor X_a. Rivaroxaban may be used for prophylaxis or treatment of women with venous thromboembolism; apixaban is currently approved for prophylaxis during elective hip or knee replacement surgeries. Additional factor X_a inhibitors are under study for use as anticoagulants.

Like direct thrombin inhibitors, factor X_a inhibitors offer greater consumer convenience than warfarin in that their use does not require regular laboratory monitoring and dosage adjustment beyond the manufacturer's standard dosage recommendations. Also similar to DTIs, there are no currently available reversal agents in the case of bleeding or if an overdose occurs with a factor X_a inhibitor.

Special Populations: Pregnancy, Lactation, and the Elderly

Coagulation disorders are more likely to occur during pregnancy, and some special considerations apply to drug treatment during pregnancy. Pregnant women have a 5-fold increased risk for VTE compared to nonpregnant women, and this risk increases to 20-fold or greater in the postpartum period.[57] Pregnant women who have an inherited or acquired thrombophilia are at a greater risk for thrombosis beyond the background-increased risk associated with pregnancy. Women at high risk for DVT and PE who are candidates for prenatal treatment with an anticoagulant are generally treated with LMWH because of these heparins' favorable effectiveness and safety profile.[35,57] Unfractionated heparin or fondaparinux can also be used.

Warfarin (Coumadin) crosses the placenta and can cause spontaneous abortion; multiple birth defects, such as central nervous system abnormalities and urinary tract abnormalities; fetal growth restriction; and stillbirth. Gross malformations, CNS defects, fetal bleeding, and fetal mortality have all been attributed to maternal warfarin use. Thus, warfarin is contraindicated during pregnancy, although it can be used by women who are breastfeeding.

Relatively little is known about the effects of the newer oral anticoagulant drugs during pregnancy or lactation. Given the insufficient data, they are not recommended for use.

The risk for thromboembolism also increases as one ages. Management of VTE or PE in elderly women can be complicated by considerations regarding the use of other medications for comorbid conditions. In particular, renal or liver impairment can significantly impact the metabolism of anticoagulant drugs.

Conclusion

Erythropoiesis and the coagulation cascade play a vital role in complete understanding of hematologic disorders. Making an accurate diagnosis, selecting the most appropriate drug, and developing an overall treatment regimen depend on knowledge of the pharmacodynamic properties of drugs used to treat these disorders (anemias as well as venous thromboembolism), the drugs' adverse-effect profiles, evidence-based guidelines for management, and overall condition of the individual. Drug therapy, whether for prophylaxis or treatment, is adjusted based on recommended monitoring parameters and individual tolerance to the drug. As additional drug therapies become available, especially for managing anticoagulation, it will be important to consider patient-specific factors when selecting drug therapies. Understanding the etiology and pathophysiology of anemias and coagulopathies, combined with appropriate diagnosis and pharmacologic selection, will help persons with hematologic disorders achieve optimal outcomes.

Resources

Organization	Description	Website
American College of Chest Physicians (ACCP)	Provides 2012 guidelines for anticoagulant therapy as well as resources for managing warfarin (Coumadin)	www.chestnet.org/Guidelines-and-Resources/Guidelines-and-Consensus-Statements/Antithrombotic-Guidelines-9th-Ed
Coumadin website	Website maintained by the manufacturer of warfarin that lists the vitamin K content in foods as well as drug–drug interactions with warfarin	www.coumadin.com/pdf/Foods_With_VitaminK.pdf
Warfarin Dosing	Website maintained by the Washington University Medical Center and the National Institutes of Health, which offers an algorithm for choosing a dose of warfarin that includes pharmacogenomic information, INR levels, and other factors	www.warfarindosing.org/Source/Home.aspx
American Heart Association (AHA)	Joint professional guidelines for use of all antithrombotic drugs can be found at this website sponsored by the AHA	Myamericanheart.org/professional/StatementGuidelines/ByTopic
Apps		
Vitamin K-iNutrient Vitamins K1, K1D, and K2	App for identifying the amount of vitamin K in foods	https://itunes.apple.com/us/app/vitamin-k-inutrient-vitamins/id393118621?mt=8
Warfarin Guide	Produced by Joshua Steinberg, MD. Steinberg has devised several evidence-based apps that are offered for free on the iTunes site. This app offers resources for warfarin management, including INR targets, and summarizes treatment duration guidelines from the ACCP.	https://itunes.apple.com/us/app/warfaringuide/id403959804?mt=8

References

1. Muno M, Vilar I, Garcia-Erce JA. An update on iron physiology. *World J Gastroenterol.* 2009;15(37):4617-4626.
2. Waldvogel-Abramowski S, Waeber G, Gassner C, et al. Physiology of iron metabolism. *Transfusion Med Hemotherap.* 2014;41(3):213-221.
3. Garratty G. Immune hemolytic anemia associated with drug therapy. *Blood Rev.* 2010;24:143.
4. Arndt PA, Garratty G. The changing spectrum of drug-induced immune hemolytic anemia. *Semin Hematol.* 2005;42:137.
5. Andersohn F, Konze C, Garbe E. Systematic review: agranulocytosis induced by nonchemotherapy drugs. *Ann Intern Med.* 2007;146(9):657-665.
6. Aster RH. Adverse drug reactions affecting blood cells. *Handb Exp Pharmacol.* 2010;196:57-76.
7. Youngster I, Arcavi L, Schechmaster R, et al. Medication and glucose-6-phosphate-dehydrogenase: an evidence-based review. *Drug Saf.* 2010;107(3):737-741.
8. DeLoughery TG. Microcytic anemia. *N Engl J Med.* 2014;371:1324.
9. Camaschella C. Iron-deficiency anemia. *N Engl J Med.* 2015; 372:1832-1843.
10. Keating GM. Ferric carboxymaltose: a review of its use in iron deficiency. *Drugs.* 2015;75(1):101-127.
11. Chertow GM, Mason PD, Vaage-Nilsen O, Ahlmen J. Update on adverse drug events associated with parenteral iron. *Nephrol Dial Transplant.* 2006;21:378.
12. Kaferle J, Strzoda CE. Evaluation of macrocytosis. *Am Fam Physician.* 2009;79(3):203-208.
13. Centers for Disease Control and Prevention. Recommendations to improve preconception health and health care—United States: a report of the CDC/ATSDR Preconception Care Work Group and the Select Panel on Preconception Care. *MMWR.* April 6, 2006. http://www.cdc.gov/mmwr/preview/mmwrhtml/rr5506a1.htm. Accessed June 13, 2014.
14. Oh RC, Brown DL. Vitamin B_{12} deficiency. *Am Fam Physician.* 2003;67:979-986.
15. Stabler SP. Vitamin B_{12} deficiency. *N Engl J Med.* 2013:368(2):149-160.
16. Lin J, Keisberg G, Safranek S. Is high-dose oral B_{12} a safe and effective alternative to a B_{12} injection? *J Fam Pract.* 2012:61(3):162-163.
17. Risitano AM. Aplastic anemia: alternative immunosuppressive treatments and eltrombopag: a report from the 2014 EBMT Educational Meeting from the

Severe Aplastic Anaemia and Infectious Diseases Working Parties. *Curr Drug Targets.* January 25, 2015. Epub ahead of print.

18. Riddel JP, Aouizerat BE, Miaskowski C, Lillicrap DP. Theories of blood coagulation. *J Pediatr Oncol Nurs.* 2007;24:123-131.
19. Goodnough LT, Schrier SL. Evaluation and management of anemia in the elderly. *Am J Hematol.* 2014; 89(1):88-96.
20. Madigan C, Malik M. Pathophysiology and therapy for hemoglobinopathies. Part 1: sickle cell disease. *Expert Rev Mol Med.* 2006;8:1-23.
21. Coates TD. Physiology and pathophysiology of iron in hemoglobin-associated diseases. *Free Rad Biol Med.* 2014;72:23-40.
22. Berdoukas V, Farmaki K, Wood JC, Coates T. Iron chelation in thalassemia: time to reconsider our comfort zones. *Expert Rev Hematol.* 2011;4:17-26.
23. Dolberg OJ, Levy Y. Idiopathic aplastic anemia: diagnosis and classification. *Autoimmun Rev.* 2014:12; 569-573.
24. Boudoulas KD, Montague CR, Goldschmidt-Clermont PJ, Cooke GE. Estradiol increases platelet aggregation in Pl(A1/A1) individuals. *Am Heart J.* 2006;152(1):136-139.
25. Hoffman M, Monroe DM. Coagulation 2006: a modern view of hemostasis. *Hematol Oncol Clin.* 2007;21:1111.
26. Rodeghiero F. Management of menorrhagia in women with inherited bleeding disorders: general principles and use of desmopressin. *Haemophilia.* 2008;14 (suppl 1):21-30.
27. Nichols WL, Hultin MB, James AH, et al. von Willebrand disease (VWD): evidence-based diagnosis and management guidelines: the National Heart, Lung, and Blood Institute.
28. (NHLBI) Expert Panel report (USA). *Haemophilia.* 2008;14(2):171-232.
29. Favaloro EJ. Von Willebrand disease and platelet disorders. *Hemophilia.* 2014;20(suppl 4):59-64.
30. Kouides PA, Byams VR, Philipp CS, et al. Multisite management study of menorrhagia with abnormal laboratory haemostasis: a prospective crossover study of intranasal desmopressin and oral tranexamic acid. *Br J Haematol.* 2009;145:212.
31. Ray S, Ray A. Non-surgical interventions for treating heavy menstrual bleeding (menorrhagia) in women with bleeding disorders. *Cochrane Database Syst Rev.* 2014;11:CD010338. doi:10.1002/14651858.CD010338.pub2.
32. Huq FY, Kadir RA. Management of pregnancy, labor, and delivery in women with inherited bleeding disorders. *Hemophilia.* 2011;17(suppl 1):20-30.
33. Heit JA. The epidemiology of venous thromboembolism in the community. *Arterios Thromb Vascul Biol.* 2008;28:370-376.
34. Goldhaber SZ. Risk factors for venous thromboembolism. *J Am Coll Cardiol.* 2010;56(1):1.
35. Kahn SR, Lim W, Dunn AS, et al. Prevention of VTE in nonsurgical patients: antithrombotic therapy and prevention of thrombosis, 9th ed.: American College of Chest Physicians evidence-based clinical practice guidelines. *Chest.* 2012;141(2 suppl):e195S-e226S.
36. Bates SM, Greer IA, Middledorp S, Veenstra DL, Prabulos AM, Vanvik PO. VTE, thrombophilia, antithrombotic therapy, and pregnancy: antithrombotic therapy and prevention of thrombosis, 9th ed.: American College of Chest Physicians evidence-based clinical practice guidelines. *Chest.* 2012;141 (2 suppl):e691S-e736S.
37. Pomp ER, Rosendaal FR, Doggen CJ. Smoking increases the risk of venous thrombosis and acts synergistically with oral contraceptive use. *Am J Hematol.* 2008;83:97.
38. Kupferminc MJ. Thrombophilia and pregnancy. *Reprod Biol Endocrinol.* 2003;1:111.
39. Cushman M, Kuller LH, Prentice R, et al. Estrogen plus progestin and risk of venous thrombosis. *JAMA.* 2004;292:1573.
40. Garcia DA, Baglin TP, Weitz JI, Samama MM. Parenteral anticoagulants: antithrombotic therapy and prevention of thrombosis, 9th ed.: American College of Chest Physicians evidence-based clinical practice guidelines. *Chest.* 2012;141(2 suppl):e24S-e43S.
41. Wells PS, Anderson DR, Rodger MA, et al. A randomized trial comparing 2 low-molecular-weight heparins for the outpatient treatment of deep vein thrombosis and pulmonary embolism. *Arch Intern Med.* 2005; 165:733.
42. Linkins LA, Dans AL, Moores LK, et al. Treatment and prevention of heparin-induced thrombocytopenia: antithrombotic therapy and prevention of thrombosis, 9th ed.: American College of Chest Physicians evidence-based clinical practice guidelines. *Chest.* 2012;141(2 suppl):e495S-e530S.
43. Di Nisio M, Middeldorp S, Buller HR. Direct thrombin inhibitors. *N Engl J Med.* 2005;353:1028-1040.
44. Ageno W, Gallus AS, Wittkowsky A, Crowther M, Hylek EM, Palareti G. Oral anticoagulant therapy: antithrombotic therapy and prevention of thrombosis,

9th ed.: American College of Chest Physicians evidence-based clinical practice guidelines. *Chest.* 2012;141(2 suppl):e44S-e88S.

45. Mahan CE. Practical aspects of treatment with target specific anticoagulants: initiation, payment and current market, transitions, and venous thromboembolism treatment. *J Thromb Thrombolysis.* 2015; 39(3): 295-303.
46. Dobesh PP, Fanikos J. New oral anticoagulants for the treatment of venous thromboembolism: understanding differences and similarities. *Drugs.* 2014;74: 2015-2032.
47. Devabhakthuni S, Yoon C, Pincus KJ. Review of the target-specific oral anticoagulants in development for treatment and prevention of venous thromboembolism. *J Pharm Pract.* 2015;1:1-15.
48. Hill CE, Duncan A. Overview of the pharmacogenetics in anticoagulation therapy. *Clin Lab Med.* 2008; 28:513-524.
49. Gage BF, Eby C, Johnson JA, et al. Use of pharmacogenetic and clinical factors to predict the therapeutic dose of warfarin. *Clin Pharmacol Ther.* 2008;84(3)326-331.
50. Daugherty N, Smith KM. Dietary supplement and selected food interactions with warfarin. *Orthopedics.* 2006;29:309-314.
51. Snaith A, Pugh L, Simpson CR, McLay JS. The potential for interaction between warfarin and coprescribed medication: a retrospective study in primary care. *Am J Cardiovasc Drugs.* 2008;8(3):207-212.
52. Anthony M, Romero K, Malone DC, Hines LE, Higgins L, Woosley RL. Warfarin interactions with substances listed in the FDA-approved label for warfarin sodium. *Clin Pharmacol Ther.* 2009;86(4):425-429.
53. Nathisuwan S, Dilokthornsakul P, Chaiyakunapruk N, Morarai T, Yodting T, Piriyachananusorn N. Assessing evidence of interaction between smoking and warfarin: a systematic review and meta-analysis. *Chest.* 2011;139(5):1130-1139.
54. Yamreudeewong W, Wong HK, Brausch LM, Pulley KR. Probable interaction between warfarin and marijuana smoking. *Ann Pharmacother.* 2009;43:1347-1353.
55. Holbrook A, Scvhulman S, Witt DM, et al. Evidence-based management of anticoagulant therapy: anticoagulant therapy: antithrombotic therapy and prevention of thrombosis, 9th ed.: American College of Chest Physicians evidence-based clinical practice guidelines. *Chest* 2012;141(2 suppl):e152S-e184S.
56. Schulman S, Kakkar AK, Goldhaber SZ, et al.; RE-COVER II trial investigators. Treatment of acute venous thromboembolism with dabigatran or warfarin and pooled analysis. *Circulation.* December 16, 2013. http://circ.ahajournals.org/content/early/2013/12/10/CIRCULATIONAHA.113.004450. Accessed July 31, 2014.
57. Schulman S, Kearon C, Kakkar AK, et al.; RE-MEDY trial investigators; RE-SONATE trial investigators. Extended use of dabigatran, warfarin, or placebo in venous thromboembolism. *N Engl J Med.* 2013; 368:709-718.
58. Marshall AL. Diagnosis, treatment and prevention of venous thromboembolism in pregnancy. *Postgrad Med.* 2014;126(7):25-34.

17 Autoimmune Conditions

Rebekah L. Ruppe

Chapter Glossary

Aminosalicylates Salts of aminosalicylic acid that act as anti-inflammatories.

Antigen-presenting cells Any cells that digest an antigen and present a portion of it on the cell surface. B cells can turn into antigen-presenting cells.

Anti-inflammatory drugs Substances that suppress the body's inflammatory response.

Antimetabolites Substances that interfere with cell growth by competing with or replacing the endogenous metabolite involved in the physiologic process.

Biologic agents Relatively new subclass within the category of disease-modifying antirheumatic drugs. These agents are synthetic drugs engineered to behave like natural immune system proteins.

Disease-modifying antirheumatic drugs (DMARDs) This term refers to a group of medications that decrease pain and/or prevent joint damage in persons with rheumatoid arthritis. They are often grouped together in contrast to anti-inflammatory agents, which reduce inflammation but do not prevent disease progression.

Glucocorticoids Adrenocortical steroid hormones with general anti-inflammatory properties.

Immunomodulator drugs Substances that modify the immune system response by competing with or mimicking the action of immune cells or products involved in the immune process.

Immunosuppressant drugs Substances that diminish immune system activity by blocking or inhibiting the function of immune cells or products involved in the immune process.

Interferons (IFNs) Glycoproteins produced by immune cells in response to pathogen exposure that regulate immune response.

Interleukins (ILs) Cytokines that are produced by white blood cells—hence the name *leukin.*

Monoclonal antibodies Antibodies cloned from a single cell, typically originating from mice, that has been exposed to a specific antigen to induce production of the desired antibody.

Pegylation Polyethylene glycol conjugation is a modification of a drug whereby PEG molecules are attached to a parent drug in specific configurations. The result is a macromolecule that because of its size has altered pharmacokinetic and pharmacodynamic properties. It improves solubility, prolongs bioavailability, slows clearance, and reduces immunogenicity.

Overview of Autoimmune Disorders

Immune system disorders can be categorized into one of three groups: (1) inflammatory diseases, in which hypersensitivity reactions cause organ or cell damage; (2) immunologic deficiency disorders, which result from a genetic or acquired deficiency in a component of the immune system; and (3) autoimmune disorders, in which autoantibodies that cause damage are generated from an aberrant immune response. Autoimmune disorders are categorized as one of two types: those that cause systemic damage to many organs (e.g., systemic lupus erythematosus [SLE]) and those that cause damage to one organ (e.g., diabetes). This chapter addresses the most common systemic autoimmune disorders. Pharmacotherapy for diabetes and thyroid disorders is addressed in specific chapters on those conditions.

While the etiology of autoimmune disorders remains unknown, it is widely accepted that both genetic and environmental factors play a role in their development. Studies of multiplex families, twin concordance, and geographic clusters suggest a variable but likely relationship between genes and environment in the pathology of autoimmune disorders.[1] Evidence indicates that inherited protein deficiencies or mutations in genes involved in immune response and regulation can increase a person's predisposition to autoimmune disorders. Specific susceptibility genes have been located in alleles of the major histocompatibility complex, which is the most gene-dense area located on the mammalian genome. This area is found in the majority of vertebrates and is integral to competent immune system and reproductive success. Autoimmune disorders most likely require multiple susceptibility genes and environmental triggers to become manifest.[2] This chapter reviews the pharmacologic treatments for individuals who experience the most common autoimmune disorders observed among women.

Gender plays a significant role in the development of autoimmunity. More than 75% of individuals with autoimmune disorders are women—a finding that supports the hypothesis that sex hormones play a role in disease susceptibility. The majority of autoimmune disorders have a skewed female-to-male ratio that ranges from 2:1 to 3:1 in the case of rheumatoid arthritis (RA) and multiple sclerosis (MS) to as high as 9:1 in persons with SLE.[3,4] Other conditions, such as type 1 diabetes and inflammatory bowel disease (IBD), occur with similar frequencies in men and women.[4] This variation suggests that sex hormones modulate (rather than induce) autoimmunity, at least in regard to these conditions.

Pathophysiology of Autoimmune Disorders

A brief review of the components of the immune system referred to in this chapter can be found in the *Immunizations* chapter. A normal-functioning immune system relies on complex physiologic mechanisms that recognize and react to invading pathogens while remaining unresponsive to self-antigens. Autoimmunity occurs when these regulatory mechanisms break down and the immune system loses tolerance to proteins or antigens that are produced by the body itself. Autoimmune disorders result when the self-directed immunologic reaction causes tissue injury. The underlying pathophysiology is production of autoantibodies that cause an adverse reaction and/or initiation of a hypersensitivity reaction that causes organ damage. Both of these initiating events are the result of an aberrant immune response to an endogenous protein.

Figure 17-1 depicts the roles of B cells and T cells in initiating the immune response and highlights one of the theories that describes how an autoimmune disorder starts. In the figure, the B cell has attached to an antigen, processed that antigen, and then presented a piece of it on the surface of the B cell. This attracts a mature T cell to couple with the B cell. The T cell helps the B cell work via release of cytokines that encourage the B cell to proliferate. This process is mutually stimulating and can continue unchecked in autoimmune disorders. The end result is an inflammatory reaction and/or production of autoantibodies. In turn, the focus of therapy is interruption of one of the signals that perpetrate the aberrant immune response process.

Cytokines are the molecular messengers that control many of the steps in the immune response. These substances are produced and released by many of the immune system cells, and are broadly organized into pro-inflammatory or anti-inflammatory categories (Figure 17-2). Individual cytokines are categorized as **interferons (IFNs)**, **interleukins (ILs)**, or growth factors.

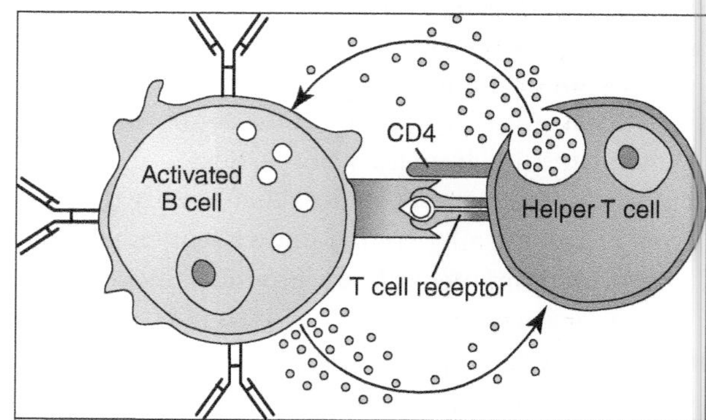

Figure 17-1 B-cell and T-cell interactions in immune system response.

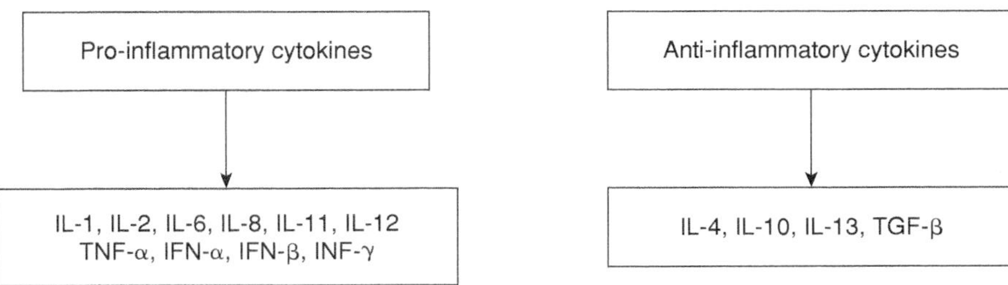

Figure 17-2 Cytokines.

Overview of Pharmacologic Agents Used to Treat Women with Autoimmune Disorders

Treatment for women with autoimmune disorders focuses on providing symptomatic relief and reducing disease progression. Pharmacologic approaches to therapy consist of three categories of agents:

- **Anti-inflammatory drugs**, which suppress nonspecific inflammatory cells (e.g., basophils, neutrophils, macrophages)
- **Immunosuppressant drugs**, which inhibit the cell and humoral-mediated immune response (T-cell and B-cell activation)
- **Biologic agents** and **immunomodulator drugs**, that manipulate specific interactions and responses within the immune system without necessarily suppressing overall activity

Different combinations of these three types of immune therapy are used to treat most autoimmune disorders. This section presents an initial overview of these drugs and their mechanisms of action. Anti-inflammatories are generally used to manage the care of individuals with mild disease states, with the use of glucocorticoids reserved for acute flares or symptomatic episodes. Immunosuppressant and immunomodulatory therapy may be used either for acute symptomatic treatment (induction of remission) or for ongoing treatment (maintenance therapy), depending on the disorder. Some therapies modify the natural course of disease and reduce disability; these disease-modifying therapies are used for management of some immune disorders even in persons who are asymptomatic. Many of these drugs are prescribed only by healthcare providers who are experienced in immunosuppressive therapy. Some are intramuscular or intravenous preparations that are only given in a healthcare setting that has facilities for managing complications. Thus, this overview for primary care providers reviews the mechanism of action and associated side effects and adverse effects. Readers who are interested in additional aspects of management will need further information and education.

Anti-inflammatory Drugs

Several different types of drugs have anti-inflammatory effects. Nonsteroidal anti-inflammatory drugs, glucocorticoids, and aminosalicylates each have a different mechanism of action in that they interupt the immune response at different biologic steps.

Glucocorticoids

Glucocorticoids (e.g., prednisone, methylprednisolone, budesonide) are potent anti-inflammatory agents that have direct effects on lymphoid cells (Table 17-1).[5–7] These agents mimic the endogenous steroid cortisol. Glucocorticoids reduce inflammation by binding to an intracellular glucocorticoid receptor. The activated receptor upregulates expression of anti-inflammatory factors and suppresses expression of pro-inflammatory proteins in the cytosol. Glucocorticoids inhibit lymphocyte proliferation and suppress the cell- and humoral-mediated immune response. In large doses, glucocorticoids reduce antibody production.[5] Glucocorticoids are categorized as short, intermediate, or long-acting.

Glucocorticoids have side effects and adverse effects that impact many organ systems. The most common side effects of glucocorticoids include hyperglycemia, weight gain and a Cushingoid appearance, anovulation, increased skin fragility, and impaired memory or attention deficits. Commonly noted adverse effects include osteoporosis, osteonecrosis, increased risk for fractures, adrenal

Table 17-1 Anti-inflammatory Drugs Commonly Used in the Treatment of Women with Autoimmune Conditions

Drug: Generic (Brand)	Indications	Side Effects/Adverse Effects	Precautions	Monitoring
Aminosalicylates				
Sulfasalazine (Azulfidine, Sulfadine)	IBD RA	Nausea, diarrhea, mouth ulcers, headache, fever, rash, hepatic impairment, myelosuppression, sulfa hypersensitivity reactions	Preexisting hepatic or renal impairment, glucose-6-phosphate dehydrogenase deficiency (G6PD)	CBC, LFTs evaluation at baseline CBC every 2–4 weeks for 3 months, then every 3 months
Glucocorticoids				
Prednisone (Deltasone), methylprednisolone (Medrol), budesonide (Entocort)	IBD RA SLE CIS	Weight gain, infection, fluid retention, hyperglycemia, hyperlipidemia, hypokalemia, osteoporosis, adrenal insufficiency, avascular necrosis femoral head, increased fracture risk, cataract	Preexisting osteoporosis or renal insufficiency, latent or active TB, recent vaccination	Blood pressure, glucose, potassium, total cholesterol evaluation at baseline Glucose dipstick every 3–6 months Bone density in high risk
Nonsteroidal Anti-inflammatories				
Ibuprofen (Motrin), naproxen (Aleve)	RA SLE	Gastrointestinal bleeding, hepatic toxicity, renal toxicity, hypertension	Preexisting renal insufficiency or liver disease, concomitant methotrexate use	CBC, creatinine LFTs evaluation at baseline CBC, LFTs yearly
5-Aminosalicylic acid (Asacol, Canasa, Colazal, Lialda, Pentasa, Rowasa)	IBD	Nausea, vomiting, headache, arthralgia, diarrhea, constipation, hepatic impairment Rare: leukopenia, acute nephritis	Current renal or hepatic impairment or history of renal disease	CBC, LFTs evaluation at baseline Consider creatinine monitoring for the first few weeks

Abbreviations: BP = blood pressure; CBC = complete blood count; CIS = clinically isolated syndrome (multiple sclerosis); IBD = inflammatory bowel disease; LFTs = liver function tests; RA = rheumatoid arthritis; SLE = systemic lupus erythematosus; UA = urinalysis.
Sources: Data from Goodin DS, Frohman EM, Garmany GP Jr, et al. Disease-modifying therapies in multiple sclerosis: report of the Therapeutics and Technology Assessment Subcommittee of the American Academy of Neurology and the MS Council for Clinical Practice Guidelines. *Neurology.* 2002;58(2):169-178. [Reaffirmed on July 19, 2008][7]; Lake DF, Briggs AD, Akporiaye ET. Immunopharmacology. In: Katzung BG, Masters SB, Trevor AJ, eds. *Basic and Clinical Pharmacology*. 13th ed. New York, NY/London, England: McGraw-Hill Medical; 2014:946-970[5]; Rhen T, Cidlowski JA. Anti-inflammatory action of glucocorticoids. *N Engl J Med.* 2005;353:1771-1723.[6]

insufficiency, myelosuppression, psychosis, and glaucoma. Thus, persons taking these medications need counseling and frequent follow-up.

Because these drugs suppress adrenal function, they must be tapered slowly upon discontinuation if used in high doses for more than a week.

Nonsteroidal Anti-inflammatory Drugs

The primary therapeutic action of nonsteroidal anti-inflammatory drugs (NSAIDs) in treating autoimmune disorders most likely involves the inhibition of prostaglandin synthesis and the downregulation of cytokine secretion. The chapter *Analgesia and Anesthesia* provides a thorough discussion of the pharmacotherapeutic actions, side effects, adverse effects, and drug–drug interactions associated with use of selective and nonselective NSAIDs.

Aminosalicylates

5-aminosalicylate acid (5-ASA) is an anti-inflammatory drug that has a topical effect on intestinal epithelium. 5-ASA is also called mesalamine (Apriso, Canasa, Pentasa) in the United States and mesalazine in European countries.

Though not entirely understood, the most likely mechanisms of action of the **aminosalicylates** relate to inhibition of interleukin 1 (IL-1) and tumor necrosis factor alpha (TNF-alpha) production; inhibition of the lipoxygenase pathway; and inhibition of nuclear factor kappa B (NF-κB) activation. NF-κB, which is normally found in the cytoplasm of all cells, controls transcription of many of the genes that initiate the inflammatory process. When this factor is inactivated, multiple inflammatory pathways are affected within both cell and humoral-mediated responses.[8]

Sulfasalazine (Azulfidine, Sulfadine) is the original combination product that includes 5-ASA. Sulfasalazine is a prodrug composed of sulfapyridine and 5-aminosalicylic acid (5-ASA). The drug is partially absorbed in the small intestine and broken down into its active sulfa and 5-ASA moieties in the colon. The 5-ASA is the therapeutic ingredient whereas most of the side effects are attributed to the sulfa portion. However, the sulfapyridine is added because 5-ASA is rapidly absorbed in the proximal gastrointestinal tract and does not get to the distal portions of the gastrointestinal where it is needed, on its own. Unfortunately, sulfa hypersensitivity reactions and side effects limit the use of sulfasalazine for many individuals.

Subsequent to the marketing of sulfasalazine, many different formulations of 5-ASA have been developed that prevent absorption of 5-ASA in the jejunum so that it can reach the ilium and colon. By changing the chemical structure of 5-ASA, direct delivery can be achieved. The newer sulfa-free 5-ASA formulations such as enteric-coated mesalamine (Asacol), olsalazine (Dipentum), balsalazide (Colazal) have similar effectiveness to sulfasalazine with fewer side effects.[8] Such drugs are delivered to specific areas of the GI tract depending on their preparation. Azo-bonded olsalazine and balsalazide are activated by bond-cleaving bacteria in the colon. Enteric-coated mesalamine disintegrates from the small bowel to the splenic fissure and is effective in treating ulcerative colitis and Crohn's disease involving the ileum or colon. Continuous-release mesalamine (Pentasa) delivers 5-ASA throughout the small bowel to the distal colon. Mesalamine multi-matrix formula (Lialda) utilizes a lipophilic/hydrophilic matrix combination with a pH-sensitive polymer coating that releases mesalamine in the colon. Mesalamine encapsulated granules (Apriso) are released in the terminal ileum and colon through the use of a proprietary extended-release mechanism.[8]

Sulfasalazine inhibits folic acid transport and therefore all persons taking this drug should also take 1 mg of folic acid per day to counteract this effect. The most common side effects of sulfasalazine are nausea, vomiting, headache, fever, and rash. Agranulocytosis is the most concerning adverse effect of sulfasalazine. If agranulocytosis occurs, it typically develops in the first 3 months of therapy.

Immunosuppressants

Immunosuppressant drugs inhibit or prevent T-cell and/or B-cell activity. Many drugs described in this chapter have immunosuppressant properties and the reader may find several different taxonomies for drugs used to treat autoimmune disorders. For the purposes of this chapter, immunosuppressant drugs refer to antimetabolites and other drugs that have immunosuppressant properties as their primary mechanism of action.

Antimetabolites

Antimetabolites are metabolite analogues that antagonize or inhibit the synthesis of nucleic acids. When nucleic acids that are essential components of RNA or DNA are not made, the proteins that the DNA and RNA code for likewise cannot be made. The three antimetabolites most commonly used for autoimmune therapy are azathioprine (Azasan, Imuran), leflunomide (Arava), and methotrexate (Rheumatrex, Trexall), (Table 17-2).[6,7]

Thiopurines

The two drugs in this class are azathioprine (Azasan, Imuran) and 6-mercaptopurine (Purinethol). Both are prodrugs of mercaptopurine, which is a synthetic analogue of purine and an inhibitor of purine synthesis. Purines are essential components of many biomolecules, including DNA and RNA. The inhibition of purine synthesis leads to decreased production of B cells and T cells. Via this mechanism of action, azathioprine inhibits cell- and humoral-mediated immune responses and is cytotoxic to stimulated lymph cells.[5]

Azathioprine is extensively metabolized and has both active and toxic metabolites. Thiopurine methyltransferase (TPMT) is the enzyme responsible for inactivating toxic metabolites of asathiopurine. Persons who have a polymorphism that makes them deficient in TPMT will have a toxic reaction to this drug such as myelosuppression or hematotoxicity. Likewise, persons who are heterozygous and have 50% enzyme activity, will tolerate half of a standard dose. The inicidence of TPMT deficiency is approximately 3 per 1000 individuals.[9] It is possible to test for TPMT and some authors recommend that all persons have this test done prior to initiating therapy with TPMT. Although genetic testing is not routine at this time, the product label for azathioprine states that genotyping for TPMT activity is available and FDA approved. Azathioprine can cause fetotoxic effects when taken during pregnancy and should not be used. Similarly, it is not recommended for use by breastfeeding women.

Side effects are relatively common. Azathioprine can cause flu-like symptoms, nausea, vomiting, and diarrhea in approximately 2% to 6.5% of recipients.[9] Adverse effects are less common and include an increased risk for infection, pancreatitis, hepatotoxicity, pancytopenia, leukopenia, thrombocytopenia, and anemia.[9] All persons who are exposed to thiopurines have a slight increased risk for subsequent development of a malignancy.

Leflunomide (Arava) and Teriflunomide (Aubagio)

Leflunomide (Arava) and its active metabolite, teriflunomide (Aubagio), inhibit the enzyme dihydroorotate dehydrogenase, which ultimately interferes with new pyrimidine synthesis, an effect that in turn prevents proliferation of activated T cells. The antiproliferative and anti-inflammatory effects of leflunomide (Arava) when used to

Table 17-2 Immunosuppressants Commonly Used to Treat Autoimmune Conditions

Drug: Generic (Brand)	Category and Indications	Side Effects/Adverse Effects	Precautions and Contraindications
Azathioprine (Azasan, Imuran)	Thiopurine that inhibits purine metabolism; used to treat MS and SLE	Rash, fever, nausea, vomiting, diarrhea, jaundice, myelosuppression, pancytopenia, liver dysfunction, lymphoproliferative disorders	Preexisting liver disease, allopurinol (increases risk of toxicity), thiopurine methyltransferase (TMPT) deficiency (increases risk of myelotoxicity)
Cyclophosphamide (Cytoxan)	Cytotoxic alkylating agent that induces cell death; used to treat SLE	Amenorrhea, nausea, vomiting, alopecia, myelosuppression, myeloproliferative disorders, bladder carcinoma, electrolyte imbalance, hemorrhagic cystitis, secondary infertility Rare: Stevens-Johnson syndrome	Preexisting renal or liver dysfunction, leukopenia, or thrombocytopenia
Cyclosporine (Sandimmune)	Immunosuppressant: Blocks transcription of IL-2 and suppresses T-cell activation; used to treat IBD, MS, and SLE	Nausea, paresthesias, tremor, headaches, gingival hypertrophy, hair growth, anemia, liver function impairment, hyperglycemia, hyperkalemia, altered mental status, seizures Rare: hypertension, renal impairment, sepsis	Multiple drug interactions, hypomagnesemia (increases seizure risk) Antibiotic prophylaxis needed with concomitant immunosuppressant use Should not be used by individuals with hypertension, renal impairment, or severe infection
Hydroxychloroquine (Plaquenil)	Immunosuppressant: Interferes with lysosome function to block production of proteins that have immune function; used to treat RA and SLE	Nausea, vomiting, diarrhea, abdominal pain, rash, nightmares, myopathy Rare: retinal toxicity/macular damage	Exposure ≥ 6.5 mg/kg per day or 10 years increases risk for retinal toxicity
Leflunomide (Arava)	Immunosuppressant: Inhibits the enzyme dihydroorotate dehydrogenase used to treat RA	Nausea, alopecia, rash, diarrhea, hypertension Rare: leukopenia, hepatitis, thrombocytopenia	Preexisting liver disease, viral hepatitis, alcoholism, severe immunodeficiency, rifampin Pregnancy (teratogenic-cholestyramine wash-out therapy prior to conception)
Methotrexate (Rheumatrex, Trexall)	Immunosuppressant: Folic acid antagonist; used to treat IBD, MS, RA, and SLE	Nausea, mucositis, liver enzyme elevations, myelosuppression, liver and renal toxicity, hepatic fibrosis, interstitial pneumonitis	Pregnancy (teratogenic) Preexisting severe renal or liver impairment, significant lung disease, alcohol abuse
Mitoxantrone (Novantrone)	Immunosuppressant that inhibits DNA replication and repair; used to treat MS	Severe local tissue damage if intravenous line infiltrates tissue; cardiotoxic; acute myelogenous leukemia; myelosuppression Hair loss, nausea, vomiting, diarrhea, urinary tract infection, menstrual irregularities, blue-green urine and sclera (up to 24 hours), acute myeloid leukemia, myelosuppression, hepatotoxicity, cardiotoxicity (risk increases with cumulative dose)	Black box warning about cardiotoxicity and risk for developing leukemia
Mycophenolate mofetil (CellCept)	Immunosuppressant: Inhibits proliferation of T-cell and B-cell lymphocytes; used to treat SLE	Leukopenia, pure red cell aplasia, diarrhea, vomiting, infection Serious: PML	Pregnancy (pregnancy loss and anomalies), renal insufficiency
Teriflunomide (Aubagio)	Immunosuppressant: Reduces the number of activated lymphocytes in the central nervous system; used to treat MS	Elevated ALT, alopecia, diarrhea, respiratory effects, nausea, paresthesias	Pregnancy (abortifacient and teratogenic; cholestyramine wash-out therapy prior to conception), infection, renal failure, peripheral neuropathy, interstitial pulmonary disease, hypertension

Abbreviations: ALT = alanine aminotransferase; BP = blood pressure; CBC = complete blood count; IBD = inflammatory bowel disease; LFTs = liver function tests; MS = multiple sclerosis; PML = progressive multifocal leukoencephalopathy; RA = rheumatoid arthritis; SLE = systemic lupus erythematosus; PML = progressive multifocal leukoencephalopathy; TPMT = thiopurine methyltransferase; TB = tuberculosis; UA = urine analysis; VS = vital signs; WBC = white blood cell.

Sources: Data from Goodin DS, Frohman EM, Garmany GP Jr, et al. Disease-modifying therapies in multiple sclerosis: report of the Therapeutics and Technology Assessment Subcommittee of the American Academy of Neurology and the MS Council for Clinical Practice Guidelines. *Neurology.* 2002;58(2):169-178. [Reaffirmed on July 19, 2008][7]; Lake DF, Briggs AD, Akporiaye ET. Immunopharmacology. In: Katzung BG, Masters SB, Trevor AJ, eds. *Basic and Clinical Pharmacology*. 13th ed. New York, NY/London, England: McGraw-Hill Medical; 2014:946-970[5]; Rhen T, Cidlowski JA. Anti-inflammatory action of glucocorticoids. *N Engl J Med.* 2005;353:1771-1723.[6]

treat rheumatoid arthritis are primarily due to suppression of cell-mediated immunity and inhibition of matrix metalloproteinase and osteoclasts.[10]

Teriflunomide (Aubagio) acts primarily on rapidly proliferating cells. Resting cells use an alternative salvage pathway for pyrimidine synthesis and are less affected by this agent.[11] The therapeutic effect of teriflunomide (Aubagio) for treating multiple sclerosis is likely due to a reduction in the number of activated lymphocytes in the central nervous system.[11]

Leflunomide and teriflunomide have FDA black box warnings that refer to the risk of fatal heptaotoxicity and teratogenicity. When this drug is used, liver function should be monitored every 6 months and the woman should be counseled to observe for signs of liver dysfunction. Both drugs have been shown to be teratogenic in animal studies. Both drugs are contraindicated for use in pregnancy. Pregnancy must be excluded prior to initiating either of these agents and the woman should have a safe form of birth control when taking one of these drugs.

Methotrexate (Rheumatrex, Trexall)

Methotrexate (Rheumatrex, Trexall) is a folic acid antagonist that has been used to treat women with malignancies for more than a half century and is discussed in the *Cancer* chapter. Indeed, this versatile drug is prescribed for a wide variety of disorders. Methotrexate inhibits the function of dihydrofolate reductase. Inhibition of dihydrofolate reductase results in functional folate deficiency. Because folate is a cofactor in DNA synthesis, cell proliferation is blocked, and cell death occurs.

The mechanism of action of low-dose methotrexate therapy used to treat autoimmune disorders is not completely understood. Many in vivo and in vitro effects that may contribute to its potent anti-inflammatory activity have been observed, including interference with adenosine-mediated inflammation, decreased cytokine and immunoglobulin G (IgG) production, and inhibited cyclooxygenase 2 (COX-2) activity.[11]

Methotrexate can be administered orally, intramuscularly, or subcutaneously. Bioavailability is better following parenteral administration when compared to oral administration, particularly when higher doses are used. Some persons respond better to parenteral administration. Individuals taking methotrexate should take a supplement of 1 mg per day of folic acid.

Methotrexate is contraindicated for women who would like to become pregnant, women who are pregnant, persons with active liver disease or excessive alcohol intake, and persons with severe renal impairment. This drug has many adverse effects and therapy is monitored carefully.

Cyclophosphamide (Cytoxan) and Cyclosporine (Sandimmune)

Cyclophosphamide (Cytoxan) is a cytotoxic alkylating agent that induces cell death by covalently bonding to the DNA of proliferating and resting lymphoid cells. Cyclophosphamide has many side effects and clinically important adverse effects. This drug is likely to cause nausea. Adverse effects that are possible following use of this drug include hair loss, cardiac toxicity, pulmonary fibrosis, bone marrow suppression and subequent cytopenias, premature amenorrhea, and permanent infertility, increased vulnerability to infection, cystitis, and increased risk of future malignancy. Cyclophosamide is teratogenic and contraindicated for pregnant women.

Cyclosporine (Sandimmune)

Cyclosporine (Sandimmune) is a peptide antibiotic that enters cells and binds to cytoplasmic cyclophilin, creating a cyclosporine–cyclophilin complex. This complex ultimately prevents T-cell activation. Cyclosporine selectively inhibits T-cell–mediated responses, including cytokine secretion.[12] Bioavailability of the drug is highly variable, with 20% to 50% of the administered drug ultimately being absorbed; moreover, due to CYP450 metabolism, the risk of drug–drug interactions with cyclosporine is high.[5] Cyclosporine has an FDA black box warning that states only healthcare providers experienced in immunosuppressive therapy should administer this drug. Cyclosporine is administered in facilities equiped with adequate laboratory and medical support resources. Cyclosporine can cause systemic hypertension and nephrotoxicity.

Hydroxychloroquine (Plaquenil)

Hydroxychloroquine (Plaquenil) is an antimalarial agent. This drug accumulates in lysosomes within cells and interferes with lysosome function. The result is decreased secretion of many proteins that have immune function. Hydroxychloroquine has an anti-inflammatory action in persons with rheumatic disease that may be attributed to its interference with antigen presentation by antigen-presenting cells, T-cell response, and deoxyribonucleotide synthesis.[13] Hydroxychloroquine has an FDA black box warning that states healthcare providers using this drug must be aware of all the information listed in the package insert prior to use.

Mitoxantrone (Novantrone)

Mitoxantrone (Novantrone) is a synthetic antineoplastic anthracenedione that inhibits DNA replication and repair and DNA-dependent RNA synthesis. As a result, mitoxantrone suppresses T-cell, B-cell, and macrophage proliferation and decreases secretion of pro-inflammatory cytokines.[14] Mitoxantrone has an FDA black box warning that states this drug should only be administered by a an experienced cancer chemotherapy physician in a facility equiped to manage complications. Mitoxantrone can cause a fatal cardiotoxicity and acute myelogenous leukemia. It is contraindicated for use during pregnancy.

Mycophenolate Mofetil (CellCept)

Mycophenolate mofetil (CellCept) is a prodrug of mycophenolic acid, a potent inhibitor of inosine-5' -monophosphate dehydrogenase. Mycophenolate mofetil inhibits proliferation of T-cell and B-cell lymphocytes and subsequent cell-mediated immune response and antibody production.[15] This drug also carries an FDA black box warning that states it should only be administered by a provider experienced in immunosuppressive therapy in a facility capable of managing complications. Mycophenolate increases one's risk for developing lymphoma or opportunistic infections. It is a teratogen and contraindicated for use by pregnant women.

Biologic Agents and Immunomodulators

In recent years, genetically engineered monoclonal antibodies and other biologic components have been developed that have selective immunomodulatory effects when used as treatments for women with autoimmune disorders. Interferons, monoclonal antibodies, and immunomodulators are listed in Table 17-3.[5,16–19]

Interferons

Interferons are cytokines that have antiviral, antiproliferative, and immunomodulatory activity. These agents inhibit protein synthesis, as well as viral penetration, translation, maturation, and release. Three major categories of interferons exist: alpha, beta, and gamma. The beta versions (IFN-βs) are type I interferons produced by fibroblasts during the normal immune response to invading pathogens.

Interferons tend to be used for a set duration. They are not absorbed orally, but rather are administered by the intramuscular or subcutaneous route. Their therapeutic action is most likely a result of reduced T-cell activation, modulated cytokine production, induction of regulatory or suppressor T cells, and inhibition of blood–brain barrier leakage. Interferons are widely used for treatment of persons with hepatitis and human papillomavirus. Additional information on their use in relation to those conditions can be found in the *Sexually Transmitted Infections* chapter.

Side effects associated with interferons include weight loss, rash, anemia, and neurologic issues of confusion, depression, and somnolence. Women should be advised that they may experience headaches, mild fever, malaise, and myalgias within the first day of IFN administration. Serious adverse effects include myelosuppression with granulocytopenia, thrombocytopenia, interstitial nephritis, pneumonia, and hepatotoxicity. Women with a history of mood disorders, cardiac arrhythmias, or current hepatic compromise should not use these drugs, and caution is advised if women are also taking methadone (Dolophine), ribavirin (Rebetol), theophylline (Theo-Dur), or zidovudine (Retrovir), since IFN co-administration can increase serum levels of these drugs. Caution is likewise recommended if interferons are used by women who also taking drugs that may induce hepatotoxicity. Women taking angiotensin-converting enzyme (ACE) inhibitors also should not use interferons.

Monoclonal Antibodies

Monoclonal antibodies are engineered antibodies that can be used to target specific areas and functions of the immune system. They are formed by replacing non-antigen-specific components of murine monoclonal antibodies with comparable regions of human antibodies. Chimeric monoclonal antibodies have less complete replacement of the murine components than do humanized monoclonal antibodies. The resulting hybrid monoclonal antibodies have less antigenicity and a longer half-life than complete murine antibodies.[5] Monoclonal antibodies are large proteins that have complex pharmacokinetic and pharmacodynamic properties. Thus there is a wide variation in individual response to these drugs.[20] Abbreviations placed at the end of the name indicate the mechanism of action. For example "-cept" refers to fusion of a receptor to par of human IgG; "-mag" refers to a monoclonal antibody; "-ximab" is a chimeric monoclonal antibody; and "-zumab" is a humanized monoclonal antibody.

Table 17-3 Immunomodulators and Biologics Commonly Used to Treat Autoimmune Disorders

Drug: Generic (Brand)	Category and Indication for Use	Side Effects/Adverse Effects	Warnings and Precautions
Abatacept (Orencia)	Immunomodulator: Selective T-cell Costimulation blocker used to treat RA	Headache, nausea, upper respiratory infection, nasopharyngitis	Chronic obstructive pulmonary disease, use with biologics (serious infections, neoplasms)
Adalimumab (Humira)	Human recombinant monoclonal antibody that act as TNF-alpha antagonist used to treat IBD and RA	Headache, rash, nausea, infusion reactions, anemia, leukopenia, lymphoma, reactivation of infection, exacerbation of congestive heart failure Rare: hepatosplenic T-cell lymphoma	Preexisting congestive heart failure, diabetes, MS, renal failure
Alemtuzumab (Lemtrada)	Monoclonal antibody used to treat relapsing MS	Infusion reactions likely Adverse effects include thyroid disorders, immune thrombocytopenia, infections, malignancies	Black box warning: Available only through restricted distribution under a Risk Evaluation Mitigation Strategy Program
Anakinra (Kineret)	Recombinant antagonist to the receptor for interleukin-1 used to treat RA	Injection site reaction, increased susceptibility to infection, headache dizziness, nausea	Asthma, chronic obstructive pulmonary disease (greater risk of pulmonary infections)
Belimumab (Benlysta)	Human monoclonal antibody that neutralizes the B-cell activating factor (BAFF) used to treat SLE	Arthralgia, infection, HA, fatigue, nausea, mild to moderate infusion reaction, hypersensitivity Rare: serious infusion reaction, mortality Serious: PML (one case report)	Depression or mood disorders Not for use in persons with severe lupus nephritis or active CNS lupus
Certolizumab pegol (Cimzia)	Pegylated humanized fragment of monoclonal antibody that act as TNF-alpha antagonist used to treat RA	HA, fatigue, nausea, rash, urinary tract infection Rare: opportunistic infection, leukopenia, neutropenia, thrombocytopenia, hepatotoxicity	Preexisting congestive heart failure, active infection, hepatitis B infection, MS
Dimethyl fumarate (Tecfidera)	Immunomodulator: Methyl ester of fumaric used to treat MS	Flushing, abdominal pain, nausea, diarrhea	Lymphopenia
Etanercept (Enbrel)	Immunomodulator recombinant fusion protein of the human TNF receptor bound to human IgG_1 Works as an anti-TNF-a agent used to treat RA	Headache, rash, nausea, infusion reactions, anemia, leukopenia, lymphoma, reactivation of infection, exacerbation of congestive heart failure Rare: new-onset demyelinating disease, exacerbation of MS, drug-induced lupus	Preexisting congestive heart failure, diabetes, MS, renal failure
Fingolimod (Gilenya)	Immunomodulator prevents migration of lymphocytes from lymph nodes; used to treat MS	Headache, flu, diarrhea, back pain, elevated liver enzymes, cough	Infection, macular edema, decreased pulmonary function, elevated serum transaminases, hypertension
Glatiramer Acetate (Copaxone)	Immunomodulator synthetic amino acid that shifts T cells from pro-inflammatory T cells to suppressor T cells; used to treat MS	Nausea, arthralgia, facial edema, pain at the injection site, postinjection reaction (within 30 minutes, benign chest pain, tachycardia, palpitations, anxiety)	Severe or prolonged post-injection reaction
Golimumab (Simponi)	Human IgG anti-TNF-a antibody used to treat RA	Injection site reaction, infection, malignancy Serious: hypersensitivity, infection (TB, bacterial sepsis, fungal, opportunistic)	Preexisting congestive heart failure, active infection, hepatitis B infection, MS
Infliximab (Remicade)	Chimeric monoclonal antibody acts as an anti-TNF-a agent used to treat IBD and RA	Infection Rare: new-onset demyelinating disease, exacerbation of MS, drug-induced lupus, hepatosplenic T-cell lymphoma	Preexisting congestive heart failure, diabetes, MS, renal failure
Interferon β-1a (Avonex, Rebif) and Interferon β-1b (Betaseron, Extavia)	Interferon used to treat MS	Injection site reaction, flu-like symptoms, fever, malaise, fatigue, nausea, anorexia. Adverse effects include dysrhythmias, seizures, depression, aggressive behavior, psychosis, suicidal ideation, hepatotoxicity, anaphylactic reaction, superimposed infection	Preexisting cardiovascular disease, seizure disorder, or depression (may exacerbate condition)
Natalizumab (Tysabri)	Humanized recombinant IgG4κ monoclonal antibody that binds to the surface of leukocytes; used to treat IBD MS	Skin irritation, arthralgia, headache, fatigue Adverse Effects: progressive multifocal leukoencephalopathy	Not for use in individuals with history of or existing PML or who have anti-JC virus antibodies; not for concomitant use with other immunosuppressants

(*continues*)

Table 17-3 Immunomodulators and Biologics Commonly Used to Treat Autoimmune Disorders (*continued*)

Drug: Generic (Brand)	Category and Indication for Use	Side Effects/Adverse Effects	Warnings and Precautions
Rituximab (Rituxan)	Monoclonal antibody that selectively destroys B cells; used to treat RA and SLE	Moderate to severe infusion reactions, severe mucocutaneous eruption, failure to response to vaccines, severe mucocutaneous reactions, hepatitis B virus reactivation, and progressive multifocal leukoencephalopathy	Preexisting cardiac arrhythmias, SLE, hepatitis B infection
Tocilizumab (Actemra)	Humanized monoclonal antibody used to treat RA	Peri-infusion reactions, hypersensitivity, hyperlipidemia, liver function abnormalities, neutropenia, thrombocytopenia Rare: gastrointestinal perforation	Preexisting neutropenia or thrombocytopenia History of GI perforation, intestinal ulcers, or diverticulitis
Tofacitinib (Xeljanz)	Immunomodulator: Inhibits production of Janus kinase enzymes that play a role in joint inflammation; used to treat RA	Diarrhea, headache hyperlipidemia, neutropenia, thrombocytopenia Serious: infection (urinary tract, respiratory, pneumonia, herpes zoster)	History of gastric perforation, severe hepatic impairment, renal transplant

Abbreviations: ALT = alanine aminotransferase; CBC = complete blood count; CNS = central nervous system; HA = headache; IBD = inflammatory bowel disease; JC = John Cunningham; LFTs = liver function tests; MS = multiple sclerosis; RA = rheumatoid arthritis; SLE = systemic lupus erythematosus; TB = tuberculosis.

Sources: Data from Goodin DS, Frohman EM, Garmany GP Jr, et al. Disease-modifying therapies in multiple sclerosis: report of the Therapeutics and Technology Assessment Subcommittee of the American Academy of Neurology and the MS Council for Clinical Practice Guidelines. *Neurology.* 2002;58(2):169-178. [Reaffirmed on July 19, 2008][7]; Lake DF, Briggs AD, Akporiaye ET. Immunopharmacology. In: Katzung BG, Masters SB, Trevor AJ, eds. *Basic and Clinical Pharmacology*. 13th ed. New York, NY/London, England: McGraw-Hill Medical; 2014:946-970[5]; McCluggage LK, Scholtz JM. Golimumab: a tumor necrosis factor alpha inhibitor for the treatment of rheumatoid arthritis. *Ann Pharmacother.* 2010;44(1):135-144[19]; Merrill JT, Ginzler EM, Wallace DJ, et al. Long-term safety profile of belimumab plus standard therapy in patients with systemic lupus erythematosus. *Arthritis Rheum.* 2012;64(10):3364-3373[17]; Saag KG, Teng GG, Patkar NM, et al. American College of Rheumatology 2008 recommendations for the use of nonbiologic and biologic disease-modifying antirheumatic drugs in rheumatoid arthritis. *Arthritis Rheum.* 2008;59(6):762-784[16]; Woodrick RS, Ruderman EM. Safety of biologic therapy in rheumatoid arthritis. *Nat Rev Rheumatol.* 2011;7(11):639-652.[18]

Natalizumab (Tysabri) is a humanized recombinant IgG4κ monoclonal antibody that binds to the surface of leukocytes, thereby blocking these cells' adhesion to vascular endothelium and subsequent transmigration of the leukocytes from the vasculature to the inflamed tissue.[21] Treatment with natalizumab has been associated with progressive multifocal leukoencephalopathy and is contraindicated for persons with history of or existing progressive multifocal leukoencephalopathy. Individuals being treated with natalizumab need to be monitored closely for signs and symptoms of progressive multifocal leukoencephalopathy. Other opportunistic infections during natalizumab therapy are rare, but herpes virus meningitis and a case of cryptosporidial gastroenteritis have been reported.[22]

Individuals meeting the strict treatment criteria can enroll in the Tysabri Outreach: Unified Commitment to Health (TOUCH) Prescribing Program to begin natalizumab therapy. The TOUCH program was developed by Biogen Idec and Elan Pharmaceuticals to closely monitor natalizumab therapy and adverse effects. This program, which was created with input from the U.S. Food and Drug Administration (FDA), registers and monitors authorized prescribers, infusion centers, and pharmacies administering natalizumab.[21]

Rituximab (Rituxan) is a monoclonal antibody that selectively destroys B cells. Possible mechanisms of action include complement-mediated cytotoxicity, antibody-mediated cytotoxicity, and induction of programmed cell death. Rituximab is used to treat leukemias, lymphomas, and autoimmune disorders characterized by a surplus of B cell activity such as rheumatoid arthritis. Rituximab has several FDA black box warnings that address the risks for fatal infusion reactions, severe mucocutaneous reactions, hepatitis B virus reactivation, and progressive multifocal leukoencephalopathy.

Belimumab (Benlysta) is a human monoclonal antibody that neutralizes the B-cell activating factor (BAFF), which is necessary for B-cell survival. By bonding to BAFF, belimumab prevents BAFF from binding to B-cell membrane receptors thereby interfering with the survival and maturation of B-cells, particularly auto-reactive ones. This mechanism of action is of particular interest in the treatment of women with SLE, as the overexpression of BAFF/BLyS is a noted feature of the disease.[23]

Anti-Tumor Necrosis Factor-Alpha Agents

Adalimumab (Humira), infliximab (Remicade), and certolizumab pegol (Cimzia) are monoclonal antibodies that act as TNF-alpha antagonists. TNF-alpha is an inflammatory cytokine involved in the pathogenesis of many chronic inflammatory diseases. Overexpression of TNF-alpha can cause an inflammatory response and local tissue damage. Blocking TNF-alpha activity results in suppression of interleukins 1 and 6 (IL-1, IL-6) and inflammatory adhesion molecules.[5]

Certolizumab pegol (Cimzia) is an interesting monoclonal antibody. Certolizumab is pegylated, which is a process that adds a polyethylene glycol (PEG) molecule to the parent drug. **Pegylation** creates a large macromolecule that has improved bioavailablility, longer duration of action, and slowed clearance. Certolizumab is used to treat Crohn's disease.

Adverse effects of anti-TNF-alpha drugs include injection side and infusion reactions and cytopenias. These drugs have an FDA black box warning that notes their use is associated with an increased risk for serious and possibly fatal infection, as well as malignancy. Rarely, some individuals may develop anti-TNF-alpha antibodies and antinuclear antibodies (ANA). Antibodies to infliximab may decrease the clinical benefit of this therapy. Concomitant administration of methotrexate (Rheumatrex, Trexall) reduces anti-infliximab antibody formation. Antibodies to adalimumab and certolizumab pegol are rare.

Immunomodulators

The area of greatest current research focuses on engineered immunomodulators that stimulate or block the immune response by imitating naturally occurring biomolecular activities in the immune cascade. Three generations of immunomodulators exist, with each generation being superior to the previous one in terms of tolerance and clinical effectiveness. The first generation includes the drug thalidomide, a prototype teratogen.

Immunomodulators are associated with increased risk of peripheral neuropathy, anemia, venous thromboembolism, and thrombocytopenia. Thus, they should be used with caution by women already at risk for these conditions. Drugs that possess potential hepatotoxicity should be used cautiously, if at all, in women taking immunomodulators.

Antigen-presenting cells are those cells that digest an antigen and present a portion of it on the cell surface. Abatacept (Orencia) is a fusion protein composed of a human immunoglobulin component and cytotoxic T lymphocyte–associated antigen 4 (CTLA-4). Abatacept binds to a receptor on antigen-presenting cells and prevents the antigen-presenting cell from binding to the T cells. Through this competitive binding, abatacept blocks T-cell activation and prevents subsequent cytokine release.[5]

Etanercept (Enbrel) is a recombinant fusion protein of the human TNF receptor bound to human IgG1. Etanercept binds competitively to TNF-alpha and TNF-β receptors.[5] Etanercept acts as a TNF antagonist and has similar effectiveness and side-effect profiles as the anti-TNF-alpha monoclonal antibodies.

Glatiramer acetate (Copaxone) is a synthetic amino acid polypeptide composed of glutamine, lysine, alanine, and tyrosine. By shifting T cells from pro-inflammatory T cells to suppressor T cells, this agent inhibits inflammation thereby avoiding an autoimmune response against myelin.[24]

Fingolimod (Gilenya) prevents migration of lymphocytes from lymph nodes thereby preventing them from participating in cell-mediated immune responses. Evidence also shows that fingolimod acts on glial cells in the CNS, which may aid in tissue repair.

Dimethyl fumarate (Tecfidera) activates the pathway involved with cellular response to oxidative stress.[25] In doing so it promotes a shift in the cytokine profile from Th_1 pro-inflammatory T cells to Th_2 suppressor T cells.

Inflammatory Bowel Disease

Inflammatory bowel disease (IBD) includes two related, but distinct gastrointestinal (GI) disorders: ulcerative colitis and Crohn's disease.[26] The latter may affect the entire GI tract from the mouth to the anus, but persons affected generally have intestinal disease, including ileitis ileocolitis, and colitis. Conversely, ulcerative colitis affects the mucosa of the large intestine and almost always involves the rectum with proximal extension that involves all or part of the colon.

The exact cause of inflammatory dysregulation in the intestine is unknown; nevertheless, a general imbalance between pro- and anti-inflammatory mediators exists. Exogenous pathogens may trigger the initial inflammatory response that goes uncontrolled, or the person's body may perceive normal intestinal flora as a pathogen. Among women with Crohn's disease, activated T cells secrete inflammatory cytokines, induce inflammatory B cells and macrophages, and recruit lymphocytes to the intestine. Transmural tissue damage results from the local cytokine activity and may result in mucosal inflammation and ulceration, structuring, fistulas, and abscess formation. In ulcerative colitis, T-cell activation may also play a role in the development of superficial mucosal inflammation—a characteristic of the disease.

Approximately 1.4 million individuals in the United States suffer from IBD, with incidence rates of 3.1 to 14.6 per 100,000 for Crohn's disease and 2.2 to 14.3 per 100,000 for ulcerative colitis.[27] There is a slight predominance of women with Crohn's disease. Multiple factors are involved in the development of IBD. Genetic studies of affected populations have identified several possible susceptibility genes, and three distinct polymorphisms of the gene *CARD15* have been associated with IBD.[28] There is a 10% lifetime risk associated with having a first-degree relative with IBD. Likely environmental factors affecting IBD incidence include appendectomy (may decrease the risk of ulcerative colitis) and cigarette smoking (mixed effect). There appears to be an inverse relationship between cigarette smoking and ulcerative colitis: Current smokers are less likely than nonsmokers to have ulcerative colitis, while ex-smokers have greater risk of disease.

There is no evidence that IBD is caused or affected by dietary factors, and there are no dietary modifications that impact the course of disease. A low-residue diet should be followed during periods of acute inflammation to decrease intestinal pain. Crohn's disease ileitis or ileocolitis is associated with indigestion and malabsorption. Vitamin B_{12} injections may be necessary for some individuals with Crohn's disease ileitis. Other supplementations may be indicated for vitamin and mineral deficiencies associated with disease therapy or surgery.

Pharmacologic Therapies for Women with Inflammatory Bowel Disease

Pharmacologic therapy is individualized and depends on disease location, severity, and coexisting complications. Most drugs fall into one of the following categories: anti-inflammatories, immunosuppressants, or immunomodulators/biologic agents (Table 17-4).[29,30]

Anti-inflammatories

Within the category of anti-inflammatory agents, aminosalicylates are first-line therapies for the induction and maintenance of remission in mild to moderate ulcerative colitis and induction therapy for distal Crohn's disease. The choice of a specific preparation depends on the disease location. Glucocorticoids are generally used to treat active IBD, particularly if it is unresponsive to first-line aminosalicylate therapy. Other immunosuppressants and immunomodulators are reserved for refractory IBD or severe Crohn's disease.

Aminosalicylates

Use of aminosalicylates for treatment of persons with Crohn's disease is controversial because studies have had mixed results.[31,32] However, these drugs are safer and have a better side-effect profile than do glucocorticoids, immunomodulators, and biologic agents. Therefore, aminosalicylates are used in clinical practice to induce remission in persons with mild Crohn's disease.

In contrast, the mainstay of therapy for ulcerative colitis has been rectal therapy with 5-aminosalicylic acid. Topical preparations such as Canasa and enemas such as Rowasa are effective in treating proctitis and distal colonic disease and are more effective in treating active ulcerative colitis or proctitis than are oral agents or topical steroid preparations.[33] There is no significant difference in effectiveness between the oral and topical preparations when used as maintenance therapy for ulcerative colitis.[34] The choice of topical preparation depends on the proximal extent of disease activity—suppositories reach approximately 10 cm, whereas enemas may reach to the splenic fissure.[33] Continued therapy for persons with ulcerative colitis may decrease future risk of colon cancer by nearly 50%.[33]

Glucocorticoids

Glucocorticoids, such as prednisone (Deltasone), methylprednisolone (Medrol), budesonide (Entocort), and hydrocortisone, are effective in rapidly reducing disease activity and inducing remission in persons with IBD. These agents are not used for maintenance therapy. Their use is generally reserved for moderate to severe active colitis or mild to moderate Crohn's disease that has not responded to aminosalicylates.[35]

Mild to moderate Crohn's disease may be treated with steroid therapy for induction of remission. Ileal-release budesonide (Entocort) is indicated for ileal or right-sided colonic Crohn's disease. Oral preparations are sufficient for therapy in all cases except unresponsive or fulminant IBD. In that setting, hospitalization and treatment with parenteral glucocorticoids are recommended. Topical steroid preparations have not been evaluated in treating distal colonic Crohn's disease.[29]

The active distal inflammation of ulcerative colitis is treated with topical preparations of budesonide or hydrocortisone. Hydrocortisone enema or foam is effective for acute therapy, and budesonide enema appears to be as effective as hydrocortisone. Once remission is achieved, the oral dose should be slowly tapered in accordance with disease activity. If the agents can be tapered successfully,

Table 17-4 Drugs Used for the Treatment of Women with Inflammatory Bowel Disease

Drug: Generic (Brand)	Dose[a]	Indications
Adalimumab (Humira)	160 mg SQ, 80 mg SQ 2 weeks later, then 40 mg SQ every 1–2 weeks starting 2 weeks later	Moderate to severe, active CD, therapy resistant/intolerant (induction and maintenance)
Azathioprine (Azasan, Imuran)	1.5–2.5 mg/kg PO once daily	Severe IBD to reduce steroid dose (induction only) Extensive UC, therapy resistant/intolerant (maintenance) Moderate to severe CD (maintenance after steroid induction, postoperative prophylaxis)
Balsalazide (Colazal)	2.25 g PO 3 times daily, then 3–6 g PO once daily	Mild to moderate UC (induction and maintenance) Colonic CD (induction only)
Budesonide, ileal release (Entocort EC)	9 mg PO once daily for 2–3 months, then taper	Ileocecal CD (induction, short-term maintenance)
Budesonide, topical enema (Entocort enema)	2 mg PR every night for 4–8 weeks	Active distal UC (induction only)
Certolizumab pegol (Cimzia)	400 mg SQ at 0, 2, and 4 weeks, then every 4 weeks	Moderate to severe, active CD (induction and maintenance)
Cyclosporine (Sandimmune)	2–4 mg/kg IV once daily	Fulminant UC, steroid refractory Fistulizing CD (induction only)
Infliximab (Remicade)	5 mg/kg IV at 0, 2, and 6 weeks, then every 8 weeks (slow infusion over 2 hours)	Moderate to severe IBD, therapy resistant/intolerant (induction and maintenance) Postoperative CD (prophylaxis)
Mesalamine, encapsulated granules (Apriso)	1.5 g PO once daily	Mild to moderate UC (maintenance)
Mesalamine, enteric coated (Asacol)	2.4–4.8 g PO daily, divided doses; then 1.6–4.8 g PO once daily, divided doses (continue at higher doses for CD)	Distal UC (induction and maintenance) Ileocolonic CD (induction only)
Mesalamine, multimatrix formulation (Lialda)	2.4–4.8 g PO once daily	Mild to moderate UC (induction and maintenance)
Mesalamine, suppository (Canasa)	500 mg suppository PR 1–2 times/day 1000 mg suppository PR once daily or every night	Active distal UC/proctitis (induction and maintenance)
Mesalamine, sustained release (Pentasa)	2–4.8 g PO in 3 divided doses once daily, then 1.4–4 g PO in divided doses once daily	Extensive UC (induction and maintenance) Active CD (induction, postoperative prophylaxis)
Mesalamine, topical enema (Rowasa)	1–4 g PR once daily or every night; then 2–4 g PR every 1, 2, or 3 days	Active distal UC/proctitis (induction and maintenance)
Methotrexate (Rheumatrex, Trexall)	25 mg IM once weekly	Active CD, steroid dependent/steroid refractory Chronic active CD (induction and maintenance)
Methylprednisolone (Medrol)	40–60 mg IV once daily	Active IBD, PO steroid refractory Severe IBD (induction only)
Natalizumab (Tysabri)	300 mg IV every 28 days (infused slowly over 1 hour)	Moderate to severe, active CD, refractory (induction and maintenance)
Olsalazine (Dipentum)	0.75–1.5 g PO 2 times daily, then 1 g PO once daily	Mild to moderate UC (induction and maintenance) Colonic CD (induction only)
Prednisone (Delacort)	40–60 mg PO once daily for 7–28 days until resolution of symptoms, then taper by 5–10 mg/week until 20 mg dose, then taper by 2.5–5 mg/week	Active IBD Active UC, 5-ASA refractory (induction only)
Sulfasalazine (Azulfidine)	1–1.5 g PO 4 times daily, then 2 to 4 g PO once daily	Mild to moderate UC (induction and maintenance) Colonic and ileocolonic CD (induction only)

Abbreviations: 5-ASA = 5-aminosalicylic acid; CD = Crohn's disease; IBD = inflammatory bowel disease; UC = ulcerative colitis.

[a] The doses listed in this table are one example of a dosing schedule. For most of these drugs, variations in dose and frequency are used in clinical practice to meet the needs of individual women.

Sources: Lichtenstein GR, Hanauer SB, Sandborn WJ, Practice Parameters Committee of American College of Gastroenterology. Management of Crohn's disease in adults. *Am J Gastroenterol.* 2009;104(2):465-483[29]; Nielsen OH, Ainsworth MA. Tumor necrosis factor inhibitors for inflammatory bowel disease. *N Engl J Med.* 2013;369:754-762.[30]

the daily dose can be reduced in 4 to 5 weeks, then further tapered until finally being discontinued after several months.[33] Inability to taper is an indication for parenteral steroid therapy.

Immunosuppressants

Azathioprine (Imuran) and 6-Mercaptopurine (Purinethol)

The thiopurines—that is, azathioprine (Azasan, Imuran) and 6-mercaptopurine (Purinethol)—are treatment options for individuals with refractory disease. For persons with chronic, severe IBD that is steroid resistant or tolerant, azathioprine or 6-mercaptopurine may provide relief of symptoms and allow for steroid tapering without relapse. These agents are not recommended as induction monotherapy, but may be used as maintenance therapy in combination with glucocorticoids after induction of remission. Combination therapy with anti-TNF-alpha may also improve rates of remission in individuals with moderate or severe Crohn's disease.[34,36]

Cyclosporine (Sandimmune)

Cyclosporine (Sandimmune) has a faster onset of action than azathioprine or 6-mercaptopurine and is effective in treating individuals with severe refractory ulcerative colitis. Its intravenous administration induces remission in severe ulcerative colitis and may provide an alternative to colectomy. Intravenous cyclosporine is effective for induction in persons who have fistulizing Crohn's disease, but oral maintenance therapy is not appropriate because disease flares are common. Azathioprine or 6-mercaptopurine must be used for maintenance therapy.[29] However, after clinical response is initially achieved, cyclosporine may be used for short-term maintenance of ulcerative colitis, until the slower-acting azathioprine or 6-mercaptopurine can take effect.

Significant toxicity may result with cyclosporine (Sandimmune) therapy. Individuals should be monitored for renal dysfunction, and if creatinine levels are elevated, cyclosporine should be given at a lower dose or discontinued.

Methotrexate (Rheumatrex, Trexall)

Methotrexate (Rheumatrex, Trexall) is indicated for treatment of women with chronic active Crohn's disease, but its use in ulcerative colitis is not supported. For individuals who are steroid dependent, methotrexate administration is effective for maintenance of remission and allows for steroid tapering.[29,37]

Immunomodulators/Biologic Agents

The biologic agents approved for treatment of women with IBD are the TNF-alpha antagonists: infliximab (Remicade), adalimumab (Humira), natalizumab (Tysabri), and certolizumab pegol (Cimzia). These agents are used for treatment of individuals with moderate to severe, refractory or fistulizing Crohn's disease.

Infliximab (Remicade)

Infliximab (Remicade) can be given as monotherapy or in combination with azathioprine (Imuran). Combination therapy is more likely to lead to glucocorticoid-free remission than either infliximab or azathioprine monotherapy (56.8% versus 44.4% [$P = 0.02$] and 30% [$P < 0.001$], respectively), with no significant differences in adverse events or serious infections.[38]

Infliximab is also indicated for treating moderate to severe, active ulcerative colitis in persons who are nonresponsive or intolerant to conventional therapies.[33] If an individual shows no initial response to infliximab, it is unlikely that another anti-TNF agent will be effective. Once remission is achieved, scheduled infliximab infusions provide effective maintenance therapy for persons with both ulcerative colitis and Crohn's disease. Antibodies to infliximab are more likely to develop following episodic therapy, which results in a reduced therapeutic response while increasing the likelihood of infusion reactions.

Adalimumab (Humira)

Adalimumab (Humira) may be used by individuals who have not used biologic therapy previously or those with prior exposure to infliximab, but the response rate is significantly lower in persons with prior infliximab use (62% versus 42%, $P < .001$).[39] Subcutaneous administration of adalimumab is a potential advantage when compared to intravenous infusion of infliximab for persons who prefer self-administration. No studies have been conducted that have compared the two therapies directly, but it appears that both medications have similar effectiveness among individuals with IBD.

Adalimumab may be given to individuals who had a poor outcome with use of infliximab such as those who lose response, develop antibodies, or experience an infusion reaction. Reported rates of development of anti-adalimumab antibodies are lower than rates of antibody development with infliximab, although individuals with anti-infliximab antibodies are more likely to develop anti-adalimumab antibodies.[40]

Certolizumab Pegol (Cimzia)

Certolizumab pegol (Cimzia) appears to have similar effectiveness as infliximab and adalimumab, although head-to-head trials have not been conducted to confirm this supposition. Like adalimumab, certolizumab is more effective in maintaining remissions in individuals without previous infliximab therapy (69% versus 44% with prior infliximab exposure); nevertheless, 50% of those with prior infliximab treatment benefited from this second-line therapy.[41]

Natalizumab (Tysabri)

Natalizumab (Tysabri) should be reserved for use as a monotherapy for those who have confirmed, active Crohn's disease intolerant or refractory to other immunomodulator therapy.[29] Some persons who use natalizumab may experience colitis or worsening Crohn's disease. Potential benefits must be weighed against risk of progressive multifocal leukoencephalopathy, which occurs in approximately 1 per 1000 individuals who use the drug.[29]

Complementary, Alternative, and Adjuvant Therapies

Alternative therapies investigated for treatment of women with IBD focus on reducing inflammation and altering the gastrointestinal environment. This approach is reasonable because disease may be triggered by an inappropriate immune response to intestinal pathogens. Studies involving probiotics, prebiotics, and synbiotics in IBD suggest that administration may restore beneficial flora, and certain strains of probiotics may serve to prevent relapse in ulcerative colitis and pouchitis.[42]

Several small studies have suggested that acupuncture, *Boswellia serrata* (frankincense), traditional Chinese medicine, and digestive herbal therapies (aloe vera and wheat grass juice) may improve measures of disease activity during exacerbations.[29] Safety and effectiveness data for these therapies are lacking, particularly when used in conjunction with conventional therapy. Although theoretically plausible, there is insufficient evidence to support the safety or effectiveness of helminth (worm) therapy in the treatment of women with inflammatory bowel disease.[43]

Special Populations

Pregnancy, Lactation, and Contraception

Medications used to treat IBD appear to be safe during pregnancy,[44] with the exception of methotrexate (Rheumatrex, Trexall), a drug with known teratogenic and abortifacient effects. Sulfasalazine (Azulfidine) therapy is not associated with increased fetal anomalies or spontaneous abortion; however, folic acid supplementation is recommended for women using sulfasalazine in pregnancy due to this agent's interference with folic acid absorption.[45] The available data on anti-TNF-alpha agents in pregnancy suggest that these drugs do not confer any increased risk for adverse pregnancy outcomes, congenital anomalies, or infections in the first year of life.[44] If disease is in remission with maintenance therapy, medication should be continued throughout pregnancy. Most disease flares during pregnancy are due to treatment withdrawal.

Sulfasalazine (Azulfidine), mesalamine (Apriso, Canasa, Pentasa), and steroids can be used during lactation. Aminosalicylates may cause watery diarrhea in breastfeeding infants, but this reaction reverses when the drug is discontinued. Slow growth has been reported in infants exposed to olsalazine (Dipentum), and this drug should be used with caution for women who are breastfeeding. Thioguanine (Tabloid) and 6-mercaptopurine (Purinethol) appear in low levels in breast milk and are considered safe for breastfeeding women.[46] Due to concerns about impaired growth, carcinogenesis, immune suppression, and neutropenia, cyclosporine (Sandimmune), cyclophosphamide, and methotrexate (Rheumatrex) should be avoided by women who are breastfeeding.

Effective contraception should be used by all women taking methotrexate and those with active disease. The choice of contraceptive is not affected by IBD itself, but rather by the potential complications of the disease or therapy. Although combined oral contraceptives are effective for women with large bowel disease, low-dose preparations may have reduced effectiveness in women with small bowel disease, malabsorption, or bowel resection. There is no evidence to suggest that the use of combined oral contraception methods increases relapse rates. A woman's disease-related risk for hepatobiliary disease or thrombosis should be considered when selecting an effective contraceptive method.[47]

Elderly

Menopause does not appear to influence or be influenced by the activity of IBD. Hormone therapy may decrease disease activity during the postmenopausal period due to the anti-inflammatory effects of estrogen.[48] Postmenopausal osteoporosis is more prevalent among women with IBD than in the general population—perhaps related to use of glucocorticoids, disease activity, or lifestyle factors. In addition, many women with IBD are physically less active due to the symptoms associated with IBD flares, and they may suffer from malnutrition related to malabsorption or long-term avoidance of dairy products. Therapy with biphosphonates in women with osteopenia improves bone mineral density, but studies evaluating use of bisphosphonates are ongoing and long-term definitive benefit has yet to be shown.

Multiple Sclerosis

Multiple sclerosis (MS) is a chronic inflammatory, demyelinating autoimmune disorder of the central nervous system. In the early, inflammatory course of MS, autoreactive T cells cross the blood–brain barrier, attacking myelin proteins and leading to local inflammation and axonal demyelination. In the earlier phases of MS, remyelination may follow, but repeated injury results in astrocyte proliferation and gliosis, forming the characteristic plaques or lesions of MS. Neurodegeneration follows, as illustrated in Figure 17-3.[67]

MS affects approximately 350,000 persons in the United States and more than 1 million worldwide.[50] The onset of disease typically occurs between 20 and 40 years, with nearly twice as many women affected as men. Due to the variability of disease onset, severity, and progression, it is difficult to predict the overall disease course of an individual with MS. Most individuals who are eventually diagnosed with MS, particularly relapsing–remitting multiple sclerosis, have an initial demyelinating episode, or clinically isolated syndrome, resulting in visual or sensory deficit. In 2010, the International Panel on the Diagnosis of Multiple Sclerosis developed and revised guidelines for diagnosing MS, to clarify the criteria needed to demonstrate dissemination of disease in time (multiple episodes) and space (multiple lesions).[51] The standardized terminology for classifying MS disease based on clinical criteria are listed in Table 17-5.[52]

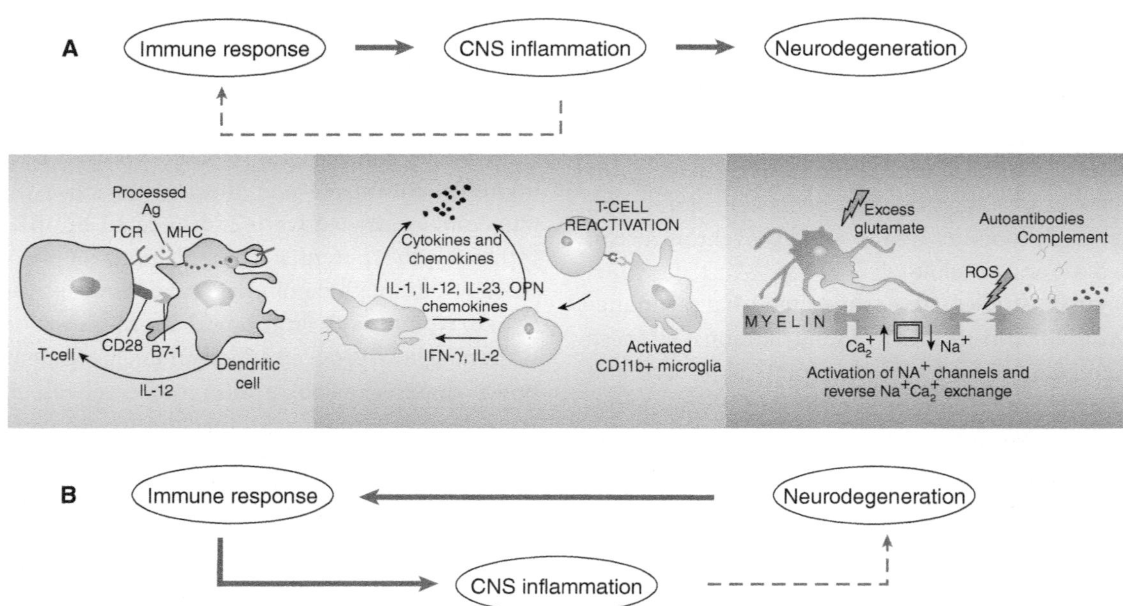

(A) The traditional neuropathological view of MS highlights CNS injury as a consequence of an autoimmune response. (B) An alternative hypothesis proposes that activation of autoimmune cells occurs as a consequence of toxic insults to CNS cells. Infections, for example, may be asymptomatic but cause cytopathic effects to target cells in the course of an antiviral response. The prolonged release of neural antigens may then induce inflammatory responses.

Figure 17-3 Models of disease pathogenesis in multiple sclerosis.

Source: Reprinted from Hauser SL, Oksenberg JR. The neurobiology of multiple sclerosis: genes, inflammation, and neurodegeneration. *Neuron*. 2006; 52(1):61-76, with permission from Elsevier.[50]

Table 17-5 Multiple Sclerosis Disease Classification

Classification	Clinical Criteria
Clinically Isolated Syndrome (CIS)	Single attack compatible with multiple sclerosis, such as optic neuritis. Many persons with an episode of CIS will develop multiple sclerosis.
Relapsing–remitting multiple sclerosis (RRMS)	Most common form of MS. Clearly defined relapses followed by full recovery with or without residual deficits and no disease progression between relapses.
Primary progressive multiple sclerosis (PPMS)	Approximately 10% of persons with MS have PPMS. Disease progresses steadily from onset with occasional plateaus, acute relapses, and only temporary minor improvements or plateaus.
Secondary progressive multiple sclerosis (SPMS)	Most persons with RRMS will eventually develop SPMS. The initial relapsing–remitting course is followed by disease progression with or without relapses, remissions, and plateaus in disease activity.

Therapy for Women with Multiple Sclerosis

The goal of MS therapy is to prevent clinical relapse and postpone neurodegeneration with the subsequent accumulation of disability. Current disease-modifying medications have had some success in reducing the number of relapses, but none has shown effectiveness in slowing disability progression in individuals with primary progressive MS. This is most likely because the effective disease-modifying therapies have primarily anti-inflammatory rather than anti-neurodegenerative effects. It is thought that control of inflammation early in the disease process may reduce damage to the axons and slow or prevent some neurodegenerative changes. However, anti-inflammatory medications become less effective as the disease progresses.

There are 12 FDA-approved disease-modifying therapies for MS. The forms of MS are often referred to as progressive or relapsing. Most drugs are approved to treat the relapsing forms of MS, which include RRMS, SPMS with relapses, and PRMS with relapses. There are no known effective medications for the progressive forms of MS, which include PPMS, SPMS without relapses, and PRMS without relapses.

Drugs used to treat MS are listed in Table 17-6.[53] Acute MS exacerbations are generally treated with glucocorticoids. Biologic agents such as interferons are the first-line therapies for women with clinically isolated syndromes and for maintenance therapy in women who have relapsing–remitting multiple sclerosis. Immunosuppressant therapy may be initiated for persons with poor response to first-line therapies or for persons with progressive forms of MS. Because existing therapies are only partially effective, combinations of drugs that could have a synergistic effect have been suggested and a few small studies have found some benefit. However, more research is needed in this area before being adopted in clinical practice.

Table 17-6 Medications Used to Treat Women with Multiple Sclerosis

Drug: Generic (Brand)	Dose[a]
Alemtuzumab (Lemtrada)	12 mg IV for 5 days followed 12 months later by 12 mg/day for 3 consecutive days
Dimethyl fumarate (Tecfidera)	240 mg PO 2 times daily
Fingolimod (Gilenya)	0.5 mg PO once daily
Glatiramer acetate (Copaxone)	20 mg SQ once daily or 40 mg SQ given 3 times/week
Interferon-β1a, intramuscular (Avonex)	30 mcg IM once weekly
Interferon-β1a, subcutaneous (Rebif)	8.8 mcg SQ 3 times/week for 2 weeks 22 mcg SQ 3 times/week for 2 weeks 44 mcg SQ 3 times/week, maintenance
Interferon-β1b (Betaseron)	0.0625 mg SQ every other day, increase every 1–2 weeks by 25%, up to 0.25 mg SQ every other day, maintenance dose
Interferon-β1b (Extavia)	0.0625 mg SQ every other day, increase every 1–2 weeks by 25%, up to 0.25 mg SQ every other day, maintenance dose
Mitoxantrone (Novantrone)	12 mg/m^2 IV once every 3 months
Natalizumab (Tysabri)	300 mg IV every 28 days (infused slowly over 1 hour)
Peginterferon-nce (Plegridy)	Initial dose: 63 mg SQ on first day; 94 mg SQ on day 15 Maintenance: 125 mg every 14 days beginning on day 29
Teriflunomide (Aubagio)	7 or 14 mg PO once daily

[a] The doses listed in this table are one example of a dosing schedule. For most of these drugs, variations in dose and frequency are used in clinical practice to meet the needs of individual women.

Sources: Data from Goodin DS, Frohman EM, Garmany GP Jr, et al. Disease-modifying therapies in multiple sclerosis: report of the Therapeutics and Technology Assessment Subcommittee of the American Academy of Neurology and the MS Council for Clinical Practice Guidelines. *Neurology*. 2002;58(2):169-178. [Reaffirmed on July 19, 2008][7]; Howley A, Kremenchutzky M. Pegylated interferons: A nurses' review of a novel multiple sclerosis therapy. *J Neuroscience Nsg*. 2014;46(2):88-96.[53]

Anti-inflammatories

Glucocorticoids

There is no evidence that the functional disease course is altered with short-term glucocorticoid administration for acute relapse. Nevertheless, brief episodes of glucocorticoid therapy can hasten recovery from an acute MS flare and acute attacks are generally treated with glucocorticoids (as long as infection has been ruled out). There is no evidence of clear benefit regarding a particular route of administration, dose, or choice of glucocorticoid for treatment of women with exacerbation in clinically definite MS.

Biologic Agents/Immunomodulators

Disease-modifying immunomodulator agents are first-line therapies for treating persons with MS. The drugs in this category include the interferons, glatiramer acetate (Copaxone) fingolimod (Gilenya), dimethyl fumarate (Tecfidera), alemtuzumab (Lemtrada), and natalizumab (Tysabri).

Interferon Beta

There are two subtypes of IFN-β: 1a (Avonex, Rebif) and 1b (Betaseron, Extavia) and a newer pegylated form, peginterferon- β1a (Plegridy). No evidence exists that suggests differences in clinical effectiveness between the two subtypes of interferon. In addition, the side-effect profiles and potential complications are quite similar between them.

IFN-β therapy has been shown to reduce the attack rate for persons with clinically isolated syndromes (CIS) and in RRMS or SPMS with relapses.[54] In a 10-year follow-up study in which the placebo group converted to IFN-β1a therapy (delayed treatment), the immediate-treatment group had significantly lower annual relapse rates from years 5 to 10 (0.14 versus 0.31; $P = 0.03$) and were more likely not to experience any relapses (59% versus 42%).[55] Very few individuals in either treatment group experienced significant disability at 10 years, and rates were no different between groups. The use of IFN-β in SPMS does not appear to ameliorate disease progression, but relapse rate and new lesions on MRI are reduced compared to placebo. The effectiveness of IFN-β for treatment of women with SPMS without relapse is not clear.

Some persons develop persistent IFN-neutralizing antibodies (NAbs), which diminish the clinical and MRI benefits of the therapy. NAbs may develop less frequently with use of IFN-β1a, particularly when this medication is administered intramuscularly.

Glatiramer Acetate (Copaxone)

Glatiramer acetate (Copaxone) generally is better tolerated than IFN-βs. Individuals with MS who receive glatiramer acetate therapy may experience a reduced clinical attack rate, fewer new lesions on MRI, and less total brain atrophy.[56] Filippi et al.[57] found that fewer new MRI lesions converted to black holes (15.6% glatiramer acetate versus 31.4% placebo; $P = 0.002$), which suggests that glatiramer acetate has a neuroprotective effect.[24] This clinical effect has yet to be confirmed, but if true, glatiramer acetate may be beneficial for long-term therapy protecting against axonal degeneration and disability accumulation. Relative to IFN-β therapy, glatiramer acetate shows comparable safety and effectiveness with no significant differences noted in disease progression or number of relapses.[58]

Fingolimod (Gilenya)

Fingolimod (Gilenya) prevents B- and T-cell lymphocyte migration and reduces rates of relapse and may improve MRI evidence of disease progression although effectiveness for disease progression has yet to be confirmed.[60–62] Compared to IFN-β1a (Avonex), fingolimod is more effective in reducing both relapses rates (0.16 versus 0.33; $P < 0.001$) and evidence of disease progression on MRI (mean number of new lesions at 12 months, 1.6 versus 2.6; $P = 0.0024$).[61] Oral administration of fingolimod provides an alternative to existing first-line therapy self-injectables. This agent's use may be limited due to cardiovascular contraindications and the need for routine laboratory testing and eye exams.

Dimethyl Fumarate (Tecfidera)

Dimethyl fumarate (Tecfidera) has anti-inflammatory and neuroprotective effects that reduce evidence of disease activity on MRI and relapse rates among individuals with RRMS.[62,63] No direct comparison studies exist with established MS therapies. A post hoc analysis of data from phase-3 placebo controlled studies[62,63] revealed consistent therapeutic effects across a variety of defined subgroups in the study population, including gender, age, relapse history, treatment history, disability score, and lesion volume.[64,65] This is an important consideration when evaluating therapy in MS, as these factors often influence prognosis and disease progression.

Alemtuzumab (Lemtrada)

Alemtuzumab is a monoclonal antibody FDA approved for treating relapsing forms of MS in 2014. Alemtuzumab carries an FDA black box warning that refers to high rates of infusion reactions and risks for malignancy and autoimmune effects. This drug is only available through restricted distribution under a Risk Evaluation Mitigation Strategy

Program. It is administered intravenously and individuals receiving this agent require premedication with corticosteroids and antiviral prophylaxis.

Natalizumab (Tysabri)

Natalizumab (Tysabri) suppresses leukocyte migration into the CNS and may reduce plaque formation by inhibiting leukocyte adhesion to endothelial cells in the vasculature and the brain. This therapy greatly reduces relapses and appearance of new lesions on MRI.

Natalizumab is recommended as a first-line monotherapy for treatment of women with relapsing forms of MS and may be appropriate as an add-on therapy for individuals with active disease despite IFN-β or glatiramer acetate therapy.

Due to the associated risk of progressive multifocal leukoencephalopathy, natalizumab has been previously considered as a second-line therapy alternative for those persons with worsening disease despite interferon or glatiramer acetate therapy. Considering risk stratification and availability of anti–JC virus antibody testing,[25] natalizumab is now considered a viable and effective first-line therapy for certain individuals with MS. Approximately 55% of individuals with MS have anti–JC virus antibodies, which increases the individual's risk for developing progressive multifocal leukoencephalopathy.[66] Despite the availability of testing for this antibody to select candidates for use of natalizumab, the clinician should carefully consider the perceived benefits and risks before initiating therapy through designated infusions centers. Persons taking natalizumab should be counseled to report signs of infection, depression, or neurologic changes.

Immunosuppressants

Mitoxantrone (Novantrone) and teriflunomide (Aubagio) are FDA-approved for treatment of individuals with MS. However, the immunosuppressant azathioprine (Imuran) has been used as an MS therapy for more than 30 years and thus, is reviewed briefly. Azathioprine reduces the incidence of relapses but does not appear to slow disease progression.[67] This drug should only be used for short periods of time since there is an accompanying risk for developing carcinoma.

Mitoxantrone (Novantrone)

Persons treated with mitoxantrone (Novantrone) should experience a reduction in clinical and MRI attack rate and may have reduced clinical disability.[14] Due to the potential cardiotoxicity of the drug and the risk for treatment-related acute leukemia, this therapy is reserved for persons with progressive disease or those with RRMS who have rapidly worsening disease and who have failed first-line immunomudulator therapies.[14] While the risk of cardiotoxicity increases with cumulative dose, this serious complication can occur at any time during therapy or after discontinuation of therapy. There is evidence to suggest mitoxantrone is a very effective induction agent when followed by first-line therapies, but prospective, long-term studies are needed to confirm the safety and effectiveness of this use.[68] At the dosing recommended for MS therapy, the maximum cumulative dose (140 mg/m^2) is generally reached in 2 to 3 years.[14] There is approximately a 12% risk of cardiotoxicity with mitoxantrone therapy and a 0.8% risk of treatment-related acute leukemia.[68]

Teriflunomide (Aubagio)

Teriflunomide (Aubagio) is a metabolite of leflunomide, which is used to treat rheumatoid arthritis. Although the mechanism of action for treating MS is unknown, teriflunomide reduces the relapse rate and thus is used to treat relapsing forms of MS.[69] This agent does not appear to reduce disability progression.

Future Therapy Considerations

Recent research in MS has focused on development of the newer oral therapies that have been approved as first-line treatments for women with relapsing forms of MS. All appear to be as effective as or more effective than self-injectables, although there are limited safety data and no long-term safety or effectiveness data specific to individuals with MS. Fumaric acid esters (dimethyl fumarate) have been used for psoriasis for more than 20 years. Leflunomide, the prodrug of teriflunomide, has been used with relative safety in rheumatoid arthritis for 15 years. Fingolimod has only a few years of surveillance, suggesting only short-term safety in MS. Comparisons of safety and effectiveness of these oral therapies to long-standing injectable therapies (IFN-βs or GA) can currently be made only through cross-comparison studies. Long-term follow-up for oral therapies and head-to-head studies are necessary to confirm their safety and effectiveness.

Complementary, Alternative, and Adjuvant Therapies

Like conventional therapy for MS, complementary, alternative, and adjuvant treatments focus on balancing the immune system and reducing inflammation. The most frequently used and recommended complemental alternative modalities are diet, essential fatty acids, vitamin/mineral supplementation, homeopathy, botanical products, and antioxidants.[70] There are no proven complementary or alternative therapies that reduce relapse rates or disease progression, and the effects of these therapies on disease-modifying therapies is unknown. Despite this fact, many individuals with MS use complementary and alternative therapies and perceive improvements in their secondary symptoms and quality of life.[70] Stress reduction and rest are generally recommended, particularly during acute attacks.

Yadav et al.[71] reviewed available evidence for complementary and alternative medicine use among individuals with MS and deduced the following: (1) oral cannabis extract decreases subjective spasticity and pain, but does not decrease objective clinical measures; (2) there is insufficient evidence to assess the effects of smoked cannabis; (3) ginkgo biloba likely reduces fatigue, but not cognitive function in MS; (4) magnetic therapy may be helpful for reducing fatigue; and (5) reflexology may help with paresthesia. The following therapies were deemed ineffective: bee stings, fish oil, and Cari Loder regimen (lofepramine plus phenylalanine with vitamin B_{12}). There was insufficient evidence to support the use of acupuncture, Chinese medicine, various herbal and naturopathic therapies, massage, chiropractic, and progressive relaxation therapy.

Special Populations

Pregnancy, Lactation, and Contraception

Limited data exist about the effects of drugs used to treat MS when used during pregnancy, and none of the FDA-approved agents are approved for use during pregnancy. The pregnancy registry for autoimmune diseases is listed in the Resources table at the end of this chapter. However, glatiramer acetate does not cross the placental barrier and has not been shown to affect fertility or fetal development. The drug also is considered compatible with breastfeeding, and given its chemical composition, gastrointestinal absorption is not likely.[72] Limited animal study data for IFN-βs show possible abortifacient effects at high doses, but no teratogenic effect. Rates of early pregnancy loss from an analysis of a global safety database and IFN-β pregnancy registries are similar to those observed in the general population.[72] Nonetheless, women using interferon therapy are advised to discontinue therapy before attempting conception.

Natalizumab (Tysabri) has a theoretical risk of increased early pregnancy loss owing to its interference with cell–cell interactions and cardiovascular complications through inhibition of $alpha_4$ integrins, but neither of these effects were reported in preclinical animal studies.[72] Because the clinical effects of natalizumab during human pregnancy are unknown, its use is based on an individual risk-benefit analysis. Due to the newborn risk for anemia, thrombocytopenia, and impaired host defense, early postnatal evaluation and monitoring is recommended.[73]

Fumaric acid esters, such as dimethyl fumarate, have been used in the treatment of psoriasis for many years with no evidence of embryotoxicity or teratogenicity, but data from human exposure are limited. Results from animal studies are conflicting, with low doses showing no effects and high doses resulting in anomalies.

Use of fingolimod (Gilenya) in pregnancy is contraindicated, and women using fingolimod should avoid pregnancy for two months after discontinuation. Similarly, teriflunomide (Aubagio) is a known teratogen. Teriflunomide has a long half-life due to its gastrointestinal reabsorption and can be found in circulation up to eight months after discontinuation. If a woman or a man desires pregnancy while taking teriflunomide, cholestyramine elimination therapy should be initiated.[72] Mitoxantrone often causes amenorrhea and has been associated with premature birth and low birth weight in animal studies.[72] Women should be advised to avoid pregnancy for at least six months after discontinuing mitoxantrone, and use of this medication is contraindicated in breastfeeding.

Of the alternative MS therapies, methylprednisolone (Medrol), intravenous immunoglobulin administration, and azathioprine (Azasan, Imuran) are likely to be safe to use in pregnancy. Prematurity and fetal growth restriction have been reported with azathioprine and cyclosporine; however, extensive use in SLE and as post-transplant therapy has shown no increase in fetal anomalies. Methylprednisolone (Medrol) should be avoided in the first trimester if possible due to reports of oral cleft anomalies. However, reports are conflicting.

No evidence exists that any contraceptive method is contraindicated for women with MS. In many cases, using a reliable contraceptive method is strongly encouraged, as risks of current pharmacotherapy or degree of disability would make pregnancy undesirable. Combined oral contraceptives may improve symptoms for women who experience worsening symptoms during menstruation.

Elderly

The relationship between multiple sclerosis and menopause has not been widely studied. Some women report exacerbations in the puerperium (a period of relative estrogen deficiency), and the same may be true for menopause. Worsening of symptoms noted during this period, however, may be related to the natural progression of MS. Relapsing–remitting MS often becomes more progressive with increasing age and duration of illness. As with other autoimmune illnesses, prior history of glucocorticoid use increases the postmenopausal risk of osteoporosis. Additionally, older women with MS often have decreased physical activity generally related to fatigue and physical limitations. Prevention strategies for postmenopausal osteoporosis among women with MS include use of calcium and vitamin D supplementation, antiresorptive agents, and hormones. Hormone therapy for perimenopausal conditions is not contraindicated for women with MS.

Rheumatoid Arthritis

Rheumatoid arthritis (RA) is an autoimmune disorder characterized by joint inflammation and progressive disability. It primarily affects synovial joints and tissues of the hands and feet, but any joint can be involved. The initial manifestation of RA is synovitis—an inflammation of the synovial fluid—which triggers an increase in cytokine and chemokine secretion. Local inflammation damages surrounding tissue. The cytokine TNF is the major player in this disease. TNF causes a massive inflammatory reaction in the synovium that results in diminished bone formation and secretion of protein-degrading enzymes, as illustrated in Figure 17-4.[74] Over time, bone and cartilage damage accumulate, resulting in joint deformity and loss of function. With the exception of cervical vertebrae, the axial skeleton is typically spared. Multisystem extra-articular manifestations and comorbidities from the disease process and its therapy can occur.

RA affects approximately 1% of adults worldwide; and occurs among all ethnic groups. The disease typically presents between 30 and 50 years and affects three times as many women as men.[75] Like other autoimmune disorders, RA is likely to occur in a genetically predisposed individual when environmental exposures trigger disease onset. RA susceptibility is associated with single-nucleotide polymorphisms in more than 30 genetic regions, with the most significant being the HLA and PTPN22 alleles.[75] The most consistently linked environmental risk factor is cigarette smoking (current or past).[75] Climate and urbanization may provide additional triggers for RA in genetically predisposed individuals.

Progression of the disease and ensuing disability is heterogeneous and unpredictable. Fewer than 20% of persons with RA will have no disability 10 to 12 years after diagnosis, while 20% to 30% will have work disability within 3 years of diagnosis; by 10 years, more than 50% will have significant work disability.[76]

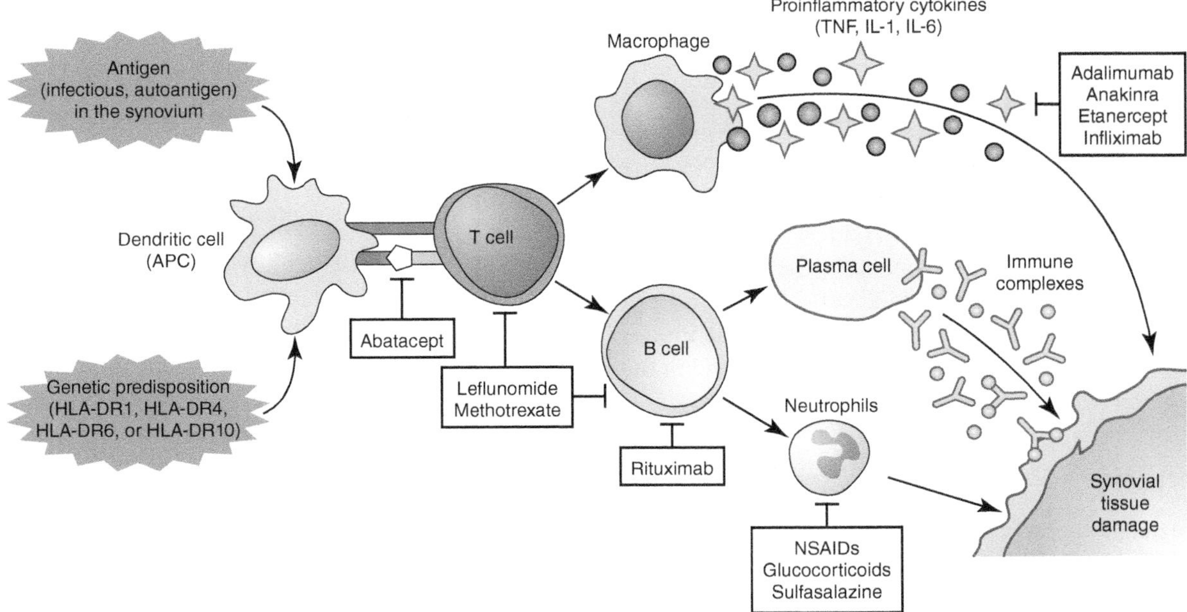

Figure 17-4 Immunopathogenesis and targeted drug therapy of rheumatoid arthritis.

RA typically presents with pain, swelling, and tenderness in joints; decreased mobility; and stiffness after periods of inactivity (morning stiffness). The individual may also report low-grade fever, anorexia, and fatigue prior to the synovial flare. Articular inflammation is generally symmetrical, involving several joints in the upper and lower extremities.

In 2010, the American College of Rheumatology (ACR) and the European League Against Rheumatism (EULAR) published new classification criteria aimed at better classifying new-onset and early-stage disease, as RA is most amenable to treatment early in the course of its development.

Therapy for Women with Rheumatoid Arthritis

Treatment of women with RA focuses on three factors: reducing joint inflammation, managing pain, and preventing joint destruction. Drugs used to treat RA are listed in (Table 17-7)[77,78] and include: (1) analgesics and NSAIDs; (2) glucocorticoids; (3) **disease-modifying antirheumatic drugs (DMARDs)**; and (4) newer biologic agents. DMARDs are a group of drugs that are unrelated structurally but that share the ability to slow disease progression in rheumatoid arthritis.

Analgesics, NSAIDs, and glucocorticoids decrease inflammation and/or pain but do not alter the disease process. DMARD drugs slow disease progression and should be initiated at diagnosis. DMARDs are often given in combinations that improve effectiveness. For example, a combination therapy with methotrexate, hydrochloroquine, and sulfasalazine is a classic "triple therapy."[75]

Table 17-7 Medications Used in the Treatment of Rheumatoid Arthritis

Drug: Generic (Brand)	Dose
Abatacept (Orencia)	500, 750, or 1000 mg[b] IV at weeks 0, 2, and 4, then every 4 weeks
Adalimumab (Humira)	40 mg SQ every 2 weeks
Azathioprine (Azasan, Imuran)	50–150 mg PO once daily
Certolizumab pegol (Cimzia)	400 mg SQ at weeks 0, 2, and 4, then 200 mg SQ every other week or 400 mg SQ every 4 weeks
Cyclosporine (Sandimmune)	2.5–5 mg/kg PO once daily
Etanercept (Enbrel)	25 mg SQ 2 times/week or 50 mg SQ weekly
Golimumab (Simponi)	50 mg SQ monthly
Hydroxychloroquine (Plaquenil)	200–400 mg PO once daily
Infliximab (Remicade)	3 mg/kg IV at weeks 0, 2, and 6, then every 8 weeks
Leflunomide (Arava)	100 mg PO once daily for 3 days, then 10–20 mg PO once daily
Methotrexate (Rheumatrex)	12–25 mg PO, IM, or SQ every week
Rituximab (Rituxan)	1000 mg IV in 2 doses, 2 weeks apart (use with methotrexate)
Sulfasalazine (Azulfidine)	3–4 g PO daily in divided doses
Tocilizumab (Actemra)	4 mg/kg IV every 4 weeks, with increase up to 8 mg/kg IV based on clinical response 162 mg SQ weekly or every 2 weeks[a]
Tofacitinib (Xeljanz)	5 mg PO 2 times daily

[a] The doses listed in this table are one example of a dosing schedule. For most of these drugs, variations in dose and frequency are used in clinical practice to meet the needs of individual women.

[b] Based on person's weight in kilograms.

Sources: Singh JA, Furst DE, Bharat A, et al. 2012 update of the 2008 American College of Rheumatology recommendations for the use of disease-modifying antirheumatic drugs and biologic agents in the treatment of rheumatoid arthritis. *Arthritis Care Res*. 2012;64(5):625-639[77]; Smolen JS, Landewe R, Breedveld FC, et al. EULAR recommendations for the management of rheumatoid arthritis with synthetic and biological disease-modifying antirheumatic drugs: 2013 update. *Ann Rheum Dis*. 2014;73(3):492-509.[78]

Nonsteroidal Anti-inflammatory Drugs

Treatment of women with RA typically involves NSAIDs to control the acute inflammation and pain of synovitis. NSAIDs are appropriate for women with symptoms during the initial diagnostic work-up and as bridge therapy until slower-acting DMARDs can take effect. NSAIDs do not alter the course of RA and should not be used as monotherapy. More information on NSAIDs can be found in the *Analgesia and Anesthesia* chapter.

Glucocorticoids

Glucocorticoid therapy is effective for reducing inflammation, joint tenderness, and pain in persons with active RA.[79] Steroids also slow the rate of joint damage over 1 to 2 years;[79] however, joint damage may increase when these drugs are discontinued. Steroids are also indicated for the control of disease activity while awaiting the onset of clinical effects of newly initiated DMRAD therapy.

Glucocorticoids may be administered orally or through local injection. When only a few joints are involved, local injection provides rapid, but temporary symptom relief. Septic arthritis must be ruled out prior to steroid injection.[7]

Despite the potential for disease modification, monotherapy with glucocorticoids is not recommended, as long-term effects are not well known. Some persons, however, will require continued low-dose steroid therapy when other treatment regimens fail. Chronic use of steroids in RA should be weighed against the potential risks associated with steroid use.

Disease-Modifying Antirheumatoid Drugs

Methotrexate (Rheumatrex), sulfasalazine, hydrochloroquine (Plaquenil), and leflunomide (Arava) were the first DMARDs used and remain the mainstay of treatment today. Newer biologic agents such as abatacept (Orencia), infliximab (Remicade), and adalimumab (Humira) have been more recently added to the pharmacotherapeutic armamentarium directed toward RA. There is marked individual variability between individuals in their response to DMARDs. In addition, the choice of drug depends on the level of disease activity, stage of therapy, and individual factors. These medications should be prescribed by specialists who care for women with autoimmune disorders.

Methotrexate (Rheumatrex, Trexall)

Methotrexate (Rheumatrex, Trexall) is the most commonly used disease-modifying antirheumatic drug and the mainstay of RA therapy for persons with moderate to severe disease. This agent is relatively inexpensive, is highly effective, and has a low risk of toxicity compared to most other disease-modifying antirheumatic drugs and biologic agents. It should be used as initial therapy, either alone or in combination, for the treatment of active RA.[77,78] Methotrexate has been shown to slow the progression of bone erosions associated with severe RA.[80] Methotrexate therapy is usually initiated with oral dosing, followed by parenteral administration if disease activity remains uncontrolled after increasing to high-dose oral therapy.

Leflunomide (Arava)

Leflunomide (Arava) is often used for individuals who have a suboptimal or intolerant response to methotrexate or in whom methotrexate use is contraindicated.[78] Leflunomide may be used as monotherapy or in combination with methotrexate. These drugs' mechanisms of action appear to be complementary, and persons on combination therapy have somewhat better response than those on either monotherapy.

Hydroxychloroquine (Plaquenil)

Hydroxychloroquine (Plaquenil) is effective for symptom relief for persons with early or mild RA. Monotherapy does not impact progression of bone erosions, but administration of this agent early in the disease process may improve long-term outcomes. Hydroxychloroquine use improves lipid profiles and glycemic control, and may reduce cardiovascular risk in individuals with RA.[81,82]

Sulfasalazine (Azulfidine)

Sulfasalazine (Azulfidine), which is given to persons with early or mild RA, has similar effectiveness to methotrexate in providing symptom relief and slowing bone erosions and is an alternative initial RA therapy for individuals with contraindications or intolerance to methotrexate.[78] Side effects of sulfasalazine are lessened with slow and gradual titration of daily dosing. This agent may be used as monotherapy or in combination with other disease-modifying antirheumatic drugs. If clinical response is not seen by 4 months, the therapy should be changed.

Immunomodulators/Biologic Agents

Biologic agents may be used as initial therapy for persons with severe RA but more commonly are used for individuals with toxicity, failure, or intolerance of traditional disease-modifying antirheumatic drug therapy. More data are available on the safety and effectiveness of anti-TNF-alpha agents than for other biologics for the treatment of women with RA.

Adalimumab (Humira), certolizumab pegol (Cimzia), etanercept (Enbrel), golimumab (Simponi), and infliximab (Remicade) are anti-TNF-alpha agents that have been shown to decrease pain, improve physical function, and reduce bone erosion in individuals with RA. There is no significant difference in effectiveness levels of these agents, but etanercept appears to have the best safety profile and lowest rate of discontinuation.[83,84]

When used as monotherapy, each agent is as effective as methotrexate and has a more rapid onset of action. Infliximab (Remicade) is recommended for combination therapy with methotrexate and when effectiveness is improved with this combination.[77,78] Adalimumab (Humira) and etanercept (Enbrel) may be used as monotherapy or in combination with methotrexate or other disease-modifying antirheumatic drugs.[78]

The choice of anti-TNF-alpha therapy generally depends on the cost and the person's preference for administration. If an individual does not have an adequate clinical response to a particular anti-TNF-alpha agent, a different anti-TNF-alpha agent may be administered or therapy with another biologic agent may be initiated.[77,78] Not all women with RA will respond to these agents, and disease flares are common when therapy is discontinued. After a sustained period of low disease activity or remission without glucocorticoids, it is acceptable to consider tapering of biologic therapy provided the individual is maintained on conventional DMARD therapy.[78]

Abatacept (Orencia) can be used as monotherapy or in combination with methotrexate in the treatment of women with severe, refractory RA. Existing data suggest that abatacept is safe and effective when used alone or in combination with methotrexate after either failure of methotrexate monotherapy or failure of another anti-TNF-therapy.[85]

Rituximab (Rituxan) is currently recommended for use with methotrexate in treating women with severe, refractory RA that has not responded to TNF-alpha antagonists.[77,78] In this context, rituximab has been shown to reduce disease activity and improve outcomes.[86] Persons receiving rituximab therapy may have slightly increased risks of infection. There have been no reports of opportunistic infections.[87]

Tocilizumab (Actemra) is an effective therapy for individuals with RA who have not responded to anti-TNF-alpha therapy or other DMARDs. Monotherapy with tocilizumab appears to be as effective as combination therapy with methotrexate[88,89] and more effective than adalimumab monotherapy.[88] Thus, this agent represents an important and effective alternative for individuals in whom methotrexate is contraindicated. Subcutaneous therapy is comparable in safety and effectiveness to intravenous therapy.[90]

Tofacitinib (Xeljanz) is approved for use in individuals with active RA who have not responded to treatment with methotrexate or other disease-modifying agents. In a systematic review and meta-analysis, Kawalec et al. found that tofacitinib, with or without methotrexate, resulted in significantly improved clinical response when compared to placebo ($P < 0.00001$) and adalimumab ($P = 0.003$), without any increased risk of adverse events.[91] This novel therapy provides an important alternative to subcutaneous or intravenous treatment of women with refractory RA.

Combination Therapy

If monotherapy with traditional disease-modifying antirheumatic drugs fails, combination therapy is recommended.[77,78] Methotrexate plus hydroxychloroquine (Plaquenil) and methotrexate plus sulfasalazine (Azulfidine) are more effective than monotherapy. Triple combination therapy with methotrexate, hydroxychloroquine, and sulfasalazine has a greater impact than dual therapy in both early and advanced RA. In their study, O'Dell et al. found a 50% improvement in RA symptoms in 40% of those participants treated with methotrexate and hydroxychloroquine, 29% treated with methotrexate and sulfasalazine, and 55% treated with triple combination therapy.[92] When compared to etanercept (Enbrel) plus methotrexate dual-agent therapy, triple-agent therapy was found to be as effective, with no significant difference between the treatment groups in terms of pain, disease progression, quality of life measures, or adverse events.[93]

Complementary, Alternative, and Adjuvant Therapies

Several nonpharmacologic therapies have been reported to improve symptoms in RA; however, studies of herbal therapies in RA treatment have yielded inconclusive results owing in part to the poor data reporting and low methodologic quality of these trials.[94] In a meta-analysis of herbal therapies, improvement in pain and stiffness was seen with gamma-linoleic acid supplementation when compared to placebo (68% versus 32% and 61% versus 39%, respectively).[95] Essential fatty acid supplementation may decrease the need for anti-inflammatory medication or dose. Proudman et al. found fish oil supplementation improved the rate of remission (hazard ratio [HR], 2.17; 95% CI, 1.07–4.42; $P = 0.03$) and reduced treatment failure (HR, 0.28; 95% CI, 0.12–0.63; $P = 0.002$) in individuals receiving methotrexate (Rheumatrex, Trexall), sulfasalazine (Azulfidine), and hydroxychloroquine (Plaquenil) when compared to placebo plus triple therapy.[96] The possible benefits of *Boswellia serrata* (frankincense) and topical capsaicin need further study.

Special Populations

Pregnancy, Lactation, and Contraception

It is reasonable to expect that a woman will experience relative disease quiescence during pregnancy due to the more anti-inflammatory cytokine profile apparent in pregnancy. DMARDs for routine use during pregnancy are limited to hydroxychloroquine (Plaquenil), glucocorticoids, NSAIDs, and sulfasalazine (Azulfidine).[97] NSAID use should be discontinued in the third trimester to limit the risk of premature closure of the fetal ductus arteriosus. Methotrexate (Rheumatrex, Trexall) and leflunomide (Arava) are known teratogens and are contraindicated during pregnancy and lactation. Due to limited data regarding the safety of biologics, regular use during pregnancy and lactation should likely be avoided,[97] although anti-TNF-alpha agents may be appropriate for use in severe RA or if flares continue despite anti-inflammatory and immunosuppressant therapy. Biologics should generally be avoided in the preconception period, but anti-TNF-alpha therapy may be continued until conception.[97,98]

Box 17-1 Rheumatoid Arthritis and Menopause

MP is a 52 year old who arrives for a routine gynecologic exam. Her last menstrual period was seven months ago. She reports frequent "hot flashes," but otherwise has no significant perimenopausal symptoms. She asks her healthcare provider what menopausal therapy would be recommended for her given her history and current medications.

MP was diagnosed with rheumatoid arthritis (RA) four years ago and is currently under the care of a rheumatologist. She was initially treated with methotrexate and has received glucocorticoids for exacerbations in the past. Her course of RA has been moderately active with intermittent periods of remission. She is currently using combination therapy, methotrexate plus etanercept, and reports minimal disability with infrequent symptom flares.

Menopausal women are at greater risk for heart disease and osteoporosis. These risks are increased with RA due to chronic inflammation of the disease, physical inactivity associated with disability, and the use of glucocorticoid therapy, which decreases bone density and affects lipid metabolism. Risk-reducing strategies for these conditions include: following a heart-healthy diet with moderate exercise as tolerated, limiting glucocorticoid exposure, screening for and managing dyslipidemia, screening and prophylactic therapy for osteopenia or osteoporosis, and consideration for hormone therapy (HT). HT is not contraindicated in RA and may be beneficial in reducing risk of heart disease and osteoporosis. Some women report RA symptom reduction with HT, which is likely due to estrogen's anti-inflammatory effects. Studies have not consistently confirmed improvement in RA symptoms with HT.

MP's healthcare provider prescribes transdermal HT for treatment of hot flashes and for osteoporosis prevention. She also recommends 1000 mg of calcium and 800 IU of vitamin D daily and will consider adding an antiresorptive agent after reviewing the results of MP's bone mineral density scan ordered today.

Owing to the shift to a pro-inflammatory cytokine profile that occurs in the postpartum period, approximately 90% of women experience disease flares after giving birth. Breastfeeding is not contraindicated in RA, but limited data are available on the use of biologic therapies during lactation. Any contraceptive method is appropriate for use by individuals with RA, provided that the woman does not have other contraindications. While some sources may advocate withholding intrauterine contraception for women on immunosuppressive therapy, there are no data to substantiate this risk or determine when it is sufficient to contraindicate this type of contraception. While the diaphragm and combined hormonal vaginal ring are not contraindicated for women with RA, some women with severe RA may have difficulty inserting these devices. Combined oral contraceptives have been associated with a decreased risk of developing RA but have not shown a therapeutic effect in the disease process.[99]

Elderly

Women with RA have increased risk for heart disease and osteoporosis during the postmenopausal years. Long-term glucocorticoid use increases risk of osteoporosis and osteoporotic fractures, while methotrexate reduces risk of cardiovascular-related death. Women with more disease activity and greater disability may be at additional risk because of worse disease and resulting physical inactivity. The effect of menopause on RA activity varies. Reported increases in disease activity after menopause may be related more to duration of illness than to hormonal changes. Some women experience improvement in pain and joint inflammation when hormone therapy is provided perimenopausally. Whether hormone therapy has a real benefit in terms of diminishing RA symptom frequency and severity is uncertain; however, hormones are not contraindicated for use for women with RA. Hormone therapy along with lifestyle changes may reduce the risk for postmenopausal heart disease and bone loss, as discussed in Box 17-1.

Systemic Lupus Erythematosus

Systemic lupus erythematosus (SLE) is a chronic, inflammatory, multisystem autoimmune disorder. The primary feature of SLE is immune dysregulation of B cells that results in abnormally increased production of autoantibodies directed toward nuclear antigens, as illustrated in Figure 17-5. Organ and tissue damage results from the deposition of immune complexes in target tissue (e.g., nephritis) or autoantibody-mediated destruction

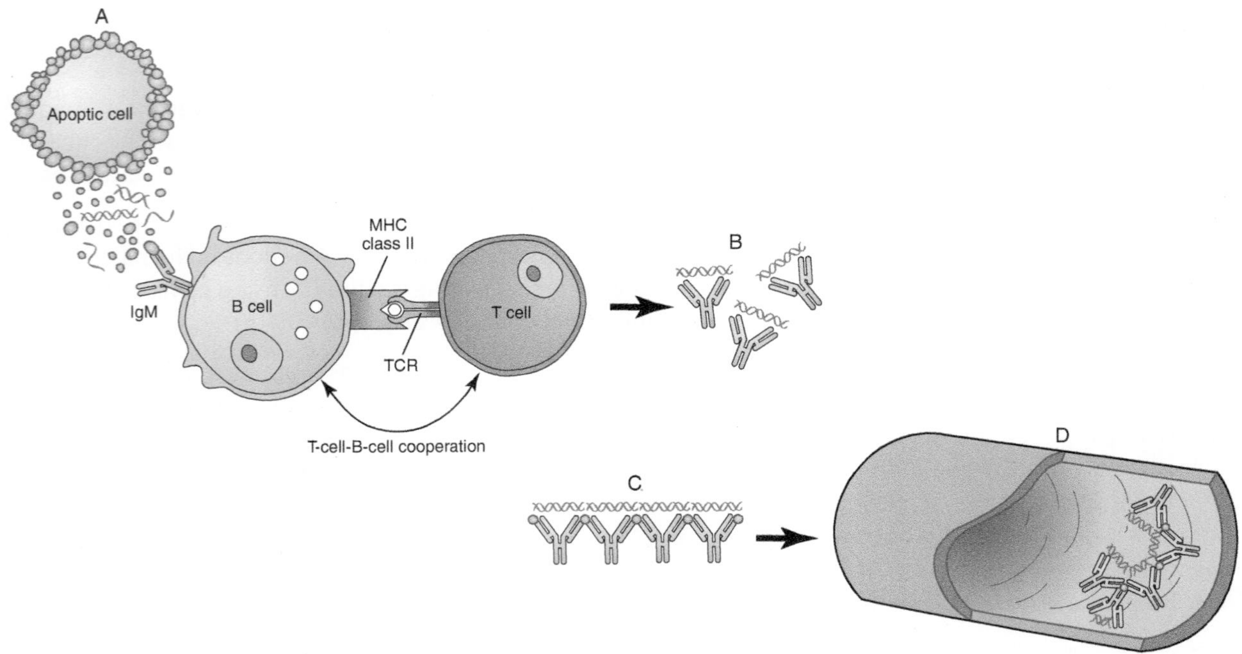

(A) Apoptic cell releases cell components. (B) Autoantiboides to nuclear antigens are formed. (C) Autoantibodies form immune complexes. (D) Immune complexes lodge in tissue such as blood vessels, skin, or glomerulus and initiate inflammation and tissue damage.

Figure 17-5 Autoantibody-mediated pathogenesis of systemic lupus erythematosus.

of host cells (e.g., hemolytic anemia). The deposition of immune complexes in vascular tissue increases the risk of premature atherosclerosis and cardiovascular events.[100]

The overall prevalence of SLE in the United States ranges from 20 to 150 cases per 100,000 population.[101] SLE is nearly 10 times more common among women than among men, and the majority of cases among women are diagnosed during the childbearing years. Interaction between susceptibility genes and environmental factors is necessary for the development of SLE. Environmental exposures—particularly those associated with oxidative stress, such as cigarette smoking, ultraviolet light, and infection—influence SLE onset and flares.[102]

SLE is a multisystem disorder with significant variations in its presentation and course. It can affect all major organ systems. The majority (90%) of individuals with SLE have constitutional symptoms (malaise, fatigue, anorexia, and low-grade fevers). Overall, however, the most common SLE manifestations are in the skin and musculoskeletal organs, such as photosensitivity, malar rash, oral ulcers, discoid rash, and arthritis.

SLE is a complex disorder characterized by periods of relative inactivity and periods of disease exacerbation (flares). Some affected individuals may have relatively quiescent disease, whereas others may have chronic activity. The majority of deaths that occur in the early stages of disease are attributed to active disease (neurologic or renal) or infection.

SLE versus Drug-Induced Lupus

Drug-induced lupus is an autoimmune syndrome that shares many of the characteristic features and symptoms of SLE. Drug-induced lupus rarely involves the central nervous or renal systems.

The cause of drug-induced lupus is not well understood. Lack of specific drug antibodies or antigen targets supports the notion that the mechanisms involved are not those of the typical drug hypersensitivity reactions. This hypothesis is further supported by the slow onset of symptom recurrence with reintroduction of the inducing drug.[103] More than 80 drugs are known to cause drug-induced lupus,

Table 17-8 Medications That Can Cause Drug-Induced Lupus

Class	Strong Risk: Generic (Brand)	Moderate or Low Risk: Generic (Brand)	Associated with Drug-Induced Lupus in Case Reports: Generic (Brand)
Antiarrhythmics	Procainamide (Pronestyl)	Quinidine (Quinaglute)	Disopyramide (Norpace) Propafenone (Rythmol)
Antihyperlipidemics			Lovastatin (Altoprev, Mevacor) Simvastatin (Zocor)
Antihypertensives	Hydralazine (Apresoline)	Methyldopa (Aldomet), Captopril (Capoten), Acebutolol (Sectral)	Beta blockers (several)
Anti-infectives		Isoniazid (INH) Minocycline (Minocin)	Nitrofurantoin (Macrodantin) Terbinafine (Lamisil)
Anti-inflammatories		Sulfasalazine (Azulfidine)	Nonsteroidal anti-inflammatory drugs
Antipsychotics/anticonvulsants	Chlorpromazine (Thorazine) Methyldopa (Aldomet)	Carbamazepine (Tegretol)	Lithium (Lithobid) Phenytoin (Dilantin)
Biologic Agents			Infliximab (Remicade) Etanercept (Enbrel)
Other		Propylthiouracil (PTU)	Fluorouracil (Carac, Efudex) Gold salts (Ridaura, Myochrysine) Hydrochlorothiazide (HydroDIURIL) Penicillamine (Cuprimine)

Sources: Data from Araujo-Fernanced S, Ajijon-Lana M, Isenberg DA. Drug-induced lupus: including anti-tumor necrosis factor and interferon induced. Lupus. 2014;23(6):545-553[106]; Lowe CG, Henderson CL, Grau RH, Hansen CB, Sontheimer RD. A systematic review of drug-induced subacute lupus erythematosus. *Br J Dermatol.* 2011;164(2):465-472[107]; Vasoo S. Drug-induced lupus: an update. *Lupus.* 2006;15(11):757-761.[105]

including antiarrhythmics, antihypertensives, antithyroid medications, antipsychotics, anticonvulsants, antirheumatics, antihyperlipidemic drugs, and antibiotics. In addition, TNF-alpha antagonists have been implicated in drug-induced lupus and are more likely to cause cutaneous and renal manifestations as well as anti-dsDNA antibodies.[103,104] Symptoms are typically mild to moderate and resolve within weeks of discontinuing the inducing drug. Severe cases, while rare, have been reported; they generally respond to short-term glucocorticoid therapy.[105-107]

Table 17-8 lists the agents most commonly associated with drug-induced lupus. Additional information about drug-induced lupus can be found in the *Drug Toxicity* chapter.

Therapy for Women with Systemic Lupus Erythematosus

The goal of SLE therapy is to control disease flares, suppress symptoms, and prevent organ damage. Treatment decisions are based on disease severity and organ involvement. In general, all persons with SLE are treated with hydroxychloroquine (Plaquenil), NSAIDs, and short-term use of other glucocorticoids. Persons with moderate disease may also use immunosuppressant agents such as azathioprine (Azasan, Imuran) or methotrexate (Rheumatrex, Trexall). Severe disease is initially treated with intensive immunosuppressant drugs such as cyclophosphamide (Cytoxan) or Mycophenolate mofetil (CellCept). Table 17-9 provides a list of medications with recommended dosing schedules.

Nonsteroidal Anti-inflammatory Drugs

SLE arthritis and arthralgia are generally relieved by NSAID therapy. NSAIDs may also be effective in treating

Table 17-9 Medications Used for Treatment of Systemic Lupus Erythematosus

Drug: Generic (Brand)	Dose[a]
Azathioprine (Azasan, Imuran)	2–3 mg/kg PO once daily
Belimumab (Benlysta)	10 mg/kg IV every 2 weeks for 3 doses, then once every 4 weeks
Cyclophosphamide (Cytoxan)	0.7–2.5 mg/kg IV monthly for 6 months 1.5–3 mg/kg PO once daily
Cyclosporine (Sandimmune)	2.5–5 mg/kg IV once daily
Hydroxychloroquine (Plaquenil)	200–400 mg PO once daily
Methylprednisolone (Medrol)	Severe: 1 g IV once daily for 3 days
Mycophenolate mofetil (CellCept)	Lupus nephritis: 1 g PO 2 times/day
NSAIDs (e.g., ibuprofen [Advil])	Toward upper limits of normal ranges
Prednisone (Deltasone)	Severe: 0.5–1 mg/kg PO once daily Mild: 0.07–0.3 mg/kg PO once daily
Topical glucocorticoids	Low potency for face, high potency for other areas

[a] The doses listed in this table are one example of a dosing schedule. For most of these drugs, variations in dose and frequency are used in clinical practice to meet the needs of individual women.

fever and mild serositis. Individuals with SLE are at greater risk of NSAID-induced aseptic meningitis, hypertension, edema, and renal dysfunction.[108]

Glucocorticoids

Topical, oral, and intravenous glucocorticoids are frequently used in treatment of SLE. Women with mild disease typically do not need systemic therapy. Systemic prednisone and methylprednisolone are generally used when the condition is severe or refractory; these agents are the foundation of therapy for life-threatening inflammation of major organ systems.[109] High-dose intravenous methylprednisolone may be given to treat women with severe, acute inflammatory manifestations, followed by an oral taper to low-dose oral maintenance therapy. Some individuals continue low-dose maintenance therapy for years.

Mild cutaneous lesions typically respond to topical steroids. Severe skin lesions may require treatment with intravenous steroids. If disease flares occur during the tapering period, another therapeutic agent such as hydroxychloroquine (Plaquenil), azathioprine (Imuran), or methotrexate (Rheumatrex, Trexall) may be added to control disease activity.

Immunosuppressants

Azathioprine (Imuran)

Azathioprine (Imuran) is an immunosuppressant usually prescribed for individuals who are steroid dependent or have SLE disease activity in multiple systems.[110] Azathioprine is widely used as a steroid-sparing agent.

Cyclophosphamide (Cytoxan)

Cyclophosphamide (Cytoxan) is used to treat severe renal and neuropsychiatric SLE. This agent is most commonly used to treat lupus nephritis in individuals who are at high risk of developing end-stage renal disease. Intravenous cyclophosphamide treatment preserves long-term renal function for the majority of women with lupus nephritis. After clinical response to pulse cyclophosphamide is achieved, it may be followed by azathioprine or mycophenolate to reduce the adverse effects associated with cyclophosphamide therapy.[1]

Cyclosporine (Sandimmune, Neoral)

Cyclosporine (Sandimmune, Neoral) is generally used for women who are intolerant to other immunosuppressive therapies or who have developed myelosuppression secondary to other immunosuppressants. It may be particularly useful in treating women who have severe or steroid-resistant SLE.[112] Individuals with SLE are at increased risk of developing accelerated atherosclerosis and should be monitored very closely for cyclosporine-induced hypertension and dyslipidemia. Cyclosporine may not be a preferred therapy for young persons with SLE because of these increased risks. This drug should be discontinued gradually, as rapid tapering is associated with disease flares.

Hydroxychloroquine (Plaquenil)

Hydroxychloroquine (Plaquenil) is the mainstay of therapy for persons with serositis, arthritis, and musculoskeletal and cutaneous manifestations of SLE and should be considered for all individuals with mild SLE.[108,109] Hydroxychloroquine has been shown to prevent future flares and organ damage.[113] Topical hydroxychloroquine reduces the severity of lesions in cutaneous SLE. This agent may be considered for use as adjunct therapy in lupus nephritis, as its use is associated with a reduced risk of renal damage. This drug has a beneficial effect on dyslipidemia and hyperglycemia as well as weak antithromboembolic effects.[109]

Methotrexate (Rheumatrex, Trexall)

Methotrexate (Rheumatrex, Trexall) is not used in women with major organ manifestations of SLE, but it may be effective for those with skin and joint disease.[109] For women with severe SLE arthritis, methotrexate may be an appropriate first-line therapy.

Mycophenolate Mofetil (CellCept)

Mycophenolate mofetil (CellCept) is used for the treatment of women with lupus nephritis. When compared to cyclophosphamide (Cytoxan), mycophenolate has similar effectiveness and similar rates of major infections. Slightly higher rates of remissions have been reported with mycophenolate treatment, but long-term outcome research is needed to show whether this therapy provides renal protection similar to cyclophosphamide therapy. Mycophenolate appears to be more effective than cyclophosphamide among Hispanic and African American individuals, and is currently preferred as a first-line nephritis therapy in these higher-prevalence groups.[111] Mycophenolate is also the preferred therapy for persons who are experiencing lupus nephritis and wish to preserve fertility, as high-dose cyclophosphamide can cause infertility in both women and men.[114]

Immunomodulators/Biologic Agents

Belimumab (Benlysta)

In 2011, belimumab (Benlysta) was approved by the FDA as the first biologic therapy for use in persons with SLE and as the first drug specifically approved for the treatment of women with SLE in more than 50 years. Belimumab is intended for use in persons with active, ANA or anti-dsDNA positive SLE who are receiving standard therapy with NSAIDs, glucocorticoids, hydroxychloroquine (Plaquenil), and immunosuppressive agents.[115] It has not been studied in persons with severe lupus nephritis or cerebritis or in persons who are taking other biologic therapies. With the exception of mild infusion reactions, there appear to be no significant differences in adverse events.[115]

Complementary, Alternative, and Adjuvant Therapies

Daily activity and lifestyle modifications may help reduce disease activity in SLE. In particular, women with this disease should minimize sun exposure and use sunscreen with at least an SPF of 15.

Exposure to sunlight or ultraviolet light can exacerbate flares of SLE disease activity. Vitamin D deficiency is common among persons with SLE.[116] Whether this is related to avoidance of sun exposure, SLE therapy, or the autoimmune process is unclear; however, vitamin D is reported to play an important role in the immune system as well as in cardiovascular and musculoskeletal systems. Ensuring adequate levels of serum vitamin D may be particularly important for persons with SLE to reduce disease activity and risk for osteoporotic fracture and cardiovascular disease.[116]

Cardiovascular disease is the leading cause of death in persons with SLE so treatments to prevent cardiovascular disease are of particular import for this population. Essential fatty acid supplementation may decrease inflammation and offer cardiovascular protection in SLE, and two randomized controlled trials have shown some benefit from use of omega-3 fatty acid supplementation.[117,118]

Dehydroepiandrosterone (DHEA) is a naturally occurring adrenal steroid hormone that has been studied for use in reducing SLE flares, albeit with mixed results. DHEA is not a suitable monotherapy but may be of benefit to some as an adjuvant therapy. Use of this supplement has a positive impact on bone mineral density and may be steroid sparing for some individuals.[119] Acne and hirsutism are common side effects experienced among women using DHEA.

Green tea polyphenols are potent antioxidant compounds that inhibit TNF-alpha–induced apoptosis and may provide epidermal protection in cutaneous manifestations of SLE. There is no evidence to suggest oral consumption has an effect on SLE-related organ damage.

Special Populations

Pregnancy, Breastfeeding, and Contraception

Treatment of women with SLE in pregnancy is generally limited to use of NSAIDs, prednisone, and hydroxychloroquine (Plaquenil). NSAIDs, with the exception of low-dose aspirin, should generally be avoided in the third trimester due to concerns about reversible oligohydramnios, possible prolonged gestation, prolonged labor, and premature closure of the patent ductus arteriosis.[120] Discontinuation of hydroxychloroquine therapy has been associated with a significant increase in disease activity and an increase in prednisone use during pregnancy. If a woman is stable on hydroxychloroquine prior to conception, she should continue that medication at the lowest possible therapeutic dose. If a woman with SLE is considering pregnancy, it is recommended that she postpone conception until the disease is stable or in remission. Active disease at conception and history of renal disease increase the likelihood of poor pregnancy outcome.[121]

If a woman has antiphospholipid (aPL) antibodies, prophylactic anticoagulant therapy with low-dose aspirin is recommended. Low-dose aspirin with low-molecular-weight heparin is used in antiphospholipid syndrome (APS). Anticoagulant therapy should be discontinued at the onset of labor and resumed postpartum—for 6 weeks in women with aPLs and indefinitely in women with APS. Glucocorticoids with or without azathioprine are preferred for the treatment of women with lupus nephritis during pregnancy.

Limited safety data exist regarding the use of belimumab in pregnancy or lactation. Animal studies have shown excretion in breast milk and transplacental transfer of the drug, which resulted in a reversible reduction in B cells and IgG in infant monkeys without signs of fetotoxicity or teratogenicity. The Belimumab Pregnancy Registry reports on pregnancy outcomes with belimumab exposure four months before and/or after conception.[122]

Contraception recommendations for women with SLE are generally no different than those for healthy women with a few exceptions. The method of contraception, including use of oral contraceptives, has no significant impact on SLE activity.[123] However, because SLE is associated with an increased risk for thromboembolic events, women with

SLE who have positive antiphospholipid antibodies have some contraceptive limitations. The United States Medical Eligibility Criteria rate combined hormonal contraception a Category 4 and progestin-only pills a Category 3 for women with SLE who also have positive antiphospholipid antibodies.[124,125] Category 4 states the contraceptive method is contraindicated and category 3 indicates theoretical or proven risks generally outweigh the advantages of the contraceptive method. While intrauterine contraception is not contraindicated for persons with SLE, appropriateness of use should be evaluated on a case-by-case basis. Women with risk factors for infection, such as use of aggressive immunosuppressant therapy, are generally poor candidates for intrauterine contraception.

Elderly

Menopause does not appear to have an effect on SLE or SLE flares. The natural history of SLE is characterized by more significant disease activity earlier in the course of illness, so menopausal women tend to have milder disease. Disease activity in SLE has not been shown to increase menopausal symptoms or to hasten the onset of menopause. Women with SLE who receive cyclophosphamide therapy have a greater risk of premature ovarian failure, however. This increased risk is related to older age when treated with cyclophosphamide and higher cumulative doses.

Due to the systemic and inflammatory nature of SLE, women with this condition have increased risk for heart disease and osteoporosis during the postmenopausal period. Hormone therapy may increase the frequency of mild flares but does not affect the rate of severe flares. Hormone therapy is contraindicated for women with SLE who have a history of thrombosis, antiphospholipid syndrome, or positive antiphospholipid antibodies (anticardiolipin antibody or lupus anticoagulant).

Late-onset lupus, which is sometimes referred to as *elderly lupus*, presents in the early menopausal years (50 to 65 years of age). The presentation and course of late-onset lupus is generally milder than the presentation and course of SLE that first occurs during the childbearing years. Treatment is based on symptom type and severity, as with earlier-onset SLE.

Conclusion

A disproportionate number of persons with autoimmune disorders are women. Thus, autoimmune conditions are a woman's issue. Fortunately, new information about these conditions is emerging in the twenty-first century, as are novel designer drugs that target the new findings. As a consequence, new drugs can be expected to enter the market on a regular basis and treatment plans are likely to become more customized based on not only gender, but also ethnic/racial background, age, and—perhaps most importantly—personal genetic composition.

Resources

Organization	Description	Website
Women's Health	Federal site that provides consumer information about autoimmune disorders and treatments, including drugs. Includes downloadable fact sheets on a variety of conditions and frequently asked questions. A separate page for healthcare providers exists, but primarily directs the clinician to health information for women.	http://womenshealth.gov/publications/our-publications/fact-sheet/autoimmune-diseases.html
American Autoimmune Related Diseases Association (AARDA)	Organization that focuses on autoimmune diseases. Although it is primarily consumer oriented, it is of note that the website is available in Spanish.	www.aarda.org Page specific to women: www.aarda.org/autoimmune-information/autoimmune-disease-in-women
Organization of Teratology Information Specialists (OTIS)	The Organization of Teratology Information Specialists is a non-profit collaboration of various information groups, primarily supported by pharmacological manufacturers. The specific OTIS autoimmune diseases study can be found on the website or by calling 877-311-8972.	www.pregnancystudies.org/ongoing-pregnancy-studies/autoimmune-studies
Consumer-oriented group		
National Multiple Sclerosis Society	Groups dedicated to a specific autoimmune disease have strong websites. Although they are primarily directed toward consumers, they often contain information about treatments that may be of value for women and providers alike.	www.nationalmssociety.org
Arthritis Foundation		www.arthritis.org
Lupus Foundation		www.lupus.org
Apps		
A myriad of apps exist for devices that offer consumer-oriented information about autoimmune disorders or mHealth tracking of symptoms and treatments. Many are free and can be suggested to women.		
@Hand: Treatment strategies in Rheumatology. The @Hand series of apps is outlined with treatment choices, benefits and risks of treatments, and when to change treatments, in addition to other features.		

References

1. Bach JF. The effect of infections on susceptibility to autoimmune and allergic diseases. *N Engl J Med.* 2002;347(12):911-920.
2. Edwards JC, Cambridge G. B-cell targeting in rheumatoid arthritis and other autoimmune diseases. *Nat Rev.* 2006;6(5):394-403.
3. Ackerman LS. Sex hormones and the genesis of autoimmunity. *Arch Dermatol.* 2006;142(3):371-376.
4. Gleicher N, Barad DH. Gender as risk factor for autoimmune diseases. *J Autoimmunity.* 2007; 28(1):1-6.
5. Lake DF, Briggs AD, Akporiaye ET. Immunopharmacology. In: Katzung BG, Masters SB, Trevor AJ, eds. *Basic and Clinical Pharmacology.* 13th ed. New York, NY/London, England: McGraw-Hill Medical; 2014:946-970.
6. Rhen T, Cidlowski JA. Anti-inflammatory action of glucocorticoids. *N Engl J Med.* 2005;353:1771-1723.
7. Goodin DS, Frohman EM, Garmany GP Jr, et al. Disease-modifying therapies in multiple sclerosis: report of the Therapeutics and Technology Assessment Subcommittee of the American Academy of Neurology and the MS Council for Clinical Practice Guidelines. *Neurology.* 2002;58(2):169-178. [Reaffirmed on July 19, 2008].
8. Wallace JL, Sharkey KA. Pharmacotherapy of inflammatory bowel disease. In: Brunton LL, Chabner BA, Knollmann BC, eds. *Goodman & Gilman's The Pharmacological Basis of Therapeutics.* 12th ed. New York: McGraw-Hill; 2011:1351-1363.
9. Teml A, Schaeffeler E, Herrlinger KR, Klotz U, Schwab M. Thiopurine treatment in inflammatory bowel disease. *Clin Pharmacokinet.* 2007;46(3):187-208
10. Doan T, Massarotti E. Rheumatoid arthritis: an overview of new and emerging therapies. *J Clin Pharmacol.* 2005;45(7):751-762.
11. Bar-Or A, Pachner A, Menguy-Vacheron F, Kaplan J, Wiendl H. Teriflunomide and its mechanism of action in multiple sclerosis. *Drugs.* 2014;74(6):659-674.
12. Griffiths B, Emery P. The treatment of lupus with cyclosporin A. *Lupus.* 2001;10(3):165-170.
13. Marmor MF, Melles RB. Hydroxychloroquine and the retina. *JAMA Opthamol.* 2014;132(10):1199-1208.
14. Goodin DS, Arnason BG, Coyle PK, Frohman EM, Paty DW. The use of mitoxantrone (Novantrone) for the treatment of multiple sclerosis: report of the Therapeutics and Technology Assessment Subcommittee of the American Academy of Neurology. *Neurology.* 2003;61(10):1332-1338.
15. Villarroel MC, Hidalgo M, Jimeno A. Mycophenolate mofetil: an update. *Drugs Today.* 2009;45(7): 521-532.
16. Saag KG, Teng GG, Patkar NM, et al. American College of Rheumatology 2008 recommendations for the use of nonbiologic and biologic disease-modifying antirheumatic drugs in rheumatoid arthritis. *Arthritis Rheum.* 2008;59(6):762-784.
17. Merrill JT, Ginzler EM, Wallace DJ, et al. Long-term safety profile of belimumab plus standard therapy in patients with systemic lupus erythematosus. *Arthritis Rheum.* 2012;64(10):3364-3373.
18. Woodrick RS, Ruderman EM. Safety of biologic therapy in rheumatoid arthritis. *Nat Rev Rheumatol.* 2011;7(11):639-652.
19. McCluggage LK, Scholtz JM. Golimumab: a tumor necrosis factor alpha inhibitor for the treatment of rheumatoid arthritis. *Ann Pharmacother.* 2010;44(1):135-144.
20. Ternant D, Bejan-Angoulvant T, Passot C, Mulleman D, Paintaud G. Clinical pharmacokineticts and pharmcodynamics of monoclonal antibodies approved to treat rheumatoid arthritis. *Clin Pharmacokinet.* 2015;June 28. [Epub ahead of print.]
21. Ransohoff RM. Natalizumab for multiple sclerosis. *N Engl J Med.* 2007;356(25):2622-2629.
22. Fine AJ, Sorbello A, Kortepeter C, Scarazzini L. Central nervous system herpes simplex and varicella zoster virus infections in natalizumab-treated patients. *Clin Infect Dis.* 2013;57(6):849-852.
23. Stohl W, Hilbert DM. The discovery and development of belimumab: the anti-BLyS-lupus connection. *Nat Biotechnol.* 2012;30(1):69-77.
24. Neuhaus O, Kieseier BC, Hartung HP. Pharmacokinetics and pharmacodynamics of the interferon-betas, glatiramer acetate, and mitoxantrone in multiple sclerosis. *J Neurol Sci.* 2007;259(1-2): 27-37.
25. Jeffery DR. Recent advances in treating multiple sclerosis: efficacy, risks and place in therapy. *Therap Adv Chronic dis.* 2013;4(1):45-51.
26. Abraham C, Cho JH. Inflammatory bowel disease. *N Engl J Med.* 2009;361:2006-2078.
27. Loftus EV Jr. Clinical epidemiology of inflammatory bowel disease: Incidence, prevalence, and environmental influences. *Gastroenterology.* 2004;126(6):1504-1517.

28. Ferguson LR, Shelling AN, Browning BL, Huebner C, Petermann I. Genes, diet and inflammatory bowel disease. *Mutation Res.* 2007;622(1-2):70-83.
29. Lichtenstein GR, Hanauer SB, Sandborn WJ, Practice Parameters Committee of American College of Gastroenterology. Management of Crohn's disease in adults. *Am J Gastroenterol.* 2009;104(2): 465-483.
30. Nielsen OH, Ainsworth MA. Tumor necrosis factor inhibitors for inflammatory bowel disease. *N Engl J Med.* 2013;369:754-762.
31. Ford AC, Kane SV, Khan KJ, et al. Efficacy of 5-aminosalicylates in Crohn's disease: systematic review and meta-analysis. *Am J Gastroenterol.* 2011; 106:617.
32. Mowat C, Cole A, Windsor A, et al. Guidelines for the management of inflammatory bowel disease in adults. *Gut.* 2011;60:571.
33. Kornbluth A, Sachar DB, Practice Parameters Committee of the American College of Gastroenterology. Ulcerative colitis practice guidelines in adults: American College of Gastroenterology, Practice Parameters Committee. *Am J Gastroenterol.* 2010;105(3):501-523.
34. Marshall JK, Thabane M, Steinhart AH, Newman JR, Anand A, Irvine EJ. Rectal 5-aminosalicylic acid for maintenance of remission in ulcerative colitis. *Cochrane Database Syst Rev.* 2012;11:CD004118.
35. Lichtenstein GR, Abreu MT, Cohen R, Tremaine W. American Gastroenterological Association Institute medical position statement on corticosteroids, immunomodulators, and infliximab in inflammatory bowel disease. *Gastroenterology.* 2006;130(3): 935-939.
36. Terdiman JP, Gruss CB, Heidelbaugh JJ, et al. American Gastroenterological Association Institute guideline on the use of thiopurines, methotrexate, and anti-TNF-alpha biologic drugs for the induction and maintenance of remission in inflammatory Crohn's disease. *Gastroenterology.* 2013;145(6):1459-1463.
37. Dassopoulos T, Sultan S, Falck-Ytter YT, Inadomi JM, Hanauer SB. American Gastroenterological Association Institute technical review on the use of thiopurines, methotrexate, and anti-TNF-alpha biologic drugs for the induction and maintenance of remission in inflammatory Crohn's disease. *Gastroenterology.* 2013;145(6):1464-1478.
38. Colombel JF, Sandborn WJ, Reinisch W, et al. Infliximab, azathioprine, or combination therapy for Crohn's disease. *N Engl J Med.* 2010;362(15): 1383-1395.
39. Lofberg R, Louis EV, Reinisch W, et al. Adalimumab produces clinical remission and reduces extraintestinal manifestations in Crohn's disease: results from CARE. *Inflamm Bowel Dis.* 2012;18(1):1-9.
40. Frederiksen MT, Ainsworth MA, Brynskov J, Thomsen OO, Bendtzen K, Steenholdt C. Antibodies against infliximab are associated with de novo development of antibodies to adalimumab and therapeutic failure in infliximab-to-adalimumab switchers with IBD. *Inflamm Bowel Dis.* 2014:20(10):1714-1721.
41. Hanauer SB, Panes J, Colombel JF, Bloomfield R, Schreiber S, Sandborn WJ. Clinical trial: impact of prior infliximab therapy on the clinical response to certolizumab pegol maintenance therapy for Crohn's disease. *Aliment Pharmacol Therap.* 2010;32(3): 384-393.
42. Hammer HF. Gut microbiota and inflammatory bowel disease. *Digestive Dis.* 2011;29(6):550-553.
43. Garg SK, Croft AM, Bager P. Helminth therapy (worms) for induction of remission in inflammatory bowel disease. *Cochrane Database Syst Rev.*2014;1: CD009400.
44. Damas OM, Deshpande AR, Avalos DJ, Abreu MT. Treating inflammatory bowel disease in pregnancy. The issues we face today. *J Crohns Colitis.* 2015; Jun 30. [Epub ahead of print.]
45. Heetun ZS, Byrnes C, Neary P, O'Morain C. Review article: reproduction in the patient with inflammatory bowel disease. *Aliment Pharmacol Therap.* 2007;26(4):513-533.
46. National Institutes of Health, Toxnet Lactmed. Thioguanine and mercaptopurine. http://toxnet.nlm.nih.gov/cgi-bin/sis/search2. Accessed March 25, 2014.
47. Zapata LB, Paulen ME, Cansino C, Marchbanks PA, Curtis KM. Contraceptive use among women with inflammatory bowel disease: a systematic review. *Contraception.* 2010;82(1):72-85.
48. Kane SV, Reddy D. Hormonal replacement therapy after menopause is protective of disease activity in women with inflammatory bowel disease. *Am J Gastroenterol.* 2008;103(5):1193-1196.
49. Palomba S, Manguso F, Orio F Jr, et al. Effectiveness of risedronate in osteoporotic postmenopausal women with inflammatory bowel disease: a prospective, parallel, open-label, two-year extension study. *Menopause.* 2008;15(4 pt 1):730-736.
50. Hauser SL, Oksenberg JR. The neurobiology of multiple sclerosis: genes, inflammation, and neurodegeneration. *Neuron.* 2006;52(1):61-76.

51. Polman CH, Reingold SC, Banwell B, et al. Diagnostic criteria for multiple sclerosis: 2010 revisions to the McDonald criteria. *Ann Neurol.* 2011;69(2):292-302.
52. Lublin FD, Reingold SC, Cohen JA, et al. Defining the clinical course of multiple sclerosis: the 2013 revisions. *Neurology.* 2014;83:278.
53. Howley A, Kremenchutzky M. Pegylated interferons: A nurses' review of a novel multiple sclerosis therapy. *J Neuroscience Nsg.* 2014;46(2):88-96.
54. Jacobs LD, Beck RW, Simon JH, et al. Intramuscular interferon beta-1a therapy initiated during a first demyelinating event in multiple sclerosis. CHAMPS Study Group. *N Engl J Med.* 2000;343(13):898-904.
55. Kinkel RP, Dontchev M, Kollman C, et al. Association between immediate initiation of intramuscular interferon beta-1a at the time of a clinically isolated syndrome and long-term outcomes: a 10-year follow-up of the Controlled High-Risk Avonex Multiple Sclerosis Prevention Study in Ongoing Neurological Surveillance. *Arch Neurol.* 2012;69(2):183-190.
56. Comi G, Filippi M, Wolinsky JS. European/Canadian multicenter, double-blind, randomized, placebo-controlled study of the effects of glatiramer acetate on magnetic resonance imaging: measured disease activity and burden in patients with relapsing multiple sclerosis. European/Canadian Glatiramer Acetate Study Group. *Ann Neurol.* 2001;49(3):290-297.
57. Filippi M, Rovaris M, Rocca MA, Sormani MP, Wolinsky JS, Comi G. Glatiramer acetate reduces the proportion of new MS lesions evolving into "black holes." *Neurology.* 2001;57(4):731-733.
58. O'Connor P, Filippi M, Arnason B, et al. 250 microg or 500 microg interferon beta-1b versus 20 mg glatiramer acetate in relapsing-remitting multiple sclerosis: a prospective, randomised, multicentre study. *Lancet Neurol.* 2009;8(10):889-897.
59. Kappos L, Radue EW, O'Connor P, et al. A placebo-controlled trial of oral fingolimod in relapsing multiple sclerosis. *N Engl J Med.* 2010;362(5):387-401.
60. Calabresi PA, Radue EW, Goodin D, et al. Safety and efficacy of fingolimod in patients with relapsing-remitting multiple sclerosis (FREEDOMS II): a double-blind, randomised, placebo-controlled, phase 3 trial. *Lancet Neurol.* 2014;13(6):545-556.
61. Cohen JA, Barkhof F, Comi G, et al. Oral fingolimod or intramuscular interferon for relapsing multiple sclerosis. *N Engl J Med.* 2010;362(5):402-415.
62. Gold R, Kappos L, Arnold DL, et al. Placebo-controlled phase 3 study of oral BG-12 for relapsing multiple sclerosis. *N Engl J Med.* 2012;367(12):1098-1107.
63. Fox RJ, Miller DH, Phillips JT, et al. Placebo-controlled phase 3 study of oral BG-12 or glatiramer in multiple sclerosis. *N Engl J Med.* 2012;367(12):1087-1097.
64. Bar-Or A, Gold R, Kappos L, et al. Clinical efficacy of BG-12 (dimethyl fumarate) in patients with relapsing-remitting multiple sclerosis: subgroup analyses of the DEFINE study. *J Neurol.* 2013;260(9):2297-2305.
65. Hutchinson M, Fox RJ, Miller DH, et al. Clinical efficacy of BG-12 (dimethyl fumarate) in patients with relapsing-remitting multiple sclerosis: subgroup analyses of the CONFIRM study. *J Neurol.* 2013; 260(9):2286-2296.
66. Bozic C, Subramanyam M, Richman S, Plavina T, Zhang A, Ticho B. Anti-JC virus (JCV) antibody prevalence in the JCV Epidemiology in MS (JEMS) trial. *Eur J Neurol.* 2014;21(2):299-304.
67. Casetta I, Iuliano G, Filippini G. Azathioprine for multiple sclerosis (review). *Cochrane Database of Syst Rev.* 2007;(4):CD003982.
68. Marriott JJ, Miyasaki JM, Gronseth G, O'Connor PW; Therapeutics, Technology Assessment Subcommittee of the American Academy of N. Evidence report: the efficacy and safety of mitoxantrone (Novantrone) in the treatment of multiple sclerosis: report of the Therapeutics and Technology Assessment Subcommittee of the American Academy of Neurology. *Neurology.* 2010;74(18):1463-1470.
69. Miller AE, Macdonell R, Comi G, et al. Teriflunomide reduces relapses with sequelae and relapses leading to hospitalizations: results from the TOWER study. *J Neurol.* 2014;261(9):1781-1788.
70. Shinto L, Calabrese C, Morris C, Sinsheimer S, Bourdette D. Complementary and alternative medicine in multiple sclerosis: survey of licensed naturopaths. *J Altern Complement Med.* 2004;10(5): 891-897.
71. Yadav V, Bever C Jr, Bowen J, et al. Summary of evidence-based guideline: complementary and alternative medicine in multiple sclerosis: report of the guideline development subcommittee of the American Academy of Neurology. *Neurology.* 2014; 82(12): 1083-1092.
72. Cree BA. Update on reproductive safety of current and emerging disease-modifying therapies for multiple sclerosis. *Multiple Sclerosis.* 2013;19(7): 835-843.
73. Schneider H, Weber CE, Hellwig K, Schroten H, Tenenbaum T. Natalizumab treatment during pregnancy: effects on the neonatal immune system. *Acta Neurol Scand.* 2013;127(1):e1-e4.

74. Gaffo A, Saag KG, Curtis JR. Treatment of rheumatoid arthritis. *Am J Health Syst Pharm.* 2006;63(24):2451-2465.
75. Scott DL, Wolfe F, Huizinga TW. Rheumatoid arthritis. *Lancet.* 2010;376(9746):1094-1108.
76. Sokka T. Work disability in early rheumatoid arthritis. *Clin Experiment Rheum.* 2003;21(5 suppl 31):S71-S74.
77. Singh JA, Furst DE, Bharat A, et al. 2012 update of the 2008 American College of Rheumatology recommendations for the use of disease-modifying antirheumatic drugs and biologic agents in the treatment of rheumatoid arthritis. *Arthritis Care Res.* 2012;64(5):625-639.
78. Smolen JS, Landewe R, Breedveld FC, et al. EULAR recommendations for the management of rheumatoid arthritis with synthetic and biological disease-modifying antirheumatic drugs: 2013 update. *Ann Rheum Dis.* 2014;73(3):492-509.
79. Gøtzsche PC, Johansen HK. Short-term low-dose corticosteroids vs placebo and nonsteroidal anti-inflammatory drugs in rheumatoid arthritis. *Cochrane Database Syst. Rev.* 2005;1:CD000189.
80. Cohen S, Cannon GW, Schiff M, et al. Two-year, blinded, randomized, controlled trial of treatment of active rheumatoid arthritis with leflunomide compared with methotrexate: Utilization of Leflunomide in the Treatment of Rheumatoid Arthritis Trial Investigator Group. *Arthritis Rheum.* 2001;44(9):1984-1992.
81. Morris SJ, Wasko MC, Antohe JL, et al. Hydroxychloroquine use associated with improvement in lipid profiles in rheumatoid arthritis patients. *Arthritis Care Res.* 2011;63(4):530-534.
82. Penn SK, Kao AH, Schott LL, et al. Hydroxychloroquine and glycemia in women with rheumatoid arthritis and systemic lupus erythematosus. *J Rheumatol.* 2010;37(6):1136-1142.
83. Aaltonen KJ, Virkki LM, Malmivaara A, Konttinen YT, Nordstrom DC, Blom M. Systematic review and meta-analysis of the efficacy and safety of existing TNF blocking agents in treatment of rheumatoid arthritis. *PloS One.* 2012;7(1):e30275.
84. Michaud TL, Rho YH, Shamliyan T, Kuntz KM, Choi HK. The comparative safety of TNF inhibitors in rheumatoid arthritis: a meta-analysis update of 44 randomized controlled trials. *Am J Med.* 2014;127(12):1208-1232.
85. Westhovens R, Kremer JM, Emery P, et al. Long-term safety and efficacy of abatacept in patients with rheumatoid arthritis and an inadequate response to methotrexate: a 7-year extended study. *Clin Experiment Rheumatol.* 2014;32(4):553-562.
86. Rigby W, Ferraccioli G, Greenwald M, et al. Effect of rituximab on physical function and quality of life in patients with rheumatoid arthritis previously untreated with methotrexate. *Arthritis Care Res.* 2011;63(5):711-720.
87. Mok CC. Rituximab for the treatment of rheumatoid arthritis: an update. *Drug Design Develop Therap.* 2014;8:87-100.
88. Dougados M, Kissel K, Sheeran T, et al. Adding tocilizumab or switching to tocilizumab monotherapy in methotrexate inadequate responders: 24-week symptomatic and structural results of a 2-year randomised controlled strategy trial in rheumatoid arthritis (ACT-RAY). *Ann Rheum Dis.* 2013;72(1):43-50.
89. Dougados M, Kissel K, Conaghan PG, et al. Clinical, radiographic and immunogenic effects after 1 year of tocilizumab-based treatment strategies in rheumatoid arthritis: the ACT-RAY study. *Ann Rheum Dis.* 2014;73(5):803-809.
90. Burmester GR, Rubbert-Roth A, Cantagrel A, et al. A randomised, double-blind, parallel-group study of the safety and efficacy of subcutaneous tocilizumab versus intravenous tocilizumab in combination with traditional disease-modifying antirheumatic drugs in patients with moderate to severe rheumatoid arthritis (SUMMACTA study). *Ann Rheum Dis.* 2014;73(1):69-74.
91. Kawalec P, Mikrut A, Wisniewska N, Pilc A. The effectiveness of tofacitinib, a novel Janus kinase inhibitor, in the treatment of rheumatoid arthritis: a systematic review and meta-analysis. *Clin Rheumatol.* 2013;32(10):1415-1424.
92. O'Dell JR, Leff R, Paulsen G, et al. Treatment of rheumatoid arthritis with methotrexate and hydroxychloroquine, methotrexate and sulfasalazine, or a combination of the three medications: results of a two-year, randomized, double-blind, placebo-controlled trial. *Arthritis Rheum.* 2002;46(5):1164-1170.
93. O'Dell JR, Mikuls TR, Taylor TH, et al. Therapies for active rheumatoid arthritis after methotrexate failure. *N Engl J Med.* 2013;369(4):307-318.

94. Cameron M, Gagnier JJ, Chrubasik S. Herbal therapy for treating rheumatoid arthritis. *Cochrane Database Syst. Rev*. 2011;2:CD002948.
95. Soeken KL, Miller SA, Ernst E. Herbal medicines for the treatment of rheumatoid arthritis: a systematic review. *Rheumatology (Oxf)*. 2003;42(5): 652-659.
96. Proudman SM, James MJ, Spargo LD, et al. Fish oil in recent onset rheumatoid arthritis: a randomised, double-blind controlled trial within algorithm-based drug use. *Ann Rheum Dis*. 2015;74(1):89-95.
97. Makol A, Wright K, Amin S. Rheumatoid arthritis and pregnancy: safety considerations in pharmacological management. *Drugs*. 2011;71(15):1973-1987.
98. Ostensen M, Forger F. Management of RA medications in pregnant patients. *Nat Rev Rheumatol*. 2009;5(7):382-390.
99. Sammaritano LR. Therapy insight: guidelines for selection of contraception in women with rheumatic diseases. *Nat Clin Pract*. 2007;3(5):273-281; quiz, 305-276.
100. Carroll MC. A protective role for innate immunity in systemic lupus erythematosus. *Nat Rev Immunol*. 2004;4(10):825-831.
101. Pons-Estel GJ, Alarcon GS, Scofield L, Reinlib L, Cooper GS. Understanding the epidemiology and progression of systemic lupus erythematosus. *Semin Arthritis Rheum*. 2010;39(4):257-268.
102. Somers EC, Richardson BC. Environmental exposures, epigenetic changes and the risk of lupus. *Lupus*. 2014;23(6):568-576.
103. Vedove CD, Del Giglio M, Schena D, Girolomoni G. Drug-induced lupus erythematosus. *Arch Dermatol Res*. 2009;301(1):99-105.
104. Marzano AV, Vezzoli P, Crosti C. Drug-induced lupus: an update on its dermatologic aspects. *Lupus*. 2009;18(11):935-940.
105. Vasoo S. Drug-induced lupus: an update. *Lupus*. 2006;15(11):757-761.
106. Araujo-Fernanced S, Ajijon-Lana M, Isenberg DA. Drug induced lupus: including anti-tumor necrosis factor and interferon induced. *Lupus*. 2014;23(6):545-553.
107. Lowe CG, Henderson CL, Grau RH, Hansen CB, Sontheimer RD. A systematic review of drug-induced subacute lupus erythematosus. *Br J Dermatol*. 2011;164(2):465-472.
108. Guidelines for referral and management of systemic lupus erythematosus in adults: American College of Rheumatology Ad Hoc Committee on Systemic Lupus Erythematosus Guidelines. *Arthritis Rheum*. 1999;42(9):1785-1796.
109. Mok CC. Emerging drug therapies for systemic lupus erythematosus. *Expert Opin Emerg Drugs*. 2006;11(4):597-608.
110. Croyle L, Morand EF. Optimizing the use of existing therapies in lupus. *Int J Rheum Dis*. 2013; 18(2):129-137.
111. Hahn BH, McMahon MA, Wilkinson A, et al. American College of Rheumatology guidelines for screening, treatment, and management of lupus nephritis. *Arthritis Care Res*. 2012;64(6):797-808.
112. Ogawa H, Kameda H, Amano K, Takeuchi T. Efficacy and safety of cyclosporine A in patients with refractory systemic lupus erythematosus in a daily clinical practice. *Lupus*. 2010;19(2):162-169.
113. Petri M. Systemic lupus erythematosus: 2006 update. *J Clin Rheumatol*. 2006;12(1):37-40.
114. Touma Z, Gladman DD, Urowitz MB, Beyene J, Uleryk EM, Shah PS. Mycophenolate mofetil for induction treatment of lupus nephritis: a systematic review and metaanalysis. *J Rheumatol*. 2011;38(1):69-78.
115. Hahn BH. Belimumab for systemic lupus erythemeatosus. *N Engl J Med*. 2013;368:1528-1535.
116. Abou-Raya A, Abou-Raya S, Helmii M. The effect of vitamin D supplementation on inflammatory and hemostatic markers and disease activity in patients with systemic lupus erythematosus: a randomized placebo-controlled trial. *J Rheumatol*. 2013;40(3):265-272.
117. Duffy EM, Meenagh GK, McMillan SA, Strain JJ, Hannigan BM, Bell AL. The clinical effect of dietary supplementation with omega-3 fish oils and/or copper in systemic lupus erythematosus. *J Rheumatol*. 2004;31(8):1551-1556.
118. Wright SA, O'Prey FM, McHenry MT, et al. A randomised interventional trial of omega-3-polyunsaturated fatty acids on endothelial function and disease activity in systemic lupus erythematosus. *Ann Rheum Dis*. 2008;67(6):841-848.
119. Greco CM, Nakajima C, Manzi S. Updated review of complementary and alternative medicine treatments for systemic lupus erythematosus. *Curr Rheumatol Rep*. 2013;15(11):378.

120. Ostensen M, Khamashta M, Lockshin M, et al. Anti-inflammatory and immunosuppressive drugs and reproduction. *Arthritis Res Therap*. 2006;8(3):209.
121. Kwok LW, Tam LS, Zhu T, Leung YY, Li E. Predictors of maternal and fetal outcomes in pregnancies of patients with systemic lupus erythematosus. *Lupus*. 2011;20(8):829-836.
122. Landy H, Powell M, Hill D, Eudy A, Petri M. Belimumab pregnancy registry: prospective cohort study of pregnancy outcomes. *Obstet Gynecol*. 2014; 123(suppl 1):62S.
123. Sanchez-Guerrero J, Uribe AG, Jimenez-Santana L, et al. A trial of contraceptive methods in women with systemic lupus erythematosus. *N Engl J Med*. 2005;353(24):2539-2549.
124. Sammaritano LR. Contraception in patients with sysetmic lupus erythematosus and antiphospholipid syndrome. *Lupus*. 2014;23:1242-1245.
125. Centers for Disease Control and Prevention. U.S. medical eligibility criteria for contraceptive use, 2010. *MMWR Recommend Rep*. 2010; 59:1-86.

18 Diabetes

Esther R. Ellsworth Bowers, Nancy Jo Reedy

Chapter Glossary

Diabetes insipidus Increased urine production resulting from inadequate vasopressin production by the pituitary gland.

Diabetes mellitus All conditions characterized by high blood glucose levels and varying degrees of glucose intolerance.

Euglycemia Normal blood glucose level.

Gestational diabetes (GDM) Insulin resistance that is initially diagnosed in pregnancy.

Glucagon Hormone secreted by the pancreas in opposition to insulin.

Gluconeogenesis Manufacture of glucose by the liver.

Glycogenolysis Breakdown of the energy storage molecule glycogen.

Glycosylation Attachment of glucose to hemoglobin, which occurs when hemoglobin is exposed to high plasma levels of glucose.

Hemoglobin A_{1c} (HbA_{1c}) Measurement of glycosylated hemoglobin.

Impaired fasting glucose (IFG) Fasting plasma glucose level between 100 mg/dL and 125 mg/dL.

Impaired glucose tolerance (IGT) Two-hour post-glucose load plasma glucose value between 140 mg/dL and 199 mg/dL.

Insulin analogue Insulin that is synthetically produced using recombinant DNA technology.

Insulin resistance Condition in which normal blood levels of insulin are insufficient to produce a normal insulin response in peripheral tissues such as muscle, liver, and adipose cells.

Insulin secretagogues Medicines that stimulate the beta cells of the pancreas to secrete insulin.

Prediabetes Impaired glucose metabolism that does not meet the criteria for type 1 or type 2 diabetes. May be impaired fasting glucose or impaired glucose tolerance.

Type 1 diabetes Condition characterized by pancreatic cell destruction that is usually the result of autoimmune destruction of these cells. Persons with type 1 diabetes always need insulin replacement. Previously called juvenile-onset diabetes and insulin-dependent diabetes.

Type 2 diabetes Condition characterized by hyperglycemia that occurs secondary to a combination of insulin resistance and insulin deficiency. May be treated with oral agents or with insulin. Previously called adult-onset diabetes and non-insulin-dependent diabetes.

Introduction

Diabetes is derived from the Greek verb *diabainein*, which means "to stand with the legs apart" or "siphon," as in urination. The two forms of diabetes that share the specific symptom of polyuria are **diabetes mellitus** and **diabetes insipidus**. *Diabetes mellitus* means "honey-sweet urine" and includes the diabetic conditions that are characterized by abnormally high levels of blood glucose and varying degrees of glucose intolerance.[1] *Diabetes insipidus* comes from a Latin word that means "without taste." Diabetes insipidus is caused by a deficiency of antidiuretic hormone secondary to pituitary dysfunction. This chapter reviews the pharmacologic management of diabetes mellitus and diabetes insipidus. **Gestational diabetes (GDM)** is addressed in the *Pregnancy* chapter.

Epidemiology and General Considerations

Diabetes is an increasing health challenge in the United States. The number of persons with diagnosed diabetes increased from 5.6 million in 1980 to 21.0 million in 2012.[2] In addition, 8.1 million persons in the United States today have undiagnosed diabetes or prediabetes as ascertained by measurements of fasting glucose and **hemoglobin A_{1c} (HbA_{1c})** values.[2] The proportion of women with prediabetes is growing at a rate nearly twice that of men.[3]

The impact of diabetes is not distributed equally across society. The incidence of diabetes is higher among non-Hispanic Blacks, American Indians, Asian/Pacific Islanders, and Hispanic/Latina American women compared to non-Hispanic Whites.[2] These populations are also the racial and ethnic minorities who have the most difficulty accessing health care and the populations most likely to experience some of the common complications of diabetes. The incidence of diabetes increases sharply with age; in 2011, 18.4% of women older than 65 years had diagnosed diabetes.[4] Women who have a history of gestational diabetes have a sevenfold increased risk for developing type 2 diabetes later in life.[5]

A number of adverse health outcomes are associated with diabetes. In fact, the diagnosis of diabetes can mark the onset of a pathophysiologic domino effect that results in both microvascular and macrovascular dysfunction.[6,7] These processes, in turn, can result in arteriosclerosis, hypertension, coronary artery disease, stroke, renal disease, blindness, and amputations, to name just a few. Although diabetes has no known cure, aggressive treatment can mitigate the development of complications and improve quality of life. Before discussing pharmacologic management of diabetes, a review of glucose metabolism and the pathophysiology of diabetes is in order.

Physiology of Glucose Metabolism

Glucose is made available for fueling metabolism via one of the following three sources: (1) intestinal absorption of food; (2) **gluconeogenesis**, which is the manufacture of glucose by the liver; and (3) **glycogenolysis**, which is the breakdown of the energy storage molecule glycogen. Under normal conditions, blood glucose levels are regulated by the hormones insulin and glucagon, which are produced and excreted by the pancreas. The goal is to maintain plasma glucose levels within a specific range. This initiates a series of interrelated events in which insulin is the main character (Figure 18-1).

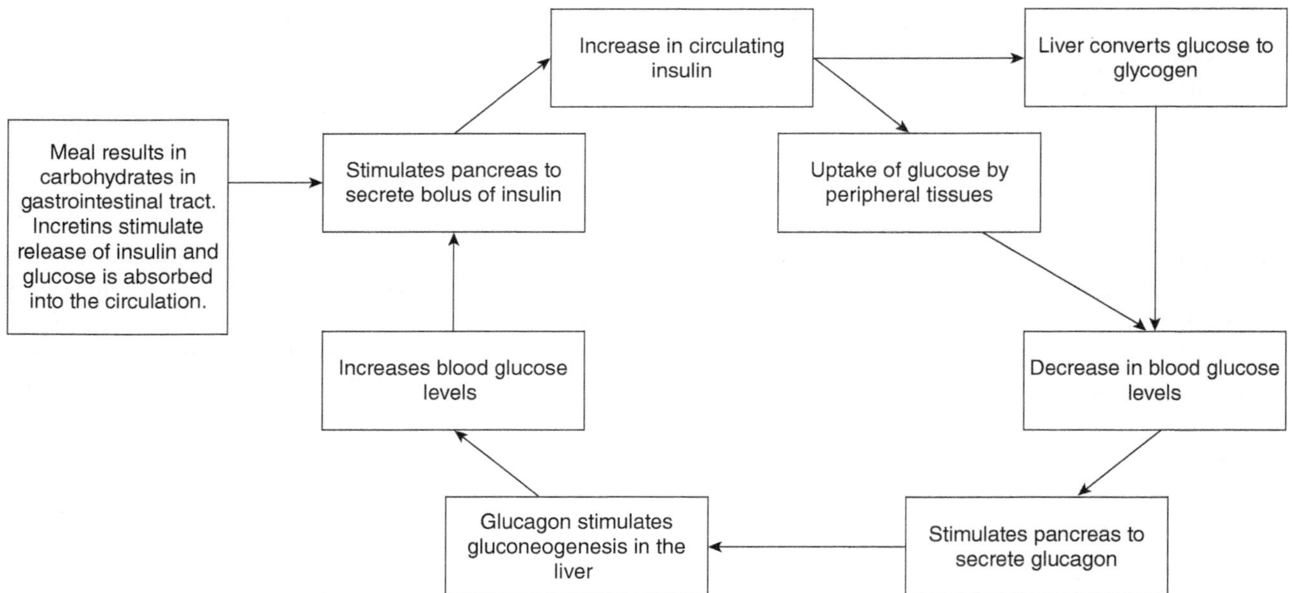

After food is ingested and blood glucose levels rise, the pancreas secretes insulin, which stimulates uptake of glucose by cells and conversion of glucose into glycogen within the liver. As blood glucose levels fall, glucagon is secreted by the pancreas. Glucagon then stimulates gluconeogenesis in the liver so blood glucose levels remain within a normal range between meals.

Figure 18-1 Regulation of glucose metabolism.

The Role of Insulin

Insulin is, in essence, an anabolic hormone that acts primarily on the liver, adipose tissue, and skeletal muscle; it has many other functions as well, some of which are still being discovered. The primary function of insulin is facilitation of glucose into peripheral tissue cells. Insulin also inhibits gluconeogenesis in the liver, stimulates glycogen formation in the liver, converts fatty acids to triglycerides, inhibits lipolysis, and stimulates protein synthesis. In addition, insulin encourages the production of nitrous oxide in the endothelial cells lining blood vessels throughout the vascular tree. In turn, nitrous oxide has multiple functions that protect against the development of atherosclerosis.[8]

Most cells in the body have cell surface receptors for insulin. Once insulin binds to the insulin receptor, glucose is taken into the cell, and different enzyme-controlled reactions occur. Interestingly, two organs do not have insulin receptors—the brain and the liver. However, the cells in these organs are permeable to glucose, and it passes into the cells of these two organs readily via diffusion.

Endogenous secretion of insulin has both a basal component and a bolus component. The basal secretion of insulin limits lipolysis and gluconeogenesis in the liver while maintaining a glucose blood level sufficient for cerebral metabolism. Non-obese, healthy adults secrete basal insulin at the rate of 0.5–1 U/hour, which maintains the plasma insulin concentration at 35–104 pmol/L. The basal insulin at normal levels results in a fasting plasma glucose of 70–110 mg/dL.[9]

Insulin secretion rises rapidly following a meal. Gastrointestinal hormones called incretins stimulate the islets of Langerhans in the pancreas to release insulin as soon as food is present in the stomach and intestine. Once glucose is absorbed into the circulation, the high levels of glucose there also stimulate production and secretion of insulin. This bolus of insulin inhibits gluconeogenesis in the liver and stimulates peripheral glucose utilization by muscle. It also prompts lipogenesis in the liver, by stimulating the production of the transcription factor known as sterol response element binding protein 1c (SREBP-1c).[10] The plasma concentrations of insulin rise to a peak of 417–556 pmol/L within 30–60 minutes of eating.

The release of bolus insulin occurs in a two-peak process, with an initial rise occurring immediately after the meal and a second rise persisting for as long as 6.5 hours, depending on the type of food consumed. The first peak of insulin is short, limiting the circulating glucose level of the quickly absorbed carbohydrates and simple sugars in the food. The second peak is longer and serves to process the blood glucose levels that occur as carbohydrates are absorbed from the gastrointestinal tract over time.

The insulin response to a meal is further affected by other factors, including the carbohydrate, fat, and protein content of the meal; the food's transit time in the gastrointestinal system; and the effect of insulin and glucagon on glucose metabolism in the peripheral tissues and the liver.[2,11] Adults who are obese but otherwise healthy show a higher rate of basal and bolus insulin response depending on the degree of obesity. Both healthy-weight and obese-weight individuals who have normal glucose metabolism will have a 2-hour postprandial blood glucose level at or below 140 mg/dL. In healthy individuals, the plasma glucose level returns to basal level within 2 to 3 hours after eating.

Glucagon

Acting in opposition to insulin is **glucagon**, a peptide hormone produced by the alpha cells within the islets of Langerhans. Glucagon is the counter-regulatory hormone to insulin. It is released when blood levels of glucose are low and acts within the liver to stimulate gluconeogenesis and glycolysis, thereby increasing blood glucose levels. It also stimulates lipolysis in adipose tissue throughout the body. Paradoxically, rising blood levels of glucose stimulate the release of insulin, and the cycle starts over.

Pathophysiology of Glucose Metabolism: Diabetes Mellitus

Type 1 diabetes is the result of autoimmune destruction of the beta cells in the islets of Langerhans within the pancreas, which results in an absolute deficiency of insulin. **Type 2 diabetes** involves dysfunction of several steps within the glucose-regulating mechanisms—insulin secretion, glucose transport, glucose production, and/or glucose utilization. Individuals with type 2 diabetes have some degree of endogenous insulin production. Because the insulin deficiency is absolute in persons with type 1 diabetes and relative in type 2 diabetes (present but with decreased ability to transport glucose into cells), the pathophysiology, progress of disease, and pharmacologic treatments of these two types of diabetes differ.

Type 1 Diabetes

Destruction of the pancreatic beta cells occurs primarily in persons with a genetic predisposition who are exposed to an environmental trigger and then produce autoantibodies. Without insulin from the beta cells or an exogenous source of insulin, blood glucose levels rise steeply. The threshold for reabsorption of glucose in the proximal renal tubules is overcome, and glycosuria results. Because glucose has a high osmolarity, water molecules stay in the urine instead of being reabsorbed. This situation leads to the three classic signs of diabetes: polyuria, polydipsia, and polyphagia. Moreover, the lack of basal insulin at adequate levels leads to release of hormone-sensitive lipase and free fatty acids. When the cells do not get glucose into the intracellular compartment, fatty acids are used to provide the energy for metabolic processes. Fatty acid breakdown produces ketones, potentially leading to diabetic ketoacidosis if this condition remains untreated.

Type 2 Diabetes

Persons with type 2 diabetes have three significant metabolic defects: (1) resistance to insulin at the level of the cell membrane, limiting insulin's ability to help glucose enter the cell; (2) hyperinsulinemia as more insulin is required to accomplish a specific lowering of blood glucose; and (3) abnormally high plasma glucagon levels, which remain elevated even during periods of hyperglycemia.[12] As the disorder progresses, many individuals with type 2 diabetes also develop a relative impairment of insulin secretion.

Because there is a degree of **insulin resistance** in the liver as well as peripheral tissue, the amount of glucose that enters liver cells is limited. The liver inaccurately perceives a deficit of glucose in the body, and all the mechanisms that increase blood glucose values surge into action (Figure 18-2). In addition, adipose cells break down stored triglycerides into free fatty acids that could be used for metabolism in the absence of glucose. The resulting high plasma level of free fatty acids helps trigger biochemical processes that lead to elevated levels of triglycerides and very low-density lipoprotein (VLDL) cholesterol, and a lower level of high-density lipoprotein (HDL) cholesterol.

Fasting plasma glucose levels higher than 140 mg/dL are a sign that beta cells in the pancreas are no longer able to increase insulin production to compensate for insulin resistance. At this point, overt type 2 diabetes can be diagnosed.[1] In some individuals with type 2 diabetes, the pancreas eventually shuts down completely, so glucose homeostasis requires management with exogenous insulin in addition to medications that reduce insulin resistance.

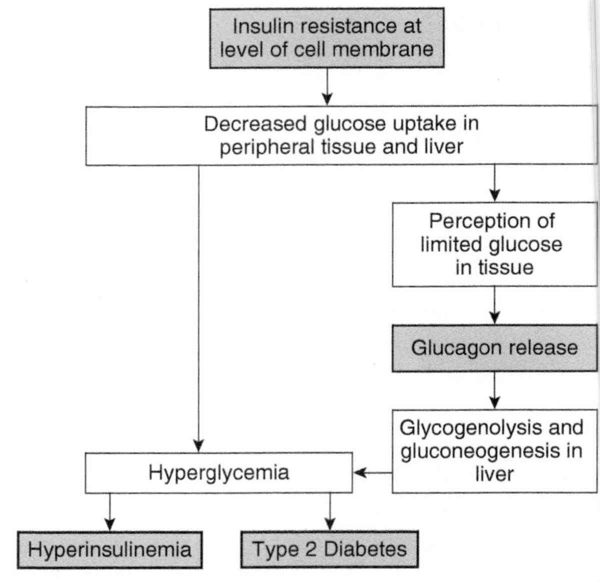

Figure 18-2 Insulin resistance model of type 2 diabetes.

The Lipocentric Model

So far, the conventional glucocentric model of type 2 diabetes has been described. However, it is becoming clear that a lipocentric model may describe the underlying pathophysiology of type 2 diabetes more completely (Figure 18-3).[10] Obesity is common in persons with type 2 diabetes and is a major contributor to insulin resistance. The pathway for obesity-related insulin resistance begins with surplus caloric intake, which prompts an elevated insulin release from the pancreas. In addition to enabling glucose transport into cells throughout the body, the insulin triggers lipogenesis in the liver. Free fatty acids produced in the liver circulate throughout the body and are deposited not only in adipose tissue, but also as "ectopic" lipids in myocytes and visceral organ tissues. Lipid deposits in skeletal muscle increase insulin resistance of the muscle, and lipid deposits in the pancreas impair insulin production, resulting in persistent hyperglycemia. As insulin resistance worsens, the body perceives a need for glucose, and adipocytes increase lipolysis, releasing additional fatty acids to circulation. It is a vicious circle: High levels of free fatty acids increase insulin resistance and pancreas suppression, the body perceives a need for glucose, and additional lipolysis occurs that further raises free fatty acid levels. The result is continually worsening insulin resistance and continually increasing hyperglycemia.

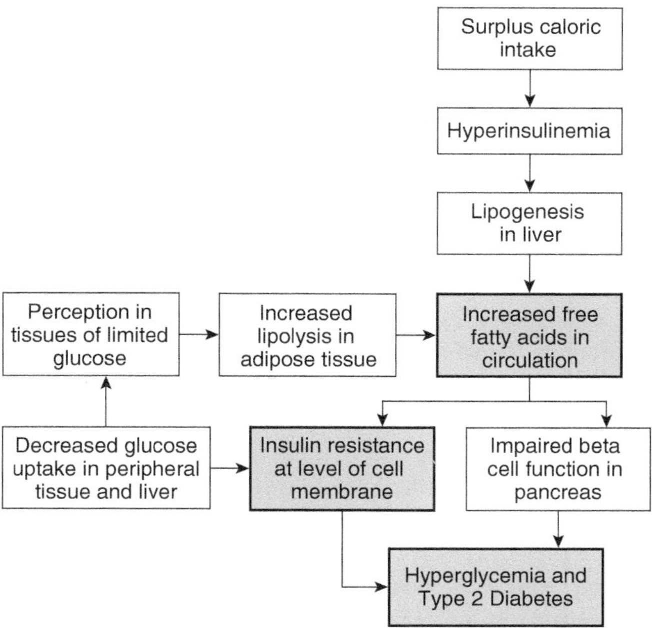

Figure 18-3 Lipocentric model of type 2 diabetes.

Prediabetes

Prediabetes, sometimes colloquially called borderline diabetes, has been described as impaired glucose metabolism that does not meet the criteria for type 1 or type 2 diabetes.[1] Prediabetes can be manifested as an **impaired fasting glucose (IFG)**, which is defined as fasting plasma glucose level between 100 mg/dL and 125 mg/dL, or an **impaired glucose tolerance (IGT)**, defined as a plasma glucose level after a 2-hour post-glucose load that is between 140 mg/dL and 199 mg/dL.[1] Some persons can have both. In 2008, the American College of Endocrinology convened a task force that changed healthcare providers' understanding of prediabetes and related health risks. According to the task force, 6% to 10% of persons with IGT progress to diabetes each year. For persons with both IFG and IGT, the cumulative risk for developing diabetes over 6 years is as high as 60%. High plasma glucose levels result in cardiovascular changes and microvascular disease before the development of type 2 diabetes. Diabetic retinopathy, hypertension, dyslipidemia, and cardiovascular disease are markedly increased in individuals with IFG or IGT.[13] In response to these risks, current algorithms from the American College of Endocrinology and the American Diabetes Association on diabetes care now include recommendations for managing prediabetes with both lifestyle changes and pharmacologic interventions.

Metabolic Syndrome

Metabolic syndrome is a constellation of disorders that increases the risk for developing both type 2 diabetes and cardiovascular disease. Insulin resistance is an integral component of metabolic syndrome, which is characterized by visceral obesity or central obesity, resistance to insulin, abnormalities in lipid metabolism, and hypertension. The pathophysiologic connections between metabolic syndrome, diabetes, and cardiovascular disease merit brief review, because this growing field of study is challenging conventional treatment of individuals with type 2 diabetes and paving the way for new pharmacologic interventions.[14]

Three of the following five criteria must be met to acquire the diagnosis of metabolic syndrome: obesity, hypertriglyceridemia, reduced HDL cholesterol, hypertension, and impaired fasting glucose.[15] Insulin resistance is the underlying pathology that links these criteria to one another. The prevalence of insulin resistance in persons with hypertension is approximately 50%; it is even higher in persons with dyslipidemia.[16] It is believed that persons with metabolic syndrome are in a state of disease evolution that includes both prediabetes and pre-atherosclerosis. Furthermore, metabolic syndrome, like diabetes, invokes an increased risk for cardiovascular disease. Treatment of women with the various abnormalities that constitute a diagnosis of metabolic syndrome can significantly decrease the risk for subsequent type 2 diabetes and the risk for cardiovascular disease.[1]

Complications of Diabetes

The adverse health consequences of hyperglycemia are perhaps even more debilitating than emergencies associated with the underlying diabetes. When the blood levels of glucose are high, the ability of glucose to chemically attach to different proteins without the stimulus of enzymatic facilitation occurs—a process called **glycosylation**. The glycosylation of proteins produces advanced glycosylation end products that attach to nerve cells, and to endothelial cells that line the interior walls of blood vessels. Nerve and endothelial cell damage starts a chain of adverse events resulting in diabetic neuropathy and macrovascular or microvascular disease.

Macrovascular disease involves dysfunction of large vessels of the body (e.g., coronary artery disease, cerebrovascular disease, and peripheral vascular disease). Once the endothelial cells are impaired, vasoconstrictive, proinflammatory, and prothrombotic mediators are released, and over time, atherosclerotic plaque develops.[17] Macrovascular disease develops more rapidly in persons with diabetes when compared to persons who do not have diabetes. Women with diabetes have a higher risk than men in particular for cardiovascular complications, and cardiovascular disease is responsible for more than 70% of the deaths attributed to diabetes.[18]

Microvascular disease results from a similar process occurring in smaller vessels of the body (e.g., diabetic retinopathy and renal failure). Many of the quality-of-life changes associated with advanced diabetes relate to microvascular disease. As more information about diabetes emerges, new pharmacologic treatments are being employed early in the disease process in hopes of preventing both macrovascular and microvascular complications.

Management Goals for Treating Diabetes

Three organizations set standards for the diagnosis and management of diabetes. The American Association of Clinical Endocrinologists (AACE), in collaboration with the American College of Endocrinology (ACE), has recently published updated guidelines for the diagnosis and management of diabetes.[19–21] The American Diabetes Association (ADA) regularly updates its *Standards of Medical Care in Diabetes*.[1] The glycemic goals of both groups are listed in Table 18-1. These organizations agree that the treatment goal for all persons with diabetes is to maintain blood glucose values as close to normal as possible, without inducing hypoglycemia.

The measurement of glycosylated hemoglobin is used to make determinations about the degree of hyperglycemia and how long it has been present. Glycosylated hemoglobin is most commonly referred to as HbA_{1c}. In the landmark U.K. Prospective Diabetes Study, the progression of type 2 diabetes was analyzed over a 10-year time frame. Researchers found a 1% increase in HbA_{1c} was associated with an 18% increase in the risk of having a cardiovascular event, a 12% to 14% increase in the risk of death, and a 37% increase in the risk of developing renal failure or retinopathy.[21] This relationship between increasing severity of hyperglycemia and increased risk for complications is the basis for current interest in interventions that tightly regulate glucose metabolism, and HbA_{1c} levels are used to guide different steps in clinical practice algorithms.[1,19]

However, trials have not supported a singular goal of tight glycemic control to reduce the risk of diabetic complications. A recent study found that glucose control may be too tight and that individuals with type 2 diabetes who maintained their HbA_{1c} lower than 6% actually had higher risks for serious cardiovascular events.[14] At this time, the HbA_{1c} goal of less than 7% or less than 6.5% and not below 6% is reasonable.

Secondary goals include prevention of complications via management of hypertension and lipids. Interventions include strict control of blood pressure. Lifestyle modification is recommended if blood pressure is higher than 120/80 mm Hg; antihypertensive medication is considered if blood pressure is higher than 130/80 mm Hg and recommended if blood pressure is higher than 140/80 mm Hg. Statin drugs are used to maintain low-density lipid (LDL) cholesterol at less than 100 mg/dL. Additional interventions include daily aspirin therapy to prevent emboli, elimination of smoking, and realistic exercise and weight loss of 5% to 10% of body weight.[1]

Management Goals for Type 1 Diabetes

The management goal for persons with type 1 diabetes is **euglycemia** and prevention of complications associated with diabetes. Lifestyle management including

Table 18-1 Glycemic Targets for Persons with Diabetes

	American Association of Clinical Endocrinologists	American Diabetes Association[a]
Fasting plasma glucose	< 110 mg/dL	70–130 mg/dL
2-hour postprandial glucose	< 140 mg/dL	< 180 mg/dL[a]
HbA_{1c}	≤ 6.5%	< 7%

Abbreviations: HbA_{1c} = hemoglobin A_{1c}.
[a] Goals should be individualized based on duration of diabetes, age/life expectancy, comorbid conditions, known cardiovascular disease, hypoglycemia unawareness, and individual patient considerations.
Sources: Data from American Association of Clinical Endocrinologists medical guidelines for clinical practice for developing a diabetes mellitus comprehensive care plan. *Endocrine Pract.* 2011;17(suppl 2):1-53[20]; American Diabetes Association. Standards of medical care in diabetes—2014. *Diab Care.* 2014;37(suppl 1):S14-S80.[1]

intensive nutrition therapy is essential in type 1 diabetes. Exogenous insulin replacement is essential for persons with this type of diabetes. The primary pharmacologic focus is on variations in the type of insulin, timing of administration, and routes of administration to maintain euglycemia while avoiding serious complications of hypoglycemia or hyperglycemia.

Management Goals for Type 2 Diabetes

The American College of Endocrinology and the American Association of Clinical Endocrinologists have published a treatment algorithm for the management of type 2 diabetes.[22] This algorithm provides management strategies to accomplish glycemic control in persons who are newly diagnosed with type 2 diabetes (naïve to therapy) and previously diagnosed persons for whom therapeutic changes are needed to accomplish treatment goals. The AACE has also published medical guidelines for comprehensive care of individuals with diabetes.[20] The ACE/AACE algorithm is similar to the more recent American Diabetes Association 2014 *Standard of Medical Care in Diabetes*.[1] The ADA's guidelines are less prescriptive and emphasize an individualized approach to treatment planning.[1] Readers who specialize in diabetes care will want to compare the two different sets of recommendations.

Nonpharmacologic Management of Diabetes

The primary nonpharmacologic interventions of diabetes are diet and lifestyle change. The ADA has promoted the most widely accepted nutrition standards, centered on diets low in fat and processed food, and rich in vegetables, fruits, and whole grains. For persons with diabetes, food is the foundation for regulating blood glucose, and medications are added to meet the remaining need for glycemic control. Some individuals with type 2 diabetes may be able to control blood sugar with diet alone; however, all individuals with type 1 diabetes and the overwhelming majority of individuals with type 2 diabetes will require additional medications to maintain glycemic control. Exercise, avoidance of tobacco products, and adequate sleep are additional lifestyle factors effective in managing diabetes.[20]

Alternative therapies such as high doses of the spice cinnamon to assist in glycemic control have been explored.[23] None of the proposed alternative or complementary therapies has been found to be effective when subjected to rigorous study.

Prediabetes

Lifestyle changes are the first intervention in prediabetes, as in other classifications of diabetes. Nutrition to accomplish a weight reduction of 5% to 10% of total body weight results in lower fat mass, reduces triglycerides and LDL levels, and lowers both blood glucose and blood pressure. Controlled sodium intake and avoidance of alcohol assist in control of blood pressure. Exercise is recommended for weight control and cardiovascular health. For individuals who do not lose weight with diet and exercise interventions, surgical weight loss may also be considered.[20]

Medications to reduce glucose levels are indicated for persons with prediabetes who do not achieve blood glucose reductions with lifestyle change, or who are at particularly high risk for developing type 2 diabetes and diabetic complications. Notable risk factors for women include a history of polycystic ovarian syndrome, cardiovascular disease, and/or gestational diabetes. Metformin (Glucophage) and acarbose (Precose) are recommended as first-line drugs because of their safety and evidence of effectiveness in preventing progression to diabetes. Metformin can be considered as soon as 6 months after prediabetes diagnosis, if lifestyle change has not effected a significant reduction in blood glucose levels.[24]

Thiazolidinediones are effective in reducing progression to diabetes, but the side effects of congestive heart failure and increased incidence of fractures argue against their use.[19] There are no data on the effectiveness of newer glycemic agents including meglitinides, glucagon-like peptide-1 (GLP-1) receptor agonists, and dipeptidyl peptidase-4 (DPP4) inhibitors for treating prediabetes.

Pharmacologic management to prevent complications of diabetes in persons with prediabetes uses the same agents recommended for individuals with type 1 or type 2 diabetes. Statin therapy is recommended to achieve the same lipid goals of LDL less than 100 mg/dL and non-HDL cholesterol less than 130 mg/dL.[25] Niacin is not recommended for lipid control because it may adversely affect glycemic control. Ezetimibe (Zetia), bile acid sequestrants, and fibrates may be used if needed.

Pharmacologic intervention is recommended for persons with blood pressure that is higher than 140/80 mm Hg. First-line antihypertensive agents used include angiotensin-converting enzyme inhibitors (ACE inhibitors) and angiotensin receptor-blocking agents (ARBs), with calcium-channel blockers as a second choice. As with other forms of diabetes, beta blockers and thiazides should be avoided because of their potential to raise blood glucose levels. Aspirin for antiplatelet therapy is recommended unless contraindicated by the presence of a hemorrhagic condition or if the person is at increased risk for gastrointestinal bleeding.

Type 1 Diabetes Insulin Therapy

The goal of insulin therapy is to simulate the normal insulin response to food, exercise, and metabolic needs of the individual. Recommendations for glycemic targets differ between the ADA and the AACE. The ADA recommends targeting therapy to a preprandial plasma glucose between 70 mg/dL and 130 mg/dL, and the AACE recommends a level less than 110 mg/dL. The recommended postprandial glucose measured 1–2 hours after a meal is less than 180 mg/dL according to the ADA and less than140 mg/dL according to AACE.[1,20] Data support both targets, but no data are available to show a preference of one set of targets over the other. HbA_{1c} levels reflect the average blood glucose level over the previous 30–90 days. The goal is to keep the HbA_{1c} lower than 7.5% for adolescents and young adults, and lower than 6.5% to 7% for adults.

Insulin therapy is monitored daily by checking for urinary ketones in the morning and at bedtime, fasting blood glucose levels in the morning, and then preprandial and postprandial glucose levels throughout the day and once more at bedtime. Additional blood glucose readings may be needed before and after exercise and if symptoms of hypoglycemia or hyperglycemia occur. Self-monitored blood glucose levels are essential to monitor the dose and effectiveness of the insulin regimen throughout the day. According to Briscoe et al., 90% of individuals who use insulin have had at least one hypoglycemic episode.[26] Care must be taken to establish a regimen that prevents hypoglycemia. The risk of hypoglycemia is increased if the woman is ill, physiologically stressed such as during pregnancy or labor, or undergoing surgery. Doses of insulin need to be adjusted in these situations and monitored very closely.

Insulin

Insulin for treating diabetes was originally made from the pancreas of cattle, pigs, horses, or fish. The structure of these insulins was very close to human insulin and well tolerated, although allergic responses did occur mostly because of impurities in the insulin preparation. Better processing improved the purity of animal insulin, but it never could match the purity of manufactured insulin. Only beef and pork insulin have been in common usage worldwide. Beef insulin was discontinued in the United States in 1998, and pork insulin was no longer manufactured or marketed in the United States beginning in January 2006. All insulin manufactured and marketed in the United States today is recombinant, genetically engineered human insulin or **insulin analogue**. Very few companies manufacture animal insulins, and their usage is limited to persons who have been successfully managed on animal insulin for many years. Persons in the United States who insist on animal insulin must import it for their personal use only. A mechanism exists within the FDA to accomplish the importation legally; information on this arrangement is available from the FDA.

Nonanimal insulins are pure insulin, albeit with some exceptions. Neutral protamine Hagedorn insulin (NPH; Humulin N, Novolin N) also contains the protein protamine, tiny amounts of zinc, and the buffer phosphate. Lispro (Humalog) and aspart (NovoLog) contain zinc and the buffer phosphate as well. Glulisine (Apidra) contains metacresol as a preservative. Such additives are suspected to be the responsible factors when hypersensitivity and allergies specific to recombinant insulins occur.

All insulin products are measured in units. The United States has implemented this standard so that all insulin is described in terms of a U-100 concentration, which is 100 units of insulin per milliliter. Regular and NPH insulin in this concentration are available over the counter without prescription. Rapid-acting and long-acting newer insulin formulations require a prescription. Higher concentrations are available by prescription for the exceptional individual who uses very high doses of insulin.

Side Effects/Adverse Effects of Insulin

Common reactions to insulin include injection-site reactions such as lipodystrophy, weight gain, pruritus, and rash. Weight gain is attributed to the anabolic effects of insulin. Peripheral edema can occur in persons on insulin therapy because insulin causes sodium retention.

Hypersensitivity Reactions

Hypersensitivity to insulin and any additives or buffers in the insulin preparation is possible. More serious reactions include severe hypoglycemia, hypokalemia, and, rarely, anaphylaxis. In persons who have renal or hepatic compromise, doses should be lowered and blood glucose monitored closely. Measurement of baseline creatinine clearance is recommended before initiating any insulin therapy. Decreased creatinine clearance indicates renal compromise and a decreased ability to metabolize insulin.

All initial insulin doses are reduced in women with low creatinine clearance. For some insulins, specific recommendations are made regarding the amount of dose adjustment per creatinine clearance.

Skin Reaction and Lipodystrophy

Local reactions are common following insulin injection via syringe or pump. Most skin reactions resolve spontaneously when injection sites are changed more frequently. Careful attention to technique will minimize skin infections.

Lipodystrophy is a loss of adipose tissue in injection sites attributed to inflammation mediated by immune complexes. Impure animal insulin has been implicated in the development of lipodystrophy, but this complication is extremely rare among individuals who use insulin analogues. Experimental treatment of severe cases has used corticosteroids and mast cell stabilizers to block the immune response.[28] Treatment of women with isolated lesions can be accomplished with a dermatologic procedure or surgical revision.

Insulin Hypersensitivity

The incidence of insulin allergy has dropped dramatically with the transition from animal insulin to recombinant and analogue insulin. The reason for the reduction in allergy is attributed to the purer product, which contains fewer impurities, additives, and animal proteins that might stimulate allergy. Hypersensitivity still may develop in response to the minor contaminants or one of the known additives—phenol, zinc, metacresol, or phosphates. A change in the type of insulin used, thereby eliminating exposure to the allergen, is recommended when such a reaction occurs. For example, lispro insulin containing phosphates could be discontinued in favor of glulisine, which has no phosphates. If the sensitivity persists, desensitization with gradually increasing doses may be tried. Antihistamines may be used in skin reactions and hypersensitivity. Severe reactions and systemic reactions are extremely rare and may require corticosteroid therapy.

Drug–Drug Interactions

Many pharmaceuticals cause hypoglycemia or hyperglycemia by influencing glucose regulatory mechanisms in the liver and pancreas. Because of this effect, insulin levels may need to be adjusted when a woman with diabetes takes another drug. Drugs of concern are listed in Table 18-2. For example, beta-adrenergic receptor antagonists (beta blockers) can potentiate hypoglycemia because they inhibit catecholamine stimulation of gluconeogenesis. In addition, beta blockers can mask hypoglycemic symptoms (i.e., tremor or palpitations). Another example of a source of drug–drug interactions is pentamidine (Pentam), which has multiphasic effects on blood glucose and increases the risk of pentamidine-associated pancreatic beta cell toxicity.

Insulin Delivery Mechanisms

Insulin is a protein that, if ingested orally, would be digested in the stomach and intestine before reaching the circulation. Insulin is therefore administered subcutaneously in multiple doses throughout the day and/or by continuous subcutaneous infusion pump. An inhaled insulin (Exubera) was approved by the FDA in 2006 but removed from the market in late 2007 due to lack of acceptance and poor sales. Exubera was very difficult to mix and manage by individuals using the product. In June 2014, a new inhaled formulation (Afrezza) that is easy to mix and use was approved by the FDA. Afrezza is given before meals and must be used in a regimen that includes a long-acting insulin. Transdermal delivery systems for insulin have

Table 18-2 Drugs That Cause Hypoglycemia or Hyperglycemia

Drugs That Cause Hypoglycemia: Generic (Brand)	Drugs That Cause Hyperglycemia: Generic (Brand)
Androgens	Atypical antipsychotics: clozapine (Clozaril), olanzapine (Zyprexa), risperidone (Risperdal)
Angiotensin-converting enzyme (ACE) inhibitors	Beta sympathomimetics
Beta-adrenergic receptor antagonists[a]	Clonidine (Catapres)
Bromocriptine (Parlodel)	Corticosteroids
Ethanol	Decongestants
Indomethacin (Indocin)	Diazoxide
Levofloxacin (Levaquin)	Diuretics
Lithium (Lithobid)	Epinephrine
Monoamine oxidase (MAO) inhibitors	Heparin
Naproxen (Aleve)	HIV protease inhibitors
Ofloxacin (Floxin)	Isoniazid (INH)
Oral hypoglycemic agents	Marijuana
Pentamidine (Pentam)	Morphine
Quinolones	Niacin
Sulfonamides	Nicotine
Sulfonylureas[a]	Phenytoin (Dilantin)
Tetracycline	Thiazides
Theophylline (Theo-Dur)	Thyroid hormones

[a] Beta-adrenergic receptor antagonists and sulfonylureas are commonly prescribed medications for persons with diabetes.

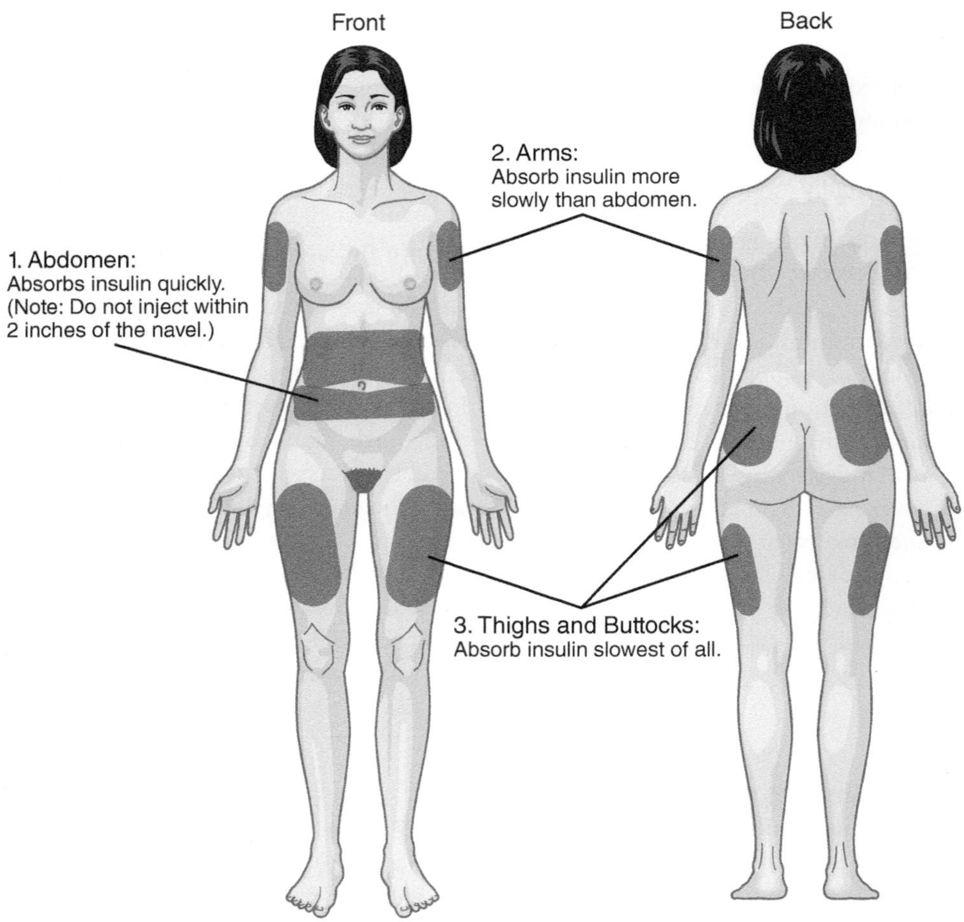
Front
Back
1. Abdomen:
Absorbs insulin quickly.
(Note: Do not inject within
2 inches of the navel.)
2. Arms:
Absorb insulin more
slowly than abdomen.
3. Thighs and Buttocks:
Absorb insulin slowest of all.

Figure 18-4 Sites for insulin injection.

been developed but are not yet ready for use. Several pharmaceutical companies are developing oral formulations of insulin, but none has progressed beyond the initial Phase 1 studies. Intravenous administration of insulin is reserved for inpatient care with intensive monitoring.

Insulin Injections

The most common method of administration of insulin is multiple injections daily. Insulin is drawn into an insulin syringe that carries clear markings for units of insulin. Short needles that assure injection in the subcutaneous tissue are needed. Intramuscular injection, in contrast, results in very rapid absorption and metabolism of the insulin. Subcutaneous injections should be placed on the abdomen, anterior thigh, buttocks, or dorsal arm. The abdomen is the preferred site of injection in the morning because the absorption of insulin is 20% to 30% faster in this site than others.[26] If the woman is unwilling or unable to use the abdominal site, a consistent area (arm, thigh, or buttock) should be chosen for injections given at specific times of day. For example, morning injections would be given in the thigh and evening injections in the buttocks. Consistent use of an area will standardize the expected absorption and enable better adjustment of insulin dose.[26] Rotation within these standard sites is needed to prevent injection-site reactions and lipodystrophy (Figure 18-4). An advantage of syringe injections is the ability to mix insulins; adjust administration times to accommodate changes in mealtimes, activity, and sleep/work schedules; and tailor the dose to anticipated food intake.

Insulin Pump

The insulin pump is a mechanism of providing continuous subcutaneous insulin administration. A needle is placed in the subcutaneous tissue of the abdomen and connected to a continuous pump, with increasingly sophisticated computer delivery calculators being used to manage dose regimens. The 24-hour basal and intermittent bolus insulin can be programmed and given automatically. The pump makes it possible to deliver insulin in fractions of units if needed, thereby facilitating tighter control of blood glucose levels. The bolus can be calculated and given for the anticipated carbohydrate intake with the upcoming meal, reduced in the situation of exercise or illness, and adjusted to various lifestyle schedules such as night employment. The disadvantage is that the pump requires careful attention because if it is kinked or empty, no insulin is given and the woman may not be aware of this fact. As a consequence, the risk of hypoglycemia is potentially increased with use of the pump. Individuals using the pump need to have backup insulin administration available in the event the pump is broken. The pump is more expensive than frequent injections, and its cost may be prohibitive for some women.

Sensor-augmented pumps are considered for women with rapid swings in their glucose levels, those who have unrecognized overnight hypoglycemia, and those who are unaware of hypoglycemia when awake.[27] With such a device, the sensor reads the blood glucose level and administers the appropriate amount of supplemental insulin. The sensor-augmented pump has been shown to be effective in reducing HbA_{1c} levels without an increase in hypoglycemia.[27]

Insulin Pens

Insulin pens are available for most insulins on the market today. The pen uses replaceable cartridges of insulin and disposable needles. For some insulins, a prefilled disposable pen is available. With this device, the woman attaches a new needle, turns the dial on the pen to select the required units, and injects the insulin into the desired site. The needle needs to remain in the subcutaneous tissue for 5 seconds to assure all the medicine is delivered. The pen is then removed, and the needle and cartridge discarded. A key advantage of the pen is its ease of use by those individuals who are sight or fine-motor impaired. In addition, the self-contained medication can be injected discreetly because it is already prepared. The disadvantage is that insulins cannot be mixed in a single syringe, potentially requiring more injections. The dose in the pen must be full or half—no other fractions are possible. In addition, pens are more expensive than individual syringe injections and may be cost prohibitive for some women. As with other insulins, the injection sites must be rotated.

Insulin Preparations

The characteristics of insulin that are of clinical import are its onset, peak time, and duration of action (Figure 18-5). Insulin preparations are categorized by duration of action—that is, they may be rapid-acting, short-acting, intermediate-acting, long-acting, and premixed formulations that are a combination of specific proportions of short-acting and intermediate-acting insulins. In most cases, the pharmacokinetics of insulin are dose dependent. Larger doses have earlier peak effects and a longer duration of activity. All insulin is metabolized in the liver, the kidney, and adipose tissue. Currently used insulins are summarized in Table 18-3, and an example of each type is described here.

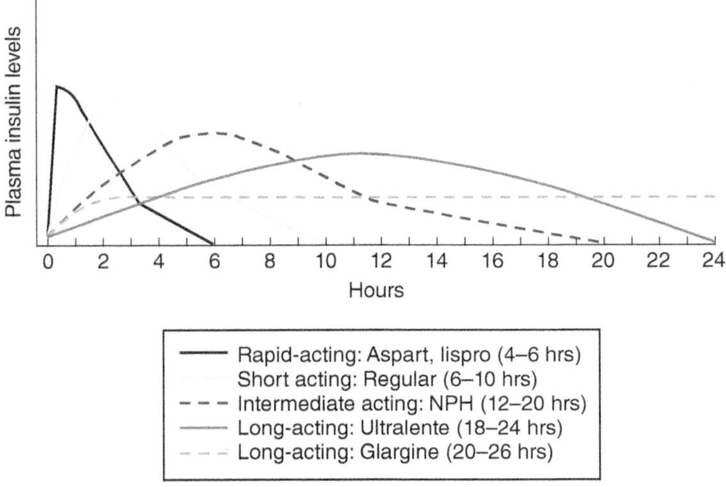

Figure 18-5 Onset, peak, and duration of action of different insulin formulations.

Table 18-3 Types of Insulin Preparations

Drug Category	Drug: Generic (Brand)	Onset	Peak	Duration	Rx/OTC	Comments
Rapid acting	Aspart (NovoLog)	10–20 minutes	1–3 hours	3–5 hours	Rx	Human
	Glulisine (Apidra)	15–30 minutes	0.5–2.5 hours	5 hours or less	Rx	Human
	Lispro (Humalog)	<15 minutes	30–90 minutes	5 hours or less	Rx	Human
Short acting	Inhaled (Afrezza)	10–15 minutes	1 hour	3 hours	Rx	Human
	Regular (Humulin R)	30–60 minutes	2–3 hours	4–6 hours	OTC	Human
	Regular (Novolin R)	30–60 minutes	2.5–5 hours	8 hours	OTC	Human
Intermediate acting	NPH (Humulin N)	1.5 hours	4–10 hours	14–18 hours	OTC	Human
	NPH (Novolin N)	1.5 hours	4–12 hours	24 hours	OTC	Human
	70% NPH and 30% regular (Humulin 70/30, Novolin 70/30)	30–60 minutes	Dual	24 hours	OTC	Human
Long acting	Detemir (Levemir)	50–120 minutes	Constant	24 hours	Rx	Insulin analogue
	Glargine (Lantus)	1 hour	Constant	24 hours	Rx	Insulin analogue
Inhalation	Insulin human [rDNA origin] (Afrezza)	12–15 minutes	53 minutes	160 minutes	Rx	Human rDNA origin

Abbreviations: OTC = over the counter; Rx = prescription only.

Rapid-Acting Insulins: Glulisine (Apidra)

Glulisine (Apidra) is a rapid-acting insulin analogue that is similar to the other two rapid-acting insulins, aspart (NovoLog) and lispro (Humalog). Glulisine is approved for use before and after food intake. This postprandial property means that the glulisine dose can be adjusted on the basis of what was actually eaten at a meal. For individuals who may not eat a planned meal at a predetermined time, the postmeal regimen reduces the risk of hypoglycemia or postprandial hyperglycemia. Glulisine inhibits gluconeogenesis and stimulates peripheral glucose uptake, thereby inhibiting lipolysis and proteolysis. The result is regulation of glucose metabolism.

Glulisine insulin is largely excreted by the kidney. The half-life of this rapid-acting insulin is 13 minutes when administered intravenously and 42 minutes when administered subcutaneously. Because it is such a rapid-acting and short-duration insulin, it is typically given with NPH insulin, which is one of the intermediate-acting insulins.

The dose of glulisine (Apidra) is 0.5–1 unit/kg/day. Glulisine is given less than 15 minutes before or less than 20 minutes after a meal. It can be given continuously via an insulin pump. No other medications can be mixed with glulisine in a pump, but NPH may be mixed with it in a syringe for immediate administration. Glulisine may also be given intravenously in an inpatient setting under close monitoring. Doses via all routes need to be decreased if the individual has renal or hepatic compromise.

Adverse reactions that are common following use of glulisine (Apidra) include those associated with all insulins. Edema, nasopharyngitis, and respiratory infections have also been associated with glulisine. Hypertension can occur in persons using this drug. Glulisine combined in a regimen with NPH insulin increases the risk for serious cardiovascular events. Glulisine should not be given to any individual who has a sensitivity to metacresol, as this additive is used as a preservative in glulisine.

Rapid-Acting Insulins: Insulin Lispro (Humalog)

Lispro (Humalog) is an insulin analogue approved for use in 1996. It is used in combination with a longer-acting insulin for type 1 diabetes, and it may be used in combination with a longer-acting insulin as a prandial dose or in combination with oral medications for persons with type 2 diabetes. Lispro is metabolized in the kidney, liver, and adipose tissue. Intravenous administration is not recommended but may be used for inpatient management. Lispro is administered less than 15 minutes before meals or in a continuous subcutaneous insulin pump. Although it may be given postprandially, it is not commonly used in this way. All doses need to be lowered for individuals with impaired renal or hepatic functions. Creatinine clearance evaluation is recommended before initiating lispro: The dose should be decreased by 25% if the creatinine clearance is between 10 mL/min and 50 mL/min, and by 50% if the creatinine clearance is less than 10 mL/min.

Rapid-Acting Insulins: Human Insulin Inhaled (Afrezza)

The rapid-acting inhaled insulin Afrezza, which is available as a powder, is used prior to meals. Because it is a short-acting preprandial insulin, it is always used in addition to a long-acting injectable insulin.

Inhaled insulin is contraindicated for individuals with lung disease or chronic respiratory disease such as asthma or chronic obstructive pulmonary disease (COPD). An FDA black box warning emphasizes the risk of bronchospasm if this drug is used by individuals who have COPD. Side effects include bronchial irritation, cough, sore throat, and sore mouth. Hypoglycemia is a risk with inhaled insulin, just as it is with all insulins.

Short-Acting Insulins: Regular Insulin (Humulin R)

Regular insulin is a human insulin made synthetically via recombinant DNA technology. This short-acting insulin is used to treat type 1 diabetes and may be the primary insulin added to oral medications for persons with type 2 diabetes who need insulin therapy. The dose of regular insulin varies depending on the application and route of administration.

Regular insulin is predominantly excreted in the urine (30–80%). The initial dose of this insulin should be decreased for women who have renal compromise. Regular insulin is the drug of choice for both diabetic ketoacidosis and hyperkalemia because it is short acting, has a rapid onset, and can be given intravenously.

Intermediate-Acting Insulins: Insulin NPH (Humulin N)

Insulin NPH (Humulin N) is an intermediate-acting insulin. Neutral protamine Hagedorn (NPH) was first created in 1936 when it was discovered that the effects of insulin could be prolonged by adding protamine.[29] The resulting formulation is excreted primarily in the urine (30–80%).

NPH insulin may be mixed with other insulins, is available in premixed syringes, and has a low cost. However, it has a more uneven peak and duration of action than other insulins so there is a greater risk of causing hypoglycemia when using this agent. Intravenous use is not recommended for NPH insulin. NPH insulin is indicated for the management of individuals with type 1 diabetes and type 2 diabetes, and it may be given concomitantly with oral medications. As with all insulin, caution needs to be used in determining the dose for individuals with renal or hepatic impairment.

Long-Acting Insulins: Insulin Glargine (Lantus)

Glargine is a human insulin analogue. Its half-life is unknown. Glargine is used as long-acting basal insulin by persons using the insulin pump. As with all basal insulin, the initial dose is calculated within the range of 0.5–1 unit/kg/day depending on the individual's age and body habitus. The onset of action is 1 hour, with a peak occurring 5 hours after administration. Glargine has the unique property of maintaining that peak for 24 hours. For this reason, it can be given at any time in a 24-hour period and has equal effectiveness with no increase in the risk of hypoglycemia. However, glargine—like all long-acting insulins—is more expensive than NPH, and it cannot be mixed with other insulins in the same syringe.

Exercise does not appear to affect the absorption of glargine. This insulin is absorbed equally from all injection sites, and there is no advantage to selecting a specific site. For very lean, insulin-sensitive individuals with type 1 diabetes, absorption is improved by splitting the dose and administering it at two sites. Glargine does not mitigate the need for bolus insulin in individuals with type 1 diabetes. It can be administered by pump but is usually given as a single daily injection.

Long-Acting Insulins: Insulin Detemir (Levemir)

Insulin detemir (Levemir) is a newer, long-acting basal insulin analogue. Detemir has a beneficial effect on weight. Specifically, individuals using this insulin have experienced a greater weight loss than those using NPH insulin.[30] Like glargine, detemir has a smoother action profile compared to NPH, reducing the risks of significant hypoglycemia. The mechanism underlying its metabolism and excretion remains unknown, and the onset, peak, and duration of its effects vary with route of administration.

Detemir can only be given subcutaneously by syringe; this insulin cannot be administered intravenously or in insulin pumps. When given subcutaneously, detemir has an onset of 1 hour, no peak, and a duration of 6 to 23 hours, depending on the dose given. For persons with type 1 diabetes, detemir is given in the usual dose of 0.5–1.0 unit/kg/day. If once-daily dosing is needed, the insulin is given with the evening meal or at bedtime. A short-acting insulin is also needed when detemir is used and is most effective if given prior to each meal. If insulin is used by an individual with type 2 diabetes, it may be taken with either oral medications or a rapid- or short-acting insulin. Detemir cannot be mixed in a syringe with other insulins, however. Individuals with impaired renal or hepatic function should use this drug in lower doses and with caution. Creatinine levels for evaluation of renal function are recommended before initiating the drug.

Individuals on insulin detemir may have difficulty recognizing hypoglycemia if they are also taking steroid medications (including those for asthma), diuretics, antihypertensive agents, sulfa drugs, or thyroid replacement medications.

Premixed Insulin

Premixed formulations of insulin typically contain 70% NPH or intermediate-acting insulin and 30% regular or short-acting insulin. These formulations are helpful for persons who have difficulty handling the small vials containing single insulins as well as persons who have poor eyesight and have difficulty measuring insulin doses.

Insulin Regimens

Historically, insulin was administered twice a day using a fixed combination of short-acting and longer-acting agents. Today, however, many persons who use insulin either administer multiple subcutaneous injections throughout the day or use an insulin pump. Insulin regimens must be tailored to the physiologic needs and daily activity of the individual, and consideration must be given to daily activity and food intake schedules. For example, if the individual exercises in the early morning or works at night, the schedule for insulin must accommodate that lifestyle. Insulin care instructions are listed in Box 18-1.

Sliding-Scale Regimen

A sliding-scale regimen involves using a fixed amount of long-acting insulin given at set times as well as fixed amounts of short-acting insulin prior to meals. The short-acting insulin may be adjusted based on the individual's blood glucose before each meal. The sliding scale refers to the relationship between insulin need and measured capillary glucose values. Blood glucose values are determined before mealtime, and the insulin is given 30–60 minutes before a meal. As the glucose level rises, the dose of regular insulin rises. The dose of insulin needed slides up or down based on the premeal glucose level.

Basal–Bolus Regimen

Unger[9] has outlined a step-by-step approach to prescribing a basal–bolus insulin regimen that is presented in Box 18-2. This is one example of a method to determine insulin doses for persons with type 1 diabetes. Many other algorithms are available, but the principles are the same. It is essential to consider the basal and bolus insulins and to

Box 18-1 Insulin Storage and Handling

Insulin is packaged in small, glass, multiuse vials that must be handled with care. Insulin does not work well if it is kept too long or if exposed to extreme temperatures. The following guidelines are recommended for all insulin preparations.

Storing Insulin

- Keep unopened bottles or unused pens in the refrigerator, but do not let them freeze. Insulin clumps into a precipitate when frozen.
- Before opening a new bottle, check the expiration date and do not use if it is too old.
- When you open a new bottle, write the date on it and do not use after 30 days.
- Insulin pens should not be kept at room temperature for more than 14 days.
- Insulin will stay fresh up to 30 days without refrigeration (and the shot is less painful if the insulin is not cold) as long as the temperature is less than 30°C (86°F) and more than 2.2°C (36°F).
- Insulin that is not refrigerated should be kept away from heat and light.
- Before using an insulin, check that it has an appropriate appearance as noted below.
- Very rapid-acting insulin, rapid-acting insulin, short-acting insulin, and glargine should be clear without any cloudiness or any particles floating in the liquid.
- Intermediate-acting insulin should look uniformly cloudy.

Handling Insulin Prior to Injection

Intermediate-acting insulins and insulin pens need to be mixed before drawing the solution into a syringe or injecting it because the concentration can become unevenly distributed in the vial or pen.

- Insulin vials: Roll the vial between two hands 10 times before drawing out the solution. Do not shake vigorously.
- Insulin pens: Roll the pen 10 times back and forth, and then point it up and down 10 times. The pen has a small glass bead that rolls back and forth to fully mix the layers of insulin.

Box 18-2 Establishing a Basal–Bolus Insulin Regimen

Step 1. Determine the total daily dose of insulin.

For adults, the total daily dose is calculated by taking the weight of the person in kilograms and multiplying it by 0.7. This calculation is adjusted for age. For example, an adolescent or adult with exceptional physical activity would need 1–2 units per kilogram per day. The ratio is reduced in the elderly (older than 65 years) to 0.5–0.7 units per kilogram per day. For this example, consider a 32-year-old woman who does not have any comorbid conditions and who weighs 80 kg. She will require 56 units of insulin per day.

Step 2. Determine the approximate starting dose of basal insulin, which will be either glargine (Lantus) or detemir (Levemir).

The day's dose is divided into two, so the morning dose will be 28 units of basal insulin and the evening dose will be 28 units of basal insulin.

Step 3. Use a simplified formula for determining baseline prandial insulin.

The baseline meal dose of insulin is calculated as 0.1 unit/kg of weight. In this case, 8 units of insulin is the standard prandial dose of a rapid-acting insulin dose.

Step 4. Allow the woman to adjust the prandial dose of insulin based on the size of the meal.

The dose of rapid-acting insulin can be increased or decreased based on the planned food intake. If the meal is small, subtract 1 or 2 units. If the meal is large or heavy in calories (pizza or pasta), add 2 units.

Step 5. Establish the insulin sensitivity factor.

The insulin sensitivity factor determines how much 1 unit of rapid-acting insulin will lower the plasma glucose level. This calculation tailors the insulin dose for the individual and is very helpful for adjusting insulin to the individual's lifestyle and schedule. The insulin sensitivity factor is equal to 1700 divided by the total daily basal insulin.

For example, suppose a woman who weighs 80 kg uses 56 units of basal insulin a day. The insulin sensitivity factor of 1700 is divided by 56; 1700/56 = 30.3, which is rounded to 30. This means each unit of insulin will lower the plasma glucose by 30 mg/dL. Prior to a meal, the woman checks her blood glucose with her meter. If the preprandial glucose is 200 and her target is 150, she needs to lower her glucose by 50 points. For an average full meal, she will add 2 units of rapid-acting insulin to the 8 units she is scheduled to take, for a total of 10 units. Additional units might be added if a large meal—or that piece of birthday cake—is anticipated.

Step 6. Allow the woman to adjust the dose of basal insulin.

One approach to adjusting basal insulin is to treat to target. The woman is advised to measure her fasting glucose in the morning and bedtime for the entire week. Every 7 days, she may adjust the basal insulin to reach the target fasting glucose of 120 agreed upon with her provider. The following chart is an example of the adjustments needed.

Average Fasting Glucose Values over 7 Days	Basal Insulin Adjustment
> 180 mg/dL	+ 8 units
140–180 mg/dL	+ 6 units
120–140 mg/dL	+ 4 units
100–120 mg/dL	+ 2 units
70–100 mg/dL	0 unit
< 70 mg/dL	– 1 unit

Source: Data from Unger J. Management of type I diabetes. *Primary Care Clin Office Pract*. 2007;34:791-808.[9]

Box 18-3 BJ Goes to College

BJ is an 18-year-old woman who has moved away from home for the first time to attend college. BJ is 5 feet, 4 inches (163 cm) tall, and her body mass index (BMI) is 23, a normal calculation. She is active on the tennis team and doing well in her studies.

BJ has had type 1 diabetes since age 3. She manages her insulin with a pump and a backup system of multiple daily injections if her pump is malfunctioning. Her insulin consists of glargine as a basal insulin and lispro for mealtime bolus. Her HbA_{1c} at last evaluation when she arrived on campus was 6.8%. BJ takes a multiple vitamin pill every day. She is not sexually active and does not use or need contraception.

BJ has been on campus for a semester when she comes to the student health center because she has a cold. She is concerned that her pump may be malfunctioning because her postprandial glucose is consistently higher than 160 mg/dL; in the past, it has usually been lower than 110 mg/dL.

On physical examination, BJ is found to have bronchitis. Upon nutritional recall, it is determined that BJ's food intake is consistent with the 1200-calorie ADA diet that she follows during the active tennis season. With further questioning about the upper respiratory infection, BJ reveals that she has treated her symptoms with an over-the-counter multi-symptom liquid medicine for colds, flu, and cough. She has not been able to go to tennis practice while she has been ill. Her random glucose value done on her arrival at 8 A.M., approximately 1 hour after her breakfast, was 174 mg/dL.

Upon further questioning, the clinician finds that BJ does not know that many of the over-the-counter medications marketed for treating colds contain sugar. In addition, BJ is consuming her usual amount of calories for her active tennis practice but has not engaged in that exercise while she has been ill.

The recommendation for BJ is to change to a cough treatment with dextromethorphan that is marketed for persons with diabetes, or a similar formulation that does not contain glucose or sorbitol; adjust her food intake until she returns to her normal exercise regimen; and increase her lispro by a few units after meals, based on her blood glucose values. BJ checks her blood glucose levels regularly, and she should find normal values within a day or so. She is instructed to return if her blood glucose values do not return to normal, if her cold symptoms worsen, or if she develops a fever.

determine the response of the individual to the dose. The individual must be willing and able to accurately perform self-monitored blood glucose testing. The insulin dose is then adjusted to enable the individual to meet the fasting and postprandial targets (Box 18-3).

Type 2 Diabetes

Pharmacologic management of women with type 2 diabetes can include both oral and injectable medications. Monotherapy with one drug may be sufficient, although multiple drug therapy will likely be required as the disease progresses over time. There are currently many classes of drugs available to lower blood glucose levels—sulfonylureas, meglitinides, biguanides, thiazolidinediones, alpha-glucosidase inhibitors, glucagon-like peptide 1 (GLP-1) receptor agonists, dipeptidyl peptidace-4 (DPP-4) inhibitors, dopamine-2 agonists, amylin mimetics, bile acid sequestrants, and sodium glucose co-transporter 2 (SGLT-2) inhibitors. Each class has a different mechanism of action (Figure 18-6), but they can be subdivided into two general categories: Sulfonylureas and meglitinides are hypoglycemic agents, whereas the others are antihyperglycemic agents (Table 18-4). If beta-cell function ceases or cannot be stimulated adequately with oral medications, insulin may be required.

The choice of pharmacologic therapy first takes into consideration the contributions of fasting and postprandial hyperglycemia to the HbA_{1c} level. The first expression of hyperglycemia in type 2 diabetes is usually an elevated postprandial glucose level. In individuals with HbA_{1c} less than 7.3%, postprandial glucose—particularly after a morning meal—contributes approximately 70% to the hyperglycemia, with fasting levels contributing 30%; as glycemia deteriorates, the contribution of the fasting glucose values increases.[31,32] The usual medications chosen for these individuals are metformin (Glucophage), a sulfonylurea, or one

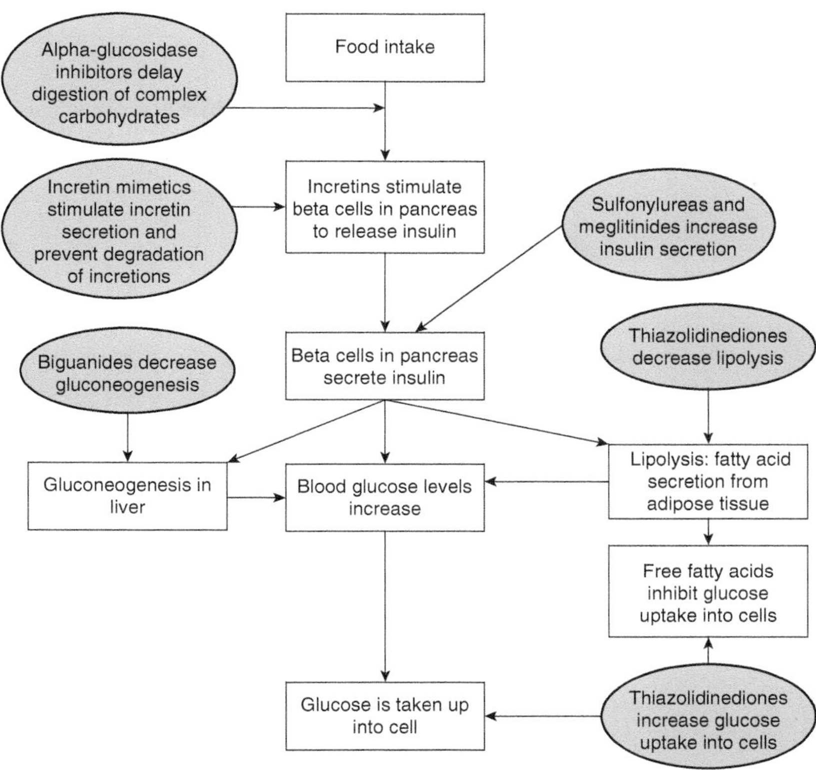

Figure 18-6 Mechanism of action of oral hypoglycemic drugs.

Table 18-4 Pharmacotherapeutic Agents for Treating Type 2 Diabetes

Drug: Generic (Brand)	Dose	Maximum Dose	Side Effects and Considerations	Effect on Weight
Sulfonylureas				
Glimepiride (Amaryl)	1–2 mg once daily with first meal of the day	8 mg daily	Sulfonylureas may cause hypoglycemia. Dizziness, headaches, and sun sensitivity have been reported in approximately 2% of users. Allergic skin rashes and GI disturbances include nausea, diarrhea, and constipation. Side effects are dose dependent and disappear after lowering and/or dividing the daily dose.	Weight gain
Glipizide (Glucotrol)	5 mg once daily before first meal	40 mg daily		Weight gain
Glipizide (Glucotrol XL)	5 mg once daily with first meal	20 mg daily		Weight gain
Glyburide (DiaBeta)	1.25–5 mg once daily with first meal	20 mg daily in divided doses		Weight gain
Glyburide (Glynase)	0.75 mg once daily	12 mg daily in divided doses		Weight gain
Meglitinides				
Nateglinide (Starlix)	120 mg 3 times daily before meals	360 mg daily	Hypoglycemia occurs in approximately 31% of users. Upper respiratory infections, headaches, nausea, diarrhea, sinusitis, are joint pain occur in as many as 6% of users.	Weight gain
Repaglinide (Prandin)	0.5–2 mg before each meal	Up to 4 mg before each meal		Weight gain
Biguanides				
Metformin (Glucophage)	500 mg twice daily or 850 mg once daily	2500–2550 mg daily	GI symptoms such as diarrhea, nausea, vomiting, abdominal bloating, and flatulence occur in as many as one-third of individuals. Some need to decrease or discontinue the medication either temporarily or permanently due to these effects. Hypoglycemia is almost unknown.	Weight neutral or loss

(*continues*)

Table 18-4 Pharmacotherapeutic Agents for Treating Type 2 Diabetes (*continued*)

Drug: Generic (Brand)	Dose	Maximum Dose	Side Effects and Considerations	Effect on Weight
Alpha-Glucosidase Inhibitors				
Acarbose (Precose)	25 mg 3 times daily with each meal	50 mg 3 times daily for women < 133 lb and 100 mg 3 times daily for women >133 lb	Abdominal pain, diarrhea, flatulence; all are reduced with time.	Weight neutral
Miglitol (Glyset)	25–50 mg with each meal	100 mg with every meal		Weight neutral
Thiazolidinediones				
Pioglitazone (Actos)	15 mg daily; can be taken in combination with insulin, metformin, and sulfonylureas	45 mg daily	No effects on lipids. Increased risk of hypoglycemia when taken with insulin.	Weight gain
Rosiglitazone (Avandia)	4 mg 1–3 times daily	8 mg daily	Increase in LDL and HDL in clinical trials. Increased risk of hypoglycemia when taken with insulin.	Weight gain
Dipeptidyl Peptidase-4 Inhibitors				
Sitagliptin phosphate (Januvia)	100 mg once daily with or without food	100 mg daily	Stuffy nose, sore throat, upper respiratory infection, and headache. Lower doses may be needed for persons with renal compromise.	Weight neutral
Sodium Glucose Transporter 2				
Canagliflozin (Invokana)	100–300 mg tablets daily before food	300 mg daily	Urinary tract infections, vulvovaginal mycotic infections. Contraindicated in persons with severe renal impairment.	Weight neutral
Empagliflozin (Jardiance)	10–25 mg tablets daily in morning	25 mg daily		Weight neutral or loss
Incretin Mimetics (Glucagon-like Peptide 1)				
Exenatide (Byetta)	5–10 mcg in prefilled pen twice daily before meals	20 mcg daily	Hypoglycemia possible if used in combination with sulfonylureas. If this effect occurs, the dose of sulfonylurea can be decreased. Nausea, vomiting, diarrhea, headache, anorexia, and acid stomach are side effects that primarily decrease over time.	Weight loss
Exenatide [extended release] (Bydureon)	2 mg SQ once a week through 2 mg single-dose pen or single-dose tray	2 mg weekly	Hypoglycemia is possible if used with insulin or sulfonylureas. A black box warning describes the risk of thyroid C-cell tumors.	Weight loss
Dulaglutide (Tricility)	0.75–1.5 mg SQ once a week in single-dose pen	1.5 mg weekly		Weight loss
Liraglutide (Victoza)	0.6–1.8 mg SQ daily in 0.6 mg, 1.2 mg, or 1.8 mg single-dose pen	1.8 mg daily		Weight loss[a]
Albiglutide (Tanzeum)	30 mg SQ once a week; may be increased to 50 mg in 30 mg or 50 mg single-dose pen	50 mg weekly		Weight loss
Amylin Mimetics				
Pramlintide (Symlin)	2.5–10 units before meals, titrated based on glucose levels and presence of nausea	10 units daily before meals	Contraindicated for individuals on potassium. Hypoglycemia is possible if uses with insulin. A black box warning describes the risk of hypoglycemia with insulin, although often co-administered.	Weight neutral or loss
Bile Acid Sequestrants				
Colesevelam (Welchol)	3750 mg PO once daily or 1875 mg PO two times daily; taken before meals in multiple-dose tablets and powders	3750 mg daily	Must be taken 4 hours after or before other medications. Has not been studied with co-administration with a dipeptidyl peptidase-4 inhibitor.	Weight neutral or loss

[a] Also marketed as Saxenda in dose from 0.6–3 mg for chronic weight management.

Source: Data from American Diabetes Association, European Association for the Study of Diabetes. Management of hyperglycemia in type 2 diabetes: a patient-centered approach: position statement of the American Diabetes Association (ADA) and the European Association for the Study of Diabetes (EASD). *Diab Care.* 2012;35(6):1364-1379.[33]

Box 18-4 Initiating Treatment for Type 2 Diabetes

JP is in for her annual examination. She is 40 years old; is 5 feet, 5 inches tall (165 cm); and weighs 205 pounds (93 kg) or a BMI of 34.1. JP has three children and had gestational diabetes during her last two pregnancies. Her youngest child is 22 years old. On examination today, it is noted that JP has an "apple" shape, indicating visceral adiposity. Her blood pressure is normal. Her laboratory findings from blood drawn a few days prior to this visit revealed an elevated lipid profile and a random blood glucose level of 190 mg/dL. The clinician suspects JP has type 2 diabetes and asks her to return in the morning and get a fasting blood glucose and HbA_{1c} drawn. Today, her fasting blood glucose level is 142 mg/dL and her HbA_{1c} is 7.2%.

JP has type 2 diabetes that requires pharmacologic treatment. She should have a baseline creatinine clearance and comprehensive metabolic panel to assure that her kidney and liver function are not compromised. She should be referred to an ophthalmologist for an eye examination and is referred to a nutritionist for diet counseling. In the past, JP would have been started on lifestyle changes and diet and then reevaluated in a few months. The current guidelines from the American College of Endocrinology and American Association of Clinical Endocrinologists, however, recommend that initial treatment include lifestyle changes, diet, and metformin because the previous stepwise path frequently results in an extended period of hyperglycemia. Because even slight elevations in HbA_{1c} are associated with complications of diabetes, early aggressive treatment of women with hyperglycemia is recommended.

JP is started on metformin (Glucophage) as monotherapy and taught how to measure and record her fasting and postprandial blood glucose levels as part of a comprehensive diabetes self-management education (DSME) program. Metformin will help lower her lipid values; it will not increase weight and is simple to monitor. However, because her HbA_{1c} is higher than 7%, JP may eventually need a sulfonylurea to become euglycemic. She will send her blood glucose values to the office weekly and schedule another appointment in 1 month to reevaluate her regimen.

of the thiazolidinediones.[20] The choice of drug balances the mechanism of action of that agent with specific characteristics of the individual (e.g., body mass index, ability to take medications several times per day, risk factors for cardiovascular disease). Individuals with an HbA_{1c} higher than 7.3% and elevated fasting glucose or elevated postprandial glucose later in the day usually require combination therapy.[20,33] In this situation, one medication is prescribed to lower the fasting glucose and an additional medication is used to treat postprandial elevations (Box 18-4).

Initial treatment and all subsequent treatment changes are usually assessed at 2- to 3-month intervals. Persons with tighter control of glycemia are less likely to develop complications.[34] Assessment includes a review of self-monitoring glucose records and HbA_{1c}. If the treatment goals are not met, additional pharmacologic therapy is prescribed and the individual is assessed again in 2–3 months to determine the effectiveness of the new regimen.

Management may need to be modified temporarily when an acute illness occurs or if a surgical procedure is needed. Individuals on oral therapy may need to be placed on insulin temporarily to enable rapid response to fluctuating glycemic status and minimize the risk of severe hyperglycemia and diabetic ketoacidosis.

Insulin Secretagogues: Sulfonylureas

Insulin secretagogues are medications that stimulate the beta cells in the pancreas to secrete insulin. The first generation of sulfonylureas includes tolazamide (Tolinase) and tolbutamide (Orinase). These agents are associated with multiple drug–drug interactions, however, so they are not used often today. In fact, several drugs of this first generation have been discontinued. The second-generation sulfonylureas have rare drug–drug interactions and include glimepiride (Amaryl), glyburide (DiaBeta, Glynase), and glipizide (Glucotrol).

Mechanism of Action

Sulfonylureas counteract the insulin resistance that is characteristic of type 2 diabetes by stimulating an increase in pancreatic insulin secretion at lower glucose thresholds and increasing insulin binding to insulin receptors. These drugs close the potassium channels of the pancreatic beta cells, which in turn opens the calcium channels, thereby enhancing the secretion of insulin. Sulfonylureas will lower HbA_{1c} levels by 1% to 2% and blood glucose levels by 60–70 mg/dL.[35] Individuals must have some functional beta cells and adequate liver and kidney function for these drugs to be effective. Over time, if pancreatic beta-cell function declines, this class of medications becomes ineffective. Maximum glucose lowering occurs at approximately 6 months and will continue for approximately 3 years, at which point blood glucose levels may begin to return to predrug levels, as pancreatic function can no longer be improved.[36]

Sulfonylureas are approved for monotherapy but may be used in combination with insulin and most other oral agents. However, they are not used in combination with meglitinides because meglitinides have a similar mechanism of action.

Because cardiovascular disease is the most frequent complication of diabetes, the role of hypoglycemic agents in lowering or increasing the risk of cardiovascular events has been the subject of many research studies.[37] Sulfonylureas have been associated with an increased risk for cardiovascular events in some observational studies. In 2001, the FDA added a special warning on the label of sulfonylurea agents that states there is an increased risk of cardiovascular mortality associated with the drug(s). To date, this association remains controversial, with some studies having shown such a relationship and others failing to find that sulfonylureas are associated with more cardiovascular events. The issue of the differing effect of the drugs on men and women is now under study, with sources suggesting that some drugs work better in women than in men.[37] Sulfonylureas are also associated with an increased risk of mortality in persons who have a myocardial infarction.[38] The theorized mechanism for this association is the effect that sulfonylureas have on ATP-dependent potassium channels in cardiac cells and cardiac vessels, which may prevent sufficient cardiac vessel dilation during a myocardial infarction.

One-third of individuals placed on sulfonylureas do not achieve their glycemic goals with these drugs alone. The most common reasons for the drug failure include dietary intake outside recommended calorie/carbohydrate levels and markedly impaired beta-cell function. For the approximately 66% of users who initially respond well to the drugs, each year 5% to 10% will develop secondary failure. By 10 years, half of all initial responders will have adequate control and half will have experienced secondary failure. The individual expected to have the best effect with sulfonylureas is older than 40 years with a diagnosis of type 2 diabetes for less than 5 years, has a normal BMI, and has not used insulin in the past.

If a sulfonylurea is being added to the regimen of an individual on insulin, the individual should have normal blood glucose levels on less than 40 units of insulin per day and have a fasting plasma glucose lower than 180 mg/dL. The optimal dose of sulfonylureas varies by the particular drug, but usually half of the maximum dose will result in the maximum glucose-lowering effect.[20] If the desired glycemic effect is not achieved above the middle range of recommended dose, a second drug should be considered.

Table 18-5 Risk of Hypoglycemia Associated with Oral Hypoglycemic Agents

No or Rare Risk: Generic (Brand)	Increased Risk: Generic (Brand)
Acarbose (Precose)	Albiglutide (Tanzeum), especially with insulin
Colesevelam (Welchol)	Chlorpropamide (Diabinese)
Exenatide (Byetta)	Glimepiride-containing products (Amaryl, Avandaryl)
Linagliptin (Tradjenta)	Glipizide-containing products (Glucotrol, Glucotrol XL, Metaglip)
Metformin (Glucophage, Glumetza)	Glyburide-containing products (DiaBeta)
Metformin/pioglitazone (ACTOplus Met)	Insulin
Metformin/rosiglitazone (Avandamet)	Nateglinide (Starlix)
Miglitol (Glyset)	Pramlintide (Symlin), if taken with insulin
Pioglitazone (Actos)	Repaglinide (Prandin)
Pramlintide (Symlin), when taken alone	Sitagliptin/metformin (Janumet)
Rosiglitazone (Avandia)	Tolbutamide
Saxagliptin (Onglyza)	
Sitagliptin (Januvia)	

Side Effects/Adverse Effects

The most common side effect of sulfonylureas is hypoglycemia secondary to overproduction of insulin. The relative risks of hypoglycemia for drugs used to treat diabetes are listed in Table 18-5. Glipizide (Glucotrol) and glimepiride (Amaryl) do not cause hypoglycemia as often as do other sulfonylureas.

Sulfonylureas do cause some weight gain secondary to stimulation of insulin activity in adipose tissue. As a consequence, they may not be the best choice for individuals who are overweight or obese. Thrombocytopenia, aplastic anemia, and pancytopenia are seen uncommonly.

Contraindications

Sulfonylureas are contraindicated for persons with a known sensitivity to any sulfonylurea or sulfonamide. Sulfonylureas are also contraindicated for use by persons taking antiviral medications due to an additive effect that increases the risk for hepatotoxicity. In addition, persons who use ethanol, methoxsalen (Oxsoralen), or

Table 18-6 Selected Drug–Drug Interactions with Oral Hypoglycemic Agents[a]

Drugs That Potentiate the Hypoglycemic Effect: Generic (Brand)	Drugs That Potentiate the Hyperglycemic Effect: Generic (Brand)
ACE inhibitors	Barbiturates
Alcohol	Calcium-channel blockers
Androgens	Corticosteroids
Beta-adrenergic receptor antagonists (beta blockers)	Diuretics
Cipro Floxin (Cipro)	Estrogen
Coumarin (Coumadin)	Isoniazid (INH)
Fluconazole (Diflucan)	Oral contraceptives
Gemfibrozil (Lopid)	Phenothiazines
Insulin	Phenytoin (Dilantin)
Itraconazole (Sporanox)	Rifampin (Rifadin)
MAO inhibitors	Sympathomimetics
Miconazole (Monistat, Lotrimin)	Thiazides
NSAIDs (Motrin, Aleve, Naproxen)	
Oral hypoglycemic agents	
Salicylates	
Sulfonamide	
Trimethoprim (Primsol)	

Abbreviations: MAO = monoamine oxidase; NSAIDs = nonsteroidal anti-inflammatory drugs.

[a] This table is not comprehensive as new information is being generated on a regular basis.

aminolevulinic acid (Levulan) should not take sulfonylureas because these combinations increase the risk of liver damage. Sulfonylurea agents can be used with caution by persons who take systemic beta blockers. Drug–drug interactions associated with sulfonylureas are listed in Table 18-6.

Meglitinides

Meglitinides were first introduced in clinical practice in 1998 and are sometimes referred to as "short-acting secretagogues." These agents work the same way that sulfonylureas work, but they bind to a different receptor on the pancreatic beta cell. The two approved agents in this category are repaglinide (Prandin) and nateglinide (Starlix). The efficacy of both repaglinide and nateglinide is similar to that of the sulfonylureas in reducing HbA_{1c} levels by 1% to 2% and blood glucose levels by 60–70 mg/dL.[35] Nateglinide is slightly less effective than repaglinide.[39]

Meglitinides have short half-lives. These agents are taken before meals to increase the insulin available for the food consumed. They are particularly helpful for persons who have fasting blood glucose values in the normal range but who become hyperglycemic after meals and for those individuals who have irregular meal schedules. If a meal is missed, the drug should not be taken.

Because meglitinides are short acting, less insulin is released overall compared to sulfonylureas. Therefore, meglitinides cause less hyperinsulinemia, and it is assumed they have less of an adverse effect on cardiovascular outcomes. That said, studies are lacking and the real association between meglitinides and cardiovascular events is unknown. Meglitinides have no significant effect on lipids.

Side Effects/Adverse Effects

Common side effects of meglitinides include nausea, dyspepsia, diarrhea, dizziness, upper respiratory symptoms, and hypoglycemia. Weight gain also is a common side effect noted with these drugs. The risk of hypoglycemia associated with meglitinides is less than the risk of hypoglycemia associated with sulfonylureas. Because of the lower risk of hypoglycemia, these drugs are especially useful for persons who are unable to manage hypoglycemia well, such as the elderly and individuals with cardiac or renal disease.

Contraindications and Adverse Reactions

Contraindications to use of meglitinides are similar to those for sulfonylureas. Specifically, these agents are contraindicated for persons with hypersensitivity to the drugs, individuals who have type 1 diabetes, and persons with diabetic ketoacidosis. Meglitinides are metabolized via the liver, so they should be used with caution by persons with liver disorders. A small portion of repaglinide is metabolized by the kidney; consequently, this drug should be used with caution by individuals with renal impairment. Serious but rare adverse reactions associated with the use of repaglinide include anaphylaxis, severe hypoglycemia, myocardial ischemia, leukopenia and thrombocytopenia, Stevens-Johnson syndrome, pancreatitis, hepatic dysfunction, and hemolytic anemia. Repaglinide should not be taken concomitantly with gemfibrozil (Lopid) secondary to a drug–drug interaction that increases the plasma levels of repaglinide up to 28-fold.

Biguanides

The first biguanide, metformin (Glucophage), was introduced into clinical practice in 1957, but was not used in the United States until 1995. Two drugs in this class, phenformin (DBI) and buformin (Silubin), were withdrawn from the market due to a high risk of lactic acidosis. Metformin has a much lower risk of lactic acidosis and has become the leading drug for persons with type 2 diabetes.

It is the second only to insulin for treating diabetes either as monotherapy or in combination with other agents.[40]

Metformin reduces hepatic glucose production and increases glucose uptake in the skeletal muscles and peripheral tissue. This drug lowers fasting blood glucose levels by 50–70 mg/dL and HbA_{1c} levels by 1% to 2%, which is comparable to the effects achieved with sulfonylureas.[35,41] Use of metformin in combination with a sulfonylurea lowers blood glucose more than either drug does alone.[41–43]

Metformin is formulated as a tablet that is taken orally and comes in both short-acting and extended-release forms. The drug is not metabolized, but rather passes unchanged through the body and is excreted 100% in the urine. The half-life in plasma is approximately 6.2 hours. A complete blood count, including red blood cell indices and a creatinine level, is recommended prior to starting metformin; it is usually rechecked at least annually. Metformin is especially helpful for persons who are overweight or obese and is the only orally administered antidiabetic agent that does not cause weight gain.

Metformin is also the only agent used to treat diabetes that improves cardiovascular outcomes (pooled odds ration [OR], 0.74; 95% confidence interval [CI], 0.62–0.89).[38] The drug has a positive effect on lipids, producing a small decrease in LDL and a slight increase in HDL, which results in an overall decrease in serum triglycerides. When persons who maintained tight glycemic control with metformin were followed for 10 years, they were found to have a 21% reduction in all diabetic complications as an aggregate, a 33% reduction in the risk for myocardial infarction, and a 27% reduction in death from any cause.[44] Metformin is superior to sulfonylureas for improving cardiovascular outcomes.[45]

Side Effects/Adverse Effects

Metformin alone is less likely to cause hypoglycemia than are the sulfonylureas or meglitinides. The most common side effects are gastrointestinal complaints such as bloating, nausea, and abdominal discomfort; they are usually mild and can be mitigated if the dose is titrated up to higher doses gradually. Other transient symptoms include anorexia, a metallic taste in the mouth, and rash. Extended-release formulations decrease the incidence of these side effects.

The two serious adverse reactions associated with metformin are lactic acidosis and megaloblastic anemia.[46] Metformin interferes with absorption of folate and vitamin B_{12}, which can, over time, cause megaloblastic anemia. If the individual has other risk factors for developing megaloblastic anemia, a cyanocobalamin assessment is recommended every 2–3 years.

Lactic acidosis is a potentially life-threatening condition. The FDA has mandated that metformin carry a black box warning for providers and users of metformin about the risk of lactic acidosis, which is rare but is fatal in more than half the cases when it does occur. However, the Cochrane Collaboration reviewed 176 studies that analyzed use of metformin and found no increased risk for lactic acidosis when the medication was used as recommended.[47]

Contraindications

Despite the Cochrane Collaboration findings, metformin is contraindicated for persons who are at risk for developing lactic acidosis (Box 18-5). In women older than 65 years, the

Box 18-5 Contraindications to Use of Metformin (Glucophage)

The incidence of lactic acidosis is approximately 3–9 per 100,000 persons who use metformin. Metformin concentrates in the intestine, where it doubles the production of lactate. The lactate subsequently passes into the portal circulation and decreases the pH in the liver. This causes a further decrease in lactate metabolism. These effects combine to increase the concentration of lactate in the circulation. Contraindications to using metformin, therefore, include disorders that might contribute to increased lactate concentrations. For example, hypoxia causes a shift to anaerobic metabolism, which produces lactate. The contraindications to use of metformin are the following:

- Renal impairment (plasma creatinine level ≥ 14 mg/dL in women)
- Cardiac or pulmonary insufficiency that is likely to result in decreased tissue perfusion or hypoxia (e.g., congestive heart failure, COPD)
- History of lactic acidosis
- Profound infection that might cause impaired perfusion of peripheral tissues (e.g., sepsis)
- Hepatic dysfunction (including alcohol-induced liver damage)
- Alcohol abuse

Temporarily discontinue metformin at the time of or before a procedure using intravenous contrast media; withhold it for 48 hours after the procedure and then restart it only when renal function is assessed as normal.

dose of metformin should be adjusted and renal function assessed more frequently than annually. Lactic acidosis is also a risk when women taking metformin undergo procedures requiring iodized contrast media. Metformin should be stopped 24 hours before the administration of iodized contrast media and restarted 48 hours later when renal function is confirmed.

Drug–Drug Interactions

Because metformin is not metabolized, clinically relevant drug–drug interactions are rare for this agent alone. Cimetidine (Tagamet) reduces renal clearance of metformin (Glucophage), which increases the blood level of metformin and increases the risk of lactic acidosis. If cimetidine must be used, renal function should be monitored carefully. Ethanol poses a risk with metformin because it may prolong hypoglycemia and increase the risk of lactic acidosis.

Thiazolidinediones

Thiazolidinediones (TZDs) are also known as glitazones. The three drugs in this category are troglitazone (Rezulin), rosiglitazone (Avandia), and pioglitazone (Actos). Troglitazone was withdrawn from the U.S. market in 2000 secondary to an increased risk for hepatotoxicity that was first noted in postmarketing research.

This class of drugs stimulates more effective use of glucose within cells in peripheral tissue via binding to an intracellular agent, peroxisomal proliferator-activated receptor (PPARγ), which activates genes involved in glucose and lipid metabolism. TZDs are considered insulin sensitizers because they improve insulin action in peripheral tissues and enhance glucose uptake in the cells. These agents decrease HbA_{1c} by 0.5% to 1.4% and reduce blood glucose values by 25–50 mg/dL.[35] TZDs work synergistically with metformin and sulfonylureas.

TZDs are metabolized in the liver and excreted primarily in urine, with some being eliminated in feces. These agents have a slow onset of action, with the first response being seen only after 2 weeks of taking the drug. At least 3 months' therapy is required to achieve the maximal benefit of the drug in an individual. When combined with another drug such as metformin (Glucophage) or insulin, the peak benefit can be seen in 4 weeks.

The primary indication for using a TZD agent is as a secondary medication for persons who have not achieved glycemic goals with insulin or metformin alone.[48] Thiazolidinediones are not used in the initial treatment of individuals with type 2 diabetes due to the increased risk of cardiovascular events and their high cost compared to other drugs. Thiazolidinediones are associated with less secondary failure than other drugs.[49] These agents are safe for individuals with renal impairment. Blood pressure is lowered in persons who take TZDs. Glycemic control is expected to last for 5 or 6 years with TZDs before these drugs begin to lose effectiveness.[35,36]

The relationship between TZDs and cardiovascular compromise is different than that noted with the other antidiabetic drugs. Specifically, TZDs increase the risk of congestive heart failure secondary to fluid retention and edema. It is postulated that TZDs may uncover latent congestive heart failure, as the TZD-related fluid retention overtaxes a circulatory system that cannot accommodate the additional fluid volume. A meta-analysis conducted by Nissen et al. convinced the FDA in 2007 that these risks warrant a black box warning.[50] Rosiglitazone now carries an FDA-mandated black box warning that this drug is associated with a significant risk of congestive heart failure. In 2009, the final results of the Rosiglitazone Evaluated for Cardiovascular Outcomes in Oral Agent Combination Therapy for Type 2 Diabetes (RECORD) trial were released. In this study, the agent did not increase the overall number of cardiovascular hospitalizations or deaths, but the risk of developing heart failure doubled in persons taking rosiglitazone compared to persons taking metformin or sulfonylureas; moreover, in persons with preexisting heart failure, there was a 26% increase in myocardial infarction.

Side Effects/Adverse Effects

The most common side effects of thiazolidinediones are edema and weight gain. Part of the weight gain can be attributed to fluid retention, but the majority is due to adiposity. Pedal edema occurs in approximately 5% of individuals who take a TZD. Caution is advised in individuals who have symptoms of congestive heart failure such as edema and in women with impaired liver function. Adverse effects including angina, pleural effusion, and pulmonary edema have all been seen with rosiglitazone. Additional side effects include anemia and headaches.

There is no risk of hypoglycemia when a thiazolidinedione is used as monotherapy; however, this risk increases significantly when pioglitazone is used in combination with other hypoglycemic agents. An increased risk for hypoglycemia also occurs when adding rosiglitazone to insulin or sulfonylurea therapy.

Women need to be warned that TZDs can induce ovulation and oral contraceptives may lose efficacy, so appropriate precautions need to be taken to avoid pregnancy.

In addition, women on rosiglitazone have a higher incidence of bone fractures than men using the drug.

Because this class of drugs is associated with an increased risk of hepatotoxicity, a baseline aminotransferase (ALT) level should be obtained. If this value is higher than 2.5 times the upper limit for the reference range, the manufacturer recommends that the TZD not be prescribed. For persons who take a TZD, the ALT level should be monitored every 3–6 months, and more often if it is elevated.[21]

Contraindications

All TZDs are contraindicated for persons with type 1 diabetes or class III or IV congestive heart failure. The primary risk with TZDs is the risk of death from congestive heart failure and myocardial ischemia. The black box warning about the increased risk of development or exacerbation of congestive heart failure is now attached to all drugs in this class, including pioglitazone. Contraindications to use of rosiglitazone include type 1 diabetes, hypersensitivity to the drug or class, congestive heart failure meeting New York Heart Association class III–IV requirements, congestive heart failure symptoms, and acute coronary symptoms.

Drug–Drug Interactions

Thiazolidinediones are primarily metabolized in the liver via CYP3A4 and CYP2C8. As a consequence, they are subject to several drug–drug interactions (Table 18-6). In particular, rifampin (Rifadin) speeds metabolism of thiazolidinediones and reduces the plasma levels, and gemfibrozil (Lopid) increases blood levels of thiazolidinediones. It is probable that the hypoglycemic effect of thiazolidinediones is decreased if other potent inducers of CYP3A4 are taken concomitantly. Drugs that are known inducers of CYP3A4 include carbamazepine (Tegretol), phenytoin (Dilantin), and St. John's wort. In contrast, these agents do not appear to alter the pharmacokinetics of other compounds.[51]

Alpha-Glucosidase Inhibitors

Alpha-glucosidase inhibitors prevent the digestion of carbohydrates, thereby reducing the number of simple sugars absorbed through the gastrointestinal system. The agents in this class that are available in the United States are acarbose (Precose) and miglitol (Glyset). These drugs are saccharides that compete with enzymes in the brush border of the small intestine, effectively preventing the action of enzymes necessary for conversion of carbohydrate to absorbable glucose. Carbohydrates are then digested in the colon.

This class of drugs is helpful particularly in controlling postprandial hyperglycemia. Alpha-glucosidase inhibitors may be used as a single-agent therapy or in combination with other hypoglycemic agents. The alpha-glucosidase inhibitors have a short-term effect on blood glucose levels and a minimal effect on HbA_{1c}. On average, they decrease HbA_{1c} by 0.7% to 1.0% and blood glucose levels by 20–30 mg/dL.[35] The effect of alpha-glucosidase inhibitors on serum lipid values and cardiovascular events is unclear, and more study of this relationship is recommended.[52]

The alpha-glucosidase inhibitors are given orally at the start of a meal. Both currently available drugs are oral tablets that are metabolized in the gastrointestinal tract. Acarbose is excreted predominantly in feces (51%) and urine (34%). Miglitol is excreted unchanged in the urine. Because of this reliance on renal excretion, a baseline creatinine level should be obtained prior to initiating therapy with one of these agents to verify adequate renal function.

Side Effects/Adverse Effects

Side effects of alpha-glucosidase inhibitors center on the gastrointestinal system and include abdominal pain, cramping, flatulence, and diarrhea. Flatulence is quite common and can reduce compliance. To minimize side effects, the dose should start low and gradually increase to an effective level.

A special consideration for alpha-glucosidase inhibitors is the management of hypoglycemia. If a woman develops hypoglycemia while taking a drug in this class, resolution requires the intake of monosaccharides in the form of glucose tablets or gel. Carbohydrates and other sugars will be blocked by the alpha-glucosidase inhibitor; thus their intake merely compounds the hypoglycemia. Hypersensitivity is possible with drugs in this class.

In addition to the common side effects noted with alpha-glucosidase inhibitors, acarbose has been linked with serious reactions including ileus, hypersensitivity to the drug, and hepatitis. Because of the risk of hepatitis, tests of liver function are recommended in addition to the baseline creatinine test. Assessment of liver function via evaluation of plasma levels of creatinine, ALT, and aspartate aminotransferase (AST) should be repeated every 3 months for a year. If these indicators of liver function remain normal, they need to be subsequently rechecked at least annually.

Contraindications

Alpha-glucosidase inhibitors are contraindicated for persons with gastrointestinal disease including inflammatory bowel disease or ulcers, those who are at risk for or have an intestinal obstruction, and those with malabsorption syndromes. The drugs should be avoided by individuals who use alcohol or take miglitol (Glyset) or pramlintide (Symlin) because of duplicate action and an increased risk of hypoglycemia.

GLP-1 Receptor Agonists

Incretins are a family of gastrointestinal hormones that induce insulin secretion in response to food ingestion. Glucagon-like peptide 1 (GLP-1) and gastric inhibitory peptide (GIP) are two of the hormones in the incretin family. Dipeptidyl peptidase-4 (DPP-4) is the enzyme responsible for degrading GLP-1 and GIP.

Unfortunately, the half-life of endogenous GLP-1 is just a few minutes, and the half-life of GIP is about 7 minutes, so although direct analogues of this hormone are effective, they have to be continuously administered intravenously or subcutaneously, which makes their clinical utility unfeasible.[53] An alternative is GLP-1 mimetics, which are GLP-1 receptor agonists resistant to degradation by DPP-4. These drugs are relatively new, and their effect on cardiovascular events is unknown at this time.[54,55] The interesting origin of exenatide (Byetta), the most common of these agents, is described in Box 18-6.

The commercially available GLP-1 mimetics include exenatide (Byetta) and weekly injectables such as liraglutide (Victoza), albiglutide (tanzeum), and an extended release exenatide (Bydureon). All of these drugs are injectable and may be administered as often as twice daily up to once weekly. Liraglutide is also administered daily subcutaneously, starting at 0.6 mg per day and potentially titrated to a maximum dose of 1.8 mg per day. If liraglutide is missed 3 days in a row, however, the dose must be restarted at 0.6 mg and titrated up again.

GLP-1 medications reduce the glucose impact of the food intake by increasing insulin secretion, suppressing glucagon secretion, and delaying gastric emptying, which leads to decreased intake and weight loss. Because their mechanism of action is triggered by food intake, exenatide must be taken only prior to a meal; if it is forgotten, the dose should not be taken at a later time of day. Others may be taken at any time during the day, although prior to a meal often is recommended.

These drugs are approved as adjunct therapy with oral medications such as metformin (Glucophage), biguanides, thiazolidinediones, and sulfonylureas. Exenatide provides a therapeutic advantage when paired with sulfonylureas, biguanides, and TZDs, although doses may be need to be adjusted with initiation of the combination therapy.[35,56] GLP-1 mimetics are currently FDA approved as monotherapy or as concurrent therapy with insulin.

GLP-1 drugs are metabolized in the kidney and excreted in urine. Prior to prescribing either agent, a baseline creatinine clearance should be obtained. A creatinine clearance less than 30 indicates a degree of renal compromise that precludes use of exenatide. The half-life of exenatide is approximately 2.4 hours; the half-life of liraglutide is approximately 13 hours. Because these drugs work in response to food intake, some of the risks of hyperglycemia and hypoglycemia that occur with other types of medications are avoided. Exenatide also suppresses release of glucagon from the pancreas in response to food intake and hyperglycemia, thereby decreasing the postprandial plasma glucose rise in response to food intake.

As with other GLP-1 drugs, there is an increased risk of severe hypoglycemia when they are administered at the same time as insulin; therefore, if used with insulin, the insulin dose must be decreased. At the time of this writing the labels for all the GLP-1 except exenatide (Byetta) carry an FDA black box warning that notes it is associated with an increased risk of thyroid C-cell tumors based on rodent studies. Women with a family history or personal history of medullary thyroid cancer or personal history of multiple endocrine neoplasia syndrome should not take liraglutide or albiglutide.

Side Effects/Adverse Effects

Gastrointestinal side effects of GLP-1 drugs include nausea, dyspepsia, vomiting, decreased appetite, and gastroesophageal reflux disease. Headaches, dizziness, and jitteriness are other reported side effects. Gastric emptying is slowed with the use of exenatide and liraglutide, so the sense of hunger is reduced. This mechanism of action has resulted in a welcome side effect of the drug—weight loss. The weight loss side effect associated with exenatide and liraglutide has made them the drugs of choice for individuals with diabetes and difficulty with weight control. It is not clear whether albiglutide (Tanzeum) will show the same weight loss effect as the other GLP-1 medications.

Exenatide has been associated with pancreatitis, and the FDA has issued a warning that anyone on the drug who exhibits signs of pancreatitis should discontinue the drug and seek medical evaluation. This decision was controversial because pancreatitis is more common in all individuals with diabetes. A recent meta-analysis was performed to evaluate the risk of pancreatitis in persons who use these drugs; this analysis could not confirm that

Box 18-6 Learning About Diabetes: From Dogs to Lizard Spit

Diabetes is a very old disease. References to the disease of sweet urine can be found in an unbroken chain of documents reaching back millennia, from an Egyptian papyrus more than 3500 years ago to modern-day resources. What may not be well known are the roles that many animals have played in the search for a cure for diabetes.

The recognition that diabetes occurs secondary to pancreatic dysfunction was discovered in 1889, when the European physician Minkowski removed the pancreas of a dog in his investigation of this organ. After the pancreas was removed, he noticed that the dog urinated more frequently and found the urine to be high in sugar content. This was the start of understanding diabetic pathophysiology.

The first compound used to treat diabetes was a preparation of canine pancreatic extract. In 1921, Frederick Banting and Charles Best kept a diabetic dog named Alpha alive for 70 days with injections of canine pancreatic extract. This success caused the duo to consider other options as treatments. Banting had been raised on a farm, so he advocated the development of concoctions made from pancreases of fetal cattle. He knew that cattle slaughtered for food would be impregnated prior to being slaughtered because pregnancy hastened their fattening. Thus, fetal calves were a source that was both plentiful and easily obtained.

In 1922, when Banting and Best had an extract that appeared pure enough, it was administered to Leonard Thompson, a 14-year-old boy who was dying of diabetes. After an initial hypersensitivity reaction, the extract was reformulated. A second dose resulted in a miraculous response, as Leonard's blood glucose levels dropped spectacularly. When Banting, Best, and colleagues published their findings, they suggested that this product of the isles of Langerhans be called "insulin." Shortly thereafter, they collaborated with Eli Lilly Company, which eventually produced an insulin made from pigs and cattle; this insulin remained the predominant type used in humans for decades.

Dogs were also involved in the discovery of drugs that treat type 2 diabetes. During World War II, Marchel Janbon, a French university pharmacologist searching for a cure for malaria, noted that dogs treated with sulfonylureas died of hypoglycemia. He quickly changed his research focus and developed sulfonylureas as a treatment for diabetes.

Since then, laboratory studies of agents that affect glucose metabolism have progressed with the sacrifice of many animals, including anglerfish, catfish, salmon, laboratory rodents, transgenic mice, and most recently Gila monsters. Exenatide (Byetta), one of the newest drugs available, is a synthetic form of a hormone found in the saliva of the Gila monster lizard (Heloderma suspectum). Studies are continuing today, and if they are successful, next up is an antidiabetic agent made from the skins of poisonous frogs.

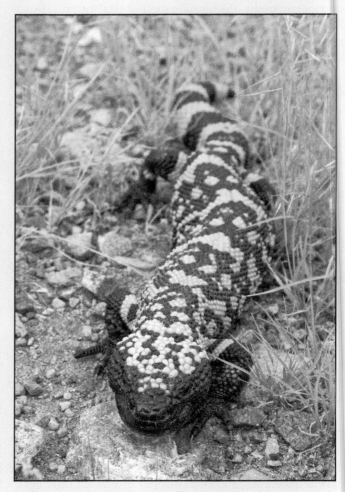

the use of incretins increased the risk. More research is needed on this topic, but caution is advised until the relationship is clear.[57]

Drug–Drug Interactions

For persons using GLP-1 medications, acetaminophen (Tylenol) and drugs that contain acetaminophen should be used with caution and monitored. Absorption of the GLP-1 medication will be delayed or decreased when acetaminophen is ingested concomitantly with the antidiabetic agent. Erythromycin (E-Mycin), metronidazole (Flagyl), and fosfomycin (Monurol) also delay and decrease absorption of GLP-1. Women taking oral contraceptives should take the contraceptive 1 hour before taking the GLP-1 medication to permit maximum absorption but need to be aware that effectiveness of contraceptives may be compromised.

Dipeptidyl Peptidase-4 Inhibitors

Dipeptidyl peptidase-4 (DPP-4) inhibitors do just as the name describes—they inhibit the degradation of the incretin GLP-1. The result is an increase in the concentration of endogenous GLP-1 and subsequent increase in insulin release from the pancreas. The unique property of DPP-4 inhibitors is that these drugs decrease glucagon and increase insulin only in response to elevated glucose. The dose–response property reduces the risk of hypoglycemia.

There are currently four drugs in this category—vildagliptin (Galvus), saxagliptin (Onglyza), linagliptin (Tradjenta), and sitagliptin (Januvia). Vildagliptin is available in Europe but not in the United States. In July 2008, the FDA requested additional clinical studies to evaluate the skin lesions and renal impairment observed in animal studies with the use of vildagliptin. The other three DPP-4 inhibitors are available in the United States.

Saxagliptin, linagliptin, and sitagliptin are oral medications given daily and can be taken with or without food. DPP-4 inhibitors are excreted predominantly in the urine (> 80%) and also in feces (13%). Because the medication is excreted by the kidney, measurement of baseline creatinine clearance is recommended prior to initiation of the drug to confirm renal function.

Sitagliptin is recommended as a monotherapy and can be used with other oral medications, although caution is needed to avoid additive effects. This agent is often used as a second drug in combination with insulin or other oral hypoglycemic agents and has a therapeutic advantage in these combinations. Synergism is expected with sulfonylureas, metformin (Glucophage), miglitol (Glyset), nateglinide (Starlix), disopyramide (Norpace), repaglinide (Prandin), pramlintide (Symlin), rosiglitazone (Avandia), glimepiride (Amaryl), and fluoxetine (Prozac). In fact, sitagliptin has a therapeutic advantage when paired with these drugs.

Side Effects/Adverse Effects

Nasopharyngitis, headache, and upper respiratory infections are the most common side effects with the DPP-4 inhibitors. Gastrointestinal discomforts include abdominal pain, diarrhea, and flatulence. Arthralgia has also been reported. Caution is recommended in individuals with impaired renal function. DPP-4 drugs increase insulin release from the pancreas, so pancreatic function is required for their effect. For this reason, this class of drugs is contraindicated in type 1 diabetes. Adverse reactions that have been reported with all three currently available DPP-4 inhibitors include Stevens-Johnson syndrome, hypersensitivity including anaphylaxis, and angioedema.

Drug–Drug Interactions

Combining beta blockers with DPP-4 inhibitors can cause an adrenergic antagonism that may alter glucose metabolism and excretion, resulting in prolonged hypoglycemia. Many drugs have an antagonistic effect when used with DPP-4 inhibitors, including angiotensin-converting enzyme (ACE) inhibitors, antihistamine/decongestant combinations, atypical antipsychotic medications, phenothiazines, isoniazid (INH), corticosteroids, estrogens, diuretics, statins, sympathomimetics, and thyroid hormones.

In addition, beta blockers mask hypoglycemia symptoms. Caution must be used when drugs that compete for the active transport mechanism used by DPP-4 inhibitors are given. These medications include adefovir (Hepsera, Preveon), cidofovir (Vistide), cimetidine (Tagamet), emtricitabine (Emtriva), and tenofovir (Viread). Androgens and MAO inhibitors have a synergistic effect that may increase the risk of hypoglycemia. Growth hormones increase insulin resistance and may increase the risk of hyperglycemia.

Sodium Glucose Transporter 2 Inhibitors

Sodium glucose transporter 2 (SGLT-2) inhibitors or glizoflozins are new agents for treatment of individuals with type 2 diabetes.[58] These drugs increase glucose excretion by blocking the renal sodium glucose transporter 2, thereby reducing the renal threshold for glucose. Thus, they increase glycosuria, which historically was a hallmark of uncontrolled diabetes. Theories of the long-term safety of this mechanism for lowering blood glucose levels are based on studies of familial renal glycosuria, a genetic condition in which SGLT-2 loses function but does not have deleterious impacts on renal sufficiency or life expectancy.

SGLT-2 inhibitors include empaglifozin (Jardiance) and canagliflozin (Invokana).[59] Dapagliflozin is under study in the United States and empaglifozin is marketed in a combination tablet with liraglutide with the brand name Glyxambi. Canagliflozin is given orally 100 mg daily before the first meal of the day. The dose may be increased to a maximum of 300 mg a day. The glomerular filtration rate (GFR) should be monitored and the drug discontinued if the estimated GFR (eGFR) is persistently less than 45 mL/min. Canagliflozin may be used as the primary single agent to treat type 2 diabetes but is typically used only after an ineffective trial of metformin. Caution has to be used with these drugs when the individual is taking other antihyperglycemic agents.

Side Effects/Adverse Effects

Common side effects of SGLT-2 inhibitors include nausea, constipation, fatigue, and increased thirst. Increased urination is common. The mechanism of action increases the risk for lower genital tract infections including bladder and urinary tract infections, vaginal mycotic infections, and vulvovaginal pruritus. Less common adverse effects include renal impairment and pancreatitis. Orthostatic hypotension is also a risk.

Contraindications

The site of action for SGLT-2 inhibitors is the kidney, so decreased renal function is a contraindication to use of these drugs. An eGFR less than 45 mL/min is a contraindication, and an eGFR of 45–59 mL/min requires caution in prescribing the drug. These drugs are not appropriate for management of type 1 diabetes and is contraindicated for individuals who are volume depleted. SGLT-2 inhibitors increase the risk of genital mycotic infections and bladder infections, so they should be used with caution by women who have a history of recurrent vaginal mycotic infections or urinary tract infections.

Drug–Drug Interactions

Caution should be used in combining SGLT-2 inhibitors with medications that may compromise renal function, such as avanafil (Stendra) or colchicine (Colcrys).

Amylin Mimetics

Amylin mimetics control glycemia by slowing gastric emptying time and suppressing postprandial secretion of glucagon. The beta cells of the pancreas secrete amylin in tandem with insulin. For this reason, individuals with poor beta-cell secretion of insulin will also have low secretion of amylin.

The only amylin mimetic available in the United States is pramlintide (Symlin). This injectable medication is used for treating individuals with either type 1 and type 2 diabetes. Its half-life is approximately 48 minutes and it is excreted renally.

Pramlintide is used only by persons already taking insulin and is not a second-line drug for individuals who are using oral medications only. Pramlintide is injected subcutaneously before full meals (at least 250 calories and 30 g of carbohydrate). The initial dose is 60 mcg before each meal, but is increased gradually until glycemic control is reached. The maximum dose is 120 mcg. The dose of pramlintide must be titrated with concomitant changes in insulin dose. When pramlintide is initiated, the rapid- or short-acting insulin taken prior to a meal should be decreased by 50%. As the pramlintide dose is further increased, the amount of insulin is decreased until glycemic control is achieved. Injection sites for insulin and pramlintide should be at least 2 inches apart to assure appropriate absorption of each drug.

Blood glucose values need to be checked before and after each meal and at bedtime when using pramlintide. Hypoglycemia can occur as long as 3 hours after injection and a meal. A key advantage associated with pramlintide is weight loss—possibly secondary to the slow gastric emptying time and the nausea experienced by some users during initiation of therapy.

Side Effects/Adverse Effects

Common side effects of pramlintide include nausea, vomiting, anorexia, arthralgia, dizziness, pharyngitis, and cough. When the dose is increased slowly over 3–7 days, the nausea side effects are minimized. Most side effects subside within a few weeks of initiation of the drug. The most significant adverse effect is severe hypoglycemia, which can occur when this drug is added to an insulin regimen.

Contraindications

Contraindications for pramlintide include having an HbA_{1c} level higher than 9%. This degree of hyperglycemia is better managed with insulin alone because pramlintide minimally affects the HbA_{1c} value. Individuals with gastroparesis or malabsorption syndromes may experience exacerbation owing to the delayed gastric emptying effect of pramlintide. Individuals with a history of severe hypoglycemia or hypoglycemia unawareness should not use this drug. Because of the intense monitoring required by the person taking pramlintide, individuals who have difficulty managing close self-monitoring should not use this medication, as the risk of severe hypoglycemia is high in these cohorts.

Pramlintide should not be administered with other drugs that slow gastric emptying, such as metoclopramide (Reglan), or that slow the absorption of food. In addition, pramlintide may delay absorption of other drugs. This drug is contraindicated if the individual is also taking solid potassium salts, such as potassium phosphate, potassium citrate (Urocit-K), potassium chloride (K-Dur, K-Tab, Klor-Con), or potassium iodide (SSKI, ThyroShield), because pramlintide slows the passage of solid potassium salts and increases the risk of ulcers and stenotic changes in the gastrointestinal tract.

Drug–Drug Interactions

Drug–drug interactions may arise when pramlintide is used concomitantly with any medication that has an anticholinergic effect. Anticholinergic drugs may further delay gastric emptying and slow medication passage through the gastrointestinal tract. Drugs of concern include tricyclic antidepressants, phenothiazines, alpha-glucosidase inhibitor oral hypoglycemics, antihistamines, and decongestants. The pramlintide-associated decrease in prokinetic activity will decrease the effectiveness of cisapride (Propulsid) and metoclopramide (Reglan). The antiarrhythmic drug disopyramide (Norpace) increases the risk of serious hypoglycemia, although the mechanism underlying this effect is unknown. Because pramlintide is associated with multiple drug interactions, clinicians prescribing this medication should review a current drug interaction list prior to initiating this drug.

Bile Acid Sequestrants

Bile acid sequestrants are not used commonly in the United States. The sole member of this class that is available in the United States is colesevelam (Welchol). Colesevelam works by binding bile acids in the gastrointestinal tract, thereby accelerating the production of hepatic bile acids. This results in increased incretin levels and decreased hepatic glucose production. One advantage associated with colesevelam is the improvement of lipid values—in fact, this medication was originally developed for lipid control. Reduction in blood glucose is a secondary effect.

Colesevelam is given once daily or twice daily with meals. No other medications, including vitamins, should be taken within 4 hours prior to the drug to allow for its absorption. Women taking colesevelam need to be on a low-fat diet; high fat consumption will decrease the overall effectiveness of colesevelam for glucose reduction.

Side Effects/Adverse Effects

The action of colesevelam decreases absorption of fat-soluble drugs. Women should be advised that contraceptives may lose effectiveness while they are taking colesevelam. Side effects include constipation and fecal impaction, dysphagia, dyspepsia, nausea, headache, hypertension, and fatigue. Hypoglycemia is possible, and women must be advised of its signs, symptoms, and management.

Contraindications

Persons with a history of bowel obstruction or hypertriglyceridemia-induced pancreatitis should not use colesevelam. Colesevelam should be used with caution in persons with elevated triglyceride levels and is contraindicated for individuals whose serum triglyceride levels are higher than 500 mg/dL. This drug is not recommended for persons with gastroparesis or other gastrointestinal motility disorders.

Drug–Drug Interactions

The key factor is to take medications 4 hours distant from colesevelam to assure absorption of the other medications. Use of colesevelam with fat-soluble medications may potentially compromise its effectiveness by blocking absorption. Caution needs to be used to assure adequate coverage with vitamins and contraception—and drugs absorbed from the GI tract or fat soluble.

Combination Therapy with Oral Agents

When monotherapy fails to maintain euglycemia in women with type 2 diabetes, the next step is to combine two or three medications that have different mechanisms of action. This is usually accomplished by adding a second medication. PrandiMet is a single-tablet combination of repaglinide and metformin. Repaglinide is a fast-acting insulin secretagogue, and metformin is an insulin sensitizer. The drug comes in two formulations: as 1 mg/500 mg or 2 mg/500 mg of repaglinide/metformin. One tablet is taken 2–3 times per day with meals. This drug is contraindicated in individuals with renal impairment and in persons who take gemfibrozil (Lopid) or itraconazole (Sporanox). Renal function should be evaluated prior to initiating therapy and assessed annually thereafter if normal at the time of initiation.

Oral Agents Plus Insulin for Treating Type 2 Diabetes

When type 2 diabetes is not well controlled with lifestyle management and oral medication, insulin is indicated. Insulin may be the second agent for an individual on one oral medication. For some individuals, a second oral medication is added, and then, if needed, insulin is added as a third agent. Insulin combined with oral medications improves glycemic control, results in less weight gain than use of insulin alone, and is effective with a relatively simple insulin regimen. The primary oral medication(s) is continued at its regular dose, and the insulin is added.

The combination of oral medications and insulin has a synergistic effect. The therapeutic effect is achieved with lower doses of these medications when they are used in combination than when each is used as monotherapy. The dose of exogenous insulin is also lower than when insulin is used as a monotherapy. Insulin as a second or third agent requires fewer injections and less complicated insulin mixtures than if insulin is administered as a single agent. The simpler regimen results in better acceptance by the individual because of the convenience of a less complicated dose and administration schedule when compared to insulin alone.

The basic process for initiating combination therapy including insulin is to leave the oral medication at the current dose and add regular insulin 10 units at bedtime—usually given by insulin pen. Careful attention to self-monitored blood glucose levels determines the next addition. If needed to control the fasting morning glucose level, NPH insulin may be added at bedtime. If the fasting and evening postprandial levels remain high, 70/30 insulins may be needed before the evening meal. Ultimately, basal insulin may be added. Insulin doses are increased weekly until the desired blood glucose results are achieved and remain consistent. Insulin is increased by 4 units per week if the blood glucose level is 180 mg/dL or higher, and increased 2 units per week if the blood glucose level is 140 mg/dL or higher but less than 180 mg/dL.[38]

Recent studies have suggested that adding insulin to metformin increases mortality from all causes by as much as 44%. Adding insulin to sulfonylureas increases mortality, albeit to a much smaller extent. These studies are new, however, and will need continued validation. Even so, the implication is clear: Caution is required in adding insulin to an oral agent, and metformin in particular warrants caution when used as the oral agent in a combined regimen.[38]

Pharmacotherapy for Diabetic Emergencies

Two emergency conditions can occur when treating persons with diabetes: hypoglycemia and hyperglycemia. Both emergencies result from potentially life-threatening blood glucose levels. Hypoglycemia (insulin shock) and hyperglycemia (sugar shock) are more common in persons with type 1 diabetes, but they may occur in persons with type 2 diabetes as well.

Hypoglycemia

Hypoglycemia is defined as a plasma glucose less than 70 mg/dL. Symptoms vary, but may include a sense of feeling bad, shakiness, palpitations, tachycardia, pallor, clamminess, dilated pupils, nausea and vomiting, and headache. Typically, mental changes occur, including impaired judgment, rage and belligerence, confusion with progression to difficulty speaking, ataxia, and coma. Focal seizures may occur in severe cases. The symptoms of hypoglycemia make it difficult for affected individuals to effectively manage advanced hypoglycemia. For this reason, it is important that everyone with diabetes and everyone who lives with a person who has diabetes be taught the signs, symptoms, and interventions to be implemented at the first signs of hypoglycemia.

Impaired Awareness of Hypoglycemia

Impaired awareness of hypoglycemia is a particularly serious complication of diabetes—most often seen in persons with type 1 diabetes. It is best understood in contrast to the low blood glucose response of persons who do not have diabetes. In such a person, the brain reliably senses hypoglycemia and responds with release of the hormones glucagon and epinephrine. These hormones prompt glucose release from the liver, which stabilizes blood glucose. The affected person notices systemic effects of epinephrine (tremors, jitters, or palpitation), perceives them as hypoglycemia, and seeks a food source. However, in persons with diabetes who have experienced recurrent hypoglycemia, the brain adapts to low glucose levels and does not signal epinephrine release.[60] Hypoglycemia can worsen until loss of consciousness occurs, without the individual being aware of the imbalance.

Impaired awareness of hypoglycemia can also occur when an individual with diabetes is taking beta blockers. The beta blockers prevent the release of epinephrine, so that the palpitations and jitteriness symptoms of hypoglycemia are inhibited. Impaired awareness of hypoglycemia is the most dangerous form of hypoglycemia and can be life threatening if a woman is alone or does not have a responsible person nearby to provide treatment in the event of diminished mental function or loss of consciousness.

Treatment of a Woman with Hypoglycemia

At the first symptom of altered glucose level, a plasma glucose level should be obtained. If the glucose is lower than 70 mg/dL, oral glucose or carbohydrate equal to 15–20 g of glucose should be given orally. Good choices of oral glucose are 3–4 oz of apple, orange, or grape juice; four crackers; one slice of bread; or 5–6 oz of regular soda. There is no advantage to providing more glucose: It is not absorbed faster and may, in fact, lead to overshooting the normal glucose level desired. Fat or protein given with the glucose (e.g., peanut butter crackers) may slow the absorption of glucose. If the woman is taking acarbose (Precose) or another alpha-glucosidase inhibitor, a monosaccharide sugar must be given because acarbose will prevent the breakdown of starch to sugar. Give glucose tablets, honey, or fruit juice to a woman who experiences hypoglycemia and is taking acarbose.

Glucagon

If a person with diabetes is unconscious, an intravenous solution with normal saline should be initiated and 2 milliliters of dextrose 50% should be given. An alternative is 1–2 mg of glucagon given intramuscularly. Glucagon is rarely used outside of a hospital setting but may be used by paramedics in the field if intravenous access cannot be obtained. Care must be taken to carefully observe anyone receiving glucagon because of the danger of severe rebound hyperglycemia. For this reason, glucagon is used almost exclusively in the hospital; if it is used in the field, the recipient is transferred immediately for inpatient evaluation and monitoring.

Hyperglycemia

Hyperglycemia is an elevated blood glucose level. Severe hyperglycemia is also called diabetic ketoacidosis (DKA). Diabetic ketoacidosis is characterized by (1) hyperglycemia (blood glucose > 200 mg/dL) with (2) metabolic acidosis (pH < 7.3) and (3) an elevated anion gap (> 12 mmol/L) and (4) positive urinary ketones. DKA is a medical emergency: It is fatal if left untreated. The symptoms of insulin-deficiency DKA occur secondary to the metabolism of triglycerides and fat when glucose is unavailable. The excess of glucagon stimulates conversion of fatty acids into ketones. Dehydration occurs secondary to glycosuria and osmotic diuresis in the kidney. Symptoms of hyperglycemia include excessive hunger and thirst, cognitive changes, nausea, and vomiting that progress to symptoms of DKA including Kussmaul hyperventilation, stupor, ketoacidosis, and coma.

Management of DKA includes emergency and intensive intervention by specialists in emergency, endocrine, and possibly intensive care medicine. Intravenous fluids are initiated with saline, and regular insulin is given. Plasma glucose and potassium levels are reassessed at least every 30 minutes until the woman is stable.

Hyperosmolar hyperglycemic state is a variation of DKA that does not usually exhibit the same degree of acidosis. This state is seen in the lactic acidosis that may develop in persons taking metformin. Dehydration is more profound than in DKA, and more fluids are needed to correct the condition. Lower doses of insulin are often required due to increased sensitivity to insulin.

Diabetes Insipidus

Diabetes insipidus (DI) is not a disease of glucose metabolism, but rather a disease of water metabolism, characterized by polyuria and polydipsia. These common symptoms result in the shared word *diabetes*, but the name is the only similarity between diabetes mellitus and diabetes insipidus.

Diabetes insipidus can be either congenital or acquired. This disorder presents in four forms: neurogenic DI, nephrogenic DI, dipsogenic DI, and gestational DI. Each form has a different physiology and, therefore, a different method of treatment.

Neurogenic DI (also called central, hypothalamic, pituitary, or neurohypophyseal DI) is caused by a deficiency of vasopressin, the antidiuretic hormone. The deficient production may be the result of damage to the posterior pituitary secondary to trauma or disease, or it can be idiopathic. Sheehan's syndrome—a serious complication of hemorrhage that results in pituitary necrosis—is a cause of neurogenic DI.

Congenital DI is a rare genetic abnormality caused by an X-linked mutation of the antidiuretic hormone V-2 receptors (80% of genetic DI). A mutation of the aquaporin 2 water channel is even rarer (10% of genetic DI). Nephrogenic DI (also called vasopressin-resistant DI) is caused by decreased or absent sensitivity of the kidneys to the effect of vasopressin. More commonly, nephrogenic DI is caused by sickle cell disease and polycystic kidney disease that damage the kidney. Lithium (Lithobid) and amphotericin B (Amphotec) can also cause nephrogenic DI.

Dipsogenic DI occurs secondary to polydipsia, resulting in abnormal intake of fluids including excess water. In this disorder, an abnormality in the brain perception of thirst exists, resulting in excess intake of water/fluids. The pituitary is unable to produce enough vasopressin to counter the excessive water intake, so polyuria results. Dipsogenic DI is seen in some women with anorexia nervosa who develop hypokalemia, because hypokalemia interferes with the action of vasopressin.

Gestagenic or gestational DI is caused by a deficiency of vasopressin that occurs only during pregnancy.[61] Vasopressin may be adversely affected by the enzyme vasopressinase, which is produced in the placenta. Administration of desmopressin acetate (DDAVP) is effective in treating this disorder. A second form of gestational DI is caused by an abnormality in the thirst mechanism. Treatment of a woman with this form of DI with desmopressin can result in water intoxication. The differential diagnosis of the two forms of gestational DI is extremely difficult and requires an endocrinologist who is familiar with the diseases. Both forms of gestational DI resolve spontaneously within 4–6 weeks postpartum.

Treatment of a Woman with Diabetes Insipidus

Treatment of a person with neurogenic DI management is based on the underlying pathology within the brain. If a mass or tumor of the pituitary is the cause, treatment or removal of the mass may resolve the DI. If a mass is not the cause, management includes replacement of the antidiuretic hormone (8-arginine vasopressin), desmopressin acetate.

Desmopressin acetate is a synthetic antidiuretic hormone analogue. It is excreted in the urine, and has a half-life of approximately 1.5–2.5 hours if given orally and approximately 3 hours if given intravenously. This drug is contraindicated in persons who have von Willebrand's disease because the drug stimulates release of the von Willebrand factor. It is also contraindicated in individuals with creatinine clearance less than 50 mL/min because of the increased risk of hyponatremia with compromised excretion. Caution should be used when prescribing DDAVP to persons with hypertension, congestive heart failure, fluid/electrolyte imbalance, or polydipsia. Desmopressin acetate should not be used with polyethylene glycol or sodium phosphate because the combination will increase the risk of seizure from hyponatremia.

In nephrogenic DI, the kidney becomes the center of management. Careful attention to fluid intake and urine output is the primary management approach with this form of DI. A low-sodium diet is prescribed that provides no more than 500–600 mg of sodium per day for adults, because the kidney's inability to concentrate urine results in high serum osmolarity. Potassium-sparing diuretics such as a thiazide, with the possible addition of an amiloride (e.g., hydrochlorothiazide [HydroDIURIL]), are necessary to help regulate sodium levels. For some individuals, a prostaglandin inhibitor is also required to maintain kidney function.

Lithium-induced nephrogenic DI can usually be reversed by discontinuing the lithium. Multiyear use of lithium may result in interstitial fibrosis of the kidney, which is irreversible. Treatment of an individual with lithium-induced DI focuses on measures intended to regulate electrolyte levels, including use of a thiazide diuretic, careful monitoring of sodium intake, and use of nonsteroidal anti-inflammatory drugs. It is not understood how the NSAIDs work in this indication, but they are beneficial to women with this form of DI.

Special Populations in Diabetes Insipidus: Pregnancy and Lactation

Medications typically taken by women with DI are not contraindicated in pregnancy. Desmopressin, in particular, is not associated with spontaneous abortion or fetal anomalies. Its dose may need to be increased in pregnancy, however, due to the placental metabolism of vasopressin. Thiazide diuretics are not contraindicated in pregnancy with DI. Women with neurogenic DI may have difficulty with milk production due to damage to the pituitary axis that resulted in the DI. Prolactin may be decreased, resulting in decreased production of breast milk. Desmopressin is excreted in breast milk, but the amounts are very small and no adverse effects have been reported.

Complementary and Alternative Treatments for Diabetes Mellitus

Dietary supplements, antioxidants, and some herbs have been recommended as effective treatments for lowering blood glucose levels. Some studies have investigated the effect of complementary therapies for preventing diabetes, and some have done so for treating type 2 diabetes. Most of the studies have been too small to generate significant results. Table 18-7 lists the most popular complementary and herbal therapies currently under investigation for treatment of individuals with type 2 diabetes.[62-65]

Table 18-7 Complementary and Alternative Therapies for Type 2 Diabetes

Where Found	Evidence	Safety
Aloe vera	MOA: Fiber may promote glucose uptake Dose: 1 Tb of aloe gel twice daily Two small studies found aloe vera may decrease fasting blood glucose levels and triglyceride levels.	Aloe leaf contraindicated as it is a cathartic Safety unknown
Alpha-lipoic acid	MOA: Antioxidant that protects against cell damage Dose: 800 mg/day in divided doses Some studies have found benefit but others have not. Sources: Liver, spinach, broccoli, and potatoes	Possible hypoglycemic reaction
American ginseng	MOA: Decreases carbohydrate absorption, increases glycogen storage, and stimulates insulin secretion Dose: 3 g before a meal Two small clinical trials found decreases in fasting blood glucose values and HbA_{1c} values.	Insomnia, headache, and anxiety are reported side effects; has many potential drug–drug interactions
Ayurvedic medicine	MOA: *Coccinia indica* appears to be insulin mimetic *Coccinia indica, Gymnema sylvestre,* holy basil, fenugreek, and the herbal formulas Ayush-82 and D-44 have a glucose-lowering effect and deserve further study. Source: Ivy gourd, creeping ivy grown on the Indian subcontinent	Safety unknown
Chinese herbal medicines	MOA: Unknown Dose: Not specified Holy basil leaves, *Xianzhen Pian, Qidan Tongmai,* traditional Chinese formulae, *Huoxue Jiangtang Pingzhi,* and *Inolter*: Have significant hypoglycemic response *Bushen Jiangtang Tang,* composite *Trichosanthis, Jiangtang Kang, Ketang Ling, Shenqi Jiangtang Yin, Xiaoke Tang,* and *Yishen Huoxue Tiaogan*: Found to be significantly better than hypoglycemic drugs.	No adverse effects reported in studies conducted
Chromium picolinate	MOA: Insulin-sensitizing effect or direct effect on insulin receptor Dose: 200 mcg/day capsule or tablet Decreased HbA_{1c} after 4 months in one study. FDA has authorized health claim that chromium picolinate may decrease insulin resistance but ADA states there is inconclusive evidence for efficacy. Source: Trace mineral found in many foods in very small amounts	Safe in low doses; high doses can cause renal failure
Cinnamon (*Cinnamomum cassia*)	MOA: Increases insulin sensitivity Dose: 1–6 g/day in divided doses Improved glucose control in one study of individuals already on sulfonylureas. Other studies have found no benefit.	Cinnamon has coumarin component; it should be taken with caution by individuals on anticoagulants
Mulberry tree (*Morus albal)*	MOA: Suppresses postprandial glucose surge Dose: *Folium moiri* extract, 5–45 mcg/mL titrated per individual Several small studies confirm effectiveness in humans; many confirm effectiveness in animals.	None reported
Nopal (*Opuntia strepacantha*)	MOA: Decreases glucose absorption and enhances insulin delivery Dose: 100–500 g daily of broiled stems A few small studies report decreases in blood glucose values following a meal with prickly pear. Additive improvement in postprandial blood glucose occurs when it is added to sulfonylureas. Sources: Member of cactus family, common food in Hispanic diets; all parts of cactus can be eaten	Diarrhea is a reported side effect
Omega-3 fatty acids	MOA: Mitigates cardiovascular disorders, decreases inflammation, and lowers triglyceride levels; lowers triglycerides but has no effect on blood glucose levels, total cholesterol, fasting blood sugars, or HbA_{1c} Some studies found increase in LDL cholesterol. Sources: Fish, fish oil, vegetable oils, walnuts, and wheat germ	Safe in moderate doses. Fish oil supplements should be used with caution, as mercury levels could be high. High doses interfere with warfarin (Coumadin) and some antihypertensive medications.
Polyphenols	MOA: Phenols may protect against cardiovascular disease and have a beneficial effect on insulin and glucose control. A few clinical trials have not found efficacy, but those studies have been too small to make definitive conclusions. Sources: Green tea and dark chocolate	Safe in moderate amounts. Green tea has caffeine, which can cause insomnia or anxiety, and small amounts of vitamin K, which could potentiate the effect of warfarin.
Sweet potato (*Ipomoea batatas*)	MOA: Decreases blood glucose by unknown action Dose: 4 g/day of the extract calapo taken from the white sweet potato Several small studies demonstrated decrease blood glucose.	Contraindicated for individuals with hypersensitivity

Abbreviations: MOA = mechanism of action.

Sources: Data from *Ayurvedic interventions for diabetes mellitus: a systematic review.* Summary, Evidence Report/Technology Assessment, no. 41. AHRQ Publication No. 01-E039. Rockville, MD: Agency for Healthcare Research and Quality; June 2001. http://www.ahrq.gov/clinic/epcsums/ayurvsum.htm. Accessed June 21, 2009[62]; Giel P, Shane-McWhorter L. Dietary supplements in the management of diabetes: potential risks and benefits. *J Am Diet Assoc.* 2008;108:S59-S65[63]; Liu JP, Zhang M, Wang W, Grimsgaard S. Chinese herbal medicines for type 2 diabetes mellitus. *Cochrane Database Syst Rev.* 2002;3:CD003642. doi:10.1002/14651858.CD003642.pub2[64]; Wang A, Wang J, Chan P. Treating type 2 diabetes mellitus with traditional Chinese and Indian medicinal herbs. *Evid Based Complement Altern Med.* 2013;345994. http://www.hindawi.com/journals/ecam/2013/343594/. Accessed October 21, 2014.[65]

Special Populations

Adolescents

The incidence of diabetes is rising dramatically in adolescents, and diabetes and adolescence are an especially difficult combination. The dramatic physiologic and psychological changes that are normal in adolescence compound the difficulty in maintaining normal glucose levels in adolescents with diabetes. The social pressures and emotional changes that characterize adolescence have resulted in an increase in the incidence of eating disorders in recent years. A new complication for young persons with diabetes is *diabulemia*, for lack of a better term.[66] Diabulemia refers to individuals, predominantly adolescents, who have both type 1 diabetes and an eating disorder. Individuals with diabulemia use bulimia and/or omit insulin to control weight. The combination of inadequate food and insufficient insulin results in significantly increased glucose levels, poor absorption of food, and subsequent weight loss and hyperglycemia. Diabetic ketoacidosis is a significant risk in this population and may be the first indication that the adolescent is using bulimia or withholding insulin for weight control purposes.

Pregnancy and Lactation

Women who have HbA_{1c} levels more than 1% above normal levels for nondiabetic women in the first 6–8 weeks of pregnancy are at increased risk for fetal malformations.[1] Achieving good glycemic control with adequate HbA_{1c} levels prior to conception significantly reduces this risk of teratogenesis. A normal HbA_{1c} is less than 5.7%, so an optimal preconception level for a woman with diabetes is less than 6.7%.

Insulin is safe for use by women during pregnancy and lactation and may be continued. Oral hypoglycemic agents such as metformin (Glucophage), glyburide, and acarbose (Precose) are also safe for use during pregnancy[67] and are beginning to be prescribed more often by teams who specialize in treating women with diabetes during pregnancy. First-generation sulfonylurea drugs should not be used in this population, however, because they cross the placenta and could induce fetal hyperinsulinemia.[68] Most of the other oral agents have not been sufficiently studied for use during pregnancy, although the common hypoglycemic agents are considered compatible with breastfeeding. Because none of the oral agents has been specifically approved for use during pregnancy by the FDA, insulin is the agent most often used to treat diabetes in women who are pregnant.

Elderly

Polypharmacy and drug–drug interactions are more frequent in the elderly. In addition, exaggerated side effects to medications and drug–disease interactions are more common in the elderly than in younger populations. Chlorpropamide (Diabinese) should not be used in elderly women because it has a prolonged half-life that is more pronounced in older adults and leads to increased risk for hypoglycemia. Metformin (Glucophage) needs to be used with caution by older adults with impaired renal function because of its associated risk of lactic acidosis. Target HbA_{1c} values are modified in the older adult population based on concomitant morbidities, quality of life, and life expectancy.

Conclusion

Diabetes has the unique distinction of being an ancient disease known since the beginning of recorded history, yet—despite decades of research and knowledge about its prevention and treatment—a disease that is increasingly afflicting persons in all age groups today. Primary care providers in the twenty-first century must be well versed in all aspects of this disease and alert to its consequences until the epidemic of obesity is resolved.

Resources

Organization	Description	Website
Diabetes Education Online	Diabetes teaching center at the University of California San Francisco; multiple web pages on management of insulin, descriptions of medications, and lists of additional online resources	http://dtc.ucsf.edu
American Diabetes Association	This site has clinical practice recommendations and a slide library, and it also lists studies currently under way	http://professional.diabetes.org/?loc=rp-slabnav
Joslin Diabetes Center	Clinical guidelines for pharmacologic management of adults with type 2 diabetes; updated September 12, 2014	www.joslin.org/docs/09_12_2014_Pharma_Guideline_emb_final.pdf
National Diabetes Education Initiative	Clinical guidelines, literature, product indications, professional resources, and a slide library	www.ndei.org

References

1. American Diabetes Association. Standards of medical care in diabetes—2014. *Diab Care.* 2014;37(suppl 1): S14-S80.
2. Centers for Disease Control and Prevention. *National diabetes statistics report, 2014.* http://www.cdc.gov/diabetes/data/statistics/2014StatisticsReport.html. Accessed January 23, 2014.
3. Bullard KM, Saydah SH, Imperatore G, et al. Secular changes in U.S. prediabetes prevalence defined by hemoglobin A(1c) and fasting plasma glucose: National Health and Nutrition Examination Surveys, 1999–2010. *Diab Care.* 2013;36(8): 2286-2293.
4. Centers for Disease Control and Prevention, National Center for Health Statistics, Division of Health Interview Statistics. Data from the National Health Interview Survey. Data computed by the Centers for Disease Control and Prevention, National Center for Chronic Disease Prevention and Health Promotion, Division of Diabetes Translation. http://www.cdc.gov/diabetes/statistics/prevalence_national.htm. Accessed June 14, 2014.
5. Bellamy L, Casas JP, Hingorani AD, Williams D. Type 2 diabetes mellitus after gestational diabetes: a systematic review and meta-analysis. *Lancet.* 2009;373(9677): 1773-1779.
6. Diabetes Control and Complications Trial Research Group. The effect of intensive treatment of diabetes on the development and progression of long-term complications in insulin-dependent diabetes mellitus. *N Engl J Med.* 1993;329(14):977-986.
7. Diabetes Control and Complications Trial Research Group. The Diabetes Control and Complications Trial/Epidemiology of Diabetes Interventions and Complications study at 30 years: summary and future directions. *Diab Care.* 2014;37(1):44-49.
8. Rajendran P, Rengarajan T, Thangavel J, et al. The vascular endothelium and human diseases. *Int J Biol Sci.* 2013;9(10):1057-1069.
9. Unger J. Management of type I diabetes. *Primary Care Clin Office Pract.* 2007;34:791-808.
10. Unger RH. Reinventing type 2 diabetes: pathogenesis, treatment, and prevention. *JAMA.* 2008;299(10): 1185-1187.
11. Skerrett PJ, Willett WC. Essentials of healthy eating: a guide. *J Midwifery Womens Health.* 2010;55(6); 492-501.
12. D'Alessio D. The role of dysregulated glucagon secretion in type 2 diabetes. *Diab Obes Metab.* 2011; 13(suppl 1):126-132.
13. Garber AJ, Handelsman Y, Einhorn D, et al. Diagnosis and management of prediabetes in the continuum of hyperglycemia: when do the risks of diabetes begin? A consensus statement from the American College of Endocrinology and the American Association of Clinical Endocrinologists. *Endocr Pract.* 2008;14(7): 933-946.
14. Action to Control Cardiovascular Risk in Diabetes Study Group (ACCORD). Long-term effects of intensive glucose lowering on cardiovascular outcomes. *N Engl J Med.* 2011;364:818-828.
15. Kassi E, Pervanidou P, Kaltsas G, Chrousos G. Metabolic syndrome: definitions and controversies. *BMC Med.* 2011;9:48.
16. Reaven GM. Relationships among insulin resistance, type 2 diabetes, essential hypertension, and cardiovascular disease: similarities and differences. *J Clin Hyperten.* 2011;13(4):238-243.
17. Laakso M, Kuusisto J. Insulin resistance and hyperglycaemia in cardiovascular disease development. *Nature Rev Endocrin.* 2014;10(5):293-302.
18. Laakso M. Cardiovascular disease in type 2 diabetes: from population to man to mechanisms. *Diab Care.* 2010;33(2):442-449.
19. AACE Diabetes Mellitus Clinical Practice Guidelines Task Force. Comprehensive diabetes management algorithm. *Endocrine Pract.* 2013;19(2):327-335.
20. AACE Diabetes Mellitus Clinical Practice Guidelines Task Force. American Association of Clinical Endocrinologists medical guidelines for clinical practice for developing a diabetes mellitus comprehensive care plan. *Endocrine Pract.* 2011;17(suppl 2):1-53.
21. Stratton IM, Adler AI, Neil HA, et al. Association of glycaemia with macrovascular and microvascular complications of type 2 diabetes (UKPDS 35): prospective observational study. *BMJ.* 2000;321:405-412.
22. Rodbard HW, Jellinger PS, Davidson JA, et al. Statement by an American Association of Clinical Endocrinologists/American College of Endocrinology consensus panel on type 2 diabetes mellitus: an algorithm for glycemic control. *Endocrine Pract.* 2009; 15(6):540-559.
23. Allen FW, Schwartzman E, Baker WL, Coleman CI, Phung OJ. Cinnamon use in type 2 diabetes: an updated systematic review and meta-analysis. *Ann Fam Med.* 2013;11(5):452-459.

24. Maruther NM, Ma Y, Delahanty LM, et al. Diabetes Prevention Program Research Group: early response to preventive strategies in the Diabetes Prevention Program. *J Gen Intern Med.* 2013;28(12):1629-1636.
25. Stone NJ, Robinson J, Lichtenstein A, et al. 2013 ACC/AHA guideline on the treatment of blood cholesterol to reduce atherosclerotic cardiovascular risk in adults: a report of the American College of Cardiology/American Heart Association Task Force on Practice Guidelines. *J Am Coll Cardiol.* 2014;63 (25 pt B):2889-2934.
26. Briscoe VJ, Davis SN. Hypoglycemia in type 1 and type 2 diabetes: physiology, pathophysiology, and management. *Clin Diab.* 2006;24(1):115-121.
27. Bergenstal RM, Tamborlane WV, Ahmann A, et al. Effectiveness of sensor-augmented insulin-pump therapy in type 1 diabetes. *N Engl J Med.* 2010; 363: 311-320.
28. Holstein A, Stege H, Kovacs P. Lipoatrophy associated with the use of insulin analogues: a new case associated with the use of insulin glargine and review of the literature. *Expert Opin Drug Saf.* 2010;9(2):225-231.
29. Felig P. Landmark perspective: protamine insulin. Hagedorn's pioneering contribution to drug delivery in the management of diabetes. *JAMA.* 1984;51: 393-396.
30. Home P, Bartley P, Russell-Jones D, et al. Insulin detemir offers improved glycemic control compared with NPH insulin in people with type 1 diabetes: a randomized clinical trial. *Diab Care.* 2004;27:1081-1087.
31. Irons BK, Minze MG. Drug treatment for type 2 diabetes mellitus in patients for whom metformin is contraindicated. *Diab Metab Syndr Obes.* 2014; 18(7): 15-24.
32. Peter R, Dunseath G, Luzio SD, Owens DR. Estimates of the relative and absolute diurnal contributions of fasting and post-prandial plasma glucose over a range of hyperglycaemia in type 2 diabetes. *Diab Metab.* 2013;39(4):337-342.
33. American Diabetes Association, European Association for the Study of Diabetes. Management of hyperglycemia in type 2 diabetes: a patient-centered approach: position statement of the American Diabetes Association (ADA) and the European Association for the Study of Diabetes (EASD). *Diab Care.* 2012;35(6):1364-1379.
34. ADVANCE Collaborative Group. Intensive blood glucose control and vascular outcomes in patients with type 2 diabetes. *N Engl J Med.* 2008;358:2540-2572.
35. Bennett WL, Wilson LM, Bolen S, et al. Oral diabetes medications for adults with type 2 diabetes: an update. Comparative Effectiveness Review No. 27. Agency for Healthcare Research and Quality publication No. 11-EHCO38-EF. March 2011. http://www.ncbi.nlm.nih.gov/books/NBK55754/. Accessed October 21, 2014.
36. Kahn SE, Haffner SM, Heise MA, et al. ADOPT Study Group: glycemic durability of rosiglitazone, metformin, or glyburide monotherapy (erratum, *N Engl J Med.* 2007;356:1387-1388). *N Engl J Med.* 2006;355:2427-2443.
37. Lyons MR, Peterson LR, McGill JB, et al. Impact of sex on the heart's metabolic and functional responses to diabetic therapies. *Am J Physiol Hearth Circ Physiol.* 2013;305(1):HI584-H1591.
38. Roumie CL, Greevy RA, Grijalva CG, et al. Association between intensification of metformin treatment with insulin vs sulfonylureas and cardiovascular events and all-cause mortality among patients with diabetes. *JAMA.* 2014;311:2288-2296.
39. Black C, Donnelly P, McIntyre L, Royale PL, Shepherd JP, Thomas S. Meglitinide analogues for type 2 diabetes mellitus. *Cochrane Database Syst Rev.* 2007;2: CD004654. doi:10.1002/14651858.CD004654.pub2.
40. Alexander GC, Schgal JL, Moloney RM, Stafford RS. National trends in treatment of type 2 diabetes mellitus, 1994-2007. *Arch Intern Med.* 2008;168(19): 2088-2094.
41. DeFronzo RA, Goodman AM. Efficacy of metformin in patients with non-insulin dependent diabetes mellitus: the Multicenter Metformin Study Group. *N. Engl J Med.* 1995;333:541-549.
42. Hermann LS, Schersten B, Bitzén PO, Kjellström T, Lindgärde F, Melander A. Therapeutic comparison of metformin and sulfonylurea, alone and in various combinations: a double-blind controlled study. *Diab Care.* 1994;17:1100-1109.
43. Saenz A, Fernandez-Esteban I, Mataiz A, Ausejo M, Roque M, Moher D. Metformin monotherapy for type 2 diabetes mellitus. *Cochrane Database Syst Rev.* 2005;3:CD002966. doi:10.1002/14651858.CD002966.pub3.
44. Holman RR, Paul SK, Bethel MA, Matthews DR, Neil HA. 10-year follow-up of intensive glucose control in type 2 diabetes. *N Engl J Med.* 2008;359: 1577-1589.
45. Schramm TK, Gialason GH, Vaag A, et al. Mortality and cardiovascular risk associated with different

insulin secretagogues compared with metformin in type 2 diabetes, with or without a previous myocardial infarction: a nationwide study. *Euro Heart J.* 2011;32:1900-1908.

46. Harrington RA, Nathan MS, Beattie P. Oral agents for the treatment of type 2 diabetes: pharmacology, toxicity, and treatment. *Ann Emerg Med.* 2001;38: 68-78.
47. Salpeter S, Greyber E, Pasternak G, Salpeter E. Risk of fatal and nonfatal lactic acidosis with metformin use in type 2 diabetes mellitus. *Cochrane Database Syst Rev.* 2010;4:CD002967.doi:10.1002/14651858. CD002967.pub4.
48. Fonseca V, Rosenstock J, Patwardhan R, Salzman A. Effect of metformin and rosiglitazone combination therapy in patients with type 2 diabetes mellitus: a randomized controlled trial. *JAMA.* 2000;283: 1695-1702.
49. St. John Sutton M, Rendell M, Dandona P, et al. A comparison of the effects of rosiglitazone and glyburide on cardiovascular function and glycemic control in patients with type 2 diabetes. *Diab Care.* 2002;25:2058-2064.
50. Nissen SE, Wolski K. Effect of rosiglitazone on the risk of myocardial infarction and death from cardiovascular causes. *N Engl J Med.* 2007;356:2457-2471.
51. Scheen AJ. Pharmacokinetic interactions with thiazolidinediones. *Clin Pharmacokinet.* 2007;46(1): 1-12.
52. Van de Laar FA, Lucassen PL, Akkermans RP, Van de Lisdonk EH, De Grauw WJ. Alpha-glucosidase inhibitors for people with impaired glucose tolerance or impaired fasting blood glucose. *Cochrane Database Syst Rev.* 2006;4:CD005061. doi:10.1002/14651858. CD005061.pub2.
53. Knop FK, Vilsbøll T, Holst JJ. Incretin-based therapy of type 2 diabetes mellitus. *Curr Protein Pept Sci.* 2009;10(1):46-55.
54. Conlon JM, Patterson S, Flatt PR. Major contributions of comparative endocrinology to the development and exploitation of the incretin concept. *J Exp Zoolog A Comp Exp Biol.* 2006;305(9):781-786.
55. Triplitt C, Chiquette E. Exenatide: from the Gila monster to the pharmacy. *J Am Pharm Assoc. (2003)* 2006;46(1):44-52.
56. Cvetković RS, Plosker GL. Exenatide: a review of its use in patients with type 2 diabetes mellitus (as an adjunct to metformin and/or a sulfonylurea). *Drugs.* 2007;67(6):935-954.
57. Li L, Shen J, Bala MM, et al. Incretin treatment and risk of pancreatitis in patients with type 2 diabetes mellitus: systematic review and meta-analysis of randomized and non-randomised studies. *BMJ.* 2014;348:g2366.
58. Chao EC. SGLT-2 inhibitors: a new mechanism for glycemic control. *Clin Diab.* 2014;32(1):4-11.
59. Stenlöf K, Cefalu WT, Kim KA, et al. Efficacy and safety of canagliflozin monotherapy in subjects with type 2 diabetes mellitus inadequately controlled with diet and exercise. *Diab Obes Metab.* 2013;15: 372-382.
60. Graveling AJ, Frier BM. Impaired awareness of hypoglycaemia: a review. *Diab Metab.* 2010;36 (suppl 3): S64-S74.
61. Aleksandrov N, Audibert F, Bedard MJ, Mahone M, Goffinet F, Kadoch IJ. Gestational diabetes insipidus: a review of an underdiagnosed condition. *J Obstet Gynecol Can.* 2010;32(3):225-231.
62. *Ayurvedic interventions for diabetes mellitus: a systematic review.* Summary, Evidence Report/Technology Assessment, no. 41. AHRQ Publication No. 01-E039. Rockville, MD: Agency for Healthcare Research and Quality; June 2001. http://www.ahrq.gov/clinic/epcsums/ayurvsum.htm. Accessed June 21, 2009.
63. Giel P, Shane-McWhorter L. Dietary supplements in the management of diabetes: potential risks and benefits. *J Am Diet Assoc.* 2008;108:S59-S65.
64. Liu JP, Zhang M, Wang W, Grimsgaard S. Chinese herbal medicines for type 2 diabetes mellitus. *Cochrane Database Syst Rev.* 2002;3:CD003642. doi: 10.1002/14651858.CD003642.pub2.
65. Wang A, Wang J, Chan P. Treating type 2 diabetes mellitus with traditional Chinese and Indian medicinal herbs. *Evid Based Complement Altern Med.* 2013;345994. http://www.hindawi.com/journals/ecam/2013/343594/. Accessed October 21, 2014.
66. Colton P, Rodin G, Bergenstal R, Parkin C. Eating disorders and diabetes: introduction and overview. *Diab Spectrum.* 2009;22(3):138-142.
67. Nicholson WK, Wilson LM, Witkop CT, et al. Therapeutic management, delivery, and postpartum risk assessment and screening in gestational diabetes. *Evid Rep Technol Assess (Full Rep).* No. 162. Report No. 08-E004. 2008;1-96. http://www.ncbi.nlm.nih.gov/books/NBK27011/. Accessed October 21, 2014.
68. Garcia-Bournissen F, Feig DS, Koren G. Maternal–fetal transport of hypoglycaemic drugs. *Clin Pharmacokinet.* 2003;42:303-313.

19 Thyroid Disorders

Michael W. Neville

Chapter Glossary

Goitrogen Any substance that interferes with thyroid function and causes goiter. The effect may be hypothyroidism or hyperthyroidism.

Graves' disease Hyperthyroidism characterized by autoimmune antibodies that are developed against the TSH receptor.

Hashimoto's disease Hypothyroidism secondary to chronic autoimmune disease.

Thyroglobulin Protein from which T_3 and T_4 are made within the thyroid gland.

Thyroid-stimulating hormone (TSH) Hormone produced and released from the anterior pituitary. This agent initiates production and release of T_3 and T_4.

Thyrotropin-releasing hormone (TRH) Hormone from the hypothalamus that stimulates production of thyroid-stimulating hormone.

Thyroxine (T_4) Prohormone composed of four atoms that is produced exclusively in the thyroid.

Thyroxine-binding globulin (TBG) Globulin that binds to T_3 and T_4 to enable their transfer through circulation.

Triiodothyronine (T_3) Active thyroid hormone composed of three iodine atoms that is produced in the thyroid and extrathyroidal tissue.

Introduction

Thyroid dysfunction is one of the most common endocrine disorders experienced by women.[1] Prescriptions for thyroid medication rank second in number after prescriptions for contraception for nonpregnant women of childbearing age in the United States.[2] The recognition and treatment of thyroid diseases are critical because thyroid hormones affect myriad body processes, including cardiovascular function, growth, and the intermediary metabolism of carbohydrates, fats, and proteins.

Physiology of Thyroid Function

The thyroid gland weighs approximately 10 to 20 grams in normal adults, making it one of the largest endocrine glands in the human body. This gland is located in the neck inferior to the thyroid cartilage and at approximately the same level as the cricoid cartilage (Figure 19-1).

The thyroid contains the only cells in the body that can absorb iodine. Iodine is an essential component of the thyroid hormones. The amount of iodine available for thyroid hormone synthesis depends on iodine obtained from one's diet because this mineral is not stored in the body. The recommended daily allowances of iodine are 65 mcg per day for children younger than 8 years, 73 mcg per day for those 9 to 13 years of age, and 95 mcg per day for all other age groups. Pregnant and lactating women should receive 160 mcg and 209 mcg per day, respectively.[3]

Thyroid hormones are formed from a large glycoprotein, **thyroglobulin**, which is produced by thyroid cells. Iodine is transported into the thyroid cells and oxidized by peroxidase enzymes to monoiodotyrosine (MIT) and diiodotyrosine (DIT). Tetraiodothyronine (T_4) is composed of two DIT molecules, whereas **triiodothyronine (T_3)** is made

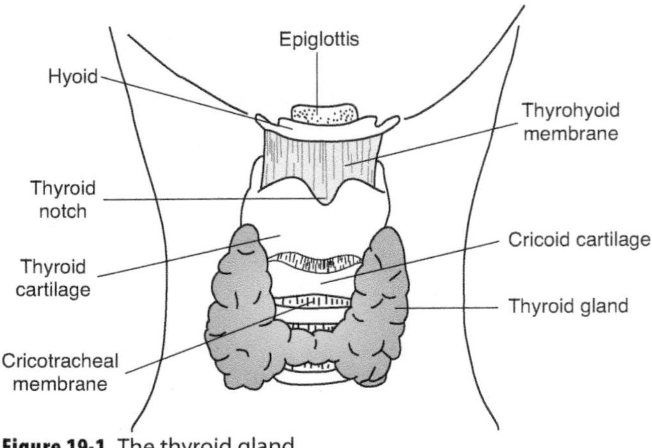

Figure 19-1 The thyroid gland.

of one MIT and one DIT.[4] T_3 is more potent than T_4 and it is the active thyroid hormone in tissue. T_4 is considered a prohormone for T_3. T_4 is converted to T_3 in cells by the deiodinase enzymes. Figure 19-2 depicts production of the two thyroid hormones within the thyroid gland.

The thyroid gland releases both T_3 and T_4 into the circulation, but the ratio of T_4 to T_3 is approximately 20 to 1. Once in the general circulation, T_3 and T_4 are bound to either **thyroxine-binding globulin (TBG)**, albumin, or transthyretin.[4] The majority of T_4 and T_3 is protein bound and not readily available for metabolism or excretion, a factor that accounts for their long half-lives in the circulation; only 0.03% and 0.3% of T_4 and T_3, respectively, are not bound to protein transporters.[4] Because a relatively small free fraction of thyroid hormone exerts metabolic effects, situations that alter thyroid hormone protein binding, such as use of drugs, can have a clinically significant effect on thyroid function. For example, estrogens and methadone increase thyroxine–TBG binding; whereas glucocorticoids and salicylates decrease thyroxine–TBG binding. Diseases can also influence protein binding. For example, liver disease increases thyroxine–TBG binding, while many acute/chronic illness can decrease thyroxine–TBG binding. Notably, pregnant women produce more TBG and thus pregnancy tends to increase thyroxine–TBG binding.[5,6]

Biosynthesis of thyroid hormones is tightly regulated in the body of a person with a normally functioning thyroid gland. The body produces 80–100 mcg of T_4 and 30–40 mcg of T_3 per day; metabolism of T_4 within peripheral tissues accounts for 80% of T_3 in the circulation.[5] The hypothalamus, pituitary, and thyroid glands interact with one another through positive and negative feedback mechanisms to maintain the plasma levels of the thyroid hormones (Figure 19-3). In brief, as the plasma level of thyroid hormones drops, the hypothalamus releases **thyrotropin-releasing hormone (TRH)**. As TRH concentrations increase within the hypothalamic–pituitary portal circulation, they eventually stimulate the release of **thyroid-stimulating hormone (TSH)** from the anterior pituitary.[5] In response to the increased TSH plasma concentration, the thyroid gland initiates production and release of T_3 and T_4. Increasing plasma concentrations of T_3 and T_4 eventually suppress the production of TRH and TSH through a classic negative feedback mechanism. Somatostatin, dopamine, and retinoids can also inhibit the effects of TRH.[5]

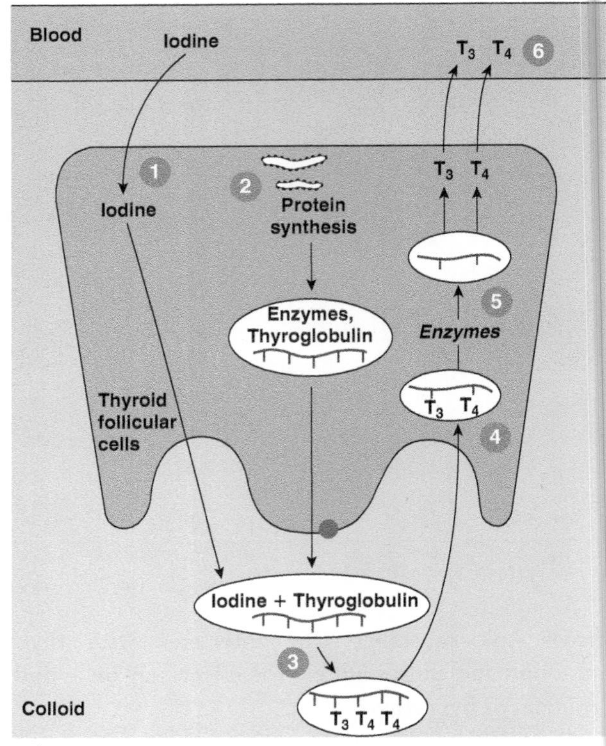

(1) Iodine is co-transported into the cell with Na^+ and transported into colloid.
(2) Follicular cell synthesizes enzymes and thyroglobulin.
(3) Enzymes add iodine to thyroglobulin to make T_3 and T_4.
(4) Thyroglobulin is taken back into the cell.
(5) Intracellular enzymes separate T_3 and T_4 from the protein.
(6) Free T_3 and T_4 enter the circulation.

Figure 19-2 Thyroid hormone synthesis and physiology.

Two important aspects of the finely tuned autoregulation of thyroid hormone production may affect pharmacologic management of persons with thyroid disorders. First is the Wolff-Chaikoff effect, which protects this part of the endocrine system from responding to large variations in dietary iodine intake.[6] Sudden large concentrations of iodine in plasma have an inhibitory effect on thyroid uptake of iodine, which decreases hormone biosynthesis, resulting in a hypothyroid effect. The sections on treatment of hypothyroidism and hyperthyroidism found later in this chapter discuss the Wolff-Chaikoff effect in clinical practice. Second, the thyroid gland has a reservoir of hormone that continues to be released if a sudden deficit of iodine in the diet occurs. This reservoir must also be accounted for when individuals are treated with drugs that suppress thyroid hormone production.

Thyroid Disease

Specific disorders of thyroid regulation usually result in a state of either hypothyroidism or hyperthyroidism. Hypothyroidism occurs in approximately 1% to 2% in women—an incidence 10 times higher than that observed in men.[7] The reason for the gender disparity is not well understood,

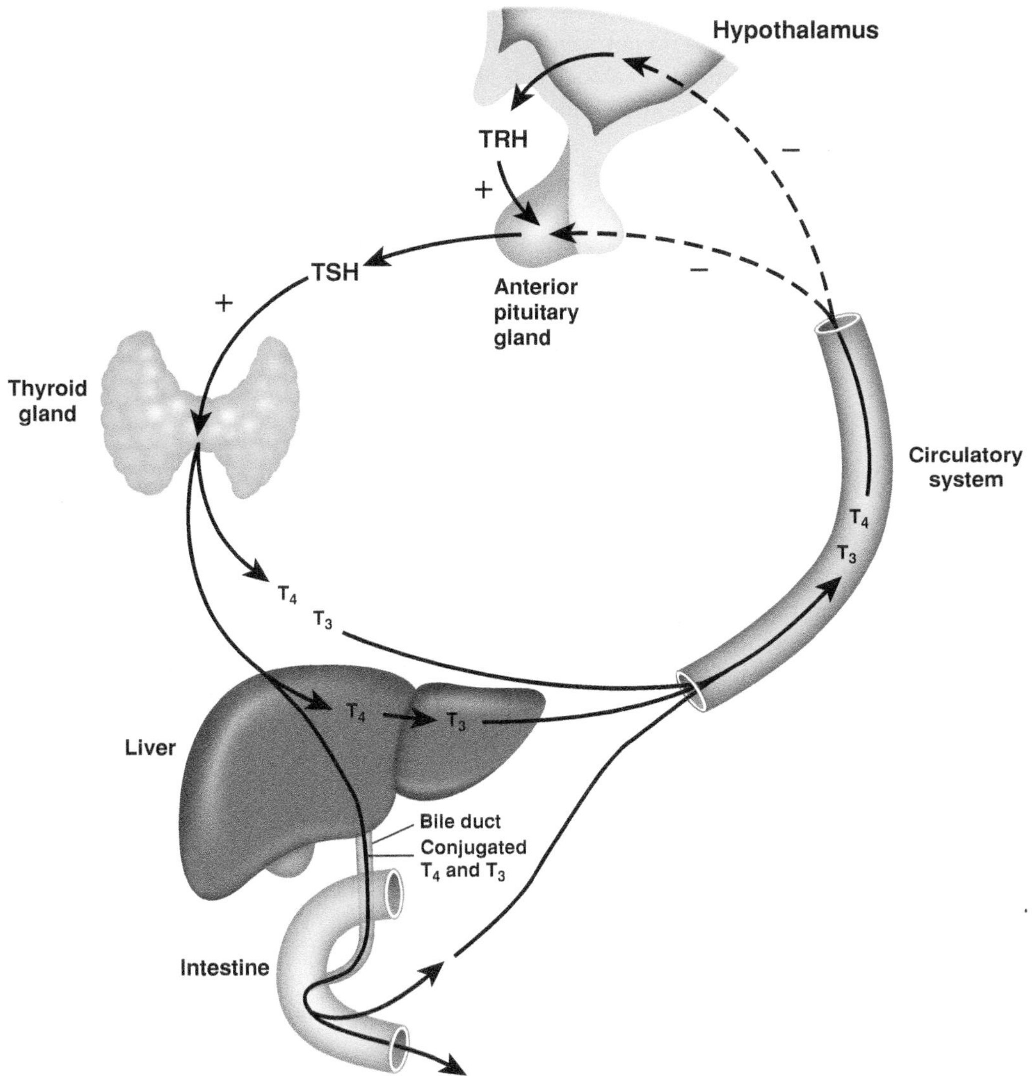

Thyrotropin-releasing hormone (TRH) increases the secretion of thyrotropin (TSH), which stimulates the synthesis and secretion of triiodothyronine (T_3) and thyroxine (T_4) by the thyroid gland. T_3 and T_4 inhibit the secretion of TSH, both directly and indirectly, by suppressing the release of TRH. T_4 is converted to T_3 in the liver and many other tissues by the action of T_4 monodeiodinases. Some T_4 and T_3 is conjugated with glucuronide and sulfate in the liver, excreted in the bile, and partially hydrolyzed in the intestine. Some T_4 and T_3 formed in the intestine may be reabsorbed. Drug interactions may occur at any of these sites.

+ = stimulatory pathway; − = inhibitory pathway.

Figure 19-3 Regulation of thyroid hormone production and pathways of thyroid hormone metabolism.

but is likely associated with the interaction between thyroid hormones and estrogen or progesterone.[8–10] Thyroid hormones are critical for generation of progesterone and estrogen; consequently, multiple adverse reproductive effects are associated with thyroid dysfunction. For example, increased levels of TRH—a feature of hypothyroidism—result in increased prolactin stimulation, which interferes with gonadotropin-releasing hormone (GnRH) production, thereby reducing fertility. Women who have polycystic ovary syndrome (PCOS) are more likely to have thyroiditis than are women who do not have PCOS.[10] Untreated thyroid disease in pregnancy is associated with an increased risk for placental abruption, miscarriage, growth restriction, and hypertensive disorders.[11]

The term *goiter* is used to define an enlarged thyroid gland. With a *diffuse goiter*, the gland is uniformly enlarged. A *nodular goiter* occurs when one or more nodules develop within the otherwise normal gland. Goiters may or may not make thyroid hormone; thus they can be associated with hypothyroidism, a euthyroid state, hyperthyroidism, thyroiditis, or rarely with thyroid cancer. Risk factors for developing a goiter include iodine deficiency, smoking, and pregnancy in areas of iodine deficiency. Conversely, alcohol use and oral contraceptives are associated with a decreased risk for developing a goiter.[12,13]

Any substance that alters thyroid function and causes a goiter is called a **goitrogen**. Several foods have been implicated in the etiology of this condition in regions where goiters are endemic. For example, thiocyanate, which is present in cassava, can cause hypothyroidism and resultant goiter. Other foods that are potential goitrogens include Brussels sprouts, soy products, rutabaga, turnips, radishes, cauliflower, cabbage, kale, and millet.[14] Some experts have suggested that these foods are not goitrogens when cooked because cooking destroys the goitrogenic compound.

Hypothyroidism

Hypothyroidism is characterized by a deficiency of T_3 and T_4 hormones. This disease may result from a primary or secondary cause. Chronic autoimmune thyroiditis, also called **Hashimoto's disease**, is the most common cause of primary hypothyroidism in the United States.[15] Other autoimmune causes include painless postpartum thyroiditis, painless sporadic thyroiditis, and painless subacute thyroiditis. In addition, surgical thyroid removal, radioiodine thyroid gland ablation, and thyroid hormone deficiency from iodine deficiency or drug-induced interference with thyroid function can cause primary hypothyroidism. For most individuals with primary hypothyroidism, the disorder is a chronic, lifelong condition that requires daily replacement of the hormone.

Secondary hypothyroidism results from pituitary disease (deficiency of TSH) or hypothalamic disease (deficiency of TRH). Secondary hypothyroidism is not a focus of this chapter.

The hallmark clinical features of hypothyroidism include fatigue, weight gain, hoarseness, hyperlipidemia, constipation, and bradycardia. Hypothyroidism is a commonly a comorbid condition in individuals who have other disorders. It is also associated with an increased risk of cardiovascular disease. Indeed, recent research suggests that even those with subclinical disease, or a TSH level within the upper limit of the reference range, may be at a greater risk for cardiovascular disease than individuals with lower TSH levels.[16]

Subclinical Hypothyroidism

Thyroid dysfunction may also be asymptomatic or subclinical. Subclinical disease usually is defined as an abnormally low or high TSH level in a person with normal circulating thyroid hormone levels.[11] The etiologies of subclinical hypothyroidism are the same as the causes of hypothyroidism. Women older than 65 years have the highest risk for subclinical disease.[16]

Hyperthyroidism

Hyperthyroidism generally results from excess concentrations of T_3 and T_4, with the most common forms being **Graves' disease** and toxic multinodular goiter.[10,17] Graves' disease occurs when autoimmune antibodies develop against the TSH receptor, which becomes chronically stimulated such that excessive thyroid hormone is produced. The signs and symptoms of hyperthyroidism include, but are not limited to, palpitations, weight loss, menstrual irregularities, and ophthalmopathy. Untreated hyperthyroidism is associated with significant morbidity and mortality. Atrial fibrillation is one of the most concerning consequences of this form of thyroid disease, as it can lead to cardiac failure.

Pharmacologic Treatment of Hypothyroidism

The goals of therapy when treating a woman with hypothyroidism are to restore normal tissue concentrations of thyroid hormones, reverse biochemical abnormalities of hypothyroidism, and provide relief of symptoms.[18]

Treatment also is designed to prevent neurologic deficits when the condition occurs in newborns and children.[9]

Levothyroxine (T_4)

Levothyroxine (Synthroid, Levothroid, Levoxyl, Tirosint) is a synthetic form of **thyroxine (T_4)** and the standard replacement therapy for persons with hypothyroidism.[18] The structural formula of levothyroxine was discovered in 1926, and the drug was first synthesized in the next year. T_4 and T_3 were originally manufactured from animal extracts or desiccated thyroid. Synthetic preparations are used exclusively today because they are much less allergenic than products obtained from animal thyroid. The advantage of levothyroxine is that it replaces the prohormone T_4, which allows the individual to convert the levothyroxine to the active hormone T_3 via physiologic mechanisms. As a consequence, plasma levels of T_3 remain stable if adequate doses of levothyroxine are given. Levothyroxine is approved for treatment of hypothyroidism and for TSH suppression in individuals with thyroid cancer or thyroid nodules. The product carries an FDA-mandated black box warning that it should not be used for weight reduction (Box 19-1).

Metabolism and Excretion

Approximately 40% to 80% of an oral dose of levothyroxine is absorbed, depending on the woman's age and the presence of foods or other drugs in her gastrointestinal tract. The bioavailability of levothyroxine is normally approximately 80% of the orally administered dose, but it can be diminished substantially by concomitant administration of foods and/or other medications.[15,18,19] Vitamins that contain iron and calcium supplements decrease absorption of levothyroxine; they should not be taken at the same time levothyroxine is taken. In addition, common breakfast beverages (e.g., coffee) used when swallowing the tablets have been linked to decreased absorption as have other dietary items such as soybeans, prunes, herbs, walnuts.[20] However, coffee and tea were not found to negatively influence absorption of a liquid formulation of Tirosint in one pharmacokinetic study.[21]

Several additional factors affect absorption. Absorption also is diminished among individuals 70 years and older, persons on high-fiber diets, and persons with lactose intolerance. Poor absorption of this agent can also occur in persons with gastrointestinal disease (e.g., celiac disease, lactose intolerance, vitamin B_{12} deficiency, *Giardia* infection), liver disease (e.g., cirrhosis, obstructive liver disease), pancreatic insufficiency, gastrointestinal surgery (e.g., jejunostomy, short bowel syndrome, jejunoileal bypass), congestive heart failure, or ingestion of multiple medications.[20]

Levothyroxine should be taken in the morning on an empty stomach, with a delay of the morning meal by 30 minutes, to improve bioavailability.[15,18] This regimen may be difficult for many individuals to manage and can negatively affect adherence. Timing or chronobiology of drug ingestion also has been called into question. A 2010 Dutch study found that participants (n = 90) who took their medication at bedtime experienced positive effects on their thyroid hormone levels when compared to taking it in the morning, suggesting that taking the drug in the evening may result in adequate bioavailability.[22] Additional studies need to be conducted to ascertain the best timing and concomitant food/beverage ingestion for the different formulations.

The plasma half-life is approximately 6 to 10 days depending on the woman's baseline hypothyroid versus euthyroid state.[5] Levothyroxine is metabolized in the liver, kidney, and other peripheral tissues and is primarily eliminated via the kidney; a small portion passes through the intestine unchanged and is eliminated via feces.

Dosing Considerations

Levothyroxine has a narrow therapeutic range, and the adverse effects of either over- or under-treatment are significant. In recognition of this fact, it is important to determine the correct dose following initiation of the drug. Because the half-life of levothyroxine is quite long, it can take several months to determine the correct dose for an

Box 19-1 Gone But Not Forgotten: Thyroid Medications for Weight Loss

In years past, some providers would prescribe levothyroxine sodium for weight loss, under the assumption that the individual had hypothyroidism without confirmatory laboratory findings. However, among individuals with a normal thyroid, there is no evidence that normal doses of levothyroxine lead to weight loss.[15] Conversely, larger doses of this drug may be associated with weight reduction, but such doses are associated with toxicity and should not be employed as weight loss agents. The FDA requires the labeling for levothyroxine (Synthroid) to include a black box warning to this effect.

individual. It takes approximately 4 to 6 weeks to achieve a steady state, and the physiologic response to a particular dose will become evident only after a steady state is reached. Persons being treated with levothyroxine are to wait 4 to 6 weeks after initiation of the drug or after a change of dose to have a serum TSH measurement obtained.

For most persons, the daily dose ranges from 50 to 200 mcg per day (Table 19-1).[23] Several different brand-name and generic formulations of levothyroxine are available; they have different bioequivalence, even though the FDA narrowed the potency standards for levothyroxine from the general standard of 90% to 110% to a more rigorous 95% to 110%.[24] This drug is available in more than 10 different tablet strengths, with color codes to reflect formulations ranging from 13 mcg to 300 mcg per tablet.[15] Tirosint was approved by the FDA in 2000; it is the only FDA-approved version of levothyroxine available in a soft gel cap. Although it is not commonly used, an intravenous formulation is also available for individuals who are unable to take levothyroxine orally.

Different formulations of levothyroxine at the same dose can result in different TSH values in one individual. Therefore individuals who have a good response using one formulation—either a brand-name or generic product—should use that formulation consistently.[18] If the formulation is changed, a follow-up serum TSH should be assessed in 4 to 6 weeks.[15,18]

Table 19-1 Thyroid Replacement Formulations

Drug	Brand Names[a]	Initial Dose[b]	Usual Dose
Levothyroxine sodium (T_4)	Levolet Levo-T Levothroid Levothyroxine sodium Levoxyl[c] Synthroid Tirosint Unithroid	1.7 mcg/kg/day	100–125 mcg per day
Liothyronine T_3	Cytomel Triostat	25 mcg daily	25–75 mg per day
Liotrix T_4 and T_3	Thyrolar	½-grain tablet daily	1- to 2-grain tablets daily

[a] These are the FDA-approved oral formulations of levothyroxine sodium.
[b] Lower doses should be considered for elderly individuals and for persons with long-standing myxedema or cardiovascular impairment.
[c] Levoxyl can rapidly swell and disintegrate, which can cause choking or gagging. It should be taken with a full glass of water and used with caution by persons with difficulty swallowing.
Sources: Data from Food and Drug Administration. *FDA Letter*. Levothyroxine sodium product information. http://www.fda.gov/Drugs/DrugSafety/PostmarketDrugSafetyInformationforPatientsandProviders/ucm161257.htm. Accessed July 17, 2014[24]; Slagle MA. Medication update: thyroid supplements, antithyroid medications. *South Med J*. 2002;95(5):520-521.[23]

Side Effects/Adverse Effects

Adverse effects of levothyroxine are uncommon. The most common problems following excessive dosing are atrial fibrillation and osteoporosis, which occur more frequently among the elderly.[18] In instances of excessive dosing, individuals may note heart palpitations, heat intolerance, diarrhea, weight loss, nervousness, tremors, or angina.[15,18] Inadequate dosing can result in progression of cardiovascular disease and detrimental effects on serum lipid profiles.[18] Tartrazine, a synthetic lemon yellow azo dye used as a food coloring that is derived from coal tar, can be found in some thyroid replacement formulations and may increase the risk of allergic reactions.[19]

Drug–Drug Interactions

The drug–drug interactions associated with thyroid supplementation are among the most important considerations in pharmacologic management of thyroid disorders. Table 19-2 lists the most common drug–drug interactions that should be taken into account in clinical practice.

Liothyronine (T_3)

To treat persons with unremitting hypothyroid symptoms who are unresponsive to T_4 monotherapy, endocrinologists may consider the empirical addition of liothyronine (Cytomel, Triostat), which is a synthetic form of T_3.[25] The plasma half-life of T_3 is 24 hours, much shorter than the half-life of T_4, and causes T_3 values to vary widely. In addition, T_3 is approximately 10 times more potent than T_4; because of this greater potency, T_3 can trigger hyperthyroid episodes.[25]

T_3 and T_4 Combinations

Liotrix is a 4:1 combination of T_4 and T_3. This drug is not widely used in clinical practice today because there is insufficient evidence showing that it is more effective than levothyroxine alone for treating hypothyroidism.[15,18,26] However, some individuals have a genetic polymorphism that prevents resolution of their symptoms when T_4 alone is used.[26] In those situations, treatment with combination therapy may be warranted.

Table 19-2 Selected Drug–Drug Interactions Associated with Levothyroxine[a]

Drug: Generic (Brand)	Clinical Effect
Interference with Absorption	
Bile acid sequestrants (e.g., cholestyramine [Questran])	Decreased effect of levothyroxine
Bisphosphonates	Decreased effect of levothyroxine
Calcium salts such as calcium carbonate (Tums) and multiple vitamins	Decreased effect of levothyroxine
Cholestyramine (Questran)	Decreased effect of levothyroxine
Chromium picolinate	Decreased effect of levothyroxine
Ciprofloxacin (Cipro)	Decreased effect of levothyroxine
Colesevelam (Welchol)	Decreased effect of levothyroxine
Ferrous sulfate (Slow-Fe)	Decreased effect of levothyroxine
Orlistat (Xenical)	Decreased effect of levothyroxine
Phosphate binders such as aluminum hydroxide	Decreased effect of levothyroxine
Proton pump inhibitors	Decreased effect of levothyroxine
Raloxifene (Evista)	Decreased effect of levothyroxine
Sevelamer (Renagel)	Decreased effect of levothyroxine
Sodium polystyrene sulfonate (Kayexalate)	Decreased effect of levothyroxine
Sucralfate (Carafate)	Decreased effect of levothyroxine
Impaired T_4-to-T_3 Conversion	
Amiodarone (Cordarone)	
Increased Metabolism and/or Clearance	
Carbamazepine (Tegretol)	Lower total and free T_3 and T_4 concentration
Nevirapine (Viramune)	Lower total and free T_3 and T_4 concentration
Phenobarbitol (Luminal)	Lower total and free T_3 and T_4 concentration
Phenytoin (Dilantin)	Lower total and free T_3 and T_4 concentration; phenytoin displaces T_3 and T_4 from protein binding sites
Primidone (Mysoline)	Lower total and free T_3 and T_4 concentration
Rifampin (Rifadin)	Lower total and free T_3 and T_4 concentration
Sertraline (Zoloft)	Lower total and free T_3 and T_4 concentration
Stavudine (Zerit)	Lower total and free T_3 and T_4 concentration
Tyrosine kinase inhibitors such as imatinib	Lower total and free T_3 and T_4 concentration
Increased Thyroxine Binding Globulin Concentrations and Lower Free T_4 Concentrations	
Estrogens	Increased levothyroxine requirements
Decreased TSH Secretion	
Bexarotene (Targretin)	Lower total and free T_3 and T_4 concentration
Dopaminergic agonists such as bromocriptine	Lower total and free T_3 and T_4 concentration
Metformin (Glucophage)	Lower total and free T_3 and T_4 concentration
Opiates	
Increased TSH Secretion	
Dopamine receptor blockers such as metoclopramide (Reglan)	Lower total and free T_3 and T_4 concentration
Ritonavir (Norvir)	Lower total and free T_3 and T_4 concentration
St. John's wort	Lower total and free T_3 and T_4 concentration
Other Mechanisms	
Antidiabetic drugs and insulin	Hyperglycemia; levothyroxine increases severity of diabetes
Digoxin (Lanoxin)	Decreased digoxin effect; dose of digoxin may need to be increased
Piracetam (Nootropyl)	Increased adverse effects such as confusion, irritability, and sleep disorders
Selective serotonin reuptake inhibitors	Reduces therapeutic effect of levothyroxine
Theophylline (Theo-Dur)	Levothyroxine increases metabolism of theophylline
Tricyclic antidepressants	Levothyroxine enhances arrhythmogenic effect of tricyclic antidepressants
Warfarin (Coumadin)	Increases clotting factor catabolism leads to increased risk for bleeding; not common if person is euthyroid on stable dose

[a] This table is not comprehensive as new information is being generated on a regular basis.

Sources: Data from Brent GA, Koenig RJ. Thyroid and anti-thyroid drugs. In: Brunton LL, Chabner BA, Knollmann BC, eds. *Goodman & Gilman's the Pharmacological Basis of Therapeutics*. 12th ed. New York: McGraw-Hill; 2011:1129-1162[5]; Garber JR, Cobin RH, Gharib H, et al. Clinical practice guidelines for hypothyroidism in adults: cosponsored by the American Association of Clinical Endocrinologists and the American Thyroid Association. *Endocr Pract*. 2012;18(6):988-1028[15]; Jonklaas J, Bianco AC, Bauer AJ, et al. Guidelines for the treatment of hypothyroidism prepared by the American Thyroid Association Task Force on Thyroid Hormone Replacement. *Thyroid*. 2014;24(12):1670-1750[18]; Slagle MA. Medication update: thyroid supplements, antithyroid medications. *South Med J*. 2002;95(5):520-521.[23]

Pharmacologic Treatment of Hyperthyroidism

In most situations, an experienced specialist such as an endocrinologist or surgeon will manage the care of a woman with hyperthyroidism. Treatment of Graves' disease is two pronged. First, beta blockers are commonly used to reduce symptoms of tachycardia, tremulousness, heat intolerance, and anxiety. Second, measures that decrease thyroid hormone synthesis—such as radioactive iodine ablation, pharmacologic doses of iodide, thionamide (sometimes called "thioamide") drugs, or surgery—may be employed.

The three primary treatments for hyperthyroidism are radioactive iodine (I^{131} or RAI), thionamide medications, and surgery (Table 19-3).[27,28]

Beta-Adrenergic Antagonists for Symptomatic Relief

The sympathetic nervous system and thyroid hormones work in concert to regulate a variety of physiologic processes. Excesses of thyroid hormones produce augmented contractility, tachycardia, and increased metabolic demand—effects similar to those seen when plasma concentrations of catecholamines are elevated. Excess triiodothyronine (T_3) has been associated with cardiomyopathy and death.[29] Although doses of propranolol of 20 to 40 mg

Table 19-3 Treatment Modalities for Hyperthyroidism

Therapy: Action and Result	Indications	Adverse Effects/Contraindications
Beta-Adrenergic Antagonists		
Mitigates the cardiovascular and other peripheral tissue effects of hyperthyroid states	Adjunct therapy for persons with Graves' disease or thyroid storm; may be the only therapy for self-limiting thyroiditis	Contraindicated for persons who have congestive heart failure, some forms of valvular heart disease, bradyarrhythmias, heart block, asthma, or chronic pulmonary obstructive disease
Thionamides		
Inhibits thyroid hormone synthesis and may have immunosuppressive effects. Propylthiouracil also inhibits peripheral conversion of T_4 to T_3. Chance of permanent remission; avoids risk of permanent hypothyroidism; low cost.	First-line therapy for Graves' disease and may be used a short-term therapy prior to RAI or surgery	*Minor:* Fever, pruritus or rash (4–6%), arthralgia (1–5%), gastrointestinal effects (1–5%), abnormal sense of taste or smell (rare)[a] *Major:* Polyarthritis (1–2%), thrombocytopenia, agranulocytosis (0.1%), immunoallergic hepatitis,[b] vasculitis (drug-induced lupus syndrome), hypoglycemia (rare)
Radioiodine (RAI)		
Radioactive iodine destroys the thyroxine-producing cells in the thyroid gland; results in permanent resolution of hyperthyroidism and may cause permanent hypothyroidism	Second-line therapy for Graves' disease	*Minor:* Transient thyroid pain *Contraindications:* Pregnancy, lactation
Thyroidectomy		
Rapid permanent cure that always results in permanent hypothyroidism if thyroid completely removed; complications can reach 13%, but are related to surgeon's experience and the surgical process	Obstructive or very large goiter; rarely used for Graves' disease	*Major:* Recurrent laryngeal nerve injury, superior laryngeal nerve injury, postoperative hypoparathyroidism, temporary hypocalcemia; vocal cord paralysis, permanent hypocalcemia, postoperative hemorrhage, wound infection
Iodide-Containing Compounds		
Inhibits release of thyroid hormone from stores in thyroid gland	Used prior to surgery and for treatment of thyroid storm	*Minor:* Can cause skin rash, flare-up of acne, or dermatitis *Major:* Multiple drug–drug interactions *Contraindications:* Pregnancy and in persons with known sensitivity to iodides, iodine-induced goiter, or dermatitis herpetiformis Use with caution in persons with Addison's disease, acute bronchitis, lactation

[a] Occurs with methimazole (Tapazole) only.
[b] Occurs with propylthiouracil (PTU) only.
Sources: Data from Bahn Chair RS, Burch HB, Cooper DS, et al.; American Thyroid Association; American Association of Clinical Endocrinologists. Hyperthyroidism and other causes of thyrotoxicosis: management guidelines of the American Thyroid Association and American Association of Clinical Endocrinologists. *Thyroid.* 2011;21(6):593-646[28]; England RJ, Kamath MB, Jabreel A, Dunne G, Atkin SL. How we do it: surgery should be considered equally with I131 and thionamide treatment as first-line therapy for thyrotoxicosis. *Clin Otolaryngol.* 2006;31(2):160-162.[27]

administered 4 times daily initially, titrated up to 480 mg per day in divided doses, have been used, cardioselective agents such as atenolol (Tenormin) may be safer alternatives.[5] Further discussion of beta blockers can be found in the chapter *Cardiovascular Conditions*.

Radioactive Iodine (RAI, I^{131})

RAI has been considered a first-line therapy for hyperthyroid conditions.[28] RAI comprises radioactive beta-particle emissions that destroy the thyroid gland tissue, thereby decreasing the synthesis of thyroid hormone. Most individuals who receive RAI eventually will develop hypothyroidism (the goal of therapy) and will require lifelong thyroid hormone supplementation, although this outcome is slightly more likely in men than in women. RAI is contraindicated for women who are pregnant, planning pregnancy within 4 to 6 months, or lactating; in persons with suspected thyroid cancer; and in those who are unable to comply with the necessary radiation safety guidelines.[28]

Dosing Considerations

The RAI dose may be a fixed-calculation dose, which results in cure rates of 64% to 75% at the end of one year, or it may be calculated individually based on the size of the thyroid and expected uptake of iodine.[28] Radioiodine is administered as a one-time dose as a capsule or oral solution. The agent is absorbed from the gastrointestinal tract and concentrates in the thyroid, where ablation occurs over a period of 6 to 18 weeks. Occasionally, an individual will require a second dose. Those individuals who are most likely to respond to single doses include persons who are younger, lack thyroid peroxidase antibodies, have smaller gland volume, and those who have a less severe case of hyperthyroidism.[30]

No consensus exists regarding the use of adjunct oral thionamides such as propylthiouracil (PTU) or methimazole (Tapazole) prior to RAI or the method for calculating the RAI dose.[31] Lithium (Lithobid), which increases iodine retention within the thyroid gland, has been used in combination with RAI for treatment of individuals with toxic nodular disease as well as Graves' disease.[32]

Side Effects/Adverse Effects

The most common side effect of RAI is thyroid tenderness and dysphagia. Adverse effects of RAI include hepatitis, arthritis, and agranulocytosis. It is estimated that fewer than 1% of women being treated for hyperthyroidism experience agranulocytosis, a condition that is more likely to occur among women taking higher doses of antithyroid medications. No single method of routine monitoring has been recommended, although some clinicians who monitored white blood cell counts every 2 to 4 weeks reported earlier detection of agranulocytosis. Regardless of the timing of diagnosis, most cases of agranulocytosis are reversible. Ophthalmopathy occurs more often in persons who receive RAI than in those who undergo thionamide therapy.[34] RAI is not associated with an increased risk for cancer, nor is it associated with decreases in fertility or birth defects in exposed fetuses. Interestingly, RAI therapy can cause thyroid storm. In this rare phenomenon, RAI increases the concentration of TSH receptor antibodies that are released from dying thyroid cells; these antibodies then precipitate the thyroid storm. RAI-associated thyroid storm is most likely to occur in the first few weeks after therapy begins.

Radiation Safety Guidelines

The most important consideration with RAI therapy is limiting radiation exposure among contacts of the person who has taken RAI. Exposure can occur via contact with saliva, urine, and radiation that is emitted from their body. Post-treatment precautions are listed in Box 19-2.[33]

Pharmacologic Doses of Iodide

Doses of inorganic iodide have been used with thionamides when rapid return to normal thyroid hormone levels is desired. Women with severe disease or those requiring urgent thyroidectomy may receive benefit from treatment with inorganic iodide. Potassium iodide (KI) and Lugol's solution have been used cautiously for fewer than 10 days with thionamide therapy, but handling these solutions may be inconvenient. Of note, combinations of potassium iodide and thionamide therapy are not routinely recommended for treatment of Graves' disease and have not been shown to be more effective than thionamide therapy alone.[35]

Thionamides: Methimazole and Propylthiouracil

Thionamide drugs—that is, methimazole (Tapazole) and propylthiouracil (Propyl-Thyracil; usually referred to as PTU)—are widely used in Japan, Australia, and Europe as a first choice for the treatment for Graves' disease, whereas RAI tends to be the first choice in the United States. Thionamides interfere with the thyroid peroxidase enzyme, which is necessary for the iodination of triiodothyronine and thyroxine. Thionamide therapies exert

Box 19-2 Post-Treatment Precautions Following Administration of Radioiodine

The number of days one should follow each of these restrictions will be based on the dose administered. This list covers doses in the range of 10 mCi to 30 mCi.

- Sleep alone in a bed that is more than 6 feet away from another person for the specified time.
- Stay at least 6 feet away from other persons for the specified time.
- Travel by public transportation is limited to a specific number of hours for each day after treatment.
- Do not kiss anyone.
- Do not have sexual activity.
- Empty the bladder frequently and increase fluids:
  - Flush each time and flush toilet paper and wipes.
  - Wash hands after each time using the toilet.
  - Dry hands on a towel not used by other persons.
- Use flushable wipes to:
  - Clean the toilet seat after use.
  - Clean the mouthpiece of the phone after use.
  - Rinse the sink to wash away saliva after brushing teeth.
- Do not share a toothbrush, razor, face cloth, towel, or any eating utensils.
- Do not cook for other persons or use plastic gloves and dispose in a specified plastic trash bag.
- Wash clothes separately from other persons' clothing.

Source: Data from American Thyroid Association Taskforce on Radioiodine Safety, Sisson JC, Freitas J, et al. Radiation safety in the treatment of patients with thyroid diseases by radioiodine 131I: practice recommendations of the American Thyroid Association. *Thyroid.* 2011;21(4):335-346.[33]

immunosuppressive effects: They reduce concentrations of antithyrotropin-receptor antibodies, intracellular adhesion molecule I, interleukin-6 and interleukin-2 receptors, helper T cells, natural killer cells, suppressor T cells, and activated intrathyroidal T cells.[36]

The goal of treatment when using thionamides is to obtain a euthyroid state within 3 to 6 weeks. Persons started on therapy should have their thyroid function tested every 4 to 6 weeks until a stable euthyroid state is achieved. Methimazole (Tapazole) is preferred over propylthiouracil (Propyl-Thyracil) as a first-line therapy except in women who are pregnant, because it can be dosed less frequently, it is less likely to cause hepatotoxicity, and compliance is better probably because of the less frequent dosing (Table 19-4).[28,36,37] The relationship between remission rates and length of thionamide therapy has been investigated, with historical trial data suggesting that longer durations of therapy result in greater remission rates. More recent findings, however, suggest that treatment for a duration of 12 to 18 months is satisfactory for a majority of persons.[36]

Table 19-4 Thionamide Dosing

Drug: Generic (Brand)	Formulations	Initial Dose (Adult)	Usual Dose (Adult)
Methimazole (Tapazole)	Trade: 5-mg, 10-mg tablets Generic: 15-mg, 20-mg tablets	15 mg per day	5–15 mg per day, up to 30–60 mg daily
Propylthiouracil (Propyl-Thyracil)	50-mg tablets	300 mg per day in three equally divided doses	100–150 mg per day in divided doses, up to 400–900 mg daily in divided doses

Metabolism and Excretion

Methimazole and propylthiouracil differ slightly with respect to their pharmacokinetic properties. Propylthiouracil is highly protein bound (approximately 75%), whereas methimazole has limited protein binding. Propylthiouracil has a shorter half-life (approximately 75 minutes), whereas methimazole's half-life is longer (approximately 6 to 9 hours). Approximately 35% of both thionamides is eliminated renally.[5]

Side Effects/Adverse Effects

The most common side effects of the thionamides include urticaria, macular rashes, gastrointestinal upset, and arthralgias, which occur among approximately 5% of persons taking either of these two medications. Skin reactions usually resolve following treatment with antihistamines. Persons who develop arthralgias should discontinue the drug because these symptoms may signal the development of polyarthritis, which is a rare adverse effect associated with a lupus-like syndrome. Side effects are dose dependent in persons taking methimazole; the relationship to dose is less clear for propylthiouracil. In general, the side-effect profile favors methimazole.[28]

Adverse effects of thionamides are listed in Table 19-3. One of the most serious adverse effects reported—agranulocytosis—occurs among 0.3% of recipients.[36] This autoimmune-mediated effect most frequently occurs in the first 3 months of therapy, although it can occur at any time. A baseline white cell blood count should be obtained for all persons prior to initiating therapy with thionamides. Routine screening during therapy is not indicated because the onset of agranulocytosis is acute and abrupt. Individuals are counseled to stop the medication and contact their provider immediately if they develop a fever and sore throat, as these are the two most common presenting symptoms associated with agranulocytosis.

Hepatic abnormalities are medication specific. Propylthiouracil can cause fulminant hepatic necrosis—an adverse effect that can appear in the first several months of therapy and may be fatal. Because asymptomatic transient increases in liver function tests can occur in persons taking propylthiouracil, routine monitoring of liver function tests is not recommended. Methimazole can rarely cause cholestasis. In either case, the medication should be stopped. Because the hepatic abnormalities have a different etiology depending on the thionamide drug involved, switching to the other drug can be recommended, albeit with caution.

The third rare, but adverse effect of these drugs is vasculitis, which appears to be a drug-induced lupus syndrome, which is reviewed in more detail in the *Drug Toxicity* chapter. Symptoms include renal dysfunction, arthritis, skin ulcerations, vasculitis rash, sinusitis, and sometimes hemoptysis.[38,39]

Drug–Drug Interactions

Hyperthyroidism itself results in increased metabolism of vitamin K–dependent clotting factors, which may require a dose reduction of anticoagulants such as warfarin (Coumadin).[5] Digoxin (Lanoxin) and beta blocker doses may require adjustment, as these drugs' metabolism may be affected by methimazole. Amiodarone (Cordarone) and bugleweed, an herbal preparation used for hyperthyroidism, may potentiate the effects of thionamide therapies and require lower doses of thionamides. Antithyroid drugs can also increase the serum concentrations of theophylline (Theo-Dur). No significant drug–food interactions have been reported with thionamide therapies.[5]

Thionamide Therapy Prior to RAI

Individuals with severe hyperthyroidism, advanced age, or cardiac complications are frequently prescribed thionamides for a few months prior to beginning RAI therapy.[5] Some clinicians believe that thionamides deplete thyroid hormones stores and reduce the chance of RAI-induced thyroid storm.[40,41] However, when Vijayakumar et al. retrospectively examined 122 participants who were given RAI and a beta blocker without thionamide pretreatment, they failed to find any episode of thyroid storm.[41]

Thyroid Storm

Thyroid storm is a rare, acute, life-threatening exacerbation of hyperthyroidism. Multiple organ systems are involved, and individuals exhibit signs and symptoms such as fever, tachycardia, nausea, vomiting, diarrhea, and tremor. Thyroid storm can progress to dehydration and coma if not treated. Persons who experience thyroid storm are admitted for hospital care. The goals for treatment of thyroid storm are fourfold: (1) decrease thyroid hormone production; (2) decrease the effect of circulating thyroid hormone; (3) provide supportive therapy; and (4) treat the underlying cause (Table 19-5). Large doses of propylthiouracil and iodide are administered concomitantly to invoke the Wolff-Chaikoff effect and inhibit release of thyroid hormone stores from the thyroid gland. In addition, cholestyramine (Questran) may be administered because it decreases thyroid hormone resorption from the small intestine. Supportive therapies include corticosteroids, which inhibit peripheral conversion of T_4 to T_3; beta-adrenergic antagonists; antipyretics; and correction of electrolyte imbalances.[28]

Table 19-5 Treatment of Thyroid Storm

Drug: Generic (Brand)	Indication
Iodine preparations Lithium carbonate (Lithobid) Propylthiouracil (PTU)	Inhibit thyroid hormone production and release from thyroid gland
Corticosteroids Propranolol (Inderal) Propylthiouracil (PTU)	Inhibit peripheral conversion of T_4 to T_3
Cholestyramine (Questran)	Increase thyroid hormone clearance
Beta-adrenergic antagonists Corticosteroids	Mitigate the hormone effect
Antipyretics Cooling blankets and ice packs Correction of electrolyte imbalances	Supportive therapy

Medications Associated with Thyroid Dysfunction

Five categories of pharmaceutical interactions are important to consider prior to prescribing either thyroid supplementation or thionamides: (1) drugs that can induce hypothyroidism or hyperthyroidism; (2) drugs that interfere with thyroid laboratory results; (3) drug–drug interactions that interfere with expected thyroid function; (4) significant drug–food interactions; and (5) drugs that contain significant amounts of iodine. Before instituting pharmacotherapy for the treatment of individuals with either hypothyroidism or hyperthyroidism, the provider should perform a comprehensive medication history to rule out drug-related causes of thyroid dysfunction.

Drugs That Alter Thyroid Function

Selected drugs that affect thyroid function are identified in Table 19-2 and Table 19-6.[42–44] Some drugs can cause clinical hyperthyroidism or hypothyroidism, with this outcome being either detrimental or useful for therapeutic purposes. For example, large doses of corticosteroids (e.g., 4 mg of dexamethasone) and beta-adrenergic antagonists (e.g., propranolol [Inderal]) can inhibit the peripheral conversion of T_4 to T_3, yet have minimal effects on thyroid function tests. As a result, these agents often are employed in the management of severe hyperthyroidism or thyroid storm to treat symptoms of tachycardia. Lithium (Lithobid) concentrates in the thyroid gland, interferes with thyroid hormone synthesis, and may induce subclinical hypothyroidism in as many as 50% of individuals. The risk appears highest among individuals who receive lithium for more than 2 years.[43] Interferon-alpha has been implicated as a transient cause of hypothyroidism in 40% to 50% of users and as a cause of hyperthyroidism in 10% to 30% of recipients.[43]

Iodine-Containing Medications

Iodine-containing medications (Table 19-7) may have a variety of effects on the thyroid gland. Short-term exposure of fewer than 7 to 10 days often inhibits thyroid hormone production, i.e., the Wolff-Chaikoff effect.[42] An iodide-induced hyperthyroidism, Jod-Basedow disease, may be observed among persons with autonomously functioning, nontoxic multinodular goiters who continue to receive iodine supplementation.[43] This phenomenon usually occurs within 3 to 8 weeks after the supplementation and may persist for several months. Its etiology is likely related to an impaired Wolff-Chaikoff mechanism. Iodide-induced hypothyroidism occurs most often in those persons with autoimmune (Hashimoto's) thyroiditis, females, and individuals with a history of thyroid disease, radioactive iodide administration, thyroid damage, partial thyroidectomy, or postpartum thyroid disease. In this case, the thyroid

Table 19-6 Selected Medications That Cause Thyroid Dysfunction

Drug: Generic (Brand)	Drug: Generic (Brand)
Decrease TSH	***Increase TSH***
Bexarotene (Targretin)	Amiodarone (Cordarone)
Bromocriptine (Parlodel)	Iodinated contrast
Dopamine (Intropin)	Metoclopramide (Reglan)
Glucocorticoids	Drug interactions that decrease absorption of levothyroxine
Levodopa (Sinemet)	
Octreotide (Sandostatin)	
Prednisone (Deltasone)	
Increase Thyroid Hormone Secretion	***Decrease Thyroid Hormone Secretion***
Amiodarone (Cordarone)	Amiodarone (Cordarone)
Iodide	Iodide-containing products
	Lithium (Lithobid)
Displace from TBG Binding, Increase Free T_4	***Increase Hepatic Metabolism, Decrease Free T_4***
Amiodarone (Cordarone)	Carbamazepine (Tegretol)
Diclofenac (Voltaren)	Phenobarbitol (Luminol)
Furosemide (Lasix)	Phenytoin (Dilantin)
Heparin	Rifampin (Rifadin)
Mefenamic acid (Ponstel)	
Nonsteroidal anti-inflammatory drugs	
Phenylbutazone (Butazolidin)	
Salicylates such as aspirin	
Decrease Serum TBG	***Increase Serum TBG***
Anabolic steroids and androgens	Estrogens
	Heroin, methadone
	Fluorouracil (Adrucil)
	Mitotane (Lysodren)
Clinical Hypothyroidism	***Clinical Hyperthyroidism***
Amiodarone (Cordarone)	Amiodarone (Cordarone)
Corticosteroids	Interferon-alpha
Interferon-alpha	
Lithium (Lithobid)	
Propanolol (Inderal)	

Abbreviations: TBG = thyroid-binding globulin; TSH = thyroid-stimulating hormone.

Sources: Data from Barbesino G. Drugs affecting thyroid function. *Thyroid*. 2010;20(7):763-770[44]; Dong BJ. How medications affect thyroid function. *West J Med*. 2000;172(2):102-106[43]; Kundra P, Burman KD. The effect of medications on thyroid function tests. *Med Clin North Am*. 2012;96(2):283-295.[42]

Table 19-7 Medications That Contain Iodine

Class	Drug: Generic (Brand)	Iodine Dose
Expectorants	Iophen Iodinated glycerol Anhydrous calcium iodide (Calcidrine)	25 mg/mL 15 mg/tablet 152 mg/5 mL
Antiasthmatic drugs	Theophylline elixir (Elixophyllin)	6.6 mg/mL
Antiarrhythmic drugs	Amiodarone (Cordarone)	75 mg/tablet
Antiamebic drugs	Iodoquinol (Yodoxin)	134 mg/tablet
Anticellulite therapy	Cellasene (brand name for combination of gingko, grape seed, clover, evening primrose, and other ingredients)	930 mcg/serving
Iodide-containing solutions	Lugol's solution Potassium iodide (Quadrinal) Saturated solution of potassium iodide (SSKI)	6.3 mg/drop 145 mg/tablet 38 mg/drop
Miscellaneous agents	Kelp	0.15 mg/tablet
Ophthalmic solutions	Echothiophate iodide (phospholine iodide) Idoxuridine solution (Herplex)	5–41 mcg/drop 18 mcg/drop
Radiology contrast agents	Iopanoic acid Intravenous preparations	333 mg/tablet 140–380 mg/mL
Topical antiseptic agents	Clioquinol cream (Alba Form HC) Iodoquinol cream (Yodoxin) Iodine tincture Iodoform gauze Povidone-iodine (Betadine)	12 mg/g 6 mg/g 40 mg/mL 4.8 mg/100 mg gauze 10 mg/mL
Vitamins	Iodine-containing vitamins	0.15 mg/tablet

Source: Adapted from Brent GA, Koenig RJ. Thyroid and anti-thyroid drugs. In: Brunton LL, Chabner BA, Knollmann BC, eds. *Goodman & Gilman's the Pharmacological Basis of Therapeutics*. 12th ed. New York: McGraw-Hill; 2011:1129-1162.[5]

gland seems to be unable to "escape" the Wolff-Chaikoff blockade.[43]

Amiodarone (Cordarone) and radiocontrast dyes are the most common medication-related causes of hypothyroidism.[43] Amiodarone is an antiarrythmic agent used for individuals with cardiac conditions. Amiodarone can cause several different thyroid dysfunction states including hypo- or hyperthyroidism. Approximately 3% to 5% of all persons in the United States who are treated with this drug will become hyperthyroid within 4 months to 3 years of therapy.[42] Amiodarone-induced hyperthyroidism is classified as one of two types: (1) induction of thyroiditis or (2) iodine-induced disease. Type 1 disease is hypothesized to be the result of direct toxicity by amiodarone on the gland. Type 2 disease occurs in individuals with Graves' disease or nontoxic multinodular goiters.

Special Populations: Pregnancy, Lactation, and the Elderly

Pregnancy induces multiple physiologic changes in the thyroid gland and thyroid hormone function.[45,46] These changes include (1) modest thyroid gland hyperplasia; (2) modified peripheral metabolism of maternal thyroid hormones; (3) estrogen-mediated increase in thyroxine-binding globulin; (4) increased dietary iodine requirements coupled with increased iodine loss via the kidney and to the fetus; and (5) transient human chorionic gonadotropin (hCG)-induced stimulation of the maternal thyroid gland. The result of these changes in women without thyroid disorders is a suppressed TSH level in the first trimester and an elevated T_4 level, yet the ratio of T_4 to T_3 remains stable and a euthyroid state is maintained.

Hypothyroidism in Pregnancy

Hypothyroidism (autoimmune/Hashimoto's disease) is the most common thyroid disorder in pregnancy. If left untreated, it may result in placental abruption, preeclampsia, preterm delivery, reduced intellectual function of the offspring, and/or fetal loss.[47] The fetal thyroid does not start synthesizing thyroid hormone until after 12 weeks' gestation, so all of the fetus's thyroid needs are supplied by the pregnant woman prior to this time (Box 19-3). Thyroid hormones are essential for normal fetal brain development. Thus, levothyroxine supplementation is recommended for all women who are diagnosed with frank hypothyroidism.

Levothyroxine is safe for use during pregnancy and while breastfeeding. To maintain the desirable TSH concentration, the dose of levothyroxine may need to be increased by 30% to 50% more than the prepregnancy dose, then reduced to the prepregnancy dose after the woman gives birth.[5] Serum TSH values are obtained every 6 weeks or so over the course of pregnancy and the dose adjusted as needed.[45–49] Endogenously produced levothyroxine is a normal constituent of breast milk, yet synthetic levothyroxine does not pass into breast milk well—the reasons for this phenomenon are not fully understood. There are no adverse effects on breastfed infants of women who take levothyroxine for hypothyroid conditions.

Subclinical Hypothyroidism During Pregnancy

Some authorities now recommend universal screening for hypothyroidism during pregnancy as a means to

Box 19-3 Hypothyroidism in Pregnancy

SL, a 28-year-old woman, comes to an ambulatory facility for a regular gynecology appointment. She mentions that she has experienced mild fatigue, nausea, and constipation—symptoms that she attributes to the "flu." The provider examines her and orders a complete blood count (CBC) with differential, serum chemistry, and a pregnancy test. SL's laboratory measures are normal except that she has a positive pregnancy test and an elevated TSH (7.2 mIU/L). The provider now must discuss a management plan with SL based on these laboratory findings.

The elevated TSH, accompanying clinical presentation, and diagnosis of pregnancy increase the probability of symptomatic hypothyroidism for SL. Human chorionic gonadotropin—the primary pregnancy hormone in the first trimester—has a stimulatory effect on the thyroid that results in a transient chemical hyperthyroidism. Therefore, it can be expected that pregnant women will have a moderately low TSH level; SL's value, however, is high.

SL plans to continue the pregnancy but is worried about taking levothyroxine (Synthroid) and asks how this drug will affect her fetus. Her provider explains that levothyroxine (Synthroid) is identical to the thyroid hormone her body makes, and that it is not just safe, but important to ensure normal development of her fetus. The fetus must obtain thyroid hormone from maternal sources because fetal production of thyroid hormone does not begin until the second trimester; even then, the majority of thyroid used by the fetus during the last months of pregnancy is supplied by the mother. SL is also told that congenital hypothyroidism is associated with abnormal brain development (cretinism), low birth weight, and other neurologic deficits. SL is informed that congenital hypothyroidism is a test included in the panel of standard newborn screening exams.

identify women with subclinical hypothyroidism. Not only is such screening controversial, but when women are diagnosed with this condition, there are differences of opinion regarding treatment. The American College of Obstetricians and Gynecologists recommends targeted testing—specifically, screening only pregnant women who are symptomatic, have a personal history of disease, or have other conditions (e.g., diabetes) associated with an increased risk of thyroidal illness.[48] This guideline is based on the lack of benefits from levothyroxine supplementation noted in those women with subclinical hypothyroidism during pregnancy.[45–49] However, a subsequent systematic review published in 2013 suggested that levothyroxine and perhaps selenium supplementation during pregnancy might decrease the incidence of untoward perinatal events and that additional study is warranted among women with subclinical disease.[50] Issues regarding diagnosis and treatment of subclinical hypothyroidism during pregnancy require further study to clarify the best course of action.

Hyperthyroidism in Pregnancy

Graves' disease is the most common reason for the development of hyperthyroidism during pregnancy. Thyroid-stimulating antibodies cross the placenta and stimulate the fetal thyroid. Thus, the fetus of a pregnant woman with untreated Graves' disease can develop thyrotoxicosis and goiter.[51] Untreated hyperthyroidism can also result in stillbirth, preterm labor, intrauterine growth restriction, preeclampsia, and heart failure.[51] In contrast, the fetus can develop hypothyroidism secondary to transplacental passage of antithyroid medications. Historically, propylthiouracil (Propyl-Thyracil) was believed to offer an advantage over methimazole (Tapazole) in pregnant and lactating women because propylthiouracil has greater protein binding, but recent trials suggest this difference is minimal. However, teratogenic risk appears to be higher for fetuses whose mothers take methimazole, so propylthiouracil is recommended in the first trimester followed by an eventual change to methimazole.[45,49] The use of the lowest effective dose may reduce teratogenic risk, and nearly 45% of women may be able to discontinue thionamides by the third trimester.[28,45,49]

Postpartum Thyroiditis

Transient postpartum thyroiditis has been reported in as many as 10% of women in the first year postpartum, with the incidence the highest between 1 and 4 months after birth. Postpartum thyroiditis can have both a hyperthyroid phase and a hypothyroid phase. No standard clinical picture has been found: Some women will have both hyperthyroid and hypothyroid phases, whereas others will exhibit only hyperthyroidism or only hypothyroidism. The most common symptoms—anxiety, fatigue, insomnia, palpitations, weight loss, and irritability—are often attributed to the normal postpartum state or postpartum depression; therefore, the thyroid dysfunction may go undetected.

Pharmacologic treatment of postpartum hypothyroidism is rarely necessary because the symptoms are usually mild. If levothyroxine (Synthroid) therapy is initiated, it should be continued for 6 to 12 months and then tapered, as 80% of women with postpartum hypothyroidism will regain normal thyroid function.

Thyroid storm can occur in the first months postpartum.[45] Women with thyrotoxicosis may be treated with beta-adrenergic antagonists for symptomatic relief and should be monitored closely because the thyroid toxic phase is transient. Antithyroid medications are not used to treat postpartum thyroid storm because the disease is self-limiting.

Thyroid Dysfunction in the Elderly

The prevalence of hypothyroidism increases as women age. Diagnosing hypothyroidism in the elderly may be difficult, however, because the symptoms are often similar to those seen during normal aging, the symptoms may mirror those seen with other diseases of old age, and physical examinations may appear normal.[52] Elderly individuals often are more sensitive to any treatment modality secondary to the increased incidence of comorbidities and use of other medications that can cause drug–drug interactions. It is recommended that persons older than 50 to 60 years who require levothyroxine replacement should receive an initial dose of 50 mcg per day; those with established cardiovascular disease should receive 12.5 to 25 mcg per day initially.[15] Postmenopausal women who take estrogen may need higher doses, as estrogen increases the production of thyroid-binding globulin, thereby lowering the fraction of free T_4 available for use.

Hyperthyroidism in elderly women is associated with an increased risk for cardiovascular disease, osteoporosis, and mortality.[52] Thionamides and beta blocker therapy are recommended before RAI is initiated in such populations. Beta blockers are recommended for the elderly who have symptomatic thyrotoxicosis.

Parathyroid Disease

The parathyroid gland is responsible for regulation of calcium levels via production and excretion of parathyroid hormone.[5] Parathyroid hormone corrects hypocalcemia by increasing bone resorption of calcium and gastrointestinal calcium absorption, and by decreasing renal excretion of calcium. In contrast, calcitonin hormone, which is secreted by the thyroid gland, decreases bone resorption of calcium and gastrointestinal calcium absorption, and increases renal excretion of calcium. The two parathyroid disorders are known as hypoparathyroidism and hyperparathyroidism.

Hypoparathyroidism

Hypoparathyroidism is a rare disorder resulting from inadequate parathyroid hormone production. This disorder may be genetically inherited or transient, but is most often acquired secondary to damage to the parathyroid gland during thyroid surgery. The iron overload found in persons with thalassemia may also cause this disorder.[53]

Therapeutic management of hypoparathyroidism primarily consists of calcium replacement and vitamin D supplementation to normalize serum calcium. Acute hypocalcemia requires hospitalization for intravenous calcium therapy. Intravenous calcium gluconate can be used in these situations and EKG monitoring is recommended.[53] Serum calcium levels should be assessed every 1 to 2 hours, then every 4 to 6 hours until the individual is stable. A transition to oral calcium and vitamin D (calcitriol) 0.5 mcg per day should begin when serum calcium is greater than 7.5 mg/dL. Individuals should be reevaluated every 1 to 2 weeks initially, and then every 3 to 6 months after the regimen is stabilized.

Hyperparathyroidism

Hyperparathyroid conditions may occur as a result of primary, secondary, or tertiary disease. The incidence is 2 to 3 cases per 1000 women.[54] Primary hyperparathyroidism is the result of excessive secretion of parathyroid hormone and is usually caused by excess parathyroid tissue generated by a parathyroid tumor, most likely an adenoma. Secondary hyperparathyroidism occurs when the parathyroid secretes abnormal amounts of hormone in response to an abnormal stimulus—that is, hypocalcemia. Causes of secondary hypoparathyroidism include vitamin D deficiency and chronic renal failure. This parathyroid condition is the one most likely to be amenable to pharmacologic treatment. Tertiary hyperparathyroidism is a condition that occurs after a long period of secondary disease that results in hypercalcemia. Ultimately, hypercalcemia is the primary underlying problem in all three types of hyperparathyroidism.

Hyperparathyroidism is usually asymptomatic and is diagnosed as a serendipitous finding in conjunction with hypercalcemia. It is classically referred to as "moans, groans, stones, and bones with psychic overtones." Symptoms, when they are present, include bone disorders, kidney stones, gastrointestinal discomfort, neuromuscular dysfunction, weakness, fatigue, anxiety, and cognitive difficulties.[54]

Treatment of hyperparathyroidism differs according to the underlying disorder. Primary and tertiary disease are usually managed surgically, whereas secondary disease is managed medically. As hyperphosphatemia and hypocalcemia are the hallmarks of secondary disease, phosphate-binding agents, low-phosphate diets, calcium supplementation, vitamin D, and calcimimetics are used as treatments.[54] Although these therapies are widely used, no interventional trial has demonstrated that phosphate reduction improves clinical outcomes. Dietary restriction of phosphate, the use of phosphate binders, and the use of calcium-based phosphate binders also have not been shown to consistently reduce serum phosphate, although calcium-based products do increase serum calcium.[55]

Treatment of Secondary Hyperparathyroidism

Phosphate Binders

A variety of medications are used to bind phosphorus. These agents are generally taken 10 to 15 minutes before a meal or during the meal to increase their effectiveness.[56] Phosphate binders include calcium (carbonate, acetate, citrate), magnesium (carbonate), and aluminum (hydroxide and carbonate).

Lanthanum carbonate (Fosrenol) is the newest orally administered phosphate binder; it was approved by the FDA in 2004 for reduction of serum phosphate in persons with stage 5 chronic kidney disease.[5] This agent dissociates in the upper gastrointestinal tract to lanthanum ions, which bind to dietary phosphate and create an insoluble complex that cannot be absorbed. The tablets are available as 500-mg, 750-mg, and 1000-mg formulations. They must be chewed or crushed completely before swallowing and should be taken with or immediately after meals. The initial daily dose is 1500 mg per day in divided doses, but a majority of subjects in clinical trials required between 1500 and 3000 mg per day. The most commonly reported adverse effects are nausea, vomiting, and abdominal pain. The risk for systemic drug–drug interactions is low because the bioavailability is poor. However, lanthanum carbonate may impair the absorption of medications such as thyroid hormones and fluoroquinolone and tetracycline antibiotics.

Lanthanum carbonate is not recommended for use by pregnant women or those who are breastfeeding, as its effects on the fetus and the breastfeeding infant are unknown. This agent should be used by elderly individuals with caution and after a review of other drugs or comorbid conditions that may affect its effectiveness.

Calcimimetics

Cinacalcet (Sensipar) was approved by the FDA in 2004 for treatment of primary and secondary hyperparathyroidism and is available in 30-mg, 60-mg, and 90-mg tablets. This agent exerts its pharmacologic effects by altering the sensitivity of the calcium-sensing receptors on the surface of the parathyroid gland, which results in improved parathyroid hormone and extracellular calcium sensitivity. Cinacalcet may be used in combination with other customary therapies (e.g., phosphate binders, calcitriol). The starting dose is 30 mg once daily, which may be titrated up to 180 mg once daily. Providers should monitor calcium and phosphorus levels within the first week of initiating therapy and the intact parathyroid levels within the first 4 weeks with the goal of maintaining them in the range of 150 to 300 pg/mL.

The most common adverse effects seen in persons who take cinacalcet include nausea, vomiting, diarrhea, myalgia, and dizziness. Cinacalcet has many potential clinically significant drug–drug interactions via its effect on CYP450 enzymes; consequently, it should not be prescribed without first performing a careful medication review.

Use of cinacalcet in pregnancy and lactation is not recommended secondary to a lack of information about this drug's effects on the fetus and the breastfeeding infant. Women who become pregnant while taking cinacalcet can contact the pregnancy registry maintained by the manufacturer. Similarly, use by elderly individuals should occur after a careful examination of other drugs being taken and any comorbid conditions that affect calcium metabolism.

Conclusion

Women with thyroid or parathyroid dysfunction are susceptible to a wide variety of complications, as these glands and their respective hormones are critical for the normal operation of many body processes. Healthcare providers have multiple pharmacologic options available to manage the derangements that may occur in these systems as a result of disease. Carefully obtained histories, physical examinations, and laboratory evaluations will help the healthcare provider provide optimal care for women with thyroid and parathyroid disorders.

Resources

Organization	Description	Website
American Thyroid Association (ATA)	ATA guidelines for treatment of hypothyroidism and hyperthyroidism in adults and pregnant women are available for download; guidelines for radiation safety are also available as well as joint guidelines from ATA and other professional organizations	www.thyroid.org/thyroid-guidelines
Endocrine Society	Guidelines for management of thyroid dysfunction during pregnancy and postpartum	www.endocrine.org/~/media/endosociety/Files/Publications/Clinical%20Practice%20Guidelines/Thyroid-Exec-Summ.pdf
Thyroid Disease Manager	Website maintained by one of the leading medical experts in thyroid disorders; it contains multiple resources for healthcare providers	www.thyroidmanager.org

References

1. Klein I. T_3 and T_4: are we missing half the picture? *Clin Cornerstone.* 2005;7(suppl 2):S5-S8.
2. Tinker SC, Broussard CS, Frey MT, Gilboa SM. Prevelance of prescription medication use among non-pregnant women of childbearing age and pregnant women in the United States: NHANES, 1999-2006. *Mat Child Health J.* 2015;19(5):1097-1106.
3. U.S. Department of Agriculture, Natural Agriculture Library. Dietary reference intakes (DRIs): recommended intakes for individuals. 2010. http://www.iom.edu/Activities/Nutrition/SummaryDRIs/~/media/Files/Activity%20Files/Nutrition/DRIs/5_Summary%20Table%20Tables%201-4.pdf. Accessed June 12, 2014.
4. Carrasco N. Thyroid hormone synthesis: thyroid iodide transport. In: Braverman LE, Cooper D. *Werner and Ingbar's the Thyroid: A Fundamental and Clinical Text.* 10th ed. Philadelphia, PA: Lippincott Williams & Wilkins; 2013:32-47.
5. Brent GA, Koenig RJ. Thyroid and anti-thyroid drugs. In: Brunton LL, Chabner BA, Knollmann BC, eds. *Goodman & Gilman's the Pharmacological Basis of Therapeutics.* 12th ed. New York: McGraw-Hill; 2011:1129-1162.
6. Burgi H. Iodine excess. *Best Pract Res Clin Endocrinol Metab.* 2010;24(1):107-115.
7. Khandelwal D, Tnadon N. Overt and subclinical hypothyroidism: who to treat and how. *Drugs.* 2012; 72(1):17-33.
8. Fortunato RS, Ferreira AC, Hecht F, Dupuy C, Carvalho DP. Sexual dimorphism and thyroid dysfunction: a mater of oxidative stress? *J Endocrinol.* 2014;221:R31-R40.
9. Poppe K, Velkeniers B, Gilnoer D. The role of thyroid autoimmunity in fertility and pregnancy. *Nat Clin Pract Endocrinol Metab.* 2008;4(7):394-405.
10. Gaberšček S, Zaletel K, Schwetz V, Pieber T, Obermayer-Pietsch B, Lerchbaum E. Mechanisms in endocrinology: thyroid and polycystic ovary syndrome. *Eur Endocrinol.* 2015;172(1):R9-R21.
11. Krassas GE, Poppe K, Glinoer D. Thyroid dysfunction and hman reproductive health. *Endocr Rev.* 2010: 31(5):702-755.
12. Jameson JL, Weetman, AP. Disorders of the thyroid gland. In: Longo DL, Fauci AS, Kaspar DL, Hauser SL, Jameson JL, Loscalzo J, eds. *Harrison's Principles of Internal Medicine.* Vol 1. 18th ed. New York: McGraw-Hill; 2012:2911-2939.
13. Knudsen N, Laurberg P, Perrild H, Bülow I, Ovesen L, Jørgensen T. Risk factors for goiter and thyroid nodules. *Thyroid.* 2002;12(10):879-888.
14. Liwanpo L, Hershman JM. Conditions and drugs interfering with thyroxine absorption. *Best Pract Res Clin Endocrinol Metab.* 2009;23(6):781-792.
15. Garber JR, Cobin RH, Gharib H, et al. Clinical practice guidelines for hypothyroidism in adults: cosponsored by the American Association of Clinical Endocrinologists and the American Thyroid Association. *Endocr Pract.* 2012;18(6):988-1028.
16. Garg A, Vanderpump MP. Subclinical thyroid disease. *Br Med Bull.* 2013;107:101-116.
17. Brent GA. Clinical practice: Graves' disease. *N Engl J Med.* 2008;358(24):2594-2605.
18. Jonklaas J, Bianco AC, Bauer AJ, et al. Guidelines for the treatment of hypothyroidism prepared by the American Thyroid Association Task Force on Thyroid Hormone Replacement. *Thyroid.* 2014;24(12): 1670-1750.
19. Liwanpo L, Hershman JM. Conditions and drugs interfering with thyroxine absorption. *Best Pract Res Clin Endocrinol Metab.* 2009;23(6):781-792.

20. Singh N, Hershman JM. Interference with the absorption of levothyroxine. *Cur Opin Endocrinol Diab Obes.* 2003;10(5):347-352.
21. Bernareggi A, Grata E, Pinorini MT, Conti A. Oral liquid formulation of levothyroxine is stable in breakfast beverages and may improve thyroid patient compliance. *Pharmaceutics.* 2013;5(4):621-633.
22. Bolk N, Visser TJ, Nijman J, Jongste IJ, Tijssen JG, Berghout A. Effects of evening vs morning levothyroxine intake: a randomized double-blind crossover trial. *Arch Intern Med.* 2010;170(22):1996-2003.
23. Slagle MA. Medication update: thyroid supplements, antithyroid medications. *South Med J.* 2002; 95(5):520-521.
24. Food and Drug Administration. *FDA Letter.* Levothyroxine sodium product information. http://www.fda.gov/Drugs/DrugSafety/PostmarketDrugSafetyInformationforPatientsandProviders/ucm161257.htm. Accessed July 17, 2014.
25. Singer AJ. Combination therapy in a hypothyroid patient intolerant of elevated thyroxine. *Clin Cornerstone.* 2005;7(suppl 2):S20-S21.
26. McDermott MT. Does combination T_4 and T_3 therapy make sense? *Endocr Pract.* 2012;18(5):750-757.
27. England RJ, Kamath MB, Jabreel A, Dunne G, Atkin SL. How we do it: surgery should be considered equally with I^{131} and thionamide treatment as first-line therapy for thyrotoxicosis. *Clin Otolaryngol.* 2006; 31(2):160-162.
28. Bahn Chair RS, Burch HB, Cooper DS, et al.; American Thyroid Association; American Association of Clinical Endocrinologists. Hyperthyroidism and other causes of thyrotoxicosis: management guidelines of the American Thyroid Association and American Association of Clinical Endocrinologists. *Thyroid.* 2011;21(6):593-646.
29. Bachman ES, Hampton TG, Dhillon H, et al. The metabolic and cardiovascular effects of hyperthyroidism are largely independent of beta-adrenergic stimulation. *Endocrinology.* 2004;145(6):2767-2774.
30. Šfiligoj D, Gaberšček S, Mekjavič J, Pirnat E, Zaletel K. Factors influencing the success of radioiodine therapy in patients with Graves' disease. *Mucl Med Commun.* 2015;36(6):560-565.
31. Bonnema SJ, Bennedbaek FN, Veje A, Marving J, Hegedüs L. Continuous methimazole therapy and its effect on the cure rate of hyperthyroidism using radioactive iodine: an evaluation by a randomized trial. *J Clin Endocrinol Metab.* 2006;91(8):2946-2951.
32. Martin NM, Patel M, Nijher GM, Misra, Murphy E, Meeran K. Adjuvant lithium improves the efficacy of radioactive iodine treatment in Graves' and toxic nodular disease. *Clin Endocrinol (Oxf).* 2012; 77(4):621-627.
33. American Thyroid Association Taskforce on Radioiodine Safety, Sisson JC, Freitas J, et al. Radiation safety in the treatment of patients with thyroid diseases by radioiodine ^{131}I: practice recommendations of the American Thyroid Association. *Thyroid.* 2011; 21(4):335-346.
34. Acharya SH, Avenell A, Phillip S, Burr J, Bevan JS, Abraham P. Radioiodine therapy for Graves' disease and the effect on opthalmopathy: a systemaic review. *Clin Endocrinol (Oxf).* 2008;69(6):943-950.
35. Takata K, Amino N, Kubota S, et al. Benefit of short-term iodide supplementation to antithyroid drug treatment of thyrotoxicosis due to Graves' disease. *Clin Endocrinol (Oxf).* 2010;72(6):845-850.
36. García-Mayor RV, Larrañaga A. Treatment of Graves' hyperthyroidism with thionamides-derived drugs: review. *Med Chem.* 2010;6(4):239-246.
37. Nakamura H, Noh JY, Itoh K, Fukata S, Miyauchi A, Hamada N. Comparison of methimazole and propylthiouracil in patients with hyperthyroidism caused by Graves' disease. *J Clin Endocrinol Metab.* 2007;92(6):2157-2162.
38. Koller E, Svoboda JBD, Jones F, Moore G. Atypical antineutrophil-cytoplasmic antibodies and vasculitis-like syndrome with aphthous ulcer and violaceous pinnae after retreatment with propylthiouracil for Graves disease. *Endocrinologist.* 2006;16(1):36-40.
39. Pillinger MH, Staud R. Propylthiouracil and antineutrophil cytoplasmic antibody associated vasculitis: the detective finds a clue. *Semin Arthritis Rheum.* 2006; 36(1):1-3.
40. Bartalena L, Bogazzi F, Pinchera A, Martino E. Treatment with thionamides before radioiodine therapy for hyperthyroidism: yes or no? *J Clin Endocrinol Metab.* 2005;90(2):1256-1257.
41. Vijayakumar V, Nusynowwitz ML, Ali S. Is it safe to treat hyperthyroid patients with I-131 without fear of thyroid storm? *Ann Nucl Med.* 2006;20(6): 383-385.
42. Kundra P, Burman KD. The effect of medications on thyroid function tests. *Med Clin North Am.* 2012;96(2):283-295.
43. Dong BJ. How medications affect thyroid function. *West J Med.* 2000;172(2):102-106.

44. Barbesino G. Drugs affecting thyroid function. *Thyroid.* 2010;20(7):763-770.
45. Stagnaro-Green A, Abalovich M, Alexander E, et al; American Thyroid Association Taskforce on Thyroid Disease During Pregnancy and Postpartum. Guidelines of the American Thyroid Association for the diagnosis and management of thyroid disease during pregnancy and postpartum. *Thyroid.* 2011;21(10):1081-1125.
46. Cooper DS, Laurberg P. Hyperthyroidism in pregnancy. *Lancet Diab Endocrinol.* 2013;1(3):238-249.
47. Carney LA, Quinlan JD, West JM. Thyroid disease in pregnancy. *Am Fam Phys.* 2014;89(4):273-278.
48. Committee on Patient Safety and Quality Improvement; Committee on Professional Liability. ACOG Committee Opinion No. 381: subclinical hypothyroidism in pregnancy. *Obstet Gynecol.* 2007; 110(4):959-960.http://www.acog.org/Resources_And_Publications/Committee_Opinions/Committee_on_Obstetric_Practice/Subclinical_Hypothyroidism_in_Pregnancy. Accessed June 17, 2014.
49. De Groot L, Abalovich M, Alexander EK, et al. Management of thyroid dysfunction during pregnancy and postpartum: an Endocrine Society clinical practice guideline. *J Clin Endocrinol Metab.* 2012;97(8): 2543-2565.
50. Reid SM, Middleton P, Cossich MC, Crowther CA, Bain E. Interventions for clinical and subclinical hypothyroidism pre-pregnancy and during pregnancy. *Cochrane Database Syst Rev.* 2013;5:CD007752. doi:10.1002/14651858.CD007752.pub3.
51. Vandana, Kumar A, Khatuja R, Mehta S. Thyroid dysfunction during pregnancy and in postpartum period: treatment and latest recommendations. *Arch Gynecol Obstet.* 2014;289(5):1137-1144.
52. Boelaert K. Thyroid dysfunction in the elderly. *Nat Rev Endocrinol.* 2013;9(4):194-204.
53. De Sanctis V, Soliman A, Fiscina B. Hypoparathyroidism: from diagnosis to treatment. *Curr Opin Endocrinol Diab Obes.* 2012;19(6):435-442.
54. Farford B, Presutti J, Morahghan T. Nonsurgical management of primary hyperparathyroidism. *Mayo Clin Proc.* 2007;82(3):351-355.
55. Block GA, Ix JH, Ketteler M, et al. Phosphate homeostasis in CKD: report of a scientific symposium sponsored by the National Kidney Foundation. *Am J Kidney Dis.* 2013;62(3):457-473.
56. de Francisco ALM. New strategies for the treatment of hyperparathyroidism incorporating calcimimetics. *Expert Opin Pharmacother.* 2008;9(5): 795-811.

20 Respiratory Conditions

Barbara W. Graves

Chapter Glossary

Antigenic drift Slow changes experienced by viruses that occur through random mutations.

Antigenic shift Rapid changes experienced when two different viruses combine to produce a new subtype that has surface antigens of the two original strains. These changes are usually associated with pandemics. Antigenic shifts result from recombination of the genomes of two viral strains.

Antitussive Cough suppressive or inhibitor of cough reflex.

Decongestants Agents that reduce swelling of mucous membranes in the nasal passages and decrease nasal congestion.

Expectorants Mucolytic drugs; agents that dissolve or thin mucus to promote expulsion of sputum from the respiratory tract.

Leukotrienes Potent endogenous inflammatory mediators that induce bronchoconstriction and airway hyperresponsiveness.

Multidrug-resistant tuberculosis Tuberculosis that is resistant to at least two drugs, isoniazid and rifampin.

Rhinitis medicamentosa Rebound congestion associated with discontinuation of or decrease in the use of topical decongestants.

Introduction

Primary care providers are usually the first contact for individuals suffering with respiratory illness. Individuals often request care for respiratory conditions, but evidence-based treatments can sometimes be different from what individuals expect. This chapter reviews the pharmacologic therapy and evidence for recommended therapies of respiratory disorders that are frequently encountered during the delivery of primary care for women.

Respiratory Anatomy and Physiology

The function of the respiratory system is gas exchange—to allow the transfer of oxygen from the alveoli to the vascular system and subsequent delivery to tissues, and removal of carbon dioxide from the vascular system into the lung. To accomplish this function, there must be inflow and outflow of air, gas exchange across the alveolar membranes, and capillary circulation around the alveoli to carry the oxygen and carbon dioxide to and from the tissues. Pulmonary ventilation refers to the mechanical movement of air in and out of the lungs. Much of the volume of air in the lungs is found in dead space areas such as the trachea and bronchi, which are not involved in gas exchange. Alveolar ventilation is the volume of air expired from the alveoli themselves.

The trachea and main bronchi are surrounded by cartilage rings that maintain patency of the upper airways (Figure 20-1).[1] As the bronchi further divide, there is progressively less cartilage; indeed, the cartilage disappears completely by the level of the bronchioles. The diameter of these terminal airways ranges from 1 to 1.5 mm. The walls of the bronchioles consist of smooth muscle that is controlled by the autonomic nervous system. These airway passages are at risk for occlusion due to their small lumen sizes.[2]

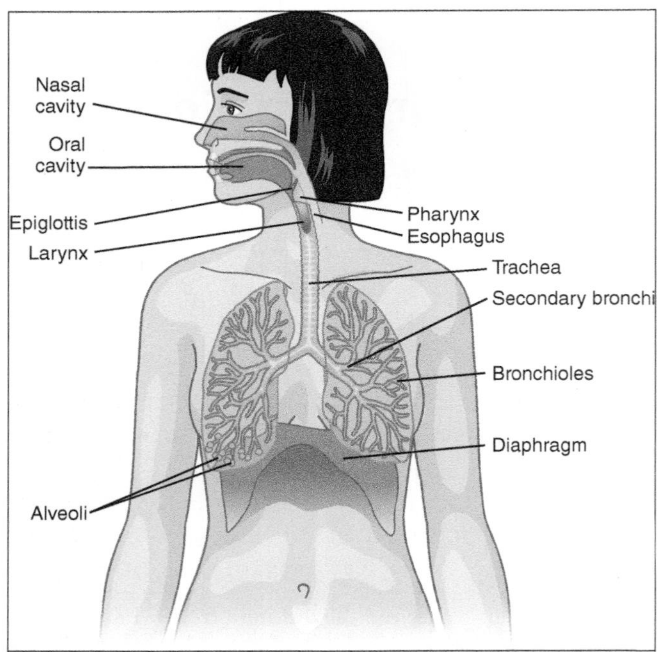

Figure 20-1 Anatomy of the respiratory tract.

Autonomic Nervous System Control of the Respiratory System

The respiratory tract responds to both sympathetic and parasympathetic stimulation. The end-organ responses to autonomic innervation are determined by both the neurotransmitter released by the postganglionic neurons and the receptor subtype displayed on the surfaces of the end-organ cells. The target organs of the parasympathetic nervous system, in addition to the sweat glands, all have the muscarinic receptors that are stimulated by the neurotransmitter acetylcholine. Two types of acetylcholine receptors are classified: muscarinic and nicotinic. Thus, drugs that stimulate acetylcholine receptors in an agonist fashion are referred to as cholinergic drugs, and those that block muscarinic or nicotinic receptors are referred to as anticholinergic drugs. Parasympathetic innervation and stimulation in the lungs cause bronchial constriction and promotion of secretions.

The sympathetic postganglionic neurons (with the exception of those innervating the sweat glands) release norepinephrine. The neurotransmitters for the sympathetic system are norepinephrine (also called noradrenaline) and epinephrine (also called adrenaline). Several adrenergic receptor subtypes exist, and the response of the target organ differs significantly depending on the receptor subtype present in that organ. For example, activation of alpha-adrenergic receptors minimally constricts the pulmonary blood vessels. Beta$_1$-adrenergic receptors are not present in the respiratory tract. In contrast, activation of beta$_2$-adrenergic receptors in the respiratory tract causes some vasodilation of the pulmonary arterioles, a more significant bronchodilation, and a vasoconstrictive effect on the nasal mucosa. Coincidentally, this is the same receptor subtype that induces uterine relaxation when stimulated by an agonist. Finally, the adrenal medulla releases epinephrine and norepinephrine. Both activate alpha$_1$- and alpha$_2$-adrenergic receptors and beta$_1$- and beta$_2$-adrenergic receptors, while norepinephrine does not activate beta$_2$ receptors.

Allergic Response of the Respiratory Tract

Mast cells are found in tissues that come in contact with the external environment, including the airway mucosa. When exposed to any of a multitude of stimuli such as antigens, anti-immunoglobulin E (IgE), or anaphylotoxins, mast cells release several inflammatory mediators, including histamine, leukotrienes, cytokines, and prostaglandins (Figure 20-2).[2,3] These substances trigger a cascade of responses in the

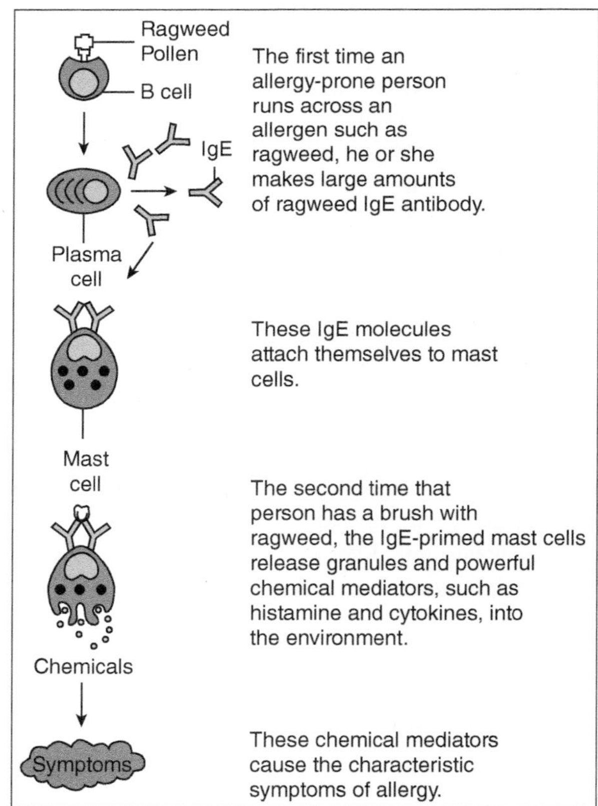

Figure 20-2 The role of mast cells in the development of an allergy.

Source: Reproduced with permission of Jeanne Kelly.

respiratory tract, including bronchoconstriction and vascular permeability. For example, **leukotrienes** are potent inflammatory mediators that induce bronchoconstriction and airway hyperresponsiveness. This, in turn, stimulates smooth muscle hypertrophy and mucus secretion. Continual stimulation of mast cells results in chronic inflammation characterized by edema, mucus plugging, and bronchial hyperreactivity.

Medications used to treat respiratory disease can be effective by treating a bacterial infection, blocking mast cell stimulation, blocking the effects of histamines or leukotrienes, or enhancing activation of $beta_2$ receptors. Anti-inflammatory medications are nonspecific agents that are used to decrease the inflammation caused by chronic stimulation $beta_2$ receptors and mast cells. Many other nonspecific medications that have little or no effect on the underlying respiratory disease often are used to counter the symptoms of respiratory illness (Box 20-1).

Upper Respiratory Infection/ Common Cold

The common cold/upper respiratory infection (URI) can be caused by more than 200 different viruses, including rhinoviruses, parainfluenza, coronaviruses, and, less often, adenoviruses or respiratory syncytial virus (RSV). The common cold is a leading cause of healthcare visits and missed days from work and school. On average, otherwise healthy adults develop two to three common cold infections per year.[4] Viruses responsible for the common cold are transmitted easily from one individual to another. Direct contact, especially hand to hand, is the most efficient mode of transmission, with significantly less virus found in aerosol emissions subsequent to coughing or sneezing.[5]

Box 20-1 Upper Respiratory Infections: To Treat or Not to Treat

Any modern pharmacy has a large amount of shelf space dedicated to various treatments for upper respiratory infections and the common cold. Despite the proliferation of such products, research indicates that most of these agents are palliative at best. Antibiotics not only are ineffective, but also are associated with increased drug resistance and expense. Because little histamine is released in such infections, antihistamines are not indicated as a treatment. Decongestants may provide mild comfort for some individuals through either topical or systemic use but are associated with unpleasant side effects. Most combination therapies include both decongestants and antihistamines. It has been said that treatment of an upper respiratory infection leaves users with some of the attributes of several of the seven dwarfs—namely, Sneezy, Sleepy, Dopey, and Grumpy. Opting not to treat an upper respiratory infection with a pharmaceutical agent is a sane choice.

Prevention and Nonpharmacologic Treatment

The primary preventive measure for the common cold is hand washing.[6] Hand-to-hand direct transmission can be decreased by the use of virucidal compounds applied to the hands. While hand treatment with 2% aqueous iodine has been shown to decrease transmission, use of this compound is unlikely to be adopted due to the staining and drying effects of iodine. Hand cleansers with ethanol alone have not been shown to be effective, although hand cleansers that have organic acids added may be more effective. Handwashing with soap and water reduces the bacterial count but is not as effective as hand cleansers with ethanol for preventing transmission of most pathogens.[7] The use of oxymetazoline (Afrin) by persons with a cold has been shown to decrease viral shedding.[8]

Pharmacologic Treatment of Upper Respiratory Infections

Upper respiratory infections include the common cold, bronchitis, influenza, and pneumonia. Many of the drugs used to treat individuals with these disorders are designed to ameliorate symptoms and are not curative. Many individuals mistakenly believe that antibiotics will cure an upper respiratory infection. In reality, not only are antibiotics ineffective for decreasing symptoms or shortening the duration of a cold, but their use can also increase the general antibiotic resistance of bacteria. Thus, when medications are recommended, it is important to help women understand how they are effective and how to best use them.

The Common Cold: Treatments for Symptomatic Relief

Medications marketed to cold sufferers include antihistamines, topical and intranasal decongestants, intranasal steroids, cough suppressants, expectorants, and mucolytics. Several meta-analyses of the effectiveness of these symptomatic treatments have been published in the *Cochrane*

Database of Systematic Reviews. At this time, there is no cure for the common cold. Although it is inappropriate to treat a cold with antibiotics, several medications can help persons with a cold feel better. Other drugs are commonly used for this purpose, but have no therapeutic benefit.

Antihistamines

Although a large meta-analysis concluded that antihistamines do not provide symptomatic relief from a cold,[9] other studies have reported a decrease in sneezing, rhinorrhea, and sometimes cough with first-generation (but not second-generation) nonsedating antihistamines.[10] Naclerio et al. demonstrated that histamine is not increased in persons with experimentally induced rhinovirus and, therefore, probably contributes little to nasal symptoms.[11] Sutter et al. theorized that the sedating and anticholinergic effects of the first-generation antihistamines, which are not present in the second-generation, nonsedating antihistamines, might alleviate some of the symptoms of the cold.[9] The combination of a first-generation antihistamine with a decongestant has been shown to decrease coughing.

Decongestants

Decongestants are sympathomimetic agents that activate alpha$_1$-adrenergic receptors on the nasal blood vessels, leading to vasoconstriction, decreased swelling of the mucous membranes, and improved nasal drainage.[12] They do not, as is commonly believed, decrease nasal secretions.[12] Decongestants are available in either systemic or topical forms, and a single dose of either a topical or systemic decongestant will diminish symptoms to some extent. Table 20-1 lists decongestants available in the United States. Use of a decongestant for 3 to 5 days often offers a significant degree of relief.

Phenylephrine (Sudafed PE) and pseudoephedrine (Sudafed) both are currently available as nonprescription oral decongestants. In recognition of the fact that pseudoephedrine is a key ingredient in the manufacture of methamphetamine, the Combat Methamphetamine Epidemic Act of 2005 was passed to ensure that pseudoephedrine is available only from pharmacists, and in limited quantities; thus it is often called a "behind-the-counter" drug.[13] While pseudoephedrine and phenylephrine have similar safety profiles, phenylephrine is more highly metabolized in the gut, and may be less effective.[14] Pseudoephedrine (Sudafed) is contraindicated for individuals who have severe hypertension, have ischemic heart disease, or are using monoamine oxidase (MAO) inhibitors (e.g., selegiline). Severe, possibly life-threatening hypertensive crisis can occur if an individual taking MAO inhibitors also takes phenylephrine or pseudoephedrine. A third nonprescriptive decongestant, phenylpropanolamine, has been removed from the market due to its association with increased risk of hemorrhagic stroke in women.

Nasal decongestants play a role in treating individuals with symptomatic rhinitis, whether it stems from an upper respiratory infection or allergic rhinitis. These agents provide symptom relief through local vasoconstriction, and they do not have the potential side effect of a hypertensive response. Short-term use to decrease congestion, especially at night, may allow for improved sleep. It is critical to counsel patients not to use topical decongestants for more than 3 days due to the risk of rebound rhinitis.[12]

Table 20-1 Decongestants

Drug: Generic (Brand)	How Supplied	Dose
Oxymetazoline 0.05% (Afrin 12 hours, Neo-Synephrine 12 hours)	Spray	2–3 sprays every 10–12 hours
Phenylephrine 0.25%–1% (Neo-Synephrine Sudafed PE, and others)	Drops	2–3 drops every 4 hours as needed
	Spray	2–3 sprays every 4 hours
	Oral	10–20 mg every 4 hours
Pseudoephedrine (Sudafed and others)	30-mg, 60-mg tablets	60 mg every 4–6 hours
	120 mg extended release	120 mg every 12 hours
Tetrahydrozoline 0.1% (Tyzine)	Drops	2–4 drops every 3 hours

Rebound Rhinitis (Rhinitis Medicamentosa)

Rebound congestion, also termed **rhinitis medicamentosa**, is an important side effect that can occur following prolonged use of topical decongestants.[12] As the profound local vasoconstrictive effect of the topical decongestant wears off, rebound swelling of the nasal mucosa and congestion develop. This phenomenon leads to continued, and at times increasing, use of the spray or drops in an attempt by the individual to relieve the congestion. When the longer-acting decongestants consisting of imidazoline derivatives such as oxymetazoline (Afrin) were introduced in the 1960s, the risk of developing rebound rhinitis was believed to be small. Further studies, however, showed that this was not the case.[15]

Research later found that healthy individuals who used either of the modern vasoconstrictors oxymetazoline or xylometazoline (e.g., Novorin, Sinutab nasal spray) for 7 to 21 days did not develop rebound rhinitis, while those with preexisting vasomotor rhinitis did.[15] Graf et al. evaluated the effects of benzalkonium chloride, which is an ingredient commonly found in decongestant preparations, versus the decongestant itself.[15] They found that both agents can induce rebound congestion, but benzalkonium chloride aggravates the severity and can induce rebound rhinitis after use for only a few days. Prolonged use for more than 30 days can lead to irreversible changes in the nasal mucosa.[16]

Once an individual has developed a dependence on nasal decongestants, it can be a challenge to discontinue them. Treatment with nasal corticosteroids at the time of decongestant withdrawal can ameliorate these symptoms.[17] Individuals who are starting use of nasal corticosteroids when they already have significant congestion also may benefit from the short-term use of imidazoline decongestants.

Combination Therapy

The majority of cold preparations are marketed as a combination of medications. In using these preparations, an individual may inadvertently consume significantly higher than recommended doses of a specific medication or, conversely, ingest subtherapeutic amounts. In addition, combination preparations often contain medications that have no benefit for the person's symptoms. For example, guaifenesin is an expectorant used in many cough preparations, but it has been shown to be of no benefit for usual cold symptoms.[18] Brand names do not necessarily indicate the specific ingredients, and reformulations are common. Therefore, professionals and consumers alike need to read the labels carefully.

Nasal Corticosteroids

Nasal administration of corticosteroids play a major role in the management of allergic rhinitis. They have no role in the symptomatic relief of nasal congestion associated with the common cold.[19]

Intranasal Ipratropium

Intranasal ipratropium (Atrovent) is an anticholinergic agent that is effective in decreasing the symptoms of cough by inhibiting vagally mediated reflexes.[20] This agent inhibits secretions from the nasal mucosa, but it has no effect on nasal congestion, sneezing, or postnasal drip. Less than 20% is absorbed systemically, and the drug quickly is metabolized into inactive metabolites. Ipratropium is safe for use during pregnancy, with no teratogenic effects reported in rats or rabbits at doses 50 to 120 times the maximum recommended adult dose. Due to the minimal systemic absorption, it is unlikely that a clinically significant amount of the drug would cross into breast milk. Adverse reactions are rare, primarily consisting of nasal dryness or epistaxis.[21] These reactions rarely lead to discontinuation of the product. Ipratropium is not commonly used by healthy women with minor conditions such as coughs associated with colds and allergies.

Cough Medicine, Expectorants, and Mucolytics

Postnasal drip is the most common etiology of the cough that accompanies the common cold. Cough medicines often are used to decrease the frequency of cough, or as a cough suppressant or **antitussive**. Other preparations, such as **expectorants** or mucolytics, are used to assist in clearing the lungs of mucus. The benefit of these agents in decreasing the symptoms of the common cold is controversial. Little evidence supports any benefit of cough medicines in ameliorating symptoms of the common cold; therefore, their use is not recommended.[22] Conversely, a combination of a first-generation antihistamine and a decongestant will lessen the cough associated with the common cold.

Analgesics

Naproxen (Naprosyn), a nonsteroidal anti-inflammatory drug (NSAID), has been reported to be effective in decreasing cough, perhaps through inhibition of the inflammatory process associated with cold symptoms.[23] A meta-analysis of a variety of NSAIDs including naproxen, however, concluded that while NSAIDs may be useful in treating aches and pains, there is no evidence that they are beneficial in treating individuals with coughs, or decreasing the duration of an upper respiratory infection.[23] Acetaminophen also provides analgesia and is effective as an antipyretic, but is inferior to ibuprofen for fever control.[4]

Complementary/Alternative Regimens

Complementary and alternative formulations promoted for treatment of the common cold fill numerous shelves in pharmacies. Herbs, homeopathic medicines, and acupuncture are all marketed for this purpose. In addition, some vitamins and minerals have been evaluated for treating colds.

Zinc

Zinc lozenges and nasal spray have grown in popularity over the last several years, since Mossad et al. reported the results of a study that demonstrated use of zinc gluconate lozenges (13.3 mg zinc) every 2 hours when awake significantly reduced the duration of cold symptoms from 7.6 days to 4.4 days ($P < .001$).[24] A more recent Cochrane review supported this finding, but advised balancing this benefit against the common side effects of bad taste, nausea, and interference with the absorption of antibiotics.[25] The same study did not find that zinc lozenges were useful for prophylaxis. The theoretical mechanism for the observed beneficial effects is the belief that zinc competes for intercellular adhesion molecule (ICAM-1) receptor sites in the nasal mucosa, thereby preventing rhinoviruses from binding to these sites.[26]

Intranasal zinc administration has a significant risk of causing irreversible anosmia—that is, loss of the sense of smell.[27] In 2009, the FDA banned nasal preparations of zinc in the United States because the risk of anosmia is unacceptably high. Based on a review of published research, the American College of Chest Physicians concluded that zinc preparations are not recommended in the treatment of common cold.[22]

Vitamin C

Vitamin C has been recommended for both prevention and treatment of the common cold, though findings from studies assessing the efficacy of vitamin C have been inconsistent. A Cochrane meta-analysis of trials evaluating the efficacy of vitamin C concluded that while there was little prophylactic benefit in the general public (relative risk [RR] = 97; 95% confidence interval [CI], 0.94–1.00), a greater benefit was demonstrated among athletes such as marathon runners, soldiers on sub-Arctic exercises, and skiers (RR = 0.48; 95% CI, 0.35–0.64).[28] No mechanism was proposed to explain these findings.

Echinacea

Results from studies of echinacea as a preventive measure and treatment for the common cold are even more conflicting. Echinacea refers to a collection of at least nine different species of American wildflowers commonly known as coneflowers. This herb is proposed to act as an immune stimulant, causing the release of tissue necrosis factor.[29] Potential side effects include allergic reactions, especially in individuals with allergies to plants such as ragweed, chrysanthemums, marigolds, and daisies. These allergic reactions may be worse than the original upper respiratory disease. The study of echinacea is complicated by the variety of species included in supplements and the inconsistent amount of active ingredient found in different products. [30] A 2014 Cochrane review concluded that echinacea was not effective in early treatment of a cold but could have a weak benefit in prophylaxis.[31] Jawad et al.[32] recently studied the effect of daily echinacea versus placebo over a 4-month period in 755 subjects. In this study population, echinacea was associated with fewer cold episodes and a shorter duration of symptoms. Given the contradictory findings, it is prudent to consider both the monetary cost and the potential for allergic reactions prior to using echinacea for either the prevention or treatment of colds.

Probiotics

There has been an increased interest in the benefits of regular consumption of probiotics as a means of warding off and ameliorating the common cold. Berggren et al.[33] performed a randomized parallel, double-blind, placebo-controlled study in which 135 subjects received probiotic supplements and 137 controls received placebos for 12 weeks. Both the incidence of colds and the symptom severity were decreased in the probiotic group. In another study, Makino et al.[34] evaluated the effects of yogurt versus milk intake in elderly individuals over an 8- to 12-week period. The risk of catching a cold was 2.6 times lower (odds ratio [OR] = 0.39; $P = 0.019$) in those who ate yogurt.

Chicken Soup

Among the traditional treatments for upper respiratory infections has been a home remedy of chicken soup. Interestingly, Rennard et al. found some antiviral effects with the ingestion of chicken soup.[35] However, there are no data supporting clinical use of this gastronomic intervention.

Menthol and Saline Irrigation

Many over-the-counter cough lozenges contain menthol. When Wise et al.[36] studied the effectiveness of menthol inhalation prior to inducing a cough challenge, they found that those subjects who received the treatment had reduced coughing when compared to a control group whose members inhaled either pine oil or air.

Saline irrigation has been shown to promote mucociliary clearance and removal of crusted mucus. Although saline sprays are often used to reduce congestion, there have not been any studies that confirmed any benefit from their application.[37]

Special Populations: Pregnancy, Lactation, and the Elderly

The nasal and respiratory tract mucosa become edematous as a response to the hormones present during pregnancy.

Thus, nasal congestion is common during pregnancy and becomes more frequent as the pregnancy progresses. With this physiologic change, the nasal symptoms of allergic rhinitis or upper respiratory infections are likely to be exacerbated.

Two major surveys have studied the extent of medication use during pregnancy. The National Birth Defect Prevention Study is a population-based, case-control study of birth defects, conducted by performing standardized interviews of mothers of case subjects with major structural birth defects and control subjects with no major birth defects between 1997 and 2001. Women are asked specific questions about medications taken during pregnancy.[38] The Boston University Slone Epidemiology Center Birth Defects Study conducts similar interviews and has presented its findings for women interviewed between 1998 and 2004.[39,40] In both of these studies, approximately 70% to 75% of pregnant women took an analgesic during pregnancy, 16% to 27% used a decongestant, 8% to 14% took an antihistamine, and 9% to 13% used some form of cough medicine. These rates of medication use during pregnancy are higher than the reported rates during the 3 months prior to conception.[39] None of the commonly used medications has been shown to be teratogenic, but without further research, it is impossible to state with confidence that they have no adverse effects on the fetus. In the absence of such studies, providers should caution pregnant women to avoid casual use of over-the-counter medications and offer suggestions for nonpharmacologic comfort measures instead.

Pharmacologic therapy poses more risks to the elderly than among younger persons. In particular, the presence of comorbidities and other medications may preclude decongestant use in older adults. Confusion and altered mental status may be more common effects of cough preparations or antihistamines. Prior to recommending over-the-counter cold preparations, a complete medical history and documentation of medications used is essential with older women. As with pregnant women, it is prudent to offer suggestions for nonpharmacologic comfort measures rather than medications.

Pharyngitis

Pharyngitis, which may or may not be associated with symptoms of the common cold, is a frequent cause of healthcare visits. Approximately 80% to 95% of these infections are viral in origin.[41] Motivations to treat them empirically include concerns about the possibility of developing adverse sequelae, including peritonsillar abscess and acute rheumatic fever, and the relief of symptoms. Despite the low incidence of a bacterial (usually group A *Streptococcus*) etiology, antibiotics are frequently prescribed without lab testing or application of specific diagnostic criteria. Crocker et al.[42] performed a retrospective cohort study evaluating adherence to accepted practice guidelines for pharyngitis in an ambulatory faculty practice. They found only 24% adherence to guidelines.[43] Given the growing concerns about overuse of antibiotics, encouragement of adherence to accepted guidelines offers a substantial opportunity to decrease nonindicated antibiotic use.

Practice guidelines for the management of pharyngitis have differed in terms of whether they recommend beginning treatment only after diagnostic testing or initiating treatment based on the symptom profile. The debate centers on the relative worth of limiting inappropriate antibiotic use versus balancing symptom relief. In 1981, Robert Centor, an emergency room physician, proposed clinical criteria that could assist in differentiating viral from bacterial pharyngitis.[43] These criteria, known as the Centor score (Table 20-2), have since been modified to take the individual's age into account due to the varying incidence of streptococcal pharyngitis based on age.[44–46]

Aalbers et al.[45] conducted a meta-analysis to determine the diagnostic accuracy of the Centor score. The predictive value of the score was improved in areas of higher prevalence and in cases of known exposure. Individual criteria, however, were inadequate in distinguishing bacterial from viral infection. Conversely, scores of 3 or higher

Table 20-2 The Centor Score

Symptoms	Points
Tonsillar exudates	1
History of fever	1
Tender anterior cervical lymphadenopathy	1
Absence of cough	1
Possible score	0–4
Additional criterion	
Age	
< 15	1
> 44	−1

Sources: Modified from Aalbers J, O'Brien KK, Chan WS, et al. Predicting streptococcal pharyngitis in adults in primary care: a systematic review of the diagnostic accuracy of symptoms and signs and validation of the Centor score. *BMC Med.* 2011;9:67. doi:10.1186/1741-7015-9-67[45]; with data from McIsaac WJ, Kellner JD, Aufricht P, Vanjaka A, Low DE. Empirical validation of guidelines for the management of pharyngitis in children and adults. *JAMA.* 2004;291(13):1587-1595.[44]

had an overall specificity of 82% and a sensitivity of 49%, and scores of 4 had a specificity of 95% and a sensitivity of 18%.[46] Given these results, treating everyone with a Centor score of 4 seems reasonable, while treating those with a score of 3 or higher could lead to the inappropriate use of antibiotics, and the use of diagnostic testing might be considered. No testing is indicated with scores of 0 to 1. The Infectious Disease Society of America[46] and the American Academy of Pediatrics/American Heart Association[47] recommend against treating pharyngitis empirically.

Group A Streptococcal Pharyngitis (Strep Throat)

Penicillin remains the drug of choice to treat group A streptococcal pharyngitis. The dose of penicillin and alternative antibiotic regimens are presented in Table 20-3. Intramuscular administration of benzathine penicillin G is an alternative for individuals who are likely not to complete the 10-day course. The majority of individuals who are allergic to penicillin can be treated safely with a narrow-spectrum cephalosporin such as cephalexin (Keflex). For those individuals with cross-allergy to both penicillin and cephalosporins, clindamycin (Cleocin) can be used—it has a 1% rate of resistance in the United States. Other options for allergic individuals include macrolides such as erythromycin (E-Mycin), clarithromycin (Biaxin), and azithromycin (Zithromax). Unfortunately, there is increasing macrolide resistance by group A *Streptococcus*, reaching as much as 12% to 15% in some population centers in the United States.[46,48]

Table 20-3 Antibiotic Treatments for Group A *Streptococcus* Pharyngitis

Drug: Generic (Brand)	Dose	Duration of Therapy
Ampicillin (Amoxil)	500 mg 3 times/day	10 days
Benzathine penicillin G	1.2 million units IM	One dose for individuals who may not be able to complete a 10-day course of oral antibiotic
Penicillin V oral	250 mg 4 times/day or 500 mg 2 times/day	10 days
For Penicillin Allergy		
Azithromycin (Zithromax)	500 mg once daily on first day followed by 250 mg once daily for 4 days	5 days
Cephalexin (Keflex)	500 mg 2 times/day	10 days
Clarithromycin (Biaxin)	250 mg 2 times/day	10 days
Clindamycin (Cleocin)	300 mg 3 times/day	10 days

Sources: Data from Shulman ST, Bisno AL, Clegg HW, et al. Clinical practice guideline for the diagnosis and management of group A streptococcal pharyngitis: 2012 update by the Infectious Diseases Society of America. *Clin Infect Dis.* 2012;55(10):1279-1282[46]; Gerber MA, Baltimore RS, Eaton CB, et al. Prevention of rheumatic fever and diagnosis and treatment of acute streptococcal pharyngitis: a scientific statement from the American Heart Association Rheumatic Fever, Endocarditis, and Kawasaki Disease Committee of the Council on Cardiovascular Disease in the Young, the Interdisciplinary Council on Functional Genomics and Translational Biology, and the Interdisciplinary Council on Quality of Care and Outcomes Research: endorsed by the American Academy of Pediatrics. *Circulation.* 2009;119(11):1541-1551.[47]

Acute Bronchitis

Bronchitis is an infection of the bronchi. Acute bronchitis usually is a secondary infection caused by a virus or bacterium; it can last for several days or weeks. By comparison, chronic bronchitis is prolonged irritation of the bronchial epithelium. Viruses cause more than 90% of cases of acute bronchitis, with the rest being caused by *Chlamydia pneumoniae, Mycoplasma pneumoniae,* or *Bordetella pertussis. Streptococcus pneumoniae, Haemophilus influenzae,* and *Moraxella catarrhalis* are much less common causes, but they may be the etiology in individuals who have chronic lung conditions.

Acute bronchitis is a frequent reason for visits to the healthcare provider and one of the most common causes of inappropriate prescribing of antibiotics.[49] Unlike the common cold, which rarely presents with systemic symptoms, acute bronchitis may cause such symptoms as fatigue and headaches, in addition to respiratory symptoms such as rhinorrhea, postnasal drip, dyspnea, and productive cough. The diagnosis of acute bronchitis should be considered for persons whose cough persists longer than 5 days.[50] The cough is accompanied by bronchial hyperreactivity and wheezing. Individuals with acute bronchitis rarely have accompanying fever, malaise, aches and pains, tachypnea, or rales. Individuals who present with a temperature higher than 100.4°F (38°C), pulse higher than 100 beats per minute, respiratory rate faster than 24 breaths per minute, or crackles on inspiration should be evaluated with a chest X ray for pneumonia,[50] and those with a paroxysmal cough, especially one followed with emesis, should be evaluated for *B. pertussis.*[50] Acute bronchitis usually resolves spontaneously within 3 weeks. Historically, treatment of acute bronchitis has consisted of medications from one of three categories: antibiotics, cough suppression/expectorants, and bronchodilators.

Antibiotics

Smith et al.[52] performed a meta-analysis of studies comparing antibiotic use with placebo for the treatment of acute bronchitis and found that antibiotics made no difference in improving night cough, frequency of productive cough, or duration of limitations on activities of daily living. Slight, albeit statistically significant decreases in the duration of cough, duration of productive cough, and a general feeling of illness were found, although the clinical significance of this finding is questionable, except possibly in persons who are elderly, are frail, and have multiple comorbidities.

Assuming that, at best, there is a modest benefit of antibiotics, given the ongoing concerns about developing antibiotic resistance, the routine use of antibiotics is not recommended for individuals with acute bronchitis who are otherwise healthy. The Centers for Disease Control and Prevention (CDC) has been working to educate providers on the inappropriate use of antibiotics for acute bronchitis.[53] Despite these efforts, providers continue to prescribe antibiotics for acute bronchitis in approximately 71% of primary care or emergency room visits.[54] Further research is necessary to provide guidance about use of antibiotics in various subsets of the population, such as smokers, persons with asthma, and individuals whose symptoms are severe.

Cough Suppressants, Expectorants, and Mucolytics

While cough medications show a notable lack of efficacy in treating the common cold, they may be more effective in treating symptoms of bronchitis by acting on one of several pathways involved in the etiology of cough (Table 20-4). For example, a medication could alter the mucoid component either by decreasing production, decreasing the viscosity, or improving ciliary function; by centrally suppressing the cough reflex; or by increasing mucus secretion, allowing such secretions to be expectorated more easily. Various other medications that are often used for the relief of chronic cough include antihistamines, antihistamine–decongestants combinations, and beta-mimetics.[51] Smith et al., following completion of their meta-analysis, concluded that there is no good evidence for or against the effectiveness of over-the-counter medications for treating an acute cough.[52]

Guaifenesin (Mucinex, Tussin), which is a component of many cough medicine formulations, is a mucociliary drug that is theorized to increase the volume and reduce the viscosity of secretions in the trachea and bronchi. Originally derived from the guaiac tree and used by Native Americans, this agent is thought to increase respiratory tract secretions and decrease mucus viscosity, although high-quality studies documenting this effect are lacking.[53] Interestingly, guaifenesin is also used by women to facilitate conception via thinning and increasing the amount of cervical mucus. To date, no studies have evaluated the effectiveness of this treatment.

Cough medications such as guaifenesin also may block the perception of the stimulus to cough—that is, the afferent limb of the reflex. A third mechanism, which is probably the most commonly employed, is suppression of the cough reflex in the central nervous system. Codeine and dextromethorphan hydrobromide (Robitussin), for example, are centrally acting cough suppressants. They are rapidly absorbed and well distributed into the central nervous system. Dextromethorphan metabolism varies according to polymorphic phenotypes, with approximately 10% of Caucasians being poor metabolizers, and it is excreted by the kidneys. The half-life is 1.4 to 3.9 hours for the drug and 3.4 to 5.6 hours for its metabolites. Codeine metabolism

Table 20-4 Medications to Treat Cough

Drug: Generic (Brand)	Dose	Level of Evidence[a]	Grade of Recommendation[b]
Mucociliary			
First-generation antihistamines	Refer to *Antihistamines* chapter	Fair	A
Guaifenesin (Mucinex, Tussin)	200–600 mg PO 4 times/day	Good	C/D
Ipratropium (Atrovent HFA) (inhaled)	40–80 mcg inhaled 4 times/day	Fair	A
Central Suppressants			
Codeine	10–20 mg PO 3–4 times/day	Fair	B
Dextromethorphan polistirex (Delsym)	30 mg PO 2 times/day	Fair	C
Unclassified			
Benzonatate (Tessalon Perles)	100–200 mg PO 3 times/day	N/A	N/A
Zinc	Variable	Fair	D

[a] Good = evidence from randomized trials; Fair = evidence from controlled trials without randomization, cohort or case-control analytic studies, or comparisons between times or places.

[b] A = good evidence to recommend the action; B = fair evidence to recommend the action; C = existing evidence is inconclusive and does not allow making a recommendation for or against the action; D = fair evidence to recommend against the action.

Sources: Data from Bolser DC. Cough suppressant and pharmacologic protussive therapy: ACCP evidence-based clinical practice guidelines. *Chest.* 2006;129(1 suppl):238S-249S[22]; Smith SM, Schroeder K, Fahey T. Over-the-counter (OTC) medications for acute cough in children and adults in ambulatory settings. *Cochrane Database Syst Rev.* 2012;8:CD001831.[53]

is also affected by polymorphic phenotype. The half-life for codeine is between 3 and 4 hours. This drug crosses the placenta and passes into breast milk. Both codeine and dextromethorphan have dissociative effects and the potential for abuse. In fact, abuse of dextromethorphan appears to be more prevalent than abuse of heroin, crack cocaine, methamphetamines, or anabolic steroids.[55]

Co-ingestion of dextromethorphan and either MAO inhibitors or selective serotonin reuptake inhibitors (SSRIs) can result in serotonin syndrome.[56] Recent research has found that most individuals do not have any risk for abuse of dextromethorphan; however, individuals who have the polymorphism that results in higher expression of CYP2D6 are extensive metabolisers of dextromethorphan and these individuals appear at the highest risk for abusing this drug. Dextromethorphan hydrobromide is available in the United States only in combination with other drugs such as promethazine (Phenergan), pseudoephedrine, or brompheniramine. Another preparation—dextromethorphan polistirex (Delsym)—is available over the counter as a single agent.

Benzonatate (Tessalon Perles) is a local anesthetic that can decrease cough. Side effects from this medication are more common when greater than the recommended dose is ingested, and may include numbness of the mouth and throat. Benzonatate is used for the treatment of opioid-resistant cough associated with lung cancer. However, no evidence has been found to support its use in treatment of acute cough.

While evidence consistently supports the effectiveness of cough suppressants in the treatment of chronic bronchitis, such agents have not been shown to be effective in treating acute bronchitis or the common cold. Despite the absence of adequate evidence of their use in acute bronchitis, the American College of Chest Physicians concluded that it is reasonable to employ these medications to reduce severe coughing.[22]

Beta$_2$ Agonists

The use of beta$_2$ agonists has been suggested to treat the bronchial reactivity and subsequent decreased airflow and wheezing associated with acute bronchitis. Beta$_2$ agonists activate the beta$_2$-adrenergic receptors, which in turn increases cyclic adenosine monophosphate (cAMP), promoting bronchodilation, reducing bronchospasm, and suppressing histamine release. A Cochrane review found that while little evidence supports the routine use of beta$_2$ agonists in the treatment of acute bronchitis, these agents may be effective in reducing coughing in those persons with evidence of airflow obstruction.[57]

Complementary and Alternative Treatments

Observational research has supported the benefit in treating bronchitis with a liquid herbal drug preparation of *Pelargonium sidoides* (EPs 7630) that is purported to have antibacterial and antiviral capabilities.[58] Further well-controlled randomized clinical trials (RCTs) are needed before conclusions can be drawn about its efficacy.

Chinese medicinal herbs are also employed to treat the symptoms of bronchitis. Various herbs are compounded depending on the specific array of symptoms for any given individual. Some of the herbs that have been studied include yu xing cao, radix Scutellaria, radix glycyrrhizae, and Shi Wei Long Dan Hua Ke Li. While a review of the literature demonstrated some benefit from such preparations, the methodologic quality of the included studies was poor. There was no standardization of purity of the herbs, their dosing, or selection of herbs to be included. None of the studies were blinded, and the outcomes were poorly defined. Little information on any adverse effects of the herbs was provided. This area is another category of herbal/pharmacologic treatment that warrants further study.[59]

Influenza

When compared to the viruses responsible for the common cold or acute bronchitis, influenza viruses cause significantly more morbidity and mortality. The onset of symptoms tends to be more acute and symptoms are more severe with these infections, including sore throat, cough and rhinitis, high fever, headaches, muscle aches, and extreme fatigue.

Two major types of influenza virus exist—influenza A and influenza B. Both viruses are spread primarily by respiratory droplet transmission. Influenza A is more prone to **antigenic shift** than influenza B, which is why influenza A is associated with pandemics. Influenza B viruses undergo less dramatic and slower antigenic changes, known as **antigenic drift**. While these distinctions are critical for epidemiologic surveillance and vaccine development, they cannot be differentiated on the basis of clinical presentation. Moreover, antibodies against one strain of influenza virus do not confer immunity to other strains.[61,62]

Following an incubation period of 1 to 4 days, symptoms (fever, headaches, muscle aches, sore throat, cough, rhinitis, and fatigue) develop abruptly. While most of the symptoms resolve after 3 to 7 days in the majority of persons, cough and malaise may continue for more than

2 weeks. Influenza can lead to complications such as viral pneumonia, secondary bacterial pneumonia, or sinusitis, and it can exacerbate comorbidities. Annual vaccination against influenza is the primary weapon against the infection and subsequent complications and is discussed in the *Immunizations* chapter.

Antiviral Medications

Antiviral medications play a role in both chemoprophylaxis and treatment for influenza. Oseltamivir (Tamiflu) and zanamivir (Relenza) are neuraminidase inhibitors, which are effective against both influenza A and B. Amantadine (Symmetrel, Symadine) and rimantadine (Flumadine) are antiviral agents that had been approved for the treatment of influenza in the past, but they should no longer be used because influenza A has high levels of resistance to these medications.[60] Mutations have been appearing in the H1N1 viruses,[62] which are a subtype of influenza virus; although these mutations have the potential to increase oseltamivir resistance, the majority of human influenza viruses were still susceptible to the medication in 2013.[63] Oseltamivir is less effective against influenza B viruses than influenza A viruses.[64] At least two new neuraminidase inhibitors, peramivir and laninamivir, have been developed and are being used in Asia, but have not yet been approved by the FDA.

In recent years, the effectiveness of neuraminidase inhibitors had been called into question. Jefferson et al.[65] performed a systematic review of randomized controlled trials to evaluate the benefits of oseltamivir in preventing transmission, relieving symptoms, and shortening the course of the illness. They concluded that the drug has a modest effect in reducing symptomatic influenza. It also reduced the duration of symptomatic illness by approximately 17 hours in adults and by 30 hours in healthy children, but no benefit was seen in children with asthma. Nausea, vomiting, and headaches were observed as side effects. Concern has also been raised about the potential for increased psychiatric adverse events while taking oseltamivir.

The CDC has critiqued these findings by noting that most of the studies included healthy adults, rather than the highest-risk populations. The CDC has also cited a number of observational studies of high-risk groups or severely ill individuals that support the benefits of oseltamivir (Tamiflu). This federal agency continues to recommend the use of antivirals by persons at high risk for complications, including children younger than 2 years, adults older than 65 years, individuals with chronic illnesses, pregnant or recently postpartum women, persons who are morbidly obese, and residents of nursing homes or other long-term care facilities.[66]

When used for treatment, both oseltamivir and zanamivir should be initiated within 2 days of the onset of symptoms. Initiation of treatment later than 2 days after the development of symptoms has no effect on the duration of uncomplicated influenza, and there are no data available concerning any potential benefit on decreasing complications. The recommended doses for oseltamivir and zanamivir are presented in Table 20-5.

Chemoprophylaxis with Antivirals

Oseltamivir and zanamivir can be used for chemoprophylaxis by individuals who have contraindications to vaccination or those at high risk for developing complications (e.g., individuals who are immunosuppressed). In this case, either antiviral should be taken daily throughout the community flu season. Chemoprophylaxis may also be appropriate for individuals who have an increased risk for

Table 20-5 Recommended Daily Dose of Influenza Antiviral Medications for Treatment and Chemoprophylaxis—United States

Drug:		Age Group (Years)	
Generic (Brand)	Indication	13–64	≥ 65
Oseltamivir (Tamiflu)[a]	Treatment, influenza A and B	75 mg 2 times/day	75 mg 2 times/day
	Chemoprophylaxis, influenza A and B	75 mg/day	75 mg/day
Zanamivir (Relenza)[b]	Treatment, influenza A and B	10 mg (2 inhalations) 2 times/day	10 mg (2 inhalations) 2 times/day
	Chemoprophylaxis, influenza A and B	10 mg (2 inhalations) 2 times/day	10 mg (2 inhalations) 2 times/day

[a] Oseltamivir is manufactured by Roche Pharmaceuticals (Tamiflu—tablet). It is approved for treatment or chemoprophylaxis of persons 1 year and older.
Source: Data from Fiore AE, Fry A, Shay D, et al. Antiviral agents for the treatment and chemoprophylaxis of influenza: recommendations of the Advisory Committee on Immunization Practices (ACIP). *MMWR Recommend Rep.* 2011;60(1):1-24.[66]
[b] Zanamivir is manufactured by GlaxoSmithKline (Relenza—inhaled powder). It is approved for treatment of persons 7 years and older and approved for chemoprophylaxis of persons 5 years and older. Zanamivir is administered through oral inhalation by using a plastic device included in the medication package. Individuals will benefit from instruction and demonstration of the correct use of the device. Zanamivir is not recommended for persons with underlying airway disease.

complications and who are vaccinated after the flu season has begun but have not yet developed antibodies (approximately 2 weeks in adults). Chemoprophylaxis may also be appropriate in the event of an influenza outbreak with a strain not included in the vaccine, or in a residential setting such as a nursing home despite adequate vaccination.

Mechanism of Action

Oseltamivir and zanamivir both inhibit neuraminidase, an enzyme required for viral replication. Oseltamivir is well absorbed after oral administration. The drug is metabolized by the liver to oseltamivir carboxylate, the active neuraminidase inhibitor. Oseltamivir carboxylate has a half-life of 6 to 10 hours and is excreted in the urine by glomerular filtration and tubular secretion.

Zanamivir is administered as inhaled powder, with 70% to 87% being deposited in the oropharynx and approximately 7% to 21% of the orally inhaled dose reaching the lungs. A small percentage of the total amount of orally inhaled zanamivir is systemically absorbed. Systemically absorbed zanamivir has a half-life of 2.5 to 5.1 hours and is excreted unchanged in the urine. Unabsorbed drug is excreted in the feces.[67]

Side Effects/Adverse Effects

Nausea and vomiting occur in approximately 10% of adults taking oseltamivir, compared to 4% to 6% of those taking placebo. In addition, neuropsychiatric symptoms such as hallucinations and delirium, which can be associated with untreated influenza, have been rarely reported in persons taking oseltamivir. Thus, individuals taking this agent should be aware of these reactions and be closely monitored for signs of unusual behavior.

Zanamivir is approved only for individuals without underlying respiratory or cardiac disease.[67] For persons with uncomplicated influenza, the frequency of adverse effects is no different for individuals inhaling zanamivir compared to individuals taking the inhaled lactose vehicle alone.[68] No specific drug interactions have been reported.

Special Populations: Pregnancy, Lactation, and the Elderly

Compared to the general population, pregnant women are at a higher risk for developing complications of influenza, including pneumonia.[66,69] It is recommended that all women who are or plan to be pregnant during flu season be vaccinated against influenza.[70] No human clinical studies have evaluated the use of oseltamivir and zanamivir in pregnancy, however, and animal studies have not found teratogenic effects. Given that influenza can be a very serious illness in pregnant women, the CDC recommends using either drug for treatment or prophylaxis if needed by a pregnant woman.[68]

Elderly persons are also likely to experience higher levels of morbidity from influenza, and both oseltamivir and zanamivir are recommended for use in this population. No reduction in the dose of oseltamivir or zanamivir is needed on the basis of age.[66]

Community-Acquired Pneumonia

Community-acquired pneumonia is an infection of the pulmonary parenchyma that is acquired in the community, as opposed to the hospital or other healthcare facilities. It is the eighth leading cause of death, and most common infectious cause of death, in the United States, and a significant cause of morbidity.[71] Approximately 31% to 49% of low-risk individuals who visit the emergency room with community-acquired pneumonia are admitted to the hospital.[72] As with influenza, prevention is an important component in the control of pneumonia. The Advisory Committee on Immunization Practices of the CDC advises that in addition to receiving influenza vaccination, the following groups should receive the pneumococcal polysaccharide vaccine: (1) individuals 65 years or older; (2) persons with high-risk conditions, including chronic cardiovascular, respiratory, renal, or liver disease; diabetes mellitus; alcoholism; or immunosuppression; (3) residents of long-term care facilities; and (4) smokers between 19 and 64 years.[73]

The pathophysiology of pneumonia involves a failure of the usual defense systems to protect the lower airways from colonization with pathogens. Microorganisms can gain access and take hold due to ineffective ciliary action, decreased mucus velocity, interference with immunoglobulin A (IgA), or an innate virulence of the pathogen. The most common route of exposure is by microaspiration. Any underlying condition that compromises an individual's defenses can increase the risk of pneumonia.

Implementation of guidelines for the management of community-acquired pneumonia has been associated with decreases in important clinical outcomes such as mortality and rate of hospitalization.[72] The decision regarding the appropriate site of care for individuals with community-acquired pneumonia is critical, and validated guidelines for determining who needs hospitalization versus who can be managed on an outpatient basis are available (Box 20-2).

Box 20-2 The Case of a Cough

DS, a 54-year-old nurse, reports having a productive cough and fatigue for 2 weeks. She has mild intermittent asthma but has been using salmeterol (Advair) for the last week, thinking her cough was related to her asthma. She was treated for rhinosinusitis 4 weeks ago with amoxicillin (Amoxil) 500 mg 3 times a day for 10 days with fair relief of her symptoms.

Further questioning reveals that this cough was not preceded by any upper respiratory symptoms. While DS feels generally "under the weather," she denies any headache, muscle aches, or pains, except pain associated with her cough. Her physical exam is significant for a temperature of 100.8°F and a respiratory rate of 28; no wheezing is auscultated, but she does have crackles on inspiration in her right lower lobe.

The differential diagnosis for DS includes bronchitis, influenza, pneumonia, and tuberculosis. When questioned about possible exposure to tuberculosis, DS reports her tuberculin skin test was negative 3 months ago, and she does not believe she has been exposed to anyone with tuberculosis. Because her major symptom is cough unrelated to systemic symptoms such as headache or malaise, she is unlikely to have influenza. Bronchitis is usually preceded by an upper respiratory infection and is rarely associated with fever or tachypnea. As DS has a low-grade fever and is tachypneic, the most likely diagnosis is community-acquired pneumonia. Following the Infectious Diseases Society of America/American Thoracic Society consensus guidelines, a chest X ray is taken, and it confirms the diagnosis.

DS's condition is compatible with outpatient therapy. Because she has recently received antibiotic treatment, she is at risk for infection with drug-resistant *S. pneumoniae*. Therefore, the best treatment is moxifloxacin (Avelox) 400 mg by mouth daily for 5 days. If she is still febrile after 3 days, the treatment should be extended to 7 days.

The organisms most commonly causing community-acquired pneumonia in ambulatory, immunocompetent adults include *Streptococcus pneumoniae*, *Mycoplasma pneumoniae*, *Haemophilus influenzae*, and *Chlamydia pneumoniae*. Respiratory viruses, including influenza, adenovirus, respiratory syncytial virus, and parainfluenza, are responsible for about as many cases as each of the previously mentioned bacteria.

Treatment of Community-Acquired Pneumonia

One concern that arises in regard to empiric treatment of community-acquired pneumonia is the increasing drug resistance of *S. pneumoniae*. From 1987 through 2005, macrolide resistance to *S. pneumoniae* increased from 0.2% to 29.6%, but it appears to have leveled off since 2000.[72] In addition to macrolide resistance, *S. pneumoniae* has developed significant beta-lactam resistance. Resistance to the fluoroquinolones—that is, ciprofloxacin (Cipro) and levofloxacin (Levaquin)—has also been noted. However, community-acquired pneumonia usually responds to appropriate regimens of amoxicillin (Amoxil), ceftriaxone (Rocephin), or cefotaxime (Claforan). Risk factors for infection with drug-resistant *S. pneumoniae*—namely, recent or repeated treatment with macrolides, fluoroquinolones, or beta-lactams; 65 years or older; residence in a long-term care facility; and daycare attendance—should be considered when choosing the most appropriate antibiotic regimen.[74] Despite the concerns regarding increasing drug resistance, most healthy adults will respond well to empiric antibiotic therapy.[75] The most recent consensus guidelines of the Infectious Diseases Society of America and the American Thoracic Society for recommended antibiotic outpatient treatment of community-acquired pneumonia as of mid-2014 are presented in Table 20-6. The treatment of hospitalized patients is beyond the scope of this chapter.

Duration of Treatment

Community-acquired pneumonia has traditionally been treated for 7 to 10 days, although this duration was not evaluated by well-controlled studies. Several studies have demonstrated comparable efficacy with shorter durations of therapy.[76] Shorter duration of therapy can improve adherence to the regimen and reduce the emergence of resistance organisms.[76] The Infectious Diseases Society of America/American Thoracic Society consensus guidelines recommend that before discontinuing therapy, individuals with community-acquired pneumonia be treated for at least 5 days, be afebrile for 48 to 72 hours, and be clinically stable.[72]

Special Populations: Pregnancy and the Elderly

The incidence of pneumonia in pregnant women is similar to the incidence in the nonpregnant population of women. Given the physiologic changes in the respiratory system during pregnancy, however, the risk of

Table 20-6 Antibiotics Recommended for Outpatient Treatment of Community-Acquired Pneumonia

Drug: Generic (Brand)	Dose
Otherwise Healthy and No Risk Factors for Drug-Resistant S. pneumoniae	
Azithromycin (Zithromax)	500 mg on day 1 and then 250 mg daily for 4 days
Clarithromycin (Biaxin)	500 mg 2 times/day for 5 days
Clarithromycin XL	1000 mg once/day for 5 days
Doxycycline	100 mg 2 times/day for 5 days
Erythromycin base	250–500 mg every 6–12 hours
Erythromycin ethylsuccinate (EES)	400–800 mg every 6–12 hours
Presence of Comorbidities[a]	
Amoxicillin (Amoxil) + a macrolide[b]	1 g 3 times/day plus a macrolide as noted above for 5 days
Amoxicillin–clavulanate (Augmentin)	2 g 2 times/day plus a macrolide as noted above for 5 days
Ceftriaxone (Rocephin), cefpodoxime (Vantin), or cefuroxime (Ceftin)	500 mg 2 times/day for 5 days
Gemifloxacin (Factive)	320 mg once daily
Levofloxacin (Levaquin)	750 mg once/day for 5 days
Moxifloxacin (Avelox)	400 mg once/daily
Regions with More Than 25% Macrolide-Resistant S. pneumoniae	
Gemifloxacin (Factive)	320 mg once daily
Levofloxacin (Levaquin)	750 mg once/day for 5 days
Moxifloxacin (Avelox)	400 mg once/daily

[a] Comorbidities include alcoholism, malignancy, immunosuppression, use of antibiotics within the previous 3 months (a different class of drugs should be selected), other risks for drug-resistant *S. pneumoniae*, or residence in a region in which prevalence of high-level macrolide-resistant *S. pneumoniae* is greater than 25%.

[b] Doxycycline (Vibramycin) is the alternative to the macrolide.

Source: Data from Mandell LA, Wunderink RG, Anzueto A, et al. Infectious Diseases Society of America/American Thoracic Society consensus guidelines on the management of community-acquired pneumonia in adults. *Clin Infect Dis.* 2007;44(suppl 2):S27-S72.[72]

complications—including need for mechanical ventilation, bacteremia, and empyema—is higher. The causative organisms are generally similar to those found in non-pregnant individuals, though varicella is another cause of community-acquired pneumonia in pregnant women. While it is a rare complication in the general population, as many as 9% of pregnant women with varicella may develop pneumonia.[77] Empiric treatment with beta-lactam and macrolide antibiotics is safe and effective in pregnant women. Fluoroquinolones and clarithromycin (Biaxin) should be avoided.[77]

Elderly individuals are at increased risk for the development of pneumonia and its complications, may present with fewer signs or symptoms than younger individuals, and are less likely to be febrile. Recommended antibiotics for the elderly are the same as for younger populations after an evaluation of other medications used and possible drug–drug interactions has been conducted.

Rhinosinusitis

Rhinosinusitis is the infection of one of the paranasal sinuses, usually following an upper respiratory infection that leads to inflammation of the sinuses; it is somewhat arbitrarily classified as acute, subacute, chronic, or recurrent (Table 20-7).[78] In 2012, 28.5 million adults were diagnosed with sinusitis, a number equivalent to approximately 12.1% of all noninstitutionalized adults.[79]

Because this disorder is accompanied by inflammation of the nasal mucosa, *rhinosinusitis* has replaced *sinusitis* as the preferred term.[80] In the vast majority of persons afflicted, the viral URI and resultant inflammation resolve spontaneously within 10 days with no complications; however, the inflammation from the preceding viral URI may prevent drainage of the sinuses, setting the stage for bacterial infection in the sinuses. At that point, a secondary acute aerobic bacterial infection (acute bacterial rhinosinusitis) develops, usually secondary to *S. pneumoniae, H. influenzae*, or *M. catarrhalis* infection. Over time, if the acute bacterial infection persists, the ongoing edema, compromised blood supply, and oxygen consumption by the aerobes, anaerobic bacteria, and coagulase-negative begin to take hold.

Acute Bacterial Rhinosinusitis

The Agency for Healthcare Research and Quality performed a meta-analysis to compare the efficacies of antibiotics and placebo in the treatment of acute bacterial rhinosinusitis.[81] Thirty-nine studies conducted between 1997 and 2004 were included, involving a total of

Table 20-7 Classification of Rhinosinusitis

Classification	Description
Acute	Symptoms last 7–10 days but less than 4 weeks, which may include purulent discharge, nasal congestion, postnasal drainage, facial pain, headache, fever, cough
Subacute	Unresolved acute rhinosinusitis, with symptoms lasting 4–12 weeks
Chronic	Symptoms lasting at least 12 weeks
Recurrent	Four or more episodes of acute rhinosinusitis per year, with resolution of symptoms between episodes

Source: Modified from Feldt B, Dion GR, Weitzel EK, McMains KC. Acute sinusitis. S Med J. 2013;106(10):577-581.[78]

15,739 subjects. Approximately two thirds of the persons recovered without receiving antibiotics, supporting the premise that antibiotics are often overused. Antibiotics did, however, decrease the likelihood of no improvement within 7 to 14 days by 25% to 30% ($P < .01$). In the short term, amoxicillin–clavulanate (Augmentin) was more effective than cephalosporins.

Three sets of guidelines have been published since 2010 addressing the diagnosis and management of acute bacterial rhinosinusitis: the Bacterial Rhinosinusitis Guidelines from the Infectious Diseases Society of America,[80] the Acute Rhinosinusitis Guidelines from the University of Michigan Health Systems,[82] and the Canadian clinical practice guidelines for acute and chronic rhinosinusitis.[83] These sets of guidelines differ in the criteria for diagnosis and first-line antibiotic therapy, as summarized in Table 20-8.

Disagreement exists about which antibiotics to select. Because of increasing antibiotic resistance, the Infectious Diseases Society of America has recommended against the use of amoxicillin (Amoxil), macrolides such as clarithromycin (Biaxin) and azithromycin (Zithromax), or TMP/SMX (Bactrim, Septra), making a strong recommendation based on moderate evidence to initiate treatment with amoxicillin–clavulanate (Augmentin). Based on their evaluation of the evidence, both the University of Michigan Health Systems and Canadian guidelines still recommend beginning treatment with ampicillin, with qualifying statements that local patterns of resistance should be considered. The three organizations agree that if there is no improvement within 72 hours of antibiotic therapy, the individual should be reevaluated and changing the antibiotic should be considered.

Table 20-8 Diagnosis and Treatment of Acute Bacterial Rhinosinusitis

Infectious Diseases Society of America	Canadian	University of Michigan Health Systems
First-Line Empiric Therapy		
Amoxicillin–clavulanate (Augmentin) 875 mg/125 mg 2 times/day[a]	Amoxicillin (Amoxil) 500 mg 2 times/day	Amoxicillin (Amoxil) 500 mg every 8 hours for 10 days
Alternative		
Doxycycline (Vibramycin) 100 mg PO 2 times/day or 200 mg once daily		Doxycycline (Vibramycin) 100 mg PO 2 times/day or 200 mg once daily Fluoroquinolones
Penicillin Allergic		
Doxycycline (Vibramycin) 100 mg 2 times/day or 200 mg once daily	Amoxicillin–clavulanate (Augmentin) 875 mg/125 mg 2 times/day	TMP/SMX (Bactrim) 800 mg/160 mg every 12 hours
Levofloxacin (Levaquin) 500 mg once daily	Azithromycin (Zithromax) 500 mg on day 1, then 250 mg on days 2–5 *Or* 500 mg per day for 3 days	
Moxifloxacin (Avelox) 400 mg once daily	TMP/SMX (Bactrim) 800 mg/160 mg every 12 hours	
Second-Line Therapy, Risk for Antibiotic Resistance		
Amoxicillin–clavulanate (Augmentin) 2000 mg/125 mg 2 times/day	Amoxicillin–clavulanate (Augmentin) 875 mg/125 mg 2 times/day Fluoroquinolones	Amoxicillin (Amoxil) 500 mg every 8 hours for 10 days
Levofloxacin (Levaquin) 500 mg once daily		Amoxicillin–clavulanate (Augmentin) 875 mg/125 mg 2 times/day *or* 2000 mg/125 mg 2 times/day
Moxifloxacin (Avelox) 400 mg once daily		Levofloxacin (Levaquin) 500–750 mg once daily
		Moxifloxacin (Avelox) 750 mg once daily
Duration of Treatment		
5–7 days	5–10 days	10–14 days, up to 3 weeks if symptoms persist

Abbreviations: TMP/SMX = trimethoprim/sulfamethoxazole.

[a] *Not* amoxicillin, fluoroquinolones, macrolides, or TMP/SMX due to increasing resistance.

Sources: Data from Chow AW, Benninger MS, Brook I, et al. IDSA clinical practice guideline for acute bacterial rhinosinusitis in children and adults. *Clin Infect Dis*. 2012;54(8):e72-e112[80]; Desrosiers M, Evans GA, Keith PK, et al. Canadian clinical practice guidelines for acute and chronic rhinosinusitis. *J Onolaryngol Head Neck Surg*. 2011;40(suppl 2):S99-S193[83]; University of Michigan Health Systems. *Acute rhinosinusitis in adults*. Ann Arbor: University of Michigan Health Systems; 2011. http://www.med.umich.edu/1info/FHP/practiceguides/Rhino/Rhino.pdf. Accessed November 24, 2014.[82]

According to the University of Michigan Health Systems and Canadian guidelines, persons who present with severe unilateral maxillary pain, swelling, and fever should be treated regardless of the duration of symptoms.[82,83] The IDSA recommends delaying treatment in otherwise healthy adults for 3 to 4 days.[80] With the exception of these severely ill individuals, watchful waiting for 7 to 10 days should not increase the incidence of complications and will avoid many unnecessary courses of antibiotics.

Given the conflicting recommendations regarding the choice of antibiotics for acute bacterial rhinosinusitis, a clinician may benefit from further guidance. Many large medical centers publish "antibiograms," which report local patterns of resistance. If a region reports low resistance to oral beta-lactam medications, then amoxicillin (Amoxil) may be a reasonable choice. The same would be true for TMP/SMX (Bactrim, Septra). Conversely, if high resistance patterns were reported, initiating treatment with amoxicillin–clavulanate would be prudent. The case presented in Box 20-3 highlights some of these clinical dilemmas.

Adjunctive Therapy

Inhaled nasal corticosteroids are potent anti-inflammatory agents and can be important adjuncts to antibiotic use in

Box 20-3 To Treat or Not to Treat? A Case of Sinusitis

AM is a 32-year-old being seen for her annual cervical cancer screening. In the process of giving an interval history, AM tells her provider that she is glad her visit was scheduled for today because she has sinusitis and needs a prescription for antibiotics, which she says always work best when she gets the symptoms of sinusitis.

In providing her history, AM reports the onset of headaches and pain over her right eye for 2 days. These symptoms appeared as she was getting over a bad head cold that included coughing and yellow-green discharge from her nose. She has been afebrile. AM is in good health and takes no medications other than birth control pills. She does not have a maxillary toothache. AM has not used any medications to treat these symptoms.

On examination, AM is found to be afebrile. She does not have maxillary sinus tenderness. The posterior pharynx is red but there is no discharge. The cervical lymph nodes are not enlarged or tender.

The provider makes a diagnosis of viral sinusitis that does not require antibiotic treatment at this time. To help AM resolve these symptoms, the provider explains how inflammation of the sinuses occurs following a viral illness and that it usually lasts 7 to 11 days but resolves spontaneously. She recommends that AM use a decongestant on a regular basis for 3 days, humidify the bedroom at night, increase fluids, and monitor for the development of more symptoms. They discuss the pros and cons of nasal sprays versus oral decongestants, and AM decides to use phenylpropanolamine (Tavist-D), which is an extended-release systemic agent she can take every 8 to 12 hours. The provider advises AM not to use antihistamines. They discuss pain control and AM is able to take NSAIDs to treat the headache and sore throat. This provider has free prescription pads from the Centers for Disease Control and Prevention's "Get Smart: Know When Antibiotics Work" campaign, and she uses it to record the recommended treatment for AM. The provider tells AM that antibiotics are indicated if her symptoms do not improve by 10 days or if they get worse in 4 days despite this treatment. AM is given the voice-mail phone number for the provider, and the pair agree that she will call in 4 days to report her progress or lack thereof. AM gives the provider the name of her pharmacy.

Four days later, AM calls to say her headache is better when she takes the decongestant but it returns when the decongestant wears off, and she now has facial pain over her right eye that has worsened. AM has the classic biphasic illness that is one of the signs of bacterial sinusitis. Bacterial sinusitis is usually caused by *H. influenzae*, *Branhamella*, *M. catarrhalis*, or *S. pneumoniae*. These bacteria are susceptible to beta-lactam antibiotics if they are not betalactamase–producing organisms. The provider reviews AM's history to make sure she is not allergic to penicillin, and then calls her pharmacy to prescribe amoxicillin–clavulanate (Augmentin) 875 mg/125 mg to be taken 2 times per day for 5 days. This agent was chosen because the clavulanate extends coverage to include efficacy against beta-lactamase–producing bacteria.

Ten days later, AM calls and leaves a message for her provider that her symptoms started resolving 3 to 4 days after she started the amoxicillin–clavulanate and she is feeling well.

the treatment of both acute and chronic sinusitis, offering faster resolution of symptoms.[84] Steroids decrease vascular permeability, inhibit release and/or formation of histamine and leukotrienes, and prevent infiltration of inflammatory cells.[85]

There is little evidence as to the benefit (or lack thereof) of oral decongestants, whose vasoconstrictive properties may provide relief of symptoms. Common side effects of these medications include increased blood pressure, central nervous system stimulation, and urinary retention.[85] Caution should be used when considering the use of oral decongestants for persons with coronary artery disease or hypertension. While over-the-counter nasal decongestants are often used to decrease congestion and have evidence supporting their short-term use for treating the symptoms of the common cold,[12] the FDA has ruled that any indication of use for sinusitis must be removed from their labeling.[86] If oral decongestants are used, their use should be limited to 3 days to avoid rebound congestion. The use of antihistamines in the treatment of acute rhinosinusitis has no supporting evidence. The only theoretical benefit might be for individuals with a significant component of allergic rhinitis as well as acute bacterial rhinosinusitis.

Subacute and Chronic Rhinosinusitis

Subacute rhinosinusitis usually occurs secondary to partial or inadequate treatment of acute rhinosinusitis. Treatment includes changing antibiotics and reinforcing completion of a 14- to 21-day course.

Chronic rhinosinusitis is a multifactorial condition that may include elements of allergy, nasal polyps, and both bacterial and fungal infection.[87] Research supports the use of inhaled nasal steroids and saline irrigation for this condition, as well as treatment for any comorbidity.[88] High doses of guaifenesin (1200 mg 2 times per day)—an expectorant found in many products such as Robitussin and sold as a single drug under the brand names Mucinex and Organidin NR. This dose of guaifenesin has been used to treat rhinosinusitis—based on its effectiveness in the treatment of chronic bronchitis. Individuals with rhinosinusitis symptoms that persist at least 8 weeks will benefit from referral to an otolaryngologist or allergist for further evaluation.

Allergic Rhinitis

Allergic rhinitis, which may be either seasonal or perennial, is characterized by nasal congestion, sneezing, rhinorrhea, itchy or watery eyes, and headache. The pathology involves both early-phase and late-phase symptoms. Early-phase symptoms such as rhinorrhea, nasal obstruction, sneezing, and pruritus are probably mediated through immunoglobulin E activation of mast cell and basophil release of histamine and leukotrienes. The late-phase reaction includes the symptoms of the early phase, with the addition of increased nasal obstruction and inflammation secondary to the recruitment of eosinophils, monocytes, and basophils.[89] It is a common condition worldwide. In the United States, allergic rhinitis affects 10% to 30% of adults, making it the fifth most common chronic disease.[90]

Increasingly, the similarities between allergic rhinitis and asthma are leading to the concept of "one airway, one disease" in approaching these conditions.[91] Both the nasal mucosa and the bronchi have similar inflammatory responses. Comorbidity is common; indeed, 80% to 90% of persons with asthma report nasal symptoms.[92,93] In addition, observational studies have demonstrated that the incidence of asthma complications is decreased by adequate treatment of allergic rhinitis.[89] Despite this interrelationship and the importance of concomitant treatment, the medications employed for these two entities are presented separately here for the sake of clarity.

The treatment of allergic rhinitis is based on the severity and frequency of symptoms and personal preferences. Management options include oral and topical antihistamines, oral and nasal decongestants, intranasal corticosteroids, intranasal cromolyn sodium, and leukotriene receptor antagonists, intranasal anticholinergics, and immunotherapy (Table 20-9).[94] Omalizumab (Xolair), an antibody that binds IgE, may be an option for the treatment of severe allergic rhinitis that is refractory to usual treatments.[95] First-line therapy involves second-generation antihistamines and/or intranasal corticosteroids.[90,96]

Antihistamines

Because of their proven safety and efficacy, second-generation antihistamines are recommended for the treatment of mild to moderate allergic rhinitis. First-generation antihistamines are associated with an unfavorable risk–benefit profile due to side effects such as sedation, dry mouth, constipation, urinary hesitancy, and tachycardia. The second-generation antihistamines are safer and have more specific H_1-receptor selectivity, faster onset, and longer duration; they also have fewer side effects than the first-generation antihistamines. Thus, they have replaced the first-generation agents as the first-line treatments for allergic rhinitis.[90,96] The *Antihistamines* chapter reviews the pharmacologic properties and uses of antihistamines in more detail.

Table 20-9 Medications for the Management of Allergic Rhinitis

Drug: Generic (Brand)	Formulation	Dose (Sprays per Nostril for Topical Medications)
Antihistamines: Oral		
Cetirizine (Zyrtec)	5-, 10-mg tablets	5–10 mg once daily
Desloratadine (Clarinex)	5-mg tablet	5 mg once daily
Fexofenadine (Allegra)	30-, 60-, 180-mg tablets	60 mg 2 times/day
Loratadine (Claritin)	10-mg tablets	10 mg once daily
Antihistamines: Topical		
Azelastine (Astelin)	137 mcg/spray	1–2 sprays each nostril 2 times/day
Nasal Corticosteroids		
Beclomethasone (Beconase AQ)	42 mcg/spray	1–2 sprays 2 times/day
Beclomethasone (Qnasl)	80 mcg/spray	2 sprays once daily
Budesonide (Rhinocort Aqua)	32 mcg/spray	1 spray daily
Ciclesonide (Omnaris)	50 mcg/spray	2 sprays daily
Flunisolide	25 mcg/spray	2 sprays 2 times/day
Fluticasone furoate (Veramyst)	50 mcg/spray	2 sprays daily
Fluticasone propionate	50 mcg/spray	2 sprays daily *or* 1 spray 2 times/day
Mometasone (Nasonex)	50 mcg/spray	2 sprays daily
Triamcinolone (Nasacort AQ)[a]	55 mcg/spray	2 sprays daily, may reduce to 1 spray daily for maintenance
Decongestants		
Oxymetazoline 0.05% (Afrin 12 hours, Neo-Synephrine 12 hours)	Spray	2–3 sprays every 10–12 hours; limit use to no more than 3–5 days
Phenylephrine 0.25%–1% (Neo-Synephrine Sudafed PE, and others)	Drops	2–3 drops every 4 hours as needed
	Spray	2–3 sprays every 4 hours
	Oral	10–20 mg every 4 hours
	30-, 60-mg tablets	60 mg every 4–6 hours
Pseudoephedrine (Sudafed and others)	120 mg ER	120 mg every 12 hours
	Drops Nasal spray	2–4 drops up to every 3 hours 3–4 sprays up to every 3 hours
Tetrahydrozoline HCl 0.1% (Tyzine)	55 mcg/spray	2 sprays daily
	55 mcg/spray	2 sprays daily
Leukotriene Receptor Agonist		
Montelukast (Singulair)	10 mg	
Anticholinergic Nasal Spray		
Ipratropium (Atrovent)	0.06%	2 sprays 3–4 times/day
Combination Formulations		
Fexofenadine 60 mg/ pseudoephedrine 120 mg (Allegra-D) (antihistamine and decongestant)		1 tablet 2 times/day
Loratadine 10 mg/ pseudoephedrine 240 mg (Claritin D) (antihistamine and decongestant)		1 tablet 2 times/day
Mast Cell Stabilizer		
Cromolyn sodium (NasalCrom)	5.2 mg/spray	1 spray 3–4 times/day

[a] Available over the counter.
Source: Data from Meltzer EO. Pharmacotherapeutic strategies for allergic rhinitis: matching treatment to symptoms, disease progression, and associated conditions. *Allergy Asthma Proc*. 2013;34(4):301-311.[94]

Azelastine (Astelin) is a topical second-generation antihistamine that is administered as an intranasal spray twice daily. The efficacy of this agent is comparable to that of the oral second-generation antihistamines, and its only commonly reported side effect is a bitter taste.[90] The Allergic Rhinitis and Its Impact on Asthma (ARIA) guidelines suggest that azelastine may be used in adults with seasonal, but not persistent, allergic rhinitis.[96]

Intranasal Corticosteroids

Intranasal corticosteroids are the mainstay of pharmacologic therapy for persons with moderate to severe symptoms or those in whom symptoms persist despite use of second-generation antihistamines.[96] All of the formulations available in the United States contain either an aqueous or a powder vehicle. These agents have potent, long-acting, anti-inflammatory effects—reducing eosinophil infiltration, suppressing the expression of cytokines, and reducing the release of histamine and leukotrienes. Although systemic corticosteroid use is associated with significant adverse effects, the minimal systemic absorption and rapid first-pass metabolism by the liver avoid such side effects with intranasal corticosteroid administration.[97] Intranasal corticosteroids are more effective for relief of the nasal symptoms of allergic rhinitis than topical antihistamines, oral antihistamines, nasal cromolyn sodium (NasalCrom), or leukotriene receptor antagonists.[90,96]

Intranasal Cromolyn Sodium

Cromolyn sodium (NasalCrom) is a mast cell stabilizer that prevents the release of histamine and other mediators of inflammation. Minimal amounts are absorbed systemically, and the drug is excreted unchanged. Cromolyn sodium is less effective than intranasal corticosteroids. One disadvantage of cromolyn sodium is that it should be administered 4–6 times per day. An advantage of this agent is that it can block symptoms even when used shortly before exposure to allergens, such as cat dander.[98]

Other Medications

Leukotrienes cause nasal congestion by increasing vascular permeability and vasodilation; in turn, medications that block leukotriene receptors are able to decrease nasal congestion. Leukotriene receptor antagonists have no effect on sneezing or itching. When used as monotherapy, they are not as effective as second-generation antihistamines or nasal steroids. The combination of leukotriene receptor antagonists and second-generation antihistamines appears to be more effective than either type of agent used alone, but not better than inhaled nasal corticosteroids.[99]

The leukotriene receptor antagonist montelukast (Singulair) was approved for the treatment of allergic rhinitis in December 2002. This drug is absorbed rapidly after oral administration and has a half-life of 2.7 to 5.5 hours. Leukotriene receptor antagonists are metabolized by the liver and excreted in the bile. Unique among the leukotriene receptor antagonists, montelukast does not have any significant drug interactions; it is the only leukotriene receptor agonist that has been studied for use in allergic rhinitis.[96] An evidence-based review concluded that montelukast was as effective as, but not more effective than, intranasal steroids in the relief of symptoms.[98] Although it is more costly, this agent may be an alternative in those women who cannot or will not use intranasal corticosteroids. Given its effect of decreasing nasal secretions, nasal ipratropium (Atrovent) may be considered as adjunctive therapy for individuals with profuse rhinorrhea.

Immunotherapy

Immunotherapy is effective for improving symptoms of allergic rhinitis and subsequent development of asthma and atopic dermatitis.[96,100] The benefits from immunotherapy persist long after the treatment ends. Both subcutaneous immunotherapy and sublingual immunotherapy are recommended in the ARIA guidelines.[96] A 2010 Cochrane review of the literature on sublingual immunotherapy concluded that sublingual immunotherapy is safe and effective in the management of allergic rhinitis.[100] In 2014, Chelladuri et al.[101] evaluated the four systematic reviews comparing subcutaneous immunotherapy and sublingual immunotherapy. These researchers concluded that subcutaneous immunotherapy is better at reducing symptoms of allergic rhinitis, but failed to find any difference in quality of life or combined symptom–medication scores. Sublingual immunotherapy produces fewer systematic reactions and may have improved compliance when compared to subcutaneous immunotherapy.[101]

Until April 2014, only subcutaneous injections of increasing doses of allergen were available in the United States. At that time, the FDA approved the use of sublingual immunotherapy for the management of grass pollen allergies.

Complementary and Alternative Therapies

The ARIA guidelines make conditional recommendations against use of homeopathy, acupuncture, butterbur or other herbal medicines, or nasal phototherapy in the treatment of allergic rhinitis.[96] In contrast, when Pfab et al.[102] reviewed the current evidence, they concluded that acupuncture has a benefit for allergic rhinitis, and may also provide benefit for other allergic conditions such as atopic dermatitis and asthma. Following a 2012 review of the literature, Hermelingmeier et al.[103] recommended nasal irrigation as adjunct therapy for allergic rhinitis.[100]

Special Populations: Pregnancy

Approximately 20% to 40% of women have allergies, and as many as 30% experience worsening symptoms during pregnancy.[104] In addition, secondary to the hormones of pregnancy, many women experience a physiologic nasal congestion, referred to as "rhinitis of pregnancy." This mucosal change can make it challenging to discriminate between rhinitis of pregnancy and other causes of rhinitis. Rhinitis of pregnancy can amplify the symptoms associated with comorbid conditions such as an upper respiratory infection, sinusitis, or allergic rhinitis.

Chlorpheniramine (Chlor-Trimeton), loratadine (Claritin), and cetirizine (Zyrtec) are believed to be safe for use in pregnancy if used at recommended doses. For those women whose symptoms are not relieved by oral antihistamines, nasal corticosteroids represent a safe option. Very little of the corticosteroid is absorbed systemically.[98,104]

Asthma

Asthma is a significant contributor to morbidity in the United States. Approximately 22 million individuals suffer from this condition.[105] Asthma affects 8% of the adult population and accounts for 14.2 million office visits and 1.8 million emergency department visits each year.[106]

Asthma is a chronic disorder of the airways that is characterized by bronchial hyperresponsiveness, inflammation, and airway obstruction. Acute symptoms usually are due to bronchospasm, but it is the inflammation that causes impaired airflow and hyperresponsiveness. Research suggests that the inflammatory process of asthma can lead to airway remodeling, which may not be prevented or treated with use of current therapies.[105]

Genetics plays a complex role in asthma. Many genes are involved in the clinical development of asthma, and polymorphisms can affect individual responses to treatment with both $beta_2$ agonists and corticosteroids. Further study of the differing phenotypes may lead to improved targeted treatments. An increasing body of evidence suggests that polymorphisms of the gene encoding the site of action of $beta_2$ agonists have an association with the clinical response to $beta_2$ agonist therapy.[89,107] Although a complete discussion of the management of asthma is beyond the scope of this chapter, a broad overview is presented for primary care providers. Readers are referred to *Expert Panel Report 3: Guidelines for the Diagnosis and Management of Asthma* (2007)[105] for a comprehensive review of current recommendations for diagnosis and management of asthma.

Stepwise Approach for Managing Asthma

Asthma is categorized as persistent or intermittent (Table 20-10), with persistent asthma further subclassified as mild, moderate, or severe. Combining the information about the classifications of asthma severity and the medications available to treat asthma, an expert panel has developed stepwise guidelines for the overall management of individuals with asthma (Figure 20-3). Drug therapy should be targeted to an individual's disease process at a given time. Neither suboptimal nor overly aggressive medication regimens are desirable, and both can lead to worsening of the asthma. Exacerbations indicate a need to step up the pharmacotherapy. Conversely, stepping down the treatment can be considered after 3 months of good control.

As with any chronic illness, drug therapy is only part of the treatment plan. Education of both the woman with asthma and her providers, avoidance of allergens, and regular follow-up also are key components of the management.

Certain comorbid conditions can aggravate an individual's asthma symptoms; conversely, treatment of

Table 20-10 Classification of Asthma Severity

Components of Severity		Classification of Asthma Severity (Youths ≥ 12 years of age and adults)			
			Persistent		
		Intermittent	Mild	Moderate	Severe
Impairment Normal FEV_1/FVC: 8–19 yr 85% 20–39 yr 80% 40–59 yr 75% 60–80 yr 70%	Symptoms	≤ 2 days/week	> 2 days/week but not daily	Daily	Throughout the day
	Nighttime awakenings	≤ 2x/month	3–4 times/month	> 1 time/week but not nightly	Often 7 times/week
	Short-acting $beta_2$-agonist use for symptom control (not prevention of EIB)	≤ 2 days/week	> 2 days/week but not > 1 time/day	Daily	Several times per day
	Interference with normal activity	None	Minor limitation	Some limitation	Extremely limited
	Lung function	• Normal FEV_1 between exacerbations • FEV_1 ≥ 80% predicted • FEV_1/FVC normal	• FEV_1 ≥ 80% predicted • FEV_1/FVC normal	• FEV_1 > 60% but < 80% predicted • FEV_1/FVC reduced 5%	• FEV_1 < 60% predicted • FEV_1/FVC reduced > 5%
Risk	Exacerbations requiring oral systemic corticosteroids	0–1/year	≥ 2/year →		
		← Consider severity and interval since last exacerbation. Frequency and severity may fluctuate over time for patients in any severity category. →			
		Relative annual risk of exacerbations may be related to FEV_1.			

Abbreviations: FEV_1 = forced expiratory volume in 1 second; FVC = forced vital capacity.

Source: Modified from National Heart, Lung, and Blood Institute. Expert Panel Report 3: Guidelines for the Diagnosis and Management of Asthma. NIH Publication No. 08-4051. Bethesda, MD: National Heart, Lung, and Blood Institute; 2007. http://www.nhlbi.nih.gov/files/docs/guidelines/asthgdln.pdf. Accessed November 22, 2014.[105]

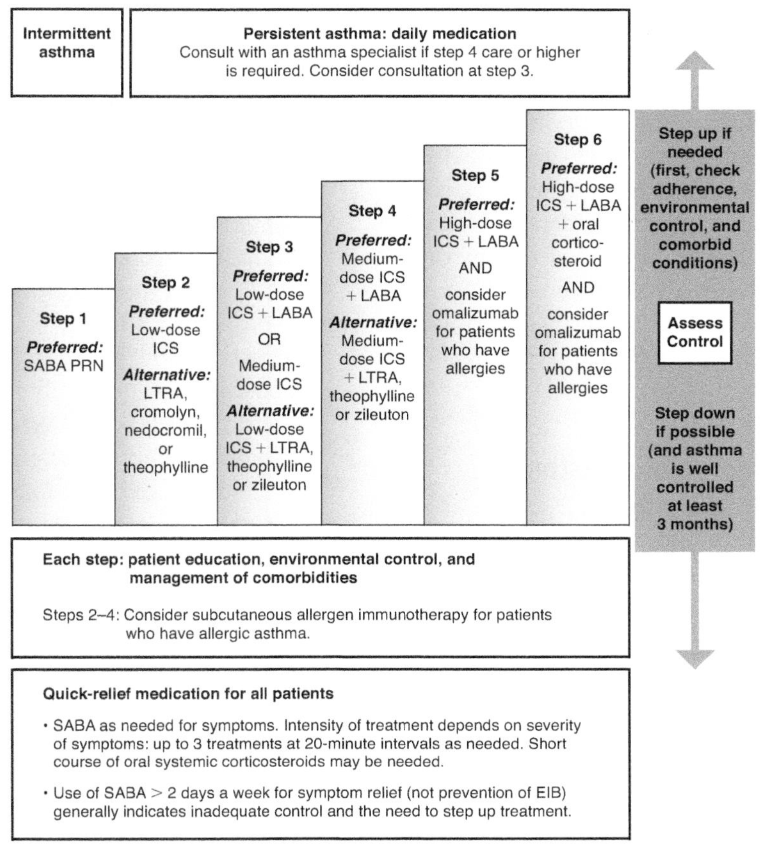

Figure 20-3 Stepwise approach for managing asthma.

Source: Modified from National Heart, Lung, and Blood Institute. Expert Panel Report 3: Guidelines for the Diagnosis and Management of Asthma. NIH Publication No. 08-4051. Bethesda, MD: National Heart, Lung, and Blood Institute; 2007. http://www.nhlbi.nih.gov/files/docs/guidelines/asthgdln.pdf. Accessed November 22, 2014.[105]

those conditions can help improve asthma management. Gastroesophageal reflux disease, rhinosinusitis, obesity, obstructive sleep apnea, and allergic bronchopulmonary aspergillosis all compromise asthma control. Chronic stress or depression may also play a role in worsening symptoms. Stress or depression may affect asthma severity directly, via increased production of pro-inflammatory mediators, or indirectly, via poorer adherence to treatment regimens. Certain medications, such as aspirin and beta blockers, are recognized precipitants of asthma, as are the sulfites found in shrimp, dried fruit, beer, and wine.

Pharmacologic Treatment of Asthma

Pharmacologic treatment is the key to asthma control and includes short-term quick-relief medications and medications that provide long-term relief of bronchospasm. The short-term or quick-acting drugs are either beta$_2$ agonists, anticholinergics, corticosteroids, or mixed formulations of beta$_2$ agonists and corticosteroids. The long-term control medications consist of inhaled corticosteroids, long-acting beta$_2$ agonists, combination formulations of inhaled corticosteroids and long-acting beta$_2$ agonists, leukotriene modifiers, and cromolyn sodium, which does not belong to any other class. Individuals with persistent asthma usually require both types of medications.

Most asthma medications are delivered directly to the lungs via metered-dose inhalers (MDIs) using hydrofluoroalkane (HFA) propellants, dry-powder inhalers (DPIs), or nebulizers. In the past, MDIs employed chlorofluorocarbons (CFCs) as propellants. However, because chlorofluorocarbons contribute to reducing the earth's ozone layer, in December of 2008, the FDA mandated that albuterol with chlorofluorocarbons (Albuterol CFC) be discontinued. Most manufacturers have since incorporated HFA as an alternative propellant; this gas does not appear to have an effect on the ozone layer. MDIs with HFA have the additional benefit of producing smaller droplets, which allow greater delivery of the medication to the lungs.

MDIs should be actuated during a slow, deep inspiration, followed by breath holding for 10 seconds. DPIs are actuated by the initiation of a rapid, deep inhalation. The delivery of the medication depends on the airflow and is lost if the individual exhales after actuating the device but before inhaling. HFA-reliant MDIs require priming and periodic cleaning. Each formulation has a slightly different requirement, which necessitates detailed reading of the instructions that come with the inhaler. Although some MDIs can be obtained on an over-the-counter basis, these formulations, which contain epinephrine, are not recommended for ongoing treatment (Box 20-4).

Quick-Relief Medications for Treating Asthma

Short-Acting Beta$_2$ Agonists

Inhaled, short-acting beta$_2$ agonists (SABAs) are the most effective medications available for the relief of bronchoconstriction and prevention of exercise-induced bronchospasm.[105] Medications used to treat asthma are listed in Table 20-11. Short-acting beta$_2$ agonists reverse bronchoconstriction and improve airflow within 3 to 5 minutes of use. The peak effect occurs in 30 minutes and the duration of action is 4 hours. These medications are inhaled via use of an MDI. A shortcoming of these devices is that a significant amount of inhaled medication is deposited in the oropharynx and does not reach the lungs.

The recommended treatment of intermittent asthma is short-acting beta$_2$ agonists as needed, but if the need exceeds use twice per week (unless for the prevention of exercise-induced bronchospasm), initiating anti-inflammatory therapy (i.e., inhaled corticosteroids) is indicated. Beta$_2$ agonists relax the smooth muscle of the airways regardless of the constricting stimulus. They may also inhibit the release of bronchoconstrictors from inflammatory cells and inhibit mast cell activation.[110] There is no evidence that regular use of short-acting beta$_2$ agonists, when compared to as-needed use, offers any benefit; in fact, routine use can lead to decreased lung function and control in some individuals.[105] An increasing body of evidence suggests that persons with the genotype Arg/Arg experience decreased lung function when treated with as-needed albuterol, such as Pro-Air HFA, Proventil HFA, or Ventolin HFA.[111]

Albuterol has been the drug most frequently used to treat bronchospasm, with approximately 52 million prescriptions for this medication filled each year in the United States. Albuterol consists of (*R*)-enantiomers and (*S*)-enantiomers, of which only the (*R*)-enantiomer is therapeutically active. In vitro studies suggest that the (*S*)-enantiomer might actually decrease smooth-muscle responsiveness. These findings prompted the development of levalbuterol (Xopenex), which contains only the active enantiomer. The majority of clinical trials have not demonstrated any clinical advantage of levalbuterol over albuterol.[105]

Adverse effects of current short-acting beta agonists are rare due to the selectivity of their beta$_2$-adrenergic agonist activity. In contrast, this is not the case for older, nonselective agents such as isoproterenol (Isuprel) or metaproterenol (Alupent). These short-acting beta$_2$ agonists may cause excessive cardiac stimulation, especially if used in excessively high doses. Consequently, these medications are not regularly used for outpatient treatment.

> **Box 20-4** Over-the-Counter Asthma Medications?
>
> For decades, individuals were able to access an over-the-counter inhaler, Primatene Mist, to treat their wheezing. Primatene Mist consisted of epinephrine propelled by chlorofluorocarbons (CFCs); thus, it was removed from the U.S. market in December 2011 along with other CFC-propellant products. Another manufacturer stepped in to fill this gap and, in 2012, began marketing the over-the-counter inhaler known as Asthmanefrin, which contained racephinephrine that was delivered as a vapor. That product was recalled in 2013 due to safety concerns, following multiple reports of chest pain, increased heart rate and blood pressure, and hemoptysis with its use.
>
> There is a consensus among asthma experts that epinephrine in over-the-counter formulations is not indicated in the management of asthma. Epinephrine stimulates both beta$_1$ and beta$_2$ receptors, leading to more side effects than prescription short-acting beta$_2$ agonists. Asthmatics who self-treat with over-the-counter inhalers treat only the symptomatic wheezing, not the underlying airway inflammation. Discussions are under way regarding the pros and cons of providing approved asthma inhalers through over-the-counter channels.[108,109]

Anticholinergics

Anticholinergics are selective antagonists of muscarinic receptors and, therefore, reverse only bronchospasm that

Table 20-11 Usual Doses of Quick-Relief Medications for Treatment of Asthma

Drug: Generic (Brand)	Dose per Activation	Adult Dose	Side Effects	Clinical Considerations
Inhaled Short-Acting Beta$_2$ Agonists: MDIs				
Albuterol HFA (ProAir HFA, Proventil HFA, Ventolin HFA)	MDI 90 mcg/puff, 200 puffs/canister	2 puffs every 4–6 hours as needed 1–2 capsules every 4–6 hours as needed	Tachycardia, skeletal muscle tremor, hypokalemia, increased lactic acid, headache, hyperglycemia. Inhaled route, in general, causes few systemic adverse effects. Persons with preexisting cardiovascular disease, especially the elderly, may have adverse cardiovascular reactions with inhaled therapy.	An increasing use or lack of expected effect indicates diminished control of asthma. Not recommended for long-term daily treatment. Regular use exceeding 2 days/week for symptom control indicates the need to step up therapy. Differences in potency exist, but all products are essentially comparable per puff. May double usual dose for mild exacerbations. Should prime the inhaler by releasing 4 actuations prior to use. Periodically clean the HFA activator, as the drug may block or plug the orifice.
Levalbuterol tartrate (Xopenex HFA)	MDI 45 mcg/puff, 200 doses/canister	2 puffs every 4–6 hours as needed		
Inhaled Short-Acting Beta$_2$ Agonists: Nebulizer Solutions				
Albuterol nebulizer solution	0.63 mg/3 mL 1.25 mg/3 mL 2.5 mg/3 mL 5 mg/mL (0.5%)	2.5-5 mg in 3 cc of saline every 4–6 hours as needed	Tachycardia, skeletal muscle tremor, hypokalemia, increased lactic acid, headache, hyperglycemia. Inhaled route, in general, causes few systemic adverse effects. Persons with preexisting cardiovascular disease, especially the elderly, may have adverse cardiovascular reactions with inhaled therapy.	May double dose for severe exacerbations. Compatible with budesonide inhalant suspension.
Levalbuterol (R-albuterol) nebulizer solution (Xopenex)	0.63 mg/3 mL 1.25 mg/0.5 mL 1.25 mg/3 mL	1.25 mg every 6–8 hours as needed		
Anticholinergics				
Ipratropium HFA MDI (Atrovent HFA) MDI	17 mcg/puff, 200 puffs/canister	2–3 puffs every 6 hours	Drying of mouth and respiratory secretions, increased wheezing in some individuals, blurred vision if sprayed in eyes.	Alternative for those who do not tolerate SABAs. Treatment of choice for bronchospasm due to beta-blocker medications.
Ipratropium HFA nebulizer	0.25 mg/mL (0.025%)	0.25 mg every 6 hours		
Combination Anticholinergic and Short-Acting Beta$_2$ Agonists				
Ipratropium with albuterol MDI (Combivent)	MDI 18 mcg/puff of ipratropium bromide and 90 mcg/puff of albuterol, 200 puffs/canister	2–3 puffs every 6 hours		Contains EDTA to prevent discoloration of the solution. This additive does not induce bronchospasm. Ipratroprium is not recommended for quick relief.
Ipratropium with albuterol nebulizer (DuoNeb)	0.5 mg/3 mL ipratropium bromide and 2.5 mg/3 mL albuterol	3 mL every 4–6 hours		

(*continues*)

Table 20-11 Usual Doses of Quick-Relief Medications for Treatment of Asthma (*continued*)

Drug: Generic (Brand)	Dose per Activation	Adult Dose	Side Effects	Clinical Considerations
Systemic Corticosteroids				
Methylprednisolone	2-, 3-, 8-, 16-, 32-mg tablets	7.5–60 mg per day administered once daily in the morning; usual duration is 3–10 days	Short-term use can cause reversible abnormalities in glucose metabolism, increased appetite, fluid retention, weight gain, mood alteration, hypertension, peptic ulcer, and rarely aseptic necrosis. Long-term use can cause adrenal axis suppression, growth suppression, dermal thinning, hypertension, diabetes, Cushing's syndrome, cataracts, muscle weakness, and—in rare instances—impaired immune function.	For short-term burst: to gain prompt control of inadequately controlled persistent asthma. Use at lowest effective dose. For long-term use, alternate-day morning dosing produces the least toxicity. Consideration should be given to coexisting conditions that could be worsened by systemic corticosteroids. No need to taper dose if used for less than 3 weeks.
Prednisolone	5-, 10-, 15-, 30-mg tablets			
Prednisone	1-, 2.5-, 5-, 10-, 20-, 50-mg tablets			

Abbreviations: CFC = chlorofluorocarbon-containing; DPI = dry-powder inhaler; EDTA = ethylenediaminetetraacetic acid; EIB = exercise-induced bronchospasm; HFA = hydrofluoroalkane; MDI = metered-dose inhaler.
Source: Modified from National Heart, Lung, and Blood Institute. *Expert Panel Report 3: Guidelines for the Diagnosis and Management of Asthma.* NIH Publication No. 08-4051. Bethesda, MD: National Heart, Lung, and Blood Institute; 2007. http://www.nhlbi.nih.gov/files/docs/guidelines/asthgdln.pdf. Accessed November 22, 2014.[105]

occurs secondary to cholinergic input. Individuals exhibit a highly variable response to these agents, which is probably secondary to individual variations in parasympathetic tone and the degree of cholinergic involvement in the bronchospasm. It appears that individuals who have psychogenic exacerbations of asthma respond well to anticholinergics.

The anticholinergic used today is ipratropium bromide (Atrovent). Following administration of this agent, bronchodilation develops slowly and lasts up to 6 hours. Tiotropium bromide (Spiriva) is used on a once-daily basis; it has been found effective in the treatment of moderate to severe asthma that is not well controlled by inhaled corticosteroids with or without long-acting beta$_2$ agonists.[112] Formulations that combine ipratropium bromide and short-acting beta$_2$ agonists generally induce better and longer-lasting bronchodilation than either agent used alone when used for acute exacerbations.

Systemic Corticosteroids

Systemic corticosteroids are also considered quick-relief medications. These agents decrease inflammation by switching off the genes that code for inflammatory factors and mucus production in the airways. They are used in conjunction with short-acting beta$_2$ agonists for moderate and severe exacerbations. Some evidence indicates that beta$_2$ agonists enhance the effect of the glucocorticoids.[110] Systemic steroids should be administered in short courses for exacerbations to minimize their adverse effects, which are related to both dose and duration of treatment; these agents should be avoided as a means of long-term control of asthma.[105]

Long-Term Therapy for Treating Asthma

Drugs used for long-term treatment of asthma are listed in Table 20-12. Inhaled corticosteroids are the mainstay for the long-term treatment of asthma.[110] These agents are the most effective long-term therapy available for persistent asthma and are associated with relatively few side effects. Other medications for the long-term control of asthma include long-acting beta$_2$ agonists, leukotriene receptor antagonists, immunomodulators, and methylxanthines. While none of these medications is as effective as inhaled corticosteroids, there may be roles for them, either when added to treatment with inhaled corticosteroids (combination therapy) or as stand-alone therapy in selected cases.

Inhaled Corticosteroids

Inhaled corticosteroids are potent anti-inflammatory agents that have several physiologic effects. Steroids inhibit the production and release of inflammatory mediators such as cytokines and leukotrienes, decrease the infiltration of eosinophils, and reduce airway edema by decreasing vascular permeability. Inhaled corticosteroids improve every measurable aspect of asthma, including pulmonary function, quality of life, prevention of exacerbations, and number of hospitalizations, emergency visits, and deaths.[105]

Doses for inhaled corticosteroids vary significantly, depending on the preparation and delivery system. Table 20-13 lists the usual low, medium, and high doses for the currently available inhaled corticosteroids. For individuals with mild or moderate asthma, increasing the dose of the inhaled corticosteroids leads to modest (at best) improvement in asthma control. Individuals with mild to moderate asthma who are started on low doses of inhaled corticosteroids show just as much improvement as those started on higher doses.[113] In addition, many individuals find that their mild to moderate asthma is adequately controlled with once-daily dosing, and those with mild, intermittent asthma may be managed with inhaled corticosteroids as needed rather than with daily therapy.[111] Individuals whose asthma has been well controlled for 2 months with high-dose inhaled corticosteroids may tolerate a 50% decrease in the dose without loss of control. Some individuals, such as smokers and African American children with poor control, have a relative insensitivity to

Table 20-12 Medications for Long-Term Control of Asthma

Drug: Generic (Brand)	Formulation and Dose	Indications/Mechanisms	Adverse Effects	Clinical Considerations
Inhaled Corticosteroids				
Beclomethasone dipropionate (Qvar)	MDI	Long-term prevention of symptoms; suppression, control, and reversal of inflammation; reduced need for oral corticosteroids	Cough, dysphonia, oral thrush (candidiasis); in high doses, systemic effects may occur	Use of spacer/holding chamber devices with non-breath-activated MDIs and mouth washing after inhalation decrease local side effects. Preparations are not absolutely interchangeable.
Budesonide (Pulmicort)	DPI			
Ciclesonide (Alvesco)	MDI			
Flunisolide HFA (Aerospan)	MDI			
Fluticasone propionate (Flovent Diskus, Flovent HFA)	DPI MDI			
Mometasone furoate (Asmanex Twisthaler)	DPI			
Immunomodulators				
Omalizumab (Xolair) Anti-IgE	Different doses based on pretreatment IgE level; maximum dose is 150 mg in one injection	Long-term control and prevention of symptoms in adults who have moderate or severe, persistent allergic asthma inadequately controlled with ICS + LABAs	Pain and bruising at injection sites; anaphylaxis, serious cardiovascular and cerebrovascular adverse events—see FDA black box warning	Monitor individuals following injection. Be prepared and equipped to identify and treat anaphylaxis that may occur. Needs to be stored under refrigeration at 2–8°C.
Leukotriene Receptor Antagonists (LTRAs)				
Montelukast tablets and granules (Singulair)	10 mg PO once/daily	Long-term control and prevention of symptoms in mild, persistent asthma in persons 1 year or older; may also be used with ICS as combination therapy in moderate, persistent asthma	No specific adverse effects have been identified; rare cases of Churg-Strauss syndrome have occurred, but the association is unclear	May attenuate EIB for some individuals but is less effective than ICS therapy. Do not use LTRA + LABA as a substitute for ICS + LABA. Administration with meals decreases bioavailability; take at least 1 hour before or 2 hours after meals.
Zafirlukast tablets (Accolate)	20 mg PO 2 times/day		Reversible hepatitis and, rarely, irreversible hepatic failure	Can inhibit the metabolism of warfarin (Coumadin). Hepatic enzymes should be monitored.

(continues)

Table 20-12 Medications for Long-Term Control of Asthma (*continued*)

Drug: Generic (Brand)	Formulation and Dose	Indications/Mechanisms	Adverse Effects	Clinical Considerations
5-Lipoxygenase Inhibitors (Leukotriene Inhibitors)				
Zileuton tablets (Zyflo)	600 mg PO 4 times/day	Long-term control and prevention of symptoms in mild, persistent asthma; may be used with ICS as combination therapy in moderate, persistent asthma	Elevation of liver enzymes has been reported; limited case reports of reversible hepatitis and hyperbilirubinemia	Inhibits the metabolism of warfarin (Coumadin) and theophylline (Theo-Dur). Monitor liver function during treatment (ALT/AST).
Zyflo CR	1200 mg 2 times/day			
Long-Acting Beta$_2$ Agonists (LABAs)				
Formoterol (Foradil)[a]	DPI: 12 mcg/dose as needed or for maintenance 2 times/day	Long-term prevention of symptoms, added to ICS; prevention of EIB Slow onset of action (15–30 minutes); duration > 12 hours	Tachycardia, skeletal muscle tremor, hypokalemia, prolongation of QT interval in overdose. Diminished bronchoprotective effect may occur within 1 week of chronic therapy. Uncommon, severe, life-threatening, or fatal exacerbation of asthma.	Should not be used as monotherapy for long-term control of asthma. May provide more effective symptom control when added to standard doses of ICS compared to increasing the ICS dose. Maximum daily dose is 100 mcg salmeterol or 24 mcg formoterol.
Salmeterol (Serevent)[a]	DPI: 50 mcg/dose as needed or maintenance 2 times/day			
Combination Corticosteroid and Long-Acting Beta$_2$ Agonists				
Budesonide/formoterol (Symbicort)	MDI: 80 mg/4.5 mg per dose *or* 160 mg /4.5 per dose; 1–2 inhalations	Long-term control of chronic asthma	Same as for LABAs. Corticosteroids are associated with oral candidiasis and adrenal suppression. Very rare anaphylactic reaction may occur in persons with milk protein allergy.	Same as for LABAs. CYP3A4 inhibitors such as ketoconazole increase concentrations of fluticasone and/or budesonide, which can result in adrenal suppression.
Fluticasone/salmeterol (Advair Discus)	500 mcg/50 mcg or 250 mcg/50 mcg or 100 mcg/50 mcg 1 inhalation 2 times/day			
Fluticasone/salmeterol (Advair HFA)	MDI: Several dosage forms available; maximum dose is 230 mcg/21 mcg 2 times/day			
Methylxanthines				
Theophylline, sustained-release tablets and capsules	300 mg once/daily in divided doses every 6 hours; maintenance dose is 400–600 mg/day	Long-term control and prevention of symptoms in mild, persistent asthma or as adjunctive with ICS, in moderate or persistent asthma	Insomnia, gastric upset, aggravation of ulcer, and reflux are common; tachycardia, nausea and vomiting, tachyarrhythmias, CNS stimulation, headache, seizures, hematemesis, hyperglycemia, and hypokalemia. Adverse effects occur at usual therapeutic doses.	Routine serum concentration monitoring is essential due to narrow therapeutic range, and individual differences in metabolic clearance. Multiple drug–drug interactions.
Anticholinergics				
Ipratropium bromide (Atrovent HFA)	17 mcg/puff, 8 inhalations every 20 minutes as needed up to 3 hours			May mix in same nebulizer with albuterol. Do not use as first-line therapy; can be added to SABA therapy for severe exacerbations. Onset of effect in 15 minutes; duration is 3–4 hours.
Ipratropium bromide with albuterol MDI (Combivent)	Each puff: 18 mcg ipratropium bromide, 90 mcg of albuterol; 8 puffs every 20 minutes as needed up to 3 hours			

Abbreviations: ALT = alanine aminotransferase; AST = aspartate aminotransferase; CNS = central nervous system; DPI = dry-powder inhaler; EIB = exercise-induced bronchospasm; HFA = hydrofluoroalkane; ICS = inhaled corticosteroids; INR = International Normalized Ratio; LABA = long-acting beta$_2$ agonist; LTRA = leukotriene receptor antagonist; MDI = metered-dose inhaler; SABA = inhaled short-acting beta$_2$ agonist.

[a] The FDA recommends that salmeterol and formoterol not be used as monotherapy for treatment of asthma secondary to an increased risk of airway responsiveness to histamine and worsening asthma morbidity that is associated with regular use of these agents.

Source: Modified from National Heart, Lung, and Blood Institute. *Expert Panel Report 3: Guidelines for the Diagnosis and Management of Asthma.* NIH Publication No. 08-4051. Bethesda, MD: National Heart, Lung, and Blood Institute; 2007. http://www.nhlbi.nih.gov/files/docs/guidelines/asthgdln.pdf. Accessed November 22, 2014.[105]

inhaled corticosteroids therapy; treatment of asthma in these individuals can be more challenging.[105,111]

The most important determinant of appropriate dosing is the individual's response to therapy. The stepwise approach to therapy emphasizes that once control of asthma is achieved, the dose of medication should be carefully titrated to the minimum dose required to maintain control, thereby reducing the potential for adverse effect.

The bioavailability of inhaled corticosteroids is significantly lower than the bioavailability of corticosteroids administered orally; in turn, inhaled corticosteroids are associated with a lower risk of serious side effects compared to oral agents. Potential systemic effects of inhaled corticosteroids include a reduction in growth velocity in children's bone mineral density,[114] immunosuppression, ocular effects, effects on hypothalamic–pituitary–adrenal (HPA) axis function, and impaired glucose metabolism.[105] There is no evidence that low- or medium-dose inhaled corticosteroid use leads to immunosuppression or altered HPA axis function.[105]

Local adverse effects of inhaled corticosteroids include oral candidiasis, dysphonia (hoarseness), and reflex cough and bronchospasm. While most persons with asthma who use inhaled corticosteroids frequently will have positive throat cultures for *Candida*, clinical thrush is much less common, especially when inhaled corticosteroids are taken at low doses. Rinsing the mouth after inhalation may help to prevent thrush, and topical or oral antifungals should be used to treat clinical infections.[105]

Long-Acting Beta$_2$ Agonists

The long-acting beta$_2$ agonists (LABAs) salmeterol (Serevent) and formoterol (Foradil) are selective beta$_2$ agonists with increased lipophilicity, which prolongs their time of retention in lung tissues. Due to this increased retention, a single dose maintains its bronchodilation action for at least 12 hours.[115] A large randomized, placebo-controlled 28-week trial of salmeterol versus placebo added to usual care was terminated early following a planned interim analysis that showed an increased risk of asthma-related deaths and combined asthma-related deaths or life-threatening events associated with salmeterol (13 deaths among 13,176 persons taking salmeterol versus 3 deaths among 13,176 persons receiving placebo).[116] A review of this and other studies prompted the FDA to issue a public health advisory

Table 20-13 Estimated Comparative Daily Doses for Inhaled Corticosteroids

Drug: Generic (Brand)	Formulations	Low Daily Dose	Medium Daily Dose	High Daily Dose[a]
Beclomethasone HFA (QVAR Auto-inhaler)	50–100 mcg/puff[b]	100–200 mcg	200–400 mcg	> 400 mcg
Budesonide (Pulmicort Flexhaler)	DPI 90, 180, or 200 mcg/puff[c]	200–400 mcg, 1–2 inhalations	> 400–600 mcg, 2–3 inhalations	> 600 mcg, > 3 inhalations
Ciclesonide (Alvesco)	80 mcg/puff 160 mcg/puff	160 mcg, 1 puff 2 times/day	320 mcg	640 mcg
Flunisolide (Flovent Diskus)	DPI 50, 100, or 250 mcg/puff	500–1000 mcg, 2–4 puffs	> 1000–2000 mcg, 4–8 puffs	> 2000 mcg, > 8 puffs
Flunisolide HFA (Flovent HFA)	MDI 44, 110, or 220 mcg/actuation	88–264 mcg, 2–6 puffs of 44 mcg	> 264–660 mcg, 2–6 puffs of 110 mcg	> 660 mcg, > 6 puffs of 110 mcg
Flunisolide HFA (Aerospan)	80 mcg/puff	320 mcg, 2 puffs 2 times/day		640 mcg, 4 puffs 2 times/day
Mometasone (Asmanex)	DPI 220 mcg/actuation	220 mcg, 1 puff	660–880 mcg, 2–3 puffs	> 880 mcg, > 4 puffs

Abbreviations: DPI = dry-powder inhaler; HFA = hydrofluoroalkane; MDI = metered-dose inhaler.

[a] Some doses may exceed those listed on the package labeling, especially in the high-dose range.

[b] MDI doses are expressed as the actuator dose (the amount of the drug leaving the actuator and delivered to the individual), which is the labeling required in the United States. This amount differs from the valve dose (the amount of drug leaving the valve, not all of which is available to the person), which is used in many European countries and in some scientific literature as the expressed dose.

[c] DPI doses are expressed as the amount of drug in the inhaler following activation.

Notes: Comparative doses are based on published comparative clinical trials. The low and medium doses reflect findings from studies in which incremental effectiveness within the low- to medium-dose ranges was established without increased systemic effect as measured by overnight cortisol excretion. The high dose is the dose that appears likely to be the threshold beyond which significant hypothalamic–pituitary–adrenal (HPA) axis suppression is produced and, by extrapolation, the risk is increased for other clinically significant systemic effects if used for prolonged periods of time.

Source: Modified from National Heart, Lung, and Blood Institute. *Expert Panel Report 3: Guidelines for the Diagnosis and Management of Asthma.* NIH Publication No. 08-4051. Bethesda, MD: National Heart, Lung, and Blood Institute; 2007. http://www.nhlbi.nih.gov/files/docs/guidelines/asthgdln.pdf. Accessed November 22, 2014.[105]

stating that long-acting $beta_2$ agonists should not be used as first-line treatments for asthma. Instead, they should be added only if the individual's asthma is not adequately controlled with low- or medium-dose corticosteroids.[117]

Combination Corticosteroids and Long-Acting $Beta_2$ Agonists

The use of both inhaled corticosteroids and long-acting $beta_2$ agonists is the preferred management regimen for moderate and severe asthma.[105] Two inhalers containing a combination of an inhaled corticosteroid and a long-acting $beta_2$ agonist are currently available: fluticasone/salmeterol (Advair) from GlaxoSmithKline and budesonide/formoterol (Symbicort) from AstraZeneca. Advair is available with three strengths of fluticasone, and Symbicort is available with two strengths of budesonide. The long-acting $beta_2$ agonist dose remains unchanged in these versions—that is, all of the Advair inhalers contain 50 mcg salmeterol and both of the Symbicort inhalers contain 4.5 mcg formoterol. Combined inhalers offer the advantage that the individual needs to use only one inhaler rather than two. When compared to increasing the dose of inhaled corticosteroids alone, the combination products have been found to improve lung function and reduce the rate of asthma exacerbations. Some evidence indicates that the combined inhalers are more effective than the same doses of inhaled corticosteroid and long-acting $beta_2$ agonist when administered separately.[118] Advair canisters have an integrated dose counter, which can help users keep track of when they need to refill their medication. Of the two long-acting $beta_2$ agonists, formoterol has a faster onset of bronchodilation, similar to that of albuterol.

While the Third Expert Panel currently does not recommend the use of long-acting $beta_2$ agonists for the treatment of acute symptoms, researchers are studying the use of budesonide/formoterol for both relief of acute symptoms and variable dosing depending on the level of symptom control.[119] If such use proves to be both safe and efficacious, it would allow women to use just one inhaler for both maintenance and rescue.

Leukotriene Receptor Antagonists

Inhaled corticosteroids do not appear to suppress leukotriene biosynthesis; leukotrienes, however, incite release of inflammatory mediators, triggering the inflammation component of asthma.[110] Two classes of leukotriene modifiers are available to address this aspect of asthma: the leukotriene receptor antagonists (LTRAs), which include montelukast (Singulair) and zafirlukast (Accolate), and the 5-lipoxygenase pathway inhibitors, which include zileuton (Zyflo). Leukotriene receptor antagonists provide for some improvement in lung function when compared to placebo, albeit consistently less than inhaled corticosteroids.[105] These drugs may offer some benefit to individuals with asthma by decreasing exercise-induced bronchospasm, but should not be used regularly for this purpose due to the risk of masking persistent asthma. A 2014 Cochrane review concluded that the combination of leukotriene receptor antagonists and inhaled corticosteroids was less effective than the combination of long-acting $beta_2$ agonists and inhaled corticosteroids.[120]

Both zileuton (Zyflo) and zafirlukast (Accolate) have been associated with liver toxicity and inhibit the metabolism of theophylline and warfarin (Coumadin); consequently, the International Normalized Ratios (INRs) of individuals receiving both medications must be monitored closely, and hepatic enzymes should be monitored if symptoms of hepatitis develop. The association between leukotriene receptor antagonists and depression or suicide was noted in postmarketing research; these medications now include warnings on their labels stating that they are associated with an increased risk of depression and insomnia.

Cromolyn Sodium and Nedocromil

Cromolyn sodium (Intal) and nedocromil (Tilade) both modulate release of mast cell mediators and eosinophil recruitment. While these agents are effective as preventive treatments for exercise-induced bronchospasm or known allergen exposure,[105] neither is currently available in the United States.

Immunomodulators

Omalizumab (Xolair) is a recombinant monoclonal antibody that inhibits the binding of IgE to mast cells and basophils, thereby decreasing the release of histamine in response to an allergen. Administration is accomplished by subcutaneous injection every 2 to 4 weeks, depending on the individual's body weight and serum IgE level. While it has not been compared to other adjunctive therapies such as leukotriene modifiers, long-acting $beta_2$ agonists, or theophylline (Theo-Dur), omalizumab is the only adjunctive therapy available for improving symptoms in individuals with severe persistent allergic asthma who are not well controlled with high-dose inhaled corticosteroids plus long-acting $beta_2$ agonists.

A review of postmarketing case reports demonstrated anaphylaxis incidence of 0.2% in persons using omalizumab.

The majority of these reactions occurred within 1 hour of administration, but a small percentage developed from 1 to 4 days after administration. These reports prompted the FDA to issue a black box warning to be carried on the drug's label. Omalizumab (Xolair) should be administered only in a setting that is prepared to treat anaphylaxis, and recipients should be informed of the signs and symptoms of anaphylaxis. Healthcare providers should observe individuals for a period of time after the drug is administered. As postmarketing case reports are made voluntarily, a higher incidence of anaphylaxis may exist.

Omalizumab is also associated with a small increased risk of serious cardiovascular and cerebrovascular adverse events. Although the most recent FDA review found no increase in the incidence of cancer in persons taking omalizumab, this risk cannot be ruled out.

Methylxanthines

Theophylline (Theo-Dur) is the most commonly used methylxanthine for the treatment of asthma. Prior to the development of cromolyn sodium and inhaled corticosteroids, theophylline was one of the first-line drugs for long-term control of persistent asthma. In addition to promoting bronchodilation, mediated by phosphodiesterase inhibition and increased cAMP, this drug shares many of the properties of caffeine.[110] Common side effects of theophylline include CNS excitation and vasoconstriction, tachycardia, peripheral vasodilation, and diuresis.

Methylxanthines are administered orally or intravenously. The metabolism of theophylline is affected by many variables, such as age, comorbidity, and other medications (Table 20-14). In addition, it has several clinically significant drug–drug and drug–food interactions and has a narrow therapeutic window; therefore, it is essential to monitor serum concentrations when this drug is prescribed. Starting doses are 10 mg/kg per day and are increased to achieve a serum concentration of 5–15 mcg/kg after at least 48 hours on the same dose, up to 300 mg/kg per day. The usual maximum daily dose is 800 mg per day. Steady-state serum concentrations between 5 and 15 mcg/mL are usually ideal. Selection of theophylline as the primary long-term control medication may be considered for individuals who cannot or will not use inhaled medication or for individuals who are unable to afford long-acting $beta_2$ agonists.

Table 20-14 Factors Affecting Serum Theophylline Levels

Factor	Decreases Theophylline Concentrations	Increases Theophylline Concentrations	Recommended Actions
Food	Decreases or delays absorption of some sustained-release preparations	Fatty food increases rate of absorption	Choose a theophylline preparation not affected by food
Diet	High protein increases metabolism	High carbohydrate decreases metabolism	Major dietary changes are not recommended for persons taking theophylline
Febrile illness		Decreases metabolism	Monitor levels and adjust accordingly
Hypoxia, heart failure		Decreases metabolism	Monitor levels and adjust accordingly
Age	Increases metabolism (1–9 years)	Decreases metabolism (< 6 months, elderly)	Monitor levels and adjust accordingly
Phenobarbital (Luminal), phenytoin (Dilantin), carbamazepine (Tegretol)	Increases metabolism		Monitor levels and adjust accordingly
Cimetidine (Tagamet)		Decreases metabolism	Use alternative
Macrolides: erythromycin (E-Mycin), clarithromycin (Biaxin)		Decreases metabolism	Use azithromycin (Zithromax) or alternate antibiotic
Ciprofloxacin (Cipro)		Decreases metabolism	Use alternative antibiotic or use ofloxacin if quinolone therapy is required
Rifampin (Rifadin)	Increases metabolism		Monitor levels and increase dose accordingly
Smoking	Increases metabolism		Advise to stop smoking; monitor levels and increase dose accordingly

Source: Modified from National Heart, Lung, and Blood Institute. *Expert Panel Report 3: Guidelines for the Diagnosis and Management of Asthma.* NIH Publication No. 08-4051. Bethesda, MD: National Heart, Lung, and Blood Institute; 2007. http://www.nhlbi.nih.gov/files/docs/guidelines/asthgdln.pdf. Accessed November 22, 2014.[105]

Anticholinergics

Ipratropium bromide (Atrovent HFA), when used in conjunction with short-acting $beta_2$ agonists, appears to improve bronchoconstriction associated with moderate or severe asthma exacerbations in the emergency setting. The long-acting anticholinergic tiotropium bromide (Spiriva), which is typically used for treating chronic obstructive pulmonary disease, has been shown to improve control of moderate to severe asthma when added to either inhaled corticosteroids alone or inhaled corticosteroids/long-acting $beta_2$ agonist combinations, at times allowing discontinuation of the long-acting $beta_2$ agonist and tapering of the inhaled corticosteroids.[112]

Special Populations: Pregnancy, Smokers, and the Elderly

Use of asthma medications is much safer for both a woman and her fetus than having poorly controlled asthma and exacerbations during pregnancy.[105,121] Adverse outcomes associated with maternal asthma include congenital malformations, preeclampsia, small for gestational age, low birth weight, preterm labor, and preterm delivery. These effects can be mediated with adequate control of the symptoms.[122] Albuterol is the medication that has been studied the most; consequently, it is the short-acting beta agonist of choice in pregnant women.

No evidence of fetal harm from any of the medications commonly used to treat asthma has been reported, with the possible exception of systemic corticosteroids. In that case, it is difficult to distinguish the effects of the oral corticosteroids from the effects of severe asthma.[121] Exposure to tobacco smoke is associated with increased symptoms and disease severity in persons with asthma. Asthma can be more difficult to treat among smokers, who are less responsive to inhaled corticosteroids.[111]

Irreversible airway obstruction from emphysema or chronic bronchitis is more likely to complicate the reversible airway obstruction of asthma among elderly persons than those in younger individuals. The elderly are also at increased risk for adverse medication effects, such as tremor or tachycardia from inhaled $beta_2$ agonists, and elevated theophylline levels due to reduced clearance. Management of comorbid conditions frequently entails reviewing a long list of medications, some of which (e.g., NSAIDs, beta blockers) may aggravate asthma. Careful attention to the diagnosis and assessment of asthma symptoms in view of all the disease processes and medications will help to decrease the risks in elderly women.[105]

Tuberculosis

Mycobacterium tuberculosis is the bacteria responsible for tuberculosis (TB). Respiratory droplets—spread by singing, coughing, sneezing, or talking, for example—transmit the bacteria. Worldwide, one third of the population is infected with TB.[123] While TB is much less common in the United States, it remains a significant public health problem. Although the incidence of and mortality from TB are dramatically lower in the United States than in developing countries, a major concern is the rise in **multidrug-resistant tuberculosis**, which is rare among U.S.-born individuals, but may be noted among foreign-born persons.

The initial treatment of active TB infection is beyond the scope of this chapter. However, primary care clinicians commonly encounter persons for whom screening for TB and the treatment of latent TB infection(LTBI) is indicated; thus, these topics are presented in this section.

Latent Tuberculosis Infection

A basic principle of the control of TB in the United States is the identification and treatment of individuals who are at high risk for developing active TB. A second principle is the prompt diagnosis and treatment of those with active disease as well as their close contacts. Latent tuberculosis infection refers to infection in individuals who have been exposed to and harbor potentially disease-causing *M. tuberculosis*, yet whose healthy immune systems effectively control the infection. Between 5% and 10% of individuals with LTBI will progress to active disease, with the greatest risk occurring in the first 2 years following exposure.[124]

Testing for latent tuberculosis and subsequent treatment of individuals with positive tests have long been essential components of the control of TB in the United States and other countries with a low incidence of TB. In recent decades, there has been a shift from widespread population-based testing to targeted testing aimed at identifying individuals at high risk who would benefit from the treatment of latent TB infection.

Two forms of tuberculosis testing are performed. The most long-standing and inexpensive means of testing is intradermal administration of 0.1 mL of five tuberculin units of purified protein derivative (PPD) into the dorsal surface of the forearm. A trained professional then measures the diameter of induration in millimeters approximately 48 to 72 hours after its placement. A second methodology employs interferon-gamma release assays (IGRAs), which are whole blood tests. The two IGRAs in use in 2015 are the Quantiferon-TB Gold In-Tube test (QFT-GIT) and the T-Spot.*TB* test. These tests must be processed within 8 to 30 hours after collection. Active tuberculosis is diagnosed by means of a chest X ray and evaluation of symptoms in individuals with a positive skin or blood test.

In the past, pharmacotherapy for the treatment of TB was referred to as "preventive therapy" or "chemoprophylaxis." Today, the more accurate term is "treatment of LTBI." Adoption of this terminology emphasizes the critical nature of this component of TB control. Table 20-15 presents the

Table 20-15 Recommended Drug Treatment Regimens for Treatment of Latent Tuberculosis Infection in Adults

Drug: Generic (Brand)	Dose	Clinical Considerations	Drug–Drug Interactions
Isoniazid (INH) 300 mg	Standard: 300 mg daily for 9 months Alternative: 300 mg PO daily for 6 months 900 mg PO 2 times/week for 9 months[b] 900 mg 2 times/week for 6 months[b]	Liver function tests at baseline in selected cases[a] and repeat measurements if baseline results are abnormal or when the woman is pregnant, in the immediate postpartum period, if the woman is at high risk for adverse reactions, or if symptoms of hepatitis are present. Hepatitis risk increases with age and alcohol consumption. Pyridoxine (vitamin B_6, 10–25 mg/day) should be administered to persons who are at increased risk for neuropathy, including in pregnancy, alcoholism, uremia, diabetes, malnutrition, HIV infection, and infants of breastfeeding women who are taking INH. May be administered concurrently with nucleoside reverse transcriptase inhibitors, protease inhibitors, or non-nucleoside reverse transcriptase inhibitors.	Multiple drug–drug interactions. Substrate for CYP2E1; inhibits CYP2A6, CYP2C19, and CYP2D6; and induces CYP2E1.
Isoniazid (INH) and rifapentine (Priftin)	INH 15 mg/kg rounded up to the nearest 50 or 100 mg; 900 mg maximum dose PO once/week for 12 doses given by DOT *and* Rifapentine 900 mg PO once/week given by DOT; dose based on weight[c]	See the clinical considerations for isoniazid above. This option is equal to the 9-month INH daily regimen in otherwise healthy adults. Not recommended for pregnant women or those at risk of becoming pregnant. Should not be used by persons with hepatic dysfunction unless under strict medical supervision. Baseline liver function tests should be obtained and then performed every 2–4 weeks during therapy. Administer with meals.	See the interactions for isoniazid above. Rifapentine is a strong inducer of CYP2C8, CYP2C9, and CYP3A4. Multiple drug–drug interactions, including warfarin (Coumadin), methadone, antidepressants, anticonvulsants, and antihypertensives.
Rifampin (Rifadin)	600 mg PO once/day for 4 months	Recommended for persons who are intolerant of INH or who have INH-resistant strains of TB. Rifampin is contraindicated or should be used with caution in persons infected with HIV and taking protease inhibitors or non-nucleoside reverse transcriptase inhibitors. Might permanently discolor soft contact lenses. Complete blood count, platelets, and liver function tests at baseline in selected cases[a] and repeat measurements if baseline results are abnormal or the person has symptoms of an adverse reaction.	Multiple drug–drug interactions. Induces CYP1A2, CYP2A6, CYP2C19, CYP2C8, CUP2C9, and CYP3A4. Decreases levels of many drugs, including methadone, warfarin (Coumadin), glucocorticoids, hormonal contraceptives, estrogens, oral hypoglycemic agents, digoxin (Lanoxin), and anticonvulsants.

Abbreviations: DOT = directly observed therapy.

[a] HIV infection, history of liver disease, alcoholism, and pregnancy.

[b] Directly observed therapy must be used with twice-weekly dosing.

[c] If more than 50 kg (110 lb), the dose is 900 mg.

Sources: Data from Centers for Disease Control and Prevention. Treatment of tuberculosis [erratum, *MMWR Recommend Rep.* 2005;53(51):1203]. *MMWR Recommend Rep.* 2003;52(RR11):1-77[125]; Centers for Disease Control and Prevention. Severe isoniazid-associated liver injuries among persons being treated for latent tuberculosis infection—United States, 2004-2008. *MMWR.* 2010;59(8):224-229[126]; Stagg HR, Zenner D, Harris RJ, Muñoz L, Lipman MC, Abubakar I. Treatment of latent tuberculosis infection: a network meta-analysis. Ann Intern Med. 2014;161(6):419-428.[127]

current pharmacotherapeutic recommendations of the CDC and the American Thoracic Society.[125–129]

Isoniazid (INH)

Isoniazid (INH) remains the mainstay for the treatment of LTBI. This bactericidal anti-infective agent is relatively inexpensive, and is nontoxic for most individuals. Isoniazid is well absorbed from the gastrointestinal tract and penetrates into all body fluids.

Side Effects/Adverse Effects

Severe side effects of isoniazid include hepatitis, which occurs in approximately 1 to 23 per 1000 exposed individuals, and peripheral neuropathy.[126] Baseline testing of liver function and bilirubin should be obtained in individuals at risk for hepatic dysfunction, such as persons with chronic hepatic disease or individuals who routinely consume alcohol. These tests are also indicated for persons with HIV infection, women who are pregnant, or women who have given birth within the prior 3 months. Persons taking isoniazid should be counseled to avoid alcohol during treatment.

Peripheral neuropathy occurs because isoniazid interferes with the metabolism of pyridoxine (vitamin B_6). This adverse effect is more commonly observed in persons with underlying conditions associated with neuropathy. Supplemental pyridoxine (vitamin B_6 25–50 mg per day) should be given to those individuals, as well as to pregnant women and individuals with seizure disorders who are taking antiepileptic medications. Concurrent administration of isoniazid and phenytoin (Dilantin) increases serum concentrations of each drug.

Rifampin (Rifadin)

Rifampin (Rifadin), a derivative of rifamycin, is a bactericidal anti-infective agent that is particularly effective against mycobacteria. Rifampin is rapidly absorbed from the gastrointestinal tract. Despite 75% of the drug being protein bound, it penetrates well into tissues and through inflamed meninges. Rifampin is as effective as—and possibly more effective than—isoniazid.[127]

Side Effects/Adverse Effects

Side effects of rifampin use include gastrointestinal upset and skin reactions. Individuals taking rifampin should be informed that the drug causes discoloration of body fluids, including sweat, urine, and tears; permanent discoloration of contact lenses may result from tear discoloration. Rare adverse effects include hepatitis and thrombocytopenia.

Drug–Drug Interactions

Rifampin is associated with many drug–drug interactions because it induces hepatic CYP 450 enzymes. It also increases the metabolism of estrogen, potentially decreasing the effectiveness of combined hormonal contraceptives.

Rifapentine (Priftin)

Rifapentine (Priftin) is a member of the same class of drugs as rifampin and has a similar mechanism of action. A combination of isoniazid with rifapentine has demonstrated better treatment effectiveness than does isoniazid alone, with lower rates of hepatotoxicity. Like rifampin, rifapentine has multiple drug–drug interactions and can lower the effectiveness of oral contraceptives.

Special Populations: Pregnancy and Lactation

Pregnant women with active TB during pregnancy should be treated for the disease rather than waiting until they give birth. Treatment of LTBI is more controversial. While the CDC states that it is acceptable to delay treatment in low-risk pregnant women until 3 months postpartum, many sources recommend that treatment be initiated at diagnosis, along with close monitoring for hepatitis. Isoniazid has been shown to be safe in pregnancy and is the preferred regimen. Rifampin (Rifadin) has also been used extensively and is probably also safe. Individuals treated for LTBI during pregnancy should receive supplemental pyridoxine (vitamin B_6) at a dose of 25 mg per day.[125] The combined regimen of isoniazid and rifapentine (Priftin) is not recommended during pregnancy.

There have been no reports of toxic effects of tuberculosis medications in breast milk, and breastfeeding is not contraindicated for lactating women receiving treatment for TB. Serum levels in breastfed infants are less than 20% of therapeutic levels and, therefore, are inadequate for treatment of the infant.[125]

Conclusion

Respiratory illness is a frequent cause of healthcare visits. Colds, bronchitis, and influenza in otherwise healthy individuals account for a significant number of these visits and may be managed with self-care counseling and perhaps recommendations for symptomatic relief such as decongestants. Primary care providers can do women a favor by educating them about the lack of a proven benefit from many of the over-the-counter medications marketed as offering relief from cold symptoms. By doing so, the provider will help women save money and avoid unwanted side effects caused by medications that are not effective.

However, not every respiratory illness is benign and self-limited. Asthma, pneumonia, and tuberculosis have serious sequelae, including mortality. It is the healthcare provider's responsibility to gather a complete history and perform a thorough physical examination to assess whether the woman is suffering from an illness associated with significant morbidity and plan for appropriate care that will minimize adverse outcomes.

Resources

Organization	Description	Website
National Institute of Allergy and Infectious Diseases	The tutorial "Understanding the Immune System" is an excellent review of the basics of the immune response that is relevant for clinical practice	www.imgt.org/IMGTeducation/Tutorials/ImmuneSystem/UK/the_immune_system.pdf
Infectious Disease Society of America (IDSA)	This professional society maintains updated links for all current practice guidelines for treatment of infectious diseases. Users can look up recommended treatments by organ system or by infectious organism. The guidelines for community-acquired pneumonia, rhinosinusitis, and streptococcal pharyngitis can be found on this site.	www.idsociety.org/IDSA_Practice_Guidelines/ www.idsociety.org/Organ_System
Centers for Disease Control and Prevention (CDC)	Guidelines for diagnosis and treatment of tuberculosis	www.cdc.gov/tb/publications/guidelines/Treatment.htm
	Guidelines for diagnosis and treatment of influenza; includes drug therapy, doses, adverse reactions, drug interactions, and practice guidelines	www.cdc.gov/flu/professionals/antivirals/index.htm
Apps		
Centers for Disease Control and Prevention (CDC)	Latent tuberculosis infection mobile application for healthcare providers; includes treatment tables and treatment options	www.cdc.gov/tb/publications/MobileLTBIApp/default.html
	Influenza mobile application for clinicians and healthcare professionals	www.cdc.gov/flu/apps/cdc-influenza-hcp.html

References

1. Clark RK. *Anatomy and Physiology: Understanding the Human Body.* Sudbury, MA: Jones and Bartlett; 2005.
2. National Institute of Allergy and Infectious Diseases. Understanding the immune system: how it works. NIH Publication No. 03-5423 2003. http://www.imgt.org/IMGTeducation/Tutorials/ImmuneSystem/UK/the_immune_system.pdf. Accessed November 24, 2014.
3. Amin K. The role of mast cells in allergic inflammation. *Respir Med.* 2012;106(1):9-14.
4. Allan GM, Arroll B. Prevention and treatment of the common cold: making sense of the evidence. *CMAJ.* 2014;186(3):190-199.
5. Arroll B. Common cold. *Clin Evid.* March 16, 2011. Online pii. 1510.
6. Jefferson T, Del Mar C, Dooley L, et al. Physical interventions to interrupt or reduce the spread of respiratory viruses. *Cochrane Database Syst Rev.* 2010;1:CD006207.
7. Turner RB, Fuls JL, Rodgers ND, Goldfarb HB, Lockhart LK, Aust LB. A randomized trial of the efficacy of hand disinfection for prevention of rhinovirus infection. *Clin Infect Dis.* 2012;54(10):1422-1426.

8. Tuladhar E, Hazeleger WC, Koopmans M, Zwietering MH, Duizer E, Beumer RR. Reducing viral contamination from finger pads: handwashing is more effective than alcohol-based hand disinfectants. *J Hosp Infect.* 2015;90(3):226-234.
9. Sutter AI, Lemiengre M, Campbell H, Mackinnon HF. Antihistamines for the common cold. *Cochrane Database Syst Rev.* 2003;3:CD001267.
10. Muether PS, Gwaltney JM Jr. Variant effect of first- and second-generation antihistamines as clues to their mechanism of action on the sneeze reflex in the common cold. *Clin Infect Dis.* 2001;33(9):1483-1488.
11. Naclerio RM, Proud D, Kagey-Sobotka A, Lichtenstein LM, Hendley JO, Gwaltney JM Jr. Is histamine responsible for the symptoms of rhinovirus colds? A look at the inflammatory mediators following infection. *Pediatr Infect Dis J.* 1988;7(3):218-222.
12. Taverner D, Latte J. Nasal decongestants for the common cold. *Cochrane Database Syst Rev.* 2007;1:CD001953.
13. Food and Drug Administration. Legal requirements for the sale and purchase of drug products containing pseudoephedrine, ephedrine, and phenylpropanolamine. 2006. http://www.fda.gov/Drugs/DrugSafety/InformationbyDrugClass/ucm072423.htm. Accessed November 24, 2014.
14. Eccles R. Substitution of phenylephrine for pseudoephedrine as a nasal decongestant: an illogical way to control methamphetamine abuse. *Br J Clin Pharmacol.* 2007;63(1):10-14.
15. Graf PM. Rhinitis medicamentosa. *Clin Allergy Immunol.* 2007;19:295-304.
16. Passàli D, Salerni L, Passàli GC, Passàli FM, Bellussi L. Nasal decongestants in the treatment of chronic nasal obstruction: efficacy and safety of use. *Expert Opin Drug Saf.* 2006;5(6):783-790.
17. Ferguson BJ, Paramaesvaran S, Rubinstein E. A study of the effect of nasal steroid sprays in perennial allergic rhinitis patients with rhinitis medicamentosa. *Otolaryngol Head Neck Surg.* 2001;125(3):253-260.
18. Dealleaume L, Tweed B, Neher JO. Do OTC remedies relieve cough in acute URIs? *J Fam Pract.* 2009; 58(10):559a-559c.
19. Hayward G, Thompson MJ, Perera R, Del Mar CB, Glasziou PP, Heneghan CJ. Corticosteroids for the common cold. *Cochrane Database Syst Rev.* 2012;8:CD008116.
20. AlBalawi ZH, Othman SS, Alfaleh K. Intranasal ipratropium bromide for the common cold. *Cochrane Database Syst Rev.* 2013;6:CD008231.
21. Mygind N. Allergic rhinitis. *Chem Immunol Allergy.* 2014;100:62-68.
22. Bolser DC. Cough suppressant and pharmacologic protussive therapy: ACCP evidence-based clinical practice guidelines. *Chest.* 2006;129(1 suppl):238S-249S.
23. Kim SY, Chang YJ, Cho HM, Hwang YW, Moon YS. Non-steroidal anti-inflammatory drugs for the common cold. *Cochrane Database Syst Rev.* 2013;6:CD006362.
24. Mossad SB, Macknin ML, Medendorp SV, Mason P. Zinc gluconate lozenges for treating the common cold: a randomized, double-blind, placebo-controlled study. *Ann Intern Med.* 1996;125(2):81-88.
25. Singh M, Das RR. Zinc for the common cold. *Cochrane Database Syst Rev.* 2013;6:CD001364.
26. Hulisz D. Efficacy of zinc against common cold viruses: an overview. *J Am Pharm Assoc.* 2004;44(5):594-603.
27. D'Cruze H, Arroll B, Kenealy T. Is intranasal zinc effective and safe for the common cold? A systematic review and meta-analysis. *J Prim Health Care.* 2009;1(2):134-139.
28. Hemila H, Chalker E. Vitamin C for preventing and treating the common cold. *Cochrane Database Syst Rev.* 2013;1:CD000980.
29. Hwang SA, Dasgupta A, Actor JK. Cytokine production by non-adherent mouse splenocyte cultures to echinacea extracts. *Clinica Chimica Acta; In J Clin Chem.* 2004;343(1-2):161-166.
30. Gilroy CM, Steiner JF, Byers T, Shapiro H, Georgian W. Echinacea and truth in labeling. *Arch Intern Med.* 2003;163(6):699-704.
31. Karsch-Völk M, Barrett B, Kiefer D, Bauer R, Ardjomand-WoelkartK, Linde K. Echinacea for preventing and treating the common cold. *Cochrane Database Syst Rev.* 2014;2:CD000530.
32. Jawad M, Schoop R, Suter A, Klein P, Eccles R. Safety and efficacy profile of echinacea purpurea to prevent common cold episodes: a randomized, double-blind, placebo-controlled trial. *Evid Based Complement Alternat Med.* 2012;2012:841315.
33. Berggren A, Lazou Ahren I, Larsson N, Onning G. Randomised, double-blind and placebo-controlled study using new probiotic lactobacilli for strengthening the body immune defence against viral infections. *Eur J Nutr.* 2011;50(3):203-210.
34. Makino S, Ikegami S, Kume A, Horiuchi H, Sasaki H, Orii N. Reducing the risk of infection in the elderly by dietary intake of yoghurt fermented with *Lactobacillus delbrueckii* ssp. *bulgaricus* OLL1073R-1. *Br J Nutr.* 2010;104(7):998-1006.

35. Rennard BO, Ertl RF, Gossman GL, Robbins RA, Rennard SI. Chicken soup inhibits neutrophil chemotaxis in vitro. *Chest.* 2000;118(4):1150-1157.
36. Wise PM, Breslin PA, Dalton P. Sweet taste and menthol increase cough reflex thresholds. *Pulmon Pharm Therapeutics.* 2012;25(3):236-241.
37. Kassel JC, King D, Spurling GK. Saline nasal irrigation for acute upper respiratory tract infections. *Cochrane Database Syst Rev.* 2010;3:CD006821.
38. Yoon PW, Rasmussen SA, Lynberg MC, et al. The National Birth Defects Prevention Study. *Public Health Rep.* 2001;116(suppl 1):32-40.
39. Werler MM, Mitchell AA, Hernandez-Diaz S, Honein MA. Use of over-the-counter medications during pregnancy. *Am J Obstet Gynecol.* 2005;193(3 Pt 1): 771-777.
40. Li Q, Mitchell A, Werier MM, Yau WP, Hernández-Díaz S. Assessment of antihistamine use in early pregnancy and birth defects. *J Allergy Clin Immunol Pract.* 2013;1(6):666-674.
41. Snellman L, Adams,W, Anderson G, et al. *Diagnosis and treatment of respiratory illness in children and adults.* Institute for Clinical Systems Improvement; 2013. http://www.guideline.gov/content.aspx?id=43792. Accessed November 24, 2014.
42. Crocker A, Alweis R, Scheirer J, Schamel S, Wasser T, Levingood K. Factors affecting adherence to evidence-based guidelines in the treatment of URI, sinusitis, and pharyngitis. *J Commun Hosp Intern Med Perspect.* 2013;3(2). doi:10.3402/jchimp.v3i2.20744.
43. Centor RM, Witherspoon JM, Dalton HP, Brody CE, Link K. The diagnosis of strep throat in adults in the emergency room. *Med Decision Making.* 1981; 1(3):239-246.
44. McIsaac WJ, Kellner JD, Aufricht P, Vanjaka A, Low DE. Empirical validation of guidelines for the management of pharyngitis in children and adults. *JAMA.* 2004;291(13):1587-1595.
45. Aalbers J, O'Brien KK, Chan WS, et al. Predicting streptococcal pharyngitis in adults in primary care: a systematic review of the diagnostic accuracy of symptoms and signs and validation of the Centor score. *BMC Med.* 2011;9:67. doi:10.1186/1741-7015-9-67.
46. Shulman ST, Bisno AL, Clegg HW, et al. Clinical practice guideline for the diagnosis and management of group A streptococcal pharyngitis: 2012 update by the Infectious Diseases Society of America. *Clin Infect Dis.* 2012;55(10):1279-1282.
47. Gerber MA, Baltimore RS, Eaton CB, et al. Prevention of rheumatic fever and diagnosis and treatment of acute streptococcal pharyngitis: a scientific statement from the American Heart Association Rheumatic Fever, Endocarditis, and Kawasaki Disease Committee of the Council on Cardiovascular Disease in the Young, the Interdisciplinary Council on Functional Genomics and Translational Biology, and the Interdisciplinary Council on Quality of Care and Outcomes Research: endorsed by the American Academy of Pediatrics. *Circulation.* 2009;119(11): 1541-1551.
48. Logan LK, McAuley JB, Shulman ST. Macrolide treatment failure in streptococcal pharyngitis resulting in acute rheumatic fever. *Pediatrics.* 2012;129(3): e798-e802.
49. Stone S, Gonzales R, Maselli J, Lowenstein SR. Antibiotic prescribing for patients with colds, upper respiratory tract infections, and bronchitis: a national study of hospital-based emergency departments. *Ann Emerg Med.* 2000;36(4):320-327.
50. Albert RH. Diagnosis and treatment of acute bronchitis. *Am Fam Phys.* 2010;82(11):1345-1350.
51. Smith SM, Fahey T, Smucny J, Becker LA. Antibiotics for acute bronchitis. *Cochrane Database Syst Rev.* 2014;3:CD000245. doi:10.1002/14651858.CD000245. pub3.
52. Smith SM, Schroeder K, Fahey T. Over-the-counter (OTC) medications for acute cough in children and adults in ambulatory settings. *Cochrane Database Syst Rev.* 2012;8:CD001831.
53. Centers for Disease Control and Prevention. Get smart: know when antibiotics work. http://www.cdc.gov/getsmart/. Accessed June 3, 2014.
54. Barnett ML, Linder JA. Antibiotic prescribing for adults with acute bronchitis in the United States, 1996–2010. *JAMA.* 2014;311(19):2020-2022.
55. Levine DA. "Pharming": the abuse of prescription and over-the-counter drugs in teens. *Curr Opin Pediatr.* 2007;19(3):27027-27034.
56. Chyka PA, Erdman AR, Manoguerra AS, et al. Dextromethorphan poisoning: an evidence-based consensus guideline for out-of-hospital management. *Clin Toxicol.* 2007;45(6):662-677.
57. Becker LA, Hom J, Villasis-Keever M, van der Wouden JC. Beta$_2$-agonists for acute bronchitis. *Cochrane Database Syst Rev.* 2011;7:CD001726. doi: 10.1002/14651858.CD001726.pub4.
58. Moyo M, Van Staden J. Medicinal properties and conservation of *Pelargonium sidoides* DC. *J Ethnopharm.* 2014;152(2):243-255.
59. Ghazi-Moghadam K, Inançli HM, Bazazy N, Plinkert PK, Efferth T, Sertel S. Phytomedicine in

otorhinolaryngology and pulmonology: clinical trials with herbal remedies. *Pharmaceuticals.* 2012; 5(8):853-874.

60. Hurt AC. The epidemiology and spread of drug resistant human influenza viruses. *Curr Opin Virol.* 2014; 8C:22-29.
61. Grohskopf LA, Shay DK, Shimabukuro TT, et al. Prevention and control of seasonal influenza with vaccines: recommendations of the Advisory Committee on Immunization Practices—United States, 2013–2014. *MMWR.* 2013;62(RR07):1-43.
62. Uyeki TM. Preventing and controlling influenza with available interventions. *N Engl J Med.* 2014;370(9): 789-791.
63. Oh DY, Hurt AC. A review of the antiviral susceptibility of human and avian influenza viruses over the last decade. *Scientifica.* 2014;2014:430629.
64. Farrukee R, Mosse J, Hurt AC. Review of the clinical effectiveness of the neuraminidase inhibitors against influenza B viruses. *Expert Rev Anti-Infect Ther.* 2013; 11(11):1135-1145.
65. Jefferson T, Jones M, Doshi P, Spencer EA, Onakpoya I, Heneghan CJ. Oseltamivir for influenza in adults and children: systematic review of clinical study reports and summary of regulatory comments. *BMJ.* 2014;348:g2545.
66. Fiore AE, Fry A, Shay D, et al. Antiviral agents for the treatment and chemoprophylaxis of influenza: recommendations of the Advisory Committee on Immunization Practices (ACIP). *MMWR Recommend Rep.* 2011;60(1):1-24.
67. Colman PM. Zanamivir: an influenza virus neuraminidase inhibitor. *Expert Rev Anti-Infect Ther.* 2005; 3(2):191-199.
68. Gravenstein S, Johnston SL, Loeschel E, Webster A. Zanamivir: a review of clinical safety in individuals at high risk of developing influenza-related complications. *Drug Saf.* 2001;24(15):1113-1125.
69. Kourtis AP, Read JS, Jamieson DJ. Pregnancy and infection. *N Engl J Med.* 2014;370(23):2211-2218.
70. Borse RH, Shrestha SS, Fiore AE, et al. Effects of vaccine program against pandemic influenza A(H1N1) virus, United States, 2009–2010. *Emerg Infect Dis.* 2013;19(3):439-448.
71. Hoyert DL, Xu JQ. *Deaths: preliminary data for 2011.* National Vital Statistics Reports, 61(6). Hyattsville, MD: National Center for Health Statistics; 2012.
72. Mandell LA, Wunderink RG, Anzueto A, et al. Infectious Diseases Society of America/American Thoracic Society consensus guidelines on the management of community-acquired pneumonia in adults. *Clin Infect Dis.* 2007;44(suppl 2):S27-S72.
73. Nuorti JP, Whitney CG. Updated recommendations for prevention of invasive pneumococcal disease among adults using the 23-valent pneumococcal polysaccharide vaccine (PPSV23). *MMWR.* 2010; 59(34):1102-1106.
74. File TM. Community-acquired pneumonia. *Lancet.* 2003;362(9400):1991-2001.
75. Remington LT, Sligl WI. Community-acquired pneumonia. *Curr Opin Pulmon Med.* 2014;20(3): 215-224.
76. Scalera NM, File TM Jr. Determining the duration of therapy for patients with community-acquired pneumonia. *Curr Infect Dis Reports.* 2013;15(2): 191-195.
77. Brito V, Niederman MS. Pneumonia complicating pregnancy. *Clin Chest Med.* 2011;32(1):121-132, ix.
78. Feldt B, Dion GR, Weitzel EK, McMains KC. Acute sinusitis. *S Med J.* 2013;106(10):577-581.
79. Blackwell DL, Lucas JW, Clarke TC. *Summary health statistics for U.S. adults: National Health Interview Survey, 2012.* National Center for Health Statistics; 2014. http://www.cdc.gov/nchs/data/series/sr_10/sr10_252.pdf. Accessed November 24, 2014.
80. Chow AW, Benninger MS, Brook I, et al. IDSA clinical practice guideline for acute bacterial rhinosinusitis in children and adults. *Clin Infect Dis.* 2012;54(8):e72-e112.
81. Ip S, Fu L, Balk E, Chew P, Devine D, Lau J. Update on acute bacterial rhinosinusitis. *Evid Rep Technol Assess.* 2005;(124):1-3.
82. University of Michigan Health Systems. *Acute rhinosinusitis in adults.* Ann Arbor: University of Michigan Health Systems; 2011. http://www.med.umich.edu/1info/FHP/practiceguides/Rhino/Rhino.pdf. Accessed November 24, 2014.
83. Desrosiers M, Evans GA, Keith PK, et al. Canadian clinical practice guidelines for acute and chronic rhinosinusitis. *J Onolaryngol Head Neck Surg.* 2011;40(suppl 2):S99-S193.
84. Hayward G, Heneghan C, Perera R, Thompson M. Intranasal corticosteroids in management of acute sinusitis: a systematic review and meta-analysis. *Ann Fam Med.* 2012;10(3):241-249.
85. Slavin RG, Spector SL, Bernstein IL, et al. The diagnosis and management of sinusitis: a practice parameter update. *J Allergy Clin Immunol.* 2005;116 (6 suppl):S13-S47.

86. Food and Drug Administration. *Cold, cough, allergy, bronchodilator, and antiasthmatic drug products for over-the-counter human use: amendment of the final monograph for over-the-counter nasal decongestant drug products.* Final rule; 2005. http://www.gpo.gov/fdsys/pkg/FR-2005-10-11/pdf/05-20304.pdf. Accessed July 23, 2015.
87. Kariyawasam HH, Scadding GK. Chronic rhinosinusitis: therapeutic efficacy of anti-inflammatory and antibiotic approaches. *Allergy Asthma Immunol Res.* 2011;3(4):226-235.
88. Jackson LL, Kountakis SE. Classification and management of rhinosinusitis and its complications. *Otolaryngol Clin North Am.* 2005;38(6):1143-1153.
89. Corren J. The connection between allergic rhinitis and bronchial asthma. *Curr Opin Pulmon Med.* 2007;13(1):13-18.
90. Tran NP, Vickery J, Blaiss MS. Management of rhinitis: allergic and non-allergic. *Allergy Asthma Immunol Res.* 2011;3(3):148-156.
91. Kariyawasam HH, Rotiroti G. Allergic rhinitis, chronic rhinosinusitis and asthma: unravelling a complex relationship. *Curr Opin Ontolaryngol.* 2013;21(1):79-86.
92. Leynaert B, Neukirch F, Demoly P, Bousquet J. Epidemiologic evidence for asthma and rhinitis comorbidity. *J Allergy Clin Immunol.* 2000;106(5 suppl):S201-S205.
93. Shaaban R, Zureik M, Soussan D, et al. Rhinitis and onset of asthma: a longitudinal population-based study. *Lancet.* 2008;372(9643):1049-1057.
94. Meltzer EO. Pharmacotherapeutic strategies for allergic rhinitis: matching treatment to symptoms, disease progression, and associated conditions. *Allergy Asthma Proc.* 2013;34(4):301-311.
95. Tsabouri S, Tseretopoulou X, Priftis K, Ntzani EE. Omalizumab for the treatment of inadequately controlled allergic rhinitis: a systematic review and meta-analysis of randomized clinical trials. *J Allergy Clin Immunol.* 2014;2(3):332-340, e1.
96. Brozek JL, Bousquet J, Baena-Cagnani CE, et al. Allergic rhinitis and its impact on asthma (ARIA) guidelines: 2010 revision. *J Allergy Clin Immunol.* 2010;126(3):466-476.
97. Brunton SA, Fromer LM. Treatment options for the management of perennial allergic rhinitis, with a focus on intranasal corticosteroids. *S Med J.* 2007;100(7):701-708.
98. Glacy J, Putnam K, Godfrey S, et al. *Treatments for Seasonal Allergic Rhinitis.* Comparative Effectiveness Review No. 120. Rockville, MD: Agency for Healthcare Research and Quality; 2013.
99. Small P, Kim H. Allergic rhinitis. *Allergy Asthma Clin Immunol.* 2011;7(suppl 1):S3.
100. Radulovic S, Calderon MA, Wilson D, Durham S. Sublingual immunotherapy for allergic rhinitis. *Cochrane Database Syst Rev.* 2010;12:CD002893.
101. Chelladurai Y, Lin SY. Effectiveness of subcutaneous versus sublingual immunotherapy for allergic rhinitis: current update. *Curr Opin Otolaryngol Head Neck Surg.* 2014;22(3):211-215.
102. Pfab F, Schalock PC, Napadow V, et al. Acupuncture for allergic disease therapy: the current state of evidence. *Exp Rev Clin Immunol.* 2014;10(7):831-841.
103. Hermelingmeier KE, Weber RK, Hellmich M, et al. Nasal irrigation as an adjunctive treatment in allergic rhinitis: a systematic review and meta-analysis. *Am J Rhinol Allergy.* 2012;26(5):e119-125.
104. Incaudo GA, Takach P. The diagnosis and treatment of allergic rhinitis during pregnancy and lactation. *Immunol Allergy Clin North Am.* 2006;26(1):137-154.
105. National Heart, Lung, and Blood Institute. *Expert Panel Report 3: Guidelines for the Diagnosis and Management of Asthma.* NIH Publication No. 08-4051. Bethesda, MD: National Heart, Lung, and Blood Institute; 2007. http://www.nhlbi.nih.gov/files/docs/guidelines/asthgdln.pdf. Accessed November 22, 2014.
106. Centers for Disease Control and Prevention, National Center for Health Statistics. FastStats asthma. 2014. http://www.cdc.gov/nchs/fastats/asthma.htm. Accessed June 30, 2014.
107. Bousquet J, Schunemann HJ, Samolinski B, et al. Allergic rhinitis and its impact on asthma (ARIA): achievements in 10 years and future needs. *J Allergy Clin Immunol.* 2012;130(5):1049-1062.
108. Milgram LJ. Asthma medications should be available "over-the-counter": con. *Ann Am Thoracic Soc.* 2014;11(6):975-979.
109. Gerald JK, Wechsler ME, Martinez FD. Asthma medications should be available for over-the-counter use: pro. *Ann Am Thoracic Soc.* 2014;11(6):969-975.
110. Barnes PJ. Biochemical basis of asthma therapy. *J Biolog Chem.* 2011;286(38):32899-32905.
111. Szefler SJ, Chinchilli VM, Israel E, et al. Key observations from the NHLBI Asthma Clinical Research Network. *Thorax.* 2012;67(5):450-455.
112. Befekadu E, Onofrei C, Colice GL. Tiotropium in asthma: a systematic review. *J Asthma Allergy.* 2014;7:11-21.

113. Alangari AA. Corticosteroids in the treatment of acute asthma. *Ann Thorac Med.* 2014;9(4):187-192.
114. Fuhlbrigge AL, Kelly HW. Inhaled corticosteroids in children: effects on bone mineral density and growth. *Lancet Resp Med.* 2014;2(6):487-496.
115. Kelly HW, Harkins MS, Boushey H. The role of inhaled long-acting beta-2 agonists in the management of asthma. *J N Med Assoc.* 2006;98(1):8-16.
116. Nelson HS, Weiss ST, Bleecker ER, Yancey SW, Dorinsky PM, SMART Study Group. The Salmeterol Multicenter Asthma Research Trial: a comparison of usual pharmacotherapy for asthma or usual pharmacotherapy plus salmeterol. *Chest.* 2006;129(1):15-26.
117. Food and Drug Administration. FDA announces new safety controls for long-acting beta agonists, medications used to treat asthma. http://www.fda.gov/NewsEvents/Newsroom/PressAnnouncements/ucm200931.htm. Accessed November 24, 2014.
118. Hirst C, Calingaert B, Stanford R, Castellsague J. Use of long-acting beta-agonists and inhaled steroids in asthma: meta-analysis of observational studies. *J Asthma.* 2010;47(4):439-446.
119. Zhong N, Lin J, Mehta P, Ngamjanyaporn P, Wu TC, Yuncus F. Real-life effectiveness of budesonide/formoterol maintenance and reliever therapy in asthma patients across Asia: SMARTASIA study. *BMC Pulmonary Med.* 2013;13:22.
120. Chauhan BF, Ducharme FM. Addition to inhaled corticosteroids of long-acting $beta_2$-agonists versus anti-leukotrienes for chronic asthma. *Cochrane Database Syst Rev.* 2014;1:CD003137. doi:10.1002/14651858.CD003137.pub5.
121. Gregersen TL, Ulrik CS. Safety of bronchodilators and corticosteroids for asthma during pregnancy: what we know and what we need to do better. *J Asthma Allergy.* 2013;6:117-125.
122. Murphy VE, Namazy JA, Powell H, et al. A meta-analysis of adverse perinatal outcomes in women with asthma. *BJOG.* 2011;118(11):1314-1323.
123. World Health Organization. *Global Tuberculosis Report.* Geneva, Switzerland: World Health Organization; 2013.
124. Centers for Disease Control and Prevention, Division of Tuberculosis Elimination. *Fact Sheet: Trends in Tuberculosis 2013.* Atlanta, GA: Centers for Disease Control and Prevention; 2013.
125. Centers for Disease Control and Prevention. Treatment of tuberculosis [erratum, *MMWR Recommend Rep.* 2005;53(51):1203]. *MMWR Recommend Rep.* 2003;52(RR11):1-77.
126. Centers for Disease Control and Prevention. Severe isoniazid-associated liver injuries among persons being treated for latent tuberculosis infection—United States, 2004–2008. *MMWR.* 2010;59(8):224-229.
127. Stagg HR, Zenner D, Harris RJ, Muñoz L, Lipman MC, Abubakar I. Treatment of latent tuberculosis infection: a network meta-analysis. *Ann Intern Med.* 2014;161(6):419-428.
128. Centers for Disease Control and Prevention, Division of Tuberculosis Elimination. *Latent Tuberculosis: A Guide for Primary Health Care Providers.* Atlanta, GA: Centers for Disease Control and Prevention; 2013.
129. Centers for Disease Control and Prevention. Recommendations for use of an isoniazid–rifapentine regimen with direct observation to treat latent *Mycobacterium tuberculosis* infection [erratum, *MMWR Morb Mortal Wkly Rep.* 2012;61:80]. *MMWR Morb Mortal Wkly Rep.* 2011;60(48):1650-1653.

21 Gastrointestinal Conditions

Patricia W. Caudle

Based on the chapter by Nancy Botehlo, Cathy L. Emeis, and Mary C. Brucker in the first edition of Pharmacology for Women's Health

Chapter Glossary

Antacids Drugs used to reduce gastric acidity for the treatment of peptic ulcer disease, gastroesophageal reflux disease, or simple pyrosis (heartburn).

Anticholinergic Agent that blocks the acetylcholine receptor, such as the one found in the stomach that enhances production of hydrochloric acid.

Antiemetic Drug that prevents or relieves nausea and vomiting. "Antiemetic" describes a function, not a chemical category. Antiemetic agents include antihistamines, benzodiazepines, and some medications from other chemical classes.

Extrapyramidal symptoms (EPS) Unintentional movements such as tardive dyskinesia, dystonia, and akathisia. EPS refers to symptoms originating in a specific part of the brain that refines and modulates movement. Drugs that antagonize dopamine receptors can cause extrapyramidal symptoms.

Laxative abuse Use of laxatives to lose weight.

Laxative dependency Overuse of laxatives resulting in the need for a laxative to have a normal bowel movement.

Milk-alkali syndrome Hypercalcemia that usually occurs secondary to overdose of calcium-containing antacids. It is characterized by kidney stones, constipation, and altered mental status, and can lead to renal failure if untreated.

Tardive dyskinesia Involuntary repetitive movements that are a side effect of dopamine antagonists. "Dyskinesia" refers to involuntary movement; "tardive" indicates that the movements may continue or appear after the drug is discontinued.

Introduction

Gastrointestinal diseases cause significant morbidity and mortality in persons of all ages. Multiple differences are found between women and men in relation to gastrointestinal function and gastrointestinal symptoms.[1] In addition, women are more likely to experience several gastrointestinal disorders such as irritable bowel syndrome, and they may respond differently to treatments as well.[2] This chapter reviews the pharmacologic treatments used for women with gastrointestinal disorders that commonly cause them to seek primary healthcare services. Upper gastrointestinal tract conditions are presented first, followed by nausea and vomiting, and finally disorders of the lower gastrointestinal tract. Autoimmune disorders that present with gastrointestinal symptoms, such as Crohn's disease, are addressed in the *Autoimmune Conditions* chapter.

The Gastrointestinal Tract

The upper gastrointestinal tract is composed of the mouth, pharynx, esophagus, and stomach (Figure 21-1). It functions primarily to ingest food and begin the digestive process through mechanical and enzymatic breakdown of the food bolus (consumed through the mouth) into smaller particles. The inner surface of the stomach has multiple rugae that disappear as the stomach becomes filled and its surface becomes smoothed. Four types of cells are found in the epithelial lining of the stomach: (1) chief cells, which secrete *pepsin*; (2) G cells, which secrete the hormone *gastrin*; (3) mucous cells, which secrete an alkaline mucus that protects the stomach lining from acid and shear stress; and (4) parietal cells, which secrete *gastric acid* and intrinsic factor, which is required for vitamin B_{12} absorption.

The parietal cells have receptors for histamine, acetylcholine, and gastrin (Figure 21-2). When any one of these receptors becomes bound to an agonist neurotransmitter, the parietal cell synthesizes and secretes gastric acid. When all three receptors are bound to agonists, large amounts of gastric acid is secreted.

Several chemical, mechanical, and neural triggers initiate secretion of gastric acid. For example, the vagus nerve secretes acetylcholine when the stomach is full; the acetylcholine then triggers the release of pepsin and gastric acid. Partially digested proteins increase the pH in the stomach, which in turn signals the G cells to secrete gastrin. Gastric acid causes the proteins to denature (unfold) and expose the peptide bonds, which can then be broken. As proteins are digested, the pH falls and gastrin production ceases. Finally, gastrin stimulates secretion of histamine from enterochromaffin-like cells that lie underneath the gastric epithelium.

Gastric acid must be actively pumped out of the parietal cells into the acidic environment of the stomach against a pH gradient. The process is powered by a *proton pump*, which is the term used to describe the hydrogen/potassium adenosine triphosphatase enzyme system that secretes gastric acid into the stomach cavity.

The contents in the stomach mix and are ultimately moved into the lower intestinal tract via peristalsis. Distention of the stomach wall by food stimulates stretch receptors and gastrin-secreting cells, which in turn increase the intensity of the peristalsis. Serotonin (5-HT), which is secreted by enterochromaffin cells (also called Kulchitsky cells), also activates peristalsis.

The lower gastrointestinal tract includes the small and large intestines and the anus. In the small intestine, proteins, carbohydrates, and fats are further digested into constituent peptides, disaccharides and monosaccharides, and triglycerides. These nutrients are subsequently absorbed by specialized enterocytes that line the numerous villi of the small intestine; these cells use a variety of mechanisms to provide uptake to the system and transport molecules from the lumen. Water, fat-soluble vitamins, and minerals also are absorbed in the small intestine. Approximately 2 liters of semi-liquid mass of digested food passes

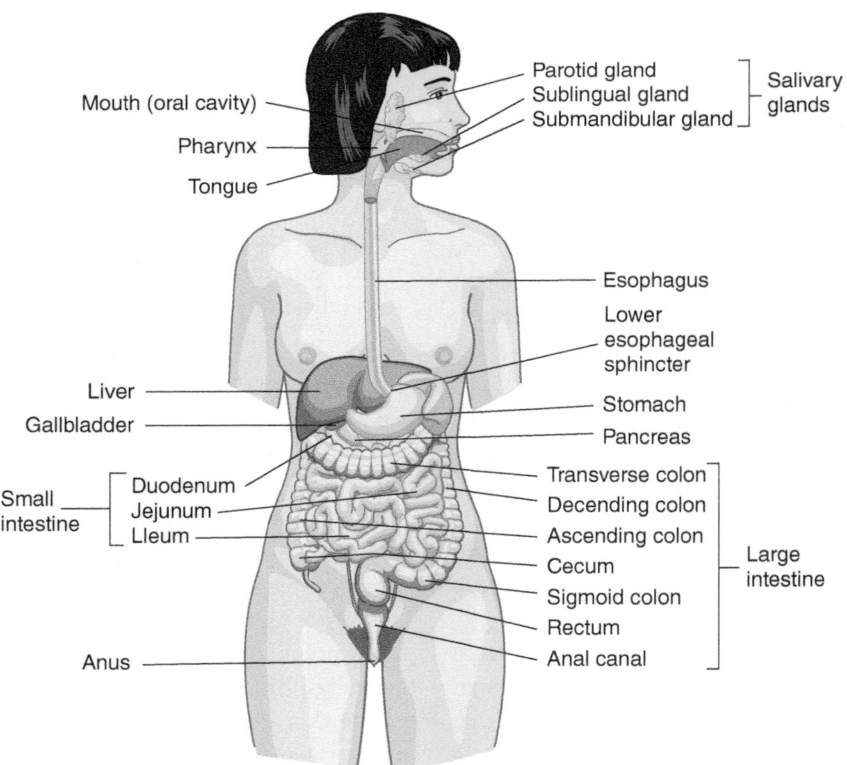

Figure 21-1 Anatomy of the gastrointestinal system.

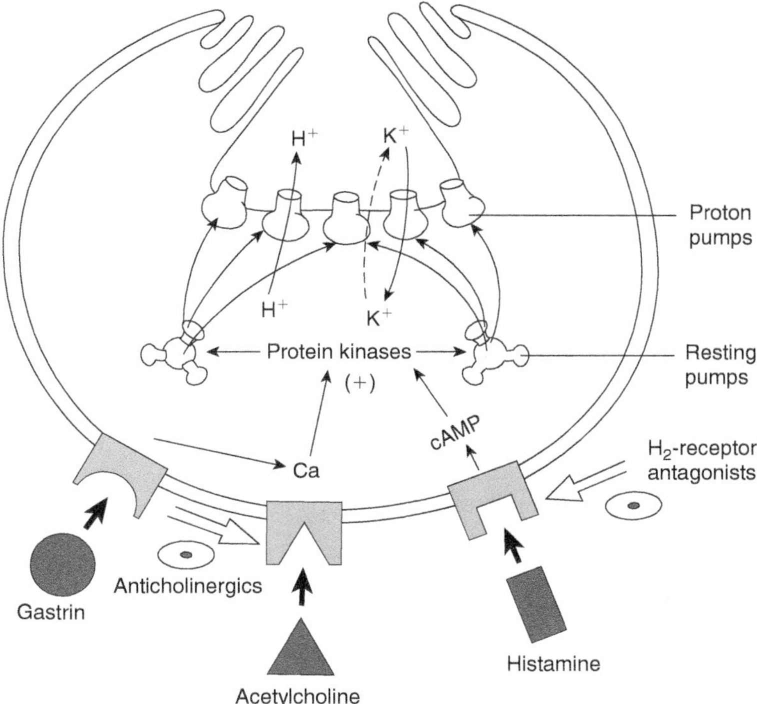

Figure 21-2 Parietal cell: stimulation of gastric acid production and secretion.

from the stomach into the lower digestive tract each day. The colon extracts a majority of the water and the rest becomes feces.

Accessory organs including the liver, gallbladder, and pancreas aid in the process of digestion (Figure 21-1). Bile secreted by the liver and stored in the gallbladder plays an important role in fat absorption, and enzymes secreted by the pancreas facilitate the breakdown of proteins, fats, and carbohydrates.

The Human Intestinal Microbiome

The human intestinal tract harbors millions of diverse microorganisms that are referred to as the gut microbiota. The collective genomes of these microorganisms are termed the gut microbiome. Although the gut microbiota is different for each individual, it displays a great deal of consistency over time in the same person. It has become increasingly clear in recent years that the gut microbiota participate in both health and disease.[3] There is a clear association between several disease states and *dysbiosis*—the term used to describe the gut microbiota when it is out of balance for a particular individual.[4] For example, gastrointestinal disorders such as irritable bowel syndrome, inflammatory bowel disease, and celiac disease are associated with dysbiosis. The balance within the gut microbiota also affects the immune response and stress response, so it may play a role in some stress-related disorders as well.[5]

Physiologic Control of Gastrointestinal Function

The gastrointestinal tract continuously absorbs substances; secretes digestive enzymes, mucus, ions, and bile; and contracts in a coordinated manner that moves material from the upper gastrointestinal tract toward the lower intestine and colon. Control of these functions is complex, but includes the actions of the epithelium, circulating hormones, the autonomic nervous system, the microbiome, and the enteric nervous system. The enteric nervous system lies within the wall of the gastrointestinal tract and is organized into two networks; the mesenteric plexus, which controls motility, and the submucosal plexus, which controls fluid transport, secretion, and blood flow. This complex organ system includes numerous defense mechanisms that prevent infection and mucosal damage from acid or digestive enzymes. Despite these defenses and the intricate system of hormonal and neural regulation, a variety of infectious, inflammatory, motile, malabsorptive, and structural disorders may occur.

Gastrointestinal Health

A healthy diet is usually the first choice for both prophylaxis and treatment of most women with gastrointestinal disorders. Dietary fiber has been touted as an important component of a healthy diet. Although it is recommended that adult women consume 25 g of plant fiber in their daily diet, most studies have found that the average diet for persons in the United States includes only approximately 15 g per day.[6] It is theorized that dietary fiber inhibits secretion of pancreatic enzymes, increases stool bulk, slows gastrointestinal transit, and stimulates growth of normal intestinal flora.

Two other potentially important dietary compounds are *prebiotics* and *probiotics*. Prebiotics are nondigested food ingredients such as oligosaccharides that act within the large intestine. Probiotics are dietary supplements, which contain microorganisms that confer a health benefit by improving the gastrointestinal microbiome balance. The most widely used probiotic bacteria are strains of *Lactobacillus acidophilus* and *Bifidobacterium*. Controversies exist regarding the usefulness of prebiotics and probiotics as therapies for gastrointestinal conditions, although a number of studies now suggest that these agents may have at least some therapeutic roles.[5]

Disorders of the Upper Gastrointestinal Tract

Dyspepsia, gastroesophageal reflux disease (GERD), and peptic ulcer disease (PUD) have much in common. Dyspepsia can be functional (epigastric pain syndrome) or meal associated (postprandial distress syndrome). All three disorders are associated with pain, bloating, early satiety, and varying degrees of nausea. Similarly, there is overlap in the medications used to treat these disorders.

Dyspepsia

The prevalence of dyspepsia in the United States is estimated to range from 25% to 40%, and this condition accounts for 3% to 5% of all primary care clinic visits.[7] Symptoms include pain in the upper abdomen that can be accompanied by bloating, early satiety, postprandial fullness, nausea, anorexia, heartburn (pyrosis), and burping or belching.[7] A variety of diverse factors are associated with dyspepsia, including foods, medications, systemic disorders, and disorders of the gastrointestinal tract. The drugs that most commonly cause dyspepsia are nonsteroidal anti-inflammatory drugs (NSAIDs), antibiotics, and estrogens. Dyspepsia may also be a symptom of GERD, although it does not always occur with GERD, nor is it pathognomonic for that disorder.

Dyspepsia can be either functional or organic. Functional dyspepsia, also known as nonulcerative dyspepsia, is the most common type of dyspepsia[7]; it is defined as persistent or recurrent pain in the upper abdomen in the absence of organic disease. Organic dyspepsia may occur secondary to peptic ulcer, GERD, or other infectious or systemic diseases. Environmental and lifestyle habits such as poor socioeconomic status, smoking, increased caffeine intake, and ingestion of NSAIDs appear to be more important in the etiology of organic dyspepsia than in functional dyspepsia.[7] The hormonal fluctuations of estrogen and progesterone associated with the menstrual cycle often make the symptoms of functional dyspepsia worse, however. First-line treatments for women with dyspepsia include over-the-counter antacids, histamine-2 (H_2) antihistamines, and proton pump inhibitors.

Alternative and complementary treatments are also used to treat dyspepsia. Peppermint oil relaxes the lower esophageal sphincter and reduces smooth muscle motility, which alleviates the symptoms of dyspepsia. Use of peppermint oil alone or in combination with caraway oil has been evaluated and appears to be modestly effective.[8] Although there are no known adverse effects associated with use of peppermint oil when taken as directed between meals, peppermint can cause dyspepsia if taken in large doses. Peppermint has theoretical drug–drug interactions with drugs metabolized by CYP1A2 and CYP2C9. Persons taking other drugs should use this agent with caution.

Peptic Ulcer Disease

Peptic ulcer disease (PUD) is an ulceration in the stomach or duodenum that occurs secondary to an imbalance between mucosal-protective factors and mucosal-damaging mechanisms. The damage may be caused by medications such as NSAIDs or corticosteroids. Nonpharmacologic risk factors include smoking, drinking alcohol, reflux of bile acids, increased acid production, age older than 40 years, male gender, and infection with the microbe *Helicobacter pylori*.

First-line medications for persons with peptic ulcer disease are H_2 antihistamines and proton pump inhibitors, with proton pump inhibitors having been shown to be more effective than H_2 antihistamines. Protective agents such as sucralfate (Carafate) and antacids are used as adjunct therapies. These agents help relieve symptoms and have some effect on healing, but are less effective than the H_2 antihistamines and proton pump inhibitors. Misoprostol (Cytotec) is effective for preventing NSAID-induced ulcers but has no effect on healing ulcers. Other treatments include antibiotics used to eradicate *H. pylori*.

Helicobacter pylori Infection

H. pylori, a gram-negative bacillus, has been associated with both duodenal and gastric ulcers. These bacilli burrow into the mucosa and weaken the protective mucous coating of the stomach and duodenum, which allows acid to enter the sensitive lining beneath. The acid and the bacteria irritate the lining of the stomach or duodenum, which causes ulcers. *H. pylori* is a common bacterium that is passed from person to person via the oral–fecal and oral–oral routes and is a known carcinogen.[6] Not every person who harbors this bacterium will develop gastritis or ulcers, but an estimated 90% to 95% of individuals with ulcers will test positive for *H. pylori*.[6,9,10] *H. pylori* does not grow easily in cultures, so it was decades before this bacterium was discovered and its role in ulcers recognized.

Several different treatment regimens for women with *H. pylori* are available, as noted in Table 21-1 and shown in Figure 21-3. The U.S. Food and Drug Administration (FDA) has approved a standard triple therapy as well as a quadruple therapy. Both have variations that are used for individuals with penicillin allergy and/or in locations associated with significant resistance to clarithromycin (Biaxin) or metronidazole (Flagyl).[10–14] All of the therapeutic regimens include a proton pump inhibitor and antibiotics; the quadruple regimen adds bismuth subsalicylate (Pepto-Bismol). The proton pump inhibitor is given to raise the pH within the stomach, which increases the effectiveness of the antibiotics. *H. pylori* is inherently resistant to sulfonamides, trimethoprim (Trimpex), and vancomycin (Vanocin). Resistance to metronidazole (Flagyl) and clarithromycin (Biaxin) is increasing, but clarithromycin is the single best antibiotic used to treat *H. pylori* if resistance is not present. Prolonging the standard triple therapy from 10 days to 14 days increases eradication rates by 5%.[12]

Nonsteroidal Anti-inflammatory Drug–Induced Peptic Ulcer Disease

NSAID use is the most frequent cause of ulcer complications in developed countries, where *H. pylori* infections are

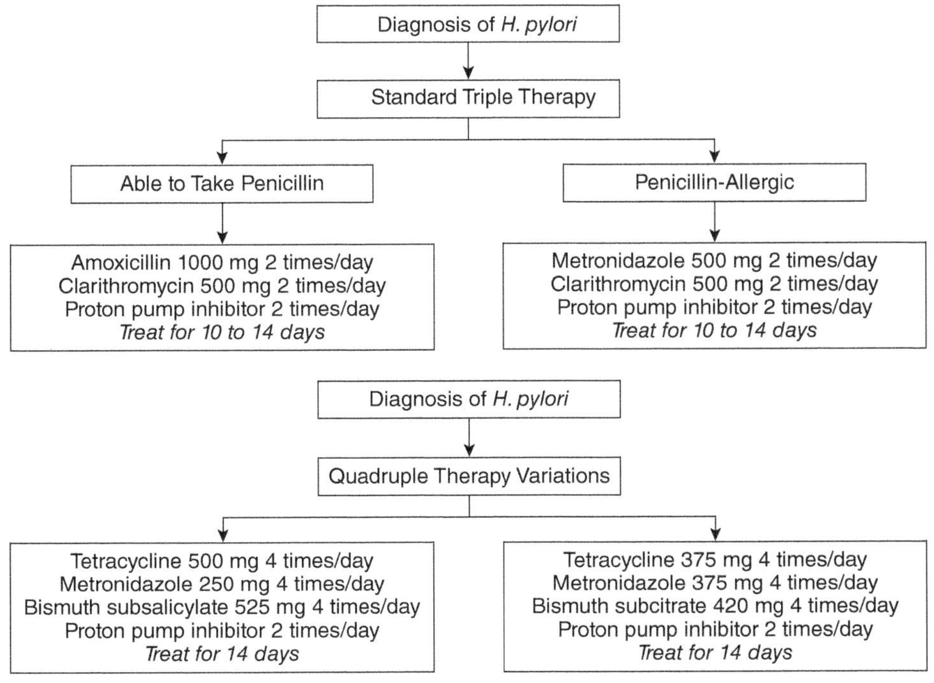

Figure 21-3 Treatment regimens for women with *H. pylori*.

Table 21-1 Medications for *H. pylori* Infection

Regimen	Treatment Duration	Eradication Rate	Clinical Considerations
Standard Triple Therapy[a]			
PPI 2 times/day *plus* clarithromycin (Biaxin) 500 mg 2 times/day *plus* amoxicillin (Amoxil) 1 g 2 times/day	7–14 days	77–85%	First-line treatment. Substitute metronidazole 500 mg 2 times/day if penicillin allergic.
Bismuth Quadruple Therapy			
PPI 2 times/day *plus* bismuth subsalicylate (Pepto-Bismol) 525 mg 4 times/day *plus* tetracycline (Sumycin) 500 mg 4 times/day *plus* metronidazole (Flagyl) 250 mg 3 times/day	10–14 days	77–90%	First-line treatment or may be used after treatment failure with standard triple therapy. May use for persons with penicillin allergy, recent exposure to clarithromycin or metronidazole, or if clarithromycin resistance is greater than 15%. Doxycycline can be substituted if tetracycline is not available.
PPI 2 times/day *plus* bismuth subcitrate 420 mg 4 times/day *plus* metronidazole (Flagyl) 375 mg 4 times/day *plus* tetracycline (Sumycin) 375 mg 4 times/day	10–14 days	70–85%	
Sequential Therapy			
PPI 2 times/day *plus* amoxicillin (Amoxil) 1 g 2 times/day for 5 days followed by PPI 2 times/day *plus* clarithromycin (Biaxin) 500 mg 2 times/day *plus* tinidazole or metronidazole (Flagyl) 500 mg 2 times/day for 5 days	10 days	78–82%	First-line therapy if penicillin allergic or clarithromycin resistance is greater than 15%. Levofloxacin 250 mg 2 times/day can be added.
Combination Products			
Prevpac: lansoprazole (Prevacid) 30 mg 3 times/day *plus* amoxicillin (Amoxil) 1 g 3 times/day *plus* clarithromycin (Biaxin) 500 mg 2 times/day	10–14 days	77%	Combination product. Indicated for persons who are allergic or intolerant to clarithromycin. Lower eradication rates. Taken with a PPI 2 times/day.
Pylera: bismuth subcitrate potassium 140 mg, metronidazole 125 mg, tetracycline hydrochloride 125 mg 3 capsules taken 4 times/day	10 days	88%	Decreased pill burden with combination product. Often used for retreatment unless it was used as a first-line therapy. Bismuth may turn the tongue or stools green or black. Taken with a PPI 2 times/day. Avoid cimetidine (Tagamet).
Other Regimens			
PPI 2 times/day *plus* clarithromycin (Biaxin) 500 mg 2 times/day *plus* metronidazole (Flagyl) 500 mg 2 times/day			Not FDA-approved.

Abbreviations: PPI = proton pump inhibitor.

[a] The FDA has approved three standard triple therapies: omeprazole, amoxicillin, and clarithromycin (OAC) for 10 days; bismuth subsalicylate, metronidazole, and tetracycline (BMT) for 14 days; and lansoprazole, amoxicillin, and clarithromycin (LAC) for 10–14 days.

Sources: Data from Chey WD, Wong BCY. Management of Helicobacter pylori infection. *Am J Gastroenterol*. 2007;102(8):1808-1825[14]; Malfertheiner P, Chan, FK, McColl KEL. Peptic ulcer disease. *Lancet*. 2009;374(9699):1449-1461[11]; McColl KE. Clinical practice: Helicobacter pylori infection. *N Engl J Med*. 2010;362(17):1597-1604[10]; Molina-Infante J, Gisbert JP. Optimizing clarithromycin-containing therapy for Helicobacter pylori in the era of antibiotic resistance. *World J Gastroenterol* 2014;20(3):10338-10347[13]; University of Texas at Austin, School of Nursing Family Nurse Practitioner Program. *Recommendations in primary care for the most efficacious and cost-effective pharmacologic treatment for* Helicobacter pylori *in non-pregnant adults*. Austin, TX: University of Texas at Austin, School of Nursing; May 2013. http://www.guideline.gov/content.aspx?id=46427. Accessed October 31, 2014.[12]

less prevalent. NSAIDs cause ulcers by suppressing gastric prostaglandin synthesis, which results in decreased mucin production, decreased bicarbonate release, and increased levels of hydrochloric acid.

Treatment for a woman with an NSAID-induced ulcer includes discontinuing the use of NSAIDs and adding an acid-suppressing drug such as an H_2 antihistamine or a proton pump inhibitor. Approximately 90% of NSAID-induced ulcers will heal if an H_2 antihistamine is taken for 8 weeks.[11] If the woman needs to continue the NSAID, then the addition of a proton pump inhibitor will be more effective in healing the ulcer than will use of an H_2 antihistamine.

Misoprostol (Cytotec), a prostaglandin analogue, has been prescribed to prevent NSAID-induced ulcers, even though the side effects of abdominal pain and diarrhea may cause individuals to discontinue use.[11,14] Another prophylactic option is a single pill marketed with the name Duexis that contains both ibuprofen (Advil) and the antihistamine famotidine (Pepcid). Duexis is designed to help those who need the pain relief of an NSAID and a medication that will prevent NSAID-induced ulcer in one simple regimen.[15]

Another combination capsule that was recently approved by the FDA for treatment of *H. pylori* infection is marketed as Pylera. Use of Pylera decreases the number of pills the woman must take in that it includes metronidazole, tetracycline, and bismuth subcitrate in one pill. During pregnancy and lactation, the treatment for *H. pylori* generally may be deferred. Regimens that do not include tetracyclines are acceptable, however.

Gastroesophageal Reflux Disease

Gastroesophageal reflux disease, also called reflux esophagitis, is characterized by heartburn and regurgitation of swallowed food caused by abnormal reflux of chyme from the stomach into the esophagus. Individuals may also experience excessive salivation and the sensation of a foreign body placed in the posterior pharynx. Other symptoms include a chronic cough, wheezing, hoarseness, sinusitis, and dental caries. These symptoms usually occur postprandially.

The resting tone of the lower esophageal sphincter normally maintains a high-pressure zone that prevents GERD. This pressure tends to be lower among persons who develop GERD and in women who are pregnant. Vomiting, coughing, lifting, or bending can contribute to the development of GERD, as can use of some medications (Table 21-2). If the chyme is highly acidic or contains bile salts and pancreatic enzymes, the refluxed matter can be erosive. Delayed gastric emptying can contribute to GERD as well. Disorders that delay emptying include gastric or duodenal ulcers, which can cause pyloric edema or pyloric strictures, and hiatal hernias, which weaken the lower esophageal sphincter.

Nonpharmacologic treatment of women with GERD includes lifestyle modifications that decrease the amount of reflux or decrease the damage to the lining of the esophagus from refluxed materials. Although there is a paucity of evidence on this subject, persons with GERD are often counseled to avoid foods and beverages that can decrease the lower esophageal sphincter pressure, including chocolate, peppermint, fried or fatty foods, caffeine, and alcoholic beverages. Decreasing the size of portions at mealtimes and eating at least 2 to 3 hours before bedtime may help to control the symptoms as well. Stopping cigarette smoking and losing weight may also help with symptoms of GERD. Cigarette smoking prolongs clearance of acid from the stomach and relaxes the baseline lower esophageal sphincter pressure, but there is no evidence that smoking cessation improves GERD symptoms.[16] Elevating the head of the bed is another effective treatment.

Table 21-2 Drugs That Can Cause or Aggravate Gastroesophageal Reflux Disease

Drug: Generic (Brand)	Drug: Generic (Brand)
Antibiotics	Iron supplements
Anticholinergics (e.g., for seasickness)	Nonsteroidal anti-inflammatory drugs
Aspirin	Progestin for abnormal menstrual bleeding or birth control
Beta-adrenergic agonists	Opioids such as codeine or hydrocodone
Bisphosphonates	Oxybutynin (Ditropan)
Bronchodilators for asthma	Sedatives for insomnia or anxiety
Calcium-channel blockers	Tetracycline
Diazepam (Valium)	Theophylline (Theo-Dur)
Dopamine-active drugs for Parkinson's disease	Tricyclic antidepressants

Drugs Used to Treat Women with Upper Gastrointestinal Disorders

Medications that decrease secretion of gastric acid or neutralize it once it is in the stomach are used to treat dyspepsia, peptic ulcer disease, and GERD. The three categories of medication used to treat GERD are antacids, antihistamines, and proton pump inhibitors. No single agent has been found to be superior to others in all cases. The choice of which agent to use varies based on the individual and clinical situation.

Antacids

Antacids are the primary treatment for women with minor gastric symptoms or to relieve heartburn (Box 21-1). These drugs are used as adjunct therapy for the relief of discomfort from peptic ulcers and to promote healing of peptic ulcers; for relief of stomach upset associated with hyperacidity; in prevention of stress ulcer bleeding; in treatment of duodenal ulcer; and in treatment of gastroesophageal reflux disease.

Antacids contain various combinations of metallic cations such as sodium bicarbonate, aluminum, calcium, or magnesium salts (Table 21-3). The overt mechanism of action is via neutralization of gastric acid, but antacids may also deliver growth factor to injured mucosa and the heavy metals are known to suppress the growth of *H. pylori*.

Mechanism of Action of Antacids

All antacids neutralize gastric acid in the stomach and increase the gastric pH. Contrary to popular belief,

Box 21-1 A Case of Heartburn

JB is a 38-year-old woman who reports that she works as a nurse on the 10-hour night shift, four nights a week. She reports being aroused from sleep several times a week by heartburn and mild regurgitation. She has used bismuth subsalicylate (Pepto-Bismol) as self-treatment with little success. She voices a concern that she may have an ulcer. JB is married and has two grade-school-aged children at home. Aside from bismuth subsalicylate, her only regular medication is Ortho Tri-cyclen Lo, which she takes daily for contraception. Her physical examination is unremarkable except for a body mass index (BMI) of 34.

Additional information is needed from JB regarding her sleep and dietary habits. Individuals who work night shifts tend to demonstrate a variety of sleeping patterns. Upon further discussion, JB reveals that after her shift she usually goes to breakfast with her coworkers; shortly after arriving home, she goes to bed.

Because of her weight and routine of sleeping shortly after eating, she is at risk for GERD. Health education about weight loss and eating light meals before sleep are first-line therapies. However, if a medication is desired, bismuth subsalicylate is not the best first choice. The salicylate in this product can interfere with absorption of orally ingested hormonal contraceptives. Instead, an inexpensive antacid such as a combination aluminum/magnesium agent (e.g., Maalox, Mylanta) would be a reasonable first choice, especially when taken remote from ingestion of her contraceptive pill.

antacids do not coat the stomach mucosal lining. Sodium bicarbonate dissociates to provide bicarbonate ions that neutralize the hydrogen ion concentration, which consequently raises blood and urinary pH. The other antacids similarly dissociate to provide a base ion and neutralize gastric hydrochloric acid. When the intragastric pH is maintained at greater than 4, the activation of pepsinogen to pepsin is decreased. Also, neutralization of gastric fluids leads to an increased lower esophageal sphincter pressure.

Antacids act rapidly and empty from the stomach quickly, with a resulting reaccumulation of acid or acid rebound. The best time to take an antacid is 1 hour after a meal or as soon as symptoms appear. Liquid formulations of antacids have greater acid-neutralizing capacity than do tablets, but tablets can be easier to use. Antacids

Table 21-3 Antacids[a,b]

Drug: Generic (Brand)	Dose Range	Contraindications	Side Effects/Adverse Effects	Clinical Considerations
Calcium carbonate[c] (Tums)	1–2 tablets PO (500–750 mg each) every 2 hours as needed; maximum dose, 7000 mg per 24 hours	Hypercalcemia, renal calculi, hypophosphatemia, persons with suspected digoxin toxicity	Constipation, anorexia, dry mouth, frequent urination, muscle twitching Milk-alkali syndrome	Should be taken with a full glass of water 1–3 hours after a meal and remote from taking other medications or vitamins. Has substantial acid-neutralizing capacity, which causes gastrin release, gastric acid secretion, and acid rebound. Not the choice for first-line therapy.
Aluminum hydroxide (Amphojel)	600–1200 mg PO between meals and at bedtime	Hypersensitivity to aluminum salts, renal impairment	Constipation, abdominal cramps, nausea, and vomiting Rare neurotoxicity in persons with renal failure; osteoporosis or kidney stones if taken for long periods of time	Binds with phosphate and decreases its absorption, which inhibits phosphate and calcium metabolism.
Magnesium hydroxide (Milk of Magnesia)	5–15 mL PO 4 times/day as needed for antacid; 30–60 mL as needed for laxative	Renal impairment; myocardial damage; heart block; colostomy or ileostomy; appendicitis; abdominal pain	Hypermagnesemia, abdominal cramps, diarrhea High serum magnesium can cause cardiac arrhythmias	More effective than aluminum antacids, but less effective than sodium bicarbonate. Use with caution by persons with renal insufficiency.

Sodium bicarbonate[d]	Effervescent powder: 1–2 tsp in glass of water after meals (4–8 g/dose) Powder: ½ tsp in a glass of water up to every 2 hours Tablets: 325 mg–2 g once/daily to 4 times/day	Persons on salt-restricted diet	Excess sodium can cause alkalosis, hypertension, congestive heart failure, edema	Component of many antacid formulations and the only compound in baking soda. Belching is common. Not recommended for treatment of PUD.
Combination Formulations				
Magnesium/aluminum combinations (Mylanta, Maalox, Gelusil)	Variable; Maalox 2–4 tsp PO 4 times/day	Hypersensitivity to aluminum salts Serious renal impairment; myocardial damage; heart block; colostomy or ileostomy; appendicitis; abdominal pain	Side effects and adverse effects of both magnesium- and aluminum-containing formulations	The magnesium component dissociates to neutralize gastric acid, while the aluminum component dissolves slowly in the stomach and provides more prolonged relief. The magnesium also has a laxative effect to counter the constipation commonly caused by aluminum.
Calcium carbonate/ sodium alginate/alginic acid (Gaviscon)	Chew 2–4 tablets 4 times daily	Hypocalcemia, hyponatremia, vomiting, concurrent use of citrate salts, renal impairment	Constipation, diarrhea, nausea, hyporeflexia, vomiting, muscle weakness	Polysaccharide that forms a layer on top of the stomach contents, which prevents regurgitation of contents.
Sucralfate (Carafate), sulfated polysaccharide/ aluminum hydroxide	1 gram 4 times/day 1 hour before each meal and before bedtime	Hypersensitivity to aluminum salts, renal impairment	Possible aluminum toxicity	Polysaccharide that forms a layer on top of the stomach contents, which prevents regurgitation of contents. Binds and delivers growth factor to injured tissue.

[a] This table is not comprehensive as new information is being generated on a regular basis.
[b] Brand names of antacids can be confusing. For example, there are several formulations of Alka-Seltzer, some of which include aspirin. Some antacids contain a combination of aluminum salts, magnesium salts, sodium salts, and calcium salts. Prescribers should know the constituents of specific brand names before recommending them.
[c] Milk-alkali syndrome has been reported when persons took a maximum dose of 4 g or more per day.
[d] Sodium bicarbonate is a component of several different brand-name products.

are available as over-the-counter (OTC) products, and no randomized trials comparing antacids head to head are available. If an antacid is chosen, the side-effect profile and drug interactions should be considered prior to use.

Side Effects/Adverse Effects

Each metal has different side effects. Magnesium causes diarrhea. Ingestion of large amounts of calcium can cause hypercalcemia, alkalosis, and renal impairment—a constellation of conditions called **milk-alkali syndrome**. Aluminum toxicity results in neurotoxicity and, although rare, can occur in persons with renal insufficiency.[17]

Drug–Drug Interactions

Antacids are associated with many drug–drug interactions.[18] Because antacids lower the pH in the stomach, drugs that are dependent on an acidic environment for their dissolution may not dissolve well when an individual takes an antacid. Conversely, drugs such as NSAIDs may dissolve more quickly in a neutral pH, which will accelerate the rate and extent of their absorption. Metallic ions can also form insoluble complexes with a drug, thereby decreasing its absorption. For example, antacids interfere with tetracycline (Sumycin) and fluoroquinolones due to this mechanism.[17]

Table 21-4 lists selected clinically important drug–drug interactions associated with antacids. Be aware, however, that antacids affect the absorption, bioavailability, and excretion of many drugs. Although these interactions may not result in detectable adverse events, individuals should refrain from using any antacid when taking other medications. When use of other medications is necessary, take the antacid at least 4 hours before or 2 hours after administration of those agents.

Table 21-4 Selected Clinically Important Drug–Drug Interactions Associated with Use of Antacids[a]

Drug: Generic (Brand)	Effect	Mechanism and Effect
Atazanavir (Reyataz)	Decreased therapeutic effect	Decreased absorption in basic or neutral pH
Bisphosphonates	No clinically significant effects	Antacids with calcium may theoretically engage in a chelation reaction and form an insoluble compound; manufacturers of bisphosphonates recommend avoiding antacids for 30 minutes after taking a bisphosphonate
Captopril (Capoten)	Decreased therapeutic effect	Decreased absorption in basic or neutral pH
Digoxin (Lanoxin)	Controversial	Decreased absorption in basic or neutral pH
Fluoroquinolones	Decreased therapeutic effect	Chelation that forms an insoluble compound
Glyburide (Diabeta, Micronase)	Neutral	Accelerated absorption but overall bioavailability remains unchanged
Ketoconazole (Nizoral)	Decreased therapeutic effect	Decreased absorption in basic or neutral pH
Iron supplements	Decreased therapeutic effect of iron, gastric upset	Chelation that forms an insoluble compound
Itraconazole (Sporanox)	Decreased therapeutic effect	Decreased absorption in basic or neutral pH
Rosuvastatin (Crestor)	Decreased therapeutic effect	Decreased absorption in basic or neutral pH
Tetracyclines	Decreased therapeutic effect	Chelation that forms an insoluble compound
Warfarin (Coumadin)	Increased risk of bleeding	Increased absorption and bioavailability of warfarin when taken with magnesium hydroxide only; other antacids are compatible with warfarin

[a] This table is not comprehensive as new information is being generated on a regular basis.

Source: Data from Ogawa R, Echizen H. Clinically significant drug interactions with antacids: an update. *Drugs.* 2011;71(14):1839-1864.[18]

Special Populations: Pregnancy, Lactation, and the Elderly

Heartburn occurs frequently during pregnancy due to the decrease in lower esophageal pressure caused by steroidal hormones, especially progesterone. Most antacids are safe to take during pregnancy because they are minimally absorbed. Magnesium trisilicate, however, should be avoided in pregnancy. Also, antacids containing sodium bicarbonate, when used in excess, may cause maternal or fetal metabolic alkalosis.[25] Antacids including sodium bicarbonate are considered safe during breastfeeding, although sodium may enter breast milk.[26]

Sodium bicarbonate is not the antacid of choice for elderly persons or for individuals on sodium-restricted diets (e.g., persons with hypertension and/or heart disease). This antacid will cause an increase in sodium and fluid retention. Excessive use can result in metabolic alkalosis, especially in individuals in whom kidney function is decreased.[26]

H_2 Antihistamines

H_2 antihistamines, also known as H_2 receptor antagonists, are excellent drugs for treating dyspepsia and are described in more detail in the *Antihistamines* chapter. These drugs have a competitive antagonist effect at the H_2 receptors of the parietal cells, thereby reducing fasting, postprandial, and nocturnal gastric acid secretion,[18] and are used as acid suppressive therapy for GERD. They may also be used in conjunction with NSAIDs in an effort to reduce dyspeptic symptoms and prevent NSAID-induced ulcers. For individuals with nocturnal GERD symptoms, administration of an H_2 antihistamine at bedtime suppresses vagally mediated, nocturnal gastric acid secretion.

All H_2 antihistamines impede gastric acid production for 6 to 24 hours and are useful for individuals who need persistent acid suppression. It usually takes 30 to 90 minutes before they are effective. The standard short-term dose for a person with nonerosive disease is an H_2 antihistamine twice daily. Examples include famotidine (Pepcid AC), cimetidine (Tagamet), ranitidine (Zantac), and nizatidine (Axid).

In 1977, cimetidine (Tagamet) became the first H_2 antihistamine approved by the FDA. Many factors need to be considered when persons are taking this medication. Among men, gynecomastia and impotence have been theorized to be a dose-related antiandrogen effect of cimetidine.[18] This drug is more likely than other H_2 antihistamines to cross the blood–brain barrier and cause depression or confusion. In addition, cimetidine has a large number of drug–drug interactions due to its effects on CYP450 metabolism. Consequently, cimetidine generally is not considered a first-line H_2 antihistamine.

Famotidine (Pepcid) is more potent than cimetidine (Tagamet), nizatidine (Axid), or ranitidine (Zantac). Famotidine does not inhibit CYP450 enzymes, so drug–drug interactions are less likely to occur with this agent.[18]

A combination drug composed of famotidine 10 mg, calcium carbonate 800 mg, and magnesium hydroxide 165 mg, is sold under two brand names: Pepcid Complete and Tums Dual Action. Initially there were concerns that the antacids in this combination would interfere with the pharmacokinetics of famotidine, as these agents often demonstrate drug–drug interactions. However, studies have failed to find any significant interactions. In fact, in this product, the antacid provides, rapid relief, while the H_2 antihistamine provides longer-lasting effects. The combination drug does interact with many other drugs, and taking the three drugs together expands the side-effect profile to include the effects of each component. It is advised that the tablets be chewed completely before swallowing.

Side Effects/Adverse Effects

H_2 antihistamines are generally well tolerated. The most commonly reported side effect is headache. Multiple small studies have reported adverse effects such as myelosuppression, thrombocytopenia, anemia, and pancytopenia as well. Because these drugs suppress production of gastric acid, malabsorption of vitamin B_{12} can occur.[19] In addition, the heart has H_2 receptors, so use of H_2 antihistamines can cause prolonged QT interval, sinus bradycardia, and hypotension.[20,21] These cardiac effects are more likely to occur if the drug is given intravenously or in very high doses. The adverse effects most commonly reported with H_2 antihistamines occur secondary to these agents blocking the H_2 receptors in the central nervous system. Confusion, somnolence, agitation, headaches, hallucinations, and dystonic reactions can occur in such circumstances.[22]

Drug–Drug Interactions

Cimetidine (Tagamet) is associated with many clinically significant drug–drug interactions because it has the dual action of inhibiting several CYP450 enzymes and decreasing renal clearance of several drugs. Caffeine levels may increase if taken with cimetidine, whereas concomitant use of St. John's wort (*Hypericum perforatum*) can decrease cimetidine levels. Antacids can reduce the effect of cimetidine, and should be taken 1–2 hours before or after cimetidine is ingested. At the current recommended over-the-counter doses (400 mg twice per day), drug–drug interactions are unlikely.

The other three H_2 antihistamines—famotidine (Pepcid), ranitidine (Zantac), and nizatidine (Axid)—are not CYP450 enzyme inhibitors to such a degree as cimetidine and are not associated with drug–drug interactions. Therefore, providers tend to recommend them more frequently.

Special Populations: Pregnancy, Lactation, and the Elderly

All H_2 antihistamines are considered safe for use by women during pregnancy and compatible with breastfeeding.[23,24] Although cimetidine (Tagamet) and famotidine (Pepcid) transfer into breast milk, they have been determined to be safe for breastfeeding women and their infants. The relative infant dose of cimetidine is 9% to 30%, which is higher than the 10% that is generally considered safe. However, there are no reports of adverse effects in infants and the American Academy of Pediatrics has listed cimetidine as safe for breastfeeding. The relative infant dose of the other antihistamines is lower than 10% and should be recommended before cimetidine if possible.

Due to the increased risk of chronic liver and kidney disease found among elderly individuals, H_2 antihistamines should be used with caution in this population. It is recommended that individuals with moderate to severe renal/hepatic impairment receive a reduced dose of H_2 antihistamines.

Proton Pump Inhibitors

Proton pump inhibitors are the most potent and long-lasting inhibitors of gastric acid production and are indicated for treatment of women with PUD, erosive gastritis, gastric ulcer prophylaxis, NSAID-associated gastropathy, GERD, heartburn, and Zollinger-Ellison syndrome. These prodrugs suppress gastric acid secretion by directly inhibiting the parietal cell H^+/K^+ ATP pump once the prodrug is converted to the active metabolite within the acidic compartment of the parietal cell.[4] Proton pump inhibitors irreversibly block the hydrogen/potassium adenosine triphosphatase enzyme; their effect lasts 2 to 3 days, until new copies of the enzymes are produced. Proton pump inhibitors suppress postprandial acid secretion best and are most effective when taken 30 to 60 minutes before a meal. Because a single dose of a proton pump inhibitor reduces 24-hour acid production by more than 90% and effectively stops food-stimulated acid production, the first dose should occur before the first meal of the day. Occasional dosing does not reliably suppress gastric acid production when compared to the recommended twice-daily dose regimen.[25] Little renal clearance occurs with proton pump inhibitors, so they may be used by individuals with renal insufficiency.

Currently, seven different proton pump inhibitors are available. Three are over-the-counter products: omeprazole (Prilosec), lansoprazole (Prevacid), and an omeprazole–sodium bicarbonate combination (Zegerid). Zegerid is an immediate-release preparation in which the sodium bicarbonate component of the combination raises gastric pH, thereby protecting the omeprazole component from acid degradation. The remaining four proton pump inhibitors are available by prescription: rabeprazole (AcipHex), pantoprazole (Protonix), esomeprazole (Nexium), and dexlansoprazole (Dexilant).[16]

Side Effects/Adverse Effects

Proton pump inhibitors are generally well tolerated, with their major side effects including headaches and diarrhea when used for short periods of time. The adverse effects of proton pump inhibitors can be grouped into two main categories: malabsorption and infection. Chronic use of proton pump inhibitors will affect the absorption of calcium, magnesium, and, in the elderly, vitamin B_{12}. Long-term use of proton pump inhibitors increases the risk for hip fracture (at 1 year: adjusted odds ratio [aOR], 1.22; 95% confidence interval [CI], 1.15–1.30; at 4 years: aOR, 1.59; 95% CI, 1.39–1.80).[26] The increased risk for hip fracture is presumed to occur secondary to malabsorption of calcium, but it may also arise because proton pump inhibitors inhibit osteoclastic vacuolar proton pumps, thereby inhibiting bone resorption. Infections linked to chronic use of proton pump inhibitors include community-acquired pneumonia,[27] *Clostridium difficile, Salmonella, Campylobacter jejuni,* and other intestinal pathogens.[28] Increased susceptibility to these organisms occurs because of the decrease in gastric acidity that would normally discourage growth of these pathogens.

Proton pump inhibitors have also been linked to acute interstitial nephritis in case reports.[29] The mechanism of action in such instances is hypothesized to be a hypersensitivity immune reaction wherein a metabolite of the proton pump inhibitor acts as an antigen.

Drug–Drug Interactions

Clinically important drug–drug interactions of proton pump inhibitors are rare. Omeprazole (Prilosec) appears to have the greatest potential for drug interactions secondary to its effects on intestinal and hepatic CYP450 enzymes. (Table 21-5).[30–33] The FDA has recommended that persons taking clopidogrel (Plavix) should avoid omeprazole because omeprazole reduces the effectiveness of clopidogrel by approximately 50%.[31] Rabeprazole (AcipHex) and pantoprazole (Protonix) have the least potential for drug–drug interactions.

Special Populations: Pregnancy, Lactation, and the Elderly

Omeprazole (Prilosec) was the first proton pump inhibitor available; there are no reports of teratogenic effects

Table 21-5 Selected Drug–Drug Interactions Associated with Use of Proton Pump Inhibitors[a]

Drug: Generic (Brand)	Clinical Effect on Drug That Interacts with Proton Pump Inhibitor
Esomeprazole (Nexium)	
Clarithromycin (Biaxin)	Increased serum level
Clopidogrel (Plavix)	Marked reduction in effectiveness; FDA black box warning to avoid using these two drugs concomitantly
Diazepam (Valium)	Decreased clearance and increased serum level
Rabeprazole (AcipHex)	
Clarithromycin (Biaxin)	Increased serum level
Fluvoxamine (Luvox)	Decreased serum levels of lansoprazole in extensive metabolizers of CYP2C19
Lansoprazole (Prevacid)	
Fluvoxamine (Luvox)	Decreased serum levels of lansoprazole in extensive metabolizers of CYP2C19
Theophylline (Theo-Dur)	Increased theophylline clearance
Omeprazole (Prilosec)	
Ciclosporin (Neoral)	Increased serum level
Citalopram (Celexa)	Increased serum level
Clarithromycin (Biaxin)	Increased serum level
Clopidogrel (Plavix)	Marked reduction in effectiveness; FDA black box warning to avoid using these two drugs concomitantly
Diazepam (Valium)	Decreased clearance and increased plasma level
Fluvoxamine (Luvox)	Decreased serum level of omeprazole in extensive metabolizers of CYP2C19
Itraconazole (Sporanox)	Reduced bioavailability secondary to increased pH and reduced absorption of itraconazole
Midazolam	Increased serum level
Nifedipine (Procardia)	Increased serum level secondary to increased absorption
Phenytoin (Dilantin)	Increased serum level
Sulfonylureas	Reduction in clearance
All Proton Pump Inhibitors	
Azoles	Decreased bioavailability of azoles
Clopidogrel (Plavix)	Marked
Digoxin (Lanoxin)	Increased serum level digoxin levels
Enteric-coated salicylates (Ecotrin)	Enteric coating may dissolve at increased rate and potentially cause gastric disturbance
Ketoconazole (Nizoral)	Reduced bioavailability secondary to increased pH and reduced absorption of ketoconazole

Methotrexate (Rheumatrex)	Elevated and prolonged serum levels of methotrexate
Protease inhibitors	Marked reduction in bioavailability secondary to loss of solubility
Warfarin (Coumadin)	Prolonged elimination and decrease in INR with all proton pump inhibitors except lansoprazole

[a] This table is not comprehensive as new information is being generated on a regular basis.
Sources: Data from Blume H, Donath F, Warnke A, Schug BS. Pharmacokinetic drug interaction profiles of proton pump inhibitors. *Drug Saf.* 2006;29(9):769-784[30]; Ogawa R, Echizen H. Drug–drug interaction profiles of proton pump inhibitors. Clin *Pharmacokinet.* 2010;49(8):509-433[32]; Wedemeyer RS, Blume H. Pharmacokinetic drug interaction profiles of proton pump inhibitors: an update. *Drug Saf.* 2014;37(4):201-211.[31]

in humans if this drug is taken during the first trimester of pregnancy.[34] Lansoprazole (Prevacid), rabeprazole (AcipHex), esomeprazole (Nexium), and pantoprazole (Protonix) are also safe for use by women during pregnancy. There is some evidence that proton pump inhibitors may be associated with an increased risk for the development of allergic conditions such as atopic dermatitis and asthma in offspring of women who use proton pump inhibitors during pregnancy.[35] However, the studies on this topic conducted to date have significant limitations, and more research is needed to determine if this association is real. Currently, the manufacturer of proton pump inhibitors recommends that breastfeeding women take these drugs with caution given they can be detected in breast milk. However, the relative infant doses appear to be less than 10% for all the proton pump inhibitors and, therefore, in practice, they are considered safe for lactating women.

Anticholinergic Agents

Anticholinergic drugs affect the parietal cells by inhibiting basal and meal-stimulated gastric acid secretion via suppression of vagal-mediated activity. Anticholinergics include atropine, scopolamine (Scopace), hyoscyamine (Levsin, Levbid), glycopyrrolate (Robinul), propantheline bromide (Pro-Banthine), and pirenzepine (Gastrozepin). All of these agents are associated with the classic anticholinergic systemic side effects, such as dry mouth, blurred vision, and urinary retention. H_2 antihistamines and proton pump inhibitors are much more effective and have fewer side effects. Anticholinergic agents have limited effectiveness and generally have no role in the treatment of women with peptic ulcer disease.

Propantheline and hyoscyamine are the exceptions. These drugs are used to treat ulcers as adjunct therapies to other medications because they decrease the motion of the muscles in the stomach, intestines, and bladder.

Special Populations: Pregnancy, Lactation, and the Elderly

Although anticholinergic agents have been used therapeutically for years, the safety of these drugs during pregnancy and breastfeeding remains unclear. Hyoscyamine (Levsin, Levbid) is considered compatible with breastfeeding.

Anticholinergic drugs should be used with caution by elderly individuals because they can cause dizziness and sedation. In addition, they are contraindicated in persons with glaucoma or difficulty urinating.

Cytoprotective Agents

Sucralfate (Carafate)

Sucralfate (Carafate) is indicated for short-term management of duodenal ulcers. Sucralfate is a complex salt of sucrose sulfate and aluminum hydroxide that binds with positively charged proteins in exudates. When combined with gastric acid, sucralfate breaks down into an aluminum salt and sucrose sulfate, which forms a viscous, paste-like, adhesive substance. This gel-like substance adheres to damaged mucosa and forms a cytoprotective coating that protects the stomach lining against damage from gastric acid, pepsin, and bile salts. Sucralfate prevents mucosal injury, reduces inflammation, and aids healing of existing ulcers. It should be administered before meals because it works best when the stomach is relatively empty. Antacids should not be taken within 30 minutes of ingestion of this agent.

Side effects of sucralfate include constipation, dry mouth, nausea, and abdominal pain. This agent should be used with caution by persons with renal impairment, because they may accumulate aluminum.

Sucralfate decreases the absorption and bioavailability of several drugs, including aminophylline, amitriptyline (Elavil), ciprofloxacin (Cipro), digoxin (Lanoxin), phenytoin (Dilantin), and theophylline (Theo-Dur). Sucralfate should not be used if fluoroquinolones are prescribed.

Bismuth Subsalicylate (Pepto-Bismol)

Bismuth is used for the treatment of women with diarrhea, PUD, and GERD. The formulation of bismuth that is commercially available in the United States is bismuth subsalicylate (Pepto-Bismol), which has an antimicrobial effect[13] that reduces the risk of duodenal ulcer recurrence caused by *H. pylori*. Bismuth combines with mucus to form a complex that coats ulcer craters, affording protection from gastric acid.

Bismuth subsalicylate can discolor the tongue and darken stools because it combines with trace amounts of sulfur in saliva and the gastrointestinal tract to form bismuth sulfide. This side effect is harmless and reversible once the drug is discontinued. Tinnitus could be an indication of toxicity. Bismuth subsalicylate may decrease the effect of tetracyclines. In contrast, persons who take bismuth subsalicylate may experience toxicity if they are concomitantly taking aspirin, warfarin (Coumadin), or oral hypoglycemics.

Misoprostol (Cytotec)

Misoprostol (Cytotec) is a prostaglandin E_1 analogue that binds to prostaglandin receptors, thereby stimulating increased production of mucus and bicarbonate. This drug also initiates increased mucosal blood flow and suppression of basal and postprandial gastric acid secretion. It is used as a prophylactic agent to prevent ulcers in individuals who take NSAIDs.[36] In essence, misoprostol is a synthetic prostaglandin used to counter NSAIDs' effect of inhibiting prostaglandin production. It is taken with food 4 times per day after meals and at bedtime.

Side effects of misoprostol are largely gastrointestinal in nature and primarily include diarrhea, gastric upset, gas, vomiting, constipation, and indigestion. Diarrhea occurs in approximately 30% of persons who use this drug. Headaches have also been reported with misoprostol use.

Special Populations: Pregnancy, Lactation, and the Elderly

Sucralfate is not absorbed, so it exhibits a local (rather than systemic) effect and is not associated with any teratogenic effects. Because it is excreted in breast milk to only a minimal extent, sucralfate is compatible with breastfeeding.

In contrast, both misoprostol (Cytotec) and bismuth subsalicylate (Pepto-Bismol) are agents that should be avoided during pregnancy. Misoprostol is a known teratogen that can cause facial paralysis of the newborn (Möbius syndrome).[37] This agent is contraindicated for use by women who are pregnant or who are trying to conceive because it increases uterine contractility and is associated with spontaneous abortions and premature labor. Misoprostol may induce vaginal bleeding in postmenopausal women. Bismuth subsalicylate should not be used during pregnancy because fetotoxicity has been reported in animals, and exposure to the salicylate component during late pregnancy may increase the risk of constriction of the fetal ductus arteriosus with resultant pulmonary hypertension. In addition, bismuth subsalicylate should be avoided during breastfeeding or at least used with caution. Although very little salicylate is transferred into breast milk, there is a known association between salicylate exposure and Reye syndrome in children, and alternative medications are available.

In elderly women, sucralfate (Carafate) may increase plasma and urine concentrations of aluminum, most likely via increased gastric absorption of the mineral contained within the agent and a decrease in renal clearance. There is a potential for bismuth subsalicylate (Pepto-Bismol) neurotoxicity if this agent is used for long periods of time, especially by persons with renal impairment.[38] Bismuth subsalicylate should also be used with caution by individuals with salicylate sensitivity or bleeding disorders. The pharmacokinetics of misoprostol is not changed in older individuals.[39]

Nausea and Vomiting

Nausea and vomiting can be a manifestation of a wide variety of conditions, including pregnancy, motion sickness, drug toxicity, radiation sickness, gastrointestinal obstruction, hepatitis, myocardial infarction, renal failure, increased intracranial pressure, asthma, Zollinger-Ellison syndrome, diabetes mellitus, thyrotoxicosis, and epilepsy.[15] Nausea and vomiting also are commonly experienced subsequent to chemotherapy and anesthesia.

Vomiting is triggered by afferent impulses to the vomiting center, a nucleus of cells within the medulla oblongata. The vomiting center can be stimulated by vestibular fibers, visceral afferents from the pharynx and gastrointestinal tract, and input from the chemoreceptor trigger zone (CTZ) located in the area postrema, an inferior part of the medulla oblongata that is located outside the blood–brain barrier.[40] A variety of neurotransmitter receptors are found in the vomiting center, CTZ, and gastrointestinal tract,

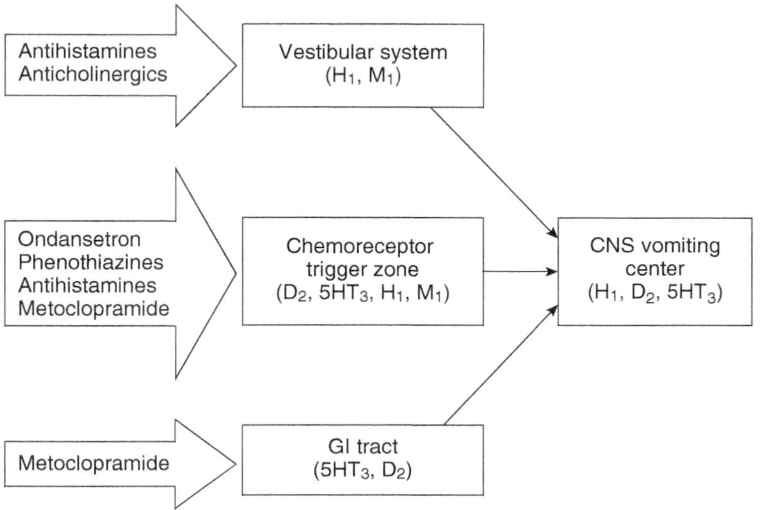

Figure 21-4 Chemoreceptor trigger zone and mechanism of action of antiemetics.

Abbreviations: $5HT_3$ = serotonin; CNS = centeral nervous system; D_2 = dopamine-2; H_1 = histamine-1; M_1 = muscarinic receptor.
Source: Modified from King TL, Murphy PA. Evidence-based approaches to managing nausea and vomiting in early pregnancy. *J Midwifery Womens Health*. 2009;54(6):430-444.[40]

including histamine (H_1), serotonin (also called 5-HT_3), dopamine (D_2), and muscarinic (M_1) receptors. These neurotransmitter receptors are the primary targets of **antiemetic** drugs (Figure 21-4).[37]

Gastroparesis

Gastroparesis—a condition of abnormal gastric motility characterized by delayed gastric emptying—is a common cause of nausea and vomiting. The most common forms of gastroparesis are associated with diabetes, occur postoperatively, or are idiopathic. Symptoms include postprandial fullness, bloating, and abdominal distention. Pharmacologic treatment includes dopamine antagonists and erythromycin (E-Mycin).

Nonpharmacologic Therapies for Nausea and Vomiting

Several nonpharmacologic therapies are used for mitigating nausea and/or vomiting. Among the most widely used interventions are ginger, pyridoxine (vitamin B_6), acupuncture, and acupressure. Therapies specific for use during pregnancy are discussed in more detail in the *Pregnancy* chapter. Some evidence indicates that ginger is more effective than placebo in decreasing the severity of nausea and vomiting.[41–43] Ginger appears to be most effective for postoperative nausea and mildly effective for nausea during pregnancy; its effect following chemotherapy is not yet well determined. Reviews of acupuncture and acupressure have yielded similar findings.[43–46]

Cannabinoids are other effective antiemetic agents. The only current medical indication for these substances is the treatment of women with nausea and vomiting associated with chemotherapy, and their use is legal in only some states. Their pharmacologic effects on opiate receptors and the cortical and vomiting centers of the brain may explain the beneficial effects of cannabinoids in such cases.[47] Their side effects include sedation, mood changes, anxiety, memory loss, fear, motor incoordination, hallucinations, euphoria, relaxation, and hunger.

Table 21-6 Antiemetics

Drug: Generic (Brand)	Dose	Major Side Effects/Contraindications	Clinical Considerations
Anticholinergics			
Scopolamine (Transderm-Scop)	Apply one patch (1.5 mg) every 72 hours	Dry mouth, blurred vision, dizziness, confusion, constipation	Primary indication is to prevent motion sickness. Has long duration of action.
H_1 Antihistamines			
Cyclizine (Cyclivert)	50 mg PO every 4–6 hours; maximum dose is 200 mg/day	Drowsiness, headache; anticholinergic symptoms such as dry mucous membranes, urinary retention, or constipation; rarely tinnitus Diphenhydramine: fatigue, vertigo, seizure, hypotension, extrasystoles, tachycardia, urinary retention, agranulocytosis, thrombocytopenia, diplopia, tinnitus, wheezing Dimenhydrinate: The most sedating of the H_1 antihistamines; do not take with other drugs that contain dimenhydrinate	Most drugs in this class are contraindicated during breastfeeding per their manufacturers. Use with caution in persons with asthma, cardiovascular disease, angle-closure glaucoma, or stenotic peptic ulcer. This is a potentially inappropriate class of medications for the elderly; can aggravate symptoms of confusion in persons with dementia.
Dimenhydrinate (Dramamine [OTC])	50–100 mg PO every 4 hours; maximum dose is 400 mg/day 50 mg every 4–6 hours IM/IV; maximum dose is 100 mg every 4 hours		
Diphenhydramine (Benadryl, Benadryl Allergy [OTC])	25–50 mg PO every 4–6 hours; maximum dose is 300 mg/day 10–50 mg IM/IV; maximum dose is 100 mg per event and 400 mg/day		
Doxylamine (Sleep Aid [OTC], Unisom)	25 mg PO daily		
Meclizine (Dramamine Less Drowsy [OTC])	25–50 mg PO taken 1 hour before travel; repeat every 24 hours as needed 25–100 mg daily in divided doses for vertigo		
Dopamine (D_2) Receptor Antagonists: Phenothiazines			
Prochlorperazine (Compazine)	5–10 mg every 4–6 hours PO/IM 2.5–10 mg IV every 3–4 hours 25 mg PR 2 times/day Maximum dose is 40 mg/day	Primary adverse effects: sedation, anticholinergic effects, extrapyramidal side effects Hypotension if given IV too quickly	Moderately effective for nausea but not effective for highly emetogenic chemotherapy.
Promethazine (Phenergan)	12.5–2.5 mg every 4–6 hours PO/IM/IV/PR		
Thiethylperazine (Torecan)	10 mg, 1–3 times/day PO/IM/per rectum		
Dopamine (D_2) Receptor Antagonists: Benzamides			
Metoclopramide (Reglan)	5–10 mg PO 4 times/day 1–2 mg/kg IV Continuous SQ dose regimens available	FDA black box warning related to irreversible extrapyramidal effects following large dose or prolonged use Agitation, anxiety, acute dystonic reactions Give 50 mg diphenhydramine (Benadryl) before dose to prevent extrapyramidal side effects	Crosses the blood–brain barrier so neurologic side effects are likely, especially in the elderly and if high doses are used.
Dopamine (D_2) Receptor Antagonists: Butyrophenones			
Droperidol	0.625–2.5 mg IM over 15 minutes, then 1.25 mg as needed	Extrapyramidal side effects, prolonged QT interval, hypotension Give 50 mg diphenhydramine (Benadryl) before dose to prevent extrapyramidal symptoms Prolonged QT interval can occur in persons who are medically ill or taking other drugs that prolong the QT interval	Major tranquilizer that potentiates the action of opioids. Short-acting. Reserve for persons who have failed other regimens.
Serotonin (5-HT_3) Receptor Antagonists			
Dolasetron (Anzemet)	0.35 mg/kg up to 12.5 mg approximately 15 minutes before a procedure, or 1.2 mg/kg PO up to 100 mg as tabs or injection 2 hours before surgery	Headache; psychomotor, cognitive, and affective disturbances; dizziness; diarrhea or constipation; rash, EKG interval changes that are not clinically significant can occur	These are the primary agents used for treating chemotherapy-induced nausea. There are no significant differences in effectiveness between the drugs in this class.

Granisetron (Granisol)	2 mg PO every hour before chemotherapy or 1 mg 2 times/day 10 mcg/kg/dose, with maximum 1 mg/dose for IV infusion	Adverse effects include fatal cardiac arrhythmias and prolonged QT interval	EKG monitoring is recommended for persons with cardiac disorders and/or electrolyte abnormalities.
Ondansetron (Zofran)	4–8 mg PO 3–4 times/day 4–8 mg over 15 minutes IV every 12 hours May be given 1 mg/hour continuously for 24 hours		
Palonosetron (Aloxi)	0.25 mg IV 30 minutes before chemotherapy		
Benzodiazepines			
Alprazolam (Xanax)	0.25–0.5 mg PO 3 times/day up to 4 mg/day	Drowsiness, sedation, amnesia, hypotension, ataxia, visual disturbances	Intrinsic antiemetic activity is controversial but these drugs are used as an adjunct to decrease anxiety, facilitate sedation, and mitigate akathisia associated with the combination of metoclopramide (Reglan) and dexamethasone (Decadron). They are also useful for treating anticipatory nausea experienced by persons receiving chemotherapy. Contraindicated during pregnancy.
Lorazepam (Ativan)	1–4 mg PO/IM/IV every 4–6 hours		
Cannabinoids			
Dronabinol (Marinol)	2.5-, 5-, and 10-mg capsules 5 mg/m^2 1–3 hours before chemotherapy, then 5 mg/m^2 every 2–4 hours after, for a total of 4–6 doses/day; maximum 15 mg/m^2/dose if needed	Vertigo; xerostomia (abnormally dry mouth); hypotension, dysphoria or euphoria; sedation; tachycardia; facial flushing; dry mouth	FDA approved for treatment of nausea, weight loss, and loss of appetite in persons using chemotherapy. Modest antiemetic properties. Administration with high-lipid meals may enhance absorption. Monitor for psychotic reactions. Additive CNS depression is possible if taken with alcohol.
Nabilone (Cesamet)	1–2 mg 2 times/day; maximum 6 mg in divided doses		

Abbreviations: CNS = central nervous system; OTC = over-the-counter.

Sources: Data from Camilleri M, Parkman HP, Mehnaz AS, Shafi MA, Abell TL, Gerson L. Clinical guideline: management of gastroparesis. *Am J Gastroenterol*. 2013;108(1):18-37[50]; Castaneto MS, Gorelick DA, Desrosiers NA, Hartman RL, Pirard S, Huestis MA. Synthetic cannabinoids: epidemiology, pharmacodynamics, and clinical implications. *Drug Alcohol Depend*. 2014;144:12-41[51]; King TL, Murphy PA. Evidence-based approaches to managing nausea and vomiting in early pregnancy. *J Midwifery Womens Health*. 2009;54(6):430-444.[40]

Antiemetic Pharmacologic Treatments

Antiemetic drugs act by blocking the muscarinic, dopamine, histamine, serotonin, and substance P receptors within the gastrointestinal tract and the central nervous system. These agents are used for a wide variety of conditions, including motion sickness, ulcers, gastritis, nausea and vomiting during pregnancy, acute gastroenteritis, postoperative nausea and vomiting, vestibular neuritis, chemotherapy-induced nausea and vomiting, and other chronic disorders. Usual doses and prescribing considerations are reviewed in Table 21-6.

First-line pharmacologic treatments for nausea and vomiting include H_1 antihistamines, anticholinergics, dopamine receptor antagonists, and serotonin receptor antagonists. The second-line treatments include corticosteroids. Benzodiazepines are used as adjunct therapy. A great deal of interindividual variability in drug effectiveness for treating nausea has been found. Because several different neurotransmitters stimulate the CTZ, adding a drug that has a different mechanism of action can be more effective than increasing the dose of an individual drug. For example, a systemic review of studies of eight different drugs compared to placebo for treatment of women with postoperative nausea found that none could be considered more effective than the others.[48]

Anticholinergics: Scopolamine

Scopolamine is a muscarinic antagonist that blocks the action of the neurotransmitter acetylcholine. It is a metabolite of plants from the Solanaceae (nightshade) family, such as jimson weed and angel's trumpet. Scopolamine is one of the most effective medications for prevention and treatment of motion sickness in women because it inhibits vestibular input to the central nervous system's vomiting center. The transdermal scopolamine patch (Transderm-Scop) has a more prolonged effect than antihistamines. This patch is applied behind the ear several hours before a trip, and its effects can last up to 3 days.

Antihistamines

H_1 antihistamines inhibit the histamine receptors in the CTZ and limit stimulation of the vomiting center by vestibular fibers. They are particularly useful for treating nausea and vomiting associated with vestibular disturbances. Meclizine (Antivert, Dramamine Less Drossy), for example, acts on the vestibular system and the CTZ. This drug has a slow onset of action and takes at least 1 hour to become effective.[49]

Antihistamines are well absorbed following oral administration. They are metabolized in the liver by the hepatic microsomal mixed-function oxygenase system. The various agents' half-lives vary, however, as some antihistamines have active metabolites and many can be administered once or twice a day at most.

Dopamine Receptor Antagonists

Drugs in three classes act as dopamine receptor antagonists: phenothiazines, benzamides, and butyrophenones.

Phenothiazines

Phenothiazines act by antagonizing dopamine (D_2) receptors in the CTZ. They have M_1 muscarine and H_1 histamine antagonist effects as well. The main side effects of phenothiazines are extrapyramidal side effects and reactions such as tardive dyskinesia. These medications have a sedative effect and can also cause orthostatic hypotension. Prochlorperazine (Compazine) is the most commonly used drug in this class of medications. Promethazine (Phenergan) antagonizes central and peripheral H_1 receptors and is also classified as a nonselective antihistamine.

Benzamides

Metoclopramide (Reglan) has several mechanisms of action, which makes this drug the most effective member of this class. Metoclopramide blocks dopamine receptors and, when given in higher doses, also blocks serotonin receptors in the CTZ. It enhances the response to acetylcholine in the gastrointestinal tract, causing enhanced motility and accelerated gastric emptying without stimulating gastric, biliary, or pancreatic secretions. It also increases lower esophageal sphincter tone. In addition to being given for nausea, metoclopramide is the only drug approved by the FDA to treat gastroparesis; reverse the gastric stasis induced by opioids; and combat nausea and vomiting associated with cancer treatment medications. Metoclopramide is generally initiated at 5 to 10 mg 3 to 4 times per day before meals; the maximum dose is 40 mg per day.[50]

Unfortunately, metoclopramide has an adverse side-effect profile of import. Notably, this drug can induce **extrapyramidal symptoms (EPS)** (also called dystonic reactions). When dopamine receptors are blocked, dopamine is unable to initiate the usual physiologic functions, and the resulting effects are similar to those seen in persons with Parkinson's disease. Symptoms include restlessness, akinesia, akathisia, **tardive dyskinesia**, dystonia (involuntary spasmodic muscle movements), oculogyric crisis, and facial grimacing. Although frightening, these symptoms are rarely life-threatening and are easily reversed by administering 50 mg of diphenhydramine (Benadryl) intravenously. Metoclopramide has an FDA-mandated black box warning that reviews the risk of tardive dyskinesia associated with this agent. Because the risk of tardive dyskinesia increases over time, chronic use of metoclopramide is not recommended. Metoclopramide can also cause galactorrhea and has been used therapeutically for this effect when lactating women need to increase their supply of breast milk. It may cause menstrual irregularities and occasionally amenorrhea as well.

Domperidone (Motilium), another dopamine antagonist, also antagonizes both peripheral and central dopamine receptors but has a less severe side-effect profile compared to metoclopramide because it does not cross the blood–brain barrier. Domperidone can cause prolonged QT interval and cardiac arrhythmias. It can be effective for treating gastroparesis but is not available in the United States except through the FDA's Expanded Access to Investigational Drugs program. An electrocardiogram is recommended before using this drug. The usual oral dose is 10 mg administered 3 to 4 times per day, given 15 to 30 minutes before meals.

Butyrophenones

Butyrophenones are tranquilizers that potentiate the action of opiates and have an antiemetic effect via dopamine receptor antagonism. Haloperidol (Haldol) and droperidol (Inapsine) block the stimulation of CTZ. Droperidol is a short-acting medication commonly used on an off-label basis to treat postoperative nausea and vomiting. This agent's label carries a black box warning that warns users about possible prolonged QT interval and ventricular arrhythmias (torsades de pointes). Haloperidol has a longer half-life, so its use is more limited. The major side effects of both drugs are extrapyramidal symptoms.

Serotonin (5-HT$_3$) Receptor Antagonists

The serotonin receptor antagonists are the newest and most effective class of antiemetic agents. They are well tolerated and have a beneficial side-effect profile; consequently, they have largely replaced dopamine antagonists for treating nausea and vomiting. The four most commonly used are ondansetron (Zofran), granisetron (Kytril), dolasetron (Anzemet), and palonosetron (Aloxi). These drugs block the serotonin receptors located on the visceral afferent nerves in the gastrointestinal tract, in the solitary tract nucleus, and in the CTZ.

Cisapride (Propulsid) is a serotonin receptor agonist that stimulates cholinergic nerves in the stomach. This drug was used for gastroparesis, functional dyspepsia, GERD, and intestinal pseudo-obstruction. Cisapride was removed from the market in 2004 and is no longer available in the United States because it was found to cause prolonged QT interval.

The most common side effects of serotonin antagonists are headache, diarrhea, and fatigue, although side effects are generally rare. Self-limiting asymptomatic prolongation of the QT interval and widening of the QRS complex have been noted with several serotonin antagonists. Hypersensitivity reactions occur but are rare. These drugs should be used with caution by individuals who have an underlying long QT syndrome.

Corticosteroids

Corticosteroids are effective and well-tolerated antiemetic choices for persons undergoing chemotherapy. These drugs enter their target cells and bind to cytoplasmic receptors. Their side effects include insomnia, increased energy, and mood changes. Corticosteroids have been used prophylactically for mild to moderate emetogenic chemotherapy. Such agents, in addition to serotonin receptor antagonists, have been used for moderate cases of chemotherapy-induced emesis.

Benzodiazepines

Benzodiazepines generally have weak antiemetic properties at best. These drugs are most often used to help prevent anticipatory nausea and vomiting, which can occur in persons receiving chemotherapy. Lorazepam (Ativan) and alprazolam (Xanax) are the drugs commonly used for chemotherapy-induced nausea and vomiting. The main side effect of benzodiazepines is sedation.

Cannabinoids

Cannabinoids are synthetic derivatives of ingredients found naturally in marijuana. Two cannabinoids are available in the United States with FDA approval for treatment of chemotherapy-induced nausea and vomiting in persons unresponsive to other drugs.[51] Although their exact mechanism of action is unknown, there may be a cannabinoid receptor that affects the CTZ. Following oral ingestion of cannabinoids, plasma levels peak in approximately 2 hours; the half-life is approximately 2 hours, but some metabolites have a half-life of up to 30 hours. These agents are metabolized via CYP450 enzymes within the liver, but no clinically important drug–drug interactions have been identified. Cannabinoid drugs should be used with caution by persons with psychiatric disorders and providers should be aware of legal prohibitions in different jurisdictions.

Special Populations: Pregnancy, Lactation, and the Elderly

The safety of antiemetic agents during pregnancy is of particular import because gestational nausea and vomiting can be debilitating and often require treatment. This subject is reviewed in more detail in the *Pregnancy* chapter. If pharmacologic agents are required for women who are breastfeeding, the antihistamines, scopolamine, and serotonin receptor antagonists are considered compatible.

Any of the antiemetics that have sedative effects (e.g., antihistamines and benzodiazepines) can promote problems with balance and have been found to increase the risk of falls and fractures in elderly individuals. Lorazepam (Ativan) has been reported to cause cognitive deficits, especially in the elderly, although discontinuation resolves the phenomenon. Because older adults have an increased risk of development of cancer, which may subsequently be treated with emetic-associated chemotherapy, antiemetic agents may be used prophylactically or post therapy while their cancer treatment is in process.

Conditions in the Lower Gastrointestinal Tract

Diarrhea and constipation are common and generally self-limiting disorders. Both, however, can be symptoms of more serious problems such as irritable bowel syndrome. Diarrhea can be either infectious or noninfectious. Given the variation in their mechanisms of action, several different classes of drugs are used to treat lower gastrointestinal tract disorders.

Diarrhea

Acute diarrhea generally is defined as the passage of stool with increased water content, frequency, and/or volume that lasts less than 14 days. Chronic diarrhea is defined as the production of loose stools with or without increased stool frequency for more than 4 weeks. Pseudo-diarrhea, or the frequent passage of small volumes of stool, is often associated with rectal urgency and accompanies irritable bowel syndrome (IBS).[52]

Acute diarrhea usually is self-limiting. Most cases are associated with infectious agents and may be accompanied by vomiting, fever, and abdominal pain. Acute infectious diarrhea is further subclassified as non-inflammatory, which is usually viral and a mild disease, or inflammatory, which can be invasive and secondary to toxin-producing bacteria.[53] Acute diarrhea can also be caused by medication, toxic ingestion, or other conditions.

Some of the medications that cause diarrhea include antibiotics, cardiac antidysrhythmics, antihypertensives, chemotherapeutic agents, NSAIDs, antidepressants, bronchodilators, antacids, and laxatives. Although oral rehydration therapy is the cornerstone of treatment for diarrhea, pharmacologic agents are used when symptoms are severe or persistent.

Traveler's Diarrhea

Traveler's diarrhea is a common illness that occurs when persons travel from resource-rich to resource-poor regions of the world. Bacteria cause approximately 85% of these cases, and the most common causative agent is enterotoxic *Escherichia coli*. Viruses cause nearly 10% of cases, with the remaining 5% to 8% of cases being caused by protozoa.[54] For individuals who are concerned that they will contract traveler's diarrhea, it is considered judicious to carry appropriate antibiotics. However, the CDC does not recommend using antimicrobial drugs for prevention of traveler's diarrhea. Antibiotics taken for prevention will not protect a person against viruses or protozoa and will eradicate the protective normal flora, which then renders the individual more susceptible to resistant bacteria.

Empiric treatment of traveler's diarrhea consists of fluoroquinolones or azithromycin.[54] When loperamide is added, the duration of illness can be shortened.[55] Trimethoprim–sulfamethoxazole (Bactrim, Septra) and doxycycline (Vibramycin) are not used because of the high resistance of microbes to these medications.

Antidiarrheal Drugs

Antidiarrheal medications can be obtained as OTC formulations or by prescription. These drugs act by inhibiting intestinal fluid secretion, increasing intestinal fluid absorption (bulking agents), and/or slowing intestinal transit time (opioids). Historically, absorbents such as charcoal, aluminum hydroxide, attapulgite, kaolin, magnesium trisilicate, pectin, and polycarbophil could be found in OTC products marketed for treatment of women with diarrhea. These agents coat the wall of the gastrointestinal tract and absorb bacteria and toxins. Evidence of their effectiveness was lacking, however, and they were withdrawn from the U.S. market in 2003. The OTC formulations currently available are bismuth subsalicylate (Pepto-Bismol) and loperamide (Imodium).

Pharmacologic and clinical information about antidiarrheal drugs are listed in Table 21-7. It is important to remember that these drugs treat the symptom of diarrhea, but do not address the underlying etiologic mechanism.

Bismuth Subsalicylate (Pepto-Bismol)

Bismuth subsalicylate (Pepto-Bismol) is FDA approved for the treatment of women with indigestion, nausea, and/or diarrhea. Its mechanism of action as an antidiarrheal has not been fully elucidated, although the clay in this product may help firm stools and absorb toxins. Bismuth subsalicylate has absorbent, antisecretory, and anti-inflammatory properties. It binds to the toxins produced by *E. coli* and stimulates absorption of fluids by the intestinal epithelium. This agent may interfere with absorption of oral anticoagulants and tetracycline. Conversely, it can enhance the effect of hypoglycemic agents. Persons who are allergic to aspirin should not use bismuth subsalicylate.

Table 21-7 Medications for Treatment of Diarrhea

Drug: Generic (Brand)	Dose	Clinical Considerations
Bismuth subsalicylate (Pepto-Bismol, Kaopectate)	524 mg tablet or caplet every 30 minutes PO, up to 8 doses in 24 hours	May cause black tongue and black stools. Contraindicated for persons with allergy to aspirin, renal insufficiency, or gout. Contraindicated for persons taking anticoagulants. Best for mild diarrhea.
Diphenoxylate (Lomotil)	2 tablets PO or 10 mL 4 times/day for no more than 48 hours	Side effects include nausea, rash, sedation, and pancreatitis. Contraindicated for persons taking MAO inhibitors as it may precipitate a hypertensive crisis.
Loperamide (Imodium)	4 mg then 2 mg PO after each stool, up to 16 mg per day	Not recommended for persons with bloody stool or fever. Use for moderate or severe diarrhea. Side effects include dry mouth, abdominal pain, distention, constipation, drowsiness, and fatigue. Adverse reactions include toxic megacolon, paralytic ileus, angioedema, and urinary retention.
Paregoric	5–10 mL PO 1–4 times/day	Extensive list of side effects and adverse effects, including CNS depression, drowsiness, dysphoria, drug dependence, pruritus, anorexia, and respiratory depression. Multiple drug–drug interactions. Use with caution during lactation.
Traveler's Diarrhea		
Azithromycin (Zithromax)	500 mg PO daily for 1–3 days	Fluoroquinolones are the antibiotics of choice for traveler's diarrhea secondary to *Campylobacter*, *Clostridium difficile*, *E. coli*, *Salmonella*, and *Shigella*. Resistant forms of *Campylobacter* have occurred in southeast Asia and the Indian subcontinent. Azithromycin is active against fluoroquinolone-resistant species.
Ciprofloxacin (Cipro)	500 mg PO 2 times/day for 3 days; single dose or 1-day therapy	
Levofloxacin (Levaquin)	500 mg PO once daily for 3 days; single dose or 1-day therapy	
Norfloxacin (Noroxin)	400 mg PO 2 times/day for 1 day	
Ofloxacin (Floxin)	200 mg PO 2 times/day for 1 day	
Metronidazole (Flagyl)	250–750 mg PO 3 times/day for 7–10 days	Recommended for treatment of *Giardia* and *Entamoeba histolytica*.
Rifaximin (Xifaxan)	200 mg PO 3 times/day for 3 days	Alternative to fluoroquinolones for persons who do not have bloody diarrhea or fever. Not approved for use against *Salmonella*, *Shigella*, or *Campylobacter*.

Abbreviations: CNS = central nervous system; MAO = monoamine oxidase.
Sources: Data from Barr W, Smith A. Acute diarrhea. *Am Fam Physician*. 2014;89(3):180-189[53]; Connor BA. Traveler's diarrhea. In: *CDC health information for international travel*. Atlanta, GA: Centers for Disease Control and Prevention; August 1, 2013. http://wwwnc.cdc.gov/travel/yellowbook/2014/chapter-2-the-pre-travel-consultation/travelers-diarrhea. Accessed May 8, 2014.[54]

Antiperistaltics

Antiperistaltic agents control diarrhea by reducing gastrointestinal motility, inhibiting watery secretions, and increasing anal sphincter tone. Diphenoxylate (Lomotil), a synthetic opiate analogue combined with atropine, directly affects the nerve endings and/or intramural ganglia of the intestinal wall. Loperamide (Imodium) may be preferred for treating chronic diarrhea because it has a longer duration of action and fewer side effects compared to diphenoxylate. Loperamide is the OTC treatment of choice for traveler's diarrhea and may be used in combination with antimicrobial therapy.[54]

Paregoric is an oral liquid that contains 2 mg/5mL of morphine in an alcohol solution. It increases smooth muscle tone in the gastrointestinal tract, which slows motility and peristalsis. Until 1973, paregoric was available over the counter, but now it is available in the United States only by prescription. Paregoric generally has been replaced by more accessible nonopiate products.

Special Populations: Pregnancy, Lactation, and the Elderly

Loperamide (Imodium) is the recommended first-line therapy for treatment of diarrhea for women during pregnancy and when breastfeeding. Diphenoxylate (Lomotil) is also safe for women during pregnancy and breastfeeding, but bismuth subsalicylate (Pepto-Bismol) is contraindicated in pregnancy because of its salicylate component and controversial effectiveness.

Diarrhea is a major cause of mortality and morbidity among the elderly. Loperamide generally is the preferred antiperistaltic agent because the usual formulation of

Table 21-8 Selected Drugs That Can Cause Constipation

Drug: Generic (Brand)	Drug: Generic (Brand)
Amitriptyline (Elavil)	Diuretics
Antacids that contain calcium or aluminum	Imipramine (Tofranil)
Anticholinergic drugs	Ipratropium (Atrovent)
Anticonvulsants, such as carbamazepine (Tegretol) and phenytoin (Dilantin)	Iron supplements
Antidepressants, such as nortriptyline (Aventyl) and SSRIs	MAO inhibitors
Antidiarrheal drugs	NSAIDs
Antihistamines that have anticholinergic properties, such as all OTC antihistamines	Opioids
Anti-Parkinson's drugs, such as selegiline (Eldepryl)	Oxybutynin (Ditropan)
Antipsychotics, such as clozapine (Clozaril)	Phenothiazines
Atropine	Pseudoephedrine (Sudafed)
Benztropine (Cogentin)	Ranitidine (Zantac)
Beta blockers	Sucralfate (Carafate)
Calcium-channel blockers, such as diltiazem (Cardizem) and nifedipine (Procardia)	Terbutaline (Brethine)
Cimetidine (Tagamet)	Trazodone (Desyrel)
Clonidine (Catapres)	Tricyclic antidepressants

Abbreviations: MAO = monoamine oxidase; NSAIDs = nonsteroidal anti-inflammatory drugs; OTC = over-the-counter; SSRIs = selective serotonin reuptake inhibitors.

diphenoxylate includes atropine, an anticholinergic that is unnecessary and may cause adverse effects in elderly persons. Treatment of women with infectious diarrhea and traveler's diarrhea, for example, is the same for individuals regardless of age.

Constipation

There is no single definition of constipation. Clinicians often assume constipation means infrequent bowel movements, but persons with constipation may describe several symptoms, including the need to strain, incomplete emptying, hard stools, infrequent stools (fewer than three stools per week), and abdominal fullness or bloating. The Bristol Stool Form Scale, which describes seven different shapes and consistencies of stool, can be used to help individuals fully describe their symptoms.[56]

Constipation occurs in 2% to 27% in adults and is twice as likely to affect females. Incidence increases with age, particularly in persons older than 65 years.[57] Some conditions associated with constipation include pregnancy, pelvic floor dysfunction, drug interactions (e.g., calcium-channel blockers and antidepressants), metabolic disorders, psychological disorders (e.g., depression, eating disorders), endocrine disorders (e.g., hypothyroidism, hypercalcemia), and dietary variations. Severe, intractable constipation may be due to inertia or anorectal dyssynergia. Dietary fiber deficiency is a contributor to constipation. The average U.S. citizen consumes 5 to 20 g of dietary fiber per day, yet an estimated 20 to 50 g of fiber per day is needed for normal bowel function.

Primary idiopathic constipation generally falls into one of three categories: (1) normal transit time; (2) slow transit time; and (3) defecatory disorders such as dyssynergia. Secondary constipation is a symptom of an underlying disorder such as cancer, or it can be a side effect of medication or drug–drug interactions. Drugs that can cause constipation are listed in Table 21-8.

Laxatives

Laxatives work via a variety of mechanisms (Figure 21-5).[58–61] Bulk-forming laxatives are hydrophilic cellulose derivatives that stimulate peristalsis by increasing the size of stool and modifying its consistency. Emollients are surfactant agents that facilitate mixing of aqueous and fatty materials, which pulls water into the stool and softens it. Emollients are not effective for treating constipation but are useful adjunct therapies to prevent straining. Lubricants coat the stool and allow easier passage; mineral oil is the only lubricant in general use. Saline cathartics retain water in the small intestine, thereby increasing the water content of stool and producing a watery stool. Cascara, senna, and magnesium stimulate peristalsis. Nonabsorbable sugars have an osmotic effect in the colon, and also lower the pH in the colon, which increases peristalsis.

All laxatives can result in bowel dependency, so they should not be used for more than 1 to 2 weeks without consulting a healthcare provider. Women who develop **laxative dependency** or **laxative abuse** need to stop using laxatives gradually (Box 21-2). Although laxatives have not been found to be effective weight loss agents, they are frequently abused for that reason. Most of these agents are available over the counter. Laxatives and anticonstipation agents should not be used concurrently and should always be taken with at least 8 oz of water or juice. Both laxatives and stool softeners can be used to treat constipation. Laxatives cause increased stool frequency, whereas stool softeners do not necessarily influence the number of bowel movements, but instead change the fecal consistency. It is important to

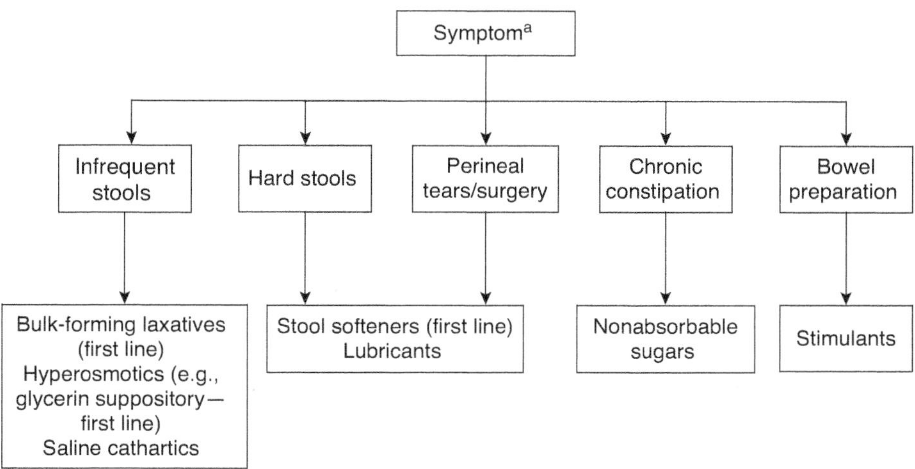

Figure 21-5 Mechanism of action of laxatives.

verify what the needs of the woman are prior to recommending a member of any particular drug category.

Drugs used to treat constipation can be divided into categories based on the amount of time it takes to produce a stool (Table 21-9). Agents that cause feces to be soft within 12 to 72 hours include bulk-forming agents, emollients, lactulose, sorbitol, and mineral oil. Drugs that will produce a stool in 6 to 12 hours include bisacodyl (Carters Little Pills, Correctol), cascara sagrada, senna (Agoral), sennosides (SenoKot), and magnesium sulfate (Epsom salt) in a low dose. Drugs that produce a watery stool in 1 to 6 hours include magnesium citrate

Table 21-9 Drugs Used to Treat Constipation

Drug: Generic (Brand)	Dose	Clinical Considerations
Bulk-Forming Laxatives		
Calcium polycarbophil (FiberCon)	500 mg/tablet: 1–2 tablets PO 2–4 times/day	Onset of action in 12–72 hours. Take each dose at the same time of day for no more than 7 days. Bulk-forming laxatives must be taken with at least 8 oz of water or they can cause a bowel obstruction. Chewable tablets must be chewed thoroughly and not swallowed whole. Calcium polycarbophil can interfere with absorption of quinolone antibiotics, tetracyclines, digoxin, and ciprofloxacin, and can cause an increased effect of glyburide. It should be avoided by persons who need to restrict calcium intake. Metamucil is contraindicated for persons with diabetes (a sugar-free product is available) or phenylketonuria.
	122 mg/caplet: 2 caplets PO 1–2 times/day	
Calcium polycarbophil (Mitrolan)	500 mg or 625 mg/tablet: 2 tablets PO 1–4 times/day	
Carboxymethylcellulose (Citrucel)	2 caplets PO 1–6 times/day; maximum dose is 20 g	
	1 tablespoon powder PO 1–3 times/day	
Psyllium (Metamucil)	1–3 tsp PO 1–4 times/day	
Emollients		
Docusate sodium (Colace)	50 or 100 mg capsules PO 1–2 times/day	Onset of action is 12–72 hours. Softens stools without increasing frequency. Unknown mechanism; probably reduces surface tension, allowing fluids to penetrate fecal mass. Do not crush or chew the capsule. Take with 6–8 oz milk or juice. Do not take Colace within 2 hours of other medications or if also using mineral oil. Contraindicated if person has nausea and vomiting or acute abdominal pain.
Docusate sodium (Peri-Colace)	50 mg docusate sodium/ 8.6 mg senna 1–2 tablets PO 1–2 times/day	Onset of action is 6–12 hours. Combination of docusate sodium and senna, which is a laxative.

(*continues*)

Table 21-9 Drugs Used to Treat Constipation (*continued*)

Drug: Generic (Brand)	Dose	Clinical Considerations
Lubricants		
Mineral oil	15–45 mL PO 1–2 times/day	Onset of action is 12–72 hours. May interfere with absorption of nutrients, vitamins, and oral contraceptives. Can cause pneumonia if aspirated. Do not take concurrently with docusate sodium. Long-term use can impair absorption of fat-soluble vitamins A, D, E, and K.
Osmotic Agents		
Lactulose (Chronulac, Kristalose)	10 or 20 g powder/packet PO 10–20 g once daily	Onset of action is 12–72 hours. Maximum dose is 40 mg/day. Can take 24–48 hours to have effect. Can cause severe diarrhea, electrolyte disorders, or metabolic acidosis if excessive doses are used. Common side effects include flatulence, diarrhea, nausea, vomiting, and abdominal bloating.
Magnesium citrate (Citroma)	1.745 g/30 mL 150–300 mL/day PO once daily or as divided dose 2 times/day	Onset of action is 1–6 hours. Maximum dose is 300 mL/day, which equals 2.8 g elemental magnesium.
Magnesium hydroxide (Milk of Magnesia)	Tablet, capsule, and liquid forms 15–30 mL PO 1–2 times/day	Onset of action is 1–6 hours. Persons with renal failure should use with caution, as frequent use can cause hypermagnesemia. Can cause diarrhea.
Magnesium sulfate (Epsom salts)	10–30 g/day PO Low dose: < 10 g/day High dose: 10–30 g/day	High-dose onset of action is 1–6 hours. Low-dose onset of action is 6–12 hours. Persons with renal failure should use with caution. Can cause hypermagnesemia.
Polyethylene glycol electrolyte solution	240 mL of solution every 10 minutes, up to 4 L until fecal discharge is clear	Fast for 2–3 hours before administering polyethylene glycol electrolyte solution.
Sorbitol	15–30 mL PO 1–2 times/day	Onset of action is 12–72 hours. Can cause abdominal cramps, flatulence, and bloating.
Stimulants		
Bisacodyl (Dulcolax)	5 mg/tablet or 10-mg suppositories 1–3 tablets PO once daily 1 suppository per rectum up to 3 times/week	Onset of action is 6–12 hours. Stimulates mucosal nerve plexus in the colon. Do not crush, chew, or cut tablets. Avoid use within 1 hour of taking an antacid or milk.
Cascara sagrada	0.5–1.5 mL of fluid extract PO once at night	
Ricinoleic acid (castor oil)	15–60 mg PO once daily	Onset of action is 1–6 hours. Can cause nausea, abdominal pain, diarrhea, and electrolyte disorders.
Senna (Senokot, Ex-lax)	8.6 mg/tablet or 8.8 mg/5 mL PO; 15 mg/5-mL granules PO 2 tablets 4 times/day or 4 tablets 2 times/day 10 mL syrup or 10 mL of granules (30 mg) PO 1–2 times/day	Onset of action is 6–12 hours. Can cause diarrhea, nausea, abdominal bloating, flatulence, or urine discoloration. Brand X-Prep has 50 g glucose per bottle and should be used with caution by persons with diabetes.
Other		
Glycerin suppository	3-g suppository	Has an osmotic action in rectum; is very safe; works within 30 minutes.
Linaclotide (Linzess)	145 mcg PO once daily	Side effects include diarrhea, gastrointestinal pain, and flatulence. Contraindicated for persons younger than 17 years. Do not break or chew the capsules.
Lubiprostone (Amitiza)	24-mg capsules PO 2 times/day	Used for treatment of chronic idiopathic constipation. Stimulates secretion of fluid from intestinal epithelial cells. The secreted fluid softens stools and increases motility. Side effects include diarrhea, nausea, and abdominal discomfort. Adverse effects include dyspnea.

Sources: Data from Bharucha AE, Pemberton JH, Locke GR III. American Gastroenterological Association technical review on constipation. *Gastroenterology*. 2013;144(1):218-238[61]; Lembo A, Camilleri M. Chronic constipation. *N Engl J Med*. 2003;349(14):1360-1368[60]; Wald A. Appropriate use of laxatives in the management of constipation. *Curr Gastroenterol Rep*. 2007;9(5):410-447.[58]

Box 21-2 Laxative Dependency and Laxative Abuse

Despite their over-the-counter status and relative safety, laxatives can be overused. Specifically, these agents are often misused in two different ways.

Laxative dependency occurs when an individual uses a laxative to treat constipation and defecate daily. The belief that defecation should occur daily can spur inappropriate use of laxatives. When laxatives are overused, the colon becomes dependent on the laxative for function and the person becomes dependent on the laxative to have a normal bowel movement. Ultimately, the muscles of the colon can become damaged. Dehydration and electrolyte imbalance are also potential risks, especially in the elderly. Laxative dependency can be resolved via slowly titrating off the laxative and increasing fluids, bulk foods, and exercise.

Laxative abuse is a different phenomenon. Women with eating disorders sometimes use purgative laxatives to lose weight. Laxative abuse can result in laxative dependency and dehydration, and eventually can cause irritable bowel syndrome or, in rare cases, liver damage.

(Citro-Mag), magnesium hydroxide (Milk of Magnesia), magnesium sulfate (Epsom salt) in a high dose, sodium phosphates (Fleet-Phospho-Soda), bisacodyl suppositories (Bisa-Lax), and polyethylene glycol-electrolyte (Pro-Lax) preparations.

Bulk-Forming Laxatives

Bulk-forming laxatives are indigestible, hydrophilic colloids that absorb water and form a bulky emollient gel that distends the colon and promotes peristalsis. Thus, their effects most closely mimic normal physiologic mechanisms. Bacterial digestion of plant fibers within the colon may lead to increased bloating and flatus. Allergies to these agents rarely exist.

Emollients and Stool Softeners

Stool softeners work by permitting water and lipids to penetrate the stool material. These agents may be administered orally or rectally and are indicated for short-term therapy only. There are rarely side effects associated with the use of stool softeners. When used concurrently with mineral oil, docusate sodium facilitates the absorption of mineral oil.

Lubricants

Mineral oil and olive oil are clear, viscous oils that lubricate fecal material and retard water absorption from stool. Such lubricants are used to prevent and treat fecal impaction in young children and debilitated adults. Neither mineral oil nor olive oil is palatable, but both may be mixed with juices. Care should be exercised when drinking a lubricant because aspiration can result in severe lipid pneumonitis.

Osmotic Agents

The colon can neither concentrate nor dilute fecal fluid because fecal water is isotonic throughout the colon. Osmotic laxatives are soluble but nonabsorbable compounds that increase stool liquidity due to an obligate increase in fecal fluid.[58] Magnesium hydroxide (Milk of Magnesia) is used for treatment of women with acute or chronic constipation and is a commonly used osmotic laxative preoperatively. However, this product should not be used for prolonged periods of time or by individuals with renal insufficiency due to a risk of hypermagnesemia.

Magnesium citrate, sodium phosphate (Glauber's salt), and magnesium sulfate (Epsom salt) are commonly used purgatives. High doses of such osmotically active agents produce prompt bowel evacuation (purgation) within 3 hours. The rapid movement of water into the distal small bowel and colon leads to a high volume of liquid stool, followed by rapid relief of constipation. Because hyperosmolar agents may lead to intravascular volume depletion and electrolyte fluctuations, they should not be used in persons who are frail, are elderly, have renal insufficiency, or have significant cardiac disease.

Lactulose (Kristalose) and sorbitol are nonabsorbable sugars metabolized by colonic bacteria, which break them down into organic acids; these organic acids then increase the osmotic pressure in the colon and slightly acidify the colonic contents, resulting in an increase in stool water content. Lactulose is contraindicated for use by individuals with galactosemia, diabetes mellitus, and colorectal electrocautery procedures.

Polyethylene glycol (GoLYTELY) is a solution that is lavaged for complete colonic cleansing prior to gastrointestinal endoscopic procedures. This balanced, isotonic solution contains an inert, nonabsorbable, osmotically active sugar (polyethylene glycol), along with sodium sulfate, sodium chloride, sodium bicarbonate, and potassium chloride. The solution is designed so that no significant intravascular fluid shift or electrolyte shift occurs. Therefore, it is safe for all populations. The solution should be ingested rapidly (4 L over 2 hours) to promote bowel cleansing.

For the treatment or prevention of chronic constipation among women, smaller doses of polyethylene glycol powder may be mixed with water or juices (17 g/8 oz) and ingested daily. In contrast to sorbitol or lactulose, polyethylene glycol does not produce significant cramps or flatus.

Stimulants

Anthraquinone is a laxative substance that occurs naturally in some plants including aloe, senna, and cascara. Aloe is the harshest anthraquinone derivative, whereas senna is the mildest. Anthraquinone derivatives are poorly absorbed. After hydrolysis in the colon, they produce a bowel movement in 6 to 12 hours when given orally and within 2 hours when given rectally. These drugs should not be used for more than 1 week because chronic use can lead to brown pigmentation of the colon known as melanosis coli.

There is controversy about the mechanism of action for anthraquinone derivatives. One theory suggests that they increase the propulsive peristaltic activity of the intestine by local irritation of the mucosa or by a more selective action on the intramural nerve plexus of intestinal smooth muscle. A competing theory indicates that there is no action on peristalsis; rather, action is restricted to the distal ileum and colon, where fluid and electrolyte secretion and absorption are altered. Long-term use of cathartics can lead to dependency and destruction of the myenteric plexus, resulting in colonic atony and dilation.

Sennosides (Ex-Lax) are a derivative of anthraquinone found in plants of the genus *Senna*. These agents work by increasing peristalsis. Electrolyte levels should be monitored if sennosides are used on a long-term basis.

Bisacodyl, another derivative of anthraquinone, can be found in such OTC agents as Correctol, Dulcolax, and Carters Little Pills. This stimulant is rarely needed in a healthy individual. Bisacodyl should not be taken within 1 hour of antacids or milk and should not be used for more than 1 week.

Ricinoleic acid (castor oil) increases peristalsis by acting as a local irritant that stimulates intestinal motility in the small intestine. This agent is most effective when administered on an empty stomach. Due to its rapid onset (2–4 hours), it should not be taken at bedtime.

Special Populations: Pregnancy, Lactation, and the Elderly

Nutritional guidance is the best intervention for pregnant women who are experiencing the common symptom of constipation. Of all the pharmacologic options, a glycerin suppository is the safest for pregnant or nursing women and is accompanied by advantages of low cost and rapid relief. Bulk-forming laxatives have little systemic absorption and can be used as a first-line therapy. All other laxatives are contraindicated for use by women during pregnancy.

Emollient stool softeners often are prescribed for postpartum women with perineal tears and are compatible with breastfeeding. When a laxative is needed, glycerin suppositories and bulk-forming laxatives should be among the first recommended because of their lack of systemic absorption.

It is estimated that 20% to 30% of individuals older than 65 years are dependent on laxatives. Hyperosmolar agents may lead to intravascular volume depletion and electrolyte fluctuations and, therefore, should not be used for those who are frail, are elderly, have renal insufficiency, or have significant cardiac disease.[62] When elderly women use lactulose (Kristalose), electrolyte levels should be monitored in individuals older than 60 years or if treatment lasts longer than 6 months. Elderly or chronically ill women may have difficulty defecating due to weak abdominal muscles; therefore, elevating the feet on a step or stool while on the commode may help with evacuation. Ricinoleic acid (castor oil) is excreted in the feces and should be used with caution in the elderly.

Hemorrhoids

Hemorrhoids are varicosities of the rectal blood vessels. Internal hemorrhoids are located above the dentate line, while external hemorrhoids are located closer to the anal verge.[63] Hemorrhoids can cause bleeding, pain, and itching. Their exact pathogenesis is not clear; however, it is speculated that internal hemorrhoids become symptomatic when their supporting structure becomes disrupted and the vascular anal cushions prolapse.[5]

One of the major causes of hemorrhoids is constipation. The incidence increases with age, with the highest prevalence being found among adults who are 45 to 65 years.[63] During pregnancy, hemorrhoids worsen because of constipation and increased venous pressure below the uterus.[64]

Hemorrhoids are classified by their point of origin: internal, external, and internal–external. They are also graded into four categories.[65] Grades 1 and 2 are usually self-treated or treated medically. Grades 3 and 4 hemorrhoids require either rubber band ligation, tissue destruction, surgical fixation, or excision.[63]

Table 21-10 Pharmacologic Treatments for Relief of Hemorrhoidal Pain

Drug: Generic (Brand)	Mechanism of Action	Preparations Available	Clinical Considerations
Local Anesthetics			
Benzocaine, benzyl alcohol, dibucaine, dyclonine, lidocaine, pramoxine, tetracaine (Nupercainal, Tronolane)	Block nerve conduction. For relief of pain, irritation, and pruritus.	Spray, ointment, cream forms are available OTC in concentrations of 0.5%, 1%, and 2.5% Use of 1% preparation is recommended	Use longer than 1 week may result in contact dermatitis. Considered compatible with breastfeeding. Systemic effects are unlikely when used according to directions.
Steroids			
Hydrocortisone (Anucort-HC, Anusol-HC, Tucks anti-itch, Westcort)	Anti-inflammatory, lysosomal membrane stabilization, antimitotic and vasoconstrictive properties.	Aerosol, cream, ointment, gel, rectal suppository forms available OTC in 0.2–2.5% concentrations	Use longer than 1 week may result in mucosal atrophy. Compatible with breastfeeding. OTC products with hydrocortisone are not recommended by the FDA for anorectal use.
Astringent/Protectant/Vasoconstriction Products			
Preparation H ointment, Tucks medicated wipes: contain astringents, protectants, or vasoconstrictors	Reduce trauma to tissues, promote hygiene.	Cream, ointment, gel, suppositories, medicated wipes	Avoid excessive or aggressive wiping with harsh toilet tissue or use of astringent cleaners. Products listed as "extra strength" or "maximum strength" usually include a local anesthetic such as pramoxine 1%.
Astringents			
Calamine, hamamelis water (witch hazel), zinc oxide	Coagulate proteins in surface skin cells, resulting in decreased cellular volume. Leave a thin layer protecting the underlying tissue. Decrease inflammation and irritation by decreasing mucus and secretions.	Cream, ointment	Witch hazel is intended for external use only.
Protectants			
Aluminum hydroxide gel, calamine, cocoa butter, cod liver oil, glycerin (external use only), shark liver oil, white petrolatum, hard fat, mineral oil, petrolatum, topical starch	Prevent water loss from the stratum corneum and decrease inflammation by forming a physical barrier.	Cream, ointment	External use only. For the protectant to be effective, it should contain at least 50% of the active ingredient.
Vasoconstrictors			
Ephedrine sulfate (Levophed), epinephrine (Adrenalin), phenylephrine HCl (Preparation H)	Stimulate alpha-adrenergic receptors in vasculature and promote constriction of blood vessels to reduce swelling.	Cream, ointment	External use only.

Abbreviations: HCl = hydrogen chloride; OTC = over the counter.

The initial treatment for women with hemorrhoids consists of a high-fiber diet that includes 25 to 30 g of fiber per day, stool softeners, and six to eight glasses of water daily. Dietary changes such as adding fiber will add bulk, soften stool, and decrease straining. Fiber supplements such as psyllium or bran will also decrease rectal itching and bleeding.[63] Witch hazel compresses (Tucks) are commonly recommended to reduce the discomfort from hemorrhoids. The majority of research has been conducted in the area of perineal pain and hemorrhoids post childbirth, and no strong evidence has been found regarding the effectiveness of any of these treatments.[66]

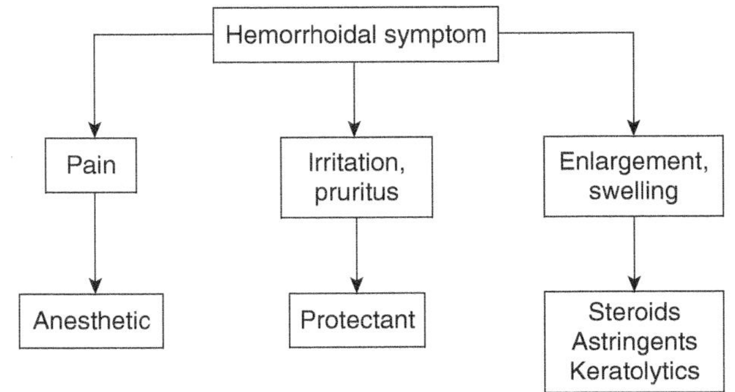

Figure 21-6 Mechanism of action of hemorrhoidal drugs.

Pharmacologic Treatments for Hemorrhoids

Many over-the-counter medications are available for the treatment of women with hemorrhoids. Such pharmacologic treatments include anesthetics, vasoconstrictors, protectants, astringents, wound-healing agents, and antiseptics (Table 21-10).[67,68] Each category has a different mechanism of action (Figure 21-6). Some authors recommend targeting the major symptom and avoiding combination agents, as they may have subtherapeutic doses.

Special Populations: Pregnancy, Lactation, and the Elderly

Women who are pregnant are at increased risk for developing hemorrhoids for several reasons: The hormonal milieu encourages development of varicosities due to relaxation of vessels; constipation is a common problem; and increased weight of the uterus results in more pressure on the vessels. Of the aforementioned pharmacologic therapies, none is contraindicated, and all are widely used during pregnancy and by women who are breastfeeding.

As individuals age, issues of sedentary lifestyle and increased weight may encourage the development of hemorrhoids. The pharmacologic treatments described in this section are all indicated for use among the elderly, although dietary changes, lifestyle changes, and weight loss also may be of value.

Drugs That Reduce Flatulence and Gas

Simethicone is a gastric defoaming agent that is marketed as a single agent such as Gas-X, but more often as an adjunctive agent combined with many popular OTC antacid formulations. Simethicone is a mixture of polydimethylsiloxane and silica gel. This agent decreases the surface tension of gas bubbles, causing them to combine more readily into larger bubbles that should facilitate elimination, but contrary to popular belief, does not reduce the quantity of gas in the gastrointestinal tract. This drug is not absorbed systemically, and adverse reactions are rare. Reports of simethicone use for the relief of flatulence and post–cesarean section abdominal discomfort exist, although evidence of its clinical effectiveness is sparse. There are no documented drug–drug interactions.

A nutritional supplement known by the brand name of Beano is widely advertised as a digestive aid to reduce gas. Beano contains alpha-galactosidase, an enzyme that breaks down the complex sugars such as oligosaccharides found in legumes and cruciferous vegetables into simple sugars, enhancing their ability to be digested and thereby reducing flatulence. The relative safety and cost of this dietary supplement suggest that it could be a reasonable agent to use for individuals who report disagreeable symptoms of gas and flatulence, especially when those symptoms are likely to be predictable.

Irritable Bowel Syndrome

Irritable bowel syndrome (IBS) is a common gastrointestinal disorder that affects 7% to 10% of persons worldwide.[69] IBS is a condition distinct from inflammatory bowel disease (IBD), which is an autoimmune disorder. Information about inflammatory bowel disease can be found in the *Autoimmune Conditions* chapter. IBS affects women more often than men, and usually appears in persons younger than 50 years. The diagnosis of IBS is made based on symptoms that include pain or discomfort and an abnormal bowel pattern at least 3 days per week that persists for 3 months without other signs of serious disease.[70] Abdominal pain is usually described as cramping that is relieved by defecation and exacerbated by eating or stress.[56] Individuals with IBS symptoms are classified according to the dominant bowel pattern they experience: constipation (IBS-C), diarrhea (IBS-D), or mixed (IBS-M).[71] Women are more likely to experience IBS-C.[70] Several comorbidities are associated with IBS, such as anxiety, depression, fibromyalgia, chronic pelvic pain, and post-traumatic stress syndrome. Persons who have experienced physical or sexual abuse are also more susceptible to IBS.

The causes of IBS are obscure and multifactorial. Theories include disordered bowel motility, mucosal barrier disruption, gut hypersensitivity, dysfunction of the neurohormonal interactions between the brain and the bowel, and stress response involving neurotransmitters.[56] IBS has occurred after acute gastroenteritis, especially after severe or prolonged diarrhea caused by a bacterial pathogen.[70] There is also evidence that genetics plays a role in its development.

Nonpharmacologic Treatment of Irritable Bowel Syndrome

When the American College of Gastroenterology IBS Task Force reviewed 20 randomized controlled trials of IBS treatments ($n = 1278$), it found that psychological therapy

Table 21-11 Medications with Evidence of Effectiveness for Treatment of Irritable Bowel Syndrome

Drug: Generic (Brand)	Target Dose	Clinical Considerations	FDA Approval for Symptoms of IBS
Constipation			
Laxatives: polyethylene glycol (MiraLax)[a]	17 g of powder dissolved in 8 oz of water once daily	Strong evidence for effectiveness. Side effects include diarrhea, bloating, and cramping. Helps increase stool frequency but does not relieve pain.	OTC product[b]
Linaclotide (Linzess)	290 mcg PO once daily	For persons with constipation despite treatment with polyethylene glycol. Side effects include diarrhea, gastrointestinal pain, and flatulence. Contraindicated in persons younger than 17 years. Do not break or chew the capsules.	Yes
Lubiprostone (Amitiza)	8 mcg PO once daily	For persons with constipation despite treatment with polyethylene glycol. Side effects include nausea.	Yes
Serotonin 5-HT_4 agonist Tegaserod (Zelnorm)	6 mg 2 times/day	Strong evidence for effectiveness. Side effects include diarrhea and abdominal pain. Adverse effects include cardiovascular ischemia and ischemic colitis. Available only for emergency use through the FDA.	Yes
Bloating			
Antispasmodic: dicyclomine (Bentyl)	20 mg PO 4 times/day as needed	Anticholinergic side effects include confusion, delirium, dry mouth, dizziness, xerostomia, blurred vision, constipation, and urinary retention. Use with caution for persons with renal impairment, hyperthyroidism, hepatic impairment, and neuropathy. Sedatives may have additive drug–drug interactions. May be inappropriate for use in elderly. Contraindicated during pregnancy and lactation. Hyoscyamine is contraindicated in persons with glaucoma, unstable cardiovascular status, gastrointestinal or genital–urinary obstruction, toxic megacolon, ulcerative colitis, or myasthenia gravis.	Yes
Hyoscyamine (Anaspaz, Hyosyne)	0.125 to 0.25 mg PO sublingually 3–4 times/day as needed; maximum dose is 1.5 mg/day		Yes
Nonabsorbable antibiotics: rifaximin (Xifaxan)	400 mg PO 3 times/day	No evidence of effectiveness; may prevent worsening of symptoms. Side effects include abdominal pain, diarrhea, and bad taste.	Off-label use
Probiotics: *Bifidobacterium infantis* 35624 *Lactobacillus*	1 capsule PO daily	Some evidence for effectiveness. No side effects reported.	OTC product[b]
Diarrhea			
Loperamide (Imodium)	2–8 mg/day PO	Strong evidence for effectiveness. Side effects include constipation.	OTC product
Serotonin 5-HT_3 antagonist: alosetron (Lotronex)	Initially 0.5 mg PO 2 times/day Up to 1 mg 2 times/day	Strong evidence for effectiveness. Side effects include constipation. Serious adverse effects include ischemic colitis. Restricted use in the United States.	Only for IBS
Pain			
Citalopram (Lexapro)	5–20 mg PO daily	Some evidence for effectiveness for pain relief IBS and symptoms. Side effects include sexual dysfunction, headache, nausea, sedation, insomnia, sweating, and withdrawal syndromes.	Off-label use
SSRIs: paroxetine (Paxil)	10–60 mg PO daily	Some evidence for reduced pain and help with psychiatric disorders. Side effects include sexual dysfunction, headache, nausea, sedation, insomnia, sweating, and withdrawal syndromes.	Off-label use
Tricyclic antidepressants: amitriptyline (Elavil)	Initially 10 mg PO once at night	Moderate evidence for effectiveness for pain relief in several RCTs. Side effects include dry mouth, dizziness, and weight gain.	Off-label use

Abbreviations: IBS = irritable bowel syndrome; OTC = over-the-counter; RCTs = randomized controlled trials; SSRIs = selective serotonin reuptake inhibitors.

[a] Many over-the-counter osmotic, irritant, or fiber laxatives are available. Studies have used lactulose (Kristalose), lubiprostone (Amitiza), and polyethylene glycol (Miralax).

[b] Not evaluated as these products are over-the-counter agents.

Sources: Data from Brandt LJ, Chey WD, Foxx-Orenstein AE, et al. An evidence-based position statement on the management of irritable bowel syndrome. *Am J Gastroenterol.* 2009;104(suppl 1):S1-S35[69]; Roisinblit KC. Irritable bowel syndrome in women. *J Midwifery Womens Health.* 2013;58(1):15-24[70]; Wald A. Irritable bowel syndrome: diarrhea. *Best Pract Res Clin Gastroenterol.* 2012;26(2012):573-580.[71]

was better than usual care. Psychological therapies considered most helpful included cognitive-behavioral therapy, dynamic psychotherapy, and hypnotherapy (Grade 1C).[69] A Cochrane review of sham acupuncture versus acupuncture RCTs as a nonpharmacologic treatment for women with IBS symptoms failed to demonstrate that true acupuncture is effective in this indication.[72] A dietary choice that is showing promise for relief of IBS symptoms is the low-FODMAP diet, which eliminates fermentable oligosaccharides, disaccharides, monosaccharides, and polyols from daily intake.[70]

Pharmacologic Treatment of Irritable Bowel Syndrome

Irritable bowel syndrome is a chronic condition; therefore the focus of treatment is relief of symptoms. Drug therapy for IBS (Table 21-11) is tailored to the person's primary symptoms. In an extensive review of the evidence surrounding treatment for women with IBS in all of its forms, antispasmodics, laxatives, antidiarrheals, 5-HT_3 antagonists, tricyclic antidepressants, serotonin reuptake inhibitors, nonabsorbable antibiotics, selective C-2 chloride-channel activators, and probiotics were all found to be helpful when used appropriately.[69] Response to any of these modalities is very individualized, however, and much remains to be discovered about the most effective treatment for IBS.

Antispasmodics

Persons with constipation or abdominal pain may benefit from use of antispasmodics; however, bowel spasm is not a proven cause of IBS. A Cochrane review of 29 RCTs (n = 2333) found that antispasmodics, including dicyclomine (Bentyl) and peppermint oil, are better than placebo for improvement of abdominal pain and symptom scores.[73] Dicyclomine is a reasonable choice because it is less likely than other agents to cause anticholinergic side effects (although they may still occur).

Laxatives

Laxatives are not generally advised for treating IBS-related constipation secondary to the risk of becoming laxative dependent. Very little research has been done concerning the effectiveness of laxative use in IBS-C. One small study found that polyethylene glycol (Miralax) increases the frequency of defecation but does not relieve abdominal pain.[69]

Serotonin 5-HT_4 Receptor Agonists

When constipation is the predominant symptom of IBS, Tegaserod (Zelnorm) has been shown to be effective in relieving constipation. However, there is a significant risk for cardiovascular ischemia with this agent. Tegaserod was voluntarily removed from the market in early 2007 because of these cardiovascular side effects. It was later returned to the U.S. market under a restricted-access program through the FDA for women who have IBS-C that does not respond to other treatments and who have no history of cardiovascular disease.[56]

Serotonin 5-HT_3 Receptor Antagonists

Alosetron (Lotronex) acts to inhibit serotonin receptors in the intestine, thereby reducing nausea, bloating, and pain. It also inhibits motility and increases bowel transit time. Unfortunately, this agent has caused severe constipation, ischemic colitis, and death. Consequently, its use is restricted to women with severe IBS-D that does not respond to other treatments.[69] Its use requires special request from the FDA.[70]

Selective C-2 Chloride-Channel Activators

Lubiprostone (Amitiza) is used for constipation and IBS-C in women. This prostanoic acid derivative stimulates the type 2 chloride channel in the bowel, which increases intestinal secretions.[70] Good evidence shows that lubiprostone is effective in controlling abdominal pain, relieving constipation and straining at stool, and improving the woman's quality of life.[67,68]

Nonabsorbable Antibiotics

The antibiotic rifaximin (Xifaxan) is used to relieve bloating, abdominal pain, and diarrhea in persons with IBS-D; its effectiveness in these indications suggests that deranged intestinal microflora must have a role in IBS.[56] Studies have shown that short-term use (2 to 3 weeks) of this nonabsorbable antibiotic is effective for relief of IBS-D symptoms.[69]

Probiotics

Probiotics, especially *Bifidobacterium infantis*, may relieve IBS symptoms and are safe in pregnancy.[69,70] The mechanism of action for these living organisms includes enhancement of the natural barrier function of the gut mucosa, strengthening of the immune system, antagonism of pathogenic bacteria, and synthesis of enzymes and beneficial metabolites.[74] More studies are needed to determine the effectiveness of probiotics in the care of women with IBS.

Antidepressants

Antidepressants are also used to help relieve symptoms of IBS despite not being FDA approved for this indication. The tricyclic antidepressants, such as nortriptyline (Pamelor), slow gastrointestinal transit time and relieve pain.[70] A Cochrane review of 8 studies (n = 517) revealed that tricyclic antidepressants compared to placebo improved abdominal pain (relative risk [RR], 1.49; 95% CI, 1.05–2.12; P = 0.03). Selective serotonin reuptake inhibitors are more effective for symptom control in persons with IBS-C.[73]

Special Populations: Pregnancy, Lactation, and the Elderly

Irritable bowel syndrome that is dominated by constipation is probably aggravated in pregnancy because of hormonal changes and physiologic changes in the bowel that increase the risks for constipation in the pregnant woman. The safest approach to the care of pregnant woman with IBS-C would be consumption of a low-FODMAP diet and probiotics. Pregnant women with IBS-D may benefit from a diet low in fat and dairy products.[70] Among the antispasmodics used to treat IBS, dicyclomine is safe during pregnancy but is not recommended for breastfeeding women because of isolated reports of neonatal apnea of the nursing infant. The use of this drug, however, may aggravate constipation.

Conclusion

Many gastrointestinal conditions disproportionately affect women. These illnesses can have a significant impact on a woman's quality of life. Pharmacotherapeutics for women with gastrointestinal conditions encompass a wide range of remedies, both nonpharmacologic and pharmacologic. Several drugs often are frequently used for these conditions, albeit with limited evidence supporting their effectiveness. Drugs such as laxatives that are considered innocuous by consumers may result in drug dependence. Until new, focused treatments emerge, clinicians need to customize treatments based on known effectiveness, cost, availability, safety, and women's preferences.

Resources

Organization	Description	Website
American College of Gastroenterology	Clinical guidelines for several gastrointestinal disorders	www.gi.org/clinical-guidelines/clinical-guidelines-sortable-list
American Gastroenterological Association	Guidelines, position statements, clinical podcasts, and research resources	www.gastro.org/practice/medical-position-statements
National Digestive Disease Information Clearinghouse (NDDIC)	Publications, podcasts, statistics, and updates on research in gastrointestinal disorders	http://digestive.niddk.nih.gov/ddiseases/pubs/gerd/index.aspx
Apps		
Bristol Stool Scale	The Bristol Stool Scale, which was developed in 1997, classifies stools into seven categories; the app helps individuals characterize stool patterns to better assist in diagnosis and management	www.bristol-stool-scale.com
Answers in Irritable Bowel Syndrome	App for medical professionals that addresses symptoms and treatments for irritable bowel syndrome; based on British Society of Gastroenterology Guidelines	https://itunes.apple.com/us/app/answersin-irritable-bowel/id347809241?mt=8

References

1. Hogan AM, Collins D, Baird AW, Winter DC. Estrogen and its role in gastrointestinal health and disease. *Int J Colorectal Dis*. 2009;24(12):1367-1375.
2. Peterson CT, Sharma V, Elmén L, Peterson SN. Immune homeostasis, dysbiosis and therapeutic modulation of the gut microbiota. *Clin Exp Immunol.* October 24, 2014. Epub ahead of print.
3. Butel MJ. Probiotics, gut microbiota and health. *Med Mal Infect*. 2014;44(1):1-8.
4. Cryan JF, Dinan TG. Mind-altering microorganisms: the impact of the gut microbiota on brain and behaviour. *Nat Rev Neurosci*. 2012;13(10):701-712.
5. American Dietetic Association. Position of the American Dietetic Association: health implications of dietary fiber. *J Am Dietetic Assoc.* 2008;108(10):1716-1731.
6. Overland MK. Dyspepsia. *Med Clin North Am.* 2014;98(3):549-564.

7. Thompson Coon J, Ernst E. Systematic review: herbal medicinal products for non-ulcer dyspepsia. *Aliment Pharmacol Ther.* 2002;16(10):1689-1699.
8. Peppermint (*Mentha x piperita*). Natural Standard Monograph. Natural Medicines Comprehensive Database. http://www.nlm.nih.gov/medlineplus/druginfo/natural/705.html. Accessed July 31, 2014.
9. Tonkic A, Tonkic M, Lehours P, Megraud, F. Epidemiology and diagnosis of *Helicobacter pylori* infection. *Helicobacter.* 2012;17(suppl 1):1-8.
10. McColl KE. Clinical practice: *Helicobacter pylori* infection. *N Engl J Med.* 2010;362(17):1597-1604.
11. Malfertheiner P, Chan, FK, McColl KEL. Peptic ulcer disease. *Lancet.* 2009;374(9699):1449-1461.
12. University of Texas at Austin, School of Nursing Family Nurse Practitioner Program. *Recommendations in primary care for the most efficacious and cost-effective pharmacologic treatment for* Helicobacter pylori *in non-pregnant adults.* Austin, TX: University of Texas at Austin, School of Nursing; May 2013. http://www.guideline.gov/content.aspx?id=46427. Accessed October 31, 2014.
13. Molina-Infante J, Gisbert JP. Optimizing clarithromycin-containing therapy for *Helicobacter pylori* in the era of antibiotic resistance. *World J Gastroenterol.* 2014;20(3):10338-10347.
14. Chey WD, Wong BCY. Management of *Helicobacter pylori* infection. *Am J Gastroenterol.* 2007;102(8):1808-1825.
15. Deeks ED. Fixed-dose ibuprofen/famotidine: a review of its use to reduce the risk of gastric and duodenal ulcers in patients requiring NSAID therapy. *Clin Drug Invest.* 2013;33(9):689-697.
16. Katz PO, Gerson LB, Vela MF. Guidelines for the diagnosis and management of gastroesophageal reflux disease. *Am J Gastroenterol.* 2013;108(3):308-328.
17. Paige NM, Nagami GT. The top 10 things nephrologists wish every primary care physician knew. *Mayo Clin Proc.* 2009;84(2):180-186.
18. Ogawa R, Echizen H. Clinically significant drug interactions with antacids: an update. *Drugs.* 2011;71(14):1839-1864.
19. Lam JR, Schneider JL, Zhao W, Corley DA. Proton pump inhibitor histamine 2 receptor antagonist use and vitamin B_{12} deficiency. *JAMA.* 2013;310(22):2435-2422.
20. Poluzzi E, Raschi E, Moretti U, De Ponti F. Drug-induced torsades de pointes: data mining of the public version of the FDA Adverse Event Reporting System (AERS). *Pharmacoepidemiol Drug Saf.* 2009;18(6):512-518.
21. Lee KW, Kayser SR, Hongo RH, Tseng ZH Scheinman MM. Famotidine and long QT syndrome. *Am J Cardiol.* 2004;93(10):1325-1327.
22. Hanlon JT, Landerman LR, Artz MB, Gray SL, Fillenbaum GG, Schmader KE. Histamine 2 receptor antagonist use and decline in cognitive function among community dwelling elderly. *Pharmacoepidemiol Drug Saf.* 2004;13(11):781-787.
23. Gilboa SM, Ailes EC, Rai RP, Anderson JA, Honein MA. Antihistamines and birth defects: a systematic review of the literature. *Expert Opin Drug Saf.* 2014;13(12):1667-1698.
24. Mahadevan U. Gastrointestinal medications in pregnancy. *Best Pract Res Clin Gastroenterol.* 2007;21(5):849-877.
25. Wolfe MM, Sachs G. Acid suppression: optimizing therapy for gastroduodenal ulcer healing, gastroesophageal reflux disease, and stress-related erosive syndrome. *Gastroenterol.* 2000;118(2 suppl 1):S9–S31.
26. Yang YX, Lewis JD, Epstein S, Metz DC. Long-term proton pump inhibitor therapy and risk for hip fracture. *JAMA.* 2006;296(24):2947-2953.
27. FDA drug safety communication: *Clostridium difficile*-associated diarrhea can be associated with stomach acid drugs known as proton pump inhibitors (PPIs). http://www.fda.gov/Drugs/DrugSafety/ucm290510.htm. Accessed February 8, 2012.
28. Janarthanan S, Ditah I, Adler DG, Ehrinpreis MN. *Clostridium difficile*-associated diarrhea and proton pump inhibitor therapy: a meta-analysis. *Am J Gastroenterol.* 2012;107(1):1001-1010.
29. Geevasinga N, Coleman PL, Webster AC, Roger SD. Proton pump inhibitors and acute interstitial nephritis. *Clin Gastroenterol Hepatol.* 2006;4(5):597-604.
30. Blume H, Donath F, Warnke A, Schug BS. Pharmacokinetic drug interaction profiles of proton pump inhibitors. *Drug Saf.* 2006;29(9):769-784.
31. Wedemeyer RS, Blume H. Pharmacokinetic drug interaction profiles of proton pump inhibitors: an update. *Drug Saf.* 2014;37(4):201-211.
32. Ogawa R, Echizen H. Drug–drug interaction profiles of proton pump inhibitors. *Clin Pharmacokinet.* 2010;49(8):509-433.
33. Information for healthcare professionals: update to the labeling of clopidogrel bisulfate (marketed as Plavix) to alert healthcare professionals about a drug interaction

with omeprazole (marketed as Prilosec and Prilosec OTC). http://www.fda.gov/Safety/MedWatch/SafetyInformation/SafetyAlertsforHumanMedicalProducts/ucm190848.htm. Accessed October 31, 2014.

34. Nikfar S, Abdollahi M, Moretti ME, Magee LA, Koren G. Use of proton pump inhibitors during pregnancy and rates of major malformations: a meta analysis. *Dig Dis Sci*. 2002;47(7):1526-1529.
35. Mulder B, Schuiling-Veninga CC, Bos HJ, De Vries TW, Jick SS, Hak E. Prenatal exposure to acid-suppressive drugs and the risk of allergic diseases in the offspring: a cohort study. *Clin Exp Allergy*. 2014;44(2):261-269.
36. Momeni M, Katz JD. Mitigating GI risks associated with the use of NSAIDs. *Pain Med*. 2013; 14(suppl 1):S18–S22.
37. Pirmez R, Freitas ME, Gasparetto EL, Araújo AP. Moebius syndrome and holoprosencephaly following exposure to misoprostol. *Pediatr Neurol*. 2010; 43(5):371-373.
38. Hemstreet BA. Use of sucralfate in renal failure. *Ann Pharmacother*. 2001;35(3):360-364.
39. Nicholson PA, Karim A, Smith M. Pharmacokinetics of misoprostol in the elderly, in patients with renal failure and when coadministered with NSAID or antipyrine, propranolol or diazepam. *J Rheumatol Suppl*. 1990;20:33-37.
40. King TL, Murphy PA. Evidence-based approaches to managing nausea and vomiting in early pregnancy. *J Midwifery Womens Health*. 2009;54(6):430-444.
41. Marx WM, Teleni L, McCarthy AL, et al. Ginger (*Zingiber officinale*) and chemotherapy-induced nausea and vomiting: a systematic literature review. *Nutr Rev*. 2013;71(4):245-254.
42. Viljoen E, Visser J, Koen N, Musekiwa A. A systematic review and meta-analysis of the effect and safety of ginger in the treatment of pregnancy-associated nausea and vomiting. *Nutr J*. 2014;13:20.
43. Chaiyakunapruk N, Kitikannakorn N, Nathisuwan S, Leeprakobboon K, Leelasettagool C. The efficacy of ginger for the prevention of postoperative nausea and vomiting: a meta-analysis. *Am J Obstet Gynecol*. 2006;194(1):95-99.
44. Cheong KB, Zhang JP, Huang Y, Zhang ZJ. The effectiveness of acupuncture in prevention and treatment of postoperative nausea and vomiting: a systematic review and meta-analysis. *PLoS One*. 2013;8(12):e82474.
45. Matthews A, Dowswell T, Haas DM, Doyle M, O'Mathúna DP. Interventions for nausea and vomiting in early pregnancy. *Cochrane Database Syst Rev*. 2010;9:CD007575. doi:10.1002/14651858.CD007575.pub2.
46. Ezzo JM, Richardson MA, Vickers A, et al. Acupuncture-point stimulation for chemotherapy-induced nausea or vomiting. *Cochrane Database Syst Rev*. 2006;2:CD002285. doi:10.1002/14651858.CD002285.pub2.
47. Parker L, Rock E, Limebeer C. Regulation of nausea and vomiting by cannabinoids. *Br J Pharmacol* [serial online]. 2011;163(7):1411-1422.
48. Carlisle J, Stevenson CA. Drugs for preventing post operative nausea and vomiting. *Cochrane Database Syst Rev*. 2006;3:CD004125. doi:10.1002/14651858.CD004125.pub2.
49. Wang Z, Lee B, Pearce D, et al. Meclizine metabolism and pharmacokinetics: formulation on its absorption. *J Clin Pharmacol*. 2012;52(9):1343-1349.
50. Camilleri M, Parkman HP, Mehnaz AS, Shafi MA, Abell TL, Gerson L. Clinical guideline: management of gastroparesis. *Am J Gastroenterol*. 2013; 108(1):18-37.
51. Castaneto MS, Gorelick DA, Desrosiers NA, Hartman RL, Pirard S, Huestis MA. Synthetic cannabinoids: epidemiology, pharmacodynamics, and clinical implications. *Drug Alcohol Depend*. 2014; 144:12-41.
52. Corinaldesi R, Stanghellini V, Barbara G, Tomassetti P, De Giorgio R. Clinical approach to diarrhea. *Int Emerg Med*. 2012; 7(supp 3):S255-S262.
53. Barr W, Smith A. Acute diarrhea. *Am Fam Physician*. 2014;89(3):180-189.
54. Connor BA. Traveler's diarrhea. In: *CDC health information for international travel*. Atlanta, GA: Centers for Disease Control and Prevention; August 1, 2013. http://wwwnc.cdc.gov/travel/yellowbook/2014/chapter-2-the-pre-travel-consultation/travelers-diarrhea. Accessed May 8, 2014.
55. Riddle MS, Arnold S, Tribble DR. Effect of adjunctive loperamide in combination with antibiotics on treatment outcomes in traveler's diarrhea: a systematic review and meta-analysis. *Clin Infect Dis*. 2008; 47(8):1007-1114.
56. Wilkins T, Pepitone C, Biju A, Schade RR. Diagnosis and management of IBS in adults. *Am Fam Physician*. 2012;86(5):419-426.
57. Gallagher P, O'Mahony D. Constipation and old age. *Best Pract Res Clin Gastroenterol*. 2009;23(6): 875-887.

58. Wald A. Appropriate use of laxatives in the management of constipation. *Curr Gastroenterol Rep.* 2007;9(5):410-447.
59. Tack J, Müller-Lissner S. Treatment of chronic constipation: current pharmacologic approaches and future directions. *Clin Gastroenterol Hepatol.* 2009;7(5):502-508; quiz 496.
60. Lembo A, Camilleri M. Chronic constipation. *N Engl J Med.* 2003;349(14):1360-1368.
61. Bharucha AE, Pemberton JH, Locke GR III. American Gastroenterological Association technical review on constipation. *Gastroenterology.* 2013;144(1):218-238.
62. Daniels G, Schmetzer M. Giving laxatives safely and effectively. *Medsurg Nurs.* 2013;22(5):290-296, 302.
63. Mounsey AL, Halladay J, Sadiq TS. Hemorrhoids. *Am Fam Physician.* 2011;84(2):204-210.
64. Longo SA, Moore RC, Canzoneri BJ, Robichaux A. Gastrointestinal conditions during pregnancy. *Clin Colon Rectal Surg.* 2010;23(2):80-88.
65. Jacobs D. Hemorrhoids. *N Engl J Med.* 2014; 371(10): 944-951.
66. Kopljar M, Balduzzi S, Patrlj L, et al. Topical treatment of hemorrhoids. *Cochrane Database Syst Rev.* 2011;11:CD009443. doi:10.1002/14651858.CD009443.
67. Lohsiriwat V. Hemorrhoids: from basic pathophysiology to clinical management. *World J Gastroenterol.* 2012;18(17):2009-2017.
68. Henderson PK, Cash BD. Common anorectal conditions: evaluation and treatment. *Curr Gastroenterol Rep.* 2014;16(10):408-412.
69. Brandt LJ, Chey WD, Foxx-Orenstein AE, et al. An evidence-based position statement on the management of irritable bowel syndrome. *Am J Gastroenterol.* 2009;104(suppl 1):S1–S35.
70. Roisinblit KC. Irritable bowel syndrome in women. *J Midwifery Womens Health.* 2013;58(1): 15-24.
71. Wald A. Irritable bowel syndrome: diarrhea. *Best Pract Res Clin Gastroenterol.* 2012;26(2012):573-580.
72. Manheimer E, Cheng K, Wieland LS, et al. Acupuncture for treatment of irritable bowel syndrome. *Cochrane Database Syst Rev.* 2012;5:CD005111. doi: 10.1002/14651858.CD005111.pub3.
73. Ruepert L, Quartero AO, de Wit NJ, van der Hejden GJ, Rubin G, Muris JW. Bulking agents, antispasmodics and antidepressants for the treatment of irritable bowel syndrome. *Cochrane Database Syst Rev.* 2011;8:CD003460. doi:10.1002/14651858.CD003460.pub3.
74. Ceapa C, Wopereis H, Rezaïki L, Kleerebezem M, Knol J, Oozeer R. Influence of fermented milk products, prebiotics and probiotics on microbiota composition and health. *Best Pract Res Clin Gastroenterol.* 2013;27(1):139-155.

© Sofimanning/Shutterstock

22 Lower Urinary Tract Disorders

Padma Kandadai, Katharine K. O'Dell

With acknowledgment to Emily E. Weber LeBrun for her contribution to the first edition of Pharmacology for Women's Health

Chapter Glossary

Detrusor urinae muscle Smooth muscle of the urinary bladder wall, which relaxes to store and contracts to expel urine.

Incompetent urethral closure mechanism Condition in which the urethra is unable to maintain a water-tight seal, resulting in urine loss almost continuously with minimal activity or urge to void; also called intrinsic sphincter deficiency.

Interstitial cystitis (IC) Specific type of painful bladder syndrome, based on the presence of findings on cystoscopy that include glomerulations or Hunner's ulcers.

Lower urinary tract symptoms Group of bladder-related symptoms including urinary urgency, frequency, nocturia, and incontinence.

Overactive bladder (OAB) Urinary urgency, usually accompanied by frequency and nocturia, with or without urge urinary incontinence, in the absence of urinary tract infection or other obvious pathology.

Painful bladder syndrome (PBS) Chronic, often waxing and waning suprapubic or retropubic pain, typically increasing with bladder filling, and in the absence of infection; it may or may not improve with emptying, and is often accompanied by lower urinary tract symptoms.

Underactive bladder (UAB) Inadequate strength and/or duration of detrusor contraction resulting in prolonged bladder emptying and/or failure to achieve complete bladder emptying in the absence of urethral obstruction; related to urodynamic diagnosis of detrusor underactivity. Also called detrusor inactivity.

Introduction

The lower urinary tract controls the complex process of storing and eliminating urine. This process typically is painless, predictable, leak proof, and consistently under cognitive control from early childhood. Reliable continence requires intact function of the entire urinary system, including the end organs (bladder and urethra), the communication tract (the spinal cord and peripheral and autonomic nerves), and the central control and coordination centers (the cortex and brain stem). This chapter reviews pharmacotherapies used to treat disorders of the lower urinary tract. Because the urinary tract is complex, misdiagnosis or inappropriate treatment may have severe adverse results. Any underlying anatomic, infectious, malignant, or neurologic pathology must be identified via taking an appropriate history, performing a physical examination, and conducting laboratory testing before pharmacologic treatment is initiated. Additionally, it is important to remember that some **lower urinary tract symptoms** may be the unwanted side effects of medications prescribed for other indications (Table 22-1). Once a thorough evaluation is completed, modifiable risks are addressed, and the woman is informed of her treatment options, many lower urinary tract symptoms can be successfully treated using pharmacotherapy.

Physiology of the Lower Urinary Tract in Women

Anatomic components of the urinary system as they relate to pharmacologic treatments are reviewed in Figure 22-1. Four components of this system facilitate continence within the bladder and urethra: (1) an intact mucoid lining that protects underlying tissue from irritants in the urine; (2) smooth muscle that is able to respond in a coordinated fashion to opposing parasympathetic and sympathetic nerve stimuli; (3) connective tissue support that maintains functional alignment; and (4) intact skeletal muscles with the sensory and motor innervation needed to affect

Table 22-1 Selected Medications and Substances with Side Effects That Can Result in Lower Urinary Tract Symptoms

Medications: Generic (Brand)	Mechanism of Action on Urinary Tract	Effect or Side Effect	Urinary Symptoms
Antihypertensives			
ACE inhibitors: benazepril, captopril, lisinopril (Zestril)	Increase bradykinin	Cough	SUI
Alpha-adrenergic antagonists: prazosin (Minipress), terazosin (Hytrin), doxazosin (Cardura)	Block alpha-adrenergic receptors	Urethral smooth muscle relaxant	SUI
Beta blockers	Block beta-adrenergic receptors	Smooth muscle relaxation; decrease urethral closure	SUI
Calcium-channel blockers: verapamil (Isoptin), nifedipine (Procardia), diltiazem (Cardizem)	Relax smooth muscle	Reduced detrusor contractility	Retention
Antidepressants			
Imipramine (Tofranil), amitriptyline (Elavil), bupropion (Wellbutrin), paroxetine (Paxil), trazodone (Desyrel)	Anticholinergics (nonmuscarinic), CNS stimulant or depressant	Impaired detrusor contractility, sedation, dizziness	Retention, overflow incontinence, constipation
Antihistamines/Decongestants			
Diphenhydramine (Benadryl), hydroxyzine (Vistaril), pseudoephedrine (Sudafed)	Alpha-agonist	Increased outlet resistance	Voiding difficulties, dyssynergia, retention
CNS Modifiers			
Antiparkinson medications: amantadine (Symmetrel), bromocriptine (Parlodel), levodopa (Sinemet)	Anticholinergic	Decreased bladder contractility	Retention
Cholinesterase inhibitors for dementia: donepezil (Aricept)	Slow breakdown of acetylcholine	Increase smooth muscle contraction	UUI
Narcotics/analgesics: opioids, NSAIDs	Analgesia	Sedation, smooth muscle relaxation, delirium	Retention, overflow, constipation
Psychotropics: lithium (Lithobid)	Mood stabilizer	Mechanism of action not clear	UUI, polyuria
Sedatives: lorazepam (Ativan), diazepam (Valium)	CNS depressant	Sedation, confusion, muscle relaxation	Functional incontinence
Skeletal muscle relaxants: baclofen (Lioresal), cyclobenzaprine (Flexeril)	Spasticity	CNS depressant	Urinary urgency, enuresis, retention, overflow
Diuretics			
Alcohol	Diuretic, irritation of bladder lining, CNS depressant	Increased urine volume, sensory nerve stimulation, sedation	Frequency, urgency, incontinence
Caffeine	Diuretic, bladder lining irritant, smooth muscle stimulant	Increased urine volume, sensory nerve stimulant	Frequency, urgency, incontinence
Diuretics: furosemide (Lasix), hydrochlorothiazide (HydroDIURIL)	Diuretic	Increased output	Frequency, urgency, incontinence

Abbreviations: ACE = angiotensin-converting enzyme; CNS = central nervous system; NSAID = nonsteroidal anti-inflammatory drug; SUI = stress urinary incontinence; UUI = urgency urinary incontinence.

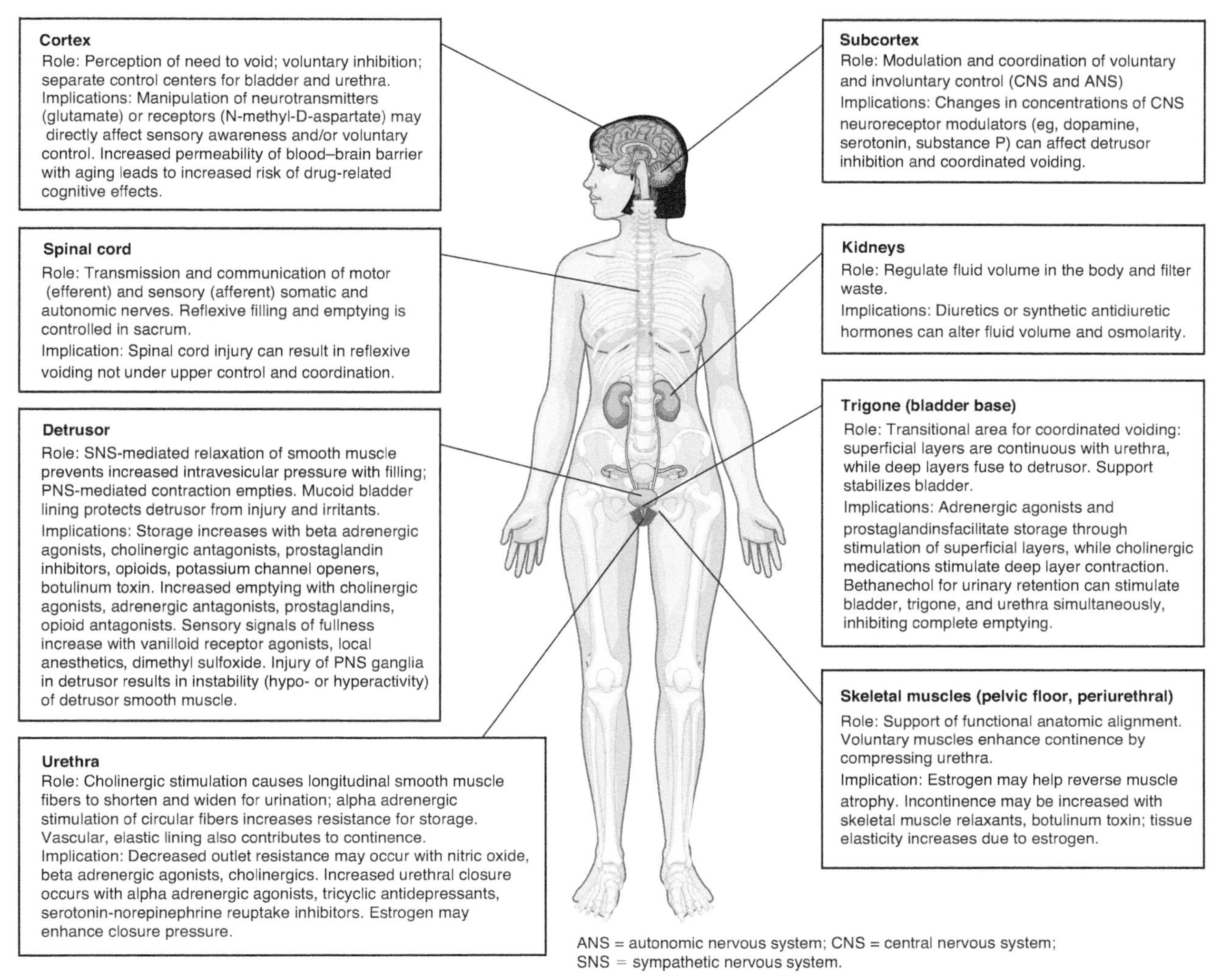

Cortex
Role: Perception of need to void; voluntary inhibition; separate control centers for bladder and urethra.
Implications: Manipulation of neurotransmitters (glutamate) or receptors (N-methyl-D-aspartate) may directly affect sensory awareness and/or voluntary control. Increased permeability of blood–brain barrier with aging leads to increased risk of drug-related cognitive effects.
Spinal cord
Role: Transmission and communication of motor (efferent) and sensory (afferent) somatic and autonomic nerves. Reflexive filling and emptying is controlled in sacrum.
Implication: Spinal cord injury can result in reflexive voiding not under upper control and coordination.
Detrusor
Role: SNS-mediated relaxation of smooth muscle prevents increased intravesicular pressure with filling; PNS-mediated contraction empties. Mucoid bladder lining protects detrusor from injury and irritants.
Implications: Storage increases with beta adrenergic agonists, cholinergic antagonists, prostaglandin inhibitors, opioids, potassium channel openers, botulinum toxin. Increased emptying with cholinergic agonists, adrenergic antagonists, prostaglandins, opioid antagonists. Sensory signals of fullness increase with vanilloid receptor agonists, local anesthetics, dimethyl sulfoxide. Injury of PNS ganglia in detrusor results in instability (hypo- or hyperactivity) of detrusor smooth muscle.
Urethra
Role: Cholinergic stimulation causes longitudinal smooth muscle fibers to shorten and widen for urination; alpha adrenergic stimulation of circular fibers increases resistance for storage. Vascular, elastic lining also contributes to continence.
Implication: Decreased outlet resistance may occur with nitric oxide, beta adrenergic agonists, cholinergics. Increased urethral closure occurs with alpha adrenergic agonists, tricyclic antidepressants, serotonin-norepinephrine reuptake inhibitors. Estrogen may enhance closure pressure.
Subcortex
Role: Modulation and coordination of voluntary and involuntary control (CNS and ANS)
Implications: Changes in concentrations of CNS neuroreceptor modulators (eg, dopamine, serotonin, substance P) can affect detrusor inhibition and coordinated voiding.
Kidneys
Role: Regulate fluid volume in the body and filter waste.
Implications: Diuretics or synthetic antidiuretic hormones can alter fluid volume and osmolarity.
Trigone (bladder base)
Role: Transitional area for coordinated voiding: superficial layers are continuous with urethra, while deep layers fuse to detrusor. Support stabilizes bladder.
Implications: Adrenergic agonists and prostaglandinsfacilitate storage through stimulation of superficial layers, while cholinergic medications stimulate deep layer contraction. Bethanechol for urinary retention can stimulate bladder, trigone, and urethra simultaneously, inhibiting complete emptying.
Skeletal muscles (pelvic floor, periurethral)
Role: Support of functional anatomic alignment. Voluntary muscles enhance continence by compressing urethra.
Implication: Estrogen may help reverse muscle atrophy. Incontinence may be increased with skeletal muscle relaxants, botulinum toxin; tissue elasticity increases due to estrogen.
ANS = autonomic nervous system; CNS = central nervous system;
SNS = sympathetic nervous system.

Figure 22-1 Anatomy and physiology of the urinary tract.

voluntary control. Disease, infection, injury, or atrophy at any level in the system, including the central nervous system (CNS), can produce problems in the storage or elimination of urine, resulting in the lower urinary tract symptoms common among women seeking healthcare services.

The dome or the body of the bladder consists of an elastic smooth muscle, the **detrusor urinae muscle**. Figure 22-2 displays the autonomic pathways related to bladder function. Urine storage is primarily mediated by activation of sympathetic motor pathways stimulated by norepinephrine. Stimulation of the beta-adrenergic receptors that predominate in the detrusor results in bladder relaxation, whereas simultaneous stimulation of the alpha-adrenergic receptors found in the urethra and bladder neck results in contraction and closure. Urethral closure is further enhanced by connective tissue support of the bladder neck, reflexive and voluntary contraction of skeletal muscles, and the mucovascular seal of the urethral lumen. During bladder filling, low-level release of norepinephrine stimulates beta-adrenergic receptors, particularly beta-3, in the smooth muscle of the bladder dome (detrusor). Higher concentrations of norepinephrine stimulate alpha-adrenergic receptors in the urethral walls and bladder base (trigone), resulting in contraction of their smooth muscle.

Urine elimination is mediated primarily by parasympathetic neurotransmitters, including acetylcholine and other noncholinergic, nonadrenergic transmitters. Stimulation of muscarinic cholinergic receptors in the detrusor results in contraction and emptying. This action is associated with simultaneous inhibition of the sympathetic pathways, resulting in relaxation of the urethral closure mechanism to facilitate emptying. Five types of muscarinic cholinergic

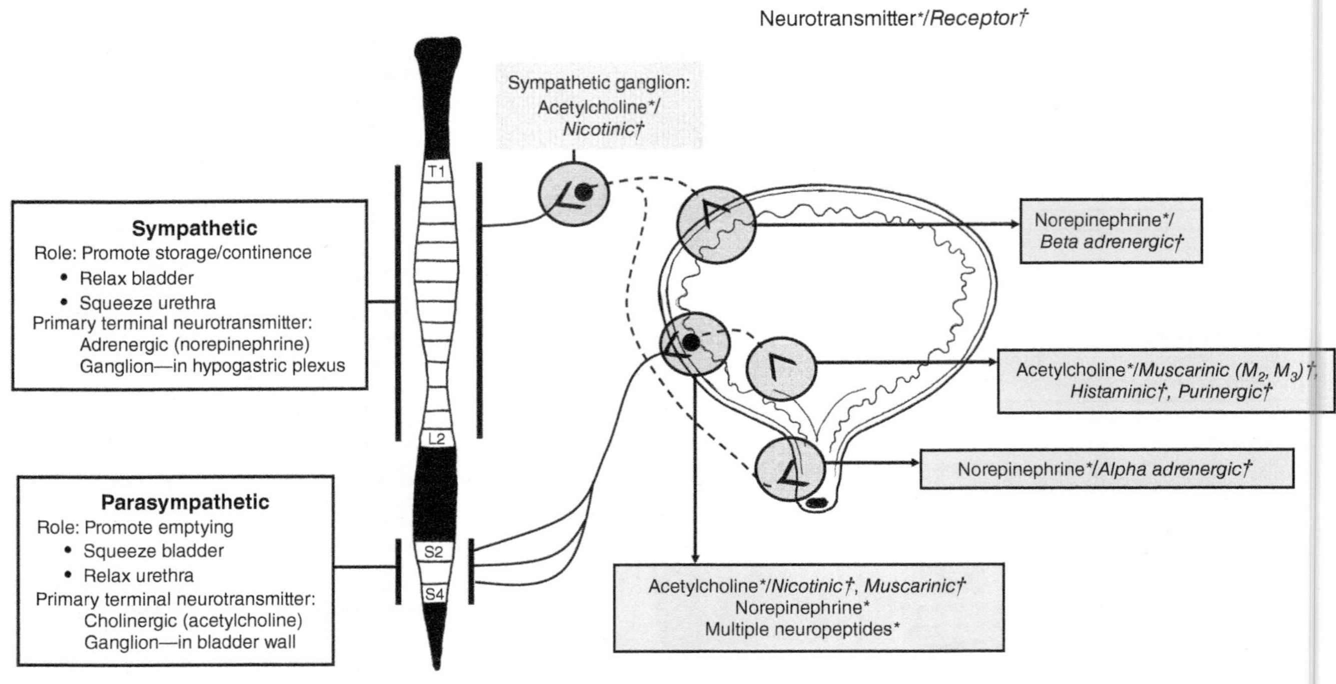

Figure 22-2 Autonomic nervous system control of the bladder.

receptors are found in the human body, referred to as M_1 through M_5. Of these five receptor types, M_2 and M_3 predominate in the detrusor, with M_3 thought to be most directly responsible for bladder emptying.[1]

Overactive Bladder

Symptoms of painless urinary urgency and frequency are often accompanied by nocturia and urge urinary incontinence (Box 22-1). Standardized terms to describe these symptoms include **overactive bladder (OAB)** with or without urge urinary incontinence. Symptoms associated with involuntary detrusor contraction during objective bladder testing (urodynamic studies) are referred to as detrusor overactivity.[2]

The incidence of OAB is obscured by the subjective nature of the symptoms, underreporting, and variations in definition. Phone interviews with 5204 adults in the United States found OAB-related symptoms were reported by approximately 5% of women younger than 25 years and by nearly 30% of those older than 75 years.[3] Men and women report similar overall prevalence of OAB, but women are more likely to experience OAB with incontinence, largely because of their anatomically shorter urethras. Continence may also be impaired secondary to external factors, including obesity and connective tissue or neuromuscular injury experienced during childbirth.

Pathophysiology of Overactive Bladder

Muscle and nerve changes may both play a role in the development of OAB and are potential targets for pharmacologic treatment.[4] Smooth muscle changes related to OAB include spontaneous or uncoordinated muscle fiber firing and abnormal responses to normal stimuli. Skeletal muscle weakness can contribute to incontinence with OAB due to loss of voluntary urethral support, resulting in mixed urinary incontinence in which both physical effort and urinary urgency result in loss of urine. Voluntary control can also be undermined by central or somatic nervous system degeneration. For example, future therapies may be designed to maintain the function of the cerebral cortex with aging, thereby preventing cognitive decline and OAB with urge urinary incontinence.

The primary mechanism of action of current first-line medications for the treatment of OAB is control of involuntary detrusor contractions via inhibition of muscarinic activity. Other, newer medications target the beta-adrenergic receptors located in the detrusor muscle.

Box 22-1 Case Study: Urinary Urgency and Incontinence

MK is a 48-year-old woman with two children. She reports occasionally missing a menses periodically over the past 2 years, along with a gradual onset of increasing problems with urinary incontinence related to urgency. Her frequent voiding (10–14 voids per day) is lifelong. She started having nocturnal enuresis starting at age 8 years, and continues to have nocturia, typically 2 to 3 times per night. Until recently, she was able to manage her urgency by voiding frequently and modifying fluid intake. However, MK has begun experiencing increasingly intense, painless urgency. Several times a week, she now leaks urine before she can reach a restroom, and she wears pads continuously. Her life is beginning to center around finding a bathroom everywhere she goes. MK rarely loses any urine with cough, sneeze, or exercise. She is a nonsmoker, has not had urinary tract infections (UTIs), and has never noticed hematuria. She has no neurologic symptoms, such as incoordination, numbness, or tremor. She currently takes no prescription or over-the-counter medications. She has no other pelvic floor problems such as dyspareunia, constipation, or fecal incontinence.

MK's physical exam is normal. Her body mass index is 24. On pelvic exam, she displays moderate pelvic floor muscle strength and no evidence of prolapse. She has minimal genital atrophy, a normal post-void residual of 50 mL, and normal urinalysis and culture.

Primary Care Treatment

As MK has no findings suggestive of a need for urgent referral because she does not demonstrate pain, sudden onset or change in symptoms, hematuria, urinary retention, or abnormal neurologic exam. Therefore, it appears she has overactive bladder and she is an appropriate candidate for initial behavioral therapy. She is instructed to try eliminating or decreasing bladder irritants such as caffeine, spices, artificial sweeteners, and alcohol. She is also told to complete intermittent intake and output bladder diaries to monitor her progress, attempt to void regularly at gradually increasing intervals, moderate fluid intake, perform correct pelvic muscle strengthening exercises, and practice using her pelvic muscles to control urgency. Over 2 months, her symptoms improve, but she continues to have unpredictable urine loss, and her bladder remains the focus of her daily life.

MK wants to try a medication. The review of her history indicates that she does not have contraindications to the use of antimuscarinic agents or any risk for drug–drug interactions. Her prescription drug plan has a tiered formulary of preferred medications. She is prescribed an inexpensive antimuscarinic agent in an extended-release formulation at the lowest recommended dose. Because MK says her biggest problem currently is restriction of her social activities due to daytime urgency, she starts taking the medication immediately on arising in the morning, anticipating that the peak effect will occur in 4 to 6 hours.

If MK does not notice satisfactory relief within the next 2 weeks of regular use, her symptoms should guide variations in her medication use. Her healthcare provider might choose to increase the dose within the recommended range, change agents, or add a second low-dose agent at bedtime if nighttime voiding problems increase. MK is also encouraged to continue using the behavioral strategies she has learned.

If medication variations do not produce satisfactory symptom relief within the next 2 months, MK will be referred to a urogynecology or urology practice for further evaluation and a review of her other options.

Pharmacologic Therapy with Antimuscarinic Anticholinergics

Optimal treatment of OAB symptoms begins with an individualized program of behavioral management strategies, including voiding diaries, fluid management, timed voiding, weight management, smoking cessation, and pelvic muscle strengthening and coordination exercises. When such behavioral strategies do not produce satisfactory symptom control, however, antimuscarinic anticholinergic medications are the first-line pharmacologic agents. The effectiveness of these agents has been reported in clinical trials that followed adults for up to 52 weeks.[5] All available agents show similar, limited benefits, but there is a dearth of data related to their long-term safety and a woman's adherence to the indicated drug

Table 22-2 Antimuscarinic Anticholinergics with FDA Approval for the Treatment of Women with Overactive Bladder

Drug: Generic (Brand)	Dose[a] Considerations	Mechanism of Action and Pharmacokinetics	Clinical Considerations
Darifenacin (Enablex)	7.5–15 mg PO daily with food	Targets M_3 receptors in the bladder. Metabolized in the liver. Half-life: 12 hours. Unlikely to cross the blood–brain barrier, limiting its CNS effects.	Clinical implications unclear; theoretical decrease in cardiac effect.
Fesoterodine (Toviaz)	4–8 mg PO daily	Nonspecific antimuscarinic agent with low affinity for other neurotransmitter receptors; unlikely to cross the blood–brain barrier, which decreases its potential adverse effects, although CNS effects have been reported. Peak action: 1–3 hours. Half-life: 7 hours. An active metabolite of tolterodine that bypasses cytochrome P450 system, so it causes only limited drug–drug interactions.	Heart rate may increase (5 beats/minute).
Oxybutynin (Ditropan IR)	2.5 mg or 5 mg PO daily, up to 5 mg 4 times/day	Targets M_1 and M_3 receptors. Mild antispasmodic and anesthetic. Metabolized in the liver. A small, lipophilic molecule that crosses the blood–brain barrier. Peak action: 1 hour. Duration: 6–10 hours.	Side effects include drowsiness.
Oxybutynin (Ditropan XL)	5, 10, 15 mg PO daily; maximum dose = 30 mg/day	Peak action: 4–6 hours. Duration: > 24 hours.	Do not chew or crush due to the internal dispensing mechanism.
Oxybutynin transdermal (Oxytrol patch) (Gelnique gel)	Patch (over-the-counter): 2 times/weekly for 3.9 mg/day dose Gel: 84 mg (3 pumps) 3% gel daily on clean, dry, intact skin (abdomen, shoulder, thigh)	A small, lipophilic molecule that is absorbed through the skin and detrusor lining. Targets M_1–M_3 receptors. Patch releases a steady dose over 3–4 days. Gel: Avoids liver first-pass and active metabolite production, which may decrease side effects such as dry mouth.	Skin irritation is a potential side effect (18%).
Solifenacin (VESIcare ER)	5–10 mg PO daily; can be taken with food	Targets M_1 and M_3 receptors. Antispasmodic. Metabolized in the liver. Long half-life: 50 hours. Unlikely to cross the blood–brain barrier.	Clinical implications of long half-life unknown.
Tolterodine IR (Detrol)	2 mg PO daily	Nonspecific antimuscarinic agent with a low affinity for other neurotransmitter receptors. GI absorption; liver metabolism through the cytochrome P340 pathway increases the drug–drug interaction risk. Unlikely to cross the blood–brain barrier; CNS effects are occasionally reported. Peak action: 1–3 hours. Half-life: 2–6 hours.	Many drug–drug interactions. Dosage adjustment is needed for persons who are concurrently taking strong CYP3A4 inhibitors such as clarithromycin (Biaxin). Contraindicated for persons with hypersensitivity to tolterodine, urinary retention, or narrow-angle glaucoma. Use with caution in persons with hepatic or renal impairment, controlled glaucoma, GI obstructive disorders, or bladder flow obstruction. Anticholinergic properties such as dizziness, drowsiness, or hallucinations may be exacerbated among older individuals. Beers criteria should be used when considering use of this medication in the elderly.
Tolterodine (Detrol LA)	2–4 mg PO daily	Peak action: 2–6 hours. Half-life: 6–8 hours.	
Trospium IR (Sanctura)	20 mg PO 2 times/day (once daily in elderly to start)	Quaternary amine agent; nonselective peripheral effect. Its minimal liver metabolism decreases the risk of drug–drug interaction. Water-soluble, larger molecule; unlikely to cross the blood–brain barrier and the majority is excreted intact into bladder. Peak action: 4–6 hours. Half-life: > 18 hours.	Take on empty stomach as fatty foods decrease activity.
Trospium XR (Sanctura)	60 mg PO daily	Extended-release formula. Peak action: 5 hours. Half-life: 35 hours.	

Abbreviations: CNS = central nervous system; ER = extended release; IR = immediate release; LA = long acting; M, M_1, M_2, M_3 = parasympathetic muscarinic receptors; XL = extended release.

[a] For women older than 65 years, start with lowest possible dose.

Source: Data from Madhuvrata P, Cody JD, Ellis G, Herbison GP, Hay-Smith EJC. Which anticholinergic drug for overactive bladder symptoms in adults. *Cochrane Database Syst Rev*. 2012;1:CD005429. doi:10.1002/14651858.CD005429.pub2.[8]

Table 22-3 Variations in Patterns of Antimuscarinic Use That May Improve Symptom Control Among Individual Women

Symptom/Problem	Suggestions
Urinary incontinence is only an occasional problem (e.g., at social gatherings or during travel)	Immediate-release agents generally work within 1 hour and may be timed for intermittent effect.
Difficulty remembering a daily medication, or prefers not to take pills/capsules/tablets	Extended-release or transdermal agents may be easier to use.
Side effects like dry mouth are intolerable	Extended-release and transdermal agents result in lower rates of dry mouth. Gum, sugarless candy, or sips of water can be used, but increasing fluid intake to more than 64 oz per day may exacerbate symptoms. Side-effect profiles vary between individuals, and trial of a different agent may eliminate the symptom. Low-dose combinations of drugs may be better tolerated than a single agent at a high dose.
Nocturia is the primary problem	Time medication use to address the symptom profile; try immediate-release agents at bedtime and extended-release formulas 2–4 hours prior to bedtime.
Medications are prohibitively expensive	Immediate-release agents tend to be less expensive; extended-release oxybutynin is available in generic form; pharmaceutical companies may offer programs to provide medications to the indigent.
Treatment helps somewhat, but symptoms persist	A trial of an additional low-dose antimuscarinic may augment symptom control without exacerbating side effects.

regimen.[6] Table 22-2 reviews the antimuscarinic agents currently approved by the U.S. Food and Drug Administration (FDA) for the treatment of OAB.[6–8]

Limited aggregated data suggest that all antimuscarinic agents demonstrate statistically significant superiority to placebo.[7] Overall, leakage episodes average 4 fewer per week (relative risk [RR] per day, −0.54; 95% confidence interval [CI], −0.67 to −0.41), while the number of voids per week averages 5 less (RR per day, −0.69; 95% CI, −0.84 to −0.54). Quality-of-life domains, including travel, social life, and emotional health, also show statistically significant improvement when these medications are prescribed. Rates of discontinuation are similar in both treatment and placebo groups, suggesting low rates of unacceptable side effects; however, this may also reflect a relatively lower rate of clinically significant changes in symptoms.

Because there are no significant differences between the antimuscarinic drugs with regard to effectiveness, the choice of a particular agent depends on factors such as side effects, drug–drug interactions, cost, and dosing frequency. Table 22-3 offers suggestions for changing antimuscarinic doses and schedules to improve an individual woman's symptoms and decrease side effects.[6,8]

Contraindications and Precautions to Use of Antimuscarinic Drugs

Table 22-4 presents a summary of contraindications to antimuscarinic drugs and precautions for their use. These agents are contraindicated for persons with hypersensitivity to tolterodine (Detrol), urinary retention, and uncontrolled narrow-angle glaucoma. These drugs should be used

Table 22-4 General Contraindications and Precautions with Use of Antimuscarinic Agents

Contraindications	Clinical Considerations
Hypersensitivity to the agent	Avoid use
Narrow-angle glaucoma, uncontrolled	Avoid use until problem is controlled; consult eye specialist prior to starting agent
Gastric retention (gastroparesis)	Avoid use until problem is resolved
Precautions	**Clinical Considerations**
Urinary retention	May be used cautiously as part of a treatment plan in some cases
Concomitant use of other anticholinergic drugs, especially in the elderly	Use with caution
Gastrointestinal disturbance (obstruction, atony, ulcerative colitis, severe constipation, ileostomy, colostomy)	Use with caution, while observing for decreasing function
Esophageal disease (reflux, esophagitis, use of medications associated with esophageal irritation such as alendronate)	Discontinue if symptoms are exacerbated
Hepatic or renal impairment	Dose adjustment advised
Myasthenia gravis	Use with caution
Extreme environmental heat	Decreased sweating may lead to heat prostration in susceptible women
Cardiac disease (arrhythmias, congestive heart failure, coronary heart disease, tachycardia, QT prolongation)	Use with caution
Hypertension	Monitor for increases in blood pressure
Concurrent use of ketoconazole (Nizoral) or other potent CYP3A4 inhibitors	Dose adjustment required
Autonomic neuropathy	Monitor symptoms
Xerostomia or associated conditions (e.g., Sjögren's syndrome)	Encourage oral hygiene and monitor status

with caution for persons with hepatic or renal impairment, controlled glaucoma, gastrointestinal (GI) obstructive disorders, or bladder flow obstruction. Contraindications and precautions for using these drugs relate in part to their metabolism and excretion. In addition, the effect of antimuscarinic agents on neurotransmitters to smooth muscle at other sites in the body can be a concern. Because related smooth muscle is present in the brain, orbit of the eye, heart, gastrointestinal tract, and urinary bladder, pathologies in these organs can be exacerbated by use of antimuscarinic agents. In older adults with cognitive decline or confusion, the potential antimuscarinic side effects of dizziness and somnolence are special concerns, especially because of the potential cumulative effects related to polypharmacy.[9] Theoretically, the larger molecular structure of quaternary amine trospium (Sanctura), which may make it less likely to cross the blood–brain barrier, make it an optimal choice for elderly persons with CNS-effect concerns, but the clinical relevance of this factor has not been demonstrated.[10]

Side Effects of Antimuscarinic Agents

All of the muscarinic receptors (M_1–M_5) are present in smooth muscle in end organs throughout the body. Symptoms resulting from this distribution may contribute to the adverse effects reported by approximately one third of individuals who use antimuscarinic therapy.[4] The M_3 receptors that predominate in the bladder, for example, are found to some extent in the exocrine glands, ocular orbits, heart, brain, and digestive tract. The most common side effects from blockade of M_3 receptors are headache, blurred vision, dry mouth, and constipation. Because of the wide distribution of receptors, even the most M_3-specific antimuscarinic agents have general side effects, which also include dental caries; other gastrointestinal symptoms such as reflux and nausea; tachycardia; sleep disturbances; confusion; and urinary retention.[9] Women taking antimuscarinic agents who live in hot climates can suffer from heatstroke if sweating is impaired. Transdermal agents may produce skin reactions and irritation.

Drug–Drug Interactions

The antimuscarinic drugs have many drug–drug interactions secondary to their effect on CYP450 enzymes. Dosage adjustment is needed for persons who are concurrently taking strong CYP3A4 inhibitors such as clarithromycin (Biaxin) or ketoconazole (Nizoral). The antimuscarinic drugs also enhance the anticholinergic effects of drugs that work through the latter mechanism of action; because of their side-effect profile, they may also enhance the sedative effect of opioids and other sedation-causing agents. A complete list of drug–drug interactions should be reviewed before prescribing any drug in the antimuscarinic category.

Choosing an Antimuscarinic Agent

Adherence to all antimuscarinic treatments for OAB has been shown to be low. In a study of 2496 California Medicaid recipients, 36.9% filled their prescription only once, and only 4% refilled at least 80% of their prescriptions over a 6-month period.[11] At 6 months, half of women had discontinued therapy; by 1 year, 75% of women had discontinued this treatment. The most commonly reported reason for discontinuation in one survey was that the medication did not work as expected.[12]

The choice among the various antimuscarinic agents is guided by limited short-term data.[8] The few comparative studies that have been completed suggest extended-release and transdermal formulas result in lower rates of dry mouth—the most common side effect.[8] Reduction of potentially bothersome side effects may be a factor in the increased adherence observed with extended-release formulations.[12] When extended-release tolterodine (Detrol) and oxybutynin (Ditropan) were compared, there was no difference in perceived improvement, leakage episodes, voids per 24 hours, or discontinuation rates, although dry mouth appeared to be more common with oxybutynin.[8] Lower doses offer similar positive effects and fewer side effects, and generally the lowest potentially effective dose should be used initially, especially in older women. Drugs administered by non-oral routes of administration avoid the risk of first pass–related drug–drug interactions, reach steady state more rapidly, and demonstrate fewer side effects, but may be more costly and may produce skin reactions in some women. The cost of any agent to an individual woman may vary markedly related to her current insurance formulary.

Additional Pharmacologic Treatment Options

Mirabegron

Mirabegron (Myrbetriq) was approved by the FDA for the treatment of OAB in 2012. This drug acts as a beta-3 adrenergic receptor agonist in the detrusor muscle of the bladder, resulting in relaxation of the bladder. It represents an alternative for persons for whom the use of antimuscarinic agents is contraindicated or unsatisfactory due to adverse effects. Results of a randomized controlled Phase 3 clinical trial showed that, compared to individuals who received placebo, those who took either 50 mg or 100 mg per day of mirabegron (Myrbetriq) had a significant decrease in daily incontinence episodes and number of voids per day. They also had significant improvements in quality-of-life measures, along with a nonsignificant increase in hypertension, compared with placebo recipients (6.1% versus 6.6%, respectively).[13] Reported side effects included hypertension, nasopharyngitis, dry mouth, headache, urinary tract infection, and upper respiratory infection.

Several precautions must be observed when prescribing mirabegron. Because beta-3 receptors are also found in the cardiovascular system, care must be taken with women who have poorly controlled cardiovascular disease such as hypertension. In addition, mirabegron is metabolized by the CYP2D6 enzyme and simultaneously inhibits the enzyme's activity, which may potentiate the activity of other drugs requiring this enzyme for metabolism, such as beta blockers, tricyclic antidepressants, opioids, warfarin (Coumadin), and several antiarrhythmic agents.

Nonspecific Oral Agents

Other medications are used on an off-label basis for OAB-related symptoms. They include desmopressin (DDAVP), a synthetic antidiuretic hormone used to treat diabetes insipidus or primary nocturnal enuresis in children, but prescribed with caution for nocturia in adults; hyoscyamine (Levsin) and dicyclomine (Bentyl), which are both nonselective anticholinergics used for irritable bowel syndrome; and tricyclic antidepressants, such as imipramine (Tofranil) and amitriptyline (Elavil). Generally, the lack of specificity and consequently increased side-effect profile of these agents result in less common use of these medications for OAB.[14]

Estrogen Therapy

The role of estrogen in the treatment of lower urinary tract symptoms in postmenopausal women is controversial. Oral conjugated equine estrogen (Premarin), either alone or with medroxyprogesterone acetate (Provera), appears to have no role in the treatment of urinary incontinence and has been found to increase incontinence in some women.[15,16] Only limited data are available on the use of vaginally inserted estrogen for OAB. However, urinary tract symptoms that are associated with genital atrophy are an FDA-approved indication for postmenopausal use of vaginal estrogen. Cochrane reviews have concluded that topical estrogen is a safe and effective treatment for symptoms of genital atrophy.[17] Topical estrogen has also been shown to slightly decrease incontinence episodes, number of daytime and nighttime voids, and urinary urgency and frequency.[16] It may take up to 3 months before improvement in urinary symptoms is noted.

If a trial of vaginal estrogen for genital atrophy is desired, three modes of topical estrogen replacement are available: vaginal creams, rings, and tablets. Endometrial stimulation and breast tenderness are more common side effects with estrogen cream, but the risk of experiencing these conditions remains low.[16,17] No studies of vaginal use of estrogen for OAB longer than 1 year have been published. The North American Menopause Society, in a separate review, concluded that cyclic progesterone and routine endometrial biopsy are not necessary during use of low-dose vaginal estrogen because there is a minimal risk of endometrial hyperplasia.[18] However, women with a history of estrogen-sensitive breast cancer were cautioned to include their oncologist in their decision-making process regarding the use of vaginal estrogen.

Intravesical Instillation

While more typically used for treatment of interstitial cystitis or painful bladder syndrome, direct instillation of medications via catheter into the bladder is also performed, often in specialty-care setting.[19] Targets of intravesical therapy are both the efferent and afferent innervations of the bladder. Agents affecting the efferent pathways include oxybutynin and atropine.[20] Intravesical instillation may be a useful route of delivery if women are suffering from significant antimuscarinic side effects. Sensory nerves and pain perception are targeted by instillation of local anesthetics.

Botulinum Toxin

In 2008, the FDA approved intravesical injection of botulinum toxin (Botox) as a treatment for neurogenic OAB in adults. The list of indications for botulinum toxin was further expanded in 2013 to include idiopathic OAB in adults who have had an inadequate response or are intolerant of anticholinergic medication. Direct injection of the toxin into the bladder wall blocks motor nerve pathways, and clinical trials have demonstrated that doses of more than 100 units are consistently better than placebo in decreasing incontinence episodes, voiding episodes, urgency, and nocturia. Higher doses are also associated with higher incidence of urinary tract infection and transient urinary retention requiring intermittent self-catheterization. Despite those caveats, quality-of-life scores were significantly improved in women who received botulinum toxin as compared to those who received placebo.[21] Injections are generally performed transurethrally using cystoscopy.

Reasons for Treatment Failure

Complete success in remedying OAB with medication alone is unlikely; that is, improvement may be maintained more effectively when behavioral change is part of the overall treatment regimen. Pharmacologic treatment can fail for a variety of reasons. First, improved objective measures such as decreased urine loss per leak or increased bladder capacity may not equate to a subjective feeling of improvement. Second, incorrect or missed additional diagnoses or omission of behavioral strategies can limit treatment effectiveness. Some women may have functional incontinence, or incontinence associated with cognitive, psychological, or physical impairments that impede toileting that is not OAB. Inadequate dosing, inability to tolerate effective dosing due to side effects, and unusual resistance to the medication due to pharmacogenetics can occur as well. For example, some women have symptoms that do not respond to antimuscarinic agents because they have atypical bladder contractions not mediated by M_3 receptors, or contractions that originate in the smooth muscle itself. All of these factors are the subject of ongoing research.[22] Finally, women with forms of stress incontinence or stress-predominant mixed incontinence may not respond to antimuscarinic drug therapy.

Nonpharmacologic Treatments for Overactive Bladder

Nerve stimulation—including intravaginal, intrarectal, or perianal functional electrical stimulation, percutaneous tibial nerve stimulation, and surgically implanted sacral nerve stimulation—may improve symptoms of OAB. Although this therapy has been shown to be effective in some women, the optimal candidates for it and the exact mechanism behind the effectiveness of peripheral nerve stimulation techniques remain unclear.

Percutaneous tibial nerve stimulation—a weekly outpatient procedure in which electrical stimulation is applied at the ankle level via an acupuncture needle—has demonstrated effectiveness similar to the antimuscarinic tolterodine (Detrol LA) for treatment of OAB symptoms.[23] The sacral nerve stimulation device (Interstim by Medtronic, Minneapolis, Minnesota) has received FDA approval for treating refractory OAB symptoms, and has been found to significantly decrease symptoms and voiding abnormalities for as long as 5 years in severely affected women.[24] Nevertheless, high-quality evidence related to optimal patterns for programming of the sacral nerve stimulation device is lacking, and additional studies are needed to understand quality-of-life implications, cost of care, and effectiveness of electrical stimulation as compared to other therapies.

Complementary Therapies

Acupuncture holds a theoretical place in treatment of OAB-related symptoms, perhaps through decrease of symptom perception via increased endorphin levels and through neuromodulation.[25] Data collected from small randomized studies have shown reductions in incontinence episodes, urgency, and frequency with such therapy.[26] The low associated risk and relative speed of effectiveness (when it appears to be effective, relief has typically been reported within 6 weeks) make acupuncture a reasonable option for some women.

The theoretical relationship between emotional stress and imbalances in autonomic neurotransmitter action supports the recommendations of structured calming and relaxation as part of a behavioral approach to OAB, and this has been assessed in a few small studies that found modest success with stress reduction techniques.[27]

Herbs are also understudied as a treatment for OAB symptoms, raising safety concerns about their use in this indication. The German Commission E Monographs suggest that herbs similar to *Scopolia* rhizome (*Scopolia* root) have anticholinergic effects and likely affect M_3 receptors, as they contain hyoscyamine and scopolamine.[28] Because research evaluating the effectiveness, dosing, and safety of these herbs is limited, general contraindications to anticholinergics should be applied when they are used.

Special Populations: Pregnancy, Lactation, and the Elderly

Transient urinary symptoms, such as urinary frequency, are ubiquitous in pregnancy but the mechanism is probably very different than the mechanisms that underlie OAB. Urinary incontinence is also common, but antimuscarinic agents are generally not used during pregnancy. There is little or no human research on use of these drugs in pregnancy, and animal studies have demonstrated some teratogenic effects. They are not recommended for lactating women, as infant risk cannot be ruled out.

Lower urinary tract symptoms increase with aging, with urgency and nocturia being reported in more than 50% of community-dwelling persons in their 80s, and daytime frequency in more than 70%.[29] Several factors are thought to contribute to the increase in bladder symptoms with aging. Physiologic changes can include diminished central sensory processing, an increased collagen-to-smooth muscle ratio in the bladder wall, and decreased numbers of muscarinic receptors. These factors play a key role both in the occurrence of lower urinary tract symptoms, and in the decreased responsiveness to pharmacologic treatment.

In addition, comorbidities such as diabetes, stroke, and neurodegenerative diseases are more common in older adults; these conditions all directly affect vascular and neuromuscular processes in the bladder. Likewise, functional decline due to muscle wasting and arthritis can make self-care and toileting increasingly difficult, increasing urinary incontinence risk. In some cases, symptoms in older adults are related to modifiable risk factors, including depression, infections, genital atrophy, certain prescription medications, endocrine abnormalities such as thyroid disorders, and stool impaction. Serious sequelae of urinary incontinence also are more prevalent in older adults, including skin breakdown, falls, fractures, social isolation, and the financial burden of supplies and care.

Many pharmacologic treatments prescribed for lower urinary tract symptoms must be used with special caution in older women.[30] Factors that affect treatment choices include age-related changes in drug absorption, distribution, metabolism, and excretion; comorbidities; polypharmacy; and increased incidence of typical contraindications to anticholinergics, such as gastrointestinal or urinary retention and reflux, uncontrolled narrow-angle glaucoma, unstable cardiovascular status and arrhythmias, hepatic and renal disease, and central nervous system compromise. Anticholinergic properties such as dizziness, drowsiness, or hallucinations may be exacerbated in the elderly; consequently, agents with such characteristics are listed as Beers criteria medications for older women.[29] The Beers criteria for Potentially Inappropriate Medication Use in Older Adults is published by the American Geriatrics Society and provides guidelines to help clinicians when prescribing for the elderly. While older adults were included in the initial trials of the oral beta$_3$-adrenergic agonist mirabegron, which was approved by the FDA in June 2012, clinical experience with this agent in elderly women is limited.[13] Use of mirabegron requires adequate liver and kidney function for its metabolism and excretion, and the drug produces the adverse effects of hypertension and urinary retention, both of which are already common in older adults. As a moderate CYP2D6 inhibitor, mirabegron may also increase serum concentrations of some medications commonly used by older individuals, such as metoprolol (Lopressor).

Stress Urinary Incontinence

Stress urinary incontinence (SUI) is the involuntary loss of urine that occurs when intra-abdominal pressure exceeds urethral resistance during physical exertion, sneezing, or laughing. It occurs predominantly in women, due to their structurally shorter urethra compared to men. SUI can be a major barrier to health-promoting exercise for many women.[31] Stress urinary incontinence is aggravated by obesity, and vaginal birth appears to increase the risk of SUI among younger women. For example, 5 years after giving birth, SUI was reported by 2.3% of women post cesarean section versus 14.2% of women post vaginal birth ($P < 0.01$); however, longer term comparisons in the incidence of stress urinary incontinence between women who have given birth vaginally and those who had a cesarean section have not shown cesarean section to be protective against this disorder.[32]

Pathophysiology

SUI results whenever bladder pressure exceeds urethral closure pressure. Even normal urethral resistance can be overcome by extreme bladder pressure, which can occur with obesity, paroxysmal cough, strenuous activity, pregnancy, or an overly full bladder. However, urethral resistance is usually sufficient to maintain continence, unless one or both of two changes occur. First, changes may occur in the urethra itself, including loss of elasticity and thinning and nonadherence of the mucovascular lining, which can result in a urethra that is structurally difficult to close. This condition is referred to as an **incompetent urethral closure mechanism** or intrinsic sphincter deficiency.[2] Second, urethral resistance can be undermined by weakened connective tissue or muscle support that becomes unable to adequately stabilize and press the urethra closed.

Several nonpharmacologic treatments may improve or cure SUI, including pelvic floor muscle strengthening and coordination exercises, vaginal pessaries, and surgical treatments.[33] These techniques can also be used in varying combinations with any effective pharmacologic agents that may be identified in the future.

Pharmacologic Interventions for Stress Urinary Incontinence

Currently, no pharmacologic agents are approved for SUI in the United States. Several drugs have been evaluated for this indication, but their ratio of risk to benefit has not proved satisfactory, as the overall direct morbidity of SUI is low. Pending the identification of safe, effective agents, a brief review of classes of agents is included here to illustrate potential targets for pharmacotherapy, based on the pathophysiology of SUI.

Adherence to pelvic floor muscle strengthening and coordination exercises increases muscle hypertrophy and remains a cornerstone of SUI therapy for women who retain voluntary control of their skeletal muscles.[34] However, these exercises are unlikely to decrease symptoms in women with high-tone muscle contraction or pain at rest, baseline high muscle strength with normal relaxation, or inability to voluntarily contract muscles due to neuromuscular abnormalities.

Adrenergic Agonists

Both alpha- and beta-adrenergic agonists have a potential role in SUI treatment. The role of alpha-adrenergic agents in this indication is clear, because they stimulate contraction of the alpha receptors that predominate in the urethra and bladder neck. However, because beta-adrenergic receptors predominate in the detrusor itself, the apparent effect of beta-adrenergic agonists is paradoxical and not completely understood.[35]

A Cochrane review reported modest symptom improvement with a variety of adrenergic agonists when compared to placebo, including phenylpropanolamine (Dexatrim), midodrine (ProAmatine), norepinephrine, clenbuterol, and terbutaline (Brethine).[35] While only 4% of women withdrew from these trials because of adverse effects, potential side effects can range from bothersome to severe, including insomnia, anxiety, restlessness, hypertension, headache, tremor, weakness, palpitations, and respiratory difficulties. Ephedrine and pseudoephedrine (Sudafed) are over-the-counter alpha agonists that have improved SUI symptoms anecdotally, but placebo-controlled trials of such agents are lacking and animal trials suggest that their use produces only minimal symptom improvement.[36]

Serotonin and Norepinephrine Agonists

Serotonin and norepinephrine agonists are generally approved for treatment of depression and neurogenic pain. They promote continence by suppressing activity of parasympathetic receptors and enhancing both sympathetic and somatic activity. One selective serotonin and norepinephrine reuptake inhibitor, duloxetine (Cymbalta), was evaluated for treatment of SUI in 2006, but its application for FDA approval for SUI indication was withdrawn due to the potential increases in suicide ideation seen among individuals taking this class of agents. This risk overshadowed the potential benefit, particularly because although statistically significant decreases in SUI incidents per day were demonstrated, SUI was not typically cured.

Tricyclic Antidepressants

Imipramine hydrochloride (Tofranil) is a tricyclic antidepressant that promotes urine storage by both decreasing bladder contractility and increasing outlet resistance.[37] Although its precise mechanism of action is unknown, it appears to block norepinephrine and serotonin reuptake, thereby affecting central and peripheral anticholinergic receptors. FDA-approved indications for imipramine are limited to treatment of depression in adults and nocturnal enuresis in children.

If imipramine (Tofranil) is prescribed, the lowest possible effective dose should be used, especially for older women or those with liver disorders. As is the case with all antidepressants, the labeling for imipramine carries a black box warning about the potential for increased suicidality and the same general contraindications for use of other anticholinergic drugs. Serious potential side effects include cardiovascular effects such as arrhythmias, heart block, hypertension, orthostatic hypotension, palpitations, and syncope. Use of imipramine in pregnancy has not been evaluated.

Related tricyclic medications, such as amitriptyline (Elavil), desipramine (Norpramin), doxepin (Sinequan), and nortriptyline (Pamelor, Aventyl), may have similar effects on urinary symptoms.

Estrogen Therapy

Estrogen has a theoretical role in improving SUI. Because estrogen receptors are present throughout the urogenital system, estrogen therapy may increase alpha-adrenergic sensitivity in the urethral smooth muscle and the vascularity needed for coaptation of the urethral mucosa.[37] However, SUI symptoms appear to increase—not decrease—when oral estrogen is used, regardless of whether progesterone is added to the treatment regimen.[18] This phenomenon may be related to the increased elasticity of estrogenized tissue, which in turn results in decreased urethral support. Future research may identify a role for estrogen in enhancing the effectiveness of dual therapy combinations (e.g., use in tandem with alpha-adrenergic agents), but at this time there is no evidence recommending use of estrogen either for prevention or treatment of SUI.[37]

Special Populations: Pregnancy, Lactation, and the Elderly

Mild SUI is the most common type of incontinence experienced during pregnancy, with increased risk for this condition being related to parity, age, and body mass. Symptoms usually improve without intervention in the postpartum period, typically within the first 3 months; continuation of bothersome urine loss for longer than 3 months postpartum warrants further evaluation. Use of botulinum toxin is contraindicated in pregnancy.

While older women often experience lower urinary tract symptoms, urinary incontinence is not considered a normal part of aging, and evaluation and treatment of this condition may markedly improve a woman's quality of life.[29] Pharmacologic therapies previously used for treatment of nocturia, including morning use of diuretics and bedtime dosing of imipramine or desmopressin, must be approached with extreme caution in older women and persons with comorbidities.[30]

Urinary Retention

Retention of urine may cause significant morbidity. Acute retention is often the result of transient urethral obstruction (e.g., following the trauma of childbirth or surgery, or due to regional anesthesia). It can result in pain and discomfort, and neuromuscular damage to the bladder from over-stretch. Acute urinary retention is typically treated with a short-term in-dwelling catheter, with resolution of the obstruction if indicated; pharmacologic management is typically not indicated.

Chronic urinary retention is more complex in terms of its definition, etiology, and management. The level of post-void residual urine likely to result in morbidity is debated, but has been previously thought to be 150 mL.[38] Nevertheless, a standard definition has not been established.[39] Women with significant urinary retention (e.g., more than 300 mL) may be asymptomatic; may experience symptoms typical of OAB, such as frequency, urgency, and incontinence; or may report classic symptoms, such as feelings of incomplete emptying, hesitancy, straining to void, and recurrent UTI.[38] Chronic retention can result in severe morbidity, including renal failure if bladder resistance is sufficient to cause ureteral reflux to the kidneys. Even where hypotonicity of the bladder results in low-pressure retention without reflux, chronic over-distention can produce increasing bladder ischemia/dysfunction and/or urinary status, with increased risks of UTI and bladder stone formation.

Disorders such as vaginal prolapse, uterine fibroids, and urethral masses appear to account for approximately 3% of cases of chronic urinary retention.[38] The remaining women with chronic urinary retention are thought to have some form of **underactive bladder (UAB)** or a condition also termed detrusor inactivity. Multiple etiologies appear to be involved in non-obstructive underactive bladder, and understanding of this indication is evolving rapidly. Etiologies may include abnormalities in neurotransmission and muscle function, both peripherally or centrally, such as those associated with atherosclerosis, diabetes, multiple sclerosis, and spinal cord injury.[40] In addition, urinary retention can occur iatrogenically, as a result of using prescribed pharmacologic agents (Table 22-5).

Table 22-5 Oral Pharmacologic Agents That Can Cause Underactive Bladder

Class	Action
Anticholinergics Tricyclic antidepressants Antimuscarinics Antihistamines	Compete with acetylcholine
Neuroleptics	Interrupt neurotransmission
Calcium-channel blockers	Impede smooth muscle function
Alpha$_1$-receptor agonists Amphetamine analogues	Increase outlet contraction
Anesthetics	Interrupt neurotransmission
Smooth muscle relaxants	Impede smooth muscle function

Nonpharmacologic Interventions for Underactive Bladder

In all women who have elevated post-void residual, it is essential to minimize bladder over-distention.[41] Intermittent self- or caregiver-assisted catheterization remains the mainstay of treatment, with this technique being performed frequently enough to keep bladder volumes at no more than 400 mL to 500 mL. In addition, bladder function may be improved with certain behavioral strategies, including smoking cessation, constipation management, scheduled voiding every 2 hours to limit over-distention, and double voiding. Physical therapy to relax any identified high-tone muscle obstruction of the urethra may be indicated for some women. The Credé's maneuver, which is suprapubic manual compression, and Valsalva voiding should be used only by women who are known to have no pathological increase in bladder pressure, to avoid increasing the risk of reflux. Sacral neuromodulation has also received FDA approval for the indication of chronic urinary retention.

Pharmacologic Agents for Underactive Bladder

Currently, no highly effective, low-risk pharmacologic agents are available specifically to treat underactive bladder and chronic retention. Potential targets for pharmacologic treatment for urinary retention include increasing the effectiveness of bladder contractions, decreasing outlet resistance, and increasing afferent-nerve sensitization. Medications currently used to treat underactive bladder and chronic retention are reviewed in Table 22-6.

Table 22-6 Pharmacologic Agents Used to Treat Women with Underactive Bladder and Chronic Urinary Retention

Drug: Generic (Brand)	Action	Clinical Considerations
Alpha-Adrenergic Antagonists		
Alfuzosin (Uroxatral) Doxazosin (Cardura, Cardura XL) Tamsulosin (Flomax) Clonidine	Relaxes the internal urinary sphincter, decreasing bladder neck tone and outlet obstruction	These drugs' only role is in the setting of outlet obstruction, as with neurologic disease. They are rarely used as solo agents for this indication. Adverse effects include fatigue, constipation, cardiac dysrhythmia, and depression.
Cholinergic/Muscarinic Receptor Agonists		
Bethanechol (Urecholine) Carbachol (Isopto)	Stimulates contraction of smooth muscle in the bladder and bowel	Effects on bladder and outlet may be simultaneous and uncoordinated; clinical effectiveness is low or inconsistent. Adverse effects include syncope, increases sweating, salivation, gastric acid, and diarrhea.

Several classes of agents may also be used—albeit with caution—for a woman with symptoms, including the antimuscarinic agents used for OAB and low-dose tricyclic antidepressants. Members of both classes may suppress excessive reflex detrusor activity, yet also decrease bladder contractility, worsening retention.[41] The severe external urinary sphincter spasticity seen with some neurologic diseases or spinal cord injuries has been treated with agents that relax skeletal muscle, such as baclofen (EnovaRX-Baclofen), botulinum toxin (Botox), and benzodiazepines. Botulinum toxin, which blocks smooth and skeletal muscle contractility, has been injected both transurethrally and transperineally to inhibit outlet obstruction related to multiple sclerosis or spinal cord injury.[42]

Complementary Therapies for Underactive Bladder

Caffeine, provided as a cup of hot tea or coffee within 30 to 60 minutes of the attempt to void, has been used as a bladder stimulant in cases of urinary retention.[43] Several herbal therapies are also described in the German Commission E Monographs as treatments for urine retention, but they predominantly function as diuretics and have no direct effect on bladder function.[28] Suggested herbs include *Phaseoli fructus sine semine* (kidney bean pods without seeds), *Levistici radix* (lovage root), and *Orthosiphonis folium* (java tea). *Urticae herba/folium* (stinging nettle herb and leaf) is a diuretic and possibly a weak antispasmodic. However, because the doses found in marketed formulations of these complementary therapies differ widely, it has proved difficult to conduct studies with standard doses. Therefore, clinical use of these herbs and botanicals is limited for treatment of urinary retention.

Box 22-2 provides a case study of a woman with chronic retention.

Urinary Tract Infection

Among community-acquired infections, urinary tract infections are one of the most common and costly types.[44] In women, a bimodal peak of incidence has been described, with one peak occurring between the ages of 18 and 24 years and a second peak being noted after age 50 years.[45] A woman's lifetime risk of UTI is estimated to be 60.4% (95% CI, 55.1–65.8). The high UTI incidence in women, and the tendency for recurrence in some women, is most likely related to a combination of anatomy, genetic factors, hormonal effects, and behavioral patterns. Risk factors for UTI differ between younger women and older women. Sexual intercourse is a prominent risk factor in premenopausal women, but is not as significant in postmenopausal women.[45]

Pathophysiology of Urinary Tract Infections

For infection to occur, virulent strains of colonizing bacteria must adhere to the bladder wall. The most common infective agents in the urinary tract include gram-negative bacilli, such as *Escherichia coli*, *Klebsiella*, *Enterobacter*, *Serratia*, *Proteus*, and *Pseudomonas*.[46] *Staphylococcus* species, including *saprophyticus*, *epidermidis*, and *aureus*, are important—but less common—pathologic organisms in the bladder. The gram-positive organisms *Streptococcus agalactiae* and *Enterococcus faecalis* are also found as urinary pathogens. These organisms may gain access to the periurethral and urethral tissues and ascend into the bladder.

In postmenopausal women, the absence of estrogen in the vagina and periurethral tissues also contributes to UTI risk. The proposed mechanism is related to the effect that estrogen deficiency has on the proliferation of lactobacilli within the vagina. In the absence of estrogen, the *Lactobacillus* population drops, which in turn leads to a loss of lactic acid production.[47] The resultant decrease in vaginal pH and loss of bacteriocin production promotes colonization of the vagina by the Enterobacteriaceae.[48]

Box 22-2 Case Study: A Woman with Residual Urine

GB is a 75-year-old woman who reports 2 years of gradually increasing problems with urination, including urgency, frequency, nocturia, dribbling, lower abdominal discomfort, and small-volume voids. Sometimes she feels as if she has to urinate but is unable to do so. At other times, GB loses urine on the way to the bathroom. She can leak with urgency and with physical exertion. She often strains to get urine out, but still feels her bladder is not really empty. She has no bowel or pelvic pain concerns, is not sexually active, and has had no recent urinary tract infections.

GB is normotensive and does not have hyperglycemia or hyperlipidemia. She underwent a hysterectomy when she was 47 years old for dysfunctional uterine bleeding and fibroids. Her current medications include trazodone (Desyrel) for sleep, fentanyl transdermal patches for osteoporotic back pain, and over-the-counter diphenhydramine hydrochloride (Benadryl), which she uses for seasonal allergies.

During GB's examination, her post-void residual is found to be elevated at 350 mL, but her urine sample is negative on office dipstick for blood, protein, nitrites, and leukocytes. She has mild atrophic genital changes, a normal-appearing urethra, and a cystocele (i.e., anterior vaginal wall prolapse) advancing to 1 cm past her introitus in the standing position while bearing down.

Primary Care Treatment

Because GB has multiple discomforts and may have had an increased post-void residual for several years, her provider assesses kidney function via a renal ultrasound and serum urea, nitrogen, and creatinine. These tests are normal. A urine clean-catch dipstick is negative for protein, blood, nitrites, and leukocytes.

GB agrees to a trial pessary treatment of her vaginal wall prolapse to see if this approach will modify her symptoms and decrease her post-void residual. With a comfortable pessary adequately supporting the prolapsed tissue, her residual remains elevated and her symptoms are only partially improved.

GB's medications include several that could potentially affect her bladder emptying (Table 22-1). Her medication use can be modified to help improve the contractile ability of her bladder—specifically, her use of diphenhydramine hydrochloride (Benadryl) and trazodone (Desyrel). In addition, GB may be able to decrease her symptoms by self-catheterizing on a regular basis. For example, she may self-catheterize in the morning after her first void and again at bedtime to see if intermittent complete emptying will reduce her urgency and frequency symptoms. If these approaches are not successful, GB will be referred to a specialist, who will order testing (e.g., urodynamic studies, cystoscopy) aimed at better understanding the etiology of her retention. Currently, however, oral medications for hypoactive bladder are used with caution, especially in older adults.

Recent work evaluating the vaginal and urinary microbiota provides corroborating evidence of the role of the native microbial environment.[49]

Infection in the urinary tract may present as asymptomatic bacteriuria, symptomatic uncomplicated cystitis, complicated cystitis, or pyelonephritis. A urinary tract infection is considered complicated if any of the following are present: upper tract involvement, recurrence, diabetes mellitus, immunocompromise, pregnancy, abnormalities of the urinary tract (congenital or acquired), kidney stone disease, hospital-acquired infection, renal failure, symptoms for 7 or more days before seeking care, or the presence of foreign bodies such as stents or indwelling catheters.

Pharmacologic Treatment of Urinary Tract Infections

Current strategies for managing uncomplicated UTIs include the empiric use of antibiotic therapy based on symptoms alone without a culture or susceptibility testing.[46] This strategy is convenient for the woman and was previously regarded as cost-effective based on the rationale that the causative organisms are predictable. However, with the growing problem of antibiotic resistance among uropathogens, this paradigm is slowly shifting, particularly for women who may have recurrent or atypical symptoms and complicating features.[47,48]

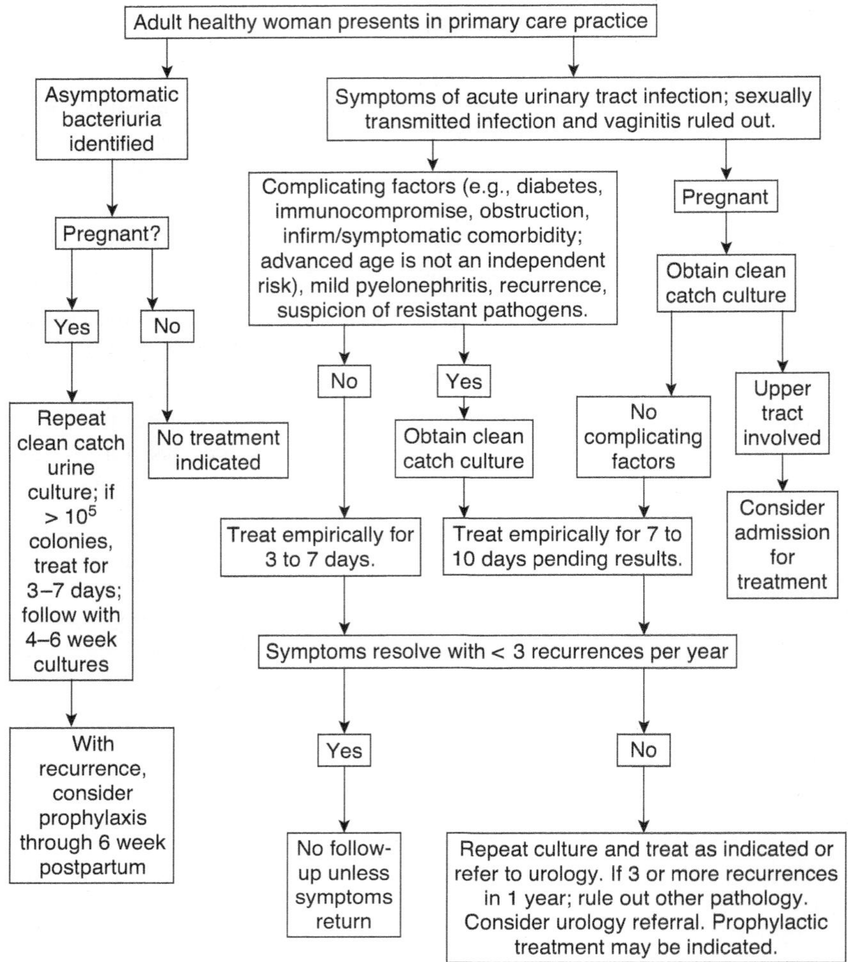

Figure 22-3 Algorithm for treatment of urinary tract infection.

Source: Data from Gupta K, Hooton TM, Naber KG, et al. International clinical practice guidelines for the treatment of acute uncomplicated cystitis and pyelonephritis in women: A 2010 update by the Infectious Diseases Society of America and the European Society for Microbiology and Infectious Diseases. *Clin Infect Dis*. 2011;52(5):e103-e120.[46]

Figure 22-3 presents a treatment algorithm compiled from current literature.[46] The decision to treat is based on the woman's clinical presentation and judgment. Traditional guidelines suggest antibiotic treatment be reserved for women with bacterial colony counts of 100,000 CFU/mL (10^5) or more who demonstrate symptoms, however, a colony count that is less than 100,000 CFU/mL may warrant treatment in some situations.[46]

Antibacterial Agents for Uncomplicated Urinary Tract Infection

Antibiotics commonly used to treat uncomplicated UTI include trimethoprim–sulfamethoxazole (TMP-SMX), nitrofurantoin, fosfomycin (Monurol), fluoroquinolones, and beta-lactam agents (Table 22-7). These agents are renally excreted and rapidly achieve high concentrations in the urine.[46] Because microbial resistance has increased dramatically in recent years due to overuse and misuse of antibiotics, appropriate prescription of antibacterial treatment for UTIs has become increasingly important.[50] Antibiotic resistance is more likely to be found among women who have had recent or recurrent antibiotic exposures or hospitalizations, and those who have diabetes mellitus.

When deciding which antibacterial agent to use, clinicians should consider the likelihood of resistance, the site of infection (e.g., pyelonephritis versus cystitis), the timing (e.g., intermittent, acute, postcoital, or recurrent), and the severity of infection (e.g., uncomplicated versus complicated).[46] An optimal initial antibiotic choice should be inexpensive, have broad-spectrum coverage,

Table 22-7 Antibiotics Commonly Used to Treat Urinary Tract Infections

Drug: Generic (Brand)	Microbial Coverage	Uncomplicated UTI Dose	Complicated UTI and Acute Pyelonephritis[a] Dose	Clinical Considerations
TMP-SMX (Bactrim, Septra, Septra DS)	*E. coli* *Klebsiella Proteus* *Enterobacter*	80 mg/400 mg PO 2 times/day for 3 days	160 mg/800 mg (one double-strength tablet) PO 2 times/day.[b]	First-choice agent if resistance in area is less than 20%. Allergic reactions are common; serious skin reactions and blood dyscrasias may occur.
Nitrofurantoin (Macrodantin, Furadantin)	*E. coli* Not active against *Proteus* or *Pseudomonas*	100 mg PO 2 times/day for 5–7 days	Do not use as empiric therapy, as resistance to this agent is high. Use is acceptable if the isolate is known to be susceptible.	First choice for uncomplicated UTI. Resistance is unlikely, but the drug is bactericidal in urine only; it has poor penetration into tissues. Administer with meals to improve absorption. Avoid using with alkalizing agents such as potassium citrate and in women with renal failure, in whom the dose reaching the bladder will be ineffective. Side effects include GI upset (especially with macrocrystals), peripheral neuropathy, and pneumonitis.
Fosfomycin (Monurol)	*E. coli* *Enterococcus* Not reliable for *Staphylococcus saprophyticus*	Single 3-g dose PO	Not recommended for treatment of complicated UTI.	First-line therapy if resistance or intolerance to TMP-SMX or nitrofurantoin. Lower effectiveness than 3 days of other agents, but resistance is rare in the United States. It may be an option for women with multiple allergies.
Ciprofloxacin (Cipro)[c]	Second-generation fluoroquinolone; broad-spectrum coverage except for anaerobes	Immediate release: 250–500 mg PO 2 times/day for 3 days	500 mg PO 2 times/day for 7 days with or without loading dose of 400 mg IV[b] *or* 1000 mg once daily for 7 days.	None of the fluoroquinolones is a first-line therapy. Use only if resistance or allergy to other first-line agents is present. Avoid in pregnancy and in women with epilepsy due to the seizure risk. Black box warning states that tendon damage/rupture may occur; elderly and steroid users are at higher risk. Side effects can include nausea, vomiting, diarrhea, hypoglycemia, abdominal pain, headache, rash, arrhythmias, angina, convulsions, GI bleeding, nephritis, and joint damage. Immediate- and extended-release formulas offer similar cure rates; cost and adherence concerns can guide treatment.
Levofloxacin (Levaquin)[c]	Third-generation fluoroquinolone; broad-spectrum coverage except for anaerobes	250 mg PO once daily 3 days	750 mg PO once daily for 5 days.[b]	
Norfloxacin (Noroxin)[c]	*E. coli* *Klebsiella* *Proteus* *Enterobacter* *Enterococcus* *Staphylococcus* *Serratia*	400 mg PO 2 times/day for 3 days	400 mg PO 2 times/day for 10–21 days.	
Ofloxacin[c]	Second-generation fluoroquinolone; broad-spectrum coverage except for anaerobes	200 mg PO every 12 hours for 3–7 days	200 mg PO every 12 hours for 10 days.	
Amoxicillin (Amoxil), ampicillin (Principen)	*E coli, Proteus, Enterococcus, Staphylococcus*	250–500 mg PO 4 times/day	Do not use as empiric therapy, as resistance is high. Use is acceptable if the isolate is known to be susceptible. Less effective and not typically used for complicated UTI. Drug of choice for enterococcal UTI: 2 g PO every 6 hours or 500 mg PO every 8 hours for 5–10 days.	Not considered first-line agents. Should be used only if resistance or allergy to first-line choices is present. Beta-lactams may be less effective than other agents due to high rates of resistance. Risks include allergies, candidal overgrowth, and pseudomembranous colitis (especially with ampicillin).

(*continues*)

Table 22-7 Antibiotics Commonly Used to Treat Urinary Tract Infections (*continued*)

Drug: Generic (Brand)	Microbial Coverage	Uncomplicated UTI Dose	Complicated UTI and Acute Pyelonephritis[a] Dose	Clinical Considerations
Cephalexin (Keflex)	*E coli, Klebsiella, Proteus, Staphylococcus*	250–500 mg PO 4 times/day for 3–5 days	Second-generation cephalosporin may be more effective in complicated cases.	Not active against enterococci. Risks include allergies and hepatic dysfunction.
Tetracycline	Gram-negative and some gram-positive coverage; *Enterococcus, Chlamydia, Mycoplasma hominis*	250–500 mg PO every 6 hours	Not commonly used.	Less commonly used. Side effects include GI upset, skin rash, candidal overgrowth, hepatic dysfunction, and nephrotoxicity. Avoid in women with renal failure and in pregnant women. Doxycycline is less likely to affect GI flora than other tetracyclines.
Doxycyline (Vibramycin)		100 mg PO 2 times/day		

Abbreviations: GI = gastrointestinal; UTI = urinary tract infection.

[a] Women with severe symptoms or suspected complications require hospitalization and intravenous antibiotic treatment, whereas women with uncomplicated pyelonephritis may be treated in an outpatient setting.

[b] If an intravenous loading dose is used, one of the following is recommended: 1 g ceftriaxone or 2–5 mg/kg gentamicin.

[c] Ciprofloxacin is a second-generation fluoroquinolone; levofloxacin is a third-generation fluoroquinolone. The difference between fluoroquinolone generations primarily reflects the expanded antimicrobial activity of the third-generation drugs. However, both generations of fluoroquinolones are becoming first-choice treatments in settings where high sulfa resistance is encountered.

Source: Data from Gupta K, Hooton TM, Naber KG, et al. International clinical practice guidelines for the treatment of acute uncomplicated cystitis and pyelonephritis in women: A 2010 update by the Infectious Diseases Society of America and the European Society for Microbiology and Infectious Diseases. *Clin Infect Dis*. 2011;52(5):e103-e120.[46]

and be predominately concentrated and excreted in urine (Box 22-3).

Trimethoprim–sulfamethoxazole (TMP-SMX, brand names Bactrim, Septra, Septra DS) was traditionally the first-choice antibiotic treatment for uncomplicated UTIs. Resistance to this drug increased sharply in the mid-1990s, however. One cross-sectional study reported that the prevalence of TMP-SMX resistance among *E. coli* increased from 9% in 1992 to 18% by 1996. Nationwide surveys indicate that resistance was about 18% in 2000.[44] Where the

Box 22-3 Case Study: Acute Dysuria

BL is a 24-year-old woman who experienced acute onset of dysuria, urgency, and frequency without urine loss. Her pain began 2 days ago and is most intense when she begins voiding and for a few seconds post voiding. BL has tried increasing fluids and drinking cranberry juice, but without achieving any relief. She denies fever, back pain, or gastrointestinal symptoms, as well as any history of UTIs. Today, she has noticed hematuria. BL has a new sexual partner, and she is concerned about sexually transmitted infections (STIs). She had a normal menses about 3 weeks before and uses combined oral contraceptives regularly.

On physical examination, BL is afebrile, in no acute distress, and has no abdominal or flank tenderness. Her pelvic exam is normal, except for mild suprapubic tenderness. Gonorrhea and chlamydia tests are obtained. A urine dipstick is positive for nitrites, leukocytes, and red blood cells, and a urine pregnancy test is negative.

Primary Care Treatment

The presumptive diagnosis for BL is uncomplicated acute cystitis. Because she has no drug allergies, BL is a good candidate for any of a variety of anti-infective agents. Based on cost and regional use, she is prescribed a 3-day course of trimethoprim–sulfamethoxazole (Bactrim, Septra, Septra DS) double-strength 160/800 mg twice a day; she is also prescribed a urinary analgesic 3 times a day for the first day, such as phenazopyridine (Pyridium), and is asked to increase her fluid intake to avoid symptomatic irritation due to concentrated urine. A urine culture and sensitivity at the initial assessment are not necessary; instead, empiric treatment is initiated. BL is instructed to take all six antibiotic doses as directed and call if her symptoms are not resolved after 48 hours. At that time, a culture could be obtained. BL is encouraged to prevent STIs by using condoms until she is in a committed, long-term monogamous relationship, and is offered appropriate STI testing.

prevalence of resistance is less than 20%, studies show that TMP-SMX (160/800 mg twice daily for 3 days) remains an effective therapeutic choice.

Nitrofurantoin monohydrate/macrocrystals (Macrodantin) 100 mg twice daily for 5 days is an effective alternative to TMP-SMX. In vitro studies confirm that it has more than 99% activity against *E. coli* isolates, but is less active against *Proteus* and *Pseudomonas* species. Recent randomized clinical trials indicate that a 5-day course of this antibiotic is as effective as the more traditional 7-day course. Chronic long-term use has been associated with pulmonary toxicity that is largely reversible once the antibiotic is discontinued.[51,52]

Fosfomycin trometanol (Monurol) 3-g in a single-dose sachet is emerging as a first-choice antibiotic in the face of growing resistance and in persons with allergies to either sulfa drugs or nitrofurantoin. In vitro studies have shown that fosfomycin exhibits high activity against multidrug-resistant organisms. This agent is generally well tolerated, with the most common side effects being gastrointestinal distress and headache. The single-dose regimen may be associated with fewer adverse effects than multi-dose alternatives.[46]

Fluoroquinolones maintain high activity against nearly all gram-negative uropathogens, but are less active against enterococci. There is concern about increasing resistance to these agents not only among uropathogens, but also among pathogenic organisms that affect other sites. This trend could potentially limit the use of this class of antibiotics for more serious infections.[46] For this reason, fluoroquinolones should be prescribed only in the setting of resistance or allergy to other first-line antibiotics.

Beta-lactam antibiotics are generally not recommended for the empiric treatment of uncomplicated UTIs. Their effectiveness is typically lower than that of the fluoroquinolones. Broad-spectrum agents have the potential to select for highly resistant organisms, such as extended-spectrum beta lactamase (ESBL)–resistant gram-negative bacilli.[46] Although narrow-spectrum beta-lactam agents may reduce this risk, available data are not adequate to settle questions about the most effective treatment regimens.[46]

Duration of Treatment

For both premenopausal and postmenopausal women, 3-day treatment is adequate for those who have an uncomplicated UTI.[53] For elderly women, expert opinion often suggests continuing antibiotics for 7 to 14 days. However, a Cochrane review concluded that short-course treatment—that is, 3 to 6 days—may be as effective as extended courses in this population.[53] Single-day doses have been associated with higher failure rates, with the exception of fosfomycin.[54]

Antibacterial Agents for Complicated Urinary Tract Infection

Women with complicated UTIs or acute pyelonephritis that does not require hospitalization should be treated empirically at the time of diagnosis. A urine culture should be obtained and drug therapy may be changed depending on culture results. The duration of therapy is 7 to 14 days in women who are able to tolerate oral medications.[46] Hospitalization may be required for women who are not able to tolerate oral intake or for pregnant women. Referral is indicated for women who have frequent recurrence, persistent hematuria, severe pyelonephritis, evidence of kidney damage, or underlying structural or functional abnormalities.

Phenazopyridine (Pyridium) for Treating Dysuria Associated with Urinary Tract Infections

Phenazopyridine (Pyridium, Uristat, Azo-Septic) acts as a urinary anesthetic and is available over the counter. Its mechanism of action on the bladder is not known. The usual dose is 200 mg 3 times daily, taken with food, typically for the initial 2 days of antibiotic therapy. Because use of phenazopyridine can mask underlying serious urinary tract disease, women should be instructed to avoid using phenazopyridine as a single treatment and use for no more than 3 days. Nonpregnant women should be instructed to notify a provider if UTI-related dysuria persists after 2 days of treatment.

Although the main indication for use of phenazopyridine is dysuria related to UTI, the drug's side effect of turning urine a bright red-orange color also makes it useful as a marker for evaluation of urinary tract dysfunction such as urinary incontinence or fistula. Other side effects, which are uncommon and mild, include headaches, vertigo, and gastrointestinal disturbances.

Pharmacologic Interventions to Prevent Urinary Tract Infections

Use of vaginal estrogen appears to play a role in preventing recurrent UTI.[55] The available data are not sufficient to identify the ideal formulation and dosing regimen.

Methenamine (Hiprex) acts as a urinary antiseptic and may have a role in preventing recurrent or chronic UTI, according to a Cochrane review.[56] This drug is converted into formaldehyde in the urine, with the conversion occurring approximately 3 hours post ingestion. Methenamine has been studied for prevention of recurrent UTI in continuous use for up to 2 years, but the study quality precludes drawing any definitive conclusions about its effectiveness.[56] This agent appears to be less effective than prophylactic treatment with nitrofurantoin (Macrodantin, Macrobid) or TMP-SMX (Bactrim, Septra), and it is not effective in women with indwelling catheters. Side effects are infrequent, but include stomatitis, nausea, vomiting, and diarrhea with accompanying abdominal pain, exacerbation of preexisting liver disease, and dysuria due to crystalluria.

The typical oral regimen for UTI prophylaxis is methenamine hippurate (Hiprex, Urex) 1 g twice daily or methenamine mandelate 1 g 4 times per day. Both agents are available as tablets, granules, and liquid suspension. Tablets can be crushed for ease of ingestion. With increasing antibiotic resistance, methenamine may become a more attractive option for UTI prevention in the future.

Prevention of Recurrent Cystitis

Recurrent UTIs are defined as three or more infections in one year.[57] Most recurrent UTIs are reinfections, in which a repeat episode of cystitis is caused by a different organism or the same organism with an intervening negative culture. By comparison, persistent infections are those in which the same organism is repeatedly cultured despite adequate and appropriate antibiotic therapy. The distinction is important because women with persistent infections may benefit from a referral to a specialist and may require more extensive evaluation of their upper and lower urinary tracts to assess for structural abnormalities, stones, or foreign bodies that may serve as reservoirs for colonization.[57]

The acute treatment for recurrent infections is the same as that for isolated episodes, and studies indicate that antibiotic courses for longer than 7 days do not provide additional benefit.[53,54] Antibiotic prophylaxis has been shown to be the superior method of preventing recurrence.[57,58] Three regimens are available: (1) acute self-treatment; (2) continuous low-dose therapy; and (3) postcoital therapy (Table 22-8).

Acute self-treatment is intended to treat, not to prevent infection. However, it may help to limit antibiotic exposure. In a study of healthy adult women who symptomatically self-diagnosed early onset of recurrent cystitis (n = 172), infection was present in 84% of suspected cases, while an additional 11% had sterile pyuria.[59] Of the women who had confirmed infection, 92% of cases resolved microscopically with a 3-day course of a fluoroquinolone. Acute self-treatment requires a cognitively aware woman who is able to recognize symptoms, so this approach may have limited utility in older populations.

Postcoital and continuous antibiotics have been shown to be highly effective when compared with placebo in meta-analyses of randomized trials.[57] Potential side effects from treatment include vaginal and oral candidiasis and gastrointestinal symptoms. Most available data are specific for 6 months' duration of therapy, although in practice this treatment period may be extended to 12 months. Infection may recur after discontinuation.

Antibiotic prophylaxis is highly effective in reducing the incidence of recurrent UTI. No antibiotic has been shown to be superior to the others in such a regimen.[57,58] Therefore, a woman's tolerance, microbial history, cost, and the potential for antibiotic resistance should guide selection of the antibiotic. Such medications can be taken either daily or 2 hours after intercourse. Duration of treatment has not been clearly determined. Some authors recommend an initial 6-month regimen, whereas others indicate that a treatment course of 2 years or more is safe and effective.[60] Chronic nitrofurantoin (Macrodantin, Macrobid) use, however, has been associated with pulmonary toxicity and hepatic dysfunction. Although most cases are reversible with discontinuation of the antibiotic, steroids and immune-suppressive treatments may be required.[52]

Minimal evidence exists to support many common recommendations for UTI prevention, including increasing fluid intake, decreasing fluid intake to avoid lowering antibiotic levels in the urine, urinating after intercourse, avoidance of douching, and wiping from front to back after toileting. Evidence does support the concept that treatment

Table 22-8 Antibiotic Regimens for Prevention of Recurrent Cystitis

Drug: Generic (Brand)	Continuous Dose	Postcoital Dose
Cephalexin (Keflex)	125–250 mg PO once daily	250 mg PO
Ciprofloxacin (Cipro)	125 mg PO once daily	125 mg PO
Nitrofurantoin[a] (Macrodantin, Macrobid)	50–100 mg PO once daily at bedtime	50–100 mg PO
Norfloxacin (Noroxin)	NA	200 mg PO
Ofloxacin	NA	100 mg PO
Trimethoprim	100 mg PO once daily	NA
Trimethoprim–sulfamethoxazole (Bactrim, Septra, Septra DS)	40/200 mg PO once daily or 3 times/week	40/200 mg PO or 80/400 mg PO

Abbreviations: NA = not applicable.
[a] Long-term use may cause pulmonary toxicity or immune-mediated liver damage.

of urinary retention and genital atrophy, avoidance of indwelling catheters, and limiting the use of spermicides can prevent UTIs.

Complementary Therapies: Cranberries and Nutritional Supplements

There is limited evidence to support or dispute the role of most complementary modalities for UTI prevention, and none that focuses on the effectiveness of these approaches for treatment of UTI. The most commonly used modalities are dietary supplements.

Cranberries and other berries in the genus *Vaccinium* contain proanthocyanidins, which have been shown to counteract bacterial virulence and prevent bacterial adhesion in urine.[61] While early clinical evidence suggested a role for cranberry products in preventing recurrent UTIs, a later Cochrane meta-analysis concluded that the studied doses of cranberry products did not reduce UTI risk overall (RR, 0.86; 95% CI, 0.71–1.04) or in any subgroup, including women with recurrent UTIs, older people, pregnant women, children with recurrent UTIs, individuals with persons with cancer or those with a neuropathic bladder or spinal injury.[62] However, dosages were not standardized, and the optimal dose to ensure maximal effectiveness may not have been determined.

The use of D-mannose has also been hypothesized to prevent UTIs based on in vitro studies demonstrating its ability to block adherence of uropathogens to the bladder epithelium.[63] While clinical studies on this topic are limited, one randomized study comparing D-mannose powder to nitrofurantoin and no prophylaxis concluded that both D-mannose and nitrofurantoin use were associated with fewer episodes of recurrent cystitis compared to no prophylaxis (P = 0.001), with no significant difference observed between D-mannose and nitrofurantoin.[64]

Dietary changes may decrease UTI risk, but their effectiveness remains understudied. Suggested dietary recommendations have included increased consumption of fresh juices, especially berry juice; fermented milk products with probiotics; onion and garlic, because of their potential antimicrobial activity; and vitamin C supplementation during acute infection in a dose of 2000 mg every 2 hours for 2 days, then 2000 mg 3 times a day for 7 days as a means of acidifying the urine.[65] *Echinacea purpurea herba* (purple coneflower) may have a role in supporting the immune system generally, although a specific role in UTI prevention has not been well studied. Other herbs with antimicrobial or diuretic properties that have been suggested for use during UTI treatment or prevention include *Hydrastis canadensis* (goldenseal), *Arctostaphylos uva-ursi* (bearberry), and *Zea mays* (corn silk). Although little research has been done to support these recommendations, the risk associated with their use is likely to be low if active infection is also treated with prescription antibiotics.[65]

Special Populations: Pregnancy, Lactation, and the Elderly

Because of the increased risk of ascending infection during pregnancy, and the resultant risk of preterm birth, pregnancy is the only time when asymptomatic bacteriuria should be treated.[66] An initial urine culture at all first prenatal visits is recommended, with follow-up treatment and culture-based surveillance throughout the pregnancy if any positive results are obtained.

Treatment of UTIs during pregnancy is reviewed in more detail in the *Pregnancy* chapter. First-line antibiotic choices for pregnant women include penicillins and cephalosporins. In the second and third trimesters, sulfonamides and nitrofurantoin may be used for UTI treatment. While a single study suggested a potential increase in the risk of birth defects related to first-trimester use of sulfonamides or nitrofurantoins,[67] such a risk has not been identified in other studies.[68] TMX-SMX (Bactrim, Septra) and nitrofurantoin (Macrodantin, Macrobid) should be used in the first trimester if there are no other suitable antibiotics. Although the American College of Obstetricians and Gynecologists states that TMP-SMX and nitrofurantoin are safe for use in the second and third trimesters and should be considered first-line agents,[68] other sources recommend avoiding these agents if possible. Nitrofurantoin should be avoided in the third trimester, as it is associated with hemolytic anemia in women and fetuses with glucose-6-phosphate dehydrogenase (G6PD) deficiency.[69] TMP-SMX may be avoided in the first trimester secondary to an antifolate effect and in the third trimester secondary to an association with kernicterus in the newborn. Overall, it is important to remember that the risks associated with these drugs are small and controversial,[70] whereas the adverse consequences of untreated UTI are well known and can be severe.

Quinolones appear to be safe for use in pregnancy.[67] A standard 3- to 7-day course of treatment is recommended for uncomplicated UTI. Upper tract infection is often treated initially with intravenous therapy until the woman is afebrile, due to the risk of preterm birth. In women at high risk for recurrent infection (e.g., those with prior infection or sickle cell trait), continuous or postcoital prophylaxis for the remainder of the pregnancy and up to 6 weeks postpartum may be warranted, typically using nitrofurantoin or cephalexin (Keflex).[69,71]

During pregnancy, group B *Streptococcus* (GBS) bacteriuria should be treated with penicillin G, cephalexin (Keflex), or clindamycin (Cleocin) for women who have a true allergy to penicillin.[68] These women should also be treated in labor, just as they would if they had been identified as colonized on third-trimester vaginal culture. Management of women who are colonized with GBS is discussed in more detail in the *Pregnancy* chapter.

Infection risk is also a concern for the elderly; older women are more likely to have asymptomatic bacteriuria, cystitis, and urosepsis. With aging, urine becomes alkaline and contains fewer antibacterial proteins—an environment that promotes bacterial colonization. On the one hand, treating all women who have asymptomatic colonization would increase the risk of resistant organisms.[72] On the other hand, decreases in immune response and thermoregulation often mask infection; UTI may manifest only as subtle changes in voiding frequency or odor. Providers must be judicious in prescribing antimicrobials for lower urinary tract symptoms in older adults, observing for cues that may indicate a transition from colonization (which should not be treated) to infection (which should).

Recurrent UTI, defined as more than three culture-positive UTIs within 12 months, may be decreased with nonpharmacologic strategies such as improved emptying (e.g., timed voiding, intermittent self-catheterization, pessary use, or surgical repair of prolapse to decrease residual urine).[72] In postmenopausal women, vaginal estrogen products have been shown to decrease UTI risk, although antibiotic suppression may be more effective.[73]

Painful Bladder Syndrome/ Interstitial Cystitis

The definition of **painful bladder syndrome (PBS)**, also known as bladder pain syndrome, continues to evolve. This condition generally includes the concern of chronic, sometimes waxing and waning, suprapubic or retropubic pain, typically increasing with bladder filling.[2,74] The pain may or may not improve with emptying, and is often accompanied by other lower urinary tract symptoms such as urgency and frequency. By definition, these symptoms occur in the absence of UTI or other obvious pathology.[75] **Interstitial cystitis (IC)** is a specific type of painful bladder syndrome, which includes symptoms occurring in women with specific findings on cystoscopy including glomerulations or Hunner's ulcers. However, these findings are nonspecific and also are seen in asymptomatic women, especially with aging.

The evolving understanding of painful bladder syndrome/interstitial cystitis results in difficulty determining the prevalence of this condition with any reliability. In women, who are thought to be more commonly affected, prevalence has been reported to range from 3% to 6%.[76] Delayed diagnosis and multiple prior unsuccessful treatments for misdiagnoses that include vaginitis and cystitis are common (Box 22-4).

Pathophysiology

Understanding of the etiology of chronic pain syndromes and their treatments is changing rapidly. Regardless of its location, chronic pain has an adverse impact on quality of life, including physical disability, psychological distress, sleep deprivation, financial burden due to lost income and costs of care, and social burden due to the negative impacts of social and sexual relationships. Women with painful bladder syndrome/interstitial cystitis share these burdens, as well as an increased risk for other pain-related syndromes such as migraine, anxiety, endometriosis, fibromyalgia, vulvodynia.[76] Twin studies demonstrate an inheritable susceptibility.[77] These findings suggest that, for many women, painful bladder syndrome/interstitial cystitis may be a pelvic manifestation of a genetically based systemic autoimmune or neuroendocrine disorder thought to underlay other related manifestations of chronic pain.

Environmental factors, such as acute UTI, radiation, or other injury, have also been implicated as promoting bladder hypersensitivity through two probable routes—neurogenic inflammation and alteration of the permeability of the bladder lining.[78]

Neurogenic inflammation is thought to result in mast cell activation, stimulation of nerve growth factor, and proliferation of sensory nerve fibers. The urothelium or bladder lining acts as a barrier to bacterial and crystal adherence and prevents urinary solutes from penetrating the bladder wall.[78] Also called the glycosaminoglycan (GAG) or mucin layer, it is predominantly composed of proteoglycans and glycoproteins. In response to injury, nerves within the detrusor itself appear to be susceptible to neuroplastic change, from myelinated alpha sensory nerves to highly sensitive nonmyelinated C nerve fibers.[78] These suspected multiple etiologies support the strategy of employing a multimodal approach to treatment.

Box 22-4 Case Study: Painful Bladder Syndrome

AW, a 46-year-old nullipara, reports having an isolated acute UTI 2 years ago that involved sudden onset of dysuria, urgency, frequency, and hematuria. She completed a 3-day course of antibiotics, and the hematuria resolved. Despite subsequent negative urine cultures, AW continues to experience chronic pelvic pain with dysuria, dyspareunia, frequency, and severe nocturia. Her symptoms lessen to some extent immediately after voiding and also seem to improve spontaneously for short periods of time, but they recur unpredictably. AW has no other positive history of urinary symptoms. She has prior diagnoses of migraine headaches and anxiety, but does not currently require pharmacologic treatment for these conditions. She is not currently sexually active and has no systemic symptoms. Her quality of life is poor, and she feels her main focus to be her bladder pain. She smokes ½ pack of cigarettes per day and drinks 2 cups of coffee per day, as well as 6 glasses of wine per week. Her physical exam demonstrates tenderness only in the suprapubic region. Her neurologic exam and post-void residual are normal. She has no anatomic abnormalities, and her sexually transmitted infection test, urinalysis, urine cytology, and culture are negative.

Treatment

The presumptive diagnosis for AW is bladder pain syndrome/interstitial cystitis. Her symptoms may continue chronically but are manageable. This diagnosis may stem from several related changes, including increased permeability of her bladder lining, inherited and acquired increased sensitivity of the nerve receptors starting in her bladder wall, and an over-response of her immune system. These changes may have been triggered by AW's acute infection, but antibiotics are not a recommended treatment now in the absence of current negative cultures. A combination of therapies is most likely to be effective.

AW starts with dietary changes to avoid caffeinated, acidic, and high-potassium foods. She discontinues smoking and alcohol. She keeps a symptom diary and measures urine volumes over 24 hours, repeating the latter process intermittently to track her progress. She works to rebuild her bladder capacity through timed voiding. AW also learns relaxation techniques and sees a cognitive-behavioral therapist, who helps her learn skills for living with chronic pain. She begins a low-dose tricyclic antidepressant at night to help her sleep, along with a 6-month trial of pentosan polysulfate (Elmiron). If these changes are not successful in decreasing her symptoms, AW will be referred to a specialist, who is likely to conduct a cystoscopic evaluation and administer intravesical treatment. AW's pharmacologic agents may be modified to include neuroleptic and/or analgesics. Once she is on an effective regimen, she may choose to return to her primary care office for maintenance care.

Treatment of Painful Bladder Syndrome/Interstitial Cystitis

As with other chronic pain syndromes, high-quality data related to the effectiveness of treatments for painful bladder syndrome/interstitial cystitis are difficult to obtain. This complexity relates to a variety of factors. For example, the existence of suspected multiple etiologies means women may have similar symptoms with differing underlying pathophysiology that would require different treatments; waxing and waning of symptoms often occurs without treatment; and the high placebo effect seen in most studies severely limits the interpretation of noncontrolled trials. Successful management of painful bladder syndrome/interstitial cystitis, therefore, typically requires a multimodal approach, including a written plan that is based on shared decision making to promote involvement of the woman and her social support system. Optimal management includes establishment of realistic goals; provision of psychological support in coping with the chronic impact of the diagnosis; regularly scheduled return visits; and stepwise interventions that start with the least invasive options and are guided by the woman's symptom diaries and assessments.[75]

Pharmacologic Treatments for Painful Bladder Syndrome

Both oral and intravesical pharmacologic agents are considered second-line therapy for painful bladder

Table 22-9 Pharmacologic Agents Used to Treat Women with Painful Bladder Syndrome/Interstitial Cystitis

Drug: Generic (Brand)	Typical Dose	Mechanism of Action	Clinical Considerations
Cystitis Agents			
Pentosan polysulfate (Elmiron)	100 mg PO 3 times/day	May decrease permeability of the bladder lining; anticoagulant and fibrinolytic effects similar to heparin	FDA approved for PBS/IC. May take up to 6 months to show an effect in some (fewer than 50%) users. No better than placebo in recent studies.
Histamine Blockers			
Cimetidine (Tagamet)	400 mg PO at bedtime	Impedes mast cell proliferation	Approved for gastric ulcer treatment. Quality of evidence is poor.
Hydroxyzine hydrochloride (Atarax, Vistaril)	25–75 mg PO once daily	Impedes mast cell proliferation; analgesic, bronchodilator, sedative, antispasmodic/emetic	Approved for anxiety and use as an antiemetic. May be useful for persons with allergy history. Also may aid sleep.
Tricyclic Antidepressants			
Amitriptyline (Elavil); nortriptyline (Aventyl)	10–25 mg PO at bedtime	Blocks absorption of serotonin and norepinephrine; sedative effect; anticholinergic effects	Approved for depression. Nortriptyline, a metabolite of amitriptyline, may have fewer side effects. Drug–drug interactions related to cytochrome P450 apply. Use with caution in elderly women.
Instillation Agents (Often Used in Nonstandardized Combinations)			
Dimethyl sulfoxide (DMSO)	50% solution in 50 mL saline for ≤ 20 minutes, weekly for 6–8 weeks, repeated as needed	Possibly anti-inflammatory, analgesic, smooth muscle relaxer, and/or mast cell inhibitor; may increase absorption of other agents	FDA approved. Low risk. Poor-quality evidence; nonresponse occurs in as many as 70% of users. Symptoms may temporarily increase after treatment before improving.
Heparin	10,000 units in 10 mL sterile water for 1 hour 3 times/week as needed	Anti-inflammatory; may directly improve bladder lining (GAG layer); promotes angiogenesis and smooth muscle growth	Off-label use. Poor-quality evidence.
Lidocaine	200 mg in sodium bicarbonate for 1 hour daily for 5 days	Topical anesthetic (bupivacaine is also used)	Offers short-term relief for acute pain; low risk but lidocaine toxicity signs include headache, sedation, and seizures.

Abbreviations: PBS/IC = painful bladder syndrome/interstitial cystitis.

syndrome/interstitial cystitis.[75] Outcome assessment focuses on improvements in symptoms, function, and quality of life. As no single optimal treatment has been identified, a combination of pharmacologic agents is often used.[75] Table 22-9 reviews the lower-risk agents suggested in the American Urological Association guidelines, which may be appropriate for use in primary care settings.[75] Additional medications used for chronic pain, including anticonvulsants such as gabapentin, may be prescribed as well.[79] Higher-risk agents, including long-term opioid use, experimental intravesical agents, the oral immunosuppressive cyclosporine A, and botulinum toxin A injected directly into the bladder wall at multiple sites, are typically reserved for subspecialty care; thus they are not reviewed here.

Complementary Therapies

Complementary and alternative treatments may offer relief for some women with painful bladder syndrome/interstitial cystitis, but evidence supporting their use is of poor quality or remains anecdotal in nature.[75,80] Modalities that are used and may play a role in symptom relief and coping include stress-reduction therapies such as meditation, yoga, hypnotherapy, and guided imagery, as well as acupuncture, trigger point injection, needling, and massage.[81]

Dietary elimination trials may seem unduly burdensome to some women, but many individuals report improvement with this low-risk option. Suggestions for this approach, which can be found on the Interstitial Cystitis Society website, may include a trial elimination of acidic (citrus), spicy, or arylalkylamine-containing foods (e.g., bananas, beer, wine, cheese, mayonnaise, aspartame, nuts, onions, raisins, sour cream, and yogurt).[82] Women who report irritation from certain foods usually notice symptoms within 2 to 4 hours after ingesting the irritant.

Nutritional supplements that have been suggested include the urinary acid neutralizer known as calcium glycerophosphate (Prelief), the amino acid L-arginine, natural muco-polysaccharides such as hyaluronic acid, chondroitin sulfate, aloe vera, and the bioflavonoid quercetin, which may have a role in inhibiting histamine release.[80,82] Naturopathic regimens are often used by symptomatic women, although evidence supporting this modality is limited.[83] Updated information on trials, support, and recommendations for women with this diagnosis is available on the Interstitial Cystitis Association website.

Special Populations: Pregnancy, Lactation, and the Elderly

Little is known about how pregnancy affects painful bladder syndrome/interstitial cystitis.[84] The majority of drugs taken orally have not been scientifically examined in human studies that show either effectiveness or safety; consequently, management should be based on use of drugs with the lowest known risks for the woman and her fetus.

In older women, pharmacologic management of chronic pain syndromes, including severe painful bladder syndrome/interstitial cystitis, warrants special consideration and possibly referral to a specialist. Optimal treatment is likely to include multiple agents and modalities for women already taking a variety of medications for significant comorbidities.[85] In addition, physiologic changes of aging are likely to result in changes in pharmacokinetics and pharmacodynamics, which may increase the risk of toxicity in older women.

Conclusion

Lower urinary tract disorders, including overactive and underactive bladder, incontinence, painful bladder syndrome, and urinary tract infections, are commonly seen in primary care practices. These conditions can severely decrease quality of life, and some are life-threatening. Because many of these disorders are chronic in nature, health education and behavioral treatments are primary interventions for amelioration of distressing symptoms. However, pharmacologic treatments also play an essential role in the armamentarium of management options. Better understanding of the normal function and pathophysiology of diseases affecting this complex system can help providers choose safe, low-cost, and effective agents, and assimilate new agents as they are developed and approved for use in this rapidly changing field.

Resources

Organization	Description	Website
American Urological Association (AUA) and Society of Urodynamics, Female Pelvic Medicine, and Urogenital Reconstruction (SUFU)	Diagnosis and treatment of overactive bladder (non-neurogenic) in adults; guidelines approved May 2014	www.sufuorg.com/docs/news/OAB-Amendment-061014.aspx
Infectious Diseases Society of America	*International Clinical Practice Guidelines for the Treatment of Acute Uncomplicated Cystitis and Pyelonephritis in Women: A 2010 Update* by the Infectious Diseases Society of America and the European Society for Microbiology and Infectious Diseases	http://cid.oxfordjournals.org/content/52/5/e103.full.pdf+html
National Kidney and Urologic Diseases Information Clearinghouse	A service of the National Institute of Diabetes and Digestive and Kidney Diseases (NIDDK), National Institutes of Health (NIH), this website has information on research, statistics, and pharmacologic treatments for a variety of urologic disorders, including bladder diaries in English and Spanish	http://kidney.niddk.nih.gov
Interstitial Cystitis Association (ICA)	The website of the ICA includes updates on current research, diagnosis, and treatment	www.ichelp.org

References

1. Unger CA, Tunitsky-Bitton E, Muffly T, Barber MD. Neuroanatomy, neurophysiology, and dysfunction of the female lower urinary tract: A review. *Female Pelvic Med Reconstr Surg.* 2014;20(2):65-75.
2. Haylen BT, de Ridder D, Freeman RM, et al. An International Urogynecological Association (IUGA)/International Continence Society (ICS) joint report on the terminology for female pelvic floor dysfunction. *Neurourol Urodynam.* 2010;29(1):4-20.
3. Stewart WF, Van Rooyen JB, Cundiff GW, et al. Prevalence and burden of overactive bladder in the United States. *World J Urol.* 2003;20(6):327-336.
4. Benson JT, Walters MD. Neurophysiology and pharmacology of the lower urinary tract. In: Walters MD, Karram MM, eds. *Urogynecology and Reconstructive*

Pelvic Surgery. 3rd ed. Philadelphia, PA: Mosby-Elsevier; 2007:31-43.

5. Rai BP, Cody JD, Alhasso A, Stewart L. Anticholinergic drugs versus non-drug active therapies for non-neurogenic overactive bladder syndrome in adults. *Cochrane Database Syst Rev*. 2012;12:CD003193. doi: 10.1002/14651858.CD003193.pub4.
6. Shamliyan T, Wyman JF, Ramakrishnan R, Sainfort F, Kane RL. Benefits and harms of pharmacologic treatment for urinary incontinence in women: a systematic review. *Ann Intern Med*. 2012;156(12):861-874.
7. Nabi G, Cody JD, Ellis G, Hay-Smith J, Herbison GP. Anticholinergic drugs versus placebo for overactive bladder syndrome in adults. *Cochrane Database Syst Rev*. 2006;4:CD003781. doi:10.1002/14651858.CD003781.pub2.
8. Madhuvrata P, Cody JD, Ellis G, Herbison GP, Hay-Smith EJC. Which anticholinergic drug for overactive bladder symptoms in adults. *Cochrane Database Syst Rev*. 2012;1:CD005429. doi:10.1002/14651858.CD005429.pub2.
9. Staskin DR. Overactive bladder in the elderly: a guide to pharmacologic management. *Drugs Aging*. 2005;22(12):1013-1028.
10. Dmochowski RR, Sand PK, Zinner NR, Staskin DR. Trospium 60 mg once daily (QD) for overactive bladder syndrome: results from a placebo-controlled interventional study. *Urology*. 2008;71(3):449-454.
11. Yu YF, Nichol MB, Yu AP, Ahn J. Persistence and adherence of medications for chronic overactive bladder/urinary incontinence in the California Medicaid Program. *Value Health*. 2005;8(4):495-505.
12. Benner JS, Nichol MB, Rovner ES, et al. Patient-reported reasons for discontinuing overactive bladder medication. *BJU Int*. 2010;105(9):1276-1282.
13. Nitti VW, Auerbach S, Martin N, Calhoun A, Lee M, Herschorn S. Results of a randomized Phase III trial of mirabegron in patients with overactive bladder. *J Urol*. 2013;189(4):1388-1395.
14. Kleeman SD, Karram MM. Overactive bladder syndrome and nocturia. In: Walters MD, Karram MM, eds. *Urogynecology and Reconstructive Pelvic Surgery*. 3rd ed. Philadelphia, PA; Mosby Elsevier; 2007: 353-376.
15. Robinson D, Toozs-Hobson P, Cardozo L. The effect of hormones on the lower urinary tract. *Menopause Int*. 2013;19(4):155-162.
16. Cody JD, Jacobs ML, Richardson K, Moehrer B, Hextall A. Oestrogen therapy for urinary incontinence in post-menopausal women. *Cochrane Database Syst Rev*. 2012;10;CD001405. doi:10.1002/14651858.CD001405.pub3.
17. Suckling JA, Kennedy R, Lethaby A, Roberts H. Local oestrogen for vaginal atrophy in postmenopausal women. *Cochrane Database Syst Rev*. 2006;4:CD001500. doi:10.1002/14651858.CD001500.pub2.
18. North American Menopause Society. Management of symptomatic vulvovaginal atrophy: 2013 position statement of the North American Menopause Society. *Menopause*. 2013;20(9):888-902.
19. Neuhaus J, Schwalenberg T. Intravesical treatments of bladder pain syndrome/interstitial cystitis. *Nat Rev Urol*. 2012;9(12):707-720.
20. Evans RJ. Intravesical therapy for overactive bladder. *Curr Bladder Dysfunc Rep*. 2006;1(1):40-44.
21. Nitti VW, Dmochowski R, Herschorn S, et al. Onabotulinum toxin A for the treatment of patients with overactive bladder and urinary incontinence: results of a Phase 3, randomized, placebo controlled trial. *J Urol*. 2013;189(6):2186-2193.
22. Dmochowski RR, Gomelsky A. Update on the treatment of overactive bladder. *Curr Opin Urol*. 2011;21(4):286-290.
23. Moossdorff-Steinhauser HF, Berghmans B. Effects of percutaneous tibial nerve stimulation on adult patients with overactive bladder syndrome: a systematic review. *Neurourol Urodyn*. 2013;32(3): 206-214.
24. Siddiqui NY, Wu JM, Amundsen CL. Efficacy and adverse events of sacral nerve stimulation for overactive bladder: a systematic review. *Neurourol Urodyn*. 2010;29(suppl 1):S18-S23.
25. O'Dell KK, McGee S. Acupuncture for urge urinary incontinence in older women: what is the evidence? *Urol Nurs*. 2005;26:23-29.
26. Emmons SL, Otto L. Acupuncture for overactive bladder: a randomized controlled trial. *Obstet Gynecol*. 2005;106(1):138-143.
27. Baker J, Costa D, Nygaard I. Mindfulness-based stress reduction for treatment of urinary urge incontinence: a pilot study. *Female Pelvic Med Reconstr Surg*. 2012;18(1):46-49.
28. Blumental M, Busse WR, eds. Bundesinstitut fur Arsneimittel und Medizinprodukte. *The Complete German Commission E Monographs: Therapeutic Guide to Herbal Medicines*. Hufford CD, trans. Austin, TX: American Botanical Council; 1998.

29. Wehrberger C, Madersbacher S, Jungwirth S, Fischer P, Tragl KH. Lower urinary tract symptoms and urinary incontinence in a geriatric cohort: a population-based analysis. *BJU Int.* 2012;110(10): 1516-1521.
30. American Geriatrics Society 2012 Beers Criteria Update Expert Panel. American Geriatrics Society updated Beers Criteria for potentially inappropriate medication use in older adults. *J Am Geriatr Soc.* 2012;60(4):616-631.
31. Asoglu MR, Selcuk S, Cam C, Cogendez E, Karateke A. Effects of urinary incontinence subtypes on women's quality of life (including sexual life) and psychosocial state. *Eur J Obstet Gynecol Reprod Biol.* 2014;176:187-190.
32. Handa VL, Pierce CB, Muñoz A, Blomquist JL. Longitudinal changes in overactive bladder and stress incontinence among parous women. *Neurourol Urodyn.* 2014;34(4):356-361.
33. Shamliyan TA, Kane RL, Wyman J, Wilt TJ. Systematic review: randomized, controlled trials of nonsurgical treatments for urinary incontinence in women. *Ann Intern Med.* 2008;148(6):459-473.
34. McLean L, Varette K, Gentilcore-Saulnier E, Harvey MA, Baker K, Sauerbrei E. Pelvic muscle training for women with stress urinary incontinences causes hypertrophy of the urethral sphincters and reduces bladder neck mobility during coughing. *Neurourol Urodyn.* 2013;32(8):1096-1102.
35. Alhasso A, Glazener CMA, Pickard R, N'Dow JMO. Adrenergic drugs for urinary incontinence in adults. *Cochrane Database Syst Rev.* 2005;3:CD001842. doi: 10.1002/14651858.CD001842.pub2.
36. Byron JK, March PA, Chew DJ, DiBartola SP. Effect of phenylpropanolamine and pseudoephedrine on the urethral pressure profile and continence scores of incontinent female dogs. *J Vet Int Med.* 2007; 21(1): 47-53.
37. Rovner ES, Wein AJ. Treatment options for stress urinary incontinence. *Rev Urol.* 2004;6(suppl 3): S29-S47.
38. Osman NI, Chapple CR, Abrams P, et al. Detrusor underactivity and the underactive bladder: a new clinical entity? A review of current terminology, definitions, epidemiology, aetiology, and diagnosis. *Eur Urol.* 2014 65(2):389-398.
39. Jeon S, Yoo EH. Predictive value of obstructive voiding symptoms and objective bladder emptying tests for urinary retention. *J Obstet Gynaecol.* 2012;32(8):770-772.
40. Miyasato, M, Yoshimura N, Chancellor MB. The other bladder syndrome: underactive bladder. *Rev Urol.* 2013;15(1):11-22.
41. Dorsher PT, McIntosh PM. Neurogenic bladder. *Adv Urol.* February 8, 2012;816274.
42. Kessler TM, La Framboise D, Trelle S, et al. Sacral neuromodulation for neurogenic lower urinary tract dysfunction: systematic review and meta-analysis. *Eur Urol.* 2010;58(6):865-874.
43. Gray M. Urinary retention: management in the acute care setting, part 2. *Am J Nurs.* 2000;100(8):36-44.
44. Foxman B. Epidemiology of urinary tract infections: incidence, morbidity, and economic costs. *Am J Med.* 2002;113(suppl 1A):5S-13S.
45. Foxman B, Somsel P, Tallman P, et al. Urinary tract infection among women aged 40 to 65: behavioral and sexual risk factors. *J Clin Epidem.* 2001; 54(7):710-718.
46. Gupta K, Hooton TM, Naber KG, et al. International clinical practice guidelines for the treatment of acute uncomplicated cystitis and pyelonephritis in women: A 2010 update by the Infectious Diseases Society of America and the European Society for Microbiology and Infectious Diseases. *Clin Infect Dis.* 2011; 52(5):e103-e120.
47. Borges S, Silva J, Teixeira P. The role of lactobacilli and probiotics in maintaining vaginal health. *Arch Gynecol Obstet.* 2014;289(3):479-489.
48. Capobianco G, Wenger JM, Meloni GB, Dessole M, Cherchi PL, Dessole S. Triple therapy with *Lactobacilli acidophili,* estriol plus pelvic floor rehabilitation for symptoms of urogenital aging in postmenopausal women. *Arch Gynecol Obstet.* 2013;289(3):601-608.
49. Kalyoussef S, Nieves E, Dinerman E, et al. *Lactobacillus* proteins are associated with the bactericidal activity against *E. coli* of female genital tract secretions. *PLoS One.* 2012;7(11):e49506.
50. Karlowsky JA, Hoban DJ, DeCorby MR, Laing NM, Zhanel GG. Fluoroquinolone-resistant urinary isolates of *Escherichia coli* from outpatients are frequently multidrug resistant. *Antimicrob Agents Chemother.* 2006;20(6):2251-2254.
51. Matthews SJ, Lancaster JW. Urinary tract infections in the elderly population. *Am J Geriatr Pharmacother.* 2011;9(5):286-309.
52. Mendez JL, Nadrous HF, Hartman TE, Ryu JH. Chronic nitrofurantoin-induced lung disease. *Mayo Clin Proc.* 2006;80(10):1298-1302.

53. Lutters M, Vogt-Ferrier NB. Antibiotic duration for treating uncomplicated, symptomatic lower urinary tract infections in elderly women. *Cochrane Database Syst Rev*. 2008;3:CD001535. doi:10.1002/14651858.CD001535.pub2.
54. Vogel T, Verreault R, Gourdeau M, Morin M, Grenier-Gosselin L, Rochette L. Optimal duration of antibiotic therapy for uncomplicated urinary tract infection in older women: a double-blind randomized controlled trial. *CMAJ*. 2004;170(4):469-473.
55. Lüthje P, Hirshberg AL, Brauner A. Estrogenic action on innate defense mechanisms in the urinary tract. *Maturitas*. 2014;77(1):32-36.
56. Lee BSB, Bhuta T, Simpson JM, Craig JC. Methenamine hippurate for preventing urinary tract infections. *Cochrane Database Syst Rev*. 2012;10:CD003265. doi:10.1002/14651858.CD003265.pub3.
57. Hickling DR, Nitti VW. Management of recurrent urinary tract infections in healthy adult women. *Rev Urol*. 2013;15(2):41-48.
58. Dason S, Dason JT, Kapoor A. Guidelines for the diagnosis and management of recurrent urinary tract infection in women. *Can Urol Assoc J*. 2011;5(5):316-322.
59. Gupta K, Hooton TM, Roberts PL, Stamm WE. Patient-initiated treatment of uncomplicated recurrent urinary tract infections in young women. *Ann Intern Med*. 2001;135(1):9-16.
60. Brumfitt W, Hamilton-Miller JM. Efficacy and safety profile of long-term nitrofurantoin in urinary infections: 18 years' experience. *J Antimicrob Chemother*. 1998;42(3):363-367.
61. Howell AB, Botto H, Combescure C, et al. Dosage effect on uropathogenic *Escherichia coli* anti-adhesion activity in urine following consumption of cranberry powder standardized for proanthocyanidin content: a multicentric randomized double blind study. *BMC Infect Dis*. 2010;10:94.
62. Jepson RG, Williams G, Craig JC. Cranberries for preventing urinary tract infections. *Cochrane Database Syst Rev*. 2012;10:CD001321. doi:10.1002/14651858.CD001321.pub5.
63. Altarac S, Papes D. Use of D-mannose in prophylaxis of recurrent urinary tract infections (UTIs) in women. *BJU Int*. 2014;113(1):9-10.
64. Kranjcec B, Papes D, Altarac S. D-Mannose powder for prophylaxis of recurrent urinary tract infections in women: a randomized clinical trial. *World J Urol*. 2014;32(1):79-84.
65. Hudson T. Treatment and prevention of bladder infections. *Altern Complement Ther*. 2006;12(6):297-302.
66. Smaill FM, Vazquez JC. Antibiotics for asymptomatic bacteriuria in pregnancy. *Cochrane Database Syst Rev*. 2007;2:CD000490. doi:10.1002/14651858.CD000490.pub2.
67. Crider KS, Cleves MA, Reefhuis J, Berry RJ, Hobbs CA, Hu DJ. Antibacterial medication use during pregnancy and risk of birth defects: National Birth Defects Prevention Study. *Arch Pediatr Adolesc Med*. 2009;163(11):978-985.
68. American College of Obstetricians and Gynecologists. Sulfonamides, nitrofurantoin, and risk of birth defects: Opinion Number 494, June 2011 (reaffirmed 2013). http://www.acog.org/Resources_And_Publications/Committee_Opinions/Committee_on_Obstetric_Practice/Sulfonamides_Nitrofurantoin_and_Risk_of_Birth_Defects. Accessed November 30, 2014.
69. Le J, Briggs GG, McKeown A, Bustillo G. Urinary tract infections during pregnancy. *Ann Pharmacother*. 2004;38(10):1692-1701.
70. Klarskov P, Andersen JT, Jimenez-Solem E, Torp-Pedersen C, Poulsen HE. Short-acting sulfonamides near term and neonatal jaundice. *Obstet Gynecol*. 2013;122(1):105-110.
71. Schneeberger C, Geerlings SE, Middleton P, Crowther CA. Interventions for preventing recurrent urinary tract infection during pregnancy. *Cochrane Database Syst Rev*. 2012;1:CD009279. doi:10.1002/14651858.CD009279.pub2.
72. Mody L, Mody L, Juthani-Mehta M. Urinary tract infections in older women: a clinical review. *JAMA*. 2014;311(8):844-854.
73. Perrotta C, Aznar M, Mejia R, Albert X, Ng CW. Oestrogens for preventing recurrent urinary tract infection in postmenopausal women. *Cochrane Database Syst Rev*. 2008;2:CD005131. doi:10.1002/14651858.CD005131.pub2.
74. Berry SH, Elliot M, Suttorp M, et al. Prevalence of symptoms of bladder pain syndrome/interstitial cystitis among adult females in the United States. *J Urol*. 2011;186:540-544.
75. Hanno PM, Burks DA, Clemens JQ, et al. Interstitial Cystitis Guidelines Panel of the American Urological Association Education and Research, Inc. AUA guidelines for the diagnosis and treatment of interstitial cystitis/bladder pain syndrome. *J Urol*. 2011;185(6):2162-2170.

76. Cheng C, Rosamilia A, Healey M. Diagnosis of interstitial cystitis/bladder pain syndrome in women with chronic pelvic pain: a prospective observational study. *Int Urogynecol J*. 2012;23(10):1361-1366.
77. Nielsen CS, Knudsen GP, Steingrimsdottir OA. Twin studies of pain. *Clin Genet*. 2012;82(4): 331-340.
78. Hurst RE, Moldwin RM, Mulholland SG. Bladder defense molecules, urothelial differentiation, urinary biomarkers, and interstitial cystitis. *Urology*. 2007;69(4 suppl):17-23.
79. Lee JW, Han DY, Jeong HJ. Bladder pain syndrome treated with triple therapy with gabapentin, amitriptyline, and a nonsteroidal anti-inflammatory drug. *Int Neurourol J*. 2010;14(4):256-260.
80. Chrysanthopoulou EL, Doumouchtsis SK. Challenges and current evidence on the management of bladder pain syndrome. *Neurourol Urodyn*. 2014;33(8): 1193-1201.
81. Anderson R, Zinkgraf K. Use and effectiveness of complementary therapies among women with interstitial cystitis. *Urol Nurs*. 2013;33(6):306-309, 311.
82. Whitmore KE. Complementary and alternative therapies as treatment approaches for interstitial cystitis. *Urology*. 2002;4(suppl 1):S28-S35.
83. O'Hare PG, Hoffmann AR, Allen P, Gordon B, Salin L, Whitmore K. Interstitial cystitis patients' use and rating of complementary and alternative medicine therapies. *Int Urogynecol J*. 2013;24(6):977-982.
84. Erickson DR, Propert KJ. Pregnancy and interstitial cystitis/painful bladder syndrome. *Urol Clin North Am*. 2007;34(1):61-69.
85. Tracy B, Sean Morrison R. Pain management in older adults. *Clin Ther*. 2013;35(11):1659-1668.

23 Sexually Transmitted Infections

Paul L. Sacamano, Hayley Mark

With acknowledgment to Jason Farley and Ashley Hanahan for their contribution to the first edition of Pharmacology for Women's Health

Chapter Glossary

Antiretroviral therapy (ART) Medications used to treat retroviruses, primarily HIV.

Expedited partner treatment (EPT) Practice of giving a woman a prescription for treatment of gonorrhea for her sexual partner without physically examining or talking with the sexual partner.

Highly active antiretroviral therapy (HAART) Use of three or more antiretroviral drug classes that have different mechanisms of action to treat HIV infection.

Postexposure prophylaxis (PEP) Short-term course of antiretroviral drugs administered after exposure to HIV to decrease the likelihood that the individual will develop the disease.

Pre-exposure prophylaxis (PrEP) Daily regimen of antiretroviral drugs administered to reduce the likelihood of infection with HIV in persons at substantial risk of HIV acquisition.

Prevention of mother-to-child transmission (PMTCT) Worldwide programs that are focused on preventing vertical (e.g., ascending) transmission of HIV from mother to child during pregnancy, labor, birth, or breastfeeding. The abbreviation has become the shorthand expression for these programs and is often part of the official title of individual programs.

Sexually transmitted disease (STD) Replacement for the term *venereal disease* (*VD*), intended to eliminate the stigma attached to that term. This term gained popularity toward the end of the twentieth century when it became apparent that an increasing number of conditions could have a sexual transmission component, such as HIV or chlamydial infection. Largely replaced today by *STI*.

Sexually transmitted infection (STI) Current term used to identify conditions that are transmitted sexually. This term is more precise than previously used terms and reflects the possibility of subclinical or latent infections.

Test of cure Repeat testing after treatment for the purpose of determining if an administered antimicrobial agent eradicated the pathogen.

Introduction

Sexually transmitted infections have been known since ancient times. Major epidemics of syphilis, or the pox, were reported periodically during the Middle Ages, and there is a hypothesis that the sailors who accompanied Columbus were infected with the same disease during their historical exploration of the New World. Important world figures from history—such as Ivan the Terrible, Lenin, Tolstoy, King Henry VIII, and Lord Randolph Churchill, as well as the American Al Capone—all have been known or strongly suspected of having syphilis.

Gonorrhea and syphilis came to be known as venereal diseases in the Middle Ages. However, it was not until after World War II that antimicrobials became available and cure of the classic venereal diseases became possible. Just as effective treatments for gonorrhea and syphilis emerged, more infections were found to have a sexual transmission component. By the 1990s, the term "venereal disease" began to fall into disuse, replaced by **sexually transmitted disease (STD)**, ostensibly in an attempt to recognize the larger number of conditions as well as decrease some of the stigma associated with the original term. Within a decade, the term **sexually transmitted infection (STI)** had replaced sexually transmitted disease. Substituting the word *infection* for *disease* enabled the use of a more precise term and allowed the acknowledgment of a number of conditions that are subclinical but still infectious. In this chapter, STI is the term of choice.

Sexually Transmitted Infections

The United States has the highest rates of STIs of any country in the industrialized world. Approximately 19 million new infections occur each year in the United States, most of which (72%) involve human papillomavirus (HPV).[1] Half of the new infections occur in persons ages 15–24 years. Along with the young, a disproportionate burden of STIs is seen in gay and bisexual men, African Americans, and women.[2]

STIs are more easily passed from men to women than from women to men, and women disproportionately bear the long-term consequences of these infections. For example, if they are inadequately treated, 20% to 40% of women infected with chlamydia or gonorrhea will develop pelvic inflammatory disease, which predisposes them to subsequent ectopic pregnancy and tubal infertility if contraception is not used. Approximately 70% of chlamydial infections and 50% of gonococcal infections in women are asymptomatic, which results in later and less frequent treatment. Pregnant women with STIs have an increased risk of miscarriage and premature birth than those without STIs. Some diseases can also be transmitted to the fetus or newborn. For example, transmission of gonorrhea and chlamydia from mother to child can cause neonatal ophthalmia or neonatal pneumonia, and herpes simplex virus transmitted through this route can cause potentially fatal neonatal viral sepsis. The prevalence and morbidity associated with STIs make this a critical topic for healthcare providers.

This chapter provides an overview of the pharmacologic therapies recommended for the major STIs that affect populations in the United States. The STIs that cause vaginitis, such as bacterial vaginosis and vaginal trichomoniasis, are discussed in depth in the *Vaginal Conditions* chapter. The STIs that are primarily dermatologic infections, such a scabies and pediculosis pubis, are addressed in the *Dermatology* chapter.

The Centers for Disease Control and Prevention (CDC) periodically publishes *Sexually Transmitted Disease Treatment Guidelines*, which are highly regarded and include additional information about management, including screening, diagnosis, and follow-up, for the reader interested in clinical management of these conditions. The CDC guidelines are developed after systematically reviewing the evidence concerning each of the major STIs, and they form the basis of the pharmacologic treatments addressed in this chapter. Because most of these drugs are antimicrobials in common usage, more detailed information about their use during pregnancy or lactation or by elderly women can be found in other chapters, especially the *Antimicrobials* chapter. To be recommended as a first-line agents for treating STIs, the antimicrobial must have microbial cure rates of at least 95%. Those that are offered as alternate regimens are often slightly less effective. Gonorrhea, hepatitis, and syphilis are reportable diseases and must be reported to the CDC by the diagnosing clinician or laboratory. The most current CDC guidelines, published in 2015, include specific information regarding risks of various STIs for women who have sex with women and transgender women. In general, treatments remain the same, but the incidence of some STIs may vary and will be noted as appropriate in the chapter.

Chlamydia Trachomatis

Introduction

Chlamydia trachomatis is a major cause of genital tract and ocular infections worldwide. It is estimated that there were 106 million new cases of genital chlamydia worldwide in 2008,[3] and total costs related to chlamydia morbidity in the United States exceed $2 billion per year.[4] In 2012, 1.4 million chlamydial infections were reported to the CDC, or nearly four times as many cases as the number of gonorrhea cases.[2]

Due to the often asymptomatic or nonspecific nature of the disease and the limited availability of testing, chlamydial infections may be undiagnosed or improperly treated. Chlamydia has become one of the leading causes of pelvic inflammatory disease (PID) in women and related infertility or ectopic pregnancy.[5] Maternal antibodies to the organism provide limited, if any, protection for the newborn.

Chlamydial infections became reportable diseases in the United States in 1986, and the reported incidence has gradually increased since that time. Chlamydia is currently the most commonly reported notifiable disease in the United States.[7] This high frequency largely is due to increased screening efforts in women and improved testing methodologies that can detect active infection. The prevalence of chlamydia among adolescents and young adults is estimated to be approximately 3.2% for women and 1.7% for men.[1] This rate does not include oropharyngeal or rectal cases. The differences in prevalence are due in part to more frequent screening of women for this infection compared to men, although men are increasingly being screened due to heightened awareness of the need and the ease of urine tests.[2] Additionally, substantial racial/ethnic and age disparities are present in the prevalence of both chlamydial and gonococcal infections, with non-Hispanic Black persons younger than 25 years having the greatest burden of disease.[2] There is a high rate of coinfection with gonorrhea and chlamydia; thus, these conditions should be suspected to coexist in any specific woman, and dual treatment is recommended.[5] Chlamydial infection is also associated with an increased risk of HIV transmission.

Pathogenesis, Microbiology, and Clinical Symptoms

C. trachomatis is a small, gram-negative bacterium with unique biologic properties that distinguish it from all other living organisms. Three chlamydial organisms are known to cause disease in humans. The family Chlamydiaceae is divided into two genera: *Chlamydia*, which includes *C. trachomatis*, and *Chlamydophila*, which includes *C. pneumoniae* (a cause of atypical pneumonia) and *C. psittaci* (the cause of parrot fever, for which humans are an incidental host).[6] Several serovars or subgroupings of *C. trachomatis* are distinguished based on a classification system that is related to their cell surface antigens. The majority of chlamydial infections of the genital tract are caused by serovars D, E, F, G, H, I, J, and K.[7]

All chlamydiae have a biphasic life cycle. The elementary body is an infectious particle that enters a cell, often a columnar epithelial cell. In the cell, the elementary body is transformed into a reticulate body, which then multiplies and fills the intracellular space. Some reticulate bodies are then transformed back into elementary bodies, which are subsequently freed from the cell. These elementary bodies start the cycle anew. The full cycle takes approximately 72 hours. Persistent infection or reinfection and associated inflammatory responses are common. In ocular and genital infections, persistent inflammation may lead to scarring, resulting in blindness or infertility.

Chlamydia is transmitted via direct, genital–genital (including anal), or oral–genital contact, or perinatally to the newborn via vertical transmission from the vagina during labor and birth. Among women, chlamydia may manifest as urethritis, Bartholin gland infection, cervicitis, salpingitis, endometritis, conjunctivitis, pharyngitis, perihepatitis (Fitz-Hugh-Curtis syndrome), proctitis, reactive arthritis (Reiter syndrome), or overt pelvic inflammatory disease.[7] Cervical infection is the most common chlamydial syndrome in women. Urethritis may accompany cervicitis and result in symptoms often associated with urinary tract infection, including poorly differentiated lower abdominal pain, frequency, and dysuria.

Treatment for Chlamydial Infection

The goals for treating chlamydia are threefold: (1) resolve symptoms; (2) decrease the risk of transmission; and (3) prevent complications. The CDC-recommended treatment regimens are presented in Table 23-1.[5] Coinfection with *C. trachomatis* frequently occurs among persons who have gonococcal infection; therefore, when treating an individual for chlamydia, presumptive treatment for gonorrhea is recommended in areas that have high gonorrhea rates.

Table 23-1 CDC-Recommended Treatment Regimens for *C. Trachomatis*[a]

Nonpregnant		Pregnant[b]	
Recommended Regimen	**Alternative Regimen**	**Recommended Regimen**	**Alternative Regimen**
Azithromycin (Zithromax) 1 g PO in a single dose *Or* Doxycycline (Vibramycin) 100 mg PO 2 times/day for 7 days	Erythromycin base 500 mg PO 4 times/day for 7 days *Or* Erythromycin ethylsuccinate (EES) 800 mg PO 4 times/day for 7 days *Or* Ofloxacin[c] (Floxin) 300 mg PO 2 times/day for 7 days *Or* Levofloxacin[c] (Levaquin) 500 mg PO once daily for 7 days	Azithromycin (Zithromax) 1 g PO single dose	Amoxicillin (Amoxil) 500 mg PO 3 times/day for 7 days *Or* Erythromycin base 250 mg PO 4 times/day for 14 days *Or* Erythromycin base 500 mg PO 4 times/day for 7 days *Or* EES 400 mg PO 4 times/day for 14 days *Or* EES 800 mg PO 4 times/day for 7 days

[a] Individuals who have chlamydial infection and also are infected with HIV should receive the same treatment regimen as those who are HIV negative.

[b] Erythromycin estolate is contraindicated during pregnancy because of drug-related hepatotoxicity.

[c] Contraindicated for persons younger than 18 years secondary to risks of bone abnormalities.

Source: Centers for Disease Control and Prevention. Sexually transmitted disease treatment guidelines, 2015. *MMWR Recomm Rep.* 2015;64(3):1-137.[5]

Because the form of *C. trachomatis* that can be killed is an obligate parasite within a cell, antimicrobials that act by breaking down the cell wall will kill the otherwise healthy cell, but not the microorganism. Thus, antibiotics such a macrolide or tetracycline that penetrates the cell are needed to treat this infection. In addition, the long life cycle explains the need for prolonged courses of treatment or an antibiotic with a long half-life. Azithromycin (Zithromax) has a half-life of 5 to 7 days and requires only one dose.[7] Intake of this medication can be directly observed in an ambulatory facility. Doxycycline (Vibramycin) requires 7 days of treatment, suggesting an increased potential for missed doses. In general, macrolides such as azithromycin have distressing gastrointestinal side effects, but studies that have compared azithromycin and doxycycline found both associated with side effects in 25% and 23% of users, respectively.[8] Levofloxacin (Levaquin) and ofloxacin (Floxin) are acceptable alternatives, but are more expensive and do not confer any additional benefits. The alternative erythromycin regimens have cure rates that are lower, which may be secondary to distressing side effects and missed doses.

Recent sex partners (within 60 days) should also be treated according to standard adult regimens. Because it is not known for certain when a person is infected, the most recent sexual partner should be treated even if the last sexual contact between the two individuals was more than 60 days prior to the diagnosis. For heterosexual couples, if the partner is not available, the clinician can offer **expedited partner treatment (EPT)** if EPT is legally permitted. The clinical practice of treating sexual partners without a formal evaluation of each partner is being increasingly promoted because it reduces rates of reinfection and is more effective than traditional partner notification programs. In addition, the CDC recommends that drug treatment for EPT is packaged and available rather than in prescription form since the partner is less likely to fill the prescription than conveniently take medication provided.[5] The key limitation to EPT is that it does not offer the sexual partner the opportunity for HIV/STI screening. EPT has an uncertain legal status but appears to be permissible in most states.

To minimize transmission, persons treated for chlamydial infection should be instructed to abstain from sexual intercourse or other sexual contact for 7 days after single-dose therapy or until completion of the treatment regimen.[5] To minimize the risk for reinfection, persons should be instructed to abstain from sexual intercourse until all of their sex partners are treated.[5]

A **test of cure** is not recommended for persons treated with the recommended or alterative regimens, unless symptoms persist, reinfection is suspected, the woman is pregnant, or adherence to the recommended regimen is in question. Resistance to azithromycin or doxycycline has not been demonstrated to date. Persistent symptoms are most often due to reinfection or other etiologic agents rather than primary failure of the antibiotic. The CDC recommends rescreening women with *C. trachomatis* infection 3 to 4 months after treatment is completed to rule out reinfection.

Complications of Chlamydial Disease

Pelvic Inflammatory Disease

Pelvic inflammatory disease includes a number of inflammatory disorders of the upper female genital tract and pelvis, ranging from endometritis, salpingitis, and tubo-ovarian abscess to pelvic peritonitis.[5] Women with mild to moderate PID often have vague, nonspecific symptoms (e.g., abnormal bleeding, dyspareunia, and vaginal discharge), which may cause the infection to go unrecognized. Both *Neisseria gonorrhoeae* and *C. trachomatis* are implicated as pathogens in many cases, but microorganisms commonly found in the vaginal flora (e.g., anaerobes, *Gardnerella vaginalis*, *Haemophilus influenzae*, enteric gram-negative rods, and *Streptococcus agalactiae*) also have been associated with PID.

Empiric treatment of persons with PID is recommended for sexually active young women and other women at risk for STIs who present with pelvic or lower abdominal pain and either cervical motion tenderness, adnexal tenderness, or uterine tenderness, when no other cause for the illness can be identified. Women who are treated for PID should be given an antibiotic that is effective against both *C. trachomatis* and *N. gonorrhea*. Most cases of mild to moderate PID can be treated on an outpatient basis with the use of broad-spectrum antibiotics, and evidence suggests that oral therapy fares well in comparison to parenteral therapy in this population. The optimal treatment regimen and long-term outcome of early treatment of women with asymptomatic or subclinical PID have not been extensively studied. If no response to oral therapy occurs within 72 hours, the woman needs to be reevaluated to confirm the diagnosis and administered parenteral antibiotics on an outpatient or in-hospital basis.[5]

The CDC recommends that in-hospital treatment for PID be considered under the following circumstances:

when surgical emergencies cannot be excluded (e.g., appendicitis); if the woman is pregnant; if no clinical response is apparent; when women are unable to follow or tolerate outpatient oral regimens; when the woman has severe illness, nausea, vomiting, or high fever; or when tubo-ovarian abscess is suspected.[5]

The CDC's recommendations for the oral and parenteral treatment for PID are presented in Tables 23-2 and 23-3. These drug therapies have recently been updated to reflect the increasing prevalence of fluoroquinolone-resistant gonorrhea in the United States.[5]

Perihepatitis

Fitz-Hugh-Curtis syndrome (perihepatitis) is an inflammation of the liver capsule; it typically occurs when women with PID develop associated peritonitis. In the presence of this syndrome, liver function tests usually are within normal limits. The condition is treated conservatively with anti-inflammatory drugs while the woman is receiving treatment for the primary infection of PID.

Lymphogranuloma Venereum

Lymphogranuloma venereum (LGV) is a genital ulcer disease caused by *C. trachomatis* (serovars L1, L2, and L3). LGV is endemic in tropical and subtropical areas of the world, including East and West Africa, India, parts of Southeast Asia, and the Caribbean, but recent outbreaks have occurred in the United States, Canada, and Europe and have been associated with HIV infection.[9] LGV is predominantly a disease of lymphatic tissue as opposed to mucosal chlamydial infection. It typically infiltrates at the initial site of infection, where a self-limited ulcer may appear.[10] Several weeks later, painful inguinal lymphadenopathy with formation and rupture of buboes (unilateral painful inguinal lymph nodes) develops. An anorectal syndrome can also occur that presents as an inflammatory mass in the rectum and retroperitoneum[10] with associated rectal discharge, anal pain, fever, constipation, and/or tenesmus (inability to completely defecate or difficulty with defecation).[5] A provider who suspects an individual has LGV is advised to follow the CDC recommendation to contact local or state health departments for specific, current management guidance. The preferred pharmacotherapeutic agent is 500 mg of doxycycline administered twice per day for 21 days. An alternative regimen is erythromycin base 500 mg administered orally 4 times per day for 21 days.

Special Populations: Pregnancy, Lactation, and the Elderly

Chlamydial infection during pregnancy can be transmitted to the newborn during the course of labor and birth.

Table 23-2 Recommended Regimens for Women with Mild to Moderately Severe Pelvic Inflammatory Disease

Recommended Regimen[a]
Ceftriaxone (Rocephin) 250 mg IM in a single dose *Plus* Doxycycline (Vibramycin) 100 mg PO 2 times/day for 14 days *With or Without* Metronidazole (Flagyl) 500 mg PO 2 times/day for 14 days *Or*
Cefoxitin (Mefoxin) 2 g IM in a single dose and probenecid 1 g PO administered concurrently in a single dose *Plus* Doxycycline (Vibramycin) 100 mg PO 2 times/day for 14 days *With or Without* Metronidazole (Flagyl) 500 mg orally 2 times/day for 14 days *Or*
Other parenteral third-generation cephalosporin (e.g., ceftizoxime or cefotaxime) *Plus* Doxycycline (Vibramycin) 100 mg PO 2 times/day for 14 days *With or Without* Metronidazole (Flagyl) 500 mg PO 2 times/day for 14 days

[a] The addition of metronidazole should be considered, as anaerobic organisms are suspected in the etiology of the majority of PID cases. Metronidazole will also treat bacterial vaginosis (BV) if present.

Source: Centers for Disease Control and Prevention. Sexually transmitted disease treatment guidelines, 2015. *MMWR Recomm Rep.* 2015;64(3):1-137.[5]

Table 23-3 Recommended Regimens for Women with Pelvic Inflammatory Disease

Regimen	Drug Combination in Regimen
First recommended parenteral regimen	Cefotetan (Cefotan) 2 g IV every 12 hours *Plus* Doxycycline (Vibramycin) 100 mg PO or IV every 12 hours *Or* Cefoxitin (Mefoxin) 2 g IV every 6 hours *Plus* Doxycycline (Vibramycin) 100 mg PO or IV every 12 hours
Second recommended parenteral regimen	Clindamycin (Cleocin) 900 mg IV every 8 hours *Plus* Gentamicin (Garamycin) loading dose IV or IM (2 mg/kg of body weight), followed by a maintenance dose (1.5 mg/kg) every 8 hours; single daily dosing may be substituted
Alternative parenteral regimen	Ampicillin/sulbactam (Unasyn) 3 g IV every 6 hours *Plus* Doxycycline (Vibramycin) 100 mg PO or IV every 12 hours

Source: Centers for Disease Control and Prevention. Sexually transmitted disease treatment guidelines, 2015. *MMWR Recomm Rep.* 2015;64(3):1-137.[5]

Infection in the newborn presents as ophthalmia neonatorum and/or atypical neonatal pneumonia. Prophylaxis and treatment for ophthalmia neonatorum are reviewed in the chapter *The Newborn*. Levofloxacin (Levaquin), ofloxacin (Floxin), doxycyline (Vibramycin), and erythromycin estolate are contraindicated during pregnancy. The cure rates of amoxicillin and erythromycin are lower than that of azithromycin; consequently, azithromycin is the only first-line regimen for treating chlamydial infection during pregnancy. Pregnant women who are treated for chlamydia should have a test of cure 3 weeks after completing therapy and then again in 3 to 4 months.[5] The test of cure should not be obtained sooner than 3 weeks because false-positive results are possible in the first 2 weeks following treatment.

Levofloxacin and ofloxacin have traditionally been contraindicated in women who are breastfeeding secondary to concerns about adverse effects on the infant's joints. Although short-term use appears to be safe, some experts recommend that the woman not breastfeed for 4 to 6 hours after taking one of the fluoroquinolones. Doxycycline presents a similar issue: It has traditionally been contraindicated secondary to concerns about staining the infant's teeth. Nevertheless, short-term use of doxycycline appears to be safe for the infant of a breastfeeding women. Because of these theoretic concerns, most clinicians will avoid these drugs in favor of azithromycin or ampicillin for women who are breastfeeding.

Gonorrhea

The organism *Neisseria gonorrhoeae* was first noted by Albert Neisser in stained smears of urethral, vaginal, and conjunctival exudate in 1879.[11] The estimated global incidence of gonorrheal infection is 106 million infected persons annually,[3] and it is the second most commonly reported infectious disease in the United States.[2] An overall marked decline of gonorrhea incidence occurred from 1975 through 2009; however, since 2009, the gonorrhea infection rate has been increasing.[2] Like other sexually transmitted diseases, gonorrhea likely is substantially underdiagnosed and underreported.[2,3] Geographical differences in the incidence of gonorrhea have been noted in the United States, with the Southern region having the highest rates of infection.[2] In medical parlance, gonorrhea is referred to as GC, an abbreviation for *gonococcus*; this abbreviation is also used in this chapter.

Complications of GC include pelvic inflammatory disease, which can cause tubal scarring and subsequent infertility or ectopic pregnancy. Gonorrhea is also associated with miscarriage and preterm birth.[2] *N. gonorrhoeae* is estimated to be the causative organism in 40% of PID cases. The gonococcus rarely becomes invasive, but when it does, the result is disseminated gonococcal infection (DGI), endocarditis, and meningitis.[12] In addition, a five-fold increase in HIV acquisition among women has been noted in the setting of incident gonorrhea infection.[13]

Substantial racial, ethnic, and age disparities are present in the prevalence of both chlamydial and gonococcal infections, with non-Hispanic Black persons younger than age 25 having the greatest burden of disease prevalence.[2]

N. gonorrhoeae is a gram-negative intracellular diplococcus that exclusively affects humans. This microorganism primarily infects the mucocutaneous surfaces of the genitourinary tract, pharynx, conjunctiva, and anus, with infections often remaining asymptomatic.

There is considerable overlap between the signs and symptoms of gonorrhea and the signs and symptoms of chlamydia infection. When symptoms occur, vaginal discharge and poorly differentiated abdominal pain or lower abdominal pain are the most frequently reported. Pain is atypical in the absence of upper tract infection.[14] Gonococcal urethritis should be considered in young, sexually active women who present with urinary symptoms such as frequency, dysuria, and pyuria.

Treatment of Individuals with Gonorrheal Infection

In the United States, gonorrhea is a nationally notifiable disease.[15] All diagnoses of gonorrhea are reported to the CDC. The CDC, in turn, coordinates treatment of individuals and sex partners through local public health departments and analyzes trends in incidence, antimicrobial resistance, and other epidemiologic data that are used to guide treatment recommendations. *N. gonorrhoeae* commonly develops resistance to antimicrobial drugs. Thus, the Gonococcal Isolate Surveillance Project was established in 1986.[2] Ongoing data collection through the CDC's Gonococcal Isolate Surveillance Project has found increasing antimicrobial resistance in the United States. Notably, fluoroquinolone-resistant gonorrhea is now widespread and oral cephalosporins are no longer effective; thus neither treatment is now recommended.

Table 23-4 presents the current CDC recommendations for treatment of persons with gonorrheal infections.[5,16] Because many isolates have demonstrated resistance to cephalosporins, dual therapy with two drugs that have a different mechanism of action is recommended. In 2011,

Table 23-4 CDC-Recommended Treatment Regimens for Women with Gonococcal Infections

Gonococcal Infection	Recommended Regimen	Alternative Regimen
Uncomplicated gonococcal infections of the cervix, urethra, and rectum[a]	Ceftriaxone (Rocephin) 250 mg IM in a single dose *Plus* Azithromycin (Zithromax) 1 g PO in a single doses	If ceftriaxone is not available: Cefixime (Suprax) 400 mg in a single PO dose *Plus* Azithromycin (Zithromax) 1 g PO in a single dose If cephalosporin allergy[b]: Gemifloxacin (Factive) 320 mg PO in a single dose *Plus* Azithromycin (Zithromax) 2 g in a single PO dose *Or* Gentamicin (Garamycin) 240 mg IM in a single dose *Plus* Azithromycin (Zithromax) 2 g in a single PO dose
Uncomplicated gonococcal infections of the pharynx[a]	Ceftriaxone (Rocephin) 250 mg IM in a single dose *Plus* Azithromycin (Zithromax) 1 g PO in a single dose	
Adults and adolescents with conjunctivitis	Ceftriaxone (Rocephin) 1 g IM in a single dose *Plus* Azithromycin (Zithromax) 1 g PO in a single dose	
Pregnancy: Uncomplicated gonococcal infections of the cervix, urethra, and rectum[a]	Ceftriaxone (Rocephin) 250 mg IM in a single dose *Plus* Azithromycin (Zithromax) 1 g PO in a single dose	If cephalosporin allergy[b]: Consultation with an infectious disease specialist is recommended

[a] These regimens are recommended for all adults and adolescents regardless of travel history or sexual behavior.
[b] Only persons with a penicillin allergy that includes severe symptoms such as anaphylaxis or angioedema should be considered also allergic to cephalosporins.
Sources: Centers for Disease Control and Prevention. Sexually transmitted disease treatment guidelines, 2015. *MMWR Recomm Rep.* 2015;64(3):1-137[5]; Centers for Disease Control and Prevention. Update to CDC's sexually transmitted diseases treatment guidelines, 2010: oral cephalosporins no longer a recommended treatment for gonococcal infections. *MMWR.* 2012;61(31):590-594.[17]

the CDC increased the recommended dose of ceftriaxone from 125 mg to 250 mg.[16] Directly observed treatment is also recommended to assure effective treatment. The CDC resources for gonorrhea treatment can be found in the Resources table at the end of this chapter.

All persons treated for gonorrhea should also be treated for chlamydia because of the high incidence of coinfection.[12] Current dual therapy achieves this goal.

Complications of Gonorrhea

A rare complication that is associated with *N. gonorrhoeae* infection is disseminated gonococcal infection (DGI).[5] This infection is more common in women than in men—a finding that is likely related to a higher incidence of asymptomatic gonococcal infection in women.[17] Hospitalization is recommended for persons with DGI, and management of this condition is beyond the scope of this chapter.

Treatment for Sexual Partners

When a woman is diagnosed with gonorrhea, both her current sex partners and her sex partners within the last 60 days before the onset of symptoms or receipt of diagnosis should be treated. EPT can be offered if the woman's sexual partner is not available and EPT is legally permitted. The prescription for EPT is oral cefixime 400 mg and azithromycin 1 gram.

Special Populations: Pregnancy, Lactation, and the Elderly

The recommendations for treatment during pregnancy are the same as for nonpregnant adults. If a pregnant woman is allergic to cephalosporins, desensitization should be instituted, as these drugs are the only antimicrobial drugs that are effective against this organism.

Infants born to women with untreated gonorrhea can become infected during the process of labor and birth. Gonorrheal infection in newborns manifests as ophthalmia neonatorum, which can cause blindness if not treated. Standard regimens for prophylaxis and treatment of newborns with ophthalmia neonatorum are reviewed in the chapter *The Newborn*.

Hepatitis

Hepatitis is an inflammatory disorder that affects the liver, the etiology of which can be infectious (e.g., viral or bacterial) or noninfectious. Five different hepatotropic viruses exist, which are named A through E. Hepatitis

Table 23-5 Overview of Viral Hepatitis

Characteristics	HAV	HBV	HCV
Type of virus	Single-strand RNA hepadnavirus	Double-stranded DNA hepadnavirus	
Mode of transmission			
Sex	Rare	Yes	Rare
Fecal–oral/food	Yes	Rare	No
Blood	Rare	Yes	Yes
Chronic infection possible	No	Yes	Yes
Incubation period (time between exposure and development of first symptoms)	2–10 weeks	6–20 weeks	4–10 weeks
Preventive vaccination available	Yes	Yes	No

Abbreviations: HAV = hepatitis A; HBV = hepatitis B; HCV = hepatitis C.
Source: Centers for Disease Control and Prevention. Sexually transmitted disease treatment guidelines, 2015. *MMWR Recomm Rep.* 2015;64(3):1-137.[5]

A (HAV), hepatitis B (HBV), and hepatitis C (HCV) are the most prevalent forms of viral hepatitis in North America. An RNA virus that requires the presence of HBV for replication causes hepatitis D; hepatitis D is uncommon in the United States. Hepatitis E is transmitted via contaminated drinking water and is also rare in the United States. Table 23-5 summarizes key differences among HAV, HBV, and HCV, which are the three sexually transmitted forms of hepatitis.

An estimated 2800 new cases of acute HAV occur in the United States each year. HAV is transmitted through fecal–oral routes, including household contacts with persons infected with HAV, ingestion of raw or contaminated foods, and international travel among both sexes. Anal sex is also a risk factor. Vaccination is the primary prevention strategy for persons who are at risk for exposure to HAV.

The incidence of HBV has been declining due to vaccination programs and has recently been estimated at 18,800 cases annually.[19] There are approximately 700,000 to 1.4 million persons with chronic HBV the United States. The most common method of HBV transmission is sexual contact or intravenous drug use. Mother-to-child vertical transmission during labor and birth is also possible.[19] The risk of developing chronic HBV infection is greatest in newborns of infected mothers (90%), but declines with age to less than 5% in adults with acute infection.[20] Previously cleared acute infections provide lifelong protective immunity. Vaccination remains the mainstay of pharmacologic prevention of hepatitis B. Current vaccination recommendations are reviewed in the *Immunizations* chapter.

Hepatitis C is the leading cause of liver transplantation in the United States. While the predominate mode of HCV transmission is intravenous drug use, sexual transmission and mother-to-child transmission during birth are also possible.[19]

Treatment of Women with Hepatitis

Treatment for Exposure to Hepatitis A and Hepatitis B

For the nonvaccinated person who is exposed to HAV, administration of hepatitis A vaccine should be initiated as soon as possible within 2 weeks of exposure.[21] It is also recommended that adults older than 40 years, those younger than 40 years who are immunocompromised, and individuals for whom the vaccine is contraindicated receive an injection of immune globulin (Gamimune). Immune globulin consists of antibodies that protect against HAV and is 85% effective if given within the first 2 weeks following exposure.

Immune globulin is recommended for household contacts and sexual contacts of persons diagnosed with HAV, travelers to countries where sanitation is a problem or where HAV is prevalent, staff in institutions where an outbreak of HAV occurs, and persons who are exposed to HAV but are allergic to the vaccine.

The serology of HBV infection is presented in Figure 23-1.[22] The recommendations for treatment of persons whose exposure to hepatitis B is not occupational are as follows: Hepatitis B immune globulin (HBIG) (0.06 mL/kg IM) should be administered as soon as possible after a nonvaccinated individual is exposed to hepatitis B (percutaneous exposure, sexual or needle-sharing contact with an HBsAg positive individual, or victim of sexual assault/abuse by an HBsAg positive individual). HBIG should be given within 24 hours of needle-stick or ocular or mucosal exposure or within 14 days of sexual exposure. The typical dose is 3–5 mL. In addition, the exposed individual should begin the HBV vaccination series with the first injection administered at a different site than that used for the injection of HGIG. If an individual previously vaccinated for HBV is exposed to hepatitis B, a vaccine booster dose is recommended. Although treatments for persons who are occupationally exposed to hepatitis B are similar, overall management includes assessment of blood levels of antibody. The specific recommendations for occupational exposure to hepatitis B can be found on the CDC website.

There is no vaccine for HCV. Also, unlike exposure to HBV, immune globulin prophylaxis for persons who are exposed to HCV is not effective. However, treatment

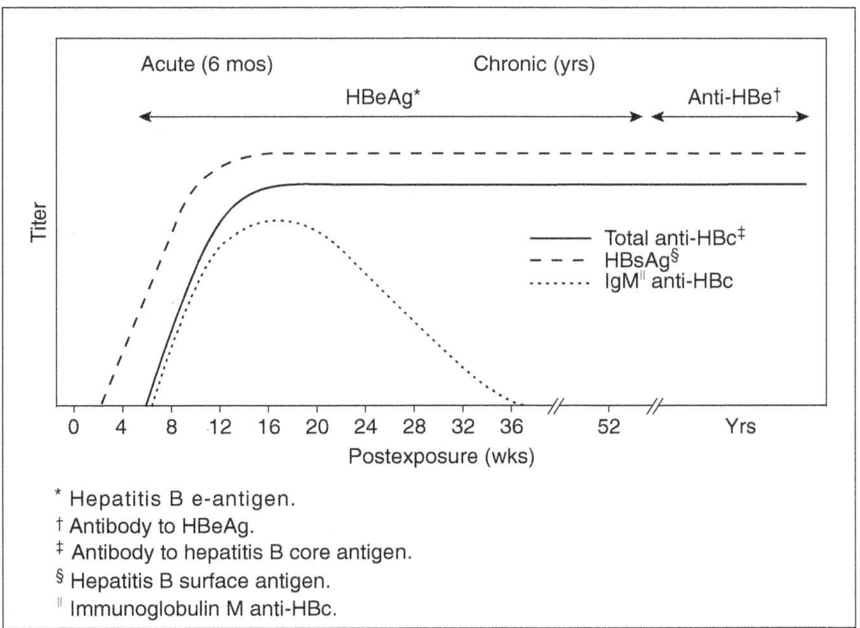

Figure 23-1 Typical serological course of acute hepatitis B virus (HBV) infection with progression to chronic HBV infection.

Source: Centers for Disease Control and Prevention. Recommendations for identification and public health management of persons with chronic hepatitis B virus infection. *MMWR.* 2008;57(RR-8):1-28.[22]

of HCV is rapidly evolving, with new pharmacologic agents greatly improving rates of viral clearance while also shortening treatment periods.

Treatment for Acute Hepatitis Infection

Infection with HAV, HBV, or HCV can be asymptomatic, a mild disease, or (rarely) a fulminant disorder. When the disease is symptomatic, the clinical symptoms of HAV, HBV, and HCV include fever, malaise, nausea and vomiting, abdominal pain, dark urine, and jaundice. There are no pharmacologic medications specific for acute hepatitis; instead, treatment is supportive in nature. For example, antiemetics may be given to reduce nausea and vomiting. If the disease is mild and managed on an outpatient basis, the person is counseled to avoid alcohol and acetaminophen (Tylenol). Other prescription medications associated with a risk of liver compromise may be discontinued temporarily. Persons with fulminant hepatitis will require hospitalization.

Treatment for Chronic Hepatitis B Infection

HBV is considered chronic when it persists for more than 6 months. In general, the goals in treating chronic hepatitis are to: (1) decrease the viral load; (2) reduce the risk of transmission; (3) prevent liver failure or cirrhosis; and (4) reduce the risk of hepatocellular carcinoma. Increased viral load measurements (i.e., measurements of HBV RNA) are associated with a higher prevalence of hepatocellular carcinoma, hepatic failure, and cirrhosis.[23] Therefore, reduction in HBV DNA and prevention of complications associated with infection are considered the gold standard when monitoring the success of HBV treatment.

Ten different genotypes of HBV are present in varying degrees in different geographic locales.[24] Knowledge of the genotype affecting the individual can be important for treatment, as some drugs are more effective for certain HBV genotypes than for others. Clinical criteria for who should be treated and choice of the best medication regimens can be complicated. In particular, special considerations apply to persons who have HBV or HCV infection and are also HIV positive that are not reviewed in this text. Ultimately, the treatment of a person with hepatitis infection is an emerging field and is best managed by experienced clinicians who specialize in gastroenterology or infectious diseases.

The pharmacologic agents used to treat chronic HBV interrupt the hepatitis B virus's life cycle in a manner that is similar to the mechanism of action of drugs used to treat HIV. In fact, some drugs used in the treatment of persons with HIV infection also are used to treat those with HBV

Table 23-6 FDA-Approved Drugs for the Treatment of Women with Hepatitis B Infection

Drug: Generic (Brand)	Indication	Dose	Clinical Considerations
Interferons			
Interferon-alpha (Intron A)	Chronic hepatitis B	5 MU once daily IM/SC for 12–24 weeks or 10 MU 3 times/week for 12–24 weeks	First-line agent for individuals without cirrhosis. Flares in liver function tests (e.g., ALT) are common. FDA black box warning states that interferons can cause life-threatening neuropsychiatric, autoimmune, ischemic, and infectious conditions. Contraindicated for persons with suicidal tendency, active psychiatric or autoimmune disorders, cirrhosis, severe systemic disorders, or cardiac disease. Influenza-like symptoms may be severe. Avoid use during pregnancy and counsel on the use of two reliable contraceptive methods.
Pegylated interferon-alfa-2b (Peg-Intron)	Chronic hepatitis B	180 mcg weekly SC	
Nucleoside Reverse Transcriptase Inhibitors			
Adefovir (Hepsera)	Chronic hepatitis B	Second-line agent 10 mg once daily PO	Abrupt discontinuation may result in severe acute HBV exacerbation. Monitor ALT for several months after stopping therapy. Lactic acidosis—a class side effect of NRTI therapy—appears to occur with greater frequency in women. Obesity and prolonged NRTI exposure may be risk factors.
Entecavir (Baraclude)	Acute hepatitis B Chronic hepatitis B	First-line agent 0.5 mg once daily PO	
Lamivudine (Epivir)	Chronic hepatitis B	100 mg once daily PO	
Telbivudine (Tyzeka)	Chronic hepatitis B	600 mg once daily PO	
Tenofovir (Viread)	Acute hepatitis B Chronic hepatitis B	First-line agent 300 mg/day PO	

Abbreviations: ALT = alanine transaminase; HBV = hepatitis B virus; NRTI = nucleoside reverse transcriptase inhibitor.

Sources: Lok AS, McMahon BJ. Practice Guidelines Committee, American Association for the Study of Liver Diseases (AASLD). Chronic hepatitis B: update 2009. *Hepatology*. 2009;50(3):1-36[20]; Wilkins T, Zimmerman D, Schade RR. Hepatitis B: Diagnosis and treatment. *Am Fam Physician*. 2010;81(8):965-972.[25]

infection. For this reason, persons coinfected with HIV and HBV require special treatment considerations, with the regimen selected being aimed at treating both viral infections concomitantly.

Seven drugs are FDA approved for treating chronic HBV (Table 23-6). The interferons include interferon alpha-2b (Intron A) and pegylated interferon-alfa (Peg-Intron). The nucleoside reverse transcriptase inhibitors (NRTIs) include lamivudine (Epivir), adefovir (Hepsera), entecavir (Baraclude), telbivudine (Tyzeca), and tenofovir (Viread).[20,25] Many of the drugs used to treat chronic hepatitis have multiple drug–drug interactions. Tables and apps for looking up these interactions are included in the Resources table at the end of this chapter.

Interferons

Interferons are proteins that act to prohibit viral penetration, translation, transcription, maturation, and release of viral agents. Inhibition of protein synthesis is the major inhibitory effect. Interferons are active against HBV, HCV, and human papillomavirus. These agents are potent cytokines that possess antiviral, immunomodulation, and antiproliferative effects that result in inhibition of viral replication.[20,25] Three major classes of human interferons have antiviral properties: alpha, beta, and gamma. Among individuals with chronic HBV infection, treatment with interferon-alpha is associated with a higher incidence of hepatitis e-antigen conversion and undetectable HBV and DNA levels. Approximately 25% to 50% of persons given interferon will experience normalization of liver enzymes and loss of hepatitis B viral DNA.[25]

Interferons are administered for a defined duration of treatment.[20,26] Oral administration of these agents does not result in absorption; however, after intramuscular or subcutaneous injection, interferon absorption exceeds 80%. Higher doses are required for coexisting delta hepatitis. The interferons are metabolized primarily in the kidney and liver and excreted in the urine.

Pegylated interferon is an interferon with a polyethylene glycol molecule attached. This structure makes the molecule larger, which delays its clearance and metabolism.[27] The net result is that pegylated interferon can be administered less often.[27]

Side effects of interferons include depression, confusion, somnolence, fatigue, weight loss, rash, anemia, hair loss, and reversible hearing loss. Headache, fever, myalgias, and malaise may occur within 6 to 12 hours of administration. Individuals with hepatic compromise, a history of cardiac arrhythmia, or autoimmune disease should not be given interferon. Caution should be exercised when giving this medication to individuals with a history of mood disorders.[20,26]

Adverse effects of interferons include myelosuppression accompanied by granulocytopenia and thrombocytopenia. Elevations of hepatic enzymes and triglycerides, alopecia, proteinuria, interstitial nephritis, pneumonia, and hepatotoxicity may occur as well.[26]

Interferons can significantly increase levels of drugs such as theophylline (Theo-Dur), zidovudine (Retrovir), methadone (Dolophine), and ribavirin (Rebetol). Caution is needed when administering interferons with other hepatotoxic drugs, such as nucleoside reverse transcriptase inhibitors (NRTIs). Hematologic abnormalities may occur when interferons are coadministered with angiotensin-converting enzyme (ACE) inhibitors.[26]

Treatment for Chronic Hepatitis C Infection

HCV has six known genotypes.[28,30] Although HCV infection is curable, past infection does not provide protective antibodies, so reinfection is possible. The treatment of persons with hepatitis C has been evolving rapidly. In the recent past, the standard treatment was pegylated interferon and ribavirin (Rebetol). However, this regimen is associated with significant side effects and adverse effects. In 2013, the FDA approved two new drugs that have direct antiviral properties: sofosbuvir (Sovaldi) and simeprevir (Olysio).[29]

The genotype of HCV must be determined to select the appropriate treatment regimen. Globally, genotype 1 is both the most common and the least responsive to treatment, followed by genotypes 2 and 3.[30] For the most current recommendations and less prevalent genotypes, refer to the guidelines jointly provided by the American Association for Study of Liver Diseases and the Infectious Diseases Society of America.[29]

The drugs used to treat chronic HCV infection have many side effects, adverse effects, and contraindications. For example, combination therapy for HCV can engender influenza-like symptoms, fevers, chills, and night sweats. In addition, HCV combination therapy may result in significant reductions in hemoglobin and hematocrit levels, which then necessitate initiation of an erythropoietin-stimulating agent. Irritability and mood swings are commonly reported among individuals undergoing HCV treatment.[31] Care of persons on these combination therapies requires expertise and an in-depth knowledge of the drugs and their interactions.[32]

Ribavirin (Rebetol)

Ribavirin (Rebetol) inhibits the replication of a wide range of RNA and DNA viruses in vitro (e.g., influenza viruses, respiratory syncytial viruses). Its mechanism of action appears to involve alteration of the cellular nucleotide pools and inhibition of viral messenger RNA synthesis, but is not clearly understood.

Ribavirin is actively absorbed in the small bowel, is metabolized by the liver, and is excreted in the urine. Food increases its plasma levels. Advanced renal insufficiency can decrease clearance of this drug by threefold.

Dose-related reversible anemia may occur in persons taking ribavirin. Fatigue, cough, rash, pruritus, nausea, insomnia, dyspnea, and depression have all been noted and may lead to early discontinuation of treatment. The aerosol form may cause conjunctivitis, irritation, and occasionally reversible decreased pulmonary function.

HCV Protease Inhibitors

HCV protease inhibitors block the function of a protein that the hepatitis C virus needs for replication. To date, the FDA has approved several HCV protease inhibitors, including simeprevir. The HCV inhibitors are coadministered with other antiviral drugs in various combinations, with the precise regimen depending on the genotype and serology of the HCV infection.

Nucleotide Analogues

Sofosbuvir (Sovaldi) is a nucleotide analogue inhibitor that eliminates the need for coadministration of interferon in some individuals, shortens treatment duration, and improves the rate of viral clearance. This drug is also administered as part of a combination regimen. Sofosbuvir is generally well tolerated. Common side effects include headache, nausea, insomnia, pruritus, rash, and diarrhea. In addition, sofosbuvir has multiple drug–drug interactions.

Special Populations: Pregnancy, Lactation, and the Elderly

Treatment of women who have chronic hepatitis and who are pregnant requires some special considerations. Perinatal transmission of either HBV or HCV can occur. Perinatal transmission is a common mode of transmission worldwide for HBV. Thus, prophylaxis to prevent maternal-to-child transmission is recommended: Immediately after birth, the newborn should receive both hepatitis B immune globulin (HBIG) and the hepatitis B vaccine.

Pharmacologic treatment of the pregnant woman is also complicated and avoided unless absolutely necessary. Interferons are contraindicated in this setting, as they are abortifacients in primates. No teratogenic or reproductive toxicity has been confirmed in humans, but because of antiproliferative activity, these drugs should be used only if the potential benefit to the mother justifies the possible risk to the fetus. The NRTIs interfere with the replication of mitochondrial DNA, but the effects of this action on a fetus are unknown; these drugs are the agents most likely to be used during pregnancy.[33]

Interferons have a high molecular weight and, therefore, are not easily transferred into human milk. No problems have been reported following administration of interferons to breastfeeding women. In contrast, caution is required if these drugs are used by elderly individuals, as such women might be at greater risk of adverse effects and drug–drug interactions if they are taking many medications or have renal or hepatic impairment.

Perinatal transmission is less common among women who have HCV infection compared to women with HBV infection.[34] Ribavirin is teratogenic, embryotoxic, and oncogenic and should not be used during pregnancy.[34] Pregnant women should not care for individuals receiving the aerosol form of ribavirin. Due to lack of available clinical trial data, combination therapy for HCV infection is contraindicated in pregnancy and women should be counseled to avoid pregnancy for 6 months post treatment. Women of childbearing potential and their sexual partners should be counseled on the importance of using barrier protection methods in addition to a reliable and effective method of contraception while combination therapy is being used. Everyone with HCV infection should be vaccinated against HAV and HBV infection.

Herpes Simplex Virus

Infections caused by the herpes simplex virus types 1 (HSV 1) and 2 (HSV-2) are highly prevalent.[35] These infections are associated with substantial morbidity, and infection with HSV-2 has been associated with a threefold increased risk of HIV acquisition in both men and women.[36] Approximately 16% of adults in the United States have antibodies to HSV-2, and 54% have antibodies to HSV-1.[35] More than two-thirds of all adults infected with the herpes virus are unaware of their infections; consequently, the majority of infections are transmitted by these individuals.[37] Classically, HSV-1 tends to be associated with oral herpes, whereas HSV-2 is associated with genital herpes. However, the type 1 virus is now linked with increasing proportions of newly diagnosed genital herpes.[38–40]

HSV-2 is transmitted both sexually (genital to genital, oral to genital, or genital to oral) and perinatally (mother to child). Longitudinal studies of serologically discordant couples indicate a transmission rate from 3% to 12% per year.[41] The frequency of transmission is influenced by gender and frequency of sexual activity. Women have higher rates of viral acquisition than men, probably due to anatomic differences because a greater mucosal surface area is exposed to the virus in the genital area of women compared with men. Soap and water and drying inactivate HSV quickly. Fomite transmission has not been documented.

Infection with HSV-2 occurs when the virus comes into contact with susceptible mucosal surfaces or abraded skin (e.g., the oropharynx, cervix, conjunctivae). Concomitant with replication at the initial site of infection, the virus travels up peripheral nerves; it then establishes latency in sensory or autonomic nerve root ganglia. The initial site of the infection depends on where the person acquired the virus. Latency can be established after both symptomatic and asymptomatic initial infection. Once an individual becomes infected, the infection persists for life. Cell-mediated responses both control HSV infections and lead to disease symptoms. Most, if not all, persons who are seropositive for HSV-2 have intermittent reactivations associated with HSV viral sheddings. Reactivations may be either symptomatic or asymptomatic. Recent research has demonstrated that there is nearly constant shedding of HSV-2 in infected individuals, rather than long quiescent, latent stages as were previously believed to occur. Thus, symptoms are not an accurate way to determine transmissibility or activation. Individuals who are immunocompromised have both more frequent and more severe reactivations.

The clinical manifestations of genital herpes differ for primary, nonprimary, and recurrent episodes and vary depending on the viral type, the woman's prior immunity, and the woman's immune status. A true primary infection is the first infection with either HSV-1 or HSV-2. The incubation period after acquisition ranges from 2 to 12 days. With primary infection, no serum antibody is present. Although often asymptomatic, some primary episodes are associated with painful lesions, itching, dysuria, and inguinal adenopathy and systemic symptoms such as fever and myalgia. Systemic symptoms appear soon after inoculation, usually peak within 3 to 4 days of the onset of lesions, and then gradually recede over the next 3 to 4 days. Dysuria, both external and internal, occurs more frequently in women (83%) than in men (44%).

Nonprimary HSV is a newly acquired infection with HSV-1 or HSV-2 in an individual previously seropositive to the other virus. Manifestations tend to be milder than with primary infection. Type-specific antibody will be present, and the severity of the episode is comparable to a recurrence.

In contrast to primary or nonprimary infection, symptoms during an HSV-2 recurrence are usually limited to the genital region. As with other HSV infections, symptoms tend to be more severe in women than in men. Recurrences may last from 2 to 6 days; be asymptomatic or associated with significant or minimal pain, itching, and dysuria; and involve few or many lesions. HSV-2 infection is more likely to recur and recurrences tend to be more severe compared with HSV-1 infection.

Approximately 70% to 90% of women with first-episode HSV-2 infection also have HSV cervicitis. Primary genital HSV cervicitis may be symptomatic or asymptomatic and involve the exocervix or endocervix. Ulcerative lesions, erythema, or friability may be present.

Antiviral therapy offers clinical benefits to the majority of individuals who are symptomatic and should be given to all persons with first-episode herpes. Options include three oral medications: acyclovir (Zovirax), valacyclovir (Valtrex), and famciclovir (Famvir). The CDC-recommended treatment guidelines for the first clinical episode and suppressive and episodic therapy of genital herpes are presented in Table 23-7.

Antiviral Therapy for Herpes

Acyclovir (Zovirax) is a nucleoside analogue that is active against herpes viruses. Through a series of cellular enzymatic actions, this drug is incorporated into the viral DNA, where it then prevents DNA replication. Acyclovir has in vitro activity against both HSV-1 and HSV-2. Treatment with this acyclovir reduces the duration of symptoms, decreases viral shedding, and promotes lesion healing.

Acyclovir (Zovirax), famciclovir (Famvir), and valacyclovir (Valtrex), when taken orally, have all been shown to be beneficial in reducing the duration of recurrent genital herpes flares. Acyclovir has only 10% to 30% bioavailability after oral administration. Valacyclovir is a prodrug of acyclovir and has better bioavailability—approximately 55%—once it is converted to acyclovir in vivo.[42] Oral famciclovir is 77% bioavailable. Studies comparing valacyclovir to acyclovir in genital HSV infection have shown the drugs to be comparable in immunocompetent individuals. Valacyclovir has the advantage of being dosed less frequently. Acyclovir resistance in immunocompromised individuals occurs occasionally.

Side effects during therapy with any of these three drugs are rare. Rare adverse effects include neutropenia, Stevens-Johnson syndrome, and hepatitis. More information on the pharmacokinetics and drug–drug interactions associated with these antiviral medications can be found in the *Antimicrobials* chapter.

The clinical effect of acyclovir on first-episode infection is substantial, as this agent reduces fever and other local symptoms within 48 hours of initiating therapy. Therapy should be initiated for all women with presumptive first-episode genital HSV who present with active lesions. While treatment of a woman's first-episode infection substantially shortens the course of primary episodes, there is no evidence that treating first episodes affects the frequency of future recurrences.

Table 23-7 CDC-Recommended Regimens for Treatment of Persons with Herpes

Treatment of Person's First Clinical Episode of Genital Herpes[a]	Suppressive Therapy for Recurrent Genital Herpes	Episodic Therapy for Recurrent Genital Herpes
Acyclovir (Zovirax) 400 mg PO 3 times/day for 7–10 days	Acyclovir (Zovirax) 400 mg PO 2 times/day	Acyclovir (Zovirax) 400 mg PO 3 times/day for 5 days
Or	*Or*	*Or*
Acyclovir (Zovirax) 200 mg PO 5 times/day for 7–10 days	Famciclovir (Famvir) 250 mg PO 2 times/day	Acyclovir (Zovirax) 800 mg PO 2 times/day for 5 days
Or	*Or*	*Or*
Famciclovir (Famvir) 250 mg PO 3 times/day for 7–10 days	Valacyclovir (Valtrex) 500 mg PO once daily	Acyclovir (Zovirax) 800 mg PO 3 times/day for 2 days
Or	*Or*	*Or*
Valacyclovir (Valtrex) 1 g PO 2 times/day for 7–10 days	Valacyclovir (Valtrex) 1.0 g PO once daily	Famciclovir (Famvir) 125 mg PO 2 times/day for 5 days
		Or
		Famciclovir (Famvir)1000 mg PO 2 times/day for 1 day
		Or
		Valacyclovir (Valtrex) 500 mg PO 2 times/day for 3 days
		Or
		Valacyclovir (Valtrex)1.0 g PO once daily for 5 days

[a] Treatment might be extended if healing is incomplete after 10 days of therapy.

Source: Data from Centers for Disease Control and Prevention. Sexually transmitted disease treatment guidelines, 2015. *MMWR Recomm Rep.* 2015; 64(3):1-137.[5]

Suppressive Antiviral Therapy

Antiviral therapy is used to suppress both clinical recurrences of genital herpes and transmission of the virus. Daily antiviral therapy is effective in preventing clinical recurrences for approximately 50% of those persons infected with HSV.[43] Overall, suppressive therapy reduces the frequency of HSV recurrence by 70% to 80%.[5] Suppressive therapy in individuals with multiple clinical outbreaks has been shown to reduce pain, depression, and anxiety associated with the infection. In addition to preventing clinical recurrences, suppressive therapy reduces viral shedding and transmission by approximately 48%.[41] Daily use of acyclovir has been shown to be safe for as long as 6 years, and daily use of valacyclovir or famciclovir is safe for at least 1 year.[44,45] In addition, suppressive therapy reduces the likelihood of transmission to a noninfected sexual partner.

Episodic Therapy

Episodic therapy is an option for some individuals with genital HSV; however, it is likely to reduce symptoms less effectively than suppressive therapy. Effective episodic treatment for recurrent herpes requires initiation of therapy within 1 day of lesion onset. The woman should be provided with the drug so she can begin therapy at the onset of symptoms.

Special Populations: Pregnancy, Lactation, and the Elderly

If a woman has an active genital lesion at the time she gives birth, the herpes virus can be transmitted to the newborn. Newborn herpes can be a fulminant systemic and life-threatening condition. Current guidelines recommend that women who know they have genital herpes begin prophylaxis with acyclovir at 36 weeks' gestation.[46] The recommended dose is reviewed in the *Pregnancy* chapter.

Acyclovir appears to be safe for use during pregnancy and lactation. The acyclovir pregnancy registry has not found any increase in birth defects in women who use this drug. Because more data are available for acyclovir than for the other two antiviral medications prescribed for HSV, this agent is formally recommended for use. However, because valacyclovir converts to acyclovir, many clinicians recommend it instead, as valacyclovir can be taken less often.

There are no changes in dosing of these antiviral agents for elderly women. Valacyclovir is recommended for treatment of individuals with postherpetic neuropathy, which is more likely in the elderly population. Dose adjustments are needed only if renal impairment is present.

Human Immunodeficiency Virus

Readers interested in a detailed discussion of the pharmacotherapy for HIV/AIDs are referred to the national AIDS website, www.AIDS.gov.

The virus that causes acquired immunodeficiency syndrome (AIDS) was first identified in 1984,[47] almost 4 years after the epidemic was first reported in the United States among homosexual men.[48] In 1987, clinical trials with the first antiretroviral drug, zidovudine (Retrovir, AZT), were prematurely terminated to obtain accelerated approval of this agent by the FDA due to the marked improvements noted in the clinical condition of recipients. Unfortunately, these improvements were soon found to be associated with worsening symptoms and the return of opportunistic infection due to the emergence of drug resistance. Zidovudine was not a cure for HIV, but it began the reframing of HIV as a chronic, manageable—albeit life-altering—disease.

Since the approval of zidovudine, the list of antiretroviral medications has grown extensively and rapidly. The two newest classes are entry inhibitors and integrase inhibitors. Prescribers initiating **antiretroviral therapy (ART)** for treatment-naïve women now consider pill burden and limitation of treatment-related side effects to be the essential factors in regimen selection. Improvements in both quantity and quality of life are allowing more individuals infected with HIV to consider family planning options and influencing the ART regimen of choice. A thorough understanding of the key issues affecting women living with HIV will assist the provider of primary and specialty women's health services to adequately address these issues.

Phylogenetic testing has tracked the origins of HIV to transmission from a primate host, which likely occurred in the early 1900s.[49] Direct evidence of the virus in humans was found in a stored biopsy sample from a person in Africa taken in 1959.

Over the years, research has shown that in heterosexual relationships, women are more likely to acquire HIV infection than are men. The increased risk of acquiring HIV infection in women has been attributed to a number of biologic and social factors, including (1) the integrity of mucosal tissue in the female genital area; (2) untreated sexually transmitted infections; (3) levels of HIV in semen; and (4) young age of sexual debut, often with older men.[50–52] Among these women are women who have sex with women (WSW) and transgender women. The latter provide an illustration of racial disparity with more than 25% of transgender women being reported to have HIV;

and more than 55% of black transgender women with the disease.[5] Statistics from 2011 reveal that women accounted for approximately 21% of the estimated 38,825 newly diagnosed HIV cases among persons 13 years of age and older in the United States.[53]

Pathophysiology of HIV Infection

The life cycle of HIV follows a series of steps that are summarized here in order of their occurrence and illustrated in Figure 23-2.[54] Specific antiviral agents work by interfering with different steps in the life cycle.

- *Attachment and entry*: The HIV virus requires specific receptors for attachment and cannot infect every cell of the body. HIV envelope proteins attach to human immune cells that have the cluster of differentiation 4 (CD4) receptor and either CXCR4 or CCR5 coreceptors. Next, the membranes fuse and the contents of the virion are released into the cell.
- *Reverse transcription*: HIV is a retrovirus and must convert its ribonucleic acid (RNA) into deoxyribonucleic acid (DNA) before it can replicate. The viral enzyme reverse transcriptase catalyzes the synthesis of double-stranded proviral DNA. Reverse transcriptase inhibitor drugs block this step.
- *Integration*: Once HIV RNA is copied into proviral DNA, the viral enzyme integrase incorporates HIV's genetic blueprint into the DNA of the host cell. Integration into the host cell DNA enables the transcription of building blocks for new virions. Integrase inhibitor drugs block this step and prevent proviral integration within the host genome.
- *Transcription and translation*: The host cell transcribes information for new viral proteins in the form of messenger RNA. Translation of the messenger RNA in the cell cytoplasm produces long viral protein sequences.
- *Assembly*: Long viral protein sequences assemble near the cell surface, where the HIV enzyme

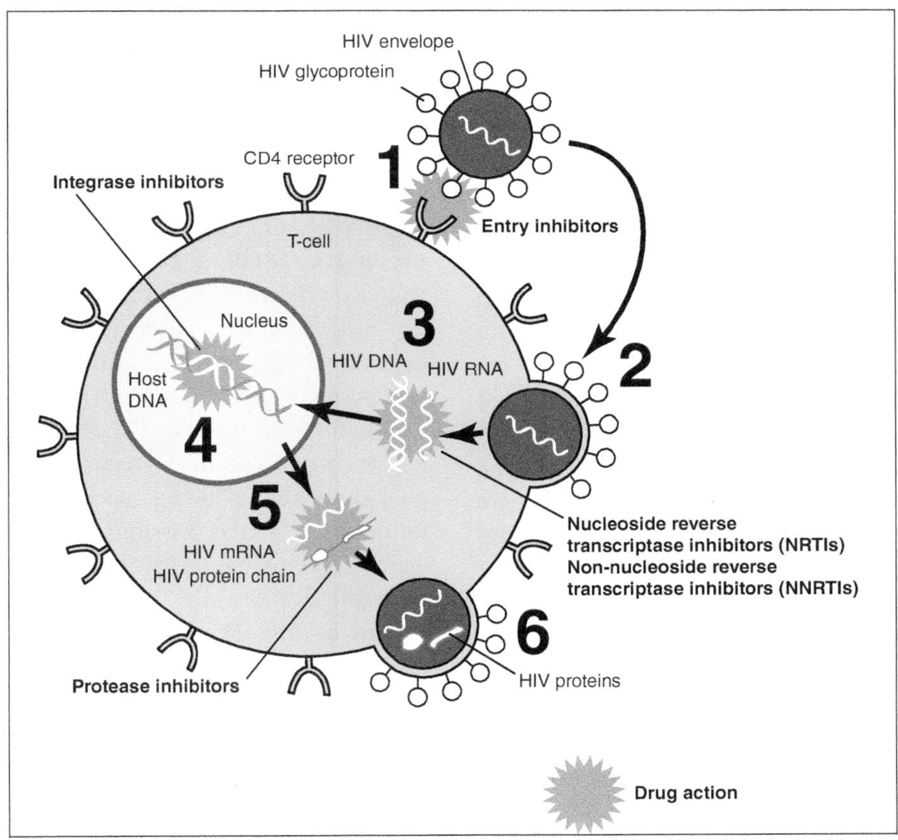

Figure 23-2 Life cycle of HIV virus and mechanism of action of anti-retroviral drugs. 1. Attachment and entry is prevented by the entry inhibitors. 2. Reverse transcription from HIV RNA to HIV DNA is prevented by NRIs and NNRTIs. 3. Integration into host cell DNA. 4. Transcription and translation is prevented by integrate inhibitors. 5. Assembly is prevented by protease inhibitors. 6. Budding and maturation.

protease cleaves them into functional viral proteins. Protease inhibitor drugs block this step, resulting in a nonviable virion.
- *Budding and maturation*: Once assembled, the new virion buds through the cell wall. Maturation occurs when the viral particle has separated and acquired the host cell wall as its own viral envelope.

Immunologic Effects of HIV Infection

Viral infection produces a robust immunologic response. As HIV viral load increases during acute infection, the body produces millions of anti-HIV antibodies. These antibodies, along with cytotoxic T cells, gradually reduce viral replication, and a viral set point for the HIV viral load of the individual is established. In general, the lower this set point, the slower the progression of HIV to AIDS. Over time and without treatment, HIV gradually depletes the number of CD4 cells and consequently increases the woman's susceptibility to opportunistic infections and malignancies.

Shortly after infection, and generally during the process of seroconversion, a person infected with HIV may develop signs and symptoms collectively known as acute retroviral syndrome. When these symptoms occur, they are similar to a mononucleosis-like illness, with fever, pharyngitis, myalgias, headache, adenopathy, and rash being the most commonly reported. Without treatment, HIV infection progresses to AIDS. AIDS is defined as the occurrence of any one of 27 AIDS-defining conditions, a CD4 count of less than 200 cells/μL, or a CD4 cell count representing less than 14% of total lymphocytes.[53] The rate of disease progression depends on a variety of factors, including the viral set point, the viral load, and access to healthcare services.

The management of HIV is a specialty practice provided by clinicians with appropriate training and experience. The best practice is to refer the woman who is HIV-positive to an HIV specialist to establish a relationship for long-term care and initiation of ART whenever possible. Clinical guidelines for the management of HIV infection are routinely updated to reflect advances in the understanding of how best to optimize health outcomes and prevent disease. The information presented here is based on the March 2014 update of the U.S. Department of Health and Human Services' guidelines. The most recent information is available at the National Institutes of Health Aids Info website, which is included in the Resources table at the end of this chapter.

Highly Active Antiretroviral Therapy

A major change in treatment of persons with HIV/AIDS has been the recommendation to initiate **highly active antiretroviral therapy (HAART)** for all persons infected with HIV, regardless of their pretreatment CD4 count. The primary goals of HAART are fourfold: (1) maximally and durably suppress HIV viral load; (2) restore or preserve immunologic function; (3) reduce HIV-related morbidity and mortality and improve quality of life; and (4) prevent HIV transmission.[55] In addition to these factors, limiting the side effects of HAART is an important consideration. In general, antiretroviral classes of medications may have the same type of side effects across the entire class of agents due to similar mechanisms of action and pharmacologic properties.

There are five categories of drugs used to treat HIV infection: (1) nucleoside/nucleoside reverse transcriptase inhibitors (NRTIs); (2) non-nucleoside reverse transcriptase inhibitors (NNRITs); (3) protease inhibitors (Pis); (4) entry inhibitors; and (5) integrase inhibitors. Table 23-8 provides an overview of the common side effects and adverse events of each class of medications, along with special considerations for women who are HIV-positive.[56–58] Additionally, potential drug–drug interactions between HAART medications and contraceptives are of import for women of childbearing age and their care providers (Box 23-1).[59] Web-based resources for checking drug–drug interactions of HIV drugs are listed in the Resources table at the end of this chapter.

Postexposure Prophylaxis

Professionals who provide care to women who are HIV-positive should be knowledgeable about **postexposure prophylaxis (PEP)** guidelines for healthcare workers who may experience occupational exposure as well as PEP for persons who experience a high-risk sexual or blood exposure. In general, PEP consists of a three-drug regimen of tenofovir-emtricitabine (Truvada) 300/200 mg once daily plus dolutegravir (Tivicay) 50 mg once daily or tenofovir-emtricitabine (Truvada) 300/200 mg once daily plus raltegravir 400 mg twice daily. Therapy should be initiated as soon as possible and less than 72 hours after exposure. Treatment continues for 4 weeks, with follow-up testing at 6 weeks, 12 weeks, and 6 months.[60–62] Women should be offered emergency contraception to prevent pregnancy. Before beginning any guideline-based PEP, the clinician should evaluate the pharmacologic principles of the drug, drug–drug interactions, dosing, and side effects in addition to appropriately weighing the risks and potential benefit of such treatment.

Pre-exposure Prophylaxis

The FDA approved the first drug for use as **pre-exposure prophylaxis (PrEP)** to prevent HIV infection in 2012.

Table 23-8 Overview of Major Side Effects and Adverse Reactions Associated with HIV Medications

Mechanism of Action/ Comments	Drug: Generic (Brand)	Clinical Considerations for Drug	Clinical Considerations for Drug Class
Nucleoside Reverse Transcriptase Inhibitors (NRTIs)			
NRTIs are faulty versions of building blocks that HIV needs to make more copies of itself. When HIV uses an NRTI instead of a normal building block, reproduction of the virus stalls.	Zidovudine, also called AZT (Retrovir)[a]	Anemia may be more pronounced in menstruating women. Side effects include mania, depression, myositis, and insomnia.	Common side effects include headache, nausea and vomiting, diarrhea, and fatigue. FDA black box warning about: Severe lactic acidosis and hepatomegaly. Associated with exacerbation of hepatitis B if discontinued and the individual is not also taking medication for treatment of people with hepatitis B. Lactic acidosis appears to occur with greater frequency in women.
	Lamivudine or 3TC (Epivir)[a]	Fewer side effects (SEs) than other NRTI drugs. Adverse effects (AEs) include pancreatitis, peripheral neuropathy, and neutropenia.	
	Emtricitabine or FTC (Emtriva)[b]	Skin discoloration is an SE specific to FTC.	
	Abacavir or ABC (Ziagen)[b]	SEs include rash, loss of appetite, and respiratory symptoms. FDA black box warning describes fatal hypersensitivity reactions, which are more likely in persons who have the *HLA-B*5701* allele. Screening for this allele is recommended before starting therapy with abacavir.	
	Tenofovir or TDF (Viread)[c]	SEs include anorexia, asthenia, and flatulence. No interactions found with ethinyl estradiol/hormonal contraceptives. Avoid during pregnancy because of potential fetal bone effects. Decreases in bone mineral density may occur, necessitating monitoring, especially of perimenopausal/postmenopausal women.	
	Stavudine or D4T (Zerit)[c]	AEs: Pancreatitis, ascending neuromuscular weakness, and peripheral neuropathy (15–20% of recipients). Contraindicated for persons with preexisting neuropathy.	
	Didanosine or DDI (Videx or Videx EC)[b]	AEs: Peripheral neuropathy, diarrhea, pancreatitis.	
Non-nucleoside Reverse Transcriptase Inhibitors (NNRTIs)			
NNRTIs bind to and disable reverse transcriptase. HIV needs this protein to make more copies of itself.	Efavirenz or EFV (Sustiva)[c]	AEs: Hallucinations and disorientation. Known teratogen during first trimester, although use after first trimester may be considered. Advocate use of a reliable contraceptive method for sexually active reproductive-aged women. Induces CYP3A4 and inhibits CYP3A4, CYP2C9, CYP2C19, and CYP2B6. May increase concentrations of ethinyl estradiol, but clinical significance is questionable.	SEs: Rash, headache, increased ALT levels.
	Intelence (Etravirine)	Inadequate study of use in pregnancy.	
	Rilpivirine (Edurant)	Inadequate study of use in pregnancy.	
	Nevirapine or NVP (Viramune)	AEs: Central nervous system (CNS) symptoms, psychiatric symptoms. FDA black box warning deals with hepatotoxicity, Stevens-Johnson syndrome, and hypersensitivity reactions. Cannot be used in women with CD4 count > 250 cells/mm^3 due to risk of severe hepatotoxicity. Several studies have noted an increase in NVP-associated rash among women. Use in pregnant women with CD4 count > 250 is warranted only if the benefits clearly outweigh the risks. In pharmacokinetic studies, women had a 13.8% lower clearance of nevirapine. Substrate for CYP3A4 and to a lesser extend CYP2B6. Induces CYP3A4 and CYP2B6. May decrease the effectiveness of estrogen-containing contraceptives.	

(*continues*)

Table 23-8 Overview of Major Side Effects and Adverse Reactions Associated with HIV Medications (*continued*)

Mechanism of Action/ Comments	Drug: Generic (Brand)	Clinical Considerations for Drug	Clinical Considerations for Drug Class
	Delavirdine or DLV (Rescriptor)[c]	May increase concentrations of ethinyl estradiol, but clinical significance is unlikely. Multiple drug–drug interactions.	
Protease Inhibitors (PIs)			
PIs disable protease, a protein that HIV needs to make more copies of itself. Protease inhibitors have been associated with changes in glucose intolerance. However, no study to date has verified an increase in gestational diabetes. All PI drugs influence liver metabolism through cytochrome P pathways (CYP) and, therefore, are involved in multiple drug–drug–herb interactions, including with *Hypericum perforatum* (St. John's wort)—an agent that decreases the effectiveness of the PI. Some studies have suggested that dietary supplements of garlic, vitamin C, milk thistle, and echinacea (coneflower) also may decrease PI effectiveness, but the clinical significance of this effect has not been demonstrated.	Loprinavir-ritonavir or LPV (Kaletra)[c]	SEs: Elevated temperature, asthenia. Pregnant women using LPV require dose adjustments during the third trimester. Inhibits CYP2D6 and possibly induces CYP1A2, CYP2C19, CYP2C9, and CYP2B6. May decrease the effectiveness of estrogen-containing contraceptives.	SEs: Gastrointestinal symptoms, hyperglycemia, fat redistribution, lipid abnormalities. AEs: Spontaneous bleeding, intracranial hemorrhage. Inhibits CYP3A4 and has multiple clinically important drug–drug interactions, many of which reduce the blood concentrations of the PI and lower its therapeutic effectiveness.
	Indinavir or IDV (Crixivan)[b]	SEs/AEs: Nephrolithiasis, blurred vision, asthenia, dizziness, rash, metallic taste, thrombocytopenia, alopecia. Inhibits CYP3A4 and may increase the effectiveness of estrogen-containing contraceptives.	
	Fosamprenavir or FOS (Lexiva)[b]	Induces CYP3A4 and may decrease the effectiveness of PI when administered with estrogen-containing contraceptives.	
	Atazanavir or ATV (Reyataz)[b]	SEs/AEs: Jaundice, arrhythmia. May increase the effectiveness of estrogen-containing contraceptives. Needs dose adjustment and ritonavir boosting when used with tenofovir.	
	Darunavir or DRV (Prezista)[b]	CYP3A4 substrate and may decrease effectiveness of estrogen-containing contraceptives.	
	Saquinavir or SQV (Fortovase)[b]	SEs/AEs: Dyspepsia. Weak inhibitor of CYP3A4 and usually used with ritonavir, resulting in possible reduction of the effectiveness of estrogen-containing contraceptives.	
	Nelfinavir or NFV (Viracept)	SE/AE: Diarrhea. Inhibits CYP32B6 and may decrease the effectiveness of estrogen-containing contraceptives.	
	Tipranavir (Aptivus)	Very limited data for use in pregnancy.	
	Ritonavir or RTV (Norvir)[b]	SEs/AEs: Paresthesia, hepatitis, pancreatitis, asthenia, taste perversion, increased triglyceride level. Currently used only in lower doses to boost the effects of other PIs. Inhibits CYP2D6 > CYP2C9 > CYP 2C19 > CYP 2A6 > CYP 2E1 and CYP 2B6. Induces GT, CYP1A2, and possibly CYP2C9, CYP2C19, and CYP2B6; may decrease the effectiveness of estrogen-containing contraceptives.	
Integrase Inhibitors			
Integrase inhibitors disable integrase, a protein that HIV uses to insert its viral genetic material into the genetic material of an infected cell.	Raltegravir (Isentress)[b]	Pharmacokinetic studies have failed to find differences between men and women.	
	Dolutegravir (Tivicay)	No studies in pregnancy reported.	
Entry Inhibitors			
Entry/fusion inhibitors work by blocking HIV entry into cells.	Enfuvirtide or T-20 (Fuzeon)[b] Maraviroc (Selzentry)[b]		

Combination Drugs		
Fixed-dose combination tablets contain two or more anti-HIV medications that can be from one or more drug classes.	Combination AZT/3TC (Combivir)[a]	See Clinical Considerations for individual agents.
	Combination TDF/FTC (Truvada)[b]	
	Combination ABC/3TC (Epzicom)[b]	
	Combination EFV/TDF/FTC (Atripla)[c]	
	Combination AZT/3TC/ABC (Trizivir)[b]	
	Combination VG/COBI/TDF/FTC (Stribild)[c]	
	Combination FTC/TDF/RPV (Complera)[c]	

[a] Recommended for use during pregnancy for preventing mother-to-child transmission.
[b] Not recommended as first-line agent in pregnancy.
[c] Avoid during pregnancy.
Note: The use of DDI in combination with D4T is not recommended due to an increased risk for mitochondrial toxicity and peripheral neuropathy.
Sources: Data from Panel on Antiretroviral Guidelines for Adults and Adolescents. Guidelines for the use of antiretroviral agents in HIV-1-infected adults and adolescents. Department of Health and Human Services; 2014. http://aidsinfo.nih.gov/ContentFiles/AdultandAdolescentGL.pdf. Accessed June 13, 2014[57]; Panel on Treatment of HIV-Infected Pregnant Women and Prevention of Perinatal Transmission. Recommendations for use of antiretroviral drugs in pregnant HIV-1-infected women for maternal health and interventions to reduce perinatal HIV transmission in the United States. March 2014. http://aidsinfo.nih.gov/contentfiles/lvguidelines/PerinatalGL.pdf. Accessed June 12, 2014[56]; Lesho EP, Gey DC. Managing issues related to antiretroviral therapy. *Am Fam Physician*. 2003;68(4):675-686.[58]

The approval was based on several large, international studies that found an approximately 60% to 99% reduced risk of HIV infection with PrEP.[62,63] Higher medication adherence was associated with greater risk reduction. Daily use of a fixed-dose combination of tenofovir disoproxil fumarate (TDF) 300 mg and emtricitabine (FTC) 200 mg (Truvada) is the only currently approved PrEP regimen.[62,63]

PrEP is recommended for adults at substantial risk of HIV infection.[62,63] For women's healthcare providers, this would include heterosexually active women whose

Box 23-1 HIV and Reproductive Health

KT, a 38-year-old nonsmoking woman, has been living with HIV for more than a decade and regularly obtains health care from a specialist in infectious medicine. However, she is seeking primary care for contraception, as she was widowed 2 years ago and now is entering a new relationship.

Identification of the best contraception option can be made only by KT herself. However, the clinician can suggest a wide range of options to KT. Condoms should be promoted because of the sexually transmitted nature of HIV.

Some potential concerns exist about theoretical risks of drug interaction between HAART and combined oral contraceptives. In addition, many of the HAART drugs have side effects related to insulin sensitivity and other metabolic dysregulation, an area of concern with systemic hormonal contraception. The method with the most advantages is likely to be the levonorgestrel intrauterine system (Mirena), which has been found to decrease menstrual flow among women with HIV while providing contraception with minimal side effects. Ultimately, the most effective method is the one that the woman will use successfully.

During KT's primary care visit, issues such as open communication with the new partner, importance of regular Pap testing, keeping vaccinations current, and general care such as routine mammograms should be discussed.

partners are HIV infected, commercial sex workers, women with a high number of sexual partners or inconsistent condom use, and intravenous drug users. Testing must be performed to exclude acute or chronic HIV infection before initiating PrEP. The approved drug(s) for PrEP is inadequate to treat HIV infection alone and can induce resistance if not used as part of a recommended combination therapy. Therefore, testing is repeated every 3 months during usage to identify incident infection. Because tenofovir can be nephrotoxic, renal function must be assessed at baseline and every 6 months. Individuals should be counseled that a high degree of adherence is required for PrEP to be effective. PrEP is one aspect of prevention that should be used along with risk reduction counseling and referrals.

Special Populations: Reproductive Age Women, Pregnancy, Lactation, and the Elderly

Management of HIV in women who need contraception requires knowledge of how contraceptive agents interact with HIV medications.[59,64-66] The effectiveness of oral contraceptives and some contraceptive implants can be reduced when taken in combination with certain ART regimens, especially those containing efavirenz or nevirapine. The United States Medical Eligibility Criteria for Contraception has reviewed the effectiveness and possible complications for each type of contraception when used by a women who has HIV infection.[66] The *Contraception* chapter reviews interactions between contraceptive agents and HIV medications in more detail. In addition, Box 23-1 presents a case study on HIV and reproductive health.[59,64,65]

Efforts directed at **prevention of mother-to-child transmission (PMTCT)** have been very successful. Fewer than 2% of infants born to mothers who are HIV-positive are infected in the United States.[56] This low transmission rate is the result of several interventions that have been broadly implemented, including testing, maternal treatment with ART during the prenatal and intrapartum periods, infant ART prophylaxis, planned cesarean section for women with viral loads greater than 1000 copies/mL, and avoidance of breastfeeding.[56]

The pharmacologic properties of HAART may differ during pregnancy compared to use in nonpregnant women. It is important to monitor for HAART-related side effects, particularly during pregnancy, and to determine any patterns of adverse outcomes that might be associated with a drug or combination of drugs. Because the incidence of resistance is high, it is important that pregnant women follow the regimen exactly as prescribed.

The Antiretroviral Pregnancy Registry is a voluntary, prospective, observational study that collects and analyzes data for any evidence of teratogenic events that might be associated with HAART use during pregnancy and postpartum. Information about the registry is listed in the Resources table at the end of the chapter. The reader is referred to the *Recommendations for Use of Antiretroviral Drugs in Pregnant HIV-1-Infected Women for Maternal Health and Interventions to Reduce Perinatal HIV Transmission in the United States*[56] to assess specific medications and the implications of HIV treatment during pregnancy.

Human Papillomavirus

Human papillomavirus (HPV) is a double-stranded DNA virus. HPV includes more than 100 genotypes that can infect cutaneous or mucosal epithelial tissues, of which 30 to 40 types infect the genital area. Genital HPV is the most common STI in the United States—at least 50% of sexually active men and women will acquire it at some point in their lives. Approximately 50% of the individuals who become infected with HPV are sexually active adolescents and young adults between 15 and 24 years of age. Among WSW, the rate has been relatively similar, suggesting female-to-female transmission and that the risk of cervical cancer exists among these women.[5]

Approximately 90% of cervical HPV infections will clear spontaneously within 2 years; 5% will persist for more than 2 years.[67] Persistent infection with HPV is a risk factor for anogenital cancers. Persistent cervical infection with selected HPV genotypes is the single most important risk factor for cervical cancer.

Approximately 13 strains of HPV are considered oncogenic. These strains are associated with 40% to 51% of vulvar cancers and 40% to 64% of vaginal cancers. In addition, HPV types 16 and 18 are associated with 70% to 76% of cervical cancers. Cancers of the anus, oropharynx, and vulva have increased substantially during recent years.[68]

Human papillomaviruses are theorized to enter the body after slight trauma to the epithelium. The virus needs terminally differentiated epithelial cells for its replication.[69] All HPV types replicate only within the cell's nucleus, but the mechanism by which HPV types transform cells is unclear. While all HPV types infect the mucous membranes of the skin, the various forms establish themselves in specific cell types.

HPV infection can be detected clinically (genital warts), cytologically (Pap test), or virologically (DNA detection).

Genital warts, also called condylomata acuminata, are typically the only visible sign of HPV infection, but they may not appear until months or even years after infection. Women are more likely than men to develop warts, and they can grow anywhere in the perineal and vaginal region. The most common method of detecting HPV is discovery of atypical cells on a routine Pap test. Because HPV is difficult to detect and difficult to treat, vaccination is the primary prevention strategy. HPV vaccination is reviewed in the *Immunizations* chapter.

Treatment of Persons with HPV Infection

Treatment is not recommended for subclinical genital HPV infection. Approximately 90% of anogenital warts are caused by the nononcogenic HPV types 6 or 11. Genital warts resolve spontaneously in 20% to 30% of women within a 3-month period. Treatment to remove the wart is recommended when symptoms need to be mitigated. Treatment may or may not lower transmission rates, and development of new lesions or recurrence at previously treated sites is common. Treatment of a woman's sexual partners is not indicated unless that person also has visible warts.

Genital warts can be removed surgically with cryoablation, laser ablation, or electrocautery. Lesions can also be treated chemically with podophyllotoxin (Podofilox), trichloroacetic acid (Tri-Chlor), or 5-fluorouracil. In addition, they can be treated with immune-mediated therapies such as imiquimod (Aldara). Treatment can be self- or provider administered. Most women require a course of therapy rather than a single treatment. The CDC-recommended treatment regimens are presented in Table 23-9.[5,70-73]

Imiquimod

Imiquimod is a cell-mediated immune response modifier that induces interferons and cytokines, which in turn enhances cell-mediated cytolytic activity against HPV-infected cells.[70] It can be self-applied by the woman. The clearance rate of imiquimod ranges from 30% to 50%, and risk of recurrence is 15%.[70] Side effects include an intense local inflammatory reaction that includes skin scabbing and severe skin irritation. Approximately 70% of recipients will experience some skin irritation. Systemic symptoms of fever and myalgias can occur. This agent should not be used intravaginally. It can also weaken condoms or vaginal diaphragms.

Imiquimod is available as a 5% or 3.75% cream. The 3.75% cream is associated with better compliance secondary to less severe side effects, but the clearance rate is slightly lower at 28%.[71] The recurrence rate is similar to that observed with the 5% cream (Aldara).[71]

Sinecatechin

Sinecatechin ointment 15% (Veregen) is an extract of green tea that has immunomodulator properties. It can be self-applied by the woman. The exact mechanism of this agent's action is unknown. The clearance rate of sinecatechin is approximately 50%, but may be higher in women than in men. The risk of genital wart recurrence over 12 weeks ranges from 5.9% to 12%, although the overall risk of recurrence is not definitively known.[70,71] Side effects of the sinecatechin ointment include skin irritation, pruritus, burning, erythema, pain, and ulceration. These effects usually occur early in the course of treatment and subside over time. Interestingly, ulceration at the site of the lesion is associated with higher clearance rates. This medication can weaken condoms or vaginal diaphragms. Sinecatechin is contraindicated for persons who are immunosuppressed, who are HIV positive, or who have genital herpes.

Podofilox

Podofilox 0.5% (Condylox 0.5%) is a purified extract of the mayapple plant (*Podophyllum petalum*).[72] It has antimitotic properties that cause necrosis of the visible wart tissue, with this effect reaching its maximal point 3 to 5 days after the medication's application.[72] The clearance rate of podofilox ranges from 45% to 80%, and risk of recurrence ranges from 5% to 30%.[70] Podofilox is generally well tolerated, but burning, pain, and local irritation occur at the site of application in 50% to 75% of recipients. Podofilox should not be applied to mucous membranes or to perianal, vaginal, or urethral lesions. This agent is flammable and should be kept away from fire. There are no known drug interactions.

Podophyllum Resin

Podophyllum resin 10% to 25% (Podocon; sometimes spelled podophyllin) is an unpurified extract of the same mayapple plant from which podofilox is obtained. Podophyllum is applied by a provider, so its use necessitates ongoing office visits for the duration of therapy. Podophyllum is available as a cream, gel, or solution. It has antimitotic properties that arrest the cell cycle during metaphase. The clearance rate of podophyllum is 62% and risk of recurrence is 26%.[70,71] This agent should not be applied to the cervix or vaginal mucosa because it can cause chemical burns and such application increases the risk of systemic absorption. Podophyllum has been associated with bone marrow suppression, neurologic defects, and death when over-applied or occluded (causing systemic absorption).[71] The treatment area should be limited to less than 10 cm^2

and no more than 0.5 mL per treatment.[5] In addition, this agent should not be used by women who might become pregnant or who are pregnant, as it is teratogenic.

Use of podophyllum has largely been replaced by podofilox and other agents because of its toxicity and adverse side-effect profile. In addition, podofilox is more effective than posophyllum.[69]

Trichloroacetic Acid and Bichloroacetic Acid

Trichloroacetic acid (Tri-Chlor) and bichloroacetic acid 80% to 90% destroy wart tissue via protein coagulation. The clearance and recurrence rates are similar to podophyllin. Repeated application is necessary but these agents can be used to treat internal lesions and those on mucous membranes. Side effects are generally benign, including local pain and skin irritation. However, these agents are very caustic to skin. They are usually applied by the clinician directly to the lesion, with an area of free skin covered with petroleum jelly around the lesion to protect unaffected areas; although, if irritation occurs, an application of sodium bicarbonate can rapidly neutralize the acidic effects. Trichloroacetic acid and bichloroacetic acid are not absorbed systemically.

Alternative Treatments for Genital Warts

Systemic treatment with interferons, topical cidofovir, intralesion injection of 5-fluorouracil, epinephrine gel, and infrared coagulation have all been applied to genital warts on an off-label basis. All of these treatments have been found to have some effectiveness, but recurrence rates are not substantially better than those of the FDA-approved therapies. Moreover, all of these options have side effects that may be more poorly tolerated than those associated with the FDA-approved therapies.

Cryoablation with liquid nitrogen or laser ablation can also be used to remove genital warts. Cryoablation is a painful procedure and associated with hypopigmentation following treatment. Laser ablation results in scar formation and hypopigmentation.

Surgical removal is used for women with extensive or large lesions. The recurrence rate following surgery is no better than the recurrence rates of medical therapies.

Special Populations: Pregnancy, Lactation, and the Elderly

No link has been found between HPV and spontaneous abortion, premature birth, or other pregnancy complications, although the hormonal changes that accompany pregnancy frequently induce warts to multiply or enlarge. In addition, the fetus/newborn can become infected via vertical transmission. HPV infection acquired through vertical transmission presents as laryngeal disease and conjunctival or mucosal lesions. Treatment may not prevent vertical transmission but can greatly improve symptoms and mitigate the growth of lesions that occurs during pregnancy. There is no evidence to support cesarean section to prevent vertical transmission.[5] Imiquimod (Aldara), sinecatechin (Veregen), podophyllum (Podocon), and podofilox (Condylox 0.5%) are contraindicated for use during pregnancy, but trichloroacetic acid and bichloroacetic acid can be safely used and are the treatments of choice for pregnant women. Similarly, due to the dearth of data available,[5] imiquimod, sinecatechin, podophyllum , and podofilox should not be used by women who are breastfeeding.

There are no specific considerations for treatment of genital warts among elderly women. Elderly individuals often have thinner epidermal layers, however, so they may be at higher risk for side effects of the pharmacotherapeutic agents.

Syphilis

Syphilis is a human bacterial infection caused by the spirochete *Treponema pallidum*. The CDC established the Syphilis Elimination Effort for the United States in 1999. Its goal was to reduce syphilis incidence to fewer than 1000 cases of primary and secondary syphilis reported per year, with an interim target of 2.2 cases per 100,000 population set for 2010.[73] As of 2013, the trend was almost a doubling of the annual number of cases to 16,663, with an annual case rate of 5.3 cases per 100,000 population.[74] The case rate for women fluctuated over the same period, but was substantially lower than the overall rate, at just 0.9 case per 100,000 population. Racial disparities are readily evident with this STI, with a 13.3 times greater rate noted among Black women compared to White women (4.0 cases per 100,000 versus 0.3 cases per 100,000, respectively).[74]

Syphilis transmission occurs primarily by sexual contact or from mother to child, although transmission can occur through nonsexual contact in communities with endemic syphilis and under poor hygiene conditions.[75] *T. pallidum* is also transmitted by blood transfusion. This pathogen can survive for several decades in humans and is capable of infecting all tissues. A slowly evolving and relatively painless disease, syphilis is associated with long asymptomatic

Table 23-9 Pharmacotherapeutic Topical Treatment Regimens for Women with External Anogenital Warts

Drug: Generic (Brand)	Instructions for Use	Clearance/Recurrence	Safe for Use in Pregnancy
External Genital Warts; Treatment Applied by Woman			
Podofilox 0.5% solution or gel (Condylox 0.5%)	Apply to visible warts with a cotton swab, or a finger 2 times/day for 3 days, then allow 4 days of no therapy. This cycle may be repeated for as many as 4 cycles. The total wart area treated should be less than 10 cm^2. The total volume of podofilox should be 0.5 mL or less per day. Allow the gel or solution to dry before returning the opposing skin surface that touches the affected area. Wash hands before and after treatment.	45–80% clearance 5–30% recurrence	No, teratogenic
Or Imiquimod 3.75% or 5% cream (Aldara)	Apply once at bedtime, 3 times/week for up to 16 weeks. Remove with soap and water 6–10 hours after the application. Wash hands before and after treatment. May weaken condoms and vaginal diaphragms.	30–50% clearance 15% recurrence	No, safety unknown
Or Sinecatechins 15% ointment (Veregen)	Apply a 0.5-cm strand of ointment to each wart 3 times/day. Do not use for more than 16 weeks. Wash hands before and after treatment. Do not wash off after application and avoid sexual contact while the ointment is present on the wart. May weaken condoms and vaginal diaphragms.	50% clearance, but may be higher in women 5.9–12% recurrence over 12 months	No, not studied
External Genital Warts; Treatment Provider Administered[a]			
Podophyllum resin 10–25% (Podocon) in a compound tincture of benzoin	This is an alternative treatment and no longer listed as a first-line agent. The treatment area must be dry before it makes contact with normal mucosa. Apply a small amount to each wart and allow to air dry. Repeat weekly, if necessary. The application should consist of less than 0.5 mL of podophyllum or focus on an area of less than 10 cm^2 of warts per session. No open lesions or wounds should be present in the area to which the agent is applied. Wash off 1–4 hours after application.	62% clearance 26% recurrence	No, teratogenic
Or Trichloroacetic acid (TCA) or bichloroacetic acid (BCA) 80–90%	May be applied weekly. Apply a small ring of petroleum jelly to the unaffected area surrounding the lesion to protect it from the caustic effects of TCA or BCA. Apply a small amount only to the warts and allow to dry. A whitened area will form under the applicator. If an excess amount is applied, the acid can be removed following application of powdered talc, sodium bicarbonate, or liquid soap.	63% clearance 35% recurrence	Yes
Vaginal Warts			
Cryotherapy with liquid nitrogen	The use of a cryo-probe in the vagina is not recommended because of the risk for vaginal perforation and fistula formation.	27% clearance 25–55% recurrence	Yes
Or TCA or BCA 8–90%	See instructions above.	63% clearance 35% recurrence	Yes
Urethral Meatal Warts			
Cryotherapy with liquid nitrogen	See instructions above.	27% clearance 25–55% recurrence	Yes
Or Podophyllum 10–25% in compound tincture of benzoin (Podocon)	See instructions above.	62% clearance 26% recurrence	No

(*continues*)

Table 23-9 Pharmacotherapeutic Topical Treatment Regimens for Women with External Anogenital Warts (*continued*)

Drug: Generic (Brand)	Instructions for Use	Clearance/Recurrence	Safe for Use in Pregnancy
Anal Warts			
Cryotherapy with liquid nitrogen	See instructions above.	27% clearance 25–55% recurrence	Yes
Or TCA or BCA 80–90%	See instructions above.	63% clearance 35% recurrence	Yes

[a] Alternative regimens include intralesional interferon *or* laser surgery.

Sources: Centers for Disease Control and Prevention. Sexually transmitted disease treatment guidelines, 2015. *MMWR Recomm Rep.* 2015;64(3):1-137[5]; Fathi R, Tsoukas MM. Genital warts and other HPV infections: established and novel therapies. *Clin Dermatol.* 2014;32(2):299-306[71]; Karnes JB, Usatine RP. Management of external genital warts. *Am Fam Physician.* 2014;90(5):312-318[70]; Lopaschuk CC. New approach to managing genital warts. *Can Fam Physician.* 2013;59(7):731-736.[72]

periods and short symptomatic periods during which the organism multiplies rapidly.

Pathogenesis, Microbiology, and Taxonomy

Historically, the understanding of *T. pallidum* pathophysiology has been limited by the inability to grow the organism in culture. *T. pallidum* is a corkscrew-shaped organism with tightly wound spirals that can be viewed with dark-field microscopy.[75] Syphilis infection is characterized by different phases that have varying signs and symptoms, depending on the duration of infection. These phases are referred to as primary, secondary, and tertiary (or late) syphilis. Syphilis infection in pregnant women can cause stillbirth or congenital infection that results in neonatal death or future disease manifestation.

Syphilis is transmitted via direct, genital–genital (including anal) or oral–genital contact, and in utero through the placenta or at the time of birth.[75] This STI is believed to be transmissible during early disease (primary and secondary syphilis).[5] The first stage of the disease, known as primary syphilis, occurs 10 to 90 days after infection and is characterized by a chancre—a painless ulceration—usually found on the genitals.[76,77] The sore is infectious and appears at the site of inoculation. A painless chancre may aid the clinician in distinguishing it from HSV infection and *Haemophilus ducreyi* (chancroid), although the presence or absence of pain is not always a reliable clinical clue.[77] This entity resolves spontaneously.

Manifestations of secondary infection, appearing weeks to a few months later, include signs such as skin rash (notably on the palms of the hands and the soles of the feet), mucocutaneous lesions, and lymphadenopathy.[78] Condylomata lata—raised, flat, papular lesions in moist areas—may occur anywhere on the genitalia, and they can be differentiated from HPV condylomata acuminata by their moist, smooth, flat appearance.[79] Meningitis is associated with syphilis and most often occurs within the first year after infection, although it can occur years later, resulting in symptoms characteristic of bacterial meningitis, including headache, confusion, nausea, vomiting, and stiff neck.[78] Similar to primary disease, the acute manifestations of secondary syphilis typically resolve spontaneously, even in the absence of therapy.

Tertiary or late infection occurs as a result of late syphilis. This stage may appear at any time from 1 to 45 years after primary infection and involve a wide variety of tissues.[79] The most concerning manifestations of late tertiary syphilis are neurosyphilis (tabes dorsalis), a slow nerve degeneration, and cardiovascular syphilis.[78] Neurosyphilis rarely develops in persons after treatment with the penicillin regimens recommended for primary and secondary syphilis.

Latent infections (i.e., those lacking clinical manifestations) are detected by serologic testing.[78] Early latent syphilis is a subcategory of latent syphilis in which symptoms are absent and the infection was acquired within the preceding 12 months. Late latent syphilis is defined as asymptomatic infection that occurred more than 12 months prior, whereas latent syphilis of unknown duration refers to cases for which the date of infection cannot be determined. A longer duration of therapy for individuals with late latent syphilis is recommended due to the knowledge that the condition has a slower metabolism and a more prolonged dividing time. Clinicians who have concerns about prolonged syphilis infections and complications should consult with a specialist prior to initiating a treatment regimen.

Treatment for Syphilis

The first-line treatment for syphilis is penicillin G (Box 23-2). This antibiotic is administered as an intramuscular or parenteral injection for treatment of all stages of syphilis and is the only therapy for syphilis during pregnancy that has documented effectiveness.[5] Only the long-acting benzathine preparation (Bicillin LA) should be used for treatment of early syphilis, because low and continuous levels of penicillin are necessary for the elimination of treponemes. The combination of benzathine penicillin and procaine penicillin (Bicillin CR) and the oral penicillin preparations are not appropriate for syphilis treatment. Be aware of the similar names of these products and avoid use of the inappropriate agent. Long-acting benzathine penicillin should be given only via the intramuscular route; intravenous administration has been associated with cardiopulmonary arrest and death. The stage and clinical manifestations of the disease determine the preparation(s) for use (i.e., benzathine, aqueous procaine, or aqueous crystalline), the dose, and the length of treatment. (Table 23-10).

All individuals who have syphilis should be tested for other STIs, including HIV, and treated as indicated.[5] In geographic areas in which the prevalence of HIV is high, individuals who have primary syphilis should be retested for HIV after 3 months if the first HIV test result was negative.[5]

Management of Sex Partners

Persons who have sexual contact with a partner who has syphilis in any stage should be evaluated clinically and serologically and treated with a recommended regimen, depending on various factors. The CDC guidelines for managing sex partners of persons infected with syphilis are presented in Box 23-3.[5]

Jarisch-Herxheimer Reaction

The Jarisch-Herxheimer reaction is an acute febrile reaction that is secondary to the sudden presence of endotoxins, cytokines, and other immune factors that are released as the spirochete is affected by penicillin. This reaction is commonly associated with using penicillin for treatment of women with syphilis. It occurs within 24 hours after penicillin administration and is frequently accompanied by myalgia and headache.[5] In most cases, the reaction is self-limited and resolves without sequelae. Persons infected with HIV are more likely to develop Jarisch-Herxheimer reaction than are persons who are not infected.

Follow-Up

Persons treated for syphilis should be evaluated at 6 and 12 months following treatment. The serologic titers should be compared to the pre-treatment titers. An estimated 15% of individuals who receive the recommended therapy for early syphilis will not achieve the two-dilution decline in their nontreponemal titers that defines an effective response at 1 year after treatment. Because it is often difficult to distinguish treatment failure from reinfection with

Box 23-2 Gone But Not Forgotten: Syphilis

Syphilis is likely the oldest known STI. In the years before antimicrobial cures and due to the stigma associated with the infection, afflicted individuals often sought to hide the telltale cutaneous signs of the disease (e.g., chancre, alopecia, rashes). Alopecia of the head was remedied by toupees; alopecia of pubic hair was disguised by merkins, or pubic wigs; and heavy makeup was used by men and women to hide blemishes. When fields of specialized medical study first emerged in the eighteenth century, one of those areas was dermatology and venereology—a title still in use today within some medical centers and in countries such as Singapore and China.

For unknown reasons, heavy metals were used as a therapy for syphilis, dating from as early as the eleventh century. Shakespeare's play *Measure for Measure* includes a phrase about hollow bones, referring to the decreased bone mineral density associated with mercury, by then a common treatment for this STI. Other drastic interventions included induction of fevers by infecting the individual with malaria under the supposition that the fever might kill the disease.

In the early twentieth century, an arsenic compound containing a synthetic antimicrobial named salvarsan was developed in the lab of Paul Ehrlich, later immortalized in the 1940 Edward G. Robinson Academy Award–nominated film, *Dr. Ehrlich's Magic Bullet*. The last two words are the term that Ehrlich coined in his attempt to develop an agent that effectively destroyed the pathogenic organism without harming the host. Although the phrase "magic bullet" entered common language, Erhlich's treatment was not especially effective, and the cure for syphilis remained elusive until the mid-twentieth century, when penicillins became available.

Table 23-10 CDC-Recommended Treatment for Syphilis in Nonpregnant Adults

Recommended Treatment	Alternative Treatments
Primary, Secondary, or Latent < 1 Year	
Benzathine penicillin G (Bicillin LA) 2.4 million units IM in one dose[a]	Penicillin allergic, nonpregnant (limited data to support): Doxycycline (Dynapen) 100 mg PO 2 times/day for 14 days *Or* Tetracycline (Sumycin) 500 mg PO 4 times/day for 14 days
Latent > 1 Year, Latent of Unknown Duration, or Tertiary without Neurologic Involvement	
Benzathine penicillin G (Bicillin CR) 7.2 million units IM total dose, administered as 3 doses of 2.4 million units IM each at 1-week intervals[a]	Penicillin allergic: consult with infectious disease specialist
Neurosyphilis (Signs, Symptoms, and/or Neurologic Findings), Syphilitic Eye Disease	
Aqueous crystalline penicillin G (Pfizerpen) 18–24 million units per day, administered as 3–4 million units IV every 4 hours or continuous infusion for 10–14 days	Alternative regimen (if compliance can be ensured): Procaine penicillin (Bicillin LA) 2.4 million units IM once daily for 14 days *Plus* Probenecid 500 mg PO 4 times/day for 10–14 days

[a] Standard benzathine penicillin (Bicillin LA) must not to be confused with combination benzathine/procaine penicillin (Bicillin CR), which is not appropriate for treatment of syphilis.
[b] Azithromycin should not be used in pregnant women.
Source: Centers for Disease Control and Prevention. Sexually transmitted disease treatment guidelines, 2015. *MMWR Recomm Rep.* 2015;64(3):1-137.[5]

T. pallidum, experts in infectious medicine usually are consulted or the woman is provided a referral in such cases.

Special Populations: Pregnancy, Lactation, and the Elderly

If a woman is infected with syphilis during pregnancy, the spirochete can be readily transmitted to the fetus. Fetal infection causes a wide array of adverse effects that range from congenital infection to stillbirth. Approximately 10% to 90% of fetuses will be infected if a woman has syphilis and becomes pregnant. The incidence of fetal infection increases as gestation increases. A newborn with congenital syphilis may be asymptomatic but can also present with low birth weight, premature birth, congenital anomalies, and/or long-term sequelae such as neurologic impairment, cataracts, or deafness.

The recommended treatment for pregnant women diagnosed with syphilis is the penicillin regimen recommended for their stage of syphilis. Treatment with penicillin can prevent the fetus from becoming infected. Unfortunately, there are no proven effective alternatives to penicillin for pregnant women. There is some evidence that a second dose of penicillin administered 1 week after the initial dose may provide additional therapeutic benefit for women who are pregnant. Pregnant women with syphilis in any stage who report penicillin allergy will need to be desensitized and treated with penicillin (Box 23-4).[5] Skin testing for penicillin allergy can be helpful.

Box 23-3 CDC Guidelines for Managing the Care of Sex Partners of Persons Infected with Syphilis

Persons who were exposed within the 90 days preceding the diagnosis of primary, secondary, or early latent syphilis in a sex partner might be infected even if seronegative; therefore, such individuals should be treated for syphilis on a presumptive basis. For purposes of partner notification and presumptive treatment of exposed sex partners, persons with syphilis of unknown duration who have high nontreponemal serologic test titers (i.e., greater than 1:32) can be assumed to have early syphilis. However, serologic titers should not be used to differe ntiate early from late latent syphilis for the purpose of selecting a treatment regimen.

Persons who were exposed more than 90 days before the diagnosis of syphilis in a sex partner should be treated presumptively if serologic test results are not available immediately and the follow-up is uncertain.

Long-term sex partners of individuals who have latent syphilis should be evaluated and treated on the basis of the clinical and laboratory evaluation findings.

For identification of at-risk sexual partners, the periods before treatment are as follows: (1) 3 months plus duration of symptoms for primary syphilis; (2) 6 months plus duration of symptoms for secondary syphilis; and (3) 1 year for early latent syphilis.

Source: Centers for Disease Control and Prevention. Sexually transmitted disease treatment guidelines, 2015. *MMWR Recomm Rep.* 2015;64(3):1-137.[5]

Box 23-4 Syphilis During Pregnancy

CM is 14 weeks' gestation and she has secondary syphilis. Her nontreponemal serologic test (RPR) and treponemal test (FTA-ABS) are positive. Her nontreponemal (VDRL) titers are 1:256. Her past history is uneventful, except she has a penicillin allergy, which is confirmed by skin testing.

Treatment of CM is complicated by her allergy to penicillin, yet syphilis has profound adverse effects for both CM and her fetus. A major cause of congenital syphilis in modern society is inappropriate or insufficient therapy. The only effective method of preventing congenital syphilis is maternal penicillin therapy.

If a woman reports a penicillin allergy and skin testing is negative, penicillin can be administered. However, CM's positive skin test indicates the need for desensitization. Protocols for desensitization have been published by the CDC, and the process should be conducted in a hospital setting because of the risk of an IgE-mediated allergic reaction. The entire desensitization usually is completed within 4 hours.

After successful desensitization, CM was treated with benzathine penicillin G 2.4 million units intramuscularly. Four weeks later, her laboratory results included VDRL 1:16. VDRL titers used to verify treatment success must demonstrate a fourfold decrease and CM;s titer indicated that the treatment was successful. Follow-up laboratory testing often does not include an RPR or a treponemal test because they often remain positive for a period of time.

Health education is an important concern for persons with sexually transmitted infections. Any sexual partner should be screened and treated. A woman with syphilis also should be assessed for other STIs, including blood-borne diseases such as hepatitis and HIV, as well as gonorrhea and chlamydia. CM should know that certain laboratory levels such as treponemal-specific tests are likely to remain positive for years, if not for life. Eventually the VDRL titers may become nondetectable, although they may be reported as weakly reactive for years as a titer of 1:1 or 1:2.

The Jarisch-Herxheimer reaction may be more common in pregnant women. Although this reaction can precipitate uterine contractions and premature labor, therapy should still be initiated. The risk of preterm labor outweighs the risks associated with untreated syphilis.[5] Antipyretics may be used, but they have not been proven to prevent this reaction.

Conclusion

Primary care clinicians have a major role in preventing, identifying, and providing services for STIs for women. STIs are extremely common, and women are more frequently and more severely affected by STIs than are men. Prompt diagnosis and treatment of persons with STIs can interrupt these infections' transmission and prevent complications. The pharmacotherapeutic management of these infections is affected by resistance, compliance, and many complicated social and cultural factors. Recent, important developments in therapy for STIs include the global emergence of fluoroquinolone resistance in gonorrhea, the introduction of new antiretroviral drugs for HIV and HCV treatment, and an understanding of the value of HSV-2 suppression for decreasing transmission to uninfected partners. Familiarity with the basic epidemiology, transmission, clinical manifestations, diagnosis, and treatment plans for STIs is crucial for women's health practitioners.

Resources

Organization	Description	Website
Sexually Transmitted Infections		
Centers for Disease Control and Prevention (CDC)	On demand printing of document, wall charts, and pocket guides. (Limited number of copies can be ordered online.)	wwwn.cdc.gov/pubs/CDCInfoOnDemand.aspx?ProgramID=122
Hepatitis		
American Association for the Study of Liver Diseases (AASLD)	Practice guidelines for treatment of persons with chronic hepatitis B and chronic hepatitis C.	www.aasld.org/publications/practice-guidelines-0
University of Liverpool hepatitis drug interactions website	Useful printable chart of drug–drug interactions associated with the hepatitis drugs.	www.hep-druginteractions.org/data/PrintableCharts/DI_col.pdf

Organization	Description	Website
HIV		
U.S. federal government AIDS website	Has information on HIV policies, treatments, side effects, and more; includes multiple resources for clinicians.	www.AIDS.gov
AIDS info	Free PDF of *Recommendations for Use of Antiretroviral Drugs in Pregnant HIV-1-Infected Women for Maternal Health and Interventions to Reduce Perinatal HIV Transmission in the United States.*	http://aidsinfo.nih.gov
Antiretroviral pregnancy registry	International pregnancy registry.	www.apregistry.com
U.S. Department of Health and Human Services	*A Guide to the Clinical Care of Women with HIV,* 2013 edition; this PDF can be downloaded from the website and provides a comprehensive review of care of women who are infected with HIV.	http://hab.hrsa.gov/deliverhivaidscare/files/womenwithaids.pdf
Infectious Diseases Society of America (IDSA)	*Primary Care Guidelines for the Management of Persons Infected with Human Immunodeficiency Virus: 2013 Update.*	www.idsociety.org/Organism
Antiretroviral Pregnancy Registry	Antiviral pregnancy registry. Persons may register online or via fax. To maintain confidentiality, no personal identifying information is collected.	www.apregistry.com
National HIV/AIDS Clinician's Consultation Center	Website of note for professionals that offers a large number of resources.	www.nccc.ucsf.edu
inPractice HIV	HIV care guidelines with complete information on all FDA-approved drugs.	www.inpractice.com
Apps		
Hep iChart	Interactive app for mobile devices to check drug–drug interactions with hepatitis drugs; available for Apple and Android devices.	
HIV iChart	Interactive app for mobile devices to check drug–drug interactions with HIV drugs; available for Apple and Android devices.	
Centers for Disease Control and Prevention (CDC)	Available from the CDC, has the complete 2015 sexually transmitted infections guidelines, including drugs and doses. At the time of this writing, this app is available only for Apple devices, but an Android app is anticipated shortly.	www.cdc.gov/std/tg2015/

References

1. Satterwhite CL, Torrone E, Meites E, et al. Sexually transmitted infections among US women and men: prevalence and incidence estimates, 2008. *Sex Transm Dis.* 2013;40(3):187-193.
2. Centers for Disease Control and Prevention. *Sexually Transmitted Disease Surveillance 2012.* Atlanta, GA: U.S. Department of Health and Human Services; 2013.
3. World Health Organization. *Baseline Report on Global Sexually Transmitted Infection Surveillance 2012.* Geneva, Switzerland: WHO Press; 2013:58.
4. Owusu-Edusei K Jr, Chesson HW, Gift TL, et al. The estimated direct medical cost of selected sexually transmitted infections in the United States, 2008. *Sex Transm Dis.* 2013;40(3):197-201.
5. Centers for Disease Control and Prevention. Sexually transmitted disease treatment guidelines, 2015. *MMWR Recomm Rep.* 2015;64(3):1-137.
6. Bush RM, Everett KD. Molecular evolution of the Chlamydiaceae. *Int J Syst Evol Microbiol.* 2001; 51:203-220.
7. Kong FY, Tabrizi SN, Law M, et al. Azithromycin versus doxycycline for the treatment of genital chlamydia infection: a meta-analysis of randomized controlled trials. *Clin Infect Dis.* 2014;59(2):193-202.
8. Stamm WE. *Chlamydia trachomatis* infections of the adult. In: Holmes K, Sparling P, Stamm W, et al., eds. *Sexually Transmitted Diseases.* 4th ed. China: McGraw-Hill, 2008:575-592.

9. Lau CY, Qurishi AK. Azithromycin versus doxycycline for genital chlamydial infections: a meta-analysis of randomized clinical trials. *Sex Transmit Dis.* 2002; 29(9):497-502.
10. Dal Conte I, Mistrangelo M, Cariti C, et al. Lymphogranuloma venereum: an old, forgotten re-emerging systemic disease. *Panminerva Medica.* 2014;56(1):73-83.
11. Mabey D, Peeling RW. Lymphogranuloma venereum. *Sex Transm Infect.* 2002;78(2):90.
12. Ligon BL. Albert Ludwig Sigesmund Neisser: discoverer of the cause of gonorrhea. *Semin Pediatr Infect Dis.* 2005;16(4):336-341.
13. Mayor MT, Roett MA, Uduhiri KA. Diagnosis and management of gonococcal infections. *Am Fam Physician.* 2012;86(10):931-938.
14. van de Wijgert JH, Morrison CS, Brown J, et al. Disentangling contributions of reproductive tract infections to HIV acquisition in African women. *Sex Transmit Dis.* 2009;36(6):357-364.
15. Miller KE. Diagnosis and treatment of Neisseria gonorrhoeae infections. *Am Fam Physician.* 2006; 73(10):1779-1784.
16. Adams DA, Jajosky RA, Kriseman J, et al. Summary of notifiable diseases—United States, 2012. *MMWR.* 2014;61(53):1-121.
17. Centers for Disease Control and Prevention. Update to CDC's sexually transmitted diseases treatment guidelines, 2010: oral cephalosporins no longer a recommended treatment for gonococcal infections. *MMWR.* 2012;61(31):590-594.
18. Bleich AT, Sheffield JS, Wendel GD Jr, Sigman A, Cunningham FG. Disseminated gonococcal infection in women. *Obstet Gynecol.* 2012;119(3):597-602.
19. Centers for Disease Control and Prevention. Viral hepatitis surveillance United States, 2011. http://www.cdc.gov/hepatitis/Statistics/2011Surveillance/index.htm. Accessed June 11, 2014.
20. Lok AS, McMahon BJ. Practice Guidelines Committee, American Association for the Study of Liver Diseases (AASLD). Chronic hepatitis B: update 2009. *Hepatology.* 2009;50(3):1-36.
21. Centers for Disease Control and Prevention. Prevention of hepatitis A through active or passive immunization: recommendations of the Advisory Committee on Immunization Practices (ACIP). *MMWR Recomm Rep.* 2006;55(RR07):1-23.
22. Centers for Disease Control and Prevention. Recommendations for identification and public health management of persons with chronic hepatitis B virus infection. *MMWR.* 2008;57(RR-8):1-28.
23. Chen CJ, Yang HI, Su J, et al.; REVEAL-HBV Study Group. Risk of hepatocellular carcinoma across a biological gradient of serum hepatitis B virus DNA level. *JAMA.* 2006;295(1):65-73.
24. Stuyver L, De Gendt S, Van Geyt C, et al. A new genotype of hepatitis B virus: complete genome and phylogenetic relatedness. *J Gen Virol.* 2000;81:67.
25. Wilkins T, Zimmerman D, Schade RR. Hepatitis B: Diagnosis and treatment. *Am Fam Physician.* 2010;81(8):965-972.
26. Buster EH, Schalam SW, Janssen HL. Peginterferon for the treatment of chronic hepatitis B in the era of nucleos(t)ide analogues. *Best Pract Res Clin Gasteroenterol.* 2008;22(6):1093-1108.
27. Howley A, Kremenchutzky M. Pegylated interferons: a nurse's review of a novel multiple sclerosis therapy. *J Neurosci Nurs.* 2014;46(2):88-96.
28. Kohli A, Shaffer A, Sherman A, Kottilil S. Treatment of hepatitis C: a systematic review. *JAMA.* 2014; 312(6):631-640.
29. AASLD, IDSA, IAS–USA. Recommendations for testing, managing, and treating hepatitis C. 2014. http://www.hcvguidelines.org. Accessed June 11, 2014.
30. Hnatyszyn HJ. Chronic hepatitis C and genotyping: the clinical significance of determining HCV genotypes. *Antiviral Ther.* 2005;10(1):1-11.
31. Farley JE, Dial DJ, Kearney M. Management of hematologic and neuropsychiatric side effects in persons undergoing treatment for chronic HCV infection. *J Nurse Pract.* 2006;2(1);38-45.
32. Strader DB, Wright T, Thomas DL, Seeff LB. Practice Guidelines Committee, American Association for the Study of Liver Diseases (AASLD). Diagnosis, management, and treatment of hepatitis C. *Hepatology.* 2004;39(4):1147-1171.
33. Borgia G, Carleo MA, Geta GB, Genitle I. Hepatitis B in pregnancy. *World J Gastroenterol.* 2012;18(34): 4677-4683.
34. Tosone G, Maraolo AE, Mascolo S, Palmiero G, Tambaro O, Oralando R. Vertical hepatitis C virus transmission: main questions and answers. *World J Hepatol.* 2014;6(8):538-548.
35. Bradley H, Markowitz, LE, Gibson T, McQuillan GM. Seroprevalence of herpes simplex virus types 1 and 2—United States 1999–2010. *JID.* 2014;209:325-333.
36. Freeman EE, Weiss HA, Glynn JR, Cross PL, Whitworth JA, Hayes RJ. Herpes simplex virus

2 infection increases HIV acquisition in men and women: systemic review and meta-analysis of longitudinal studies. *AIDS*. 2006;20(1):73-83.

37. Mertz GJ. Asymptomatic shedding of herpes simplex virus 1 and 2: implications for prevention of transmission. *J Infect Dis*. 2008;198(8):1098-1100.
38. Belshe RB, Leone PA, Bernstein DI, et al. Efficacy results of a trial of a herpes simplex vaccine. *New Engl J Med*. 2012;366(1):34-43.
39. Bernstein DI, Bellamy AR, Hook EQ III, et al. Epidemiology, clinical presentation, and antibody response to primary infection with herpes simplex virus type 1 and type 2 in young women. *Clin Infect Dis*. 2013;56(3):344-351.
40. Ryder N, Jin F, McNulty AM, Grulich AE, Donovan B. Increasing role of herpes simplex virus type 1 in first episode anogenital herpes in heterosexual women and younger men who have sex with men, 1992–2006. *Sex Transm Infect*. 2009;85(6):416-419.
41. Corey L, Wald A, Patel R, et al. Once-daily valacyclovir to reduce the risk of transmission of genital herpes. *New Engl J Med*. 2004;350(1):11-20.
42. James SH, Prichard MN. Current and future therapies for herpes simplex virus infections: mechanism of action and drug resistance. *Curr Opin Virol*. 2014;8:54-61.
43. Cernik C, Gallina K, Brodell RT. The treatment of herpes simplex infections: an evidence-based review. *Arch Intern Med*. 2008;168(11):1137-1144.
44. Goldberg LH, Kaufman R, Kurtz TO, et al. Acyclovir Study Group. Long-term suppression of recurrent genital herpes with acyclovir: a 5-year benchmark. *Arch Dermatol*. 1993;129(5):582-587.
45. Fife KH, Crumpacker CS, Mertz GJ, Hill EL, Boone GS; Acyclovir Study Group. Recurrence and resistance patterns of herpes simplex virus following cessation of ≥6 years of chronic suppression with acyclovir. *J Infect Dis*. 1994;169(6):1338-1341.
46. Hollier LM, Wendel GD. Third trimester antiviral prophylaxis for preventing maternal genital herpes simplex virus (HSV) recurrences and neonatal infection. *Cochrane Database Syst Rev*. 2008;1:CD004946.
47. Broder S, Gallo RC. A pathogenic retrovirus (HTLV-III) linked to AIDS. *N Engl J Med*. 1984;311(20):1292-1297.
48. Gottlieb MS, Schroff R, Schanker HM, et al. *Pneumocystis carinii* pneumonia and mucosal candidiasis in previously healthy homosexual men: evidence of a new acquired cellular immunodeficiency. *N Engl J Med*. 1981;305(24):1425-1431.
49. Worobey M, Gemmel M, Teuwen DE, et al. Direct evidence of extensive diversity of HIV-1 in Kinshasa by 1960. *Nature*. 2008;455(7213):661-664.
50. Pitchenik AE, Fischl MA, Dickinson GM, et al. Opportunistic infections and Kaposi's sarcoma among Haitians: evidence of a new acquired immunodeficiency state. *Ann Intern Med*. 1983;98(3):277-284.
51. Karim QA, Sibeko S, Baxter C. Preventing HIV infection in women: a global health imperative. *Clin Infect Dis*. 2010;50(suppl 3):S122-S129.
52. Ferreira VH, Kafka JK, Kaushic C. Influence of common mucosal co-factors on HIV infection in the female genital tract. *Am J Reprod Immun*. 2014;71(6):543-554.
53. Centers for Disease Control and Prevention. HIV surveillance report, 2011. Vol. 23. February 2013. http://www.cdc.gov/hiv/topics/surveillance/resources/reports/. Accessed June 12, 2014.
54. The HIV life cycle. *Education Materials AIDSinfo*. http://aidsinfo.nih.gov/education-materials/fact-sheets/19/73/the-hiv-life-cycle. Accessed March 21, 2015.
55. Centers for Disease Control and Prevention. Revised recommendations for HIV testing of adults, adolescents, and pregnant women in health-care settings. *MMWR*. 2006;55(RR14):1-17.
56. Panel on Treatment of HIV-Infected Pregnant Women and Prevention of Perinatal Transmission. Recommendations for use of antiretroviral drugs in pregnant HIV-1-infected women for maternal health and interventions to reduce perinatal HIV transmission in the United States. March 2014. http://aidsinfo.nih.gov/contentfiles/lvguidelines/PerinatalGL.pdf. Accessed June 12, 2014.
57. Panel on Antiretroviral Guidelines for Adults and Adolescents. Guidelines for the use of antiretroviral agents in HIV-1-infected adults and adolescents. Department of Health and Human Services; 2014. http://aidsinfo.nih.gov/ContentFiles/AdultandAdolescentGL.pdf. Accessed June 13, 2014.
58. Lesho EP, Gey DC. Managing issues related to antiretroviral therapy. *Am Fam Physician*. 2003;68(4):675-686.
59. Tittle V, Bull L, Boffito M, Nwokolo. Pharmacokinetic and pharmacodynamic drug interactions between antiretrovirals and oral contraceptives. *Clin Pharmacokinet*. 2015;54(1):23-34.
60. Kuhar DT, Henderson DK, Struble KA, et al. Updated US Public Health Service guidelines for the management of occupational exposures to human immunodeficiency virus and recommendations

for postexposure prophylaxis. *Infect Control Hosp Epidemiol.* 2013;34(9):875-892.

61. World Health Organization. Guidelines on post-exposure prophylaxis for HIV and the use of co-trimoxazole prophylaxis for HIV-related infections among adults, adolescents and children: recommendations for a public health approach. http://apps.who.int.ucsf.idm.oclc.org/iris/bitstream/10665/145719/1/9789241508193_eng.pdf?ua=1. Accessed on March 09, 2015.
62. Marrazzo JM, del Rio C, Holtgrave DR, et al. HIV prevention in clinical care settings: 2014 recommendations of the International Antiviral Society-USA Panel. *JAMA.* 2014; 312(4):390-409.
63. U.S. Public Health Service. Preexposure prophylaxis for the prevention of HIV infection in the United States—2014 clinical practice guideline. 2014. http://www.cdc.gov/hiv/prevention/research/prep/. Accessed June 13, 2014.
64. Lehtovirta P, Paavonen J, Heikinheimo O. Experience with the levonorgestrel-releasing intrauterine system among HIV infected women. *Contraception.* 2007;75(1):37-39.
65. U.S. Department of Health and Human Services, Health Resources and Services. A *Guide to the Clinical Care of Women with HIV—2013 Edition.* Rockville, MD: U.S. Department of Health and Human Services; 2013.
66. Update to CDC's U.S. Medical Eligibility Criteria for Contraceptive use 2010: revised recommendations for the use of hormonal contraception among women at high risk for HIV infection or infected with HIV. *MMWR.* 2012;61(24);449-452.
67. Centers for Disease Control and Prevention. Tracking the hidden epidemic: trends in STDs in the United States 2000. http://www.cdc.gov/std/Trends2000/trends 2000.pdf. Accessed June 13, 2014.
68. Chaturvedi AK. Beyond cervical cancer: burden of other HPV-related cancers among men and women. *J Adolesc Health.* 2010;46(4 suppl):S20-S26.
69. Kahn JA. HPV vaccination for the prevention of cervical intraepithelial neoplasia. *N Engl J Med.* 2009;361(3):271-278.
70. Karnes JB, Usatine RP. Management of external genital warts. *Am Fam Physician.* 2014;90(5):312-318.
71. Fathi R, Tsoukas MM. Genital warts and other HPV infections: established and novel therapies. *Clin Dermatol.* 2014;32(2):299-306.
72. Lopaschuk CC. New approach to managing genital warts. *Can Fam Physician.* 2013;59(7):731-736.
73. Centers for Disease Control and Prevention. The national plan to eliminate syphilis from the United States, 2006. http://www.cdc.gov/stopsyphilis/seeplan2006.pdf. Accessed June 9, 2014.
74. Patton ME, Su JR, Nelson R, Weinstock H. Primary and secondary syphilis—United States, 2005–2013. *MMWR.* 2014;63(18):402-406.
75. Peeling RW, Mabey DCW. Focus: syphilis. *Nature Rev Microb.* 2004;2(6):448-449.
76. Mattei PL, Beachkofsky TM, Gilson RT, Wisco OJ. Syphilis: a reemerging infection. *Am Fam Physician.* 2012;86(5):433-440.
77. Kent ME, Romanelli F. Reexamining syphilis: an update on epidemiology, clinical manifestations, and management. *Ann Pharmacother.* 2008;42(2):226-236.
78. Centers for Disease Control and Prevention. STD surveillance case definitions. 2014. http://www.cdc.gov/std/stats/CaseDefinitions-2014.pdf. Accessed June 10, 2014.
79. Musher DM. Biology of *Treponema pallidum.* In: Holmes KK, Mardh PA, Sparling PF, et al., eds. *Sexually Transmitted Disease.* New York: McGraw-Hill; 2008:205-222.

24 The Central Nervous System

William P. Fehder, Tekoa L. King

Chapter Glossary

Absence seizures Brief periods of unconsciousness that may or may not be accompanied by involuntary movement.

Akinesia Motor hypoactivity or muscular paralysis.

Bradykinesia Slowness of movements.

Catamenial seizure patterns Seizure exacerbation in relation to the menstrual cycle.

Dyskinesias Impaired ability to execute voluntary muscle movement. Also called extrapyramidal symptoms.

Extrapyramidal symptoms Disorders of movement associated with depletion of dopamine in the synapses of the extrapyramidal neurons on the pyramidal tract. Also called dyskinesias.

Focal seizures Seizures that originate within the neural networks of the cerebral cortex limited to one hemisphere. Formerly known as partial seizures.

Generalized seizures Seizures that involve both hemispheres of the cerebral cortex.

Inhibitory interneurons Multipolar neurons that become the connection between afferent neurons and efferent neurons. The cell body of the inhibitory interneuron is always in the central nervous system.

Muscarinic One of the two types of acetylcholine receptors; the other is nicotinic.

Neocortex Outermost layer of the cerebral hemispheres. It is approximately 2 to 4 mm thick and is the center for higher mental functions. It is the gray matter composed of neuronal cell bodies that surrounds the deeper white matter of the cerebrum. It consists of six horizontal layers.

Nonlinear kinetics Small increases in the dose of a drug that result in a much larger increase in plasma concentrations. For example, if the dose of phenytoin (Dilantin) is increased 50% from 300 mg/day to 450 mg/day, a tenfold increase in steady-state plasma concentration occurs. When the pharmacokinetics of a drug is linear, increases in dose result in a proportional increase in plasma concentrations.

Pyramidal neurons Type of neuron in the central nervous system that has a triangular-shaped cell body and a very long axon that extends through the layers of the cerebral cortex to form the corticospinal tract. The pyramidal neurons are excitatory and control motor function.

Pyramidal tract Collection of pyramidal neuron axons that extend from the cortex to the spinal cord. Also known as corticospinal tract.

Introduction

Health practitioners have used both naturally occurring and synthetic substances to alter processes within the central nervous system (CNS) for many years. This chapter reviews the disorders that originate in the central nervous system that are likely to be encountered by primary care providers. The pathophysiology and pharmacologic treatments for epilepsy, Parkinson's disease, Alzheimer's disease, attention-deficit disorder, restless leg syndrome, sleep disorders, and migraine headaches are reviewed, with special emphasis on how these disorders affect women. Although this may appear to be a diverse collection of disorders, all of these conditions share commonalities with regard to the neurotransmitter systems affected in the central nervous system, and there is significant overlap among these disorders in the drugs used to treat them. Psychiatric disorders and pharmacotherapeutics are discussed in the *Mental Health* chapter.

Anatomy and Physiology of the Cerebral Cortex

The human cerebrum is the largest and most highly developed portion of the human brain. The cerebrum consists of an outer thin layer of gray matter, which covers the inner core of myelinated nerves that make up the white matter. The cerebrum has an outer layer, called the cerebral cortex, as well as a subcortical layer, which consists of white matter. The outermost layer of the cerebral cortex is the **neocortex**, which, in terms of the evolution of the brain, developed most recently. The neocortex is the center for higher mental functions. Approximately 2 to 4 mm thick, it contains billions of neuronal cell bodies and unmyelinated fibers that are arranged horizontally in six horizontal layers.[1]

The two primary types of cells in the neocortex are excitatory **pyramidal neurons** and **inhibitory interneurons**. The pyramidal neurons have triangularly shaped cell bodies—hence their name. These neurons have many dendrites that receive input and one very long axial dendrite (axon) that provides output to other neurons. The axons extend over a distance vertically to other layers of the neocortex or the white matter before branching into terminal dendrites (Figure 24-1). The pyramidal neurons release the neurotransmitter glutamate.

The inhibitory neurons connect afferent neurons and efferent neurons in neural pathways. They interrupt or restrict activity paths. The axons of the inhibitory

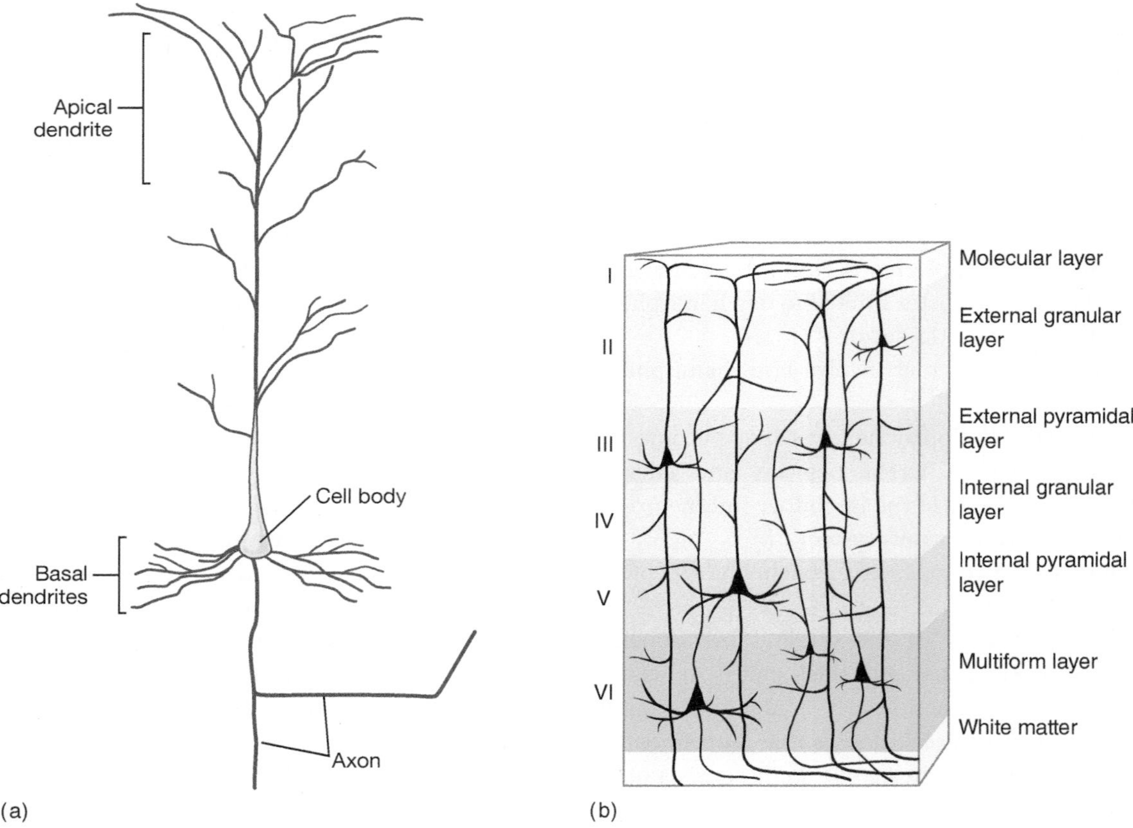

Figure 24-1 (a) The anatomy of the pyramidal neuron and (b) extrapyramidal tracts of the cerebral cortex.

interneuron release the neurotransmitter gamma-amino butyric acid (GABA).

The neurons in the neocortex are also arranged vertically in functional columns. The neurons in a column will have a certain common set of physiologic properties and function.[1] Thus, the cerebral cortex and much of the brain are organized both vertically in columns and tracts, permitting precise control of sensory and motor functions, and horizontally in association areas, which permits higher levels of processing.

Localized, discrete areas of the cerebral cortex on the surface of the brain have been extensively mapped (somatotopic maps) to establish the anatomy of motor and sensory pathways to and from the peripheral nervous system. Functional areas such as speech and memory centers (Brodmann areas) have also been identified in the cerebral cortex. The motor pathways from the cerebral cortex to the peripheral nervous system consist of large pyramidal neurons with long axons extending to the spinal cord, known as the **pyramidal tract** or corticospinal tract.

The cerebral white matter located beneath the cerebral cortex contains myelinated nerve fibers bundled into tracts that transmit nerve impulses to and from the cerebral cortex in three directions—between hemispheres (commissural tracts), between functional areas (association tracts), and in communication with lower areas of the central and peripheral nervous systems (projection tracts). Thus, there is a great deal of interconnection and coordination among the various components of the nervous system.

The regulation of neuronal activity in the CNS is based on a balance between excitatory neurons that use glutamate as their primary neurotransmitter and inhibitory neurons that use GABA as their primary neurotransmitter. The summation of the excitatory and inhibitory neuronal influences on postsynaptic neurons determines whether an electric threshold is reached and an impulse in the form of an action potential is generated.

Headaches

Approximately 90% of all individuals will experience a headache at some time in their life. Although most headaches are benign and fleeting, some may be serious and life threatening.[2] The International Classification of Headache Disorders (ICHD) was developed by the International Headache Society to assist clinicians in the diagnosis and classification of headache disorders.[3] The ICHD divides headaches into two broad categories: primary headache disorders, which do not have an anatomic or physiologic explanation, and secondary headaches, which occur as a result of another disease or disorder. The Resources table at the end of this chapter includes the website for the current ICHD-II and the beta version of ICHD-III, both of which list the extensive classifications of headache diagnoses and diagnostic criteria.

Most primary headaches fall into the categories of migraine, cluster, or tension-type headaches, all of which are reviewed in this chapter. Secondary headaches similarly have multiple etiologies. Acute withdrawal of drugs such as caffeine and alcohol and the misuse of certain migraine medications can cause a type of secondary headache. Disorders such as rhinosinusitis, vascular problems, infectious diseases, tempomandibular joint disorders, and intracranial neoplasms often cause headaches as well.[2] Finally, several vascular disorders—including stroke, carotid dissection, subdural hematoma, subarachnoid hemorrhage, dural venous thrombosis, temporal arteritis, and intracranial hemorrhage—can present with sudden-onset, intense headaches called "thunderclap headaches."

Many nonpharmacologic methods of treatment for headaches have demonstrated effectiveness, including acupuncture, trigger point injections, relaxation training, biofeedback, stress-management therapy.[4] Pharmacologic treatment for headaches can be abortive or preventive, with different classes of drugs being used for these two types of treatments.

Medication-Overuse Headache

Interestingly, headaches may be the result of overuse of medications used to treat primary or secondary headaches. Table 24-1 lists the medications that are likely to cause a medication-overuse headache if taken too often.[5–7] Triptans and ergotamine (Cafergot) are the most common cause of medication-overuse headache in the United States today. The headache associated with ergotamine appears to be one of the most severe of this type of headache.

Treatment of medication-overuse headaches initially begins with a tapered withdrawal of opiates or barbiturates and an abrupt withdrawal of other offending medications. Nonpharmacologic support in the form of short-term cognitive therapy may help as well as pharmacologic treatments for withdrawal symptoms such as antiemetics for nausea or beta blockers for restlessness. Depending on the severity of the problem, short-term hospitalization may be of value for some individuals.

Table 24-1 Medication-Overuse Headaches

Drug: Generic (Brand)	Diagnostic Criteria and Clinical Considerations
Acetaminophen (Tylenol)	Regular overuse for ≥ 10 days per month for > 3 months. Withdrawal is of longer duration than withdrawal from triptan medication-overuse headache.
Analgesics with butalbital	Can occur if used more than 5 days per month. Diagnosed following regular overuse for ≥ 10 days per month for > 3 months.
Analgesics with caffeine	Regular overuse for ≥ 10 days per month for > 3 months.
Barbiturates	Can occur if used more than 5 days per month. Risk is higher in women than in men.
Ergotamine (Cafregot)	Regular overuse for ≥ 10 days per month for > 3 months. Chronic use of ergotamine can cause a physical dependency.
Nonsteroidal anti-inflammatory drugs	Regular overuse for ≥ 15 days per month for ≥ 3 months.
Opiates	Can occur if used more than 8 days per month. Regular overuse for ≥ 10 days per month for > 3 months.
Triptans	Can occur if used more than 10 days per month. Regular overuse for ≥ 10 days per month for > 3 months.

Sources: Data from Cheung V, Maoozergar F, Dilli E. Medication overuse headache. *Curr Neurol Neurosci Rep.* 2015;15(1):509[6]; Evers S, Marziniak M. Clinical feathers, pathophysiology, and treatment of medication-overuse headache. *Lancet Neurol.* 2012;9(4):391-401[5]; Saper JR, Da Silva AN. Medication overuse headache: history, features, prevention and management strategies. *CNS Drugs.* 2013;27:867-877.[7]

Migraine Headaches

Migraines are a neurologic disorder characterized by recurring attacks that are usually severe and accompanied by altered body perceptions and aura, nausea, vomiting, and photophobia. Migraines have varied presentations: Some persons do not have the classic aura, while others have the altered sensation but no headache. Onset typically begins in adolescence or young adulthood before 30 years. Onset after 50 years is rare.

Migraine headaches are debilitating and represent a significant cost in terms of healthcare dollars spent, absence from work, and pain and suffering.[8] The results of large population surveys suggest migraine headaches are undertreated.[8] Although women may suffer from any form of headache, the incidence of migraine headaches has a 3:1 female-to-male ratio. The prevalence of migraine headaches in the United States is 18.2% in women and 6.5% in men.[8]

Migraines can be episodic or chronic. The four primary subtypes are: (1) migraine without aura; (2) migraine with aura; (3) chronic migraine; and (4) complicated migraines.[3] When migraines become chronic and occur daily, the headaches are referred to as transformed migraine. It usually takes several years for episodic migraines to evolve into daily transformed migraine.

Migraines are affected by reproductive hormones. Sixty percent of women who have migraines will have a subcategory called menstrually associated migraine. These women cyclically develop a migraine headache from 1 to 3 days before their menses to 3 days after the menses starts[9] (Box 24-1). They usually experience a remission during pregnancy and after menopause but often have more frequent headaches in the perimenopausal period.

Migraine headaches generally proceed through four stages. The prodrome stage, which starts up to 24 hours before the headache occurs, is characterized by increased or decreased perception, irritability, food cravings, fluid retention, and a variety of nondescript symptoms. The second stage is the development of an aura, which precedes the headache by an hour and may continue as the headache begins. Auras are characterized by flashing lights, numbness, or tingling and occur in 15% to 20% of persons who have migraines. The third stage is the period of disability secondary to the severe headache, which can last 4 to 72 hours. The final prodrome stage is a period of fatigue, muscle weakness, food intolerance, and another round of nondescript symptoms that are highly individualized. Diagnosis of migraines is based on specific criteria listed in the ICHD.[3]

Etiology of Migraine Headaches

Migraine is a neurovascular disorder, albeit one that is not yet completely characterized. Migraine is probably initiated as an event of cortical spreading depression in which a slowly propagating wave of transient neuronal depolarization is followed by repolarization. Cortical spreading depolarization causes the migraine aura and may serve as the trigger for the headache.[10,11] The resultant changes in cerebral blood flow, release of inflammatory mediators, and effects such as irritation of the meninges cause the pain of a migraine headache.[10] It is not clear yet if the neuronal event or blood vessel changes start the process. The neurotransmitter serotonin is an important player involved in the migraine process. Of particular importance are three serotonin receptor (5-HT_1) subtypes that influence cerebral vasodilation and trigeminal nerve stimulation—namely,

Box 24-1 A Case of Acute Headache Pain

MD, a 25-year-old female, presents to the urgent care center complaining of a headache. She describes the headache as unilateral and throbbing in quality. She characterizes the pain as an 8 on a 10-point scale. She states that this headache has been present for about 6 hours and has been unrelieved by acetaminophen (Tylenol). She denies any visual disturbances but states that bright lights and noise make the pain worse. MD typically gets a headache with the onset of her menses; this headache lasts anywhere from 5 to 48 hours. Her pain is intense enough that she often misses at least 1 day of work every month because of the headache. She has tried Excedrin (a combination formulation of acetaminophen, aspirin, and caffeine) to treat the pain in the past, without success.

After conducting a physical examination, the healthcare provider diagnoses MD with menstrually associated migraine. Several options are available to MD. Conventional abortive therapies such as nonsteroidal anti-inflammatory drugs (NSAIDs), triptans, or ergotamines may be helpful.

Abortive therapy with a long-acting triptan such as naratriptan (Amerge) or frovatriptan (Frova) can also be used as prophylaxis. When used prophylactically, these drugs are usually started 2 days before the onset of menses and continued for 5 to 6 days. NSAIDs have also been used prophylactically, starting 7 days prior to menses and continuing for 13 to 14 days. However, this dosing schedule may contribute to rebound headaches in some women. If menstrual cycles are not regular, this method of prophylaxis is not practical.

Estrogen supplementation may be useful when estrogen withdrawal triggers migraine. It may take the form of 100-mcg estrogen patches, started 2 days prior to menses and continued for 7 days. Combination monophasic oral contraceptives (COCs) such as Mircette, which has 10 mcg of estrogen during the last 5 days of the placebo week, may help prevent estrogen withdrawal migraines. Continuous-dose COCs such as (Seasonale) or (Seasonique) may also be useful in reducing the number of headaches. Women who have migraines with auras should not use COCs.

After reviewing the treatment options, MD selects naratriptan, 2.5 mg, to be repeated in 4 hours if there is no relief. She also plans to change her current contraception to a continuous 3-month option to reduce the number of menstrual cycles and use naratriptan prophylactically when she anticipates menses.

5-HT_{1B}, 5-HT_{1D}, and 5-HT_{1F}. In addition, vulnerability to migraines demonstrates a strong genetic component.

Treatment for Migraine Headaches

Treatment of migraine headaches includes both abortive therapy and prophylactic therapy. Abortive therapy should be combined with prophylactic therapy for persons who experience more than two or three headaches per month. Traditional treatment follows a classic series of steps wherein the potency of the medication is increased if less potent regimens prove to be ineffective. In step care, everyone starts with the same medications when the migraine starts. This approach can delay effective treatment for persons with severe pain. In contrast, the stratified care approach starts with a medication that is based on individual characteristics and level of disability. Stratified care has been definitively proven to be more efficacious in reducing the disability time and headache response 2 hours after initiating therapy.[12] The only potential disadvantage of stratified care is that more side effects of medication occur with this regimen. Adverse effects do not occur more frequently.

Abortive Treatment of Migraine Headaches

Abortive therapy for migraine headaches is aimed at achieving pain relief as rapidly as possible after onset of symptoms. Control of associated symptoms such as nausea and vomiting may also be needed. Mild to moderate migraine headaches may be successfully treated by acetaminophen (Tylenol), aspirin, or nonsteroidal anti-inflammatory drugs (NSAIDs) alone or in combination with caffeine. Occasionally, opioids may also be necessary for treatment of more severe migraines. However, because of the unique nature of migraine pain, drugs specifically designed to treat the underlying cause of pain are commonly used—triptans, isometheptene, ergotamine derivatives, and combination products. Detailed information on management of acute migraines is available in several published guidelines.[13–15]

Serotonin Agonists: Triptans

Triptans are the typical first-line abortive therapy for migraines. These medications are serotonin (5-HT$_{1B}$ and 5-HT$_{1D}$) receptor agonists. Triptans activate serotonin receptors located in the extracerebral and intracranial blood vessels to reverse cranial vessel constriction. Although all of the seven available triptans have similar chemical structures, they vary with regard to onset and duration of action, incidence of recurrent headache, and affinity for specific receptor agonists. Therefore, failure of one agent does not preclude successful use of an alternative triptan. The triptans most likely to be effective in the randomized clinical trials (RCTs) that have compared these agents head-to-head were rizatriptan (Maxalt), eletriptan (Relpax), and almotriptan (Axert), with eletriptan being most likely to provide short-term and sustained benefits.[16] Sumatriptan (Imitrex) offers the most variety in routes of administration. Variations among the triptans are detailed in Table 24-2.

Side Effects/Adverse Effects

Common side effects of triptans include flushing, tingling, sensation of heat, vertigo, fatigue, transient chest pain,

Table 24-2 Medications Used to Treat Migraine Headaches

Triptan: Generic (Brand)	Dose	Maximum per 24 Hours	Time to Peak Effect	Onset of Action	Duration of Effect	Clinical Considerations
Almotriptan (Axert)	6.5-, 12.5-mg tablets PO, 1 tablet every 2 hours	25 mg	1–3 hours	30–120 minutes		Not contraindicated if person is also using MAO inhibitors. Better tolerated than sumatriptan. Slow onset of action.
Eletriptan (Relpax)	20-, 40-mg tablets, 1 tablet PO every 2 hours	80 mg	1.5 hours	< 120 minutes	24 hours	Metabolized by CYP3A4. Do not use within 72 hours of CYP3A4 inhibitor. Bioavailability is increased by high-fat meal.
Frovatriptan (Frova)	2.5 mg PO, may repeat in 2 hours	7.5 mg	2–3 hours	120–180 minutes		Can be safely combined with MAO inhibitors. Slowest onset of action.
Naratriptan (Amerge)	1-, 2.5-mg tablets 2.5 mg PO every 4 hours	5 mg	2 hours	60–180 minutes		Can be safely combined with MAO inhibitors. Fewer headache recurrences than with sumatriptan.
Rizatriptan (Maxalt)	5-, 10-mg tablets 1 tablet PO every 2 hours	30 mg	1 hour	30–120 minutes		Orally disintegrating tablet available
Sumatriptan (Imitrex), intranasal	5 mg per spray 1 spray in both nostrils every 2 hours	40 mg	2 hours	30–60 minutes	1–1.5 hours	Faster onset than with tablet forms
Sumatriptan (Imitrex), oral	25-, 50-,100-mg tablets, 1 tablet PO every 2 hours, may repeat in 2 hours	200 mg	4 hours	20–60 minutes	2.5 hours	Incidence of recurrent headache within 24 hours is 40%
Sumatriptan (Imitrex), SQ	6 mg, may repeat in 1 hour	12 mg	2 hours	15 minutes	1.5–2 hours	Most rapid onset of action
Zolmitriptan (Zomig), nasal spray	2.5 mg PO	5 mg	2–4 hours	45 minutes		Orally disintegrating tablet available. Food has no significant effect on absorption. Fewer side effects than sumatriptan and naratriptan.
Zolmitriptan (Zomig), oral	1.25–2.5 mg PO	5 mg	2–4 hours	45 minutes		

Abbreviations: MAO = monoamine oxidase.

pruritus, dry mouth, and paresthesias. Sumatriptan has the highest rate of warmth, burning, and tingling sensations among the triptans.[17] Transient erythema may occur with injection. The intranasal formulations leave a bad taste in the person's mouth. Hypersensitivity to triptans is rare, but anaphylactic reactions have occurred.

Serious adverse effects of triptans occur secondary to their vasoconstricting properties and include coronary artery spasms, myocardial infarction or ischemia, hypertension, ventricular tachycardia and/or fibrillation, seizures, and transient ischemia attacks.

Contraindications

All triptans are contraindicated for individuals with uncontrolled hypertension, coronary artery disease, peripheral vascular disease, hepatic dysfunction, or any history of ischemic conditions. Individuals with renal impairment should use rizatriptan and sumatriptan with caution.

Drug–Drug Interactions

Triptans should not be used concurrently with ergotamine derivatives. Dosing of triptans and ergotamines should be separated by at least 24 hours to avoid the possibility of a prolonged vasospastic reaction. Different triptans should not be used in combination with one another because of the risk of vasospastic reactions. Triptans can also cause serotonin syndrome if taken concurrently with other serotonergic agonists such as selective serotonin reuptake inhibitors (SSRIs) or metoclopramide (Reglan), although the incidence of this complication appears to be rare.[17] The triptans are metabolized by monoamine oxidase (MAO), so concurrent use of MAO inhibitors can also cause toxicity. Additional drug interactions associated with triptans are summarized in Table 24-3.

Table 24-3 Selected Drug–Drug Interactions Associated with Triptans[a]

Drug: Generic (Brand)	Effect
All Triptans and	
Ergotrate derivatives	Increased incidence of vasospastic reactions
Almotriptan (Axert) and	
MAO inhibitors	Decreased clearance of almotriptan
Potent CYP3A4 inhibitors—ketoconazole, macrolides, protease inhibitors	Increased plasma concentrations of almotriptan
Eletriptan (Relpax) and	
Potent CYP3A4 inhibitors—ketoconazole, macrolides, protease inhibitors	Increased plasma concentrations of eletriptan; do not take within 72 hours of these drugs
Frovatriptan (Frova) and	
Oral contraceptives	Increased plasma concentrations of frovatriptan
Propranolol (Inderal)	Increased plasma concentrations of frovatriptan
Naratriptan (Amerge) and	
Oral contraceptives	Increased plasma concentrations of naratriptan
Sibutramine (Meridia)	Increased plasma concentrations of naratriptan
SSRIs, SNRIs	Increased levels of SSRIs and subsequent risk of serotonin syndrome
Rizatriptan (Maxalt) and	
Propranolol (Inderal)	Increased plasma concentrations of rizatriptan
MAO inhibitors	Increased plasma concentrations of rizatriptan
Sibutramine (Meridia)	Increased plasma concentrations of rizatriptan
Sumatriptan (Imitrex) and	
SSRIs, SNRIs	Increased risk of serotonin syndrome
MAO inhibitors	Increased plasma concentrations of sumatriptan
Zolmitriptan (Zomig) and	
Acetaminophen (Tylenol)	Delayed maximum concentration of acetaminophen
Cimetidine (Tagamet)	Doubled half-life of zolmitriptan
MAO inhibitors	Increased plasma concentrations of zolmitriptan
Oral contraceptives	Increased plasma concentration but delayed time to maximum concentration of zolmitriptan
Propranolol (Inderal)	Increased plasma concentrations of zolmitriptan
Isometheptene/Acetaminophen/Dichloralphenazone (Midrin) and	
MAO inhibitors	Increased plasma concentrations of isometheptene
All Ergotrate Derivatives and	
Triptans	Increases incidence of vasospastic reactions
Dihydroergotamine (Migranal) and	
Azoles	Increased cerebral and peripheral ischemia through induction of CYP3A4
Macrolide antibiotics	Increased cerebral and peripheral ischemia through induction of CYP3A4
Protease inhibitors	Increased cerebral and peripheral ischemia through induction of CYP3A4

Abbreviations: MAO = monoamine oxidase; SNRI = serotonin-norepinephrine reuptake inhibitor; SSRI = selective serotonin reuptake inhibitor.

[a] This table is not comprehensive as new information is being generated on a regular basis.

Table 24-4 Isometheptene Combination Products for Treatment of Migraines

Drug: Generic (Brand)	Dose	Maximum Dose	Clinical Considerations
Isometheptene/ acetaminophen/ caffeine (Podrin)	500 mg acetaminophen/20 mg caffeine/130 mg isometheptene 1–2 caplets PO to start, followed by 1 caplet every hour until relief is obtained	5 caplets/ 12 hours	Contraindicated for persons with glaucoma, heart disease, renal or hepatic impairment, or concurrent MAO inhibitor therapy. Acetaminophen has a black box warning about hepatotoxicity. Several clinically significant drug–drug interactions may occur. Avoid taking with ergotamines and pimozide. Dichloralphenazone is a prodrug that converts to chloral hydrate (sedative) and antipyrine (analgesic). May cause some drowsiness or dizziness.
Isometheptene/ acetaminophen/ dichloralphenazone (Nodolor)	325 mg acetaminophen/65 mg isometheptene/100 mg dichloralphenazone 1–2 caplets PO to start, followed by 1 caplet every hour until relief is obtained	8 caplets/ 24 hours	

Abbreviations: MAO = monoamine oxidase.

Isometheptene

Isometheptene is a sympathomimetic agent that causes vasoconstriction of the cerebral and cranial arterioles. It is available in combination formulations with acetaminophen and caffeine (Podrin) or with acetaminophen and dichloralphenazone (Nodolor) (Table 24-4). These combination formulations are contraindicated for individuals with glaucoma; severe renal or hepatic disease; coronary artery or other vascular diseases, or hypertension; and for persons taking MAO inhibitors. These agents are considered reasonable alternatives to triptans.[17]

Ergotamine Derivatives

Ergotamine was the etiology of an epidemic in the Middle Ages that caused countless deaths, a story that became the subject of many famous pieces of artwork from that time period. Persons who ate bread made of rye, wheat, and barley that was infected with the *Claviceps purpurea* fungus developed ergotism, which is also known as St. Anthony's fire.[18] This fungus contained ergot, which has remarkable vasoconstrictor effects and convulsive symptoms. The convulsive symptoms associated with its use include nausea, vomiting, spasms, and hallucinations similar to those produced by lysergic acid diethylamide (LSD), a derivative of ergot. The vasoconstrictor effects cause gangrene.

Ergotamine derivatives include ergotamine tartrate (Cafergot) and dihydroergotamine (Migranal) (Table 24-5). Ergotamines have lost favor as a first-line treatment for migraines in recent years secondary to their adverse-effect profile. However, they are effective if administered at the earliest sign of migraine. Their chief advantage is low cost.

Mechanism of Action

The exact mechanism by which ergotamine derivatives abort migraine attacks is unknown. Ergotamines are alpha-adrenergic antagonists. They are also serotonin receptor agonists and act directly on cranial arteries to promote vasoconstriction. Recent evidence also suggests that ergotamines exert an agonist effect at 5-HT_{1B} and 5-HT_{1D} receptors and may also block inflammation of the trigeminal vascular system.[19]

Ergotamine tartrate (Ergomar)—the prototype ergotamine—is available in oral, sublingual, rectal, and inhaled preparations. Its bioavailability is increased when the drug is delivered via the inhaled or rectal route. The half-life of ergotamine tartrate is approximately 2 hours, although effects of the drug may persist for 24 hours. Dihydroergotamine (Migranal) is available in only parenteral and inhaled forms because of its extensive hepatic first-pass effects.

Side Effects/Adverse Effects

Adverse effects of ergotamine are uncommon but include an increase in nausea and vomiting, which may be reduced by concomitant administration of a prokinetic drug such as metoclopramide (Reglan). Weakness, myalgias, numbness or tingling of the fingers and toes, angina-like pain, tachycardia, and bradycardia have also been reported. Dihydroergotamine is less likely to cause nausea and vomiting, but does cause diarrhea.

In overdose or chronic use scenarios, ergotamines can cause ergotism, a serious disorder associated with acute peripheral ischemia. Constriction of the peripheral arteries results in muscle pain; intermittent claudication; pale, cold extremities; and numbness. Gangrene of extremities can develop if this condition is not recognized and treated. Individuals should be instructed to immediately discontinue any ergot and seek immediate medical attention should such signs or symptoms occur.

Contraindications

Ergotamines are contraindicated for women during pregnancy and for those with coronary artery disease, peripheral

Table 24-5 Ergotamines

Drug: Generic (Brand)	Dose	Maximum Dose	Time to Peak Effect	Onset of Action	Duration of Effect	Clinical Considerations
Dihydroergotamine mesylate[a] (Migranal)	Nasal spray 0.5 mg/spray	4 sprays in each nostril/attack or 6 sprays/day or 8 sprays/week	15–45 minutes	15–30 minutes	8 hours	All ergotamine formulations are contraindicated during pregnancy and for persons with peripheral artery disease, coronary heart disease, hypertension, or impaired renal or hepatic function. Nausea and vomiting are common (10% of users). Numbness and tingling in the toes may occur. Risk of rebound headache. FDA black box warning states that ergot alkaloids should not be taken concurrently with potent inhibitors of CYP3A4, which include azole drugs, HIV protease inhibitors, and macrolide antibiotics. Other peripheral vasoconstricting drugs such as triptans or beta blockers, and serotonin receptor agonists should also be avoided. Dihydroergotamine has fewer side effects than ergotamine.
Ergotamine/caffeine[a] (Cafergot)	1 mg ergotamine/100-mg caffeine 2 tablets PO at onset, 1 tablet PO every 30 minutes	6 tablets per attack	2 hours	Variable, depending on duration of headache prior to administration, but faster than ergotamine tartrate than with addition of caffeine	Variable	
Ergotamine/caffeine suppository[a]	2 mg ergotrate/100-mg caffeine rectal suppository	2 per attack or 10 mg (5 suppositories)/week	1 hour		Variable	
Ergotamine sublingual (Ergomar)[a]	2 mg, 1 tablet under tongue at first sign of migraine and let dissolve, then 2 mg sublingual every 30 minutes	6 mg/24 hours or 10 mg/week	Variable	Variable	Variable	
Ergotamine tartrate (Ergomar)[a]	2-mg tablets, use 1 PO every 30 min	6 mg	2 hours	Variable, depending on duration of headache prior to administration	Variable	

[a] Ergotism is possible if this medication is taken concurrently with macrolide antibiotics or other CY3A4 inhibitors. The drug is contraindicated during pregnancy and for persons with peripheral artery disease, coronary heart disease, hypertension, or impaired renal or hepatic function. Do not take with other peripheral vasoconstricting drugs such as triptans or beta blockers.

vascular disease, sepsis, uncontrolled hypertension, and renal or hepatic impairment.

Drug–Drug Interactions

Ergotamines have multiple clinically significant drug–drug interactions, as they are metabolized via CYP450 enzymes. Drugs that inhibit CYP3A4 will inhibit metabolism of ergotamine. This can result in ergotism, which can be severely disabling. The FDA has mandated that ergotamines' labels carry a black box warning stating that these drugs are contraindicated for persons using protease inhibitors, azole antifungals, and some macrolide antibiotics. In addition, these drugs should never be used in combination other serotonin receptor agonists such as triptans or SSRIs. The third category of concern is concomitant use of other alpha or beta agonists, because ergotamines will potentiate the vasoconstricting effect of the alpha or beta agonists. Dosing of triptans and ergotamines should be separated by at least 24 hours to avoid the possibility of a prolonged vasospastic reaction. Persons taking ergotamines should also avoid grapefruit juice because it can cause increased blood levels of ergotamine.

Prophylactic Treatment of Migraine Headaches

The goal of preventive migraine therapy is to reduce attack frequency, duration, and severity; improve responsiveness to treatment of acute attacks; and improve function and reduce disability. Preventive therapy should be considered for individuals who experience more than 6 headache days per month, or at least 3 headache days with severe impairment.[20]

Many agents are useful for migraine prevention. Table 24-6 summarizes the first-line agents used for migraine prophylaxis. Published practice guidelines from the United States Headache Consortium are available to help clinicians individualize preventive treatment appropriately.[14,15,20]

Triptans may also be used as short-term preventive agents for women with menstrually associated migraines. Therapy is most effective when started 2 to 3 days before menses and continued until 3 days after the onset. Triptans with longer half-lives, such as naratriptan (Amerge) and frovatriptan (Frova) twice daily, have demonstrated effectiveness for short-term prophylaxis.

Table 24-6 Drugs Used as Prevention Therapy for Migraine Headaches

Drug: Generic (Brand)	Dose and Administration	Advantages	Side Effects/ Adverse Effects	Clinical Considerations
Antiepileptics				
Divalproex (Depakote)	250–500 mg PO 2 times/day Clinical effectiveness at 500–1500 mg/day	Very effective; mild to moderate side effects	Fatigue, weight gain, tremor, hair loss, liver toxicity, pancreatitis, memory impairment, cognitive dysfunction. Teratogenic. All AEDs increase the risk for suicidality.	Established effectiveness. Avoid during pregnancy and in persons with liver impairment.
Topiramate (Topamax)	50 mg PO 2 times/day			
Valproate	Clinical effectiveness at 800–1500 PO mg/day			
Tricyclic Antidepressants				
Amitriptyline (Elavil)	10–150 mg PO/day	Mild to moderate side effects. Most effective in persons with mixed migraine and tension headaches.	Drowsiness, weight gain, anticholinergic symptoms. Lowered seizure threshold may cause dysrhythmias in excessive doses.	Probably effective. Avoid in persons with acute-angle glaucoma or seizures.
Beta Blockers				
Atenolol (Tenormin)	100 mg PO once daily	Atenolol and nadolol are probably effective. Metoprolol, propranolol, and timolol have established effectiveness. Inexpensive; useful in persons with coexisting cardiovascular disease.	Mild to moderate side effects. Fatigue, exercise intolerance, depression, insomnia. Can take several weeks to become effective.	Avoid in persons with asthma, uncontrolled diabetes, hypotension, and heart block
Metoprolol (Lopressor)	100 mg/day PO in 2 divided doses			
Nadolol (Corgard)	80 mg PO once daily			
Propranolol (Inderal)	80–240 mg/day PO			
Timolol (Blocadren)	10–15 mg PO 2 times/day			
ACE Inhibitors				
Lisinopril (Zestril)	20 mg/day PO	Inexpensive; generally well tolerated and effective	Increased incidence of cough. Teratogenic.	Possibly effective. Avoid in pregnancy.
Angiotensin Receptor Blockers				
Candesartan (Atacand)	16 mg/day PO	Reduces need for rescue therapy	Teratogenic.	Possibly effective. Avoid in pregnancy.

Abbreviations: ACE = angiotensin-converting enzyme; AED = antiepileptic drug.

Tension-Type Headaches

Tension-type headaches affect more than 40% of adults worldwide and, therefore, are the most common form of headache.[21] These headaches are bilateral and have a pressing or tightening quality, with mild to moderate intensity; routine activity does not aggravate them.[3] The exact pathophysiology is unclear.

Over-the-counter (OTC) NSAIDs or acetaminophen (Tylenol) are generally effective for relieving the pain of a tension headache. The dose of simple analgesics used in studies that showed effectiveness is generally 1000 mg of acetaminophen, 400 mg of ibuprofen (Advil), or 25 mg of ketoprofen.[22] Use of these agents should be limited to no more than 2 times per week to avoid medication-overuse rebound headaches.

If simple analgesics are not effective, adjunctive use of a sedative antihistamine such as diphenhydramine (Benadryl) or promethazine (Phenergan) can be used. An OTC combination formulation of aspirin (500 mg) or acetaminophen (1000 mg) with caffeine (Excedrin) or a prescription formulation of aspirin 325 mg, caffeine 40 mg, and butalbital 50 mg (Fiorinal) can be more effective than analgesics alone. However, the combination drugs that include caffeine are likely to cause a medication-overuse headache if taken too often. Products with butalbital are especially likely to cause rebound headaches and should not be used more than 4 times per month. These agents are generally no longer recommended.[23]

When tension-type headaches are chronic, preventive therapies are needed. Nonpharmacologic preventative treatments such as biofeedback, relaxation techniques, and cognitive-behavioral therapy have all shown some effectiveness in this indication. Botulinum toxin A injections and trigger point injections with lidocaine both appear to have a modest effect in reducing the number of chronic headaches per month.[24,25] However, the mainstay pharmacologic treatment is the tricyclic antidepressant amitriptyline, which is usually given as 10 to 12.4 mg once daily. The dose can be increased to a maximum of 100 to 125 mg daily if necessary.[21]

Cluster Headaches

Cluster headaches are unilateral, generally temporal or periorbital, and severe. They tend to last 15 to 180 minutes and are often accompanied by autonomic symptoms such as restlessness, agitation, tearing, nasal stuffiness, orbital swelling, or drooping eyelid.[26] Cluster headaches are the least likely to be seen in primary care, with incidence of approximately 1 per 1000 persons. They are slightly more common in men than in women. Abortive therapy for cluster headaches includes oxygen and a triptan such as sumatriptan (Imitrex) or zolmitriptan (Zomig). Although less evidence supports its effectiveness, ergotamine and octreotide (Sandostatin; administered subcutaneously) have also been used.[26] Verapamil at a minimum dosage of 240 mg per day is the first-line treatment for prophylaxis of cluster headaches.

Special Populations: Pregnancy, Lactation, and the Elderly

Although there is no evidence of harm to human fetuses following in utero exposure to triptans, animal studies have yielded evidence of teratogenesis. As a consequence, triptans are generally avoided during pregnancy. The manufacturer's pregnancy registry for sumatriptan collected data for 558 infants who were exposed to this drug and found no increase in major congenital anomalies or pattern of specific anomalies.[27] The pregnancy registry was then closed. At this time, sumatriptan is considered acceptable for use by women during pregnancy if simpler analgesics are not effective.

Triptans may be excreted in breast milk, although adverse effects on the infant have not been well studied. Sumatriptan is approved by the American Academy of Pediatrics for use with breastfeeding.[28]

Ergotamines are contraindicated for use during pregnancy because these drugs induce uterine contractions, which can cause fetal harm or miscarriage. Ergotamine tartrate has been linked to vomiting, diarrhea, and convulsions in the neonate when used in lactating women at levels required to suppress migraines.[28]

Migraines are rare after menopause, and evidence is limited on the use of triptans by persons in this age group. Triptans should be used cautiously because of the increased risk of comorbidities such as coronary artery disease, hypertension, or other cardiovascular conditions that may be exacerbated by triptans. Ergotamines should be used cautiously by postmenopausal women because there is an increased risk of comorbidities, such as coronary artery disease, hypertension, or other cardiovascular conditions, that may be worsened by ergotamines.

Sleep Disorders

Sleep disorders are subcategorized into insomnia, daytime sleepiness, or disrupted sleep. Sleep disturbances such as sleep apnea or narcolepsy are primary sleep disturbance diagnoses. Sleep disturbance can also be a symptom of another medical condition such as hyperthyroidism, restless leg syndrome, periodic leg movement disorder, depression, or substance abuse.[29] Insomnia occurs more frequently in women than in men and is commonly associated with the menstrual cycle, pregnancy, postpartum, and menopause.[29–31] The incidence of sleep disturbances increases as women age.

The relationship between sleep disturbance and depression is a good example of how sleep disturbances can affect one's health. This relationship is probably bidirectional, in that sleep disturbances make depression worse, and vice versa. Therefore, identifying and treating insomnia or sleep disturbances can be an important primary or adjunct therapy for a range of conditions.[32]

Once a diagnosis has been made and treatment is determined to be necessary, a large number of nonpharmacologic and pharmacologic therapies are available to treat sleep disturbances. Nonpharmacologic therapies may be preferred, but they take effect more slowly and few studies have documented the effectiveness of these interventions. Nonetheless, behavioral therapies such as stimulus control and sleep restriction during the day appear to be as efficacious as some of the medications used in the short term, and more efficacious for long-term treatment. Other nonpharmacologic therapies that are often recommended but for which there is limited evidence of effectiveness include meditation, hypnotherapy, and biofeedback.

Table 24-7 Selected Drugs Used as Sleep Aids

Drug: Generic (Brand)	Dose Range	Onset of Action	Half-life	FDA Approved for Treating Insomnia
Benzodiazepines				
Estazolam (ProSom)	1–2 mg	Slow	10–24 hours	Yes, short-term
Flurazepam (Dalmane)	15–30 mg	Rapid	40–114 hours	Yes, short-term
Quazepam (Doral)	7.5–15 mg	Intermediate	28–114 hours	Yes
Temazepam (Restoril)	7.5–30 mg	Slow	3.5–18.4 hours	Yes, short-term
Triazolam (Halcion)	0.125–0.5 mg	Intermediate	2.3 hours	Yes, short-term
Non-benzodiazepine Sedatives				
Eszopiclone (Lunesta)	1–3 mg	30 minutes	6–9 hours	Yes
Zaleplon (Sonata)	5–20 mg	Rapid	1 hour	Yes, short-term, up to 5 weeks
Zolpidem, extended release (Ambien CR)	6.25 mg (females) or 6.25–12.5 mg (males)	30 minutes	1.4–4.5 hours	Yes
Zolpidem IR (Ambien)	5 mg (females) or 5–10 mg (males)		1.4–4.5 hours	Yes, short-term
Zolpidem, sublingual tablet (Edluar)	5 mg (females) or 5–10 mg (males)		1.4–6.7 hours	Yes, short-term
Zolpidem, sublingual tablet (Intermezzo)	1.75 mg (female) or 3.5 mg (male)		1.4–6.7 hours	Yes for middle-of-the-night insomnia
Melatonin Agonists				
Ramelteon (Rozerem)	8 mg	30 minutes	1–3 hours	Yes
Antidepressants				
Doxepin (Silenor)	3–6 mg	—	15 hours	Yes
Trazodone (Oleptro)	25–200 mg	1–3 hours	7–10 hours	No, off-label use
Over-the-Counter Antihistamines				
Diphenhydramine (Benadryl)	25–200 mg	2 minutes	7–12 hours	Yes
Doxylamine (Unisom)	25 mg	2–4 minutes	10–12 hours	Yes

The current FDA-approved medications for sleep disorders include several benzodiazepines, non-benzodiazepine sedating agents, a melatonin receptor agonist (Ramelteon), and doxepin (Silenor). Most are approved for a duration of less than 35 days. Eszopiclone (Lunesta) is the exception: No restriction is placed on the duration of therapy for this agent. Barbiturates also have FDA approval for treating sleep disorders, but these medications are not recommended for the treatment of insomnia due to the weak evidence, problematic side-effect profiles, narrow therapeutic indexes, and high risk for dependence.[33] Given their limited use, these agents will not be discussed in this chapter.

Some non–FDA-approved medications may also be used in the treatment of insomnia; these include sedating antidepressants, antipsychotics, anticonvulsants, antihistamines, melatonin, and numerous herbal agents. Table 24-7 reviews drugs commonly used as sleep aids.

Drugs That Cause Sleep Disturbance

Several medications can cause sleep disturbances. Nicotine and caffeine are well-known stimulants. Bronchodilators, central nervous system stimulants, pseudoephedrine, methyldopa (Aldomet), beta blockers, alpha-adrenergic blockers, and cholinesterase inhibitors are all stimulants that can interfere with sleep.[29,34] Less well known are the sleep disturbances caused by some medications that are sedating. SSRIs, SNRIs, MAO inhibitors, and bupropion (Wellbutrin) alter sleep patterns and can cause sleep that is not restful.[33]

Hormone Therapy for Sleep Disturbances

Hormone therapy deserves special mention. Such therapy has traditionally been recommended for menopause-related insomnia; however, it has limited effectiveness when objective measures of sleep are studied. The various estrogen and progesterone components have differential effects on sleep.[35] Hormone therapy is effective for treatment of menopause-related vasomotor symptoms, including night sweats, and may have an indirect positive effect on sleep via this mechanism of action; however, the exact mechanisms by which hormones may improve sleep disorders remain unknown.[35] Similarly, antidepressants can have an indirect effect on sleep by improving menopausal symptoms such as vasomotor symptoms, mood swings, or pain, and are considered a possible option for women who do not want to use hormone therapy.[35]

Antihistamines

As their name implies, antihistamines block the action of the neurotransmitter histamine, and their anticholinergic side effects include sedation and dry mouth.[34] The antihistamines diphenhydramine (Benadryl) and doxylamine (Unisom) are widely available on an OTC basis, and many women prefer to try one of them before accepting a prescription sleep aid. Although antihistamines can be effective for short-term or occasional use, they tend to lose their effectiveness as hypnotics within 1 or 2 weeks as the individual develops tolerance.[36] If the antihistamine is discontinued following prolonged use, rebound insomnia may occur.

In addition, diphenhydramine (Bendadryl) can induce sleepiness the next day after it is used secondary to its long half-life. This drug can cause increased intraocular pressure, urinary retention, and other classic anticholinergic effects such as dry mouth, constipation, blurred vision, and rarely delirium.

Benzodiazepines

The benzodiazepine receptor agonists are classified into two categories: (1) those that are hypnotics, which include alprazolam (Xanax), clonazepam (Klonopin), diazepam (Valium), flurazepam (Dalmane), lorazepam (Ativan), temazepam (Restoril), and triazolam (Halcion); and (2) those that act at benzodiazepine receptors but have a non-benzodiazepine structure, which include eszopiclone (Lunesta), zaleplon (Sonata), and zolpidem (Ambien).[37]

For most individuals, benzodiazepines can be very helpful in providing restful sleep, calming anxiety, and treating occasional panic attacks. All benzodiazepines are Schedule IV controlled substances and require a written prescription because of their risk for addiction as well as their value as street drugs. The risk for addiction appears to be highest among persons with a preexisting substance abuse problem or psychiatric disorder.[37,38]

Benzodiazepines are frequently categorized based on their half-life as short, intermediate, or long acting. The short-acting benzodiazepines such as alprazolam (Xanax) are most closely associated with dependence because they take effect quickly and wear off suddenly, causing withdrawal symptoms including shakiness, nausea, and rebound anxiety.[38,39] The longer-acting clonazepam (Klonopin) has some mood-stabilizing effect and tends to be metabolized slowly, without rebound effects. The effects of diazepam (Valium), another long-acting benzodiazepine, can last for several days.[40,41]

Side effects of benzodiazepines include ataxia, daytime sedation, cognitive impairment, motor incoordination, memory loss, and rebound insomnia. All of these effects are more pronounced in elderly individuals. Occasional paradoxical effects of benzodiazepines can include increased anxiety, suicidal thoughts, and mania. This group of medications often requires ongoing increases in doses to obtain the desired effect.[33,40] In 2007, the FDA requested that manufacturers of all benzodiazepines include language on the medication label about risks for allergic reactions and complex sleep behaviors including sleep-driving.[33] Benzodiazepines must be tapered slowly after prolonged use to avoid rebound effects.[42] Moreover, although these drugs are rarely lethal when used alone, overdoses can prove lethal if they are taken concurrently with alcohol or other CNS depressants.[38,39]

Most benzodiazepines are metabolized in the liver via the CYP450 enzyme system and may have high plasma levels if taken concomitantly with CYP450 inhibitors such as azole antibiotics, clarithromycin (Biaxin), and erythromycin (E-Mycin). Omeprazole (Prilosec) increases the plasma levels of diazepam (Valium). Conversely, CYP450 inducers such as rifampin (Rifadin), phenytoin (Dilantin), and carbamazepine (Tegretol) can decrease effectiveness of benzodiazepines. Of import is the potential combination of certain antidepressants (including fluoxetine [Prozac]) and alprazolam (Xanax). Depression is often accompanied by insomnia, and if both of these drugs are taken together, the plasma levels of alprazolam can be significantly increased.[43]

Non-benzodiazepines: The "Z Drugs"

The search for the perfect sleep medication has led to the development of several new brand-name drugs in recent years. These agents are heavily advertised in the popular media. Zolpidem (Ambien) was the first non-benzodiazepine introduced, followed by zaleplon (Sonata) and eszopiclone (Lunesta). In 2009, the FDA approved zolpidem tartrate for treating insomnia.

The non-benzodiazepines, which are informally referred to as "Z drugs," are structurally different from the benzodiazepine drugs. These agents are agonists for the same GABAergic receptors in the central nervous system; however, they are more selective for one GABA receptor configuration and have a shorter half-life and duration of action, which explains why they have fewer side effects and adverse effects.[44]

Side effects of the Z drugs may include somnolence, headache, dizziness, nausea, rebound insomnia, and anterograde amnesia. In addition, these agents may cause residual effects during the daytime or complex sleep-related behaviors, including sleep-driving or sleep-eating.[44,45] The risks of tolerance, dependence, and withdrawal persist with the Z drugs; however, rates are lower than traditional benzodiazepimes.[44]

The Z drugs are metabolized via CYP450 enzymes and, therefore, are subject to several drug–drug interactions. As with the benzodiazepines, CYP450 inhibitors can increase plasma levels and therapeutic effects of the Z drugs, while CYP450 inducers can interfere with their effectiveness. Dose reductions may be required if one of these agents is taken concomitantly with erythromycin, ketoconazole, or cimetidine, whereas the dose may need to be increased if rifampin (Rifadin) is being administered simultaneously with a Z drug.[44] There has been minimal research on the safety of the non-benzodiazepines during pregnancy and lactation.

Tricyclic Antidepressants

The tricyclic antidepressant (TCA) group includes two drugs that are often used for sleep. Low-dose amitriptyline (Elavil) has long been used for the treatment of gynecologic pain conditions; however, there is minimal evidence for use in vulvodynia.[46] At slightly higher doses, it can also be helpful to induce sleep. Doxepin (Silenor) is another TCA that is used more often for sleep than for depression. Both amitriptyline and doxepin are available as inexpensive generic preparations.[47]

The tetracyclic antidepressant trazodone (Desyrel) is often prescribed by psychiatric clinicians.[40,48] Trazodone is known for its ability to cause priapism among men, and it has been cited as a possible factor in case reports of clitoral pain among women. Overall, the safety and effectiveness of trazodone make it a useful hypnotic, especially in those persons with a history of substance abuse.[48]

Melatonin and Ramelteon

Many women are interested in using natural aids to help restore normal sleep cycles. Recent research on the endocrine hormone melatonin indicates that it may be helpful in regulating circadian rhythms and restoring a normal sleep–wake cycle. Melatonin is produced by the pineal gland and helps maintain circadian rhythm. It is available as an OTC food supplement, and some persons find it effective in inducing sleep or relieving the discomforts of jet lag.[47,49] The most common side effects reported with this agent are nausea, drowsiness, headache, and dizziness.[50] Melatonin has not been studied for its safety in pregnancy and lactation.

In addition to OTC melatonin, ramelteon (Rozerem) is a selective melatonin agonist at the MT_1 and MT_2 receptors. It is approved for insomnia related to difficulty initiating sleep. Common side effects include somnolence, dizziness, nausea, fatigue, and headache.[51] Ramelteon has not been associated with tolerance or abuse, so it may be appropriate for persons who do not want to take a controlled substance or for persons with a history of substance abuse. Administration with fatty foods should be avoided.

Seizures: An Overview

When a dysregulation of the balance between excitatory and inhibitory neuronal influences occurs, pathologic conditions such as epilepsy, Parkinson's disease, or Alzheimer's disease may arise. Behavioral manifestations of a seizure are determined by the site in the cortex at which the seizure arises. The long pyramid-shaped neurons appear to play a significant role in many types of epilepsy. The axons of pyramidal cells have collateral branches that make local connections between association areas of the cerebral cortex. Many of these axon connections are excitatory in nature, and this arrangement can result in an abnormal synchronous discharge of large numbers of neurons during an epileptic seizure. A small focus of excitatory neural activity can spread horizontally and vertically through the brain by synchronous discharge of increasing numbers of neurons, producing one of several types of seizure activity depending on the extent and areas of the brain recruited. Seizure activity can be partial or generalized seizures.[52]

Types of Seizures

Nonepileptic seizures, such as those provoked by abnormal metabolic conditions or drugs, must be differentiated from epileptic seizures. Similarly, the seizure associated with preeclampsia/eclampsia is different and addressed in the *Labor* chapter. Abnormal physical and metabolic conditions can cause seizures that are referred to as provoked seizures. Electrolyte imbalances, such as hypocalcemia, water intoxication, uremia, hypoglycemia, hypoxia, and alkalosis, can all cause seizure. The rapid withdrawal of sedative-hypnotic drugs such as alcohol, barbiturates, benzodiazepines, and antiepileptic drugs may precipitate seizure activity. Conversely, some drugs lower the threshold for seizures and may increase the risk that a seizure will occur (Table 24-8).[53]

Table 24-8 Drugs That May Lower the Seizure Threshold

Category	Drugs: Generic (Brand)
Antiasthmatics	Aminophylline, theophylline (Theo-Dur), albuterol
Antibiotics	Isoniazid (INH), lindane (Kwell, Kwellada lotion 1%), metronidazole (Flagyl), nalidixic acid (NegGram), penicillins, fluconazole (Diflucan)
Antidepressants	Tricyclic antidepressants, serotonin-specific agents, bupropion (Wellbutrin)
Hormones	Insulin, prednisone, estrogen
Immunosuppressants	Chlorambucil (Leukeran), cyclosporine (Sandimmune)
Local anesthetics	Lidocaine, bupivacaine, procaine
Opioids	Fentanyl (Sublimaze), meperidine (Demerol), pentazocine (Talwin), propoxyphene (Darvocet), tramadol (Ultram)
Psychostimulants	Amphetamines, cocaine, methylphenidate (Ritalin), phenylpropanolamine, heroin
Neuroleptics	Clozapine, phenothiazines, butyrophenones
Other	Anticholinergics, anticholinesterases, antihistamines, baclofen (Lioresal, Kemstro), heavy metals, hyperbaric oxygen, lithium (Lithobid), mefenamic acid, oral hypoglycemics, oxytocin

Source: Modified from Bromfield EB. Epilepsy and the elderly. In: Schachter SC, Schomer DL, eds. *The Comprehensive Evaluation and Treatment of Epilepsy.* San Diego, CA: Academic Press; 1997:233-254.[53]

Epilepsy

Classification and Diagnosis

The specific type of medication that is useful for the treatment of epileptic seizures depends on the nature of the seizure and its underlying pathophysiology. Attempts to classify seizure disorders were first proposed in 1970 by Gastaut and later redefined in 1989 by the Commission on Classification and Terminology of the International League Against Epilepsy.[54] The classification system used today was updated in 2010 and can be found in the Resources table at the end of this chapter.

Seizures that begin at some point of the cerebral cortex limited to one hemisphere are now classified as **focal seizures**, whereas seizures that originate at some point and rapidly engage bilaterally distributed neuronal networks are termed **generalized seizures**. The hormonal changes associated with menstruation produce **catamenial seizure patterns** in approximately one-third of women with epilepsy. "Catamenial" is derived from the Greek word *katamenios*, which means "monthly." The catamenial seizure pattern has been defined as increased seizure frequency that begins either immediately before or during menses.[57] Women with this type of epilepsy may experience exacerbations of their seizures during ovulation or around the time of menstruation.

Initiating Drug Therapy

The decision to start an individual on antiepileptic medication is complex because it must balance the risks of seizures, including the rare risk of death, against the risks of medications that often have significant adverse effects. The goal of drug treatment in epilepsy is to identify a single medication that is effective in eliminating or reducing the symptoms, thereby avoiding the side effects of multiple-drug therapy or treating the woman with a sequence of ineffective single medications. Because these drugs do have adverse effects, one of the primary concerns in choosing an agent is the side-effect profile. Despite the problems associated with these drugs, between 60% and 70% of persons with a new diagnosis of epilepsy are able to become seizure free when taking an appropriate medication used as monotherapy. Furthermore, most individuals who achieve complete seizure control can successfully discontinue their medication.[58]

There are no pharmacologic agents available at this time that protect against the development of epilepsy or cure it.[59]

Thus, there remains a role for novel nonpharmacologic approaches, such as neurosurgery and vagus nerve stimulators for individuals who have intractable epilepsy as well as for persons who are unable to tolerate antiepileptic drugs.

Antiepileptic Drugs

The term *antiepileptic drug* (AED) is used interchangeably with *anticonvulsant.* The AEDs are classified into five chemical groups: hydantoins, barbiturates, succinimides, oxazolidinediones, and acetylureas. A sixth "miscellaneous" classification of AEDs includes drugs from many different chemical families. Several new drugs for epilepsy were introduced in the 1990s. Thus, in clinical practice, the drugs used to treat epilepsy are commonly classified into the older, traditional AEDs and the newer AEDs. The newer AEDs were initially approved as add-on therapy for individuals who had refractory seizures despite treatment with one of the older AEDs (Box 24-2).[60] The use of the newer AEDs as replacements for older ones is a subject of debate, in that evidence is lacking that the newer AEDs are more effective. Some evidence-based guidelines advocate for the use of the newer AEDs because they have fewer side effects and fewer drug–drug interactions.[61] These drugs are increasingly being used for other conditions such as bipolar disorder, depression, chronic pain, and migraine headaches, all of which affect women more often than men. The newer AEDs are also used to treat menopausal hot flashes and pelvic pain. Thus a basic understanding of how these drugs work is of import for clinicians who care for women of all ages.

Mechanism of Action

Most AEDs prevent seizure activity by altering the balance of excitation and inhibition of neurons via one of three basic mechanisms: (1) modulation of the voltage-gated calcium and sodium channels that perpetrate conduction of the impulse along the axon; (2) enhancement of the neurotransmitter GABA that inhibits stimulation of the postsynaptic neuron; or (3) attenuation of brain excitation via inhibition of glutamate, which is the most abundant excitatory neurotransmitter in the brain (Figure 24-2).

Box 24-2 New Drug Evaluation for Effectiveness of Antiepileptic Drugs

When a new drug is developed for treating persons who have a serious medical condition that requires medication, the new drug cannot be tested for effectiveness in a randomized controlled trial that includes a placebo group because it is unethical to withhold treatment from persons with serious medical disorders. The story of how the new AEDs were evaluated is a good illustration of some of the problems involved in testing new drugs.

Eight "new AEDs" were tested in randomized controlled trials, each of which enrolled two groups of participants. The first group was treated with a traditional AED only. The second group was treated with a traditional AED and one of the newer AEDs added. Persons in both groups were followed for 8 to 12 weeks. If the group whose members took the new AED had 50% fewer seizures from their baseline rate of seizure activity, the new AED was determined to be effective. Although this design might sound reasonable, several methodological problems emerged with its use.

Because this study design was able to evaluate the new AED only in the role of adjunct medication, the FDA approved these drugs only as adjunct medications. Moreover, such a study design is likely to underestimate effectiveness and overestimate toxicity. The individuals who were enrolled in the study had more seizures than most persons with epilepsy, and responder rates are often less than 50%. Therefore, the new AEDs that were effective in combination with traditional AEDs were not fully evaluated for effectiveness in a standard clinical population. Also, upon close reading of the studies, it appears that these drugs were titrated down much more rapidly than is currently recommended, and the sudden decreases in plasma levels were responsible for many of the toxicities that were noted in the studies.

What is a clinician to do? Monotherapy has several important advantages. Notably, it is safer and has fewer drug–drug interactions. In addition, monotherapy is less expensive and compliance is higher. Therefore, many of the newer AEDs are used on an off-label basis as monotherapies, and as would be expected, they appear to be both efficacious and safe.

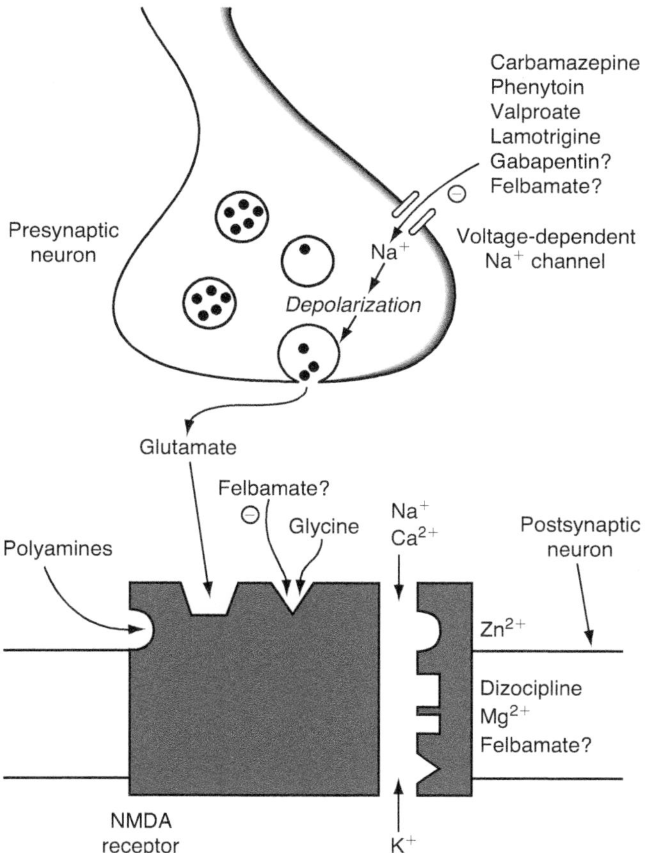

Figure 24-2 Mechanisms of action of common antiepileptic drugs.

Some AEDs are theorized to work, at least in part, by reducing the ability of the sodium channels in the axonal membrane to recover from inactivation after an action potential, thereby prolonging the refractory period. This is the proposed mechanism of action by which carbamazepine (Tegretol), lamotrigine (Lamictal), phenytoin (Dilantin), topiramate (Topamax), valproic acid (Depakene), and zonisamide (Zonegran) inhibit the high-frequency neuronal firing characteristic of partial seizures.

Benzodiazepines and barbiturates are agonists for the $GABA_A$ receptor binding site on the postsynaptic neuron. Binding to this receptor promotes the influx of chloride ions, which hyperpolarizes the neuron and raises the seizure threshold. Tiagabine (Gabitril) inhibits the reuptake of GABA by the presynaptic neuron, thereby ensuring the postsynaptic neuron remains hyperpolarized and is less likely to fire and cause a seizure. Similarly, vigabatrin (Sabril) interferes with the enzyme that degrades GABA, thereby promoting its duration of action.

Other AEDs inhibit the voltage-gated calcium channels that are located primarily in the presynaptic terminal membrane. Ordinarily, upon arrival of a nerve impulse, these calcium channels open and permit the passage of calcium ions into the presynaptic nerve, triggering a release of neurotransmitter in proportion to the number of calcium ions entering the terminal. Inhibition of the influx of calcium ions results in a decrease in neurotransmitter release that, in turn, reduces the likelihood that the postsynaptic neuron will fire. This mechanism is how ethosuximide (Zarontin) and valproate (Depacon, Depakene, Depakote) are thought to inhibit **absence seizures**.

Although gabapentin (Neurontin) and pregabalin (Lyrica) are analogues of GABA, they produce their effects by inhibiting the voltage-gated calcium presynaptic channels, thereby decreasing the release of glutamate—the primary excitatory neurotransmitter in the CNS.

All of the older AEDs—and to a lesser extent, some of the newer AEDs—interfere with folate metabolism via a mechanism that has not been fully elucidated. Folate supplementation is recommended for all women of childbearing age who are taking any AED.

Adverse Effects

All of the antiepileptic drugs have clinically significant side effects and adverse effects. Table 24-9 summarizes the side-effect profiles of the various drugs used to treat epilepsy, including one very important adverse effect—suicidal ideation and/or suicidal behavior. The FDA has mandated that a black box warning be placed on the label of the AEDs that are associated with a risk of suicidality (Box 24-3).

Some persons have a genetic disposition to develop a painful and debilitating condition called porphyria that can be triggered by several AEDs. Porphyria is a metabolic disorder characterized by a deficiency of porphobilinogen deaminase. This enzyme is involved in an intermediary step of heme production. The deficiency of porphobilinogen deaminase is triggered by the presence of an AED. The symptoms occur secondary to a buildup of porphobilinogen; they include abdominal pain, constipation, and muscle weakness.

Anticonvulsant hypersensitivity syndrome is a condition that typically begins within 2 to 8 weeks of initiation of therapy with AEDs.[61] This syndrome usually starts with a fever and develops into a rash, swollen lymph nodes, and sometimes pharyngitis. The most serious reactions involve hepatic, hematologic, renal, or pulmonary impairment. Anticonvulsant hypersensitivity syndrome is associated with the aromatic AEDs—phenytoin

Table 24-9 Side-Effect and Adverse-Effect Profiles of Antiepileptic Drugs

Drug: Generic (Brand)	Generation of AED	Initial Common Side Effect	Weight	Incidence of Fatigue (%)	Skin Rash	AED Hypersensitivity Syndrome	Cognitive Impairment	Suicidality	Porphyria	Other
Carbamazepine (Carbatrol, Tegretol)	Old	Diplopia, blurred vision, vertigo, and ataxia; rash; leukopenia in 10% that resolves in approximately 4 months	Weight gain	4.2	High risk	Yes	Some	Yes		Hyponatremia; irreversible agranulocytosis. Contraindicated for persons with hematologic disorders. Decreased bone density and osteoporosis, increased risk for fracture. Stevens-Johnson syndrome.[a]
Eslicarbazepine (Aptiom)	New	Dizziness, nausea, diplopia		5.2	Low risk	Yes	Possible	Yes		Hyponatremia, Stevens-Johnson syndrome, aplastic anemia
Ethosuximide (Zarontin)	Old	Nausea and vomiting, drowsiness, ataxia, hiccups		Unknown	Unknown			Yes	Yes	Aggression, irritability, hyperactivity, blood dyscrasias, hyponatremia, Stevens-Johnson syndrome, aplastic anemia, agranulocytosis
Ezogabine (Potiga)	New	Urinary retention, dizziness, somnolence, blue skin discoloration, confusion, abnormal coordination, diplopia	Weight gain	Common	Low risk	Yes	Yes	Yes		Retinal discoloration and vision loss. Skin discoloration described as blue, gray-blue, or brown of lips, nail beds, or face and legs. Suicidal thoughts. Psychotic symptoms and confusion may occur. QT interval prolongation may occur.
Felbamate (Felbatol)	New	Irritability, insomnia	Weight loss	10–20	Low risk			Higher risk		Anorexia, nausea, insomnia, aplastic anemia, hepatic failure
Gabapentin (Neurontin)	New	Drowsiness, fatigue	Weight gain	29	Low risk		Minimal	Yes		Decreased bone density and osteoporosis, increased risk for fracture
Lamotrigine (Lamictal)	New	Dizziness, blurred vision, insomnia, headaches	Weight neutral	6	High risk	Yes	Minimal	Yes		Stevens-Johnson syndrome
Levetiracetam (Keppra)	New	Ataxia, abnormal gait, agitation, hostility, anxiety, depression	Unclear, possibly weight neutral	27.3	Low risk		Minimal	Higher risk		Leukopenia, psychosis, withdrawal seizures
Oxcarbazepine (Trileptal)	New	Sedation, dizziness		5	High risk	Yes	Minimal	Yes		Hyponatremia

Perampanel (Fycompa)	New	Aggression, anxiety, dizziness, headache, nausea, dry mouth, gait disorder, insomnia, irregular heartbeat	Weight gain	10	Low risk	Yes		Yes		Serious or life-threatening psychiatric and behavioral outcomes, including aggression, hostility, irritability, anger and homicidal ideation
Phenobarbital (Luminal)	Old	Initial sedation; nystagmus and ataxia if overdose		10	High risk	Yes	Potentially significant	Yes		Decreased bone density and osteoporosis, increased risk for fracture, risk of dependence
Phenytoin (Dilantin)	Old	Gingivitis in 20% of persons, nystagmus, double vision, rash, sedation	Weight neutral	10.2	High risk	Yes	Possible	Yes	Yes	Decreased bone density and osteoporosis, increased risk for fracture, Sevens-Johnson syndrome
Pregabalin (Lyrica)	New	Dizziness, somnolence, ataxia, confusion, abnormal thinking, diplopia	Weight gain	8	Low risk	Yes	Possible	Yes		Angioedema, peripheral edema
Primidone (Mysoline)	Old	Drowsiness, dizziness, ataxia, nausea, and vomiting	Weight neutral	Common	High risk	Yes	Potentially significant	Yes	Yes	Increased risk of osteoporosis with long-term use
Rufinamide (Banzel)	New	Sedation, diarrhea, nausea, headache, somnolence	Weight neutral or weight loss	9–16	Low risk		Yes	Yes		Contraindicated for persons with familial short QT syndrome
Tiagabine (Gabitril)	New	Nausea, vomiting abdominal pain, impaired concentration	Weight gain	4.8	Low risk		Minimal	Higher risk		Sevens-Johnson syndrome, hepatic impairment
Topiramate (Topamax)	New	Dizziness, slowed cognition, nervousness, confusion, memory difficulty	Weight loss	12.1	Low risk		Potentially significant	Higher risk		Closed-angle glaucoma, metabolic acidosis, nephrolithiasis
Valproate sodium (Depacon), valproic acid (Depakene)	Old	Nausea and vomiting, heartburn, weight gain, irregular menses	Significant weight gain	4.2	Low risk	No	Some	Yes		Decreased bone density and osteoporosis, increased risk for fracture, hepatic failure, pancreatitis, teratogenic effects following in utero exposure
Vigabatrin	New	Fatigue, dizziness, diplopia	Weight gain	33.1				Higher risk		Irreversible bilateral visual field loss
Zonisamide (Zonegran)	New	Fatigue, nervousness, dizziness, confusion, anorexia	Weight loss	23	High risk	Yes	Some	Higher risk		Contraindicated for persons who are allergic to sulfa

[a] Increased risk in persons of Asian descent with *HLA-B*1502* and/or *HLA-A*3101* polymorphism.

Sources: Data from Asconape JJ. Some common issues in the use of antiepileptic drugs. *Semin Neurol.* 2002;22(1):27-39[63]; Knowles SR, Dewhurst N, Shear NH. Anticonvulsant hypersensitivity syndrome: an update. *Expert Opin Drug Saf.* 2012;11(5):767-778[62]; Siniscalchi A, Gallelli L, Russo E, De Sarro G. A review on antiepileptic drugs-dependent fatigue: pathophysiological mechanisms and incidence. *Eur J Pharmacol.* 2013;718(1-3):10-16.[64]

Box 24-3 Antiepileptic Drugs and Risk of Suicide

What is the connection between AED drugs and suicide? One of the pathogenic mechanisms that predisposes a person to seizures also predisposes an individual to mood disorders, anxiety, and suicide. A decreased level of serotonin in the central nervous system is the culprit, but the exact mechanism by which AEDs increase these risks is not well elucidated.

Although persons who take AEDs have an increased risk for suicidality, which includes suicide ideation, suicide attempt, and completed suicide, this risk is actually low in absolute numbers. The FDA analyzed the pooled results of several studies of 11 AEDs and found that the risk of suicide was 4.3 per 1000 persons who took AEDs versus 2.2 per 1000 persons who took a placebo.

Healthcare providers who prescribe these drugs need to balance the risk of suicidality with the clinical need for the drug. In addition, providers are encouraged to monitor for unusual changes in behavior and notify individuals and their families of this risk.

Information given to persons who take these agents states that they should not change the medication regimen without having input from their healthcare provider and that they monitor for symptoms of suicide, which include the following:

- Talking or thinking about wanting to hurt oneself or end one's life
- Withdrawing from friends and family
- Becoming depressed or having depression get worse
- Becoming preoccupied with death and dying
- Giving away prized possessions

Persons using AEDs are encouraged to contact their healthcare provider if any of these behaviors occur.

(Dilantin), phenobarbital (Luminal), primidone (Mysoline), carbamazepine (Tegretol), and lamotrigine (Lamictal). The cross-reactivity between these and other AEDs is high. Valproate sodium (Depacon) is considered a safe alternative for treatment for persons with anticonvulsant hypersensitivity syndrome.

Drug–Drug Interactions

The AEDs are inducers, inhibitors, and substrates for various CYP450 enzymes, including those that metabolize AEDs. Thus the potential for drug–drug interactions is quite high with these agents. The older AEDs in particular have multiple drug–drug interactions that are clinically important considerations when caring for a person who is taking an AED.[62–64] Table 24-10 provides an overview of the drug–drug interactions associated with AEDs, including the very important effects these drugs have on the effectiveness of hormonal contraceptives. Table 24-11 summarizes specific interactions. The interactions with CYP450 enzyme–inducing AEDs are particularly significant for women using hormonal contraceptive agents because metabolism of the contraceptive is enhanced through this synergistic effect, which lowers plasma levels and contraceptive effectiveness.[65] The AEDs that are CYP450 inhibitors will cause a decrease in metabolism of other drugs and higher plasma levels of those drugs.

Traditional Antiepileptic Drugs

Phenobarbital (Luminal) was first used to treat epilepsy in 1912, and phenytoin (Dilantin) was first used for this indication in 1932. Both of these drugs remain in use today. The other three traditional antiepileptic drugs have been used for several decades. All five of the older antiepileptic drugs are effective and inexpensive, but their uncomfortable side effects and multiple drug–drug interactions have been the impetus for developing newer drugs to treat epilepsy. Doses, indications, side effects, and important clinical considerations are presented in Table 24-12.

Table 24-10 Overview of Drug–Drug Interactions Associated with Antiepileptic Drugs[a]

Drug: Generic (Brand)	CYP450 Drug–Drug Interactions	Potential for Drug–Drug Interactions	Reduced Effectiveness of Combined Oral Contraceptives
Carbamazepine (Carbatrol, Tegretol)	Inducer	High	Yes
Eslicarbazepine (Aptiom)			Yes
Ethosuximide (Zarontin)	No or minimal effect	Low	No
Felbamate (Felbatol)	Inhibitor	High	Yes
Gabapentin (Neurontin)	No or minimal effect	Low	No
Lamotrigine (Lamictal)	No or minimal effect	Intermediate	Combined oral contraceptives decrease the effectiveness of lamotrigine
Levetiracetam (Keppra)	No or minimal effect	Low	No
Oxcarbazepine (Trileptal)	No or minimal effect	Intermediate	Yes
Phenytoin (Dilantin)	Inducer	High	Yes
Phenobarbital (Luminal)	Inducer	High	Yes
Pregabalin (Lyrica)			No
Primidone (Mysoline)	Inducer	High	Yes
Tiagabine (Gabitril)	No or minimal effect	Intermediate	No
Topiramate (Topamax)	No or minimal effect	Intermediate	Yes
Valproate sodium (Depacon), valproic acid (Depakene), divalproex (Depakote, Depakote ER)	Inhibitor	High	No
Vigabatrin (Sabril)		Low	No
Zonisamide (Zonegran)	No or minimal effect	Intermediate	No

[a] This table is not comprehensive as new information is being generated on a regular basis.

Sources: Data from Asconape JJ. Some common issues in the use of antiepileptic drugs. *Semin Neurol.* 2002;22(1):27-39[63]; Perucca E. Clinically relevant drug interactions with antiepileptic drugs. *Br J Clin Pharmacol.* 2006;61(3):246-255.[65]

Table 24-11 Selected Drug–Drug Interactions of Commonly Used Antiepileptic Drugs[a]

Drug: Generic (Brand)	Antiepileptic Drug: Generic (Brand)	Effect of Interaction
Amiodarone (Cordarone)	Phenytoin (Dilantin)	Increased level of AED and possible toxicity
Antacids	Phenytoin (Dilantin), carbamazepine (Tegretol), gabapentin (Neurontin), phenobarbital (Luminal)	Reduced absorption of AED leading to decreased effectiveness
Benzodiazepines	Carbamazepine (Tegretol), phenytoin (Dilantin), phenobarbital (Luminal)	Decreased plasma levels of benzodiazepines
Carbamazepine (Tegretol)	Phenytoin (Dilantin)	Decreased plasma levels of phenytoin and increased seizure risk
	Valproate (Depacon, Depakene, Depakote)	Increased plasma levels of active metabolite of carbamazepine. Can reach toxic levels. Valproate should not be used concomitantly with carbamazepine.
Beta blockers, such as propranolol (Inderal)	Enzyme-inducing AEDs[†]	Decreased plasma levels of beta blockers. These AEDs may be contraindicated in persons needing antihypertensive medications.
Chloramphenicol (Chloromycetin)	Phenobarbital (Luminal)	Increased metabolism of chloramphenicol
	Phenytoin (Dilantin), phenobarbital (Luminal)	Increased plasma levels of AEDs, possible toxic effect
Cimetidine (Tagamet)	Phenytoin (Dilantin), gabapentin (Neurontin)	Increased plasma levels of AED
Clarithromycin (Biaxin)	Phenytoin (Dilantin)	Increased plasma levels of phenytoin
Erythromycin (E-Mycin)	Carbamazepine (Carbatrol, Tegretol)	Increased plasma level of carbamazepine
Digoxin (Lanoxin)	Phenytoin (Dilantin)	Decreased plasma levels of digoxin
Fluconazole (Diflucan)	Phenytoin (Dilantin), valproate (Depacon, Depakene, Depakote)	Increased plasma levels of phenytoin

(*continues*)

Table 24-11 Selected Drug–Drug Interactions of Commonly Used Antiepileptic Drugs[a] (*continued*)

Drug: Generic (Brand)	Antiepileptic Drug: Generic (Brand)	Effect of Interaction
Fluoxetine (Prozac)	Carbamazepine (Carbatrol, Tegretol)	Increased level of AED
Folate	Phenytoin (Dilantin)	Bidirectional interaction: decreased plasma levels of phenytoin and decreased plasma levels of folate.
Isoniazid (INH)	Phenytoin (Dilantin), carbamazepine (Carbatrol, Tegretol), ethosuximide (Zarontin), valproate (Depacon, Depakene, Depakote)	Increased plasma levels of AED and possible toxicity
Ketoconazole (Nizoral)	Carbamazepine (Carbatrol, Tegretol)	Increased plasma level of carbamazepine and potential toxicity
Lipid-lowering drugs	Phenytoin (Dilantin)	Decreased plasma levels of lipid-lowering agents
Metronidazole (Flagyl)	Enzyme-inducing AEDs[b]	Decreased effectiveness of metronidazole
	Carbamazepine (Carbatrol, Tegretol)	Increased plasma level of carbamazepine
	Phenytoin (Dilantin)	Decreased effectiveness of oral contraceptives
Phenobarbital (Luminal)	Phenytoin (Dilantin)	Decreased plasma levels of phenytoin and increased seizure risk
Rifampin (Rifadin)	Phenytoin (Dilantin)	Decreased plasma levels of phenytoin and increased seizure risk
St. John's wort	Carbamazepine (Carbatrol, Tegretol), phenytoin (Dilantin)	Decreased plasma levels of phenytoin and carbamazepine
Sulfonamides	Phenytoin (Dilantin)	Increased plasma levels of phenytoin
Tricyclic antidepressants	Enzyme-inducing AEDs[b]	Bidirectional interaction: tricyclic antidepressant plasma levels decrease and AED plasma levels increase
Valproate (Depakene, Depakote, Depacon)	Phenytoin (Dilantin)	Valproate displaces phenytoin on plasma protein-binding sites, which causes increased plasma levels of active phenytoin
	Oral contraceptives	Enhanced metabolism of valproate
Warfarin (Coumadin)	Phenytoin (Dilantin)	Decreased plasma levels of warfarin

Abbreviations: AED = antiepileptic drug.

[a] This list is not comprehensive as new information is being generated on a regular basis.

[b] Enzyme-inducing AEDs include carbamazepine (Carbatrol, Tegretol), felbamate (Felbatol), oxcarbazepine (Trileptal), phenobarbital (Luminal), phenytoin (Dilantin), primidone (Mysoline), and topiramate (Topamax).

[c] Felbamate appears to induce metabolism of progesterone component of combined oral contraceptives only; its clinical effect on contraceptive effectiveness is unclear. There is also preliminary evidence showing that lamotrigine induces metabolism of progestin.

Table 24-12 First-Generation Antiepileptic Drugs[a]

Drug: Generic (Brand)	Formulations	Therapeutic Indication	Dose	Clinical Considerations
Carbamazepine (Carbatrol, Tegretol)	Oral: 200-mg tablets, 100-mg chewable tablets; oral suspension 100 mg/5 mL Extended-release (12-h4) capsules: Carbatrol or Tegretol XR 100-, 200-, 300-, and 400-mg capsules	Partial and generalized tonic–clonic seizures First-line treatment for focal-onset seizures Off-label use: Chronic pain syndromes Bipolar disorder (under brand name Equetro)	Initial therapy 100–200 mg/day PO, increasing weekly in 100- to 200-mg increments to target dose of 600–800 mg/day (may require doses as high as 1600–2400 mg/day)	Recent food intake slows absorption but may make larger doses more tolerable, so it is recommended that carbamazepine be taken with food. Extended-release capsules permit 12-hour dosing, but missed doses are more likely to result in breakthrough seizures.
Ethosuximide (Zarontin)	250-mg capsules; 250-mg/5-mL elixir	Absence seizures	250 mg 2 times/day PO	Increase in 250-mg increments until seizures are controlled. Usual maintenance dose is 20 mg/kg/day.
Phenobarbital (Luminal)	Tablets: 15, 30, 60, 100 mg Oral solution: 15, 20 mg/5 mL Parenteral solution: 20 mg/5 mL for IM or IV	Generalized tonic–clonic seizures, partial seizures	Adult dose: 1–3 mg/kg/day PO in divided doses Usual dose: 50–100 mg PO 2–3 times/day	Titration to full dose is not necessary due to the slow accumulation over 2–3 weeks to reach the steady-state level
Phenytoin (Dilantin)	Parenteral: 50 mg/mL for IV administration Oral: 30-mg, 100-mg capsules	Generalized tonic–clonic seizures, partial seizures	Status epilepticus: Start at 10–20 mg/kg IV as a loading dose	Large oral doses can be taken with meals to avoid gastric discomfort. Extended-release capsules are most appropriate for large single daily doses.

Phenytoin (Dilantin) (*continued*)	Chewable tablets: 50 mg; oral suspension 125 mg/5 mL Extended-release capsules (Phenytek): 200 mg or 300 mg	Off-label use: Neuropathic pain, motion sickness, cardiac arrhythmias	Nonacute situations: 150 mg 2 times/day PO, increasing to 300–400 mg per day as tolerated	Brands differ in their rates of absorption; changing brands or formulations may result in underdosage or overdosage symptoms. Decreases effectiveness of oral contraceptive agents.
Primidone (Mysoline)	Tablets: 50, 250 mg	Generalized tonic–clonic seizures, partial seizures; more effective than phenobarbital	Usual dose: 750–1500 mg/day PO in divided doses, up to a maximum of 2 g/day	
Valproate sodium (Depacon), valproic acid (Depakene), divalproex (Depakote, Depakote ER)	Valproate sodium: IV solution Valproic acid: capsules, 250 mg; syrup, 250 mg/5 mL Divalproex: 125-, 250-, 500-mg enteric-coated tablets Divalproex ER: 250, 500 mg	Generalized tonic–clonic seizures, partial seizures, absence seizures Off-label use: Neuropathic pain	10–20 mg/kg/day in adults	Initial dose 5–15 mg/kg/day increasing to maintenance levels. Enteric-coated tablets (Depakote) avoid gastric upset. Individuals taking enzyme-inducing drugs such as phenobarbital may require higher doses.

[a] Except absence seizures.

Phenytoin (Dilantin)

Phenytoin (Dilantin) is the oldest nonsedative antiseizure drug. The major mechanism of action is through binding to the postsynaptic sodium channel, which prolongs the inactivated state of the sodium channel and stabilizes neuronal membranes. Phenytoin has some presynaptic actions that inhibit the release of the excitatory neurotransmitter glutamate and promote the release of the inhibitory neurotransmitter GABA.[66] These effects may explain some of the toxic symptoms associated with high levels of phenytoin.

Phenytoin is available as rapid-release tablets and extended-release capsules. The absorption varies between preparations made by different manufacturers, so plasma phenytoin levels may vary when the individual switches from a medication produced by one manufacturer to a formulation produced by another manufacturer. The time to peak absorption can vary from 3 to 12 hours. Ideally, individuals should be treated with the same drug from a single manufacturer, although changes can be made if the person is monitored for seizure control or onset of toxicities. A soluble phosphate prodrug fosphenytoin (Cerebyx) is well absorbed after intramuscular injection. Fosphenytoin is converted in the body to phenytoin and is available for both intramuscular and intravenous use.

Phenytoin is metabolized by liver enzymes to inactive metabolites that are then excreted by the kidneys. The half-life of phenytoin ranges from 12 hours to more than 36 hours due to the variations in metabolism. At blood levels within a therapeutic range, the liver enzymes responsible for metabolizing phenytoin become saturated, so small additional doses may produce large increases in phenytoin blood levels and a longer half-life. These unusual **nonlinear kinetics** result in a small and unpredictable therapeutic index for the medication. Although the average half-life at mid-therapeutic range is about 24 hours, much longer half-lives occur at the higher concentration ranges.

Phenytoin is extensively bound to protein (87–93%) in the plasma—primarily to albumin. Only the unbound fraction is pharmacologically active because the protein-bound fraction cannot cross the blood–brain barrier. Approximately 90% of phenytoin is found in the bound form in the body if there is an adequate albumin concentration and no other drugs are competing for albumin binding sites.

Side Effects/Adverse Effects

Twenty percent of persons on chronic phenytoin therapy develop gingival hyperplasia that includes swollen, tender, and bleeding gums. The overgrowth involves altered collagen metabolism and can be minimized with good oral hygiene such as flossing and gum massage.

At excessively high doses, phenytoin can lose its selectivity for seizure suppression and begin to elicit more diverse CNS symptoms, including nystagmus (involuntary eye movements), excessive sedation, cognitive impairment, diplopia (double vision), ataxia (staggering), and behavioral changes.

Endocrine effects include inhibition of antidiuretic hormone (ADH) release, inhibition of insulin secretion resulting in hyperglycemia, and glycosuria. Softening of bones or osteomalacia occurs because phenytoin interferes with vitamin D metabolism, resulting in decreased calcium absorption. Phenytoin also increases vitamin K metabolism, which can result in increased bleeding tendencies in neonates of mothers who take this agent during pregnancy. Lower vitamin K levels can interfere with the production of proteins important for calcium metabolism in bone, resulting in vitamin D–resistant osteomalacia.

Between 2% and 5% of individuals taking phenytoin develop a hypersensitive morbilliform (measles-like) rash that can progress to more serious skin reactions such as exfoliative dermatitis or Stevens-Johnson syndrome.

Drug–Drug Interactions

Phenytoin is an inducer of CYP1A2, CYP2C19, and CYP3A4 and has numerous drug–drug interactions. Toxic blood levels of this drug can also occur as the result of competition for albumin binding. Valproic acid (Depakene) competes for binding sites in this manner and is well known to increase plasma phenytoin concentrations.

Carbamazepine (Tegretol)

Carbamazepine (Tegretol) is closely related chemically to the tricyclic antidepressants. It has a widely variable rate of absorption, with time to full absorption ranging from 4 to 8 hours after ingestion. The rate of absorption is slowed by recent food intake. Extended-release forms of the drug permit twice-daily dosing for many persons and help to avoid adverse effects. Carbamazepine has an active metabolite that may contribute to its effectiveness as an AED.

Side Effects/Adverse Effects

Carbamazepine is not sedating when given within the usual dose range. However, acute alcohol intoxication can have an additive effect in persons who take carbamazepine; this combination can cause CNS and respiratory depression or, conversely, hyperirritability and convulsions. Gradual increases of the dose of carbamazepine over time may permit individuals to develop tolerance to the drug, alleviating CNS symptoms.

Approximately 10% of persons treated with carbamazepine develop rash. Severe skin reactions such as erythema multiforme and Stevens-Johnson syndrome occur rarely and require withdrawal of the drug.

Drug–Drug Interactions

Carbamazepine is a potent inducer of several CYP450 enzymes. Interestingly, during the initial phase of treatment, the half-life of this agent is approximately 40 hours. With continued treatment, the half-life decreases to about 15 hours because the drug induces the CYP450 enzymes that metabolize it, so metabolism speeds up. Doses sometimes have to be increased to compensate for this effect.

Phenobarbital (Luminal)

Phenobarbital (Luminal) is the oldest available AED and is considered one of the safest antiseizure drugs. The advantage of phenobarbital over other barbiturates is that it has a maximal antiseizure effect at a dose lower than that required for hypnosis.

Absorption of orally administered phenobarbital is slow. It takes several hours for the peak plasma concentration to be reached after a single dose of the drug. The half-life of phenobarbital is approximately 4 days, resulting in a slow time to plateau plasma concentration of 2 to 3 weeks if a loading dose is not given.

Side Effects/Adverse Effects

Sedation is the most common and most troubling side effect of phenobarbital. Phenobarbital intensifies the CNS depression caused by other drugs such as alcohol, benzodiazepines, opioids, and antihistamines. This drug interaction can result in severe respiratory depression and coma; therefore, persons on phenobarbital therapy should be warned to avoid other CNS depressants. Elderly individuals may experience confusion and agitation with phenobarbital therapy and are especially prone to adverse drug–drug interactions. Therefore, this drug is avoided whenever possible in this population.[67]

Phenobarbital, like all barbiturates, can cause physical dependence and should not be abruptly withdrawn. Sudden withdrawal of the drug can precipitate status epilepticus.

Drug–Drug Interactions

Like the other older AEDs, phenobarbital is metabolized by CYP450 enzymes and is a potent inducer of those enzymes as well. Therefore, drugs that are metabolized by CYP450 enzymes are degraded more rapidly when administered with phenobarbital. Most notable among these drugs are the hormonal contraceptives, oral anticoagulants, and some other AEDs, especially carbamazepine (Tegretol).

Primidone (Mysoline)

Primidone (Mysoline), also known as 2-desoxyphenobarbital, is metabolized into two compounds: phenobarbital and phenylethylmalonamide (PEMA). All three compounds are active AEDs. Primidone has more CNS toxic effects at lower doses than phenobarbital, so it should be administered in gradual increments. Some individuals experience transient side effects such as drowsiness, dizziness, ataxia, nausea, and vomiting to such a debilitating degree that they are unwilling to take another dose. Initial dosing at bedtime often minimizes the side effects until tolerance develops.

Ethosuximide (Zarontin)

First introduced in 1958, ethosuximide (Zarontin) remains the drug of choice for absence seizures due to its safety and effectiveness. Phensuximide (Milontin) and methsuximide (Celontin) are two other members of the succinimide family of AEDs that are not extensively used due to their toxicity profile.

Ethosuximide is well absorbed after oral administration, reaching a peak concentration in the plasma after about 3 hours. The drug becomes distributed evenly throughout most of the tissues of the body, except for adipose tissue.

Side Effects/Adverse Effects

Behavioral changes such as aggression, hyperactivity, and irritability occur occasionally. Psychotic episodes including anxiety, depression, and hallucinations occur mostly in persons with a history of prior mental illness.

Drug–Drug Interactions

Although ethosuximide is metabolized by CYP3A, it does not induce its own metabolism, nor does it induce or inhibit the metabolism of other drugs by these enzymes. However, other drugs known to be CYP3A inducers, such as rifampin (Rifadin), do speed up ethosuximide metabolism, resulting in lower serum levels of this drug.

Valproate Sodium (Depakene) and Valproic Acid (Depacon)

Valproic acid (Depakene) and valproate sodium (Depacon) can be used singly or in a derivative combination formulation called divalproex sodium (Depakote, Depakote ER). The active ingredient in all three formulations is valproate ion, which is effective against myoclonic seizures, tonic–clonic seizures, and partial seizures. The mechanism of action of valproate is not known.

Valproate is readily absorbed after oral administration, becomes widely distributed throughout the body, and is metabolized in the liver through the action of cytochrome P450 enzymes. Valproate has two active metabolites, each having its own antiseizure activity.

Side Effects/Adverse Effects

Most commonly, valproate sodium causes nausea, vomiting, abdominal pain, and heartburn. These effects are dose related, occur in approximately 16% of individuals, and may be due to direct gastric irritation by valproate sodium. Taking valproate sodium in an enteric-coated formulation or with meals may decrease these gastrointestinal effects, which are usually transient. Substantial weight gain is the problem most often associated with valproate, which is hypothesized to occur secondary to disordered fat metabolism rather than increased appetite.[68] The label for valproate sodium carries an FDA-mandated black box warning that it has caused fatal hepatotoxicity.[69]

Drug–Drug Interactions

Although valproate does not itself induce liver enzymes, it is sensitive to the action of other enzyme-modifying drugs. Drugs that are enzyme inducers, such as many other AEDs, when taken with valproate, will increase its metabolism, resulting in lower serum concentrations and a greater likelihood of seizures occurring.

Second-Generation Antiepileptic Drugs

The newer antiepileptic drugs are generally better than the first-generation AEDs in controlling seizures and have fewer drug–drug interactions. At the same time, these drugs also have potential adverse effects that require careful monitoring. Doses, indications, side effects, and clinical considerations for second-generation AEDs are presented in Table 24-13.

Lamotrigine (Lamictal)

Lamotrigine (Lamictal) is most often used as adjunctive therapy with other antiseizure medications. Therefore, maintenance doses are tailored to the type of interaction possible with various AEDs. Lamotrigine is well absorbed, and its absorption is not affected by food or antacids. Because lamotrigine is approximately 55% protein bound, this agent is not vulnerable to the drug–drug interactions that occur when drugs compete for plasma proteins. Lamotrigine is metabolized via glucuronic acid conjugation in the liver and excreted via the kidneys.

Side Effects/Adverse Effects

The FDA has specified schedules for initiation of lamotrigine therapy in an attempt to minimize the major adverse reaction of skin rashes. The FDA studies have found the rashes, which can lead to hospitalization and life-threatening Stevens-Johnson syndrome, may occur secondary to overly rapid titration of initial therapy.

Table 24-13 Second-Generation Antiepileptic Drugs

Drug: Generic (Brand)	Formulations	Therapeutic Indication	Dose
Eslicarbazepine (Aptiom)	200-, 400-, 600-, and 800-mg tablets	Prodrug of oxcarbazepine. Both drugs are converted to a common active metabolite. Approved by the FDA in November 2013. Indicated as an adjunct treatment for focal seizures.	Start at 400 mg PO/day, increase to 800 mg (recommended maintenance dose) Maximum dose: 1200 mg/day
Ezogabine (Potiga)	50-, 200-, 300-, and 400-mg tablets	Adjunct treatment of focal seizures in persons 18 years and older who have responded inadequately to alternative treatments and for whom the benefits outweigh the risk of retinal abnormalities and potential decline in visual acuity	Initial dose: 100 mg PO 3 times/day, increase by no more than 50 mg 3 times/day up to a maintenance dosage of 200–400 mg 3 times/day
Felbamate (Felbatol)	400- and 600-mg tablets; 600 mg/5 mL suspension	Adjunct for refractory seizures	Average dose: 3600 mg/day PO Increase dose by 15 mg/dose in 1- to 2-week intervals
Gabapentin (Neurontin)	100-, 300-, 400-, 600-, and 800-mg tablets; 100-, 300-, and 400-mg capsules; 250 mg/5 mL solution	Adjunct against generalized tonic–clonic seizures and partial seizures Off-label use: Chronic pain, peripheral neuropathy, postherpetic neuralgia	900–1800 mg/day PO in 3 divided doses Start at 300 mg/day and then advance by 300 mg/day until effective dose is reached
Lamotrigine (Lamictal)	25-, 100-, 150-, and 200-mg tablets; 2-, 5-, and 25-mg chewable tablets	Partial seizures	300–500 mg/day PO in 2 divided doses
Lamotrigine (Lamictal) added to valproate		Adjunctive therapy with other antiseizure medications	100–200 mg/day PO in 2 divided doses 25 mg every other day for 2 weeks, then 25 mg/day for 2 weeks, then increase dose by 25–50 mg/day every 1–2 weeks
Levetiracetam (Keppra)	250-, 500-, 750-, and 1000-mg tablets	Adjunct for refractory seizures	500 mg/day PO Maximum dose: 3000 mg/day
Oxcarbazepine (Trileptal)	150-, 300-, and 600-mg tablets; 300 mg/5 mL oral suspension		Start at 300 mg PO 2 times/day, increasing by a maximum of 600 mg/week, up to a maximum of 2400 mg/day Often used as adjunctive therapy
Perampanel (Fycompa)	2-, 4-, 6-, 8-, 10-, and 12-mg tablets	Adjunctive treatment of focal seizures in persons 12 years and older	Start at 2 mg PO daily at bedtime or 4 mg PO if on enzyme-inducing AEDs May increase dose weekly by 2 mg daily PO to a dose of 4–12 mg once daily at bedtime
Pregabalin (Lyrica)	25-, 50-, 75-, 100-, 150-, 200-, 225-, and 300-mg capsules		150–600 mg/day PO in 2–3 divided doses Start at 50 mg 3 times/day PO or 75 mg 2 times/day Maximum dose: 600 mg/day
Rufinamide (Banzel)	200 mg/mL, 400 mg/mL, and 40 mg/mL oral suspension	Adjunctive treatment for Lennox-Gastaut syndrome seizures in children older than 4 years and adults	Adults: Initial dose 400–800 mg/day PO in 2 divided doses Increase by 400–800 mg PO every other day until maximum dose of 3200 mg/day PO in 2 equally divided doses per day
Tiagabine (Gabitril)	2-, 4-, 12-, and 16-mg tablets	Adjunct for refractory seizures	32–56 mg/day PO in 2–4 divided doses Start at 4 mg per day in 2–4 divided doses, increasing by 4 mg/day after 1 week, then increasing by 4–8 mg/day each week Maximum dose: 56 mg/day PO Give with food to minimize gastric upset
Topiramate (Topamax)	25-, 50-, 100-, and 200-mg tablets; 15- and 25-mg sprinkles	Generalized tonic–clonic seizures, adjunct for partial seizures, atonic myotonic and atypical absence seizures	200–600 mg/day PO Start at 50 mg per day, increasing slowly to avoid adverse effects
Zonisamide (Zonegran)	25-, 50-, and 100-mg capsules	Adjunct for refractory seizures	100–600 mg PO divided 1–2 times/day Start at 100 mg and increase every 2 weeks to maximum dose of 600 mg/day

Topiramate (Topamax)

Topiramate (Topamax) is approved by the FDA as a monotherapeutic agent for generalized tonic–clonic seizures.

Side Effects/Adverse Effects

Dose-related adverse effects of topiramate usually occur within the first 4 weeks of therapy and can include fatigue, somnolence, dizziness, slowed cognition, paresthesias, nervousness, and confusion. The cognitive effects, which are most common, present as memory difficulty, word-finding difficulty, and slowed cognition. Weight loss has been observed among individuals using topiramate. Those who lost weight had improved lipid profiles, glycemic control, and blood pressure. Topiramate can also cause metabolic acidosis, renal calculi, and a rare ocular condition characterized by acute myopia and glaucoma that requires withdrawal from the drug.

Drug–Drug Interactions

Although the level of liver enzyme induction is less with topiramate than with the potent enzyme inducers such as carbamazepine (Tegretol), topiramate does speed the metabolism of the estrogen component of combination oral contraceptives. It also decreases plasma concentrations of digoxin.

Gabapentin (Neurontin) and Pregabalin (Lyrica)

Gabapentin (Neurontin) is a GABA molecule bound to a cyclohexane ring. It is highly lipid soluble and, therefore, readily crosses the blood–brain barrier. Pregabalin (Lyrica) is also a GABA analogue and closely related to gabapentin. Gabapentin and pregabalin are not metabolized in the body and do not induce hepatic enzymes. Both drugs are excreted unchanged in the urine. Because they do not induce hepatic enzymes and are not bound to plasma proteins, the drugs have virtually no known drug–drug interactions.

Side Effects/Adverse Effects

Behavioral changes such as aggression, anger, and oppositional behavior have occurred in developmentally delayed persons and in those with attention-deficit disorder. Adverse reactions are not dose related, and some individuals do not tolerate even small doses of gabapentin.

Felbamate, Levetiracetam, Tiagabine, and Zonisamide

Felbamate (Felbatol), levetiracetam (Keppra), tiagabine (Gabitril), and zonisamide (Zonegran) are used as adjunct medications when monotherapy is not effective.

Felbamate (Felbatol) can cause fatal aplastic anemia, usually within the first year of therapy. It is reserved for use as a third medication for those persons who have severe epilepsy that is unresponsive to previous drugs.

Adverse effects of levetiracetam (Keppra) mostly occur during the first 4 weeks of therapy and include ataxia, abnormal gait, and incoordination. Reported behavioral symptoms include agitation, hostility, anxiety, apathy, emotional lability, depersonalization, and depression. Reduction of the dose usually improves the behavioral problems.

Tiagabine (Gabitril) is extensively oxidized via the CYP450 enzyme system. When tiagabine is coadministered with enzyme-inducing AEDs, the half-life of tiagabine is reduced from 5–8 hours to 2–3 hours due to increased clearance of the drug. Tiagabine itself neither induces nor inhibits CYP450 enzymes, and it is given in low enough doses that it does not displace other drugs from protein-binding sites.

Zonisamide (Zonegran) does not induce or inhibit CYP450 enzymes, so it does not cause any significant alteration in the metabolism of other drugs.

Benzodiazepines for Treating Seizures

The benzodiazepines act as inhibitory neurotransmitters by binding to a specific binding site on the GABA receptor. Benzodiazepines have no action at the GABA receptor in the absence of GABA itself. Rather, the benzodiazepines enhance the action of GABA at its binding site. The GABA receptor permits a greater influx of chloride ions at lower GABA concentrations when the benzodiazepine occupies a site on the receptor, so use of benzodiazepines promotes the neuro-inhibition produced by GABA. The potency of a specific benzodiazepine correlates with its binding affinity at the benzodiazepine sites on neuronal GABA receptors.

Although benzodiazepines are effective against almost every type of seizure, the individual drugs vary in their effectiveness in different types of epilepsy (Table 24-14). Long-term benzodiazepine treatment results in the phenomenon of tolerance, in which increasing doses of the drug are required to induce the same effect. Tolerance also increases the risk of rebound seizures upon withdrawal of the drug. Thus, the major role for benzodiazepines as AEDs is as a first-line therapy for status epilepticus and seizure clusters—these drugs have a rapid onset and proven effectiveness in this indication. Status epilepticus is a life-threatening condition in which the brain is in a state of persistent seizure that manifests as one continuous seizure lasting 30 minutes or longer (Box 24-4).[70]

Table 24-14 Benzodiazepines Used to Treat Seizures

Drug: Generic (Brand)	Formulations	Dose	Clinical Considerations
Clobazam (Onfi)	Oral: 5-, 10-, and 20-mg tablets	Persons weighing < 30 kg: Initial dose of 5 mg PO once daily for first week, then 10 mg 2 times/day Persons weighing > 30 kg: Titrate initially at 5 mg PO 2 times/day, to a maintenance dose of 20 mg 2 times/day Persons older than 65 years: Titrate slowly	Clobazam has been approved as an adjunctive treatment for seizures associated with Lennox-Gastaut syndrome in persons 2 years or older. Avoid rapid discontinuance, which may exacerbate seizures. An additive effect with alcohol can significantly increase plasma levels of clobazam (Frisium).
Clonazepam (Klonopin)	Oral: 0.5-, 1-, and 2-mg tablets; 0.125-, 0.25-, 0.5-, and 2-mg dispersible tablets placed on tongue for absorption	Up to 8 mg/day PO in 2–3 divided doses	Not available in parenteral form in the United States
Diazepam (Valium)	Oral: 2-, 5-, and 10-mg tablets; oral solution: 5 mg/5 mL; parenteral solution: 5 mg/5 mL and 5 mg/mL; rectal gel (Diastat): 2.5, 5, 10, and 20 mg	Initial dose for status epilepticus 10–20 mg IV, 5–10 mg every few hours *Or* 10 mg PR, may repeat once if necessary	Rapid redistribution from brain to muscle tissue results in a short half-life. Diazepam can be followed by longer-acting AEDs such as phenytoin (Dilantin).
Lorazepam (Ativan)	Oral: 0.5-, 1-, and 2-mg tablets; parenteral solution: 2 mg/mL or 4 mg/mL for IV or IM	Initial dose for status epilepticus: 0.1 mg/kg up to 4 mg IV at 2 mg/minute. Repeat after 10–15 minutes if necessary.	Longer duration of action and greater potency makes it the agent of choice in adults with status epilepticus

Diazepam (Valium), Lorazepam (Ativan), and Clonazepam (Klonapin)

Diazepam (Valium) was the first benzodiazepine used as an AED and has become the standard drug for therapy of status epilepticus. It is available in oral, parenteral, and rectal (Diastat) forms. Diazepam rapidly enters the brain, but then its concentration decreases due to its redistribution to other tissues of the body. The initial half-life is only 1 hour, resulting in a short duration of action in the brain. Lorazepam (Ativan) has a greater potency and longer duration of action than diazepam and has become the agent of choice for initial treatment of status epilepticus in adults.[70]

Clonazepam (Klonopin) is a benzodiazepine that is often prescribed to treat anxiety and can also be used as an AED. It is useful for treating both acute seizures and chronic epilepsy. Clonazepam is available only in an oral formulation in the United States; therefore, it is not used in this country to treat status epilepticus. The dose of clonazepam for treating chronic epilepsy in adults is as high as 8 mg per day in two or three divided doses.

Approximately 50% of adults experience lethargy and drowsiness as an adverse effect of clonazepam, but tolerance to the drug over time decreases this effect. Other adverse effects include nystagmus, which is fairly common. Due to the high rates of adverse effects seen with clonazepam, this agent is usually reserved for the most difficult epileptic

Box 24-4 Emergency Treatment of Seizures

Status epilepticus is defined as either more than 30 minutes of continuous seizure activity or two or more sequential seizures without full recovery of consciousness between seizures. Status epilepticus is regarded as a medical emergency, with overall mortality rates of 30%.

Diazepam (Valium) has been used to treat status epilepticus due to its relative effectiveness and low likelihood of inducing respiratory depression. However, the anticonvulsant effect of a single intravenous dose of diazepam is approximately 20 minutes. A dose of 10 to 20 mg administered intravenously is followed by a continuous intravenous infusion at a rate of 20 mg per hour.

Lorazepam (Ativan) is associated with a slightly increased risk of respiratory depression compared to diazepam. The duration of anticonvulsant effect of a single dose of lorazepam is more than 6 hours; therefore, it is becoming the favored treatment for status epilepticus. An initial dose of 4 mg is given intravenously, and it is repeated once after 10 to 15 minutes if needed.

conditions. Furthermore, tolerance to its antiseizure effects usually develops after 1 to 6 months of administration, after which some persons do not respond to clonazepam at any dose.[70]

Special Considerations for Women Taking Antiepileptic Drugs

Catamenial Epilepsy

Nadkarni et al.[61] summarized recent findings about catamenial seizures as follows: 20% to 35% of women with such seizures experience an increase in seizure frequency with changing hormonal levels; 3% to 25% experience a decrease; and 60% to 85% experience no change in seizure frequency. Three distinct patterns have been described: perimenstrual, periovulatory, and luteal. The changes that occur may be due to hormonal fluctuations, altered protein binding that affects AED plasma levels, and perhaps other unexplained effects. The combination of progesterone with an AED can be helpful for some women with catamenial seizures.[70] Alloprogesterone, a metabolite of progesterone, has potent antiseizure properties.

Antiepileptic Drugs and Contraception

Many AEDs induce the liver enzymes that are responsible for metabolizing combined oral contraceptives (COC), which results in degradation of the contraceptive agent, decreased contraceptive effectiveness, and an increased likelihood of unplanned pregnancy.[71] Estrogen acts as a proconvulsant factor, whereas progesterone is a seizure inhibitor. Thus, complex interactions occur between hormonal contraceptives and AEDs, and providing effective contraception for women who want to use a hormonal birth control method can be challenging. The U.S. medical eligibility criteria (MEC) for contraceptive use state that combined oral contraceptives, the contraceptive patch, and the contraceptive ring are not recommended for use by women using CYP450 enzyme-inducing AEDs (Table 24-10).[72] Progestin-only pills are likewise not recommended. Some experts do not recommend progestin implants but the MEC state the advantages may outweigh the theoretical risks for women using CYP450 enzyme-inducing AEDs. The DMPA injection and intrauterine devices provide safe and effective contraception for these women.[72]

For women who do use combined oral contraceptives, the dose should contain at least 50 mg of estrogen. Effectiveness may also be improved through use of a tricycle regimen that avoids the usual 7-day pill-free interval.[73] If the woman is relying on medroxyprogesterone (DPMA) injections for contraception, some neurologists recommend that the injections be given every 10 weeks instead of every 12 weeks.[73] Because both DMPA and some AEDs increase the risk for osteoporosis, this combination should be used be considered cautiously.

Lamotrigine (Lamictal) has a unique dual interaction with combined oral contraceptives; while it only moderately increases the metabolism and clearance of the COC, lamotrigine itself is metabolized to a greater extent during the 21-day cycle of contraceptive use, leading to a possible loss of antiepileptic effectiveness. There is a prominent rebound of serum levels of lamotrigine during the 7-day period when no COC is taken.

Antiepileptic Drugs and Osteoporosis

Carbamazepine (Tegretol), phenytoin (Dilantin), and valproate (Depacon, Depakene, Depakote) are associated with lower levels of calcium and an increased risk for fracture.[74] Therefore, all women taking these drugs should ensure they have a daily intake of 1200 mg of calcium and 600 IU of vitamin D. Women who take AEDs for more than 5 years should undergo a bone density scan.

Antiepileptic Drugs During Pregnancy

Older AEDs taken during the first trimester of pregnancy are associated with a twofold to threefold increase in the risk for both major and minor congenital malformations (6% in women with epilepsy versus 2% in the general population).[74] This risk also increases when multiple AEDs are administered together and may be dose related.[75] It was originally unclear whether the increase in teratogenic effects occurs secondary to epilepsy or secondary to AEDs, but recent research clarified that AEDs are the culprit. Valproate (Depacon, Depakene, Depakote) increases the risk for major congenital malformations when used as either monotherapy or part of a polytherapy regimen (6% to 10.2% incidence of major congenital malformations) and is associated with a reduction in IQ and cognitive skills in the offspring.[76] Additionally, some evidence suggests that carbamazepine (Tegretol) increases the risk for posterior cleft palate, and lamotrigine (Lamictal) in high doses is associated with an increased risk for congenital malformations. However, clinicians should not recommend discontinuing any AED for women who present for initial prenatal care and who are taking an AED. Rather, these women should be referred to a specialist for counseling and possible changes in their medication regimen.

Prospective pregnancy registries as listed in the Resources table at the end of this chapter have been established to determine the true risk rates associated with individual agents, and specific risks are now known (Table 24-15).[77–81] Clusters of congenital malformations such as craniofacial malformations, microcephalus, mental retardation, and hypoplasia of the distal phalanges are associated with phenytoin (Dilantin) and are often referred to as "fetal hydantoin syndrome." AEDs that act as folic acid antagonists, such as phenytoin (Dilantin), carbamazepine (Tegretol), valproic acid (Depakene), and barbiturates, increase the risk of neural tube defects. It is not clear whether folic acid supplementation will decrease the incidence of neural tube defects in women taking these AEDs. Current recommendations for folic acid supplementation vary. It is recommended that all women take 0.4 mg per day of folic acid starting before conception and continuing through 3 months before conception until the end of the first trimester. Some organizations recommend 4 mg per day of folic acid for women taking AEDs although the higher doses have not been conclusively shown to be protective for women taking AEDs.

Table 24-15 Rates of Congenital Malformations in Offspring of Women Using Antiepileptic Drugs During Pregnancy

Drug: Generic (Brand)	Teratogenic Effect
Carbamazepine (Tegretol)	2.5–4% risk of major malformations[a] (specifically posterior cleft palate, neural tube defects)
Diazepam (Valium)	Small increased risk of pyloric stenosis and alimentary tract atresia
Lamotrigine (Lamictal)	1.4–2.7% risk of major malformations, primarily oral clefts; risk is not dose dependent
Phenobarbital	6.5% incidence of major malformations; increased incidence of cardiac malformations; exposure during third trimester may lower IQ score of offspring by 0.5 standard deviation
Phenytoin (Dilantin)	Fetal hydantoin syndrome; neural tube defects; slight decrease in IQ scores in offspring
Valproate, valproic acid (Depacon, Depakene)	10.73–13% risk of major malformations (including neural tube defects, facial cleft palate, and possibly hypospadias). Risk may be dose dependent; it increases at doses greater than 800–1000 mg/day. Lower IQ scores in offspring (9–10 points). Polypharmacy is associated with an increased risk relative to monotherapy.

[a] Major malformation is an abnormality of an essential anatomic structure present at birth that interferes significantly with function and/or requires major intervention. The major malformations most commonly associated with AEDs include heart defects, cleft palate, urogenital defects, and neural tube defects.

Sources: Data from Meador KJ. Effects of in utero antiepileptic drug exposure. *Epilepsy Curr.* 2008;8(6):143-147[77]; Meador KJ, Bake GA, Browning N, et al.; NEAD Study Group. Cognitive function at 3 years of age after fetal exposure to antiepileptic drugs. *N Engl J Med.* 2009;360(16):1597-1605[79]; Pennell PB. Antiepileptic drugs during pregnancy: what is known and which AEDs seem to be safest? [Review]. *Epilepsia.* 2008;49(suppl 9):43-55.[81]

Antiepileptic Drugs During Lactation

The majority of AEDs are lipophilic and likely to become concentrated in breast milk. Although milk/plasma ratios and concentrations of many of the AEDs in breast milk are known, the effect of these medications on the newborn remains unclear. That said, discontinuing AEDs during lactation is not recommended, as clinical experience suggests adverse outcomes are rare. Long-term developmental outcomes of children who are exposed to AEDs via breast milk are not adversely affected.[82] Nevertheless, some drugs, such as lamotrigine (Lamictal), levetiracetam (Keppra), and carbamazepine (Tegretol), reach serum concentrations in the newborn that are potentially therapeutic; these infants should be observed carefully for apnea, rash, drowsiness, or poor sucking. Valproate (Depakene) and phenytoin (Dilantin) have poor transfer to breast milk and low milk/plasma ratios.

Benzodiazepines and barbiturates are associated with sedation in the newborn and should be used with caution by nursing mothers.

The Mature Woman

Women frequently experience an increase in seizures during the perimenopausal period and a decrease in seizures when they are postmenopausal.[83] This effect is especially common in women who demonstrate the catamenial epilepsy pattern. Hormone therapy is also associated with increased seizure activity. Because postmenopausal women have a higher risk for fracture if they fall or are injured, clinicians caring for women during the postmenopausal years who take AEDs should focus on interventions that decrease fracture risks and consult with neurologists to find the best treatments for menopausal symptoms.

Restless Leg Syndrome

Restless leg syndrome (RLS) is a sensorimotor disorder that affects up to 10% of the general population and is more prevalent in women and the elderly. Although remissions occur, RLS is considered a chronic and progressive disorder. *Restless limb syndrome* may better describe the disorder, as the legs, abdomen, and face can be affected, unilaterally or bilaterally. Women diagnosed with RLS should be reassured the disorder is not a precursor to Parkinson's disease.

Although not clearly understood, the etiology of RLS appears to be, in part, a dopaminergic dysfunction in the substantia nigra of the basal ganglia. Anemia can contribute to this dysfunction by limiting the brain's iron metabolism of coenzymes and enzymes ultimately necessary for the production of dopamine, a phenomenon called the "iron–dopamine connection."

A clinical diagnosis of restless leg syndrome is made when all four of the following criteria are met: (1) There is an urge to move the legs accompanied by dyskinesias; (2) the dyskinesias worsen when the person is at rest, especially when sitting or lying down; (3) the dyskinesias are partially or totally relieved by movement; and (4) symptoms exhibit a circadian pattern, becoming worse in the evening and into the night, and improving during the morning hours.[84]

Restless leg syndrome is categorized as primary (or idiopathic) or secondary. Primary RLS is subdivided into early onset (45 years or younger), which is characterized by a slow progression of the disorder and thought to be familial, and late onset (older than 45 years), which has a more aggressive progression. Secondary RLS may occur in persons with medical conditions that are associated with anemia, such as pregnancy, iron deficiency, and end-stage renal disease. The symptoms of primary and secondary RLS are the same; therefore, a medical work-up to rule out the causes of secondary RLS is recommended.

Treatment of Restless Leg Syndrome

An algorithm for the treatment of RLS symptoms, whether primary or secondary, was devised by the Medical Advisory Board of the Restless Leg Syndrome Foundation in 2004.[85] Definitions for treatment include (1) intermittent RLS, which requires treatment as necessary; (2) daily RLS, which requires daily treatment; and (3) refractory RLS, which requires treatment adjustment or adjunct.

Dopaminergic Agents

The first line of pharmacologic treatment for primary RLS is a dopamine agonist such as ropinirole (Requip), pramipexole (Mirapex), or rotigotine (Neupro). All three are non-ergoline dopamine agonists that are believed to stimulate dopamine (D_2) receptors. Rotigotine is available as a transdermal patch that has the advantages of 24-hour dosage and avoidance of the first-pass effect. The first line of treatment for secondary RLS is to diagnose and treat the causative medical disorder (e.g., iron therapy for anemia). Pharmacologic treatments for RLS are listed in Table 24-16.[86–88]

Side Effects/Adverse Effects

Although nausea and other gastrointestinal upsets are the most commonly reported side effects of ropinirole and pramipexole, increased somnolence can occur during daily activities such as driving.

Hallucinations, syncope, orthostatic hypotension, lack of impulse control, and increased compulsive behavior related to such events as gambling, sexual urges, and eating are rare adverse effects. These are all reasons to decrease dosing or discontinue medication. Should the medications need to be discontinued for nonemergent reasons, weaning the woman off them is recommended to avoid theoretic neuroleptic malignant syndrome.

Dopaminergic agents, especially levodopa (Sinemet), are associated with "augmentation," a condition in which symptoms are worsened secondary to use of the dopaminergic agent. Augmentation occurs as a paradoxical response to the medication such that the individual experiences worsening symptoms when the dose is increased. A second form of augmentation takes the form of a shorter latency period from rest to symptom onset, spread to previously unaffected body parts, increased intensity of symptoms, or shorter duration of relief following treatment. Augmentation in either form is generally treated by switching to a different agent or trying combination agents.

Special Populations: Pregnancy and Lactation

Dopaminergic agents are generally not recommended during pregnancy due to possible teratogenic effects in animals. These medications should not be used by breastfeeding women, as the amount of the drug secreted into breast milk and its effect on the newborn are unknown. Dopamine is also known as prolactin-inhibiting factor, which could impair lactogenesis.

Other Pharmacologic Treatments for Restless Leg Syndrome

In addition to ropinirole (Requip) and pramipexole (Mirapex), opioids, sedative-hypnotics, and anticonvulsants have been used as adjunctive therapies for RLS. Opioids are an effective alternative for persons with RLS that is not treated effectively with dopaminergic agents. Opioids can be used intermittently. Sedative-hypnotics can

Table 24-16 Pharmacotherapy for Restless Leg Syndrome

Drug: Generic (Brand)	Dose	Advantages	Clinical Considerations
Dopamine Precursors			
Carbidopa/levodopa (Sinemet)	1/2 or 1 tablet of 25/100 (mg carbidopa/mg levodopa) PO 1 hour before symptom onset, not to exceed a dose of 50/200	Can be used on a one-time basis or as needed. Useful for persons with intermittent RLS, as dopamine receptor agonists take longer to have an effect.	May develop augmentation, a worsening of symptoms prior to the next expected dose. Therapeutic value is reduced if taken with high-protein food. Can cause insomnia, sleepiness, and gastrointestinal distress.
Dopamine Receptor Agonists (Ergot Derived)			
Cabergoline (Dostinex)		Associated with cardiac valve fibrosis; not recommended for RLS	
Dopamine Receptor Agonists (Non-ergoline)			
Pramipexole (Mirapex)	Initial dose: 0.125 mg Mean effective dose: 0.375 mg Maximum dose: 0.75 mg	Decreases periodic limb movements and mitigates consequences of RLS symptoms	Can cause nausea, orthostatic hypotension, and augmentation. Associated with impulse-control disorders.
Ropinirole (Requip)	Initial dose: 0.25 mg Average dose: 1.0–2.5 mg/day Maximum dose: 4 mg/day		
Rotigotine (Neupro)	Initial dose: 1 mg/24 hours Maximum dose: 3 mg/24 hours	Supplied as a transdermal patch: 1, 2, 3, 4, 6, and 8 mg/24 hours	
Codeine	15–30 mg Maximum dose: 120 mg/day	Opioids offer an effective alternative for persons whose RLS is not effectively treated with or cannot be treated by dopaminergic agents. They can be used on an intermittent basis or can be used successfully for daily therapy. A wide range of potencies are available.	Can cause constipation, urinary retention, sleepiness, or cognitive changes. Tolerance and dependence are possible with higher doses of stronger agents, especially those with a shorter half-life.
Propoxyphene (Darvon)	65 to 130 mg/day Maximum dose: 260–390 mg/day		
Hydrocodone (Vicodin)	5–10 mg/day Maximum dose: 20–30 mg/day		
Oxycodone (Percocet, Roxicodone, OxyContin)	5–10 mg/day; maximum dose: 15–20 mg/day Extended release: 10 mg/day; maximum dose: 20–30 mg/day		
Tramadol (Ultram)	50–100 mg/day Maximum dose: 300–400 mg/day		
Methadone	5–10 mg/day Maximum dose: 20–40 mg/day		
Gabapentin (Neurontin)	100–300 mg/day Maximum dose: 2400 mg/day	Anticonvulsants offer an effective alternative for those persons whose RLS is not effectively treated with dopaminergic agents	Disadvantages vary depending on the agent, but include nausea, sedation, dizziness, dermatologic conditions, hepatic disorders, and bone marrow suppression. Increases the risk for suicidality.
Clonazepam (Klonopin)	0.25 mg/day Maximum dose: 2 mg/day	Sleeping aids are most effective for improving sleep quality if RLS symptoms occur at night. May be used alone if the person is intolerant of dopaminergic drugs.	Can cause daytime sleepiness and cognitive impairment
Oxazepam (Serax)	10 mg/day Maximum dose: 40 mg/day		
Temazepam (Restoril)	7.5–30 mg at bedtime Maximum duration: 1 month		
Zolpidem (Ambien)	5 mg/day Maximum dose: 20 mg/day		
Triazolam (Halcion)	0.125 mg/day Maximum dose: 0.25 mg/day.		

Source: Modified from Hensley JG. Leg cramps and restless legs syndrome during pregnancy. *J Midwifery Womens Health*. 2009; 54(3):211-218.

improve sleep quality for persons who have symptoms at night. Gabapentin (Neurontin) is the most studied anticonvulsant and appears to be as effective for controlling symptoms and has fewer drug–drug interactions. Gabapentin has mild sedative properties and can be used to facilitate sleep in persons with RLS who have concomitant sleep disturbances.

Adult Attention-Deficit/Hyperactivity Disorder

Attention-deficit/hyperactivity disorder (ADHD) is a syndrome that is often first observed in childhood; it is characterized by difficulty in sustaining attention, excessive motor activity, and impulsiveness. ADHD is also often associated with underachievement in school and may continue into adulthood in a modified form. In the United States, approximately 40% to 70% of children with this disorder will have symptoms that persist into adolescence and adulthood.[89] The prevalence of adult attention-deficit/hyperactivity disorder (AADHD) is difficult to determine, as many affected individuals have coping skills that allow them to be functional members of society.

Treatment for AADHD includes medication and some form of stress management such as biofeedback or meditation. Stimulants and antidepressants are the two categories of drugs used to treat AADHD. In addition, several atypical antidepressants have been used with some success. Medications help retain focus and attention but are not effective as monotherapy in helping individuals with AADHD manage daily activities; thus, cognitive and behavioral interventions are an essential element in the overall treatment regimen for AADHD.

Amphetamines

Amphetamines, which are also called sympathomimetic drugs, act as agonists at adrenergic receptors in the autonomic nervous system and are the first-line of treatment for AADHD. Approximately 75% of individuals with AADHD have improved symptoms when given sympathomimetic drugs. In addition to methylphenidate (Ritalin, Ritalin-SR), dextroamphetamine (Dexedrine) and amphetamine/dextroamphetamine (Adderall) are considered to be preferred medications for AADHD. Although the exact mechanism of action of these agents remains elusive, they are thought to block the reuptake of norepinephrine and increase the release of norepinephrine and dopamine, thereby inducing sympathetic nervous system activation. Table 24-17 reviews the doses, side effects, and dosing considerations for the drugs used to treat AADHD.

Table 24-17 Medications Used to Treat Adult Attention-Deficit/Hyperactivity Disorder

Drug: Generic (Brand)	Formulations	Dose	Side Effects/Adverse Effects
Stimulants			
Amphetamine/ dextroamphetamine (Adderall, Adderall XR)	5-, 10-, 20-, and 30-mg tablets; 5-, 10-, 15-, 20-, 25-, and 30-mg extended-release capsules	5–40 mg PO in the morning or 2 times/day Extended-release capsules: 20–60 mg/day PO Maximum dose: 60 mg/day at a rate of 10 mg/week	Increased heart rate, blood pressure, decreased appetite, weight loss, disturbed sleep. Hypertension is not a contraindication, but blood pressure should be monitored carefully. FDA black box warning highlights the potential for abuse and dependence. FDA black box warning indicates that misuse can cause sudden death.
Dextroamphetamine (Dexedrine)	5-mg tablets; 5-, 10-, and 15-mg extended-release capsules	5–60 mg PO/day in 2-3 divided doses Maximum dose: 60 mg/day if needed	Schedule II controlled substance; prescription cannot be refilled, and a written copy of the prescription is required. Increased heart rate, blood pressure, decreased appetite, weight loss, disturbed sleep. Hypertension is not a contraindication but blood pressure should be monitored carefully. FDA black box warning highlights the potential for abuse and dependence. FDA black box warning indicates that misuse can cause sudden death.

(*continues*)

Table 24-17 Medications Used to Treat Adult Attention-Deficit/Hyperactivity Disorder (*continued*)

Drug: Generic (Brand)	Formulations	Dose	Side Effects/Adverse Effects
Dexmethylphenidate (Focalin)	2.5-, 5-, and 10-mg tablets; 5-, 10-, 15-, and 20-mg extended-release capsules	2.5–10 mg PO 2 times/day Extended release: 10–20 mg each morning Maximum dose: 20 mg/day	Increased heart rate, blood pressure, decreased appetite, weight loss, disturbed sleep. Hypertension is not a contraindication, but blood pressure should be monitored carefully. FDA black box warning highlights the potential for abuse and dependence. FDA black box warning indicates that misuse can cause sudden death.
Methylphenidate (Concerta, Metadate, Methylin, Ritalin) Methylphenidate transdermal (Daytrana)	5-, 10-, and 20-mg tablets; 18-, 27-, 36-, and 54-mg controlled-release tablets Transdermal: 10-, 15-, 20-, and 30-mg per 9-hour patches	5–15 mg PO 2–3 times/day; controlled release: 18–72 mg/day Transdermal: 10–30 mg/9-hour patch each day Maximum dose: 30 mg/9-hour patch/day	Schedule II controlled substance; abuse and dependence are possible. Increased heart rate, blood pressure; decreased appetite; weight loss; disturbed sleep. Hypertension is not a contraindication, but blood pressure should be monitored carefully. FDA black box warning highlights the potential for abuse and dependence.
Nonstimulants			
Atomoxetine (Strattera)	10-, 18-, 25-, 40-, 60-, 80-, and 100-mg capsules	80 mg PO in the morning Maximum dose: 100 mg/day Larger doses may be divided into 2 times/day	SNRI; does not have the stimulant properties of amphetamines. Well tolerated. Rare adverse effects: Hepatotoxicity, suicidal ideation. FDA black box warning highlights the risk of suicidal ideation in children and adolescents.
Bupropion (Budeprion SR, Budeprion XL, Wellbutrin)	75- and 100-mg tablets; 100-, 150-, 200-, and 300-mg extended-release tablets	100 mg PO 3 times/day Extended release: 200 mg in the morning and 100 mg in the evening	Contraindicated in persons with a history of seizures. FDA black box warning highlights the risk of suicidal ideation.
Imipramine (Tofranil)	10-, 25-, and 50-mg tablets	10–25 mg PO/day to start; then increase to 100–150 mg/day	Rare prolonged QT syndrome. ECG should be obtained before initiating therapy. Drowsiness, sexual dysfunction, weight gain, postural hypotension, and anticholinergic effects are common. FDA black box warning highlights the risk of suicidal ideation.
Nortriptyline (Norpramin)	10-, 25-, 50-, and 75-mg capsules	10–25 mg PO/day to start; then increase to 100–150 mg/day	Rare prolonged QT syndrome. ECG should be obtained before initiating therapy. Drowsiness, sexual dysfunction, weight gain, postural hypotension, and anticholinergic effects are common. FDA black box warning highlights the risk of suicidal ideation.

Abbreviations: ECG = electrocardiogram; SNRI = serotonin–norepinephrine reuptake inhibitor.

Antidepressants

Tricyclic antidepressants inhibit the uptake of norepinephrine and serotonin. Nortriptyline (Pamelor) and desipramine (Norpramin) are preferred because they have greater effects on norepinephrine. Bupropion (Wellbutrin) is an atypical antidepressant that also appears to work well in women with AADHD.

Special Populations: Pregnancy and Lactation

In light of the high incidence of adolescent pregnancy as well as the increased recognition of ADHD, it is of note that little has been published regarding ADHD during pregnancy. One brief report cautioned that use of the common medications presented unknown risks, although no teratogenic effects had been reported.[90] A study of the transfer of dexamphetamine into breast milk revealed less than a 10% maternal concentration in the milk, suggesting this medication may be safe during breastfeeding. However, only four women participated in the study; thus, more research is needed in this area.[91]

Parkinson's Disease

Several nervous system degenerative disorders are characterized by an irreversible, progressive destruction of neurons from specific regions of the brain, including

Parkinson's disease, Alzheimer's disease, and myasthenia gravis. Multiple sclerosis is also characterized by myelin sheaths that surround nerve axons but the genesis of multiple sclerosis is an autoimmune process and therefore, it is addressed in the *Autoimmune Conditions* chapter. Parkinson's disease affects men and women equally, and the lifetime risk for onset of Parkinson's disease is 2%.

Some evidence indicates that estrogen promotes the development and differentiation of dopaminergic neurons.[92] Premenopausal women with Parkinson's disease occasionally report increased symptoms during menstruation, when the body has lower levels of circulating estrogen. One study found that postmenopausal women receiving conjugated estrogen had better symptom control on the same dose of antiparkinson drugs than when they were not taking the hormone.[93] Although only sparse evidence is available, this is clearly an area that deserves further research.

Pathophysiology of Parkinson's Disease

The pathologic change responsible for Parkinson's disease is progressive destruction of dopamine-secreting neurons in the basal ganglia of the brain. The basal ganglia comprise groups of neurons located deep within the cerebrum and midbrain that serve as an accessory motor system communicating bidirectionally with the cerebral cortex and the corticospinal motor system (pyramidal tract). They act as a modulator that regulates the flow of signals down from the motor cortex to the motor neurons of the spinal cord. Disorders of movement that occur secondary to basal ganglia impairment are termed **extrapyramidal symptoms** because although the pyramidal tract remains intact and functional, it lacks adequate modification from the extrapyramidal system.

Dopamine is the inhibitory neurotransmitter and acetylcholine is the excitatory neurotransmitter in this area of the brain. Four major dopamine pathways are present in the brain: nigrostriatal, mesolimbic, mesocortical, and tuberoinfundibular. Decreased dopamine in the nigrostriatal tract causes the altered movement symptoms of Parkinson's disease, and dopamine deficiencies in the other three tracts is the probable etiology of the neuropsychiatric pathology seen in persons with Parkinson's disease.

The movement disorders (**dyskinesias**) associated with Parkinson's disease have four characteristic features: (1) **bradykinesia** (slowness and poverty of movement); (2) muscular rigidity; (3) tremor while at rest that decreases with voluntary movement; and (4) impaired posture and balance that result in gait disturbance and falling.[94,95] These symptoms appear only when 65% to 80% of the dopamine is depleted.

Dopamine Metabolism

Because Parkinson's disease is caused by a relative lack of dopamine, pharmacologic treatments for this condition are aimed at altering different phases of dopamine metabolism and physiology.

Dopamine is synthesized by dopaminergic neurons in a series of steps starting with the amino acid tyrosine, which is acted upon by tyrosine hydroxylase to produce first L-dihydroxyphenylalanine (L-dopa) and then dopamine. The dopamine is subsequently stored in vesicles and released into a synapse when the presynaptic neuron is depolarized by entry of calcium ions. Dopamine binds to one of two important receptors to produce an effector response in the postsynaptic neuron—the D_1 or D_2 receptor. The action of dopamine is terminated either by reuptake of the dopamine into the presynaptic or postsynaptic nerve terminal or by its breakdown by the sequential action of two enzymes, catechol-*O*-methyltransferase (COMT) and monoamine oxidase (MAO). Drugs used to treat Parkinson's disease work in one of the following three ways: (1) replace dopamine in the brain; (2) decrease the amount of acetylcholine; or (3) provide neuroprotection. (Table 24-18).

Drugs That Cause Dyskinesias

Dyskinesias can be an adverse reaction to medications. Commonly used drugs that cause dyskinesias include antipsychotics such as chlorpromazine (Thorazine) and haloperidol (Haldol); tricyclic antidepressants; and antiemetics such as promethazine (Phenergan), prochlorperazine (Compazine), and metoclopramide (Reglan). The common mechanism of action is antagonism of dopamine, which leads to inhibition of postsynaptic impulses.

Dopaminergic Therapy: Levodopa

Levodopa (Sinemet), also called L-dopa, is the metabolic precursor of dopamine and the most effective treatment currently available for the treatment of Parkinson's disease. Dopamine itself does not cross the blood–brain barrier, so it cannot be administered peripherally. More than 90% of individuals with Parkinson's disease respond favorably to the administration of levodopa, however. Orally administered levodopa is absorbed from the small intestine and crosses the blood–brain barrier by means of special transport mechanisms for aromatic amino acids. In the brain, it is converted to dopamine. It is this dopamine that is responsible for the therapeutic action of levodopa in Parkinson's disease therapy, as L-dopa has no effect on its own.

Table 24-18 Medications Used to Treat Parkinson's Disease

Drug: Generic (Brand)	Formulations	Dose	Clinical Considerations
Anticholinergic Agents			
Diphenhydramine (Benadryl)	25- and 50-mg capsules; 12.5 mg/5 mL solution	25–50 mg PO 3–4 times/day Maximum dose: Single dose of 100 mg or 400 mg/day	Anticholinergic. Treats dystonic reactions.
Benztropine (Cogentin)	0.5-, 1-, and 2-mg tablets	1–2 mg PO 2 times/day Maximum dose: 6 mg/day (4 mg in elderly)	Anticholinergic. SE: Confusion, dry mouth, nausea. AE: memory impairment, hallucinations, more common in elderly.
Trihexyphenidyl (Artane)	2- and 5-mg tablets; 2 mg/5 mL elixir	6–10 mg PO/day in 3 divided doses Maximum dose: 15 mg/day	
Dopamine Agonists			
Amantadine (Symmetrel)	100-mg tablets; 50 mg/5 mL syrup	100 mg PO 2 times/day Maximum dose: 400 mg/day	Antiviral agent with mild dopamine agonist activity. Low toxicity and useful for younger persons; toxic effects more likely in the elderly. SE: Confusion, nausea, ankle edema. AE: Hallucinations, neuroleptic malignant syndrome.
Bromocriptine (Parlodel)	2.5-mg tablets; 5-mg capsules	1.25–30 mg PO 2–3 times/day; increase by 2.5 mg/day every 2–4 weeks Maximum dose: 100 mg/day	Dopamine agonist. SE: Nausea, vomiting, orthostatic hypotension, hallucinations, dizziness, peripheral edema with chronic use, confusion, sleepiness. Initiate with low dose and increase slowly to minimize SE.
Pramipexole (Mirapex)	0.125-, 0.25-, 0.5-, 0.75-, 1-, and 1.5-mg tablets	0.5–1.5 mg PO 3 times/day	
Ropinirole (Requip)	0.25-, 0.5-, 1-, 2-, 3-, 4-, and 5-mg tablets	3 mg PO 3 times/day	
Dopamine Replacement			
Carbidopa/levodopa (Sinemet 25/100)	10/100-, 25/100-, 25/250-mg tablets; 50/200-mg controlled-release tablets	Normal dosage range for levodopa (in combination with carbidopa): 200–1200 mg/day PO in 2–3 divided doses Initial dose: 10 mg carbidopa/100 mg levodopa 3–4 times/day *or* 25 mg carbidopa/100 mg levodopa 3 times/day; increase by 1 tablet/day every 24–48 hours	Dopamine replacement
Entacapone (Comtan)	200-mg tablets	200 mg per dose Maximum dose: 1600 mg/day	Used as adjunctive treatment with each dose of carbidopa/levodopa
MAO Inhibitors			
Selegiline (Eldepryl, Zelapar)	5-mg capsules; 1.25-mg dispersible tablets (Zelapar)	5 mg PO 2 times/day Maximum dose: 10 mg/day	MAO inhibitor; enhances effect of levodopa. Food restrictions. Do not use with SSRIs or TCA antidepressants. SE: Nausea and headaches; amphetamine metabolites may cause insomnia; may increase SE of levodopa. AE: Confusion in elderly.
Other			
Tolcapone (Tasmar)	100- and 200-mg tablets	100 mg PO 3 times/day Maximum dose: 200 mg 3 times/day	COMT inhibitor used as adjunctive treatment with carbidopa/levodopa. SE: Dyskinesia, hallucinations, nausea, orthostatic hypotension.

Abbreviations: AE = adverse effects; COMT = catechol-*O*-methyltransferase; MAO = monoamine oxidase; SE = side effects; SSRI = selective serotonin reuptake inhibitor; TCA = tricyclic antidepressant.

Levodopa is also decarboxylated by enzymes in the intestines and liver into dopamine that then enters the peripheral circulation. This peripheral conversion results in a low availability of the drug entering the brain because, as noted earlier, dopamine does not cross the blood–brain barrier. The presence of dopamine in the peripheral circulation causes undesirable effects such as nausea, orthostatic hypotension, and cardiac arrhythmias. Therefore, levodopa is usually administered with a peripherally acting decarboxylase inhibitor such as carbidopa. This combination of levodopa and carbidopa prevents much of the peripheral conversion of levodopa, resulting in increased drug availability in the brain while avoiding the undesirable peripheral effects of dopamine. For these reasons, levodopa is most commonly prescribed in a combined form containing 25 mg carbidopa and 100 mg levodopa (Sinemet 25/100).

Side Effects/Adverse Effects

Levodopa therapy often has dramatic effects on the signs and symptoms of early Parkinson's disease, with almost complete improvement of tremor, rigidity, and bradykinesia occurring and long-lasting benefits arising possibly due to storage and release of the exogenous dopamine. In later stages of the disease, this buffering effect is lost, and dramatic changes in motor ability occur secondary to each dose of levodopa, termed the *on-off phenomenon.* When this phenomenon occurs, each dose of levodopa may improve symptoms for only 1 to 2 hours, after which rigidity and akinesia rapidly return. Increasing the dose and frequency of dosing is limited by the possibility that a hyperdopaminergic state will induce dyskinesias. The use of sustained-release formulations or changing the dosing schedule from every 4 to 6 hours to every 2 hours, while providing the same total daily dose, sometimes helps with the on-off symptoms.

Rapid initial titration of levodopa or high doses of the pharmaceutical may result in dyskinesias. Excessive and abnormal involuntary movements such as head bobbing, tics, and grimacing develop in as many as 80% of individuals treated with the drug during the first year of therapy. Reduction of the dose can decrease dyskinesias but may lead to increased symptoms of Parkinson's disease. Elderly individuals with preexisting cognitive problems are susceptible to confusion and hallucinations requiring dose reduction, which can make treatment ineffective. Levodopa-induced psychosis can be effectively treated with atypical antipsychotic agents such as clozapine (Clozaril) that do not tend to worsen Parkinson's disease symptoms, such as might occur with phenothiazine antipsychotics.

Drug Interactions

Individuals taking nonspecific MAO inhibitors for depression such as phenelzine (Nardil) and tranylcypromine (Parnate) can experience a life-threatening hypertensive crisis and hyperpyrexia if they receive catecholamines such as dopamine. These drugs should be stopped at least 2 weeks before starting L-dopa administration.

Abrupt withdrawal of dopaminergic agents such as levodopa can precipitate neuroleptic malignant syndrome. Taking a dose of levodopa on a full stomach may delay absorption due to competition with other amino acids for the transport mechanism in the small intestine. Pyridoxine (vitamin B_6) enhances decarboxylase activity, which may increase the peripheral transformation of levodopa into dopamine, thereby decreasing its availability in the brain. Phenothiazine antipsychotic drugs decrease the therapeutic effects of levodopa and are also capable of inducing Parkinsonian symptoms on their own.

Amantadine (Symmetrel)

Amantadine (Symmetrel) is used in the initial therapy of mild Parkinson's disease and may also be helpful as an adjunct agent in individuals receiving levodopa who have symptom fluctuations or dyskinesias. Amantadine is thought to enhance dopamine release from the presynaptic storage vesicles and is used as an early treatment to delay the initiation of levodopa therapy.[96]

Dopamine Receptor Agonists

Bromocriptine (Parlodel)

Bromocriptine (Parlodel) is an older dopamine receptor agonist derived from ergot. It acts as an agonist at the D_2 receptor and is the drug used when amantadine is no longer useful. Initial treatment with bromocriptine can cause profound hypotension, so the medication should be started at a low dose. Bromocriptine can induce transient nausea and fatigue as well, so it can sometimes require weeks to months to slowly adjust the dose up to the therapeutically necessary levels. This agent is most often prescribed for persons who are already receiving levodopa to reduce motor fluctuations, such as those associated with on-off symptoms, or to decrease the dose of levodopa to avoid dyskinesias.

Ropinirole (Requip) and Pramipexole (Mirapex)

Two newer agents, ropinirole (Requip) and pramipexole (Mirapex), are more selective for the D_2 receptor sites, better tolerated, and more quickly titrated. Both drugs also are less apt to cause nausea and fatigue. These selective dopamine agonists are being increasingly used as initial monotherapy for Parkinson's disease. They have the advantage of better tolerance and less likelihood of on-off phenomena due to their longer half-lives when compared to levodopa.

Acetylcholine Muscarinic Receptor Antagonists

Several acetylcholine **muscarinic** receptor antagonists, also called anticholinergic drugs, are currently used to treat early Parkinson's disease or as adjunctive therapy coadministered with dopamine agonists. These drugs include benztropine (Cogentin), diphenhydramine (Benadryl), and trihexyphenidyl (Artane). Their ability to cause smooth muscle relaxation makes them particularly useful for treating muscle rigidity and **akinesia**.

Side Effects/Adverse Effects

The side effects of the acetylcholine muscarinic receptor antagonists result from their anticholinergic properties and include sedation, mental confusion, constipation, urinary retention, and blurred vision. Anticholinergic drugs can have an additive effect with any drug or agent that causes sedation. Adverse effects may include confusion, hallucinations, mydriasis, and photophobia. These drugs are contraindicated for persons who have narrow-angle glaucoma or a history of urinary retention.

Neuroprotection: Catechol-*O*-Methyltransferase Inhibitors

Catechol-*O*-methyltransferase is one of the two enzymes responsible for the catabolism of levodopa and dopamine. Its inhibition prolongs both the half-life of levodopa, permitting more of the drug to reach the brain, and the effect of dopamine in the synapse within the brain.

Entacapone (Comtan), a COMT inhibitor, is available as a single pill combined with levodopa/carbidopa in several fixed-dose combinations. Tolcapone (Tasmar) is a potent COMT inhibitor whose label carries a FDA black box warning about an increased risk for hepatotoxicity and acute liver failure. Both of the COMT inhibitors are used as adjunctive therapies with levodopa/carbidopa and have similar side effects as levodopa/carbidopa, including nausea, orthostatic hypotension, vivid dreams, confusion, and hallucinations.

Selective MAO-B Inhibitors

Two isoenzymes of MAO are responsible for metabolism of catecholamines: MAO-A and MAO-B. Both are present in periphery, but only MAO-B is found in the striatum; this isoenzyme is responsible for most of the metabolism of dopamine in the brain. Selegiline (Eldepryl) is an irreversible selective MAO-B inhibitor. Unlike nonspecific MAO inhibitors, selegiline does not inhibit peripheral catecholamine metabolism and does not potentiate catecholamines or tyramine as long as daily doses do not exceed 10 mg. Selegiline has a modest effect in relieving Parkinson's disease symptoms, presumably by retarding the breakdown of dopamine in the striatum. It appears to have a neuroprotective effect and, if started early in the course of the disease, can delay progression. Metabolites of selegiline include amphetamine and methamphetamine, which may cause insomnia, anxiety, and other adverse symptoms.

Special Populations: Pregnancy and Lactation

Relatively few persons are diagnosed with Parkinson's disease before the age of 50 years; therefore not a lot of data is available regarding the use of antiparkinson drugs taken by women during pregnancy and lactation. Anecdotal reports have been published indicating worsening of Parkinson's symptoms occurs in women who are untreated during pregnancy.[97] Among the medications used to treat Parkinson's disease, only amantadine (Symmetrel) is associated with an increased risk of complications during pregnancy and fetal osseous abnormalities, although animal studies would urge caution with the use of selegiline.[98]

The data regarding breastfeeding while taking Parkinson's drugs are even more sparse. The potential risks of these drugs must be weighed by the mother against the known benefits of feeding her child breast milk.

Alzheimer's Disease

Alzheimer's disease is a neurodegenerative condition that results from a progressive destruction of neurons in the cerebral cortex associated with memory and abstract reasoning (i.e., the hippocampus and the association areas of the cortex). Degenerating neuronal processes and neurofibrillary tangles lead to accumulation of senile plaques consisting of the protein β-amyloid. Neuronal loss results in a reduction of neurotransmitters in the areas of the brain that experience the most destructive effects—especially acetylcholine. Thus treatments for Alzheimer's disease focus on increasing the availability of acetylcholine in the brain. Attempts to increase the concentration of acetylcholine by administration of its synthetic pathway precursors such as choline and phosphatidyl choline (lecithin), however, have not proved consistently successful. Clearly, much work remains to be done in the evaluation of all agents, including nutritional supplements as an aid to memory among the elderly.

Pharmacologic interventions for Alzheimer's disease currently concentrate on drugs that inhibit acetylcholinesterase, the intrasynaptic enzyme that breaks down acetylcholine. Acetylcholinesterase inhibitors have proved moderately successful in treating early symptoms of Alzheimer's disease and have also been used in combination with nutritional supplements such as choline with modest results.[99]

Drugs Used for Alzheimer's Disease

The FDA has approved four anticholinesterase-inhibiting drugs for use in the treatment of Alzheimer's disease. Tacrine (Cognex) is associated with significant side effects, such as abdominal cramping, nausea, diarrhea, and anorexia, all of which are dose related. Approximately 30% of individuals taking this drug at therapeutic levels experience these symptoms. Furthermore, the risk of hepatotoxicity is greater with tacrine and has led to reduction in clinical use.[100] The three other drugs in this class—donepezil (Aricept), rivastigmine (Exelon), and galantamine (Razadyne)—have less effect on peripheral tissues and are associated with fewer of the side effects that are most pronounced with tacrine.[101]

Other pharmacologic approaches to altering brain neurotransmitters for the treatment of Alzheimer's disease remain in the development stage. However, one new drug, memantine (Namenda), has been approved and is currently in use. Memantine is an *N*-methyl-D-aspartic acid (NMDA) glutamate receptor antagonist that appears to reduce neurologic excitotoxicity and might reduce the rate of clinical deterioration by that mechanism.[8] It has mild and reversible side effects that include headache and dizziness and is useful for those persons with moderate to severe Alzheimer's disease.

The dosing considerations for all of the drugs used to treat Alzheimer's disease are summarized in Table 24-19.

Table 24-19 Medications Used to Treat Alzheimer's Disease

Drug: Generic (Brand)	Formulations	Dose
Donepezil (Aricept)	5- and 10-mg tablets; 5-mg dispersible tablets	5–10 mg PO at bedtime
Galantamine (Razadyne)	4-, 8-, and 12-mg tablets; 4 mg/mL liquid; 8-, 16-, and 24-mg extended-release capsules	8–12 mg PO 2 times/day Maximum dose: 24 mg/day
Memantine (Namenda)	5- and 10-mg tablets; 2 mg/mL solution	10 mg PO 2 times/day Maximum dose: 20 mg/day
Rivastigmine (Exelon)	1.5-, 3-, 4.5-, and 6-mg capsules; 2 mg/mL liquid; 4.6- and 9.5-mg/24 hour-transdermal patch	3–6 mg PO 2 times/day Maximum dose: 12 mg/day
Tacrine (Cognex)	10-, 20-, 30-, and 40-mg capsules	20–40 mg PO 4 times/day Maximum dose: 40 mg 4 times/day

Myasthenia Gravis

Myasthenia gravis is a progressive incurable disorder characterized by the loss of acetylcholine receptors. It name comes from the Latin *gravis*, meaning "serious," and the Greek *mys*, meaning "muscle," and *asthenēs*, meaning "weakness." Thus, myasthenia gravis is characterized by skeletal weakness and fatigue that become worse with exertion but are milder when the individual is resting. In this autoimmune disorder, circulating autoantibodies block acetylcholine receptors at the postsynaptic neuromuscular junction. The most serious complication of the disorder is weakness of the respiratory muscles, which sets the stage for pneumonia. Myasthenia gravis tends to occur more often in women when it is diagnosed during early adulthood (20–30 years) and more often in men when it is diagnosed in persons older than 50 years.

Anticholinesterase inhibitors are the mainstay of medical treatment for myasthenia gravis. These drugs prevent cholinesterase from inactivating acetylcholine. Corticosteroids and immunosuppressants may be used to suppress the abnormal immune response. Because the thymus is frequently involved in producing the destructive antibodies, surgical removal of the thymus gland is also a common treatment.

Neostigmine (Prostigmin) and pyridostigmine (Mestinon) are two examples of the anticholinesterase drugs used to treat myasthenia gravis. Their side effects include nausea, vomiting, diarrhea, urinary frequency, and increased bronchial secretions. These agents should be used with caution by persons with bronchial asthma or those who are taking a cardiac glycoside. All of these agents are classified into FDA Pregnancy Category C secondary to documented fetal harm in animal studies, but no studies have been done on humans.

Conclusion

Diseases that affect the central nervous system are of particular import for women. The reproductive hormones estrogen and progesterone affect the function of most neurotransmitters that are involved in this collection of disorders. Pharmacologic treatment of nervous system disorders is typically aimed at regulating neuronal transmission imbalances primarily at the synaptic level. The drugs available are not always able to be targeted to just the specific imbalance, however, so they may produce global effects on many body systems, resulting in numerous side effects. Newer drugs have fewer side effects due to their greater specificity.

The most productive area of new research related to the central nervous system disorders most likely will be in the area of neuroprotection or the prevention of neuronal damage. Combinations of neuroprotective drugs and dietary supplements may hold the greatest hope for the future.

Resources

Organization	Description	Website
International Headache Society (HIS)	Diagnostic criteria for different types of headaches can be found on this website. Both the current ICHD-II version and the beta version of ICHD-III are available.	www.ihs-classification.org/en
International League Against Epilepsy	Provides the current classification of epilepsy, along with multiple guidelines and reports on treatment of epilepsy	www.ilae.org
Antiepileptic Pregnancy Registry	Supported by Massachusetts General Hospital, this website has gathered data about the pregnancy risks of many AEDs	www.aedpregnancyregistry.org
National Parkinson Foundation (NPF)	Contains NPF white papers, professional resources, and professional training	www.parkinson.org/professionals.aspx

References

1. Marin-Padilla M. The mammalian neocortex new pyramidal neuron: a new conception. *Frontiers Neuroanat.* 2014;7(51):1-8.
2. Bernstein JA, Fox RW, Martin VT, Lockey RF. Headache and facial pain: differential diagnosis and treatment. *J Allergy Clin Immunol: In Pract.* 2013; 1:242-251.
3. Headache Classification Committee of the International Headache Society. The international classification of headache disorders. 3rd ed. (beta version). *Cephalalgia.* 2013;33(9):629-808.
4. Yu S, Han X. Update on chronic tension-type headache. *Curr Pain Headache Rep.* 2015;19(1):469.
5. Evers S, Marziniak M. Clinical feathers, pathophysiology, and treatment of medication-overuse headache. *Lancet Neurol.* 2012;9(4):391-401.
6. Cheung V, Maoozergar F, Dilli E. Medication overuse headache. *Curr Neurol Neurosci Rep.* 2015;15(1):509.
7. Saper JR, Da Silva AN. Medication overuse headache: history, features, prevention and management strategies. *CNS Drugs.* 2013;27:867-877.
8. Lipton RB, Walter F, Diamond S, Diamond M, Reed M. Prevalence and burden of migraine in the United States: data from the American Migraine Study II. *Headache.* 2001;41(7):646-657.
9. Martin VT. Menstrual migraine: a review of prophylactic therapies. *Curr Pain Headache Rep.* 2004; 8:229-237.
10. Goadsby PJ. Pathophysiology of migraine. *Ann Indian Acad Neurol.* 2012;15(suppl 1):S15-S22.
11. Eikermann-Haerter K, Ayata C. Cortical spreading depression and migraine. *Curr Neurol Neurosci Rep.* 2010;10:176-173.
12. Lipton RB, Steward WF, Stone AM, Lainez MJ, Sawyer JP. Stratified care vs step care strategies for migraine: the Disability in Strategies of Care (DISC) study: a randomized trial. *JAMA.* 2000;284(20):2599-2605.
13. Loder E, Burch R, Rissoli P. The 2012 AHS/AAN guidelines for prevention of episodic migraine: a summary and comparison with other recent clinical practice guidelines. *Headache.* 2012;52(6):930-945.
14. Silberstein SD, Holland S, Freitag F, Dodick DW, Argoff C, Ashman E. Evidence-based guideline update: pharmacologic treatment for episodic migraine prevention in adults: report of the quality standards subcommittee of the American Academy of Neurology and the American Headache Society. *Neurology.* 2012;78(17):1337-1345.
15. Holland S, Silberstein SD, Freitag F, Dodick DW, Argoff C, Ashman E. Evidence-based guideline update: NSAIDs and other complementary treatments for episodic migraine prevention in adults: report of the quality standards subcommittee of the American Academy of Neurology and the American Headache Society. *Neurology.* 2012;78(17): 1346-1353.
16. Thorlund K, Mills EJ, Wu P, et al. Comparative efficacy of triptans for the abortive treatment of migraine: a multiple treatment comparison meta-analysis. *Cephalalgia.* 2014;34(4):258-267.
17. Gilmore B, Michael M. Treatment of acute migraine headache. *Am Fam Phys.* 2011;83(3):271-280.

18. Tfelt-Hansen P, Saxena PR, Dahlöf C, et al. Ergotamine in the acute treatment of migraine: a review and European consensus. *Brain.* 2000;123(pt 1):9-18.
19. Silbertein SD, McCrory DC. Ergotamine and dihydroergotamine: history, pharmacology, and efficacy. *Headache.* 2003;43(2):144-166.
20. Estimalik E, Tepper S. Preventive treatment in migraine and the new US guidelines. *Neuropsychiatr Dis Treat.* 2013;9:709-720.
21. Hainer BL. Approach to acute headache in adults. *Am Fam Phys.* 2013;87(10):682-687.
22. Moore RA, Derry S, Wiffen PJ, Straube S, Bendtsen L. Evidence for efficacy of acute treatment of episodic tension-type headache: methodological critique of randomized trials of oral treatments. *Pain.* 2014; 155(11):2220-2228.
23. Bendtsen L, Evers S, Linde M, Mitsikostas DD, Sandrini G, Schoenen J. EFNS guideline on the treatment of tension-type headache: report of an EFNS task force. *Eur J Neurol.* 2010;17(11): 1318-1325.
24. Karadaş Ö, Gül HL, Inan LE. Lidocaine injection of pericranial myofascial trigger points in the treatment of frequent episodic tension-type headache. *J Headache Pain.* 2013;14:44.
25. Jackson JL, Kuriyama A, Hayashino Y. Botulinum toxin A for prophylactic treatment of migraine and tension headaches in adults: a meta-analysis. *JAMA.* 2012;307(16):1736-1745.
26. Weaver-Agostoni J. Cluster headache. *Am Fam Phys.* 2013;88(2):122-128.
27. Cunnington M, Ephross S, Churchill P. The safety of sumatriptan and naratriptan in pregnancy: what have we learned? *Headache.* 2009;49(10):1414-1422.
28. American Academy of Pediatrics. Transfer of drugs and other chemicals into human milk. *Pediatrics.* 2001;108:776-789.
29. Schutte-Rodin S, Broch L, Buysse D, Dorsey C, Sateia M. Clinical guideline for the evaluation and management of chronic insomnia in adults. *J Clin Sleep Med.* 2008;4(5):487-504.
30. Pavlova M, Sheikh LS. Sleep in women. *Semin Neurol.* 2011;31(4):397-403.
31. Krishnan V, Collop NA. Gender differences in sleep disorders. *Curr Opin Pulm Med.* 2006;12(6):283-289.
32. Staner L. Comorbidity of insomnia and depression. *Sleep Med Rev.* 2010;14(10):35-46.
33. Schwartz TL, Goradia V. Managing insomnia: an overview of insomnia and pharmacologic treatment strategies in use and on the horizon. *Drugs Context.* 2013;212257.
34. Buysse DJ, Germain A, Moul D, Nofzinger EA. Insomnia. *FOCUS.* 2005;3(4):568-584.
35. Joffe H, Massler A, Sharkey KM. Evaluation and management of sleep disturbance during the menopause transition. *Semin Reprod Med.* 2012;28(5): 404-421.
36. Vande Griend JP, Anderson SL. Histamine-1 receptor antagonism for treatment of insomnia. *J Am Pharm Assoc.* 2012;52:e210-e219.
37. Arnedt JT, Conroy DA, Brower KJ. Treatment options for sleep disturbances during alcohol recovery. *J Addict Dis.* 2007;26(4):41-54.
38. Testa A, Giannuzzi R, Sollazzo F, Petrongolo L, Bernardini L, Dain S. Psychiatric emergencies (part II): psychiatric disorders coexisting with organic diseases. *Eur Rev Med Pharmacol Sci.* 2013;17(suppl 1): 65-85.
39. Tan KR, Rudolph U, Lüscher C. Hooked on benzodiazepines: $GABA_A$ receptor subtypes and addiction. *Trends Neurosci.* 2011;34(4):188-197.
40. Roehrs T, Roth T. Insomnia pharmacotherapy. *Neurotherapeutics.* 2012;9:728-738.
41. Nardi AE, Perna G. Clonazepam in the treatment of psychiatric disorders: an update. *Int Clin Psychopharmacol.* 2006;21(3):131-142.
42. Cunnington D, Junge MF, Fernando AT. Insomnia: prevalence, consequences, and effective treatment. *Med J Aust.* 2013;199(8):S36-S40.
43. Proctor A, Bianchi MT. Clinical pharmacology in sleep medicine. *ISRN Pharmacol.* 2012;2012:914168.
44. Gunja N. The clinical and forensic toxicology of Z-drugs. *J Med Toxicol.* 2013;9(2):155-162.
45. Gunja N. In the Zzz zone: the effects of Z-drugs on human performance and driving. *J Med Toxicol.* 2013;9(2):163-171.
46. Brown CS, Wan J, Bachmann G, Rosen R. Self-management, amitriptyline, and amitriptyline plus triamcinolone in the management of vulvodynia. *J Womens Health.* 2009;18(2):163-169.
47. Morin CM, Benca C. Chronic insomnia. *Lancet.* 2012;379(9821):1129-1141.
48. Friedmann PD, Rose JS, Swift R, Stout RL, Millman RP, Stein MD. Trazodone for sleep disturbance after alcohol detoxification: a double-blind, placebo-controlled trial. *Alcohol Clin Exp Res.* 2008;32(9):1652-1660.
49. Zhdanova IV. Melatonin as a hypnotic: pro. *Sleep Med Rev.* 2005;9(1):51-65.

50. Buscemi N, Vandermeer B, Hooton N. The efficacy and safety of exogenous melatonin for primary sleep disorder: a meta-analysis. *J Gen Intern Med.* 2005; 20(12):1151-1158.
51. Zammit G, Erman M, Wang-Weigand S, et al. Evaluation of the efficacy and safety of ramelteon in subjects with chronic insomnia. *J Clin Sleep Med.* 2007; 3(5):495-504.
52. Badawy RA, Vogrin SJ, Lai A, Cook MJ. Patterns of cortical hyperexcitability in adolescent/adult-onset generalized epilepsies. *Epilepsia.* 2013;54(5): 871-878.
53. Bromfield EB. Epilepsy and the elderly. In: Schachter SC, Schomer DL, eds. *The Comprehensive Evaluation and Treatment of Epilepsy.* San Diego, CA: Academic Press; 1997:233-254.
54. Terminology CoCa. Proposal for revised classification of epilepsies and epileptic syndromes. Commission on Classification and Terminology of the International League against Epilepsy. *Epilepsia.* 1989; 30(4):389-399.
55. Berg AT, Berkovic SF, Brodie MJ, et al. Revised terminology and concepts for organization of seizures and epilepsies: report of the ILAE Commission on Classification and Terminology, 2005-2009. *Epilepsia.* 2010;51(4):676-685.
56. Berg AT, Scheffer IE. New concepts in classification of the epilepsies: entering the 21st century. *Epilepsia.* 2011;52(6):1058-1062.
57. Badawy RA, Vogrin SJ, Lai A, Cook MJ. Are patterns of cortical hyperexcitability altered in catamenial epilepsy? *Ann Neurol.* 2013;74(5):743-757.
58. Shorvon S, Luciano AL. Prognosis of chronic and newly diagnosed epilepsy: revisiting temporal aspects. *Curr Opin Neurol.* 2007;20(2):208-212.
59. Hitiris N, Brodie MJ. Modern antiepileptic drugs: guidelines and beyond. *Curr Opin Neurol.* 2006; 19(2):175-180.
60. LaRoche SM, Helmers SL. The new antiepileptic drugs: scientific review. *JAMA.* 2004;291(5):605-614.
61. Nadkarni S, LaJoie J, Devinsky O. Current treatments of epilepsy. *Neurology.* 2005;64(12 suppl 3):S2-S11.
62. Knowles SR, Dewhurst N, Shear NH. Anticonvulsant hypersensitivity syndrome: an update. *Expert Opin Drug Saf.* 2012;11(5):767-778.
63. Asconape JJ. Some common issues in the use of antiepileptic drugs. *Semin Neurol.* 2002;22(1):27-39.
64. Siniscalchi A, Gallelli L, Russo E, De Sarro G. A review on antiepileptic drugs-dependent fatigue: pathophysiological mechanisms and incidence. *Eur J Pharmacol.* 2013;718(1-3):10-16.
65. Perucca E. Clinically relevant drug interactions with antiepileptic drugs. *Br J Clin Pharmacol.* 2006; 61(3):246-255.
66. Czapinski P, Blaszczyk B, Czuczwar SJ. Mechanisms of action of antiepileptic drugs. *Curr Top Med Chem.* 2005;5(1):3-14.
67. Pugh MJV, Van Cott AC, Cramer JA, et al.; Treatment In Geriatric Epilepsy Research (TIGER) team. Trends in antiepileptic drug prescribing for older patients with new-onset epilepsy: 2000–2004. *Neurology.* 2008;70(20 pt 2):2171-2178.
68. Belcastro V, D'Egidio C, Striano P, Verroti A. metabolic and endocrine effects of valproic acid chronic treatment. *Epilepsy Res.* 2013;107(1-2):1-8.
69. Nanau RM, Neuman MG. Adverse drug reactions caused by valproic acid. *Clin Biochem.* 2013; 46(15): 1323-1338.
70. Glauser T, Ben-Menachem E, Bourgeois B, et al. ILAE treatment guidelines: evidence-based analysis of antiepileptic drug efficacy and effectiveness as initial monotherapy for epileptic seizures and syndromes. *Epilepsia.* 2006;47(7):1094-1120.
71. Guillemette T, Yount S. Contraception and antiepileptic drugs. *J Midwifery Womens Health.* 2012;57(3): 290-295.
72. Centers for Disease Control and Prevention. U.S. medical eligibility criteria for contraceptive use. *MMWR.* June 18, 2010;59(RR04):1-6. http://www.cdc.gov/mmwr/preview/mmwrhtml/rr5904a1.htm?s_cid=rr5904a1_e. Accessed Jaunuary 14, 2015.
73. Johnston CA, Crawford PM. Anti-epileptic drugs and hormonal treatments. *Curr Treat Options Neurol.* 2014;16(5):288-295.
74. Sidhu J, Job S, Singh S, Philipson R. The pharmacokinetic and pharmacodynamic consequences of the co-administration of lamotrigine and a combined oral contraceptive in healthy female subjects. *Br J Clin Pharmacol.* 2006;61(2):191-199.
75. Adab N, Tudur SC, Vinten J, Williamson PR, Winterbottom JB. Common antiepileptic drugs in pregnancy in women with epilepsy. *Cochrane Database Syst Rev.* 2004;3:CD004848. doi:10.1002/14651858.CD004848.
76. Bromley R, Weston J, Adab N, et al. Treatment for epilepsy in pregnancy: neurodevelopmental outcomes in the child. *Cochrane Database Syst Rev.* 2014; 10: CD010236. doi:10.1002/14651858.CD010236.pub2.

77. Meador KJ. Effects of in utero antiepileptic drug exposure. *Epilepsy Curr.* 2008;8(6):143-147.
78. Harden CL. Antiepileptic drug teratogenesis: what are the risks for congenital malformations and adverse cognitive outcomes? *Int Rev Neurobiol.* 2008; 83:205-213.
79. Meador KJ, Bake GA, Browning N, et al.; NEAD Study Group. Cognitive function at 3 years of age after fetal exposure to antiepileptic drugs. *N Engl J Med.* 2009;360(16):1597-1605.
80. Harden CL, Hopp J, Ting TY, et al. Practice parameter update: management issues for women with epilepsy—focus on pregnancy (an evidence-based review): obstetrical complications and change in seizure frequency. Report of the Quality Standards Subcommittee and Therapeutics and Technology Assessment Subcommittee of the American Academy of Neurology and American Epilepsy Society. *Neurology.* April 27, 2009. http://www.neurology.org/content/73/2/126.full.pdf+html?sid=b5ebc098-7125-4c56-887d-ccd31fc08f33. Accessed July 2, 2014.
81. Pennell PB. Antiepileptic drugs during pregnancy: what is known and which AEDs seem to be safest? [Review]. *Epilepsia.* 2008;49(suppl 9):43-55.
82. Meador KJ. Breastfeeding and antiepileptic drugs. *JAMA.* 2014;311(17):1797-1798.
83. Harden CL. Issues for mature women with epilepsy. *Int Rev Neurobiol.* 2008;83:385-395.
84. Allen R, Picchietti D, Hening W, Trenkwalder C, Walters A, Montplaisi J. Restless legs syndrome: diagnostic criteria, special considerations, and epidemiology. A report from the restless legs syndrome diagnosis and epidemiologic workshop at the National Institutes of Health. *Sleep Med.* 2003;4(2):101-109.
85. Sibler MH, Ehrenber BL, Allen RP, et al. An algorithm for the management of restless legs syndrome. *Mayo Clinic Proc.* 2004;79(7):916-922.
86. Hensley JG. Leg cramps and restless legs syndrome during pregnancy. *J Midwifery Womens Health.* 2009; 54(3):211-218.
87. Allen RP. Controversies and challenges in defining the etiology and pathophysiology of restless legs syndrome. *Am J Med.* 2007;120(1A):S13-S21.
88. Scholz H, Trenkwalder C, Kohnen R, Riemann D, Kriston L, Hornyak M. Dopamine agonists for the treatment of restless legs syndrome. *Cochrane Database Syst Rev.* 2011;3:CD006009. doi:10.1002/14651858.CD006009.pub2.
89. Ramsay JR, Rostain AL. Adult ADHD research: current status and future directions. *J Atten Disord.* 2008; 11(6):624-627.
90. Humphreys C, Garcia-Bournissen F, Ito S, Koren G. Exposure to attention deficit hyperactivity disorder medications during pregnancy. *Can Fam Physician.* 2007;53(7):1153-1155.
91. Ilett KF, Hackett LP, Kristensen JH, Kohan R. Transfer of dexamphetamine into breast milk during treatment for attention deficit hyperactivity disorder. *Br J Clin Pharmacol.* 2007;63(3):371-375.
92. Morale MC, Serra PA, L'Episcopo F, et al. Estrogen, neuroinflammation and neuroprotection in Parkinson's disease: glia dictates resistance versus vulnerability to neurodegeneration. *Neuroscience.* 2006; 138(3):869-878.
93. Henderson VW. The neurology of menopause. *Neurologist.* 2006;12(3):149-159.
94. Lang AE, Lozano AM. Parkinson's disease: first of two parts. *N Engl J Med.* 1998;339(15):1044-1053.
95. Lang AE, Lozano AM. Parkinson's disease: second of two parts. *N Engl J Med.* 1998;339(16):1130-1143.
96. Lees A. Alternatives to levodopa in the initial treatment of early Parkinson's disease. *Drugs Aging.* 2005; 22(9):731-740.
97. Golbe LI. Parkinson's disease and pregnancy. *Neurology.* 1987;37(7):1245-1249.
98. Hagell P, Odin P, Vinge E. Pregnancy in Parkinson's disease: a review of the literature and a case report. *Mov Disord.* 1998;13(1):34-38.
99. Ott BR, Owens NJ. Complementary and alternative medicines for Alzheimer's disease. *J Geriatr Psychiatry Neurol.* 1998;11(4):163-173.
100. Bonner LT, Peskind ER. Pharmacologic treatments of dementia. *Med Clin North Am.* 2002;86(3):657-674.
101. Doggrell SA, Evans S. Treatment of dementia with neurotransmission modulation. *Expert Opin Investig Drugs.* 2003;12(10):1633-1654.

© Sofimanning/Shutterstock

25 Mental Health

Nicole K. Early

Based on the chapter by Ruth Johnson and Vivian Gamblian in the first edition of Pharmacology for Women's Health

With acknowledgment to Nell Tharpe for her contribution to this chapter

Chapter Glossary

Anxiolytics Drugs used to treat anxiety. Many are sedative-hypnotic drugs from the barbiturate or benzodiazepine class.

Desensitization Resistance of a receptor to agonist neurotransmitters or agonist drugs; the reason why the initial side effects of a drug gradually disappear.

Downregulation Disappearance of a receptor from the post-synaptic nerve, which renders the nerve less able to be stimulated by agonist neurotransmitters or agonist drugs.

Dysthymia Chronic, mild form of unipolar depression that is characterized by low-level depression and lack of enjoyment in life or pessimism.

Floppy baby syndrome Syndrome noted at birth in which the neonate has the following characteristics: hypothermia, lethargy, hypotonia, poor respiratory effort, and difficulty feeding. It is associated with maternal use of benzodiazepines shortly before birth.

Hypnotics Class of drugs that induce sleep.

Monoamine oxidase (MAO) Enzyme that degrades neurotransmitters intracellularly, thereby decreasing the amount of neurotransmitter that can be released into the synapse.

Psychotropic Any of the psychoactive drugs used to treat individuals with mental illness.

Sedatives Class of drugs that have a calming or tranquilizing effect. Used to reduce anxiety.

Sedative-hypnotic drugs Descriptor for barbiturates and benzodiazepines, which have overlapping functions on the mental health disorders continuum.

Selective serotonin reuptake inhibitor (SSRI) Class of antidepressants that inhibit reuptake of serotonin into the presynaptic cell, which increases the amount of serotonin in the synapse. SSRIs have a weak affinity for norepinephrine and dopamine receptors.

Serotonin–norepinephrine reuptake inhibitor (SNRI) Class of antidepressants that inhibit reuptake of serotonin and of norepinephrine into the presynaptic cell, which increases the amount of serotonin and norepinephrine in the synapse.

Serotonin syndrome Triad of clinical changes of mental status, autonomic hyperactivity, and neuromuscular abnormalities caused by excess serotonin in the synapses in the central nervous system. It is a predictable adverse drug reaction secondary to excess serotonin in neural synapses within the central nervous system and periphery. *Serotonin toxicity* is the preferred term, but it is not yet used widely in clinical practice.

Introduction

According to the World Health Organization, "Mental health is a state of well-being in which the individual realizes his or her own abilities, can cope with the normal stresses of life, can work productively and fruitfully, and is able to make a contribution to his or her community."[1] In contrast, the term *mental disorder* refers to all diagnosable conditions characterized by alterations in thinking, mood, or behavior. Although the terms *mental illness* and *mental disorder* are synonymous, *mental disorder* is the preferred term today. An estimated 26.2% of adults in the United States suffer from a diagnosable mental disorder.[2]

The overall rates of mental disorders in men and women are roughly equal; however, there is a striking gender difference in the patterns of illness. Women are twice as likely as men to suffer from depression, anxiety, and post-traumatic stress disorder (PTSD).[3] Perinatal depression affects roughly 8% to 11% of women in the first postpartum year,[4] and women account for 90% of all individuals with an eating disorder.[4] Women are also more likely than men to make suicide attempts, although they are less likely than men to die by suicide.[5] Additionally, the course of some disorders in women is often different than the course of the same disorder in men; in particular, hormone fluctuations may increase the frequency and severity of episodes of mood disorders or depression.

This chapter reviews **psychotropic** medications and discusses their effective use in a primary women's health-care practice. The emphasis is on depression and anxiety, the two most common mood disorders frequently encountered in primary care practice.[2] Although the diagnosis and management of women with specific mental disorders are beyond the scope of this chapter, resources for diagnostic criteria, referral to psychiatric specialists, and additional web-based resources are listed at the end of this chapter. The interested reader is also referred to primary care texts and professional association guidelines.[6,7]

Treatment of Women with Psychiatric Conditions in Primary Care

Mental disorders are relatively common in the general population, but the number of psychiatric providers who treat these disorders are limited, especially those with prescriptive authority. Overall, more than half of the persons in the United States who are prescribed a medication for a mental disorder are treated by a primary care provider,[8] and it is generally recognized that primary care providers have an important role in treatment of individuals with common mental disorders.[9,10] Prompt intervention can prevent symptoms from worsening and lessen the impact of illness. In addition, women who are hesitant to see a specialist may more readily accept treatment from their primary care provider.

Treatment of women's mental disorders in the primary care setting should take place within a practice structure that provides for consultation and collaboration with appropriate psychiatric providers and referral for specialized care when indicated. A variety of conditions require care by a psychiatric professional, including severe major depression (especially persons with suicidal thoughts with or without a plan), bipolar disorder (especially bipolar I disorder), psychotic disorders (including schizophrenia and postpartum psychosis), anorexia nervosa, and bulimia nervosa.[10]

Nevertheless, a primary care provider can offer valuable assistance to women with psychiatric conditions that require treatment from a psychiatric provider. In contrast to the intensely client-focused process of individual psychotherapy, primary care clinicians who are accustomed to offering family-centered care can support a woman's decision making and help her incorporate her values in planning her treatment. In addition to having regular contact with the woman, the primary care provider can provide monitoring for potential drug–drug interactions, discuss the risks of teratogenicity associated with various agents, offer health education regarding contraception, and provide treatment of the woman for her comorbid conditions.[11]

If a woman is perceived as being unable to keep herself or her family safe, the situation becomes an emergency. These circumstances include any episode of psychosis or mania wherein the woman's insight is poor and the risk of harm is correspondingly high. When a woman appears to pose a danger to herself or others, the clinician becomes responsible for ensuring her safety, which may require obtaining an on-site mental health consultation, referral to an emergency room for care, and/or notification of authorities about possible harm to others.[10]

When discussing drug treatment options, including woman-specific risks and benefits, it is important to remember that mental disorders, by definition, impair thought processes and can interfere with both memory and reasoning.[12] In addition, most psychotropic medications have side effects and drug–drug interactions that are clinically significant; these factors should be reviewed as part of the informed consent process. Considerations prior to initiating therapy include review of FDA black box warnings, the effects of drugs during pregnancy, and disclosure of off-label use if the drug does not have Food and Drug Administration (FDA) approval for the indication.

Neurobiology of Mood Disorders

While psychotropic medications have been used empirically for many years, it is only recently that research has identified the specific actions of particular medications on human neurochemistry. Norepinephrine, dopamine, serotonin, glutamate, and gamma-aminobutyric acid (GABA) are all neurotransmitters known to have an effect on mood. Norepinephrine, dopamine, and serotonin are monoamines derived from tryptophan or L-tyrosine, both of which are amino acids. Figure 25-1 illustrates the actions and relationships among the three primary neurotransmitters, and Table 25-1 summarizes the agonist functions of neurotransmitters involved in mental disorders and the means by which psychotropic drugs stimulate these effects.[13,14]

Neurotransmitters have complex and interrelated effects on many physiologic functions. Despite this complexity, they have a relatively simple life cycle:

1. All of these neurotransmitters are synthesized in a presynaptic neuron.
2. These agents are released into the synaptic space, where they have an agonist or antagonist action on the postsynaptic neuron.
3. The neurotransmitters move from the synaptic space back into the presynaptic neuron. This action, referred to as "reuptake," depends on a protein transporter on the presynaptic neuron cell membrane.
4. Once the agents are back in the presynaptic neuron, the neurotransmitters are either enzymatically degraded or recycled into vesicles for release into the synaptic space again.

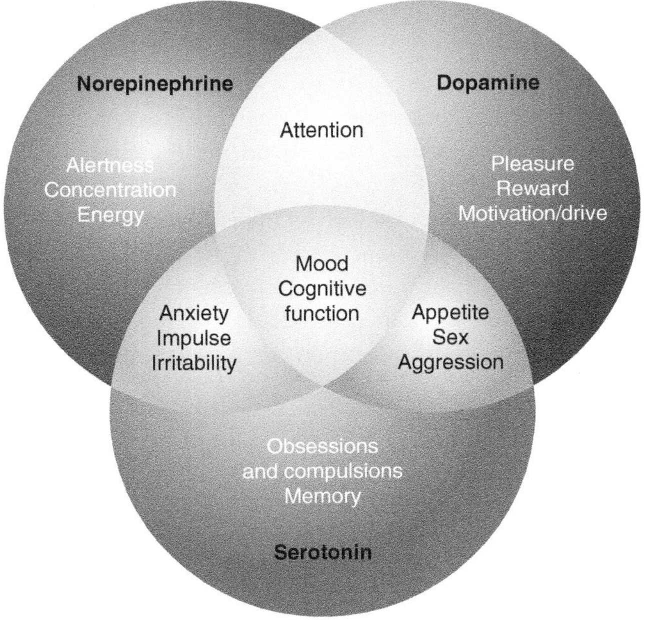

Figure 25-1 Roles of dopamine, norepinephrine, and serotonin.

Table 25-1 Biologic Functions of Key Neurotransmitters

Neurotransmitter	Agonist Function	Antagonist Action
Excitatory Neurotransmitters: Stimulate neuronal action potential		
Acetylcholine[a]	Triggers skeletal muscle and smooth muscle of parasympathetic system contraction	Dry mouth, blurred vision, constipation, ataxia, increased body temperature, urinary retention
Dopamine	Controls movement, posture, gastrointestinal motility, and primitive emotions; modulates mood; plays a role in positive reinforcement	Extrapyramidal symptoms, dystonic reaction, increased prolactin levels, psychosis, insomnia, psychomotor agitation
Inhibitory Neurotransmitters: Inhibit neuronal action potential		
Gamma-aminobutyric acid (GABA)	Central nervous system depressant; causes presynaptic inhibition that slows nerve conduction and transmission	None known
Glutamate	Precursor to GABA; responsible for memory formation and learning	Blurred vision, fainting, confusion, or dizziness
Histamine	Bronchoconstriction, vasodilation, gastric acid secretion, smooth muscle relaxation	Sedation, hypotension, weight gain, allergic symptoms
Norepinephrine	Memory, information processing, emotions, psychomotor function, blood pressure, heart rate, bladder emptying	Tachycardia, tremors, sexual dysfunction
Serotonin	Appetite and eating behaviors; regulates anxiety, movements, gastrointestinal motility, sexual function, and sleep	Sexual dysfunction, anxiety, obsessions and compulsions, headache, hypotension

[a] Acetylcholine is antagonized by many of the psychotropic drugs. When the normal function of acetylcholine is suppressed, a classic set of symptoms referred to as "anticholinergic effects" can manifest.

The drugs that affect these neurotransmitters alter one of these steps as shown in Figure 25-2.

The Monoamine-Deficiency Hypothesis

One of the earliest theories proposed to explain the mechanism of action of antidepressants is the monoamine-deficiency hypothesis. According to this theory, persons with depression have a deficiency of one or both of the monoamines norepinephrine and serotonin in the synaptic cleft.[15] The theory is overly simple and does not account

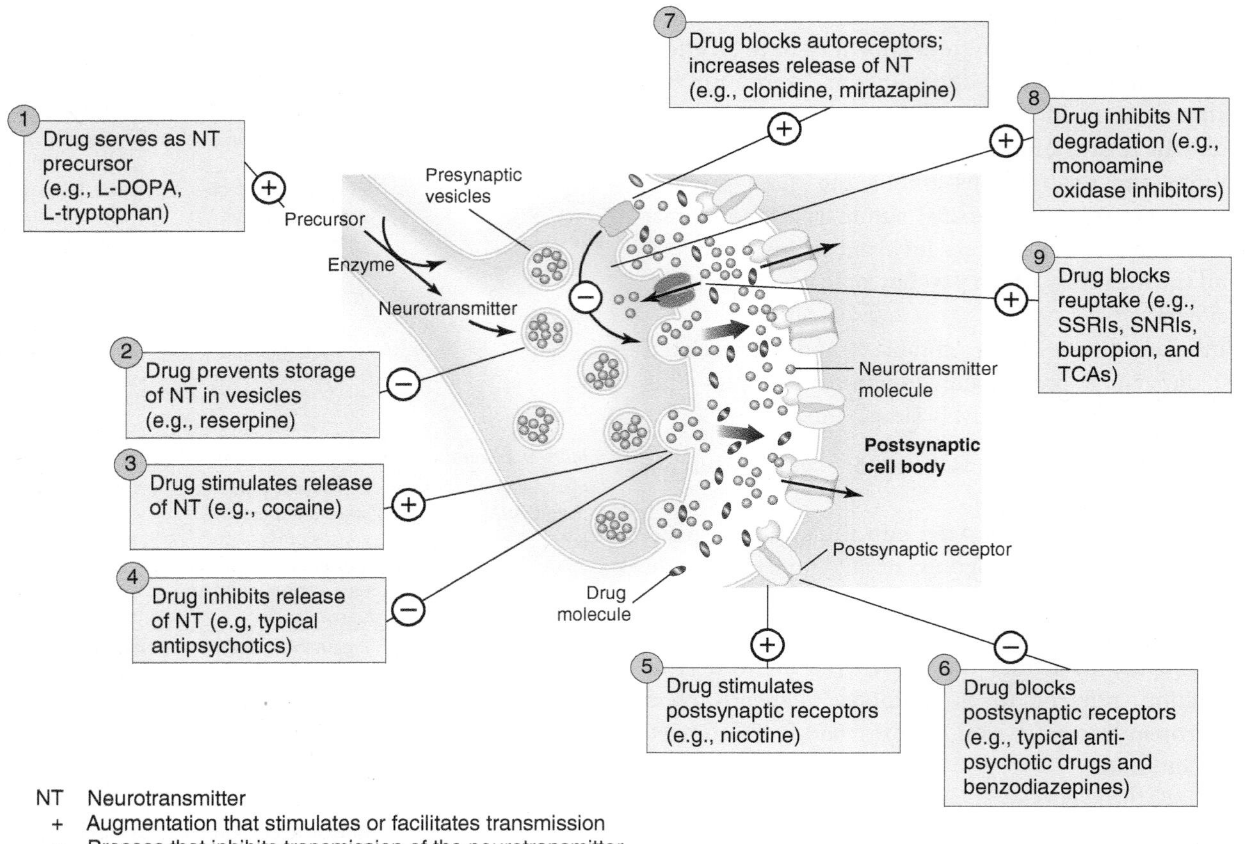

Figure 25-2 The effect of psychotropic drugs on neurotransmitter action.

for the complex interactions between the norepinephrine and serotonin systems or the role of other players such as dopamine, genetics, stress hormones, and reproductive hormones. Nevertheless, it has served as an important foundation for much of the initial research on mood disorders and continues to be evaluated as new technologies lead to novel methods of assessing brain function.[16]

Role of Gender

The fact that women are twice as likely as men to have major depression suggests that there is a biologic difference in the underlying neuropathology of this disorder. However, the biologic mechanisms responsible for the gender differences in mental disorders are just beginning to be elucidated. The complex interplay between genetic predisposition, psychosocial events such as role stress or victimization, and disadvantaged social status plays a role as well, but the specific influence of each of these various factors has not yet been determined. Women are most susceptible to developing a mental disorder during the childbearing years. Estrogen and progesterone, which control major reproductive transitions such as menstruation, childbirth, and menopause, are associated with an increased occurrence or intensity of some mood disorders.[17,18] In addition, the drugs used to treat these disorders appear to work somewhat differently in women compared to men.

Role of Genetics

Genetic polymorphisms in neurotransmitter receptors appear to play a significant role in both vulnerability to psychiatric disorders and response to psychotropic medications.[19,20] Although genetic variants and their effects have been identified and research into new drug targets is under way, as yet there are no clinical applications available. More work is needed in this area.

Overview of Mood Disorders and Psychotropic Drugs

There are two widely used classification schemes for mental disorders: The International Classification of Diseases (ICD-10) is produced by the World Health Organization, and the *Diagnostic and Statistical Manual of Mental Disorders, Fifth Edition* (*DSM-5*) is produced by the American Psychiatric Association. The two schemes are largely comparable, and the *DSM* is the taxonomy preferred by most mental health practitioners in the United States. Four *DSM* categories—mood disorders, anxiety disorders, sleep disorders, and eating disorders—are addressed in this chapter.[21,22] Substance abuse disorders are addressed in the *Smoking Cessation* and *Drugs of Abuse* chapters. Personality disorders, schizophrenia, psychotic disorders, delirium, and impulse control disorders require psychiatric management and are not addressed in this text. Table 25-2 presents a brief description of the mental disorders reviewed in this chapter.

Psychotropic Drugs

Like the conditions for which they are indicated, psychotropic medications are categorized in several ways. These drugs may be identified according to their original use (e.g., anticonvulsants, antipsychotics), by their chemical structure (e.g., tricyclic antidepressants), by their intended chemical action (e.g., monoamine oxidase [MAO] inhibitors), or by a combination term (e.g., anticonvulsant mood stabilizers). Sometimes the manufacturer invents a category de novo—such as **selective serotonin reuptake inhibitor (SSRI)** or **serotonin–norepinephrine reuptake inhibitor (SNRI)**—and it is incorporated into general usage among the professionals to whom the drug is marketed. This chapter uses the terminology that is most generally accepted by mental health professionals; a lexicon that may vary slightly from the terms used by neurologists, internists, or researchers who refer to the same medications. Before reviewing the psychotropic drugs, a brief discussion of drugs that cause neuropsychiatric symptoms is in order.

Drugs That Have Neuropsychiatric Side Effects

Several medications can cause symptoms of mental disorders (Table 25-3). The medications that are most often associated with development of depression are glucocorticoids, interferon, propranolol (Inderal), and oral contraceptives.[23]

Table 25-2 Common Psychiatric Disorders

Disorder	Description
Acute stress disorder	Development of acute anxiety, dissociative symptoms, and decreased emotional responsiveness within 3 days to 1 month of a traumatic event that was experienced as a terrifying event. Individuals with acute stress disorder experience at least one of the following symptoms: negative mood or intrusion symptoms, dissociative/avoidance symptoms, or arousal symptoms.
Anxiety disorders	Pathologic fears and anxieties. Generalized anxiety disorder, panic disorder, and post-traumatic stress disorder are common anxiety disorders that affect women.
Anorexia nervosa	Eating disorder characterized by low body weight, disturbed body image, and obsessive fear of gaining weight. Anorexia nervosa is a psychiatric disorder.
Binge-eating disorder	Eating disorder that does not meet the full criteria for anorexia or bulimia.
Bipolar disorders	Also known as manic depressive illness. Mental disorders that cause unusual shifts in mood, energy, activity levels, and the ability to conduct daily activities. Bipolar disorders are subclassified as bipolar I, bipolar II, cyclothymia, and bipolar disorder not otherwise specified.
Bipolar I	Bipolar disorder characterized by one or more episodes of abnormally elevated mood. Bipolar I is the classic cyclic expression of manic moods followed by depression. Persons with bipolar I can also experience mixed episodes.
Bipolar II	Bipolar disorder with more frequent and intense depressive symptoms when compared to the occurrences of manic episodes. Manic episodes are hypomania rather than full manic episodes.
Bipolar not otherwise specified (NOS)	Mood disorder with bipolar features that do not fit another bipolar category.
Bulimia nervosa	Eating disorder characterized by recurrent binge eating, which is followed by compulsive behaviors. The most common is self-induced vomiting.
Cyclothymia	Hypomania with periods of depression that have never met the criteria for major depressive, manic, or hypomanic episodes.
Depressive disorders	Conditions generally characterized by sadness, feelings of worthlessness and lack of desire to participate in activities that previously were associated with enjoyment. A group of disorders that are further subclassified based on the primary symptomatology. Examples include dysthymia (persistent depressive disorder), major depressive disorder, and seasonal affective disorder.
Dysthymia	Chronic, mild form of unipolar depression that is characterized by low-level depression and lack of enjoyment in life or pessimism.
Eating disorders	Abnormal eating disorders characterized by serious health implications and associated with psychological etiology. The three primary eating disorders are anorexia nervosa, bulimia nervosa, and binge-eating disorder. An additional category called "eating disorder not otherwise specified" is used to refer to individuals who have an eating disorder that does

(*continues*)

Table 25-2 Common Psychiatric Disorders (*continued*)

Disorder	Description
Eating disorders (*continued*)	not meet the full criteria for anorexia or bulimia. Both anorexia and bulimia are further divided: Anorexia is categorized as binge–purge subtype or restricting subtype; bulimia includes purging and non-purging subtypes.
Generalized anxiety disorder (GAD)	Excessive anxiety and worry about life circumstances that are difficult to control. The anxiety is unrealistic, generalized, and persistent. It is present on more days than not over at least a 6-month time period.
Major depressive disorder	Depressive disorder characterized by an overwhelming pervasive and persistent low mood or feeling of sadness that is accompanied by loss of pleasure in normally enjoyable activities and low self-esteem.
Mania	From the Greek *uavia*, which means "to rage or be furious." A condition of extreme elevated or irritated mood and the behaviors associated with this mood. May be characterized by grandiose thoughts or a flood of good ideas. Most often associated with bipolar disorder. Mania is a continuum of intensity, with hypomania (mild mania) at one end and mania with psychotic features at the other end. Mania can occur simultaneously with depressive thoughts; a woman in such a mixed state is at particularly high risk for suicide. Corticosteroids can sometimes induce a manic episode.
Manic episode	Period of days to weeks marked by unusually high energy, euphoria, hyperactivity, or impaired judgment.
Mental disorder	A behavioral or psychological syndrome that occurs and is associated with distinct disability or significantly increased suffering. There is no single definition for the precise boundaries for the concept of mental disorder.
Mood disorders	Set of conditions wherein a disturbance in one's emotional mood is the primary underlying feature. In addition to depressive disorders and bipolar disorders, premenstrual dysphoric disorder is now classified as a mood disorder.
Obsessive–compulsive disorder	Form of anxiety disorder characterized by involuntary intrusive thoughts and dysfunctional beliefs.
Panic disorder	Form of anxiety disorder characterized by recurring, severe, unexpected, panic attacks.
Phobia	Form of anxiety disorder characterized by irrational, persistent fear of specific situations, persons, activities, or items.
Post-traumatic stress disorder (PTSD)	Form of anxiety disorder that develops after exposure to a traumatic event or highly unsafe experience. PTSD is characterized by reliving a traumatic event, symptoms of avoidance or numbing, and feeling on edge, with symptoms persisting for longer than 1 month following the event.
Psychosis	From the Greek *psyche*, which means "mind" or "soul," and *osis*, which means "abnormal condition." A state of delusional thinking that is characterized by hallucinations or delusional beliefs and/or disordered thinking. May be accompanied by unusual behavior and personality changes. Impaired ability to manage activities of daily living is often present.

Table 25-3 Selected List of Medications That Have Neuropsychiatric Side Effects

Drug: Generic (Brand)	Neuropsychiatric Effects
Acyclovir (Zovirax)	Depression
Adrenocorticoids	Anxiety, panic attack, depression, hallucinations, mania, psychoses
Amphetamines	Psychosis
Anticholinergic agents	Psychosis, cognitive impairment
Anticonvulsants	Depression
Antidepressants such as SSRIs, SNRIs, and TCAs	Suicidal ideation
Antihistamines	Agitation, anxiety, nervousness, confusion, hallucinations
Barbiturates	Depression, suicidal ideation, hallucinations; excitement or violent behavior (paradoxical effect of some sedatives
Benzodiazepines	Depression, psychosis
Beta blockers	Anxiety, agitation, depression
Bromocriptine (Parlodel)	Hallucinations
Calcium-channel blockers	Depression
Carbidopa/levodopa (L-dopa)	Psychosis, depression
Corticosteroids	Psychosis, mood disorders, delirium, depression
Dopamine agonists	Extrapyramidal symptoms, hallucinations, depression
Dextromethorphan	Psychosis
Fluoroquinolone antibiotics	Depression, psychosis
Hormonal preparations	Depression
Interferon	Depression
Isoniazid (INH)	Delirium, psychosis
Methamphetamine (Desoxyn)	Psychosis, exacerbation of tics, insomnia
Methyldopa	Depression
Methylphenidate (Ritalin, Concerta)	Suicidal thoughts, hallucinations, anxiety, depression
Metoclopramide (Reglan)	Extrapyramidal effects, anxiety, toxic psychosis
Phenylpropanolamine (found in cold medications)	Psychosis, paranoia, mania, confusion
Pseudoephedrine	Anxiety, hallucinations
Statins	Depression
Valproic acid (Depakote, Depakene)	Depression, hallucinations

Abbreviations: SNRI = serotonin–norepinephrine reuptake inhibitor; SSRI = selective serotonin reuptake inhibitor; TCA = tricyclic antidepressant.

Pharmacologic Treatment of Women with Depression

Antidepressant medications are among the most frequently prescribed drugs in the United States. In addition to being used to treat **dysthymia** and depression, antidepressants are increasingly being used to treat several other conditions, including perimenstrual disorders; to treat vasomotor symptoms and sleep disturbances; as an aid to smoking cessation; and as an adjunct in the management of women with chronic pain conditions such as vulvodynia and neuropathic pain.[24–26] An overview of the classes of these drugs and their indications, as well as examples of common off-label uses, is presented in Table 25-4.

Mechanism of Action

Antidepressants generate a variety of effects within the body, and they have a complicated mechanism of action that has important clinical implications. These drugs have an immediate effect on inhibiting reuptake of serotonin or norepinephrine (or both) into the presynaptic cell, but clinical relief of depression symptoms does not occur for at least the first 2 to 3 weeks after treatment is initiated.

The physiology that explains this clinical puzzle is not yet fully understood in humans. However, certain aspects are known in clinical use. When treatment begins, the antidepressant causes an increase in serotonergic or norepinephrine actions throughout the body, and most of the early side effects such as gastrointestinal upset, headache, and jitteriness are attributable to this neurotransmitter rush. After approximately 2 weeks, the postsynaptic neurons that have receptors for these neurotransmitters begin to decrease their receptiveness—a process called **desensitization**. In addition, some of these receptors undergo **downregulation**, in which they disappear from the postsynaptic neuron membrane. When desensitization and downregulation occur, the troublesome side effects recede or are resolved. Because desensitization and downregulation eliminate the negative feedback systems that initiate reuptake of the neurotransmitter into the presynaptic neuron, the concentration of the neurotransmitter within the synaptic space increases, and the effectiveness of the medication begins to become apparent.

Most antidepressants are equally effective for treating depression.[27,28] Their differences are primarily apparent in their individual side-effect profiles, secondary to their effects on different neurotransmitters.[29] Side effects of

Table 25-4 Classifications of Antidepressant Drugs

Category	Drug: Generic (Brand)	FDA-Approved Use	Off-Label Uses
5-HT_2 receptor antagonists	Trazodone (Desyrel)	Depression	Insomnia
5-HT_3 receptor antagonists	Vortioxetine (Brintellix)	Major depression	
Dopamine reuptake inhibitors	Bupropion (Wellbutrin, Wellbutrin SR, Wellbutrin XL, Zyban)	Major depression, seasonal affective disorder, smoking cessation	Dysthymia, ADHD adjunct, mood stabilizer
Monoamine oxidase (MAO) inhibitors	Phenelzine (Nardil)	Depression	Agoraphobia, panic disorder, bulimia, social phobia
	Tranylcypromine (Parnate)	Major depression	
	Selegiline patch (Emsam)	Major depression	
Noradrenergic antagonists	Mirtazapine (Remeron)	Major depression	Anxiety, dysthymia, OCD, panic disorder
Serotonin–norepinephrine reuptake inhibitors (SNRIs)	Desvenlafaxine (Pristiq)	Major depression	Similar to venlafaxine
	Duloxetine (Cymbalta)	Major depression, GAD, diabetic peripheral neuropathy, fibromyalgia, chronic musculoskeletal pain	Pain, urinary incontinence
	Levomilnacipran (Fetzima)	Major depression	
	Milnacipran (Savella)	Fibromyalgia	Depression
	Venlafaxine (Effexor, Effexor XR)	Major depression, panic disorder, GAD, social phobia	ADHD, binge-eating disorder, bipolar depression, dysthymia, vasomotor symptoms, OCD, PTSD, PMDD, tension-type headache

(continues)

Table 25-4 Classifications of Antidepressant Drugs (*continued*)

Category	Drug: Generic (Brand)	FDA-Approved Use	Off-Label Uses
Selective serotonin reuptake inhibitors (SSRIs)	Citalopram (Celexa)	Depression	Alcoholism, anxiety disorder, OCD, bulimia, fibromyalgia, chronic fatigue, panic disorder, vasomotor symptoms, PMDD
	Escitalopram (Lexapro)	Major depressive disorder, GAD	Anxiety disorder, OCD, bulimia, fibromyalgia, chronic fatigue, panic disorder, vasomotor symptoms, PMDD
	Fluoxetine (Prozac, Sarafem)	Major depressive disorder, bipolar depression, bulimia, OCD, panic disorder, PMDD	Body dysmorphic disorder, chronic fatigue syndromes, dysthymia, fibromyalgia, pain syndromes, PTSD, vasomotor symptoms
	Fluvoxamine (Luvox CR)	OCD	Depression, eating disorder, panic disorder, social phobia
	Paroxetine (Paxil)	Vasomotor symptoms, GAD, major depression, OCD, panic disorder	
	Sertraline (Zoloft)	Major depression, OCD, panic disorder, PTSD, PMDD, social phobia	Bipolar depression, dysthymia, GAD, night eating syndrome
	Vilazodone (Viibryd)	Major depression	
Tricyclic antidepressants (TCAs)	Amitriptyline (Elavil)	Depression	Headache, irritable bowel syndrome, pain, neuropathy
	Clomipramine (Anafranil)	OCD	Depression, OCD, chronic pain, panic disorder, delusional disorder
	Desipramine (Norpramin)	Depression	ADHD, diabetic neuropathy
	Doxepin (Sinequan)	Anxiety, depression, isomnia, alcoholism	Urticaria
	Imipramine (Tofranil)	Depression	Diabetic neuropathy, panic disorder
	Nortriptyline (Pamelor)	Depression	ADHD, nicotine dependence, neurogenic bladder, postherpetic neuralgia

Abbreviations: ADHD = attention-deficit/hyperactivity disorder; GAD = general anxiety disorder; OCD = obsessive–compulsive disorder; PMDD = premenstrual dysphoric disorder; PTSD = post-traumatic stress disorder.

commonly used antidepressants are summarized in Table 25-5.[27,30–32]

Antidepressants and Suicidal Behavior

Although the medications described in this chapter are generally well tolerated, they can, albeit rarely, trigger life-threatening illness. Two of these complications, suicidal behavior and serotonin syndrome, are associated with most of the antidepressant drugs discussed in this chapter.

Antidepressants and Suicidal Behavior

In 2004, the FDA recommended a change to the product labeling for antidepressants to note their association with an increased risk of suicidal thinking and behavior in children and adolescents during the initial few months of treatment. In 2007, this warning was extended to young adults between 18 and 24 years of age. The history and text of the black box warning are presented in Box 25-1.[33]

Serotonin Syndrome

High plasma levels of serotonin can cause **serotonin syndrome**, wherein excess serotonergic activity in the central nervous syndrome very quickly results in a life-threatening constellation of symptoms. The clinical picture of serotonin syndrome includes gastrointestinal upset, chills, shakes, increased muscle rigidity or jerking, confusion, restlessness, and delirium, and it may progress to rhabdomyolysis, pulmonary hypertension, and coma.[34]

Serotonin syndrome can occur following a significant overdose of a serotonergic antidepressant or following a normal dose in the presence of other medications that have a drug–drug reaction with the antidepressant. Concentrations of serotonin also become elevated following administration of agents that provide the amino acid L-tryptophan, which is the precursor of serotonin. For example, monoamine (MAO) inhibitors limit metabolism

Table 25-5 Antidepressant Drugs: Side-Effect Profiles

Drug: Generic (Brand)	Anticholinergic	Sedation	Gastrointestinal Distress	Weight Gain	Orthostatic Hypotension	QT Prolongation	Sexual Dysfunction	FDA Black Box Warning About Suicidality
Monoamine Oxidase (MAO) Inhibitors								
Phenelzine (Nardil)	1+	2+	1+[a]	2+	3+	0	4+	Yes
Selegiline (Emsam)	1+	0	0[a]	0	1+	0	0	Yes
Tranylcypromine (Parnate)	1+	1+	1+[a]	1+	2+	1+	4+	Yes
Selective Serotonin Reuptake Inhibitors (SSRIs)								
Citalopram (Celexa)	0	0	1+[a]	1+	1+	1+[b]	3+	Yes
Escitalopram (Lexapro)	0	0	1+[a]	1+	1+	1+	3+	Yes
Fluoxetine (Prozac, Sarafem)	0	0	1+[a]	1+	1+	1+	3+	Yes
Fluvoxamine (Luvox)	0	1+	1+[a]	1+	1+	1+	3+	Yes
Paroxetine (Paxil)	1+	1+	1+[a]	1+	2+	1+	4+	Yes
Sertraline (Zoloft)	0	0	2+[a]	2+	1+	1+	3+	Yes
Vilazodone (Viibryd)	0	0	1+[a]	1+	1+	1+	3+	Yes
Vortioxetine (Brintellix)	Rare	Rare	3+[a]	Rare	Rare	Rare	1+	Yes
Serotonin–Norepinephrine Reuptake Inhibitors (SNRIs)								
Desvenlafaxine[c] (Pristiq)	0	1+	2+ initially[a]	0	0	0	3+	Yes
Duloxetine (Cymbalta)	0	0	2+ initially[a]	0	0	1+	3+	Yes
Levomilnacipran[c] (Fetzima)	1+	0	2+[a]	0	2+	1+	0	Yes
Milnacipran[c] (Savella)	1+	1+	2+[a]	0	0	0	0	Yes
Venlafaxine[c] (Effexor)	0	1+	2+ Initially[a]	0	0	1+	3+	Yes
Tricyclic Antidepressants (TCAs)								
Amitriptyline (Elavil)	4+	4+	1+	1+	3+	3+	3–4+	Yes
Amoxapine (Asendin)	2+	2+	0	0	2+	2+	ND	Yes
Clomipramine (Anafranil)	4+	4+	1+	1+	2+	2+	4+	Yes
Desipramine (Norpramin)	1+	2+	0	1+	2+	3+	ND	Yes
Doxepin (Sinequan)	3+	3+	0	4+	2+	3+	3+	Yes
Imipramine (Tofranil)	3+	3+	1+	0	4+	3+	3+	Yes
Maprotiline (Ludiomil)	2+	4+	0		2+	3+	ND	Yes
Nortriptyline (Pamelor)	2+	2+	0	1+	1+	3+	ND	Yes
Protriptyline (Vivactil)	2+	1+	1+	1+	2+	3+	3–4+	Yes
Trimipramine (Surmontil)	4+	4+	0	4+	3+	1+	ND	Yes
Other Agents								
Bupropion (Wellbutrin)	0	0	1+	0	0	1+	0	Yes
Mirtazapine (Remeron)	1+	4+	0	4+	0	4+	1+	Yes
Trazodone (Desyrel)	0	3+	1+	1+	3+	1+	0	Yes

0 = absent or rare; 1+ = slight risk; 2+ = low risk; 3+ = moderate risk; 4+ = high risk; ND = no data.

[a] All of the MAO inhibitors, SSRIs, and SNRIs may cause mild nausea when the dose is initiated or increased.

[b] Based on case reports of prolonged QT syndrome, the maximum dose of citalopram is 20 mg for persons who have an *a priori* risk for elevated citalopram serum concentration based on drug–drug interactions or pharmacogenomic variations in metabolism.

[c] These SNRIs may cause a dose-related increase in diastolic blood pressure and heart rate; they may require regular monitoring of blood pressure.

Sources: Data from American Psychiatric Association. *Practice Guideline for the Treatment of Patients with Major Depressive Disorder*. 3rd ed. Arlington, VA: American Psychiatric Association; 2010[27]; Ferguson JM. SSRI antidepressant medications: adverse effects and tolerability. *Primary Care Companion J Clin Psychiatry*. 2001;3(1):22-27[31]; Joffe RT. Dosing and monitoring guidelines for mood disorders. *Prim Psychiatry*. 2003;10(11):67-74[30]; Mann JJ. Medical management of depression. *N Engl J Med*. 2005;353(17):1819-1834.[32]

Box 25-1 Antidepressants and Increased Risk for Suicidality

In 2004, the FDA mandated a black box warning to appear on the labels of most antidepressants that notifies prescribers of an increased risk for suicidality (suicidal ideation or suicidal behavior) in children who are prescribed these drugs. Prior to issuing this warning, a meta-analysis of 372 randomized trials of antidepressants and found suicidal behavior in 4% of those who received antidepressants versus 2% of those who did not receive the antidepressants. Subgroup analysis found the increased rate of suicidal behavior to be highest among children and adolescents. Following additional analyses, the warning was modified in 2007 and extended to include young adults. The current text of the FDA black box warning follows:

> Antidepressants increased the risk compared to placebo of suicidal thinking and behavior (suicidality) in children, adolescents, and young adults in short-term studies of major depressive disorder (MDD) and other psychiatric disorders. Anyone considering the use of [insert established name] or any other antidepressant in a child, adolescent, or young adult must balance this risk with the clinical need. Short-term studies did not show an increase in the risk of suicidality with antidepressants compared to placebo in adults beyond age 24; there was a reduction in risk with antidepressants compared to placebo in adults aged 65 and older. Depression and certain other psychiatric disorders are themselves associated with increases in the risk of suicide. Patients of all ages who are started on antidepressant therapy should be monitored appropriately and observed closely for clinical worsening, suicidality, or unusual changes in behavior. Families and caregivers should be advised of the need for close observation and communication with the prescriber.[33]

The psychotropic medications that carry this black box warning include all of the SSRIs, SNRIs, MAO inhibitors, and TCAs; some anticonvulsants; and trazodone (Desyrel) and nefazodone (Serzone). It is recommended that persons taking these agents be closely monitored for suicidal thinking or unusual behavior.

Table 25-6 Drug Interactions That Can Induce Serotonin Syndrome

Category	Drugs or Drug Classes
Antidepressants	MAO inhibitors, SSRIs, SNRIs, trazodone, nefazodone, buspirone, clomipramine
Antiemetics	Ondansetron (Zofran), metoclopramide (Reglan), granisetron (Kytril)
Antimigraine agents	Triptans such as sumatriptan (Imitrex), rizatriptan (Maxalt), naratriptan (Amerge), zolmitriptan (Zomig), eletriptan (Relpax), almotriptan (Axert), and frovatriptan (Frova)
Botanicals/herbs	St. John's wort, dietary supplements containing tryptophan, *Panax ginseng*
CNS stimulants	Amphetamines
Cough/cold remedies	Dextromethorphan
Drugs of abuse	Ecstasy, LSD
L-Tryptophan	Increases serotonin synthesis
Mood stabilizers	Lithium (Lithobid), valproate (Depakene)
Opiates	Opiates such as meperidine (Demerol), tramadol (Ultram), fentanyl (Duragesic), and pentazocine in any formulation including transdermal patches

Abbreviations: CNS = central nervous system; MAO = monoamine oxidase; SNRI = serotonin–norepinephrine reuptake inhibitor; SSRI = selective serotonin reuptake inhibitor.

of serotonin, lithium increases serotonin release, and SSRIs inhibit reuptake of serotonin. Examples of drugs other than antidepressants that are associated with serotonin syndrome are listed in Table 25-6.

While serotonin syndrome is a life-threatening condition, prompt recognition and treatment typically results in resolution of symptoms within 24 hours. Treatment consists of discontinuing the offending agent(s), administering activated charcoal for large or intentional overdose, and maintaining normothermia. Muscle rigidity, agitation, and seizures are treated, if necessary, with benzodiazepines such as alprazolam (Xanax), clonazepam (Klonopin), diazepam (Valium), and lorazepam (Ativan).[34]

Depression or Bipolar Disorder?

Antidepressant drugs can worsen the course of bipolar illness and increase the risk of a manic episode, impulsive behavior or agitation, and rapid-cycling bipolar disorder. These adverse effects are more likely to occur in women.[35] Perhaps more seriously, antidepressants can induce suicidal ideation or psychosis for an individual with bipolar disorder. Thus, when a woman presents with symptoms of depression, it is critical that bipolar disorder be eliminated from the differential diagnosis before antidepressant medication is recommended through careful screening and identification of clinical signs and symptoms.

Clinical Effects

Once the diagnosis of major depressive disorder is made, there are a few clinically important effects common to all antidepressants. First, since 2004, the labels for all antidepressant medications have carried an FDA-mandated black box warning that describes an increased risk of suicidal thinking and behavior in children, adolescents, and young adults up to 25 years who are prescribed these drugs. Counseling prior to initiation of therapy and early monitoring after initiation of therapy are focused on suicidality, safety, and efficacy. Second, antidepressants do not take effect quickly. During the first 2 weeks of treatment, side effects including gastrointestinal upset, headache, irritability, sleepiness, orthostatic changes, or difficulty sitting still (akathisia) may be prominent.

Approximately 50% of all individuals who take an antidepressant will respond partially to the initial medication used. However, only 30% of those treated will experience a complete remission with use of one drug alone.[36] Treatment of people with depression occurs in three phases:

- The acute phase (a minimum of 6 to 12 weeks) focuses on attaining remission. In general, it takes 4 to 8 weeks to assess a woman's response to a specific intervention. The maximum effect of a medication is usually evident by 8 to 12 weeks, and if the symptoms are not sufficiently relieved, the agent can be changed or augmented with an additional agent.
- The continuation phase (4 to 9 months) is directed at preventing relapse. It is recommended that the individual continue to take the medication for at least 4 to 9 months after complete remission of the illness.[27] Ending treatment sooner increases the likelihood of a relapse within the year.[27]
- The maintenance phase is focused on prevention of a recurrence or new episode of major depression.[27]

Although there is limited evidence for this effect, one peculiarity of pharmacologic treatment of women with psychiatric disorders is that blood relatives often seem to respond similarly to the same medications, even if their diagnoses are different. Conversely, unrelated persons with similar symptoms may need different medications. If members of a woman's family are taking psychotropic medication, it is helpful to know what drugs have been effective and, to start with that regimen, unless other information or circumstances dictate otherwise.

Monoamine Oxidase Inhibitors

The monoamine oxidase inhibitors were the first antidepressant drugs to be discovered; as is typical of medical discoveries, the discovery was an accident.[37] There was a great deal of initial excitement when the mood-elevating effects of these drugs were noted, but unfortunately the MAO inhibitors have some serious adverse effects and demonstrate more drug–drug interactions than do the antidepressants in other classes.[27,38,39] They were supplanted first by the TCAs and later by the SSRIs and SNRIs. The MAO inhibitors appear to be the most effective for individuals with atypical or resistant depression and/or anxiety. They are also used for persons who do not find tricyclic antidepressants effective and should be prescribed by a mental health specialist. Doses and clinical considerations for prescribing MAO inhibitors are listed in Table 25-7.

Table 25-7 Monoamine Oxidase Inhibitors

Drug: Generic (Brand)	Usual Starting Dose	Target Dose/Day	Range for Dose/Day	Clinical Considerations
Phenelzine (Nardil)	15 mg PO	30–90 mg PO	15–90 mg PO	When discontinuing, dose must be tapered over several weeks. When switching to another class of antidepressant, allow 14 days (4–5 half-lives) before starting the other drug. Allow 5 weeks if switching from fluoxetine to an MAO inhibitor. All of the labels for these drugs carry the FDA black box warning about suicidality. Multiple drug–drug interactions may occur. There is a risk of serotonin syndrome if MAO inhibitors are used with other drugs that affect serotonin reuptake. Thus these drugs should not be use d concomitantly with SSRIs or SNRIs, TCAs, lithium, tramadol, or linezolid. Persons using MAO inhibitors must follow a low-tyramine diet.
Selegiline (Emsam)	10 mg PO (5 mg 2 times/day) Transdermal: 6 mg/24 hours once daily	15–90 mg PO Transdermal: titrate in increments of 3 mg/24 hours every 2 weeks	7.5–90 mg PO Transdermal: maximum or 12 mg/24 hours	
Tranylcypromine (Parnate)	10 mg PO	30–60 mg PO	10–60 mg PO	

Abbreviations: MAO = monoamine oxidase; SNRI = serotonin–norepinephrine reuptake inhibitor; SSRI = selective serotonin reuptake inhibitor; TCA = tricyclic antidepressant.

Mechanism of Action

The MAO inhibitors irreversibly inhibit **monoamine oxidase (MAO)**, which is the enzyme responsible for degrading norepinephrine, dopamine, and serotonin after they are returned to the presynaptic neuron. When MAO is inhibited, more neurotransmitter becomes available for release by the presynaptic neuron. Because this effect is irreversible, the duration of this action can continue for 2 to 3 weeks after discontinuation of the drug. For this reason, a washout period of at least 14 days is recommended between discontinuing an MAO inhibitor and starting another antidepressant or between discontinuation of the MAO inhibitor and resumption of a normal diet.[27]

The Story of Cheese and Monoamine Oxidase Inhibitors

Many clinicians know that individuals taking MAO inhibitors cannot eat specific foods, but the reason is not as well publicized. MAO breaks down tyramine in the liver. Tyramine is a naturally occurring amine found in cheeses, meats, red wine, and pickled foods; it releases norepinephrine from the presynaptic neuron into the neural synapse.[39–41] When monoamine is inhibited and the individual eats foods that have tyramine, the subsequently elevated level of tyramine in the body causes elevated norepinephrine levels in the synaptic spaces of peripheral adrenergic neurons, which can result in a hypertensive crisis.[39–41] Individuals who take MAO inhibitors should adhere to a low-tyramine diet, as summarized in Table 25-8.[39–41] There is one exception, which is the transdermal formulation of selegiline (Emsam), approved for treatment of women with major depression by the FDA in 2006: The 6 mg/24 hours dose of transdermal selegiline can be used without dietary restrictions.[40]

Side Effects/Adverse Effects

The most common side effects of MAO inhibitors are insomnia and overeating; the latter causes weight gain. Dizziness, daytime somnolence, sedation, headache, movement problems, constipation, anorgasmia, and orthostatic hypotension are also possible.

The adverse side effects of import associated with MAO inhibitors are hypertensive crisis and serotonin syndrome. These drugs increase the amount of norepinephrine and/or serotonin in the presynaptic neurons of the peripheral autonomic nervous system, just as they do in the CNS.[39–41] Thus MAO inhibitors can precipitate a hypertensive crisis or serotonin syndrome if taken in overdose.

Table 25-8 Dietary Guidelines for Persons Taking Oral Monoamine Oxidase Inhibitors

Foods to Avoid	Foods That Are Allowed
Cheese	
Cheese: all matured or aged cheese Casseroles made with cheese	Fresh cheese: cottage cheese, cream cheese, ricotta cheese, processed cheese slices; fresh milk products, such as sour cream, yogurt, and ice cream
Meat and Fish	
Dried, aged, smoked, fermented, spoiled, and/or improperly stored meat, poultry or fish, sausage, salami, mortadella	Fresh or processed meat, poultry and fish, appropriately stored pickled or smoked fish, hot dogs
Vegetables	
Broad bean pods or fava bean pods	Other fruits and vegetables
Kimchee, sauerkraut	Peanuts
Fruits	
Banana peel	Banana pulp and all other fruits
Other	
Nutritional supplements containing tyramine	Canned or bottled beer or other alcohol can be consumed because they have low levels of tyramine, but excessive consumption may result in moderate to higher levels, Therefore, no more than two 4-oz glasses of red or white wine or 2 bottled or canned beers per day.
Unpasteurized or draft beer	
Marmite or vegemite	Brewer's and baker's yeast
Fermented soy products: soy sauce	Soy milk, tofu

[a] The list of specific foods that should be avoided and those that can be eaten in small amounts varies, as the amount of tyramine and individual responses are not absolutely known. Thus, individuals taking MAO inhibitors should consult with a dietician or clinician who has expertise in this field.

Sources: Data from Grady MM, Stahl SM. Practical guide for prescribing MAOIs: debunking myths and removing barriers. *CNS Spectrums.* 2012;17(1):2-10[39]; Nandagopal JJ, DelBello MP. Selegiline transdermal system: a novel treatment option for major depressive disorder. *Expert Opin Pharmacother*. 2009;10(10):1665-1673[40]; Shulman K, Hermann N, Walker SE. Current place of monoamine oxidase inhibitors in the treatment of depression. *CNS Drugs*. 2013;27(10):789-797.[41]

Drug–Drug Interactions

MAO inhibitors are associated with multiple drug–drug interactions, which fall into one of two categories: those that can precipitate a hypertensive crisis and those that cause serotonin syndrome (Table 25-9).

Tricyclic Antidepressants

The tricyclic antidepressants are so called because their chemical structure features three rings of atoms. This

Table 25-9 Selected Drug–Drug Interactions Associated with Monoamine Oxidase Inhibitors[a]

Drug: Generic (Brand)	Increased Risk of Hypertensive Crisis	Increased Risk of Serotonin Syndrome	Other Adverse Effects
Alpha-1 agonists	Yes		
Amphetamines	Yes	Yes	
Analgesics/opioids			
Meperidine (Demerol)	Yes	Yes	
Methadone		Yes	
Tramadol (Ultram)		Yes	
Anticonvulsants			Decreases drug exposure
Carbamazepine (Tegretol)		Yes	
Oxcarbazepine		Yes	
Antidepressants			
Bupropion (Wellbutrin)	Yes		Hyperthermia, coma, seizures
Other MAO inhibitors	Yes		
SNRIs	Yes	Yes	
SSRIs		Yes	
TCAs	Yes		
Antihistamines			Hypotension
Antihypertensives			Hypotension
Antiparkinson drugs		Yes	
Armodafinil (Nuvigil)	Yes		
Buspirone (BuSpar)	Yes		
Central nervous systems depressants			Increased sedation
Decongestants and over-the-counter cold remedies (phenylephrine and pseudoephedrine)	Yes	Yes	Psychosis
Disulfiram			Severe toxicity, coma and circulatory collapse
Diuretics			Hypotension
Levodopa (L-dopa)	Yes		Headache, hyperexcitability
Local anesthetics containing vasoconstrictors	Yes		
Modafinil (Provigil)	Yes		
Sedatives			Increased sedation
St. John's wort		Yes	
Sympathomimetic agents			
Dopamine	Yes		
Epinephrine	Yes		
Methylphenidate (Concerta)			
Phenylalanine	Yes		
Reserpine	Yes		
Tryptophan	Yes		

Abbreviations: MAO = monoamine oxidase; SNRI = serotonin-norepinephrine reuptake inhibitor; SSRI = selective serotonin reuptake inhibitor; TCA = tricyclic antidepressant.

[a] This table is not comprehensive as new information is being generated on a regular basis.

class of drugs, like the MAO inhibitors, affects several neurotransmitters, which makes them highly effective but also highly likely to generate adverse effects. Due to these adverse effects, this class of drugs has fallen out of favor for first-line treatment of individuals with depression.[27] These agents are still used (either alone or in combination with other agents) to treat depression, pain, and insomnia. The tertiary amine TCAs, doxepin (Sinequan) and amitriptyline (Elavil) have been used for the treatment of individuals with insomnia. All of the TCAs that are presented in Table 25-10 appear equally effective, with their differences based on their individual side-effect profiles.[27]

Mechanism of Action

The TCAs bind to presynaptic transport proteins, thereby inhibiting reuptake of neurotransmitters that are in the synapse. These agents are not discriminating in their binding; that is, they bind to the transport proteins for a host of neurotransmitters. TCAs inhibit acetylcholine, histamine, and some alpha-adrenergic receptors. Some of these drugs are better at blocking the transport protein

Table 25-10 Tricyclic Antidepressants

Drug: Generic (Brand)	Usual Starting Dose	Usual Adult Dose
Amitriptyline (Elavil)	25–75 mg PO as necessary	100–300 mg PO/day
Amoxapine (Asendin)	50 mg PO 1–3 times/day	100–400 mg PO/day
Clomipramine (Anafranil)	25–75 mg PO once/day	100–250 mg PO/day
Desipramine (Norpramin)	25–50 mg PO/day	100–300 mg PO/day
Doxepin (Sinequan)	25–75 mg PO once/day	100–300 mg PO/day
Imipramine (Tofranil)	25–75 mg PO once/day	100–300 mg PO/day
Maprotiline (Ludiomil)	25–75 mg PO once/day	100–225 mg PO/day
Nortriptyline (Pamelor)	25–50 mg PO once/day	50–150 mg PO/day
Protriptyline (Vivactil)	10–20 mg PO in 3–4 divided doses/day	15–60 mg PO/day
Trimipramine (Surmontil)	25–50 mg PO once/day	75–300 mg PO/day

for norepinephrine versus the transport protein for other neurotransmitters, and some are more selective for the serotonin transport protein. These differences do not affect their antidepressant efficacy, but they do affect the incidence and pattern of side effects.

TCAs are metabolized in the liver by several CYP450 enzymes. Genetic polymorphisms of the CYP450 system are probably responsible for the noted wide variations in blood levels of TCAs.[42] Persons who are either poor metabolizers or ultra-rapid metabolizers can have TCA drug concentrations outside the therapeutic range and experience either therapeutic failure or drug toxicity.[42] Some researchers have proposed genotyping for CYP2D6 prior to initiating therapy with TCAs to identify poor metabolizers and ultra-metabolizers, as knowing this status could then facilitate individualized dosing. The FDA has mandated that pharmacogenomic biomarkers be noted on the product labels of some of the drugs in this class.

Side Effects/Adverse Effects

The most common side effects of TCAs relate to the anticholinergic effects secondary to increased acetylcholine concentrations in the neural synapse and include dry mouth, urinary retention, constipation, dizziness, impaired memory, and confusion. Sedation and weight gain are related to histamine increase, and orthostatic hypotension may occur secondary to blockade of the reuptake of alpha-adrenergic neurotransmitters.[27,43]

The adverse effects of TCAs are the problems that really limit their use. The alpha-adrenergic blockade in combination with blockade of fast sodium channels in myocardial cells increases the risk of cardiac arrhythmias and prolonged QT interval. In addition, the TCAs have a narrow therapeutic window and are often lethal if an overdose is taken.[27,43]

Drug–Drug Interactions

TCAs are involved in many drug–drug interactions (Table 25-11). Desipramine and nortriptyline are the least likely drugs in this class to cause drug–drug interactions.[43]

Table 25-11 Selected Drug–Drug Interactions of Tricyclic Antidepressants[a]

Interacting Drugs: Generic (Brand)	Effect
Antipsychotics	May increase blood concentration of TCAs
Cimetidine (Tagamet)	May increase TCA levels and increase risk of anticholinergic side effects
Cisapride (Propulsid)	Contraindicated with some TCAs due to risk of arrhythmias and QT prolongation
Clonidine (Catapres)	TCA limits hypotensive effects of clonidine
CNS depressants	Additive depressant effect
CYP2D6 inhibitors	May increase blood concentration of TCAs
Monoamine oxidase inhibitors	Symptoms of serotonin syndrome
Quinidine (Apo-Quinidine)	May decrease clearance of the TCA
SSRIs	CYP2D6 inhibitors may increase TCA blood concentration
Thyroid agents	Accelerate therapeutic effects of TCAs, but may increase risk of arrhythmias
Methylphenidate (Ritalin)	Increased TCA levels and increased risk of cardiotoxicity

Abbreviations: CNS = central nervous system; SSRI = selective serotonin reuptake inhibitor; TCA = tricyclic antidepressant.

[a] This table is not comprehensive as new information is being generated on a regular basis.

Selective Serotonin Reuptake Inhibitors

Selective serotonin reuptake inhibitors are by far the most commonly prescribed class of antidepressants. Fluoxetine (Prozac) was the first drug designed to act on a single neurotransmitter, serotonin. Since its introduction into clinical practice in 1987, fluoxetine has revolutionized the treatment of women with depression as a "clean" drug with a single targeted neurochemical action and, therefore, limited adverse effects.[44] Over time, additional SSRIs have been refined in an attempt to decrease the side-effect profile of this class and expand their usefulness (Table 25-12).

All of the SSRIs, with the exception of fluvoxamine (Luvox) which is approved for OCD, have been approved by the FDA for the treatment of a woman with depression. The drug manufacturers have sponsored studies to gain FDA approval of SSRIs for the treatment of women with other disorders. For example, sertraline (Zoloft) is now approved to treat PTSD, and escitalopram (Lexapro) is approved to treat generalized anxiety disorder. Because the studies usually test the drugs against placebo and not against one another, all of the SSRIs may have similar effectiveness; however, slight differences in receptor affinity may cause a different response with individual agents. Therefore, the clinician's first choice of SSRI for a specific woman may be based on other factors besides effectiveness alone.[27]

Mechanism of Action

As their name implies, SSRIs increase the concentration of serotonin in the synapse by inhibiting its reuptake into the presynaptic cell. There are several receptors for serotonin that these agents may affect. As a result, each drug in the

Table 25-12 Selective Serotonin Reuptake Inhibitors Used in Primary Care Settings

Drug: Generic (Brand)	Dose	Elimination Half-Life	Clinical Considerations
Citalopram (Celexa)	20–40 mg PO/day	35 hours	Dose increase limited due to risk of QT prolongation
Escitalopram (Lexapro)	5–20 mg PO/day	27–32 hours	Least likely to have drug–drug interactions
Fluoxetine[a] (Prozac, Sarafem)	20–80 mg PO/day	4–6 days	Tends to be energizing; recommend taking in the morning
Fluvoxamine (Luvox)	50–300 mg PO/day	15–26 hours	FDA approved for treating OCD; used off-label for treating depression
Paroxetine (Paxil, Paxil CR)	IR: 20–60 mg PO/day CR: 12.5–62.5 mg/day	21 hours	Tends to be sedating; more likely to cause weight gain; withdrawal syndrome can be severe
Sertraline (Zoloft)	50–200 mg PO/day	26 hours	Some anxiolytic effects; may improve symptoms of hypersomnia
Vilazodone (Viibryd)	10-40 mg PO/day	25 hours	Also binds to 5-HT_{1A} receptors and is a 5-HT_{1A} receptor partial agonist

Abbreviations: OCD = obsessive–compulsive disorder.

[a] Dosing for premenstrual dysphoric disorder is 20-60 mg once daily either continuously or intermittently (initiate 14 days prior to menses and continue through the first full day of menses).

SSRI family has a slightly different side-effect profile based on its action on different serotonin receptors and the elimination half-life of the drug.

Fluoxetine is typically somewhat energizing and is associated with uncomfortable side effects more often than the other SSRIs, with one notable exception: It has fewer anticholinergic effects.[44] Fluoxetine is typically taken in the morning and can help with focus and attention. This drug has the longest half-life of the SSRIs and may take longer to reach a steady state; similarly, it tends to wear off gradually and does not appear to have untoward effects when tapering the dose down. Paroxetine (Paxil) has a half-life of less than 24 hours and is more likely to induce a discontinuation syndrome, which is characterized by flu-like symptoms, insomnia, nausea, and hyperarousal.[45]

Side Effects/Adverse Effects

SSRIs have a wide therapeutic index. Unlike with TCAs, up to five times the usual dose of an SSRI may be taken without significant ill effects if the individual is otherwise healthy and without genetic polymorphisms that alter the normal metabolism of these drugs.[46] While usually well tolerated, the SSRIs can cause nausea, headache, jitteriness, dizziness, anhedonia, sweating, photosensitivity, and strange, vivid dreams. These effects generally decrease after a few weeks of treatment, and initial doses can be titrated upward as these effects begin to subside. Weight gain or loss, if any, may occur early or late in treatment. Sexual side effects, including decreased libido and delayed orgasm, tend not to decrease over time. Paroxetine is associated with the greatest amount of weight gain and sexual dysfunction, whereas sertraline is associated with diarrhea more often than are the other SSRIs.[47]

Adverse effects of SSRIs may include an increase in suicidal ideation but not completed suicide in children, adolescents, and young adults. Conversely, these drugs decrease suicide ideation in adults. If an individual has an underlying bipolar illness, antidepressant therapy can induce mania or suicidality.

Overdose with SSRIs can cause serotonin syndrome, although the incidence is rare. Most individuals who overdose have mild symptoms of generalized toxicity such as nausea and vomiting, dizziness, blurred vision, tachycardia, and rarely CNS toxicity.[48]

SSRI use can induce serotonin syndrome when these agents added to other serotonergic drugs and substances, and numerous drugs and drug combinations have been associated with serotonin syndrome. An SSRI should not be prescribed until 2 weeks after any MAO inhibitor antidepressant has been discontinued to avoid hypertensive crisis.

SSRIs increase the risk of gastrointestinal hemorrhage. If they are combined with aspirin or nonsteroidal anti-inflammatory drugs (NSAIDs), this risk is further increased, although the absolute number of individuals affected is small.[49]

Serotonin Discontinuation Syndrome

Serotonin discontinuation syndrome is not well understood, but appears to be related to the adaptation that neural cells undergo during therapy with SSRIs. This adaptation leaves the brain unable to quickly adjust to the absence of the drug. Typical symptoms include dizziness, tremor, confusion, and flu-like symptoms. Due to its short half-life, paroxetine is the SSRI most likely to cause a discontinuation syndrome; fluoxetine is the SSRI least likely to cause discontinuation syndrome due to its long half-life.[45]

Table 25-13 Selected Drug–Drug Interactions Associated with Selective Serotonin Reuptake Inhibitors[a,b]

Drug: Generic (Brand)	**Effect**
Antiarrhythmics	Increase the risk of cardiac arrhythmias
Anticoagulants	Increased risk of bleeding with fluoxetine (Prozac), paroxetine (Paxil)
Benzodiazepines	Increased blood levels of benzodiazepines leading to sedation, and confusion; most noted with fluvoxamine (Luvox) and fluoxetine (Prozac)
Beta blockers	Increased levels of beta blockers, causing bradycardia and ECG abnormalities with fluoxetine (Prozac) and fluvoxamine (Luvox)
Bupropion (Wellbutrin)	Increased risk of seizure
Buspirone (BuSpar)	Enhanced effect of SSRI with fluoxetine (Prozac)
Calcium-channel blockers	Increased blood levels of calcium-channel blockers and hypotension
Carbamazepine (Tegretol)	Increased blood levels of carbamazepine and toxicity with fluoxetine (Prozac), sertraline (Zoloft), and fluvoxamine (Luvox)
Cimetidine (Tagamet)	Increased blood levels of paroxetine (Paxil), citalopram (Celexa), and venlafaxine (Effexor)
Clozapine (Clozaril)	Increased blood levels of clozapine and risk of seizures with fluvoxamine (Luvox)
Cyclosporine (Sandimmune, Neoral)	Increased blood levels of cyclosporine
Dextromethorphan	Visual hallucinations with fluoxetine (Prozac)
Diazepam (Valium)	Decreased clearance of diazepam with fluvoxamine (Luvox) and sertraline (Zoloft)
Digoxin (Lanoxin)	Increased levels of digoxin and digoxin toxicity
Haloperidol (Haldol)	Increased blood levels of haloperidol and extrapyramidal symptoms with fluoxetine (Prozac) and fluvoxamine (Luvox)
Insulin	Fluvoxamine (Luvox) can decrease blood glucose levels with fluoxetine (Prozac)
Lithium (Lithobid)	Neurotoxicity, confusion, ataxia, and seizures with fluoxetine (Prozac); increased serotoninergic effect with fluvoxamine (Luvox) that causes seizures, nausea, and tremor
MAO inhibitors	Serotonin syndrome, potentially fatal hypertensive crisis is risk with all SSRIs
Methadone (Dolophine)	Increased blood levels of methadone with fluvoxamine (Luvox)
Nefazodone (Serzone)	Increased blood level of nefazodone and anxiety
Phenytoin (Dilantin)	Increased blood levels of phenytoin and toxicity with fluoxetine (Prozac)
Theophylline (Theo-Dur)	Increased blood levels of theophylline and anxiety
Tolbutamide (Orinase)	Decreased blood glucose levels with fluvoxamine (Luvox)
Tranquilizers	Increased blood levels of tranquilizer
Trazodone (Desyrel)	Increased blood level of trazodone and anxiety with fluoxetine (Prozac)
Tricyclic antidepressants	Increased TCA blood levels and cardiac arrhythmias with all SSRIs
Valproate (Depakote, Depakene)	Increased blood levels of valproate with fluoxetine (Prozac)
Venlafaxine (Effexor)	Increased blood levels of venlafaxine

Abbreviations: MAO = monoamine oxidase; SSRI = selective serotonin reuptake inhibitor; TCA = tricyclic antidepressant.

[a] This table is not comprehensive as new information is being generated on a regular basis.

[b] Because of the risk of additional drug–drug interactions with various CYP interactions, it is crucial that a thorough assessment be done when selecting an SSRI or adding additional medications.

Drug–Drug Interactions

The SSRIs are primarily metabolized via the CYP450 enzyme system, and are often CYP450 enzyme inhibitors that may cause increased blood levels of other drugs. Thus, these drugs are associated with a wide variety of drug–drug interactions (Table 25-13). Fluoxetine (Prozac) and paroxetine (Paxil) are stronger CYP450 inhibitors, whereas sertraline (Zoloft) and citalopram (Celexa) are less potent and less likely to induce clinically significant drug–drug interactions with coadministered drugs. Escitalopram (Lexapro) has minimal CYP inhibition and is least likely to have drug–drug interactions.[47,50,51]

Serotonin–Norepinephrine Reuptake Inhibitors

The serotonin–norepinephrine reuptake inhibitors are designed to enhance both serotonin and norepinephrine action (Table 25-14). These agents work by inhibiting the reuptake of serotonin and norepinephrine in the neuronal synapse, and some also inhibit reuptake of dopamine. Depending on a woman's symptoms, history of treatment, cost, or availability, an SNRI may be chosen for first-line treatment. Venlafaxine (Effexor), desvenlafaxine (Pristiq), levomilnacipran (Fetzima), and duloxetine (Cymbalta) are FDA approved for treating depression. Milnacipran (Savella) is also an SNRI; however, it is FDA approved only for the treatment of women with fibromyalgia.

There is debate regarding whether SNRIs are more effective than SSRIs for treating individuals with depression.[46] The SNRI venlafaxine has been shown to be more effective at increased doses, at improving remission rates; however, this drug is more likely to be discontinued secondary to side effects than are the other SSRIs or SNRIs. SNRIs have been shown to be more effective as an analgesic and may be more effective in relieving vasomotor symptoms associated with hormone fluctuations.

Table 25-14 Serotonin–Norepinephrine Reuptake Inhibitors

Drug: Generic (Brand)	Dose	Elimination Half-Life	Clinical Considerations
Desvenlafaxine (Pristiq)	50 mg PO/day	10–11 hours	Active metabolite of venlafaxine that does not require dose titration; relieves vasomotor symptoms
Duloxetine (Cymbalta)	30–120 mg PO/day	12 hours	May cause nausea, appetite loss, somnolence, insomnia
Levomilnacipran (Fetzima)	20–120 mg PO/day	12 hours	Active enantiomer of milnacipran
Venlafaxine (Effexor)	IR: 75–325 mg PO/day (use 2–3 doses) Effexor XR: 37.5–225 mg PO/day	5 hours	May cause hypertension, increased intraocular pressure, mydriasis

Side Effects/Adverse Effects

Side effects of SNRIs are similar to those of the SSRIs; likewise, they tend to fade with use over time. SNRIs appear to be more toxic in overdose than SSRIs. Adverse effects of SNRIs include excess sweating, asthenia, or syndrome of inappropriate antidiuretic hormone secretion (SIADH). These agents may cause hypertension and/or increased heart rate; consequently, blood pressure and pulse should be monitored during therapy.[52] Like other antidepressants, the SNRIs may trigger mania, suicidal thoughts, or seizures, and their labels carry the same FDA black box warning that is printed on the labels of SSRIs regarding suicidal ideation. Discontinuation symptoms can be significant (particularly with venlafaxine [Effexor]), so doses need to be tapered down prior to discontinuation.[45]

Drug–Drug Interactions

Like SSRIs, the SNRIs are metabolized by the liver through the CYP450 system, so they are subject to potential drug–drug interactions. SNRIs can cause serotonin syndrome when combined with other agents with serotonergic properties.[51] Venlafaxine (Effexor) has also been associated with severe arrhythmias in individuals who are poor metabolizers of CYP2D6.[48] Duloxetine (Cymbalta) is a moderate inhibitor of CYP2D6 and should be used with caution by individuals who take TCAs, antipsychotics, or type 1C antiarrhythmic drugs.[50,51]

Clinical Considerations

The SNRIs often are helpful for women whose illness includes somatic symptoms or chronic pain. These agents are all available in formulations that can be taken once daily, and they tend to be nonsedating. Like the SSRIs, the SNRIs take time to become effective. The same precautions and course of treatment apply to the SNRIs as to other antidepressants.

Atypical Antidepressant Drugs

Several atypical antidepressants exist that have mechanisms of action slightly different from those of the SSRIs, SNRIs, TCAs, or MAO inhibitors (Table 25-15). These drugs can also be used for medical conditions other than depression.

Bupropion (Wellbutrin)

The atypical antidepressant bupropion (Wellbutrin) has several characteristics that make it a popular first-line choice for many individuals or an option for women who have experienced unfavorable side effects with other antidepressants. Bupropion is not sedating and may improve attention and alertness; it does not cause weight gain or loss of sexual desire; and it may take effect more quickly

Table 25-15 Atypical Antidepressants

Drug: Generic (Brand)	Dose	Elimination Half-Life	Clinical Considerations
Bupropion (Wellbutrin SR, Wellbutrin XL, Budeprion SR, Forfivo XL, Aplenzin)	Wellbutrin XL: 200–450 mg PO/day (in divided doses) Budeprion SR: 150–400 mg PO/day (in divided doses) Forfivo XL: 450 mg PO/day Aplenzin: 174–522 mg PO/day	21 hours	Can cause seizures; contraindicated in those with seizure disorders
Mirtazapine (Remeron)	15–60 mg PO/day	20–40 hours	Lower doses can cause somnolence, weight gain
Trazodone (Oleptro)	150–600 mg PO/day (in divided doses)	7–10 hours	Low doses of 25–150 mg are often used to treat insomnia, but lack antidepressant effects
Vortioxetine (Brintellix)	5–20 mg PO/day	66 hours	Inhibits serotonin reuptake, but also is a serotonin agonist

than other antidepressants. It has also been used (under the brand Zyban) to help decrease the craving for nicotine, an indication that is discussed in more detail in the *Smoking Cessation* chapter.

Although bupropion has been used empirically for years, its exact mechanism of action remains uncertain; its antidepressant effects are presumed to be related to inhibition of presynaptic dopamine and norepinephrine reuptake transporters.[53] Bupropion has no serotonin activity and, therefore, has none of the side effects associated with serotonin agonists.[54] However, this drug can cause seizures and as a result, it is contraindicated for individuals with known or suspected seizure disorders, bipolar disorder, or history of an eating disorder. The risk of seizures is dose related, so when initiating or restarting the medication, the dose should be gradually titrated upward to minimize seizure risk.[53,54] Other potential side effects of bupropion include insomnia due to excessive neural activation, nausea, and headache.[54] This medication should be used cautiously with other drugs that lower seizure thresholds, including other antidepressants, antiparkinson drugs, and some antipsychotics (Table 25-16).[54]

While bupropion (Wellbutrin) can be useful as an antidepressant, it does not relieve anxiety; however, this agent may be helpful in treating panic disorder.[27] Various formulations of bupropion are available, including an extended-release formulation with less significant peak plasma levels that can be used for individuals who prefer once-daily dosing.

Table 25-16 Selected Drug–Drug Interactions Associated with Bupropion[a]

Drug: Generic (Brand)	Clinical Effect
Alcohol	Adverse neuropsychiatric reactions
Amantadine (Symmetrel)	Increases risk of CNS side effects
Antiarrhythmics: flecainide (Tambocor)	Increases plasma levels of antiarrhythmic drugs
Antipsychotics: risperidone (Risperdal)	Bupropion inhibits CYP2D6, which decreases metabolism of these drugs and potentiates their effect. Also increases risk for seizure.
Antiseizure medications: phenobarbital (Luminal), phenytoin (Dilantin), carbamazepine (Tegretol)	Hepatic metabolism of bupropion inhibited, which increases adverse effects of bupropion
Beta blockers	Bupropion inhibits CYP2D6, which decreases the metabolism of these drugs. Increased risk for hypotension, bradycardia, and atrioventricular block.
Cimetidine (Tagamet)	Increases drug level of bupropion
Clopidogrel (Plavix)	Increases drug level of bupropion
Codeine	Decreases codeine efficacy
Cyclophosphamide (Cytoxan)	Increases drug level of bupropion
Levodopa (Sinemet)	Increases bupropion-related side effects
MAO inhibitors	Increases drug levels of bupropion. Use of bupropion within 14 days of using an MAO inhibitor is contraindicated.
Meperidine (Demerol)	Increases meperidine levels and risk of respiratory depression
Metronidazole (Flagyl)	Increases risk of seizure
Orphenadrine (Norflex)	Increases drug level of bupropion
Phenothiazines	Increased phenothiazine levels, prolonged QT interval, and cardiac arrhythmias
Quinolones, all	Increase risk of seizure
Rifampin (Rifadin)/isoniazid (INH)	Decreased efficacy of bupropion; isoniazid increases risk of seizure
Selective serotonin reuptake inhibitors (SSRIs)	Increase serotonin levels and increase risk for seizure (additive effect)
Steroids: oral contraceptives and hormone replacement therapy, tamoxifen	Increase drug level of bupropion. Decreases active tamoxifen metabolite levels.
Theophylline (Theo-Dur)	Lower seizure threshold and increased risk of arrhythmias (additive effect)
Tramadol (Ultram)	Increases tramadol levels
Tricyclic antidepressants: amitriptyline (Elavil), desipramine (Norpramin)	Bupropion inhibits CYP2D6, and decreases metabolism of these drugs and potentiates their effects
Venlafaxine (Effexor)	Increases risk of seizure
Warfarin (Coumadin)	Increases risk of bleeding

[a] This table is not comprehensive as new information is being generated on a regular basis.

Trazodone (Desyrel) and Mirtazapine (Remeron)

Trazodone (Desyrel) and mirtazapine (Remeron) are multifunctional drugs, in that they are antagonists for the serotonin receptor subtype 5-HT_2 and have effects on other neurotransmitter receptors. Trazodone inhibits the reuptake of serotonin; its major metabolite is an agonist for several of the serotonin receptor subtypes. Mirtazapine has antagonist activity at alpha-2 adrenergic receptors, 5-HT_3 receptors, and histamine-1 receptors.

Both trazodone and mirtazapine act as potent antihistamines, which accounts for their side effects of dry mouth and sedation.[55] These agents have some cardiovascular effects, including orthostatic hypotension and risk of QT prolongation. In addition, mirtazapine may increase cholesterol levels in some persons. A few case reports describe cardiac arrhythmias developing in individuals taking trazodone, but the association is unclear.

Both mirtazapine and trazodone are often is taken at bedtime to enhance sleep. Mirtazapine is an unusual medication in that it tends to produce its strongest side effects at low doses. The sleepiness and weight gain that are common when starting this agent usually disappear as the dose is raised.[55]

Antidepressant Discontinuation Syndrome

The term *antidepressant discontinuation syndrome* refers to the collection of symptoms that persons can experience if an antidepressant medication is discontinued abruptly. Commonly reported symptoms include flu-like symptoms, nausea and vomiting, insomnia, imbalance, tremors, vertigo, dizziness and confusion, or hyperarousal. Persons who stop MAO inhibitors abruptly may exhibit psychosis. The underlying pathophysiology relates to a deficiency of synaptic neurotransmitter and down-regulated receptors that can remain hypoactive for several days. The disorder is more common when antidepressants with short half-lives, such as paroxetine (Paxil), are discontinued. Restarting the medication and then instituting a slow taper will resolve the symptoms.

Bipolar Disorder

Bipolar disorder is a chronic and recurrent mental disorder with a lifetime prevalence of approximately 4%.[56] Elevated mood is the cardinal sign that distinguishes bipolar disorder from depression; manic episodes that alternate with hypomania and depression are the leading cause of impairment and death in individuals with bipolar disorder. Bipolar disorder is subcategorized as bipolar I, bipolar II, cyclothymic, or mixed features bipolar disorder. Persons with bipolar I disorder have manic episodes, hypomania, and depression. Bipollar II disorder is characterized by major depression and hypomania but no manic episodes. Mixed features bipolar disorder is less well characterized.

The diagnosis of this disorder in primary care settings is difficult. Affected individuals rarely report manic episodes, and a single cross-sectional interview may not elicit the history needed to identify the manic and depressive symptoms. Longitudinal contact with an individual and interviews with family members can help identify information that will aid diagnosis. Treatment is the purview of mental health specialists, so only a brief introduction to the disorder is included in this chapter. The interested reader is referred to reviews of the topic and the resources listed at the end of this chapter.[57]

Mood-stabilizing drugs are the mainstay of pharmacologic treatment of women with bipolar I and bipolar II disorders; these drug include lithium (Lithobid) and the antiepileptic drug valproic acid (Depakote, Depakane). Other antiepileptic drugs and antipsychotic medications that reduce the risk of a manic episode can also be used to treat bipolar disorder.

To date, the FDA has approved approximately 10 drugs for treatment of bipolar disorder. Monotherapy with a mood stabilizer is usually the initial therapeutic regimen. The current controversy is about the addition of antidepressants to help individuals who are not sufficiently treated with a mood-stabilizing drug.[58,59] The risk that antidepressants might cause a manic event or more rapid cycling has been an important concern in clinical practice. However, the incidence of inducing mania when an individual with bipolar illness takes an antidepressant is not clear and remains under study.[58,59] A combination product consisting of fluoxetine/olanzapine (Symbyax) is FDA approved for treating bipolar-related depression. If a person with bipolar disorder uses an antidepressant, the antidepressant should never be used as monotherapy but only in combination with a drug that reduces or mitigates manic episodes.[59]

Lithium (Lithobid)

Lithium (Lithobid) has been prescribed by many psychiatrists over the years to treat a variety of illnesses. Prior to its use in mental health, this agent was used for the treatment of women with gout and was noted to have mood-stabilizing properties. In 1949, the Australian psychiatrist John Cade proposed using lithium to treat mania.[60]

The mechanism of action of lithium remains unknown. Various preparations of lithium salts are used to treat bipolar disorders, particularly in persons with predominantly manic symptoms. Lithium has a narrow therapeutic window and plasma levels should be regularly monitored.

Side Effects/Adverse Effects

The side effects of lithium are numerous and onerous. Nausea and vomiting, diarrhea, and muscle tremor are common initial problems that are usually treated with dose changes and taking the medication at night. Headache, poor memory, confusion, acne, weight gain, and impaired motor performance are other common side effects of lithium.[61]

Lithium can affect the kidney in two ways. Tubular dysfunction reduces the kidney's ability to concentrate urine, so polyuria and its companions, polydipsia and nocturia, occur in 15% to 40% of individuals taking lithium.[62] This is the most common renal complication of lithium therapy. If addressed early, it is reversible once the drug is discontinued, but it can become irreversible once structural damage occurs.[62,63]

Lithium also induces the formation of thyroid antibodies and may result in the subsequent development of hypothyroidism and goiter.[64] Lithium-induced hypothyroidism is much more likely to occur in women compared to men and occurs among approximately 14% of women who use this medication. Dehydration or heat stress can elevate lithium blood levels and produce toxic effects that include somnolence, cardiac arrhythmias, seizure, and kidney or liver damage.[64]

Lithium exhibits protective effects against suicide after about 6 to 8 weeks of treatment. Rapid discontinuation of this agent, however, may significantly increase suicide risk.

Drug–Drug Interactions

Lithium is involved in numerous drug–drug interactions. Its use with other drugs that affect kidney function is particularly concerning. All diuretics and NSAIDs should be used with caution by persons taking lithium, and kidney function monitored to avoid additive effects.[64] Drugs that can elevate serum lithium levels include NSAIDs, angiotensin-converting enzyme (ACE) inhibitors, and thiazide diuretics.[64] Agents that speed lithium metabolism and excretion, including caffeine, may reduce serum lithium levels.[64]

Antiepileptic Drugs

Antiepileptic drugs (AEDs) that are effective as mood stabilizers include carbamazepine (Tegretol), valproic acid (Depakote, Depakene), and lamotrigine (Lamictal). Newer agents, with less proven efficacy, include gabapentin (Neurontin), pregabalin (Lyrica), oxcarbazepine (Trileptal), and topiramate (Topamax). Lamotrigine has been associated with a rare side effect, Stevens-Johnson syndrome, especially if rapid changes in serum levels or overdose occurs. Each of the antiepileptic drugs has a unique side-effect profile. General pharmacologic management of women using these drugs is reviewed in the *Central Nervous System* chapter.

Other Treatments for Mood Disorders

Electroconvulsive Therapy

Both the old word *electroshock* and the modern term *electroconvulsive therapy* (ECT) can sound ominous to women and their clinicians alike. But as currently practiced—under light general anesthesia and without generalized seizure activity—the brief electrical stimulation of focused areas of the brain can provide relief of severe and otherwise intractable psychiatric illness. In the United States, ECT is most often used when multiple medication trials have failed or when an individual's medical condition precludes risking the interactions of multiple medications. ECT can also produce symptom relief more rapidly than pharmaceuticals, sometimes after a single treatment, which can be a major advantage if a woman has severe symptoms.[65]

Light Therapy

Bright light exposure is most widely recognized as a treatment for seasonal affective disorder. However, it is increasingly being used as an adjunct treatment to improve mood and stabilize circadian rhythms in non-seasonal mood disorders and other diagnoses.[66] Bright light exposure has been studied in combination with medication, manipulation of sleep–wake cycles, melatonin, and aerobic exercise and has been associated with elevation of mood. Irritability and hypomania have been reported so the same precautions should be taken as when antidepressant medications are prescribed.[66]

Complementary and Alternative Therapies

Essential Fatty Acids

The essential fatty acids have been studied as a treatment for depression and bipolar disorder with conflicting results.[67,68] While essential fatty acid treatment may be helpful as either primary or adjunctive treatment in a variety of disorders, standardized sources and doses for specific situations have yet to be developed.

St. John's Wort

The plant *Hypericum perforatum* (St. John's wort) produces flavonoids in its buds that may be used to self-treat depressive symptoms, despite controlled trials that have not found such preparations to be more helpful than placebo. Although substances isolated from St. John's wort have been extensively studied to determine their potential mechanisms of action, their exact effects on neurotransmission remain unclear. An additional concern is that St. John's wort products affect the metabolism of a variety of commonly prescribed medications, including common anti-inflammatory agents such as ibuprofen (Advil), some antibiotics, cardiovascular drugs [including digoxin (Lanoxin), warfarin (Coumadin), and nifedipine (Procardia)], CNS agents [including antidepressants, benzodiazepines, and opiates], hypoglycemic drugs, oral contraceptives, proton pump inhibitors, allergy medications, and certain statins. Clinicians should regard *Hypericum* preparations with the same cautions accorded to any other drug category and consider their risks and potential benefits carefully.

Anxiety Disorders

Anxiety disorders are at least as common as mood disorders, but women who are anxious are likely to be overlooked and under-diagnosed by primary care providers.[69] Anxiety disorders include generalized anxiety disorder, panic disorder, obsessive–compulsive disorder, phobias, acute stress disorder, and PTSD. The suffering caused by panic, phobias, and generalized anxiety disorder can be disabling. Women with an anxiety disorder should be referred to a mental health specialist if they have been resistant to two or more treatment regimens, if they have a high risk of suicide, or if the primary care provider does not feel he or she can adequately manage the care of the woman.

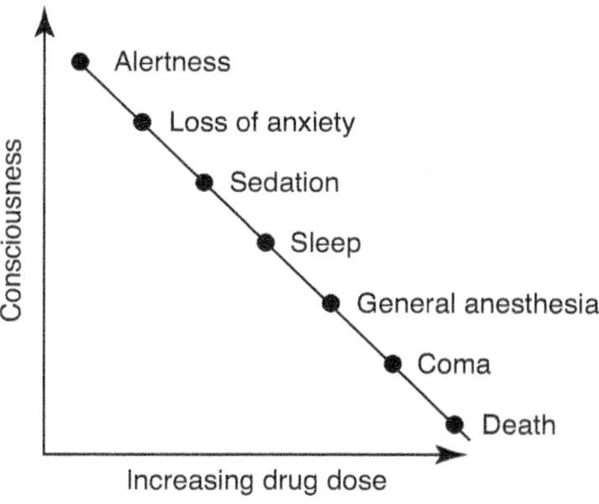

Figure 25-3 Relationship between drug dose and consciousness.

The first-line drugs for most anxiety disorders are either an SSRI or SNRI with adjunctive use of benzodiazepines. Drugs from other classes are used for treating these disorders as well. The FDA-approved drugs for anxiety disorders are presented in Table 25-17; Table 25-18 reviews those agents used on an off-label basis for treating anxiety. Table 25-19 summarizes the benzodiazepines used to treat anxiety.

Table 25-17 FDA-Approved Medications for Anxiety Disorders

Drug: Generic (Brand)	FDA-Approved Indications	Dose	Common Side Effects	Clinical Considerations
Selective Serotonin Reuptake Inhibitors (SSRIs)[a]				
Escitalopram (Lexapro)	GAD	Initial dose: 10 mg PO/day; increase to 20 mg/day if necessary; single dose any time of day. 10 mg of escitalopram may be comparable in efficacy to 40 mg of citalopram with fewer side effects. Give an adequate trial of 10 mg PO prior to giving 20 mg. Maximum dose: 30–40 mg.	Sexual dysfunction, GI symptoms, dry mouth, insomnia, sedation, agitation, tremors, headache, dizziness, sweating, bruising, and rare bleeding; rare hyponatremia	Fewer GI symptoms than citalopram
Fluoxetine (Prozac)	GAD, OCD, panic disorder	Initial dose: 5 mg PO/day in the morning; then increase by 5 mg PO/week up to 20 mg/day. Wait a month to assess drug effects before increasing dose; increase by 20 mg per month. Maximum dose: 80 mg/day.	Initial agitation/sleep disturbance, sedation at high doses, sexual dysfunction[69]	No need to taper for discontinuation
Fluvoxamine maleate (Luvox)	OCD; off-label use for PTSD and social anxiety			
Paroxetine (Paxil, Paxil CR)	GAD, PTSD, OCD, panic disorder, social anxiety	Panic disorder: initial dose, 10 mg PO/day (12.5 mg/day CR); wait a few weeks to assess drug effects before increasing dose, but can increase by 10 mg PO/day (12.5 mg/day CR) once a week; maximum dose: 60 mg PO/day (75 mg/day CR); single dose. Other anxiety disorders: initial dose, 20 mg PO/day (25 mg/day CR); increase by 10 mg PO/day (12.5 mg/day CR) once a week as needed; maximum dose: 60 mg PO/day (75 mg/day CR); single dose.	Sedation, weight gain, sexual dysfunction	Most sedating SSRI and most potential for weight gain; difficult discontinuation[69]; a favorite first choice for GAD and PTSD

(*continues*)

Table 25-17 FDA-Approved Medications for Anxiety Disorders (*continued*)

Drug: Generic (Brand)	FDA-Approved Indications	Dose	Common Side Effects	Clinical Considerations
Sertraline (Zoloft)	OCD, panic disorder, PTSD, PMDD, social anxiety; off-label use for eating disorders, GAD	Initial dose: 25 mg PO/day; increase to 50 mg PO/day after 1 week; wait a few weeks to assess drug effects before increasing dose; maximum dose: 200 mg PO/day; single dose. Anxiety associated with PMDD: 25–50 mg PO in luteal phase of menstrual cycle; onset is 4.5–8 hours.	GI distress, weight gain, sexual dysfunction	Good first-choice SSRI
Tricyclic Antidepressants (Mixed Serotonin and Norepinephrine Reuptake Inhibitors)[a]				
Clomipramine (Anafranil)	OCD	Initial dose: 25 mg PO/day; increase over 2 weeks to 100 mg/day; maximum dose: 250 mg PO/day at night. Treatment for OCD may often require doses at the high end of the range (e.g., 200–250 mg PO/day).	GI upset, sedation	Take with meals; more side effects than SSRIs
Doxepin (Sinequan)	Anxiety	Initial dose: 25 mg PO/day at bedtime; increase by 25 mg PO every 3–7 days. 75 mg PO/day; increase gradually. Maximum dose: 300 mg PO/day.	Sedation	Helpful for anxiety with skin/hair/scalp/nail issues
Serotonin–Norepinephrine Reuptake Inhibitors (SNRIs)[a]				
Duloxetine (Cymbalta)	GAD	For generalized anxiety, initial 60 mg PO once daily; maximum dose: 120 mg PO/day	Nausea	Weight neutral; fewer sexual side effects; hepatotoxicity
Venlafaxine (Effexor XR)	GAD, panic disorder, social anxiety; off-label use for OCD	Initial dose: 37.5 mg PO once daily; may increase to 75 mg PO once daily after 1 week and then increase by ≤ 75 mg once daily at intervals of ≥ 4 days. Maximum dose: 375 mg/day.	Less sexual dysfunction than SSRIs	Difficult discontinuation; monitor for hypertension; helpful for pain syndromes
Other Non-benzodiazepines				
Buspirone (BuSpar)	Anxiety and short-term relief of anxiety symptoms	Initial dose: 15 mg PO 2 times/day; increase in 5 mg/day increments every 2–3 days until desired efficacy is reached; Max dose 60 mg/day	Nausea, dizziness, restlessness, insomnia	Generally not as effective for monotherapy as other agents; recommended to augment SSRIs to reduce sexual dysfunction
Hydroxyzine (Vistaril)	GAD	50–100 mg PO 4 times/day	Sedation, dizziness	Can be agitating; take driving precautions
Meprobamate	Anxiety			

Abbreviations: GAD = generalized anxiety disorder; GI = gastrointestinal; OCD = obsessive–compulsive disorder; PMDD = premenstrual dysphoric disorder; PTSD = post-traumatic stress disorder.

[a] All drugs in these classes carry a black box warning regarding increased risk of suicidality in children, adolescents, and young adults.

Source: Modified from Karsnitz DB, Ward S. Spectrum of anxiety disorders: diagnosis and pharmacologic treatment. *J Midwifery Womens Health*. 2011;56(3):266-281.[69]

Table 25-18 Non-FDA-Approved Medications Commonly Used for Anxiety Disorders

Drug: Generic (Brand)	Classification	Clinical Use	Most Common Side Effects	Clinical Considerations
Clonidine (Catapres)	Centrally active alpha-1 adrenergic antagonist, antihypertensive	Performance anxiety, hyperarousal PTSD	Dry mouth, sedation, constipation, headache, fatigue[81]	Contraindicated with use of other antihypertensives.[81] Avoid abrupt discontinuation.[81] Taper dose gradually in women with hypertension.[81]
Gabapentin (Neurontin)	Anticonvulsant	Anxiety	Sedation, dizziness, nystagmus, tremor dyspepsia, diarrhea, dry mouth, constipation, weight gain, blurred vision	Useful for anxiety syndromes in individuals with bipolar disorder. Good choice for individuals with anxiety accompanied by pain syndromes. Relatively few drug–drug interactions.
Guanfacine (Tenex)	Centrally acting alpha-2A agonist; antihypertensive	Nightmares in PTSD	Sedation, dizziness, dry mouth, constipation fatigue, weakness	If guanfacine is terminated abruptly, rebound hypertension may occur within 24 days

Mirtazapine (Remeron)	Alpha-2 antagonist; dual serotonin and norepinephrine agent; antidepressant	GAD, PTSD, panic disorders	Sedation, weight gain, dry mouth; can increase cholesterol levels	Side effects are worse at lower doses, but tend to resolve as dose increases. Breaking a 15-mg tablet in half and administering a 7.5-mg PO dose may actually increase sedation. Some women require more than 45 mg daily, including up to 90 mg in difficult situations with women who tolerate these doses.
Prazosin (Minipress)	Centrally active alpha-1 adrenergic antagonist, antihypertensive	Nightmares in PTSD	First dose—syncope[81]	Use with caution in individuals taking other antihypertensives
Propranolol (Inderal)	Beta blocker	Performance anxiety; prevention of PTSD in individuals with symptoms of acute stress disorder	Hypotension, bronchospasm, bradycardia, sexual dysfunction	Use with caution for individuals with asthma, diabetes or comorbid depression
Trazodone (Deseril)	Serotonin-2 antagonists reuptake inhibitor	Insomnia in PTSD, panic disorder, GAD	Sedation, weight gain, orthostatic hypertension, dry mouth, dissociative feeling[81]	Falls are common in the elderly.[81] Black box warning: Suicidality in children, adolescents, and young adults up to 25 years.[66]

Abbreviations: GAD = generalized anxiety disorder; PTSD = post-traumatic stress disorder.
Source: Modified from Karsnitz DB, Ward S. Spectrum of anxiety disorders: diagnosis and pharmacologic treatment. *J Midwifery Womens Health*. 2011;56(3):266-281.[69]

Table 25-19 Benzodiazepines Used for Anxiety[a,b]

Drug: Generic (Brand)	FDA Approved for Anxiety Disorders	Dose	Onset	Half-Life	Classification	Clinical Considerations
Alprazolam (Xanax)	Anxiety, GAD, panic disorder	0.25–0.5 mg PO 3 times/day; maximum dose: 0.5–4 mg/day	15–30 minutes	12–15 hours	Intermediate acting	Withdrawal symptoms can be severe; multiple drug interactions
Alprazolam ER (Xanax ER)	Anxiety, GAD, panic disorder	0.5–6 mg PO once daily	15–30 minutes	12–15 hours	Intermediate acting	
Chlorazepate (Tranxene-T)	Anxiety disorders	7.5–15 mg PO 2–4 times/day; maximum dose: 60 mg	15–30 minutes	36–200 hours	Long acting	Has an active metabolite; residual effects may be present for several days. Multiple drug interactions.
Chlordiazepoxide (Librium)	Anxiety disorders	5–25 mg PO 3–4 times/day; maximum dose: 15–100 mg	15–30 minutes	24–96 hours	Long acting	Has an active metabolite; residual effects may be present for a few days. Dose should be tapered if discontinued after regular use. Multiple drug interactions.
Clonazepam (Klonopin)	Panic disorder	0.5 mg PO 3 times/day; maximum dose: 20 mg PO/day	15–30 minutes	18–50 hours	Intermediate acting	Used off-label for anxiety; recommended for treatment of women with epilepsy and panic disorder. Has risk of stimulating suicidal behavior. If discontinued after regular use, the dose should be tapered slowly.
Diazepam (Valium)	Anxiety disorders	2–10 mg PO 2–4 times/day; maximum dose: 4–40 mg	≤ 15 minutes	50–100 hours	Long acting	Has several active metabolites; residual effects may be present for a few days. Multiple drug interactions.
Lorazepam (Ativan)	Situational anxiety	0.5–2 mg PO 3–4 times/day; maximum dose: 2–6 mg/day	15–30 minutes	10–14 hours	Intermediate acting	Few drug interactions
Oxazepam (Doral)	Anxiety disorders	10–30 mg PO 3–4 times/day; maximum dose: 30–120 mg/day	30–60 minutes	5–15 hours	Intermediate acting	Few drug interactions

Abbreviations: GAD = generalized anxiety disorder.
[a] All of the benzodiazepines are listed as potentially inappropriate for older adults based on Beer's criteria, as they can have prolonged effects in elderly individuals.
[b] Benzodiazepines should not be used by women during pregnancy or while breastfeeding.

Drugs that mitigate anxiety are called **anxiolytics** or **sedatives**. Barbiturates and benzodiazepines are the classic **sedative-hypnotic drugs** that are also anxiolytics. Figure 25-3 presents the progression from alertness to death that illustrates why sedative-hypnotics can be used as anxiolytics. The anxiolytic drugs enhance the effects of GABA, the primary inhibitory neurotransmitter throughout the CNS. The result is general reduced neuron excitability.

The oldest known anxiolytic is alcohol. Of course, as one author states, "It is difficult to administer in accurate doses, and has a very poor therapeutic index. It has no medical use."[14]

Barbiturates

The barbiturates are the oldest sedative-hypnotic drugs. These drugs are subcategorized on the basis of their structure, which defines their mechanism of action. Thus they are ultra-short acting, short/intermediate acting, or long acting. Barbiturates are excellent anxiolytic drugs but they have marked adverse effects, including cognitive clouding, impaired judgment, and slowed reflexes. They can be addicting, and their abuse potential is high. Overdose can result in coma and death. These drugs are largely used to induce anesthesia and to prevent seizures. They are reviewed in more detail in the *Central Nervous System* chapter.

Benzodiazepines

Today, most anxiety disorders are treated with benzodiazepines for ameliorating acute symptoms while waiting for antidepressants to become effective or for acute periodic management of a woman with an anxiety attack. Thus, because these agents have a small potential for addiction, they are not generally used as monotherapy for anxiety disorders and are recommended for short time periods only.[70,71] Benzodiazepines provide relief from physical symptoms of anxiety, and they reduce the worry and feelings of tension associated with anxiety.[70] These drugs are not effective for treating depression, which is a common comorbidity with anxiety.

Mechanism of Action

Benzodiazepines have an agonist action on the complexes they form with GABA receptors in the central nervous system, thereby enhancing the effects of GABA. The various agents in this class have different onsets of action and duration. The duration of action is determined by the method of metabolism and the presence or absence of an active metabolite. Because benzodiazepines are lipid soluble, the parent drug may become deposited in fat (an inert deposit), then be slowly released back into the woman's circulation. This factor explains why some individuals experience residual or drug hangover effects.

The benzodiazepines used to treat anxiety are summarized in Table 25-19. Those that are used to treat insomnia are presented in the *Central Nervous System* chapter.

The long-acting benzodiazepines undergo phase I and phase II metabolism, with the phase I metabolite being an active anxiolytic. In contrast, the short-acting benzodiazepines undergo phase I metabolism only, and their metabolite is inactive pharmacologically.

Side Effects/Adverse Effects

Benzodiazepines have several potential adverse effects, including sedation and impaired dexterity, although these effects are much less severe than those seen with use of barbiturates.[70] Another adverse effect of this medication class is the withdrawal syndrome that occurs following discontinuation. If benzodiazepines are used regularly for a period of time, the dose should be tapered slowly. These symptoms may persist even when the woman slowly weans off the medication. Benzodiazepines also have an abuse potential that is not present with the antidepressants that are used in treating GAD.[71]

Drug–Drug Interactions

Drug–drug interactions with the benzodiazepines occur secondary to the effects of other drugs that are CYP3A4 inducers or inhibitors, as the benzodiazepines are metabolized by this enzyme. Alprazolam (Xanax) and diazepam (Valium) should not be used concomitantly with antifungal azole drugs. Cimetidine (Tagamet), oral contraceptives, disulfiram, isoniazid (INH), and propranolol inhibit metabolism of the benzodiazepines that undergo phase II metabolism. Oxazepam (Doral) and lorazepam (Ativan) have fewer drug–drug interactions because they are not metabolized via the same pathway. All the benzodiazepines will potentiate the central nervous system depression exerted by other CNS depressants such as alcohol or other sedative-hypnotics.

Buspirone

Buspirone (BuSpar) appears to be a partial agonist for serotonin receptors and has some antagonist action at the dopamine receptors without affecting benzodiazepine–GABA receptors. Its exact mechanism of action is unknown, however. Nonetheless, this unusual agent is highly effective for treating generalized anxiety and is FDA approved for treating GAD. The onset of action is longer than that for the benzodiazepines and similar to that for the SSRIs—approximately 4 weeks. Buspirone does not have a risk of dependence or withdrawal.

Generalized Anxiety Disorder

The mainstay pharmacologic treatments for generalized anxiety disorder are SSRIs and SNRIs, with benzodiazepines being reserved for initial treatment or for acute episodes. However, multiple drugs with different mechanisms of action are FDA approved for treating GAD. Buspirone (BuSpar) and pregabalin have been shown to be effective in several randomized controlled trials. Pregabalin is a GABA analogue calcium-channel modulator anticonvulsant. It is used on an off-label basis for treating anxiety in the United States but is approved for this purpose in other countries.

Acute Stress Disorder and Post-Traumatic Stress Disorder

Hypervigilance—a constant state of autonomic arousal—is the hallmark of anxiety produced by traumatic stress. A woman with acute stress–related anxiety may feel edgy and irritable, be emotionally numb, and be unable to focus or concentrate on tasks. In extreme cases, she may dissociate from reality and feel as if she were an observer in her own life, unable to engage with others. Disordered sleep, either insomnia or unrefreshing hypersomnia, is almost universal among persons with this type of anxiety, and dreams may be especially troubling.[72]

There is minimal evidence to support the use of pharmacotherapy to treat acute stress disorder; however, cognitive-behavioral therapy has been effective in reducing symptoms. If the individual does not have access to cognitive-behavioral therapy, a short course of pharmacotherapy may be appropriate.[73] Treatment options include benzodiazepines and a variety of antidepressants, as well as short-term psychotherapy. Acute stress symptoms may begin to resolve as soon as a few days after the traumatic experience, but a significant minority of persons will continue to suffer for more than a month after the danger has passed. At that time, the illness can be reclassified as PTSD.[72]

PTSD is often characterized by sleep disturbances that may interfere with daytime function. As a result, benzodiazepines are often used combat the symptoms of anxiety and sleep disturbance that can be prominent after a trauma.[74] This usage is concerning because these agents may cause retrograde amnesia that can interfere with the psychotherapy process. These agents should be avoided due to the risk of side effects, except in the most severe situations.[72] Antidepressants are also used to treat PTSD, but realizing their full efficacy may take months and often requires higher doses than those used for depression.[72] Studies that have evaluated use of psychotropic drugs for treating PTSD have generally found SSRIs to be the best first-line agents.[75]

Propranolol (Inderal) has been investigated as a potential agent to prevent the development of PTSD; however, recent studies did not find a reduction in new-onset PTSD when this medication was prescribed.[76] Neither benzodiazepines nor antidepressants have been shown to be helpful in preventing PTSD; however, they appear to help relieve symptoms of PTSD.[72]

Eating Disorders

Eating disorders are characterized by persistent disturbances in eating that threaten physical and psychological function. These disorders include anorexia nervosa, avoidant/restrictive food intake disorder, binge-eating disorder, bulimia nervosa, pica, and rumination disorder. Anorexia is categorized as binge–purge subtype or restricting subtype.

The term *eating disorder* may be misleading. Women who have anorexia nervosa rarely have true anorexia or loss of appetite, but instead perceive themselves as overweight and exercise rigid control to decrease intake. Those individuals with bulimia nervosa or binge-eating disorder also have skewed body perception and tend to eat normally, but experience periods of loss of control during which they overeat. For most individuals, eating disorders first occur during adolescence.[77]

The etiology of the various eating disorders is unclear, although numerous theories have been suggested. Psychological intervention remains the most common strategy for treatment, but has questionable effectiveness. Most pharmacologic agents that are used for women with these conditions are used as adjuncts in combination with behavior psychology or psychotherapy.[77]

Pharmacologic Treatments for Eating Disorders

Limited evidence exists for use of pharmacologic agents to treat anorexia nervosa; in turn, there are no recommendations for specific drugs that are effective in managing this disease. In contrast, a stronger link has been found between the use of antidepressants and bulimia nervosa. Fluoxetine (Prozac) administered as a 60 mg/day dose for 6 to 18 weeks has been found to successfully mitigate symptoms.[77] Other SSRIs can be used, as can TCAs.[78] Bupropion (Wellbutrin) should not be used to treat bulimia as it can cause seizures in this population. Binge eating can be treated with a wide variety of antidepressants, although the SSRIs are the first-line medications, with specific agents being chosen based on their tolerability and safety profiles. The choice of the drug category reflects the assumption that there is an association between binge-eating disorder and depression.[79]

In summary, although eating disorders have been recognized for years, effective treatments remain elusive and current treatment options are associated with low rates of remission.[77]

Psychosis

Psychosis is usually defined as a psychiatric disorder characterized by loss of contact with reality. Symptoms can include delirium, hallucinations, agitation, and thought disorganization. Psychosis is a symptom and can manifest in persons with a number of psychiatric disorders, including schizophrenia, depression with psychotic features, delusional disorder, or postpartum psychosis. These symptoms can also arise in persons with a wide variety of medical disorders, such as vitamin B_{12} deficiency, hepatic encephalopathy, mercury poisoning, and fluid and electrolyte disturbances. Psychotic symptoms can be a medical emergency, and an individual who has any psychotic symptoms is best treated by an expert in the field. A brief review of the various antipsychotic drugs is presented here for the primary care provider who may care for an individual who is taking one of these agents.

Antipsychotic Drugs

The antipsychotic or neuroleptic drugs were developed to treat psychotic conditions such as schizophrenia. Antipsychotics target dopamine receptors in the brain to varying degrees and are classified as high potency, intermediate potency, or low potency based on their affinity to various neurotransmitter receptors.

First-Generation Antipsychotic Drugs

The first-generation antipsychotics—which include haloperidol (Haldol), chlorpromazine (Thorazine), prochlorperazine (Compazine), promethazine (Phenergan), and perphenazine (Trilafon)—have a high incidence of extrapyramidal symptoms (EPS) involving the neurons in the spinal cord that govern reflexes, locomotion, and complex movements.[81] EPS include dystonias, parkinsonism, and tardive dyskinesia, and their severity has led to the development of second- and third-generation agents that are referred to as novel or atypical antipsychotics. These newer agents, most of which were developed within the last 15 years, have more favorable side-effect profiles.[82]

Novel Antipsychotic Drugs

The novel antipsychotics are often used to stabilize mood and calm the racing thoughts of mania or to boost the action of antidepressants. These drugs are also prescribed for psychotic episodes of PTSD, depression, and impulsive or aggressive behavior. In very low doses, some of these agents are used as **hypnotics**.

Despite their improved tolerability, novel antipsychotics have a number of significant side effects that disproportionately affect women.[81] Most of the novel antipsychotics—including clozapine (Clozaril), olanzapine (Zyprexa), quetiapine (Seroquel), ziprasidone (Geodon), and risperidone (Risperdal)—can induce significant weight gain, metabolic syndrome, and hyperprolactinemia. Clozapine and olanzapine are particularly likely to cause an increase in appetite. One of the newest antipsychotics, aripiprazole (Abilify), is often prescribed for women because it is usually weight neutral, but long-term studies remain to be done.[82] Whenever any of the newer antipsychotic agents are prescribed, baseline serum values for glucose tolerance, electrolytes, prolactin levels, thyroid, and liver function should be established and followed, along with waist measurements and body mass index.[83] Clozapine also requires frequent monitoring of white blood cell and granulocyte counts so that doses can be titrated to minimize the risk of agranulocytosis.[84]

Some drug side effects can be mistaken for symptoms of anxiety; dizziness, fainting, nausea, and palpitations may actually be caused by arrhythmias associated with QT prolongation.[83] Anticholinergic drug effects can reduce peristalsis and cause constipation and dry mouth or blurred vision.[84] Exogenous estrogen therapy may potentiate the hyperprolactinemic effect of antipsychotics.[84]

Drugs That Cause Psychotic Symptoms

Psychosis symptoms are an unfortunate adverse effect of many drugs as listed in Table 25-20. The class of prescription medications most often associated with psychosis

Table 25-20 Drugs That Can Induce Psychotic Symptoms

Class	Drug: Generic (Brand)	Description
Angiotensin-converting enzyme inhibitors		Mania, anxiety, hallucinations
Analgesics	Meperidine (Demerol)	Delirium, hallucinations, nightmares, agitation, euphoria, dementia; usually dose related
Anticholinergics	Atropine, scopolamine	Most likely in elderly persons; memory loss, disorientation, delirium, visual hallucinations, paranoia
Antidepressants: MAO inhibitors	Phenelzine (Nardil)	Mania, hypomania, suicidality
Antidepressants: SSRIs	Venlafaxine (Effexor)	Mania, hypomania, hallucinations, suicidality
Antidepressants: TCAs	Bupropion (Wellbutrin), others if they trigger a manic switch	Mania, delirium, hallucinations; anticholinergic effect can cause delirium among elderly persons
Antiretrovirals	Zidovudine (Retrovir)	Mania, psychosis
Antiepileptics	Zonisamide (Zonegran), other anticonvulsants at high doses	Delirium, mania; zonisamide is associated with visual hallucinations
Barbiturates	Phenobarbitol (Luminal)	Visual hallucinations, hyperactivity, disinhibition; most likely among children or elderly persons
Benzodiazepines	Alprazolam (Xanax), Zolpidem (Ambien)	Paranoia, visual hallucinations, delirium; women may have higher risk; may be dose related
Beta-adrenergic blockers	Metoprolol (Lopressor)	Delirium, hallucinations with oral or ophthalmic preparations
Antimalarials	Mefloquine (Lariam), chloroquine (Aralen)	Delirium, hallucinations
Antiparkinson drugs	Levodopa (Sinemet), amantadine (Symmetrel), pramipexole (Mirapex)	Delirium, hallucinations
Antivirals	Abacavir (Ziagen), acyclovir (Zovirax), efavirenz (Sustiva), nevirapine (Viramune)	Delirium, hallucinations
Cardiovascular drugs	Digoxin (Lanoxin), disopyramide (Norpace), propafenone (Rythmol)	Delirium, hallucinations
Corticosteroids	Prednisone, dexamethasone	Delirium, hallucinations, mania; may be dose related
Decongestants	Dextromethorphan (Robitussin), pseudoephedrine (Sudafed)	Delirium, hallucinations
Fluoroquinolone antibiotics	Ciprofloxacin (Cipro)	Delirium, hallucinations, paranoia
Histamine-1 antagonists	Diphenhydramine (Benadryl)	Delirium, hallucinations; first generation
Interferons	Interferon alfa-2a/2b	Delirium, hallucinations
Nonsteroidal anti-inflammatory drugs	Indomethacin (Indocin)	Confusion, depression, paranoia
Procaine	Procaine penicillin G	Fear of imminent death, hallucinations, delusions, mania
Salicylates	Aspirin	Agitation, hallucinations, paranoia

Abbreviations: SSRI = selective serotonin reuptake inhibitor; TCA = tricyclic antidepressant.

is corticosteroids. Steroid psychosis is dose dependent and more likely to occur in women than in men. Overall, approximately 25% of persons taking corticosteroids will develop psychiatric symptoms, and approximately 5% will manifest symptoms of psychosis.[86]

Hormonal Pharmacotherapeutic Agents and Psychotropic Drugs

The gonadal steroids affect neurotransmission. Consequently, clinicians who prescribe estrogen or progesterone products must consider that these agents may potentially affect the mental status of women who use them, and that they can affect the effectiveness of psychotropic medications used by women with psychiatric disorders. Primary care providers should work collaboratively with the mental health prescriber to review possible medication interactions when prescribing hormone preparations or contraception for women who take psychotropic drugs. Table 25-21 summarizes some of the clinically relevant interactions. Some evidence suggests that combined oral contraceptives appear to potentiate the effects of SSRI and TCA antidepressants.[86]

Oral contraceptives have also been studied as antidepressants themselves and as adjuncts to other medication, with varying outcomes.[87] Perhaps the most encouraging use of oral contraceptives as psychotropics is to stabilize hormone levels to prevent premenstrual worsening of depression.[88]

Table 25-21 Interactions of Psychotropic Medications and Combination Oral Contraceptives

Drugs That *Decrease* COCs' Effectiveness
Carbamazepine (Tegretol)
Lamotrigine (Lamictal)
Modafinil (Provigil)
Oxcarbazepine (Trileptal)
Phenobarbital (Luminal)
Phenytoin (Dilantin)
Primidone (Mysoline)
Topiramate (Topamax)
Drugs with *Increased* Serum Levels in the Presence of COCs
Alprazolam (Xanax)
Diazepam (Valium)
Drugs with *Decreased* Serum Levels in the Presence of COCs
Lamotrigine (Lamictal)
Lorazepam (Ativan)
Oxazepam (Serax)

Special Populations: Mental Disorders During Pregnancy

Between 10% and 25% of pregnant women meet the clinical criteria for major depression.[90] Untreated major depression during pregnancy has been associated with pregnancy loss, intrauterine growth restriction, preterm birth, increased use of cigarettes and alcohol, and impaired maternal–infant bonding.[91] Multiple studies have documented that depressed women are more likely to use substances of abuse or attempt suicide, and they are less likely to take care of themselves or obtain prenatal care.[91] Maternal mental illness during pregnancy has also been found to be the strongest predictor of mental illness postpartum. The depression and anxiety that affect 10% to 15% of women in the early weeks after childbirth can seriously impair a woman's ability to care for her family. Infants of depressed mothers tend to develop impaired cognitive function and behavioral problems, although the etiologic relationship between maternal depression and adverse health consequences in offspring has not been fully established.[90]

As compared to the documented risks of untreated mental illness during pregnancy, information on the relative risks associated with psychotropic medications is less than robust. Healthcare professionals seeking to advise women must rely largely on case studies, observational studies in which the observers are not blinded to the medication status of the subjects, and retrospective studies that rely on maternal or clinician recall.

All psychotropic agents need to be evaluated for both teratogenic and fetotoxic effects. Birth defects may occur at any point throughout pregnancy; however, the most significant abnormalities (including neural tube defects, cardiovascular defects, and facial abnormalities) are often due to disturbances during organogenesis, which occurs 3 to 8 weeks following conception.[92]

Selective Serotonin Reuptake Inhibitors and Selective Norepinephrine Reuptake Inhibitors

SSRIs as a group do not appear to be teratogenic or associated with perinatal death.[93,94] Paroxetine (Paxil) may have an association with a small increased risk for congenital heart defects, but study results are conflicting and an etiologic relationship has not been clearly established.[94,95] The American College of Obstetricians and Gynecologists has recommended that paroxetine be avoided by women who are planning to become pregnancy and by those who are pregnant.[89]

Use of SSRIs late in pregnancy is associated with a small increased risk for persistent pulmonary hypertension (odds ratio [OR], 2.5; 95% confidence interval [CI], 1.3–4.7).[96] The absolute risk is approximately 2 per 1000 live births.[96] It is important to recognize that the background rate of persistent pulmonary hypertension is quite low—1 to 2 per 1000 live births.[97] Even if this association is confirmed, with a sixfold increase in relative risk for SSRI use after 20 weeks' gestation, it would be expected that 98.8% of exposed neonates would not have persistent pulmonary hypertension.[97] However, this condition is very serious, and can even be life threatening (mortality rates of 10% to 20% despite treatment).

Neonatal complications of in utero exposure to SSRIs include poor neonatal adjustment syndrome, which is similar to the symptoms experienced by adults who discontinue these drugs after a period of regular use.[98] Symptoms include agitation, irritability, poor feeding, insomnia, respiratory distress, hypoglycemia, and hypothermia. Studies have noted wide variations in their incidence—ranging from 5% to 85% of exposed neonates—and the symptoms are generally mild, lasting 1 to 2 weeks.[99] More recent observational studies have found associations between prenatal SSRI use and autism and/or developmental delays in offspring.[100,101] The findings in this field of research are currently conflicting and challenging to interpret.

SNRIs do not appear to have teratogenic effects but may be associated with preeclampsia.[102] Short-term neonatal adverse effects of maternal use of SNRIs appear to be similar to those found in neonates exposed to SSRIs in utero.

In summary, it is challenging to provide thorough, informed consent and to help pregnant women balance the risks associated with untreated depression with as-yet-uncertain levels of risk to the fetus from use of antidepressants.[103] Women who choose to continue SSRIs in pregnancy may need dose adjustments over time, as clearance increases in late pregnancy. If a woman and her clinician have decided that the benefits of SSRI use outweigh the risks in her individual case, it is important to ensure that the dose is therapeutic, because otherwise risks are incurred through inadequate management of the woman's symptoms.

Tricyclic Antidepressants

Tricyclic antidepressants have not been associated with congenital anomalies. These drugs are not widely used in pregnancy, however, because their side-effect profiles limit their tolerability in many women. When a TCA is required, nortriptyline may be preferred in pregnancy due to its lessened anticholinergic effects. However, neonatal abstinence effects such as jitteriness, irritability, and rarely seizures have also been reported for TCAs used in pregnancy, and rebound cholinergic hyperactivity in the newborn has occurred, resulting urinary retention and functional bowel obstruction.[104]

Bupropion (Wellbutrin)

Bupropion (Wellbutrin) is chemically unique among antidepressant classes. One study identified a positive association between in utero exposure to bupropion and ventricle septal defects in the neonate (adjusted OR, 2.5; 95% CI, 1.3–5.0).[105] This increased risk was small, and other cardiovascular defects were not found to be associated with bupropion exposure. In addition, this study did not find bupropion exposure to be associated with neural tube defects or craniofacial defects.

Benzodiazepines

Older studies of the benzodiazepines—lorazepam, alprazolam, clonazepam, diazepam, and oxazepam—suggested a risk of oral clefts in the neonate when these agents were taken in the first trimester, and these drugs have generally been contraindicated during pregnancy. More recent studies have yielded conflicting results.[106] Benzodiazepine use in pregnancy may be associated with preterm labor and low birth weight, but this finding has not been corroborated.[107] It is certain that newborns exposed to benzodiazepines in utero do undergo a withdrawal syndrome. Specifically, **floppy baby syndrome**—characterized by lack of tone,

Box 25-2 Case Study: Use of Lithium During Pregnancy

GF is a 38-year-old G1P0 with a long history of bipolar disorder who presented for her initial prenatal visit at 7 weeks' gestation. She was stable and functioning well for the past 10 years at the same dose of lithium carbonate (Lithobid) 500 mg orally 3 times per day. GF was concerned because she had heard that lithium can harm her baby. However, in the years before she began lithium treatment, she had experienced several severe manic episodes followed by significant depressive episodes, including at least one suicide attempt. She was essentially asymptomatic after reaching her maintenance dose on lithium and wanted to know if she should stop taking her medication once she became pregnant.

GF was counseled that the primary teratogenic risk associated with lithium is for cardiac abnormalities. At 7 weeks' gestation, cardiac development had already been essentially completed. GF was counseled that she had approximately a 1–2/1000 chance of having a baby unaffected by Ebstein's anomaly. She was prescribed a multivitamin containing 400 mcg of folic acid and began regular prenatal care. She was offered a perinatal ultrasound and fetal echocardiogram at 18 weeks, which she accepted. She decided to continue both her lithium and her pregnancy, and was able to maintain stable moods throughout the third trimester on her usual dose. Her fetal echocardiogram and ultrasound were found to be normal. At 36 weeks, weekly lithium serum levels were assessed and found to be in the therapeutic range.

When GF entered labor at 39 weeks, her lithium was discontinued. Eighteen hours later, she gave birth to a healthy male infant with Apgar scores of 7 and 9, who was appropriate for gestational age at 7 pounds, 6 ounces. Lithium was restarted the next morning at 500 mg orally twice a day and was then titrated using serum lithium levels for the first 4 days postpartum. GF continued her lithium in the postpartum period and maintained a stable mood, other than mild baby blues on day 3.

sluggishness, and sucking challenges—is present in the immediate postpartum period.[107]

Buspirone (BuSpar)

Few data are available regarding use of buspirone (BuSpar) in pregnancy; in turn, this agent should not be used or should be used with caution in pregnant women. Although animal data suggest there is little risk to the fetus, published data regarding human exposure are extremely limited. Hydroxyzine (Vistaril) is an effective agent for short-term relief of anxiety during pregnancy and does not appear to increase the risk of fetal anomalies when used at normal doses.

Lithium (Lithobid)

Pregnancy in the context of bipolar disorder is a particular pharmacologic challenge, as commonly used pharmacotherapeutics (with the exception of first-generation antipsychotics) either are known to be teratogenic or have very little data regarding their use in pregnancy (Box 25-2). Lithium is a first-line drug for both acute and maintenance treatment of women with bipolar disorder and is associated with a small absolute risk of human cardiovascular malformations. In utero exposure to lithium in the first trimester is associated with ventricular hypoplasia and Ebstein's anomaly, in which the fetus's tricuspid valve is downwardly displaced. The increased relative risk is 10 to 20 times that seen in the general population. Although the relative risk is increased substantially, the condition is uncommon, and, therefore, the absolute risk of this event becomes approximately 1 to 2 in 1000 pregnancies.[108,109] Lithium has also been associated with premature birth, polyhydramnios, diabetes insipidus, and neonatal lithium toxicity. Signs of lithium toxicity in the neonate include floppy baby syndrome, thyroid abnormalities, cyanosis, hypotonia, and diabetes insipidus.

The American College of Obstetricians and Gynecologists recommends that women at low risk for relapse be tapered off lithium prior to conceiving.[89] Those who are at moderate risk should be tapered off lithium before organogenesis and then restarted on this medication after the first trimester. Those who have severe disease should remain on lithium and be counseled accordingly.

Maternal toxicity may also occur, particularly during labor, if maternal dosing requirements for lithium have increased over the course of pregnancy to maintain therapeutic levels. A prudent choice is to withhold lithium once labor starts and reduce the dose immediately postpartum to that used prior to conception, and to monitor lithium levels every few days in the immediate postpartum period.[108,109]

Antiepileptic Drugs

Antiepileptic drugs—primarily valproate (Depakene) and carbamazepine (Tegretol)—have been used effectively to stabilize mood in bipolar disorder, but both increase the likelihood of neural tube disorders and other congenital malformations among the children of women with epilepsy. It is recommended that women who take these medications during pregnancy also take a supplement of folic acid at 4 mg/day.[89] However, a retrospective case-control study examining the effects of folate supplementation (in a multivitamin formulation) in the first trimester of pregnancy in women who also used carbamazepine, phenytoin, phenobarbital, or primidone found no decrease in the risk for congenital anomalies in the women who used supplements as compared to those who did not.[109]

Valproate (Depakene) is a known human teratogen. Along with spina bifida, which occurs in 1% to 2% of infants exposed to this agent between 17 and 30 days after fertilization, a characteristic pattern of minor facial abnormalities has been observed; urogenital tract malformations and alterations in the digits are also associated with use of valproate and valproic acid during pregnancy.[109] In addition, valproate appears to have neurobehavioral effects in children; those exposed in utero have a higher incidence of lower IQ scores and need for special education. Neonatal abstinence symptoms are also seen in newborns whose mothers take valproate during pregnancy, with higher incidences corresponding to higher doses of valproate in third trimester.[110]

Carbamazepine (Tegretol) exposure in utero is associated with a 1% risk of spina bifida. Carbamazepine, a folic acid antagonist, is associated with an increased risk of minor craniofacial defects, fingernail hypoplasia, and, in some studies but not in others, developmental delay. This agent has also been associated with vitamin K deficiency, which potentially increases the risk of neonatal bleeding; women who take carbamazepine are often advised to supplement with an additional 20 mg of vitamin K daily during pregnancy.[110]

Lamotrigine (Lamictal) is approved for mood stabilization, and monotherapy with this drug does not appear to pose a major risk for fetal loss or congenital malformations.[110] No data to date suggest that lamotrigine might have neurobehavioral effects on fetuses, but human data for pregnancy are limited.

Antipsychotic Drugs

First-generation antipsychotic agents such as chlorpromazine and prochlorperazine have been used effectively in pregnancy as both acute antimania treatments and monotherapy or adjunctive therapy for bipolar disorder. There is no evidence that these agents have teratogenic effects, although neonates exposed in utero to them may have transient extrapyramidal symptoms, which are followed by normal motor development.[110] Atypical antipsychotics such as risperidone (Risperdal), olanzapine (Zyprexa), and quetiapine (Seroquel) often cause obesity and other metabolic complications in women. These agents have been shown to have an effect for infants as well, in that infants exposed to the atypical antipsychotics are more likely to have an increased birth weight, demonstrate reduced insulin sensitivity, and experience neonatal hypoglycemia. As a result of these metabolic complications, first-generation antipsychotics may be more appropriate in pregnancy. All antipsychotics are associated with an increased risk of neonatal complications, and care should be taken to discuss the individual risks and benefits with each woman.

Peripartum Depression

Postpartum or peripartum depression (PPD) can occur anytime within the first year postpartum and affects approximately 15% to 20 % of all women who have given birth. PPD is defined as a major depressive disorder that occurs within 1 month of childbirth. Its name was changed to peripartum depression in *DSM-5* to reflect the fact that symptoms may start either during pregnancy or in the postpartum period.

Untreated peripartum depression is associated with multiple adverse infant outcomes, including heightened arousal and poor self-regulation in infancy, negative maternal–infant interactions, impaired child development, and poor cognitive function.[111] It is not clear if treatment of women with PPD improves infant development, but considering the serious effects of untreated disease, most research in this area has focused on identification of effective therapies.

Studies have been conducted in which women at risk for postpartum depression were treated prophylactically with antidepressants during pregnancy. However, these studies were small and not of rigorous design. Thus

Table 25-22 Pharmacologic Treatment for Postpartum Depression

Drug: Generic (Brand)	Starting Dose	Maintenance Dose and Maximum Dose	Clinical Considerations	Implications for Breastfeeding
Selective Serotonin Reuptake Inhibitors				
Citalopram (Celexa)	10–20 mg PO/day	20–40 mg PO/day; maximum dose: 60 mg/day	SE: nausea, vomiting, dizziness. Few drug–drug interactions.	May produce detectable serum levels in some infants. Case reports of newborn somnolence reported.
Escitalopram (Lexapro)[a]	10 mg PO/day	5–20 mg PO/day	Active metabolite of citalopram and has the same SE; however, escitalopram is more potent and generally better tolerated.	Serum level in infants is less than 5% of maternal weight-adjusted doses. Case reports of newborn somnolence reported.
Fluoxetine (Prozac)[a]	10–20 mg PO/day	20 mg PO/day; maximum dose: 80 mg/day	Long half-life of both drug and active metabolite. SE: dizziness, nausea, anorexia, anxiety, sexual dysfunction.	Serum level in infants is similar to the equivalent serum level in adults in infants who are symptomatic. Case reports of colic, irritability, poor feeding, and drowsiness.
Fluvoxamine (Luvox)[a]	50 mg PO/day	50–100 mg PO 2 times/day; maximum dose: 300 mg/day	No active metabolites. SE: Can be sedating, nausea common, sexual dysfunction. Drug–drug interactions with Coumadin (warfarin).	Levels not detected in infant. No adverse effects reported.
Paroxetine (Paxil)[a]	10–20 mg PO/day	20 mg PO/day in divided doses; maximum dose: 60 mg/day	No active metabolites. SE: More anticholinergic effects than other SSRIs, sedating, sexual dysfunction. Avoid use in adolescents. Serum levels increased by cimetidine (Tagamet).	Low or undetectable levels in infant serum. No adverse effects reported.
Sertraline (Zoloft)[a]	25–50 mg PO/day	50–100 mg PO/day; maximum dose: 200 mg PO/day	Weakly active metabolite. SE: Not sedating, diarrhea. Bioavailability increased with food.	Low or undetectable levels in infant serum. No adverse effects reported.

(*continues*)

Table 25-22 Pharmacologic Treatment for Postpartum Depression (*continued*)

Drug: Generic (Brand)	Starting Dose	Maintenance Dose and Maximum Dose	Clinical Considerations	Implications for Breastfeeding
Tricyclic Antidepressants				
Amitriptyline (Elavil)	25–50 mg PO/day	25–100 mg PO/day; maximum dose: 300 mg PO/day	SE: Highly sedating, and anticholinergic effects	Low or undetectable levels in infant serum. No adverse effects reported.
Desipramine (Norpramin)	25–50 mg PO/day	50–200 mg PO/day; maximum dose: 300 mg/day	SE: Sedation, weight gain, anticholinergic effects, orthostatic hypotension. May be energizing, so usually given at night. Baseline ECG recommended.	Low or undetectable levels in infant serum. No adverse effects reported.
Nortriptyline (Aventyl, Pamelor)[a]	10–25 mg PO/day	75–100 mg PO/day; maximum dose: 150 mg/day	Twice as potent as other TCAs. SE: Sedation, weight gain, anticholinergic effects, orthostatic hypotension. Baseline ECG recommended.[b]	Low or undetectable levels in infant serum. No adverse effects reported.
Other				
Bupropion (Wellbutrin SR, Zyban)[a]	100 mg PO 2 times/day	150 mg PO 2 times/day; maximum dose: 400 mg in divided doses	Active metabolite. SE: Agitation, dry mouth, headache dizziness, nausea. No sexual side effects. Increased risk of seizure for persons with bulimia. Dosing must titrate up.	Low or undetectable levels in infant serum. No adverse effects reported.
Mirtazapine (Remeron)	15 mg PO/day	15–45 mg PO/day; maximum dose: 45 mg/day	SE: Dry mouth, somnolence, nausea, dizziness. Low incidence of sexual dysfunction. Administer at night.	Low serum levels for infants, especially for those older than 2 months
Nefazodone (Serzone)[a]	50–100 mg PO/day	200 mg PO 2 times/day; maximum dose: 600 mg/day	SE: Dry mouth, somnolence, nausea, dizziness	Low but variable serum levels, especially for those infants older than 2 months. Few case reports of adverse effects in newborn (premature infant).
Serotonin–Norepinephrine Reuptake Inhibitors				
Venlafaxine (Effexor)	37 mg PO 2 times/day	75 mg PO 2 times/day; maximum dose: 375 mg/day in divided doses	SE: Hypertension, diaphoresis, anxiety, headache, jitteriness, nausea, insomnia, sexual dysfunction. Particularly helpful for refractory depression.	Undetectable or low serum levels of drug. Metabolite is measurable at levels similar to those in adults. Drug level may be higher in breast milk than in maternal serum.
Venlafaxine (Effexor, Effexor SR)	37.5–75 mg PO 4 times/day	150 mg PO/day; maximum dose: 225 mg/day	SE: hypertension, diaphoresis, anxiety, headache, jitteriness, nausea, insomnia, sexual dysfunction. Particularly helpful for refractory depression.	Undetectable or low serum levels of drug. Metabolite is measurable at levels similar to those in adults. Drug level may be higher in breast milk than in maternal serum.

Abbreviations: SE = side effects; SSRI = selective serotonin reuptake inhibitor; TCA = tricyclic antidepressant.
[a] Multiple drug–drug interactions because it is an inhibitor of CYP450 enzymes.
[b] If the ECG shows conduction defects, consider a non-tricyclic antidepressant.

prophylaxis with antidepressants has not been definitively proved effective, nor has it been definitively determined to be ineffective.

Prior to initiating treatment with an antidepressant, it is critical that postpartum depression be diagnosed accurately and other disorders ruled out. Symptoms of depression are also symptoms of bipolar disorder, and antidepressants can trigger a manic episode, if the problem is bipolar disorder rather than depression. Such an assessment should always include questions to the woman about thoughts of harming herself or her infant. Positive comments are indications of possible postpartum psychosis and require immediate psychiatric evaluation and possibly hospitalization for inpatient care.

Many antidepressants can be used for women with PPD (Table 25-22).[111] If the woman has successfully used an antidepressant prior to pregnancy, that agent should be restarted. For women who are naïve to antidepressant therapy, SSRIs are generally the first choice, as they have low toxicity and are easy to administer. Fluoxetine (Prozac) was one of the first medications used for this indication and remains a mainstay of treatment. Tricyclic antidepressants are also effective but have more undesirable side effects. Although head-to-head drug studies to determine which single first-line agent is most effective are lacking, sertraline (Zoloft) and paroxetine (Paxil) are often recommended for initial therapy if the woman has no prior history of antidepressant use because they have negligible effects on the newborn.[112]

The drug regimen for treating postpartum depression is split into three phases: acute initial dosing, continuation dosing, and maintenance dosing. Because women are especially sensitive to the side effects of these drugs during the postpartum period, they are usually started at half the recommended starting dose for the first 4 days, with the dose then increased weekly until full remission is evident. It is generally recommended that drug therapy continue for 9 to 12 months, at which time the drug is gradually titrated downward until discontinuation. Maintenance treatment is recommended for women who have had more than three episodes of major depression within 3 years.

Nonpharmacologic treatments that have been proposed for peripartum depression include dietary manipulation, such as increased omega-3 acids, protein, B vitamins, St. John's wort, kava, traditional Chinese medicine, massage, and acupuncture. Although small studies have evaluated some of these options, overall evidence of their effectiveness remains lacking.

Use of antidepressants during lactation is an important issue. No data suggest that any of the aforementioned agents are contraindicated for the breastfeeding dyad. Clinical considerations specific to the newborn who is being breastfed can be found in the *Breastfeeding* chapter.

Postpartum Psychosis

Postpartum psychosis is an entity distinct from the blues or postpartum depression. Postpartum psychosis occurs in approximately 1 in 500 to 1000 women in the postpartum period. This disorder has a rapid onset and usually appears in the first 2 weeks after giving birth. A woman with this condition experiences hallucinations and delusions and may report hearing voices. Any woman who has serious compulsions to harm herself or her child/children should immediately receive expert psychiatric intervention, including admission for inpatient care and the use of antipsychotic pharmacologic agents.[112,113]

Pseudocyesis

A woman's belief that she is pregnant, when there is no evidence of pregnancy, is termed pseudocyesis. This condition is psychological and becoming rare in developed countries, perhaps due to the ubiquitous early ultrasound. However, treatment of a woman with pseudocyesis is best managed by a mental health professional. Pharmaceutical therapy has not been found to be of value in this situation.[114]

Special Populations: Mood Disorders and Elderly Women

Although mental illness is most likely to be diagnosed during the childbearing years, the years just prior to menopause are a time of particular risk for new-onset mental illness.[115] Treatment during these years requires a three-pronged approach that includes ensuring sleep, improving mood, and reducing vasomotor symptoms.[116] Primary care clinicians are ideally positioned to ensure that all three aspects of treatment are addressed to achieve optimal health for their clients.

Treating elderly women presents a number of challenges. Advancing age, comorbid conditions, and use of other medications make medicating psychiatric illness more complex. Drugs are often metabolized more slowly, increasing the risk of toxic reactions, and side effects are often more prominent in older clients. When psychotropic medications are added to a regimen that includes treatment of mature individuals with other common, drug interactions are a serious concern. Geriatric psychopharmacology is still an emerging field, with limited information available on the use and safety of medications that have chiefly been studied in younger populations.[117] Primary care clinicians need to be particularly cautious and work closely with other prescribers when treating older women for mental disorders.

Conclusion

Women's primary healthcare providers are a vital resource in the identification and treatment of a woman with mental illness. By integrating the care of women's minds with the care of their bodies, primary clinicians can help women achieve healthy outcomes.

Resources

Organization	Description	Website
American Psychiatric Association	APA practice guidelines for depression, anxiety, stress disorder, post-traumatic stress disorder, bipolar disorder, panic disorder, eating disorders, and suicidal behaviors	www.psychiatryonline.org/guidelines
American Psychological Association	Monographs, journal articles, and videos that address all the common psychiatric disorders	www.apa.org
Institute for Clinical Systems Improvement	Guidelines for Major Depression in Adults and Primary Care	www.icsi.org/guidelines__more/catalog_guidelines_and_more/catalog_guidelines/catalog_behavioral_health_guidelines/depression
Apps		
American Psychological Association	*DSM-5* Diagnostic Criteria; mobile app that lists the *DSM-5* diagnostic criteria for many disorders and includes the ICD-9 and ICD-10 codes	Available for purchase on iTunes
Zur Institute	Mental Health Apps: The Pocket Therapist; links to mobile apps that address multiple psychiatric disorders	www.zurinstitute.com/mentalhealthapps_resources.html#addiction
Psych on Demand	Mobile app that includes assessment and diagnostic requirements for many psychiatric disorders	Available for purchase on iTunes

References

1. World Health Organization. *World Health Report 2001—Mental Health: New Understanding, New Hope.* Geneva, Switzerland: World Health Organization; 2001.
2. Kessler RC, Chiu WT, Demler O, Walters EE. Prevalence, severity, and comorbidity of twelve-month *DSM-IV* disorders in the National Comorbidity Survey Replication (NCS-R). *Arch Gen Psychiatry.* 2005;62(6):617-627.
3. Kessler RC, Berglund PA, Demler O, Jin R, Merikangas KR, Walters EE. Lifetime prevalence and age-of-onset distributions of *DSM-IV* disorders in the National Comorbidity Survey Replication. *Arch Gen Psychiatry.* 2005;62(6):593-600.
4. American Psychiatric Association. *Diagnostic and Statistical Manual of Mental Disorders, Fifth Edition (DSM-5).* Arlington, VA: American Psychiatric Association; 2013.
5. Crosby AE, Han B, Ortega LAG, Parks SE, Gfoerer J; Centers for Disease Control and Prevention. Suicidal thoughts and behaviors among adults aged ≥18 years—United States, 2008–2009. *MMWR Surveill Summ.* 2011;60(13):1-22. http://www.cdc.gov/mmwr/preview/mmwrhtml/ss6013a1.htm?s_cid=ss6013a1_e.
6. Hackley B, Kriebs JM, Rousseau ME. *Primary Care of Women: A Guide for Midwives and Women's Health Providers.* Sudbury, MA: Jones and Bartlett; 2007.
7. Gaynes BN, Gavin N, Meltzer-Brody S, et al. Perinatal depression: prevalence, screening accuracy, and screening outcomes. *Evid Rep Technol Assess (Summ).* 2005;119:1-8.
8. Mark TL, Levit KR, Buck JA. Datapoints: psychotropic drug prescriptions by medical specialty. *Psychiatr Serv.* 2009;60(9):1167.
9. World Health Organization. Depression. October 2012. http://www.who.int.ucsf.idm.oclc.org/mediacentre/factsheets/fs369/en/. Accessed January 3, 2015.
10. Hackley B, Sharma C, Kedzior A, Sreenivasan S. Managing mental health conditions in primary care. *J Midwifery Womens Health.* 2010;55(1):9-19.
11. Lester H, Tritter JQ, Sorohan H. Patients' and health professionals' views on primary care for people with serious mental illness: focus group study. *BMJ.* 2005;330(7500):1122.
12. Frank B, Gupta S, McGlynn DJ. Psychotropic medications and informed consent: a review. *Ann Clin Psychiatry.* 2008;20(2):87-95.
13. Blier P. Neurotransmitter targeting in the treatment of depression. *J Clin Psychiatry.* 2013;74(suppl 2):19-24.
14. Meyer JS, Quenzer LF. *PsychopharmacologyDrugs, the Brain, and Behavior.* Sunderland, MA: Finauer Associates; 2005.
15. Hirschfeld RMA. History and evolution of the monoamine hypothesis of depression. *J Clin Psychiatry.* 2000;61(suppl 6):4-6.
16. Lanni C, Govoni S, Lucchelli A, Boselli C. Depression and antidepressants: molecular and cellular aspects. *Cell Mol Life Sci.* 2009;66:2985-3008.
17. Accort E, Freeman MP, Allen JB. Women and major depressive disorder: clinical perspectives on causal pathways. *J Womens Health.* 2008;17(10):1583-1600.
18. Watson CS, Alyea RA, Cunningham KA, Jeng Y. Estrogens of multiple classes and their role in mental health disease mechanisms. *Int J Womens Health.* 2010;2:153-166.

19. Reynolds GP, McGowan OO, Dalton CF. Pharmacogenomics in psychiatry: the relevance of receptor and transporter polymorphisms. *Br J Clin Pharmacol.* 2014;77(4):654-672.
20. Tang H, McGowan OO, Reynolds GP. Polymorphisms of serotonin neurotransmission and their effects on antipsychotic drug action. *Pharmacogenomics.* 2014;15(12):1599-1609.
21. World Health Organization. International statistical classification of diseases and related health problems. 10th ed. World Health Organization; 2010. http://apps.who.int/classifications/icd10/browse/2010/en#/F32. Accessed June 2, 2014.
22. Greenberg AJ, Freeman MP, Markowitz JC, et al. Practice guideline for the treatment of patients with major depressive disorder. 3rd ed. American Psychiatric Association; 2010. http://psychiatryonline.org/guidelines. Accessed January 4, 2014.
23. Huffman JC, Stern TA. Neuropsychiatric consequences of cardiovascular medications. *Dialogues Clin Neurosci.* 2007;9(1):29-45.
24. Nekovarova T, Yamamotova A, Vales K, et al. Common mechanisms of pain and depression: are antidepressants also analgesics. *Fron Behav Neuroscience.* 2014;8(99):1-12.
25. Marjoribanks J, Brown J, O'Brien PMS, Wyatt K. Selective serotonin reuptake inhibitors for premenstrual syndrome. *Cochrane Database Syst Rev.* 2013;6: CD001396. doi:10.1002/14651858.CD001396.pub3.
26. Hall E, Frey BN, Soares CN. Non-hormonal treatment strategies for vasomotor symptoms: a critical review. *Drugs.* 2011;71(3):287-304.
27. American Psychiatric Association. *Practice Guideline for the Treatment of Patients with Major Depressive Disorder.* 3rd ed. Arlington, VA: American Psychiatric Association; 2010.
28. Gartlehner G, Hansen RA, Morgan LC, et al. Comparative benefits and harms of second-generation antidepressants for treating major depressive disorder: an updated meta-analysis. *Ann Intern Med.* 2011;155:772.
29. Work Group on Major Depressive Disorder. Practice guideline for the treatment of patients with major depressive disorder. *Am J Psychiatry.* 2010; 167(suppl):1-152.
30. Joffe RT. Dosing and monitoring guidelines for mood disorders. *Prim Psychiatry.* 2003;10(11):67-74.
31. Ferguson JM. SSRI antidepressant medications: adverse effects and tolerability. *Primary Care Companion J Clin Psychiatry.* 2001;3(1):22-27.
32. Mann JJ. Medical management of depression. *N Engl J Med.* 2005;353(17):1819-1834.
33. Food and Drug Administration. Suicidality and antidepressant drugs: revisions to product labeling. http://www.fda.gov/downloads/Drugs/DrugSafety/InformationbyDrugClass/UCM173233.pdf. Accessed January 6, 2015.
34. Boyer EW, Shannon M. The serotonin syndrome [Erratum: *N Engl J Med.* 2007;356(23):2437]. *N Engl J Med.* 2005;352(11):1112-1120. Review.
35. Muzina DJ, Kemp DE, McIntyre RS. Differentiating bipolar disorders from major depressive disorders: treatment implications. *Ann Clin Psychiatry.* 2007; 19(4):305-312.
36. Arroll B, Macgillivray S, Ogston S, et al. Efficacy and tolerability of tricyclic antidepressants and SSRIs compared with placebo for treatment of depression in primary care: a meta-analysis. *Ann Fam Med.* 2005;3(5):449-456.
37. López-Muñoz F, Baumeister AA, Hawkins MF, Álamo C. The role of serendipity in the discovery of the clinical effects of psychotic drugs: beyond the myth. *Actas Esp Psiquiatr.* 2012;40(1):34-42.
38. Stahl SM, Felker A. Monoamine oxidase inhibitors: a modern guide to an unrequited class of antidepressants. *CNS Spectr.* 2008;13(10):855-870.
39. Grady MM, Stahl SM. Practical guide for prescribing MAOIs: debunking myths and removing barriers. *CNS Spectrums.* 2012;17(1):2-10.
40. Nandagopal JJ, DelBello MP. Selegiline transdermal system: a novel treatment option for major depressive disorder. *Expert Opin Pharmacother.* 2009;10(10):1665-1673.
41. Shulman K, Hermann N, Walker SE. Current place of monoamine oxidase inhibitors in the treatment of depression. *CNS Drugs.* 2013;27(10): 789-797.
42. Hicks JK, Swen JJ, Thorn CF, et al. Clinical pharmacogenetics implementation consortium guideline for CYP2D6 and CYP2C19 genotypes and dosing of tricyclic antidepressants. *Clin Pharmacol Ther.* 2013;93(5):402-408.
43. Gillman PK. Tricyclic antidepressant pharmacology and therapeutic drug interactions updated. *Br J Pharmacol.* 2007;151(6):737-748.
44. Brambilla P, Cipriani A, Hotopf M, Barbui C. Side-effect profile of fluoxetine in comparison with other SSRIs, tricyclic and newer antidepressants: a meta-analysis of clinical trial data. *Pharmacopsychiatry.* 2005;38(2):69-77.

45. Renoir T. Selective serotonin reuptake inhibitor antidepressant treatment discontinuation syndrome: a review of the clinical evidence and the possible mechanisms involved. *Front Pharmacol.* 2013;4(45):1-10.
46. Thase ME. Are SNRIs more effective than SSRIs? A review of the current state of the controversy. *Psychopharmacol Bull.* 2008;41(2):58-85.
47. Sanchez C, Reines EH, Montgomery SA. A comparative review of escitalopram, paroxetine, and sertraline: are they all alike? *Int Clin Psychopharmacol.* 2013;29:185-196.
48. Horstmann S, Binder EB. Pharmacogenomics of antidepressant drugs. *Pharmacol Ther.* 2009;124:57-73.
49. Loke YK, Trivedi AN, Singh S. Meta-analysis: gastrointestinal bleeding due to interaction between selective serotonin uptake inhibitors and non-steroidal anti-inflammatory drugs. *Aliment Pharmacol Ther.* 2008;27(1):31-40.
50. Spina E, Santoro V, D'Arrigo C. Clinically relevant pharmacokinetic drug interactions with second-generation antidepressants: an update. *Clin Ther.* 2008;30(7):1206-1227.
51. Spina E, Trifiro G, Caraci F. Clinically significant drug interactions with newer antidepressants. *CNS Drugs.* 2012;26(1):39-67.
52. Lieberman DZ, Massey SH. Desvenlafaxine in major depressive disorder: an evidence-based review of its place in therapy. *Core Evidence.* 2009;4:67-82.
53. Foley KF, DeSanty KP, Kast RE. Bupropion: pharmacology and therapeutic applications. *Expert Rev Neurother.* 2006;6(9):1249-1265.
54. Jefferson JW, Pradko JF, Muir KT. Bupropion for major depressive disorder: pharmacokinetic and formulation considerations. *Clin Ther.* 2005;27:1685-1695.
55. Agency for Healthcare Research and Quality. Second-generation antidepressants in the pharmacologic treatment of adult depression: an update of the 2007 comparative effectiveness review. Agency for Healthcare Research and Quality; 2011. http://www.effectivehealthcare.ahrq.gov/ehc/products/210/863/CER46_Antidepressants-update_20111206.pdf. Accessed June 6, 2014.
56. Belmaker RH. Treatment of bipolar depression. *N Engl J Med.* 2007;356(17):1771-1713.
57. Cruellar AK, Johnson SL, Winters R. Distinctions between bipolar and unipolar depression. *Clin Psych Rev.* 2005;25:307-339.
58. Kemp DE. Managing the side effects associated with commonly used treatments for bipolar depression. *J Affect Disord.* 2014;169(suppl 1):S34-S44.
59. Geddes JR, Miklowitz DJ. Treatment of bipolar disorder. *Lancet.* 2013;381(9878):1672-1682.
60. Cole N, Parker G. Cade's identification of lithium for manic-depressive illness: the prospector who found a gold nugget. *J Nerv Ment Dis.* 2012;200:1101-1104.
61. Malhi GS, Tanious M. Optimal frequency of lithium administration in the treatment of bipolar disorder: clinical and dosing considerations. *CNS Drugs.* 2011;25(4):289-298.
62. Raedler TJ. Will lithium damage my kidneys? *J Psychiatry Neurosci.* 2012;37(3):E5-E6.
63. Young AH, Hammond JM. Lithium in mood disorders: increasing evidence base, declining use? *Br J Psychiatry.* 2007;191:474-476.
64. Grandjean EM, Aubry JM. Lithium: updated human knowledge using an evidence-based approach: part III: clinical safety. *CNS Drugs.* 2009;23:397-418.
65. Andrade C, Thyagagarajan S. The influence of name on the acceptability of ECT: the importance of political correctness. *J ECT.* 2007;23(2):75.
66. Pail G, Huf W, Pjrek E, et al. Bright-light therapy in the treatment of mood disorders. *Neuropsychobiology.* 2011;64:152-162.
67. Grosso G, Galvano F, Marventano S, et al. Omega-3 fatty acids and depression: scientific evidence and biological mechanisms. *Oxid Med Cell Longev.* 2014;313570.
68. Sarris J, Lake J, Hoenders R. Bipolar disorder and complementary medicine: current evidence, safety issues, and clinical considerations. *J Altern Complement Med.* 2011;17(10):881-890.
69. Karsnitz DB, Ward S. Spectrum of anxiety disorders: diagnosis and pharmacologic treatment. *J Midwifery Womens Health.* 2011;56(3):266-281.
70. Bandelow B, Boerner RJ, Kasper S, et al. Diagnosis and treatment of generalized anxiety disorder *Dtsch Arztebl Int.* 2013;110(17):300-310.
71. Canadian Agency for Drugs and Technologies in Health. Short-and long-term use of benzodiazepines in patients with generalized anxiety disorder: a review of guidelines. July 28, 2014. http://www.cadth.ca/en/publication/4718. Accessed January 10, 2015.
72. Davidson JR, Feltner DE, Dugar A. Management of generalized anxiety disorder in primary care: identifying the challenges and unmet needs. *Prim Care Companion J Clin Psychiatry.* 2010;12(2):PCC.09r00772.
73. Frommberger U, Angenendt J, Berger M. Post-traumatic stress disorder: a diagnostic and therapeutic challenge. *Dtsch Arztebl Int.* 2014;111(5):59-65.

74. Kavan MG, Elsasser GN, Barone EJ. The physician's role in managing acute stress disorder. *Am Fam Physician*. 2012;86(7):643-649.
75. Cohen H, Kaplan Z, Koresh O, et al. Early post-stressor intervention with propranolol is ineffective in preventing posttraumatic stress responses in an animal model for PTSD. *Eur Neuropsychopharmacol*. 2011;21(3):230-240.
76. Germain A, Buysse DJ, Nofzinger E. Sleep-specific mechanisms underlying posttraumatic stress disorder: integrative review and neurobiological hypotheses. *Sleep Med Rev*. 2008;12(3):185-195.
77. Stein DJ, Ipser JC, Seedat S. Pharmacotherapy for post traumatic stress disorder (PTSD). *Cochrane Database Syst Rev*. 2006;1:CD002795. doi:10.1002/14651858.CD002795.pub2.
78. Berkman ND, Bulik CM, Brownley KA, et al. *Management of Eating Disorders*. Evidence Report/Technology Assessment No. 135. (Prepared by the RTI International–University of North Carolina Evidence-Based Practice Center under Contract No. 290-02-0016.) AHRQ Publication No. 06-E010. Rockville, MD: Agency for Healthcare Research and Quality; April 2006. http://archive.ahrq.gov/downloads/pub/evidence/pdf/eatingdisorders/eatdis.pdf. Accessed January 4, 2015.
79. Bacaltchuk J, Hay PPJ. Antidepressants versus placebo for people with bulimia nervosa. *Cochrane Database Syst Rev*. 2003;4:CD003391. doi:10.1002/14651858.CD003391.
80. Araujo DM, Santos GF, Nardi AE. Binge eating disorder and depression: a systematic review. *World J Biol Psychiatry*. 2010 Mar;11(2 Pt 2):199-207.
81. Reas DL, Grilo CM. Review and meta-analysis of pharmacotherapy for binge-eating disorder. *Obesity (Silver Spring)*. 2008;16(8):2024-2038.
82. Zhang JP, Gallego JA, Robinson DG, et al. Efficacy and safety of individual second-generation vs. first-generation antipsychotics in first-episode psychosis: a systematic review and meta-analysis. *Int J Neuropsychopharmacol*. 2013;16(6):1205-1218.
83. Maher AR, Theodore G. Summary of the comparative effectiveness review on off-label use of atypical antipsychotics. *J Manag Care Pharm*. 2012;18(5 suppl B):S1-S20.
84. Kiraly B, Gunning K, Leiser J. Primary care issues in patients with mental illness. *Am Fam Physician*. 2008;78(3):355-362.
85. Gallego JA, Nielsen J, De Hert M, Kane JM, Correll CU. Safety and tolerability of antipsychotic polypharmacy. *Expert Opin Drug Saf*. 2012;11(4):527-542.
86. Dubovsky A, Arvikar S, Stern TA, Axelrod L. The neuropsychiatric complications of glucocorticoid use: steroid psychosis revisited. *Psychosomatics*. 2012;53:103-115.
87. Gentile S. The role of estrogen therapy in postpartum psychiatric disorders: an update. *CNS Spect*. 2005;10(12):944-952.
88. Joffe H, Petrillo L, Viguera AC, et al. Treatment of premenstrual worsening of depression with adjunctive oral contraceptive pills: a preliminary report. *J Clin Psychiatry*. 2007;68(12):1954-1962.
89. American College of Obstetricians and Gynecologists. Use of psychiatric medications during pregnancy and lactation. *Obstet Gynecol*. 2008;111(4):1001-1120.
90. Wisner KL, Sit DK, Hanusa BH, et al. Major depression and antidepressant treatment: impact on pregnancy and neonatal outcomes. *Am J Psychiatry*. 2009;166(5):557-566.
91. Marcus SM. Depression during pregnancy: rates, risks and consequences—Motherisk Update 2008. *Can J Clin Pharmacol*. 2009;16(1):e15-e22.
92. U.S. Department of Health and Human Services, Food and Drug Administration. Reviewer guidance: evaluating the risks of drug exposure in human pregnancies. April 2005. http://www.fda.gov/downloads/scienceresearch/specialtopics/womenshealthresearch/ucm133359.pdf. Accessed June 9, 2014.
93. Koren G, Nordeng HM. Selective serotonin reuptake inhibitors and malformations: case closed? *Semin Fetal Neonatal Med*. 2013;18(1):19-22.
94. Stephansson O, Kieler H, Haglund B, et al. Selective serotonin reuptake inhibitors during pregnancy and risk of stillbirth and infant mortality. *JAMA*. 2013;309:48.
95. Malm H, Artama M, Gissler M, Ritvanen A. Selective serotonin reuptake inhibitors and risk for major congenital anomalies. *Obstet Gynecol*. 2011;118:111.
96. Grigoriadis S, VonderPorten EH, Mamisashvili L, et al. The effect of prenatal antidepressant exposure on neonatal adaptation: a systematic review and meta-analysis. *J Clin Psychiatry*. 2013;74:e309.
97. Chambers CD, Hernández-Díaz S, Van Marter LJ, et al. Selective serotonin reuptake inhibitors and persistent pulmonary hypertension of the newborn. *N Engl J Med*. 2006;354(6):579-587.
98. Moses-Kolko EL, Bogen D, Perel J, et al. Neonatal signs after late in utero exposure to serotonin reuptake inhibitors: literature review and implications for clinical applications. *JAMA*. 2005;293:2372.
99. Hayes RM, Wu P, Shelton RC, et al. Maternal antidepressant use and adverse outcomes: a cohort study

of 228,876 pregnancies. *Am J Obstet Gynecol.* 2012; 207:49.e1.

100. Harrington RA, Lee LC, Crum RM, et al. Prenatal SSRI use and offspring with autism spectrum disorder or developmental delay. *Pediatrics.* 2014;133:e1241.
101. Hviid A, Melbye M, Pasternak B. Use of selective serotonin reuptake inhibitors during pregnancy and risk of autism. *N Engl J Med.* 2013;369(25):2406.
102. Palmsten K, Setoguchi S, Margulis AV, et al. Elevated risk of preeclampsia in pregnant women with depression: depression or antidepressants? *Am J Epidemiol.* 2012;175:988.
103. Kieviet N, Dolman KM, Honig A. The use of psychotropic medication during pregnancy: how about the newborn? *Neuropsychiatr Dis Treat* 2013;9:1257-1266.
104. Gentile S. Tricyclic antidepressants in pregnancy and puerperium. *Expert Opin Drug Saf.* 2014; 13(12): 207-225.
105. Louik C, Kerr S, Mitchell AA. First-trimester exposure to bupropion and risk of cardiac malformations. *Pharmacoepidemiol Drug Saf.* 2014;23(10):1066-1075.
106. Ban L, West J, Gibson JE, et al. First trimester exposure to anxiolytic and hypnotic drugs and the risks of major congenital anomalies: a United Kingdom populations-based cohort stud. *PLoS One.* 2014;9(6):e100996.
107. Wilkner BN, Stiller CO, Bergman U, Asker C, Kallen B. Use of benzodiazepines and benzodiazepine receptor agonists during pregnancy: neonatal outcome and congenital malformations. *Pharmacoepidemiol Drug Saf.* 2007;16(11):1203-1210.
108. Giles JJ, Bannigan JG. Teratogenic and developmental effects of lithium. *Curr Pharm Des.* 2006;12(12): 1531-1541.
109. Hernández-Díaz S, Werler MM, Walker AM, Mitchell AA. Folic acid antagonists during pregnancy and the risk of birth defects. *N Engl J Med.* 2000;343(22):1608-1614.
110. Burt VK, Rasgon N. Special considerations in treating bipolar disorder in women. *Bipolar Disord.* 2004;6(1):2-13.
111. Hirst KP, Moutier CY. Postpartum major depression. *Am Fam Phys.* 2010;82:926-933.
112. Spinelli MG. Postpartum psychosis: detection of risk and management. *Am J Psychiatry.* 2009;166(4): 405-408.
113. Guille C, Newman R, Fryml LD, Lifton CK, Epperson CN. Management of postpartum depression. *J Midwifery Womens Health.* 2013;58(6):643-653.
114. Seeman MV. Pseudocyesis, delusional pregnancy, and psychosis: the birth of a delusion. *World J Clin Cases.* 2014;2(8);338-344.
115. Cohen LS, Soares CN, Vitonis AF, Otto MW, Harlow BL. Risk for new onset of depression during the menopausal transition: the Harvard study of moods and cycles. *Arch Gen Psychiatry.* 2006;63(4):385-390.
116. Ameratunga D, Goldin J, Hickey M. Sleep disturbance in menopause. *Int Med Journal.* 2012;42(7):742-747.
117. Meyers BS, Jeste DV. Geriatric psychopharmacology: evolution of a discipline. *J Clin Psychiatry.* 2010;71(11):1416-1424.

26 Dermatology

Barbara VanDersarl Slocum

Based on the chapter by Jan M. Kriebs in the first edition of Pharmacology for Women's Health

With acknowledgment to Marianne (Teri) Stone-Godena for her contribution to this chapter

Chapter Glossary

Calcineurin inhibitors Immunosuppressant agents that are theorized to act by selectively inhibiting inflammation through action on T-cell activation.

Cosmeceutical Portmanteau derived from the terms *cosmetic* and *pharmaceutical;* descriptor for agents that have therapeutic effects as well as esthetic effects.

Emollients Moisturizers composed of chemical agents designed to soften the epidermis by increasing hydration of the skin.

Humectant Ingredient that absorbs water and promotes maintenance of moisture on the skin.

Protectant Drug such as petroleum jelly that provides a protective barrier for the skin.

Retinoids Natural or synthetic derivatives of vitamin A that are widely used in pharmacotherapeutics in dermatology.

Sun protection factor (SPF) Measure of the degree of ultraviolet radiation (sunlight) required to produce a burn on skin that is protected with sunscreen.

Sunscreen Agent that blocks ultraviolet rays, usually ultraviolet A rays. Its effectiveness is measured with the sun protection factor (SPF) rating.

Introduction

The skin is the largest organ of the body, accounting for 15% of an adult's body weight. When skin problems are identified, clinicians may rapidly refer the person to a dermatologist. Although some conditions require the evaluation and management skills of a specialist, a primary care clinician can diagnose and treat many skin conditions. This chapter focuses primarily on the common skin disorders that affect women.

Anatomy and Physiology of the Skin

The skin is composed of the epidermis, dermis, and hypodermis. The dermis and hypodermis is also referred to as subcutaneous tissue. The functions of the skin include protection of the body, temperature regulation, sensation, and metabolism, especially for vitamin D. In addition to variations of color and texture, skin is subject to normal maturational changes, allergic stimuli, injury, and infection.

The epidermis, which functions primarily as a protective covering, is formed by stratified layers of squamous epithelial cells (Figure 26-1). As keratinocytes—the dominant cell type—move upward through the layers of epidermis, they progressively acquire more keratin, harden, and ultimately die. The outer layer of dead and dying cells becomes abraded and is shed, in a process known as desquamation. Other cells found in the epidermis are melanocytes, Langerhans cells, and Merkel cells. Melanocytes are the source of the pigment known as melanin, which the melanocytes transfer to the keratinocytes via melanosomes that move along the dendrite of a melanocyte to a keratinocyte. Melanin protects the body against the effects of ultraviolet radiation. Langerhans cells are macrophages; they respond to antigens on the skin and facilitate recognition by lymphocytes. Merkel cells are sensory receptors.[1]

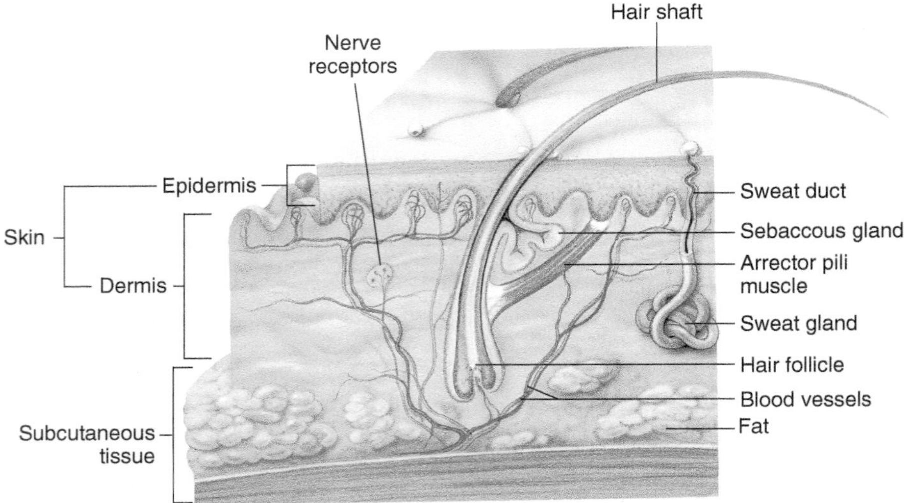

Figure 26-1 The skin and its anatomic components.

The dermis is the most superficial vascular layer and the source of the skin's elasticity. A thin basement membrane divides the dermis from the epidermis. The dermis is composed of collagen, elastin, and ground substance, all of which are derived from fibroblasts. Macrophages present in the dermis assist in prevention of infections. The thickness of the dermis varies with location on the body; indeed, this layer is the most variable component of the skin. Below the dermis is a layer of subcutaneous fatty tissue.

Various appendages to the skin arise from the subcutaneous and dermal layers. These appendages include sweat glands, sebaceous glands, and hair follicles. Both sweat glands and sebaceous glands are exocrine in nature, discharging their products (sweat and sebum) directly through ducts onto the skin. The sweat glands assist in temperature regulation as well as the excretion of salts and waste products such as ammonia. Sebaceous glands secrete an oily substance known as sebum, which lubricates skin.

Skin Changes

Skin changes are common and can be temporary and/or inconsequential. In other cases, however, they may be indicative of life-threatening cancers. Standard nomenclature exists to describe skin changes in terms of type, color, shape, distribution, and appearance. The importance of assessing these characteristics in forming a diagnosis, planning treatment, and assessing response to changes in the skin cannot be overemphasized. Table 26-1 lists terms and descriptions for common skin manifestations categorized by type, color, appearance, and shape.

Table 26-1 Terms and Descriptions for Common Skin Manifestations

Term	Description
Type	
Macule	Flat, well-circumscribed change in skin color
Nodule	Solid lesion that may involve dermis or subcutaneous tissue, larger in size than a papule
Papule	Solid superficial raised lesion, < 1 cm
Plaque	Solid, superficial raised lesion, ≥ 1 cm in diameter
Vesicle	Fluid-filled lesion at epidermal surface, < 0.5 cm
Wheal (urticaria)	Raised edematous tissue, involving the epidermis or dermis, irregular in size, shape, and color
Color	
Brown	Hypermelanosis
Red	Erythema, violaceous, purpura (does not blanch)
White	Leukoderma, hypomelanosis
Other colors	Also can be characteristic of various conditions or diseases
Appearance	
Crusting	Dried serum, blood, or pus covering a lesion
Excoriation	Skin torn or irritated by scratching
Fissure	Linear tear in epidermis/dermis
Scaling	Accumulated epidermal tissue
Thickening	In relationship to surrounding tissue
Ulcer	Loss of epidermis and part of dermis, usually round or oval
Shape	
Annular	Central clearing surrounded by a raised lesion
General	Linear, oval, round, clustered
Reticulated	Lacy
Serpentine	Snakelike, curving

Sources: Data from Farnam K, Chang C, Teuber S, Gershwin ME. Nonallergic drug hypersensitivity reactions. *Int Arch Allergy Immunol.* 2012;159(4):327-345[23]; Pichler WJ, Adam J, Daubner B, et al. Drug hypersensitivity reactions: pathomechanism and clinical symptoms. *Med Clinic N Am.* 2010;94:645-66[43]; Wang H, Wang HS, Liu ZP. Agents that induce pseudo-allergic reaction. *Drug Discov Ther.* 2011;5(5):211-219.[30]

Dermatologic Reactions to Medications

Many medications produce unintended responses in the skin and mucous membranes. These changes are distinguished by type of lesion, location and pattern, timing, and duration. Skin changes may be localized or general, present only on a limited area of the body or more broadly, or cause alopecia, itching, or a sunburn-like rash. In many cases, removal of the allergen and supportive care to ease symptoms are the only interventions; in others, use of another drug, such as the application of a cortisone cream or sunscreen, may be required. Examples of the types of skin changes and medications associated with each are listed in Table 26-2. Box 26-1 provides a clinical illustration of a serious but rare cutaneous reaction.

Common Skin Changes Experienced by Women

Skin changes occur throughout women's lifetimes. Many skin disorders are age specific. In turn, the drugs used to treat skin disorders have different clinical effects in persons of different ages and under different circumstances, including variations in the hormonal milieu as found during pregnancy and lactation.

Pregnancy

Skin undergoes changes during pregnancy that may affect the course of dermatologic problems. Sebaceous gland secretions increase, which has a variable effect on acne and other skin eruptions. Increased sweat gland function can cause skin irritation or rashes. The increased vascular dilation that occurs during pregnancy may facilitate absorption of topical medications, such that more is absorbed compared to the amount that reaches a nonpregnant woman's circulation. Pregnancy can also cause striae gravidarum, which is characterized by marked areas of thinned skin. Increased production of melanin results in areas of hyperpigmentation that can darken moles. Assessment of changes in pre-existing areas of hyperpigmentation during pregnancy is usually deferred until the pregnancy is over and pregnancy-related changes recede.

Lactation

Breastfeeding women also can experience dermatologic problems, especially involving the breasts. One of the primary reasons that women discontinue breastfeeding is nipple pain. Other breast dermatoses that can be observed among lactating women are atopic dermatitis, contact dermatitis (allergic or irritant), psoriasis, bacterial and fungal infections, and even viral infections.

Table 26-2 Examples of Adverse Dermatologic Reactions to Medications[a]

Drug or Drug Category: Generic (Brand)	Dermatologic Reaction	Clinical Manifestations
Anticoagulants Antimetabolites Norethindrone	Alopecia	Hair loss
Androgenic agents Contraceptive hormones Corticosteroids	Acneform	Cysts, pustules
Bacitracin (Neosporin) Chlorhexidine (Hibiclens)	Contact dermatitis	Erythematous, pruritic, papular eruptions localized to area
Barbiturates Epinephrine Iodine Penicillin Phenytoin (Dilantin) Sulfas Tetracyclines	Fixed drug eruptions	Localized erythematous, macules that reoccur in the same location (e.g., ears, upper thigh) with repeated exposure to the medication
Quinidine (Quinaglute) Thiazides	Lichenoid	Firm scaling plaques
Anticonvulsants Barbiturates Insulin Salicylates Sulfas Tetracyclines	Morbilliform	Separated, edematous, erythematous papules
Antihistamines Diuretics Fluoroquinolones NSAIDs Sulfas Thiazides Tricyclic antidepressants	Photosensitization	May contain all or any of the following: erythema, papules, edema, blistering in exposed areas
Anticoagulants Corticosteroids Penicillin Sulfas	Purpura	Red or purple discoloration from bleeding under the skin
Vancomycin (Vancocin) Other antibiotics producing powerful antihistamine responses	Red man syndrome	Flushing, pruritus accompanied by hypotension and muscle weakness
NSAIDs Penicillins Phenytoin (Dilantin) Sulfas	Stevens-Johnson syndrome	Papules, bullae, and vesicles, including mucous membrane lesions occurring within weeks of exposure to the allergen
Barbiturates Meperidine (Demerol) Nitrofurantoin (Macrobid) Penicillin Tetracyclines	Urticaria	Raised skin wheals

Abbreviations: NSAIDs = nonsteroidal anti-inflammatory drugs.
[a] This table is not comprehensive as new information is being generated on a regular basis.

Box 26-1 Case Study: A Serious Dermatologic Condition

C.F. is a 35-year-old woman who was treated with trimethoprim–sulfamethoxazole (Bactrim) for a mild respiratory infection one week ago. This week she returned to the office reporting difficulty swallowing because of painful ulcers in her mouth for the last 24 hours. Her physical examination revealed mucosal desquamation of her oral cavity as well as a skin rash consisting of several round lesions on her breasts and abdomen. She was diagnosed with Stevens-Johnson syndrome (SJS) and referred for immediate care by a specialist for this potentially life-threatening condition.[2]

Although SJS is considered to be a mild form of toxic epidermal necrolysis, it can progress and be fatal. SJS is usually an adverse drug reaction, although in rarer situations an infection can be the etiologic culprit. Most individuals who develop SJS as an adverse drug reaction do so after they have taken sulfonamides; these persons usually have been found to have a slow acetylator genotype. Slow accelerators produce higher levels of sulfonamide hydroxylamine via the CYP450 enzyme metabolism, and these metabolites are theorized to have direct toxic effects.[3]

Usual treatment is palliative, involving hospitalization, intravenous fluids, and symptomatic therapies. Steroid therapy may be useful.[4] Because ophthalmic complications are common, it is wise to have an ophthalmologist as a member of the healthcare team. C.F.'s prognosis is good because less than 10% of her body is affected. In such cases, it is estimated that her risk of mortality is less than 5%; conversely, if large portions of the body are involved, the diagnosis is changed to toxic epidermal necrolysis with a mortality risk of 30% to 40%. Stevens-Johnson syndrome illustrates that cutaneous eruptions are not always a minor condition.[5]

The Elderly

As the population in the United States ages, geriatric dermatology is becoming a healthcare specialty. Intrinsic aging refers to normal changes associated with maturation, whereas extrinsic aging is produced by outside factors such as the environment.

As skin thins and dries, it becomes less elastic, and wrinkles develop. Receptors for estrogen, progesterone, and androgens are all found in the skin. Following menopause, decreases in estrogen extend to receptors in both fibroblasts and keratinocytes.[7] Skin collagen also decreases owing to the loss of sex steroid stimulation, causing thinning and weakening of the tissue. Intrinsic skin aging is characterized by thinner, more lax tissue, finer lines, and fewer pigment changes.[8]

Photoaging refers to the damage done to skin as a result of a lifetime of exposure to the ultraviolet (UV) radiation in sunlight. Thus the normal skin aging process for women includes hormonal changes as well as possible skin damage from exposure to weather, sunlight, and/or smoking. Smoking accelerates skin aging and wrinkling. Although supplementation with exogenous hormones can reverse some hormonally driven changes, it has no effect on extrinsic causes of skin aging such as sun damage.[9]

The loss of subcutaneous fat coupled with decreased levels of collagen leaves surface blood vessels less protected and increases the risk of bruising. Dilated small blood vessels produce spider veins, particularly on the face and lower extremities. Some conditions, such as xerosis, pruritus, and eczema, are more common among older individuals.[10]

A variety of additional changes occur in aging skin. Melanocytes tend to decline by as much as 15% per decade, while Langerhans cells decrease in both density and responsiveness in the older adult. The immune response is decreased, and wound healing is delayed.[11] Some diseases such as diabetes mellitus and HIV have dermatologic expressions that confound diagnosis and treatment.

The skin changes associated with aging affect the response to medications. The lower levels of lipids in older women's skin affect absorption of some topical medications. In addition, the decreased vascularity and increased keratin in elderly individuals' skin inhibits absorption of topical medications. Both kidney and liver function tend to decline with age, which further delays metabolism of medications.

As individuals live longer, chronic diseases become more common. These chronic conditions may include diseases of the skin. In this chapter, when appropriate, drug information specific to caring for the elderly is included.

The Cornerstone of Dermatology: The Common Drugs

Skin conditions may have different etiologies, but often present with similar symptoms, such as inflammation and/or pruritus. Thus, among the treatments for women with various skin disorders, steroids and antihistamines hold a special place as the general first-line therapies. Moreover, topical therapy tends to be integral in dermatologic treatment plans.

Topical Therapy

Compared to oral therapy, topical agents frequently have lower levels of systemic absorption, plasma concentration, and bioavailability. Topical administration also avoids the first-pass effect of oral therapy, in which passage of a drug through the gastrointestinal system into the portal circulation and liver decreases the initial bioavailability of the medication. The choice of a vehicle for topical drugs controls the degree and speed of absorption. For example, transdermal patches provide a steady dose of medication without peaks and troughs. This pharmacokinetic effect may decrease the incidence of some side effects or adverse effects. During pregnancy and lactation, a drug that is delivered topically will be less well absorbed into the maternal bloodstream compared to the absorption of a drug administered orally and thus, fetal or infant exposure to that drug is less.

Topical delivery of medication is influenced by a variety of factors, including both the active and inactive components of a topical agent, the degree of adherence to the skin, the level of absorption, and any general moisturizing or drying effect of the medication on different components of the skin's layers (Figure 26-2). Tolerability of topical medications depends on the woman's skin type, thickness, and sensitivity, and is generally assessed by degree of erythema, dryness, peeling, or other adverse local effects that may occur.

Both the active medication and the vehicle in which it is administered can affect the tolerability of an agent. Table 26-3 lists the inactive components or vehicles most commonly associated with topical preparations. In general, drying preparations are intended for use in acute inflammation, and hydrating preparations are appropriate for chronic inflammation. Skin **protectants** are formulations

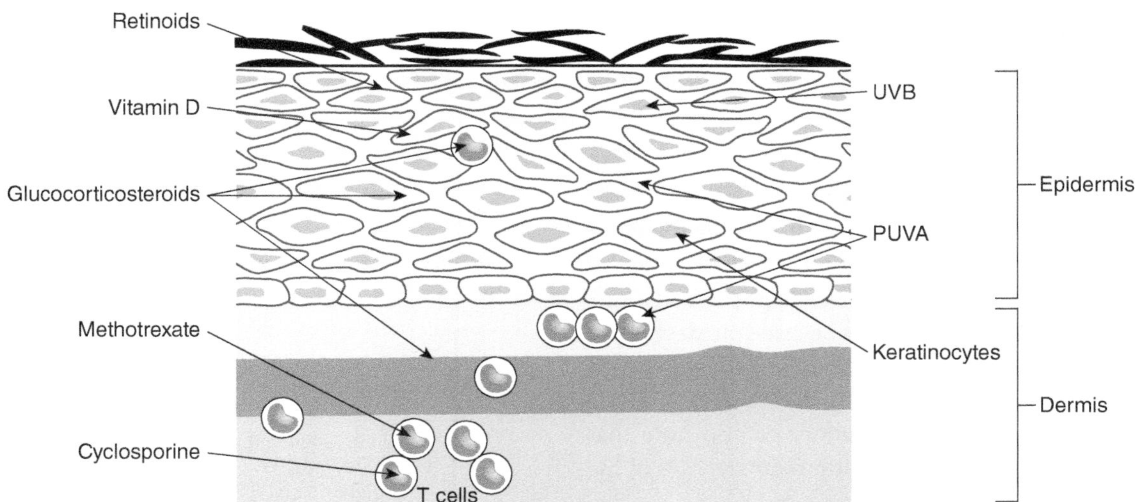

The skin is a multicellular organ containing numerous cells and structures as well as circulating T cells that are targets for dermatologic drugs.

Figure 26-2 Skin as a pharmacologic target.

Table 26-3 Vehicles Used for Topical Medications

Vehicle	Description
Cream	Emulsion of oil in water; absorbs well, lubricating.
Emulsion	Stable mixture of oil, water, and surfactant; often categorized as water in oil or oil in water. Micro-emulsions are commonly used with cosmetics.
Foam	Gas bubbles suspended in substance to enhance spread of the agent.
Gel	Water or alcohol base with polymer as a thickener; less well absorbed than other agents.
Lotion	Suspended powder in water or water and oil; easy to apply, cooling; less potent than creams, gels, or ointments.
Oil	Viscous liquid or liquefiable substance that is often used as a vehicle for botanicals or other agents. Easily spread on skin and may form protective cover; thinner than a cream or ointment, so it does not remain as stable as those vehicles.
Ointment	Oil-based, thick, adherent to skin, lubricating. Most effective medium for hydration and absorption, so the potency of a drug will be highest when it is formulated in an ointment.
Paste	Semisolid preparation containing a high proportion of finely powdered material.
Powder	Solid that has been pulverized into tiny loose particles to be combined with a pharmacologic agent and spread on the skin.
Soak	Agent dissolved in water; least hydrating of all vehicles.
Solution	Dissolved substance in water, alcohol, or glycol; more drying than other agents, but more hydrating than soaks or lotions.
Spray	Drug in the form of dispersed droplets contained in water or another liquid; delivered via a dedicated device in a fine mist.
Tape	Occlusive dressing with medication (e.g., steroid) impregnated within the tape.

that protect injured or exposed skin surfaces from harmful stimuli. Protectants may provide relief to these skin surfaces and allow natural healing to occur.

The Rule of Nines provides a way to approximate the relative surface area to be treated. Originally developed as a method of describing the percentage of body surface injured by burns, it can also be used in describing the distribution of skin lesions or area to be treated and in calculating the percent of body surface area that needs treatment (Figure 26-3). Some authorities also note that each palm and the groin make up approximately 1% of the body surface.

Topical Steroids

Topical glucocorticoids can be prescribed in several levels of potency (class I–VII), with class I being the most powerful. Topical steroids produce significant relief for as many as 80% of individuals using them.[12] When choosing a prescription, both the strength of the medication and the carrier (e.g., ointment, lotion, solution) should be considered. In general, only dermatology specialists prescribe the most potent steroid drugs, although these agents are included in Table 26-4 for the sake of completeness. The lowest effective potency and frequency of application should be prescribed initially for acute treatment, based on the severity of the woman's symptoms. Selection of steroid potency must consider the anatomic location of the lesion, the size of the involved area, and the age of the individual. For example, very young and elderly women will require lower doses. In general, fluorinated steroids should not be used on sensitive skin areas such as eyelids, face, neck, axilla, and groin/genitals because they are absorbed rapidly and are therefore associated with an increased risk for adverse side effects of steroid application. Milder preparations are used when treating large surface areas, sensitive skin areas, and when treating young and older women.

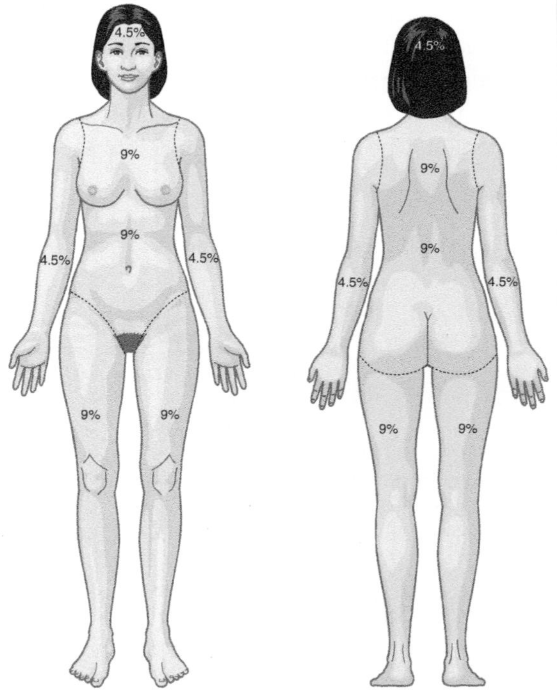

Figure 26-3 The Rule of Nines.

Table 26-4 Topical Steroids: From Least to Most Potent by Class

Potency (I Is Most Potent)	Generic Name	Brand Names/Percent Active Ingredient/Vehicle
VII	Hydrocortisone widely available as generic	LactiCare/1.0-AC/lotion LactiCare/2.5-AC/lotion
		Hytone/2.5/cream, lotion, ointment
	Hydrocortisone acetate	Epifoam/1.0/foam spray
VI	Desonide	DesOwen/0.05/cream, lotion
	Flurandrenolide	Cordran SP/0.025/cream
	Fluocinolone acetonide	Capex/0.01/shampoo Derma-Smoothe/0.01/oil
	Prednicarbate	Aclovate/0.05/cream, ointment
	Triamcinolone acetonide	Aristocort A/0.025/cream
V	Betamethasone valerate cream	Betatrex/0.1/cream
	Clocortolone pivalate	Cloderm/0.1/cream
	Desonide	DesOwen/0.05/ointment Tridesilon/0.05/ointment
	Fluocinolone acetonide	Synalar/0.025/cream Synemol/0.025/cream
	Flurandrenolide	Cordran SP/0.05/cream
		Cordran/0.5/ lotion
		Cordran/0.025/ointment
	Hydrocortisone butyrate	Locoid/0.1/cream Locoid Lipocream/0.1/ointment, solution
	Hydrocortisone valerate	Westcort/0.2/cream
	Triamcinolone acetamide	Aristocort/0.1/cream Kenalog/0.1/cream, lotion
IV	Amcinonide	Cyclocort/0.1/cream
	Betamethasone valerate	Luxiq/0.12/foam
	Fluocinolone acetonide	Synalar/0.025/ointment
	Flurandrenolide	Cordran/0.05/ointment
	Mometasone furoate	Elocon/0.1/cream, lotion
	Prednicarbate	Dermatop-E/0.1/ointment
	Triamcinolone acetonide	Aristocort A/0.1/ointment Kenalog/0.1/ointment
III	Amcinonide	Cyclocort/0.1/cream, lotion
	Betamethasone dipropionate	Alphatrex/0.05/cream, ointment Diprosone/0.05/cream, lotion
	Betamethasone valerate	Betatrex/0.1/ointment
	Fluticasone propionate	Cutivate/0.005/ointment
	Mometasone furoate	Elocon/0.1/ointment
	Triamcinolone acetonide	Aristocort A/0.5/cream Kenalog/0.5/cream
II	Amcinonide	Cyclocort/0.1/ointment
	Augmented betamethasone dipropionate	Diprolene AF/0.05/cream
	Betamethasone dipropionate	Diprosone/0.1/aerosol Diprosone/0.05/ointment
	Desoximetasone	Topicort/0.25/cream
	Diflorasone diacetate	Psorcon-E/0.05/cream, ointment
	Fluocinonide	Lidex-E/0.05/cream Lidex/0.05/cream, gel, ointment, solution
	Halcinonide	Halog/0.1/cream, ointment, solution Halog-E/0.1/cream
	Mometasone furoate	Elocon/0.1/ointment
I	Augmented betamethasone dipropionate	Diprolene/0.05/gel, lotion, ointment
	Clobetasol propionate	Cormax/0.05/cream, ointment, scalp solution Olux/0.05/foam Temovate-E/0.05/cream Temovate/0.05/gel, ointment
	Diflorasone diacetate	Psorcon/0.05/ointment
	Flurandrenolide	Cordran/0.05/tape
	Halobetasol propionate	Ultravate/0.05/cream, ointment

The steroid classes vary by carrier (e.g., cream versus lotion) and by percentage of active ingredient, even for products with the same generic or trade name. Thus, the prescriber must pay careful attention to both factors to avoid prescribing errors. For example, one systematic review found once-daily steroid therapy similar in effectiveness to more frequent dosing, and the once-daily regimen is more cost-effective and less likely to produce adverse effects. [13] However, the authors noted that differences in pricing and potency made direct comparisons of products difficult.[13]

Side Effects and Adverse Effects of Topical Steroids

Over time, use of high-potency topical steroids can cause atrophy of the skin, striae, hypopigmentation, decreased immune function in the skin cells, worsening rosacea and facial telangiectasia, and (rarely) glaucoma following periocular use. Adrenal suppression is an uncommon, albeit serious, effect of topical preparations. Allergic responses to the medication or the vehicle are contraindications to topical use.

Special Populations: Pregnancy, Lactation, and the Elderly

While low-dose topical steroid use in pregnancy has not been associated with an increased risk of fetal malformations, these agents have been reported to increase the risk of stretch marks.[14] Current guidelines recommend use of the lowest possible dose for the shortest duration when topical steroids are prescribed to pregnant women. Mild topical steroids appear to be compatible with breastfeeding.[7,15] No specific recommendations or precautions appear to be needed with use of these drugs among older women.

Oral Steroids

In rare situations such as severe inflammation secondary to exposure to poison ivy or poison oak, topical steroid therapy is inadequate. When an oral steroid is required, it is usually prescribed either as a dose pack of methylprednisolone (Medrol) or as a tapered prednisone dose (Table 26-5). Oral steroids generally should be taken with food in the morning. A commonly used 10-day tapered regimen consists of prednisone 40 mg orally for 3 days, then 20 mg for 3 days, then 10 mg for 4 days. If the Medrol dose pack does not resolve the skin condition, a consultation/referral with a specialist is indicated.

Side Effects and Adverse Effects of Oral Steroids

Oral steroids are associated with several adverse effects. Adrenal insufficiency is a rare, but significant risk of prolonged steroid therapy; both higher doses and longer regimens may induce this effect. Hypotension, dehydration, hypoglycemia, and mental confusion are symptoms of acute adrenal insufficiency. Oral prednisone should not be given for more than 7 days without reducing the dose sequentially (tapering), to avoid triggering adrenal insufficiency.

Oral steroid use can cause osteonecrosis, most often of the femoral head. This rare adverse effect is most commonly associated with high doses and prolonged use. Although these treatment regimens are not common for dermatologic conditions, all clinicians who prescribe oral steroids must be aware of the potential for osteonecrosis. Other adverse effects of oral steroids when used for a prolonged period of time include immunosuppression, Kaposi's sarcoma, neuropsychiatric symptoms, glaucoma, and acute myopathy. Hypersensitivity and anaphylactic reactions have been reported following use of oral steroids, albeit rarely.

Persons taking immunosuppressive doses of oral steroids should not be given live attenuated vaccines as the steroid suppresses the immune response slightly, thereby increasing the risk of developing the vaccine-related disease. Killed vaccines may be given but they may be less effective if the individual is using oral steroids.

Special Populations: Pregnancy, Lactation, and the Elderly

The pharmacokinetics of prednisone and methylprednisolone appear to differ, including during pregnancy.[16] Nevertheless, both drugs increase the risk of orofacial defects in the fetus when taken in the first trimester of pregnancy, although the risk is low and these agents are used when necessary following thorough counseling.[17] In general, it appears the background risk for oral clefts is approximately 1 per 1000 pregnancies and this risk increases to 3 to 6 per 1000 pregnancies in women who use oral steroids during

Table 26-5 Prescribing a Methylprednisolone (Medrol) Dose Pack

Day 1	Six 4-mg tablets PO
Day 2	Five 4-mg tablets PO
Day 3	Four 4-mg tablets PO
Day 4	Three 4-mg tablets PO
Day 5	Two 4-mg tablets PO
Day 6	One 4-mg tablet PO

the first trimester.[17] Limited studies indicate that these agents can be found in low amounts in breast milk but are compatible with breastfeeding.[15]

Few data exist regarding the specific risks of oral steroid use among older women. A 2014 study noted that individuals older than 65 years who used corticosteroids had a higher risk (odds ratio [OR], 1.26; 95% confidence interval [CI], 1.07–1.50) of readmission when compared to a cohort group.[18]

Antihistamines

Itching commonly is experienced in conjunction with a variety of skin conditions as well as many systemic diseases. In every case, itching should not be treated without an assessment of its possible causes. If there is no apparent dermatologic source of the irritation, laboratory testing may include a complete blood count; assessment of thyroid, liver, and kidney function; and measurement of blood glucose.[19] This general panel will assist in identifying infectious, endocrine, and metabolic causes underlying the symptoms. Other possible screens would include stool samples for ova and parasites (indicating a helminthic condition) and imaging to identify malignant processes such as lymphoma.[20]

Treatment of a woman with pruritus most commonly includes topical or systemic therapy with antihistamines such as the classic diphenhydramine (Benadryl) as listed in Table 26-6. Other agents include **emollients**, low-potency steroids, calamine, camphor or menthol, and anesthetics

Table 26-6 Antihistamines Used as Dermatologic Drugs[a]

			Selected Drug Interactions		
Name: Generic (Brand)	**Dose**	**Side Effects**	**Other Drug**	**Potential Response**	**Clinical Considerations**
Sedating					
Chlorpheniramine maleate (Chlor-Trimeton)	4 mg PO at bedtime	Drowsiness, decreased mental capacity, dry mouth	Topiramate (Topamax)	Increases topiramate (Topamax) side effects of sweating	Oral syrups containing chlorpheniramine maleate frequently contain other ingredients, including alcohol; increases risk of drowsiness
			Potassium supplements in solid forms	Increases irritation of gastric lining	
			Alcohol	Potentiates effects of alcohol (sedation, confusion, dizziness)	
Diphenhydramine hydrochloride (Benadryl)	25–50 mg PO 3–4 times/day	Drowsiness, decreased mental capacity, dry mouth	Alcohol and other CNS depressants, including opioids	Potentiates CNS depression	Increase the risk of drowsiness, although paradoxical effects have been noted in which individuals—usually young—are excited rather than sedated
			MAO inhibitors	Potentiates anticholinergic activity and increases drying effect	
Hydroxyzine (Vistaril, Atarax)	25 mg PO 3–4 times/day	Drowsiness, allergic response, tremor, headache, rash	Topiramate (Topamax)	Increases topiramate side effects of sweating	Often used for sedative or antianxiety effects
			Potassium supplements in solid forms	Increases irritation of gastric lining	
Nonsedating					
Cetirizine (Zyrtec)	10 mg PO	Drowsiness, nervousness, dry mouth, dry skin, nausea, allergic reaction, seizure, irregular heartbeat	No major drug interactions		Use with caution for women with liver or kidney insufficiency
			Alcohol	Potentiates effects of alcohol (sedation, confusion, dizziness)	
Fexofenadine (Allegra)	60 mg PO 2 times/day	Headache, dysmenorrhea, back pain	No major drug interactions but grapefruit, orange, and apple juice should be avoided	Decreases levels of fexofenadine	Use with caution for women with liver or kidney insufficiency
Loratadine (Claritin)	10 mg PO daily	Drowsiness, nervousness, dry mouth, sedation, fatigue	No major drug or food interactions		Use with caution for women with liver or kidney insufficiency

Abbreviations: MAO = monoamine oxidase; CNS = central nervous system.

[a] This table is not comprehensive as new information is being generated on a regular basis.

such as pramoxine (PrameGel, Procto-Foam). All of these drugs are recommended for temporary relief of the symptom, but do not necessarily treat the underlying etiology. The reader is referred to the *Antihistamines* chapter, which reviews this class of drugs in more detail. Herbal or botanic remedies, such as witch hazel, chamomile, aloe vera, and nutritional supplementation with vitamins D and E and linoleic acid are also used, although the effectiveness of these complementary and alternative remedies remains unproven.[21]

Special Populations: Pregnancy, Lactation, and the Elderly

Chlorpheniramine (Chlor-Trimeton), diphenhydramine (Benadryl), and cetirizine (Zyrtec) are safe for use during pregnancy. Although limited human data exist about hydroxyzine (Vistaril) and loratadine (Claritin), these agents also are considered safe for use in pregnancy. Fexofenadine (Allegra) has been associated with some teratogenic effects in animals but there is no human data available, thus it also is considered safe for use in pregnancy when needed.[14] In general, more safety data are available for use of first-generation antihistamines during pregnancy, and thus they are considered the first-line agents.

Large doses of any of the antihistamines, including nonsedating second-generation agents such as fexofenadine and loratadine, may be associated with neonatal sedation and decreased breast milk production. However, none of these medications is contraindicated for use during lactation.[7,15]

Older women are more likely to experience the sedative effects of antihistamines. These agents should be used with caution by elderly individuals. In addition, the elderly are at higher risk for renal dysfunction than their younger counterparts; given this factor, caution should be exercised when prescribing or recommending these agents for the more mature woman.

Skin Conditions

This chapter focuses on common conditions of the integumentary system. Some skin disorders, such as folliculitis and those that predominantly affect the vulvar area, are addressed in the *Vulvar Disorders* chapter. Rashes and eruptions secondary to use of specific drugs are discussed throughout the text. Skin conditions addressed in this chapter include skin damage, dermatitis, papulosquamous conditions, acne, hirsutism, alopecia, parasitic infections, and the use of cosmeceuticals in the treatment of women.

Skin Damage: Sunscreen, Burns, and Actinic Keratosis

Skin color is defined in terms of photo type—a measure of tanning ability. These types range from I (pale, white, always burns/never tans) to VI (dark brown or black, never burns/tans easily), based on the Fitzpatrick skin type scale. Skin color is relevant not only for ease of vitamin D synthesis, but also for risks of photoaging and skin damage. In general, more darkly pigmented skin is thicker and more elastic in nature.

Exposure to ultraviolet radiation, whether from the sun or from artificial light tanning sources, causes long-term damage to the skin. In addition, prolonged exposure to the sun is associated with an increased risk of developing melanoma. UV radiation refers to high-frequency, short-wavelength light that is not within the visible spectrum of the human eye. Such radiation is divided into three categories—UVA, UVB, and UVC—based on the length of the light waves. UVA reaches the earth's surface largely unaffected by atmospheric condition or location on the planet. By comparison, only approximately 10% of UVB reaches the earth's surface, with the precise amount being affected by latitude and elevation, degree of cloud cover, and proximity to industrial areas. UVC is absorbed by the atmosphere, including ozone, oxygen, carbon dioxide, and water vapor. Both UVA and UVB produce tissue injury. UVA penetrates more deeply into the skin and is the cause of photoaging, whereas UVB primarily affects the upper skin layers and is the cause of sunburns.[4] The mechanisms by which UV affects the skin include breakdown of collagen, promotion of free radicals, interference with intracellular repairs, and suppression of immune responses.

Among the visible effects of skin damage are photoaging, pigment changes (freckles, liver spots), wrinkling, actinic keratosis, and seborrheic keratosis. UV exposure is a major factor in the development of skin cancers—that is, melanoma, basal cell, and squamous cell carcinomas.

Sunscreens

A **sunscreen** is any topical product applied to the skin that blocks UV radiation. Sunscreens are classified as a drug by the U.S. Food and Drug Administration (FDA).

Sunscreens reflect light and provide a barrier to 99% of the UV light. Commonly used light-blocking ingredients in sunscreens include titanium dioxide and zinc oxide, which are inert substances that are not absorbed into the skin. Other ingredients in sunscreens include dibenzoyl methanes, cinnamates, salicylates, benzophenone, and para-aminobenzoic acid (PABA), which has derivatives padimate A and O and glyceryl PABA that can be added as well.[9] Benzophenone and dibenzoyl methanes are effective against UVA.

Contact dermatitis, photoallergic responses, and urticaria may occur following exposure to sunscreen ingredients, although these reactions are less common with newer preparations that do not contain PABA, methyl PABA, or benzophenone-10.

The possibility of decreased vitamin D absorption exists following prolonged use of sunscreens, but evidence does not support an increase in osteoporosis or other adverse effects related to a potential decrease vitamin D synthesis.[22] Because UV exposure is a known carcinogen, unprotected exposure to skin to increase vitamin D is no longer recommended as a means to promote bone health.[23] Currently, the Institute of Medicine (IOM) recommends that women maintain skeletal health through consumption of a balanced diet that contains the recommended daily allowance (RDA) of 600 IU of vitamin D for individuals between 1 and 70 years of age, and 800 IU for adults older than 70 years.[23]

Sunscreens are labeled using a **sun protection factor (SPF)** rating. Although not perfect, SPF ratings provide consumers with guidance regarding which products are more protective than others. For example, a woman who usually suffers a burn when exposed to the sun for 10 minutes can obtain protection for approximately 150 minutes after applying a thick dose of sunscreen that has an SFP factor of 15. This calculation is performed by multiplying the SPF factor by the usual sunburn time. However, this protection can be diminished by sweating or swimming. Additionally, no product may claim it protects users for more than 2 hours without repeat application, unless it receives explicit FDA approval for this claim.[11]

Controversies continue to exist about the SPF rating scale. Skin is influenced by genetics and age, but SPF ratings have generally been tested only among adult white individuals, raising some questions about their applicability to individuals of other racial or ethnic groups. Personal factors also influence the use of sunscreens. Some women, for example, may apply the sunscreen more thickly than other women might. Some products today are being marketed with exceptionally high SPF factors, such as SPF 50 and SPF 70; these sunscreens are often described as "broad-spectrum" agents. According to the FDA, the term "broad spectrum" should be limited to those products that protect the skin from both UVA and UVB exposure. Most sunburns are caused by UVB rays, but long-term skin damage is associated with UVA exposure. The FDA further notes there is no research to support sunscreen ratings higher than SPF 50.[11]

In the United States, sunscreen labeling also includes a "Skin Cancer/Skin Aging Alert" on all products that are not broad spectrum or that have an SPF in the range of 2 to 14. Essentially, the alert informs a consumer that sun exposure increases the risk of cancer and early aging and indicates this product will provide protection only from the former, not the latter.[11]

Terms such as "water proof," "sweat proof," and "sunblock" are no longer approved labeling, but "water resistant" remains acceptable. In conjunction with the "water resistant" label, the sunscreen company is allowed to say the product maintains the indicated SPF for 40 to 80 minutes. Also, items such as sunscreen wipes, powders, shampoos, and body washes are no longer eligible to use the term "sunscreen" on their labels. Although spray products are popular, especially for use among children, these agents are under current FDA review due to concerns about the potential risks when they are inhaled, particularly among young children.

Box 26-2 provides general guidelines for consumers regarding sun exposure.

Box 26-2 Consumer Sun Safety Guidelines

- Apply SPF 15 or higher sunscreen 15 to 30 minutes before any exposure.
- Limit sun exposure during peak hours (10 A.M. to 2 P.M.).
- Wear protective clothing: long-sleeve, collared shirt, long pants, wide-brimmed hat.
- Reapply sunscreen every 1 to 2 hours, or more often if swimming, toweling off, or sweating.
- Apply adequate sunscreen, approximately 1.25 to 1.5 fluid ounces, with each application for an adult-sized body.
- Apply sunscreen with a higher SPF and/or with greater frequency near water, snow, sand, or high altitude because there is a greater risk of a burn in these environments.

Minor Burns

Burns are graded by the degree of damage to the skin and by the extent of body coverage affected, regardless of their etiology. First-degree burns are superficial, with the skin remaining intact. These burns are usually treated with ice or cold water initially to decrease heat, a mild painkiller, and a topical anesthetic spray such as benzocaine or an herbal product. Herbal products include aloe vera gel, which can be applied for relief of pain and heat 3 to 4 times daily, as can tea tree oil, which is applied 2 to 3 times daily for pain relief. A meta-analysis of aloe vera studies found a reduction in mean healing time in users of these products compared to healing time in members of a control group (P = .006); however, as the authors noted, the lack of standardization of products makes evaluation difficult.[24] Propolis, a resinous mixture that honeybees collect from trees, is believed to have effects including immune modulation and antioxidant, anti-inflammatory, and antibacterial properties.[25]

Topical Anesthetics for Treating Women with Minor Burns

Applications of anesthetic medication to the skin are used not only for minor burns, but also for cuts and scrapes, and in some instances prior to surgical procedures. Topical application or anesthetics such as lidocaine (Xylocaine) usually produces an analgesic rather than anesthetic effect, because the absorption is limited in comparison to delivery by injection. Topical anesthetics should be applied only to intact skin to prevent excessive absorption. The minimal amount needed to induce analgesia should be applied, and prolonged or frequent use should be discouraged. Application of topical anesthetics to the eye or to mucous membranes should be avoided, as absorption is increased from these tissues.

Mild skin irritation and burning on application are common side effects of topical anesthetics. Common drug interactions include decreased antibacterial potency of sulfa drugs and increased cardiovascular risk for persons taking St. John's wort, although it is unclear to what degree these risks are present with correct use of topical treatments.

Eutectic mixture of local anesthetics (EMLA) cream was the first topically applied anesthetic in general use. This drug is available over the counter in some countries. One to two grams per 10 cm^2 area is applied. A drawback to the use of EMLA is the long time period (1 hour) between application and effective anesthesia, and the necessity of maintaining an occlusive covering during that period. Systematic toxicity is rare, as is hypersensitivity. However, skin diseases that disrupt the epidermis will increase absorption.[26] Lidocaine is available as cream, gel, or spray solution in concentrations up to 5%.

A lidocaine patch (Lidoderm) also is available for management of pain from herpes zoster and for chronic pain in various anatomic locations. It is applied for up to 12 hours daily on intact skin, followed by a 12-hour waiting period before applying a new patch. Serious allergic responses to the lidocaine patch that may require emergency care include itching, shortness of breath, swelling, dizziness, faintness, tremor, tinnitus, and slowed pulse.

Liposomal carriers are phospholipid-based materials that promote absorption of the anesthetic agent through the skin. A systematic review of 25 randomized controlled trials (RCTs) found that liposome-encapsulated lidocaine, tetracaine, and liposome-encapsulated tetracaine are at least as effective as EMLA and offer lower-cost alternatives.[27] Liposome-encapsulated lidocaine and EMLA were found to be comparable in terms of their pain relief effectiveness, using qualitative pain scores. Tetracaine and liposome-encapsulated tetracaine were more effective than EMLA using weighted mean difference in 100-mm visual analog scale scores. However, other studies have found EMLA to be more effective than the other options. These differences may be secondary to different research methodologies rather than clinically significant differences.

A gel or solution made of lidocaine, epinephrine, and tetracaine (LET solution) can be used for minor laceration repairs. LET solution should not be applied to any part of the body with an end-arterial supply, such as the nose or fingers, due to possible damage from vasoconstriction. Application to large areas or to mucous membranes increases the risk of central nervous system or cardiovascular toxicity. Following the onset of action, a local injection of anesthetic can be used to ensure longer-acting relief. Both LET and EMLA have demonstrated effectiveness for pretreatments before laceration repairs in small studies.[28]

Tetracaine hydrochloride cream (Pontocaine) or gel produces PABA as a metabolite. Consequently, persons with hypersensitivity reactions to PABA—an ingredient found in many sunscreens—should not use tetracaine products.

Benzocaine 20% spray (Endocaine, Hurricaine) can be recommended for over-the-counter relief of minor cuts, stings, sunburn, and similar pain. This agent can be applied 3 to 4 times daily, by spraying the agent onto the skin from a distance of 12 inches away from the skin. This spray is intended for short-term use; when it is used externally on intact skin, the risk of hypersensitivity or allergic response is minimal.

Second- or Third-Degree Burns

Second-degree burns, which include blistering, effect the epidermis and part of the dermis. These burns are partial-thickness burns. In addition to keeping the area clean and dry and leaving the blister intact, topical medication can be used for these burns, just as it is for first-degree burns. A topical antibiotic can be applied to open areas to prevent secondary bacterial infection.

Third-degree, full-thickness burns destroy the epidermis and dermis, and extend into the subcutaneous tissue below the skin. Expert treatment to decrease scarring and risk of infection is needed. The percentage of body surface affected also contributes to burn severity and decision making about office versus hospital treatment.

Silver sulfadiazine cream 1% (Silvadene) is a topical sulfa antimicrobial used to treat both second- and third-degree burns. This cream is applied 1 to 2 times a day to the affected area in a thin coat. Side effects include irritation or burning at the site, rash, and skin discoloration. More serious adverse events, such as hypersensitivity, skin damage, urinary problems, leukopenia, and bleeding, have also been reported.

Special Populations: Pregnancy, Lactation, and the Elderly

Active ingredients in sunscreens, such as topical PABA, have minimal absorption and are considered safe for use during pregnancy and lactation, although no human research on this topic has been published.[29] Silver sulfadiazine should be avoided at and near term because maternal absorption may increase the risk of neonatal kernicterus. While the World Health Organization (WHO) has identified silver sulfadiazine cream as safe during breastfeeding, there are no data available on Silvadene specifically. In addition, no evidence exists regarding the safety of propolis supplements during pregnancy or breastfeeding, and some of these products may contain a high alcohol content.

In small doses, both lidocaine and epinephrine are safe for use during pregnancy and lactation.[14,17] However, both agents cross the placenta, potentially leading to spiral artery vasoconstriction and fetal tachycardia if large doses are used.[14] It is well known that sulfonamides are excreted in breast milk; for this reason, the manufacturer recommends either discontinuation of the drug or discontinuation of nursing when these agents are used by a woman who is breastfeeding.[7,15]

There is some suggestion that zinc oxide or PABA-free sunscreens may induce fewer allergic reactions and, therefore, are better choices for elderly women as well as for women with sensitive skin. There have been no special considerations recommended for older women in terms of topical anesthetic or sulfonamide use.

Actinic Keratosis

Actinic keratosis, a precancerous condition found on exposed skin, is the result of UV damage. The skin appearance is flat, dry, and variable in color; it may also have multiple crusty patches. Approximately 1% to 5% of all actinic keratosis proceed to squamous cell carcinoma. Actinic keratosis can be removed surgically or treated medically. One of several products, including 5- imiquimod (Aldara), fluorouracil (Efudex), or retinoids, can be used to treat actinic keratosis medically.

Imiquimod (Aldara)

Imiquimod (Aldara) is a topical immune modulator that acts by inducing interferons alpha and gamma, tumor necrosis factor, and interleukin. A single packet is applied 2 to 3 times per week for up to 16 weeks. During use of imiquimod, sun exposure should be avoided. Adverse effects include erythema, oozing and swelling of tissue, and increased scaly or crusted skin in the treated area. Two studies have found that 3-times-weekly application for 4 weeks, with a 4-week rest period between treatment cycles, resulted in all lesions clearing among 50% to 69% of individuals.[30] In one of these studies, 75% of the persons in remission continued to be free of lesions at the 12-week mark.[31] An RCT comparing imiquimod to 5-FU and cryosurgery found that sustained remission of actinic keratosis over 12 months was achieved in 73% of individuals receiving imiquimod, versus 33% using 5-FU and 4% who had cryosurgery.[32]

5-Fluorouracil (Efudex)

5-Fluorouracil (Efudex) is an antimetabolite that is available in several formulations—5% cream, 2% solution, 1% cream or solution, or 0.5% micronized cream. This agent blocks DNA synthesis within cells to prevent cell proliferation. The 5% cream is applied twice daily for up to 6 weeks. The micronized 0.5% cream (Carac) is applied once daily. Inflammatory responses may be induced with application of 5-fluorouracil. A comparison of daily versus weekly dosing found twice-daily treatment to be significantly more effective (P = .01) 24 weeks after treatment.[33] This agent should not be applied to mucus membranes as it can induce local inflammation and ulceration.

Multiple adverse drug effects may be experienced by women using 5-FU, although most are related to systemic use, rather than topical application. Most common among these effects are nausea and diarrhea. However, a rare but serious side effect with systemic use has been cardiotoxicity. Adverse effects associated with topical use include delayed-type hypersensitivity reactions.

Special Populations: Pregnancy, Lactation, and the Elderly

It is unclear if imiquimod (Aldara) is safe to use during pregnancy. Although nonpregnant women with actinic keratosis, basal cell carcinoma, and genital/perianal warts are often treated with this medication, the risks versus benefits of its use must be considered for pregnant and nursing women.[14,17]

Reproductive-age women must be on effective birth control if using 5-fluorouracil (Efudex), as this agent is known to cause birth defects. It is critical to caution a woman that if her male partner is using this agent and she becomes pregnant, the fetus is at risk for birth defects. Additionally, breastfeeding is not recommended while using 5-fluorouracil.[7,15]

Imiquimod has been suggested as a possible substitute for surgery for melanomas when elderly women are poor surgical candidates. Older women in good health have not been found to have difficulty in using this agent, even in the high doses associated with cancer treatments.[34]

Skin Cancers

Skin cancers are the most common type of cancer in the United States.[35] More than 90% of skin cancers are related to exposure to ultraviolet light. The most common of these cancers are basal and squamous cell tumors; women with these types are treated by surgical excision. Superficial radiation therapy may be considered for basal cell and squamous cell carcinoma treatment among individuals older than 65 years.

The rarest of the skin cancers is melanoma, but it is the most deadly, causing the majority of deaths associated with skin cancer. The number of persons with skin cancer continues to rise, with current projections suggesting that by 2015, 1 in every 50 persons in the United States will have a melanoma in his or her lifetime.[35] Currently, melanoma is the sixth most frequently diagnosed cancer among women in the United States.[35] Cumulative sun exposure and number of sunburns increase the risk of melanoma; in fact, a single blistering sunburn during or prior to adolescence will double a woman's risk. Unfortunately, more than five sunburns over the course of a lifetime also double an individual's melanoma risk.[36]

Standard treatment for a melanoma is surgical excision, usually followed by radiation therapy and/or chemotherapy. Optimal treatment is prevention through liberal use of sunscreens or, in lieu of prevention, early diagnosis, often through a woman practicing regular skin self-examination. Women should consult a healthcare provider if they have any lesion that appears different from others on the skin, regardless of its color, size, or shape, or they have a lesion that crusts, bleeds, or fails to heal.

Atopic Dermatitis (Eczema) and Xerosis (Dry Skin)

Dermatitis is an umbrella term that indicates an inflammation of the skin. There have been long-term debates among the dermatology community regarding standardizing terminology for dermatitis. For example, *eczema* is occasionally used as another term for dermatitis in general; in this chapter, as in other sources, this term is used as a synonym for atopic dermatitis.

Atopic dermatitis, or eczema, is the product of both genetic influences and inflammatory responses. This condition is a chronic disease, usually characterized by relapses or flares. It is typically seen initially in early childhood and is often associated with a personal or family history of childhood asthma. As much as 17% of the U.S. population has symptoms of eczema or atopic dermatitis.[37] Approximately 25% of all individuals with eczema have chronic symptoms without remission.[38] Criteria for the diagnosis include dry pruritic skin, primarily in flexural areas (e.g., elbow, neck creases), often thickened and with pronounced texture. Vesicles may or may not be present.[39] When signs of infection are present, topical or oral antibiotics usually are prescribed, and the woman is referred for long-term follow-up with a dermatologist.

Xerosis (Dry Skin)

Xerosis (dry skin) may precipitate recurrences of the atopic dermatitis. Dehydration, or decreased water storage in the stratum corneum of the skin, also precipitates symptoms of xerosis. Aging, excessive washing, and exposure to extreme weather conditions can further contribute to the problem.

Emollients and Moisturizers

First-line treatment of women with dry skin is often initiated by the woman herself using over-the-counter agents. Moisturizers, emollients, lubricants, and protectors are the terms used to describe products available for treatment of dry skin. Most sources agree that moisturizers soften the stratum corneum and increase hydration, making these outermost layers of the epidermis more pliant. In addition, these agents provide a temporary barrier, allowing time for natural skin repair to occur. Today's moisturizers may include botanicals, metabolites of collagen, and vitamins. Moisturizers often have an added **humectant**—an ingredient like glycerin or urea that facilitates absorption of water, thereby moisturizing the area to which the humectant is applied. Moisturizers may also contain emollients. Emollients are products that soften the skin, most likely by filling spaces between the corneocytes and assist in smoothing rough skin and replacing natural skin lipids, thus improving desquamated skin. The major component of an emollient is oil, contained in a water emulsion. Lubricants are oily agents that reduce friction, heat, or chafing between solid substances. Some emollients are also called protectants because of their ability to provide a barrier over the skin. Petroleum jelly is an example of an agent that can be an emollient or even a lubricant depending upon if it is applied with other agents or alone as a thick coating.

Most agents recommended for women with atopic dermatitis are in the form of creams and identification of the best product for an individual woman may be a matter of trial and error. Products containing urea (e.g., Aqua Care, Carmol) or ammonium lactate (e.g., Lac-Hydrin) are often recommended.[40] The most common side effect of the use of emollients and moisturizers is stinging or other skin sensations. True allergies are rare. However, cosmetic moisturizers may contain fragrances to which an individual may have a reaction.

Aqua Care and Carmol are over-the-counter (OTC) preparations of 10% urea, which acts as a humectant. The lotion is applied twice daily. Carmol-HC, which is available by prescription, contains hydrocortisone to decrease inflammation and should be used only for inflammatory skin conditions. Ammonium lactate (Lac-Hydrin 12%) cream or ointment is available by prescription and over-the-counter as AmLactin 12%; the two formulations contain the same ingredients. Ammonium lactate is applied twice daily to affected areas, and improvement should be expected within 1 week. Application to abraded or inflamed skin may cause stinging or burning and should be avoided.

In one study, skin lubrication to reduce dryness reduced the need for corticosteroid treatment by as much as 50%.[41] A thick cream or ointment should be recommended, rather than a lotion. Lotions contain more water compared to creams, and therefore, they are more likely to dehydrate the skin. Common hydrating products that may be recommended include dimethicone, glycerin, colloidal oatmeal, and petrolatum. Generic versions of all these products are available; common brand names include Cetaphil (dimethicone and glycerin), Eucerin (colloidal oatmeal, glycerin, and lanolin, among other components), and Aquaphor (petrolatum product). Additionally, ceramide creams (CeraVe, Cetaphil Restoraderm) may be beneficial for women with eczema.[42]

Steroid Therapy

Steroid therapy is indicated to suppress symptoms of atopic dermatitis, although use may be best limited to flares when moisturizing treatments are ineffective. A low-potency steroid may be topically applied by women who have mild to moderate atopic dermatitis (Table 26-4). High-potency steroids may be needed—including oral or injectable forms—if the woman has severe eczema.

In addition to their daily use as first-line management of acute symptoms, topical steroids can be applied once or twice weekly as therapy for maintenance. Berth-Jones et al. evaluated fluticasone (Cutivate) as twice-weekly maintenance dosing and found the cream preparation to be more effective than the ointment formulation; both were more effective than use of an emollient alone in preventing recurrences during a 20-week trial. In that study, persons who used the fluticasone cream were 5.8 times less likely to experience a recurrence than those who used the emollient only (95% CI, 3.1–10.8; $P < .0001$), and persons who used the fluticasone ointment were 1.9 times less likely to experience a recurrence than those who used the emollient only (95% CI, 1.2–3.2; $P = .01$).[43]

Although oral steroids may be used for the treatment of women with particularly severe atopic dermatitis flares, they are not reviewed in depth in this chapter. Women who need oral steroids will be cared for by dermatologic specialists. Several major risks are associated with long-term oral steroid use, including adrenal insufficiency, decreased bone density, glaucoma, diabetes, and mood changes, and osteonecrosis, among others.

Calcineurin Inhibitors

Calcineurin inhibitors are immunosuppressants that inhibit cytokines and reduce inflammation. These drugs bind to intracellular proteins that combine with calcineurin to inhibit cytokine release and, therefore, the activation of T cells. Tacrolimus (Protopic) is similar in effectiveness to high-potency steroids; pimecrolimus (Elidel) is milder in effect.[44] Topical tacrolimus and pimecrolimus usually are prescribed when steroids are not effective in reducing symptoms or when they are not well tolerated. In contrast to the topical steroids, these pharmaceuticals do not increase the risk of skin damage or glaucoma. When 0.1% tacrolimus is used for persistent facial or periocular lesions, studies have demonstrated marked reduction of symptoms.[45] Tacrolimus 0.03% has also been shown to be effective, but over time users noticed a reduction in improvement with this lower dose.[34]

Studies also have evaluated the effectiveness of tacrolimus (Protopic) when a steroid, such as betamethasone, is added to the treatment regimen. Small studies reported by Nakahara et al. and by Furue et al. found relative improvement in symptoms with the steroid–calcineurin inhibitor combination, particularly with regard to skin thickening and lichenification.[46,47] Furue et al. demonstrated the effectiveness of tacrolimus plus a glucocorticoid in a 6-month trial of twice-weekly maintenance therapy.[47] When combination topical therapies are applied, the steroid is applied first; the second preparation is then applied 15 minutes later so that the vascular dilating effects of the steroid enhances absorption of the second medication.

Calcineurin inhibitors are not innocuous medications. In 2006, the FDA mandated that their labels include a black box warning because of potential risk of cancers associated with their use. Later research, however, has called these precautions into question. Both tacrolimus (Protopic) and pimecrolimus (Elidel) should be utilized as a second-line therapy—that is, only if other therapies have failed—and should be used for a short time only. Table 26-7 provides prescribing information for these agents.

Other Treatments for Women with Atopic Dermatitis

In the event that a woman with atopic dermatitis does not respond to the usual treatments, other drugs may be used, including systemic immunosuppressants such as methotrexate (Rheumatrex). Under these circumstances, referral to a specialist is indicated.

In addition to pharmacologic management, counseling should include information about identifying and avoiding environmental stimuli and allergens that cause symptoms, treatment of secondary infections, and use of antihistamines for women who need symptomatic relief, especially when the itching interferes with sleep. Table 26-6 lists common antihistamine choices; antihistamine dosing may need to be at the upper end of the range for best effect in treating atopic dermatitis. A Cochrane review failed to find any study of sufficient rigor and power to associate antihistamines as effective monotherapy for the treatment of individuals with atopic dermatitis.[48] Antihistamines are simply palliative measures, not therapeutic agents that will resolve the condition.

Special Populations: Pregnancy, Lactation, and the Elderly

For treatment of women with atopic dermatitis, topical emollients are considered safe for use during pregnancy and lactation.[49] It is theorized that poor systemic absorption of topical calcineurin inhibitors occurs; therefore, as a last resort, application on small surfaces is considered safe during pregnancy.[14] Topical use in breastfeeding women should be limited, and the medication should never be applied to the areola or nipples as significant oral absorption by the infant could occur.[7] Calcineurin inhibitors generally are effective treatments for atopic dermatitis for older women, and have fewer side effects or adverse effects when compared to steroids.

Allergic Dermatitis and Irritant Dermatitis

When dermatitis is caused by direct exposure or contact with a substance, the individual can have either an allergic response or an irritant response. The pattern of symptoms can be similar for both types of dermatitis, but treatment should be coupled with identification of the trigger substance to avoid recurrence (Box 26-3).

Table 26-7 Topical Calcineurin Inhibitors

Drug: Generic (Brand)	Formulation and Dose	Side Effects/Adverse Effects	Contraindications
Pimecrolimus (Elidel)	1% cream twice daily—for eczema, contact dermatitis Apply to affected area in a thin layer	Skin irritation, burning, erythema, pharyngitis, flulike symptoms, headache Increased risk of cancer	Allergy Not indicated for long-term use
Tacrolimus (Protopic)	0.1% ointment 2 times/day (0.03% ointment is available for pediatric use and can be used if needed) Apply to affected area in a thin layer	Skin irritation, burning, erythema, pharyngitis, flulike symptoms, headache Elevated liver enzymes Increased risk of cancer FDA black box warning states that tacrolimus may increase risk of malignancies and serious infections	Allergy Not approved for long-term use

Box 26-3 A Case of Itchy Palms

An old myth exists that says if the palm of the right hand is itchy, it means that money is coming—but do not scratch it, because doing so stops any payments. If the left palm is itchy, money will need to be paid, so continue to scratch. This case study concerns a woman who had bilateral itchy palms.

KJ is a 30-year-old woman who presented with an irregular, erythematous, highly pruritic rash on the palms of her hands. She currently is taking multivitamins and combination oral contraceptives; she also finished a course of metronidazole (Flagyl) for treatment of *Trichomonas* vaginalis 3 days ago. She denies any significant health conditions.

One of the major challenges in treatment of persons with dermatologic symptoms is making the correct diagnosis. Because KJ has recently been treated with metronidazole, one condition to be included in the differential diagnosis is drug side effects. In this case, however, metronidazole is most likely to be associated with fixed drug reactions that most commonly occur up to 8 hours after drug exposure. The hands are a possible site where the reaction to metronidazole might occur, but the timing of the rash makes that etiology unlikely.

Palmar rashes also are associated with treponemal infections. KJ is sexually active. Her recent diagnosis of *Trichomonas* vaginalis requires further discussion because it suggests that she is not well protected from sexual transmission of disease. Thus, it is likely that screening to rule out syphilis would be indicted. Rocky Mountain spotted fever also is a possibility, but was ruled out in KJ's case by following a thorough history.

After a careful physical exam and consideration of her history, it became apparent that KJ had contact dermatitis. She currently is working as a produce manager at a supermarket, where she spends much of her day placing food on displays, including nonorganic fruits and vegetables that have been sprayed with pesticides.

A common consumer mistake is to use a topical antihistamine in a situation like this one. However, irritated skin often does not absorb the drug effectively, so that the woman may actually experience more irritation. Alternatively, a systemic antihistamine is a very reasonable option.

KJ responded well to an over-the-counter hydrocortisone cream and nighttime oral ingestion of diphenhydramine hydrochloride (Benadryl). Within 24 hours, she noticed an improvement in the rash. Her test for syphilis was found to be negative.

KJ was advised to use gloves when touching produce in the future. It was also suggested that she discuss issues of pesticides with her company to prevent similar situations among her coworkers as well as potential problems for the supermarket's consumers.

The classic skin allergy is the one occurring after exposure to poison ivy. Poison ivy produces urushiol, a powerful allergen. Other common allergies include nickel, chemicals, and preservatives found in clothing and household products as well as antibiotics and topical medications. The primary symptom of an allergic response is intense itching. In the area of involvement, erythema, papules, and vesicles may accompany pruritis. Although most allergic dermatitis is caused by an acute exposure, chronic exposure to an irritating substance may lead to the development of similar symptoms.

Treatment for mild allergic responses includes the identification and removal of the offending agent. Additionally, application of drying agents such as calamine (a liquid mixture of zinc oxide and iron), soothing lotions such as Aveeno (a combination of colloidal oatmeal, glycerin, and allantoin), and topical steroid creams of moderate potency can relieve symptoms (Table 26-4). While topical antihistamines may often be used, they are typically ineffective for this indication.

The choice of therapy can be made empirically based on location of the reaction, the severity of symptoms, and the woman's preference. More severe events may require an oral steroid, either as a dose pack of methylprednisolone (Medrol; Table 26-5) or as a tapered prednisone dose.

Unlike allergens, irritants are more likely to be substances to which the woman has chronic exposure. As abrasion or chemicals damage skin, for example, the resultant inflammatory response produces the symptoms. While itching may occur, pain, redness, dryness, and fissures are more commonly observed in irritant dermatitis. A systematic review by Saary et al. found barrier creams, such as those containing the silicon polymer dimethicone (e.g., Cetaphil, Remedy Skin Repair, Johnson's baby cream); lipid-rich moisturizers; cotton glove liners; and the use of fabric softeners could potentially control irritants and prevent future skin reactions.[50] However, additional research is needed to determine the effectiveness of these measures.

Seborrheic Dermatitis

Seborrheic dermatitis appears as reddened, flaky, occasionally greasy skin on the scalp, face, especially in the naso-labial folds, and chest. When it appears on the scalp it is colloquially termed dandruff. Infantile or neonatal seborrheic dermatitis is often known as cradle cap. Like tinea versicolor, seborrheic dermatitis is associated with *Malassezia* spp. rather than dermatophytes. This condition is chronic and requires persistent treatment to control symptoms. Treatment of women with seborrheic dermatitis varies according to the age group and the location of the lesions, and is focused on symptomatic relief versus cure. Ketoconazole is one drug that is FDA approved for treatment of seborrheic dermatitis; however, a variety of products are effective, including selenium sulfide shampoo (Selsun Blue) and other topical antifungals such as terbinafine (Lamisil).[51] These products are applied twice daily to the affected areas, and their use is preferred to topical corticosteroids because use may be prolonged. Treatment for adults with seborrhea in folds and creases consists of comfort measures such as Burow's solution for topical relief from itching. Low to moderate potency steroid lotions may be used 1 or 2 times per day to decrease inflammation during an acute flare but are felt to exacerbate flares if used chronically.

Calcineurin inhibitors such as pimecrolimus cream (Elidel) and tacrolimus cream (Protopic) may be used. These agents are pharmaceuticals that have an immune modulating effect.[52] Pimecrolimus cream has demonstrated effectiveness in the management of severe facial seborrheic dermatitis when applied twice daily for several weeks ($P = .0156$; 95% CI, 0.129–1.197 compared to vehicle alone). A small study of tacrolimus found 61% reported total clearance of symptoms during use.[53] Prophylaxis to prevent recurrences can be provided with ketoconazole shampoo weekly or topical miconazole (Monistat) twice a month.[51]

Systemic ketoconazole or fluconazole (Diflucan) may be valuable if seborrheic dermatitis is severe or unresponsive or if there is evidence of a fungal overgrowth. Systemic terbinafine (Lamisil) has been shown to defer recurrences for up to 3 months.[54] Systemic itraconazole 200 mg taken on 2 consecutive days monthly has been shown to be an effective maintenance regimen. A small study demonstrated absence of recurrence over a 12-month period using this regimen.[55] Itraconazole persists in tissue due to its lipophilic nature; additionally, it exhibits anti-inflammatory action.

Treatment with ultraviolet light improves seborrheic lesions, which is the likely explanation for improvement of the condition during the summer. Tea tree oil has been proposed as a natural treatment for seborrheic dermatitis and is the active ingredient in many dandruff shampoos. However, because it is an essential oil, there is the risk of contact dermatitis, especially if a strong solution is applied to the area. Both tea tree oil and cinnamic acid have antifungal properties and have potential value, although more research is needed to assess the effectiveness of these complementary therapies.[51]

Prevention of reoccurrence of seborrheic dermatitis consists of frequent removal of sebum with soap and water. Zinc- or coal tar-containing shampoos, zinc soap, or benzoyl peroxide washes may be useful in controlling seborrhea. Education includes cautioning the woman to rinse thoroughly after application of these agents and to apply moisturizer to the area. Individuals should be warned that these agents may bleach clothing and bed linens.

Special Populations: Pregnancy and Lactation

Women who have seborrheic dermatitis can be advised that terbinafine appears to be compatible with pregnancy based on animal data. Tropical ketoconazole and itraconazole also are considered compatible with pregnancy based on limited data. Topical ketoconazole should be used by a breastfeeding woman rather than itraconazole because the latter accumulates even in low doses in breast milk.[7,14,15,17]

Intertrigo

A rash or inflammation of the body folds or intertriginous areas of the skin represents another type of dermatitis, intertrigo. Also commonly called chafing, intertrigo most frequently occurs in areas of warm, moist skin. A diaper rash is an intertrigo, as are rashes experienced by individuals who are overweight, suffer from diabetes, or use prosthetic devices against their skin. The elderly, especially those with incontinence, are at increased risk for intertrigo.[51] This condition may have a bacterial, fungal, or viral infection associated with it, especially if there is broken skin that allows entry of the offending agent. Discussion of secondary infections and their treatments can be found in following sections.

Treatment of a Woman with Uncomplicated Intertrigo

Treatment of simple intertrigo includes protectants such as petroleum jelly or astringents like zinc oxide cream. If an infection is suspected, therapy should be specific to the agent in question. Persistent intertrigo infections tend to be fungal or yeast. For fungal infection, antifungal azole creams such as clotrimazole 1% are often used while Nystatin cream or powder is most frequently used for yeast. Other treatments include palliative use of glucocorticoid over-the-counter cream for symptoms. However, fluorinated steroids (Table 26-4) are contraindicated for use in body folds because of the potential development of striae.[14] When a women presents with chronic groin dermatitis she should be advised to wear loose cotton underwear and loose skirts or dresses, and avoid pantyhose and fabrics that trap heat and moisture. Protectants and creams used to treat intertrigo tend to be water resistant, so it is suggested to apply them using a vehicle such as a tissue or towel to avoid difficulty washing them from hands. The main treatment for women with intertrigo is to keep the area as dry as possible.

Special Populations: Pregnancy, Lactation, and the Elderly

Protectants and topical azoles are agents that are compatible with pregnancy and lactation.[7,14,15,17] No special considerations have been suggested for use with mature women.

Papulosquamous Disorders: Psoriasis

Psoriasis is a chronic skin disorder that affects both genders and persons of all races. In the United States, the incidence is approximately 2% to 3%, with onset most common between ages 15 and 20 years, and a second peak occurring after age 55 years.[37] In individuals with psoriasis, overgrowth of keratinocytes and accompanying inflammation occur as a result of a breakdown in the immune system, in which T cells are stimulated and migrate to skin tissue.[13] Normally, it takes approximately one month for skin cells to mature and shed. For women with psoriasis, the cells may mature in a few days; because the lower layer of skin cells divides more rapidly than normal, dead cells accumulate in thick patches on the epidermis.

Several genes that predispose an individual to develop psoriasis have been identified, as well as environmental triggers that stimulate the onset of symptoms. Among the factors associated with psoriasis are skin infections or injury, medications, stress, and alcohol use. In particular, smoking appears to increase the likelihood of a psoriasis diagnosis; conversely, smoking cessation may decrease the severity of symptoms.[56,57]

Plaque psoriasis is the most common type of psoriasis, accounting for approximately 80% of all diagnoses. This condition is characterized by reddened papules and plaques with distinctly outlined silvery, flaking patches of skin, presenting symmetrically. The elbows, knees, and scalp are commonly affected; palms and soles may also be affected. Inverse psoriasis is found in folds of skin, such as the axillae, gluteal cleft, groin, and antecubital and popliteal fossae. Guttate (from Latin for *drop)* or eruptive psoriasis generally appears after streptococcal infections. In contrast to plaque psoriasis, guttate psoriasis appears as erythematous papules or so-called droplet-like spread across the trunk and extremities.[58] Guttate psoriasis generally has a limited course but is more common in women than in men, and women affected with this variant often later manifest plaque psoriasis.

Treatment of Psoriasis

Treatment of psoriasis is determined both by type and severity. Mild psoriasis (affecting less than 3% of the total body surface) can be treated in a stepwise fashion beginning with topical medications. The progression of therapy is from topical treatments, to light therapy with sunlight or UV radiation, to systemic treatment.

Steroids work rapidly but become less effective over time and can cause tissue atrophy. Tazarotene (Tazorac), a retinoid gel, is FDA approved for psoriasis. A pea-sized amount of this medication is applied to a lesion (an area equivalent to the size of an open hand) nightly. Care should be taken to keep the medication limited to the plaques.

Severe psoriasis may be treated with systemic therapies including methotrexate (Rheumatrex), cyclosporine (Neoral), and oral retinoids. These treatments are best prescribed by a specialist.

Guttate psoriasis is generally treated with UVB light therapy, although long-term antibiotics have been considered, given the relationship between disease onset and skin infections. Either penicillin VK 1 g per day or erythromycin (E-Mycin) 1 g per day can be administered for as long as 14 days. There is no evidence that treatment beyond the usual course of antibiotics improves outcomes.[59]

Topical drug therapy for psoriasis includes many modalities. Topical steroids (Table 26-4), often combined with emollients to soften the skin and create a barrier to prevent infection, are the first line of therapy. Other treatments for women with psoriasis include calcipotriene (Dovonex), salicylic acid creams or ointments, and tar products. The calcineurin inhibitors tacrolimus (Protopic) and pimecrolimus (Elidel) (Table 26-7) are used in more delicate tissue areas, such as the face and skinfolds, or when steroid-sparing regimens are preferred. Treatments for vulvar psoriasis are presented in the *Vulvar Disorders* chapter.

Retinoids

Retinoids have been suggested as an alternative therapy. These are vitamin A analogs and, although their exact mechanism of action is unknown, several actions have been suggested including blocking production of procollagen; decreasing the number of inflammatory mediators; and unblocking clogged pores; and working synergistically with antimicrobials, facilitating their transfer into the cells so they can attack bacteria. Common side effects include alopecia, skin dryness, and peeling. Alterations in lipid metabolism, pancreatitis, depression, and pseudotumor cerebri are less common, but serious adverse effects. Tretinoin (Retin-A, Renova), a topical retinoid preparation, is not FDA approved for treatment of individuals with psoriasis, though tazarotene (Tazorac, Avage), another retinoid gel, does have FDA approval for this indication. Acitretin (Soriatane) is an oral retinoid that may be used on an off-label basis for persons with severe psoriasis at a dose of 25–50 mg once daily.

Calcipotriene (Dovonex)

Calcipotriene (Dovonex 0.005%), a vitamin D preparation, is available by prescription as an ointment or a solution. This agent is applied once or twice daily to the affected area for a maximum of 8 weeks. Calcipotriene acts by slowing skin cell proliferation, although its exact mechanism of action is unknown. Itching, skin irritation, redness, or peeling may occur with use of this medication. Hypercalcemia may occur as well, and use of calcipotriene can cause kidney stones to reoccur in susceptible individuals. This medication also induces sensitivity to sunlight. Pigment changes and skin thinning are rare side effects.

Calcipotriene also is available as a combination therapy with betamethasone under the brand name Taclonex; this preparation may work more rapidly to achieve reduction in psoriasis symptoms than either product alone. Douglas et al. demonstrated a 74.4% reduction in lesion thickness over 4 weeks with the calcipotriene/betamethasone combination, compared to a 61.3% reduction with betamethasone alone (P = .0001) and a 55.3% reduction with calcipotriene alone (P = .0001).[60] This dual-agent preparation should be applied daily for 4 weeks, after which calcipotriene alone can be continued. The maximum weekly dose should be limited to 100 g.

Salicylic Acid

Salicylic acid (SalAc, Dermal Zone, and multiple other brand names), a nonsteroidal anti-inflammatory drug, is used as a keratinolytic agent, usually in combination with a steroid. For example, the formulation that is marketed under the brand name Diprosalic consists of betamethasone and salicylic acid. The salicylic acid breaks down keratin, thereby improving absorption of the steroidal component. Concentrations of 2% to 3% in a variety of formulations are available over the counter; higher concentrations are available by prescription. If a woman has used over-the-counter products without complete resolution of psoriatic plaques, a formulation of 6% or less can be prescribed. Higher concentrations tend to destroy tissue and should not be used for this purpose. Salicylic acid should not be applied to irritated or inflamed skin, as it may worsen the irritation. Persons with bleeding problems, diabetes mellitus, and renal or hepatic disease should use nonsteroidal medications with caution.

Coal Tar

Tar, especially coal tar, is used as an occlusive and emollient product and slows the proliferation of skin cells. Over-the-counter products contain concentrations ranging from 0.5% to 5% active ingredient. Psoriasin ointment (2% coal tar in a petrolatum base with other inactive ingredients) and Psoriasin gel (1.25% coal tar in aloe vera gel with other ingredients) are examples of the many products designed for skin application. Shampoos with tar, such as Tegrin, Neutrogena T/Gel, and Denorex, are available for scalp treatment. Coal tar has few side effects, although rash, redness, or irritation may occur. Tar increases sun sensitivity; drug interactions include tetracycline and tretinoin. Women should be cautioned about the risk of staining with the use of tar products.

Biologic Immune Modulators (Biologics)

Tacrolimus (Protopic), an immune modulator, should be reserved for a woman with psoriasis that is unresponsive to other agents and is prescribed by a specialist familiar with its use, because it potentially may increase the risk for malignancies and opportunistic infections. Other biologic immune modulators used to treat psoriasis include alefacept (Amevive), adalimumab (Humira), etanercept (Enbrel), infliximab (Remicade), and ustekinumab (Stelara). Biologics act to stimulate the body's immune system and block the production of T cells or tumor necrosis factor alpha, thereby affecting the progression of psoriatic plaques. These products are all administered by injection or infusion (e.g., infliximab). Side effects of this class of drugs include a flulike syndrome and injection-site inflammation.

Other Treatments: Antimetabolites, Immunosuppressants, and Biologics

Persons with more severe psoriasis may require ultraviolet light therapy, methotrexate (Rheumatrex, Trexall), cyclosporine (Sandimmune), or immunomodulating biologic agents. These treatments are managed by a dermatologic specialist. Methotrexate (Rheumatrex), an antimetabolite and antifolate agent, acts to decrease the production of new skin cells by interfering with cellular metabolism. Cyclosporine (Neoral), an immune suppressant, inhibits lymphocytes, thereby decreasing T-cell infiltration of the dermis. Both methotrexate and cyclosporine have demonstrated similar effectiveness in treating severe psoriasis.[61]

Special Populations: Pregnancy, Lactation, and the Elderly

Treatment plans for women with psoriasis may include a variety of drugs. Among the possible therapies, there is no evidence about the safety of topical salicylates in pregnancy or breastfeeding. Limited use of these agents for a short period of time appears to be compatible with pregnancy, although systemic salicylates should be avoided.[14] There are insufficient data available regarding the effects of maternal ingestion of coal tar on fetal development, but if a woman did use this agent during pregnancy, no additional action/intervention is required.[14]

All systemic retinoids are contraindicated in pregnancy, and women should be on an effective birth control method prior to initiation of such therapy. Topical retinoid application appears to be safe, but most studies do not support the use of any retinoid, including topical ones during pregnancy.[14,17] Notably, acitretin (Soriatane) is not recommended for reproductive-age women because pregnancy is contraindicated for 3 years after completion of therapy.[14] Methotrexate (Rheumatrex) is an antifolate agent that can be an abortifacient, so it is contraindicated for use during pregnancy and lactation.[7,14,15,17] Cyclosporine (Neoral) has not been shown to have any deleterious effects on a fetus, but has been shown to cause maternal hypertension; thus its use is not advised in pregnancy.[14]

Coal tar use while breastfeeding is not recommended.[7] Biologics are considered compatible with pregnancy, although they are relatively new and the data on them are sparse. These medications are likely to be safe in lactation, although breastfeeding infants who are exposed to infliximab through breastfeeding must avoid live vaccine immunizations for the first 6 months of life.[7,14,15] If a woman elects to breastfeed while taking cyclosporine, the infant needs be monitored for possible toxicity via measurement of blood plasma levels.[7]

The agents used for treatment of women with psoriasis do not appear to be limited by the age of a woman; thus, there are no suggestions to treat older individuals differently based on age. Cyclosporine, however, should be used with caution by a woman of any age who has renal disease—a condition that is more common among older women.

Acne Vulgaris

Acne vulgaris is the term applied to persistent comedones, nodules, or pustules developing from the pilosebaceous follicles; it is known as a skin disorder of the appendages. The pathogenesis of acne vulgaris involves four factors: (1) androgen-mediated hyperstimulation of sebaceous gland activity, which causes increased sebum production; (2) hyperkeratinization, which leads to blockage of the follicular gland, which in turn mixes with sebum to become impacted within the gland; (3) inflammation that occurs when the follicular epithelium around the mass ruptures; and (4) presence of *Propionibacterium acnes*, which is the dominant bacterium that causes acne vulgaris. The degree of inflammation depends on the individual immune responsiveness. Clinically, acne vulgaris can be non-inflammatory, which includes open comedones (blackheads) and closed comedones, or inflammatory, which includes pustules and papules. Acne is also categorized as mild, moderate, or severe—a distinction that guides recommended treatment options. The head, neck, and upper trunk are the most common locations for eruptions.

Treatment is divided into preventive/drying and antibacterial categories, and is recommended based on the severity of the outbreak. The use of hormonal contraception offers an additional therapeutic option for managing the symptoms of acne and is especially useful for sexually active women of reproductive age who want contraception.

Several authors describe a stepwise recommendation for choosing the appropriate therapy, recommending topical benzoyl peroxide (Benoxyl, Benzagel) and topical retinoids for mild acne (unless the woman is pregnant), topical antibiotics with or without retinoids for mild to moderate acne, systemic antibiotics for moderate to severe inflammatory disease, and isotretinoin (Accutane) for the most severe cases of nodular acne in non-pregnant women. Spironolactone, an antiandrogenic agent, also has been suggested as a therapy. The drugs used are based on both disease severity and the effectiveness of treatment.[62] A secondary goal of this treatment structure is to avoid the prolonged or unnecessary use of antibiotics that may induce resistance in *P. acnes*.

Prevention of Acne

Oral Contraceptives

The use of combination oral contraceptives to treat a woman with mild acne, or even to prevent outbreaks, is based on these drugs' ability to suppress androgen expression through increased sex hormone–binding globulin. Ethinyl estradiol/triphasic norgestimate (Ortho Tri-Cyclen), 20 mcg ethinyl estradiol/levonorgestrel (Alesse), and ethinyl estradiol/drospirenone (Yaz) all have FDA-approved indications for the treatment of acne, but other combined oral contraceptives with similarly low androgen–progesterone ratios have comparable overall effects even though the manufacturer may not have sought FDA approval for this indication.[63] Triphasic norgestimate/ethynyl estradiol has been shown to reduce both total lesions (mean reduction 46.4% versus 33.9% with placebo; $P = .001$) and inflammatory lesions (mean reduction 51.4% versus 34.6%; $P = .01$).[64] Both drospirenone-containing contraceptives and contraceptives containing 20 mcg ethinyl estradiol have comparable benefits.[65,66] At this time, the effect of other non-oral combined hormonal contraceptive products on acne has not been studied.

Special Populations: Pregnancy, Lactation, and the Elderly

Although combination oral contraceptives have not been causally linked with teratogenic effects or miscarriages, it is illogical to recommend their use during pregnancy. Oral contraceptives are safe for use by breastfeeding women although some authors do not recommend starting oral contraceptives that contain estrogen until breastfeeding is well established. More information about oral contraceptives can be found in the *Contraception* chapter. Combination oral contraceptives are reasonable for most women of reproductive age who desire contraception. Use of estrogen and progestin drugs are discussed in the chapter *The Mature Woman*, however, such use is rare to treat the older woman with acne.

Treatment of a Woman with Mild Acne

Face Washes

Benzoyl peroxide acts to dry and peel away the desquamated epidermis, thereby opening the sebaceous glands, as well as being an antimicrobial agent. It is used in both noninflammatory and inflammatory acne. Benzoyl peroxide is the most cost-effective therapy available for mild acne; indeed, it is as effective as other regimens, although it may have an unacceptable side-effect profile of increased skin irritation.[67]

Azelaic acid (Azelex, Finacea) is a dicarboxylic acid that occurs naturally in the skin. This agent acts to decrease keratin production and is an antibacterial agent that has been shown to be as effective as tretinoin, benzoyl peroxide, or topical erythromycin (Akne-Mycin) in treating mild to moderate acne.[60] Four to six weeks of treatment with either of these agents is required for an improvement in symptoms to be evident.

Salicylic acid, a product also recommended for treatment of women with psoriasis, also may be suggested for women with mild acne. This agent acts as an exfoliant for the outer layers of the stratum corneum. For any facial wash, a rash or worsening symptoms of skin irritation require that the clinician be notified, as a contact allergy may be developing. These agents are usually categorized as anti-infectives.

Retinoids

Retinoids are vitamin A derivatives that act by normalizing keratinocyte development, reducing inflammation, inhibiting immune factors, and decreasing sebum production, thereby preventing comedone formation. The retinoids promote the development of smooth skin and they are, therefore, included in some anti-aging skin care products. Topical preparations, including tretinoin (Retin-A), adapalene (Differin), and tazarotene (Tazorac, Avage), have 40% to 70% effectiveness in reducing the incidence of comedones and inflammation. Before beginning any topical retinoid treatment, the woman should discontinue other topical treatments and confirm that she is not pregnant. Table 26-8 provides a list of topical retinoid and oral retinoid preparations. The oral retinoids are only used for treatment of severe acne.

Special Populations: Pregnancy, Lactation, and the Elderly

Benzoyl peroxide may seem an innocuous option for many pregnant women suffering from acne, but it should be used with caution and in limited areas of the body.[14,17] Azelaic acid appears to be safer than benzoyl peroxide for use in pregnancy, but there are fewer data available on its use in this population.[14] All systemic retinoids are contraindicated during pregnancy, and all women should be on an effective birth control method prior to initiation of therapy. Topical application does appear to be safe, but most studies do not support the use of any retinoid in pregnancy, including topicals.[14,17] Azelaic acid

Table 26-8 Retinoid Therapy

Drug: Generic (Brand)	Route	Dosing	Side Effects/Adverse Effects	Special Considerations
Topical Retinoids				
Adapalene (Differin gel)	Apply 1–2 times/day in a thin layer	Gel: 0.3% Cream, solution: 0.1%	Photosensitivity, local skin irritation including redness, edema, peeling skin, dryness, itching	Contraindicated during pregnancy. Lowest strength prescription retinoid and best tolerated. Use with caution with other potentially irritating products or open skin lesions.
Tazarotene (Tazorac)	Apply 1–2 times/day	Gel: 0.05%, 0.1% Cream: 0.05%	Photosensitivity; skin irritation including redness, edema, peeling skin, and itching; hyperlipidemia	Contraindicated during pregnancy. Most potent topical treatment for acne associated with skin irritation. Apply for 5–15 minutes and then wash off. Weak evidence for teratogenicity. Use with caution with irritated or open skin.
Tretinoin (Retin-A, Renova, Avita cream)	Apply daily at bedtime	Cream or gel: 0.01%, 0.025%, 0.05% Solution: 0.05%	Photosensitivity; local skin irritation including redness, edema, and peeling skin; leukocytosis	Contraindicated during pregnancy or with skin lesions or sunburn. Avoid use in extreme weather.
Tretinoin (Retin-A micro)	Apply daily at bedtime	Gel: 0.04%, 0.1% Active ingredient encapsulated in microspheres	Photosensitivity; local skin irritation including redness, edema, and peeling skin; leukocytosis	Contraindicated during pregnancy or with skin lesions or sunburn. Avoid use in extreme weather.
Oral Retinoids				
Acitretin (Soriatane)	Oral	25–50 mg PO daily with main meal	Hair loss, skin dryness and peeling, night blindness, alterations in lipid metabolism, pancreatitis, depression, pseudotumor cerebri	Contraindicated during pregnancy. Contraindicated for persons with impaired liver/kidney function, elevated lipid levels, and current use of methotrexate or tetracyclines.
Isotretinoin (Accutane)	Oral	0.5 mg/kg to 1.0 mg/kg PO daily in divided doses with food; maximum total dose: 120–150 mg/kg	Dry skin, lips, eyes; itching; photosensitivity; peeling; decreased night vision; vascular fragility (nose bleeds or bleeding gums); elevated triglycerides, hepatotoxicity, hearing loss, pancreatitis, pseudotumor cerebri; anemia, tachycardia, depression, headaches, jaundice, nausea, vomiting or diarrhea, stomach pain, irritable bowel condition, rectal bleeding, loss of appetite	Contraindicated during pregnancy. Use with caution for persons with paraben allergy, diabetes, depression, liver disease, cardiac disease, or asthma.
Micronized isotretinoin	Oral	0.4 mg/kg PO daily	Dry skin, lips, eyes; itching; photosensitivity; peeling; decreased night vision; vascular fragility (nose bleeds or bleeding gums); nausea; vomiting or diarrhea; stomach pain; chest pain, vasculitis, hyperglycemia, thyrotoxicosis, lipid abnormalities, inflammatory bowel disease, pancreatitis, leukocytopenia, anemia, headache, musculoskeletal pain	Contraindicated during pregnancy.

and benzoyl peroxide are believed to be compatible with breastfeeding.[7,15] Use of face washes or retinoids among elderly women does not appear to be different than that among other adults, but few studies have explored geriatric prescriptions.

Treatment of a Woman with Moderate Acne

Topical Anti-infectives

Topical antibiotics, including clindamycin (Cleocin-T, Clinda-Derm), erythromycin (A/T/S 2%, Erycette, Benzamycin), and metronidazole (Flagyl), are widely available in generic formulations and are used for the treatment of mild to moderate acne. Benzoyl peroxide and azelaic acid also demonstrate antimicrobial effects. Table 26-9 lists the doses and adverse effects of these drugs.

Combinations of benzoyl peroxide and clindamycin (Cleocin) or erythromycin (E-Mycin) are more effective than either agent used individually, both in decreasing inflammatory lesions and in producing overall improvement as assessed by both providers and consumers.[68] Similarly, combination therapy with clindamycin/tretinoin gel (Ziana gel) yields superior results than when either component is used individually to treat moderate acne. A report of two randomized trials found improved reduction in both inflammatory (P = .005) and non-inflammatory (P = .0004) lesions.[69] Ozolins et al. compared five topical and oral regimens for management of mild to moderate acne.[70] In this report, benzoyl peroxide/erythromycin combination topical treatment was as effective as either oral oxytetracycline or minocycline, and was more cost-effective than the single agents.

The use of a combination product for 6 to 8 weeks is now standard practice when treating a woman with moderate acne vulgaris. With the exception of benzoyl peroxide and azelaic acid, antimicrobial therapy for acne—whether topical or oral—carries a risk of increasing antibiotic resistance. Individual antibiotic products are associated with a higher risk of resistance developing when used alone due to selective pressure.

Clindamycin cream (Cleocin-T, Clinda-Derm) is a lincosamide antibiotic. It is bacteriostatic, interfering with bacterial protein synthesis. When used topically for acne, this preparation is directly antibacterial, with a small likelihood of side effects other than local irritation. Therapeutic results can take 12 weeks to become apparent.

Table 26-9 Topical Anti-infective Agents

Drug: Generic (Brand)	Dose	Formulations	Side Effects/Adverse Effects	Special Considerations
Azelaic acid (Azelex, Finacea)	Apply 2 times/day	Cream: 20% Gel: 15%	Itching, stinging, burning; may cause hypopigmentation	
Bacitracin (Baciguent)	Apply 1–3 times/day	Ointment	Contact dermatitis	Use with caution for persons with myasthenia gravis.
Benzoyl peroxide	Facial wash: apply 1–2 times/day	Gel: 2.5%, 5%, 10% 5% mixed with glycolic acid Solution: 5% mixed with erythromycin	Local irritation, photosensitivity, dryness	Do not use simultaneously with retinoids. Bleaching agent; avoid contact with hair and clothing.
Clindamycin (Cleocin-T)	Apply 2 times/day	Gel, lotion, solution: 10%	Dry skin, redness, peeling itching, oiliness Rarely with topical application: gastrointestinal upset, diarrhea, colitis, shortness of breath	Contraindicated for persons with history of ulcerative colitis or antibiotic-associated colitis.
Erythromycin (Erycette, A/T/S 2%, Benzamycin)	Apply 1–2 times/day	Gel, ointment: 2% Solution: 1.5%, 2%	Stinging, burning, dryness, peeling, redness	
Mupirocin (Bactroban)	Apply 3 times/day	Ointment: 2%	Burning, itching, headache, nausea, rash	
Neomycin (Myciguent)	Apply 1–3 times/day	Ointment	Skin irritation, burning, rash, ototoxicity	Use with caution for persons with impaired renal function.
Polymyxin B/neomycin (Neosporin cream)	10,000 units/g; 3.5 mg/g, respectively; apply 1–3 times/day	Cream	Skin irritation, rash, allergic response	Contraindicated for persons with myasthenia gravis.
Polymyxin B/Bacitracin/ neomycin (Neosporin ointment)	400 units/g; 3.5 mg/g and 5000 units/g, respectively; apply 1–3 times/day	Ointment		

Metronidazole gel (Flagyl gel) is a nitroimidazole, approved for use in rosacea, although it can also be prescribed for acne vulgaris. The metabolites of this drug are active and bactericidal. Contraindications to oral metronidazole include anticoagulant therapy, because this product potentiates the effect of warfarin (Coumadin). Detailed information about metronidazole can be found in the *Antimicrobials* chapter. The topical gel should be used with caution in women with a history of clotting disorders based on the risks associated with oral administration of the agent. While complications are less likely with a topical preparation, metronidazole can easily be avoided by using another approved topical treatment. In general, metronidazole gel is used for 3 weeks before improvement typically is seen, and the skin will continue to improve for as much as 6 months after treatment is discontinued.

Oral Anti-infectives

Erythromycin (E-Mycin) and tetracyclines are used to treat moderate to severe acne or when simpler treatments have failed. The tetracyclines cause less antibiotic resistance than erythromycin and, therefore, are favored as first-line therapy.[71] Table 26-10 lists many of the oral antibiotics used for skin conditions, including those prescribed for acne. The table includes dose ranges, uses, side effects, and warnings. More information about all anti-infectives can be found in the *Antimicrobials* chapter.

Among members of the tetracycline family used to treat acne are tetracycline, minocycline (Minocin), and doxycycline (Vibramycin). These bacteriostatic antibiotics can be used to treat a broad spectrum of gram-positive and gram-negative bacteria. Tetracycline drugs inhibit the inflammatory properties of normal bacterial flora—an action that contributes to their benefit in treating acne.[72] Members of this drug category are considered bacteriostatic because they interrupt protein synthesis. Subantimicrobial doses of doxycycline have been shown to be effective in treating moderate acne; in one study, the reported total decrease in lesions was 52% versus 18% with placebo ($P = .01$).[73]

The tetracyclines have multiple drug–drug interactions, the most common of which are discussed in the *Antimicrobials* chapter. When tetracyclines are taken simultaneously with agents that contain calcium, magnesium, aluminum, or iron, the absorption of tetracycline is inhibited and, in turn, its effectiveness is decreased. Sustained-release forms of doxycycline (Atridox, Oracea) and minocycline (Solodyn) are now available and may have fewer gastrointestinal effects for some women.

Erythromycin is used in the treatment of moderate acne. This macrolide antibiotic has a fairly narrow spectrum of action and is commonly prescribed in conjunction with benzoyl peroxide. Generally, this agent is prescribed orally as enteric-coated tablets because the base drug dissolves rapidly in the stomach. Combination oral contraceptives often are used as a treatment for women with acne; antibiotics may be used as well.[74] The concern that antibiotics might decrease the effectiveness of combination oral contraceptives appears to be based on conflicting evidence; research on this topic remains sparse. Archer has reported that pharmacokinetic data do not support an association between antibiotics and combination oral contraceptives, with the exception of rifampin (Rifadin).[73] While the failure rate in women taking combined oral contraceptives with tetracycline is higher than the failure rate with perfect use, it is still within the expected range for women with typical use.[75]

Metabolism of most antibiotics occurs in the liver via the CYP450 enzyme pathway. Erythromycin inhibits CYP3A4 and CYP1A2; consequently, it is involved in many drug–drug interactions. Notably, one of its most common drug–drug interactions is with carbamazepine (Tegretol). The effect of erythromycin on the enzymes that metabolize carbamazepine is substantial, and carbamazepine toxicity can occur, including major neurological deviations and rare, but possible cardiotoxicity. Because of this risk, these two drugs should not be taken concurrently. Drug–herb interactions involving erythromycin are also possible.[76] Providers are advised both to ask women about their use of complementary and alternative medications and to check for possible interactions between those products and prescribed medications.

Spironolactone

Spironolactone, a potassium-sparing diuretic, is a medication that has been used on an off-label basis to treat acne and hirsutism for decades.[77] While the exact mechanism of action is not understood, it is believed that this medication decreases sebum production by affecting the androgen receptor in the sebaceous glands. This ultimately leads to a decrease in acne formation. The usual dosing is 25 to 200 mg per day in 2 divided doses.

Adverse drug events noted with spironolactone include hyperkalemia, hypotension, diuresis, dehydration, rash, diarrhea, somnolence, and headache. Menstrual irregularities are not uncommon with use and are usually dose related. Because the medication is potassium sparing, women with renal insufficiency, hyperkalemia, or known

Table 26-10 Oral Anti-infective Agents Used to Treat Acne

Drug: Generic (Brand)	Dose Range	Indication	Side Effects/Adverse Effects	Special Considerations
Azithromycin (Zithromax)	500 mg as 1 dose then 250 mg daily for 5 days	MRSA	Diarrhea, nausea, severe allergic response including anaphylaxis or Stevens-Johnson syndrome	Use caution for persons with pneumonia, impaired liver or kidney function, or prolonged QT interval.
Erythromycin	250–750 mg 2 times/day	Acne	Gastrointestinal upset, decreased liver function, anaphylaxis, cardiac dysrhythmia	Diarrhea associated with use may indicate *Clostridium difficile* infection. Simultaneous use of clindamycin is contraindicated.
Clindamycin hydrochloride (Cleocin)	150–450 mg every 6 hours	MRSA	Rash, diarrhea, nausea, jaundice, pseudomembranous colitis	Simultaneous use of erythromycin is contraindicated. Use with caution for persons with history of colitis or atopy.
Cefaclor (Ceclor, Ceclor CD)	250–500 mg every 8 hours ER-375 mg every 12 hours	Skin or subcutaneous infections	Nausea, diarrhea, rash, arthralgia	Use with caution for persons with penicillin sensitivity or history of colitis.
Cefadroxil monohydrate (Duricef)	1 g/day	Skin or subcutaneous infections	Diarrhea, nausea, rash	Use with caution for persons with penicillin sensitivity or history of colitis.
Cephalexin (Keflex)	250 mg every 6 hours or 500 mg every 12 hours	Skin or subcutaneous infections	Nausea, diarrhea, increased liver enzymes	Use with caution for persons with penicillin sensitivity or history of colitis.
Ciprofloxacin (Cipro)	400–750 mg orally, every 8–12 hours	Adverse skin infections	Rash, diarrhea, nausea, dizziness, headache, tendinitis, peripheral neuropathy	Use with caution for persons with alkaline urine, seizure disorder, renal impairment, or exposure to excessive sunlight.
Levofloxacin (Levaquin)	500–750 mg daily	Adverse skin infections	Nausea, diarrhea, constipation, headache, hypoglycemia, prolonged QT interval, liver failure, anemias, tendon rupture, acute renal failure	Use with caution for persons with CNS disorders, steroid use, diabetes, or impaired renal function.
Amoxicillin/ clavulanate (Augmentin)	250 mg every 8 hours or 500 mg every 12 hours	*Staphylococcus aureus, Escherichia coli, Klebsiella* spp.	Nausea, diarrhea, vaginitis, headache, transient elevation of liver functions, transient anemia	Use with caution for persons with liver dysfunction. Contraindicated if prior liver symptoms occurred with Augmentin.
Dicloxacillin sodium (Dynapen)	250–500 mg every 6 hours	*Staphylococcus*	Nausea, gastrointestinal upset (take 1 hour before or 2 hours after eating)	
Trimethoprim–sulfamethoxazole (Bactrim)	1 DS 2 times/day	MRSA	Gastrointestinal distress, urticaria, rash, aplastic anemia, agranulocytosis, hepatic disease	Contraindicated during pregnancy in third trimester. Contraindicated for persons with folate deficiency. Use with caution for persons with G6PD deficiency or asthma.
Doxycycline (Vibramycin, Atridox)	100 mg 2 times/day	Acne vulgaris	Photosensitivity, lightheadedness, vertigo, gastrointestinal upset, diarrhea, vaginitis, pseudotumor cerebri, hepatotoxicity, CNS symptoms	In pregnancy, fetal tooth damage and bone damage are possible. Use with caution in persons with renal or liver impairment or SLE.
	50–100 mg 2 times/day	Acne rosacea		
	100 mg 2 times/day for 7 days	MRSA		
Minocycline (Minocin, Solodyn)	100 mg 2 times/day	Acne vulgaris Acne rosacea MRSA		
Tetracycline	250–500 mg 2 times/day	Acne vulgaris Acne rosacea		

Abbreviations: CNS = central nervous system; G6PD = glucose-6-phosphate dehydrogenase; MRSA = methicillin-resistant *Staphylococcus aureus*; SLE = systemic lupus erythematosus.

electrolyte imbalances are not candidates to use this agent. Some providers require women to have their potassium levels measured after 2 to 4 weeks of use to confirm safe levels, and then monitored annually with continued use. Women who experience signs of hypotension related to the diuretic effect of the medication should discontinue the drug.[77] Note that the common combined oral contraceptives known as Yasmin and Yaz contain the progestin drospirenone, an analog of spironolactone and are discussed in more detail in *Contraception* chapter.

Special Populations: Pregnancy, Lactation, and the Elderly

Beta-lactam antibiotics and most topical anti-infective agents are considered safe for use during pregnancy, although their dosing may need to be adjusted to accommodate for the increased rate of drug elimination. In contrast, tetracycline is contraindicated after 15 weeks' gestation because of the risks of fetal tooth and bone malformation.[14] Women who breastfeed while taking antibiotics should watch for infant complications such as diarrhea, dehydration, and thrush.[7] As mentioned earlier in this section, retinoids are contraindicated in pregnancy. Spironolactone should not to be used by pregnant women or those who are planning a pregnancy, because this agent is known to cause feminization in male fetuses.[14,17] Spironolactone is considered to be compatible with breastfeeding, but (theoretically) may decrease the maternal milk supply.[7] No special considerations with treatment of moderate acne vulgaris have been noted based on a woman's age.

Treatment of a Woman with Severe Acne Vulgaris

Isotretinoin (Accutane)

Oral isotretinoin (Accutane) is a naturally occurring vitamin A metabolite and the only acne vulgaris treatment that acts to correct all four pathologic mechanisms. Persons who need isotretinoin treatment should be cared for by a dermatologist or other provider skilled in the management of severe acne. This pharmaceutical is associated serious adverse reactions that can affect the individual who uses it. Because of these risks, clinicians who prescribe isotretinoin, wholesalers that distribute it, pharmacists who dispense it, and persons who take it are required by the FDA to be part of a risk management program called iPLEDGE[78] (Box 26-4).

Isotretinoin is highly lipophilic, and its absorption is enhanced if the drug is taken with a high-fat meal. Given the high risk of congenital abnormalities when isotretinoin is taken during pregnancy, women of childbearing age who take isotretinoin are counseled to use two methods of birth control simultaneously, and they are further advised not to donate blood while taking this medication.

Common side effects of isotretinoin include muscle aches (which occur in approximately 16% of persons who take this drug), dryness of the eyes, and dry skin and oral mucosa. Adverse effects include hyperlipidemia, an increased risk of depression, rarely psychosis or suicidal ideation, pseudotumor cerebri (especially if the agent is used in conjunction with tetracyclines), pancreatitis, hepatotoxicity, irritable bowel syndrome, decreased night vision, and hearing loss.

Isotretinoin is metabolized by the CYP450 enzymes. Clinically significant drug–drug interactions occur if it is taken concurrently with carbamazepine (Tegretol), vitamin A, methotrexate (Rheumatrex, Trexall), or a tetracycline. Use of isotretinoin may be associated with a decreased effectiveness of any hormonal contraceptive method, although this effect is individual and variable.[79]

Special Populations: Pregnancy, Lactation, and the Elderly

The most important contraindication to isotretinoin is pregnancy, because the risk of congenital malformations is high and includes craniofacial, cardiac, and central nervous system injuries.[80] Additional contraindications include breastfeeding and reproductive-age women at risk of pregnancy, such as those not using any form of contraception. There is no evidence available regarding the effect of isotretinoin during lactation.

Current studies, especially among the elderly, are being conducted to explore if any association exists between isotretinoin and behavioral changes, decrease in folate, and even potential increase in degenerative diseases. However, no strong evidence of such associations is available at this time.

Hirsutism and Alopecia

Hirsutism and alopecia usually are categorized as disorders of skin appendages. Hair growth occurs in three phases: (1) anagen—growth; (2) catagen—involution and transition between growth and resting; and (3) telogen—resting phase.[91] On the scalp, anagen lasts about 3 years and telogen lasts approximately 3 months. Because the hair follicles are not in the same cycle at the same time, humans continually lose and regrow hair. Most humans have approximately 5% to 15% of hair in the telogen phase at any one time.

Hirsutism

Hirsutism, or excessive hair growth, occurs when the anagen phase is extended and hair follicles become abnormally enlarged. Hirsutism can be an indication of a pathologic condition, such as polycystic ovary syndrome, Cushing's syndrome, and prolactin disorders, or it may be idiopathic and a simple cosmetic concern. Because hirsutism develops secondary to androgen action on hair follicles, disorders characterized by excessive androgen production must be ruled out before making the diagnosis of idiopathic hirsutism.

Nonpharmacologic treatments for hirsutism include bleaching, shaving, laser, chemical depilatories, waxing, and electrolysis. OTC chemical depilatories and waxing work but often cause skin irritation. Pharmacologic treatments for hirsutism include medications directed at the underlying pathology and medications that are specific for treating excessive hair growth.

Box 26-4 Isotretinoin

Soon after its discovery, isotretinoin (Accutane) was developed as a chemotherapeutic drug, and it remains an established cancer treatment even today. Isotretinoin kills rapidly dividing cells—a hallmark of cancer cells—which explains its utility in this indication.

In the 1930s, high doses of vitamin A were used to treat acne. The pharmaceutical company Hoffmann-La Roche conducted multiple studies and eventually created isotretinoin, which is a retinoid or vitamin A derivative. Isotretinoin was approved by the FDA in 1982 for treatment of acne.

The lethal action of isotretinoin on dividing cells became obviously problematic when it was used during pregnancy. The first report of an infant born with malformations that appeared to occur secondary to maternal use of isotretinoin during pregnancy was published in 1983. In 1984, the FDA issued a black box warning that recommended use of contraception 1 month prior to initiation of isotretinoin therapy and evidence of a negative pregnancy test prior to prescription of the drug.

Over time, additional adverse effects were revealed. In 2007, the FDA issued an additional black box warning that recommended users of isotretinoin be monitored for signs of depression or suicide ideation. In addition, pregnancies continued to occur among users of isotretinoin despite use of educational handouts and participation in voluntary risk management programs.

Today, all parties involved in prescribing or receiving this drug must register with the iPLEDGE program. The iPLEDGE program is a computer-based risk management program that helps prescribers and individuals who take the drug comply with monthly requirements that are reported to the program. Women wholesalers, pharmacists, and healthcare providers participate in the program's reporting requirements. All women who use isotretinoin are required to take the following steps:

1. Register with the iPLEDGE program and access it monthly to reply to questions about the program's requirements.
2. Obtain baseline liver function values and two negative pregnancy tests before receiving the first prescription.
3. Use two forms of contraception for 1 month prior to starting therapy, during therapy with isotretinoin, and for 2 months after discontinuing the drug. The primary contraceptive agent must be tubal sterilization, partner's vasectomy, or hormonal contraception (combined oral contraceptives or patch, vaginal ring, or implantable device). The secondary contraceptive must be a latex condom, diaphragm, cervical cap, or vaginal sponge.
4. Sign an informed consent form.
5. Review the medication guide and present evidence of a recent pregnancy test with negative results each month when the prescription is renewed. No more than a 30-day supply is prescribed.
6. Fill the prescription within 7 days of a negative pregnancy test and within 30 days of being issued the prescription.
7. Refrain from donating blood until 1 month after the drug is discontinued.
8. Agree not to share the drug or obtain it over the Internet.

Eflornithine (Vaniqa) was initially studied as a chemotherapeutic agent, but was found to have greater value in the treatment of African trypanosomiasis and potential use as part of a treatment regimen to reduce the incidence of recurrence of colon polyps. In the area of dermatology, however, eflornithine has been found to inhibit unwanted facial hair growth by irreversibly inhibiting ornithine decarboxylase, an enzyme involved in controlling hair growth and proliferation.[81] Eflornithine is marketed under the brand name Vaniqa as a cream with an active ingredient concentration of 13.9%. This cream is used as an adjunct in combination with nonpharmacologic methods of treatment. It is applied in a thin layer to the face and under the chin twice daily, with 8 hours elapsing between each application. After being massaged thoroughly until it is no longer visible, the area should not be washed for at least 4 hours. Hair growth returns approximately 8 weeks after the drug is discontinued. In clinical trials, older women obtained positive results similar to those obtained by younger women with use of eflornithine.

Eflornithine rarely causes side effects, but those reported include swollen patches of skin, headache, ingrown hairs, and itching, burning, or tingling rash. Contact dermatitis, nausea, and herpes simplex are rare. Eflornithine has no known drug–drug interactions.

Other medications used on an off-label basis to slow or stop hair growth include combined oral contraceptives and the antiandrogens spironolactone (Aldactone) and flutamide (Eulexin). Combination oral contraceptives are often the first drug of choice for reproductive-age women who also want contraception.[82] Treatment with antiandrogens takes approximately 18 months to achieve full effectiveness. Individuals using flutamide need to have liver function monitored. Spironolactone can cause hyperkalemia, but it is a rare side effect.

Ketoconazole (Nizoral) is also effective for treating hirsutism but is not commonly used because of its severe side effects including alopecia, abdominal pain, and hepatotoxicity. This agent is reserved for persons who have not responded to other drugs. Persons taking ketoconazole will need liver function tests on a regular basis while using this medication and should be screened carefully for use of other drugs because ketoconazole is associated with several drug–drug interactions. Additional information about this drug can be found in the *Antimicrobials* chapter.

Special Populations: Pregnancy, Lactation, and the Elderly

While women may be concerned about unwanted facial hair during pregnancy, it is best to avoid treatments for hirsutism while pregnant or breastfeeding.[14] Additionally, spironolactone should not be used by women who are seeking a pregnancy or who are pregnant because it is known to cause feminization in male fetuses. Reproductive-age women should use a reliable contraceptive method if taking spironolactone.[14,17] This medication appears to be safe in conjunction with breastfeeding, but (theoretically) may decrease the maternal milk supply.[7] No special considerations based on age have been reported in terms of treatment of women with hirsutism.

Alopecia

Alopecia, or thin hair, is known to occur in persons who have a genetic predisposition for hair loss; it often becomes evident during times of significant stress. *Alopecia areata* refers to hair loss in specific areas; *alopecia areata universalis* (also called *anagen effluvium*) describes the phenomenon of hair loss over the entire body (e.g., as associated with chemotherapy); and *telogen effluvium* is a sudden loss of hair in which the follicles are normal but growth is disturbed, as is commonly seen a few months after giving birth.

The etiology of alopecia is often elusive and may be a function of androgenicity or androgenetic alopecia, aging, genetics, metabolic disease, or anxiety. Androgenic alopecia, also known as female pattern baldness, is hair loss that occurs in the presence of androgen dihydrotestosterone, which increases as women age. Androgenic alopecia is caused by progressive shortening of the anagen stage and is the most common etiology of alopecia.[84]

Alternatively, alopecia may be idiopathic. In cases for which the etiology is known, treatment or removal of the underlying cause (e.g., diabetes) may aid in reversing the hair loss or thinning. Table 26-11 lists drugs that can cause hair growth or loss.[83] Traction alopecia is loss of hair resulting from trauma to the hair follicles associated with such behaviors as tight banding of hair or cornrows. This condition resolves with discontinuation of the causative behaviors. Telogen effluvium occurs when a number of follicles enter telogen prematurely and then shed their hair follicles. Drugs, fever, parturition, major illness, anorexia, and anemia can cause this type of alopecia and usual treatment is palliative. Hair loss typically starts 2 to 3 months after the inciting event with telogen effluvium; regrowth then follows, but usually takes several months. Female alopecia areata can be the result of an autoimmune condition characterized by sudden loss of patches of hair and the majority of women recover within 1 to 2 years with or without treatment.

Table 26-11 Selected Drugs Associated with Hirsutism or Alopecia[a]

Drugs Associated with Hirsutism: Generic (Brand)	Drugs Associated with Alopecia: Generic (Brand)
Anabolic steroids	Amiodarone (Cordarone)
Danazol (Danocrine)	Angiotensin-converting enzyme inhibitors
Glucocorticoids	Anticoagulants
Metoclopramide (Reglan)	Antifungal drugs
Methyldopa (Aldomet)	Acyclovir (Zovirax)
Phenothiazines	Beta blockers (propranolol and metoprolol)
Phenytoin (Dilantin)	Carbamazepine (Tegretol)
Progestins	Chemotherapeutic agents
Reserpine (Serpasil)	Heparin
Testosterone	Ibuprofen (Advil)
	Isoniazid (INH)
	Isotretinoin (Accutane)
	Lamotrigine (Lamictal)
	Levodopa (Larodopa)
	Lithium (Lithobid)
	Lopid (Gemfibrozil)
	Naproxen (Aleve)
	Phenytoin (Dilantin)
	Tricyclic antidepressants
	Valproic acid (Depakene)

[a] This table is not comprehensive as new information is being generated on a regular basis.

The majority of hair regrowth cosmetics are found in the form of shampoos or conditioners and occasionally oral formulations. Among the most popular OTC brands is Nioxin, a line of hair products that propose to act as an antiandrogenic product. However, no research supports these products' use for hair thinning or alopecia. Hair Genesis is a brand containing saw palmetto, a botanical with some preliminary findings that suggest it may be more effective than placebo; larger studies are needed to confirm this relationship.[85]

Medications for women with alopecia either affect the hair follicles via nonhormonal mechanisms or modify the action of androgen on the hair follicles by altering production, transport, or metabolism of androgens. Minoxidil (Rogaine) is an agent that is effective in stopping or slowing hair loss and promoting hair growth in men and women, primarily those with androgenically associated hair loss. Minoxidil prolongs the anagen stage of hair development and causes follicles at rest to grow. In a study published in 1994, women who used 2% minoxidil were up to twice as likely to report hair regrowth when compared to a control group of women who used a placebo agent.[86] Minoxidil is FDA approved for OTC use in a 5% formulation for men and a 2% formulation for women and men.[87] It is available in various vehicles such as sprays, foams, or liquids, with the recommended dose being 1 mL/spray twice daily. The mechanism of action for minoxidil remains unknown.

The most common side effect of minoxidil is itching on the scalp and dryness. Propylene glycol is likely the etiological agent for this scalp irritation.[83] Minoxidil is a vasodilator and a powerful antihypertensive agent. If taken orally, it can cause dizziness and cardiac arrhythmias. New hair growth will be lost when minoxidil is discontinued.

Finasteride (Propecia) and dutasteride (Avodart) inhibit type II 5-alpha-reductase, the enzyme that converts testosterone to dihydrotestosterone (DHT). These agents are not FDA approved to treat hair loss in women, but are more commonly used in Europe for this indication compared to the United States.[83] There is no evidence as to whether these drugs are of value for postmenopausal women with thinning hair.

Hair regrowth is not limited to the scalp. In late 2008, the FDA issued approval of bimatoprost ophthalmic solution 0.03% (Latisse) to treat inadequate eye lashes. Bimatoprost initially was used for management of borderline glaucoma. However, when this prostaglandin analog was used, a side effect of increased eyelash length, thickness, and darkness was found. This agent is packaged as a 3-mL bottle with sterile applicators and directions for one application nightly. Side effects and adverse effects include conjunctivitis, reversible darkening of the eyelid skin, and potentially irreversible increased brown pigmentation of the iris. Once the agent is discontinued, the eyelashes will return to pretreatment condition within a few weeks or months.

Special Populations: Pregnancy, Lactation, and the Elderly

Minoxidil and bimatoprost cannot be recommended as safe during pregnancy because of a lack of data; however, they are believed to be relatively safe for use by breastfeeding women.[7,14,15,17] Finasteride (Propecia) and dutasteride (Avodart) are contraindicated for use in pregnancy and should not even be handled by pregnant women because they can be absorbed topically and can cause birth defects in fetal reproductive organs, especially in male fetuses.[14,17] There is no indication that age modifies treatment plans for alopecia.

Infections of the Skin and Cutaneous Tissue

Bacterial skin infections can range from pyodermas (surface lesions) to cellulitis. These conditions primarily are caused by *Staphylococcus aureus*, and less commonly by *Streptococcus* species. *Pseudomonas aeruginosa* and *Candida* species can also be etiologic agents. *Impetigo* is a term commonly applied to describe shallow vesicles and pustules that develop in scattered areas of the face and extremities and that crust before healing. *Folliculitis* refers to infections at the hair follicle, which are characterized by redness and pustule development; it is discussed in the *Vulvar Disorders* chapter. *Furuncles* are nodules that form following folliculitis. *Carbuncles* (boils) are subcutaneous abscesses; this term is used when large lesions or groups of boils appear.

Infections limited to the epidermis and dermis, such as folliculitis, can be treated with topical antibacterial agents. Over-the-counter products can be used for occasional mild recurrences of bacterial infections. These products include bacitracin, neomycin, or a combination product such as polymyxin B/neomycin sulfate (Neosporin). Mupirocin (Bactroban) is commonly prescribed because it has little cross-resistance, due to the unique mechanism of action by which it binds to RNA during bacterial protein synthesis. Severe or persistent infections can be treated with oral antibiotics. Whenever skin infections do not resolve following use of a first-line treatment, the possibility of methicillin-resistant *Staphylococcus aureus* (MRSA) should be considered.

Furuncles and Carbuncles

Bacterial skin infections can be managed initially with warm compresses to promote localization and drainage; surgical incision and drainage may be needed if the lesions are fluctuant, regardless of their size. When antibiotic therapy is used, dicloxacillin (Dynapen), which is penicillinase resistant, is FDA approved to treat *Staphylococcus* infections and should be the first choice. A 7- to 10-day course usually is an adequate treatment course. Cephalexin (Keflex) and other first-generation cephalosporins can be used to treat most gram-positive organisms and gram-negative aerobes. Persistent infections and women with immune compromise should be treated with a second- or third-generation cephalosporin, and parenteral treatment should be considered. Clindamycin (Cleocin) and erythromycin (E-Mycin) are the drugs of choice for uncomplicated skin and subcutaneous infections for those women who are penicillin or cephalosporin allergic.[88] Carbuncles represent a deeper and more extensive infection and require longer courses of therapy at doses in the high end of the dosing range for the particular agent.

Cellulitis

Deeper infections of the soft tissue, which appear as poorly demarcated, swollen, erythematous, tender areas, are termed cellulitis. Skin disruption coupled with skin colonization or infection predispose women to develop cellulitis. Beta-hemolytic streptococci and *S. aureus* microbes are the most common pathogens found with cellutitis.[88] Women with significant disease should be evaluated for in-hospital parenteral therapy.

Methicillin-Resistant Staphylococcus aureus

Methicillin-resistant *S. aureus (MRSA)* can either colonize or infect the affected individual. Screening for MRSA colonization is not routine, but is recommended in communities where there is a high incidence of infection. When colonization is identified and treatment is appropriate, pseudomonic acid A, commonly known as mupirocin ointment (Bactroban), can be used. The ointment is applied to the lower nares, the most common carrier location, for a week.

Community acquired MRSA (CA-MRSA), unlike its nosocomial cousin, typically manifests as pustules, boils, and open infectious lesions. A MRSA skin lesion may be erythematous and painful, with or without drainage. When culturing skin lesions, it is essential to specify that sensitivities are desired even if the identified species is MRSA. Many laboratories have not yet recognized that agents other than vancomycin (Vancocin) are available for treatment of skin disease from CA-MRSA.

Empiric therapy for CA-MRSA, whether diagnosed or suspected, can include clindamycin hydrochloride (Cleocin), the long-acting tetracyclines doxycycline (Vibramycin) and minocycline (Minocin), and trimethoprim–sulfamethoxazole, which is often abbreviated as TMP-SMX (Bactrim, Septra). None of these treatments is FDA approved specifically for MRSA, but each has been reported to be effective against CA-MRSA.[89]

Clindamycin hydrochloride (Cleocin), a bacteriostatic lincosamide, is metabolized via CYP450 enzymes in the liver and, therefore, is associated with a higher risk of development of *Clostridium difficile* colitis than other antibiotics. Individuals should be cautioned to report any gastrointestinal disturbance and not to self-medicate to treat diarrhea. Clindamycin interacts with kaolin, a component of some antidiarrheal agents, which will decrease its effectiveness.[90]

Doxycycline (Vibramycin) and minocycline (Minocin) should not be used as first-line therapy unless sensitivity is documented because a high rate of resistance to these antibiotics has developed, particularly among gram-positive aerobes, including *S. aureus*. The tetracyclines are poorly metabolized and are excreted unchanged. Drug–drug interactions are discussed in the *Antimicrobials* chapter.

Absorption of the tetracyclines is decreased when these agents are administered simultaneously with antacids and iron-containing compounds.

TMP-SMX (Bactrim, Septra) is a combination of an antibacterial sulfonamide and a folic acid inhibitor. Its use as a treatment for MRSA is based on limited data, but this combination usually is employed when other agents are contraindicated. TMP-SMX should not be given to women who have folate deficiency. Multiple drug–drug interactions have been reported. Notably, cyclosporine (Neoral), methotrexate (Rheumatrex), warfarin (Coumadin), and thiazide diuretics should not be taken concomitantly with sulfonamides. Use with tricyclic antidepressants and antiseizure medications causes an increased risk of cardiotoxicity and should be avoided. Phenytoin (Dilantin) toxicity can occur when phenytoin is used with TMP-SMX. Oral antidiabetic medications may have greater hypoglycemic effect when administered concurrently with TMP-SMX.

Fungal Skin Infections

Dermatophytes

Tinea corporis, tinea cruris, and tinea pedis are superficial skin infections caused by dermatophytes (*Trichophyton* spp., *Microsporum* spp.). These microorganisms are spread through direct inoculation, including autoinoculation, and through fomites such as bed sheets or towels that carry scales shed from the lesions.

Tinea corporis (ringworm) initially appears as a flat, reddened area. As the infection spreads across the skin, the appearance becomes annular with a raised, scaly edge and central clearing. Isolated papules may remain in the central area.

Tinea cruris is found in the groin area. Initially it may have a moist, reddened appearance. Subsequently, central hyperpigmentation and a raised, papular, flaking edge develops. Occasionally, intense pruritus is associated with the infection.

Tinea can be confirmed at the point of care by performing a microscopic exam of skin scrapings treated with potassium hydroxide (KOH, also known as a KOH prep), which will demonstrate hyphae. This inexpensive rapid testing can differentiate between tinea and other possible skin disorders.

Both tinea corporis and tinea cruris are treated with topical antifungals for a period of 2 to 4 weeks. The use of corticosteroids should be discouraged. While the steroids may initially appear to improve the rash, their use will result in a worsening dermatitis, characterized by increased irritations, erosions, and pustular leasions.[91]

Tinea pedis (athlete's foot) is found in the intertriginous spaces on the plantar aspects of the feet. This condition is prone to secondary bacterial infections if left untreated. An inflammatory response at the site of infection suggests the need for antibacterial treatment as well as antifungal therapy. Any of the various topical antifungals will be efficacious. They can be procured over the counter or by prescription. Most topical antifungals are applied twice daily for 4 to 6 weeks (Table 26-10). All of the topical antifungals have the same mechanism of action: They attack the fungal cell wall. Severe or widespread infection can be treated with oral ketoconazole (Nizoral), itraconazole (Sporanox), terbinafine (Lamisil), griseofulvin (Gris-PEG), or fluconazole (Diflucan) weekly for at least 4 weeks. Tinea pedis is likely to recur; women should be cautioned to maintain good hygiene (wear shower shoes at the gym, dormitories, and pool) and dry feet carefully after showering.

Tinea versicolor (also known as pityriasis versicolor) is a chronic infection in which lesions are primarily found on the trunk, neck, and arms. The causative agent of the fungus is *Malassezia* species. The lesions are round or oval and slightly raised; they may be hypopigmented or hyperpigmented, depending on the woman's skin. In persistent cases, the lesions may coalesce into large patches. This fungal infection can be confirmed in the office by performing a KOH prep. Hyphae and spores will be present and are often referred to as having the look of "spaghetti and meatballs" on the slide. Onset of tinea versicolor is most common in adolescents and young adults. Following treatment, the skin will remain relatively less able to tan until the skin cells have gone through a complete replacement cycle. Relapses after treatment are common, particularly in summer and in warmer moist climates. Individuals should be reassured that the condition is not related to hygiene and is not communicable.

Treatment for tinea versicolor consists of a topical antifungal, usually ketoconazole 2% cream by prescription, or miconazole (Monistat) or clotrimazole dermal (Lotrimin). Dermal and vaginal preparations differ in the vehicle used, reflecting differences in absorption rates from various tissues. The choice of medication is based on the size of the affected area, as the prescription-only products come in a larger tube than the OTC products. Ketoconazole (Nizoral) is used once daily for 2 weeks, while the OTC products are used twice daily. Selenium sulfide shampoo (Selsun Blue) can be recommended, particularly if the affected area extends above the hair line. While oral therapy was a treatment in the past, it is no longer recommended. First-line treatment should be topical. If topical treatment is not effective, itraconazole (Sporanox) may be considered.[14]

Onychomycosis

Onychomycosis is a fungal infection of the nail and nail bed. Dermatophytes and *Candida* species are the most common organisms involved. Onychomycosis is often a secondary infection following tinea pedis.[53] When long-term oral antifungal therapy is needed, treatment usually is managed by a dermatologist or skin specialist, because of the potential severe adverse events. Topical preparations are unlikely to be useful for this condition in the form of monotherapy. Ciclopirox (Penlac) has been used for mild to moderate cases and is applied to the affected nail daily; once weekly, the nail is cleaned with alcohol to remove the buildup. Treatment duration can last from 6 to 12 months.[92] Ciclopirox inhibits intracellular transport of proteins and disrupts DNA and RNA synthesis. Itraconazole (Sporanox), fluconazole (Diflucan), and terbinafine (Lamisil) all can be prescribed based on effectiveness and cost considerations for an individual. The typical course of treatment lasts 6 weeks for fingernail infections and up to 12 weeks for toenail infections. Combination therapy using ciclopirox for several months plus a standard course of terbinafine, an oral antifungal, has been shown to improve outcomes significantly (mycological cure rate 88.2% combination therapy, 64.7% terbinafine only, $P = .05$).[93]

Topical Antifungal Therapy

Imidazole and triazole antifungals act primarily by disrupting the fungal cell membrane, with their secondary actions including inhibition of lipid synthesis and of exudative/peroxidative enzyme activity. These agents are only minimally absorbed. Whenever treatment with a topical antifungal agent is reasonable, it should be preferred to the oral regimen.

Oral Antifungal Therapy

Many individuals prefer the convenience associated with oral antifungal therapy (Table 26-12). However, the oral antifungals have significant adverse events associated with their use. These medications are metabolized in the liver, then eliminated primarily through renal excretion. Monitoring liver function tests is a common recommendation, as hepatitis is one of the major risks associated with such agents. The azoles, in particular, have many drug interactions, primarily related to drug metabolism and are discussed in more detail in the *Antimicrobials* chapter. One author lists them among the red flag drugs responsible for as many as 80% of clinically significant drug interactions.[94] Women taking these medications orally need to know that they should remind all their providers that the drug has been prescribed.

Special Populations: Pregnancy, Lactation, and the Elderly

Topical anti-infective agents generally are compatible with pregnancy, with the exception of tetracycline, a macrolide that should be avoided in pregnancy because of its effect on fetal teeth and bone. Topical antifungal agents are generally safe in pregnancy and breastfeeding when used for a limited period of time.[7,14,15,17] Nystatin is the drug of choice in pregnancy.[7] Limited data are available for ciclopirox and terbinafine, so their use should be limited in pregnancy. Oral antifungal agents are not recommended in pregnancy due to limited data on their use in this population.[14] Additionally, oral griseofulvin (Gris-PEG) is contraindicated while breastfeeding.[7] No modifications of treatment plans have been recommended for healthy older women.

Ectoparasites and Skin Infestations and Bites/Stings

Scabies

Scabies (*Sarcoptes scabiei*) is a common skin infestation caused by a microscopic mite that can be found worldwide. Infection is associated with crowding, sharing personal items such as clothing, and close physical contact. Older persons and anyone who has a weakened immune system is at risk of severe infestation. Healthcare workers are often exposed in the work setting. Symptoms include the appearance of burrows, particularly on the webbing between digits and in intertriginous areas or areas where there is constriction from clothing and severe itching. Intense irritation and itching as a result of hypersensitivity to the mites may lead to open sores. Presence of mites or eggs on KOH exam can immediately confirm the diagnosis. Symptoms take 4 or more weeks to develop following first exposure, as sensitization occurs. With reinfection, irritation may begin within 24 hours of exposure. Itching tends to be most severe at night and may cause sleep disturbances. Severe infestations in elderly individuals and immunocompromised persons may develop into crusted (Norwegian) scabies.

Pruritus may persist for several weeks after effective treatment. Persistent symptoms may also indicate incomplete treatment, overtreatment, resistance to the selected agent, or reinfection. Allergic reactions may be treated with an antihistamine and emollients. Reinfection requires retreatment—perhaps with a different agent—and

Table 26-12 Treatment of Skin Conditions with Antifungal Agents[a]

Drug: Generic (Brand)	Route of Administration/Dose	Side Effects/Adverse Effects	Special Considerations
Ciclopirox (Penlac, Loprox)	Topical gel 0.77%, shampoo 1% Gel applied every day for onychomycosis	Irritation, redness at site of application	Use caution for persons with diabetes or immune suppression.
Clotrimazole (Lotrimin, Gyne-Lotrimin)	Topical: cream, lotion, solution Apply 2 times/day	Skin irritation, erythema	
Clotrimazole/ betamethasone dipropionate (Lotrisone)	Topical cream Apply 2 times/day	Skin irritation, edema, erythema, secondary infection, paresthesia	
Econazole nitrate 1% (Spectazole)	Topical cream: Apply 1–2 times/day	Itching, erythema	
Fluconazole (Diflucan)	Oral 100 mg, 150 mg, 200 mg 150 mg PO once weekly for 4 weeks	Rash, nausea, vomiting, elevated liver enzymes	
Griseofulvin (Gris-PEG Fulvicin)	Oral: 330 mg PO once daily for onychomycosis	Rash, urticaria, edema, paresthesia, nausea, diarrhea, headache; development of leukopenia or hepatic toxicity	Contraindicated during pregnancy. Interacts with warfarin; many other drug interactions.
Itraconazole (Sporanox)	Oral: 200 mg PO every day for 1 week in divided doses (100 mg PO 2 times/day) Increase by 100 mg/day if needed Maximum dose: 400 mg/day	Congestive heart failure, photosensitivity, rash including Stevens-Johnson syndrome, lipid abnormalities, gastrointestinal symptoms, pseudomembranous colitis, hepatotoxicity, anaphylaxis, headache, dizziness, neuropathy	Contraindicated during pregnancy, congestive heart failure, and renal or liver disease. Many drug interactions.
Ketoconazole (Nizoral)	Topical 2% cream or shampoo	Pruritus, abdominal pain, nausea, vomiting; hepatotoxicity (rare); anaphylaxis (rare)	Many drug interactions.
Miconazole (Monistat)	Topical 2% cream	Pruritus	
Nystatin (Mycostatin)	Topical cream, ointment, powder: Apply 2 times/day		
Selenium sulfide (Selsun Blue)	Topical: Once daily for 7 days	Skin irritation	Contraindicated during pregnancy.
Terbinafine hydrochloride (Lamisil)	Topical: 1% gel, cream, solution Oral: 250 mg daily (onychomycosis only)	Headache, gastrointestinal, itching, taste disturbance; severe skin reactions including Stevens-Johnson syndrome, hepatotoxicity	Use caution for persons with kidney or liver disease, systemic lupus erythematosus, or immunodeficiency.

[a] This table is not comprehensive as new information is being generated on a regular basis.

education to ensure correct application of the medication and completion of environmental care instructions.[95]

All personal clothing, household linens, and surfaces (such as furniture) with which the scabies-infected person has had contact within the prior 3 days must be cleaned. Items that cannot tolerate hot-water washing should be sealed in a plastic bag for 2 weeks, dry cleaned, or placed in a hot dryer for more than 30 minutes. Furniture and carpets must be vacuumed and the vacuum bag immediately discarded. Seemingly unaffected family members should be treated prophylactically.

Treatments for Scabies

Table 26-13 summarizes the treatments for scabies. Permethrin cream 5% (Elimite), lindane (Kwell), and crotamiton (Eurax) are the three drugs approved by the FDA for treating scabies. Permethrin cream is the recommended first-line topical therapy. It is applied to the entire body below the neck for 8 to 14 hours before washing thoroughly; a repeat dose should then be applied in 7 to 14 days. Permethrin kills mites and lice by disrupting nerve cell membranes. Allergy to chrysanthemum plants is a contraindication to the use of permethrin—it is a derivative of these plants. Irritation, itching, or erythema may be exacerbated after treatment. In its meta-analysis of scabies therapy, the Cochrane Collaboration included 20 small trials and identified permethrin as the most effective topical agent, when compared to lindane and crotamiton.[96]

Crotamiton 10% cream or lotion is applied from the neck down; a second application is applied 24 hours later.

Washing is delayed for 48 hours after the second dose. This agent is not as effective as permethrin.

Today, lindane 1% cream (Kwell) is recommended only as a second-line therapy because of its potential side and adverse effects. Lindane acts as a CNS stimulant and an environmental pollutant. Because it has a long half-life, its use in the environment is of considerable concern, and it has been banned as a pesticide in more than 50 countries and some states (e.g., California). This agent has demonstrated neurotoxicity in humans and is contraindicated for persons who have a seizure disorder or skin lesions that would increase absorption of lindane. The FDA requires that lindane labels carry a black box warning notifying consumers of the risk of neurotoxicity.

Malathion 0.5% lotion (Ovide) is a pesticide whose use is suggested by the Centers for Disease Control and Prevention (CDC) but that is less effective than permethrin. Like permethrin, malathion acts on the nervous system of lice and mites. A contact hypersensitivity reaction can occur following its use. Use of heat to dry hair or exposure to open flames should be avoided, as the lotion is flammable.

Ivermectin (Stromectol) administered orally can be used to treat women with severe cases and those distinguished by open crusted lesions (Norwegian scabies). Like the other products used for treatment of mites, it is a neurotoxin, although it does not appear to cross the blood–brain barrier unless it is used for long periods or at high doses.

Treatment of crusted scabies requires two to three oral doses of ivermectin (Stromectol), usually in conjunction with topical permethrin or lindane, and it may also require use of a keratolytic agent and vigorous scrubbing prior to topical treatment.[75] All current sexual partners and family members with whom the woman has had close, prolonged, personal contact also should be treated.

Lice

Pediculus humanus capitis (head lice), *Pediculus humanus corporis* (body lice), and *Phthirus pubis* (crab lice or pubic lice) are most commonly transmitted via sexual contact, although sharing linens, clothing, or towels may cause nonsexual transmission of these parasites. Usually, the afflicted

Table 26-13 Treatments for Scabies and Lice

Drug: Generic (Brand)	Dose	Side Effects and Clinical Considerations
Benzyl alcohol (Ulesfia)	Head lice: 5% lotion—apply for 10 minutes, then wash off; reapply for 10 minutes, then wash off. May repeat in 1 week if needed.	Side effects: Irritation to skin and numbness at site of application.
Crotamiton (Eurax)	Scabies or lice: 10% cream—apply to whole body from neck down. Leave for 24 hours, then wash off, before reapplying for a second dose. Wash off the second dose 48 hours after application.	Side effects are uncommon; severe allergic reactions are rare. Has an antipruritic effect but diphenhyramine (Bendadryl) or calamine lotion are safer choices for itching until parasites are eliminated.
Ivermectin (Stromectol)	Scabies or lice: 3-mg tablets. 200 mcg/kg PO repeated in 14 days and second dose 14 days later if needed.	Seizures, muscle spasm, aplastic anemia. Absorption improved if taken with a fatty meal.
Lindane (Kwell)	Scabies or lice: 1% lotion or shampoo—apply in a thin coat to whole body from neck down for 8–12 hours, then rinse off. Most adults will need 30 mL. Shampoo: Apply to dry pubic hair and surrounding areas; allow to set for 4 minutes, lather for 4 minutes, then rinse; repeat in 7 days as needed.	Not recommended for first-line therapy. Seizures, muscle spasm, aplastic anemia.
Malathion (Ovide)	Scabies or lice: Apply for 8–12 hours to hair and scalp; let dry. Lotion is flammable—do not use electrical heat sources like a hair dryer or curlers when applying this lotion or apply it near open flames.	May induce stinging to the skin or scalp. Severe allergic reactions are rare.
Permethrin (Elimite)	Scabies: 5% cream—apply, then rinse off after 8–14 hours, followed by a second administration 1 week after the first application.	Itching and stinging on application.
Permethrin lotion (Nix)	Lice: Apply to the affected area and wash off after 10 minutes. Will continue to kill newly hatched lice for several days. May reapply in 9–10 days.	Treatment failure is common secondary to increasing resistance. Adverse drug events are uncommon.
Pyrethrin/butoxide (RID)	Lice: Apply to affected area and leave on for 5 minutes. Rinse off and reapply in 5–10 days because pyrethrins kill only live lice; they do not kill the eggs.	

woman will report nits (white louse egg cases resembling dandruff), moving lice, or genital itching.

Treatments for Lice

Permethrin 1% lotion (Nix) and pyrethrin with piperonyl butoxide (Rid) are FDA approved for treating head lice, and both are available as OTC preparations (Table 26-13). Resistance to this class of drugs has been increasing, however. Accordingly, women should be instructed to observe carefully for incomplete resolution or recurrences. In 2009, the FDA approved benzyl alcohol lotion for treatment of head lice.

Malathion 0.5% lotion (Ovide) applied for 8–12 hours and ivermectin (Stromectol) 250 mcg/kg orally in a single dose can be used as alternatives to permethrin (Nix) or pyrethrin/piperonyl butoxide (Rid) if there is hypersensitivity to the first-line therapies, but they are not desirable first-line therapies. Lindane (Kwell) is a neurotoxin that interferes with gamma-aminobutyric acid (GABA) neurotransmission, resulting in potential negative effects to the kidney, liver, and nervous system. Because of the risks associated with lindane (Kwell), its label carries a black box warning and an accompanying medication guide is included to help women understand the potential adverse effects. Lindane is only used in cases of resistance to other medications, when the need for this medication outweighs the risks.[67]

Correct application of lindane (Kwell) is critical. The individual should be instructed to take a warm bath or shower, dry off thoroughly, and then apply the lotion or cream to the whole body excluding the face, nose, and mouth. The scalp and groin should be included in the application. Mucosal surfaces should be avoided.

When shampoos are used, regardless of which product, manufacturers recommend washing the infested area and toweling it dry before applying and thoroughly saturating the bodily hair with the pediculicide shampoo. Permethrin or pyrethrin/piperonyl butoxide is left on for 10 minutes, after which time it should be thoroughly rinsed off with water and the area dried with a clean towel. Even after treatment, dead nits will still be attached to hair shafts. Nits may be removed with fingernails or a fine-toothed comb. Clean underwear, clothing, and bed clothing should be used, and retreatment in 7 to 10 days is recommended to ensure that all nits have been killed. Because the eggs may live up to 6 days, the treatment should be applied for the time recommended on the package for any of these agents. Hair conditioners or combination shampoo/conditioner should be avoided prior to applying medication to hair, and hair should not be rewashed for 1 to 2 days afterwards. Dead lice and nits can be removed from the hair using a fine-toothed comb, which should subsequently be soaked in hot water (temperature ≥ 130°F) for 5 minutes.

To prevent self-reinfection and transmission to others, close contacts of an infested individual, including family and close friends as well as sex partners, need to be treated. All clothing and bedding used within 3 days of first finding the lice should be dry cleaned or washed in very hot water (temperature = 125–130°F). Once clothing and bedding are washed, the laundered items need to be dried at a high setting for at least 20 minutes and ironed to rid them of any lice. Pubic lice die within 24 hours of being separated from the host. The floor and furniture should be vacuumed, but whole-house fumigation is not required.

Lice found in the hair or eyelashes and body lice are transmitted through close contact, or sharing combs, brushes, or clothing with an infected person. Itching usually is the first symptom. Treatment with permethrin or pyrethrin is the first-line therapy.

Fleas and Ticks

Fleas and ticks are common pests in households where animals live and in outdoor areas across the United States. Most individuals will notice flea bites on the ankles and lower calves; ticks may attach to any part of the body that is exposed.

The common flea species are primarily the cause of irritation, although some species can transmit diseases. Bubonic plague is a flea-borne illness, and cases have been reported, albeit rarely, in the United States. Occasionally, humans, like pets, will develop an allergic dermatitis in response to flea bites. Treatment includes topical lotions such as those discussed earlier for pruritus and topical antibiotics for secondary infection.

Ticks are primarily a source of painful sores at the site of a bite, but can cause a number of illnesses in humans; among the most common are Lyme disease and Rocky Mountain spotted fever. Lyme disease is the single most common tick-borne disease in the United States. When a tick can be reliably identified as *Ixodes scapularis* and has been attached for more than 36 hours, a single 200-mg dose of doxycycline (Vibramycin) can be given as prophylaxis within 72 hours in areas with high incidence of Lyme disease.[97]

Prevention is the best way to deal with possible exposure to fleas and ticks in the outdoors. *N,N*-diethyl-*m*-toluamide (DEET) can be found in many bug repellent formulations at 20% or greater concentrations and will last several hours after being applied to the skin. Permethrin-containing products are safe and can be applied to clothing, but not to skin, to prevent bug bites.

The key to treating both flea and tick infestations is treatment of the house and of pets, which are the common hosts and often the source of human exposure. Veterinary products and household fumigation products for fleas can be easily obtained.

Other Insect and Arachnoid Stings and Bites

Bees, wasps, spiders, bedbugs, and other small animals can produce irritating stings or bites. Unless a person is severely allergic to the venom, management focuses on removing any stinger left behind by a flying insect and treating the symptoms of pain or itching. Ice may relieve the initial painful reaction; antipruritics should then be applied, and a mild painkiller such as acetaminophen or ibuprofen given. Diphenhydramine (Benadryl) or a similar antihistamine may relieve the body's allergic response.

Persons who are aware that they have severe allergies to insect or spider bites should have a prescription for an epinephrine 1:1000 0.3-mg auto-injector (Epi-Pen) and carry it with them at all times.

Special Populations: Pregnancy, Lactation, and the Elderly

Several pesticides are available to women who have interactions with skin parasites. Both lindane and ivermectin are contraindicated for pregnant and lactating women and for young children. Compared with other available treatments, they have an unacceptably high risk of neurologic injury. At this time, permethrin, topical sulfur, benzyl benzoate, and crotamiton are the only medications that should be used by pregnant women with scabies.[14,17] Additionally, permethrin is the drug of choice to treat scabies in breastfeeding women, while lindane and malathion are contraindicated in this population.[7,15] While few data are available regarding use of DEET in pregnancy or lactation, this product appears to be safe later in pregnancy and among breastfeeding women.[7,14,15,17] Additionally, using DEET is less of a pregnancy risk than contracting an illness, such as West Nile virus.

Use of ivermectin by elderly women is controversial, as some studies have suggested increased risk of death with prolonged use by the older individual, whereas other studies have failed to replicate these findings.[98] No special considerations are needed with use of permethrin cream or malathion among older woman. The risk of neurotoxicity is increased among elderly women when compared to younger cohorts with the use of lindane, however, so this agent should be avoided for older women.[99]

Cosmeceuticals

A **cosmeceutical** is a cosmetic skin product with pharmaceutical properties. The U.S. federal government does not recognize the term "cosmeceutical"; rather, "cosmeceutical" is a portmanteau first coined in the 1970s that is now making its way into the popular vocabulary. Agents often mentioned as cosmeceuticals include nutritional supplements such as antioxidant vitamins as well as FDA-approved prescription drugs like retinoids. Other frequently named cosmeceuticals include phytoestrogenic foods and other botanicals.[88] Among the most common botanicals included this category are pomegranates, grape seed, horse chestnut, chamomile, comfrey, allantoin, and aloe. Some research has been conducted, but large rigorous clinical trials of these agents for specific dermatology indications have not been reported and are needed.

The growth of cosmeceuticals has underscored the emergence of a new field within dermatology. A quarter of a century ago, facial rejuvenation was the turf of cosmetic surgeons and plastic surgeons—professionals who were educated in subspecialties within the field of surgery. Today, however, dermatologists may limit their practices to cosmetics and medical aesthetics (also called esthetics). These clinicians and other providers who care for women are able to use pharmacologic agents to treat issues such as wrinkles and facial hair.

Wrinkles and Frown Lines

Facial Washes

Hydroxyl acids exfoliate the outer layers of stratum corneum. These agents may be recommended for treatment of women with mild acne or psoriasis, but they are more often used for so-called "chemical peels" because after exfoliation the stratum corneum becomes thinner, looks more luminous, and may be more elastic as with younger, healthy skin. However, the skin also may be more susceptible to irritation and burns.

Salicylic acid is a beta hydroxyl acid and, in contrast to alpha hydroxyl acids, penetrates sebaceous substance in hair follicles and acts as an exfoliant for the pores. This wash also decreases the density of microcomedones and has a stronger comedolytic effect than the alpha hydroxyl acids. It also has some anti-inflammatory effects. Alpha hydroxyl acids (AHA) are widely used by aestheticians.

Botulinum Toxin (Botox, Dysport)

More than 50 years ago, botulinum toxin type A was found to block acetylcholine release at the neuromuscular junction and inhibit a muscle from contracting for a period of several months. Currently, botulinum toxin (Botox, Dysport) is FDA approved to treat a number of medical conditions including migraines, spastic limbs, spastic bladder, excessive sweating, cervical dystonia, strabismus, and blepharospasm. In addition, botulinum toxin is used cosmetically to diminish wrinkles. The initial brand was Botox, which has since become a household name owing to its use by celebrities. An alternative brand, Dysport, received FDA approval in late 2008. Both agents are composed of *Clostridium botulinum* toxin A, although their concentrations are slightly different.

Botulinum toxin is the most lethal poison yet discovered.[100] Although the dose used for cosmetic purposes poses little risk, there have been several cases of botulism—that is, botulinum poisoning—primarily stemming from misuse of this product by untrained individuals. In 2009, the FDA initiated a black box warning that reviews the symptoms of botulism, which can be life-threatening, when the agent spreads beyond the area in which it was injected. This warning applies to both Botox and Dysport for all their indications, including cosmetic use.

Botulinum dosing depends on where the toxin is to be administered and what it is being administered for, as it can be mixed with other agents to create a synergistic effect. Cosmetic use of botulinum toxin generally is repeated every 3 to 4 months. Drug interactions are possible with other agents such as curare, but not with commonly used drugs. While many providers choose not to perform cosmetic injections, women may present with the side effects of poorly administered botulinum (Botox or Dysport). It is important to be able to recognize the side effects of these agents, as many women may not have an appropriate clinician perform the procedure. Some of these symptoms may not present until a few weeks after treatment and may be challenging to diagnose as a botulinum side effect. Even when botulinum toxin is administered with the proper technique, the medication can shift from the original injection site and cause complications in other body regions. As with any procedure that breaks the surface of the skin, infection is a risk. Additionally, allergic reactions including rash, itching, arrhythmia, and shortness of breath may occur. The medication may also cause drooping of the skin in the area of injection, which may appear to be a stroke-like effect. In rare cases, the recipient may have problems with speech and swallowing.[100]

Other treatments for wrinkles include injectable fillers to soften deep folds in the skin. In 2006, the FDA approved a hyaluronic acid preparation with the brand name of Juvéderm. This drug is used predominantly to fill smile lines and to augment lips, especially as they lose shape during aging. Some hyaluronic acid fillers are absorbed within 6 to 9 months, and newer products can last up to 2 years, but all require repeated treatments. An alternative nonanimal hyaluronic acid filler is Restylane, which is used in the same manner. Restylane is a gel created from *Streptococcus* bacteria.

Solar Lentigines, Freckles, and Other Areas of Hyperpigmentation

Skin whiteners have been popular for centuries. In some parts of the world, lighter skin is sought for cultural reasons.[101] Mercury was once used for this purpose, to the detriment of many unsuspecting individuals. In the United States, most women using whiteners today desire to diminish areas of hyperpigmentation such as solar lentigines (old age spots, liver spots) and freckles.

Alpha-hydroxy acids (AHAs) are naturally occurring or synthetic acids. In concentrations between 5% and 10%, these agents are found in OTC preparations. Higher concentrations require prescriptions, and concentrations of more than 50% are used for chemical peels by professional aestheticians. Although some evidence indicates that AHAs can decrease hyperpigmentation, these products also carry a risk of side effects that may include increased photosensitivity and even increased risk of hyperpigmentation. AHAs may be found in creams, lotions, and peels. These agents generally act as exfoliants and have been suggested for treatment of mild wrinkles secondary to photoaging.

Hydroquinone (Esoterica, Solaquin) is an agent that is known to inhibit melanin production. For many years, this agent was available over the counter in a 2% concentration or by prescription as a 4% concentration. It was often—and inappropriately—called a skin bleaching agent. In reality, hydroquinone does not bleach the skin, but rather disrupts hyperpigmentation due to melanin buildup. Although concerns have been raised regarding the potential carcinogenicity of this drug, few side effects have been reported with topical use, although it may increase the risk of photosensitivity. The usual dose is to apply cream twice daily to the affected area. The FDA recommended removal of this agent from the market in both OTC and prescription formulations, and it is no longer available in several American jurisdictions and is even banned in a number of countries.[102] It has not been formally removed from the U.S. marketplace, however, but instead is the subject of studies under the auspices of the National Toxicology Program.[103]

A newer skin lightening agent called lumixyl, or decapeptide-12, is proposed to inhibit tyrosinase, the enzyme responsible for initiating the overproduction of melanin that can cause uneven pigmentation and dark spots. Several studies have suggested that lumixyl may be effective as a skin whitener, especially in conjunction with sunscreens and other topical agents.[104,105]

Several other agents have been suggested as cosmetic whiteners or brighteners. Tretinoin, a retinoic acid, has been proposed to inhibit pre-melanin synthesis, but the agent makes skin more sensitive to ultraviolet A and B rays. Other proposed skin whiteners that may act as inhibitors of melanin (although studies are sparse) include arbutin, or hydroquinone-beta-d-glucoside, a natural product found in the leaves of several plants such as cranberry, pears, and blueberry; kojic acid, a by-product of manufacturing of the alcoholic drink sake; and azelaic acid, an agent found in wheat, rye, and barley. Antioxidants such as vitamin C and glutathione may aid in preventing oxidative damage to the skin, and the latter has been proposed to interfere with melanin production. *Cinnamomum subavenium* is a Chinese herb that may inhibit tyrosinase, an enzyme necessary for production of melanin. All of these treatments for women with hyperpigmentation need further study. If they are used, the general recommendation is to use one agent at a time and not combine them in case side effects are increased synergistically.[106]

The market for cosmetics and cosmeceuticals continues to grow at a rapid pace.[107] It might seem incongruous to the primary care provider who is accustomed to prescribing drugs as therapeutic agents that individuals may request prescriptions for cosmetic treatments. Nevertheless, even medications used for cosmetic reasons have potential risks, and the issue of informed consent for these agents, as well as all others, is paramount.

Special Populations: Pregnancy, Lactation, and the Elderly

Although cosmeceuticals are believed to be safe in pregnancy and breastfeeding, most providers will not perform elective cosmetic injections on a pregnant or breastfeeding woman.[7,14,15,17] No safety data have been reported for use of whiteners by a woman who is pregnant or breastfeeding. Therefore, it is best practice to recommend a good concealer, daily use of sunscreen, and avoidance of sun exposure until after birth and nursing have ceased. There are no documented special considerations for older women.

Conclusion

In addition to providing a protective covering for a woman's body, the skin serves a number of metabolic and sensory functions. The breadth of conditions that affect the skin, which range from normal maturation to injury to allergy and infection, presents a challenge for women's health-care providers. Correct diagnosis begins with an accurate description of the lesion or skin disturbance, determination of whether the onset is acute or chronic, and identification of any predisposing factors. Many of the conditions described in this chapter can be treated in the ambulatory setting if the provider is willing to use assessment skills. Confidence to recognize and manage common skin problems is an essential instrument today in the delivery of primary care to women.

Resources

Organization	Description	Website
American Academy of Dermatology	Includes the most frequently used clinical guidelines in the delivery of health care to individuals with various dermatologic conditions; some materials are limited to members	www.aad.org
Centers for Disease Control and Prevention	Federal government site that is constantly updated; it includes webpages and materials on such areas as MRSA infections, psoriasis, and other conditions, in a topical index arranged alphabetically	www.cdc.gov
iPLEDGE	Computer-based risk management program to prevent fetal exposure to isotretinoin; all women of reproductive age who are taking isotretinoin must register with the iPLEDGE program	www.ipledgeprogram.com
Apps		
More than 200 distinct dermatology apps exist on the Internet. Most of them are free, although not all are peer-reviewed. The main focus is on diagnosis rather than treatment. Following are some of the more popular apps.		

Organization	Description	Website
Apps		
Skin Scanning	Ability to take a photo and, using set guidelines, suggest a diagnosis	Multiple apps for this function exist, including Skin Scan, Minescraft Skin Scanner, Doctor Mole, and Skin Scanner. All can be located through use of a browser exploring dermatology apps.
iRash	Similar to scanning for skin cancer, but focuses on rashes	https://itunes.apple.com/us/app/irash/id344019104?mt=8

References

1. Butnaru CA, Kanitakis J. Structure of normal human skin. *Eur J Dermatol.* 2002;12(6):II-IV.
2. Mockenhaupt M. The current understanding of Stevens-Johnson syndrome and toxic epidermal necrolysis. *Expert Rev Clin Immunol.* 2011;7(6): 803-815.
3. Lonjou C, Thomas L, Borot N, et al. A marker for Stevens-Johnson syndrome: ethnicity matters. *Pharmacogenomics J.* 2006;6(4):265-268.
4. Law EH, Leung M. Steroids in Stevens-Johnson syndrome/toxic epidermal necrolysis: current evidence and implications for future research. *Ann Pharmacother.* 2015:49(3):335-342.
5. Mockenhaupt M. Stevens-Johnson syndrome and toxic epidermal necrolysis: clinical patterns, diagnostic considerations, etiology, and therapeutic management. *Semin Cutan Med Surg.* 2014;33(1):10-16.
6. Barrett ME, Heller MM, Fullerton Stone H, Murase JE. Dermatoses of the breast in lactation. *Dermatol Ther.* 2013;26(4):331-336.
7. Butler DC, Heller MM, Murase JE. Safety of dermatologic medications in pregnancy and lactation: Part II. Lactation. *J Am Acad Dermatol.* 2014;70(3):417-428.
8. Salasche S. Epidemiology of actinic keratoses and squamous cell carcinoma. *J Am Acad Dermatol.* 2000;42(1 pt 2):S4-S7.
9. Rigel DS. The effect of sunscreen on melanoma risk. *Dermatol Clin.* 2002;20(4):601-606.
10. Salasche S. Epidemiology of actinic keratoses and squamous cell carcinoma. *J Am Acad Dermatol.* 2000;42(1 pt 2):S4-S7.
11. U.S. Food and Drug Administration. FDA sheds light on sunscreens. http://www.fda.gov/ForConsumers/ConsumerUpdates/ucm258416.htm. Accessed November 25, 2014.
12. Hoare C, Li Wan Po A, Williams H. Systematic review of treatments for atopic eczema. *Health Technol Assess.* 2000;4(37):1-191.
13. Green C, Colquitt JL, Kirby J, Davidson P. Topical corticosteroids for atopic eczema: clinical and cost effectiveness of once-daily vs. more frequent use. *Br J Dermatol.* 2005;152:130.
14. Murase JE, Heller MM, Butler DC. Safety of dermatologic medications in pregnancy and lactation. Part I: pregnancy. *J Am Acad Dermatol.* 2014;70(3):401-414.
15. National Library of Medicine. LactMed: a TOXNET database. http://toxnet.nlm.nih.gov/newtoxnet/lactmed.htm. Accessed November 28, 2014.
16. Pacheco LD, Ghulmiyyah LM, Snodgrass WR, Hankins GD. Pharmacokinetics of corticosteroids during pregnancy. *Am J Perinatol.* 2007;24(2):79-82.
17. Park-Wyllie L, Mazzota P, Pastuszak A et al. Birth defects after maternal exposure to corticosteroids: prospective cohort study and meta-analysis of epidemiological studies. *Teratology.* 2000;62(6):385-92.
18. Pavon JM, Zhao Y, McConnell E, Hastings SN. Identifying risk of readmission in hospitalized elderly adults through inpatient medication exposure. *J Am Geriatr Soc.* 2014;62(6):1116-1121.
19. Heymann WR. Itch. *J Am Acad Dermatol.* 2006; 54(4):705-706.
20. Farage MA, Miller KW, Elsner P, Maibach HI. Functional and physiologic characteristics of aging skin. *Aging Clin Exp Res.* 2008;20(3):195-200.
21. Millikan LE. Alternative therapy in pruritus. *Dermatol Ther.* 2003;16:175-180
22. Lautenschlager S, Wulf HC, Pittelkow MR. Photoprotection. *Lancet.* 2007;370:528-537.
23. American Academy of Dermatology. Position statement on vitamin D. https://www.aad.org/Forms/Policies/Uploads/PS/PS-Vitamin%20D%20Postition%20Statement.pdf. Accessed November 30, 2014.
24. Maenthaisong R, Chaiyakunapruk N, Niruntraporn S, Kongkaew C. The efficacy of aloe vera used for burn wound healing: a systematic review. *Burns.* 2007;33(6):713-718.
25. Sforcin JM. Propolis and the immune system: a review. *J Ethnopharmacol.* 2007;113(2):1-14.

26. Huang W, Vidimos A. Topical anesthetics in dermatology. *J Am Acad Dermatol.* 2000;43(2):286-298.
27. Eidelman A, Weiss JM, Lau J, Carr DB. Topical anesthesia for dermal instrumentation: a systematic review of randomized controlled trials. *Ann Emerg Med.* 2005;46:343-351.
28. Singer AJ, Stark MJ. LET versus EMLA for pretreating lacerations: a randomized trial. *Acad Emerg Med.* 2001;8(3):223-230.
29. Bozzo P, Chua-Gocheco A, Einarson A. Safety of skin care products during pregnancy. *Can Fam Physician.* 2011;57(6):665-667.
30. Stockfleth E, Sterry W, Carey-Yard M, Bichel J. Multicentre, open-label study using imiquimod 5% cream in one or two 4-week courses of treatment for multiple actinic keratoses on the head. *Br J Dermatol.* 2007;157(suppl 2):41-46.
31. Rivers JK, Rosoph L, Provost N, Bissonette R. Open-label study to assess the safety and efficacy of imiquimod 5% cream applied once daily three times per week in cycles for treatment of actinic keratoses on the head. *J Cutan Med Surg.* 2008;12(3): 97-111.
32. Krawtchenko N, Roewert-Huber J, Ulrich M, Mann I, Sterry W, Stockfleth E. A randomized study of topical 5% imiquimod vs. topical 5-fluorouracil vs. cryosurgery in immunocompetent patients with actinic keratoses: a comparison of clinical and histologic outcomes including 1-year follow-up. *Br J Dermatol.* 2007;157(suppl 2):34-40.
33. Jury CS, Ramraka-Jones VS, Gudi V, Herd RM. A randomized trial of topical 5% 5-fluorouracil (Efudix cream) in the treatment of actinic keratoses comparing daily versus weekly treatment. *Br J Dermatol.* 2005;153(4):808-810.
34. Lorenzen S, Pauligk C, Homann N, Schmalenberg H, Jäger E, Al-Batran SE. Feasibility of perioperative chemotherapy with infusional 5-FU, leucovorin, and oxaliplatin with (FLOT) or without (FLO) docetaxel in elderly patients with locally advanced esophagogastric cancer. *Br J Cancer.* 2013;108(3):519-526.
35. Rigel DS, Russak J, Friedman R. The evolution of melanoma diagnosis: 25 years beyond the ABCDs. *CA: A Cancer J Clin.* 2010;60(5):301-316.
36. Pfahlberg A, Kölmel KF, Gefeller O, Febim Study Group. Timing of excessive ultraviolet radiation and melanoma: epidemiology does not support the existence of a critical period of high susceptibility to solar ultraviolet radiation-induced melanoma. *Br J Dermatol.* 2001;144(3):471-475.
37. Hanefin JM, Reed ML, Eczema Prevalence and Impact Working Group. A population-based survey of eczema prevalence in the United States. *Dermatitis.* 2007;18(2):82-91.
38. Roberts W. Dermatologic problems of older women. *Dermatol Clin.* 2006;24:271-280.
39. Williams, HC. Clinical practice: atopic dermatitis. *N Engl J Med.* 2005;352:2314-2324.
40. Loden M. Role of topical emollients and moisturizers in the treatment of dry skin barrier disorders. *Am J Clin Dermatol.* 2003;4(11):771-788.
41. Lucky AW, Leach AD, Laskazruski P, Wench H. Use of an emollient as a steroid sparing agent in the treatment of mild to moderate atopic dermatitis in children. *Pediatr Dermatol.* 1997;14:321-324.
42. Draelos Z. The effect of ceramide-containing skin care products on eczema resolution duration. *Cutis.* 2008;81(1):87-91.
43. Berth-Jones J, Damstra RJ, Golsch S, et al. Twice weekly fluticasone propionate added to emollient maintenance treatment to reduce risk of relapse in atopic dermatitis: randomised, double blind, parallel group study. *BMJ.* 2003;326:1367.
44. Ashcroft DM, Dimmock P, Garside R, et al. Efficacy and tolerability of topical pimecrolimus and tacrolimus in the treatment of atopic dermatitis: meta-analysis of randomised controlled trials. *BMJ.* 2005;330: 516-521.
45. Kawakami T, Soma Y, Morita E, et al. Safe and effective treatment of refractory facial lesions in atopic dermatitis using topical tacrolimus following corticosteroid discontinuation. *Dermatology.* 2001;203:32-37.
46. Nakahara T, Koga T, Fukagawa S, Uchi H, Furue M. Intermittent topical corticosteroid/tacrolimus sequential therapy improves lichenification and chronic papules more efficiently than intermittent topical corticosteroid/emollient sequential therapy in patients with atopic dermatitis. *J Dermatol.* 2004;31:524-528.
47. Furue M, Terao H, Moroi Y, et al. Dosage and adverse effects of topical tacrolimus and steroids in daily management of atopic dermatitis. *J Dermatol.* 2004;31:277-283.
48. Apfelbacher CJ, van Zuuren EJ, Fedorowicz Z, Jupiter A, Matterne U, Weisshaar E. Oral H1 antihistamines as monotherapy for eczema. *Cochrane Database Syst Rev.* 2013;2:CD007770. doi:10.1002/14651858.CD007770.
49. Gelmetti C. Therapeutic moisturizers as adjuvant therapy for psoriasis patients. *Am J Clin Dermatol.* 2009;10(suppl 1):7-12.

50. Saary J, Qureshi R, Palda V, et al. A systematic review of contact dermatitis treatment and prevention. *J Am Acad Dermatol.* 2005;53:845.
51. Gupta AK, Nicol K, Batra R. The role of antifungal agents in the treatment of seborrheic dermatitis. *Am J Clin Dermatol.* 2004;5(6):417-422.
52. Warshaw EM, Wohlhuter RJ, Liu A, et al. Results of a randomized, double-blind, vehicle-controlled efficacy trial of pimecrolimus cream 1% for the treatment of moderate to severe facial seborrheic dermatitis. *J Am Acad Dermatol.* 2007;57(2):257-264.
53. Haneke E, Roseeuw D. The scope of onychomycosis: epidemiology and clinical features. *Int J Dermatol.* 1999;38(suppl 2):7-12.
54. Scapparo E, Quadri G, Virno G, Orific C, Milani M. Evaluation of the efficacy and tolerability of oral terbinafine (Dsakil) in patients with seborrhoeic dermatitis: a multicentre randomized, investigator-blinded, placebo-controlled trial. *Br J Dermatol.* 2001;144:854-857.
55. Baysal V, Yildrim M, Ozcanli C, Ceyhan AM. Itraconazole in the treatment of seborrheic dermatitis: a new treatment modality. *Int J Dermatol.* 2004;43(1):63-66.
56. Agency for Heathcare Research and Quality. National Guideline Clearinghouse: psoriasis. http://www.guideline.gov/browse/by-topic-detail.aspx?id=26919&ct=1. Accessed November 30, 2014.
57. Lebwohl M, Callen JP. Obesity, smoking and psoriasis. *JAMA.* 2006;295(2):208-210.
58. Lebwohl M. Psoriasis. *Lancet.* 2003;361:1197-1204.
59. Owen CM, Chalmers R, O'Sullivan T, Griffiths CEM. Antistreptococcal interventions for guttate and chronic plaque psoriasis. *Cochrane Database Syst Rev.* 2000;2:CD001976. doi:10.1002/14651858.CD001976.
60. Douglas WS, Poulin Y, Decroix J, et al. A new calcipotriol/betamethasone formulation with rapid onset of action was superior to monotherapy with betamethasone dipropionate or calcipotriol in psoriasis vulgaris. *Acta Dermato-Venereologica.* 2002; 82(2):131-135.
61. Heydendael VMR, Spuls PI, Opmeer BC, et al. Methotrexate versus cyclosporine in moderate-to-severe chronic plaque psoriasis. *N Engl J Med.* 2003; 349:658-665.
62. Haider A, Shaw JC. Treatment of acne vulgaris. *JAMA.* 2004;292:726-735.
63. Huber J, Walch K. Treating acne with oral contraceptives: use of lower doses. *Contraception.* 2006; 73(1):23-29.
64. Redmond GP, Olson WH, Lippman JS, Kafrissen ME, Jones TM, Jorizzo J. L. Norgestimate and ethinyl estradiol in the treatment of acne vulgaris: a randomized, placebo-controlled trial. *Obstet Gynecol.* 1997;89(4):615-622.
65. Thorneycroft IH, Gollnick H, Schellschmidt I. Superiority of a combined contraceptive containing drospirenone to a triphasic preparation containing norgestimate in acne treatment. *Cutis.* 2004; 74:123-130.
66. Winkler UH, Ferguson H, Mulders JAPA. Cycle control, quality of life and acne with two low-dose oral contraceptives containing 20 μg ethinyl estradiol. *Contraception.* 2004;69:469-476.
67. Ozolins M, Eady EA, Avery A, et al. Randomised controlled multiple treatment comparison to provide a cost-effectiveness rationale for the selection of antimicrobial therapy in acne. *Health Technol Assess.* 2005;9(1): iii-212.
68. Leyden JJ, Hickman JG, Jarratt MT, Stewart DM, Levy SF. The efficacy and safety of a combination benzoyl peroxide/clindamycin gel compared with benzoyl peroxide alone and a benzoyl peroxide/erythromycin combination product. *J Cutan Med Surg.* 2001;5(1): 37-42.
69. Leyden JJ, Krochmal L, Yaroshinsky A. Two randomized, double-blind, controlled trials of 2219 subjects to compare the combination clindamycin/tretinoin hydrogel with each agent alone and vehicle for the treatment of acne vulgaris. *J Am Acad Dermatol.* 2006;54:73-81.
70. Ozolins M, Eady EA, Cunliffe WJ, et al. Comparison of five antimicrobial regimens for the treatment of mild to moderate inflammatory facial acne vulgaris in the community: randomised controlled trial. *Lancet.* 2004;364:2188-2195.
71. Cooper AJ. Systematic review of *Propionibacterium acnes* resistance to systemic antibiotics. *Med J Aust.* 1998;169:259-261.
72. Webster G, del Rosso JQ. Anti-inflammatory activity of tetracyclines. *Dermatol Clin.* 2007;25:133-135.
73. Skidmore R, Kovach R, Walker C, et al. Effects of subantimicrobial-dose doxycycline in the treatment of moderate acne. *Arch Dermatol.* 2003;139:459-464.
74. Lam C, Zaenglein AL. Contraceptive use in acne. *Clin Dermatol.* 2014;32(4):502-515.
75. Archer JSM, Archer MD. Oral contraceptive efficacy and antibiotic interaction: a myth debunked. *J Am Acad Dermatol.* 2002;46(6):917-923.
76. Pai MP, Momary KM, Rodvold KA. Antibiotic drug interactions. *Med Clin North Am.* 2006;90:1223-1255.
77. Lessner E, Fisher S, Kobraei K, et al. Spironolactone and topical retinoids in adult female cyclical acne. *J Drugs Dermatol.* 2014;13(2):126-129.

78. Werner CA, Papic MJ, Ferris LK, et al. Women's experiences with isotretinoin risk reduction counseling. *JAMA Dermatol.* 2014;150(4):366-371.
79. Hendrix CW, Jackson KA, Whitmore E, et al. The effect of isotretinoin on the pharmacokinetics and pharmacodynamics of ethinyl estradiol and norethindrone. *Clin Pharmacol Ther.* 2004;75(5):464-475.
80. Bérard A, Azoulay L, Koren G, Blais L, Perrault S, Oraichi D. Isotretinoin, pregnancies, abortions, and birth defects: a population-based perspective. *Br J Clin Pharmacol.* 2007;63(2):196-205.
81. Hunter MH, Carek PJ. Evaluation and treatment of women with hirsutism. *Am Fam Physician.* 2003;67:2565-2572.
82. Blume-Peytavi U, Hahn S. Medical treatment of hirsutism. *Dermatol Therap.* 2008;21(5):329-339.
83. Shapiro J. Hair loss in women. *N Engl J Med.* 2007; 357:1620-1630.
84. Camacho-Martines F. Hair loss in women. *Semin Cutan Med Surg.* 2009;28:19-32.
85. Prager N, Bickett K, French N, Marcovici G. A randomized, double-blind, placebo-controlled trial to determine the effectiveness of botanically derived inhibitors of 5-alpha-reductase in the treatment of androgenetic alopecia. *J Altern Complement Med.* 2006;12(2):199.
86. Bandaranayake I, Mirmirani P. Hair loss remedies: separating fact from fiction. *Cutis.* 2004;73:107-114.
87. DeVillez RL, Jacobs JP, Szpunar CA, Warner ML. Androgenetic alopecia in the female: treatment with 2% topical minoxidil solution. *Arch Dermatol.* 1994;130:303-307.
88. Rayner C, Munckhof WJ. Antibiotics currently used in the treatment of infections caused by *Staphylococcus aureus. Internal Med J.* 2005;35(suppl 2):S1-S16.
89. Centers for Disease Control and Prevention. Methicillin-resistant *Staphylococcus aureus* (MRSA). http://www.cdc.gov/mrsa/. Accessed December 1, 2014.
90. Fleisher D, Li C, Zhou Y, Pao LH, Karim A. Drug, meal and formulation interactions influencing drug absorption after oral administration: clinical implications. *Clin Pharmacokinet.* 1999;36(3):233-254.
91. Gupta RA. Management of superficial fungal infections. *Am J Clin Dermatol.* 2004;5(4):227-237.
92. Baran R, Kaoukhov A. Topical antifungal drugs for the treatment of onychomycosis: an overview of current strategies for monotherapy and combination therapy. *J Eur Acac Dermatol Venereol.* 2005;19:25-29.
93. Avner S, Nir N, Henri T. Combination of oral terbinafine and topical ciclopirox compared to oral terbinafine for the treatment of onychomycosis. *J Dermatol Treat.* 2005;16:327-330.
94. Berranco VP. Update on clinically significant drug interactions in dermatology. *J Am Acad Dermatol.* 2006; 54(4):676-684.
95. Chosidow O. Scabies. *N Engl J Med.* 2006;354(16): 1718-1727.
96. Strong M, Johnstone P. Interventions for treating scabies. *Cochrane Database Syst Rev.* 2007;3:CD000320. doi:10.1002/14651858.CD000320.pub2.
97. Wormser GP, Dattwyler RJ, Shapiro ED, et al. The clinical assessment, treatment, and prevention of Lyme disease, human granulocytic anaplasmosis, and babesiosis: clinical practice guidelines by the Infectious Diseases Society of America. *Clin Infect Dis.* 2006;43:1089-1134.
98. Diazgranados JA, Costa JL. Deaths after ivermectin treatment. *Lancet.* 1997;349:1698.
99. Wooltorton E. Concerns over lindane treatment for scabies and lice. *CMAJ.* 2003;168(11):1447.
100. Barbano R. Risks of erasing wrinkles: buyer beware. *Neurology.* 2006;67:E17-E18.
101. Mendoza RL. The skin whitening industry in the Philippines. *J Public Health Policy.* 2014;35(2): 219-238.
102. Desmedt B, Van Hoeck E, Rogiers V, et al. Characterization of suspected illegal skin whitening cosmetics. *J Pharm Biomed Anal.* 2014;90:85-91.
103. U.S. Food and Drug Administration. Hydroquinone studies under the National Toxicology Program (NTP). http://www.fda.gov/AboutFDA/CentersOffices/OfficeofMedicalProductsandTobacco/CDER/ucm203112.htm. Accessed November 25, 2014.
104. Kassim AT, Hussain M, Goldberg DJ. Open-label evaluation of the skin-brightening efficacy of a skin-brightening system using decapeptide-12. *J Cosmet Laser Ther.* 2012;14(2):117-121.
105. Bhatia A, Hsu JTS, Hantash BM. Combined topical delivery and dermal infusion of decapeptide-12 accelerates resolution of post-inflammatory hyperpigmentation in skin of color. *J Drugs Dermatol.* 2014; 13(1):84-85.
106. Watanabe F, Hashizume E, Chan GP, Kamimura A. Skin-whitening and skin-condition-improving effects of topical oxidized glutathione: a double-blind and placebo-controlled clinical trial in healthy women. *Clin Cosmet Investig Dermatol.* 2014;7: 267-274.
107. Gao XH, Zhang L, Wei H, Chen HD. Efficacy and safety of innovative cosmeceuticals. *Clin Dermatol.* 2008;26(4):367-374.

© Sofimanning/Shutterstock

27

Ophthalmic and Otic Disorders

Alexa A. Gorwoda

Based on the chapter by Patrick J. M. Murphy and Therese M. Horan in the first edition of Pharmacology for Women's Health

Chapter Glossary

Cerumen Earwax.

Closed-angle glaucoma Condition that occurs when the pupil dilates to such an extent that the iris leans against the cornea and blocks the outflow of aqueous humor.

Cycloplegic drugs Pharmaceuticals that paralyze the ciliary body and prevent the lens from changing shape. They are used during eye examinations and surgery on the eye.

Dry eye Condition that results from inadequate levels of tear film.

Exophthalmos Bulging of the eye anteriorly out of the orbit.

Fixed-dose combinations Medications that contain two different drugs, usually a beta blocker and prostaglandin analogue, in one formulation.

Glaucoma Group of disorders characterized by vision loss that is secondary to damage to the optic nerve. This damage occurs when pressure in the aqueous humor increases and interferes with the blood flow to the optic nerve.

Miotics Drugs that cause constriction of the pupil.

Mydriasis Excessive dilation of the pupil.

Nystagmus Involuntary eye movement.

Open-angle glaucoma Increased intraocular pressure that results from a blockage in the trabecular meshwork or Schlemm's canal.

Ophthalmia neonatorum Gonorrheal conjunctivitis. Contracted by a newborn during vaginal birth if the woman is infected with *Neisseria gonorrhoeae.*

Otalgia Ear pain or earache.

Sympathomimetic mydriatic drugs Pharmaceuticals that cause the iris's radial muscle to contract, which results in pupil dilation. Sympathomimetic mydriatics do not paralyze the ciliary muscle and consequently do not prevent lens movement or refocusing during the examination.

Introduction

The use of pharmaceuticals to treat disorders affecting the eye and the ear often involves specialized approaches to pharmacotherapy. Although many of the medications discussed in this chapter are presented in detail in other chapters, the route of administration, pharmacokinetics, and pharmacodynamics of a drug may all be modified when the agent is used to treat an ophthalmic or otic condition. Ophthalmic medications are frequently used to treat conjunctivitis, dry eye, and glaucoma. Drugs used for otic disorders include treatments for acute otitis media and otitis externa.

Structure of the Eye

Medications used to treat ophthalmic disorders primarily act in the anterior chamber of the eye, affecting the ciliary body, trabecular meshwork and Schlemm's canal, iris, and aqueous humor. Therefore, a brief review of the anatomy of the eye is in order (Figure 27-1).

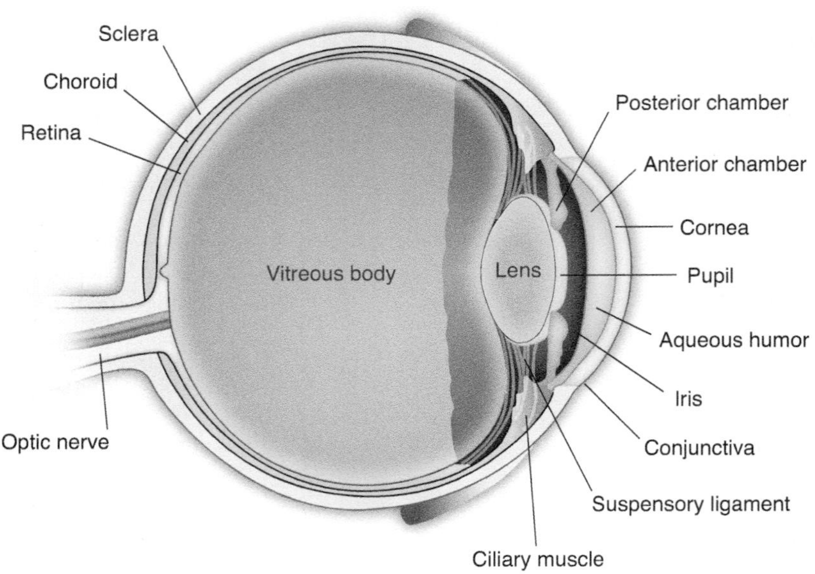

Figure 27-1 Anatomy of the eye.

The eye is an irregular sphere. Its wall consists of three layers: the sclera, the choroid, and the retina. The conjunctiva is the squamous epithelial membrane that lines the eyelids and covers the sclera. The sclera is the outermost layer of the eye; it is made of tough, white connective tissue and surrounds the sphere of the eyeball except for where the cornea lies. The choroid is a vascular, dark brown membrane that lies between the retina and the sclera. Anteriorly, the choroid differentiates into the ciliary body. The ciliary body surrounds the lens and is composed of the ciliary muscle, which controls the shape of the lens, and the ciliary processes, which contain the capillaries, which themselves secrete the fluid that makes up the aqueous humor. The lens is a transparent crystalline curved structure located behind the iris and pupil; it is attached to the ciliary body by ligaments.

The aqueous humor is the watery fluid that circulates in the anterior and posterior chambers of the eye. The aqueous humor transports oxygen and nutrients to the lens and cornea, facilitates the removal of wastes, and maintains the convex shape of the cornea. The aqueous humor is secreted by the ciliary processes in the posterior chamber, traverses around the iris and through the pupil into the anterior chamber, and ultimately drains into the venous system primarily through the trabecular meshwork and Schlemm's canal.

Under normal physiologic conditions, an intraocular pressure of 10–20 mm Hg results from the presence of the aqueous humor. A constant intraocular pressure is maintained when the rate of aqueous humor production by the ciliary body is equivalent to the rate of drainage through the trabecular meshwork. Antiglaucoma medications are able to decrease intraocular pressure by either decreasing aqueous humor production or increasing aqueous humor outflow. While the majority of outflow occurs through Schlemm's canal, a fraction (< 20%) of the aqueous humor drains through the iris root (i.e., the uveoscleral pathway), which is subject to pharmacotherapeutic modulation.

Autonomic Nervous System Innervation

Regions of the eye are innervated by both the sympathetic and the parasympathetic nervous systems. Activation of muscarinic cholinergic receptors in the ciliary muscle causes contraction, thereby focusing the lens for near vision, while activation of muscarinic receptors in the iris sphincter muscle results in pupil constriction, also called miosis. Drugs that cause pupil constriction are called **miotics**. Contraction of the ciliary muscle leads to increased opening of pores in the trabecular meshwork, which increases aqueous humor outflow and subsequently reduces intraocular pressure. Alpha1-adrenergic receptor activation in the iris radial muscle causes muscle contraction, resulting in **mydriasis** (excessive dilation of the pupil), which facilitates increased outflow of aqueous humor. Aqueous humor outflow may also be increased in the uveoscleral pathway by activation of the sympathetic nervous system. Beta$_1$- and beta$_2$-adrenergic receptors are present on the ciliary epithelium that covers the ciliary processes, and their stimulation facilitates aqueous humor secretion. Inhibition of beta receptors decreases secretion, leading to a lowering of intraocular pressure.

The eye produces a wide range of pharmacokinetically significant enzymes, including acetylcholinesterase, carbonic anhydrase, catechol-*O*-methyltransferase (COMT), and monoamine oxidase (MAO), all of which affect drug metabolism. Several medications discussed in this chapter are metabolized by these enzymes, either from an active drug to an inactive metabolite or from an inactive prodrug to an active compound.

Effects of Ocular Physiology on Pharmacokinetic Properties

The pharmacokinetics of topically administered ophthalmic medications deserves special comment. The eye has several barriers and efflux pumps that make drug delivery to various parts of the eye challenging.[1] Most agents intended for ophthalmic use are prepared in an aqueous formulation and absorbed into the tear film and epithelium via passive diffusion. Hydrophobic gels and ointments may be used to extend the duration that a medication remains on the eye surface.[1] Following topical administration, high concentrations of ophthalmic drugs amass in the aqueous humor and are subsequently distributed through the trabecular meshwork. These drugs may be absorbed into the bloodstream through the nasal mucosa and, in turn, distributed systemically throughout the body. Topically administered ophthalmic drugs that are absorbed into the bloodstream through this pathway bypass first-pass metabolism in the liver, which may lead to high serum drug concentrations. Gentle eyelid closure following drug application increases drug exposure to the eye and decreases systemic absorption. Instructions for self-administration of topical ophthalmic medications are presented in Box 27-1.

Box 27-1 Self-Administration of Topical Ophthalmic Medications

1. Prior to administration, wash hands with soap and water.
2. If the medication is formulated as a suspension, thoroughly shake the bottle.
3. The dropper tip should be treated as a sterile applicator, and it should not touch the eye or come into contact with any surface.
4. With the head tilted back, depress the lower eyelid and gently squeeze the dropper, releasing one drop into the eye at a time. Rest with the eyes closed for at least 1–2 minutes before administering the next drop of the same medication.
5. Excess medication can be wiped away from the eye with a clean tissue.
6. To allow maximum absorption, 10–15 minutes should transpire between topical administrations of different medications.

Conjunctivitis

Conjunctivitis is an inflammation of the conjunctiva (i.e., the mucous membrane that lines the inside surface of the eyelid and surrounding tissue) and is the most common diagnosis among individuals who present with unilateral or bilateral red eyes and accompanying discharge. Conjunctivitis can be infectious (viral or bacterial) or non-infectious (allergic, mechanical irritation, toxic exposure, neoplastic, or immune-mediated). In addition, conjunctivitis can be acute or chronic. It can be a primary disorder, or it may occur secondary to a systemic infection such as gonorrhea or chlamydia. Conjunctivitis is typically benign and self-limiting, although a few forms can result in vision impairment if not treated. Both viral and bacterial diseases are highly contagious, and all forms can be uncomfortable. This chapter reviews the most common types of both infectious and non-infectious conjunctivitis, which include viral, bacterial, and allergic conjunctivitis.

Viral Conjunctivitis

Viral conjunctivitis, also called "pink-eye," is the most common cause of infectious conjunctivitis in both children and adults.[2] Although adenovirus is the most common etiology of this infection, viral conjunctivitis may also be caused by herpes or varicella. Other viruses, such as Epstein-Barr virus, influenza virus, and human immunodeficiency virus (HIV), are rare etiologies of conjunctivitis.

This disorder has an abrupt onset and can be unilateral or bilateral or, more commonly, sequentially bilateral.[3]

The discharge of viral conjunctivitis is watery and may produce a burning (rather than itching) sensation. The clinical course of viral conjunctivitis typically mirrors that of the common cold, with symptoms potentially continuing for 2–3 weeks. Viral conjunctivitis does not require systemic therapy and is generally self-limiting.

Treatment for viral conjunctivitis is directed at lessening symptoms rather than at eradicating the underlying pathogen (Table 27-1). Non-antibiotic topical lubricants and antihistamine/vasoconstrictor combination medications may provide symptomatic relief.[4] Topical steroids may be prescribed to treat severe symptoms, but they can prolong viral replication and, therefore, are not a standard first-line treatment. Rationally prescribing any of these medications is important to avoid unwarranted use of topical antibacterial agents, which will not expedite healing but may hasten the development of antibiotic drug resistance. Topical treatments may themselves produce irritation and increase redness and discharge.

Conjunctivitis Secondary to Cytomegalovirus or Herpes Simplex Virus

Conjunctivitis caused by cytomegalovirus (CMV) or herpes simplex virus (HSV) type 1 or 2 is usually initially unilateral. Symptoms can include blurry vision, photophobia, pain, redness, and tearing. Corneal ulcers and vision impairment is possible if these infections are untreated. Ganciclovir (Cytovene), trifluridine (Viroptic), and vidarabine (Vira-A) are topically administered antivirals used to treat these viral ophthalmic infections. Only trace amounts of the drugs are systemically absorbed. Trifluridine and topical acyclovir (Zovirax) cause epithelial toxicity if used for more than 2 weeks. Although ganciclovir is less toxic, all of the topical antiviral medications can cause epithelial toxicity.[3] Ganciclovir is indicated for sight-threatening CMV infections such as CMV retinitis, which may occur among individuals who are immunocompromised.

Topical or oral antiviral medications can also be used to treat conjunctivitis secondary to HSV. Trifluridine (Viroptic) and vidarabine (Vira-A) can be used for keratoconjunctivitis and recurrent epithelial keratitis. The most common side effect is localized burning and discomfort at the site of administration. Although topical and oral antiviral agents are equally effective, oral agents such as acyclovir (Zovirax), famciclovir (Famvir), or valacyclovir (Valtrex) are generally preferred to avoid the epithelial toxicity that topical agents can induce. Corticosteroids should be avoided as they can potentiate replication of the virus.

Bacterial Conjunctivitis

Bacterial conjunctivitis is the second most frequent form of conjunctivitis and is most often caused by *Staphylococcus aureus, Streptococcus pneumoniae, Haemophilus influenzae,* or *Moraxella catarrhalis.*[2] Primary modes of transmission are contaminated fingers, contaminated fomites, and oculogenital spread. Bacterial conjunctivitis is more often observed in children than in adults. The discharge of bacterial conjunctivitis is purulent and typically globular and opaque.

Although bacterial conjunctivitis is generally self-limiting, drug therapy shortens the clinical course of the disease and decreases communicable transmission (Table 27-2). A meta-analysis of clinical and microbiologic remission found that topical antibiotics significantly improve early (days 2–5) clinical remission rates (relative risk [RR], 1.24; 95% confidence interval [CI], 1.05–1.45) and microbial remission rates (RR, 1.77; 95% CI, 1.23–2.54); however, this benefit is marginal for later clinical and microbial remission (days 6–10).[5] A decrease in discharge and less redness and irritation should be noted within 2 days of initiating treatment. Obtaining cultures is seldom necessary, and resistance to first-line pharmacotherapy is unusual. Common side effects of topical antibacterial drugs include localized irritation and inflammation. The pharmacokinetic profiles of ointments tend to make them good vehicles for drug delivery, but adults may prefer drops, as ointments blur vision for 15–20 minutes. There are no major differences in the effectiveness of the various broad-spectrum antibiotic formulations used to treat bacterial conjunctivitis.[2]

First-line treatments include erythromycin ophthalmic ointment (Ilotycin), sulfacetamide ophthalmic drops (Sulf-10, Sulamyd), and polymyxin B–trimethoprim drops (Polytrim).[2] All three of these preparations contain broad-spectrum antimicrobial drugs that are effective against the common bacterial conjunctivitis pathogens. Erythromycin is a bacteriostatic inhibitor of protein synthesis. Polymyxin B–trimethoprim is a bacterial agent that alters the permeability of bacterial cytoplasmic membrane, thereby promoting leakage of intracellular constituents. Both erythromycin and polymyxin B–trimethoprim are preferred topical treatments for pregnant and breastfeeding women.

Other antibacterial drugs frequently employed for the treatment of conjunctivitis include bacitracin ointment (AK Tracin), azithromycin drops (ASA Site), and fluoroquinolone drops. Aminoglycoside (e.g., gentamicin) drops are not recommended because of their lack of gram-positive antibacterial spectrum coverage and potential toxicity.

Table 27-1 Pharmacotherapy for Viral Conjunctivitis

Drug: Generic (Brand)	Formulation	Dose	Clinical Considerations
H_1 Receptor Antagonists (Antihistamines): Oral Formulations			
Cetirizine (Zyrtec)	5-mg, 10-mg tablets	5–10 mg once/day	May be preferred if person is averse to ophthalmic application; slower to act. More likely to elicit systemic effects (e.g., headache, somnolence, xerostomia, and nervousness) than are ocular formulations.
Desloratadine (Clarinex)	5-mg tablets	5 mg once/day	
Fexofenadine (Allegra)	30-mg, 60-mg tablets	60 mg 2 times/day	
Loratadine (Claritin)	10-mg tablets	10 mg once/day	
H_1 Receptor Antagonists (Antihistamines): Topical Formulations			
Emedastine (Emadine)	0.05% solution	1 drop 4 times/day	Ocular stinging.
Levocabastine (Livostin)	0.05% suspension	1 drop 4 times/day	Ocular stinging.
Vasoconstrictors			
Naphazoline (Clear Eyes)	0.012% solution	1–2 drops 4 times/day	Ocular stinging; hypertension; palpitations.
Oxymetazoline (Visine LR)	0.25% solution	1–2 drops 4 times/day	Ocular stinging; hypertension; palpitations.
Phenylephrine (Neo-Synephrine)	0.12% solution	1–2 drops 4 times/day	Ocular stinging; hypertension; palpitations.
Tetrahydrozoline (Visine Moisturizing)	0.05% solution	1–2 drops 4 times/day	Ocular stinging; hypertension; palpitations.
Mast Cell Stabilizers			
Cromolyn (Opticrom)	4% solution	1–2 drops every 4–6 hours	Ocular stinging.
Lodoxamide (Alomide)	0.1% solution	1–2 drops 4 times/day	Ocular stinging.
Nedocromil (Alocril)	2% solution	1–2 drops 2 times/day	Ocular stinging.
Pemirolast (Alamast)	0.1% solution	1–2 drops 4 times/day	Ocular stinging.
Dual-Acting Topical Combination H_1 Receptor Antagonists/Vasoconstrictors			
Pheniramine/naphazoline (Visine-A)	0.3% (pheniramine) and 0.025% (naphazoline)	1–2 drops 4 times/day	Ocular stinging; limited to 4 times/day administration for less than 2 weeks to avoid rebound congestion and hyperemia.
Dual-Acting H_1 Receptor Antagonists/Mast Cell Stabilizers			
Azelastine (Optivar)	0.05% solution	1 drop 2 times/day	Stinging and headache.
Bepotastine (Bepreve)	1.5% solution	1 drop 2 times/day	Taste abnormality, ocular irritation, and headache.
Epinastine (Elestat)	0.05% solution	1 drop 2 times/day	Stinging and headache.
Ketotifen (Zaditor)	0.025% solution	1 drop 2 or 3 times/day	Stinging and headache.
Olopatadine (Patanol)	0.1% solution	1 drop 2 times/day	Stinging and headache.
Pain Relievers: Topical Nonsteroidal Anti-inflammatory Drugs			
Ketorolac (Acular)	0.5% solution	1 drop 4 times/day	Headache, gastrointestinal pain; contraindicated for pregnant women during third trimester.
Antiviral Agents for Herpes Simplex Virus Types 1 and 2			
Acyclovir (Zovirax)	Ophthalmic ointment	1 drop to both eyes 9 times/day	Epithelial toxicity is likely if used more than 10 days; oral acyclovir is generally preferred.
Acyclovir (Zovirax)	400-mg tablet	1 tablet 5 times/day for 7–10 days	Oral acyclovir enters the tear film in concentrations that effectively treat the virus.
Famciclovir (Famvir)	250-mg tablet	1 tablet 3 times/day	
Ganciclovir (Cytovene)	0.15% gel	Treat 3–5 times/day	Less toxic than trifluridine.
Trifluridine (Viroptic)	1% solution	Apply 1 drop 5–8 times per day or every 2 hours while awake; after re-epithelialization has occurred, apply every 4 hours for another 7 days	Trifluridine can cause epithelial toxicity if used for more than 2 weeks.
Valacyclovir (Valtrex)	500-mg tablet	One tablet PO 2 or 3 times/day	Prodrug of acyclovir; higher bioavailability than acyclovir and equally effective.
Vidarabine (Vira-A)	3% ointment	Apply ½ inch of ointment to lower conjunctival sac 5 times/day; after re-epithelialization has occurred, apply 2 times/day for another 7 days; recommended to avoid recurrence	

Table 27-2 Pharmacotherapy for Bacterial Conjunctivitis

Drug: Generic (Brand)	Formulation	Dose	Clinical Considerations
First-Line Medications			
Erythromycin (Ilotycin)	0.5% ointment	Apply thin layer (1.25 cm) every 4–8 hours	Commonly administered to newborns after birth for prophylaxis against *Neisseria* and *Chlamydia* ocular inoculation during birth.
Polymyxin B–trimethoprim drops (Polytrim)	Trimethoprim 1 mg/10,000 units polymyxin B per mL	1–2 drops 4 times/day	Preferred treatment during pregnancy. Polymyxin B is effective against gram-negative organisms, and trimethoprim is effective against gram-positive organisms. Side effects are rare.
Sulfacetamide (Sulf-10, Sulamyd)	10% solution or 10% ointment	1–2 drops Small amount 4 times/day and once at night	Contraindicated for persons who have sulfa allergy.
Second-Line Medications			
Azithromycin drops (Aza Site)	2.5 mL in 5-mL bottle contains 25 mL of azithromycin and 1% sterile ophthalmic solution	Days 1–2: 1 drop 2 times/day Days 3–5: 1 drop once/day	Requires less-frequent dosing than other antibacterial agents; significantly more expensive.
Bacitracin (AK Tracin)	500 units/g	Apply thin layer (1.25 cm) 2–3 times/day	Local irritation possible.
Polymyxin B–bacitracin drops (Polysporin)	5000 U per g of bacitracin/1000 U per g of polymyxin B	1–2 drops every 3–4 hours for 7 days	Effective against gram-positive and gram-negative organisms; nontoxic to epithelial tissue.
Fluoroquinolones			
Besifloxacin (Besivance)	0.6% ophthalmic suspension	1 drop in both eyes 3 times/day for 7 days	Newest fluoroquinolone to be approved for treating conjunctivitis. Bottle needs to be inverted and shaken once before applying drops to eye.
Ofloxacin (Ocuflox)	0.3% solution	Days 1–2: 1–2 drops every 3 hours Days 3–7: 1–2 drops 4 times/day	The fluoroquinolones are indicated for moderate to severe conjunctivitis. They are highly effective against gram-negative organisms but lack full coverage against *Streptococcus* coverage. They should not be used fewer than 4 times per day, as suboptimal therapeutic levels encourage antibiotic resistance. Treatment for 5–7 days maximum.
Ciprofloxacin (Ciloxan)	0.3% solution	Days 1–2: 1–2 drops every 3 hours Days 3–7: 1–2 drops 4 times/day	
Levofloxacin (Iquix)	0.5% solution	Days 1–2: 1–2 drops every 3 hours Days 3–7: 1–2 drops 4 times/day	
Gatifloxacin (Zymar) (Zymaxid)	0.3% solution	Days 1–2: 1–2 drops every 3 hours Days 3–7: 1–2 drops 4 times/day	

Chlamydial and Gonococcal Conjunctivitis

Two forms of bacterial conjunctivitis—chlamydial and gonococcal—deserve special attention, as these infections can result in loss of vision if not treated promptly and appropriately. Gonococcal conjunctivitis is associated with a high risk of corneal perforation. Its treatment is presented in Table 27-3.[6,7] Treatment is also recommended for sexual partners. Additional information about treatment of both chlamydia and gonorrhea can be found in the *Sexually Transmitted Infections* chapter.

Table 27-3 Pharmacotherapy for Chlamydial and Gonococcal Conjunctivitis

Drug: Generic (Brand)	Formulation	Dose	Clinical Considerations
Neisseria gonorrhoeae			Dual therapy for chlamydia is recommended.
Azithromycin (Zithromax) PLUS	1-g tablet	1 g PO as a single dose	
Ceftriaxone (Rocephin) *plus*	1-g injectable	1 g IM as a one-time dose	
Chlamydia			Dual therapy for gonorrhea is recommended.
Azithromycin (ZIthromax) *or*	1-g tablet	1 tablet PO as a single dose	
Doxycycline (Vibramycin) *or*	100-mg tablet	1 tablet PO 2 times/day for 7 days	Contraindicated during pregnancy; pregnant women should be treated with azithromycin, erythromycin (E-Mycin), or amoxicillin (Amoxil).
Erythromycin base (E-Mycin)	500 mg	1 tablet PO 4 times/day for 7 days	

When conjunctivitis is secondary to chlamydia, it occurs in one of three forms: adult inclusion conjunctivitis, trachoma, or neonatal ophthalmia neonatorum. Adult inclusion conjunctivitis is usually unilateral with a mucopurulent discharge, and genital infection is concomitant. Adults should be treated with systemic antibiotics that also eradicate gonorrhea, as coinfection is common.[6,7] Treatment is recommended for sexual partners.

Trachoma is a chronic or recurrent ocular infection that causes scarring of the eyelids. Trachoma is the most common source of blindness in the world, and although this disease has been eradicated in the United States, it is often seen in rural Asia and Africa.[8] Topical treatment is not effective. Antibiotics recommended by the World Health Organization (WHO) can be found in the WHO documents that address trachoma and the recent Cochrane review of antibiotic treatment for trachoma.[8,9]

Ophthalmia Neonatorum

Ophthalmia neonatorum is conjunctivitis secondary to chlamydia or gonorrhea, which occurs in newborns and presents within the first 15 days of life. Ophthalmia neonatorum can result in blindness if it is not treated, although blindness is more likely when the offending organism is *N. Gonorrhea* and quite rare when it is *C. trachomatis*. The German physician Carl Siegmund Franz Crede introduced prophylaxis treatment with 2% silver nitrate in 1881.[10] The silver nitrate was administered to both conjunctiva in the first few hours after birth. Newborn prophylaxis programs are today a routine component of early newborn care; indeed, newborn prophylaxis is legally mandated in most states in the United States. Treatments available for newborn prophylaxis are reviewed in more detail in the chapter *The Newborn*.

Allergic Conjunctivitis

Allergic conjunctivitis is a common comorbidity of allergic rhinitis. This condition is caused by direct contact of allergens to the eye, resulting in immunoglobulin E (IgE) activation, mast-cell degranulation, and histamine release. Both H_1 and H_2 histamine receptors are activated in response to histamines, and H_1 receptors in particular contribute to the symptoms of conjunctivitis. Allergic conjunctivitis is relatively benign and not sight threatening. As many as 20% of the population may be affected annually. Many of these individuals seek pharmacotherapy for symptomatic relief. Those afflicted typically have a history of experiencing seasonal or perennial allergies with an ophthalmic watery discharge and itching sensation.

Although the principal intervention for allergic conjunctivitis is avoidance of the causal allergen, pharmacotherapy can play an important role in lessening symptoms. Artificial tears, antihistamines, vasoconstrictors, and mast cell stabilizers are all used in a stepwise approach to treatment. Artificial tears lubricate the eye to prevent dry eye and irritation. Vasoconstrictors function as ocular decongestants. Antihistamines and mast cell stabilizers inhibit the allergic response. Although glucocorticoids have well-known anti-inflammatory properties, these agents are associated with major complications; consequently, their use is generally limited to prescription by ophthalmologists for treatment under unusual conditions.

Topical dual-agent formulations consisting of an antihistamine and a vasoconstrictor are highly effective short-term treatments for managing acute episodes of allergic conjunctivitis. They are available as over-the-counter (OTC) medications. One example is the combination of the antihistamine pheniramine (Neo-Synephrine) and the vasoconstrictor naphazoline (Clear Eyes). The antihistamine blocks the effects of histamine on the H_1 histamine receptors and further blocks constitutive histamine receptor activity. Vasoconstrictors act by activating alpha$_1$-adrenergic receptors in the arterioles of the conjunctiva, thereby producing vasoconstriction and decongestion. Use of a combined antihistamine/vasoconstrictor should be limited to administration 4 times per day for less than 2 weeks to avoid rebound congestion and hyperemia. The combination of an antihistamine and a vasoconstrictor in a topical formulation produces better effects than either topical medication alone.

Orally administered second-generation antihistamines such as fexofenadine (Allegra), loratadine (Claritin), desloratadine (Clarinex), and cetirizine (Zyrtec) provide an alternative approach to treating allergic conjunctivitis. These drugs selectively inhibit H_1 histamine receptors and are substantially less sedating than nonselective H_1/H_2 antihistamines. Such agents may be preferred by individuals who are averse to ophthalmic application of drops or ointments; however, oral antihistamines act more slowly and are more likely to elicit systemic side effects (e.g., headache, somnolence, xerostomia, and nervousness). Artificial tears may also be employed as an adjunct to either oral or topical medications.

Extended Therapy for Seasonal or Perennial Allergic Conjunctivitis

When treatment is necessary for more than 2 weeks or if the individual experiences frequent acute attacks of allergic conjunctivitis, a combination of a topical antihistamine and a mast cell stabilizer is preferred.[11] The therapeutic effects of such a regimen may take as long as 2 weeks to become fully effective, but treatment may begin prophylactically in anticipation of an acute attack (e.g., exposure to a known allergen). Oral second-generation antihistamines and topical mast cell stabilizers alone are also viable treatment approaches, particularly if administered prophylactically.

The combination of a mast cell stabilizer and an antihistamine facilitates blockage of both the early and late stages of the allergic response. Mast cell stabilizers prevent mast-cell degranulation, thereby preventing the initial release of histamine. Antihistamines block the activation of H_1 receptors occurring at the end of the atopy (i.e., the signaling cascade). Dual-acting drugs such as bepotastine (Bepreve), olopatadine (Patanol), azelastine (Optivar), epinastine (Elestat), and ketotifen (Zaditor) produce both selective histamine H_1 antagonism and mast cell stabilization and are widely used for chronic allergic conjunctivitis. Of these dual-acting agents, olopatadine is generally regarded as the first-line drug of choice. These medications do not affect alpha$_1$-adrenergic receptors, and they do not produce vasoconstriction. Dosing is typically twice daily, and these agents may produce optic stinging and headache as adverse effects.

Nedocromil (Alocril), pemirolast (Alamast), and cromolyn (Opticrom) act primarily as mast cell stabilizers with minimal antihistaminergic effects. While these medications are safe and efficacious, they typically require more frequent (i.e., 4 times per day) dosing and have a prolonged onset of action of 1–2 weeks before therapeutic effects are observed.

The effectiveness of oral antihistamines in treating individuals with symptoms of allergic conjunctivitis generally is less than the effectiveness of topical antihistamine/mast cell stabilizer medications; however, the oral medications may be preferred if the individual is additionally experiencing non-ophthalmic allergic symptoms, such as sneezing and rhinorrhea associated with seasonal allergic rhinitis. Oral antihistamines more often produce xerostomia and decreased tear production, which may be treated by use of artificial tears.

If other treatment approaches are unsuccessful, topical nonsteroidal anti-inflammatory drugs (NSAIDs) such as ketorolac (Acular) may be an appropriate alternative to lessen ocular itching. Ketorolac does not improve wound healing and has been shown to be less effective than olopatadine (Patanol). Ketorolac may require up to 2 weeks to achieve maximal effectiveness.

Noninfectious–Nonallergic Conjunctivitis, Dry Eye, and Red Eye

Dry eyes resulting from inadequate levels of tear film are particularly common among women. Current treatment for **dry eye** disease is aimed at increasing or supplementing tear production, slowing tear evaporation, and reducing tear resorption. First-line treatments include tear supplementation and environmental coping strategies such as humidifier use and discontinuation—if possible—of systemic or ophthalmic medications known to contribute to dryness.[12] Non-antibiotic topical artificial tear lubricants are available in an array of OTC formulations, including water-soluble polymer drops and lipid-based nonreactive ointments. Like the antibacterial ophthalmic preparations, these ointments have a more protracted duration of action but may blur vision. Artificial tears may also be used to counter decreased tear production resulting from oral antihistamines. Persons typically respond well to the use of artificial tears, which can be administered as adjuncts to ophthalmic drops or ointments. Such medications may be used frequently and produce minimal side effects. The preservatives in these topical medications may cause stinging, which can be remedied by switching products. Preservative-free formulations are also available, but are more expensive.

If tear supplementation and environmental modifications do not adequately relieve symptoms, other medications—including topical cyclosporine (Restasis), topical glucocorticoids, and oral antioxidants—may be considered. Topical cyclosporine is an immunosuppressive agent that has been found to improve signs and symptoms of dry eyes significantly for some persons.[13] Available as a 0.05% emulsion, it may take up to 6 weeks to achieve noticeable improvement in symptoms. Cyclosporine can cause an occasional, temporary burning sensation in the eye. With topical use, no systemic toxicity has been reported. An important consideration with use of cyclosporine is the expense of this therapy.

Low-dose topical glucocorticoid eye drops such as dexamethasone (Maxidex) and prednisolone (Blephamide) can also help to relieve symptoms of dry eye.[14] However, these drugs should be used only for short periods of time or less than 30 days due to the significant adverse effects associated with their continued use, which include cataracts and glaucoma.

Both human and animal studies have shown some benefit of using oral omega-3 and omega-6 fatty acids and oral antioxidants to improve and prevent dry eye.[15,16]

Supplementation is a relatively safe and cost-effective option to consider. Other effective treatment modalities, such as topical sodium hyaluronate, topical vitamin A, and autologous serum tears, should be provided by an ophthalmologist after referral when other options have failed.[17,18]

Cycloplegic and Mydriatic Drugs Used During Eye Examinations

Ophthalmic anticholinergic **cycloplegic drugs** (cycloplegics) and **sympathomimetic mydriatic drugs** (mydriatics) are ophthalmic medications used during diagnostic eye exams and ocular surgery. These agents are administered topically and act on the autonomic nervous system within the eye. Both anticholinergic cycloplegics and sympathomimetic mydriatics facilitate pupil dilatation (mydriasis). Additionally, anticholinergic cycloplegics paralyze the ciliary muscle, thereby preventing the lens from adjusting. None of these drugs are indicated for treatment of women with known ophthalmic conditions, but instead are used clinically for measurement of refraction, intraocular examination, eye surgery, and adjunctive therapy for anterior uveitis. Because of their differing mechanisms of action, anticholinergic and sympathomimetic drugs may be combined to produce greater mydriasis than that observed with a single agent.

Anticholinergic Cycloplegic Drugs

Anticholinergic cycloplegic drugs inhibit muscarinic receptor activation by blocking their interaction with acetylcholine (Table 27-4). Anticholinergic medications cause mydriasis by blocking muscarinic receptors of the iris sphincter muscle, which in turn inhibits iris muscle contraction and prevents reflex pupil constriction during an ocular examination. Mydriasis enables the examiner to more fully observe the interior of the eye. The five topically administered anticholinergic cycloplegics—atropine (Atropisol), cyclopentolate (AK-Pentolate), homatropine (Isopto Homatropine), scopolamine (Isopto Hyoscine), and tropicamide (Mydriacyl)—have similar efficacies and side effect profiles; however, their durations of action vary.[19]

Side Effects/Adverse Effects

The most common side effects of cycloplegics include photophobia secondary to pupil dilation, blurred vision secondary to ciliary muscle paralysis, and inhibited lens movement. Mydriasis may cause the iris to occlude the

Table 27-4 Mydriatic and Cycloplegic Drugs

Drug: Generic (Brand)	Formulation	Dose	Duration of Action	Clinical Considerations
Anticholinergic Cycloplegic Drugs				
Atropine (Atropisol)	2% solution 1% solution 0.5% solution	1 drop before exam	Long (5–12 days)	Photophobia and blurred vision; closed-angle glaucoma secondary to mydriasis. Classic anticholinergic symptoms (dry mouth, blurred vision, constipation, urinary retention, tachycardia, and mental clouding).
Cyclopentolate (AK-Pentolate)	2% solution 1% solution 0.5% solution	1 drop before exam	Short (1 day)	
Homatropine (Isopto Homatropine)	5% solution 2% solution	1–2 drops before exam	Intermediate (1–3 days)	
Scopolamine (Isopto Hyoscine)	0.25% solution	1–2 drops before exam	Intermediate (1–3 days)	
Tropicamide (Mydriacyl)	1% solution 0.5% solution	1–2 drops before exam	Very short (< 1 day)	
Sympathomimetic Mydriatic Drugs				
Phenylephrine (Neo-Synephrine)	10% solution for uveitis 2.5% solution	1 drop before exam	Very short (< 1 day)	Photophobia and intense pain in response to bright light; closed-angle glaucoma secondary to mydriasis. Sympathetic nervous system activation (hypertension, dysrhythmias, and tremor).

trabecular meshwork, which can precipitate a rapid elevation in intraocular pressure and acute closed-angle glaucoma. At therapeutic concentrations, cycloplegics may be absorbed into systemic circulation and produce both peripheral and central nervous system (CNS) effects. Systemic effects present as the classic anticholinergic symptoms of dry mouth, blurred vision, constipation, urinary retention, tachycardia, and mental clouding.

Sympathomimetic Mydriatic Drugs

Phenylephrine (Neo-Synephrine) is a potent, direct-acting alpha$_1$-adrenergic receptor agonist with weak beta-adrenergic receptor activity. It stimulates the iris radial muscle to cause contraction, which results in pupil dilation. Sympathomimetic mydriatics do not paralyze the ciliary muscle and consequently do not prevent lens movement or refocusing during the examination.

Side Effects/Adverse Effects

Sympathomimetic mydriatic drugs, like the anticholinergic cycloplegics, can cause acute closed-angle glaucoma secondary to mydriasis. Additional side effects include photophobia and intense pain in response to bright light. Systemic absorption of phenylephrine may result in sympathetic nervous system activation, resulting in hypertension, dysrhythmias, and tremor.

Glaucoma

Glaucoma includes a collection of ophthalmic disorders characterized by visual field loss and optic nerve damage. The term **glaucoma** comes from the Greek word *glaukos*, which means "bluish gray." It was first used by Hippocrates in referring to the color of the cornea when increased intraocular pressure exists.[20] Glaucoma often occurs secondary to elevated intraocular pressure caused by impaired outflow of aqueous humor in the anterior chamber. It is one of the leading causes of preventable blindness in the United States and is most common among women and men 60 years or older.[21] The initial diagnosis of glaucoma is made by an ophthalmologist.

The two principal forms of glaucoma are **open-angle glaucoma** and **closed-angle glaucoma** (Figure 27-2). Primary open-angle glaucoma accounts for more than 90% of glaucoma. More than 2 million persons were estimated to have glaucoma in 2000, with an increase of 50% in this number predicted to occur by 2020 due to the aging of the population.[22] Glaucoma is six times more prevalent in African Americans than in whites, and African Americans are more likely than whites to develop blindness.[18]

Glaucoma is a chronic and often bilateral disorder that may be painless and progress undiagnosed for years until peripheral vision loss begins to occur. Open-angle glaucoma results from a blockage in either the trabecular

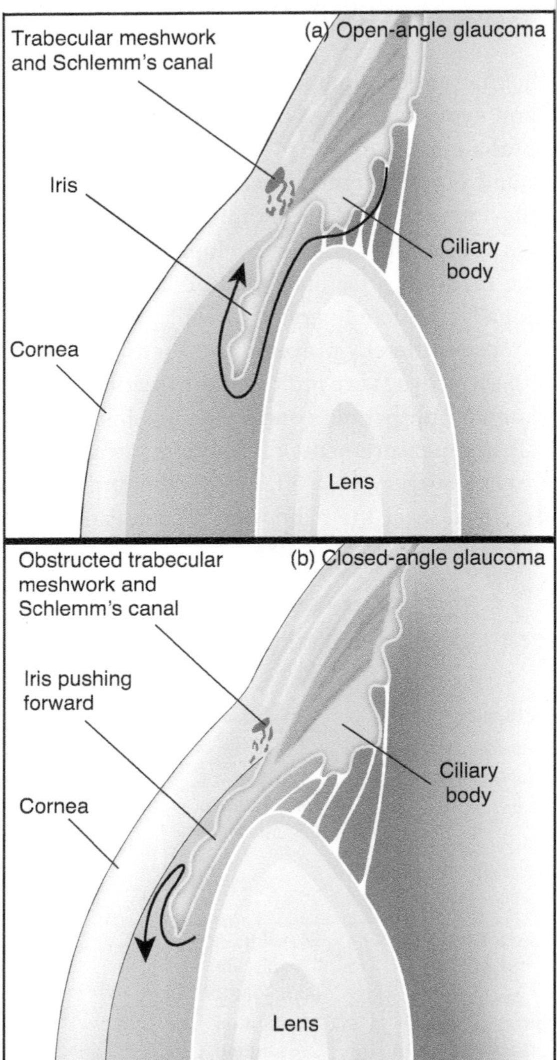

Aqueous humor movement is represented by the arrow. In open-angle glaucoma (a), the trabecular meshwork and Schlemm's canal are accessible. In closed-angle glaucoma (b), the iris occludes the trabecular meshwork and Schlemm's canal, preventing aqueous humor outflow.

Figure 27-2 Illustration of impaired aqueous humor flow in open-angle glaucoma and closed-angle glaucoma.

meshwork or Schlemm's canal, which prevents aqueous humor outflow and drainage. In contrast to closed-angle glaucoma, the pupil does not dilate or cause a blockage of aqueous humor circulation. Open-angle glaucoma may also develop in persons with disorders such as diabetes mellitus and hypertension or as a complication of eye surgery.

Closed-angle glaucoma is also referred to as narrow-angle glaucoma. This type of glaucoma develops when the pupil dilates to such an extent that the iris abuts the cornea and blocks outflow of aqueous humor through Schlemm's canal. This disorder is more common in Asians and Asian Americans. Acute closed-angle glaucoma is an emergent condition that develops rapidly, may cause exceptional pain, and can lead to complete and irreversible blindness if untreated within 5 days.

The primary risk factor for both forms of glaucoma is increased intraocular pressure.[23] Although it is an important consideration, elevated intraocular pressure measured by tonometry is not in itself definitive for diagnosing chronic glaucoma. A person with primary open-angle glaucoma may be asymptomatic and have an intraocular pressure within normal limits (i.e., 10–20 mm Hg). Some individuals may have an extremely elevated intraocular pressure (> 30 mm Hg) but no evidence of optic nerve damage. Genetic testing may assist in screening because several new gene loci have been identified as being associated with glaucoma.[24,25] Age and family history of glaucoma are additional established risk factors. A study published in 2012 demonstrated an association between caffeine consumption and elevated intraocular pressure, but to date caffeine consumption has not been proven to be a risk factor for glaucoma.[26]

Open-Angle Glaucoma

The goal of therapy for open-angle glaucoma is to inhibit disease progression, visual field deterioration, and further optic nerve damage by decreasing intraocular pressure.[24,27,28] This type of glaucoma is typically managed with topical applications such as eye drops, ointments, and emulsions of beta-adrenergic receptor blockers, also commonly termed beta blockers in this chapter; prostaglandin analogues; carbonic anhydrase inhibitors; and alpha$_2$ agonists. All of these agents decrease intraocular pressure by decreasing aqueous humor volume.[29] Such medications decrease intraocular pressure by either inhibiting aqueous humor production or increasing outflow. Although not curative, long-term pharmacotherapy for open-angle glaucoma can decrease or prevent further nerve damage. Surgical intervention lowers intraocular pressure more than primary medication but is associated with more eye discomfort, complications, and greater cost, making pharmacotherapy the preferred treatment for most women.[30]

The goal of the initial course of treatment is to decrease intraocular pressure by approximately 20% from the baseline. In persons exhibiting normotensive glaucoma or advanced optic neuropathy, intraocular pressure should be reduced from the baseline intraocular pressure by 30% or more. The two most commonly identified first-line treatment regimens utilize monotherapy of either a beta blocker or a prostaglandin analogue. If both beta blockers and prostaglandin analogues are contraindicated, a carbonic anhydrase inhibitor or alpha$_2$ agonist should be considered as a second-line agent. If single-agent drug therapy is not sufficient to lower intraocular pressure to the target level, switching to an alternative medication or combination drug therapy should be considered. While individuals may obtain some benefit from trying a different drug in the same drug class, many practitioners prefer to switch to an agent from another drug class.[31–33]

The evaluation period for an initial treatment is 2–4 months because some medications require 6–8 weeks to produce their maximum therapeutic effects. Individuals should be initially evaluated for therapeutic response and any side effects after 2–4 weeks of treatment, at which time the dose may be adjusted or a different first-line medication may be prescribed. If subsequent reevaluation indicates the adjustment in treatment produced unacceptable side effects or an insufficient decrease in intraocular pressure, it is possible to modify the dose or drug, or consider selecting a second-line medication.

Multidrug pharmacotherapy typically involves two to four topically administered medications from different drug classes. In addition to **fixed-dose combinations**, a single-agent beta blocker is often prescribed with either a prostaglandin or carbonic anhydrase inhibitor. Multidrug treatment regimens, although effective, have several potential drawbacks, including expense, inconvenience of administration, and additive side effects, all of which should be considered and discussed before these regimens are prescribed.

Closed-Angle Glaucoma

Acute closed-angle glaucoma treatment often requires an immediate initial medical and subsequent surgical approach.[34] Initial pharmacotherapy is used to facilitate pupil constriction and mitigate intraocular pressure-associated pain. The goal of subsequent laser or conventional ophthalmic surgery is to increase the flow of fluid and decrease intraocular pressure. Pharmacotherapy includes rapidly acting, systemically administered osmotic diuretics as well as topically administered ocular medications used in treating open-angle glaucoma. Topical medication should be continued to manage intraocular pressure until surgery can be performed.

Ocular Hypertension and Normotensive Open-Angle Glaucoma

There is considerable debate as to whether an individual who has not experienced optic nerve damage should be treated solely based on a finding of an abnormally high intraocular pressure. Approximately two thirds of persons with elevated intraocular pressure do not exhibit visual impairment. These individuals are referred to as having ocular hypertension, and ongoing studies are evaluating the utility of beginning early treatment in such persons.[34] The Early Manifest Glaucoma Trial demonstrated that early treatment decreases disease progression by half (hazard ratio, 0.50; 95% CI, 0.35–0.71).[35,36] However, the 6-year follow-up to the same study found that persons with early glaucoma in the original control group had no changes in intraocular pressure over the 6-year period, bringing into question the need for medical treatment in early stages of the disease. More research is warranted to determine when treatment should be initiated.[37]

In contrast, 10% to 15% of persons displaying glaucoma-associated optic nerve damage possess an intraocular pressure within normal limits (baseline < 21 mm Hg). Persons displaying this normal-tension glaucoma have nonetheless been shown to benefit from treatments targeting intraocular pressure reduction; for example, they show a decrease in the progression of visual field loss. Therapeutic goals and treatment approaches for managing ocular hypertension and normotensive open-angle glaucoma pharmacotherapy are comparable to the goals and treatment approaches used for primary open-angle glaucoma.

Closed-Angle Glaucoma Pharmacotherapy

Acute closed-angle glaucoma treatment often requires an immediate initial medical and subsequent surgical approach.[39] Initial pharmacotherapy is used to facilitate pupil constriction and mitigate intraocular pressure associated pain. The goal of subsequent laser or conventional ophthalmic surgery is to increase the flow of fluid and decrease intraocular pressure. Pharmacotherapy includes rapidly acting, systemically-administered osmotic diuretics as well as topically administered ocular medications used in treating open-angle glaucoma (e.g., beta blockers, prostaglandin analogues, and carbonic anhydrase inhibitors).

Topical medication should be continued to manage intraocular pressure until surgery can be performed.

Glaucoma Over the Lifespan

Studies investigating glaucoma and lifetime estrogen and progesterone exposure—including that associated with pregnancies, births, menstruation years, and the use of oral contraceptives—have not found a significant correlation or increased risk for elevated intraocular pressure.[39] One study did observe an association between postmenopausal hormone use and decreased intraocular pressure, suggesting hormone use may actually decrease the risk of open-angle glaucoma.[40]

Antiglaucoma Drugs

Pharmacotherapy for both open-angle glaucoma and closed-angle glaucoma is directed at decreasing intraocular pressure by altering aqueous humor production or outflow (Table 27-5). By controlling intraocular pressure, further optic nerve damage and visual field loss can be slowed and prevented.[41] Currently, five major classes of drugs are used for the treatment of glaucoma: (1) beta-adrenoreceptor antagonists; (2) prostaglandin analogues; (3) carbonic anhydrase inhibitors; (4) cholinergics (acetylcholine receptor agonists); and (5) adrenoceptor agonists.[33] Beta-adrenergic receptor blockers have been the most frequently used topical treatment, but recently prostaglandin analogues have increasingly replaced beta blockers in this indication. Prostaglandin analogues are equally or more effective than beta blockers and possess better tolerated side-effect profiles.[42] Carbonic anhydrase inhibitors, alpha$_2$-adrenergic receptor agonists, nonselective sympathomimetics, cholinergic and anticholinesterase miotics, and osmotic diuretics may also be utilized depending on the individual's specific condition. The different mechanisms of actions of these drug classes permit therapeutically advantageous combination drug therapy when monotherapy does not produce the desired outcome. The profound difference in the time frame of disease progression—5–15 years for primary open-angle glaucoma versus 1–5 days for acute closed-angle glaucoma—necessitates differences in treatment methodologies and relative urgency.

Table 27-5 Antiglaucoma Medications

Drug: Generic (Brand)	Formulation and Dose	Clinical Considerations
$Beta_1$ Receptor Antagonists		
Betaxolol (Betoptic)	0.5% solution or 0.25% suspension 1–2 drops 2 times/day	Avoid abrupt withdrawal. Ocular irritation, dry eyes, and conjunctivitis; increased risk of bradycardia and hypotension; tolerance may develop. Contraindicated in second and third trimesters of pregnancy.
Levobetaxolol (Betaxon)	0.5% solution 1 drop 2 times/day	
Mixed $Beta_1$/$Beta_2$-Adrenergic Antagonists		
Carteolol (Ocupress)	1% solution 1 drop 2 times/day	For all $beta_1$/$beta_2$-acting drugs: Contraindicated in persons with bradycardia and atrioventricular heart block. Use with caution in persons with asthma or chronic obstructive pulmonary disease. Carteolol produces least ocular burning; metipranolol produces greatest ocular burning. Contraindicated in second and third trimesters of pregnancy.
Levobunolol (Betagan)	0.5% solution 1 drop once/day or 2 times/day 0.25% suspension 1 drop 2 times/day	
Metipranolol (OptiPranolol)	0.3% solution 1 drop 2 times/day	
Timolol (Timoptic) (Istalol) (Betimol)	0.5% solution or 0.25% solution 1 drop once/day or 2 times/day 0.5% gel or 0.25% gel 1 drop once/day	
Prostaglandin $F_{2\alpha}$ Analogues		
Bimatoprost (Lumigan)	0.01% solution 1 drop once/day	Localized irritation, redness, and hyperemia; administer in evening to decrease sensation of ocular pain. Harmless iris discoloration; latanoprost produces greatest iris discoloration. Lengthening and darkening of eyelashes. Hyperemia occurs more commonly with bimatoprost and travoprost.
Latanoprost (Xalatan)	0.005% solution 1 drop once/day	
Tafluprost (Zioptan)	0.0015% solution 1 drop once/day	
Travoprost (Travatan)	0.004% solution 1 drop once/day	
Unoprostone (Rescula)	0.15% solution 1 drop once/day or 2 times/day	
Carbonic Anhydrase Inhibitors: Topical Formulations		
Brinzolamide (Azopt)	1% suspension 1 drop 2 times/day or 3 times/day	Produce substantially fewer systemic side effects than oral formulations; localized irritation, taste distortion; more ocular stinging with dorzolamide. All carbonic anhydrase inhibitors are sulfonamides and are contraindicated for persons with a sulfa allergy.
Dorzolamide (Trusopt)	2% solution 1 drop 2 times/day or 3 times/day	
Carbonic Anhydrase Inhibitors: Oral Formulations		
Acetazolamide (Diamox)	Tablets: 125 mg, 250 mg 250 mg every 6–24 hours	Fatigue and paresthesias; myopia, appetite loss, gastrointestinal disturbances, blood dyscrasias, kidney stones; dichlorphenamide less well tolerated than others. All carbonic anhydrase inhibitors are sulfonamides and are contraindicated for persons with a sulfa allergy.
Dichlorphenamide (Daranide)	Tablet: 50 mg 50–100 mg 2 times/day initially, then 25–50 mg once/day to 3 times/day for maintenance dose	
Methazolamide (Neptazane)	Tablets: 50 mg 50–100 mg 2 times/day or 3 times/day initially, then 25–50 mg for maintenance 2 times/day or 3 times/day	
$Alpha_2$ Receptor Agonists		
Apraclonidine (Iopidine)	1% solution, 0.5% solution 1 drop 2 times/day or 3 times/day	Localized irritation, hyperemia, headache; hypotension. Apraclonidine indicated for short-term use only. Respiratory arrest and fatigue (greatest concern in children with brimonidine).
Brimonidine (Alphagan)	0.15% solution, 0.1% solution 1 drop 2 times/day or 3 times/day	
Combination Medications		
Dorzolamide/timolol (Cosopt)	2%/0.5% solution 1 drop 2 times/day	Similar to once-daily administration of latanoprost; give 10 minutes apart if given with other eye drops.
Brimonidine/timolol (Combigan)	0.2%/0.5% solution 1 drop 2 times/day	Ocular stinging/burning, headache, dry mouth.
Brimonidine/brinzolamide (Simbrinza)	0.2%/1% suspension 1 drop 3 times/day	Blurred vision, dry mouth, eye irritation.
Nonselective Sympathomimetics		
Dipivefrin (Propine)	0.1% solution 1 drop once/day or 2 times/day	Contraindicated in closed-angle glaucoma; mydriasis; systemic effects including increased heart rate, blood pressure, and arrhythmias.
Epinephryl Borate (Eppy/N)	2% solution, 0.25% solution 1–2 drops once/day or 2 times/day	

(*continues*)

Table 27-5 Antiglaucoma Medications (*continued*)

Drug: Generic (Brand)	Formulation and Dose	Clinical Considerations
Direct-Acting Cholinergic Receptor Agonists (Cholinergic Miotics)		
Carbachol (Carboptic) (Isopto Carbachol) (Miostat)	3% solution 2.25% solution 1.5% solution 0.75% solution 1 drop 2 times/day or 3 times/day	Myopia, headaches, irritation, and red eye; bradycardia and bronchospasm; should be avoided by persons with iritis or asthma.
Pilocarpine (Isopto Carpine) (Pilopine)	1% solution 2% solution 4% solution 1 drop every 4–12 hours 4% gel 0.5-inch ribbon once/day	
Anticholinesterase Inhibitors (Anticholinesterase Miotics)		
Echothiophate (Phospholine)	0.25% solution 0.03% solution 1–2 drops once/day or 2 times/day	Myopia, headache; bradycardia, and bronchospasm; has potential to promote cataract formation.
Osmotic Diuretics (Only for Acute Closed-Angle Glaucoma)		
Glycerin (Ophthalgan)	50% solution 75% solution	Peripheral edema, electrolyte imbalances, tremors, dizziness, headaches, use with caution if renal impairment or cardiovascular disease.
Mannitol (Osmitrol)	20% solution	

Beta-Adrenergic Receptor Antagonists (Beta Blockers)

Beta-adrenergic receptor antagonists have been the drugs of choice for treating primary open-angle glaucoma and continue to be commonly used for this indication.[43] These agents decrease aqueous humor production in the ciliary body, thereby lowering intraocular pressure. They may be used as part of the initial management of acute closed-angle glaucoma. The six topically administered medications approved for treatment of glaucoma include the $beta_1$-selective drugs betaxolol (Betoptic) and levobetaxolol (Betaxon) and the nonselective $beta_1$/$beta_2$ antagonists carteolol (Ocupress), levobunolol (Betagan), metipranolol (OptiPranolol), and timolol (Timoptic).

Beta blockers inhibit the beta-adrenergic receptors of the ciliary epithelium, which results in a decrease in aqueous humor production, which in turn lowers intraocular pressure. Although the overwhelming majority of beta receptors in this tissue are of the $beta_2$ subtype, the $beta_1$-selective antagonists have been shown to be equally effective and the exact mechanism of action is not well elucidated. Ophthalmic beta blockers have a long duration of action, which permits them to be administered as single drops either once or twice daily. These drugs have been shown to decrease intraocular pressure by 20% to 30% from pretreatment levels.[44] Tolerance to ophthalmic beta blockers may develop with chronic use. As such, periodic monitoring of intraocular pressure is required, and there is the potential need to switch to a medication of a different class or to employ combination drug therapy. Differences between members of the drug class include cost, frequency of administration, and the frequency of systemic side effects.

Side Effects/Adverse Effects

Beta blockers have relatively minor localized side effects, including ocular irritation, dry eyes, and conjunctivitis. These effects are generally equivalent among the drugs. Fewer ocular side effects are typically reported with beta blockers than with second-line treatment modalities, such as epinephrine or pilocarpine.[43]

Disseminated sympatholytic side effects are possible, due in part to the lack of first-pass metabolism following systemic drug absorption. The nonselective $beta_1$/$beta_2$ antagonists in particular are contraindicated for persons with bradycardia and atrioventricular heart block. They should be used with caution by persons with asthma or chronic obstructive pulmonary disease (COPD) as well as by persons with congestive heart failure (CHF), who are likely to be treated with oral beta blockers. Ophthalmic beta blockers have the potential to inhibit cardiac $beta_1$ and pulmonary $beta_2$ receptors, so they may cause or exacerbate conditions associated with those receptor sites.[45] The $beta_1$-selective drugs betaxolol and levobetaxolol are less likely to cause bronchospasm and are the preferred beta blockers for individuals with asthma or COPD; however, they have been reported to cause greater local irritation. Concurrent use of topical ophthalmic beta blockers and oral cardiac beta blockers should be avoided, as this combination poses an increased risk of bradycardia and hypotension. Systemic side effects decrease in intensity following the first 2 weeks of therapy.

Pregnancy and Lactation

Currently available evidence suggests beta blockers are generally safe during pregnancy; however, neonatal hypoglycemia, bradycardia, and arrhythmia have all been reported following maternal use of ophthalmic beta blockers during pregnancy, at parturition, or during breastfeeding.[46] Expert panel recommendations indicate that beta blockers, including betaxolol (Betoptic) and timolol (Timoptic), should be avoided during the second and third trimesters.

Prostaglandin Analogues

Prostaglandin $F_{2\alpha}$ analogues represent a newer drug class and have increasingly become the preferred treatment approach for primary open-angle glaucoma.[42] They may be administered once daily as monotherapy and can reduce intraocular pressure by 40% to 60%. These drugs increase the outflow of aqueous humor through the uveoscleral pathway and relaxation of the ciliary muscle. Relaxation occurs by several mechanisms, some of which are not fully understood. Prostaglandin analogues may be given in combination with beta blockers if either type of drug alone is unable to decrease intraocular pressure sufficiently.

The five ophthalmic prostaglandin analogues are latanoprost (Xalatan), travoprost (Travatan), unoprostone (Rescula), bimatoprost (Lumigan), and tafluprost (Zioptan). These medications are administered topically once daily and are generally well tolerated with minimal systemic side effects. Latanoprost was the first member of the class and is the most frequently prescribed of all antiglaucoma medications. Bimatoprost and travoprost have been shown to be effective when used by African Americans with primary open-angle glaucoma.[47] Tafluprost is formulated without any preservatives, so it must be refrigerated. This drug is found in single-dose packets that should not be used more than once.[48]

Side Effects/Adverse Effects

Prostaglandin analogues are well tolerated, and systemic reactions are not common. A few notable localized adverse effects exist, including irritation and redness, the physically harmless discoloration (browning) of the iris, and lengthening and darkening of the eyelashes. The irritation and redness typically dissipate during the first month of therapy and may be further decreased by administering the medication before bedtime. Among the five prostaglandin analogues, latanoprost (Xalatan) is the best tolerated.[49] Discoloration of the iris occurs most often with this agent, however, and is often permanent.

For some women, the side effect of lengthening and darkening of eyelashes is desired. Bimatoprost also is marketed as the brand-name drug Latisse and has been widely advertised directly to consumers with the FDA indication for cosmetic treatment of hypotrichosis (thin eyelashes). This agent also has been used successfully for women who have experienced alopecia areata or hair loss subsequent to chemotherapy. As with latanoprost, an adverse effect of bimatoprost can be permanent darkening of the iris. In addition, treatment is relatively expensive, and eyelashes begin to recede to pretreatment state with a few weeks after drug discontinuation. Cosmetic use is also discussed in the *Dermatology* chapter.

The most frequently reported adverse effect of prostaglandin analogues is hyperemia, which typically occurs with bimatoprost (Lumigan) and travoprost (Travatan). Some persons who have an insufficient intraocular pressure reduction following latanoprost treatment have been shown to be responsive to bimatoprost.[50]

Pregnancy and Lactation

There are currently no well-controlled antiglaucoma prostaglandin studies in pregnant women. An observational study of 11 women indicated no systemic or neonatal side effects as a consequence of topically administered latanoprost.[46,51] However, adverse fetal effects have been reported in animal studies of latanoprost. Also, based on the known uterine actions of orally administered prostaglandins, the question of whether prostaglandin analogues should be contraindicated during pregnancy remains unresolved.[52]

Carbonic Anhydrase Inhibitors

Carbonic anhydrase inhibitors are second-line antiglaucoma medications that are available for both topical and oral administration. In addition to being used as a treatment for individuals who are not responsive to first-line medications, carbonic anhydrase inhibitors may be used for the initial management of acute closed-angle glaucoma as part of multidrug therapy. These medications are also used perioperatively for decreasing intraocular pressure prior to eye surgery. Individuals younger than 40 years experience fewer side effects from the medications than older persons do.

While the oral drugs were the first to be developed, the topically administered agents have overwhelmingly replaced them in recent years due to their improved side-effect profiles. The efficacy of topical carbonic anhydrase inhibitors is similar to that observed with timolol (Timoptic).

Like beta blockers, carbonic anhydrase inhibitors reduce intraocular pressure by inhibiting production of aqueous humor. Carbonic anhydrase is an enzyme found in the epithelial cells of the ciliary processes that converts water and carbon dioxide to bicarbonate. Thus carbonic anhydrase inhibitors prevent the enzymatic production of bicarbonate necessary for fluid transport and aqueous humor production.

The topical formulations include dorzolamide (Trusopt) and brinzolamide (Azopt). Dorzolamide is more often used, both as a single agent and in combination with other antiglaucoma drugs. Topical carbonic anhydrase inhibitors require dosing 2 or 3 times per day, which is substantially less convenient than the once-daily dosing offered with prostaglandin analogues and some beta blockers.

Dorzolamide is available in a fixed-dose formulation with the beta blocker timolol (Cosopt). Twice-a-day dosing of the dorzolamide/timolol fixed-combination therapy results in safety and effectiveness similar to once-daily administration of latanoprost (Xalatan).[53] Both treatments reduce diurnal intraocular pressure from baseline ($P < 0.0001$), and there is no statistical difference in intraocular pressure between treatments or in the incidence of adverse events. Dorzolamide/timolol has shown teratogenic effects in animal studies and should be used with caution during pregnancy.

Side Effects/Adverse Effects

Both topical and oral medications are sulfonamides and, therefore, are contraindicated for persons with a known sulfa allergy. The topically administered carbonic anhydrase inhibitors are generally well tolerated and produce substantially fewer systemic effects than the orally administered formulations; however, topical formulations are more likely to cause localized reactions, including eye irritation and the sensation of a bitter taste shortly after drug administration. Incidents of ocular stinging and burning occur less frequently with brinzolamide, due to the neutral pH of the medication.

Oral Formulations

The orally administered drugs include acetazolamide (Diamox), methazolamide (Neptazane), and dichlorphenamide (Daranide). The systemic side effects of these formulations have substantially limited their use, and they are no longer recommended for long-term therapy. Oral carbonic anhydrase inhibitors are known to have adverse effects on the nervous system and may cause fatigue and paresthesias. Additional side effects include myopia, loss of appetite, gastrointestinal disturbances, blood dyscrasias, and kidney stones. The orally administered carbonic anhydrase inhibitors have diuretic properties, which may result in an electrolyte imbalance and require monitoring. These agents cross the placenta and are excreted in breast milk. They are not commonly used during pregnancy or lactation.

Alpha$_2$-Adrenergic Receptor Agonists

Brimonidine (Alphagan) and apraclonidine (Iopidine) are alpha$_2$-adrenergic receptor agonists. These drugs inhibit production of aqueous humor and are used as second-line antiglaucoma therapies. Of the two agents, brimonidine is used more often, either as monotherapy if the individual is unresponsive to first-line open-angle glaucoma treatment or as a component in a multidrug regimen. The effectiveness of this drug approaches that of timolol (Timoptic); specifically, brimonidine produces a decrease in intraocular pressure of approximately 15% to 25%. Brimonidine (Alphagan) may also produce a beneficial neuroprotective effect via an unidentified mechanism that is independent of intraocular pressure reduction.[54] Apraclonidine is used only on a short-term basis and perioperatively for eye surgery. Both medications are administered topically 3 times daily.

The most common side effects of the alpha$_2$-adrenergic receptor agonists include ocular irritation, red eye, hyperemia, and headache. These drugs produce few systemic cardiovascular effects. Although equally or more effective than the beta blockers, alpha$_2$-adrenergic agents are generally less tolerated by individuals and are not considered first-line treatment.[55] Brimonidine (Alphagan) is the more lipophilic of the two agents. It crosses the blood–brain barrier and elicits alpha$_2$-mediated effects in the brain, including hypotension and fatigue. This drug should be used with caution. Well-controlled studies in pregnant women have not been completed with either medication.

Combination Products

Combination products are becoming more widely available in the United States. The current combinations include the carbonic anhydrase inhibitor/beta blocker dorzolamide/timolol (Cosopt), the alpha agonist/beta blocker brimonidine/timolol (Combigan), and the carbonic anhydrase inhibitor/alpha agonist brimonidine/brinzolamide (Simbrinza).[56] These combination products should not be used as initial treatment. For women requiring treatment with two of these drug classes, the combination products are more convenient and generally more cost-effective.[57] Side effects that are commonly noted in one or both of the drug classes may be experienced by persons using combination products. Combination products containing prostaglandin analogues are currently being researched and are available in Canada but have not yet been approved in the United States.[58]

Nonselective Adrenergic Receptor Agonists (Sympathomimetics)

Activators of the sympathetic nervous system in the eye have been shown to be useful as a third-line antiglaucoma treatment approach capable of lowering intraocular pressure.[59] Paradoxically, a nonselective adrenergic receptor agonist may be used in consort with a beta-adrenergic receptor antagonist to lower intraocular pressure. Adrenergic receptor agonists are presumed to decrease intraocular pressure by increasing uveoscleral outflow and by modifying blood flow to the ciliary body.

The most commonly used medication in this class is dipivefrin (Propine). This highly soluble prodrug is administered topically twice daily. Once absorbed into the eye, it is rapidly hydrolyzed by enzymes such as acetylcholinesterase and carbonic anhydrase into the active drug epinephrine. Epinephrine stimulates ophthalmic alpha$_1$-adrenergic receptors, causing mydriasis, which in turn results in an increase in aqueous humor outflow.

Side Effects/Adverse Effects

Epinephrine is primarily metabolized by ocular enzymes such as COMT and MAO; however, a pharmacologically significant amount of the drug can enter the systemic circulation, which causes an increase in blood pressure, arrhythmias, and tachycardia. Because mydriasis exacerbates closed-angle glaucoma, nonselective adrenergic receptor agonists are contraindicated for persons with this condition.

Cholinergic Receptor Agonists (Cholinergic Miotics)

Activation of muscarinic (M_3) cholinergic receptors in the eye causes pupil constriction (i.e., miosis) and contraction of the ciliary muscle, thus stretching the trabecular meshwork and permitting greater outflow of aqueous humor. Topically administered direct-acting cholinergic receptor agonists, also referred to as *cholinergic miotics*, include pilocarpine (Isopto Carpine) and carbachol (Carboptic). Cholinergic miotics mimic the effects of acetylcholine in the eye and have been shown to be effective for the management of both open- and closed-angle glaucoma. Cholinergic miotics were among the first classes of medications to be used to lower intraocular pressure and can reduce intraocular pressure by 20% to 30%. However, their use has substantially declined with the advent of ophthalmic beta blockers and prostaglandin analogues.[60] Pilocarpine is the best-tolerated cholinergic miotic.

Cholinergic miotics have relatively short half-lives and require administration 3 or 4 times per day. The combination therapy of a beta blocker such as metipranolol (OptiPranolol) and cholinergic miotic such as pilocarpine (Salagen) can produce a synergistic effect.

Side Effects/Adverse Effects

Miotics have several common side effects including myopia, ciliary spasm leading to headaches, irritation, and red eye. Although these drugs generally produce fewer systemic effects than the first-line antiglaucoma medications, the frequency with which persons using them experience discomfort from the localized side effects makes them a second- or third-line medication. Cholinergic miotics should be avoided by persons with iritis due to their potential for worsening inflammation. Systemic effects, when present, result in generalized parasympathetic activation and include bradycardia and bronchospasm. As such, these drugs are contraindicated for persons with asthma.

Anticholinesterase Inhibitors (Anticholinesterase Miotics)

Ocular acetylcholinesterase regulates the parasympathetic response in the eye by degrading acetylcholine and thereby dissipating muscarinic cholinergic receptor activation. Cholinesterase inhibition prevents acetylcholine degradation through this pathway and allows the neurotransmitter to have a prolonged effect via continued interaction with muscarinic receptors. Consequently, anticholinesterase inhibitors may be regarded as indirect-acting cholinergic activators.

The one drug in this class used for treating glaucoma is echothiophate (Phospholine). Echothiophate irreversibly inhibits cholinesterases, resulting in an extended duration of action of acetylcholine. It is administered topically once every 12–48 hours and is indicated for treating primary open-angle glaucoma in persons who are not responsive to first- or other second-line drug regimens. Anticholinesterase miotics cause intraocular pressure reductions equivalent to those achieved using direct-acting cholinergic miotics.[61]

Echothiophate (Phospholine) shares many therapeutic effects and adverse effects with the direct-acting muscarinic agonists. Myopia and headache may develop, as well as increased systemic parasympathetic activity at high doses. Due to the longer half-life of echothiophate, this drug has a greater potential to promote the formation of cataracts. It is more often used by persons who have had lenses removed.

Osmotic Diuretics

The ophthalmic uses of osmotic diuretics are limited to treatment of acute closed-angle glaucoma emergencies and preoperative administration before eye surgery. These drugs are not used for chronic antiglaucoma therapy. Ophthalmic osmotic diuretics include oral formulations of glycerin (Ophthalgan) and isosorbide (Isordil) and an intravenous infusion of mannitol (Osmitrol). These drugs rapidly lower intraocular pressure by creating an osmotic gradient between intraocular fluid (i.e., both aqueous humor and vitreous humor) and the blood, drawing intraocular fluid from the eye into the vasculature.[62] Such medications produce their maximum effects within 0.5 to 1 hour and should be used with caution by individuals with renal or cardiovascular disease. Side effects include peripheral edema, electrolyte imbalances, tremors, dizziness, and headache.

Macular Degeneration

Macular degeneration, or more frequently termed age-related macular degeneration (AMD or ARMD) is a disease of aging in which retinal damage results in loss of visual acuity in the macula, or center of the visual field. This condition is divided into two types: wet and dry. The categorization is based on the etiology. Dry disease—the most common type—occurs when drusen (cellular debris) accumulates between the retina and choroid. The more severe form is the wet type, in which blood vessels develop from the choroid and retinal detachment is common. Symptoms include lack of visual acuity, inability to identify faces, and problems reading. Risk factors include age, genetic predisposition, hypertension, hypercholesterolemia, obesity, and smoking.

There is no single cure for either type of macular degeneration. Surgical (laser) treatment has been suggested, but pharmaceuticals are commonly employed for therapy. Statins have been proposed as a therapy, but a meta-analysis failed to find evidence supporting their use for this indication.[63] The most common pharmacologic treatment is vitamin supplements. Studies have failed to find an association between vitamin and mineral intake and development of AMD. Nevertheless, a meta-analysis found that supplementation consisting of carotenoids, vitamin C, vitamin E, selenium, and zinc was associated with a delay in progression as measured by loss of reading letters (adjusted odds ratio [OR], 0.77; 95% CI, 0.62–0.96), although it was noted the findings were primarily based on one large study conducted in the United States among well-nourished individuals.[64] Thus, the generalizability of these findings is unclear. Vitamin and mineral supplementation remain a common AMD treatment due to their widespread availability and low cost.

Drugs That Can Cause Ocular Disorders

Some drugs can cause glaucoma or exacerbate preexisting glaucoma. Others can cause **nystagmus**, optic neuritis, **exophthalmos**, or blurred vision. Interestingly, the eyelids are most frequently involved in drug-induced ocular effects and respond with inflammation or dermatitis.[65] A comprehensive review of drug-induced ocular disorders is not possible; therefore the interested reader is referred to published reviews.[17,65–71] Drugs commonly recognized as causes of ocular disorders are listed in Table 27-6.[65–71]

Otic Drugs

The most common conditions that affect the ear are infections in the inner or outer ear canals. The second most common family of conditions that affect the otic system are vestibular disorders, which have a wide range of etiologies. Interestingly, many pharmacotherapeutic agents can cause otic problems such as tinnitus and ototoxicity.

Table 27-6 Drugs That Can Cause Ocular Disorders[a]

Drug: Generic (Brand)	**Ocular Disorders**
Adrenergic agents used to dilate pupils during eye exams	Angle-closure glaucoma
Allopurinol (Zyloprim)	Retinal hemorrhage
Aminoglycosides	Ptosis, extraocular muscle paresis, papilledema
Amiodarone (Cordarone)	Optic neuropathy
Antihistamines	Narrow-angle glaucoma
Antipsychotics[b]	Mydriasis, pigmentary retinopathy, cataracts
Barbiturates	Nystagmus
Benzodiazepines	Disturbance in eye movement
Beta-adrenergic receptor agonists	Dry eye and increased intraocular pressure
Bisphosphonates	Intraocular inflammation
Carbamazepine (Tegretol)	Ocular dystonia, impaired color perception and contrast discrimination
Cidofovir (Vistide)	Intraocular inflammation
Cimetidine (Tagamet)	Narrow-angle glaucoma
Clomiphene citrate (Clomid)	Blurred vision, light flashes
Clonidine (Catapres)	Myosis
Digoxin (Lanoxin)	Scotomas, optic neuritis
Ethambutol (EMB, Myambutol)	Loss of visual acuity or color vision
Glucocorticoids	Angle-closure glaucoma and cataract following long-term use, exophthalmos, cataracts, cranial nerve palsy, papilledema
Hydralazine (Apresoline)	Lacrimation, blurred vision
Hydrochlorothiazide (Maxzide, Dyazide)	Angle-closure glaucoma
Ibuprofen (Advil)	Altered color vision, blurred vision
Ipratropium bromide (Atrovent)	Angle-closure glaucoma
Isoniazid (INH)	Optic neuritis
Linezolid (Zyvox)	Optic neuropathy
Lithium (Lithobid)	Exophthalmos
Metronidazole (Flagyl)	Myopia
Nifedipine (Procardia)	Periorbital edema or eyelid edema
Opiates	Nystagmus
Phenothiazines	Photo toxic retinopathy, nystagmus, cataracts
Phenytoin (Dilantin)	Nystagmus
Quinolones	Bull's eye maculopathy
Ranitidine (Zantac)	Narrow-angle glaucoma
Rifabutin (Mycobutin)	Intraocular inflammation
Salbutamol (Albuterol)	Angle-closure glaucoma
Selective serotonin reuptake inhibitors (SSRIs)	Angle-closure glaucoma
Sulfonamides	Periorbital edema or eyelid edema, Stevens-Johnson syndrome with acute dry-eye syndrome, phototoxic reaction of eyelid skin
Tamoxifen (Nolvadex)	Retinopathy
Tetracyclines	Conjunctival deposits, myopia, papilledema, phototoxic reaction of eyelid skin
Thiazide diuretics	Yellow coloring of vision, myopia
Topiramate (Topamax)	Angle-closure glaucoma
Tricyclic antidepressants	Disturbance of ocular movement, reduced tear formation
Trimethoprim/sulfamethoxazole (TMX/SMX [Bactrim, Septra DS])	Angle-closure glaucoma
Warfarin (Coumadin)	Retinal hemorrhage
Vitamin A overdose	Ptosis, paresis of extraocular muscles
Vitamin D overdose	Calcium deposits in cornea

[a] This table is not comprehensive as new information is being generated on a regular basis.

[b] More commonly seen with typical antipsychotics.

Source: Data from Li J, Tripathi RC, Tripathi BJ. Drug-induced ocular disorders. *Drug Safety*. 2008;31(2):127-141[65]; Abdollahi M, Shafiee A, Bathaiee FS, Sharifzadeh M, Nikfar S. Drug-induced toxic reactions in the eye: an overview. *J Infus Nurs*. 2004;27(6):386-398.[69]

Before reviewing otic treatments, a review of the structure of the ear is in order.

Structure of the Ear

There are three major divisions of the ear—the outer ear, the middle ear, and the inner ear. The outer and the middle ear are often involved in conditions requiring pharmacotherapeutic intervention (Figure 27-3). The outer ear consists of the auricle and external auditory canal. It collects sound waves and channeling them to the tympanic membrane. The external auditory canal maintains a level of **cerumen** (earwax) that aids in the protection against microbial infection. The middle ear conveys auditory vibrations from the tympanic membrane to the inner ear. The Eustachian tube, which connects the middle ear to the nasopharynx, is lined with ciliated epithelial cells; these cells aid in the transit of microbes out of the middle ear. The inner ear includes the semicircular canals and cochlea, which are involved in balance and serve as the sense organ for hearing.

Otitis media, an infection of the middle ear, is the most common infection of the ear. External otitis, often called swimmer's ear, is seen in persons of all ages. Another condition that affects the ear and is treated with pharmacotherapeutic agents is impacted cerumen. Instructions for self-administration of otic drops are presented in Box 27-2.

Box 27-2 Self-Administration of Otic Drops

The optimal method for applying ear drops is as follows:

1. Prior to administration, wash hands with soap and water.
2. Treat the dropper tip as a sterile instrument, being careful not to touch it to the ear or any other surface.
3. Warm the dropper bottle with the hands to prevent discomfort and minimize dizziness.
4. Gently clean the external auditory canal as much as possible prior to drop administration.
5. Tilt head to the unaffected side and allow drops to be released. Gently wiggle the ear to allow for improved absorption and distribution within the external auditory canal if desired.
6. Maintain this position for 2–3 minutes following drug administration to maximize absorption.
7. If edema in the external auditory canal is inhibiting drop administration, a wick may be used to resolve symptoms more quickly. Discontinue use of the wick once the edema subsides.
8. Visually inspect and clean the canal every 2–5 days.
9. To allow for improved absorption and distribution within the external auditory canal, treat a small plug of cotton with the drops and insert the cotton into the ear.

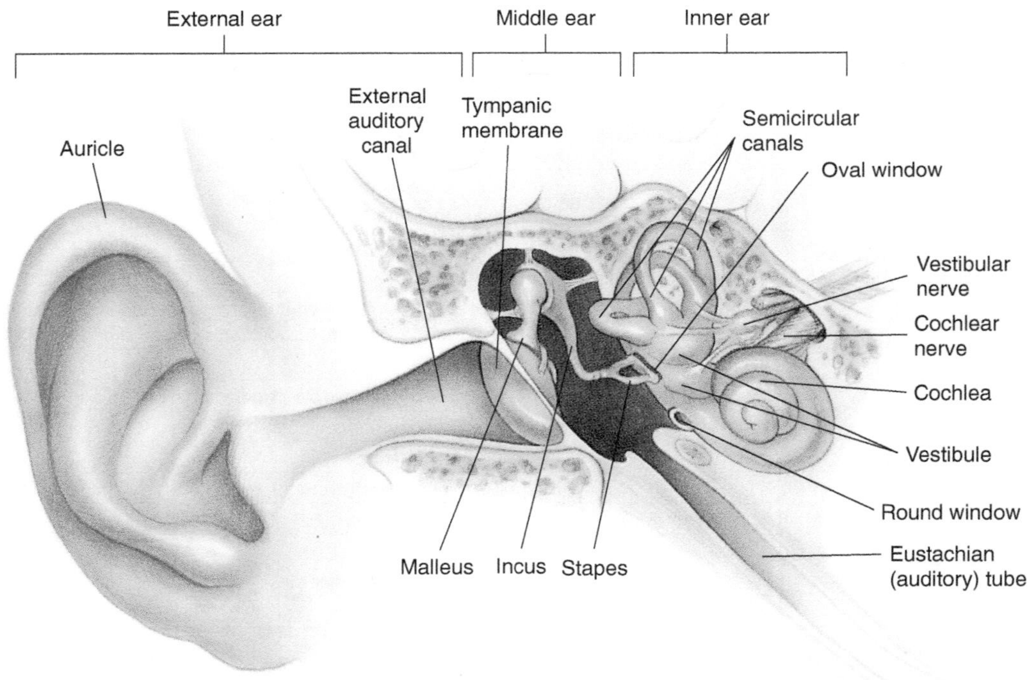

Figure 27-3 Anatomy of the ear.

Acute Otitis Media

The large majority of publications on treatment of otitis media refer to children; thus the information we have on etiology and treatment is based on data gathered primarily from pediatric populations. Acute otitis media is an infectious disease caused by a bacterium, virus, or mixed combination of pathogens; it frequently occurs following an upper respiratory infection. The microbes that are most often implicated in the etiology of acute otitis media are *Streptococcus pneumoniae* (> 40%), *Haemophilus influenzae* (> 20%), and *Moraxella catarrhalis* (> 10%).[72]

Acute otitis media is clinically diagnosed by a sudden onset of symptoms that include ear pain (**otalgia**), fever, irritability, sleeplessness, purulent discharge, middle ear effusion, and signs of middle ear inflammation. Systemic and local symptoms of acute otitis media typically last 1–3 days in individuals receiving antibacterial pharmacotherapy. Symptoms last slightly longer if antibacterial drugs are not used. Middle ear effusion may not subside for several weeks following successful acute otitis media resolution.

The increase in antibiotic resistance and questions about when it is appropriate to prescribe antibacterial drugs for acute otitis media have been the subject of substantial debate[73] (Table 27-7). Factors to weigh in considering observation in lieu of antibacterial pharmacotherapy include age, diagnostic certainty (i.e., certain versus presumed acute otitis media diagnosis), severity of illness, and assurance of follow-up.

Otalgia is a common symptom of acute otitis media, and management of acute otitis media should include assessment for pain. Regardless of whether antibacterial drugs are used, treatment for pain should commence promptly. Standard analgesics include ibuprofen (Advil), acetaminophen (Tylenol), and codeine. Homeopathic remedies, naturopathic herbal extracts, and external application of heat or cold have all been proposed as alternative approaches to palliative care, but their clinical effectiveness is yet to be determined. However, one observational study that compared the outcomes of homeopathic remedies and conventional medications for acute respiratory and ear complaints found that both were equally effective at 7 days, the homeopathic group had a more rapid response to treatment, and the conventional medication group had more adverse drug reactions.[75]

When antibacterial treatment is determined to be appropriate, administration of high-dose amoxicillin is the first-line treatment. Amoxicillin (Amoxil) is a safe and inexpensive antibacterial drug with effectiveness against

Table 27-7 Commonly Used Ear Medications[a]

Drug: Generic (Brand)	Dose	Clinical Considerations
Acute Otitis Media		
Amoxicillin (Amoxil)	875 mg PO 3 times times/day for 5 days	First-line treatment.
Amoxicillin/clavulanate (Augmentin)	875 mg PO 2 times/day for 7 days	Second-line treatment.
Ceftriaxone (Rocephin)	1 g IM per day for 1–3 days	Third-line treatment for infections that are resistant to amoxicillin.
Trimethoprim/sulfamethoxazole (Bactrim DS, Septra)	1 double-strength tablet PO 2 times/day for 7–10 days	
Azithromycin (Zithromax)	500 mg for 1 dose, then 250 mg/day for 4 days	For persons with penicillin allergy.
Cefuroxime (Ceftin)	500 mg PO 2 times/day for 7 days	
Otitis Externa		
Ciprofloxacin with hydrocortisone (Cipro HC Otic)	3 drops 2 times/day for 7 days	Combination antibiotic and steroid decreases inflammation.
Ofloxacin (Floxin Otic)	10 drops once/day into affected ear for 7 days	Highly effective and least irritating. If a systemic antibiotic is needed, give ciprofloxacin (Cipro) 500 mg PO 2 times/day for 7 days. Avoid benzocaine as a topical anesthetic because it can cause an allergic response. Use acetaminophen (Tylenol) or an NSAID for pain relief.
Polymyxin B neomycin, hydrocortisone (Cortisporin)	4–6 drops 3 times/day	Do not use if perforated tympanic membrane. Not effective against *P aeruginosa* or *Staphylococcus* spp.

Abbreviations: NSAID = nonsteroidal anti-inflammatory drug.

[a] This table presents the most commonly used medications for otic disorders and is not all-inclusive.

Source: Data from Bouchard ME. Common conditions of the eye and ear. In: Hackley B, Kriebs J, Rousseau ME, eds. *Primary Care of Women: A Guide for Midwives and Women's Health Providers*. Sudbury, MA: Jones and Bartlett; 2007:339-382.[74]

the most common acute otitis media pathogens and intermediate-resistant pneumococci. If amoxicillin is not effective, a course of high-dose amoxicillin/clavulanate (Augmentin) is suggested. Three doses of intramuscular ceftriaxone (Rocephin) is an alternative treatment regimen.

Acute External Otitis

Acute external otitis (swimmer's ear) is an inflammation of the outer ear typically caused by *Pseudomonas aeruginosa* and *Staphylococcus aureus*; it occurs secondary to superficial tissue damage and excessive moisture. The infection may infiltrate the tissues surrounding the external auditory canal, requiring more extensive therapy. Persons with external otitis develop sudden otalgia, otic pruritus, impaired hearing, and purulent discharge. Most report decreased symptoms following 3 days of initiating treatment and resolution within 2 weeks.

Topical medications such as ear drops and gentle cleaning typically provide efficacious antibacterial treatment. Three to four drops are administered 4 times per day for 3 days beyond the cessation of symptoms. Otalgia may be treated with systemic analgesics such as codeine and NSAIDs.[76] Reevaluation is unnecessary unless the symptoms fail to resolve within 2 weeks of treatment.

Superficial otitis externa infections can be treated with a combination of a 2% acetic acid solution and hydrocortisone.[77] Acetic acid inhibits bacterial growth by acidifying the outer ear, creating an inhospitable environment through direct lowering of the pH. The anti-inflammatory effects of hydrocortisone minimize pain and irritation. Acetic acid is inexpensive, efficacious against almost all bacteria, and does not result in otic sensitization. One potential adverse effect of this medication is irritation of the external auditory canal, which may be lessened by administration of hydrocortisone. The combination therapy of acetic acid and hydrocortisone may also be given prophylactically with minimal adverse consequences.

When acetic acid is too irritating, or if the expected treatment duration is greater than 1 week, a combination antibiotic/steroid cream is equally effective and preferred.[78] Ciprofloxacin with hydrocortisone (Cipro HC Otic) or polymyxin B neomycin/hydrocortisone (Cortisporin) can be used in such cases.[79] All otic pathogens are susceptible to fluoroquinolones, whereas polymyxin B may be ineffective against *P. aeruginosa* and is known to be ineffective against *Staphylococcus* spp.[80,81] Aminoglycosides (e.g., gentamicin and tobramycin) produce minimal irritation, yet are potentially ototoxic. Fluoroquinolone otic solutions (e.g., ciprofloxacin) and ofloxacin drops (Ocuflox) are highly effective and produce the least amount of irritation; however, they are the most expensive treatment option and pose the potential risk of accelerating antibacterial drug resistance. All of these antibiotics offer similar efficacy when used to treat uncomplicated cases of external otitis.[82]

Oral antibacterial therapy should be used only if the infection spreads beyond the external auditory canal.[76] Fluoroquinolones, including ciprofloxacin, are prescribed for adults. Systemic administration of fluoroquinolones is contraindicated for individuals 18 years or younger due to the rare adverse effect of tendon rupture that is associated with this drug.[83]

Impacted Cerumen

When wax builds up and occludes the ear canal, pain and hearing loss can develop. Wax can be softened to facilitate its removal via installation of a wax emulsifier for a few days. Wax emulsifiers can be found over the counter under the brand names Debrox Drops, Murine Ear Drops, and Auro Ear Drops. Wax emulsifiers are composed of glycerine, propylene glycol, and carbamide peroxide. The glycerin softens the cerumen, and the carbamide peroxide releases hydrogen peroxide and oxygen when exposed to moisture. The oxygen has a weak antibacterial effect, and the effervescence that occurs from the production of hydrogen peroxide and oxygen has a mechanical effect of loosening the cerumen from the wall of the ear canal.

The popular alternative approach of using ear candles to remove cerumen should be discouraged, as it is neither effective nor consistently safe. The purported mechanism that burning a hollow candle with one end in the ear canal creates negative pressure to draw cerumen out has been invalidated. Furthermore, ear candling may result in serious injury.[84,85]

Drugs That Cause Otic Disorders

Drugs can cause disorders of the ear and hearing. For example, there is a well-known association between aspirin and tinnitus, and recently associations between NSAID and acetaminophen (Tylenol) use and hearing loss have been found.[86–88] Many drugs can cause ototoxicity through various mechanisms (Table 27-8). Ototoxicity refers to functional impairment and cellular degeneration of the tissues of the inner ear caused by therapeutic agents.

Table 27-8 Ototoxic Medications[a]

Antibiotics: Generic (Brand)	Chemotherapeutic Agents: Generic (Brand)	Antimalarial Agents: Generic (Brand)
Amikacin (Amikin)	Bumetanide (Bumex)	Chloroquine (Aralen)
Azithromycin (Zithromax)	Carboplatin (Paraplatin)	Hydrochloroquine (Plaquenil)
Capreomycin (Capastat Sulfate)	Cisplatin (Platinol)	Mefloquine (Lariam)
Chloramphenicol (Chloromycetin)	Ethacrynic acid (Edecrin)	Quinacrine (Atabrine)
Gentamicin (Garamycin)	Furosemide (Lasix)	
Erythromycin (E-Mycin)	Loop diuretics	
Metronidazole (Flagyl)	Vincristine (Oncovin)	
Neomycin (Neo-Fradin Cortisporin, Neosporin)		
Streptomycin		
Tobramycin (Nebcin, TobraDex)		
Vancomycin (Vanocin)		
Quinine sulfate (Qualaquin)		

[a] This table is not comprehensive as new information is being generated on a regular basis.

The cochlea, vestibulum, and stria vascularis are the primary sites affected. The drugs most likely to be ototoxic are the aminoglycoside antibiotics, macrolide antibiotics, loop diuretics, antimalarial agents, and platinum-based chemotherapeutic drugs. Drugs that are not ototoxic when taken as monotherapy can sometimes be ototoxic when taken concomitantly with another drug. Ototoxicity is most likely to affect older persons.

Aminoglycoside-induced ototoxicity results from a unique mechanism of action. The aminoglycoside drug binds with available iron and forms a complex. This complex catalyzes the formation of reactive oxygen species, which in turn promote apoptosis and cell death.[89] Although a detailed description of the mechanisms and treatments of drug-induced ototoxicity are beyond the scope of this chapter, the reader can find detailed information in published reviews on the subject.[89–91]

Conclusion

Ocular and otic conditions are commonly encountered in primary care settings. Primary care providers should be aware of drugs that can cause ocular or otic adverse effects and know how to best prevent complications from multidrug use; they should also recognize the agents most commonly prescribed by ophthalmology specialists for conditions such as glaucoma. The majority of ocular and otic conditions experienced by women are self-limited and resolve without treatment, but sometimes such symptoms are harbingers of a rare, serious condition. Given this risk, women with ocular and otic symptoms always require a thorough evaluation prior to prescribing medications.

Resources

Organization	Description	Website
American Academy of Ophthalmology	National organization of ophthalmologists; includes some consumer-oriented information	www.aao.org/aao
Apps		
Sightbook	App that includes 10 different vision tests that consumers can perform themselves, including the Amsler grid for macular degeneration	https://itunes.apple.com/us/app/sightbook/id468016180?mt=8
visualFields easy	App for consumer to ascertain if visual fields are normal, and it has been used in research among vulnerable populations with good results	https://itunes.apple.com/us/app/visualfields-easy/id495389227?mt=8
uHear (and many others)	One of many apps available for self-testing hearing; accessories for those who are hearing impaired (e.g., conducting television sounds through earphones connected to tablet, allowing louder sounds) or even how to learn sign language	https://itunes.apple.com/us/app/uhear/id309811822?mt=8

References

1. Acjpiro D, Ajampit L, Piccerelle P, Andrieu V. Recent advances in ocular drug delivery. *Drug Devel Ind Pharm.* 2013;39(11):1599-1617.
2. Azari AA, Barnes NP. Conjunctivitis: a systematic review of diagnosis and treatment. *JAMA.* 2013; 310(16):1721-1729.
3. American Academy of Ophthalmology, Cornea/ External Disease Panel. *Preferred Practice Pattern Guidelines: Conjunctivitis—Limited Revision.* San Francisco, CA: American Academy of Ophthalmology; 2011.
4. Wilkins MR, Khan S, Bunce C, Khawaja A, Siriwardena D, Larkin DF. A randomised placebo-controlled trial of topical steroid in presumed viral conjunctivitis. *Br J Ophthalmol.* 2011;95(9):1299-1303.
5. Sheikh A, Hurwitz B, van Schayck CP, McLean S, Nurmatov U. Antibiotics versus placebo for acute bacterial conjunctivitis. *Cochrane Database Syst Rev.* 2012;9:CD001211. doi:10.1002/14651858.CD001211. pub3.
6. Mishori R, McClaskey EL, WinklerPrins VJ. *Chlamydia trachomatis* infections: screening, diagnosis, and management. *Am Fam Physician.* 2012;86(12): 1127-1132.
7. Centers for Disease Control and Prevention. Sexually transmitted disease treatment guidelines, 2015. *MMWR.* 2015;64(RR3):1-137.
8. Mabey D, Fraser-Hurt N, Powell C. Antibiotics for trachoma. *Cochrane Database Syst Rev.* 2005;2: CD001860.
9. World Health Organization. Trachoma control: a guide for programme managers. World Health Organization; 2006:1–53. http://www.who.int/blindness/publications/disease_control/en/. Accessed September 25, 2014.
10. Darling EK, McDonald H. A meta-analysis of the efficacy of ocular prophylactic agents used for the prevention of gonococcal and chlamydial ophthalmia neonatorum. *J Midwifery Womens Health.* 2010:55: 319-327.
11. Bielory L, Friedlaender MH. Allergic conjunctivitis. *Immunol Allergy Clin North Am.* 2008;28:43, 58, vi.
12. Management and therapy of dry eye disease: report of the Management and Therapy Subcommittee of the International Dry Eye Workshop (2007). *Ocul Surf.* 2007;5:163.
13. Perry HD, Solomon R, Donnenfeld ED, et al. Evaluation of topical cyclosporine for the treatment of dry eye disease. *Arch Ophthalmol.* 2008;126(8): 1046-1050.
14. Avunduk AM, Avunduk MC, Varnell ED, Kaufman HE. The comparison of efficacies of topical corticosteroids and nonsteroidal anti-inflammatory drops on dry eye patients: a clinical and immunocytochemical study. *Am J Ophthalmol.* 2003;136(4): 593-602.
15. Miljanović B, Trivedi KA, Dana MR, Gibard JP, Buring JE, Schaumberg DA. Relation between dietary n-3 and n-6 fatty acids and clinically diagnosed dry eye syndrome in women. *Am J Clin Nutr.* 2005;82(4): 887-893.
16. Wojtowicz JC, Butovich I, Uchiyama E, Aronowicz J, Agee S, McCulley JP. Pilot, prospective, randomized, double-masked, placebo-controlled clinical trial of an omega-3 supplement for dry eye. Cornea. 2011;30: 308-314.
17. Vogel R, Crockett RS, Oden N, et al. Demonstration of efficacy in the treatment of dry eye disease with 0.18% sodium hyaluronate ophthalmic solution (Vismed, Rejena). *Am J Ophthalmol.* 2010;149(4):594-601.
18. Pan Q, Angelina A, Zambrano A, et al. Autologous serum eye drops for dry eye. *Cochrane Database Syst Rev.* 2013;8:CD009327. doi:10.1002/14651858. CD009327.pub2.
19. Fan DS, Rao SK, Ng JS, Yu CB, Lam DS. Comparative study on the safety and efficacy of different cycloplegic agents in children with darkly pigmented irides. *Clin Experiment Ophthalmol.* 2004;32(5):462-467.
20. Tripathi RC, Tripathi BJ, Haggerty C. Drug-induced glaucomas: mechanism and management. *Drug Safety.* 2003;26(11):749-767.
21. Klein R, Klein BE. The prevalence of age-related eye diseases and visual impairment in aging: current estimates. *Invest Ophthalmol Vis Sci.* 2013;54(14): ORSF5-ORSF13.
22. Akpek EK, Smith RA. Overview of age-related ocular conditions. *Am J Manag Care.* 2013;19(5 suppl): S67-S75.
23. Quigley HA. Glaucoma. *Lancet.* 2011;377(9774): 1367-1377.
24. Kwon YH, Fingert JH, Kuehn MH, Alward WLM. Primary open-angle glaucoma. *N Engl J Med.* 2009; 360(11):1113-1124.
25. Ramdas WD, van Koolwijk LM, Lemij HG, et al. Common genetic variants associated with open-angle glaucoma. *Hum Mol Genet.* 2011;20(12):2464-2471.

26. Jiwani AZ, Rhee DJ, Brauner SC, et al. Effects of caffeinated coffee consumption on intraocular pressure, ocular perfusion pressure, and ocular pulse amplitude: a randomized controlled trial. *Eye (Lond).* 2012;26(8):1122-1130.
27. Peters D, Bengtsson B, Heijl A. Factors associated with lifetime risk of open-angle glaucoma blindness. *Acta Ophthalmol.* 2013;92(5):421-425.
28. Lascaratos G, Garway-Heath DF, Burton R, et al. The United Kingdom Glaucoma Treatment Study: a multicenter, randomized, double-masked, placebo-controlled trial: baseline characteristics. *Ophthalmology.* 2013;120(12):2540-2545.
29. Weinreb RN, Aung T, Medeiros FA. The pathophysiology and treatment of glaucoma: a review. *JAMA* 2014; 311(18):1901-1911.
30. Burr J, Azuara-Blanco A, Avenell A, Tuulonen A. Medical versus surgical interventions for open angle glaucoma. *Cochrane Database Syst Rev.* 2012; 9:CD004399. doi:10.1002/14651858.CD004399.pub3.
31. Law SK. Switching within glaucoma medication class. *Curr Opin Ophthalmol.* 2009;20(2):100-115.
32. Distelhorst JS, Hughes GM. Open-angle glaucoma. *Am Fam Physician.* 2003;67(9):1937-1944.
33. Marquis RE, Whitson JT. Management of glaucoma: focus on pharmacological therapy. *Drugs Aging.* 2005; 22(1):1-21.
34. Grover DS, Smith O. Recent clinical pearls from clinical trials in glaucoma. *Curr Opin Ophthalmol.* 2012;23(2):127-134.
35. Leske MC, Heijl A, Hussein M, et al. Factors for glaucoma progression and the effect of treatment: the Early Manifest Glaucoma Trial. *Arch Ophthalmol.* 2003;121(1):48-56.
36. Leske MC, Heijl A, Hyman L, Bengtsson B, Komaroff E. Factors for progression and glaucoma treatment: the Early Manifest Glaucoma Trial. *Curr Opin Ophthalmol.* 2004;15(2):102-106.
37. Hyman L, Heijl A, Leske MC, Bengtsson B, Yang Z. Early Manifest Glaucoma Trial Group. Natural history of intraocular pressure in the early manifest glaucoma trial: a 6-year follow-up. *Arch Ophthalmol.* 2010;128(5):601-607.
38. American Academy of Ophthalmology Glaucoma Panel. *Preferred Practice Pattern Guidelines: Primary Angle Closure.* San Francisco, CA: American Academy of Ophthalmology; 2010.
39. Abramov Y, Borik S, Yahalom C, et al. Does postmenopausal hormone replacement therapy affect intraocular pressure? *J Glaucoma.* 2005;14(4):271-275.
40. Newman-Casey PA, Talwar N, Nan B, et al. The potential association between postmenopausal hormone use and primary open-angle glaucoma. *JAMA Ophthalmol.* 2014;132(3):298-303.
41. Boland MV, Ervin AM, Friedman DS, et al. Comparative effectiveness of treatments for open-angle glaucoma: a systematic review for the U.S. Preventive Services Task Force. *Ann Intern Med.* 2013;158(4): 271-279.
42. van der Valk R, Webers CA, Lumley T, Hendrikse F, Prins MH, Schouten JS. A network meta-analysis combined direct and indirect comparisons between glaucoma drugs to rank effectiveness in lowering intraocular pressure. *J Clin Epidemiol.* 2009;62(12): 1279-1283.
43. Sambhara D, Aref AA. Glaucoma management: relative value and place in therapy of available drug treatments. *Ther Adv Chronic Dis.* 2014;5(1): 30-43.
44. Mundorf TK, Ogawa T, Naka H, Novack GD, Crocket RS, US Istalol Study Group. A 12-month, multicenter, randomized, double-masked, parallel-group comparison of timolol-LA once daily and timolol maleate ophthalmic solution twice daily in the treatment of adults with glaucoma or ocular hypertension. *Clin Ther.* 2004;26(4):541-551.
45. Han JA, Frishman WH, Wu Sun S, Palmiero PM, Petrillo R. Cardiovascular and respiratory considerations with pharmacotherapy of glaucoma and ocular hypertension. *Cardiol Rev.* 2008;16(2):95-108.
46. Salim S. Glaucoma in pregnancy. *Curr Opin Ophthalmol.* 2014;25(2):93-97.
47. Noecker RJ, Earl ML, Mundorf TK, Silverstein SM, Phillips MP. Comparing bimatoprost and travoprost in black Americans. *Curr Med Res Opin.* 2006; 22(11):2175-2180.
48. Tafluprost (Zioptan): a new topical prostaglandin for glaucoma. *Med Lett Drugs Ther.* 2012;54(1388): 31-32.
49. Orme M, Collins S, Dakin H, Kelly S, Loftus J. Mixed treatment comparison and meta-regression of the efficacy and safety of prostaglandin analogues and comparators for primary open-angle glaucoma and ocular hypertension. *Curr Med Res Opin.* 2010;26(3): 511-528.
50. Bournias TE, Lee D, Gross R, Mattox C. Ocular hypotensive efficacy of bimatoprost when used as a replacement for latanoprost in the treatment of glaucoma and ocular hypertension. *J Ocul Pharmacol Ther.* 2003;19(3):193-203.

51. De Santis M, Lucchese A, Carducci B, et al. Latanoprost exposure in pregnancy. *Am J Ophthalmol.* 2004;138(2):305-306.
52. Fiscella G, Jensen MK. Precautions in use and handling of travoprost. *Am J Health Syst Pharm.* 2003;60(5):484-485; author reply 485.
53. Mulaney J, Sonty S, Ahmad A, Stewart JA, Stewart WC. Comparison of daytime efficacy and safety of dorzolamide/timolol maleate fixed combination versus latanoprost. *Eur J Ophthalmol.* 2008;18(4):556-562.
54. Evans DW, Hosking SL, Gherghel D, Bartlett JD. Contrast sensitivity improves after brimonidine therapy in primary open angle glaucoma: a case for neuroprotection. *Br J Ophthalmol.* 2003;87(12):1463-1465.
55. Krupin T, Liebmann JM, Greenfield DS, et al. A randomized trial of brimonidine versus timolol in preserving visual function: results from the Low-Pressure Glaucoma Treatment Study. *Am J Ophthalmol.* 2011;151(4):671-681.
56. Brinzolamide/brimonidine (Simbrinza) for glaucoma. *Med Lett Drugs Ther.* 2013;55(1421):57-58.
57. Higginbotham EJ, Olander KW, Kim EE, et al. Fixed combination of latanoprost and timolol vs individual components for primary open-angle glaucoma or ocular hypertension: a randomized, double-masked study. *Arch Ophthalmol.* 2010;128(2):165-172.
58. Tanna AP, Rademaker AW, Stewart WC, Feldman RM. Meta-analysis of the efficacy and safety of beta-2-adrenergic agonists, adrenergic antagonists, and topical carbonic anhydrase inhibitors with prostaglandin analogs. *Arch Ophthalmol.* 2010;128(7):825-833.
59. Widengård I, Mäepea O, Alm A. Effects of latanoprost and dipivefrin, alone or combined, on intraocular pressure and on blood–aqueous barrier permeability. *Br J Ophthalmol.* 1998;82(4):404-406.
60. Gandolfi SA, Rossetti L, Cimino L, Mora P, Tardini M, Orzalesi N. Replacing maximum-tolerated medications with latanoprost versus adding latanoprost to maximum-tolerated medications: a two-center randomized prospective trial. *J Glaucoma.* 2003;12(4):347-353.
61. Kaplan-Messas A, Naveh N, Avni I, Marshall J. Ocular hypotensive effects of cholinergic and adrenergic drugs may be influenced by prostaglandins E2 in the human and rabbit eye. *Eur J Ophthalmol.* 2003;13(1):18-23.
62. Hoh ST, Aung T, Chew PT. Medical management of angle closure glaucoma. *Semin Ophthalmol.* 2002;17(2):79-83.
63. Gehlbach P, Li T, Hatef E. Statins for age-related macular degeneration. *Cochrane Database Syst Rev.* 2012; 3:CD006927. doi:10.1002/14651858.CD006927.pub3.
64. Evans JR, Lawrenson JG. Antioxidant vitamin and mineral supplements for slowing the progression of age-related macular degeneration. *Cochrane Database Syst Rev.* 2012;11:CD000254. doi:10.1002/14651858.CD000254.pub3.
65. Li J, Tripathi RC, Tripathi BJ. Drug-induced ocular disorders. *Drug Safety.* 2008;31(2):127-141.
66. Santaella RM, Fraunfelder FW. Ocular adverse effects associated with systemic medications: recognition and management. *Drugs.* 2007;67(1):75-93.
67. Lachkar Y, Bouassida W. Drug-induced acute angle closure glaucoma. *Curr Opin Ophthalmol.* 2007;18(2):129-133.
68. Pula JH, Kao AM, Kattah JC. Neuro-ophthalmologic side-effects of systemic medications. *Curr Opin Ophthalmol.* 2013;24(6):540-549.
69. Abdollahi M, Shafiee A, Bathaiee FS, Sharifzadeh M, Nikfar S. Drug-induced toxic reactions in the eye: an overview. *J Infus Nurs.* 2004;27(6):386-398.
70. Moorthy RS, London NJ, Garg SJ, Cunningham ET Jr. Drug-induced uveitis. *Curr Opin Ophthalmol.* 2013;24(6):589-597.
71. Richa S, Yazbek JC. Ocular adverse effects of common psychotropic agents: a review. *CNS Drugs.* 2010;24(6):501-526.
72. Hendley JO. Clinical practice: otitis media. *N Engl J Med.* 2002;347(15):1169-1174.
73. American Academy of Pediatrics, Subcommittee on Management of Acute Otitis Media. Diagnosis and management of acute otitis media. *Pediatrics.* 2004;113(5):1451-1465.
74. Bouchard ME. Common conditions of the eye and ear. In: Hackley B, Kriebs J, Rousseau ME, eds. *Primary Care of Women: A Guide for Midwives and Women's Health Providers.* Sudbury, MA: Jones and Bartlett; 2007:339-382.
75. Haidvogl M, Riley DS, Heger M, et al. Homeopathic and conventional treatment for acute respiratory and ear complaints: a comparative study on outcome in the primary care setting. *BMC Complement Altern Med.* 2007;7:7.

76. Rosenfeld RM, Schwartz SR, Cannon CR, et al. Clinical practice guideline: acute otitis externa. *Otolaryngol Head Neck Surg.* 2014;150(2):161-168.
77. Sander R. Otitis externa: a practical guide to treatment and prevention. *Am Fam Physician.* 2001;63(5): 927–936, 941-942.
78. Kaushik V, Malik T, Saeed SR. Interventions for acute otitis externa. *Cochrane Database Syst Rev.* 2010;1:CD004740. doi:10.1002/14651858.CD004740.pub2.
79. van Balen FA, Smit WM, Zuithoff NP, Verheij TJ. Clinical efficacy of three common treatments in acute otitis externa in primary care: randomised controlled trial. *BMJ.* 2003;327(7425):1201-1205.
80. Dohar JE, Roland P, Wall GM, McLean C, Stroman DW. Differences in bacteriologic treatment failures in acute otitis externa between ciprofloxacin/dexamethasone and neomycin/polymyxin B/hydrocortisone: results of a combined analysis. *Curr Med Res Opin.* 2009;25(2):287-291.
81. Drehobl M, Guerrero JL, Lacarte PR, Goldstein G, Mata FS, Luber S. Comparison of efficacy and safety of ciprofloxacin otic solution 0.2% versus polymyxin B–neomycin–hydrocortisone in the treatment of acute diffuse otitis externa. *Curr Med Res Opin.* 2008;24(12):3531-3542.
82. Rosenfeld RM, Singer M, Wasserman JM, Stinnett SS. Systematic review of topical antimicrobial therapy for acute otitis externa. *Otolaryngol Head Neck Surg.* 2006;134(4 suppl):S24-S48.
83. Kowatari K, Nakashima K, Ono A, Yoshihara M, Amano M, Toh S. Levofloxacin-induced bilateral Achilles tendon rupture: a case report and review of the literature. *J Orthop Sci.* 2004;9(2):186-190.
84. Ernst E. Ear candles: a triumph of ignorance over science. *J Laryngol Otol.* 2004;118(1):1-2.
85. Seely DR, Quigley SM, Langman AW. Ear candles: efficacy and safety. *Laryngoscope.* 1996;106(10): 1226-1229.
86. Cazals Y. Auditory sensori-neural alterations induced by salicylate. *Prog Neurobiol.* 2000;62(6):583-631.
87. Curhan SG, Shargorodsky J, Eavey R, Curhan GC. Analgesic use and the risk of hearing loss in women. *Am J Epidemiol.* 2012;176(6):544-554.
88. Seligmann H, Podoshin L, Ben-David J, Fradis M, Goldsher M. Drug-induced tinnitus and other hearing disorders. *Drug Safety.* 1996;14(3):198-212.
89. Rybak LP, Ramkumar V. Ototoxicity. *Kidney Int.* 2007;72(8):931-935.
90. Roland PS. New developments in our understanding of ototoxicity. *Ear Nose Throat J.* 2004;83 (9 suppl 4):15-16; discussion 16-17.
91. Yorgason JG, Fayad JN, Kalinec F. Understanding drug ototoxicity: molecular insights for prevention and clinical management. *Expert Opin Drug Safety.* 2006;5(3):383-399.

28
Cancer

Joyce L. King

With acknowledgment to Lori Smith for her contribution to the first edition of Pharmacology for Women's Health

Chapter Glossary

Adjuvant therapy Treatment that is administered after curative surgical intervention or radiation therapy in women who have a high rate of disease recurrence.

Chemotherapeutic agent Anticancer drug that is classified on the basis of their mechanism of action.

Combination chemotherapy Use of multiple chemotherapeutic agents, often with effects at various points within the cell cycle in an attempt to increase effectiveness.

Human epidermal growth factor receptors (HER1 through HER4) Proteins that promote the growth of cancer cells. Cancers that are HER2 positive tend to be more aggressive.

MicroRNA genes Single-stranded RNA molecules that regulate gene expression. These RNA strands usually down-regulate gene expression.

Monoclonal antibody Monospecific antibody that is produced using recombinant technologies. The antibodies are made from immune cells that are cloned from a parent immune cell. When monoclonal antibodies are used as pharmacologic agents, their names always end in "-mab."

Oncogenes Genes that are capable of turning normal cells into cancer cells. For an oncogene to cause cancer, an additional step is usually required, which could be a mutation in another gene or an environmental factor such as a viral infection.

Proto-oncogene Gene that codes for a protein that regulates cell growth or cell differentiation. When a mutation occurs in a proto-oncogene, it can become an oncogene.

Tumor suppressor genes Genes that code for a protein that promotes apoptosis or inhibits progression of the cell cycle. Tumor suppressor proteins repair DNA damage. If tumor suppressor genes are inhibited, the repair work does not occur and the damaged cell will continue to replicate.

Women and Cancer

Cancer has no prejudice with regard to age, race, ethnicity, or gender. More than 500,000 women are diagnosed with cancer annually, and more than 250,000 women will die each year as a result of this disorder. Although the survival rates of persons diagnosed with cancer have improved overall during the last four decades, the improvement is less pronounced among women than among men.[1]

This chapter addresses reproductive organ cancers that affect women. Although women can develop cancer in any tissue, cancer specific to the reproductive organs is the most likely to occur. Breast cancer is the most frequently diagnosed cancer among women, while lung cancer is the variant that most often causes death. The most common cancer specific to the female genital tract is endometrial cancer, which accounts for approximately 6% of all cancers affecting women. Other gynecologic malignancies include cancers of the cervix, fallopian tube, ovary, peritoneum, vagina, and vulva, as well as gestational trophoblastic disease.[1] Breast cancer overwhelmingly occurs among women, albeit not exclusively. For the purposes of this chapter, however, it will be considered a woman's cancer.

Primary care providers routinely and appropriately screen for cancer. Yet there is no such entity as "a touch of cancer." When cancer is found, specialists in oncology provide the expert care. Although management of cancer is directed by an oncology team, the woman's general health care often remains the purview of the primary provider. This chapter provides an overview of chemotherapy and summarizes information about the cancers that most commonly affect women, with an emphasis on information important for the primary care provider to know. Helping to manage side effects of chemotherapy can be an essential contribution of the primary care clinician; thus, pharmacologic therapies to help mitigate chemotherapy side effects are included here.

Characteristics of Neoplastic Cells

Normal cell growth is determined by growth-stimulating signals as well as by the space available for cells to fill. Eventually, all normal cells undergo a signaling process called apoptosis, which initiates the process of cellular death.[2] Malignant cells, however, do not respond to the signals promoting apoptosis; as a consequence, they achieve a type of immortality that allows them to continue to replicate indefinitely during the life of the host. Normal cells tend to stop growing after approximately 50 generations of cellular division, whereas malignant cells lack this characteristic. Depending on histologic type, malignant cells can spread locally or via the lymphatic and circulatory systems.

The word neoplasia is derived from the Latin *neo*, meaning "new," and the Greek *plasis*, meaning "molding" or "growth"; this term for "new growth" is used to describe tissues that demonstrate excessive growth that is not consistent with normal growth patterns. Neoplasms are subclassified as benign, malignant, or borderline malignant. The primary differentiation between benign tumors (also called solid tumors) and malignant tumors (also termed cancer) is that benign tumors do not invade adjacent tissues. Malignant tumors are able to proliferate, invade, and metastasize to distant sites or organs.

No single etiology that causes carcinogenesis, or the creation of cancer, has been identified. Rather, many substances have been shown to have carcinogenic effects, including certain drugs that are used to treat specific disorders. For example, an alkylating agent may be used to treat ovarian cancer, but due to its toxicity may cause leukemia. Other examples of drugs that may have carcinogenic effects are anabolic steroids that are associated with liver cancer, estrogens that induce endometrial cancer, and immunosuppressive drugs that can cause lymphoma and skin cancer. Environmental exposures may also trigger carcinogenesis. Contact with coal tars has been shown to cause skin cancer, while pesticide exposure is associated with development of reproductive cancers.

The abnormal behavior of malignant cells involves irreversible genomic changes that alter critical gatekeeper genes such as **oncogenes**, **tumor suppressor genes**, or **microRNA genes**. Alterations in these genes have been identified in essentially every form of human cancer and are believed to be the initiator of neoplastic growth.[3–5] A **proto-oncogene** is a normal gene that codes for a protein involved in cell growth and cell division. A small mutation can alter the proto-oncogene and change it into an oncogene, which then causes abnormal proliferation of cells. Tumor suppressor genes are responsible for retarding cellular division, repairing DNA errors, and triggering apoptosis. Therefore, when a mutation in a tumor suppressor gene occurs, cells are able to divide rapidly, DNA remains altered, and apoptosis or cellular death is delayed. MicroRNA genes code for a single RNA strand that regulates gene expression.

Sometimes cells develop abnormal characteristics that are not malignant but may develop into malignancies. An example of this type of precursor lesion is high-grade cervical dysplasia, which has the propensity to evolve into squamous cell carcinoma. Unopposed estrogen exposure can lead to atypical endometrial increase in growth of cells, also called hyperplasia or a precursor associated with endometrial cancer.

Genetics and Cancer

Cancer is a genetic disorder. Although the vast majority of cancers arise secondary to a genetic mutation in somatic cells, approximately 5% to 10% of all cancers occur secondary to inherited genetic mutations. The latter disorders are referred to as familial cancer syndrome or hereditary cancer. Two cancer susceptibility syndromes account for the majority of inherited gynecologic cancers: hereditary breast–ovarian cancer syndrome (HBOS) and Lynch syndrome, which may also be termed hereditary nonpolyposis colorectal cancer (HNPCC) syndrome.[6]

Approximately 6% to 13% of ovarian cancer and 5% to 7% of breast cancer is due to genetic mutations in the *BRCA-1* and *BRCA-2* genes. Both of these genes are tumor suppressor genes that help repair damaged DNA.[6] Women who have a *BRCA-1* or *BRCA-2* mutation also have a 35% to 60% lifetime risk of developing ovarian cancer.[6]

Lynch syndrome is a disorder that has been linked with multiple cancers, including colon cancer and other gastrointestinal tumors as well as endometrial, ovarian, and hepatobiliary tract neoplasms. This syndrome is associated with 2% to 3% of all colon cancers and 2% of ovarian cancers.[7] Lynch syndrome is related to mutations in the *MSH2, MLH1, PMS1, PMS2,* and *MSH6* genes that function as DNA repair genes, excising errors that occurs during DNA replication.[7,8] The lifetime risk of colorectal cancer for an individual with Lynch syndrome is 50% to 82% and the lifetime risk of developing endometrial cancer for that woman is approximately 21% to 57%.[7] Both HBOS and Lynch syndrome are inherited in an autosomal dominant pattern.[7]

Although cancer is a genetic disease, not every individual with genetic mutations will develop the condition. Environmental carcinogens usually are important factors. For example, if not exposed to a carcinogen, a woman who has a mutation in her *BRCA-1* or *BRCA-2* gene may never develop an occult cancer, although she retains a 50% chance of passing the genetic mutation on to her offspring.

General Considerations for Use of Chemotherapeutics

While the term "chemotherapy" was historically coined to refer to chemicals (*chemo*) that treat any disease (*therapy*), today this term refers to anticancer drugs that are classified on the basis of their mechanism of action. There are three main—albeit different—goals when treating women with gynecologic malignancies: cure, control, and palliation. Treatment goals depend on multiple factors, including stage at diagnosis, tumor histology, performance status, age, comorbidities, overall health status, and the woman's desire for treatment.

Staging of cancer is of particular importance in developing management plans. Staging is a standardized method of evaluating the extent of cancer in the body and provides information about prognosis, which can guide treatment. Two organizations provide guidance for staging gynecologic cancers: The International Federation of Gynecologists and Obstetricians (FIGO) and the American Joint Committee on Cancer (AJCC) publish staging criteria for gynecologic cancers.[9,10] More information about staging of gynecologic cancers can be found in the Resources table at the end of this chapter.

Cancer stage usually is identified by numbers 0 through IV and most often is subcategorized by TNM levels, which denote such issues as tumor size (T), lymph node involvement (N), and metastasis (M).[9] Staging can also be divided into a clinical stage and a pathologic stage. Although staging remains important, today information such as hormone sensitivity of the tumor, pathology of the sentinel nodes, and risk status also influence the plan of treatment for an individual woman.

Choice of a specific **chemotherapeutic agent** is increasingly being directed by evidence-based research. The National Comprehensive Cancer Network (NCCN) is an alliance of 21 cancer centers that develops evidence-based guidelines for specific cancers.[11] These guidelines are constantly updated as the results of clinical trials become available. Because of the complexity involved in developing the best plan for an individual, treatment is not easily standardized as it is for other conditions. This chapter discusses commonly used chemotherapeutic agents without reference to specific regimens.

Drug Resistance

Drug resistance can be a major obstacle when using chemotherapeutic agents.[12] Two types of drug resistance exist—acquired resistance and intrinsic resistance. Acquired resistance arises secondary to a biochemical change in the cancer cells that occurs subsequent to the introduction of a specific chemotherapeutic agent.[12] Intrinsic resistance occurs when a tumor fails to respond to initial treatment with the cytotoxic agent. Tumors can display pleiotropic resistance—that is, multiple drug resistance—to one or more single agents or even entire drug classes, compromising the action of certain chemotherapeutic agents.[12]

Chemotherapeutic Drug Classes

Chemotherapeutic drugs are either cell cycle specific or cell cycle nonspecific. To understand these distinctions, a brief review of the cell cycle is in order. All cells, normal and malignant, must undergo a four-step sequential cellular replication if they are to survive (Figure 28-1). During the mitotic (M) phase, cellular division occurs. During the postmitotic G_1 phase, cellular activity continues, and RNA synthesis, and DNA repair occur. At this time, the cell will either differentiate and enter the G_0 resting phase, or continue the cell cycle. If the cell enters G_0, which is a period of quiescence, it may reenter the cell cycle at a later time. The synthesis (S) phase is the period in which DNA replication takes place. Following the S phase, a cell enters the

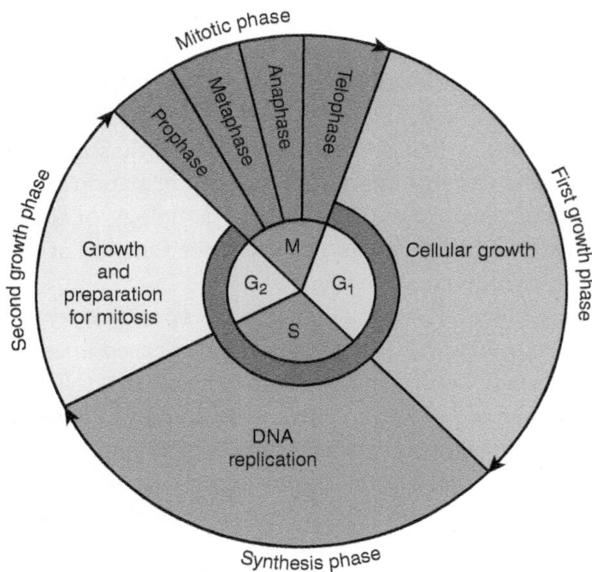

M = Mitotic phase; G_1 = Initial growth phase; G_0 is period of quiescence; S = DNA synthesis; G_2 = Second growth phase.

Figure 28-1 The cell cycle.

G_2 phase, a short period of time when a cell has twice the amount of DNA found in a normal cell. From the G_2 phase, a cell reenters the M phase and completes the cell cycle.

Cell Cycle–Specific Drugs

Drugs that are cell cycle specific are frequently used for treating women with gynecologic malignancies. Such drugs are chosen because they act on the cell during phases when the cell is replicating. Examples of cell cycle–specific agents include etoposide (VP-16), which acts during the G_2 phase; methotrexate (Rheumatrex) and 5-fluorouracil (Adrucil), which act during the S phase; and vinca alkaloids that halt mitosis and are active during the M phase.

Cell Cycle–Nonspecific Drugs

Cell cycle–nonspecific agents can act on cells during any stage of the cell cycle. Examples of such drugs include cisplatin (Platinol), carboplatin (Paraplatin), cyclophosphamide (Cytoxan), doxorubicin (Adriamycin), and mitomycin (Mutamycin).

During the treatment of a particular gynecologic malignancy, **combination chemotherapy** may be used, utilizing both cell cycle–specific and –nonspecific agents. Combination chemotherapy allows for simultaneous treatment of cells during differing phases of the cell cycle and has been shown to be more effective than single-agent therapy.

Chemotherapeutic Drugs' Mechanisms of Action

Chemotherapeutic drugs are further classified on the basis of their mechanism of action, chemical structure, or molecular target.[13,14] Sometimes the classification reflects the original plant source from which the drug is derived.[15] Chemotherapeutic drugs used to treat gynecologic cancers are listed in Table 28-1.

Alkylating Agents

Alkylating agents chemically interact with DNA by attaching an alkyl group to DNA to cause arrest of mitosis during metaphase by forming single- or double-strand breaks of DNA.[16] These drugs are cell cycle nonspecific. Cross-resistance to other drugs within this class is common because the alkylating agents have similar mechanisms of action.

Antitumor Antibiotics

Antitumor antibiotics are a class of chemotherapeutic drugs that are isolated during the fermentation process of naturally occurring fungi such as the *Streptomyces* species.[17] Members of this class of drugs, which are cell cycle nonspecific, cause free radical formation that damages DNA, RNA, and proteins. They also cause metal ion chelation and tumor cell membrane alteration.

Antimetabolites

Antimetabolites are a cell cycle–specific class of drugs that act on proliferating cells, primarily during the S phase. These agents are most effective against rapidly growing tumors that have short doubling times and large growth fractions. A longer duration of exposure to the drug is generally more effective when treating tumors with antimetabolites because of their cell cycle–specific mechanism of action. This class of chemotherapeutic agents is further subclassified into purine analogues, fluorinated pyrimidines, ribonucleotide reductase inhibitors, and folic acid antagonists.

Plant Alkaloids

Several types of alkaloid drugs derived from a variety of plants have differing mechanisms of action, and are generally classified on the basis of their mechanisms of action versus their plant origin. For instance, the Madagascar periwinkle *Catharanthus roseus* is the source of vinca alkaloids such as vinblastine (Velban).[16] These agents cause mitotic arrest at metaphase. Extracts of the roots and rhizomes of *Podophyllum peltatum*, also known as the mandrake plant, are the constituents of the cytotoxic agent

Table 28-1 Selected Cytotoxic Agents: Pharmacologic Class, Indications, and Major Toxicities

Drug: Generic (Brand)	Indication: Type of Cancer	Side Effects/Adverse Effects
Alkylating Agents		
Altretamine (Hexalen)	Recurrent ovarian	All alkylating agents are toxic to tissues that have a high growth fraction; as a consequence, these drugs may have toxic effects on bone marrow, resulting in neutropenia, thrombocytopenia, and anemia. These agents are also toxic to the GI mucosa and to germinal epithelium. Other toxic effects include hair loss and nausea and vomiting.
Carboplatin (Paraplatin)	Cervical, endometrial, EOC, GC, GTD, vaginal vulvar	
Cisplatin (Platinol)	Cervical, endometrial, EOC, GC, GTD, vaginal vulvar	
Melphalan (Alkeran)	Cervical, EOC	
Oxaliplatin (Eloxatin)	EOC	
Thiotepa (Thioplex)	Breast, ovarian, bladder	
Chlorambucil (Leukeran)	EOC, GTD	Bone marrow suppression; an FDA-mandated black box warning reviews the risk of bone marrow suppression, adverse effects on fertility, and teratogenic potential. May cause acute myelocytic leukemia and secondary malignancies.
Cyclophosphamide (Cytoxan)	Breast, ovarian, and several other malignancies	Hemorrhagic cystitis with ifosfamide and cyclophosphamide. Renal damage can be reduced by adequate hydration.
Ifosfamide (Ifex)	Cervical, EOC, sarcoma	
Plant Alkaloids		
Docetaxel (Taxotere)	Breast, EOC	Significant neutropenia is very common. Severe hypersensitivity (hypotension, bronchospasm, generalized rash) can occur. Fluid retention may cause generalized edema, dyspnea at rest, pleural effusion, or pronounced abdominal distention. Other side effects include anemia, nausea, diarrhea, stomatitis, fever, and neurosensory symptoms (paresthesias, pain). Etoposide can cause peripheral neuropathy following repeated infusions (may not be reversible). It is also associated with hypotension, bradycardia, second- and third-degree heart block, and rarely fatal myocardial infarction. Muscle and joint pain has also occurred. Hair loss, nausea and vomiting, diarrhea, and mucositis are common.
Etoposide (Etopophos, VePesid)	EOC, GTD, GC, sarcoma	
Paclitaxel (Taxol, Onxol)	Ovarian, breast, endometrial	
Vinblastine (Velban)	Breast, GC, GTD	
Vincristine (Oncovin)	Breast, GC, GTD	
Vinorelbine (Navelbine)	EOC, cervical	
Topoisomerase-1 Inhibitors		
Irinotecan (Camptosar)	EOC	Bone marrow suppression is the dose-limiting side effect (neutropenia occurs in 98% of those treated). Other side effects include hair loss, nausea, vomiting, diarrhea, stomatitis, abdominal pain, and headache.
Topotecan (Hycamtin)	Ovarian	
Hormonal Agents		
Anastrozole (Arimidex)	Breast	Aromatase inhibitor. The most common side effects are mild but can include hot flashes, vaginal dryness, musculoskeletal pain, and headache.
Exemestane (Aromasin)	Breast	Aromatase inhibitor. The most common side effects are fatigue, nausea, hot flushes, depression, and weight gain.
Fluoxymesterone (Halotestin)	Breast	The doses of these drugs, when used for breast cancer, are high; therefore virilization is a common side effect. Adverse effects include severe hypercalcemia.
Testosterone	Breast	
Testolactone (Teslac)	Breast	
Fulvestrant (Faslodex)	Breast	The most common side effects are GI disturbances, hot flushes, headaches, pharyngitis, and bone and back pain.
Letrozole (Femara)	Breast	Aromatase inhibitor. The most common side effects are musculoskeletal pain and nausea.
Megestrol acetate (Megace)	Endometrial, breast, ESS	Thromboembolism is uncommon. There is no increased risk for endometrial cancer.
Raloxifene (Evista)	Breast	Estrogen agonist antagonist/Selective estrogen receptor modulator. Side effects are similar to those associated with tamoxifen, although raloxifene does not increase the risk for endometrial cancer.
Tamoxifen (Nolvadex)	Breast, EOC	Estrogen agonist antagonist/Selective estrogen receptor modulator. The most common side effects are hot flashes, fluid retention, vaginal discharge, nausea, vomiting, and irregular vaginal bleeding. There is an increased risk of thromboembolic events (e.g., deep vein thrombosis, pulmonary embolism, and stroke). Tamoxifen acts as an estrogen agonist in the uterus, increasing the risk for endometrial cancer.
Toremifene (Fareston)	Metastatic breast cancer	Major toxicities are similar to those associated with tamoxifen.

(continues)

Table 28-1 Selected Cytotoxic Agents: Pharmacologic Class, Indications, and Major Toxicities (*continued*)

Drug: Generic (Brand)	Indication: Type of Cancer	Side Effects/Adverse Effects
Monoclonal Antibodies		
Bevacizumab (Avastin)	EOC	The major adverse effect is cardiac damage that can lead to ventricular dysfunction and congestive heart failure. Many individuals experience flulike symptoms during the first infusion. Infrequently, some persons may have a serious hypersensitivity reaction. Trastuzumab does not cause bone marrow suppression or hair loss.
Trastuzumab (Herceptin)	Metastatic breast	
Antimetabolites		
Capecitabine (Xeloda)	Metastatic colorectal and breast	Severe diarrhea is common and can be dose limiting. Other common side effects include nausea and vomiting, stomatitis, and numbness, tingling, pain, swelling, and erythema of the palms and soles. Can cause leucopenia, but severe bone marrow suppression is uncommon. Hair loss has not been reported.
Fluorouracil (5-FU)	Colon, rectal, breast, stomach, and pancreatic	The most common dose-limiting toxicities are neutropenia and oral and GI ulceration. Other side effects include hair loss, hyperpigmentation, and neurologic deficits.
Gemcitabine (Gemzar)	Recurrent ovarian, metastatic breast, and uterine sarcomas	The main dose-limiting response, if myelosuppression occurs, is neutropenia. GI effects may include nausea, vomiting, diarrhea, and mucositis. Pulmonary adverse effects are rare but reported. Flu-type syndrome is reported in some women.
Hydroxyurea (Hydrea)		Inhibits the production of DNA. Side effects include nausea and vomiting, diarrhea, constipation, mucositis, and myelosuppression. Concern that hydroxyurea can increase the risk of leukemia limits its use, although studies that corroborate this association are lacking.
Methotrexate (Rheumatrex, Trexall)	GTD, noncancers such as ectopic pregnancy and rheumatoid arthritis	This antifolate has minimal side effects at therapeutic doses. An FDA-mandated black box warning focuses on toxic effects that may cause death, including renal, kidney, and liver toxicity; bone marrow suppression; hemorrhagic enteritis; and pneumonitis.
Antitumor Antibiotics		
Actinomycin D (Dactinomycin)	GTD	May be used in combination therapy. Myelosuppression is the main effect that causes changes in dosing. GI toxicity, alopecia, and skin ulceration secondary to action as a vesicant have been reported.
Bleomycin (Mithracin)	Ovarian	Main toxic effects are pulmonary adverse effects such as pneumonitis, especially among the elderly. Rashes also are common. Neutropenia is not a common effect.
Doxorubicin (Adriamycin)	Endometrial, breast	Cardiotoxicity is most pronounced among women 70 years and older and with cumulative dosing. GI side effects tend to be mild, but alopecia is to be expected.
Liposomal doxorubicin (Doxil)	Recurrent epithelial ovarian carcinoma	Minimal GI, alopecia, and cardiotoxicity effects. Increased risk of stomatitis and palmar–plantar erythrodysesthesia for women using this drug compared to others in same drug category.
Mitomycin-C (Mutamycin)		Myelosuppression is the main effect that causes changes in dosing. GI toxicity, alopecia, and skin ulceration are secondary to its action as a vesicant have been reported.

Abbreviations: EOC = epithelial ovarian carcinoma; ESS = endometrial stromal sarcoma; GC = germ cell tumor; GI = gastrointestinal; GTD = gestational trophoblastic disease.

epipodophyllotoxin (etoposide, VP-16). This drug blocks the cell cycle in the late S phase by causing damage to the DNA. Taxanes, such as paclitaxel (Taxol) and docetaxel (Taxotere), are derived from the bark of *Taxus brevifolia* and *Taxus baccata*, respectively.[17] These mitotic spindle inhibitors interfere with mitosis.

Topoisomerase-1 Inhibitors

Topoisomerase-1 is an enzyme that is necessary for DNA replication, repair, and transcription. When DNA activity is blocked by topoisomerase-1 inhibitors, DNA strands break and cell death occurs. Topoisomerase-1 inhibitors are cell cycle specific. Examples of such drugs that are used in the treatment of gynecologic malignancies include topotecan (Hycamtin) and irinotecan (Camptosar), both of which are derived from the wood stem of the *Camptotheca acuminate* tree.

Hormonal Agents

Hormonal agents are effective for treatment of hormone-dependent tumors and are used to treat certain gynecologic malignancies, such as ovarian and endometrial carcinomas, as well as breast cancer. Hormonal agents have multiple mechanisms of action. Some are used to suppress production of a specific hormone naturally produced by the human body. For example, aromatase inhibitors prevent androgens from being converted into estrogen in postmenopausal women, thereby blocking the effect of estrogen in promoting tumor growth. Other hormonal agents block the hormone receptors on the surface of the tumor cell. Still others substitute chemically similar substances that are inactive for the active hormones. Hormonal agents used to treat cancer include progestins, antiestrogens, aromatase inhibitors, androgens, antiandrogens, and estrogen antagonists/agonists (EAAs), also known as selective estrogen receptor modulators (SERMs).

Monoclonal Antibodies

In 1893, W. B. Coley published an article advocating the treatment of cancer with injections of killed bacteria.[18] Coley noticed that individuals with solid tumors who subsequently developed a high fever and bacterial infection caused by *Streptococcus pyogenes* often experienced a regression of the cancerous tumor. He postulated that induction of the immune system by the bacterial infection facilitated or caused an immune response against the tumor. Coley subsequently invented an infusion of killed bacteria, called Coley's toxins, that successfully induced remissions in several individuals with severe tumors. The advent of radiotherapy eventually eclipsed this initial foray into immunotherapy, and the approach was not pursued again until the late twentieth century.

Today, cancer immunotherapy is the subject of a large number of research investigations. In 1997, the U.S. Food and Drug Administration (FDA) approved the first **monoclonal antibody** for use in cancer, thereby bringing immunotherapy back into focus in the war against cancer. Monoclonal antibodies are a form of passive immunization.[19] These tumor-specific antibodies are effective for only a short duration of time, however, and they must be provided in large amounts. Two types of monoclonal antibodies are used in cancer therapy—naked and conjugated. Naked monoclonal antibodies lack a drug or radioactive substance attachment, whereas conjugated monoclonal antibodies are attached to a chemotherapeutic agent, radioactive substance, or toxin.[19] The standard chemotherapeutic drugs interfere with mitosis, DNA synthesis, and DNA repair systems. The immunotherapeutic agents capitalize on immune response processes to retard tumor growth and/or induce apoptosis. The different mechanisms of action have correspondingly different side effects and adverse effects.[20]

Examples of monoclonal antibodies used in the treatment of gynecologic malignancies include trastuzumab (Herceptin) and bevacizumab (Avastin), which are used to treat breast cancer. Trastuzumab is used for the treatment of breast cancer characterized by an over-expression of the **human epidermal growth factor receptors (HER1 through HER4)**. These transmembrane receptors normally regulate cell growth and survival when they are activated.[21] Trastuzumab, however, binds to HER2 receptors and prevents activation of their agonist effect.[21] Bevacizumab, a monoclonal antibody, binds to vascular endothelial growth factor (VEGF), a substance necessary for the production of new blood vessels, in an attempt to halt angiogenesis.[22]

Breast Cancer

According to the American Cancer Society, the 5-year survival rate for women diagnosed with localized breast cancer has increased from 80% in the 1950s to 99% today, with some variation based upon staging of the cancer.[1,10] Breast cancer staging ranges from stage 0, which is ductal carcinoma in situ without spread to regional lymph or distant metastases, to stage IV, which includes a tumor of any size and distant metastases.[10] The improvement in survival time for breast cancer has been attributed to earlier detection through more widespread and more effective screening as well as to improved treatments.[23]

Surgery and radiotherapy are used to treat tumors in the breast, chest wall, and regional lymph nodes, while chemotherapy drugs and hormonal agents are used as **adjuvant therapy** to reduce metastasis and recurrences. Trastuzumab (Herceptin) is recommended as adjuvant therapy for women with HER2-positive invasive breast cancer.[20, 24] The National Comprehensive Cancer Network publishes clinical practice guidelines that list current recommended regimens for treating women with breast cancer.[25]

The majority of breast cancers express estrogen receptors that facilitate cell growth when estrogen binds to the receptor. For women whose tumors are estrogen receptor positive, agents that inhibit the growth of those tumors by competitive antagonism of estrogen at its receptor site generally are recommended to reduce the likelihood of recurrence and to prolong disease-free survival. The standard hormonal treatment is tamoxifen (Nolvadex), an EAA (SERM) agent.

Tamoxifen's mechanism of action is complex because EAAs have partial estrogen-agonist effects as well as act as estrogen-antagonist effects. The agonist effects can have additional benefits such as prevention of bone loss in postmenopausal women, but they can be detrimental when they increase the risk of estrogen-related uterine cancer and thromboembolism.[26,27]

Aromatase inhibitors can be an alternative to tamoxifen. These drugs suppress estrogen levels in postmenopausal women by inhibiting aromatase, the enzyme responsible for the synthesis of estrogen from androgenic substrates in peripheral tissues. Unlike tamoxifen, aromatase inhibitors have no agonist activity.[28] Therefore, these agents are not associated with adverse estrogenic effects—but they also lack the agonist (positive) effect on bone.

Chemoprevention

There is no question that prevention of a disease is a far better choice than treatment after the disease develops. Due to the relatively high incidence of breast cancer and its known response to chemotherapy, research has been conducted in the area of chemoprevention of breast cancer. Although this method seems promising, some major clinical questions persist regarding use of chemotherapeutics to decrease the risk of the disease, as described in Box 28-1.[27,29,30]

Box 28-1 To Treat or Not to Treat: The Role of Chemoprevention

Treatment of cancer, although clearly important, is of less value than primary prevention of the disease. After more than 20 years of use as adjuvant chemotherapy, the drug tamoxifen was approved by the FDA in 1998 for use as a chemopreventive agent for breast cancer. In 2007, a second EAA, raloxifene (Evista), was approved for the indication of breast cancer chemoprevention. For both drugs, studies found that the risk of breast cancer was reduced by more than 40% among high-risk women who used these agents prophylactically in the postmenopausal period. Unfortunately, neither drug is without side effects and adverse effects.

Some authorities suggest raloxifene is the better choice because thromboembolic events and endometrial hyperplasia occur less often with this drug than with tamoxifen. In either case, major questions remain unanswered regarding who should be characterized as "high risk," which women will benefit the most from chemoprevention, how long these agents should be used, and how long the protection lasts.

Cervical Cancer

Human papillomavirus (HPV) infection is the most important risk factor for the development of both preinvasive and invasive cervical cancer. The FDA has approved the use of human papilloma quadrivalent recombinant vaccines for the prevention of HPV infection caused by HPV types 6, 11, 16, and 18 in girls and women. More information about HPV vaccines is available in the *Sexually Transmitted Infections* and *Immunizations* chapters.

The FIGO clinical practice guidelines and staging criteria are most frequently used to stage cervical cancers.[9] Staging of cervical carcinoma ranges from stage I to stage IV.[9] Stage I cancer is confined to the cervix and associated with a 5-year survival rate of 95% or higher. Stage IV includes mucosal involvement of the bladder or rectum, or distant disease, and has a 5-year survival rate of 20% to 30%. Each stage has a subdivision of A or B based on extension of the tumor. Chemotherapy is used to treat cervical cancer in two scenarios: (1) as primary treatment for women who present with stage IVB or recurrent disease and (2) in women with stage IIB, III, or IVA disease in conjunction with radiation therapy.[31]

Endometrial Cancer

The most common gynecologic malignancy among women in the United States is endometrial carcinoma, which accounts for 6% of all cancers affecting women.[1] Ninety percent of women with endometrial cancer initially present with vaginal bleeding, most commonly in the postmenopausal period.[32] In the United States, uterine sarcomas represent fewer than 5% of uterine cancers and include malignant mixed Müllerian tumors, leiomyosarcomas, and other classifications such as endometrial stromal sarcomas.

FIGO staging of endometrial and ovarian carcinoma ranges from stage I to stage IV. For endometrial carcinoma, the tumor is confined to the corpus uteri in stage I; it invades the bladder and/or bowel mucosa and/or demonstrates distant metastasis in stage IV. For ovarian carcinoma, the tumor is confined to the ovaries in stage I and extends to the bladder and/or bowel mucosa and/or shows distant metastasis in stage IV.[9]

Most women with endometrial cancer present with early endometrial cancer (stage I), and are treated surgically with a hysterectomy. For women who present with advanced or metastatic disease, however, radiation, brachytherapy, or radiation seed implantation with or without surgery or chemotherapy may be recommended.

Gestational Trophoblastic Disease

Gestational trophoblastic disease (GTD) comprises a spectrum of rare, highly curable tumors that arise from placental tissue. These include hydatidiform moles, benign non-neoplastic trophoblastic lesions, and gestational trophoblastic neoplasia (GTN). The different GTD disorders are classified on the basis of histology and malignant or nonmalignant characteristics (Table 28-2).

Although the etiology remains uncertain, at some early point in the pregnancy, trophoblastic cells that normally would form the placenta proliferate and villous stroma becomes edematous. The latter changes evolve into the grapelike clusters that characterize a hydatidiform mole. Hydatidiform moles are categorized as either complete hydatidiform mole or incomplete hydatidiform mole based on the degree and extent of the changes. Complete and partial hydatidiform moles can develop into nonmetastatic or metastatic gestational trophoblastic neoplasia.[33]

Gestational Trophoblastic Neoplasia

Complete hydatidiform moles are the type of mole most likely to develop into GTN. In turn, GTN comprises a group of tumors that include choriocarcinoma, placental site trophoblastic tumor, epithelioid trophoblastic tumor, and invasive mole. Any of these conditions can occur subsequent to a normal pregnancy or a molar pregnancy. The most common GTN tumors are invasive moles and gestational choriocarcinoma, based on characteristics of the disease. Invasive moles penetrate the myometrium but tend not to metastasize to distant organs. Chemotherapy is highly effective against these tumors, and cure rates range from 80% to 100% depending on the extent of the disease.[34] Choriocarcinoma, however, usually develops systemic metastases if not aggressively treated early.

Once GTN is diagnosed, surgical treatment in the form of a hysterectomy is a common first-line treatment. Chemotherapy is recommended with or without surgery. For women with low-risk disease, the most common chemotherapeutic agent is the folic acid antagonist, methotrexate (Rheumatrex, Trexall), although some oncologists prescribe pulsed actinomycin D (Dactinomycin). Women who have high-risk GTN, including those who are older that 40 years, have an hCG level of 10^5 or higher, and

Table 28-2 Gestational Trophoblastic Tumors

Tumor Type	Description	Benign versus Malignant
Hydatidiform mole	Placental villi swollen in fluid-filled clusters. Hydatidiform moles are not cancerous, but they can develop into GTN. They are subdivided into two categories—partial and complete.	A hydatidiform mole is considered malignant when serum beta-hCG levels continue to rise after surgical removal (assuming a normal pregnancy is not present). This occurs in 15–20% of hydatidiform moles.
Partial hydatidiform mole	Partial hydatidiform moles occur when two sperm fertilize an egg. The tumor contains some fetal tissue but no fetus.	Persistent trophoblastic disease occurs in 1–5% of partial moles.
Complete hydatidiform mole	A complete hydatidiform mole develops when 1 or 2 sperm fertilize an egg that does not have maternal DNA. This hydatidiform mole is completely paternal genetic material, and there is no fetal tissue.	Persistent trophoblastic disease, indicating malignancy, occurs in 15–20% of complete molar pregnancies.
Gestational Trophoblastic Neoplasia		
Invasive mole	Hydatidiform mole that grows into the uterine myometrium.	Invasive moles are malignant. Approximately 15% metastasize to distant organs, usually the lungs.
Choriocarcinoma	Choriocarcinoma can develop de novo in other organs such as ovaries or chest. Most often associated with a complete hydatidiform mole.	Highly metastatic if untreated.
Placental-site trophoblastic tumor and epithelioid trophoblastic tumor	Rare gestational trophoblastic neoplasms. Unlike choriocarcinoma, these trophoblastic tumors can develop long after a gestational event.	Approximately 15–25% become malignant with distant metastases.

Abbreviations: GTN = gestational trophoblastic neoplasia; hCG = human chorionic gonadotropin.
Source: Data from Berkowitz RS, Goldstein DP. Clinical practice: molar pregnancy. *N Engl J Med.* 2009;360(16):1639-1645.[33]

women diagnosed with multiple metastases, are treated with combination chemotherapy.

A woman who has one molar pregnancy has a 1% to 2% risk of experiencing another. Pregnancy after chemotherapy has not been found to confer an increased risk of adverse outcomes.[34]

Ovarian Cancer

Ovarian cancer is the leading cause of death from a gynecologic malignancy in the United States.[1] Symptoms of this disease are vague, which makes its diagnosis challenging. The most common symptoms include bloating, pelvic and/or abdominal pain, urinary symptoms such as frequency or urgency, early satiety, and difficulty eating. Most women (75%) have stage III or IV disease at initial diagnosis; overall, approximately 44% of women diagnosed with the disease will survive for 5 years and fewer than 20% will be cured.[35]

Women with ovarian cancer are initially treated surgically with a total hysterectomy and bilateral oophorectomy. Ovarian malignancies encompass multiple histopathologic subtypes. The majority develop from ovarian epithelial cells (epithelial ovarian carcinoma), but a small proportion develop from other types of cells within the ovary. Upon final histopathologic diagnosis, an appropriate treatment plan is individualized for each woman and different drug combinations are used.

A number of cytotoxic agents can be used for treating epithelial ovarian cancer. The standard agents for treating this disease are platinum compounds, such as cisplatin and carboplatin, along with a taxane such as paclitaxel (Taxol) or docetaxel (Taxotere). Women are considered platinum sensitive if they experience no recurrence of the disease more than 6 months after their last dose of the platinum agent. Women who are considered platinum resistant have (1) disease progression while on an initial platinum-based chemotherapy regimen; (2) continued stable disease while on initial treatment; or (3) relapse within 6 months after a combination regimen.

Vulvar and Vaginal Cancer

Vaginal and vulvar cancers are the least common gynecologic malignancies. Squamous cell carcinomas account for 85% of vaginal cancers and are known to metastasize to the lungs and liver in many women. Conversely, adenocarcinoma represents 15% of vaginal cancers and is most often seen in women 17 to 21 years, with common sites of metastasis being the lungs and supraclavicular and pelvic lymph nodes. Less commonly occurring vaginal cancers include melanoma, sarcoma, and adenosquamous types.

Women with a history of in utero diethylstilbestrol (DES) exposure present with vaginal adenosis, which can progress into a vaginal or cervical adenocarcinoma.[36–38] Although rare, these clear cell adenocarcinomas occur more frequently in women with a history of in utero DES exposure and this risk may continue throughout their lifespan.[36–38] DES was removed from the market in the 1970s, and as the cohort of exposed women has aged, their relative risks for different cancers continue to be elucidated. Thus, it is important for clinicians caring for women of all ages to remember the DES story (Box 28-2).

Vulvar cancer can occur at any age but is most often seen in women who are postmenopausal.[39] Many vulvar cancers are preceded by condylomas or dysplasias, and HPV is the causative factor in the development of many genital tract malignanies.[40] Cellular types include basal cell carcinoma, verrucous carcinoma, sarcoma, histiocytosis X, and malignant melanoma. Treatment options for both vulvar and vaginal cancers depend on the cellular classification and stage of the disease, but include surgery, radiation, and chemotherapy. Cisplatin (Platinol) with or without fluorouracil (Adrucil) is the chemotherapeutic regimen most often used.

Major Chemotherapeutic Side Effects and Adverse Effects

Chemotherapeutic agents have an array of toxic side effects and adverse effects that are collectively referred to as chemotherapy toxicities. Some, such as alopecia, do not have pharmacologic treatments; these effects are not addressed here. Readers interested in supportive treatments for all cancer toxicities can find more information in the Resources table at the end of this chapter.

In general, highly proliferative cells, such as those in the gastrointestinal tract and bone marrow, are the cells that—in addition to tumor cells—are most affected by chemotherapeutic agents.[14] Bone marrow suppression becomes evident after mature blood components are normally removed from the system and results in varying degrees of cytopenia, including anemia, neutropenia, and thrombocytopenia. White blood cells, especially neutrophils, have the shortest lifespan (6 to 12 hours), which is why neutropenia is the most common form of myelosuppression induced by chemotherapeutic agents. Platelets normally live 5 to 10 days, and when they are depleted, thrombocytopenia

Box 28-2 Gone But Not Forgotten: Diethylstilbestrol (DES)

Diethylstilbestrol is a nonsteroidal estrogen that was discovered more than seven decades ago in England. In the early 1940s, this drug received FDA approval as a treatment for gonorrhea, atrophic vaginitis, and menopause, as well as a lactation suppression agent. Gradually, DES gained popularity for off-label use to treat threatened abortion and as a prophylactic intervention for women with a history of previous spontaneous abortion. In 1947, this indication was added to the list by the FDA. By the mid-1950s, research found that DES was not effective to prevent pregnancy loss, yet the drug continued to be used, although the number of prescriptions decreased. The peak years of DES use were between 1941 and 1971. In 1971, researchers found DES causes a rare form of vaginal tumor called clear cell carcinoma and the FDA withdrew approval for use of DES for any pregnancy indications. However, DES retained FDA approval for treatment of lactation suppression until 1978, and treatment of advanced breast cancer until the 1990s. DES continued to be used off-label for post-coital contraception until 1975 when the FDA added a strong note to the product label stating DES should not be used for post-coital contraception.

Many agents have been discovered to be ineffective and disappeared from the market. Although use of DES in early pregnancy ceased, this drug's effects last for a lifetime—actually, potentially across multiple generations. Women who took DES have an increased risk of breast cancer—a classic example of how endocrine disruption in the fetal environment induces epigenetic effects. Persons exposed to DES in utero are commonly called DES daughters and DES sons. DES daughters have an increased risk of clear cell vaginal adenocarcinoma, a relatively rare cancer. They also have an increased risk of breast cancer, clear cell cancers of the cervix and vagina, infertility, and pregnancy complications such as preterm birth. Long-term effects for DES sons suggest increased risks of epididymal cysts, hypospadias, and perhaps autoimmune disorders. Research continues to be ongoing regarding the second generation as these individuals age.

Research today on the grandchildren of women who took DES during pregnancy suggests that it is possible DES will continue to plague families, as the children of DES daughters and DES sons may have untoward health outcomes. However, longitudinal studies are needed to identify any third-generation effects and to establish how much longer this drug, even though it is no longer available, will continue to impact future generations.

can become evident. Red blood cells normally live approximately 120 days, but an individual with cancer can become anemic in many ways other than experiencing bone marrow suppression; anemia, therefore, is a common problem for women using these treatment regimens.

All of the epithelial cells that line the gastrointestinal tract have a rapid turnover time. Mucositis and diarrhea are both manifestations of chemotherapy-associated gastrointestinal toxicities. These side effects and adverse effects are most likely to be the symptoms that a primary care clinician can help treat. The Multinational Association of Supportive Care in Cancer listed in the Resources table at the end of this chapter is an international coalition of professional associations in oncology that updates clinical practice guidelines pertinent to care of chemotherapy side effects and adverse effects.

All of the symptoms reviewed here can arise secondary to any number of disorders. Therefore, the first step in evaluating an individual on chemotherapy who presents with one of the following symptoms is to identify and treat other causes before using agents specifically recommended for chemotherapy toxicities.

Anemia

Despite the fact that red blood cells have a longer lifespan than other blood components, anemia is a common hematologic abnormality in persons receiving chemotherapy. While chemotherapeutic drugs primarily cause anemia by reducing the number of circulating erythrocytes, additional etiologies include malnutrition secondary to mucositis, hemolysis, renal dysfunction, and bone marrow metastases. Many women are already anemic when chemotherapy is initiated. If the cause is determined to be myelosuppression, anemia can be treated with iron supplementation, a blood transfusion, or an erythropoiesis-stimulating drug.[41]

Erythropoietin, which is produced in the kidney, regulates red blood cell production. In 1993, the FDA approved the use of human recombinant erythropoietin-stimulating agents such as epoetin alfa (Procrit, Eprex, and Epogen) for the treatment of chemotherapy-induced anemia.[41] Initial studies and a meta-analysis found that erythropoietin-stimulating agents increase hemoglobin levels, decrease the need for blood transfusion, and reduce fatigue.[42] Unfortunately, more recent studies have found that epoetin alfa increases the risk of thromboembolic disease, promotes tumor growth, and may be associated with decreased survival.[42]

In 2007, the FDA issued a black box warning for erythropoietin that cautions about the potential for tumor promotion and thromboembolic events. An FDA advisory panel in 2008 recommended that this drug be used at the lowest dose feasible and only for individuals with a hemoglobin level less than 11 g/dL.[43]

Constipation

Constipation, like all other chemotherapy side effects, can be the result of an underlying medical condition, medications, such as antiemetics or opioids, or the chemotherapy drugs themselves. The most serious complication associated with constipation is bowel obstruction. Symptoms of bowel obstruction include nausea, vomiting, abdominal distention, decreased or no flatus, decreased or no bowel movements, and cramp-like abdominal pain.

Unless contraindicated, medications such as psyllium (Metamucil), senna (SenoKot), bisacodyl (Dulcolax), docusate sodium (Colace), glycerin suppository, magnesium hydroxide (Milk of Magnesia), lactulose (Chronulac), and sorbitol and sodium phosphate (Fleet's enema) are reasonable treatments for constipation.

Because the drugs for constipation work via different mechanisms of action, some may be more effective than others for women experiencing chemotherapy-associated constipation. In contrast, others—such as bulk laxatives, which have a side effect of bloating and pain—may not be recommended following abdominal surgery. In addition, all laxatives are contraindicated for persons with intestinal obstruction and should be used with caution if the woman is not able to maintain hydration. Specific doses and regimens for these drugs are discussed in more detail in the *Gastrointestinal Conditions* chapter.

Diarrhea

Chemotherapeutic drugs can have a direct effect on the gastrointestinal mucosa, causing inflammation, edema, and ulceration. The immunosuppressive drugs that are frequently used during cancer treatment render the woman vulnerable to opportunistic infections within the gastrointestinal tract; such infections can, in turn, cause diarrhea.

Diarrhea is classified as osmotic, secretory, exudative, or secondary to motility disturbances; chemotherapy-associated diarrhea is often secretory and/or exudative in nature.[44] 5-Fluorouracil and topoisomerase-1 inhibitors such as irinotecan (Camptosar) are highly likely to cause diarrhea.[44–46]

Loperamide

The American Society of Clinical Oncology recommends loperamide (Imodium) as the first-line pharmacologic treatment for chemotherapy-associated diarrhea. Loperamide is a synthetic opioid derivative that slows intestinal motility. The slower transit, in turn, allows for increased absorption of fluid.[44,47–49] Loperamide is not absorbed systemically and is excreted in the feces unchanged.[46] The recommended dose of this medication is 4 mg after the first incidence of diarrhea, followed by 2 mg after each loose stool or every 4 hours. The maximum dose is 20 mg per day.

Octreotide

Octreotide (Sandostatin), administered intravenously or subcutaneously, is usually the second pharmacologic agent employed if the symptoms of chemotherapy-associated diarrhea are not relieved after using loperamide.[45] Octreotide is associated with multiple side effects and adverse effects, including hypertension, sinus bradycardia, arrhythmia, fatigue, malaise, fever, pruritus, and hyperglycemia. Thus it is used only when loperamide is not effective.

Other Therapies for Diarrhea

Some authorities recommend tincture of opium or budesonide (Entocort EC) for diarrhea that is refractory to loperamide. Complicated diarrhea can be treated with antibiotics based on the assumption that an infection is involved.[47] Agents that have been proposed as treatments for chemotherapy-associated diarrhea but that lack evidence for their use include charcoal, probiotics, and glutamate.

Fatigue

One of the most common and distressing side effects of cancer and cancer treatment is fatigue, which can occur secondary to anemia, depression, pain, or the cancer itself. Multiple randomized trials have assessed both pharmacologic and nonpharmacologic treatments for fatigue.[50] Several studies have shown that both cognitive-behavioral therapy and exercise are effective nonpharmacologic methods to reduce fatigue. A Cochrane meta-analysis of 27 randomized trials found that methylphenidate (Ritalin) and erythropoietin have a modest positive effect on cancer-related fatigue, but paroxetine (Prozac) and progestational steroids are no better than placebo in this indication.[51]

Hypersensitivity Reactions

Approximately 5% to 40% of women treated with an intravenous infusion of a chemotherapeutic drug for a malignancy will have some form of hypersensitivity reaction to the agent used during treatment.[52] Hypersensitivity reactions are common following administration of L-asparaginase, taxanes, and procarbazine.[52,53] Hypersensitivity reactions to platinum occurs in approximately 5% to 20% of persons treated, and it has been reported that 12% of individuals exposed to carboplatin may experience an allergic reaction.

Prophylaxis with an antihistamine, corticosteroid, or both is common practice; however, premedication does not prevent all hypersensitivity reactions and will not prevent anaphylaxis. Premedication prior to an infusion of paclitaxel often includes dexamethasone (Decadron), diphenhydramine (Benadryl), and an H_2 antagonist such as cimetidine (Tagamet) (Table 28-3). If a hypersensitivity reaction occurs, the medication is discontinued. Additional administration of an antihistamine, a steroid, or possibly epinephrine is usually sufficient to reverse the process.[52]

Mucositis

Mucositis refers to damage to the mucosa, secondary to cancer therapy, that occurs in the oral, pharyngeal, laryngeal, and esophageal regions.[54] This adverse effect occurs in approximately 20% to 40% of persons who receive conventional chemotherapy and approximately 80% of persons who receive high-dose chemotherapy. Mucositis generally presents as erythema or ulceration of the oral mucosa. The buccal and labial mucosa, oral soft palate and floor, and ventral surface of the tongue are the areas most commonly affected, with symptoms arising approximately 5 to 7 days after chemotherapy administration.

The 2014 Multinational Association of Supportive Care in Cancer guidelines include treatments for mucositis secondary to specific chemotherapy regimens.[53] Due to its desiccant effects, milk of magnesia (MOM) should be avoided. Cold liquids and ice chips may be implemented for comfort. Pharmacologic management may include the use of 2% viscous lidocaine or a 50/50 mixture of attapulgite/diphenhydramine (Kaopectate/Benadryl) to be used as needed.[55] Systemic analgesics can be administered to minimize pain.[56]

Table 28-3 Example Premedication Regimen for Prevention of a Hypersensitivity Reaction

Drug: Generic (Brand)	Dose
Cimetedine (Tagamet)	300 mg IV 30 minutes before administration
Dexamethasone (Decadron)	20 mg orally 12 and 6 hours before and 20 mg IV just before administration of chemotherapy
Diphenhydramine (Benadryl)	50 mg IV 30 minutes before administration of chemotherapy

Neutropenia

Neutrophils are phagocytes that are highly important in immune function and infection prevention. Neutropenia—depletion of neutrophils—is the most common dose-limiting factor in adjusting chemotherapy dosing schedules. Depending on the chemotherapeutic agent used, neutropenia generally appears 6 to 12 days after drug administration; in most cases, the person with neutropenia recovers within 21 to 24 days. Neutropenia and the more serious form known as febrile neutropenia occur in 24% and 14% of all persons receiving chemotherapy, respectively.[57] Agents such as carboplatin (Paraplatin) and paclitaxel (Taxol) are associated with higher incidences of neutropenia owing to their myelosuppressive characteristics.

Filgrastim, Pegfilgrastim, and Sargramostim

Granulocyte colony-stimulating factor (G-CSF) and granulocyte–macrophage colony-stimulating factor (GM-CSF) are naturally occurring growth hormones involved in the maturation of blood cell components, available commercially as filgrastim (Neupogen) or pegfilgrastim (Neulasta); these agents stimulate the production of neutrophils. GM-CSF, which is available as sargramostim (Leukine), stimulates production of neutrophils, eosinophils, monocytes, and macrophages.[58] All of these agents reduce the duration and severity of neutropenia, and current national guidelines from the National Comprehensive Cancer Network recommend that they be used prophylactically for persons whose risk of developing febrile neutropenia is 20% or higher.[59]

Side effects and adverse effects of pegfilgrastim include bone pain, urticaria, angioedema, anaphylaxis, sickle cell crisis, acute respiratory distress syndrome (ARDS), splenomegaly, and (rarely) splenic rupture that may be fatal. Pegfilgrastim has been found to be teratogenic in animals, although no teratogenic effects have been reported among humans. Caution should be used in women who are breastfeeding while receiving this drug because it is unknown if the medication is excreted in breast milk. Pegfilgrastim is contraindicated for persons who are hypersensitive to *Escherichia coli*–derived proteins, pegfilgrastim, or filgrastim.

The development of neutropenia increases the risk of developing certain bacterial and fungal infections that can potentially be life threatening. If a woman receiving chemotherapy has a one-time oral temperature of 38.3°C (101.0°F) or a temperature elevation of 38°C (100.4°F) or above for more than 2 hours, she should be evaluated for possible infection. Common bacterial infections are those that affect the skin, such as *Staphylococcus aureus* and infections involving the gastrointestinal tract, such as *E. coli* and *Klebsiella pneumoniae*. Fungal infections such as *Candida* and *Aspergillus* are common among women with neutropenia who have been treated with antibiotics, and these infections require prompt treatment with the usual antifungal drugs.

Nausea and Vomiting

Approximately 70% to 80% of all persons who are undergoing chemotherapeutic treatment will experience nausea and/or vomiting, with nausea more frequent than emesis. Women are more likely than men to experience chemotherapy-induced nausea and vomiting.[60]

Chemotherapy-induced nausea and vomiting is classified into three categories: (1) acute onset, occurring within 24 hours after administration of chemotherapy; (2) delayed onset, occurring 24 hours to several days after treatment; and (3) anticipatory, whereby the nausea and vomiting are triggered by taste, odors, and anxiety due to a previous experience of nausea and vomiting following a chemotherapy treatment.[61] When nausea and vomiting occur despite administration of antiemetics, the condition is termed breakthrough nausea and vomiting. Antiemetic regimens have been designed for each of these categories.

In addition, chemotherapeutic drugs have an inherent emetogenicity that varies between agents. This emetogenicity is the primary consideration in developing treatment plans to eradicate or mitigate nausea and vomiting. The Multinational Association of Supportive Care in Cancer has assigned chemotherapeutic drugs to one of four emetogenicity classifications (Table 28-4).[60–62]

The mechanism of action underlying chemotherapy-induced nausea and vomiting is fairly straightforward: Chemotherapeutic drugs stimulate the enterochromaffin cells in the gastrointestinal tract to release serotonin. Once serotonin binds to serotonin receptors, the vagal afferent pathway is stimulated, which activates the vomiting center in the central nervous system. The areas of the brain where the vagal pathway terminates have receptors for several neurotransmitters that play a role in the emetic response, including neurokinin-1, serotonin, histamine, and dopamine.[60]

Thus, it is not surprising that several classes of antiemetic drugs that have different molecular targets are used to treat this condition.[63] In particular, combining drugs that have different mechanisms of action can potentiate the individual effects of one agent. Vomiting can be prevented in 70% to 80% of individuals who receive a chemotherapy drug with high emetic potential via the combined use of a serotonin receptor (5-HT_3) antagonist, neurokinin-1 receptor (NK_1) antagonist, and steroids.[61] Commonly used drugs and doses are listed in Table 28-5.[60–66] The pharmacokinetics and general side effects and adverse effects of these agents are reviewed in more detail in the *Gastrointestinal Conditions* chapter.

Dopamine Receptor Antagonists

When administered in high doses, the dopamine receptor antagonists can cause extrapyramidal reactions, disorientation, and sedation, all of which limit their use for treating chemotherapy-induced nausea and vomiting. These drugs are generally used to treat acute or established nausea and vomiting.

Serotonin Receptor Antagonists

A combination of a serotonin receptor antagonist in addition to dexamethasone (Decadron) is recommended for pre-chemotherapy treatment to prevent acute nausea and vomiting by several professional associations.[62,64–66] The serotonin receptor antagonists have few side effects or adverse effects other than headache and occasionally diarrhea.

The first-generation serotonin receptor antagonists have equal effectiveness when used in recommended doses but are not as effective as the second-generation serotonin receptor antagonists in preventing delayed emesis.[62] The second-generation drugs have antiemetic activity in both central and gastrointestinal sites, stronger potency, and a longer half-life than the first-generation drugs.[62] Palonosetron (Aloxi) may be more effective in controlling delayed emesis than other agents in this general class, as it induces prolonged inhibition of the target receptors.

Glucocorticoids

Dexamethasone (Decadron) has been used for many years to help mitigate acute and delayed chemotherapy-induced nausea and vomiting. This drug is recommended as part of a combination regimen with a serotonin receptor antagonist for both highly emetic and moderately emetic chemotherapeutic agents.

Table 28-4 Emetogenicity of Chemotherapeutic Drugs

High Emetic Risk (> 90%)[a]: Generic (Brand)	Moderate Emetic Risk (30–90%)[a]: Generic (Brand)	Low Emetic Risk (10–30%)[a]: Generic (Brand)	Minimal Emetic Risk (< 10%): Generic (Brand)
Intravenous			
Carmustine (Becenum)	Carboplatin (Paraplat)	5-Fluorouracil (Adrucil)	2-Chlorodeoxyadenosine
Cisplatin (Platinol)	Cyclophosphamide (Cytoxan) < 500 mg/m^2	Bortezomib (Velcade)	Bevacizumab (Avastin)
Cyclophosphamide (Cytoxan) 1500 mg/m^2	Cytarabine (Cytosar-U) > 1 g/m^2	Cetuximab (Erbitux)	Bleomycin (Mithracin)
Dacarbazine (Dtic-Dome)	Daunorubicin (Cerubidine)	Cytarabine (Cytosar-U) 100 mg/m^2	Busulfan (Busulfex, Myleran)
Mechlorethamine (Mustargen)	Doxorubicin (Adriamycin)	Docetaxel (Taxotere)	Fludarabine (Fludara)
Streptozotocin (Zanosar)	Epirubicin (Ellence)	Etoposide (VePesid)	Vinblastine (Velban)
	Idarubicin (Idamycin PFS)	Gemcitabine (Gemzar)	Vincristine (Oncovin)
	Ifosfamide (Ifex)	Methotrexate (Rheumatrex, Trexall)	Vinorelbine (Navelbine)
	Irinotecan (Camptosar)	Mitomycin (Mutamycin)	
	Oxaliplatin (Eloxatin)	Mitoxantrone	
		Paclitaxel (Taxol, Onxol)	
		Pemetrexed (Alimta)	
		Teniposide (Vumon)	
		Topotecan (Hycamtin)	
		Trastuzumab (Herceptin)	
Oral			
Hexamethylmelamine (Hexalen)	Cyclophosphamide (Cytoxan)	Capecitabine (Xeloda)	6-Thioguanine (Tabloid)
Procarbazine (Matulane)	Etoposide (Toposar)	Fludarabine (Fludara)	Chlorambucil (Leukeran)
	Imatinib (Gleevec)		Erlotinib (Tarceva)
	Temozolomide (Temodar)		Gefitinib (Iressa)
	Vinorelbine (Navelbine)		Hydroxyurea (Hydrea)
			L-Phenylalanine mustard (Alkeran)

[a] Percentage is the risk of vomiting if no antiemetic drug is administered.
Sources: Data from Hesketh PJ. Chemotherapy-induced nausea and vomiting. *N Engl J Med*. 2008;358(23):2482-2494[60]; Navari RM. Management of chemotherapy-induced nausea and vomiting. *Drugs*. 2013;73(2):249–262[62]; Rolia F, Herrstedt J, Aapro M, et al. Guideline update for MASCC and ESMO in the prevention of chemotherapy- and radiotherapy-induced nausea and vomiting: results of the Perugia consensus conference. *Ann Oncol*. 2010;21(suppl 5):v232-v243.[61]

Table 28-5 Antiemetic Drugs for Treating Nausea and Vomiting Associated with Chemotherapy Treatment

Drug: Generic (Brand)	Emesis Prevention Dose Before Chemotherapy	Emesis Prevention Dose After Chemotherapy	Clinical Considerations
First-Generation Serotonin Receptor Antagonists			
Dolasetron (Anzemet)	100 mg PO	100 mg PO once daily on days 2 and 3 for MEC with potential for delayed N&V	SE: Headache, fatigue, dizziness AE: Potential risk for serotonin syndrome; FDA black box warning about increased risk for cardiac arrhythmias and prolonged QT interval Only used orally Multiple drug–drug interactions
Granisetron (Kytril)	2 mg PO daily *or* 1 mg PO 2 times/day or transdermal patch applied 24–48 hours prior to dose of chemotherapy	1–2 mg PO daily *or* 1 mg PO 2 times/day	SE: Headache, nausea, weakness, constipation AE: Potential risk for serotonin syndrome Multiple drug–drug interactions
Ondansetron (Zofran)	16–24 mg PO *or* 8–16 mg IV; IV dose should not exceed 16 mg	8 mg PO every 8 hours for 1–3 days after chemotherapy for delayed N&V	SE: Headache, fatigue, constipation, dizziness AE: Potential risk for serotonin syndrome; FDA black box warning about risk for prolonged QT interval when used intravenously Requires lower dosing for women who are older

(continues)

Table 28-5 Antiemetic Drugs for Treating Nausea and Vomiting Associated with Chemotherapy Treatment (*continued*)

Drug: Generic (Brand)	Emesis Prevention Dose Before Chemotherapy	Emesis Prevention Dose After Chemotherapy	Clinical Considerations
Second-Generation Serotonin Receptor Antagonists			
Palonosetron (Aloxi)	0.25 mg IV given 30 minutes prior to chemotherapy		SE: headache AE: Potential risk for serotonin syndrome; increases QT interval Multiple drug–drug interactions
Tropisetron (Navoban)	5 mg IV or PO		
Dopamine/Serotonin Receptor Antagonists			
Metoclopramide (Reglan)	1–2 mg/kg IV (infuse over 1–2 minutes) given 30 minutes prior to chemotherapy		Used for prevention of acute N&V and prevention of delayed N&V AE: Increased risk for extrapyramidal symptoms
Histamine Receptor Antagonists			
Prochlorperazine (Compazine)	5–10 mg (PO, IM, IV), then every 6 hours as needed; maximum dose is 40 mg/day	5–10 mg (PO, IM, IV), then every 6 hours as needed; maximum dose 40 mg/day	SE: Anticholinergic effects, orthostatic hypotension, sedation AE: Increased risk for extrapyramidal symptoms, hyperprolactinemia, blood dyscrasias
Neurokinin-1 Receptor Antagonists			
Aprepitant (Emend)	125 mg PO given 1 hour prior to chemotherapy	80 mg PO on days 2 and 3 following chemotherapy	Aprepitant and fosaprepitant are used in combination with other antiemetics Aprepitant/fosaprepitant is a substrate inducer and inhibits several CYP450 enzymes
Fosaprepitant (Emend)	115-mg dose given IV on day 1 only		
Glucocorticoids			
Dexamethasone (Decadron)[a]	12 mg PO or IV every day	8 mg PO daily on days 2–4 with aprepitant for HEC drugs	Side effects and adverse effects include insomnia, hyperglycemia, epigastric discomfort, weight gain, and acne; dose may be decreased or eliminated based on individual response
Cannabinoids			
Dronabinol (Marinol)	5 mg/m^2 PO every 24 hours; dose may be increased to maximum of 15 mg/m^2	5 mg/m2/dose every 2–4 hours after chemotherapy, for a total of 4–6 doses/day	Used to treat N&V refractory to other antiemetics
Nabilone (Cesamet)	1–2 mg PO 2 times/day; maximum dose is 6 mg in divided doses	2–3 mg per day for entire chemotherapy course and up to 48 hours after last dose	
Benzodiazepines			
Lorazepam (Ativan)	0.5–2 mg PO or IV every 4–6 hours on days 1–4	0.5–2 mg PO or IV every 4–6 hours on days 1–4	Used as adjunct rather than primary drug for anticipatory or delayed nausea and vomiting
Antipsychotics			
Olanzapine (Zyprexa)	10 mg PO on days 1–4	10 mg PO on days 1–4	SE: Sedation, increased serum prolactin, increased appetite, dyspepsia, constipation AE: Hypertension, extrapyramidal reaction in higher doses Multiple drug–drug interactions FDA black box warning about increased mortality among older women with dementia and delirium/coma post injection

Abbreviations: AE = adverse effects; HEC = highly emetic chemotherapy; MEC = moderately emetic chemotherapy; N&V = nausea and vomiting; SE = side effects.

[a] Use may vary depending on whether the chemotherapeutic agent is considered highly or moderately emetogenic.

Sources: Data from Navari RM. Management of chemotherapy-induced nausea and vomiting. *Drugs*. 2013;73(2):249-262[62]; Rolia F, Herrstedt J, Aapro M, et al. Guideline update for MASCC and ESMO in the prevention of chemotherapy- and radiotherapy-induced nausea and vomiting: results of the Perugia consensus conference. *Ann Oncol*. 2010;21(suppl 5):v232-v243.[61]

Neurokinin-1 Receptor Antagonists

Aprepitant (Emend) blocks the emetic effects of substance P, which triggers the emetic response in the vomiting center. Aprepitant is added to the combination of a serotonin receptor antagonist and dexamethasone (Decadron) to prevent nausea and vomiting from chemotherapeutic drugs that have a high emetic risk.[62,66] Use of aprepitant is optional when individuals are receiving medications with a moderate emetic risk and is not used for those drugs that have a low emetic risk.[66] Fosaprepitant (Emend) is a prodrug that is converted to aprepitant within 30 minutes of administration and has the same pharmacologic characteristics as aprepitant.

Olanzapine

Olanzapine (Zyprexa) is an antipsychotic drug that inhibits dopamine, histamine, serotonin, and acetylcholine receptors; as a consequence, it is highly effective for treating nausea and vomiting. Olanzapine can be used in combination with dexamethasone (Decadron) and a serotonin receptor antagonist in place of the combination of a dexamethasone/serotonin receptor antagonist and neurokinin-1 receptor antagonist for highly emetic chemotherapeutic agents.[66] Although olanzapine is included in professional association antiemetic guidelines, it is used on an off-label basis for this purpose.

Cannabinoids

Tetrahydrocannabinol (THC), which is the active ingredient in cannabinoids, is a broad-spectrum antiemetic agent. Its effectiveness is similar to that of conventional antiemetics, but because THC has psychoactive effects, it is used only when other regimens are not effective.

Preventive Therapy Prior to Chemotherapy Administration

The National Comprehensive Cancer Network antiemetic recommendations state that persons who are receiving agents in the high emetic risk category should be given aprepitant (Emend), a 5-HT_3 receptor antagonist, and dexamethasone (Decadron) prior to chemotherapy and should receive aprepitant and dexamethasone post chemotherapy for the prevention of delayed emesis.[62] Supplemental contraception has been advocated for women who are using hormonal contraceptive methods while taking aprepitant because of the potential for increased metabolism of the oral contraceptive hormones.

Nephrotoxicity and Neurotoxicity

Many chemotherapeutic agents and their metabolites are excreted renally, putting the renal system and urinary tract at risk of injury when such drugs are prescribed. Manifestations of neurotoxicity include peripheral neuropathy, autonomic dysfunction, ototoxicity, retinal toxicity, and seizures. Peripheral neuropathy is the most common neurotoxicity. Symptoms are generally described as stocking-glove distribution paresthesias of the feet, legs, arms, and hands, which can ultimately result in loss of deep tendon reflexes (DTR) and vibratory sensation. The two chemotherapeutic agents most frequently associated with neurotoxicity are cisplatin (Platinol) and paclitaxel (Taxol).

Antiseizure medications such as gabapentin (Neurontin), topiramate (Topamax), pregabalin (Lyrica), carbamazepine (Tegretol), and phenytoin (Dilantin) can be effective for the treatment of nerve pain, but produce their own medication-related side effects of drowsiness and dizziness. Topical lidocaine patches may also be used for this indication, with the woman placing the patch over the area of most severe pain. Antidepressants, such as venlafaxine (Effexor), duloxetine (Cymbalta), selective serotonin reuptake inhibitors (SSRIs), amitriptyline (Elavil), and nortriptyline (Pamelor), have also been used to treat peripheral neuropathy; these agents have the additional advantage of having antidepressant effects.

Pain

Persons with cancer can experience intense pain. Cancer-related pain can be acute or chronic, and it can occur secondary to either the disease or the treatment. In 1996, the World Health Organization (WHO) published a three-step analgesic ladder to assist practitioners in managing cancer pain and to promote better use of opioids.[67] Today, the WHO ladder is used as an initial guide for all severe pain but there has been a great deal of additional research on managing cancer-related pain.[68–70]

In brief, WHO's three-step ladder includes use of (1) non-opioids for mild pain; (2) moderate opioids, such as tramadol (Ultram) or codeine, for moderate pain; and (3) strong opioids, such as morphine, for severe pain. In addition, WHO recommends regular dosing rather than per-request dosing so that blood levels of the pain medication remain consistent and pain is better controlled. Current guidelines suggest that moving more quickly to strong opioids may be indicated for individuals in some situations.[68,69]

Morphine is the cornerstone of treatment of moderate or severe pain. Unfortunately, this medication has multiple side effects and adverse effects, and some individuals do not get adequate pain relief from morphine secondary to genetic polymorphisms. Thus, therapy for cancer pain is individualized with regard to the specific opioid, route of administration, and dose. Additional information about the pharmacologic effects of opioids can be found in the *Analgesia and Anesthesia* chapter.

Adjuvant Analgesia

Adjuvant analgesics, also called co-analgesics, are medications that have a side effect of analgesia but whose primary indication is for the treatment of a medical condition.[70] Adjuvant analgesics can have a synergistic effect when added to opioids or other conventional analgesics. They are often used for managing neuropathic pain. Medications used as adjuvant analgesics include serotonin–norepinephrine reuptake inhibitors (SNRIs), tricyclic antidepressants, anticonvulsants, local anesthetics, steroids, cannabis, gamma-aminobutyric acid (GABA) receptor inhibitors, and bupropion (Wellbutrin). The use of adjuvants extends the therapeutic index of the opioids and allows lower doses of these medications to be prescribed, thereby decreasing the side effects and adverse effects of opioids.[71]

SNRIs, tricyclic antidepressants, and anticonvulsants are generally the first-line adjuvant options for treating neuropathic pain. Steroids and calcitonin are the first-line adjuvant options for bone pain. Readers interested in dosing and additional details can access information from the National Comprehensive Cancer Network (listed in the Resources table at the end of this chapter).

Thrombocytopenia

Individuals with platelet counts lower than 20,000/mm^3 have a significantly increased risk of spontaneous hemorrhage. Common hemorrhagic sites are the skull and the gastrointestinal tract. Women with thrombocytopenia may experience abdominal or extremity petechiae, epistaxis, oral bleeding (gingival), hematuria, rectal bleeding, or bloody stools. Oprelvekin (Neumega), which is a synthetically derived form of interleukin-11, is administered prophylactically to prevent thrombocytopenia. Oprelvekin stimulates bone marrow production of megakaryocytes—the cells that serve as precursors of platelets.

The most commonly occurring side effects associated with oprelvekin are tachycardia, fever, headache, nausea and vomiting, and insomnia. Adverse effects include neutropenic fever, syncope, atrial fibrillation, fever and pneumonia, edema, dyspnea, tachycardia, conjunctival infection, palpitations, atrial arrhythmias, and pleural effusions.[58] Postmarketing reports of allergic reactions such as anaphylaxis have resulted in an FDA black box warning on oprelvekin's label that hypersensitivity reactions including anaphylaxis may occur with use of this drug. Additional adverse effects include optic disc edema, ventricular arrhythmia, capillary leak syndrome, and renal failure.

Chemotherapy Drug–Drug Interactions

Combination chemotherapy is chosen carefully because of the high potential for adverse drug–drug interactions to occur. Although a thorough review of the many drug–drug interactions associated with chemotherapeutic agents is beyond the scope of this chapter, some important examples are mentioned here. First, some chemotherapeutic agents cannot be combined with other chemotherapeutic agents. For example, concomitant use of cisplatin (Platinol) and methotrexate (Rheumatrex, Trexall) can result in renal damage, because both agents are excreted by the kidney. Sequencing of cisplatin and paclitaxel (Taxol) can be synergistic or antagonistic, depending on which drug is administered first.[72]

In the primary care arena, some drug interactions are more common among chemotherapeutic agents and medications used for comorbid conditions.[72] For example, many chemotherapeutic agents can reduce the metabolism of warfarin (Coumadin) and increase the chance of bleeding or hemorrhage. Similarly, drugs that have an independent effect of prolonging the QT interval need to be used with caution if chemotherapeutic drugs are administered. Selective serotonin reuptake inhibitors may potentially reduce the effectiveness of concomitant administration of tamoxifen (Nolvadex).[73]

Finally, interactions between chemotherapeutic drugs and foods or supplements can be important. Although individuals may consume foods high in antioxidants in an attempt to advance their healthy habits, chemotherapeutics that act by destruction of DNA theoretically may have decreased effectiveness when taken with antioxidants such as vitamin A, C, or E. Therefore, the importance of exploring potential interactions is of utmost importance when caring for women taking chemotherapeutic agents.

Complementary and Alternative Therapy

Complementary and alternative medicine (CAM) is often used to treat cancer- and chemotherapy-related symptoms. For example, studies have shown that acupuncture may be a helpful adjunct for reducing hot flashes, fatigue, arthralgias, and neuropathies.[75] Meditation practices such as Transcendental Meditation, mindfulness meditation, and yoga may reduce anxiety, stress, and depression, although studies on the use of these modalities for cancer symptom management are lacking.[75]

Alternative treatments for nausea and vomiting are perhaps the best studied. Ginger root preparations may reduce nausea and vomiting, although the ideal dose has not been determined.[76] A review of seven randomized clinical trials provided limited evidence that Chinese medicinal herbs may reduce the proportion of persons who experience chemotherapy-induced nausea and vomiting. In addition, these compounds are associated with a decrease in the incidence of leukopenia and an increase in the number of T lymphocytes in persons being treated for cancer.[77]

Although no evidence of harm arising from the use of these compounds has been found, individuals should be cautioned about the use of botanicals due to mounting evidence of botanical–drug interactions.[72] Several reports cite drug–herb interactions involving *Hypericum perforatum* (St. John's wort) and *Allium sativum*, where the herb behaves as a CYP450 inhibitor or inducer, which potentiates toxicity or decreases chemotherapy effectiveness.[78] The use of antioxidants remains controversial as well. There is limited human research on this topic, but many preclinical studies indicate vitamins C and E, as well as coenzyme Q10, are beneficial for reducing tumor size and chemotherapy-related toxicities.[78]

Special Populations: Pregnancy, Lactation, and the Elderly

Chemotherapy-Induced Ovarian Failure

Ovarian failure may be caused by the administration of certain chemotherapeutic agents. Factors related to the development of this toxicity include age, agent used, total cumulative dose, and length of time since treatment. Sterility may be temporary or permanent and should be discussed in great detail with a woman and her partner. Alkylating agents have been found to damage fertility, and chemotherapeutic agents such as busulfan (Busulfex), melphalan (Alkeran), cyclophosphamide (Cytoxan), cisplatin (Platinol), chlorambucil (Leukeran), mechlorethamine (Mustargen), carmustine (BiCNU), lomustine (CeeNU), cytarabine (Cytosar-U), ifosfamide (Ifex), vinblastine (Velban), and procarbazine (Matulane) are known to be gonadotoxic.[79,80]

Chemotherapy During Pregnancy

A concern unique to women is a cancer diagnosis during pregnancy. Chemotherapy may be recommended if delay in treatment until after birth is not prudent and pregnancy termination is not desired. When caring for a pregnant woman with cancer, a multidisciplinary team that includes an oncologist, perinatologist, and neonatologist among others is needed to coordinate care and improve the outcome for both the mother and the fetus/neonate. The decision to use chemotherapy during pregnancy must always be balanced against the effect of treatment delay on maternal survival.

If possible, chemotherapy should be avoided during the first trimester because most chemotherapy agents administered during this time increase the incidence of spontaneous miscarriage, fetal death, and major malformations. Use of chemotherapy in the second and third trimesters appears to be relatively safe, although it confers an increased risk of fetal growth restriction.[81] It is recommended that low-molecular-weight and highly diffusible drugs, such as the antimetabolites (e.g., methotrexate [Rheumatrex]), be avoided in such circumstances, as these drugs have properties that favor transfer across the placenta to fetus. Chemotherapy should not be given near term because spontaneous delivery may occur before the mother's bone marrow has recovered, increasing the risk for hemorrhage and infection due to maternal neutropenia and thrombocytopenia.[81] Chemotherapy administered shortly before birth results in the presence of the drugs in the newborn, who will have limited ability to metabolize and excrete drugs due to immaturity of the liver and kidneys; this is especially true for premature infants.[81]

Breastfeeding is contraindicated while the woman is undergoing chemotherapy. Neonatal neutropenia has been reported in an infant whose mother was being treated with cyclophosphamide (Cytoxan). The amount of drug that passes into breast milk varies, reflecting both the dose and timing of chemotherapy. For most chemotherapy agents, no specific breastfeeding information is available, although concerns exist. In summary, then, it is recommended that they be avoided in breastfeeding mothers.

Pregnancy After Cancer

Much has been accomplished in the treatment of childhood cancers. Most cancer treatment regimens used in young children or adolescents consist of radiation, chemotherapy, and sometimes surgery. The Childhood Cancer Survivor Study reported that there is an increased risk of premature ovarian failure in those women who had cancer when compared to their siblings (8% versus 0.8%; relative risk [RR], 13.21; 95% confidence interval [CI], 3.26–53.51; $P < .001$).[82] Among the more than 1900 women in the study who had more than 4000 births, the only adverse pregnancy outcome reported was small for gestational age infants. There was no increased risk in congenital anomalies among childhood cancer survivors.[82]

Women who have experienced a gynecologic malignancy and who retain fertility may opt not to pursue conception, but for those who do, the data on subsequent cancer risks are limited. Among the considerations is whether pregnancy itself will increase risk of cancer recurrence, although anecdotal reports on this point appear reassuring.[83] Pregnancy concerns that have been suggested include potential increase in risk of preterm birth or intrauterine growth restriction; congenital anomalies secondary to previous treatments appear to be remote, although there are not enough data to estimate the risks of these events.

Use of Perimenopausal Hormones

The controversies surrounding postmenopausal use of hormones are discussed in detail in the chapter *The Mature Woman*. However, for cancer survivors, hormone therapy is even more controversial. In general, women who have receptor-positive estrogen or progesterone cancers have been counseled against using hormones. However, there is a paucity of rigorous studies on this topic.

A randomized clinical trial called HABITs was conducted to explore whether women, with any type of receptor status, who had been treated for breast cancer were more likely to have recurrences when treated with perimenopausal hormones. Of the 221 women in the hormone therapy arm, 39 developed a new breast cancer, compared to 17 of the 221 women in the control group who developed breast cancer (hazard ratio [HR], 2.4; 95% CI, 1.3–4.2). Cumulative incidences were 22.2% in the hormone therapy arm and 8.0% in the control arm at the 5-year point. The study was halted early because of these findings, which indicate hormone therapy increases the risk for recurrent breast cancer and, therefore, is not recommended for women who are breast cancer survivors.[84] Although this study was limited to survivors of breast cancer, limited data exist regarding women with other types of cancers and hormone therapy.

Conclusion

Gynecologic malignancies alter an individual's life path irrevocably. All healthcare providers involved in the care of a woman with a gynecologic malignancy should be knowledgeable about evaluation and management of the side effects experienced during treatments. Working collaboratively to care for women may not only assist individuals during the treatment process, but also increase the support provided to these women—support that women with these disorders so clearly need.

Resources

Organization	Description	Website
American Cancer Society	Cancer facts and statistics and cancer staging information that reviews the meaning of the TNM classification system	www.cancer.org www.cancer.org/treatment/understanding yourdiagnosis/staging
American Joint Committee on Cancer (AJCC)	Staging information for healthcare providers	https://cancerstaging.org/Pages/default.aspx
International Federation of Gynecologists and Obstetricians (FIGO)	Staging guidelines for endometrial vaginal, fallopian tube, and ovarian cancer	www.sgo.org/wp-content/uploads/2012/09/FIGO-Ovarian-Cancer-Staging_1.10.14.pdf www.cancer.gov/cancertopics/pdq/treatment/endometrial/HealthProfessional/page3
National Cancer Institute	Many resources available, including cancer staging information and a list of all chemotherapeutic drugs, along with their indications, contraindications, side effects, and adverse effects	www.cancer.gov www.cancer.gov/cancertopics/druginfo/carboplatin

National Comprehensive Cancer Network	This site has all the NCCN clinical practice guidelines for management of different cancers available for download and offers resources for managing chemotherapy side effects and a comprehensive review of individual chemotherapeutic drugs	www.nccn.org
Multinational Association of Supportive Care in Cancer	Guidelines and tools for treatment of nausea and vomiting, mucositis, and skin toxicities, including tools for patients	www.mascc.org
Oncology Nursing Society	Putting evidence into practice (PEP) topics that summarize the evidence for many treatments of chemotherapy side effects	www.ons.org/practice-resources/pep
World Health Organization Cancer Pain Relief	A 1996 monograph that reviews the WHO pain ladder steps and the role of opioids in treating cancer pain	http://whqlibdoc.who.int/publications/9241544821.pdf

References

1. American Cancer Society. *Cancer facts and figures, 2014.* Atlanta, GA: American Cancer Society; 2014. http://www.cancer.org/acs/groups/content/@research/documents/webcontent/acspc-042151.pdf. Accessed December 26, 2014.
2. Elmore S. Apoptosis: a review of programmed cell death. *Toxicol Pathol.* 2007;35(4):495-516.
3. Guo XE, Ngo B, Modrek AS, Lee WH. Targeting tumor suppressor networks for cancer therapeutics. *Curr Drug Targets.* 2014;15(1):2-16.
4. Tlsty TD, Coussens LM. Tumor stroma and regulation of cancer development. *Annu Rev Pathol Mech Dis.* 2006;1:119-150.
5. Croce CM. Molecular origins of cancer: oncogenes and cancer. *N Engl J Med.* 2008;358(5):502-511.
6. Ballinger LL. Hereditary gynecologic cancers: risk assessment, counseling, testing and management. *Obstet Clin North Am.* 2012;39(2);165-181.
7. Lu KH. Hereditary gynecologic cancers: differential diagnosis, surveillance, management, and surgical prophylaxis. *Fam Cancer.* 2008;7(1):53-58.
8. Lynch HT, Lynch PM, Lanspa SJ, Cnyder CL, Lynch JF, Boland CR. Review of the Lynch syndrome: history, molecular genetics, screening, differential diagnosis, and medicolegal ramifications. *Clin Genet.* 2009; 76(1):1-18.
9. Mutch DG. The new FIGO staging system for cancers of the vulva, cervix, endometrium, and sarcomas. *Gynecol Oncol.* 2009;115(3):325-328.
10. Edge S, Byrd DR, eds. American Joint Committee on *Cancer. Cancer Staging Manual.* 7th ed. New York, NY: Springer Healthcare; 2011.
11. National Comprehensive Cancer Network. Clinical practice guidelines in oncology. http://nccn.org/professionals/physician_gls/f_guidelines.asp. Accessed June 12, 2014.
12. Wilson TR, Johnston PG, Longley DB. Anti-apoptotic mechanisms of drug resistance in cancer. *Curr Cancer Drug Targets.* 2009;9(3):307-319.
13. Lyman GH. Impact of chemotherapy dose intensity on cancer patient outcomes. *J Natl Compr Cancer Netw.* 2009;7(1):99-108.
14. Espinosa E, Zamora P, Feliu F, González Barón M. Classification of anticancer drugs: a new system based on therapeutic targets. *Can Treat Rev.* 2003; 29(6):515-523.
15. Frandsen G, Pennington SS. *Abrams' Clinical Drug Therapy.* 10th ed. Philadelphia, PA: Lippincott Williams & Wilkins; 2014.
16. Noble RL. The discovery of the vinca alkaloids: chemotherapeutic agents against cancer. *Biochem Cell Biol.* 1990;68(12):1344-1351.
17. Denmain A, Sanchez S. Microbial drug discovery: 80 years of progress. *J Antibiot.* 2009;62(1):5-16.
18. Coley WB. The treatment of malignant tumors by repeated inoculations of erysipelas: with a report of ten original cases. *Am J Med Sci.* 1893;105(5):487-511.
19. Fumito I, Chang AE. Cancer immunotherapy: current status and future directions. *Surg Oncol Clin North Am.* 2013;22(4):765-783.
20. Ma WW, Adjei AA. Novel agents on the horizon for cancer therapy. *CA Cancer J Clin.* 2009;59(2):111-137.
21. Hudis CA. Trastuzumab: mechanism of action and use in clinical practice. *N Engl J Med.* 2007;357(1):39-51.
22. Weiner LM, Dhodapkar MV, Ferrone S. Monoclonal antibodies for cancer immunotherapy. *Lancet.* 2009; 373(9668):1033-1040.
23. Caplan L. Delay in breast cancer: implications for stage at diagnosis and survival. *Front Public Health.* 2014;2:87 ecollection.
24. Nandy A, Gangopadhyay S, Mukhopadhyay A. Individualizing breast cancer treatment: the dawn of personalized medicine. *Experiment Cell Res.* 2014;320(1):1-11.

25. NCCN Clinical Practice Guidelines in Oncology. Breast cancer, version 3.2014. http://www.nccn.org. Accessed June 12, 2014.
26. McArthur HL, Hudis CA. Adjuvant chemotherapy for early-stage breast cancer. *Hematol Oncol Clin North Am.* 2007;21(2):207-222.
27. Gabriel EM, Jatoi I. Breast cancer chemoprevention. *Expert Rev Anticancer Ther.* 2012;12(2):223-228.
28. Ingle JN. Postmenopausal women with hormone receptor-positive breast cancer: balancing benefit and toxicity from aromatase inhibitors. *Breast.* 2013; 22(suppl 2):S180-S183.
29. Cummings SR, Tice JA, Bauer S, et al. Prevention of breast cancer in postmenopausal women: approaches to estimating and reducing risk. *J Natl Cancer Inst.* 2009;101(6):384-398.
30. Thomsen A, Kolesar JM. Chemoprevention of breast cancer. *Am J Health Syst Pharm.* 2008;65(23): 2221-2228.
31. Downs L. Advances in cervical cancer treatment. *Gynecol Oncol.* 2011;121(3):431-433.
32. Espindola D, Kennedy KA, Fischer EG. Management of abnormal uterine bleeding and the pathology of endometrial hyperplasia. *Obstet Gyn Clin.* 2007;34(4): 717-737.
33. Berkowitz RS, Goldstein DP. Clinical practice: molar pregnancy. *N Engl J Med.* 2009;360(16):1639-1645.
34. Taylor F, Grew T, Everard J, et al. The outcome of patients with low risk gestational trophoblastic neoplasia treated with single agent intramuscular methotrexate and oral folinic acid. *Eur J Cancer.* 2013; 49(15):3184-3190.
35. Siegel R, Ma J, Zou Z, Jemal A. Cancer statistics, 2014. *CA Cancer J Clin.* 2014;64(1):9-29.
36. Reed CE, Fenton SE. Exposure to diethylstilbestrol during sensitive life stages: a legacy of heritable health effects. *Birth Defects Res C Embryo Today.* 2013; 99(2):134-146.
37. Gibson DA, Saunders PT. Endocrine disruption of oestrogen action and female reproductive tract cancers. *Endocr Relat Cancer.* 2014;21(2):T13-T31.
38. Hilakivi-Clarke L. Maternal exposure to diethylstilbestrol during pregnancy and increased breast cancer risk in daughters. *Breast Cancer Res.* 2014;16(2):208.
39. Deppe G, Mert I, Winer IS. Management of squamous cell vulvar cancer: review. *J Obstet Gynecol Res.* 2014; 40(5):1217-1225.
40. Rodrigues IS, Lavorato-Rocha, AM, de M Maia B, et al. Epithelial-mesenchymal transition-like events in vulvar cancer and its relation with HPV. *BJC.* 2013; 109(1):184-194.
41. Bormanis J, Quirt I, Chang J, et al. Erythropoiesis-stimulating agents (ESAs): do they still have a role in chemotherapy-induced anemia (CIA)? *Crit Rev Oncol Hematol.* 2013;87(2):132-139.
42. Tonia T, Mettler A, Robert N. et al. Erythropoietin or darbepoetin for patients with cancer. *Cochrane Database Syst Rev.* 2012:CD003407.
43. Khuri FR. Weighing the hazards of erythropoiesis stimulation in patients with cancer. *N Engl J Med.* 2007;356(24):2445-2448.
44. Richardson G, Dobish R. Chemotherapy induced diarrhea. *J Oncol Pharm Pract.* 2007;13(4): 181-198.
45. Gibson RJ, Keefe DM. Cancer chemotherapy-induced diarrhoea and constipation: mechanisms of damage and prevention strategies. *Support Care Cancer.* 2006; 14(9):890-900.
46. Andreyev J, Ross P, Donnellan C, et al. Guidance on the management of diarrhoea during cancer chemotherapy. *Lancet Oncol.* 2014;15(10):e447-e460.
47. Shaw C, Taylor L. Treatment-related diarrhea in patients with cancer. *Clin J Oncol Nurs.* 2012;16(4): 412-416.
48. Muehlbauer PM, Thorpe D, Davis A, Drabot R, Rawlings BL, Kiker E. Putting evidence into practice: evidence-based interventions to prevent, manage, and treat chemotherapy- and radiotherapy-induced diarrhea *Clin J Oncol Nurs.* 2009;13(3):336-341.
49. Benson AB III, Ajani JA, Catalano RB, et al. Recommended guidelines for the treatment of cancer treatment-induced diarrhea. *J Clin Oncol.* 2004; 22: 2918-2926.
50. Neefjes ECW, van der Vorst M, Blauwhoff-Buskermolen S, Verheul H. Aiming for a better understanding and management of cancer-related fatigue. *Oncologist.* 2013;18(10):1135-1143.
51. Minton O, Stone P, Richardson A, Sharpe M, Hotopf M. Drug therapy for the management of cancer-related fatigue. *Cochrane Database Syst Rev.* 2008;1:CD006704.
52. Syrigou E, Makrilia N, Koti L, Saif MW, Syrigos KN. Hypersensitivity reactions to antineoplastic agents: an overview. *Anti-Cancer Drugs.* 2009;20(1):1-6.
53. Lenz JJ. Management and preparedness for infusion and hypersensitivity reactions. *Oncologist.* 2007; 12(5):601-609.
54. Lalla RV, Bowen J, Barasch A, et al. MASCC/ISOO clinical practice guidelines for the management of mucositis secondary to cancer therapy. *Cancer.* 2014;120(10):1453-1461.
55. Harris DJ, Eilers J, Harriman A, Cashavelly BJ, Maxwell C. Putting evidence into practice:

evidence-based interventions for the management of oral mucositis. *Clin J Oncol Nurs.* 2008;12(1): 141-152.
56. Lalla RV, Sonis ST, Peterson DE. Management of oral mucositis in patients who have cancer. *Dent Clin North Am.* 2008;52(1):61-77.
57. Crawford J, Dale DC, Lyman GH. Chemotherapy-induced neutropenia: risks, consequences, and new directions for its management. *Cancer.* 2004; 100(2):228-237.
58. Lyman GH, Shayne M. Granulocyte colony-stimulating factors: finding the right indication. *Curr Opin Oncol.* 2007;19(4):299-307.
59. Saloustros E, Tryfonidis K, Georgoulias V. Prophylactic and therapeutic strategies in chemotherapy-induced neutropenia. *Expert Opin Pharmacother.* 2011;12(6):851-863.
60. Hesketh PJ. Chemotherapy-induced nausea and vomiting. *N Engl J Med.* 2008;358(23):2482-2494.
61. Rolia F, Herrstedt J, Aapro M, et al. Guideline update for MASCC and ESMO in the prevention of chemotherapy- and radiotherapy-induced nausea and vomiting: results of the Perugia consensus conference. *Ann Oncol.* 2010;21(suppl 5):v232-v243.
62. Navari RM. Management of chemotherapy-induced nausea and vomiting. *Drugs.* 2013;73(2):249-262.
63. Jordan K, Schmoll HJ, Aapro MS. Comparative activity of antiemetic drugs. *Crit Rev Oncol Hematol.* 2007; 61(2):162-175.
64. Tageja M, Groninger H. Chemotherapy-induced nausea and vomiting #285. *J Palliat Med.* 2014; 17(12):1400-1402.
65. Basch E, Prestrud AA, Hesketh PJ, et al. Antiemetic American Society Clinical Oncology clinical practice guideline update. *J Clin Oncol.* 2011;29(31): 4189-4198.
66. NCCN Clinical Practice Guidelines in Oncology version 2.2014. Antiemesis. National Comprehensive Cancer Network (NCCN). http://www.nccn.org/professionals/physician_gls/PDF/antiemesis.pdf. Accessed December 28, 2014.
67. World Health Organization. *Cancer Pain Relief: With a Guide to Opioid Availability.* 2nd ed. Geneva, Switzerland: World Health Organization; 1996.
68. Fielding F, Sanford TM, Davis MP. Achieving effective control in cancer pain: a review of current guidelines. *Int J Palliat Nurs.* 2013;19(12):584-588.
69. Ripamonti CI, Santini D, Maranzano E, Berti M, Roila F. Management of cancer pain: ESMO clinical practice guidelines. *Ann Oncol.* 2012;23(suppl 7): vii139-vii154.
70. Mercadante S. Management of cancer pain. *Intern Emerg Med.* 2010;5(suppl 1):S31-S35.
71. Khan MI, Walsh D, Brito-Dellan N. Opioid and adjuvant analgesics: compared and contrasted. *Am J Hospice Palliat Med.* 2011;28(5):378-383.
72. van Leeuwen RWF, Swart EL, Boven E, Boom FA, Schuitenmaker MG, Hugtenburg JG. Potential drug interactions in cancer therapy: a prevalence study using an advanced screening method. *Ann Oncol.* 2011;22(10):2334-2341.
73. Lash TL, Pedersen L, Cronin-Fenton D, et al. Tamoxifen's protection against breast cancer recurrence is not reduced by concurrent use of the SSRI citalopram. *Br J Cancer.* 2008;99(4):616-621.
74. Tyler T. Drug interactions in metastatic breast cancer. *J Oncol Pharm Pract.* 2010;17(3):236-245.
75. Blaes AH, Kreitzer MJ, Torkelson C, Haddad T. Non-pharmacologic complementary therapies in symptom management for breast cancer survivors. *Semin Oncol.* 2011;38(3):394-402.
76. Boon H, Wong J. Botanical medicine and cancer: a review of the safety and efficacy. *Expert Opin Pharmacother.* 2004;5(12):2485-2501.
77. Zhang M, Liu X, Li J, He L, Tripathy D. Chinese medicinal herbs to treat the side-effect of chemotherapy in breast cancer patients. *Cochrane Database Syst Rev.* 2007;2:CD004921.
78. Hardy ML. Dietary supplement use in cancer care: help or harm. *Hematol Oncol Clin North Am.* 2008;22(4):581-617.
79. Blumenfeld Z. Chemotherapy and fertility. *Best Pract Res Clin Obstet Gynaecol.* 2012;26(3):379-390.
80. Gadducci A, Cosio S, Genazzani AR. Ovarian function and childbearing issues in breast cancer survivors. *Gynecol Endocrinol.* 2007;23(11):625-631.
81. Amant F, Han SN, Gziri MM, Dekrem J, Van Calsteren K. Chemotherapy during pregnancy. *Curr Opin Oncol.* 2012;24(5):580-586.
82. Green DM, Sklar CA, Boice JD Jr, et al. Ovarian failure and reproductive outcomes after childhood cancer treatment: results from the Childhood Cancer Survivor Study. *J Clin Oncol.* 2009;27(14):2374-2381.
83. Chabbert-Buffet N, Uzan C, Gligorov J, Delaloge S, Rouzier R, Uzan S. Pregnancy after breast cancer: a need for global patient care, starting before adjuvant therapy. *Surg Oncol.* 2009; 19(1):e47-e55.
84. Holmberg L, Iversen OE, Rudenstam CM, et al.; HABITS Study Group. Increased risk of recurrence after hormone replacement therapy in breast cancer survivors. *J Natl Cancer Inst.* 2008;100(7): 475-482.

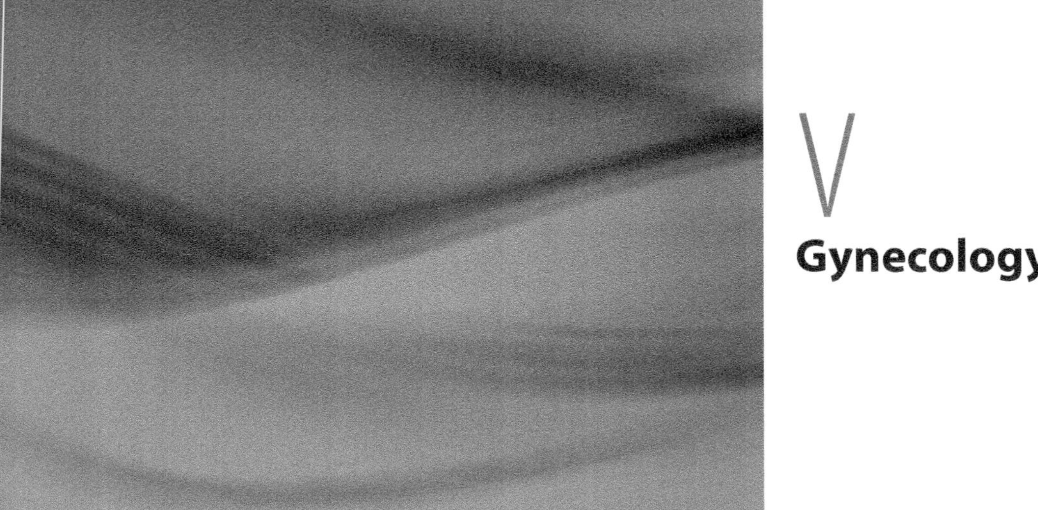

V Gynecology

Most discussions of the etymology of the term *gynecology* note that the word indicates the study of women, or the study of diseases of women. However, currently the term connotes a branch of health care involving women and conditions associated with reproductive organs. These conditions are not always pathologic. For example, *Contraception* not only addresses potential side and adverse effects associated with hormonal contraceptives but also the growing list of noncontraceptive benefits of such drugs.

Of course, some gynecologic conditions are abnormal. *Pelvic and Menstrual Disorders* reviews treatment of women with pelvic infections and menstrual irregularities, among others. Many disparate conditions presented in this chapter use the same drugs as remedies. *Vaginal Conditions* addresses the management of individuals with vaginal infections as well as changes due to hormonal milieus that benefit from targeted treatments. *Vulvar Disorders* includes treatment of those with changes in pigmentation as well as symptoms such as pruritus that can cause major concerns to women. Another issue for women involves sexual dysfunction, which may be treated by pharmacologic agents albeit if also may be caused by other medications; these agents are discussed in *Sexual Dysfunction*. The last chapter in this section, *The Mature Woman*, discusses a normal condition in which women will find themselves spending a third of their lives, namely postmenopause, and drugs often used by those women.

29 Contraception

Patricia Aikins Murphy, Christina E. Elmore

Chapter Glossary

Combined hormonal contraception Contraceptive methods (e.g., pills, patches) that contain both an estrogen and a progestin.

Combined oral contraceptives (COCs) Contraceptive pills with estrogen and progestin as the primary components.

Effectiveness Ability of a drug or treatment to produce a result in real-life circumstances. In contraception, it is a synonym for *typical use*.

Efficacy In pharmacology, the maximum ability of a drug or treatment to produce a result regardless of dose as demonstrated under optimal or ideal circumstances. In the context of contraception, it is a synonym for *perfect use*.

Emergency contraception Use of contraceptives (usually oral hormonal contraceptives or an intrauterine device) by a woman after unprotected intercourse.

Extended cycling Use of combined oral contraceptives for longer than 21 days to postpone withdrawal bleeding (pseudo-menses).

Implantable contraceptives Long-term hormonal contraceptives that are placed, or implanted, into a woman for continuous release over a period of years.

Injectable contraceptives Long-term progestins that are administered by injection and provide contraceptive protection for several weeks.

Intrauterine contraceptives Products (also called devices or systems) that reside in situ in the uterus and provide contraceptive methods for several years.

Long-acting reversible contraceptives (LARCs) Contraceptive methods that are effective for an extended period with minimal or no user action.

Phasic formulations Combined oral contraceptives containing the same daily dose of ethinyl estradiol and a progestin during the 21 days of active pills (monophasic) or different amounts (multiphasic). Multiphasic formulations can be further described, such as biphasic that has two different amounts, triphasic that has three different amounts.

Progestin-only methods Hormonal contraceptives that do not have an estrogen component.

Short-acting reversible contraceptives (SARCs) Contraceptive methods that have shorter durations of action and depend on user action for sustained effectiveness.

Spermicide Chemical agent that kills sperm as its contraceptive mechanism of action.

Transdermal contraceptive patch Contraceptive method that provides delivery of hormones through a transdermal product.

Vaginal contraceptive rings Contraceptive method that provides delivery of hormones through a device inserted into vagina.

Introduction

Women have practiced contraception since ancient times. Observations that animals grazing on certain plants did not reproduce likely led to use of the same herbs and plants to prevent conception in women.[1] With the advent of the industrial age, contraceptive devices began to be manufactured from rubber, and a political debate began in the 1800s that continues today regarding access to contraception.

The roots of hormonal contraception date back to the early twentieth century, when estrogens were first administered to animals to prevent pregnancy.[2] Later, scientists began synthesizing exogenous estrogen and progestins from known organic compounds, paving the way for production of modern oral contraceptive pill.[1]

This chapter reviews pharmacologically based contraception, both hormonal and nonhormonal, including the various methods' mechanism of action, initiation, efficacy, adverse effects, common side effects, and availability. Because certain methods, such as **combined hormonal contraception** and progestin-only contraception, share some commonalities, factors similar to each are presented first. Specifics about the individual methods are discussed in the following sections.

Among all the pharmaceutical contraceptives, duration of action is of particular interest: Indeed, contraceptive methods today often are categorized on this basis. **Long-acting reversible contraceptives (LARCs)** are birth control methods that provide effective contraception for an extended period of time without requiring frequent user action. **Short-acting reversible contraceptives (SARCs)** are methods that have shorter durations of action and depend on user adherence for sustained success. Unintended pregnancy rates are reduced when LARC methods are used.[3] Figure 29-1 illustrates the currently available pharmacologic-based contraceptives and indicates the amount of user interaction required to use them.

Background

The effectiveness of a particular contraceptive product depends on many factors including a priori fertility status, and the efficacy and effectiveness of the method. In addition, there are different methods for calculating a contraceptive failure rate.

Definition of Pregnancy

Since 1978, the U.S. Department of Health and Human Services (DHHS) has defined pregnancy as "the period of time from confirmation of implantation until the expulsion or extraction of the fetus."[4] The American College of Obstetricians and Gynecologists similarly defines pregnancy as "The state of a female after conception and until termination of the gestation," noting that "conception is the implantation of the blastocyst."[5] There has been much debate about when pregnancy begins biologically, especially in legislation related to abortion, and some women have a definition based on their personal beliefs. However, the accepted medical definition of pregnancy remains that which was formulated by DHHS and the American College of Obstetricians and Gynecologists.

The risk of pregnancy from a single act of intercourse is low. Researchers estimate that if 100 women have unprotected intercourse during week 2 or 3 of their menstrual cycle, approximately 8 will become pregnant. However,

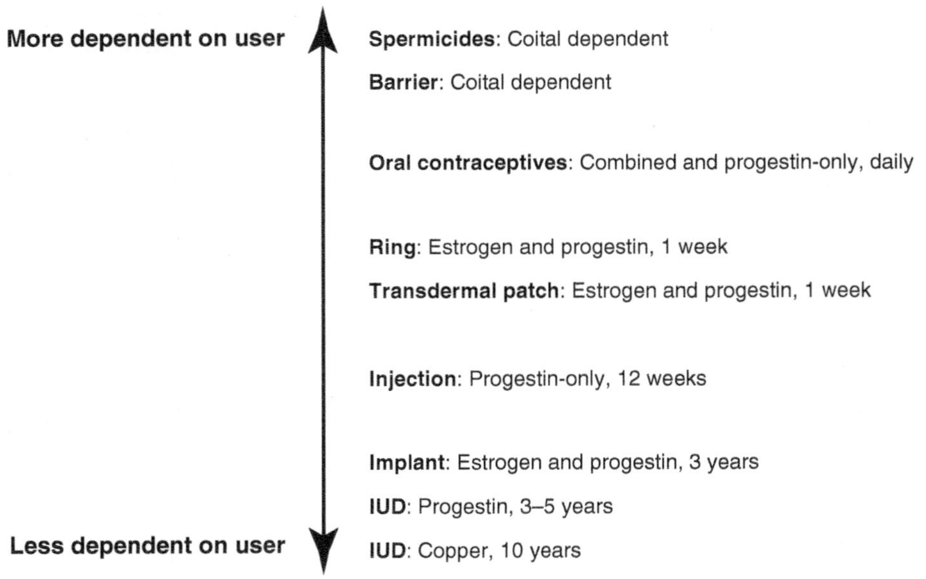

More dependent on user

Spermicides: Coital dependent

Barrier: Coital dependent

Oral contraceptives: Combined and progestin-only, daily

Ring: Estrogen and progestin, 1 week

Transdermal patch: Estrogen and progestin, 1 week

Injection: Progestin-only, 12 weeks

Implant: Estrogen and progestin, 3 years

IUD: Progestin, 3–5 years

IUD: Copper, 10 years

Less dependent on user

Figure 29-1 Selected contraceptive methods based on degree of user interaction and duration of action.

the closer intercourse occurs to ovulation, the higher the risk.[6] A number of other factors also affect fecundity, or the physiologic ability to reproduce. For example, older women are less fecund than younger women; this decline in fecundity begins in the late 20s for women, and a similar decline begins in the late 30s for men.[7] Thus, all methods of contraception will appear to be more effective in reducing the risk of pregnancy among older (less fecund) couples. In addition, studies have reported differences in the risk of pregnancy according to a woman's motivation to avoid pregnancy. Relationship status, sexual activity, adherence to the contraceptive method, and accuracy of pregnancy reporting all affect the reported risk of pregnancy.

Becoming pregnant also depends on many steps that occur over several days. First ovulation must occur, followed by fertilization of a viable ovum. Fertilization is the process by which a single sperm penetrates the layers of an egg or oocyte to form a new cell. This action can take as long as 24 hours and usually occurs in the fallopian tubes. A narrow window of 12 to 24 hours exists during which the egg can be fertilized after ovulation; otherwise, the egg dissolves. Implantation of the fertilized egg in the uterine lining begins at approximately day 5 after fertilization and is usually complete by approximately 14 days after fertilization. Studies estimate that between one-third and one-half of all fertilized eggs are not successfully implanted; moreover, after implantation, approximately 15% of pregnancies end in spontaneous abortion (miscarriage).[8]

Efficacy and Effectiveness of Contraceptive Methods

The contraceptive methods available today each have different success rates that are based on a combination of the method's theoretic effectiveness, use effectiveness, and failure rate. The term **efficacy** refers to how well a contraceptive method works when used consistently as prescribed.[9] Failure related to a method's efficacy may occur even when the method is used perfectly (known as perfect use); such events are termed method failures. The term **effectiveness** refers to how well a contraceptive method works in conditions of typical use or under real-life circumstances. Failure rates related to effectiveness include all pregnancies that occur whether the method is or is not used properly. Because all methods have inherent method failure rates, not all failures involve user failures.

Contraceptive Failure Rates

Contraceptive failure rates for all methods decrease over time: Most occur during early usage of the method, in part because those women who are more fertile and those who use contraception inconsistently will become pregnant sooner. Failure rates for contraceptive methods are calculated in two ways: the Pearl index and the Kaplan Meier rate.

The Pearl index, named after biologist Richard Pearl, has remained popular for decades in part because of the simplicity of the calculation. The formula for this index is the number of pregnancies divided by total years in which a woman is exposed to pregnancy risk. However, the Pearl index is based on the flawed assumption that the risk of pregnancy is constant over time. Moreover, the index addresses only accidental pregnancy, not the number of women lost to follow-up, number of women experiencing adverse reactions, or the number of women dissatisfied with the method. Thus, the Pearl index is not considered the best measure of contraceptive efficacy, although it has long been the FDA standard used for new drug applications.

In contrast, the Kaplan Meier rate calculates a separate rate for each month of use, as opposed to the entire study period. With this method, it is possible to derive 6- or 12-month cumulative rates and to account for discontinuation of contraception for reasons other than pregnancy. This calculation is preferred by scientific journals. Table 29-1 lists the failure rates for all methods of contraception using the Kaplan Meier formula.[10]

Guidelines for Prescribing and Managing Contraceptives

Medical Eligibility Criteria and Selected Practice Recommendations for Contraceptive Use

The origin of medical eligibility criteria (MEC) for contraceptive use can be found in a 1996 World Health Organization (WHO) publication. Today, these criteria are regularly updated recommendations intended to assist countries in the development of guidelines specific to their populations and health systems. The Centers for Disease Control and Prevention (CDC) released guidelines in 2010 for hormonal methods and the copper intrauterine device that were developed for healthcare providers in the United States.[11] These medical eligibility criteria list health conditions that can interfere with successful use of a contraceptive method and health conditions in which contraceptive methods are contraindicated.

The MEC categorizes contraceptives into one of four groups as listed in Table 29-2. These widely used categories are referred to throughout this chapter. Some conditions have a theoretical or actual risk associated with

Table 29-1 Percentage of Women Experiencing an Unintended Pregnancy During the First Year of Typical Use and the First Year of Perfect Use of Contraception and the Percentage Continuing Use at the End of the First Year, United States

	Percentage of Women Experiencing an Unintended Pregnancy Within the First Year of Use		Percentage of Women Continuing Use at One Year[c]
Method	**Typical Use[a]**	**Perfect Use[b]**	
No method[d]	85	85	
Spermicides[e]	28	18	42
Fertility awareness-based methods	24		47
StandardDays method[f]		5	
TwoDay method[f]		4	
Ovulation method[f]		3	
Symptothermal method		0.4	
Withdrawal	22	4	46
Sponge			36
Parous women	24	20	
Nulliparous women	12	9	
Condom[g]			
Female (fc)	21	5	41
Male	18	2	43
Diaphragm[h]	12	6	57
Combined pill and progestin-only pill	9	0.3	67
Evra patch	9	0.3	67
NuvaRing	9	0.3	67
DMPA	6	0.2	56
Intrauterine contraceptives			
ParaGard (copper T)	0.8	0.6	78
Mirena (LNG)	0.2	0.2	80
Implanon	0.05	0.05	84
Female sterilization	0.5	0.5	100
Male sterilization	0.15	0.10	100

Emergency Contraceptives: Emergency contraceptive pills or insertion of a copper intrauterine contraceptive after unprotected intercourse substantially reduces the risk of pregnancy.[i]

Lactational Amenorrhea Method: LAM is a highly effective, *temporary* method of contraception.[j]

[a] Among *typical* couples who initiate use of a method (not necessarily for the first time), the percentage who experience an accidental pregnancy during the first year if they do not stop use for any other reason. Estimates of the probability of pregnancy during the first year of typical use for spermicides and the diaphragm are taken from the 1995 National Survey of Family Growth, corrected for underreporting of abortion; estimates for fertility awareness-based methods, withdrawal, the male condom, the pill, and DMPA are taken from the 1995 and 2002 National Survey of Family Growth, corrected for underreporting of abortion. See the text for the derivation of estimates for the other methods.

[b] Among couples who initiate use of a method (not necessarily for the first time) and who use it *perfectly* (both consistently and correctly), the percentage who experience an accidental pregnancy during the first year if they do not stop use for any other reason. See the text for the derivation of the estimate for each method.

[c] Among couples attempting to avoid pregnancy, the percentage who continue to use a method for 1 year.

[d] The percentages becoming pregnant in columns (2) and (3) are based on data from populations where contraception is not used and from women who cease using contraception so as to become pregnant. Among such populations, about 89% become pregnant within 1 year. This estimate was lowered slightly (to 85%) to represent the percentage who would become pregnant within 1 year among women now relying on reversible methods of contraception if they abandoned contraception altogether.

[e] Foams, creams, gels, vaginal suppositories, and vaginal film.

[f] The Ovulation and TwoDay methods are based on evaluation of cervical mucus. The StandardDays method avoids intercourse on cycle days 8 through 19. The Symptothermal method is a double-check method based on evaluation of cervical mucus to determine the first fertile day and evaluation of cervical mucus and temperature to determine the last fertile day.

[g] Without spermicides.

[h] With spermicidal cream or jelly.

[i] Ella, Plan B One-Step, and Next Choice are the only dedicated products specifically marketed for emergency contraception. The label for Plan B One-Step (one dose is 1 white pill) says to take the pill within 72 hours after unprotected intercourse. Research has shown that that all of the brands listed here are effective when used within 120 hours after unprotected sex. The label for Next Choice (one dose is 1 peach pill) says to take one pill within 72 hours after unprotected intercourse and another pill 12 hours later. Research has shown that that both pills can be taken at the same time with no decrease in efficacy or increase in side effects and that they are effective when used within 120 hours after unprotected sex. The Food and Drug Administration has, in addition, declared the following 19 brands of oral contraceptives to be safe and effective for emergency contraception: Ogestrel (one dose is 2 white pills); Nordette (one dose is 4 light-orange pills); Cryselle, Levora, Low-Ogestrel, Lo/Ovral, or Quasence (one dose is 4 white pills); Jolessa, Portia, Seasonale, or Trivora (one dose is 4 pink pills); Seasonique (one dose is 4 light-blue-green pills); Enpresse (one dose is 4 orange pills); Lessina (one dose is 5 pink pills); Aviane or LoSeasonique (one dose is 5 orange pills); Lutera or Sronyx (one dose is 5 white pills); and Lybrel (one dose is 6 yellow pills).

[j] To maintain effective protection against pregnancy, another method of contraception must be used as soon as menstruation resumes, the frequency or duration of breastfeeds is reduced, bottle feeds are introduced, or the infant reaches 6 months of age.

Source: Reprinted from Trussell J. Contraceptive failure in the United States. *Contraception*. 2011;83(5):397-404, with permission from Elsevier.

Table 29-2 Centers for Disease Control and Prevention's Medical Eligibility Criteria Categories for Contraceptive Use

Category	Description
1	Condition for which there is no restriction for the use of the contraceptive method.
2	Condition for which the advantages of using the method generally outweigh the theoretical or proven risks.
3	Condition for which the theoretical or proven risks generally outweigh the advantages of using the method.
4	Condition that represents an unacceptable health risk if the contraceptive method is used.

Source: Reproduced from Centers for Disease Control and Prevention. U S. medical eligibility criteria for contraceptive use, 2010. *MMWR Recommend Rep.* 2010;59:1-86.[11]

contraceptive use, yet the condition also has a higher risk for adverse health outcomes during pregnancy. Therefore, the guidelines note where the risks associated with contraceptive use are lower than the risk of becoming pregnant for women with particular disorders. The CDC's MEC focuses on who *cannot* use a particular contraceptive method; however the typical healthy woman rarely has an absolute contraindication to a method, and choice ultimately is primarily based on her lifestyle and desire. The optimal contraceptive method is the one that a woman chooses and will use consistently and correctly.

In 2002, in addition to the MEC, the WHO published *Selected Practice Recommendations for Contraceptive Use* (SPR). While the MEC concentrates on who should not use a method, the SPR document focuses on evidence-based best practices associated with how to use the method. Similar to the MEC, the SPR are broad and regularly updated guidelines. The SPR specific to the United States was published by CDC in 2013.[12]

Drug–Herb and Drug–Drug Interactions

Drug–herb and drug–drug interactions have emerged as a major concern in clinical pharmacotherapeutics today. The CYP3A4 enzyme, in particular, is responsible for approximately 60% of P450 enzyme-mediated metabolism of therapeutic drugs,[13] including contraceptive steroid hormones. Thus, in addition to identifying criteria for eligibility for a contraceptive method based on a woman's health condition, the MEC lists drugs that can impair contraceptive effectiveness.[11] Table 29-3 lists the drugs identified by the U.S. MEC as potential drug–drug interactions for combined hormonal contraceptive products. For all of these drugs, complete guidance and clarification are available from the full discussion in the MEC guidelines.

Drugs such as many antiepileptic medications induce the CYP3A4 enzymes that metabolize contraceptive hormones and the resultant lower level of hormone can lead to contraceptive failure[14,15] (Box 29-1). Some herbs and natural compounds isolated from herbs have also been identified as inducers of various CYP enzymes,[16] and St. John's wort in particular has been shown to induce metabolism of contraceptive hormones.[17] Non–enzyme-inducing antiepileptic drugs (AEDs) such as valproate, benzodiazepines, ethosuximide (Zarontin), levetiracetam (Keppra), tiagabine (Gabitril), and zonisamide (Zonegran) do not show any interactions with the **combined oral contraceptives (COCs)**.[14]

According to the U.S. MEC, broad-spectrum antibiotics such as penicillins and tetracyclines are placed in category 1 for use with COCs, in contrast to common myths

Table 29-3 Drugs That Decrease Effectiveness of Hormonal Contraceptive Formulations[a]

Drug: Generic (Brand)	Medical Eligibility Criteria
Anti-seizure Medications	
Barbiturates	3
Carbamazepine (Tegretol)	3
Eslicarbazepine (Aptiom)	3
Lamotrigine (Lamictal)	3
Oxcarbazepine (Trileptal)	3
Perampanel (Fycompa) in dosage > 12 mg/day)	3
Phenytoin (Dilantin)	3
Topiramate (Topamax) in dosage of > 200 mg/day	3
HIV Medications	
Nucleoside reverse transcriptase inhibitors (NRTIs)	1
Non-nucleoside reverse transcriptase inhibitors (NNRTIs)	2
Ritonavir-boosted protease inhibitors	3
Antibiotics	
Rifampicin or rifabutin (Rifadin)	3

[a]Includes combined oral contraceptive pills, progestin-only pills, transdermal contraceptive patch, and combined hormonal vaginal ring.

Source: Centers for Disease Control and Prevention. U S. medical eligibility criteria for contraceptive use, 2010. *MMWR Recommend Rep.* 2010;59:1-86.[11]

Box 29-1 A Challenge in Primary Care

NB, a 17-year-old nulligravida, is being seen for a regular visit, and she requests pills for contraception. Her past history includes a diagnosed seizure disorder that is controlled with phenytoin (Dilantin). Her last seizure was 6 months ago, and she is under the continuing care of a neurologist. NB's physical examination is unremarkable, including normal vital signs and BMI.

Prescribing combined oral contraceptives is challenging in this situation. Combined oral contraceptives will not cause a physiological change in NB's seizure disorder. Rather, the issue of concern is the potential for drug–drug interactions. Contraceptive efficacy of oral contraceptives can be decreased if taken concurrently with phenytoin; therefore, contraceptive failure is more likely than if NB did not take this agent. In addition, phenytoin is not metabolized as rapidly and serum levels increase when it is taken concomitantly with COCs; therefore, serum levels of phenytoin can become excessive. The same issues theoretically apply to the use of the transdermal patch (Ortho Evra) and ring (NuvaRing).

However, NB is at risk for an unwanted pregnancy as well as possible teratogenic effects from the antiepileptic medication. Depot medroxyprogesterone acetate (DMPA) may be a reasonable option for her, especially since it can also decrease seizure activity. If prescribed, as for all adolescents, NB should receive counseling about dietary and exercise options to increase bone density. Although NB is nulliparous, that factor alone is not a contraindication to an intrauterine contraceptive agent. Therefore NB can also be offered the choice of one of the intrauterine devices.

Consultation with NB's neurologist may be of great value. Non–enzyme-inducing antiepileptic agents such as gabapentin (Neurontin) or pregabalin (Lyrica), do not appear to have the same drug–drug interactions associated with phenytoin. Should the seizure activity be controlled with the use of these drugs, NB may be able to use her first choice, combined oral contraceptives.

that these antibiotics lower contraceptive effectiveness. The U.S. MEC specifically classify protease inhibitors, certain anticonvulsants, and rifampicin/rifabutin (Rifadin) as category 3 for combined hormonal contraceptives and the **progestin-only method** of pills.[11]

The majority of **injectable contraceptives** and implantable intrauterine contraceptives in common use by women are classified as category 1 or 2. These contraceptive formulations rarely have drug–drug interactions.

Updates to the U.S Medical Eligibility Criteria for Contraception

Periodically, the CDC issues revised recommendations to the MEC. To date, these updates have focused on contraception for women who have specific conditions or disorders. In 2011, the CDC released additional contraceptive guidelines for postpartum women; in the following year, the agency issued contraceptive guidelines for women who are at high risk of becoming infected with human immunodeficiency virus (HIV) or who already are infected with the virus.[18,19] Additional updates may be expected as new information in the area of contraception emerges.

Overview of Hormonal Contraception

Hormones and Pregnancy

All hormonal contraceptives act to interfere with the cascade of events that lead to ovulation and fertilization. Therefore, a brief review of the normal phenomena is in order. On the first day of each menstrual cycle, low blood levels of estrogen and progesterone permit secretion of gonadotropin-releasing hormone (GnRH) from the hypothalamus, which in turn stimulates release of follicle-stimulating hormone (FSH) from the pituitary. A cohort of follicles in the ovary responds to the influx of FSH with accelerated growth and secretion of estrogen. Estrogen levels rise and stimulate proliferation of the uterine endometrium. When the estrogen level exceeds a threshold, it triggers release of luteinizing hormone (LH) from the pituitary. Ovulation occurs within 36 hours of the onset of the LH surge and the follicle walls then collapse.

Over the next several days, progesterone becomes the primary hormone, and the majority of progesterone secreted during the cycle being produced at this time; progesterone levels peak approximately 8 days after ovulation. Progesterone promotes a secretory endometrium—changes that are important for implantation of a fertilized egg. When conception does not occur, the thickened endometrium loses its hormonal support, becomes ischemic, and is subsequently shed during menstruation.

In addition to the events of ovulation, the capacity for conception is affected by changes in the cervical mucus and endometrial lining. The rapidly increasing estrogen

Table 29-4 Hormonal Contraceptive Methods by Type of Agents

Hormones	Contraceptive Methods
Estrogen and progestin	Combined oral contraceptives (various formulations and brands)
	Transdermal patch (ethinyl estradiol/norelgestromin [Ortho Evra, Xulane])
	Vaginal ring (ethinyl estradiol/etonogestrel [NuvaRing])
Progestin only	Injectable/subcutaneous (depot medroxyprogesterone acetate [DMPA])
	Implants (etonogestrel [Nexplanon])
	Intrauterine devices (levonorgestrel [Mirena, Liletta, Skyla])

production by the dominant follicle causes an increase in thin, watery cervical mucus secretion that facilitates sperm transport, whereas rising progesterone levels after ovulation changes cervical mucus to a thick and sticky consistency that inhibits sperm transport.

Types of Hormonal Contraceptives

Hormonal contraceptives contain either estrogen and a progestin or progestin only. Table 29-4 lists specific products that use one of these hormonal components.

Initiation of Hormonal Contraceptives

Traditionally, all hormonal contraceptives, and especially oral contraceptives, have been initiated in association with the date of the last menstrual period, either on the first day, on the fifth day, or as the "Sunday Start," which refers to starting the contraception the first Sunday following the onset of bleeding. The rationale for this approach was to initiate hormones before follicle development, and to reduce the incidence of unscheduled bleeding. In addition, the risk of ovulation within the first 5 days of the menstrual period is low. In general, if the method is started more than 5 days after the beginning of menstrual bleeding, ovulation may not be effectively suppressed. In that case, a backup method of contraception is suggested.[20]

An alternative, the "Quick Start" method, initiates the hormonal contraceptive—whether it be oral, transdermal, implant, injectable, or intrauterine—at any point in the cycle, as long as the woman is not pregnant. The Quick Start approach takes advantage of the woman's motivation to begin contraception and eliminates the need for complicated instructions regarding when to start the method. Evaluating whether a woman is not pregnant generally includes a history exploring the information found in Box 29-2. Most practices also will perform a point-of-care pregnancy test. Contrary to original expectations that Quick Start would result in more unscheduled bleeding, initiation of a hormonal contraceptive method with the Quick Start method does not increase the incidence of unscheduled bleeding or spotting during the first cycle, nor is Quick Start associated with higher rates of pregnancy.[21]

A woman interested in the Quick Start method should be advised to use an additional form of contraception for the first week of use of the method.

Switching Hormonal Contraceptive Methods

Unfortunately, much remains unknown in the area of hormonal contraception. For example, it was only a few decades ago that women were advised to use a backup method such as a **spermicide** and condom during every act of intercourse for a full month after initiating use of contraceptive pills or intrauterine devices (IUDs). Based on current knowledge of physiology of the menstrual cycle, the average woman who is not already using a hormonal method is now advised to use a backup method for 7 days after initiation of a combined hormonal contraception.

Many women switch methods from one to another for a variety of reasons, including side effects, costs, and lifestyle issues. A period of time without contraceptive coverage may be avoided if certain methods overlap. Table 29-5 provides a guide for switching contraceptive methods to minimize a gap in pregnancy prevention.[22,23] Note that overlapping also avoids the need for a backup in these situations. Switching from pills, patches, **vaginal contraceptive rings**, and implants to the nonhormonal copper IUD can be done up to 5 days after discontinuation of the former methods or up to 16 weeks after the last contraceptive injection. Should a woman with a levonorgestrel IUD desire to switch to a copper IUD, the latter can be inserted immediately after

Box 29-2 General Criteria Indicating That a Woman Is Not Pregnant

- No sexual intercourse since the last menses
- Correct and consistent use of another reliable method of contraception, including lactational amenorrhea method
- 7 days or fewer after first- or second-trimester abortion/miscarriage
- 7 days or fewer after start of normal menses
- 28 days or fewer after giving birth

Table 29-5 When to Start a New Hormonal Method When Switching from Another Method to Minimize Risk of Pregnancy

Current Method	New Method					
	COC or POP	**Transdermal Patch**	**Vaginal Ring**	**Progestin Injection**	**Implant**	**LNG IUD**
COC or POP		1 day before pill discontinued	The day after taking any pill	7 days before pill discontinued	4 days before pill discontinued	7 days before pill discontinued
Transdermal Patch	1 day before patch discontinued		Insert ring same day as patch discontinued	7 days before patch discontinued	4 days before patch discontinued	7 days before patch discontinued
Vaginal Ring	1 day before ring discontinued	2 days before ring discontinued		7 days before ring discontinued	4 days before ring discontinued	7 days before ring discontinued
Progestin Injection	Any day within 15 weeks of injection	Any day within 15 weeks of injection	Any day within 15 weeks of injection		Any day within 15 weeks of injection	Any day within 15 weeks of injection
Implant	7 days before implant discontinued	7 days before implant discontinued	7 days before implant discontinued	7 days before implant discontinued		
LNG IUD	7 days before removing LNG IUD	7 days before removing LNG IUD	7 days before removing LNG IUD	7 days before removing LNG IUD	4 days before removing LNG IUD	

Abbreviations: COC = combined oral contraception; LNG IUD = levonorgestrel intrauterine device; POP = progestin-only pill.
Sources: Data from Lesnewski R, Prine L, Ginzburg R. Preventing gaps when switching contraceptives. *Am Fam Physician.* 2011;83(5):567-570[22]; Reproductive Health Access Project. How to switch birth control methods, 2013. http://www.reproductiveaccess.org/wp-content/uploads/2014/12/switching_bc.pdf. Accessed February 14, 2015.[23]

the first device is removed, but in this case use of a backup method is advised for 7 days.

Obesity and the Use of Combined Hormonal Contraceptives

Obesity may lower the effectiveness of certain contraceptives. Some older studies suggested that women who are overweight and obese may have an increased risk of unintended pregnancy while using hormonal contraception in comparison to women with normal body mass indices (BMI).[24–27] Two national surveillance systems also found a two- to three-fold increase in apparent contraceptive failure based on increasing BMI.[28] One older study that reported 5 of the 15 of the pregnancies reported in clinical trials of the contraceptive patch occurred in the 3% of users who weighed more than 90 kg (198 pounds).[29] This finding led the FDA to require product labeling for the patch that warns, "Contraceptive effectiveness may be decreased in women weighing over 198 pounds." Other studies have failed to demonstrate any association between obesity and contraceptive failure.[30,31] Some reasons why the results of studies are conflicting may be related to whether hormonal contraceptive use was measured as typical or perfect use. In addition, adherence to method use instructions may be an important confounding factor.[32]

Pharmacokinetic studies have demonstrated differences in hormone levels between obese and normal-weight women using hormonal contraception, but little difference in ovarian activity has been found in studies conducted among women using vaginal rings,[33,34] injectable contraceptives,[35] implants,[36,37] or combined oral contraceptives.[38] In addition, a recent systematic review failed to demonstrate a consistent association between BMI and hormonal contraceptive failure.[39] The authors noted, however, that the evidence was limited for any individual contraceptive method, and the overall quality of evidence was low. The researchers also noted that the use of BMI as a measure, rather than weight alone, better addresses potential pharmacokinetic and pharmacodynamic changes related to body composition and fat. In the five studies that used BMI as a measure, only one showed a higher pregnancy risk in overweight or obese women using oral contraceptives.[40] The authors further concluded that the effectiveness of subdermal implants and injectable contraceptives which also use the same hormonal method of action, seem to be unaffected by body mass.

In summary, there is no definitive proof of a direct association between weight or BMI and contraceptive failure, nor are there evidence-based guidelines for management of hormonal contraception for women who are in the overweight or obese BMI categories. The CDC's MEC classify all hormonal contraceptives as category 2 for women who are obese; there are no contraindications to use of any method in otherwise healthy women who are overweight or obese.[11]

Combined Hormonal Contraceptives

Combined hormonal contraceptives contain both estrogen and a progestin and are categorized separately from progestin-only agents. Originally this category was populated only by combined oral contraceptives, colloquially called "the pill." The COC method remains one of the most widely used options for reversible contraception. More than 80% of women surveyed from 2006 to 2010 and who were of reproductive age and who had sexual intercourse reported using COCs at some point.[41] More recently, other combined hormonal contraceptives have emerged that include LARC methods such as implants and the transdermal patch. Thus, the current term "combined hormonal contraceptives" refers to all contraceptive products that contain estrogen and a progestin.

Mechanism of Action

The primary mechanism of action of all of the combined hormonal contraceptives is prevention of ovulation. Estrogen primarily inhibits release of follicle-stimulating hormone, and the progestin component of COCs inhibits release of luteinizing hormone. The estrogen component offers additional contraceptive efficacy by inhibiting the development of a dominant follicle. Estrogen stabilizes the endometrium to provide better cycle control, as evidenced by less frequency of unscheduled bleeding when compared to progestin-only methods. Estrogen also potentiates the action of progestins; thus, the addition of estrogen allows reductions in progestin dosage. Low levels of estrogen and progestin also inhibit proliferation of the endometrium, and progestins contribute to production of implantation-inhospitable cervical mucus. The hormones are also theorized to inhibit the ability of the sperm to fertilize an egg and to delay sperm transport through the reproductive tract.

Box 29-3 Selected Noncontraceptive Benefits Associated with Combined Hormonal Contraceptives

- Acne improved
- Bone mineral density improved, especially among older women
- Dysmenorrhea decreased
- Endometrial, ovarian, and colorectal cancer risk decreased
- Leiomyomata bleeding and pain decreased
- Menstrual bleeding changed based on method for lifestyle considerations (e.g., amenorrhea, regularity of menses)
- Premenstrual discomforts decreased based on method (e.g., premenstrual headaches)

Benefits

Much has been written about the adverse effects of combined hormonal contraception. Nevertheless, hormonal contraceptive methods have several advantages in addition to prevention of pregnancy.[42] For women with some medical disorders, an unintended pregnancy may expose the woman to a high risk of morbidity or even mortality. Some important noncontraceptive benefits are listed in Box 29-3.

Eligibility for Use of Combined Hormonal Contraceptives and Contraindications

The U.S. MEC identify a list of medical conditions that may predispose a woman to adverse effects from COCs.[11] In the past, many adverse effects have been attributed to hormonal contraceptives, such as altered glucose tolerance, cholecystitis, and liver tumors; these problems were associated with the higher hormone levels used in early contraceptive pill formulations and rarely occur with contemporary low-dose formulations. The most concerning adverse effects that may limit eligibility for current versions of combined hormonal contraceptives are related to thrombotic events such as myocardial infarction or stroke, which are associated with the estrogen component in these contraceptives. Contemporary low-dose hormonal contraceptives do not appreciably increase these risks among healthy women who do not smoke and who do not have underlying damage from hypertension or have other cardiovascular risk factors.[43,44] Women with migraines accompanied by aura have a higher risk of ischemic stroke that is compounded by use of estrogen-containing contraceptives.[45] Current practice guidelines simultaneously call for better cardiac screening and advocate against prescribing hormonal contraceptives for women who are at risk for cardiovascular disorders.[12]

As compared to nonpregnant women who do not use hormonal contraceptive methods, the risk of thromboembolism is also higher among users of combined hormonal contraceptives.[46] Although some women with comorbidities or genetic predisposition have an increased risk for thrombophlebitis when using a combined hormonal contraceptive, this population of women have a higher risk of such events when pregnant.[46] The majority of studies that have found an increased risk of thromboembolic disease were conducted with women on COCs, although any combined hormonal method may confer a higher risk of thromboembolic disease. Women who have a known risk of thromboembolism should not take COCs.

Certain conditions, such as factor V Leiden mutation, which is often asymptomatic and undiagnosed until the occurrence of an untoward event, may account for many cases of venous thromboembolism (VTE) among COC users, although the incidence of these events remains very small (approximately 4 to 5 cases per 100,000 women per year).[47] Screening for such disorders would require testing large numbers of healthy women and result in a high cost to detect an uncommon condition and prevent a very small number of events. Most experts do not recommend laboratory screening for these inherited disorders, but instead advocate screening first by history and not pursuing additional testing unless the woman or a close family member has a history of unexplained thromboembolism.[11]

Some studies have implicated selected progestins—specifically, desogestrel, norgestimate, drospirenone, and gestodene, which is not available in the United States,—in the development of venous thromboembolism. These progestins are discussed in the *Steroid Hormones* chapter. The original findings suggesting their association with VTE were subsequently reevaluated in a number of reports, and any observed increase in risk due to the gonanes when first introduced to the marketplace was determined to be either so small as to be not meaningful or the result of bias and confounding in the original studies.[48]

Increases in angiotensin II and aldosterone activity associated with estrogens and progestins may adversely affect blood pressure in susceptible women. If due solely to the estrogen component, this effect is reversible upon discontinuation of the contraceptive. Drospirenone has an antimineralocorticoid activity, and contraceptives containing this progestin should not be prescribed to women using other potassium-sparing drugs such as angiotensin-converting enzyme (ACE) inhibitors, potassium sparing diuretics, or nonsteroidal anti-inflammatory drugs (NSAIDs) on a chronic basis, without evaluating potassium levels.

Common Side Effects of Combined Hormonal Contraceptives

Side effects are frequently reported by users of combined hormonal contraceptives, but not all of the reported symptoms are secondary to the contraceptive product. A double-blind, placebo-controlled trial showed that many side effects traditionally thought to be due to the hormone content of COCs actually occurred with the same frequency among pill and placebo users.[49] Thus, reports of side effects should not be automatically attributed to contraceptive hormones, but rather should be evaluated and managed appropriately. It is also important to note that metabolism of contraceptive steroids can vary from woman to woman, and side effects will not be experienced by every woman, even those taking the same dosage of these hormones.

Few evidence-based data exist regarding management of women with side effects determined to be related to the contraceptive product. In general, most side effects will subside within the first months of use as the woman adjusts to the different hormone levels. Changing to another product to alter the hormone dosing is an option if expectant management fails; individual patterns in drug metabolism may make certain formulations more tolerable for individual women even if larger studies do not show an overall benefit from this approach.

Altered bleeding patterns, such as spotting and breakthrough bleeding, are common in the first few months of combined hormonal contraceptive use as the endometrium adjusts to the hormone dose, specifically the progestin. Approximately 10% to 30% of users will experience unscheduled bleeding in the first month of use, but only 10% or fewer will experience this effect by the third month of contraceptive use. Women who smoke have higher rates of unscheduled bleeding, especially if they use low-dose methods containing 20 mcg of ethinyl estradiol (EE).[50]

Missing a dose of a combined oral contraceptive is also associated with spotting and bleeding. In contrast, withdrawal bleeding during the hormone-free interval may be less or absent with contemporary low-dose hormonal contraceptives.

Nausea is often related to the estrogen component of the hormonal contraceptive. Many clinicians advise women who experience nausea to take their pills at bedtime, yet there is no evidence that this practice is of value, although it also does no harm. The nausea may be a local gastric effect or operate at the level of the central nervous system. Progestins may contribute to decreased peristalsis, constipation, or bloating.[10] In most cases, the symptoms resolve after a few months of use. Vomiting and diarrhea secondary to another gastrointestinal disorder may interfere with absorption of contraceptive steroids, and women should be advised to use backup contraception during and for a week after such an illness or to consider use of **emergency contraception**, if appropriate.[12]

Breast tenderness and increased vaginal discharge are other commonly reported side effects in the first few months of hormonal contraceptive use; they are likely related to both the estrogen and progestin components. Lower doses of estrogen produced fewer such symptoms in one study.[51]

Although it may be tempting to attribute various symptoms to the use of hormonal contraceptives, each symptom should be evaluated in the same manner as would be appropriate for any woman. For example, occasional headaches are commonly reported by women who use hormonal contraceptives and are of little clinical significance. In contrast, new-onset, severe, or worsening headaches need to be evaluated promptly.

Depression, mood alterations, and changes in libido are occasionally reported with combined hormonal contraception use. There is no evidence of an overall increased risk of clinical depression in women who use hormonal contraception; however, it is important to remember that depression is not uncommon in reproductive-aged women in general. Some women may experience a decrease in libido due to lower levels of free testosterone.[52–54]

Studies have suggested a small beneficial effect of drospirenone-containing hormonal contraceptives on symptoms of premenstrual syndrome and premenstrual dysphoric disorder.[55] Based on such data, in 2006 Yaz, a combined oral contraception containing drospirenone in 24-day dosing, became the first oral contraceptive to receive an FDA indication as a treatment for women with premenstrual dysphoric disorder (PMDD).

Skin changes such as darkened patches on the face may occur due to estrogen stimulation of melanocytes; these may fade when estrogen is discontinued, but may not fade completely in some women. Such changes may develop in users of the transdermal patch under the patch site as well. Some women may also experience a worsening of acne or hirsutism, but in general combined hormonal contraceptives decrease androgen production and increase sex hormone–binding globulins, which bind testosterone and androgen, thereby reducing the levels of free testosterone that worsens acne and hirsutism. Some oral contraceptive formulations have FDA indications for treatment of acne, but all combined hormonal contraceptives act in a similar fashion and should be effective in ameliorating acne.[56]

Combined Oral Contraceptives

The oldest type of the combined hormonal contraceptives is the combined oral contraceptive. The vast majority of combined oral contraceptives available in the United States contain 20 to 35 mcg of ethinyl estradiol as the estrogen component. Mestranol, which is metabolized to ethinyl estradiol continues to be found in a few formulations, but is rarely prescribed. A newer formulation contains estradiol valerate,[57] and a few formulations contain 50 mcg ethinyl estradiol, although these higher dose pills are no longer commonly prescribed. A few of the combined oral contraceptive on the market in biphasic or multiphasic formulations include 10 mcg of ethinyl estradiol for some of the unit doses. Metabolism of ethinyl estradiol varies significantly from woman to woman; thus, some women will experience side effects from the same dose that produces few clinical effects in other women. Table 29-6 lists oral contraceptives available in the United States. Although the progestin-only pill is technically not a combined oral contraceptive, it is included in the table for ease of comparison.

Oral contraceptive progestins in the COCs available in the United States include the estranes (norethindrone, norethindrone acetate, ethynodiol diacetate); the gonanes (norgestrel, levonorgestrel, desogestrel, norgestimate), which include a non-ethinylated subgroup containing dienogest (similar to norethindrone); and a 17-alpha spironolactone derivative drospirenone.[59] Most authorities assert that the clinical effects of the various progestins in contemporary hormonal contraceptives are essentially the same; dosages of the different progestins have been adjusted to account for their biological effects and clinical differences are minimal for most women.[60] However, individual differences in progestin metabolism may lead

Table 29-6 Oral Contraceptive Formulations Available in the United States, April 2014

Product (Brand Name)	First Phase	Second Phase	Third Phase	Fourth Phase
Progestin-Only Pills				
Camila Errin Jolivette Micronor Nora-be NorQD	0.35 mg norethindrone continuously	None	None	None
Monophasic 10 mcg Pill				
Lo Loestrin Fe	10 mcg ethinyl estradiol with 1 mg norethindrone for 24 days	10 mcg ethinyl estradiol for 2 days	Hormone-free tablets for 2 days.[a] Hormone-free tablets contain 75 mg ferrous fumarate.	
Monophasic 20 mcg Pills				
Aviane Lessina Levlite Lutera	20 mcg ethinyl estradiol with 0.1 mg levonorgestrel for 21 days	Hormone-free tablets for 7 days[a]		
Lybrel	20 mcg ethinyl estradiol with 0.09 mg levonorgestrel for continuous dosing	None		
Minastrin 24 Fe	20 mcg ethinyl estradiol and 1 mg norethindrone acetate for 24 days	4 hormone-free tablets contain 75 mg ferrous fumarate[a]		
Junel 1/20 Loestrin 1/20 Microgestin 1/20	20 mcg ethinyl estradiol with 1 mg norethindrone acetate for 21 days	0.35 mg norethindrone continuously		
Junel 1/20 Fe Loestrin-FE 1/20 Microgestin 1/20 Fe	20 mcg ethinyl estradiol with 1 mg norethindrone acetate for 21 days	7 hormone-free tablets contain 75 mg ferrous fumarate[a]		
Loryna Yaz	20 mcg ethinyl estradiol with 3 mg drospirenone for 24 days	Hormone-free tablets for 4 days[a]		
Beyaz[c]	20 mcg ethinyl estradiol with 3 mg drospirenone for 24 days	Hormone-free tablets for 4 days[a]		
Monophasic 25 mcg Pills				
Generess Fe	25 mcg ethinyl estradiol and 0.8 mg norethindrone	Hormone-free tablets for 4 days[a]		
Monophasic 30 mcg Pills				
Cryselle Lo-Ovral Low-Ogestrel	30 mcg ethinyl estradiol with 0.3 mg norgestrel for 21 days	Hormone-free tablets for 7 days[a]		
Altavera Levlen Levora Nordette Portia	30 mcg ethinyl estradiol with 0.15 mg levonorgestrel for 21 days	Hormone-free tablets for 7 days[a]		
Introvale Jolessa Quasense Seasonale	30 mcg ethinyl estradiol with 0.15 mg levonorgestrel for 84 days	Hormone-free tablets for 7 days[a]		
Junel 1.5/30 Loestrin 1.5/30 Microgestin 1.5/30	30 mcg ethinyl estradiol with 1.5 mg norethindrone acetate for 21 days	Hormone-free tablets for 7 days[a]		

Junel 1.5/30 Fe Loestrin 1.5/30 FE Microgestin 1.5/30 Fe	30 mcg ethinyl estradiol with 1.5 mg norethindrone acetate for 21 days	Hormone-free tablets for 7 days.[a] Hormone-free tablets contain 75 mg ferrous fumarate.		
Apri Desogen Ortho-Cept Reclipsen	30 mcg ethinyl estradiol with 0.15 mg desogestrel for 21 days	Hormone-free tablets for 7 days[a]		
Ocella Syeda Yasmin	30 mcg ethinyl estradiol with 3 mg drospirenone for 21 days	Hormone-free tablets for 7 days[a]		
Safyral[c]	30 mcg ethinyl estradiol with 3 mg drospirenone for 21 days	Hormone-free tablets for 7 days[a]		
Monophasic 35 mcg Pills				
Necon 1/35 Norinyl 1+35 Nortrel 1/35 Ortho-Novum 1/35	35 mcg ethinyl estradiol with 1 mg norethindrone for 21 days	Hormone-free tablets for 7 days[a]		
Brevicon ModiCon Necon 0.5/35 Nortrel 0.5/35	35 mcg ethinyl estradiol with 0.5 mg norethindrone for 21 days	Hormone-free tablets for 7 days[a]		
Balziva	35 mcg ethinyl estradiol with 0.4 mg norethindrone for 21 days	Hormone-free tablets for 7 days[a]		
Femcon Fe Ovcon 35 Fe[d]	35 mcg ethinyl estradiol with 0.4 mg norethindrone for 21 days	Hormone-free tablets for 7 days.[a] Hormone-free tablets contain 75 mg ferrous fumarate.		
MonoNessa Ortho-Cyclen Previfem Sprintec	35 mcg ethinyl estradiol with 0.25 mg norgestimate for 21 days	Hormone-free tablets for 7 days[a]		
Kelnor 1/35 Zovia 1/35E	35 mcg ethinyl estradiol with 1 mg ethynodiol diacetate for 21 days	Hormone-free tablets for 7 days[a]		
Multiphasic Formulations				
Kariva Mircette	20 mcg ethinyl estradiol with 0.15 mg desogestrel for 21days	Hormone-free tablets for 2 days	10 mcg ethinyl estradiol for 5 days	
Camrese Seasonique	30 mcg ethinyl estradiol with 0.15 mg levonorgestrel for 84 days	10 mcg ethinyl estradiol for 7 days	None	
Camrese Lo Lo Seasonique	20 mcg ethinyl estradiol and 0.1 mg levonorgestrel for 84 days	10 mcg ethinyl estradiol for 7 days	None	
Quartette	20 mcg ethinyl estradiol with 0.15 mg levonorgestrel for 42 days	25 mcg ethinyl estradiol with 0.15 mg levonorgestrel for 21 days	30 mcg ethinyl estradiol with 0.15 mg levonorgestrel for 21 days	10 mcg ethinyl estradiol for 7 days
Estrostep-FE Tilia FE Tri-Legest Fe	20 mcg ethinyl estradiol with 1 mg norethindrone acetate for 5 days	30 mcg ethinyl estradiol with 1 mg norethindrone acetate for 7 days	35 mcg ethinyl estradiol with 1 mg norethindrone acetate for 9 days	Hormone-free tablet with 75 mg ferrous fumarate for 7 days
Ortho Tri-Cyclen Lo	25 mcg ethinyl estradiol with 0.18 mg norgestimate for 7 days	25 mcg ethinyl estradiol with 0.215 mg norgestimate for 7 days	25 mcg ethinyl estradiol with 0.25 mg norgestimate for 7 days	Hormone-free tablets for 7 days[a]
Cyclessa Velivet	25 mcg ethinyl estradiol with 0.1 mg desogestrel for 7 days	25 mcg ethinyl estradiol with 0.125 mg desogestrel for 7 days	25 mcg ethinyl estradiol with 0.150 mg desogestrel for 7 days	Hormone-free tablets for 7 days[a]

(*continues*)

Table 29-6 Oral Contraceptive Formulations Available in the United States, April 2014 (*continued*)

Product (Brand Name)	First Phase	Second Phase	Third Phase	Fourth Phase
Enpresse Tri-Levlen Trivora	30 mcg ethinyl estradiol with 0.05 mg levonorgestrel for 6 days	40 mcg ethinyl estradiol with 0.075 mg levonorgestrel for 5 days	20 mcg ethinyl estradiol with 0.125 mg levonorgestrel for 10 days	Hormone-free tablets for 7 days[a]
Ortho Tri-Cyclen Trinessa Tri-Previfem Tri-Sprintec	35 mcg ethinyl estradiol with 0.18 mg norgestimate for 7 days	35 mcg ethinyl estradiol with 0.215 mg norgestimate for 7 days	35 mcg ethinyl estradiol with 0.25 mg norgestimate for 7 days	Hormone-free tablets for 7 days[a]
Necon 7/7/7 Nortrel 7/7/7 Ortho-Novum 7/7/7	35 mcg ethinyl estradiol with 0.5 mg norethindrone for 7 days	035 mcg ethinyl estradiol with 0.75 mg norethindrone for 7 days	35 mcg ethinyl estradiol with 1 mg norethindrone days	Hormone-free tablets for 7 days[a]
Aranelle Leena Tri-Norinyl	35 mcg ethinyl estradiol with 0.5 mg norethindrone for 7 days	35 mcg ethinyl estradiol with 1 mg norethindrone for 7 days	35 mcg ethinyl estradiol with 0.5 mg norethindrone for 7 days	Hormone-free tablets for 7 days[a]
Necon 10/11-28	35 mcg ethinyl estradiol/0.5 mg norethindrone for 21days	35 mcg ethinyl estradiol/1 mg norethindrone for 11days	Hormone-free tablets for 7 days	
50 mcg Pills				
Necon 1/50 Norinyl 1+50	50 mcg mestranolb with 1 mg norethindrone	1 mg norethindrone		
Ogestrel	50 mcg ethinyl estradiol with 0.5 mg norgestrel	0.5 mg norgestrel		
Zovia 1/50	50 mcg ethinyl estradiol with 1 mg ethynodiol diacetate	1 mg ethynodiol diacetate		
Ovcon 50	50 mcg ethinyl estradiol with 1 mg norethindrone	1 mg norethindrone		
Other Formulations				
Natazia	3 mg estradiol valerate for 2 days	2 mg estradiol valerate with 2 mg dienogest for 5 days	2 mg estradiol valerate for 17 days with 3 mg dienogest for 17 days	1 mg estradiol valerate for 2 days followed by hormone-free tablet for 2 days

[a] Hormone-free interval may be a certain number of inert tablets or a pill-free interval. The woman can eliminate the hormone-free interval by starting a new pack right away.
[b] Mestranol must be converted to ethinyl estradiol in the body. Animal studies have suggested that mestranol is weaker, but this has not been confirmed in human studies.[58]
[c] 28 tablets contain 0.451 mg levomefolate calcium
[d] Also available as a chewable tablet.

to differences in side effects and preferences for certain progestins, although these differences cannot be predicted in advance.

Early formulations of the pill contained doses of estrogens that were 3-4 times higher and doses of progestins that were 10 times higher than in currently used formulations. High rates of undesirable side effects and cardiovascular complications led to attempts to drive the dosages lower. With today's low dosages, evidence suggests that suppression of ovarian activity is less complete than with higher-dose formulations, and it is likely that contemporary dosing cannot be lowered further without reducing contraceptive effectiveness.

Variations in formulations, such as the **phasic formulations** have been introduced in recent years, with the intention of minimizing the total hormonal load while maximizing ovarian suppression and lowering the incidence of common side effects. Monophasic formulations maintain the same dosage of ethinyl estradiol (10, 20, 30, or 35 mcg) and progestin for 21 days, followed by a 7-day hormone-free interval. Many brands provide inert or placebo pills that the woman takes during this interval, with some formulations adding iron to the pills taken during the traditional placebo week. Newer monophasic formulations tend to extend the time for which active pills are taken or shorten the hormone-free interval.

Multiphasic formulations have different formulations. Biphasic formulations provide two separate dosing levels of the ethinyl estradiol or the progestin component for 21 days, followed by a hormone-free interval. These regimens were developed to reduce the total steroid dose during the 21 days of active pills while maintaining adequate cycle control and reducing breakthrough bleeding. Biphasic formulations begin with a lower progestin dose for the first 1 to 10 days of the active pill cycle, followed by a higher progestin dose for the remainder of the 21 days. Triphasic formulations also modulate the hormone dosing over the 21-day interval by providing three different dosing levels. Some formulations change only the ethinyl estradiol dosing, some change just the progestin dosing, and some alter both the estrogen and progestin doses over the course of 21 days. Quadriphasic formulations have four different doses of the hormones over 28 days.

Studies have shown that with a 7-day hormone-free interval, FSH begins to increase on cycle days 3 to 4, permitting follicular growth. The reinitiation of pharmacologically active pills causes the follicles to degenerate.[61] When the hormone-free interval exceeds 7 days, the chance of follicle growth and possible breakthrough ovulation appear to be higher.

Some evidence indicates that continuous hormone use will more effectively prevent ovarian follicle development and ovulation.[61] Newer formulations are designed to shorten or eliminate the hormone-free interval with the aim of increasing suppression of ovarian activity. **Extended cycling** is a an approach in which a woman either takes a daily pill for 84 days before she has a pill-free interval, usually lasting 7 days, or uses pills continuously. To date, no large-scale studies have reported improvements in effectiveness based on these variations in pill-taking regimens. A systematic review found that effectiveness, safety profiles, and adherence were similar; menstrual symptoms were improved in the extended-cycle groups; and bleeding patterns were either similar or improved in the extended-cycle groups.[62] Although continuous regimens appear to be safe, longer-term data are needed to confirm this perception.[63]

Specially formulated products are not necessary to eliminate or shorten the hormone-free interval; rather, women can start a new package of pills immediately after finishing the active pills in one pack to achieve the same effect. The only disadvantage to this method is that over each 12-week period, instead of three packages of oral contraceptives, a woman will need to purchase four packages—an action that may cause problems with insurance reimbursement or budgetary constraints. Similarly, shortening the hormone-free interval to 2 to 4 days does not require dedicated products. A monthly bleeding episode is not physiologically necessary in women using hormonal contraception, and many women appreciate the convenience. Some others may prefer to experience monthly bleeding even when they understand that the bleeding associated with COCs is due to the artificial progesterone withdrawal and not a natural menstrual cycle.[64]

Most 21-day pills also are available in a 28-day pack, in which the last week of pills is inert or may contain iron. These noncontraceptive pills are used as reminders to facilitate adherence and avoid delays in restarting the agents, although they tend to cost more than the 21-day packs.

If a woman misses an active pill, she should take an active hormonal pill as soon as possible. Figure 29-2 shows the U.S. selected practice recommendation algorithm for missed COCs. Figure 29-3 describes the U.S. selected practice recommendation algorithm for management of nausea, vomiting, or diarrhea while taking oral contraceptive pills.

Box 29-4 provides a case study of a woman with some common side effects.

Transdermal Patch

Only one **transdermal contraceptive patch** product is available in the United States at the present time, although others are in development. The patch is marketed under the brand name Evra or Ortho Evra; a generic, Xulane, was introduced in 2014.

Transdermal delivery of contraceptive hormones avoids hepatic first-pass metabolism, allowing for lower total hormone doses to be used than are present in oral formulations. However, this route of administration does not bypass the liver entirely, and hepatic metabolism of the drug is not altered. Transdermal delivery also avoids gastrointestinal symptoms related to pill ingestion and provides a more steady-state release of hormones, thereby avoiding the typical peaks and troughs that occur with daily ingestion of a pill. Because the patch is changed just once weekly, there also is a decreased risk of being without contraceptive coverage such as occurs with a missed daily pill, although the risk does exist if the patch is not replaced as appropriate. Transdermal delivery does not counteract the estrogen-induced increase in sex hormone–binding globulin, which results in lower levels of free testosterone; thus, the patch would be expected to have similar beneficial effects on acne as oral contraceptives.

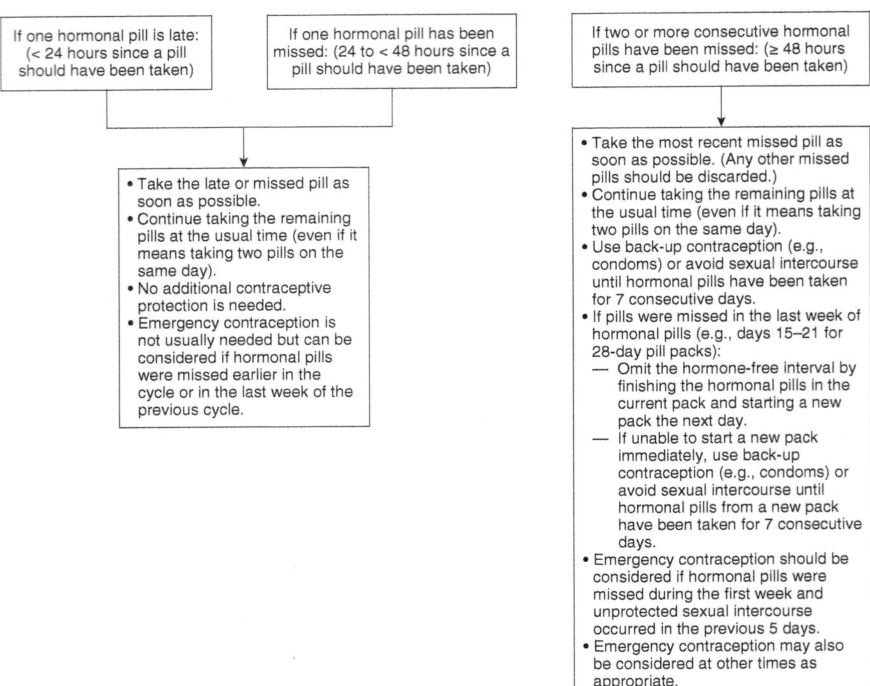

Figure 29-2 Selected practice recommendations for missed combined oral contraceptives.

Source: Reproduced from Division of Reproductive Health, Health Promotion, Centers for Disease Control and Prevention. U.S. selected practice recommendations for contraceptive use, 2013: adapted from the World Health Organization selected practice recommendations for contraceptive use. 2nd ed. *MMWR Recommend Rep.* 2013;62:1-60.[12]

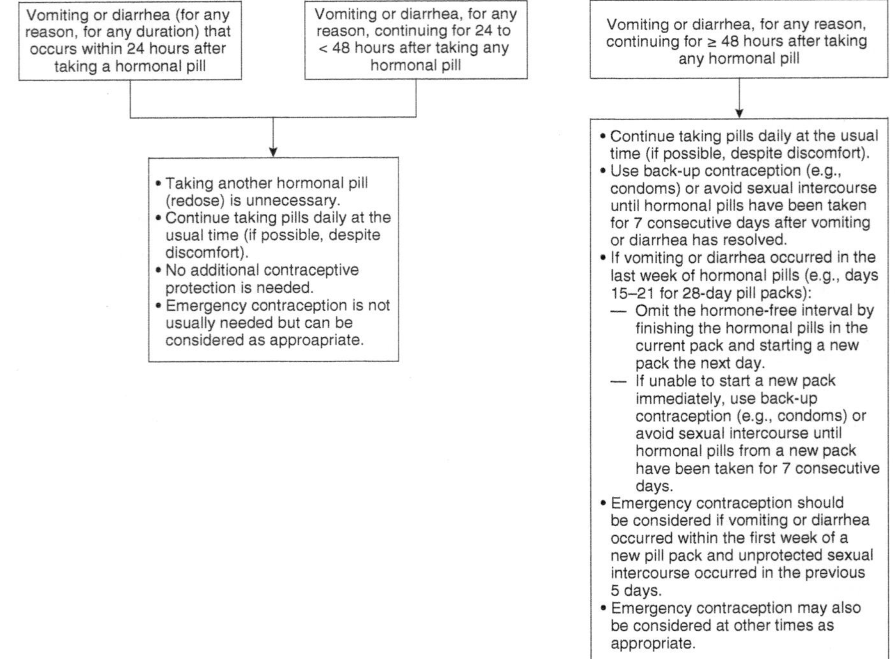

Figure 29-3 Recommendations after gastrointestinal conditions when using combined oral contraceptives.

Source: Reproduced from Division of Reproductive Health, Health Promotion, Centers for Disease Control and Prevention. U.S. selected practice recommendations for contraceptive use, 2013: adapted from the World Health Organization selected practice recommendations for contraceptive use. 2nd ed. *MMWR Recommend Rep.* 2013;62:1-60.[12]

Box 29-4 Troublesome Side Effects

JN is a 26-year-old woman who began taking combined oral contraceptive pills 2 months ago. She calls her provider to report that she is taking the pills correctly, but she is requesting to switch to another brand of pills because she has frequent nausea and is experiencing intermenstrual bleeding/spotting.

JN clearly is seeking relief from troublesome symptoms that she attributes to the oral contraceptives. Unless they are addressed, it is possible that JN may discontinue the method entirely, and even potentially risk pregnancy.

In the past, women often have been told that unpredictable bleeding may occur for up to 3 months after initiation. With the lower-dose agents commonly used today, irregular bleeding may sometimes occur for up to 6 months—information that JN needs to know. Empirically based advice, such as taking pills at bedtime to decrease nausea, has little evidence to support it, but such actions can be mentioned because they are relatively risk free. Also, there is no clinical evidence that another combined oral contraceptive brand will be a remedy for irregular bleeding and/or nausea. Although many brand names exist, only a few formulations are actually available.

Counseling JN about the normalcy of these early side effects may help her continue the method, especially since it is a highly effective one. However, after counseling, JN may consider another contraceptive method entirely.

The transdermal product is a thin, beige patch, approximately 4.5 cm square. It has an outer protective layer of polyester, and an adhesive layer that contains the medication (a protective liner is removed prior to application). This layer is placed on clean, dry skin of the buttock, abdomen, upper outer arm, or upper torso. The patch should not be placed over irritated or infected skin. While the patch has not been associated with increased risk of breast cancer, it should not be placed on the breasts to avoid potential or imagined increase in such risk. The user should be certain not to apply the patch over skin that is covered with lotion, cream, oil, reside from shampoo or conditioner, or other substances that could interfere with adherence.

Each patch is designed to adhere for 7 days; a month's supply contains 3 patches (21 days of hormone dosing). Each patch delivers 20 mcg of ethinyl estradiol and 150 mcg norelgestromin (the primary active metabolite of norgestimate) daily into the systemic circulation. After 3 weeks of use, or 3 patches, a 7-day hormone-free week is advised according to package labeling, although eliminating or shortening the hormone-free interval can be considered as off-label use of extended cycling. Pharmacokinetic parameters are similar at the various recommended placement sites, and serum levels remain stable under varied conditions of heat, humidity, and exercise.

Hormone levels for contraceptive efficacy are reached after 48 hours; forgetting to restart the patch after a hormone-free interval of several days raises the theoretical risk of unintended pregnancy.[65] Unprotected intercourse during this time requires emergency contraception. Once the patch has been restarted, clinical recommendations are to use a backup method for 7 days, although the exact length of time that this measure is necessary is not clear; backup protection is not needed if it is started within 5 days of the first day of the last menstrual period. During the second and third weeks of patch use, late placement of a new patch by 1 to 2 days does not substantially increase the risk of follicle activity, and serum levels of the contraceptive hormones remain within acceptable ranges.[12] This phenomenon is sometimes termed "patch forgiveness" (Figure 29-4). If a patch is partially or completed detached, adequate contraceptive hormone levels cannot be assured. If the patch adheres well after reapplication, it can be used; otherwise, it should be replaced (Figure 29-5). Use of a backup method or emergency contraception may be indicated if the period of detachment is unknown or exceeds 1 to 2 days.

Users of the transdermal patch may be more likely to experience breast tenderness than women using oral formulations.[66,67] However, in any case, this symptom tends to be time limited to the first few months of use of the method.

Because of the pharmacodynamics of transdermal delivery systems, 20 mcg of ethinyl estradiol in the patch cannot be compared to 20 mcg ethinyl estradiol in a pill. Pharmacokinetic studies have shown that the area under the curve and average concentration at steady state for ethinyl estradiol are approximately 60% higher in women using the patch than in women using an oral contraceptive containing 35 mcg ethinyl estradiol. Alternatively, this relationship may be stated as the peak concentration of ethinyl estradiol being approximately 25% lower in women using the patch.[68] Whether these pharmacokinetic differences affect the risk of serious adverse events is not known. Increased estrogen exposure may theoretically increase the risk of

Patch EE
Patch NGMN
Mean ethinyl estridiol concentration (pg/mL)
Mean norgestimate concentration (ng/mL)
1st patch applied
Day 8: 2nd patch applied
Day 15: Scheduled patch change day
2-day forgiveness
Time (days)

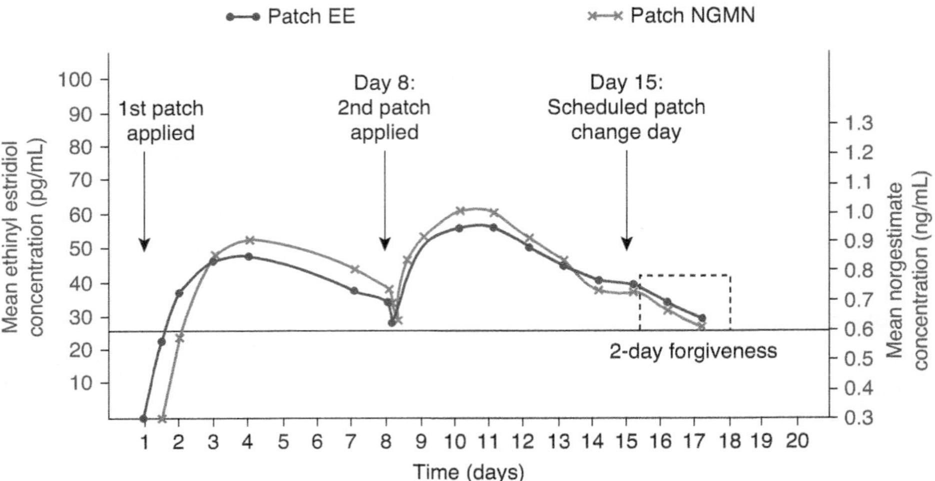

Figure 29-4 Transdermal contraceptive patch and dosing reserve.

Source: Data from Abrams LS, Skee D, Natarajan J, Wong F. An overview of the pharmokinetics of a contraceptive patch. *Int J Gynecol Obstet.* 2000;70(suppl 2):B78-B82.[65]

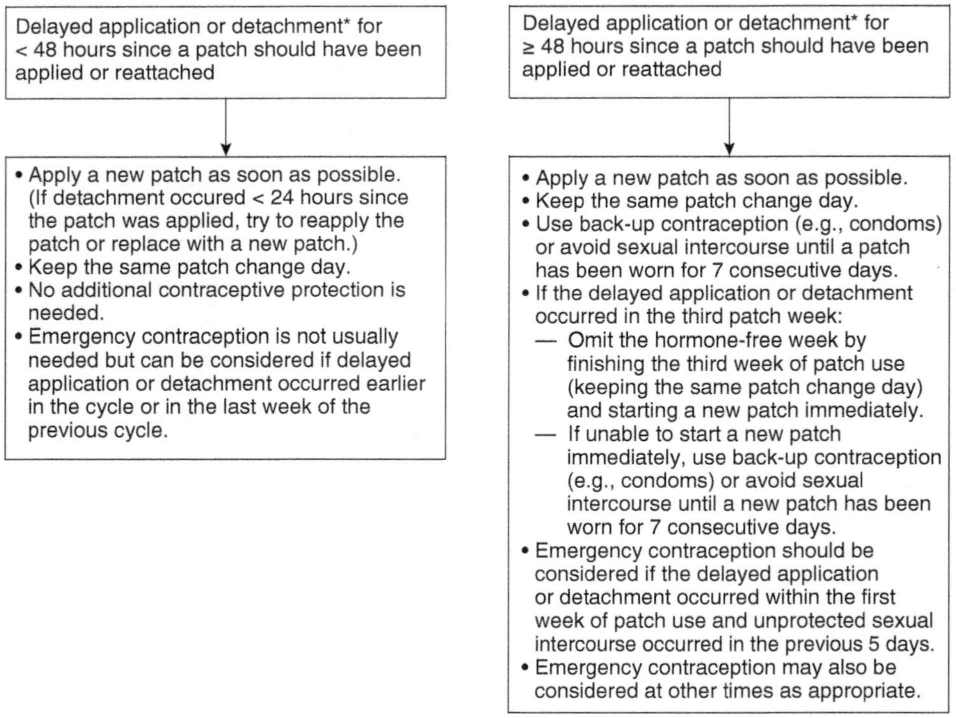

Delayed application or detachment* for < 48 hours since a patch should have been applied or reattached
• Apply a new patch as soon as possible. (If detachment occured < 24 hours since the patch was applied, try to reapply the patch or replace with a new patch.)
• Keep the same patch change day.
• No additional contraceptive protection is needed.
• Emergency contraception is not usually needed but can be considered if delayed application or detachment occurred earlier in the cycle or in the last week of the previous cycle.
Delayed application or detachment* for ≥ 48 hours since a patch should have been applied or reattached
• Apply a new patch as soon as possible.
• Keep the same patch change day.
• Use back-up contraception (e.g., condoms) or avoid sexual intercourse until a patch has been worn for 7 consecutive days.
• If the delayed application or detachment occurred in the third patch week:
— Omit the hormone-free week by finishing the third week of patch use (keeping the same patch change day) and starting a new patch immediately.
— If unable to start a new patch immediately, use back-up contraception (e.g., condoms) or avoid sexual intercourse until a new patch has been worn for 7 consecutive days.
• Emergency contraception should be considered if the delayed application or detachment occurred within the first week of patch use and unprotected sexual intercourse occurred in the previous 5 days.
• Emergency contraception may also be considered at other times as appropriate.

Figure 29-5 Recommendations to manage detachment or delayed application of combined hormonal patch.

Source: Reproduced from Division of Reproductive Health, Health Promotion, Centers for Disease Control and Prevention. U.S. selected practice recommendations for contraceptive use, 2013: adapted from the World Health Organization selected practice recommendations for contraceptive use. 2nd ed. *MMWR Recommend Rep.* 2013;62:1-60.[12]

adverse events, including venous thromboembolism, but existing studies have not found such an association.[69,70]

The FDA has required labeling for the transdermal contraceptive patch warning of a possible increase in the risk of blood clots when using this product. However, VTE is rare, and the increased risk, based on absolute risks, would be in the range of 5 to 10 additional cases per 10,000 women per year.[71] Other conditions that influence advisability of use of the patch can be found in the summary table at the end of this section concerning combined hormonal contraceptives (Table 29-7).

Intravaginal Ring

One vaginal contraceptive ring product (NuvaRing) is available in the United States, although others are in development. The flexible ring is made of ethylene vinyl acetate (a plastic used in many healthcare products); it has an outer diameter of 54 mm and is approximately 4 mm thick. The ring is inserted in the vagina by the woman and remains for 3 weeks. Maximum serum concentrations of hormones are reached approximately 1 week after insertion of the ring, and then concentrations decrease over time. After a 7-day hormone-free interval, or sooner if a shorter hormone-free interval is desired, a new ring is inserted.

Contraceptive hormones are embedded in the ring and deliver 15 mcg ethinyl estradiol and 120 mcg etonogestrel daily across the vaginal mucosa and into the systemic circulation. The ring releases the hormones in steady concentrations throughout the day. Contraceptive pills have occasionally been administered vaginally as well—for example, in women with significant nausea and vomiting; this approach offers similar effectiveness as taking the pill orally and is associated with a reduction in the incidence of side effects.[72]

Some women remove the ring during intercourse or for other reasons during the 21-day hormonal period. If it is removed for more than 3 hours, it should be replaced and backup contraception used for the next 7 days. Figure 29-6 describes the U.S. selected practice recommendation algorithm for management when a woman has delayed insertion of the contraceptive vaginal ring. Studies of ovarian

Table 29-7 U.S. Medical Eligibility Categories 3 and 4 for Combined Hormonal Contraceptives (Pill, Patch, and Ring)

Condition	Category	Comments
Anticonvulsant therapy, such as phenytoin (Dilantin), carbamazepine (Tegretol), barbiturates, lamotrigine (Lamictal), primidone (Mysoline), topiramate (Topamax), oxcarbazepine (Trileptal)	3	Anticonvulsants can decrease the effectiveness of combined hormonal contraception. Category 3 for lamotrigine applies only to when lamotrigine is used as monotherapy. When lamotrigine is combined with other anticonvulsants, the combination does not decrease effectiveness of combined hormonal contraception.
Bariatric surgery, history with malabsorptive procedures	3	Category 3 for combined oral contraceptives only. Condition exposes woman to increased risk as result of an unintended pregnancy.
Breast cancer, current	3,4	Category 3 if past and no evidence of current disease for 5 years; category 4 if current breast cancer. Note: Condition exposes woman to increased risk as result of an unintended pregnancy.
Breastfeeding for < 1 month postpartum	3	The evidence regarding the effect of combined hormonal contraceptives on breast milk production is conflicting. Nonetheless, the best evidence to date suggests any effect is greatest in the early postpartum period when milk flow is being established.
Cardiovascular disease, multiple risk factors such as smoking, diabetes, and hypertension	3,4	When multiple risk factors that singly increase the risk for cardiovascular disease are present, use of combined hormonal contraceptives may increase her risk to an unacceptable level. Note: Simply adding up 2 or 3 risk factors is not indicated. The presence of two risk factors that are a category 2 may not substantially increase the risk. Women with multiple cardiovascular risks should be evaluated by an expert prior to initiation of combined hormonal contraception.
Cirrhosis, severe (decompensated)	4	Condition exposes woman to increased risk as result of an unintended pregnancy.
DVT/PE history	3,4	Category associated with risk of recurrence. If low risk, category 3; if high risk, category 4.
DVT/PE, acute	4	
DVT risk after major surgery with prolonged immobilization	4	Category 2 if no prolonged immobilization.
Diabetes with nephropathy, retinopathy, neuropathy, other vascular disease or diabetes of > 20 years' duration	3,4	Category associated with severity of disease. Note: Condition exposes woman to increased risk as result of an unintended pregnancy.

(*continues*)

Table 29-7 U.S. Medical Eligibility Categories 3 and 4 for Combined Hormonal Contraceptives (Pill, Patch, and Ring) *(continued)*

Condition	Category	Comments
Gallbladder disease, symptomatic	2,3	Category 2 if treated by cholecystectomy; category 3 if treated medically or if current disease present.
Headaches, migraine	3,4	Category 3 for continuation if migraines without aura and woman < 35 years; category 3 for initiation and category 4 for continuation of method for women for women ≥ 35 years; category 4 for initiation or continuation for any women with migraines with aura.
Human immunodeficiency virus, ARV therapy with ritonavir-boosted protease inhibitors	3	ARV drugs can either decrease or increase the bioavailability of steroid hormones in hormonal contraception. Evidence suggests ritonavir-boosted protease inhibitors decrease effectiveness of hormonal contraception and decrease effectiveness of the ARV.
Hyperlipidemia	2,3	Category 2 or 3 based on severity.
Hypertension	3,4	Category 3 if adequately controlled, but additional guidance is available from the source; category 3 if BP is 140–159/90–99 mm Hg; category 4 if BP is 160/100 mm Hg or higher, or if vascular disease is present.
Inflammatory bowel disease	2,3	Category 2 or 3 based on severity.
Ischemic heart disease	4	
Liver tumors, hepatocellular adenoma or malignant tumor	4	
Peripartum cardiomyopathy	3,4	Category associated with severity and duration. Condition exposes woman to increased risk as result of an unintended pregnancy.
Postpartum < 21 days	3	Theoretic concern that there is an association between combined hormonal contraceptives and an increased risk for thrombosis in the first 3 weeks postpartum.
Rifampin (Rifadin) or rifabutin (Mycobutin) therapy	3	These antimicrobial drugs are likely to reduce the effectiveness of combined hormonal contraception.
Smoking at 35 years or older	3,4	Category 3 if ≤ 15 cigarettes smoked daily; category 4 if ≥ 15 cigarettes smoked daily.
Solid-organ transplantation, complicated	4	Note: Condition exposes woman to increased risk as result of an unintended pregnancy.
Stroke/history of cerebral accident	4	Note: Condition exposes woman to increased risk as result of an unintended pregnancy.
Systemic with erythematosus, positive or unknown antiphospholipid antibodies	4	Category 2 if lupus with thrombocytopenia immunosuppressive treatment or none of the above. Note: Condition exposes woman to increased risk as result of an unintended pregnancy.
Thrombogenic mutations	4	Note: Condition exposes woman to increased risk as result of an unintended pregnancy.
Valvular heart disease, complicated	4	Note: Condition exposes woman to increased risk as result of an unintended pregnancy.
Viral hepatitis, acute or flare	3,4	Category only for initiation of method based on severity of disease.

Abbreviations: ARV = antiretroviral; BP = blood pressure; DVT = deep vein thrombosis; PE = pulmonary embolism.
Source: Data from Centers for Disease Control and Prevention. U.S. medical eligibility criteria for contraceptive use, 2010. *MMWR Recommend Rep.* 2010;59:1-86.[11]

function during NuvaRing use indicate that it takes several days after removing the ring for a dominant follicle to develop[73]; thus, the longer the hormone-free interval, the higher the risk of ovulation.

The vaginal ring has been studied in the context of extended cycling or continuous use.[74] When it is used in extended cycles of 49 days, 91 days, or year-round patterns, many women will have an increase in unscheduled spotting days. However, the amount of bleeding is small and may be tolerable for women who wish to avoid menstrual periods. This usage pattern will require more rings annually and may introduce financial constraints.

Increased vaginal discharge experienced by some women who use the intravaginal ring is likely due to the estrogen component and is not associated with vaginal conditions or infections. Use of the contraceptive ring is not associated with cervical or cytological abnormalities or bacteriological changes in vaginal flora, even though women may report increased discharge.

Summary of MEC Categories 3 and 4 for Pills, Patches, and Rings

Combined hormonal contraceptives are a popular approach to contraception, and the majority of women can safely use these agents. However, some women, especially those with significant medical conditions, should be advised to avoid this form of contraception. Table 29-7 provides a summary of the MEC categories 3 and 4 for combined hormonal methods.

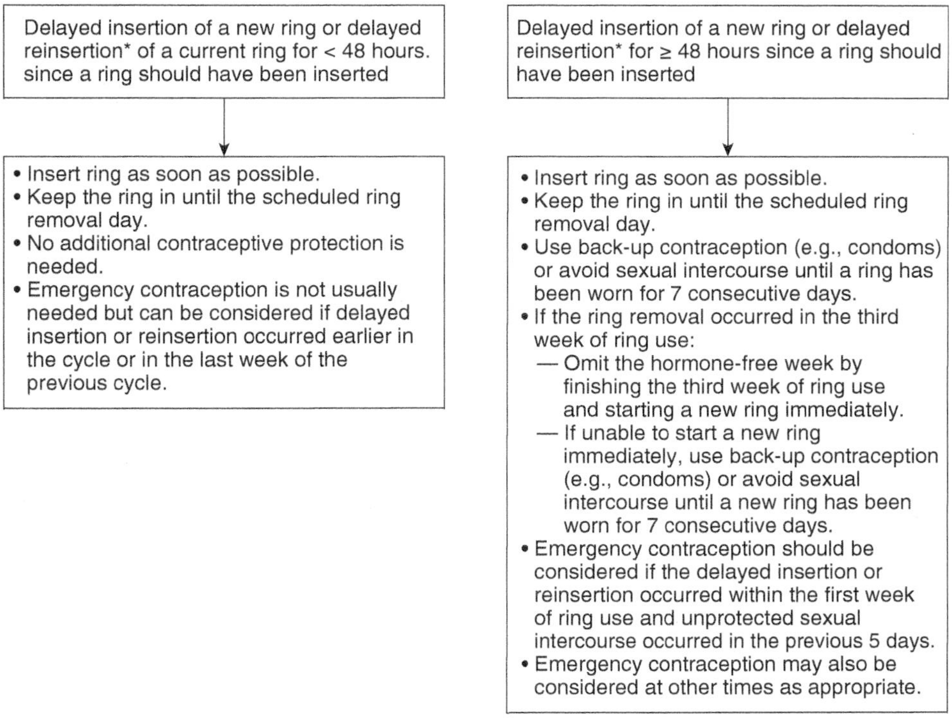

Delayed insertion of a new ring or delayed reinsertion* of a current ring for < 48 hours. since a ring should have been inserted	Delayed insertion of a new ring or delayed reinsertion* for ≥ 48 hours since a ring should have been inserted
• Insert ring as soon as possible. • Keep the ring in until the scheduled ring removal day. • No additional contraceptive protection is needed. • Emergency contraception is not usually needed but can be considered if delayed insertion or reinsertion occurred earlier in the cycle or in the last week of the previous cycle.	• Insert ring as soon as possible. • Keep the ring in until the scheduled ring removal day. • Use back-up contraception (e.g., condoms) or avoid sexual intercourse until a ring has been worn for 7 consecutive days. • If the ring removal occurred in the third week of ring use: — Omit the hormone-free week by finishing the third week of ring use and starting a new ring immediately. — If unable to start a new ring immediately, use back-up contraception (e.g., condoms) or avoid sexual intercourse until a new ring has been worn for 7 consecutive days. • Emergency contraception should be considered if the delayed insertion or reinsertion occurred within the first week of ring use and unprotected sexual intercourse occurred in the previous 5 days. • Emergency contraception may also be considered at other times as appropriate.

Figure 29-6 Recommendations to manage delayed insertion or reinsertion of combined hormonal ring.

Source: Reproduced from Division of Reproductive Health, Health Promotion, Centers for Disease Control and Prevention. U.S. selected practice recommendations for contraceptive use, 2013: adapted from the World Health Organization selected practice recommendations for contraceptive use. 2nd ed. *MMWR Recommend Rep.* 2013;62:1-60.[12]

Progestin-Only Contraceptives

Progestin-only methods include progestin-only pills, implants, intrauterine devices, and injectable methods.

Mechanism of Action

Progestins have a negative feedback effect on the hypothalamic–pituitary axis, thereby suppressing the LH surge and FSH peak necessary for ovulation.[58] However, ovulation is not consistently prevented in users of progestin-only contraceptives, and some women will ovulate and have regular cycles while using this method of birth control. Other effects associated with the method appear to provide additional contraceptive effectiveness, such as thickening of cervical mucus with subsequent inhibition of sperm migration secondary to progestins.[58] Progestins also produce a thinly developed endometrium, which may inhibit implantation—a physiological change that is also associated with irregular, unpredictable bleeding and amenorrhea. The progestin's effect on cervical mucus occurs within a few hours of administration and lasts approximately 20 hours after the last administration. Therefore, to maintain the overall mechanisms of action, it is important that the progestin-only pill be taken at the same time every day, as the cervical mucus effect wanes in approximately 24 hours.

Initiation

As with COCs, women may Quick Start progestin-only methods at any time as long as they are reasonably certain they are not pregnant. The woman should be assessed for the need for emergency contraception; if there are any doubts about a possible early pregnancy, a pregnancy test can be done 2 to 3 weeks after beginning the contraceptive. In the event that pregnancy is diagnosed, progestin-only oral contraceptives can be discontinued promptly; however, that is not true for injectables, and intrauterine contraceptives require removal by a healthcare professional.

Efficacy and Effectiveness

In the first year of use, the probability of pregnancy is estimated to be similar between users of progestin-only pills

(POPs) and users of COCs. Women who are fully breastfeeding enjoy the most effectiveness, nearly 100%, due to the hormonal effects of lactation, which also provide a degree of contraceptive benefit.

Eligibility

Serious adverse effects are unlikely in women who take progestin-only hormonal contraception, and those that occur are generally secondary to allergic reactions to progestins. However, progestin-only methods in general raise concerns about an increased likelihood of ectopic pregnancy should a contraceptive failure occur. The thickening of mucus and slowing of tubal motility associated with this method could theoretically contribute to a tubal pregnancy. Because the use of POPs is effective in preventing pregnancy, the *overall* rate of ectopic pregnancy in POP users is not increased above the expected rate of approximately 2%; if a woman taking POPs becomes pregnant, however, the likelihood that the pregnancy is ectopic is approximately 10%.[75]

Some older studies raised concerns that POP methods might increase the risk of development of diabetes in women who experienced gestational diabetes in pregnancy.[76] Evidence for this relationship to date is limited and inconsistent. Consequently, the CDC's MEC classify all progestin-only methods as category 1 for women with a history of gestational diabetes.[11]

Because the progestin-only methods lack the estrogen component of the contraceptive pill, ovarian follicular activity is not inhibited as well as ovulation is inhibited. In turn, benign follicular cysts of the ovary are more common with progestin-only methods (10–20%) but are usually asymptomatic and resolve spontaneously.[77]

Common Side Effects of Progestin-Only Contraceptives

Breast tenderness, headaches, changes in vaginal discharge, and other minor side effects may be experienced by a user of any type of hormonal contraceptive. A variety of treatments, such as dietary restrictions and botanical treatments, have been suggested to treat these side effects, but there is no evidence supporting the effectiveness of these interventions.

An effect of any progestin method is the production of a thinly developed endometrium, which is associated with irregular and unpredictable bleeding and amenorrhea. Approximately 40% of women taking progestin-only pills will have normal ovulatory cycles; most will have irregular periods of bleeding or spotting, or amenorrhea.[78]

Progestin-Only Oral Contraceptives

Progestin-only pills (POPs) are sometimes referred to as "mini-pills," but this term risks confusion with very-low-dose combination pills and should be avoided. POPs are highly effective, with only 9% of women experiencing unwanted pregnancies within the first year with typical use. Norethindrone is the progestin used in POPs available in the United States.

Forty-eight hours of POP use will produce contraceptive effects by thickening the cervical mucus.[12] No backup method is required if the method is started within the first 5 days since last menstrual period; otherwise, backup methods should be used for 2 days following initiation of the pills. Missing progestin-only pills is a prime reason for unintended pregnancy. Expert opinion is that missing a pill by 3 hours or more creates a risk of unintended pregnancy due to diminishing of the cervical mucus effect. A woman who misses a pill should take one pill as soon as possible, and then resume daily pill administration as before, even if that means taking two pills in one day. She should abstain from intercourse or use additional protection until resumption of pill routine has been completed for 2 consecutive days to reestablish the cervical mucus effect.[12]

Table 29-8 lists the health conditions identified by the MEC as either category 3 or 4 for POPs.

Progestin-Only Injectable

Two injectable contraceptives are available in the United States; both are progestin-only methods. Depot medroxyprogesterone acetate (DMPA) is marketed as the brand name Depo-Provera. It contains 150 mg DMPA and is given as a deep intramuscular injection every 12 (11–13) weeks. There is also a medroxyprogesterone acetate injectable suspension that is given as a subcutaneous injection; it is marketed as Depo-subQ Provera 104. Aside from the lower dosage, the subcutaneous delivery system allows for the potential for self-injection, rather than needing to visit a provider's office for injections. There is no evidence that the incidence of common side effects is less with this version, and the newer formulation may not be covered by all insurance plans.

DMPA is extremely effective: The probability of pregnancy is approximately 0.2% in perfect users and 6% in the more typical users. The product labeling recommends reinjection every 11 to 13 weeks. Some studies of the 150 mg intramuscular formulation have suggested that contraceptive efficacy is maintained longer; the CDC SPR states that a repeat DMPA injection can be given up to 2 weeks late which is 15 weeks from the last injection.[12]

Table 29-8 U.S. Medical Eligibility Categories 3 and 4 for Progestin-Only Pills

Condition	Category	Comments
Anticonvulsant therapy such as phenytoin (Dilantin), carbamazepine (Tegretol), barbiturates, primidone (Mysoline), topiramate (Topamax), oxcarbazepine (Trileptal)	3	Anticonvulsants can decrease the effectiveness of progestin-only pills.
Bariatric surgery, history with malabsorptive procedures	3	Note: Condition exposes woman to increased risk as result of an unintended pregnancy.
Breast cancer, current	3,4	Category 3 if past and no evidence of current disease for 5 years; category 4 if current. Note: Condition exposes woman to increased risk as result of an unintended pregnancy.
Cirrhosis, severe (decompensated)	3	Note: Condition exposes woman to increased risk as result of an unintended pregnancy.
Headaches, migraine with aura	3	Category 3 for continuation for any woman with migraines with aura.
Human immunodeficiency virus, ARV therapy, ritonavir-boosted protease inhibitors	3	ARV drugs can either decrease or increase the bioavailability of steroid hormones in hormonal contraception. Evidence suggests ritonavir-boosted protease inhibitors decrease effectiveness of hormonal contraception and decrease effectiveness of the ARV.
Ischemic heart disease	3	For continuation only.
Liver tumors, hepatocellular adenoma or malignant disease	3	Malignant disease exposes woman to increased risk as result of an unintended pregnancy.
Rifampin (Rifadin) or rifabutin (Mycobutin) therapy	3	These antimicrobial drugs are likely to reduce the effectiveness of progestin-only contraceptives.
Stroke/history of cerebral accident	3	For continuation only. Note: Condition exposes woman to increased risk as result of an unintended pregnancy.
Systemic lupus erythematosus, positive or unknown antiphospholipid antibodies	3	Category 2 if lupus with thrombocytopenia immunosuppressive treatment or none of the above. Note: Condition exposes woman to increased risk as result of an unintended pregnancy.

Abbreviations: ARV = antiretroviral.
Source: Data from Centers for Disease Control and Prevention. U.S. medical eligibility criteria for contraceptive use, 2010. *MMWR Recommend Rep.* 2010;59:1-86.[11]

In fact, some women will not resume ovulation for several months after discontinuing injectable contraceptives. This outcome cannot be predicted, however, and standard clinical recommendations state that effectiveness wanes if reinjection is delayed. Anecdotally, some women report self-administration of DMPA or administration by a worker in the community. This off-label use is intended to facilitate injections by removing the necessary office visit, but there are no data regarding its effectiveness.

Unscheduled bleeding is common in the first few cycles of use of progestin-only injectables; initially heavy or prolonged bleeding is reported by many women. Heavy bleeding can be treated with oral estrogens or combined oral contraceptives for 10 to 20 days or a nonsteroidal anti-inflammatory drug daily for 5 to 7 days.[12]

Some women note marked weight gain when using DMPA. Progestins may contribute to decreased peristalsis, constipation, or bloating. Women using DMPA appear to gain more weight than users of progestin implants or COCs.[79,80] This weight increase in users of DMPA occurs principally as the result of an increase in fat and may be related to the medication's effect in increasing appetite rather than fluid retention. The weight gain seems to be more common among overweight adolescents and certain ethnic groups. However, there is no evidence that obesity alters the efficacy of DMPA.[81]

In 2004, the FDA announced the addition of a black box warning, highlighting the possibility that prolonged use of injectables might result in the loss of bone density.[82] The warning also states that women who are able to use alternative forms of birth control should switch methods after 2 years of DMPA. Recent reevaluations of data about bone density suggest that the black box warning may be too strict or at least over-interpreted. Bone loss does not appear to be permanent, and several studies suggest similar bone mass density (BMD) in DMPA users as in nonusers. Many experts state bone density should not prevent practitioners from prescribing DMPA or continuing its use beyond 2 years; such theoretical concerns should be balanced against the real risks of unintended pregnancy.[83] Table 29-9 lists the health conditions identified by the MEC as either category 3 or 4 in relation to injectable progestin contraceptives.

Progestin-Only Implants

Implantable contraceptives are small rods or capsules containing a progestin that are inserted under the skin of the upper arm where they continuously release the progestins into the circulation. This method has the advantage of

Table 29-9 U.S. Medical Eligibility Categories 3 and 4 for Injectable Progestin Contraceptives (*continued*)

Condition	Category	Comments
Breast cancer, current or past and no evidence of disease for 5 years	3,4	Category 3 if past and no evidence of current disease for 5 years; category 4 if current. Note: Condition exposes woman to increased risk as result of an unintended pregnancy.
Cardiovascular disease, multiple risk factors such as smoking, diabetes, and hypertension	3,4	When multiple risk factors that singly increase the risk for cardiovascular disease are present, use of combined hormonal contraceptives may increase her risk to an unacceptable level. Note: simply adding up 2 or 3 risk factors is not indicated. The presence of two risk factors that are a category 2 may not substantially increase the risk. Women with multiple cardiovascular risks should be evaluated by an expert prior to initiation of combined hormonal contraception.
Cirrhosis, severe (decompensated)	3	Note: Condition exposes woman to increased risk as result of an unintended pregnancy
Diabetes with nephropathy, retinopathy, neuropathy, vascular disease, or duration of disease > 20 years	3	Note: Condition exposes woman to increased risk as result of an unintended pregnancy
Headaches, migraine with aura	3	Category 3 for continuation for any women with migraines with aura.
Hypertension, BP 160/100 mm Hg or higher; or vascular disease	3	Use of injectable contraceptives is associated with a small increased risk for cardiovascular events.
Ischemic heart disease	3	
Liver tumors, hepatocellular adenoma or malignant disease	3	Malignant disease exposes woman to increased risk as result of an unintended pregnancy.
Rheumatoid arthritis	2,3	Category 2 or 3 based on severity of disease.
Stroke/history of cerebral accident	3	Note: Condition exposes woman to increased risk as result of an unintended pregnancy.
Systemic lupus erythematosus, positive or unknown antiphospholipid antibodies	3	Note: Condition exposes woman to increased risk as result of an unintended pregnancy.
Systemic lupus erythematosus, severe thrombocytopenia	3	Initiation only. Note: Condition exposes woman to increased risk as result of an unintended pregnancy.
Unexplained vaginal bleeding	3	In the presence of bleeding, suspicious for serious condition before evaluation.

Abbreviations: BP = blood pressure.
Source: Data from Centers for Disease Control and Prevention. U.S. medical eligibility criteria for contraceptive use, 2010. *MMWR Recommend Rep.* 2010;59:1-86.[11]

not being coitus dependent, not requiring daily or periodic action on the part of the user, and being highly effective.

The first implantable contraceptive that was developed was Norplant, which contained six small flexible capsules, each of which had 36 mg levonorgestrel, and was approved for 5 years of continuous use. Jadelle, or Norplant II, has two capsules, each containing 150 mg of levonorgestrel. Neither of these products is currently marketed in the United States. Implanon was the next to be developed, and has recently been replaced by the radio-opaque version containing etonogestrel, which is Nexplanon. While many providers still have Implanon in stock, it is being phased out and replaced with Nexplanon in the United States. Nexplanon consists of one capsule containing 68 mg etonogestrel and has been approved for contraceptive protection for 3 years.

The etonogestrel implant effectively inhibits ovulation. In clinical trials, the earliest evidence of ovulation after appropriate insertion of the implant occurred in the third year of use. Etonogestrel levels in the serum reach a level compatible with ovulation inhibition within 8 hours after insertion.[84] Increased viscosity of cervical mucus likely is the reason that even with evidence of returned ovulation, pregnancy is still unlikely. As is true of all progestin-only contraceptives, the endometrial effect is associated with irregular bleeding or amenorrhea. Once the implant is removed, serum levels of etonogestrel fall rapidly and are undetectable within a week.[84]

Clinical trials that preceded FDA approval reported no pregnancies in women who used the etonogestrel implant. Since its approval and more widespread use, however, unintended pregnancies have been reported. Some are likely method failures, including those related to interactions with other medications, and some are related to failure to properly insert the device according to recommendations. The estimated method failure rate is approximately 1 per 1000 insertions. Studies show that obese women have lower plasma levels of etonogestrel than normal-weight women in the first months of use, but more data are needed to determine if this finding equates to decreased contraceptive effectiveness.

The etonogestrel implant is a progestin contraceptive method and therefore ovulation may occur. However the etonogestrel implant has very high contraceptive effectiveness, which makes the likelihood of ectopic pregnancy very low overall.[85]

Hormonal side effects such as breast pain, headaches, dizziness, acne, and mood swings have been reported by less than 12% of users in clinical trials. Acne improved in 61% of users in one study,[60] and dysmenorrhea improved in 91% of users.

With the absence of ovulation, irregular bleeding activity is common. Amenorrhea is the most common pattern, but any pattern of frequent, irregular, prolonged bleeding, or spotting is possible, and the patterns are unpredictable over time. Nonsteroidal anti-inflammatory drugs or oral estrogen has been recommended to treat women with heavy bleeding, but there are limited data as to the effectiveness of such measures.[86] Table 29-10 lists the health conditions identified by the MEC as either category 3 or 4 for progestin-only implants.

Table 29-10 U.S. Medical Eligibility Categories 3 and 4 for Implanted Progestin Contraceptives

Condition	Category	Comments
Breast cancer, current or past and no evidence of disease for 5 years	3,4	Category 3 if past and no evidence of current disease for 5 years; category 4 if current. Note: Condition exposes woman to increased risk as result of an unintended pregnancy.
Cirrhosis, severe (decompensated)	3	Note: Condition exposes woman to increased risk as result of an unintended pregnancy.
Headaches, migraine with aura	3	Category 3 for continuation for any women with migraines with aura.
Ischemic heart disease	3	Category 3 for continuation only.
Liver tumors, hepatocellular adenoma or malignant disease	3	Malignant disease exposes woman to increased risk as result of an unintended pregnancy.
Stroke/history of cerebral accident	3	Category 3 for continuation. Note: Condition exposes woman to increased risk as result of an unintended pregnancy.
Systemic lupus erythematosus, positive or unknown antiphospholipid antibodies	3	Note: Condition exposes woman to increased risk as result of an unintended pregnancy.
Unexplained vaginal bleeding	3	In the presence of bleeding, suspicious for serious condition before evaluation.

Source: Data from Centers for Disease Control and Prevention. U.S. medical eligibility criteria for contraceptive use, 2010. *MMWR Recommend Rep.* 2010;59:1-86.[11]

Intrauterine Progestin-Only Contraception

Intrauterine contraceptives are among the most effective contraceptive methods in use today and serve as a prototype of a long-acting reversible contraceptive, although they preceded use of that term. These small devices are inserted into the uterus by a trained clinician. Once inserted, the devices are not coitus dependent, nor do they require daily action on the part of the user for contraceptive effect. They provide from 5 to 10 years of effective contraception, depending on the device.

Recent years have seen renewed interest in intrauterine contraception. Whereas early IUDs were made primarily of inert materials, contemporary intrauterine contraceptives include additional active materials that are intended to improve their effectiveness. The primary mechanism of action for IUDs is to prevent contraception through inhibition of sperm, changes in tubal transport, or destruction of the ovum. Essentially, IUDs work primarily to prevent sperm and ovum from meeting. There may be some effects of copper ions on endometrial receptivity, although the primary contraceptive action occurs before implantation.[87,88]

Three brand named intrauterine devices that use hormones for contraception are currently available in the United States: the Mirena IUD, the Liletta IUD, and the Skyla IUD. These devices have a T-shaped polyethylene frame and a reservoir around the stem that contains 52 mg (Mirena and Liletta) or 13.5 mg (Skyla) of the progestin levonorgestrel. Devices with other hormonal doses are in development. The reservoir is covered by a silicone membrane, and levonorgestrel is released into the uterine cavity at a rate of 18.5 to 20 mcg per day (Mirena and Liletta) or 14 mcg per day (Skyla). Mirena is effective for 5 years, and Skyla and Liletta currently are approved as effective for 3 years.

The levonorgestrel-releasing IUDs result in atrophy of the endometrial glands, which in turn may inhibit sperm survival. The progestin effect decreases endometrial thickness and secretions, while thickening cervical mucus and possibly altering sperm penetration.[87] Studies have suggested that IUDs may lower the risk of endometrial cancer most likely due to endometrial changes[89] and possibly cervical cancer,[90] but definitive studies documenting this relationship are lacking. The progestin-releasing system also has several noncontraceptive uses—for example, treating heavy uterine bleeding from fibroids or heavy menses, as well as protecting the endometrium as part of hormone therapy in menopause.

Intrauterine contraception is an option for most reproductive-aged women. Women with an allergy to any of the constituents of the device (copper, progestin)

should not use it, nor should women who have a rare genetic disease that is associated with increased deposits of copper in the body (Wilson's disease). Intrauterine contraception is not contraindicated in women who have a history of sexually transmitted infection (STI), but women at continued high risk for acquiring STIs may not be the best candidates for this method.[11] Devices may be inserted up to day 7 of the menstrual cycle, due to an acceptably low risk of ovulation. Prophylactic antibiotics are not needed for insertion of intrauterine contraceptive devices in healthy women.[12]

Typical-use pregnancy rates in the first year are less than 1%. These rates rival those associated with tubal sterilization. Should a woman become pregnant when using an intrauterine contraceptive device, the risks of miscarriage, preterm birth, and infection are substantial and if the device should be removed as soon as possible.[12]

Concerns that IUD use could lead to tubal infertility have been evaluated, in a study that demonstrated tubal infertility is strongly associated with previous chlamydia infection; IUDs in isolation are not associated with infertility.[91] Whether the IUD string can contribute to ascending pelvic infection in women who acquire an STI is unknown, but current CDC guidelines do not mandate IUD removal in women diagnosed with an STI.[11,12]

The progestin-releasing IUDs are associated with frequent spotting for the first several months of use, followed by very light menses or amenorrhea. There are no data on effective treatment options for this side effect; notably, the administration of estrogen to alleviate such effects may interfere with the desired atrophic effect on the endometrium. Benign follicular cysts of the ovary can occur with any progestin-only method and have been observed among users of Mirena. Hormonal side effects such as breast pain, headaches, dizziness, acne, and mood swings also have been reported. Table 29-11 lists the health conditions identified by the MEC as either category 3 or 4 for progestin-only intrauterine contraception.

Table 29-11 U.S. Medical Eligibility Categories 3 and 4 for Levonorgestrel (Hormonal) Intrauterine Contraceptives

Condition	Category	Comments
Anatomic abnormalities, distorted uterine cavity	4	Any congenital or acquired uterine abnormality that distorts the uterine cavity in a manner that is incompatible with IUD insertion and retention.
Breast cancer, current	3,4	Category 3 if past and no evidence of current disease for 5 years; category 4 if current. Note: Condition exposes woman to increased risk as result of an unintended pregnancy.
Cervical cancer, awaiting treatment	4	Category 4 for initiation only. Concern is for the increased risk of infection and bleeding at insertion.
Cirrhosis, severe (decompensated)	3	Note: Condition exposes woman to increased risk as result of an unintended pregnancy.
Endometrial cancer	4	Category 4 for initiation only. Note: Condition exposes woman to increased risk as result of an unintended pregnancy.
Gestational trophoblastic disease	3,4	Category 3 if decreasing or undetectable β-hCG laboratory findings; category 4 if persistent levels or malignant disease.
Headaches with aura, any age	3	Category 3 for continuation only.
Hepatocellular adenoma	3	No evidence is available about contraception use in women with hepatocellular adenoma, but combined oral contraceptive use is associated with development and growth of this tumor.
History of cholestasis	3	Only if related in past to use of combined oral contraceptives.
Human immunodeficiency virus, AIDS	2,3	Category 3 for initiation in a woman who has AIDs; category 2 if well on ARV therapy.
Human immunodeficiency virus, ARV therapy	2,3	Category 3 for initiation only if woman is not well on ARV therapy; category 2 if well on ARV therapy.
Ischemic heart disease, current	3	Category 3 for initiation only. Note: Condition exposes woman to increased risk as result of an unintended pregnancy.
PID, current	4	Category 4 for initiation. Treat PID with appropriate antibiotics. The IUD does not usually need to be removed if the woman wishes to continue using it.
Post abortion, immediate septic	4	IUD insertion might worsen the condition.
Pregnancy	4	IUD is not indicated for any woman during pregnancy secondary to the risk for spontaneous abortion and/or serious pelvic infection.
Puerperal sepsis	4	IUD insertion might worsen the condition.
STIs, current purulent cervicitis, chlamydial infection, or gonorrhea	4	Category 4 for initiation only. Treat STI with appropriate antibiotics. The IUD does not usually need to be removed if the woman wishes to continue using it.
STIs, increased risk	2,3	If the woman has a very high risk for exposure to gonorrhea or chlamydia, the category is 3.
Solid-organ transplantation, complicated	3	Category 3 for initiation only. Note: Condition exposes woman to increased risk as result of an unintended pregnancy.

Condition	Category	Comments
Systemic lupus erythematosus, positive or unknown antiphospholipid antibodies	3	Category 2 if lupus with severe thrombocytopenia, immunosuppressive treatment, or none of the above. Note: Condition exposes woman to increased risk as result of an unintended pregnancy.
Tuberculosis, pelvic	3,4	Category 4 for initiation; category 3 for continuation
Unexplained vaginal bleeding	4	If pregnancy or an underlying pathologic condition such as pelvic malignancy is suspected, it must be evaluated and the MEC category adjusted after evaluation. The IUD does not need to be removed before evaluation.

Abbreviations: ARV = antiretroviral; IUD = intrauterine device; MEC = medical eligibility criteria; PID = pelvic inflammatory disease; STI = sexually transmitted infection.
Source: Data from Centers for Disease Control and Prevention. U.S. medical eligibility criteria for contraceptive use, 2010. *MMWR Recommend Rep.* 2010;59:1-86.[11]

Copper Intrauterine Device

Another medicated IUD does not use hormones, but instead uses a mineral—namely, copper. The copper IUD (ParaGard T380A or Cu IUCD) is a T-shaped polyethylene device. The body is wound with 176 mg of copper wire, and each of the arms has a copper "collar" containing approximately 68 mg of copper. The copper-containing IUDs inhibit sperm function via the release of copper ions into the uterine and tubal fluids and also alter the cervical mucus.[58] Changes in the endometrium may also inhibit

Table 29-12 U.S. Medical Eligibility Categories 3 and 4 for Copper Intrauterine Contraceptives

Condition	Category	Comments
Anatomic abnormalities, distorted uterine cavity	4	Any congenital or acquired uterine abnormality that distorts the uterine cavity in a manner that is incompatible with IUD insertion.
Cervical cancer, awaiting treatment	4	Category 4 for initiation only.
DVT/PE, acute	3	
Endometrial cancer	4	Category 4 for initiation only. Note: Condition exposes woman to increased risk as result of an unintended pregnancy.
Gestational trophoblastic disease	3,4	Category 3 if decreasing or undetectable β-hCG laboratory findings; category 4 if persistent levels or malignant disease.
History of cholestasis	3	Only if related in past to use of combined oral contraceptives.
Human immunodeficiency virus, AIDS	3	Category 3 for initiation only. Note: Condition exposes woman to increased risk as result of an unintended pregnancy.
Human immunodeficiency virus, ARV therapy	2,3	Category 3 for initiation only if woman is not well on ARV therapy; category 2 if well on ARV therapy.
Ischemic heart disease, current	3	Category 3 for continuation only.
Pelvic inflammatory disease, current	4	Category 4 for initiation only.
Post abortion, immediate septic	4	IUD insertion might worsen the condition.
Pregnancy	4	IUD is not indicated for any woman during pregnancy secondary to the risk for spontaneous abortion and/or serious pelvic infection.
Puerperal sepsis	4	Insertion of IUD might worsen this condition.
STIs, current purulent cervicitis, chlamydial infection, or gonorrhea	4	Category 4 for initiation only. Treat STI with appropriate antibiotics. The IUD does not usually need to be removed if the woman wishes to continue using it.
STIs, increased risk	2,3	If the woman has a very high risk for exposure to gonorrhea or chlamydia, the category is 3.
Solid-organ transplantation, complicated	3	Category 3 for initiation only. Note: Condition exposes woman to increased risk as result of an unintended pregnancy.
Systemic lupus erythematosus, severe thrombocytopenia	3	Category 3 for initiation only. Note: Condition exposes woman to increased risk as result of an unintended pregnancy.
Tuberculosis, pelvic	3,4	Category 4 for initiation; category 3 for continuation. Note: Condition exposes woman to increased risk as result of an unintended pregnancy.
Unexplained vaginal bleeding	4	Category 4 for initiation only in the presence of bleeding suspicious for serious condition before evaluation.

Abbreviations: ARV = antiretroviral; DVT = deep vein thrombosis; IUD = intrauterine device; PE = pulmonary embolism; STI = sexually transmitted infection.
Source: Data from Centers for Disease Control and Prevention. U.S. medical eligibility criteria for contraceptive use, 2010. *MMWR Recommend Rep.* 2010;59:1-86.[11]

Box 29-5 A Case of the Missing Strings

MB is a 38-year-old G3 P2103 who comes into your office reporting she is unable to find the strings of her ParaGard since just before her last menses. That menses, which was normal in character and amount, began 5 days ago. MB's history reveals that she has hypertension treated with medications. She expelled a previous intrauterine contraceptive device several years ago and then used combined oral contraceptives (COCs) until she became hypertensive. Two months ago she had a ParaGard inserted. Her physical examination is normal except for a body mass index (BMI) of 36 and a blood pressure of 138/80 mm Hg. Upon pelvic examination, the IUD strings are not visible, nor is the device felt during the bimanual examination.

Although pregnancy is unlikely, most clinicians would perform a point-of-care pregnancy test to provide reassurance to the clinician and the woman alike. Regarding possible expulsion, the provider should not attempt to blindly explore the uterine cavity in a quest to find the intrauterine device. However, gentle rotation of a cotton-tipped applicator in the cervical os may locate the strings if they have simply curled within the cervical os. If the strings cannot be located, a sonogram should be obtained. If the ParaGard is visualized in situ on sonogram with a fundal position, there should be a discussion with MB about her desires. Fundal placement provides contraceptive protection, but she will be unable to verify appropriate placement; that condition may be concerning, especially since she has already expelled one IUD. If she chooses to have the IUD removed, the procedure should be done under ultrasound visualization.

Alternative contraceptive options for MB are limited if she does not want to choose condoms or one of the barrier methods. Hypertension and obesity are associated with an increased risk for cardiovascular disease, yet those conditions also can negatively influence a pregnancy, which is a possible consequence of using some of the less effective methods. MB might consider a progestin-only method such as a POP or implant. Depot medroxyprogesterone acetate (DMPA) may be available or might be avoided because of the potential side effect of weight gain. MB might also opt for permanent sterilization for herself or her partner.

sperm migration; copper IUDs increase the number of leukocytes in the endometrium, producing a chronic inflammatory response in the endometrium.

Like levonorgestrel IUDs, copper IUDs may be inserted up to day 7 of the cycle. However, the risk of an existing pregnancy remains low until approximately day 12 of the cycle for the copper IUD, and it has an additional indication for use as emergency contraception.[12] The ParaGard device is FDA approved for 10 years of continuous use. In the first year of use, the pregnancy rate is less than 1% (0.7 per 100 women), and it falls even lower in years 2 through 10.

Copper-containing IUDs are associated with increased cramping and menstrual flow. Blood loss increases by approximately 55% in copper IUD users.[92] Over several years of use, serum ferritin levels may drop; however, decreases in hemoglobin values in copper IUD users were not sufficient in studies to induce anemia in previously non-anemic women.[12,93] Among women at high risk of iron-deficiency anemia, assessment may be warranted. Use of nonsteroidal anti-inflammatory drugs or prostaglandin synthesis inhibitors effectively treats women with both cramping and heavy menses.[12] Treatment should begin at the onset of menses and continue for 3 days.

Table 29-12 lists the health conditions identified by the MEC as either category 3 or 4 for copper IUDs. Box 29-5 describes a woman who is having a problem with her IUD.

Physical Barrier Contraceptive Methods

Barrier methods of contraception include male and female condoms, diaphragms, sponges, and cervical caps. By themselves, they are not strictly seen as pharmacologic agents. However, most barriers, such as the vaginal sponge, use both physical and chemical barriers, as they are used in conjunction with a spermicide (usually nonoxynol-9). Given the focus of this text on pharmacologic contraception, only a brief overview of barrier methods is provided here; more information on spermicides follows.

Many condoms and other barriers are made of latex, an agent manufactured from a milky fluid obtained from the rubber tree (*Hevea brasiliensis*). The natural rubber proteins may induce latex allergy, so alternative latex-free condoms are available, including natural skin condoms made from lamb intestines and synthetics such as polyurethane. Some vaginal and cervical barrier devices (e.g., Lea's shield and FemCap) are latex free and composed of medical-grade silicone. The sponge that is available in the United States is made of polyurethane foam; it also functions as a reservoir for 1000 mg of nonoxynol-9, which is gradually released over 24 hours. Effective use assumes that the individual has both the knowledge and the dexterity required to properly use, insert, and remove the device. The CDC's MEC classify barrier methods as category 1 or 2, except for those that are used in conjunction with spermicides; in these cases, the methods are classified as category 3 or 4 only for women at high risk for HIV/AIDS.[11]

Common Side Effects and Adverse Effects

Symptoms of latex allergy include irritant contact dermatitis, allergic dermatitis, and generalized hypersensitivity including anaphylaxis. Diaphragms have been associated with an increased risk of urinary tract infection.[11]

Availability

Male and female condoms can be purchased over the counter. Male latex condoms are less expensive than synthetics and natural skin male condoms. Female condoms are generally made of synthetic material, although a natural latex version is now available. Diaphragms must be fit by a clinician, so their costs include the fitting visit as well as the device. Lea's shield and FemCap are available through Planned Parenthood clinics and certain providers.

Spermicides

Spermicides are chemical substances used as contraceptives: They are intended to inactivate or kill sperm in the woman's reproductive tract, thereby preventing fertilization. They are generally used in conjunction with physical barriers intended to prevent sperm from entering the upper reproductive tract, where fertilization occurs, but they can be used in a film or cream separately. Use of spermicide as a sole contraceptive method has declined dramatically over years and is currently at a low level of use.[41]

All spermicides currently marketed in the United States contain nonoxynol-9 (N-9), although other products and spermicides such as menfegol, benzalkonium chloride, octoxynol are available in various countries and some can be obtained via the Internet. Spermicides share a number of characteristics with vaginal microbicides. These agents include surfactants such as nonoxynol-9, octoxynol-9, menfegol, and benzalkonium chloride, that disrupt the cell membranes of sperm and some pathogens, and an antimicrobial compound known as C31G which is an equimolar mixture of alkyl dimethyl glycine and alkyl dimethyl amine oxide. Buffering agents maintain acidity in the vagina in the presence of alkaline seminal fluid. Several randomized controlled trials have evaluated the use of topical microbicides for reducing the risk of HIV or STI acquisition,[94] and to date, there is not sufficient evidence to support this use.

Mechanism of Action

Nonoxynol-9 and similar spermicides are surfactants, which are designed to dissolve lipids in the sperm cell membrane, thereby inactivating or killing the sperm. Because they are toxic to cell membranes, they also have the potential to disrupt cervical and vaginal epithelium. These agents may alter vaginal flora as well, predisposing users to urinary tract infections.[95]

Various formulations may be used to deliver the spermicide: jellies, foams, creams, or soluble films. Suppositories and tablets that are designed to melt or foam after insertion in the vagina are also available; these products contain carbon dioxide, which forms bubbles to help disperse the product. Spermicides can be used alone or with other barrier devices such as condoms, diaphragms, and cervical caps. Various formulations may need different amount s of time for dispersion of the N-9 product. For example, film or suppositories need approximately 10 to 15 minutes to melt. Duration of activity once inserted in the vagina is also unclear. Some product instructions state that protection will last for 6 to 8 hours, although some experts have expressed concern about the accuracy of that statement and suggested that tablets and suppositories may have only 1 hour of effectiveness after insertion.[96]

N-9 is generally formulated as 50 to 150 mg per unit dose. The contraceptive sponge contains approximately 1000 mg of N-9, but after being moistened it gradually releases 125 to 150 mg of spermicide over 24 hours of use. General instructions on use are the same for all N-9 products, although all of the products were on the market before FDA oversight and the instructions are not evidence based.

A spermicide, BufferGel, that acts as a buffering agent has recently been studied in clinical trials.[97] Because of the natural acidity of the vagina, acid-sensitive sperm are immobilized and the alkalinity of semen acts to counter this effect. Buffering compounds maintain the acidic environment in the vagina and provide a contraceptive effect. Such products, however, are not yet available in the United States.

Efficacy and Effectiveness

Few rigorous studies have been conducted on the contraceptive effectiveness of spermicides alone. Typical-use pregnancy rates range as high as 28%. Spermicides used alone are less effective in preventing pregnancy than other contraceptive methods, but use of spermicide remains superior to using no method at all.

Side Effects/Adverse Effects

Nonoxynol-9 is an irritant to human tissue, and frequent use is associated with increased reports of vaginal irritation. The risk of damage to epithelial tissue in the vagina increases with frequency of use and dose. Despite assumptions that the surfactant activity might also disrupt other organisms and possibly prevent sexually transmitted infection, N-9 has not been proven to reduce STIs among sex workers or women attending STI clinics.[94] The CDC's MEC currently label use of the spermicide N-9 as a category 4 for persons with HIV/AIDS. Current contraindications for the use of N-9–based spermicides include STI protection, multiple daily acts of intercourse, individuals at high risk for HIV acquisition, and rectal administration. However, for women at low risk of HIV acquisition, N-9 is an appropriate contraceptive option and is intended to be used with other female barrier methods such as diaphragms and condoms.

Data from clinical trials describe the likelihood of developing certain genital infections over a period of 6 to 7 months of use. With spermicide use, a 13% to 17% risk exists of developing a yeast infection, a 8% to 12% probability of developing bacterial vaginosis, and a 19% to 27% chance of developing general vulvovaginal irritation. Urinary tract symptoms have been reported among 11% to 15% of women using N-9 spermicides (although less than 6% of these cases proved to be urinary tract infections by culture). Because these studies had no comparison groups, it is not clear if the rates found among spermicide users are different from those among the general population of sexually active women.[98]

Availability

Spermicides containing N-9 are widely available as over-the-counter products. These agents do not require a prescription or provider visit. Advantages for women include their ready accessibility, the ability to exert personal control over contraception, and the low cost. Spermicides are coitus dependent in that they must be applied at each act of intercourse.

Other Pharmacologic Contraceptive Methods

In addition to regular use of contraception, hormones and other pharmaceutical agents are used in the area of pregnancy prevention. Drugs currently used for emergency contraception as well as medical abortion are discussed in this section.

Emergency Contraception

Emergency contraception (EC) is a woman's only reliable option for preventing pregnancy after unprotected intercourse. There are two methods: oral medication taken within 72 to 120 hours of unprotected intercourse (depending on the drug) or insertion of a copper-containing intrauterine device. At one time, the oral agents were called "morning after" pills, but this term implies—incorrectly—that they must be used only within 24 hours of exposure.

Oral Emergency Contraception

The first type of oral emergency contraception that was used was the Yuzpe regimen, containing both ethinyl estradiol and levonorgestrel, The Yuzpe method has been prescribed for decades and can be followed by taking a specified number of pills from specific brands of oral contraceptives. In 1998, a dedicated product for emergency contraception (Preven), containing ethinyl estradiol and levonorgestrel, was approved by the FDA. It is no longer marketed because levonorgestrel-only formulations were found to be more effective and have fewer side effects than the combined drug.

Levonorgestrel-only emergency contraception was approved as a prescription product by the FDA in 1999 was and then approved as an over-the-counter medication in 2006; however, a prescription was required for women younger than 18 years. A lengthy legal challenge over the age restrictions finally ended in 2013, when the FDA approved this emergency contraception method as a nonprescription product for all women of childbearing potential.[99]

An antiprogestin, ulipristal acetate (ella), was approved for emergency contraception in the United States in 2010. Another antiprogesterone, mifepristone (Mifeprex), is used for medication abortion and originally known as RU 486. This agent also is an effective postcoital contraceptive but was not approved for emergency contraception at the time of publication.

Studies have examined whether other progestins such as norethindrone can be used as emergency contraception and suggest that such products are also somewhat effective.[100] However, there are no dedicated emergency contraception products using any progestins other than levonorgestrel.

Mechanism of Action

The hypothesized mechanism of action for oral emergency contraception is the inhibition or delay of ovulation. Other effects have also been noted, including thickening of cervical mucus, slowing of tubal motility, interference with sperm transport, deficient luteal function, and changes in the endometrium that make it inhospitable to implantation.[101] Observations that a dose of estrogen and levonorgestrel caused changes in the endometrium that interfered with implantation led to the introduction of the Yuzpe regimen, but recent studies have not found an effect of altered endometrial receptivity that interferes with implantation.[101]

Dosing Considerations

Levonorgestrel is an approved progestin in many current oral contraceptives. For emergency contraception, the current maximum dose is 0.15 mg per day, taken either in a single dose or divided in two doses taken 12 hours apart. While dosing with combined oral contraceptives can be used for emergency contraception if levonorgestrel-only methods are not available, the latter method is preferable because it is more effective and has fewer side effects.

Ulipristal acetate is a prescription product and the dose is a single 30 mg taken orally. Women who use ulipristal acetate should not start a progesterone-containing contraceptive for 5 days following use of this emergency contraception product.

Efficacy and Effectiveness

Oral emergency contraception prevents pregnancy during the days between intercourse and implantation; it is ineffective after implantation has occurred. Recent research suggests that levonorgestrel prevents approximately 50% of expected pregnancies in women using the method within 72 hours of intercourse.[102] Effectiveness is best if the emergency contraception is taken as directed as soon as possible after unprotected intercourse. Ulipristal acetate prevents almost two-thirds of pregnancies, and its effectiveness has been demonstrated up to 120 hours after unprotected intercourse.[101,102]

Eligibility and Contraindications

The MEC for contraceptive use applies to daily use of hormonal contraception. Contraindications to the use of hormonal contraceptives do not apply to emergency contraception. Cardiovascular disease, thrombophilic disorders, migraine, liver disease and breastfeeding are conditions in which the theoretical risks of remaining pregnant outweigh the risks of using the levonorgestrel or estrogen/progestin forms of emergency contraception.

The MEC does not have data on ulipristal acetate because it was not yet FDA-approved when the MEC were published in 2010. Ulipristal acetate is contraindicated for women who are younger than 16 years and should not be used by breastfeeding women per manufacturers instructions. It is not recommended for women with poorly controlled asthma or hepatic dysfunction. Table 29-13 summarizes the formulations and dosing for oral hormonal emergency contraception.

Table 29-13 Oral Hormonal Emergency Contraception

Emergency Contraception Regimen	Recommended Dosage	Instructions for Use
Levonorgestrel only (Plan B)	1.5 mg levonorgestrel	Take in 2 doses of 0.75 mg each, 12 hours apart, or take 1.5 mg (both tablets) at once
Ulipristal acetate (ella)	30 mg tablet	Taken as a single dose as soon as possible but up to 120 hours after unprotected intercourse
Yuzpe regimen	200 mcg ethinyl estradiol plus 1 mg levonorgestrel	Take in 2 doses 12 hours apart, beginning as soon as possible after unprotected intercourse

Side Effects

Irregular bleeding is common the first month following use of all regimens. Side effects with oral emergency contraception use tend to be mild to moderate and resolve quickly. The Yuzpe regimen is associated with nausea in approximately 20% of women and vomiting in approximately 9% of women. Approximately 12% to 20% of women taking levonorgestrel-only regimens will experience headaches, painful menstruation, or nausea. In clinical trials of ulipristal acetate, the most frequently reported side effects were abdominal pain and nausea/vomiting (13%).[101] Three hours is probably sufficient for absorption of the hormone dose. If a woman experiences vomiting, a repeat dosing is not needed if the vomiting occurs 3 hours or more after administration.[12]

Antiemetics can be given to prevent nausea and vomiting. Most clinicians give them to women using the estrogen-progestin formulations and recommend prophylactic dosing. Meclizine 50 mg taken orally one hour before the first dose of estrogen/progestin reduces nausea and may induce some sedation. Metoclopramide (Reglan) 10 mg taken orally one hour before taking the estrogen/progestin has also been used effectively. Levonorgestrel and ulipristal acetate are better tolerated and women using these formulations may take the antiemetic as needed.

Concerns have been voiced that an emergency contraception failure may raise the risk of ectopic pregnancy due to effects on thickening cervical mucus and slowing tubal motility, but there are no data to date that support this concern.[102]

Recurrent use of emergency contraception is suggested as signaling a need for further counseling and may be harmful for women with health conditions classified as category 2, 3, or 4 for combined hormonal or progestin-only contraceptive use.[103]

Drug–Drug Interactions

Ulipristal acetate and levonorgestrel should not be used concomitantly with drugs that are CYP3A4 inducers. Drugs that induce CYP3A4 and decrease the effectiveness of the emergency contraceptive agent include topiramate (Topamax), phenytoin (Dilantin) carbamazepine (Tegretol), felbamate (Felbatol), oxcarbazepine (Trileptal), rifampin (Rifadin), barbiturates, and St. John's wort. In contrast, drugs that inhibit CYP3A4 can increase concentrations of ulipristal, including itraconazole (Sporanox) and ketoconazole (Nizoral). Ulipristal absorption is reduced when the gastric pH is altered, so women using this drug should not take proton-pump inhibitors or antacids.

Availability

Pharmacy availability of emergency contraception is not universal. A number of healthcare professionals and institutions decline to prescribe or provide these products and/or cite a religious objection to providing the service, and they are protected by several federal and state laws. Providers are advised to be aware of pharmacies in the community that facilitate access to oral emergency contraception. Ulipristal acetate (ella) is usually is more expensive than levonorgestrel emergency contraception, although the former may be covered by insurance when the latter is not.

Copper IUD for Emergency Contraception

Although intrauterine contraceptive devices have previously been discussed, it is important to include the copper-bearing devices in this section as they can be used for postcoital contraception. Copper IUDs can be inserted up to 5 days after an episode of unprotected intercourse. This use was first reported by Lippes and Tatum in 1976.[104]

Mechanism of Action

The copper in the intrauterine device has toxic effects on ovum and sperm; thus, its effectiveness in inhibiting fertilization is immediate following insertion. The copper ions, as a secondary mode of action, may inhibit endometrial receptivity if fertilization has already occurred.[88,101]

Efficacy and Effectiveness

In a review of 20 studies and more than 8000 insertions, the failure rate for copper IUD insertion as a postcoital contraceptive was estimated at 0.1%.[102] This rate is far lower than the failure rate for the Yuzpe and progestin-only regimens described previously.

Eligibility and Contraindications

Contraindications to IUD use include uterine abnormalities, active pelvic infection, and copper allergy.

Medication (Pharmaceutical) Abortion

For women with unintended pregnancy, termination of the pregnancy is a legal option. Surgical abortion may not be available for many women, or medication options may be preferred. Three drugs are currently used in the United States for medical termination of a pregnancy.

Mechanism of Action

Mifepristone (Mifeprex) is an antiprogestin and blocks the action of progesterone, which is necessary for the maintenance of pregnancy. Thus, this agent causes the uterine lining to shed.

Methotrexate is an antimetabolite and an antifolate agent that interferes with the growth of rapidly dividing cells and is used to treat certain conditions such as neoplastic disease, psoriasis, and rheumatoid arthritis. It is occasionally employed to terminate pregnancy as well. This agent acts on the cytotrophoblast rather than the embryo and also is effective in treating extrauterine pregnancies. It is a pharmaceutical treatment for ectopic pregnancy.

Misoprostol (Cytotec) is a prostaglandin analogue that produces a softening of the cervix and uterine contractions, which result in the expulsion of uterine contents. Misoprostol is approved for the prevention and treatment of stomach ulcers.

Dosing and Efficacy/Effectiveness

In 2000, the FDA approved the use of mifepristone in conjunction with misoprostol for the termination of early pregnancy. The FDA-approved regimen, which is based on older research, calls for oral dosing with 600 mg of mifepristone, followed 2 days later by 400 mcg of misoprostol to terminate a pregnancy of no more than 49 days' gestation. A number of alternative, evidence-based regimens are also used in the United States. In most practices, the dose of mifepristone is 200 mg orally. Misoprostol is then administered orally (400 mcg) or vaginally (800 mcg) 1, 2, or 3 days later depending on the institutional protocols. Approximately 95% of women will experience a complete abortion following this regimen; the rate of success is somewhat less in later gestation. Effective termination of pregnancies up to 63 days' gestation has also been demonstrated.[105]

Methotrexate is usually administered by injection (50 mg/m^2), followed by administration 3 to 7 days later of vaginal misoprostol. Similar to the case with misoprostol, 95% of women using this method will abort completely if the pregnancy is less than 49 days' gestation, but in 20% to 30% of cases it may take longer than the mifepristone regimen (as long as 1 to 5 weeks).[105,106]

No standard protocol for misoprostol alone exists in the termination of early pregnancy, and the drug is not approved for this use. Studies have evaluated several dosing regimens, most providing 600 to 800 mcg vaginally at periodic intervals, with effectiveness ranging from 65% to 90%.[107]

Eligibility and Contraindications

Use of mifepristone is contraindicated for women with confirmed or suspected ectopic pregnancy, with history of allergy to mifepristone, or with chronic use of corticosteroids, chronic adrenal failure, coagulopathy or current therapy with anticoagulants, and inherited porphyria. Methotrexate (Rheumatrex, Trexall) is contraindicated for women with a history of allergy or intolerance to methotrexate, coagulopathy or current severe anemia, acute or chronic renal or hepatic disease, acute inflammatory bowel disease, or uncontrolled seizure disorders. In addition to contraindications existing for each of the specific drugs, these agents are contraindicated for women with a history of allergy or intolerance to them. Intrauterine devices should be removed before medication abortion regimens are initiated.

Side Effects/Adverse Effects

Reported side effects of medication abortion regimens are sometimes difficult to distinguish from the abortion itself. These effects include nausea, vomiting, diarrhea, dizziness, headache, fever, chills, and cramping. In some cases, the abortion may be incomplete, or the uterine bleeding following abortion may be prolonged; approximately 2% to 10% of women will require intervention for these events.[108] Additional side effects of methotrexate include oral ulcers. Uterine and abdominal pain is managed with analgesics and opiates. There is no evidence that mifepristone is associated with birth defects in the case of failed abortion, but methotrexate has been associated with birth defects when given in high doses. Misoprostol is associated with a birth defect known as Mobius syndrome, although the causal relationship is unclear and the actual risk is low.

Infection with *Clostridium sordelli*, a gram-positive, toxin-producing anaerobe, has been known to occur in women after medical abortion, although any specific connection remains unclear. The Society of Family Planning has published guidelines for reducing the risk of abortion-associated infection.[109]

Special Populations

Pregnancy and Lactation

Clearly the issue of using contraceptives during pregnancy is a moot one, given that the indication for the agents is to prevent pregnancy. However, contraception is an important topic among women during the postpartum period, especially women who are breastfeeding and continue to do so for at least the first year of their children's lives.[110–112] The issues of initiation, eligibility, and continuation of contraceptives for these women are covered in detail in the *Postpartum* chapter.

Midlife Women

The MEC do not list a woman's age as a consideration of category 3 or 4, except in the case of combined hormonal contraception for women who have either headaches without aura or smoking. With both conditions, use of combined methods is not recommended when the woman is 35 years or older.

Midlife women experiencing menstrual irregularities may use hormonal contraception as a therapeutic intervention as well as a contraceptive one. Additional information about this use can be found in the *Pelvic and Menstrual Disorders* chapter.

Contraception is indicated for women during their reproductive years. However, the perimenopausal period can present a clinical quandary. Although fecundity is decreased during this time frame, it does not mean a woman is unable to become pregnant. Menopause is a retrospective diagnosis, and many women are at risk of pregnancy for several years, as menses may cease for several months, only to resume spontaneously. Additional information about women and use of steroid hormones during menopause is found in the chapter *The Mature Woman.*

The Future: Hormonal Contraception for Men

No hormonal contraceptive methods are currently available for men in the United States. In part, this is because development of hormonal contraceptives for men must target the continuous production of sperm over a period of several weeks, as opposed to targeting ovulation and a fertile period in women. Research on hormonal control of male fertility has evaluated the contraceptive efficacy of interfering with the hormonal support necessary for the development, maturation, function, and transport of sperm. Suppression of LH and FSH in men via administration of a progestin inhibits the production of sperm in the testes. However, testosterone production is also inhibited, and most regimens under consideration require adding back synthetic testosterone to reverse the adverse effects on libido and ejaculatory function. A number of drug combinations show potential, but none is approved at this time for use in the United States.[113]

Conclusion

A number of options for contraception are currently available to women in the United States. Nonetheless, of the 6.6 million pregnancies that occur each year in this country, approximately half (51%) are unintended. Half of those unintended pregnancies occur among couples who were actively practicing contraception; the remainder occur among couples who were not using a birth control method at the time of conception.[114,115] Because approximately 1 million pregnancies each year are the result of contraceptive failure, health education for all women not seeking pregnancy is a critically important responsibility of clinicians. Effective contraception depends on thorough counseling regarding contraceptive options, listening to women's desires, assisting women with selection of appropriate methods, and performing follow-up to ensure adherence with a method or method change.

Resources

Organization	Description	Website
Centers for Disease Control and Prevention	Federal site that contains the full Medical Eligibility for Hormonal Contraception table; this information is available as an app	www.cdc.gov
Guttmacher Institute	Organization that, among other interests, has a focus on contraception and abortion; website includes interactive data about the topics in different locales	www.guttmacher.org
Planned Parenthood Federation of America	Website primarily dedicated to providing information to consumers	www.plannedparenthood.org
Apps		
A myriad of apps exist for devices in the area of consumer-oriented contraceptive information. Among them are apps that send email/text messages to remind women about taking pills or changing patches, implants, IUDs, and other contraceptives. Most of these apps are free. For healthcare providers, the MEC is available for free from CDC: www.cdc.gov/mobile/healthcareproviderapps.html.		
Other Resources		
Managing Contraception	Facebook and Twitter companions to the popular text and meetings Contraceptive Technology	www.facebook.com/managingcontraception
Public Broadcasting Service (PBS)	Website devoted to the 2003 American Experience film, *The Pill*, that includes ancillary information such as a historical gallery	www.pbs.org/wgbh/amex/pill
U.S. Department of Health and Human Services, Office of Population Affairs	Federally funded family planning information, training, and grant funding; consumer and provider information available on website	www.hhs.gov/opa

References

1. Christin-Maitre S. History of oral contraceptive drugs and their use worldwide. *Best Pract Res Clin Endocrinol Metab.* 2013;27:3-12.
2. Ellertson C. History and efficacy of emergency contraception: beyond Coca-Cola. *Fam Plann Perspect.* 1996;28:44-48.
3. Winner B, Peipert JF, Zhao Q, et al. Effectiveness of long-acting reversible contraception. *N Engl J Med.* 2012;366:1998-2007.
4. DHHS Code of Federal Regulations 45 CFR 46.203. In: Services DoHaH, ed. 1978.
5. Hughes EC. Gametogenesis and fertilization. In: American College of Obstetricians and Gynecologists, ed. *Obstetric-Gynecologic Terminology.* Philadelphia: Davis; 1972.
6. Stirnemann JJ, Samson A, Bernard JP, Thalabard JC. Day-specific probabilities of conception in fertile

cycles resulting in spontaneous pregnancies. *Hum Reprod.* 2013;28:1110-1116.

7. Dunson DB, Colombo B, Baird DD. Changes with age in the level and duration of fertility in the menstrual cycle. *Hum Reprod.* 2002;17:1399-1403.
8. Mukherjee S, Velez Edwards DR, Baird DD, Savitz DA, Hartmann KE. Risk of miscarriage among black women and white women in a U.S. prospective cohort study. *Am J Epidemiol.* 2013;177:1271-1278.
9. Singal AG, Higgins PD, Waljee AK. A primer on effectiveness and efficacy trials. *Clin Translational Gastroenterol.* 2014;5:e45.
10. Trussell J. Choosing a contraceptive: efficacy, safety and personal considerations. In: Hatcher RA, Trussell J, Nelson AL, Cates W, Kowal D, Policar M, eds. *Contraceptive Technology.* 20th ed. New York: Ardent Media; 2011:19-41.
11. Centers for Disease Control and Prevention. U.S. medical eligibility criteria for contraceptive use, 2010. *MMWR Recommend Rep.* 2010;59:1-86.
12. Division of Reproductive Health, Health Promotion, Centers for Disease Control and Prevention. U.S. selected practice recommendations for contraceptive use, 2013: adapted from the World Health Organization selected practice recommendations for contraceptive use. 2nd ed. *MMWR Recommend Rep.* 2013;62:1-60.
13. Johnston CA, Crawford PM. Anti-epileptic drugs and hormonal treatments. *Curr Treat Opt Neurol.* 2014;16:288.
14. Tseng A, Hills-Nieminen C. Drug interactions between antiretrovirals and hormonal contraceptives. *Expert Opin Drug Metab Toxicol.* 2013;9:559-572.
15. Taylor J, Pemberton MN. Antibiotics and oral contraceptives: new considerations for dental practice. *Br Dental J.* 2012;212:481-483.
16. Ioannides C. Pharmacokinetic interactions between herbal remedies and medicinal drugs. *Xenobiotica.* 2002;32:451-478.
17. Murphy PA, Kern SE, Stanczyk FZ, Westhoff CL. Interaction of St. John's wort with oral contraceptives: effects on the pharmacokinetics of norethindrone and ethinyl estradiol, ovarian activity and breakthrough bleeding. *Contraception.* 2005;71:402-408.
18. Centers for Disease Control and Prevention. Update to CDC's U.S. medical eligibility criteria for contraceptive use, 2010: revised recommendations for the use of contraceptive methods during the postpartum period. *MMWR.* 2011;60:878-883.
19. Centers for Disease Control and Prevention. Update to CDC's U.S. medical eligibility criteria for contraceptive use, 2010: revised recommendations for the use of hormonal contraception among women at high risk for HIV infection or infected with HIV. *MMWR.* 2012;61(24):449-452.
20. Brahmi D, Curtis KM. When can a woman start combined hormonal contraceptives (CHCs)? A systematic review. *Contraception.* 2013;87:524-538.
21. Westhoff C, Morroni C, Kerns J, Murphy PA. Bleeding patterns after immediate vs. conventional oral contraceptive initiation: a randomized, controlled trial. *Fertil Steril.* 2003;79:322-329.
22. Lesnewski R, Prine L, Ginzburg R. Preventing gaps when switching contraceptives. *Am Fam Physician.* 2011;83(5):567-570.
23. Reproductive Health Access Project. How to switch birth control methods, 2013. http://www.reproductiveaccess.org/wp-content/uploads/2014/12/switching_bc.pdf. Accessed February 14, 2015.
24. Brunner LR, Hogue CJ. The role of body weight in oral contraceptive failure: results from the 1995 National Survey of Family Growth. *Ann Epidemiol.* 2005; 15: 492-499.
25. Brunner Huber LR, Hogue CJ. The association between body weight, unintended pregnancy resulting in a livebirth, and contraception at the time of conception. *Matern Child Health J.* 2005;9:413-420.
26. Holt VL, Scholes D, Wicklund KG, Cushing-Haugen KL, Daling JR. Body mass index, weight, and oral contraceptive failure risk. *Obstet Gynecol.* 2005;105:46-52.
27. Gallo MF, Lopez LM, Grimes DA, Carayon F, Schulz KF, Helmerhorst FM. Combination contraceptives: effects on weight. *Cochrane Database Syst Rev.* 2014; 1:CD003987.
28. Brunner Huber LR, Hogue CJ, Stein AD, Drews C, Zieman M. Body mass index and risk for oral contraceptive failure: a case-cohort study in South Carolina. *Ann Epidemiol.* 2006;16:637-643.
29. Zieman M, Guillebaud J, Weisberg E, Shangold GA, Fisher AC, Creasy GW. Contraceptive efficacy and cycle control with the Ortho Evra/Evra transdermal system: the analysis of pooled data. *Fertil Steril.* 2002; 77:S13-S18.
30. Brunner Huber LR, Toth JL. Obesity and oral contraceptive failure: findings from the 2002 National Survey of Family Growth. *Am J Epidemiol.* 2007;166: 1306-1311.
31. Vessey M. Oral contraceptive failures and body weight: findings in a large cohort study. *J Fam Plann Reprod Health Care.* 2001;27:90-91.
32. Trussell J, Schwarz EB, Guthrie K. Obesity and oral contraceptive pill failure. *Contraception.* 2009;79: 334-338.
33. Westhoff CL, Torgal AH, Mayeda ER, et al. Pharmacokinetics and ovarian suppression during use of

a contraceptive vaginal ring in normal-weight and obese women. *Am J Obstet Gynecol.* 2012;207:39.
34. Dragoman M, Petrie K, Torgal A, Thomas T, Cremers S, Westhoff CL. Contraceptive vaginal ring effectiveness is maintained during 6 weeks of use: a prospective study of normal BMI and obese women. *Contraception.* 2013;87:432-436.
35. Segall-Gutierrez P, Taylor D, Liu X, Stanzcyk F, Azen S, Mishell DR Jr. Follicular development and ovulation in extremely obese women receiving depo-medroxyprogesterone acetate subcutaneously. *Contraception.* 2010;81:487-495.
36. Mornar S, Chan LN, Mistretta S, Neustadt A, Martins S, Gilliam M. Pharmacokinetics of the etonogestrel contraceptive implant in obese women. *Am J Obstet Gynecol.* 2012;207:110.
37. Xu H, Wade JA, Peipert JF, Zhao Q, Madden T, Secura GM. Contraceptive failure rates of etonogestrel subdermal implants in overweight and obese women. *Obstet Gynecol.* 2012;120:21-26.
38. Westhoff CL, Hait HI, Reape KZ. Body weight does not impact pregnancy rates during use of a low-dose extended-regimen 91-day oral contraceptive. *Contraception.* 2012;85:235-239.
39. Lopez LM, Grimes DA, Chen M, et al. Hormonal contraceptives for contraception in overweight or obese women. *Cochrane Database Syst Rev.* 2013;4: CD008452.
40. Burkman RT, Fisher AC, Wan GJ, Barnowski CE, LaGuardia KD. Association between efficacy and body weight or body mass index for two low-dose oral contraceptives. *Contraception.* 2009;79:424-427.
41. Daniels K, Mosher W, Jones J. Contraceptive methods women have ever used: United States 1982–2010. National Health Statistics reports. No. 62, February 14, 2014. Available from: http://www.cdc.gov/nchs/data/nhsr/nhsr062.pdf. Accessed July 3, 2015. Hyattsville, MD: National Center for Health Statistics; 2013.
42. Wyatt KD, Anderson RT, Creedon D, et al. Women's values in contraceptive choice: a systematic review of relevant attributes included in decision aids. *BMC Womens Health.* 2014;14(1):28.
43. Balci K, Utku U, Asil T, Celik Y. Ischemic stroke in young adults: risk factors, subtypes, and prognosis. *Neurologist.* 2011;17(1):16-20.
44. Lalude OO. Risk of cardiovascular events with hormonal contraception: insights from the Danish cohort study. *Curr Cardiol Rep.* 2013;15:374.
45. Sacco S, Ricci S, Carolei A. Migraine and vascular diseases: a review of the evidence and potential implications for management. *Cephalalgia.* 2012;32:785-795.
46. Lidegaard O, Nielsen LH, Skovlund CW, Skjeldestad FE, Lokkegaard E. Risk of venous thromboembolism from use of oral contraceptives containing different progestogens and oestrogen doses: Danish cohort study, 2001–9. *BMJ.* 2011;343:d6423.
47. Grimes DA, Stuart GS, Levi EE. Screening women for oral contraception: can family history identify inherited thrombophilias? *Obstet Gynecol.* 2012;120: 889-895.
48. Bitzer J, Amy JJ, Beerthuizen R, et al. Statement on combined hormonal contraceptives containing third- or fourth-generation progestogens or cyproterone acetate, and the associated risk of thromboembolism. *J Fam Plan Reprod Health Care.* 2013;39:156-159.
49. Redmond G, Godwin AJ, Olson W, Lippman JS. Use of placebo controls in an oral contraceptive trial: methodological issues and adverse event incidence. *Contraception.* 1999;60:81-85.
50. Hickey M, Agarwal S. Unscheduled bleeding in combined oral contraceptive users: focus on extended-cycle and continuous-use regimens. *J Fam Plan Reprod Health Care.* 2009;35:245-248.
51. Rosenberg MJ, Meyers A, Roy V. Efficacy, cycle control, and side effects of low- and lower-dose oral contraceptives: a randomized trial of 20 micrograms and 35 micrograms estrogen preparations. *Contraception.* 1999;60:321-329.
52. Graham CA, Bancroft J, Doll HA, Greco T, Tanner A. Does oral contraceptive-induced reduction in free testosterone adversely affect the sexuality or mood of women? *Psychoneuroendocrinology.* 2007;32:246-255.
53. Graham CA, Ramos R, Bancroft J, Maglaya C, Farley TM. The effects of steroidal contraceptives on the well-being and sexuality of women: a double-blind, placebo-controlled, two-centre study of combined and progestogen-only methods. *Contraception.* 1995;52:363-369.
54. Burrows LJ, Basha M, Goldstein AT. The effects of hormonal contraceptives on female sexuality: a review. *J Sex Med.* 2012;9:2213-2223.
55. Lopez LM, Kaptein AA, Helmerhorst FM. Oral contraceptives containing drospirenone for premenstrual syndrome. *Cochrane Database Syst Rev.* 2012; 2: CD006586.
56. Huber J, Walch K. Treating acne with oral contraceptives: use of lower doses. *Contraception.* 2006;73:23-29.
57. Kiley JW, Shulman LP. Estradiol valerate and dienogest: a new approach to oral contraception. *Int J Womens Health.* 2011;3:281-286.
58. Fritz M, Speroff L. *Clinical Gynecologic Endocrinology and Infertility.* 8th ed. Philadelphia: Lippincott, Williams & Wilkins; 2011.

59. Stanczyk FZ, Hapgood JP, Winer S, Mishell DR Jr. Progestogens used in postmenopausal hormone therapy: differences in their pharmacological properties, intracellular actions, and clinical effects. *Endocrine Rev.* 2013;34:171-208.
60. Lawrie TA, Helmerhorst FM, Maitra NK, Kulier R, Bloemenkamp K, Gulmezoglu AM. Types of progestogens in combined oral contraception: effectiveness and side-effects. *Cochrane Database Syst Rev.* 2011: CD004861.
61. Sulak PJ. Continuous oral contraception: changing times. *Best Pract Res Clin Obstet Gynaecol.* 2008;22:355-374.
62. Edelman AB, Gallo MF, Jensen JT, Nichols MD, Schulz KF, Grimes DA. Continuous or extended cycle vs. cyclic use of combined oral contraceptives for contraception. *Cochrane Database Syst Rev.* 2005;3:CD004695.
63. Panicker S, Mann S, Shawe J, Stephenson J. Evolution of extended use of the combined oral contraceptive pill. *J Fam Plan Reprod Health Care.* 2014;40:133-141.
64. Bonnema RA, Spencer AL. The new extended-cycle levonorgestrel-ethinyl estradiol oral contraceptives. *Clin Med Insights Reprod Health.* 2011;5:49-54.
65. Abrams LS, Skee D, Natarajan J, Wong F. An overview of the pharmokinetics of a contraceptive patch. *Int J Gynecol Obstet.* 2000;70(suppl 2):B78-B82.
66. Lopez LM, Grimes DA, Gallo MF, Stockton LL, Schulz KF. Skin patch and vaginal ring versus combined oral contraceptives for contraception. *Cochrane Database Syst Rev.* 2013;4:CD003552.
67. Audet MC, Moreau M, Koltun WD, et al. Evaluation of contraceptive efficacy and cycle control of a transdermal contraceptive patch vs an oral contraceptive: a randomized controlled trial. *JAMA.* 2001;285: 2347-2354.
68. van den Heuvel MW, van Bragt AJ, Alnabawy AK, Kaptein MC. Comparison of ethinylestradiol pharmacokinetics in three hormonal contraceptive formulations: the vaginal ring, the transdermal patch and an oral contraceptive. *Contraception.* 2005;72:168-174.
69. Sidney S, Cheetham TC, Connell FA, et al. Recent combined hormonal contraceptives (CHCs) and the risk of thromboembolism and other cardiovascular events in new users. *Contraception.* 2013;87:93-100.
70. Kaunitz AM, Archer DF, Mishell DR Jr, Foegh M. Safety and tolerability of a new low-dose contraceptive patch in obese and nonobese women. *Am J Obstet Gynecol.* 2014;212(3):318.e1-8.
71. Raymond EG, Burke AE, Espey E. Combined hormonal contraceptives and venous thromboembolism: putting the risks into perspective. *Obstet Gynecol.* 2012;119:1039-1044.
72. Ziaei S, Rajaei L, Faghihzadeh S, Lamyian M. Comparative study and evaluation of side effects of low-dose contraceptive pills administered by the oral and vaginal route. *Contraception.* 2002;65:329-331.
73. Mulders TM, Dieben TO, Bennink HJ. Ovarian function with a novel combined contraceptive vaginal ring. *Hum Reprod.* 2002;17:2594-2599.
74. Jacobson JC, Likis FE, Murphy PA. Extended and continuous combined contraceptive regimens for menstrual suppression. *J Midwifery Womens Health.* 2012;57:585-592.
75. Hatcher RA, Trussel J, Nelson AL, Cates W, Kowal D, Policar MS. *Contraceptive Technology.* 20th ed. New York: Ardent Media; 2011.
76. Damm P, Mathiesen ER, Petersen KR, Kjos S. Contraception after gestational diabetes. *Diab Care.* 2007; 30(suppl 2):S236-S241.
77. Group ECW. Ovarian and endometrial function during hormonal contraception. *Hum Reprod.* 2001; 16: 1527-1535.
78. Smith OP, Critchley HO. Progestogen only contraception and endometrial break through bleeding. *Angiogenesis.* 2005;8:117-126.
79. Dal'ava N, Bahamondes L, Bahamondes MV, Bottura BF, Monteiro I. Body weight and body composition of depot medroxyprogesterone acetate users. *Contraception.* 2014;90(2):182-187.
80. Lopez LM, Edelman A, Chen M, Otterness C, Trussell J, Helmerhorst FM. Progestin-only contraceptives: effects on weight. *Cochrane Database Syst Rev.* 2013; 7:CD008815.
81. Robinson JA, Burke AE. Obesity and hormonal contraceptive efficacy. *Womens Health.* 2013;9:453-466.
82. Food and Drug Administration. Depo-Provera (medroxyprogesterone acetate injectable suspension). 2004. http://www.accessdata.fda.gov/drugsatfda_docs/label/2004/20246s025lbl.pdf. Accessed February 14, 2015.
83. American College of Obstetricians and Gynecologists. Committee Opinion No. 602: Depot medroxyprogesterone acetate and bone effects. *Obstet Gynecol.* 2014;123:1398-1402.
84. Schnabel P, Merki-Feld GS, Malvy A, Duijkers I, Mommers E, van den Heuvel MW. Bioequivalence and x-ray visibility of a radiopaque etonogestrel implant versus a non-radiopaque implant: a 3-year, randomized, double-blind study. *Clin Drug Investig.* 2012;32:413-422.
85. Funk S, Miller MM, Mishell DR Jr, et al. Safety and efficacy of Implanon, a single-rod implantable

contraceptive containing etonogestrel. *Contraception.* 2005;71:319-326.

86. World Health Organization. *Selected Practice Recommendations for Contraceptive Use.* 2nd ed. Geneva: World Health Organization; 2005.
87. American College of Obstetricians and Gynecologists. ACOG Practice Bulletin No. 121: Long-acting reversible contraception: implants and intrauterine devices. *Obstet Gynecol.* 2011;118:184-196.
88. Gemzell-Danielsson K, Berger C, Lalitkumar PGL. Emergency contraception: mechanisms of action. *Contraception.* 2013;87:300-308.
89. Benshushan A, Paltiel O, Rojansky N, Brzezinski A, Laufer N. IUD use and the risk of endometrial cancer. *Eur J Obstet Gynecol Reprod Biol.* 2002;105:166-169.
90. Castellsague X, Diaz M, Vaccarella S, et al. Intrauterine device use, cervical infection with human papillomavirus, and risk of cervical cancer: a pooled analysis of 26 epidemiological studies. *Lancet Oncol.* 2011;12:1023-1031.
91. Hubacher D, Lara-Ricalde R, Taylor DJ, Guerra-Infante F, Guzman-Rodriguez R. Use of copper intrauterine devices and the risk of tubal infertility among nulligravid women. *N Engl J Med.* 2001;345:561-567.
92. Milsom I, Andersson K, Jonasson K, Lindstedt G, Rybo G. The influence of the Gyne-T 380S IUD on menstrual blood loss and iron status. *Contraception.* 1995;52:175-179.
93. Lowe RF, Prata N. Hemoglobin and serum ferritin levels in women using copper-releasing or levonorgestrel-releasing intrauterine devices: a systematic review. *Contraception.* 2013;87:486-496.
94. Obiero J, Mwethera PG, Wiysonge CS. Topical microbicides for prevention of sexually transmitted infections. *Cochrane Database Syst Rev.* 2012;6:CD007961.
95. Scholes D, Hooton TM, Roberts PL, Stapleton AE, Gupta K, Stamm WE. Risk factors for recurrent urinary tract infection in young women. *J Infect Dis.* 2000;182:1177-1182.
96. Speroff L, Darney P. *A Clinical Guide for Contraception.* 5th ed. Philadelphia: Wolters Kluwer; 2011.
97. Abdool Karim SS, Richardson BA, Ramjee G, et al. Safety and effectiveness of BufferGel and 0.5% PRO2000 gel for the prevention of HIV infection in women. *AIDS.* 2011;25:957-966.
98. Raymond EG, Chen PL, Luoto J, Group ST. Contraceptive effectiveness and safety of five nonoxynol-9 spermicides: a randomized trial. *Obstet Gynecol.* 2004;103:430-439.
99. FDA approves Plan B One-Step emergency contraceptive for use without a prescription for all women of child-bearing potential. 2013. http://www.fda.gov/NewsEvents/Newsroom/PressAnnouncements/ucm358082.htm. Accessed February 14, 2015.
100. Ellertson C, Webb A, Blanchard K, et al. Modifying the Yuzpe regimen of emergency contraception: a multicenter randomized controlled trial. *Obstet Gynecol.* 2003;101:1160-1167.
101. Murphy PA. Update on emergency contraception. *J Midwifery Womens Health.* 2012;57:593-602.
102. Glasier A. Emergency contraception: clinical outcomes. *Contraception.* 2013;87:309-313.
103. World Health Organization. Medical eligibility criteria for contraceptive use. 4th ed. http://whqlibdoc.who.int/publications/2010/9789241563888_eng.pdf?ua=1. Accessed February 14, 2015.
104. Lippes J, Malik T, Tatum HJ. The postcoital copper-T. *Adv Plan Parent.* 1976;11:24-29.
105. Kulier R, Kapp N, Gülmezoglu AM, Hofmeyr GJ, Cheng L, Campana A. Medical methods for first trimester abortion. Cochrane Database of Systematic Reviews 2011;11:CD002855.
106. Shaw KA, Topp NJ, Shaw JG, Blumenthal PD. Mifepristone–misoprostol dosing interval and effect on induction abortion times: a systematic review. *Obstet Gynecol.* 2013;121:1335-1347.
107. Borgatta L, Mullally B, Vragovic O, Gittinger E, Chen A. Misoprostol as the primary agent for medical abortion in a low-income urban setting. *Contraception.* 2004;70:121-126.
108. Kruse B, Poppema S, Creinin MD, Paul M. Management of side effects and complications in medical abortion. *Am J Obstet Gynecol.* 2000;183:S65-S75.
109. Achilles SL, Reeves MF. Prevention of infection after induced abortion: release date October 2010: SFP guideline 20102. *Contraception.* 2011;83:295-309.
110. Kapp N, Curtis KM. Combined oral contraceptive use among breastfeeding women: a systematic review. *Contraception.* 2010;82:10-16.
111. World Health Organization. *Combined Hormonal Contraceptive Use During the Postpartum Period.* Geneva, Switzerland: World Health Organization; 2010.
112. Kapp N, Curtis K, Nanda K. Progestogen-only contraceptive use among breastfeeding women: a systematic review. *Contraception.* 2010;82:17-37.
113. Chao J, Page ST, Anderson RA. Male contraception. *Best Pract Res Clin Obstet Gynecol.* 2014;28(6):845-857.
114. Finer LB, Zolna MR. Shifts in intended and unintended pregnancies in the United States, 2001–2008. *Am J Public Health.* 2014;104(suppl 1):S43-S48.
115. Unintended pregnancy in the United States. January 2015. http://www.guttmacher.org/pubs/FB-Unintended-Pregnancy-US.html. Accessed February 14, 2015.

30 Pelvic and Menstrual Disorders

Dawn Durain, William F. McCool

Based on the chapter by Kerri Durnell Schuiling and Mary C. Brucker in the first edition of Pharmacology for Women's Health

Chapter Glossary

Coxibs Drugs that selectively inhibit the COX-2 isoform of cyclooxygenase, thereby inhibiting the production of pro-inflammatory prostaglandins without inhibiting the COX-1 isoform.

Cyclooxygenase (COX) Enzyme that converts arachidonic acid to prostaglandin.

Estrogen agonists/antagonists (EAAs) Drugs that act as agonists, antagonists, or mixed agonists/antagonists for estrogen receptors. Formerly known as selective estrogen receptor modulators.

Gonadotropin-releasing hormone (GnRH) agonists Drugs that attach to the gonadotropin-releasing hormone receptor in the pituitary.

Gonadotropin-releasing hormone (GnRH) analogues Nonsteroidal agents that suppress ovarian estrogen production.

Selective estrogen receptor modulators (SERMs) Class of drugs that act as agonists, antagonists, or mixed agonist/antagonists for estrogen receptors. This is an older term that is increasingly being replaced by estrogen agonist/antagonists (EAAs).

Introduction

A century ago, women availed themselves of patent "cures," such as the popular Lydia Pinkham tonic if experiencing an illness. Claims for her remedy encompassed treatment of a wide variety of ills including kidney disease, depression, insomnia, gastrointestinal conditions, and others. However, the majority of women who used Lydia Pinkham's tonic were seeking relief from menstrual disorders, pelvic disease, and/or infertility. Of course, Pinkham's tonic did not fulfill all of its grandiose claims—even today, modern healthcare providers can find it challenging to treat some of these conditions.

Menstrual and pelvic disorders are common conditions that may occur independent of each other or concomitantly. For example, dysmenorrhea often is part of the constellation of symptoms that occur with chronic pelvic pain. For women with menstrual variations or pelvic disease, therapy may be directed at a single symptom or a specific condition, such as endometriosis. Oftentimes, treatments for different disorders include use of the same drugs, such as analgesics, hormones, and receptor agonists/antagonists.

This chapter focuses on both symptoms and disease conditions. Symptoms of menstrual disorders and pelvic pain are discussed first, followed by a review of specific conditions. Several menstrual abnormalities can be treated pharmacologically. Among these are episodes of dysmenorrhea, abnormal uterine bleeding, amenorrhea, and mood disorders related to menstrual cycles. Unlike the other chapters that separately discuss pharmacologic management of women who are pregnant, lactating, or of advanced age in separate sections, the conditions in this chapter generally are exclusive to women who are neither pregnant nor breastfeeding. However, the clinician should always consider, and exclude, pregnancy, especially if the woman reports any menstrual disruption.

Dysmenorrhea

The term dysmenorrhea refers to painful menstruation. Most women experience some degree of dysmenorrhea at some point during their lives. Dysmenorrhea is categorized as either primary or secondary. Primary dysmenorrhea is painful menstruation for which there is no identifiable pathology and which usually is associated with the onset of normal ovulatory cycles.[1,2] The initial onset of primary dysmenorrhea usually occurs shortly after menarche, and frequently backache, nausea and vomiting, and diarrhea accompany the pain.[3] Primary dysmenorrhea occurs most often during adolescence or early adulthood.[2,3]

Secondary dysmenorrhea is menstrual pain associated with identifiable pathology. This entity is more likely to present after years of relatively painless menses and often has an acyclic or chronic component.[4] Common causes of secondary dysmenorrhea include uterine leiomyomata (also known as fibroids), adenomyosis, endometriosis, and pelvic inflammatory disease (PID). Pharmacologic treatment for dysmenorrhea depends on the etiology, although nonsteroidal anti-inflammatory drugs (NSAIDs) frequently are used to treat the pain associated with any of the underlying causes.

The painful abnormal uterine cramping that occurs during primary dysmenorrhea is secondary to overproduction of prostaglandins within the endometrium, with elevated levels of vasopressin also potentially involved.[1,3] Prostaglandins are paracrine hormones that function as inflammatory modulators. Prostaglandins in the uterine muscle stimulate myometrial contractions and ischemia, thereby producing the classic cramping pain of dysmenorrhea.[1] Elevated levels of vasopressin can produce dysrhythmic uterine contractions that reduce uterine blood flow, thereby causing myometrial hypoxia (Figure 30-1).[3]

Pharmacologic Treatments Dysmenorrhea

Antispasmodics have been proposed for treatment of dysmenorrhea but few studies have been conducted assessing use of these agents. Instead, the drugs most often used in the management of primary dysmenorrhea, such as nonsteroidal anti-inflammatory drugs (NSAIDs) are given for pain relief. Other treatments include hormonal contraceptives; estrogen agonists/antagonists (EAAs), which are also known as selective estrogen receptor modulators (SERMs); and various complementary and alternative therapies.

Nonsteroidal Anti-inflammatory Drugs

Nonsteroidal anti-inflammatory drugs are the most common pharmacologic treatment for women with dysmenorrhea. Aspirin is a NSAID, although it has some unusual properties and will be addressed separately. Currently, there is insufficient evidence to determine which NSAID is the most effective and safest option for treating dysmenorrhea, although ibuprofen (Advil, Motrin) often is considered the gold standard because of its proven effectiveness in providing pain relief, low risk of side effects during short-term use, and wide availability in many inexpensive generic formulations (Box 30-1).[2,5,6]

In addition to ibuprofen, other NSAIDs commonly used to treat dysmenorrhea include diclofenac potassium (Cataflam), ketoprofen (Orudis, Orudis KT), naproxen (Naprosyn), and naproxen sodium (Aleve). All of the

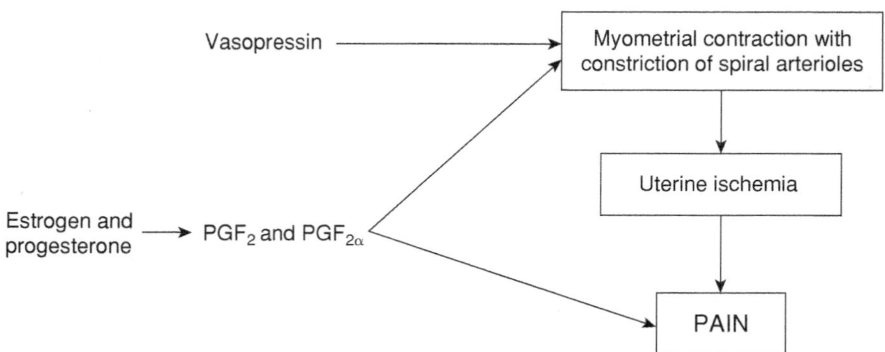

The prostaglandins PGF$_2$ and PGF$_{2\alpha}$ stimulate myometrial contraction and sensitize the afferent nerves to pain, thereby contributing to dysmenorrhea in two ways.

Figure 30-1 Pathophysiology of primary dysmenorrhea.

Table 30-1 Nonsteroidal Anti-inflammatory Drugs Used to Treat a Woman with Primary Dysmenorrhea

Drug: Generic (Brand)	Dose	Onset of Action	Peak Effect	Duration
Acetylsalicylic acid (aspirin)	325–650 mg PO every 3–4 hours Maximum dose 4 g/day	15–20 minutes	1–3 hours	3–6 hours
Diclofenac potassium (Cataflam)	50 mg PO *or* 100 mg PO loading dose followed by 50 mg every 8 hours	30 minutes	2–3 hours	8 hours
Ibuprofen (Advil, Motrin, Midol IB)	400-800 mg PO every 4–6 hours	30 minutes	1–2 hours	4–6 hours
Ketoprofen (Orudis, Orudis KT)	25–50 mg PO every 6–8 hours Maximum dose 300 mg/daily	30 minutes	2 hours	Up to 6 hours
Naproxen (Naprosyn)	500 mg PO for first dose then 250 mg every 6–8 hours as needed	30–60 minutes	2–4 hours	6–8 hours
Naproxen sodium (Aleve)	440 mg PO first dose then 220 mg every 2 times/day	1 hour	1–4 hours	7 hours
Naproxen sodium (Naprelan)	Sustained-release formulation 375-mg or 500-mg tablets; dose is 1000 mg PO once daily	30–60 minutes	Peak unknown	Unknown

aforementioned agents are available in over-the-counter (OTC) formulations (Table 30-1).

Although a full description of the mechanism of action of NSAIDs can be found in the chapter *Analgesia and Anesthesia*, some functions of this class of analgesics are specific to the reproductive tract. The primary mechanism of action of NSAIDs is inhibition of **cyclooxygenase (COX)**, the enzyme that converts arachidonic acid to prostaglandin. When COX is removed from the physiologic pathway, inhibition of PG synthesis occurs, which in

Box 30-1 An Adolescent with Dysmenorrhea

KS, a 15-year-old high school student who is healthy and not sexually active with males or females presents for an ambulatory care visit. She reports "horrible cramps with my periods" for the last 3 months, requiring that she stay home from school for 1–2 days every month. She does not understand why "this is happening now" and questions what she can do. She experienced menarche 18 months prior to this visit and her menses occur every 28–31 days, lasting 4–5 days. Her best friend had dysmenorrhea, but has noticed that it has lessened since she started taking combined oral contraceptives.

Many adolescents and their parents are perplexed that dysmenorrhea occurs not with menarche, but several months thereafter. This is a common timing because the first cycles following the onset of menarche, are often anovulatory and unpredictable. When dysmenorrhea occurs, it generally indicates an ovulatory cycle is occurring. Therefore, one of the first actions is to provide health counseling and reassurance of normalcy for this young woman.

Nonsteroidal anti-inflammatory drugs would be the most logical first-line treatment. Such a drug may be initiated shortly before expected menses or with the first sign of pain or bleeding, usually in a dose of 400–800 mg of ibuprofen (Advil) every 6–8 hours is recommended. There is lack of evidence that any one regimen is superior to the others.

Appropriate to her developmental age, this young woman has a "best friend." Therefore, she is asking about combined oral contraceptives (COCs) because her friend is using them. COCs are another reasonable treatment for dysmenorrhea and may offer this young woman some additional attractive noncontraceptive benefits, such as, improved acne, and potential long-term benefits of protection from endometrial and ovarian cancers. If KF is considering heterosexual activity, the contraceptive protection with COCs will be of value to her. There is no indication that one brand or type (e.g., monophasic, continuous) is better than another. However, the healthcare provider should recognize that most jurisdictions allow adolescents to give personal consent for care only in cases of sexually transmitted diseases, pregnancy, or contraception. Therefore, if KF is not sexually active or does not desire to be sexually active, parental consent for this off-label use of COCs may be required.

Regardless of which treatment is chosen, KF should be told that the menstrual flow may decrease due to the treatment. If she does not experience relief within the next two or three menses, she should return for follow-up.

turn results in decreased hypercontractility of the uterus or decreased dysmenorrhea.[2] Several small studies suggest that NSAIDs decrease the volume of the menstrual flow, although reports of this effect are subjective and, therefore, not amenable to quantification.[7] NSAIDs also have direct analgesic properties in the central nervous system.[2,8]

Of the two main isoforms of the COX enzyme, COX-1 and COX-2, COX-1 is synthesized constitutively and, therefore, is present in all tissues at all times. COX-1 generates prostaglandins that are involved in maintenance of homeostasis, including gastrointestinal mucosal protection, platelet function, regulation of blood flow to the kidney and stomach, and regulation of gastric acid secretion. COX-2, which is inducible, mediates pain and inflammation at the site of tissue damage.[9]

The therapeutic effects of NSAIDs are due primarily to their ability to inhibit production of COX-2. Because inhibition of COX-1 and COX-2 also can suppress ovulation, NSAIDs are not recommended for use by women who are trying to achieve a pregnancy.[10] NSAIDs are metabolized primarily in the liver, and their metabolites are excreted mainly by the kidneys.

Side Effects/Adverse Effects

The most common side effect of NSAIDs is gastric irritation, which can be ameliorated to some degree by taking the medication with food. Serious side effects are gastrointestinal related and include ulceration, gastrointestinal bleeding, and potential perforation. The risks for adverse reactions appear to increase with age and in individuals who have a history of gastrointestinal ulcers, smoking, or alcoholism. Women with the aforementioned history should use NSAIDs with caution and should avoid them entirely if they have ongoing health problems that increase the risk of gastrointestinal irritation. Women who are using selective serotonin reuptake inhibitors (SSRIs) may be at a moderately increased risk of serious upper gastrointestinal events with concurrent NSAID use and also should use NSAIDs with caution.[11] General contraindications to the use of NSAIDs include kidney impairment, liver disease, and active or chronic inflammation or ulceration of the gastrointestinal tract.

The majority of NSAIDs are nonselective—that is, they inhibit both COX-1 and COX-2. However, the **coxibs** are selective COX-2 inhibitors. Because the selective COX-2 inhibitors do not affect COX-1 function, their side-effect profile differs from the one associated with nonselective NSAIDs.

Although initially some COX-2 selective drugs (e.g., celecoxib [Celebrex]) seemed promising candidates as treatments for women with dysmenorrhea, their associated cardiovascular risks appear to outweigh the benefits for most women.[12] Rofecoxib (Vioxx) and valdecoxib (Bextra) were withdrawn from the marketplace in 2004 and 2005, respectively, because of their adverse cardiovascular effects. Today, coxibs are generally not recommended for the treatment of women with dysmenorrhea. In addition, little information is available about use of coxibs in women who are breastfeeding, so alternative NSAID agents, particularly ibuprofen, should be chosen for the breastfeeding woman experiencing dysmenorrhea.[13]

NSAIDs interact with many drugs, as discussed in the *Analgesia and Anesthesia* chapter, so it is critical to know the full details of a woman's pharmacologic history and current use, including prescription medications, OTC products, complementary and herbal preparations, and any other street or recreational drugs, before recommending NSAIDs. For example, NSAIDs decrease the effectiveness of angiotensin-converting enzyme (ACE) inhibitors (antihypertensives) and may prolong prothrombin time if taken with anticoagulants. Women taking NSAIDs should avoid alcohol use because of an increased risk of gastric irritation when NSAIDs and alcohol are used concomitantly.

Acetylsalicylic Acid (Aspirin)

Acetylsalicylic acid (ASA) is an NSAID that has properties which are different from those of other NSAIDs and, therefore, requires separate discussion. The commonalities shared by aspirin and NSAIDs include analgesic, anti-inflammatory, and antipyretic properties. One major difference is that aspirin inhibits platelet aggregation for the life of the platelet, which accounts for some of the adverse side effects observed such as gastrointestinal bleeding. However, this antiplatelet effect is also the reason why aspirin is indicated for other purposes, such as cardiovascular protection.[14]

Aspirin is indicated for treatment of women with mild to moderate pain and may be used to treat dysmenorrhea. If heavy bleeding accompanies the cramping, then aspirin should be avoided because of its antiplatelet effects. Aspirin is contraindicated for anyone with allergies to the agent and should not be used by individuals with bleeding disorders, gastric irritation, or ulcers, or by those who have vitamin K deficiencies. This agent should be used with caution by anyone with asthma, NSAID-induced bronchospasm, or impaired renal function. It should never be prescribed if there is suspicion that the individual (especially if younger than 20 years) has influenza or varicella due to its association with the development of Reye's syndrome. Therefore, adolescents with dysmenorrhea should avoid ASA. Aspirin also should be avoided by persons anticipating surgery within 1 week of taking the medication.

Adverse effects of aspirin include aspirin toxicity, gastric irritation, occult bleeding, and salicylism. A number of drug–drug interactions associated with aspirin exist, such as increased bleeding with oral anticoagulants and increased risk of gastrointestinal ulcers if taken concomitantly with steroids. Salicylates are ototoxic at high blood levels and, therefore, should be discontinued if the individual develops dizziness, tinnitus, or difficulty hearing. Most of the adverse effects of aspirin are associated with long-term use, and the risk for treating women with dysmenorrhea by using aspirin is low. Information regarding doses can be found in Table 30-1.

Hormonal Contraceptives

Combination oral contraceptives (COCs) and other combined hormonal contraceptives often are used to treat dysmenorrhea because they decrease PG synthesis by the endometrial tissues during menstruation.[15] Continuously cycled COCs also result in fewer days of bleeding and, therefore, less opportunity for dysmenorrhea. The off-label use of COCs for dysmenorrhea can provide relief for the women who use them.[16] The Cochrane Collaboration meta-analysis conducted by Wong established that COCs can successfully treat primary dysmenorrhea but did not find a difference in effectiveness amongst the various types of COCs.[15]

Progestin-only contraceptive methods may also be employed as treatment modalities for dysmenorrhea.[17] Progestin-only methods provide time-limited amenorrhea and, therefore, relief from the dysmenorrhea accompanying menstruation.

Considering the added benefit of contraceptive provision, contraceptives may well be considered a first-line approach to treatment of heterosexually active women who have dysmenorrhea and who do not desire a pregnancy. Further discussion about the mechanisms of action, effects, and contraindications of hormonal contraception can be found in the *Contraception* chapter.

Complementary Therapies

A variety of herbal preparations and formulations are marketed for treatment of women with dysmenorrhea. However, there are few well-controlled studies in humans that demonstrate the effectiveness of herbal preparations. Providers unfamiliar with the use of herbs should consult with skilled clinicians such as naturopathic doctors or herbalists who are recognized to prescribe or use these modalities. The *Complementary and Alternative Therapies* chapter addresses use of herbal remedies for treating dysmenorrhea.

The majority of randomized, controlled trials (RCTs) that evaluated the effectiveness of dietary and herbal therapies for treating dysmenorrhea have assessed thiamine (vitamin B_1), vitamin B_6 (pyridoxine), vitamin E, magnesium, omega-3 fatty acids (fish oil), and guaifenesin[18] (Table 30-2).

Table 30-2 Dietary Supplements and Vitamins Used to Treat Women with Dysmenorrhea

Drug: Generic (Brand)	Dose	Available Forms
Guaifenesin	2400 mg/day PO for 2 days[a]	Tablets
Magnesium (MagMin, Maginex, Magnesiocard)	Unclear	Tablets
Omega-3 fatty acids	2 g/daily PO	Liquid
Thiamine hydrochloride (vitamin B_1)	100 mg/daily PO	Elixir Injections Tablets
Tocopherol (vitamin E)	200 IU 2 times/day PO or 2500 IU once daily PO for 5 days	Capsules Drops Liquid Tablets

[a] Guaifenesin comes in many formulations, including long-acting preparations and combination preparations. Generic tablets that contain guaifenesin only are available in 100-mg, 200-mg, and 400-mg tablets and caplets; extended-release tablets contain 600 mg and 1200 mg; liquid preparations have 100 mg/5mL.

Guaifenesin

Guaifenesin is a common expectorant found in many OTC preparations marketed for treating cough. This old drug was originally derived from the resin of guaiacum trees and used in the 16th century as an analgesic. A small RCT that included 25 women assessed the effects of guaifenesin on the participants' dysmenorrhea. Although the findings were not statistically significant, trending demonstrated that the women in the study preferred using guaifenesin over placebo.[19] The theoretical mechanism of action is that guaifenesin thins secretions, which includes vaginal secretions, perhaps decreasing the accompanying dysmenorrhea. However, there are no studies published to date that clearly support its use.

Magnesium

Magnesium is theorized to reduce PGs and decrease muscle contractility.[1] Several older small studies, all with fewer than 50 participants, have found that a magnesium supplement may be used as a treatment for dysmenorrhea.[20–22] The clinical benefits were theorized to be due to both the direct muscle relaxant effects of magnesium and inhibition of the biosynthesis of PGF2 alpha. The true mechanism of action of magnesium is not known; thus the dose, preparation, and regimen to use in the treatment of women with dysmenorrhea are unclear, and further studies are needed.[1]

Omega-3 Fatty Acids (Fish Oil)

Omega-3 polyunsaturated fatty acids are potentially potent anti-inflammatory agents, so they may be effective in combating dysmenorrhea. The theoretic mechanism related to the development of dysmenorrhea is an imbalance between omega-3 fatty acids, from which anti-inflammatory, vasodilator eicosanoids are derived, and omega-6 fatty acids, which increase levels of inflammatory, vasoconstrictor eicosanoids.[23] Diets of women residing in North America typically include fewer omega-3 fatty acid sources (e.g., oily fish) than sources of omega-6 fatty acids (e.g., arachidonic acid).

Some studies suggest that fish oil relieves dysmenorrhea better than placebo, and women whose diets are higher in fish may have less pain during their menses than those with diets low in the fatty acids.[24] Like vitamin E, omega-3 fatty acids may reduce platelet aggregation, so they should be used cautiously by women who are also taking drugs that have anticoagulant properties. In summary, omega-3 fatty acids have potential as treatments for dysmenorrhea because they are effective anti-inflammatory agents and decrease the production of PGs.[25] More studies are warranted to clarify the level of their effectiveness, as well as to determine the optimal dose and route of administration.

Thiamine (Vitamin B_1)

There is some suggestion that vitamin B_1 is most useful for women who have a vitamin B_1 deficiency. Symptoms of a vitamin B_1 deficiency include muscle cramps, fatigue, and reduced pain tolerance.[1] An open trial conducted more than 50 years ago found that 90% of women who took 100 mg of niacin daily when they were actively cramping reported reduced symptoms; however, more rigorous studies have not since been reported.[18]

Tocopherol (Vitamin E)

Vitamin E is used to treat women with dysmenorrhea because it inhibits PG synthesis and promotes vasodilator and uterine muscle relaxation.[3] Small RCTs have suggested that use of vitamin E may decrease dysmenorrhea as well as blood loss more effectively than placebo.[26,27] A precautionary note about vitamin E supplementation is that it may increase the risk of bleeding, especially among women who are taking other medications such as warfarin (Coumadin) or aspirin.

Nonpharmacologic Treatments for Dysmenorrhea

A growing body of information is focused on nonpharmacologic treatments for dysmenorrhea, such as transcutaneous electrical nerve stimulation (TENS), spinal manipulation, acupuncture, and exercise. These interventions are noted only because they may be used in clinical practice to augment or substitute for drugs. In general, larger and more rigorous studies are indicated to ascertain whether they are effective ways to treat women with dysmenorrhea.[28–34]

Abnormal Uterine Bleeding

Abnormal uterine bleeding (AUB) is a term that denotes excessive bleeding during the menses or bleeding that occurs outside the parameters of a normal menstrual cycle.[35] Other terms have been used in the past to further define the specific conditions, such as *menorrhagia*, *metrorrhagia*, and *menometrorrhagia*. The use of these labels is currently discouraged in favor of terms that more clearly and specifically define the occurrence of the abnormal bleeding in relation to frequency, duration, and volume of blood loss.[36,37] A variety of conditions can cause abnormal uterine bleeding, including anovulation, systemic disease, reproductive tract pathology such as sexually transmitted infections, trauma, and drug use or poor nutrition. Some pharmacologic agents have among their side effects a negative influence on normal menses (Table 30-3). Management is directed toward identifying and treating the underlying cause of the AUB.

Acute hemorrhage requires in-hospital treatment and should be individualized based on etiology and a woman's status. Pharmacologic treatments for acute hemorrhage are beyond the scope of this chapter.

Abnormal bleeding may occur in the absence of uterine pathology. Some experts believe abnormal uterine bleeding can be one of two types: ovulatory and

Table 30-3 Selected Drugs That Can Cause Abnormal Vaginal Bleeding

Drug Category	Common Drugs: Generic (Brand)
Agents commonly abused	Alcohol Amphetamines[a] Cannabis Heroin
Alkylating agents	Procarbazine
Anticoagulants	Coumadin (Heparin)
Antidepressants	Tricyclics—e.g., amitriptyline (Elavil)[a] MAO inhibitors—e.g., phenelzine (Nardil)
Antidopaminergics	Droperidol (Inapsine)
Antihistamines	Cimetidine (Tagamet)[a]
Antihypertensives	Methyldopa (Aldomet) Reserpine (Serpasil)[a]
Antitubercular agents	Isoniazid (INH)[a]
Benzodiazepines	Diazepam (Valium)[a]
Butyrophenone antipsychotics	Haloperidol (Haldol)[a]
Diuretics	Spironolactone (Aldactone)[a]
Hormones	Thyroid, estrogen,[a] progesterone,[a] testosterone[a]
Opiates	Methadone Morphine[a]
Phenothiazines	Chlorpromazine (Thorazine) Prochlorperazine (Compazine) Promethazine (Phenergan)
Sedative-hypnotics	Chlordiazepoxide (Librium)

[a] Also associated with galactorrhea.

anovulatory.[35] Pregnancy must first be ruled out in all women of childbearing age who present with uterine bleeding. The goal of treating abnormal bleeding is to normalize the bleeding, correct anemia if present, prevent or diagnose early cancer, and restore quality of life. Treatment is either emergent, requiring hospitalization, or nonemergent and can be effectively undertaken in the office setting. This section focuses on nonemergent treatment.

Age and Abnormal Uterine Bleeding

The approach to accurate assessment and treatment of a woman with AUB varies according to a woman's reproductive status. A brief description of abnormal bleeding patterns and related etiologies in the context of reproductive status provides a framework for differential diagnosis and the appropriate pharmacologic treatment.

Adolescence

Anovulation is frequently the cause of AUB in adolescents from 13 to 17 years, particularly in the 1 to 2 years after menarche. The second most common cause of abnormal bleeding in adolescents is undiagnosed coagulopathies, including von Willebrand's disease, leukemia, or aplastic anemia.[35] Congenital malformations of the uterus or outflow tract may also be the cause of abnormal vaginal bleeding. These conditions become more apparent in the period of time around menarche.

Reproductive Years

Complications of pregnancy can be the cause of abnormal bleeding, which is why it is essential to rule out pregnancy whenever a woman with reproductive potential has AUB. Other causes of AUB during these years include uterine fibroids, endometrial hyperplasia, and anovulation associated with polycystic ovary syndrome.

Perimenopause

As the reproductive system begins its normal transition toward menopause, anovulation, which can be accompanied by abnormal bleeding patterns, occurs with increasing frequency. Menses that are light or absent (amenorrhea) are not uncommon. However, unusually heavy or prolonger menses and bleeding between menses are not normal; further evaluation is warranted in such a case. Because ovulation is unpredictable during the perimenopausal period, pregnancy should always be ruled out prior to treatment.

Postmenopausal Period

Postmenopausal bleeding is never considered normal, and cancer must always be considered as a diagnosis. Bleeding may be due to the endometrium becoming atrophic; however, this diagnosis can be made only after verifying that endometrial cancer or other pathologies are not present.

Treatment of a Woman with Abnormal Uterine Bleeding

Overall, anovulatory bleeding is the most common reason for AUB in all age groups. Anovulation is associated with a level of progesterone that is insufficient to offset estrogen stimulation of the endometrium. The result may be uterine hyperplasia, which causes bleeding that is initially shorter than normal and eventually becomes prolonged and heavy as hyperplasia of the endometrium becomes more pronounced. The most common etiological condition for chronic anovulation is polycystic ovary syndrome (PCOS).[35]

In clinical practice, a progesterone challenge is a commonly used test to determine whether appropriate

Box 30-2 Progesterone Challenge Test

Indication

In the case of secondary amenorrhea with a negative pregnancy test, a progesterone challenge should result in vaginal bleeding if adequate estrogen is present.

Progesterone Options

- Medroxyprogesterone (Provera), 10 mg PO every day for 7–10 days
- Micronized progesterone (Prometrium), 300–400 mg PO every day at bedtime for 10 days
- Norethindrone (Aygestin), 5 mg PO every day for 7–10 days
- Progesterone, 5 mg PO every day for 7–10 days

Interpretation

Withdrawal bleeding that occurs within 2–7 days after last dose validates adequate endogenous estrogen production and signifies the patency of the outflow tract.

endogenous estrogen production is occurring. If a woman has an intact hypothalamus–pituitary–ovarian axis and is not pregnant, bleeding should result within a few days after cessation of the progesterone treatment. This progesterone withdrawal typically is used to induce bleeding among women who are amenorrheic or to regulate menses when a woman is experiencing AUB. If withdrawal bleeding occurs following the administration of a progestogen and the possibility of a pituitary tumor is ruled out, the diagnosis is anovulation, and treatment is as outlined in this section. To administer a progesterone challenge, the clinician can prescribe a variety of agents (Box 30-2). If micronized progesterone is used, it should be taken in the evening because it is known to cause drowsiness, and clinicians should remember that this agent is contraindicated for individuals with peanut allergies because the drug formulation contains peanut oil. Women need to be informed that cyclic progestins prescribed as a progestin challenge test do not provide contraception.

Combined Oral Contraceptives

When a woman is experiencing chronic AUB, regardless of whether she is anovulatory or ovulatory, initial treatment typically is a prescription for combination oral contraceptives. If the bleeding is not acute, the COCs are taken in the usual manner. Usually after 3 months of treatment with COCs, the endometrium will be of normal thickness and subsequent withdrawal of the progesterone will stimulate a normal bleeding episode.[35]

In 2012, a COC consisting of estradiol valerate and dienogest was approved for use in the treatment of a woman with heavy menstrual bleeding.[38] This unique contraceptive is designed with an "estrogen step-down and progestin step-up" formulation in a four-phase design. It also has a shortened, two-day hormone-free interval. Clinical trials remain ongoing with this contraceptive agent; however, preliminary data suggest it may be superior to other COCs and to NSAIDs for the control of heavy menstrual bleeding.[38]

During the use of any hormonal method as treatment modality, if the bleeding remains abnormally heavy or irregular, further investigation is necessary to determine its etiology. Although evidence is not yet well established, the use of any combined hormonal method, such as the contraceptive patch or ring, might also remedy this bleeding pattern for women who prefer a non-oral treatment approach.

Cyclic Progestins

Cyclic progestin therapy instead of combined hormonal contraceptives also may be used to treat heavy or prolonged bleeding associated with chronic anovulation (Table 30-4).

Table 30-4 Progestin Therapy for Treatment of Women with Heavy Menstrual Bleeding

Drug: Generic (Brand)	Dose	Schedule
Aqueous progesterone—progesterone in oil	5–10 mg/day IM for 6–8 days	Must take on consecutive days
Depot medroxyprogesterone acetate (DMPA)	150 mg IM	Administered every 12 weeks
Levonorgestrel intrauterine contraceptive system (LNG-IUS, Mirena, Skyla)	The Mirena and Lilette LNG-IUS contains 52 mg levonorgestrel at time of insertion; Skyla contains 13.5 mg	Mirena approved for contraception for up to 5 years; Skyla and Liletta for 3 years
Medroxyprogesterone acetate (Provera)	5–10 mg PO/day for 5–10 days	Begin on day 16 or 21 of the menstrual cycle
Norethindrone acetate (Aygestin)	2.5–10 mg PO	Start day 5 of the menstrual cycle and end on day 25
Oral micronized progesterone (Prometrium Crinone)[a]	400 mg PO for 10 days	Take in the evening—may cause drowsiness

[a] Contraindicated for women who are allergic to peanuts since it contains peanut oil.

If withdrawal bleeding does not occur within 7 days of stopping the progestogen, further evaluation is merited. Progestin-only contraceptive methods used for this indication, however, do confer contraceptive benefit and may be an appropriate option for women desiring treatment for AUB and contraception. Contraindications to progestins are discussed in the *Steroid Hormones* chapter.

Side Effects/Adverse Effects

Adverse effects commonly associated with use of progestins include headache, irregular bleeding, amenorrhea, bloating, and weight changes. Some women report moodiness. More serious side effects include changes in or loss of vision, cerebrovascular disorders, and increases in blood pressure. If any of the latter signs or symptoms occur, the progestogen should be discontinued immediately. Progestins should not be prescribed if pregnancy is suspected, although there is no documented teratogenic effect.

High-Dose Estrogen

If the cause of the heavy bleeding is anovulation, use of high-dose estrogen usually will end an acute bleeding episode. This hormonal treatment allows time for evaluation of underlying causes and is not considered a long-term treatment. Nausea is a common side effect of high-dose estrogen; therefore, prescribing an antiemetic may be necessary.

Frequently, conjugated equine estrogen (CEE; Premarin) is prescribed as 25 mg administered intravenously every 4 to 6 hours. After the bleeding stops, oral conjugated estrogen in a dose of 2.5–5 mg may be given; it is followed by the addition of 10 mg of medroxyprogesterone acetate (Provera) for the last 10 to 14 days of therapy to initiate withdrawal bleeding.[39] Some clinicians prescribe two or three daily doses of combination oral contraceptives, but most side effects are dose dependent, so this approach is used less often today.

Many women with AUB are treated for an additional period of time, usually approximately 3 months, after which, if there is no improvement, reevaluation is necessary. Information regarding drugs for such long-term management can be found in Table 30-5.

Studies comparing the effectiveness of various doses of estrogens or determining how best to taper the doses are lacking. High-dose estrogen can precipitate a thromboembolic event and, therefore, is contraindicated in women with a history of thrombosis or family history of idiopathic thromboembolism.[35]

Table 30-5 Selected Medical Therapies for Long-Term Management of a Woman with Menorrhagia

Drug: Generic (Brand)	Dose
Combined hormonal contraceptives	Use oral, patch, or ring as usual
Cyclic medroxyprogesterone acetate	10 mg/day PO for 10–14 days every 30–40 days, with or without conjugated equine estrogen[a]
Depot medroxyprogesterone (DMPA)	150 mg IM every 3 months
Levonorgestrel intrauterine contraceptive system (LNG-IUS)	Insert as usual
Nonsteroidal anti-inflammatory drugs	As needed for pain
Oral micronized progesterone[b]	300 mg for 10–14 days, PO every 30–40 days

[a] High doses of estrogen can precipitate a thrombotic event and are contraindicated for women with a history of thrombosis or family history of idiopathic venous thromboembolism.
[b] Contraindicated for women with peanut allergies.

Nonsteroidal Anti-inflammatory Drugs

NSAIDs are effective for treating ovulatory bleeding that is unusually heavy or prolonged. The bleeding may be of sudden onset or a result of several months with heavier bleeding each cycle. It is theorized that NSAIDs may decrease the amount of bleeding because they inhibit production of specific vasodilator prostaglandins.[7] Controversy exists over when to initiate NSAID therapy so as to decrease bleeding, with some clinicians suggesting that women start the agent up to 3 days prior to the onset of the menses, others recommending that it be started with the onset of bleeding, and still others advocating that the drugs be given when menses begins. Evidence is lacking as to which method should be used. Doses are listed in Table 30-6.

Systemic Progestins

Systemic progestins, in addition to being useful for the treatment of women with anovulatory AUB, are also useful

Table 30-6 Nonsteroidal Anti-inflammatory Drugs Used to Treat Menorrhagia

Drug: Generic (Brand)	Dose
Ibuprofen (Advil)	600–800 mg 3 times/day PO for 3–5 days
Mefenamic acid (Ponstel)	500 mg 3 times/day PO for 3–5 days
Naproxen sodium (Aleve)	550 mg loading dose, then 275 mg every 6 hours for 3–5 days PO

for treating ovulatory AUB, although studies suggest their use offers no advantages over other pharmacologic therapies, including NSAIDs, progesterone-releasing intrauterine systems, or danazol (Danocrine).[39] It generally is conceded that progestogen therapy during days 5–26 of the menstrual cycle results in markedly less bleeding.[40] However, women usually find systemic treatment, with its accompanying side effects of bloating and moodiness, less appealing than localized systems, such as the progesterone-releasing intrauterine system, which produce markedly fewer side effects. Amenorrhea due to endometrial atrophy occurs with long-term use of continuous progestin therapy. Progestins are not as effective as estrogen in treating acute bleeding episodes but are effective for long-term treatment for chronic anovulation. These agents should not be prescribed if the woman believes she may be pregnant.

Progestin-Releasing Intrauterine Systems

The levonorgestrel-releasing intrauterine systems (LNG-IUS) release levonorgestrel, a potent progestin, in low daily doses into the uterine cavity, thereby directly targeting the endometrium (Table 30-5). As a result, endometrial proliferation is suppressed, which in turn significantly decreases menstrual flow. Several studies have found that the LNG-IUS (e.g., Mirena) is an effective treatment for heavy menstrual bleeding related to anovulation or leiomyomas, at least compared to medical regimens.[41] Research has demonstrated that women using LNG-IUS experience a marked reduction in bleeding, and following 3 months of use, they often indicate their menstrual flow has become light. This method is satisfying to the user, can be cost-effective, and is more effective than oral treatment modalities. Decreased flow is less pronounced with the lower-dose LNG-IUS, Skyla, than with Mirena; consequently, Skyla is not presently approved for the treatment of women with heavy menstrual bleeding. In 2015, a new LNG-IUS was approved by the FDA. This contraceptive, Lilette, although similar to Mirena, currently has an indication only for contraception.

Continuous use of the Mirena LNG-IUS can effectively suppress endometrial proliferation for at least 5 years.[42] The most common side effects of progesterone-releasing intrauterine systems are related to the levonorgestrel component and include mood changes, acne, breast tenderness, hirsutism, and weight change, although these side effects occur to a lesser degree compared to systemic delivery of levonorgestrel.[42] Some intermenstrual spotting, which is a normal side effect frequently experienced with any IUS or IUD, may occur. The *Contraception* chapter provides an in-depth discussion of the risks and benefits associated with using an intrauterine agent.

Androgens

Danazol (Danocrine) is a weak androgen that has been found in some studies to be more effective than NSAIDs, progestogens, or COCs for the treatment of women with heavy menstrual bleeding.[35] A 2007 Cochrane Collaboration meta-analysis of danazol for treatment of women with this abnormal bleeding pattern supported positive findings from earlier RCTs, but the authors noted that the confidence intervals of the studies reviewed were wide and the results imprecise.[43] Women on danazol also reported more adverse effects compared to those taking NSAIDs (odds ratio [OR], 7.0; 95% confidence interval [CI], 1.7–28.2) or progestogens (OR, 4.05; 95% CI, 1.6–10.2), including androgenic side effects such as hot flashes, hirsutism, and acne, which are not acceptable to most women.[35,43] It appears from current studies that danazol may be effective in treating dysmenorrhea, but its use in this indication is limited because of its side effects.

Gonadotropin-Releasing Hormone Agonists

Gonadotropin-releasing hormone (GnRH) agonists attach to the gonadotropin-releasing hormone receptor in the pituitary, which stimulates the synthesis and release of follicle-stimulating hormone (FSH) and luteinizing hormone (LH); the FSH and LH then facilitate regulation of the menstrual cycle via their natural biologic functions. GnRH agonists are a synthetic form of GnRH. Native GnRH is released in a pulsatile fashion, causing stimulation of the release of gonadotropins. When these agents are administered constantly, an exacerbation of symptoms—a flare tends to occur first. Within a few weeks, the GnRH receptors retract into the pituitary cell—a process called downregulation. At that point, these drugs effectively suppress pituitary production of FSH and LH, which results in hypoestrogenemia amenorrhea and decreases in uterine and leiomyoma volume.[35]

Typically, the GnRH agonists have been used to treat prostatic and breast cancer. They are also useful for the treatment of women with endometriosis and leiomyomata. Often the formulation is depot in nature, indicating that the drug should be injected or implanted allowing it to be slowly absorbed into the circulation.

GnRH agonist therapy generally is reserved for episodes of acute menorrhagia caused by leiomyomas. Such treatment enables the woman's hemoglobin to return to normal prior to surgery or other types of intervention. Information

Table 30-7 Gonadotropin-Releasing Hormone Agonists Used to Treat Heavy Menstrual Bleeding[a]

Drug: Generic (Brand)	Dose/Route and Course of Treatment
Goserelin (Zoladex)	Administered via implant. To thin the endometrium, the following schedule is suggested: • One to two 3.6-mg SQ depots 4 weeks apart • Surgery is done week 4 after the first dose and within 2–4 weeks after the second dose if two are used
Leuprolide acetate (Lupron Depot—3 month or 4 month)	Use depot formulation: 3.75 mg IM as a single monthly injection for 3 months or 11.25 mg IM once
Nafarelin acetate (Synarel)	Primarily used to treat endometriosis; however, its mechanism of action decreases heavy bleeding. Dose: 400 mcg/day: one spray (200 mcg) into one nostril in the morning and one spray into the other nostril in the evening. Start treatment between days 2 and 4 of the menstrual cycle. Treatment is recommended for maximum of 6 months.

[a] If anemia is present due to the heavy menstrual bleeding, iron supplements and attention to dietary iron sources also are recommended.

about doses for GnRH agonist therapy is provided in Table 30-7.

Leuprolide Acetate

Leuprolide acetate (Lupron Depot) is a luteinizing hormone agonist that occupies pituitary GnRH receptors and desensitizes them.[44] This agent is available in either 3- or 4-month doses. It is contraindicated in pregnancy and among women who have undiagnosed vaginal bleeding. Leuprolide acetate should be used cautiously by women who are lactating. Adverse effects may include dizziness, headache, blurred vision, lethargy, peripheral edema, thrombophlebitis, and myocardial infarction. Women using leuprolide may experience urinary frequency and hematuria that can be an indication of urinary obstruction or other abnormality; if either condition occurs, they should be referred to a specialist. Hot flashes, sweats, and bone pain may also accompany use of leuprolide acetate.[44]

Nafarelin Acetate

Nafarelin acetate (Synarel) is a potent GnRH analogue that initially stimulates LH and FSH release from the pituitary, whereas prolonged use causes desensitization of the GnRH receptor and then decreased LH and FSH secretion.[44] The desired therapeutic effect is diminished bleeding from endometrial tissue that is no longer stimulated by LH and FSH.

Women who have undiagnosed vaginal bleeding, women who are pregnant, and women who are lactating should not take nafarelin acetate. Side effects include headaches, sleep disorders, and some dizziness. The androgenic side effects of nafarelin can cause acne, hirsutism, and weight gain. Hypoestrogenic side effects may include vasomotor reactions such as hot flashes, sweating, and emotional lability. A significant adverse effect for women who use the drug on a long-term basis is decreased bone density; therefore, any woman who has osteoporosis or osteopenia should not take nafarelin. Treatment is generally limited to 6 months because of the risk of osteoporosis. If treatment is longer than 6 months, concomitant therapy with low doses of estrogen and progesterone is recommended to prevent bone loss.

Goserelin Acetate

Goserelin acetate (Zoladex) is a potent inhibitor of pituitary gonadotropin secretion. Its initial administration produces a rise in FSH and LH, which in turn stimulates testosterone production, leading to a flare reaction. After 2 to 4 weeks of therapy, women taking goserelin have lowered serum estradiol levels that effectively reduce the size and function of the ovaries.[35] The uterus and mammary glands also decrease in size.

Goserelin is contraindicated in women who have undiagnosed vaginal bleeding, are sensitive to any GnRH drugs, or are pregnant or lactating. Adverse effects may include insomnia, lethargy, emotional lability, cardiac arrhythmia, nausea, and anorexia. Hot flashes, dysmenorrhea, and urinary tract and vaginal infections have also been reported.

Antifibrinolytic Agents

A final approach to abnormally heavy menstrual bleeding focuses on the desired endpoint of hemostasis at the level of the endometrium. Various hemostatic agents have been used in the past to control bleeding in surgical situations; however, the use of such agents to control menstrual bleeding remains a somewhat new approach in the United States. In 2009, the FDA approved tranexamic acid (Lysteda) for the treatment of women with heavy menstrual bleeding. Tranexamic acid is an antifibrinolytic agent that decreases blood loss by blocking plasma-binding sites and preventing fibrinolysis. The result is a significant decrease in menstrual bleeding compared to placebo. Comparisons to hormonal treatments have not yet been established.[45]

In addition to the reported gastrointestinal upset side effects of this drug, it is important to remember that thrombosis is a significant potential pharmacodynamic adverse effect. Consequently, concurrent use of hormonal contraceptives is not recommended, nor are other drugs commonly used by menstruating women, such as NSAIDs.[45] Tranexamic acid is also clearly contraindicated in women otherwise at risk of thromboembolic events.

Tranexamic acid does not resolve any underlying structural or hormonal causes of heavy menstrual bleeding and it may be costly, but it does provide important time-limited and reversible relief for some women. The recommended dose of this drug, which is supplied in 650-mg tablets, is 2 tablets 3 times a day during menstruation only, for up to 5 days.[44,45]

Premenstrual Syndrome and Premenstrual Dysphoric Disorder

Premenstrual syndrome (PMS) is common among reproductive-aged women, from adolescence to midlife. The distinct pattern of emotional, cognitive, behavioral, and physical symptoms affiliated with PMS occurs during the luteal phase of the menstrual cycle and spontaneously subsides within a few days of the onset of menses.[35] Premenstrual dysphoric disorder (PMDD) is a diagnostic label from the American Psychological Association,[46] which describes PMDD as a depressive disorder with symptoms that are much more severe than those experienced with PMS and includes predominant severity of emotional symptoms.[46,47] Symptoms experienced by women who have either PMS or PMDD include abdominal bloating and pain, irritability, moodiness, depression, decreased ability to concentrate, fatigue, headache, and breast tenderness and pain.[35,48] It is estimated that approximately 85% of menstruating women have one or more of these symptoms, and as many as 10% report symptoms so severe they are disabling.[46] Additionally, approximately 8% of women who are ovulating experience PMDD.[49]

The etiology of PMS/PMDD remains unclear, but most authorities suspect gonadal hormones are involved because ovulation suppression frequently results in improvement. Initial treatment is often nonpharmacologic; however, if symptoms remain unrelieved, then symptom-specific drugs are prescribed. Treatment is by necessity individualized and symptom specific. Selective serotonin reuptake inhibitors are considered the first-line treatment for PMS/PMDD, while drugs such as anxiolytics, ovulation suppressants, and diuretics are recommended for specific symptoms.[50] Additional information about psychotropic drugs can be found in the *Mental Health* chapter.

Selective Serotonin Reuptake Inhibitors

Selective serotonin reuptake inhibitors (SSRIs) (fluoxetine [Prozac], paroxetine [Paxil], sertraline [Zoloft], and citalopram [Celexa]) are considered first-line drugs for severe PMS and for PMDD.[50] Fluoxetine can be found in two popular forms: a green and white pill marketed under the brand name Prozac, or a pink and purple tablet, directly advertised to consumers under the name Sarafem. Other than coloring and outside packaging, the agents are the same. It has been suggested that rebranding the drug enabled women to avoid any perceived stigma associated with use of antidepressants; others have suggested it allows the manufacturer to set different prices for the drug.[51]

The SSRIs inhibit serotonin transporters, thereby preventing reuptake of serotonin into the presynaptic neurons, which increases the synaptic concentration. Because the symptoms of PMS/PMDD occur during the luteal phase with remittance at the onset of menses, many authorities suggest that treatment can be limited to the luteal phase.[52]

There does appear to be a difference in the involvement of the serotonergic system in PMDD relative to other depressive orders. The response to SSRIs is much more rapid among women with PMDD than among women who have other depressive disorders.[52] Another distinction is that SSRIs are effective for PMDD even when administered only during the luteal phase.[52]

A wide variety of SSRIs are effective in treating severe PMS and PMDD. Some of the more common SSRIs used to treat PMS/PMDD are discussed here, and information about doses and the extensive drug–drug interactions associated with these agents are provided in alphabetical order in Table 30-8.

Fluoxetine Hydrochloride (Prozac)

Fluoxetine hydrochloride (Prozac, Sarafem) is indicated for the treatment of women with symptoms such as anger/irritability, depression, and affect lability related to PMDD. When taken during the luteal phase, fluoxetine significantly ameliorates mood-related symptoms associated with PMDD; however, it has little effect on associated physical symptoms such as leg and joint pain.[52] Fluoxetine

Table 30-8 Drugs Used for Treatment of Women with Severe Premenstrual Syndrome and Premenstrual Dysphoric Disorder

Drug: Generic (Brand)	Category	Indication	Dose	Onset/Peak of Action
Alprazolam (Xanax XR)[a]	Benzodiazepine	Anxiety and other affective symptoms	PMS dose: 0.25 mg PO 3 times/day PMDD dose: 0.375–1.5 mg PO once daily	30 min/1–2 hours
Bromocriptine mesylate (Parlodel)	Dopamine receptor agonist	Mastalgia	Up to 2.5 mg PO 3 times/day	Varies/1–3 hours
Citalopram hydrobromide (Celexa)	SSRI	Premenstrual dysphoric disorder	20 mg/day PO as a single dose. Increase to 40 mg/day only if clearly needed and no response. For use only during luteal phase.	Onset: 4 hours
Clomipramine hydrochloride (Anafranil)	Tricyclic antidepressant	All symptoms, anticholinergic effects	25–75 mg/day PO	Slow onset
Fluoxetine hydrochloride (Sarafem)	SSRI	Premenstrual dysphoric disorder	20 mg/day PO starting 14 days prior to menses and continue until first day of menses. Do not exceed 80 mg/day.	Onset: 6–8 hours
Ibuprofen (Advil)	NSAID	Pain/mastalgia	600–1000 mg/day PO	Onset: 0.5–1 hour; duration: 4–6 hours
Paroxetine hydrochloride (Paxil)	SSRI	Premenstrual dysphoric disorder	12.5 mg/day PO as a single dose in the morning. Range 12.5–25 mg/day. May be given daily or only during luteal phase of cycle.	Onset: 5 hours
Sertraline hydrochloride (Zoloft)	SSRI	Premenstrual dysphoric disorder	50 mg/day PO or only during luteal phase of menstrual cycle	Onset: 4.5–8 hours
Spironolactone (Aldactone)	Diuretic	Water retention	100 mg PO once daily	24–48 hours/ 48–72 hours

Abbreviations: NSAID = nonsteroidal anti-inflammatory drug; SSRI = selective serotonin reuptake inhibitor.
[a] Alprazolam is a controlled Schedule IV substance.

is contraindicated for individuals with hypersensitivity to the medication. This agent should be used cautiously by women who have impaired liver or renal function, diabetes mellitus, or a history of seizures or suicide attempts. Although information about its use during lactation is generally lacking, fluoxetine is considered by the American Academy of Pediatrics to be a drug that may be of concern for use during lactation.[53]

Adverse effects of fluoxetine include headache, nervousness, drowsiness, seizures, and dizziness. Hot flashes may occur with use. Dermatologic adverse effects include sweating, rash, pruritus, and contact dermatitis. Gastrointestinal adverse effects include nausea, vomiting, diarrhea, anorexia, dry mouth, and constipation, and some women will notice taste changes. Some women using fluoxetine note an increase in dysmenorrhea, sexual dysfunction in the form of loss of libido, and urinary frequency. Weight changes are not uncommon.

Fluoxetine should never be taken with monoamine oxidase (MAO) inhibitors or within 14 days of the administration of an MAO inhibitor because this drug–drug interaction can be fatal.[54] Increased serum concentrations of tricyclic antidepressants (TCAs) occur if taken concomitantly with fluoxetine. Smoking decreases the effectiveness of fluoxetine, and this agent should not be combined with alcohol. Avoidance of other serotonergic drugs when taking fluoxetine is critical because of the risk of serotonin syndrome (hypertension, hyperthermia, and mental status changes).

Paroxetine (Paxil)

Paroxetine (Paxil) provides an antidepressant effect and is FDA approved to treat depressive symptoms associated with PMDD.[55] It is contraindicated for any woman who is also using MAO inhibitors or thioridazine (Mellaril). Adverse effects include somnolence, dizziness, insomnia, headache, and sometimes anxiety. Sweating and rash may occur. Nausea, dry mouth, constipation, and diarrhea are notable gastrointestinal side effects.[54]

Paroxetine interacts with digoxin (Lanoxin) and phenytoin (Dilantin) by decreasing the therapeutic effects of these drugs. If paroxetine is used with procyclidine (Kemadrin), tryptophan, or warfarin (Coumadin), it can increase the serum concentrations of these drugs, with toxicity as a potential outcome.[54]

Sertraline Hydrochloride (Zoloft)

The therapeutic actions of sertraline hydrochloride (Zoloft) are the same as the therapeutic effects of other

SSRIs. Sertraline is indicated for treatment of women with mood-related symptoms of PMDD. It is contraindicated for anyone who has hypersensitivity to SSRIs or specifically to sertraline. This drug should be used with caution by individuals with impaired liver or renal function. Side effects include general CNS effects such as headache, nervousness, drowsiness, insomnia, and fatigue. This drug may cause nausea and vomiting, diarrhea, and dry mouth. Sertraline also may increase the risk of developing dysmenorrhea.

Sertraline should never be used concomitantly with MAO inhibitors, and at least 14 days should elapse between MAO inhibitor and sertraline use. There is a possible risk of abnormal heart rhythms if sertraline is used with the antipsychotic pimozide (Orap), and these two drugs should not be used concurrently. Food increases the absorption rate of sertraline. If sertraline is taken by a woman who is also using St. John's wort, there is a risk of a serotonin syndrome, a condition in which toxic levels of serotonin can cause symptoms that range from mild (e.g., diarrhea) to severe (e.g., seizures) symptoms.[54]

Citalopram Hydrobromide (Celexa)

Citalopram hydrobromide (Celexa), an SSRI, is used on an off-label basis to treat PMDD.[35] It is contraindicated for anyone who is using MAO inhibitors or other SSRIs and should not be used concomitantly with pimozide (Orap). Citalopram should be used with caution by individuals with hepatic or renal impairment, and its side effects are the same as those associated with other SSRIs.

If citalopram is taken with MAO inhibitors, the serum concentration of citalopram can increase, which in turn increases the risk of toxicity. There should be a 14-day window following cessation of MAO inhibitors prior to administering citalopram. Increased citalopram serum concentrations can develop in persons who also are also taking azole antifungals or macrolide antibiotics.[54] There is a possibility of severe adverse effects if this agent is used concomitantly with TCAs, erythromycin (E-Mycin), or beta blockers. Citalopram may increase the bleeding time of persons on warfarin (Coumadin). It should not be taken with pimozide (Orap), as this combination can cause fatal heart arrhythmias.

Other Pharmacologic Agents

In addition to the drugs already reviewed for treatment of women with PMS/PMDD, there are a variety of other pharmacologic agents from various drug classes that can be prescribed. These agents have varying degrees of effectiveness and some have side effect profiles that limit use.

Clomipramine Hydrochloride (Anafranil)

Clomipramine hydrochloride (Anafranil) is a tricyclic antidepressant. TCAs affect the neurotransmitters serotonin and norepinephrine by inhibiting their reuptake into the presynaptic neurons.[54] These drugs are also antagonists of histamine receptors, a mechanism of action that contributes to their notable side effects of weight gain and drowsiness. TCAs are absorbed in the gastrointestinal tract following oral administration. They are highly lipophilic and protein bound.[54]

TCAs are used to treat depression and are less costly than newer drugs, such as some of the selective serotonin reuptake inhibitors. However, the side effects of TCAs are more serious than those associated with SSRIs, so TCAs are not prescribed as often for PMS/PMDD.

TCAs are contraindicated for anyone with a cardiac disorder because of their direct alpha-adrenergic blocking effect.[54] They should be used with caution by women who have glaucoma or urinary incontinence. TCAs should not be prescribed to anyone who is also taking MAO inhibitors.[54] These drugs are excreted in small amounts in breast milk, so caution should be used when prescribing a TCA to a breastfeeding woman.

Side effects of clomipramine include sedation and anticholinergic effects such as dry mouth, constipation, urinary hesitancy, and urinary retention. Other side effects include weight gain, drowsiness, and loss of libido. As with all drugs affecting the CNS, the dose of clomipramine should be titrated slowly when increasing or decreasing the dose. The therapeutic window is very narrow, so great caution should be taken when prescribing this agent for PMDD if depression with suicidal ideology is apparent.

The most significant drug interactions are those that increase the blood levels of clomipramine, increasing the risk of toxicity and cardiac arrhythmias. The *Mental Health* chapter includes discussion of a number of drug–drug interactions that are associated with TCAs.

Drospirenone

Drospirenone, a unique progestin and an analogue of spironolactone, is a component of some combined oral contraceptives (e.g., Yasmin). These agents were the first oral contraceptives to be approved for the treatment of women with premenstrual syndrome and provide a safe, acceptable, and effective treatment for PMS and PMDD.[56]

As it is a component of a combined oral contraceptive, more information on drospirenone can be found in the *Contraception* chapter.

It is important to note that any combined oral contraceptive with a shortened hormone-free interval may provide benefit to women with PMS and PMDD due to the lack of a "withdrawal" time frame. Similarly, any combined hormonal contraceptive may be used in a continuous fashion with no hormone-free interval. Caution is recommended in using COCs for women at high risk of developing blood clots or otherwise at risk with regard to COC use.

Tamoxifen to Treat a Woman with PMS-Related Mastalgia

Tamoxifen, a selective estrogen receptor modulator, is a drug most commonly used for women to treat or prevent breast cancer. It has also been studied as a relief measure for mastalgia at a dose of 10–20 mg daily.[57] In spite of its effectiveness in treating mastalgia, this agent has a significant side-effect profile, including "menopause-like" symptoms such as hot flashes and vaginal dryness; consequently, it is not considered a preferred drug for this indication.

Spironolactone to Treat a Woman with PMS-Associated Water Retention

Spironolactone (Aldactone) is a potassium-sparing diuretic and aldosterone antagonist that can provide relief from water retention. The use of this agent for the treatment of women with PMS is an off-label indication. In recent years, spironolactone has largely been abandoned for more effective treatments with a more acceptable side-effect profile.

Alprazolam to Treat a Woman with PMS-Associated Anxiety

Alprazolam (Xanax) is a benzodiazepine and anxiolytic used to treat anxiety disorders; its mechanism of action is not well understood. Studies suggest an involvement with the gamma-aminobutyric acid (GABAergic) neural pathway system.[58] Although alprazolam is used off-label to treat women with PMS and PMDD, this drug has been used successfully to treat symptoms of profound anxiety among women who suffer from a severe form of either condition.[35] The dose for treating anxiety associated with PMS is less than the dose for treating anxiety associated with PMDD. This drug is potentially addictive and the most commonly abused benzodiazepine; therefore, it is considered a second-line treatment for women with PMS/PMDD.[58]

Alprazolam is contraindicated for individuals with hypersensitivity to benzodiazepines or those who have acute narrow-angle glaucoma. Moreover, it should not be used during lactation because breastfeeding infants whose mothers use the drug may become lethargic and suffer weight loss. Adverse effects in women include mild drowsiness, particularly when the drug is initiated; lightheadedness; headache; and restlessness.[35]

Historic but Ineffective Methods of Treatment

Bromocriptine mesylate (Parlodel), an antiparkinson drug and a dopamine agonist receptor, was once used as a lactation suppressant given to women postpartum who did not want to breastfeed. It was also a treatment for PMS-related mastalgia. Bromocriptine is no longer used for these conditions due to either ineffectiveness or a range of side effects.

Progesterone acetate has been widely prescribed for the treatment of women with PMS. Unfortunately, few studies demonstrate its effectiveness, and some experts suggest that progesterone actually worsens some of the physical and emotional symptoms associated with PMS.[48]

With the exception of combined oral contraceptives containing the progestin drospireonone,[56] COCs are not consistent in their effectiveness for treating PMS or PMD. Progesterone-only methods may actually worsen the symptoms associated with PMS in some women, while ameliorating the physical symptoms for others.[48,59] Overall, their use—particularly for women with severe PMS and those with PMDD—is very limited.

Complementary and Alternative Treatments for PMS and PMDD

Several lifestyle modifications can be suggested to ease many of the symptoms of PMS and PMDD, yet data on their effectiveness are generally lacking, although many have biologic plausibility. Routine exercise improves many symptoms of PMS, possibly by releasing endorphins, which may help to elevate mood. Dietary modifications also have great potential in improving many of the symptoms. Diets high in complex carbohydrates could reduce food cravings, and foods high in tryptophan could elevate brain levels of serotonin and help improve mood. Reducing sodium consumption could reduce water retention and weight gain. Lowering caffeine intake as part of the diet could aid in improving sleep and reduce irritability. Multiple studies have been conducted on various interventions, but most of the

Table 30-9 Complementary and Alternative Treatments for Women with Premenstrual Syndrome and/or Premenstrual Dysphoric Disorder

Agent	Dose	Symptoms Relieved
Nutritional Supplements		
Calcium carbonate	1200–1600 mg/day PO	Negative mood, water retention, and food cravings
Magnesium	200–500 mg/day PO taken either cyclically or only during luteal phase	Bloating
Vitamin B_6	25–100 mg/day PO	Mastalgia, swollen breasts, pain, bloating, and depression
Herbal Products		
Chasteberry (*Vitex agnus castus*)	20–40 mg/day PO	Effective for short term use Relieves breast engorgement and core symptoms
Evening primrose oil	500 mg/day to 1000 mg 3 times/day PO	No evidence for effectiveness but purported use is to treat breast tenderness
St. John's wort (*Hypericum perforatum*)[a]	300 mg/day PO	Mood disturbances

[a] Rare but severe phototoxicity reported with use. Significant drug reactions can also occur, including reduced levels of oral contraceptives, theophylline, cyclosporine, antiretroviral drugs, digoxin, buspirone, and carbamazepine.

research involves small numbers; thus more rigorous studies are needed.

Vitamins and Dietary Supplements

Vitamin supplements including calcium and magnesium have been studied for their ability to reduce many of the physical symptoms of PMS. Some symptoms of hypocalcemia (depression, muscle cramps, and personality disturbances) mimic those of PMS. Several clinical trials have found calcium supplementation to be effective in reducing PMS symptoms such as anxiety, depression, irritability, mood swings, headache, fluid retention, and menstrual cramps.[60–62] A dose of 1200 mg of calcium carbonate (Tums) daily, in divided doses taken 2 to 4 times per day, is the typical dose used in most of these trials.

Similar to calcium, magnesium levels also fluctuate with the menstrual cycle. Magnesium is involved in many cellular pathways that directly influence PMS. In addition, magnesium deficiency has been linked to PMS.[63] A dose of 200 to 360 mg magnesium per day in divided doses during the luteal phase is the typical dose used for treating PMS. A Cochrane Collaboration meta-analysis that included three small RCTs comparing magnesium to placebo found magnesium was effective in relieving pain and decreased the need for additional medication, but noted that more studies in this area are needed.[18]

A systematic review of the effectiveness of pyridoxine (vitamin B_6) for treatment of women with PMS included nine clinical trials (n = 940 women) and suggested that this vitamin may improve several PMS symptoms; most of the trials, however, were of low quality. Larger and more sophisticated (in terms of design) studies are needed to verify this effect. The mechanism of pyridoxine's possible benefit is unclear but could relate to its role as a necessary cofactor for dopamine production in the brain.

Supplementation with other vitamins, such as vitamins E and D, has also been investigated for possible benefits in treating PMS.[64,65] Table 30-9 provides doses and other information about complementary and alternative modality (CAM) treatments purported to be effective in the treatment of women with PMS or PMDD.

Pelvic Pain

Dysmenorrhea is pain that accompanies menses, yet some women have pain independent of their menstrual cycles. The etiology of pelvic pain is challenging because the nature of the pain can be diffuse and difficult to localize. Pelvic pain is a symptom, not a disease, and it may stem from a variety of causes, such as gastrointestinal conditions or disorders within the reproductive tract.

Pelvic pain is subdivided into two types: acute and chronic. Regardless of the type of pelvic pain or underlying pathology, the first consideration always should be adequate pain relief for the woman. In many situations, nonpharmacologic pain relief strategies and pharmaceutical agents can be employed, especially if the woman is undergoing painful but necessary examinations to identify the exact causative factor.

Acute Pelvic Pain

Because pelvic pain may be caused by infections (e.g., urinary tract), muscle strain, or other factors, most pharmacotherapeutic interventions for conditions related to acute pelvic pain are discussed in specific chapters elsewhere in this text. For example, obstetric/gynecologic causes of acute pelvic pain include ectopic pregnancy, as discussed in the *Pregnancy* chapter, and salpingitis associated with pelvic infections, as described in the *Sexually Transmitted Infections* chapter. Some etiologies, such as ovarian torsion, require surgical intervention.

Chronic Pelvic Pain

Chronic pelvic pain is an enigmatic symptom that may signal one of several pathologies or, perhaps, no identifiable entity at all. Nevertheless, it is cited as the main indication for 12% of hysterectomies performed in the United States.[66] Some sources suggest that chronic pelvic pain often may be misdiagnosed. In one study, more than one-third of women presenting with a diagnosis of chronic pelvic pain actually had irritable bowel syndrome.[67] Some women with painful bladder syndrome or interstitial cystitis are first evaluated for chronic pelvic pain.

The generally accepted definition of chronic pelvic pain relates to duration as opposed to intensity. Three months of pain is usually the time required for persistent pain to be termed "chronic," although this criterion is not standardized. Some sources mandate a 6-month period, and the pain may be of constant low-level intensity or of varying degrees of discomfort. The woman may describe pain as originating in a variety of areas, including the vagina, uterus, bladder, gastrointestinal tract, or spine.

Treatments for a Woman with Pelvic Pain

Currently the most commonly used interventions for pelvic pain include laparoscopy, which is performed to assess and exclude serious pathology, as well as analgesics, hormonal therapy, and surgery to interrupt nerve pathways. A Cochrane Collaboration review included 21 RCTs that focused on pain relief and increase in quality of life.[68] The participants included women with chronic pelvic pain but without primary dysmenorrhea, endometriosis, chronic pelvic inflammatory disease, or irritable bowel syndrome. Although counseling and a multidisciplinary approach demonstrated value, among the drugs used, only medroxyprogesterone acetate (MPA; oral Provera and injectable DMPA) and goserelin (Zoladex) appeared to be of value.

Goserelin is a GnRH analogue that is chemically similar to native GnRH but possesses an extended half-life. The usual dose is 3.6 mg administered subcutaneously as an implant every 28 days. Goserelin rapidly binds to the GnRH receptor cells in the pituitary gland, leading to an initial increase in production of luteinizing hormone and, therefore, an initial increase in the production of corresponding sex hormones—and, in turn, a flare effect that can be worse than the original symptoms. However, after 2 to 3 weeks, production of LH is reduced due to receptor downregulation.

Goserelin is not widely used for several reasons: the flare effect, its overall expense, and the time limitation of 6 months imposed on its use. Thus, there is no clear and effective single drug that a clinician can prescribe for chronic pelvic pain. Most women suffering from chronic pelvic pain are treated for specific symptoms, such as dysmenorrhea or infertility or subfertility, which may respond to various pharmacologic treatments.

Infertility

Women with pelvic pain or abnormal menstrual conditions also commonly experience infertility. Infertility is defined as failure to achieve a pregnancy after 12 months of appropriately timed unprotected intercourse. Infertility has many causes, with 55% of cases being attributed to female factors, 35% to male factors, and 10% to an unexplained causes.[35] Ovulatory disorders are an identified cause of female infertility, and PCOS is the most common cause of infrequent or inconsistent ovulation and anovulation.[35]

The successful treatment of women with infertility is continuously improving, with new methods and new drugs being discovered on a regular basis. Many of these drugs are extremely potent and have adverse effects, necessitating specific guidelines to assure the woman's safety and to avoid superfecundity. It is recommended that clinicians who are not specialists in infertility collaborate and consult with specialists in the field of infertility before prescribing any fertility regimen.

Infertility and Thyroid Disorders

Thyroid deficiency can cause ovulatory dysfunction.[69] Signs of hypothyroidism include menstrual irregularities both in cycle regularity and bleeding patterns. For women with hypothyroidism, a euthyroid status usually is achieved with thyroxine supplementation, with spontaneous ovulatory cycles typically resuming after such therapy is established.[70]

Synthetic thyroid replacement compounds are used instead of natural hormones because the bioavailability of the natural compounds varies.[71] Thyroid hormone is contraindicated for women with a history of an acute myocardial infarction (MI). Thyroid hormone also decreases the effectiveness of digoxin (Lanoxin). Thyroid levels need to be monitored when thyroid replacement drugs are prescribed. Additional information about thyroid disease and pharmacologic treatments can be found in the *Thyroid Disorders* chapter.

Infertility and Amenorrhea

Amenorrhea is categorized as either primary or secondary. Primary amenorrhea is defined as an absence of menses by age 14 years with accompanying delayed maturation of secondary sex characteristics, or absence of menses by age 16 years regardless of the presence of secondary sex characteristics. Secondary amenorrhea describes women who have a cessation of menses after having previously menstruated regularly, and who are not pregnant. Once pregnancy is ruled out in a woman with amenorrhea, then a prolactin level, a thyroid-stimulating hormone level, and a progesterone challenge are the usual diagnostic steps in determining the cause of the amenorrhea.

Pharmacologic Treatments for a Woman with Infertility

Ovulatory disorders account for 30% to 40% of all cases of female infertility.[69] However, ovulatory induction and superovulation are the most widely used treatments for infertility, especially because well-established agents have existed for the last several decades.[70,72] Ovarian stimulation is accomplished by either the administration of exogenous gonadotropins or the augmentation of endogenous FSH with clomiphene citrate (Clomid).[35,72] Table 30-10 provides common doses and additional information about fertility drugs. The World Health Organization (WHO) and the European Society for Human Reproduction and Embryology developed a classification system of ovulatory disorders that assists in the identification of associated health risks and defining options for treatment.[73]

Clomiphene Citrate

Clomiphene citrate (Clomid, Milophene, Serophene) is an estrogen agonist/antagonist that has been the first line of treatment for ovulatory disorders for more than 40 years, resulting in a fecundity rate of 15%.[35] This agent is indicated for treatment of women with ovulatory failure who have normal liver function and normal endogenous estrogen levels. Clomiphene citrate decreases the number of available estrogen receptors, which falsely signals the hypothalamus and pituitary to increase FSH and LH secretion. This action, in turn, stimulates the ovary.[35]

Clomiphene citrate is contraindicated for any woman who suspects she is pregnant or who has AUB of undetermined etiology, an ovarian cyst, uncontrolled renal or thyroid dysfunction, or organic intracranial lesions. It should be used with caution during lactation. Women taking

Table 30-10 Fertility Drugs

Drug: Generic (Brand)	Dose/Route and Course of Treatment
Clomiphene citrate (Clomid, Milophene, Serophene)	Ovulatory failure: Initial treatment: 50 mg PO for 5 days started anytime if no recent bleeding or on fifth day of cycle if uterine bleeding occurs Second course: If ovulation does not occur after first course, administer 100 mg/day PO for 5 days; start this course as early as 30 days after the previous one Third course: Repeat second-course regimen, and if no response, further treatment with clomiphene is not recommended Male sterility: 50–400 mg/day PO for 2–12 months (controversial)
Follitropin alpha (Gonal-F)	Follicle development: 150 IU/day SQ on days 2 or 3 and continue for 10 days For women whose endogenous gonadotropin levels are suppressed, initiate at 225 IU/day SQ. Adjust dose after 5 days based on response. Dose should be adjusted no more than every 3–5 days and by no more than 75–150 IU at each adjustment. Maximum dose 450 IU/day Given in conjunction with hCG Spermatogenesis: 150 IU SQ 3 times/week in conjunction with hCG May increase to 300 IU prn 3 times/week as needed. May administer up to 18 months for adequate effect.
Follitropin beta (Follistatin)	Ovulation induction: Same as for follitropin alpha. Follicle development: 150–225 IU/day SQ or IM for at least 4 days of treatment. Adjust dose based on ovarian response. Given in conjunction with hCG
Human chorionic gonadotropin (hCG) (Chorex-5, Chorex-10, Choron 10, Pregnyl, Profasi)	5000–10,000 units IM, 1 day following the last dose of menotropins
Human menopausal gonadotropin (hMG)	Ovulation induction: 75 IU/day SQ, increase by 37.5 IU/day after 14 days; may increase again after 7 days. Do not exceed 35 days of treatment.
Letrozole (Femara)	2.5–5 mg/daily PO for 5 days
Menotropins[a] (Pergonal, Humegon, Menopur, Repronex)	225 units IM; then 150 units/day for 10 days up to maximum of 450 units IM/day for no longer than 12 days

[a] To achieve ovulation, menotropins must be followed by the administration of hCG.

this agent should be informed it can cause abdominal bloating, nausea, visual disturbances, insomnia, and ovarian hyperstimulation.

Clomiphene Citrate Challenge Test

Because a number of women today are choosing to delay childbearing, an increasing number are presenting with infertility due to advancing age and diminished ovarian reserve. A number of tests and diagnostic measures may be used to determine ovarian reserve, including a test based on clomephine citrate itself—the so-called clomiphene citrate challenge test.[74] In this test, a daily dose of 100 mg of clomiphene citrate is administered from days 5 to 9 of the menstrual cycle. An abnormal test is indicated by the absence of FSH suppression.[74] Tests of ovarian reserve are often used to predict failure of in vitro fertilization: An abnormal clomiphene citrate challenge test is associated with a significant reduction in pregnancy rates for women who have an infertility diagnosis.

Aromatase Inhibitors

Aromatase inhibitors have become an increasingly popular first step for ovarian stimulation and may replace clomiphene citrate for this indication in the future.[75] Inhibition of aromatase leads to a decrease in estrogen production, which in turn increases the secretion of FSH; this stimulates the ovaries, resulting in follicular development.[75]

FDA approved for the treatment of women with hormonal-responsive breast cancer, letrozole (Femara) is the most widely used aromatase inhibitor.[75] Its off-label use for infertility treatment has been shown to result in a thicker endometrium, increased pregnancy rates, and less cost than clomiphene citrate.[75] Side effects include hot flashes, headache, depression, and sometimes vaginal bleeding. Women should not use this drug if there is any suspicion of pregnancy or impaired liver function. Myocardial infarction and thromboembolism are the major adverse reactions to aromatase inhibitors.

Gonadotropin-Releasing Hormone

Synthetically produced gonadotropin-releasing hormone (leuprolide acetate [Lupron]) may be used to stimulate ovulation. If the woman has functional pituitary activity and an ovary that can produce a luteinizing hormone (LH) surge, GnRH can be used in pulsatile doses to stimulate ovulation.

Menotropins

Menotropins (Pergonal, Humegon, Repronex), also known as human menopausal gonadotropin (hMG), comprise a combination of FSH and LH that is derived from the urine of menopausal women; these agents are standardized in terms of their LH and FSH content. Menotropins can promote ovarian follicle development and stimulate ovulation when their use is followed by administration of hCG.[44]

The greatest risks associated with FSH analogues such as menotropins are multiple births and arterial thromboembolism. Adverse effects include dizziness, arterial thromboembolism, nausea, vomiting, and abdominal bloating. Ovarian enlargement may be a sign of ovarian hyperstimulation syndrome; the drug should be discontinued in such a case. Severe symptoms of ovarian hyperstimulation may require hospitalization and removal of excess fluid in the abdominal cavity. If a woman taking any of the FSH analogues experiences abdominal bloating and pain, she should seek care immediately.

Menotropins are ineffective if the woman has primary ovarian failure; thus, if she has a high gonadotropin level—a finding indicative of primary ovarian failure—these agents are contraindicated. Menotropins also are contraindicated for women who have overt thyroid or adrenal dysfunction, AUB of unknown etiology, PCOS, or suspected pregnancy. Table 30-10 provides information about doses.

Follitropins

Follitropin alpha (Gonal-F) and follitropin beta (Follistim) are recombinant-DNA, synthetically manufactured FSH. Follitropins do not have LH or contaminant urinary proteins, and there is more batch-to-batch consistency in these products. Follitropins have a greater stimulatory effect on ovarian follicles and a slightly higher pregnancy rate compared to menotropins. These drugs are also more widely available than menotropins.

Human Chorionic Gonadotropins

Human chorionic gonadotropin (hCG) (Chorex-5, Profasi) is used to stimulate ovarian function and to stimulate the corpus luteum to produce progesterone and androgens.[44] To induce ovulation, hCG is administered the day following the last dose of menotropins. This drug should be used with caution by women who have epilepsy, migraines, asthma, cardiac disease, or renal disease, and by those who are breastfeeding. Human chorionic gonadotropin is contraindicated for women with known sensitivity to chorionic gonadotropins, precocious puberty, or any androgen-dependent carcinoma. If there is any suspicion that the woman is pregnant, hCG should not be used.

Complementary and Alternative Therapies for Infertility

Guaifenesin

Guaiacol glyceryl ether (guaifenesin [Robitussin, Mucinex]) is an expectorant used to treat upper respiratory infections and pulmonary disease. Some experts have suggested that it might be useful in the treatment of women with infertility because of its ability to thin secretions.[76,77] A few small studies have suggested that it may thin cervical secretions, such that women using guaifenesin may achieve pregnancy more readily than those who do not use the agent.[77] Some clinicians have suggested that women should use guaifenesin concurrently with clomiphene citrate.[77] The recommended dose is guaifenesin 600 mg orally, twice a day, begun 5 days prior to ovulation and stopping once ovulation occurs. If a woman is taking clomiphene, it is suggested that she begin guaifenesin the day after her last dose of clomiphene. It is possible that guaifenesin will have the same thinning effect on with thick semen; however, studies to confirm this effect are lacking.

Vitamin C

Vitamin C is involved in recycling vitamin E and glutathione. Glutathione plays a role in the development of the zygote; it is present in the oocyte and in the tubal fluid. In one RCT, vitamin C supplementation at a dose of 750 mg per day was given to women with luteal-phase defects, and this treatment resulted in improved pregnancy rates.[78] In another RCT that enrolled 620 women, high doses of vitamin C supplementation (1, 5, or 10 g per day) were given PO during the luteal phase to women undergoing in vitro fertilization prior to embryo transfer but no differences in pregnancy rate or implantation rates were observed.[79]

Multivitamins

It is difficult to assess the role of multivitamin supplementation in fertility. Few useful studies exist, although some do show promise for this therapy.[80] In one observational study, multivitamin supplementation was associated with less infertility due to anovulation in a cohort of healthy women (n = 18,555) who were followed for 8 years.[81] The women who took multivitamins had approximately a one-third lower risk of developing ovulatory infertility compared to non-multivitamin users. Women taking B vitamins (B_1, B_2, B_6, B_{12}, folic acid, and niacin) at least 3 times per week had a decrease in ovulatory infertility. It is thought that folic acid may be the most influential vitamin influencing infertility.

Male Infertility

Although this text is focused on care of women, infertility may be related to both male and female partners. Indeed, male factor is the sole cause of infertility in 35% of infertile couples, and it may be a contributing factor in many more cases. Infertility in men may be caused by many problems, including anatomic or structural problems, abnormal sperm production or function, or sexual, hormonal, and genetic conditions. Other causes of male infertility include erectile dysfunction and decreased testosterone production. Treatment depends on the cause of the infertility. Unfortunately, with few exceptions, male infertility is not yet amenable to medical treatment.[82,83] Studies suggest that genetics is more frequently the cause of infertility in men. This section focuses on medications that are occasionally used to treat male infertility.

Polycystic Ovary Syndrome

Polycystic ovary syndrome (PCOS) is the most common known cause of anovulation, with its accompanying menstrual irregularities affecting between 5% and 8% of all women.[35,69] PCOS is a multifaceted disorder, and central to its pathogenesis are hyperandrogenemia and hyperinsulinemia, which are the primary targets for treatment.[35,69] Hyperandrogenemia can cause hirsutism, alopecia, acne, virilization, and menstrual irregularity and infertility. Women with PCOS are frequently overweight, which is believed to be due to insulin resistance that accompanies the syndrome. If an obese woman desires pregnancy and is diagnosed with PCOS, she is first encouraged to lose weight. Weight loss alone has been shown to reverse the deleterious effects of obesity, and often ovarian function improves.[84]

PCOS is associated with a classic ovarian morphology.[35] The polycystic ovary has 12 or more follicles measuring 2 to 9 mm in diameter and/or increased ovarian volume to more than 10 cm^3. The diagnosis of PCOS may be made on the basis of only one ovary having the aforementioned appearance.[85] Several pharmacologic treatments designed to restore ovulation and fertility among women with PCOS are available.

Clomiphene Citrate (Clomid)

Clomiphene citrate (Clomid) remains the first line of intervention for medically induced ovulation for women with PCOS. A functional hypothalamus–pituitary–ovarian axis is required for clomiphene citrate to be effective. It is believed that this agent binds to and inhibits stimulation of estrogen receptors in the hypothalamus, which decreases the normal hypothalamus–estrogen feedback loop.[86] This effect increases GnRH levels, which in turn increases pituitary secretion of gonadotropins and promotes ovarian follicle development. Unfortunately, among obese women with PCOS and insulin resistance, the success rate of clomiphene citrate alone in inducing ovulation is relatively low.[86]

Metformin Hydrochloride (Glucophage)

Metformin hydrochloride (Fortamet, Glucophage, Riomet) is a member of a group of hypoglycemia-inducing drugs used for treating diabetes mellitus. Metformin acts primarily by decreasing hepatic glucose production and increasing glucose utilization in peripheral tissues.[86] More details about metformin can be found in the *Diabetes* chapter. Insulin-sensitizing agents such as metformin may be used prior to administration of clomiphene citrate, administered at the same time as clomiphene citrate, or prescribed as monotherapy for women with PCOS who are resistant to clomiphene citrate.[86] Ovulation rates increase among women with PCOS who use metformin,[86] which is available in both short- and long-acting formulations.

Metformin is contraindicated for women who have heart disorders, type 1 diabetes, renal disease, or conditions predisposing them to renal dysfunction, liver disease, or serious hepatic impairment. The safety of this agent has not been established for use by breastfeeding women. Adverse effects of metformin include diarrhea, abdominal bloating, nausea, and a metallic taste. Anorexia can occur. The most serious adverse effect is lactic acidosis. Studies comparing the use of clomiphene citrate alone, metformin alone, and clomiphene citrate with metformin found that the combined regimen of clomiphene citrate and metformin significantly increases the success of ovulation induction when compared to use of either agent individually.[87]

Aromatase Inhibitors

Aromatase inhibitors such as letrozole (Femara) are being used with increasing frequency and increasing success as first-line treatments for anovulation. A few studies have found that letrozole is superior to clomiphene citrate.[88] The potential benefit of combining metformin with letrozole in a therapeutic regimen for PCOS is that this combination would provide insulin control along with an increase in FSH secretion and regular ovulation and menstruation.

Endometriosis

Endometriosis is a condition that is associated with chronic pelvic pain and dysmenorrhea as well as infertility. The classic definition of endometriosis, also termed *adenomyosis externa*, is the presence of endometrial tissue outside of the endometrial cavity (Figure 30-2). Adenomyosis is a separate condition that is characterized by the presence of endometrial glands and stroma within the myometrium, although symptoms and pharmacologic treatments are similar for both conditions. Endometriosis often is associated with primary or secondary infertility, although the most common initial symptom is pelvic pain. The pelvic pain may be specific to dyspareunia, or it may include severe dysmenorrhea. Most women with severe endometriosis are cared for by gynecologists who have expertise in this area.

Endometriosis has been a known gynecologic entity since the 1920s, and it is estimated that as many as 10% of adult women suffer from this condition. Yet much about endometriosis remains a mystery. For example, a variety of hypotheses about the etiology of this condition have been proposed, including retrograde menstruation, polygenic causes, or autoimmune influences, among others. The only definitive diagnosis is one made during surgical or laparoscopic visualization. The American Society for Reproductive Medicine has established a classification system for endometriosis based on size, depth, and location of endometriosis implants and adhesions.[89]

The two most common symptoms associated with endometriosis are pelvic pain and subfertility or infertility. In an ironic twist, one of the most basic interventions to promote regression of the disease process and to ameliorate pain is for the woman to become pregnant. Pregnancy, with its accompanying endometrial quiescence, will delay progression of the disease and may retard pain, although recurrence is common. Yet subfertility or infertility precludes this treatment for many, if not most, women. Moreover, this intervention is not of value for women who do not desire pregnancy.

The pharmacologic agents most frequently used to promote endometrial quiescence include contraception methods such as combined hormonal contraceptives

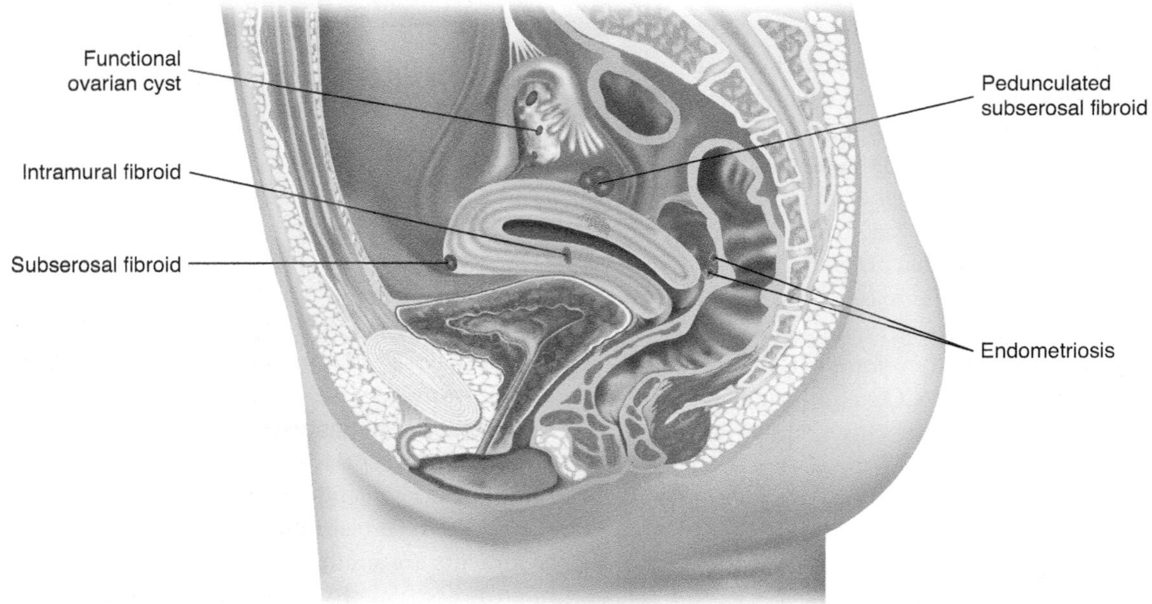

Figure 30-2 Pelvic sites associated with pelvic pain.

and medroxyprogesterone acetate (MPA; DPMA).[90,91] If a woman desires treatment of endometriosis-associated infertility, medroxyprogesterone acetate usually is best avoided because of the length of amenorrhea that persists after its discontinuation. Two specific drug categories are used to treat endometriosis: synthetic testosterone and various GnRH agonists.

Danazol

Danazol (Danocrine) is a derivative of 17 alpha-ethinyl testosterone, which has multiple anti-gonadotropin properties that create a high-androgen/low-estrogen environment hostile to endometrial growth. Danazol was the first medication to receive FDA approval as a treatment for women with endometriosis. This fat-soluble drug increases androgens and decreases secretion of endogenous estradiol. Gonadotropin levels are usually not changed, although LH may be slightly elevated. Because danazol changes the hormonal milieu, pregnancy is prevented; however, the drug is not intended to be a contraceptive. Danazol has been primarily used to treat women with endometriosis, fibrocystic breast disease, or menorrhagia, although the last indication is an off-label use. This drug is metabolized in the liver and should be used with caution by women with compromised liver function. The usual treatment regimen for danazol is to initiate therapy with a dose of 800 mg daily PO in four divided doses and, if used for pain relief and satisfactory response is attained, to continue at 200–800 mg daily in two to four divided doses.

Although danazol has been available for more than three decades, its use appears to be diminishing because of side effects that make it relatively unattractive to women. The androgenic adverse effects include amenorrhea, acne, weight gain, hirsutism, and, for a few women, a masculine-sounding voice. Most treatment regimens are limited to 6 months in an attempt to minimize the side effects. Currently, more clinicians prescribe GnRH analogues for endometriosis than prescribe danazol.

GnRH Analogues

GnRH analogues, such as leuprolide acetate (Lupron), buserelin (Suprefact), and nafarelin (Synarel), are nonsteroidal agents that suppress ovarian estrogen production. Although these agents tend to initially cause an initial flare effect and increase in symptoms, downregulation occurs with continuous administration, a reversible state of hypogonadism being the ultimate result.

Pharmacologic treatment for endometriosis is often combined with surgical intervention. The most common surgery is ablation of endometrial implants ("powder burns") and lysis of adhesions, although the long-term effectiveness of pharmacologic and surgical treatments is not well established. Recurrence rates are estimated to be as high as 40% over a 5-year period. Many women with severe disease ultimately have a hysterectomy and bilateral salpingo-oophorectomy for definitive treatment.

Leiomyomata (Uterine Fibroids)

Leiomyomata is the most common benign tumor found among women. Leiomyomata are also referred to "myoma" or "fibroids" and these terms are used interchangeably. The incidence of uterine fibroids is estimated to be as high as 35% among normal, healthy women, with 50% of them remaining asymptomatic.[92] As women age, the uterus and ovaries naturally decrease in size, as do uterine leiomyomata. Therefore, many fibroids are never problematic and are often an incidental finding during a physical exam, imaging studies, or surgery. However, 50% of women with fibroids do experience symptoms that range from being a minor problem to a major, life-altering condition. The most common symptoms include dysmenorrhea, AUB, and pelvic pain. Fibroids also are associated with subfertility/infertility.[93]

Fibroids may occur either inside or outside the body of the uterus (Figure 30-3). African American women are more likely than women of other races and ethnicities to have multiple and larger fibroids that are symptomatic, regardless of age. The reasons for this difference remain unknown. The incidence of fibroids peaks during the perimenopausal years, so women tend to seek care for leiomyomata more often during this period.[93]

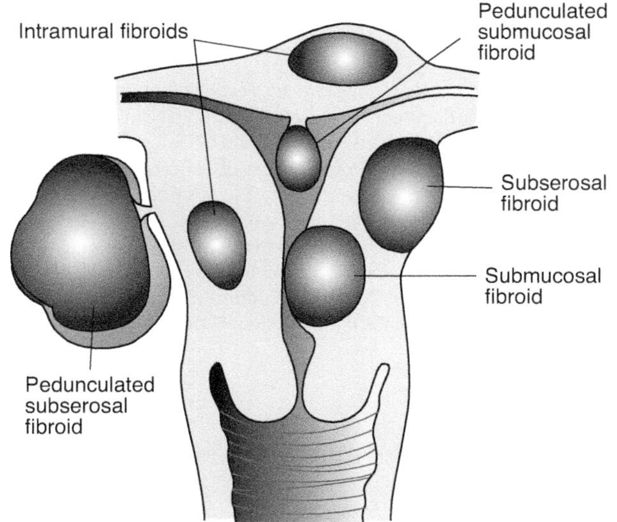

Figure 30-3 Different types of uterine fibroids.

Treatment of Women with Leiomyomata

Initial treatment of a woman with fibroids is based on symptoms. Women with dysmenorrhea usually are treated with analgesics. In addition to dysmenorrhea, fibroids can cause AUB. Both current COCs and the LNG-IUS contraceptives use low doses of hormones and inhibition of hormonal production with either estrogen or progesterone, or both, has been theorized to be an effective treatment for fibroids. Previously, concerns had been voiced that fibroids might be estrogen dependent, such that use of combined oral contraceptives would cause growth of the uterine tumor. However, currently available COCs actually have been linked to a reduction in the development of symptomatic fibroids,[94] and there is no indication that use of COCs for treatment of women with menorrhagia results in an increase in fibroid size. The levonorgestrel intrauterine system (LNG-IUS [Mirena]) has been found to be effective in decreasing bleeding in women with fibroids as well as in women without fibroids, but this contraceptive system does not decrease the size of the fibroid per se.[95,96]

GnRH agonists have also been suggested as a method to decrease the size of fibroids and, in turn, the symptoms associated with them. However, GnRH agonists have uncomfortable side effects, and women in the past often were faced with a choice between the effects of the fibroids or the side effects of the treatment. Today, GnRH is more commonly used to decrease the size of the fibroid in anticipation of an easier operative intervention. A course of therapy for 3 to 4 months prior to either a myomectomy or a hysterectomy is associated with shorter operative time, smaller incisions, increased operative options (e.g., vaginal versus abdominal hysterectomy), and less blood loss.[97]

Estrogen agonists/antagonists (EAAs), also known as **selective estrogen receptor modulators (SERMs)**, have been used by some researchers for treatment of women with fibroids. Tamoxifen (Nolvadex), raloxifene (Evista), and asoprisnil have been suggested as possible therapies due to their antiestrogen properties, but more research is needed to assess the effectiveness of these agents.[98] Asoprisnil is a selective progesterone-receptor modulator that is currently under investigation for treatment of progesterone-sensitive fibroids.

Mifepristone (Mifeprex, formerly RU-486) is an antiprogestin that is also a progesterone receptor modulator. This agent, combined with misoprostol, is used as a medical abortifacient and is discussed in more depth in the *Contraception* chapter. However, as a progesterone receptor modulator, mifepristone can decrease the size of fibroids. In 2004, a systematic review was published that evaluated the use of mifepristone for treatment of women with symptoms associated with uterine fibroids. Mifepristone did reduce the volume of the leiomyomas. It also decreased the incidence of dysmenorrhea, menorrhagia, and pelvic pressure. Unfortunately, 28% of the women screened by endometrial biopsy demonstrated the presence of endometrial hyperplasia, causing routine use of the drug to be called into question.[99] A RCT published in 2008 found similar positive results with use of mifepristone to ameliorate symptoms of fibroids, based on a dose of either 5 or 10 mg per day, with only a 2% risk of endometrial hyperplasia. This study suggests that the risk of endometrial hyperplasia, although present, is dose dependent.[100] Ulipristal acetate (Ella), another progesterone receptor modulator that is currently used as emergency contraception, is also being studied as a possible therapy for the treatment of women with fibroids but has not been approved for such use at this time.[101]

A hysterectomy is the definitive treatment for leiomyomata, yet a woman may choose a myomectomy in order to maintain possible fertility. Uterine artery embolization is less invasive than abdominal myomectomy, although no type of surgery for fibroids has been found to be a definitive cure for fibroid-related subfertility. No treatment is without side effects and, with the exception of hysterectomy, the possibility of fibroid recurrence exists.[102,103]

Conclusion

Women can have a variety of gynecologic conditions and concerning presentations. Prominent among them are menstrual disorders, pelvic disease, and infertility. Several conditions, such as endometriosis, polycystic ovarian syndrome, and leiomyomata, are distinct entities with shared gynecologic symptoms. In most cases, pharmacologic treatments are targeted to the symptoms, and many of the pharmacologic treatments overlap. Often definitive studies are lacking regarding the effectiveness of treatments. However, the advent of new drugs and the development of new delivery systems, such as intrauterine systems, may herald research opportunities from which future treatments will emerge. Until the unlikely day that a Lydia Pinkham–type, all-encompassing treatment is found, modern healthcare providers need to be aware of multiple pharmacologic agents for the multiple gynecologic conditions that women may experience.

Resources

Apps

A myriad of apps exist for mobile devices that provide consumer-oriented information as well as provider-specific data. The apps identified here are currently available for free, although they may be limited by platform (e.g., Android). These apps usually are available via iTunes or Google Play. Some women will prefer a specific app to others; the same is true with providers.

Menstrual Cycle Disruptions

iPeriod Period Tracker, Menstrual Calendar, Monthly Cycles Period Tracker, Menstruation and Ovulation, Period Log Free—Menstrual Calendar, Free Menstrual Calendar, LoveCycles, Period Plus, Glow, My Cycles, Pink Pad Period and Fertility Tracker, MyDays—Period and Ovulation, Period Tracker!, Period Log—Menstrual Calendar, Cotton Plop, MonthyPal, Period Calendar, Menstrual Cycle Monitor, Only for Women, Petals (Menstrual Period Calendar), Clue—Period Tracker, Period Planner Lite, Day After, Period Pace: Menstrual Cycle Log, MeLady, My Menstrual Diary, Ladytimer Free Ovulation, Fertility Cycle—Period and Ovulation Calendar, Simple Period (Free Period Calendar), The Secret Diary Lite, WomanLog, Cycles, My Period Tracker, Menstrual Cycle Monitor, Menstruation and Fertility—Lite, My Drops Timer, Period Tracker Lite, Period Diary Supreme Lite, Period View, First Response Tracker, Heavy Menstrual Bleeding

Exercises and Therapies for Pelvic Pain/Dysmenorrhea

Pain Coach, KegelTunes: Guided Kegel Exercises, Birdi—Pelvic Floor Training, Exercises for a Healthy Back and Pelvic Floor, KegelMate, Kegel Trainer Lite, Pelvic Floor First, EcoAtlas Pelvic Floor, iURO Pelvic Floor

Female Infertility

Infertility Survival Kit, My Mobile Fertility, FertileThoughts, Freedom Fertility Pharmacy, Pregnancy Due Date & Fertility Calculator, Attain Fertility Predictor, Fertility View—Fertility and IVF Support, Fertility App, iVF4U, Fertility: Increase Your Chances of Conceiving, Fertility Journey, Jetanin, What to Expect: Fertility, Glow, Kindara Fertility Tracker, Ovulation Calculator, Basal Body Temperature Chart & Period Calendar—to Help You Get Pregnant with the Fertility Awareness Method of Natural Family Planning, Cincinnati Fertility, Main Line Fertility, My Mobile Fertility, My Hopeful Journey Organizer, Infertility Survival Kit, OvuView, myInfertility, Freedom Fertility Mobile

Polycystic Ovary Syndrome

PCOS Diva, PCOS Fertility

Endometriosis

For providers: Endo App, Endometriosis App, Management of Women with Endometriosis

Uterine Fibroids

British Fibroid Trust Android App

References

1. Doty E, Attaran M. Managing primary dysmenorrhea. *J Pediatr Adolesc Gynecol.* 2006;19:341-344.
2. Harel Z. Dysmenorrhea in adolescents and young adults: etiology and management. *J Pediatr Adolesc Gynecol.* 2006;19(6):363-371.
3. Dawood MY. Primary dysmenorrhea: advances in pathogenesis and management. *Obstet Gynecol.* 2006;108:428-441.
4. Proctor M, Farquhar C. Diagnosis and management of dysmenorrhea. *BMJ.* 2006;332:1134-1138.
5. Marjoribanks J, Proctor M, Farquhar C, Derks RS. Nonsteroidal anti-inflammatory drugs for dysmenorrhoea. *Cochrane Database Syst Rev.* 2010;1:CD001751.
6. Zahradnik HP, Hanjalic-Beck A, Groth K. Nonsteroidal anti-inflammatory drugs and hormonal contraceptives for pain relief from dysmenorrhea: a review. *Contraception.* 2010;81:185.
7. Proctor M, Farquhar C. Diagnosis and management of dysmenorrhea. *BMJ.* 2006;332:1134-1138.
8. Lethaby A, Duckitt K, Farquhar C. Non-steroidal anti-inflammatory drugs for heavy menstrual bleeding. *Cochrane Database Syst Rev.* 2013;1:CD000400.
9. Weberschock TB, Muller SM, Boehncke S, Boehncke WH. Tolerance to coxibs in patients with intolerance to non-steroidal anti-inflammatory drugs (NSAIDs): a systematic structured review of the literature. *Arch Dermatol.* 2007;299:169-175.
10. Gaytan M, Morales C, Bellido C, Sanchez-Criado JE, Gaytan F. Non-steroidal anti-inflammatory drugs (NSAIDs) and ovulation: lessons from morphology. *Histol Histopathol.* 2006;221:541-556.
11. Helin-Salmivaara A, Huttunen T, Gronroos JM, Klaukka T, Huupponen R. Risk of serious upper gastrointestinal events with concurrent use of NSAIDs and SSRIs: a case-control study in the general population. *Eur J Clin Pharmacol.* 2007;63:403-408.
12. DeMaria AN, Weir MR. Coxibs: beyond the GI tract: renal and cardiovascular issues. *J Pain Symptom Manage.* 2003;25:S41-S49.
13. National Library of Medicine Toxnet Lactmed. Ibuprofen. http://toxnet.nlm.nih.gov/cgi-bin/sis/search2/f?./temp/~yfGTf8:1. Accessed March 15, 2015.
14. Seshasai SR, Wijesuriya S, Sivakumaran R, et al. Effect of aspirin on vascular and nonvascular outcomes: meta-analysis of randomized controlled trials. *Arch Intern Med.* 2012;172(3):209.
15. Wong CL, Farquhar C, Roberts H, Proctor M. Oral contraceptive pill for primary dysmenorrhoea. *Cochrane Database Syst Rev.* 2009;4:CD002120.
16. Machado RB, de Melo NR, Maia H Jr. Bleeding patterns and menstrual-related symptoms with the continuous use of a contraceptive combination of ethinylestradiol and drospirenone: a randomized study. *Contraception.* 2010;81:215.
17. Hubacher D, Lopez L, Steiner MJ, Dorflinger L. Menstrual pattern changes from levonorgestrel subdermal implants and DMPA: systematic review and evidence-based comparisons. *Contraception.* 2009; 80:113.
18. Proctor M, Murphy PA. Herbal and dietary therapies for primary and secondary dysmenorrhoea. *Cochrane Database Syst Rev.* 2001;2:CD002124.
19. Marsden JS, Strickland CD, Clements TL. Guaifenesin as a treatment for primary dysmenorrhea. *J Am Board Fam Pract.* 2004;17:240-246.
20. Seifert B, Wagler P, Dartsch S, Schmidt U, Nieder J. Magnesium: a new therapeutic alternative in primary dysmenorrhea. *Zentraldl Gynakol.* 1989; 111(11):755-760.
21. Fontana-Klaiber H, Hogg B. Therapeutic effects of magnesium in dysmenorrhea. *Schweiz Rundsch Med Prax.* 1990;79(16):491-494.
22. Benassi L, Barletta FP, Baroncini L, et al. Effectiveness of magnesium pidolate in the prophylactic treatment of primary dysmenorrhea. *Clin Exp Obstet Gynecol.* 1992;19(3):175-179.
23. Sampalis F, Bunea R, Pelland M, Kowalski O, Duguet N, Dupuis S. Evaluation of the effects of Neptune Krill Oil on the management of premenstrual syndrome and dysmenorrhea. *Alternative Med Rev.* 2003;8:171-179.
24. Harel Z, Biro FM, Kottenhahn RK, Rosenthal SL. Supplementation with omega-3 polyunsaturated fatty acids in the management of dysmenorrhea in adolescents. *Am J Obstet Gynecol.* 1996;174:1335-1338.
25. Calder PC. *N*-3 polyunsaturated fatty acids inflammation and inflammatory diseases. *Am J Clin Nutr.* 2006;83:1505S-1519S.
26. Ziaei S, Fughihzadeh S, Sohrabuand F, Lamyian M, Emamgholy T. A randomized placebo-controlled trial to determine the effect of vitamin E in the

treatment of primary dysmenorrhea. *BJOG.* 2001; 108(11):1181-1183.

27. Ziaei SZM, Zakeri M, Kazemnejad A. A randomized controlled trial of vitamin E in the treatment of primary dysmenorrhea. *BJOG.* 2005;112(4): 466-469.
28. Proctor M, Farquhar C, Stones W, He L, Zhu X, Brown J. Transcutaneous electrical nerve stimulation for primary dysmenorrhoea. *Cochrane Database Syst Rev.* 2002;1:CD002123.
29. Proctor M, Hing W, Johnson TC, Murphy PA, Brown J. Spinal manipulation for dysmenorrhoea. *Cochrane Database Syst Rev.* 2006;3:CD002119.
30. Witt CM, Reinhold T, Brinkhaus B, Roll S, Jena S, Willich SN. Acupuncture in patients with dysmenorrhea: a randomized study on clinical effectiveness and cost-effectiveness in usual care. *Am J Obstet Gynecol.* 2008;198:166e161-166e168.
31. Jiang HR, Ni S, Li JL, et al. Systematic review of randomized clinical trials of acupressure therapy for primary dysmenorrhea. *Evid Based Complement Alternat Med.* 2013;2013:169692.
32. Brown J, Brown S. Exercise for dysmenorrhoea. *Cochrane Database Syst Rev.* 2010;2:CD004142.
33. Rakhshaee Z. Effect of three yoga poses (cobra cat and fish poses) in women with primary dysmenorrhea: a randomized clinical trial. *J Pediatr Adolesc Gynecol.* 2011;24:192.
34. Mirbagher-Ajorpaz N. The effects of acupressure on primary dysmenorrhea. *Complement Ther Clin Pract.* 2011;17(1):3-36.
35. Fritz M, Speroff L. *Clinical Gynecologic Endocrinology and Infertility.* Philadelphia, PA: Wolters Kluwer; 2011.
36. ACOG Practice Bulletin Number 128. *Obstet Gynecol.* 2012;120(1):1-8.
37. Munro M. IJGO FIGO Classification system (PALM COEIN) for causes of AUB. *Int J Gynecol Obstet.* 2011;113:3-13.
38. Micks EA. Treatment of heavy menstrual bleeding with the estradiol valerate and dienogest oral contraceptive pill. *Adv Ther.* 2013;30(1):1-13.
39. Faucher M, Schuiling K. Normal and abnormal uterine bleeding. In: Schuiling KD, Likis F, eds. *Women's Gynecologic Health.* 2nd ed. Burlington, MA: Jones & Bartlett Learning; 2013:609-647.
40. Lethaby A, Irvine GA, Cameron IT. Cyclical progestogens for heavy menstrual bleeding. *Cochrane Database Syst Rev.* 2008;1:CD001016.
41. Matteson KA. Nonsurgical management of heavy menstrual bleeding. *Obstet Gynecol.* 2013;121(3): 632-643.
42. Shaaban MM, Zakherah MS, El-Nashar SA, Sayed GH. Levonorgestrel-releasing intrauterine system compared to low dose combined oral contraceptive pills for idiopathic menorrhagia: a randomized clinical trial. *Contraception.* 2011;83:48.
43. Beaumont HH, Augood C, Duckitt K, Lethaby A. Danazol for heavy menstrual bleeding. *Cochrane Database Syst Rev.* 2007;3:CD001017.
44. Parker KL, Schimmer BP. Introduction to endocrinology: hypothalamus pituitary axis. In: Bruton L, Chabman B, Knollman BC, eds. *Goodman Gilman's The Pharmacological Basis of Therapeutics.* 12th ed. New York: McGraw-Hill; 2013:1101-1128.
45. Lukes AS, Moore KA, Muse KN, et al. Tranexamic acid treatment for HMB. *Obstet Gynecol.* 2010; 116(4):865-875.
46. American Psychiatric Association. *Diagnostic and Statistical Manual of Mental Disorders.* 5th ed. Arlington, VA: American Psychiatric Publishing; 2013.
47. Hartlage SA, Breaux CA, Yonkers KA. Addressing concerns about the inclusion of premenstrual dysphoric disorder in *DSM*-5. *J Clin Psychiatry.* 2014; 75(1):70-76.
48. Halbreich U, O'Brien PM, Eriksson E, Backstrom T, Yonkers KA, Freeman EW. Are there differential symptom profiles that improve in response to different pharmacological treatments of premenstrual syndrome/premenstrual dysphoric disorder? *CNS Drugs.* 2006;20:523-547.
49. Wittchen HU, Becker E, Lieb R, Krause P. Prevalence incidence and stability of premenstrual dysphoric disorder in the community. *Psychol Med.* 2002; 32: 119-132.
50. Yonkers KA, Shaughn O'Brien PM, Eriksson E. Premenstrual syndrome. *Lancet.* 2008;371(9619): 1200-1210.
51. Greenslit N. Pharmaceutical branding: identity individuality and illness. *Mol Interv.* 2002;2:342-345.
52. Marjoribanks J, Brown J, O'Brien PMS, Wyatt K. Selective serotonin reuptake inhibitors for premenstrual syndrome. *Cochrane Database Syst Rev.* 2013; 6:CD001396.
53. Sachs HC, Committee on Drugs. The transfer of drugs and therapeutics into human breast milk: an update on selected topics. *Pediatrics.* 2013;132:e796-e809.

54. Meyer, J. Pharmacotherapy of psychosis and mania. In: Bruton L, Chabman B, Knollman BC, eds. *Goodman Gilman's The Pharmacological Basis of Therapeutics*. 12th ed. New York: McGraw-Hill; 2013:417-456.
55. Jarvis CI, Lynch AM, Morin AK. Management strategies for premenstrual syndrome/premenstrual dysphoric disorder. *Ann Pharmacother*. 2008;42:967-978.
56. Lopez LM, Kaptein AA, Helmerhorst FM. Oral contraceptives containing drospirenone for premenstrual syndrome. *Cochrane Database Syst Rev*. 2012;2:CD006586.
57. Srivastava A, Mansel RE, Arvind N, Prasad K, Dhar A, Chabra A. Evidence-based management of mastalgia: a meta-analysis of randomised trials. *Breast*. 2007;16:503-512.
58. Singh A, Kumar A. Protective effect of alprazolam against sleep deprivation-induced behavior alternations and oxidative damage in mice. *Neurosci Res*. 2008;60(4):372-379.
59. Freeman EW. An overview of 4 studies of a continuous OC on PMDD and PMS. *Contraception*. 2012;85:437.
60. Wyatt K, Dimmock P, Jones P, Obhrai M, O'Brien S. Efficacy of progesterone and progestogens in management of premenstrual syndrome: systematic review. *BMJ*. 2001;323:776-780.
61. Thys-Jacobs S, Ceccarelli S, Bierman A, Weisman H, Cohen MA, Alvir J. Calcium supplementation in premenstrual syndrome. *J Gen Intern Med*. 1989;4:183-189.
62. Penland JG, Johnson PE. Dietary calcium and magnesium effects on menstrual cycle symptoms. *Am J Obstet Gynecol*. 1993;168:1417-1423.
63. Quaranta S, Buscaglia MA, Meroni MG. Pilot study of the efficacy and safety of a modified release magnesium 250 mg tablet (Sincromag) for the treatment of premenstrual syndrome. *Clin Drug Investig*. 2007;27:51-58.
64. London RS, Murphy L, Kitlowski KE, Reynold MA. Efficacy of alpha-tocopherol in the treatment of the premenstrual syndrome. *J Reprod Med*. 1987;32(6):400-404.
65. Bertone-Johnson ER, Hankinson SE, Bendih A, Johnson SR, Willett WC, Manson JE. Calcium and vitamin D intake and risks of incident premenstrual syndrome. *Arch Intern Med*. 2005;165: 1246-1252.
66. Lamvu G. Role of hysterectomy in the treatment of pelvic pain. *Obstet Gynecol*. 2011;117(5): 1175-1178.
67. Williams RE, Hartmann KE, Sandler RS, Miller WC, Savitz LA, Steege JF. Recognition and treatment of irritable bowel syndrome among women with chronic pelvic pain. *Am J Obstet Gynecol*. 2005; 192(3):761-767.
68. Cheong YC, Smotra G, Williams ACDC. Nonsurgical interventions for the management of chronic pelvic pain. *Cochrane Database Syst Rev*. 2014;3:CD008797.
69. Ben-Shlomo I, Younis JS. Basic research in PCOS: are we reaching new frontiers? *Reprod BioMed Online*. 2014;28:669-683.
70. Garber JR, Cobin RH, Hossein G. Clinical practice guidelines for hypothyroidism in adults: cosponsored by the American Association of Clinical Endocrinologists and the American Thyroid Association. *Endocr Pract*. 2012;18(6):e1.
71. Biondi B, Wartofsky L. Treatment with thyroid hormones. *Endocr Rev*. 2014;35:433-512.
72. Luciano A, Lanzone A, Goverde AJ. Management of female infertility from hormonal causes. *Int J Gynecol Obstet*. 2013;123:S9-S17.
73. World Health Organization. Advances in fertility regulation. *World Health Organ Tech Rep Ser*. 1973; 1-42.
74. Hendriks DJ, Mol BW, Bancsi LF, te Velde ER, Broekmans FJ. The clomiphene citrate challenge test for the prediction of poor ovarian response and nonpregnancy in patients undergoing in vitro fertilization: a systematic review. *Fertil Steril*. 2006;86(4):807-818.
75. Franik S, Kremer JAM, Nelen WLDM, Farquhar C. Aromatase inhibitors for subfertile women with polycystic ovary syndrome. *Cochrane Database Syst Rev*. 2014;2:CD010287.
76. Check JH. Diagnosis and treatment of cervical mucus abnormalities. *Clin Exp Obstet Gynecol*. 2006;33:140-142.
77. Check JH, Adelson HG, Wu CH. Improvement of cervical factor with guaifenesin. *Fertil Steril*. 1982;37(5):707-708.
78. Henmi H, Endo T, Kitajima Y, Manase K, Hata H, Kudo R. Effects of ascorbic acid supplementation on serum progesterone levels in patients with a luteal phase defect. *Fertil Steril*. 2003;80(2): 459-461.

79. Griesinger G, Franke K, Kinast C, et al. Ascorbic acid supplementation during luteal phase in IVF. *J Assist Reprod Genetics*. 2002;19(4):164-168.
80. Buhling KJ, Grajecki D. The effect of micronutrient supplements on female fertility. *Curr Opin Obstet Gynecol*. 2013;25:173-180.
81. Chavarro JE, Rich-Edwards JW, Rosner BA, Willett WC. Use of multivitamins intake of B vitamins and risk of ovulatory infertility. *Fertil Steril*. 2008;89(3):668-676.
82. Bhasin S. Approach to the infertile man. *J Clin Endocrinol Metab*. 2007;92:1995-2004.
83. Gudeloglu A, Brahmbhatt JV, Parekattil MD. Medical management of male infertility in the absence of a specific etiology. *Semin Reprod Med*. 2014;32:313-318.
84. Harrison C. Exercise therapy in polycystic ovary. *Hum Reprod*. 2011;17(2):171-183.
85. Balen AH, Laven JS, Tan SL, Dewailly D. Ultrasound assessment of the polycystic ovary: international consensus definitions. *Hum Reprod*. 2003;9:505-514.
86. Legro RS, Siva SA, Ehrmann DA. Diagnosis and treatment of polycystic ovary syndrome: an Endocrine Society clinical practice guideline. *J Clin Endocrinol Metab*. 2013;98(12):4565-4592.
87. Berger JJ, Bates GW. Optimal management of subfertility in polycystic ovary syndrome. *Int J Womens Health*. 2014;6:613-621.
88. Legro RS, Brzyski RS, Diamond MP, et al. Letrozole versus clomiphene for infertility in the polycystic ovary syndrome. *N Engl J Med*. 2014;371(2):119-129.
89. Schuiling KD, Likis F, eds. *Women's Gynecologic Health*. 2nd ed. Burlington, MA: Jones & Bartlett Learning; 2013.
90. Vercellini P, Barbara G, Somigliana E, Bianchi S, Abbiati A, Fedele L. Comparison of contraceptive ring and patch for the treatment of symptomatic endometriosis. *Fertil Steril*. 2010;93(7):2150-2161.
91. Davis LJ, Kennedy SS, Moore J, Prentice A. Oral contraceptives for pain associated with endometriosis. *Cochrane Database Syst Rev*. 2007;3:CD001019.
92. Parker W. Etiology, symptomatology, and diagnosis of uterine myomas. *Fertil Steril*. 2007;87(4):725-736.
93. Parker W. Uterine myomas: management. *Fertil Steril*. 2007;88(2):255-271.
94. Huber JC, Bentz EK, Ott J, Tempfer CB. Non-contraceptive benefits of oral contraceptives. *Expert Opin Pharmacother*. 2008;9(13):2317-2325.
95. Zapata LB, Whiteman MK, Tepper NK, Jamieson DJ, Marchbanks PA, Curtis KM. Intrauterine device use among women with uterine fibroids: a systematic review. *Contraception*. 2010;82:41.
96. Magalhaes J, Aldrighi JM, de Lima GR. Uterine volume and menstrual patterns in users of the levonorgestrel-releasing intrauterine system with idiopathic menorrhagia or menorrhagia due to leiomyomas. *Contraception*. 2007;75:193.
97. Lethaby A, Vollenhoeven B, Sowter M. Efficacy of pre-operative gonadotropin releasing analogues for women with uterine fibroids undergoing hysterectomy or myomectomy: a systematic review. *BJOG*. 2002;109(10):1097-1108.
98. Wilkens J, Chwalisz K, Han C, et al. Effects of the selective progesterone receptor modulator asoprisnil on uterine artery blood flow, ovarian activity, and clinical symptoms in patients with uterine leiomyomata scheduled for hysterectomy. *J Clin Endocrinol Metab*. 2008;93:4664.
99. Steinaer J, Pritts EA, Jackson R, Jacoby AF. Systematic review of mifepristone for the treatment of uterine leiomyomata. *Obstet Gynecol*. 2004;103(6):1331-1336.
100. Carbonell Esteve JL, Acosta R, Heredia B, Perez Y, Castaneda MC, Hernanndez AV. Mifepristone for the treatment of uterine leiomyomas: a randomized controlled trial. *Obstet Gynecol*. 2008;112(5):1029-1036.
101. Donnez J, Tatarchuk TF, Bouchard P, et al. Ulipristal acetate versus placebo for fibroid treatment before surgery. *N Engl J Med*. 2012;366(5):409.
102. Marjoribanks J, Lethaby A, Farquhar C. Surgery versus medical therapy for heavy menstrual bleeding. *Cochrane Database Syst Rev*. 2006;2:CD003855.
103. Khan AT, Shehmar M, Gupta JK. Uterine fibroids: current perspective. *Int J Womens Health*. 2014;6:95-114.

31 Vaginal Conditions

Sharon M. Bond, Mary C. Brucker

Based on the chapter by Jane Mashburn in the first edition of Pharmacology for Women's Health

Chapter Glossary

Atrophic vaginitis Inflammatory condition characterized by burning, itching, dysuria, and a sensation of dryness, accompanied by dyspareunia, which occurs as a result of decreased vaginal estrogen and vulvovaginal atrophy.

Bacterial vaginosis (BV) Noninfectious vaginal condition that occurs in association with an overgrowth of anaerobic organisms and diminished, absent, or ineffective hydrogen-peroxide producing species of lactobacilli.

Desquamative inflammatory vaginitis (DIV) Rare inflammatory, noninfectious vaginitis characterized by profuse and purulent-appearing discharge, introital and vaginal erythema, and vaginal burning/dyspareunia.

Trichomoniasis *Trichomonas* vaginitis (TV); condition caused by sexual transmission of *Trichomonas vaginalis*, an anaerobic protozoan organism.

Vaginal microbiome Collection of microbial organisms that inhabit the vagina, organize its environment, and respond to fluctuations in hormonal levels, menstrual cycles, aging, pathogenic substances, foreign bodies, medications, stress, and aging; also known as the vaginal ecosystem.

Vulvovaginal candidiasis (VVC) Condition caused by *Candida* species, characterized by symptoms such as itching, irritation, burning, dysuria, and dyspareunia, and often accompanied by a thick, white, adherent discharge.

Vaginal Conditions

Symptomatic vaginal discharge is one of the most common reasons why women visit a primary care or gynecology practice.[1] This chapter focuses on conditions in which vaginal discharge is the characteristic sign. Traditionally, three classic conditions are placed in this category: bacterial vaginosis (BV), trichomoniasis, and vulvovaginal candidiasis (VVC). This chapter also addresses atrophic vaginitis and a rare condition known as desquamative inflammatory vaginitis (DIV).

In order of prevalence, the most frequent types of vaginal conditions diagnosed in the United States are bacterial vaginosis, vulvovaginal candidiasis, and trichomoniasis (also called trichomoniasis vaginitis). Diagnosis of these conditions requires a systematic approach that includes a complete health history; physical examination, including speculum examination; use of pH and amine testing; microscopy; Gram stain; Nugent scoring; point-of-care testing aids; and cultures, when indicated.[1,2] Table 31-1 provides a clinical review of the differential diagnosis for each of the common vaginal conditions. Because some women do not develop the classic symptoms, it is important that clinicians perform a full assessment for any woman who reports an unusual vaginal discharge, rather than simply making a diagnosis based on just the history or description of the discharge and symptoms. Occasionally, more than one pathogen may be present; after treatment of the first microorganism, a second condition may then emerge.

Table 31-1 Differential Diagnosis of Common Vaginal Conditions

	Normal	Bacterial Vaginosis	Trichomonas Vaginitis	Candidiasis	Irritant Contact, Allergic, Dermatologic	Atrophic Vaginitis
Etiology	Occasional vaginal secretions	Overgrowth of anaerobic organisms	Parasitic protozoa transmitted by sexual contact	*Candida* species	Allergens/chemical irritants, epithelial abnormalities such as vulvar vestibulitis, lichen planus	Diminished vaginal estrogen due to menopause, breastfeeding
Color of vaginal secretions	Clear or cloudy	Gray/white	Yellow/green, or any color	White/yellow	Clear or cloudy; may be none if condition is of dermatologic origin	Gray/yellow
Odor	None	Positive amine test; fishy	Malodorous	Usually none	None	None
Consistency of vaginal secretions	Usually thin, pooling in posterior fornix	Thin, homogenous	Frothy, bubbly	Thick, adherent plaques; may be without visible discharge	Usually thin	Scant, sticky
Complaint (s)	Variable amount	Malodorous discharge, pruritus; may be asymptomatic	Pruritus, burning, dyspareunia, or no symptoms	Pruritus, burning, dyspareunia	Burning, tenderness, itching, dyspareunia	Dyspareunia, burning
Physical observations	No abnormalities; physiologic leukorrhea	Pooling of discharge at introitus, lack of inflammatory signs such as erythema or edema	Erythema, edema, cervicitis, strawberry cervix; discharge can be profuse	Erythema, edema; sometimes no visible vaginal or vulvar signs	Erythema, edema, vestibular erosions	Pale vaginal color, minimal rugae, diminished labia minora, introital narrowing, erythema if symptomatic
pH	3.5–4.5	> 4.5	5.2–7.0	3.8–4.5	3.8–4.5	5.5–7.0
Microscopic findings	Abundant mature epithelial cells, normal flora, presence of lactobacilli	More than 20% of epithelial cells as clue cells; absent or limited lactobacilli	Trichomonads, heavy WBCs, RBCs if cervicitis	Pseudohyphae, budding spores, few lactobacilli	Nonspecific inflammation, immature epithelial cells, WBCs, minimal or absent lactobacilli	Minimal cellular content with parabasal cells dominant, no lactobacilli, many WBCs
Clinical considerations	Education, reassurance	Associated with multiple untoward obstetric and gynecologic conditions, recurrence rates of approximately 30%; partner treatment not indicated	Treatment often occurs at discretion of the provider for asymptomatic women or if incidental finding; partner treatment indicated	Treatment varies depending on whether it is classified as uncomplicated or complicated; reduce risk factors and predisposing conditions	Remove allergen; decrease use of perfumed products; use topical corticosteroids if of dermatologic origin	Topical estrogen; risk of vaginal candidiasis may increase with estrogen use

Abbreviations: RBCs = red blood cells; WBCs = white blood cells.

Sources: Data from Edwards L. Dermatologic causes of vaginitis: a clinical review. *Dermatol Clin.* 2010;28(4):727-735[4]; Workowski KA, Berman S; Centers for Disease Control and Prevention. Sexually transmitted diseases treatment guidelines, 2010. *MMWR Recommend Rep.* 2010;59(RR-12):1-110.[3]

The Vaginal Microbiome

Vaginal secretions are composed of a mixture of shed vaginal epithelium, cervical mucus, vaginal transudate, and scant material from the Skene and Bartholin glands. The unique combinations of organisms normally present in the vagina are theorized to protect a woman by providing an initial line of defense against infection. The normal vagina contains a mixture of heterogeneous microorganisms including *Lactobacilli acidophilus*, *Staphylococcus epidermidis*, and *Corynebacteria*, as well as small amounts of anaerobic microorganisms, such as *Gardnerella*, *Mobiluncus*, *Peptostreptococcus*, *Bacteroides*, *Escherichia coli*, *Streptococcus*, and anaerobic lactobacilli.[5] This community of microorganisms is collectively known as the **vaginal microbiome** or vaginal ecosystem. The growth of opportunistic and pathogenic organisms becomes facilitated when this host environment is altered by use of antibiotics, vaginal lubricants, hormonal contraceptives, douching, and other behavioral and intrinsic factors.[6]

Vaginal secretions vary throughout the menstrual cycle and increase in amount around ovulation, during the premenstrual period, during pregnancy, and when sexual arousal occurs. Physiologic vaginal secretions are usually clear or cloudy and nonirritating in nature, although they may leave a yellow cast on clothing after drying. An increase in the amount of vaginal secretion, known as leukorrhea, is classically described as a thin or thick white discharge resulting from congestion of the vaginal mucosa and an increase in polymorphonuclear leukocytes visible under microscopy.[7] Leukorrhea can be categorized as either normal (physiologic) leukorrhea, as is found during pregnancy or menstruation, or inflammatory leukorrhea, as is noted in the presence of vaginal infection.

Vaginal epithelial cells contain glycogen. When glycogen from shed vaginal epithelial cells is metabolized by lactobacilli, lactic acid is produced. Lactic acid maintains the pH of the vagina between 3.5 and 4.5—a factor that is hypothesized to prevent overgrowth of pathogenic organisms under normal conditions. Under the right circumstances, however, an overgrowth of some normal inhabitants or acquisition of a sexually transmitted infection (STI) can disrupt the vaginal microbiome, resulting in untoward vaginal symptoms and infection. The association between vaginitis and lactic acid remains theoretical, as postmenopausal women and prepubertal girls do not typically develop vaginitis, yet both groups lack lactobacilli in the vaginal environment.[7] Additionally, some studies have noted that women with minimal lactobacilli species who are otherwise healthy do not consistently report vaginitis or infection.[5]

Bacterial Vaginosis

Approximately 22% to 55% of women who present with symptoms of a vaginal condition have **bacterial vaginosis (BV)**.[1,8,9] This condition was initially termed "nonspecific vaginitis." Later, when the microorganism *Gardnerella vaginalis* was considered to be the single etiologic agent, the disorder became known simply as *Gardnerella*. Eventually, it was found that other microorganisms were involved; the more general term "bacterial vaginosis" was then created. The term "vaginosis" is used instead of "vaginitis" to indicate that this condition is not an inflammatory disease.

When the vaginal pH becomes more alkaline, normally occurring anaerobic and facultative organisms such as *Gardnerella vaginalis*, *Corynebacterium*, and *Escherichia coli* may overgrow and produce the characteristic symptoms of BV, including the fishy-type malodor that results from production of putrescine and cadaverine in the vagina.[10]

Bacterial vaginosis is enigmatic for several reasons, including the lack of a single pathogen as the cause and the observation that the symptoms for many women are transitory. A woman may schedule an appointment for care, only to note that the discharge and other symptoms have dissipated before she is seen. This resolution is associated with a spontaneous reappearance of a healthy vaginal ecosystem.[11]

While the majority of women with BV are asymptomatic, a significant proportion of women experience recurring and chronic symptoms. The condition has long been associated with multiple adverse gynecologic and obstetric sequelae, such as spontaneous abortion, upper genital tract disease, preterm birth, and postpartum endometritis, among others;[8] however, screening for BV and treatment of women with asymptomatic BV is controversial (Box 3-1).[12–14]

Treatment of Women with Symptomatic Bacterial Vaginosis

The Centers for Disease Control and Prevention (CDC) recommends that all symptomatic women be tested for BV; if positive, they should be treated.[3] Table 31-2 lists recommended treatments for BV under different circumstances. A woman with uncomplicated BV can be treated equally effectively with oral or vaginal medications, although the latter is associated with fewer gastrointestinal effects.[15–17] Although no universal definition exists for recurrent BV, three episodes in a 12-month period often is used as the criterion in the literature.[16]

Metronidazole

Metronidazole (Flagyl) is a synthetic antiprotozoal and antimicrobial agent in the nitroimidazole class. This agent can be administered orally or intravaginally in a topical formulation. Metronidazole is effective against gram-positive anaerobes *Clostridium* and *Peptostreptococcus*

Box 31-1 To Treat or Not to Treat: Asymptomatic Bacterial Vaginosis

Many women improve without treatment, and treatment itself is associated with subsequent development of vaginal yeast. Although BV is more prevalent in women with infertility, a systematic review and meta-analysis found that there was no association between BV and conception rates in general or conception rates after in vitro fertilization.[12] The situation is similar for pregnant women. Approximately one third of pregnant women in the United States have BV and women who have BV when pregnant have higher rates of preterm birth.[13] However, many studies and meta-analyses have found that treatment of asymptomatic BV during pregnancy does not reduce the risk of adverse outcomes.[14] Women who are symptomatic during pregnancy should be treated.

At this time, screening is only recommended for one clinical situation: Women who are undergoing gynecologic procedures such as surgical abortion or hysterectomy should be screened and treated for BV prior to the procedure to decrease the incidence of postoperative infection.[3,15]

species, gram-negative anaerobes such as *Bacteroides*, and protozoa such as *Trichomonas vaginalis*. Resistance to metronidazole is rare worldwide, and it is most commonly reported among gram-negative anaerobes found outside the United States.[19]

The majority of the adverse effects associated with metronidazole are gastrointestinal, including nausea, metallic taste in the mouth, and dry mouth. Headaches have been reported, as have vomiting and diarrhea. Rarely, neurotoxic symptoms occur; if they do present, the drug should be discontinued immediately because they may become permanent. Metronidazole (Flagyl) should be used with caution by women with central nervous system disorders because of the potential for neurotoxicity, and by women with hepatic disease because the drug is primarily metabolized through the liver.

The package labeling for metronidazole discusses a disulfiram effect when an individual concomitantly ingests alcohol at the same time or within 3 days of the time when metronidazole is administered. A disulfiram effect also is known as an anti-abuse effect, but has been called into question for this drug.[20,21] However, combining metronidazole with alcohol has been reported to result in mental confusion and psychosis in some cases. Metronidazole has multiple drug interactions, as discussed in the *Antimicrobials* chapter.

Women reporting intolerance to oral doses of metronidazole can be treated with clindamycin (Cleocin) or vaginal metronidazole. If a woman reports she is allergic to metronidazole, she should not use this drug in any form.[3]

Clindamycin (Cleocin) is an acceptable alternative to metronidazole. Because an oil base is used in the manufacturing process for clindamycin, latex condoms

Table 31-2 Recommended Treatments for a Woman with Bacterial Vaginosis

Drug: Generic (Brand)	Dose	Duration
Uncomplicated BV		
Clindamycin cream 2% (Cleocin vaginal, Clindesse vaginal)	One full applicator (5 g) intravaginally once daily	7 days
Metronidazole (Flagyl)	500 mg by mouth 2 times/day	7 days
Metronidazole gel 0.75% (MetroGel)	One full applicator (5 g) intravaginally once daily	5 days
Alternative Regimens		
Clindamycin (Cleocin)	300 mg by mouth 2 times/day	3 days
Clindamycin ovules (Cleocin ovules)	100 mg intravaginally at bedtime	3 days
Tinidazole (Tindamax)	2 g by mouth once daily	2 days
Tinidazole (Tindamax)	1 g by mouth once daily	5 days
During Pregnancy		
Clindamycin (Cleocin)	300 mg by mouth 2 times/day	7 days
Metronidazole (Flagyl)	500 mg by mouth 2 times/day	7 days
Metronidazole (Flagyl)	250 mg by mouth 3 times/day	7 days
Recurrent BV		
Metronidazole (Flagyl) *followed by* vaginal boric acid capsules	500 mg by mouth 600 mg intravaginally	7 days 21 days
Metronidazole gel 0.75% (Flagyl)	One applicator daily intravaginally	10 days[a]
Tinidazole (Tindamax)[b]	500 mg by mouth 2 times/day	14 days

[a] Followed by 2 times/week applications for 4–6 months.
[b] Off-label use.

Sources: Data from Forsum U, Holst E, Larsson PG, Vasquez A, Jakobsson T, Mattsby-Baltzer I. Bacterial vaginosis: a microbiological and immunological enigma. *APMIS.* 2005;113(2):81-90[11]; Reichman O, Akins R, Sobel JD. Boric acid addition to suppressive antimicrobial therapy for recurrent bacterial vaginitis. *Sex Transm Dis.* 2006;36(11):732-734[18]; Workowski KA, Berman S; Centers for Disease Control and Prevention. Sexually transmitted diseases treatment guidelines, 2010. *MMWR Recommend Rep.* 2010;59(RR-12):1-110.[3]

and diaphragms may be weakened for as long as 5 days following use of vaginal formulations.[3]

The FDA has also approved oral tinidazole (Tindamax) for treatment of BV. Tinidazole is a second generation nitroimidazole and it has a longer half-life than metronidazole (12 to 14 hours versus 6 to 7 hours) and fewer side effects. The effectiveness of tinidazole is similar to the effectiveness of metronidazole but it is not better. Tinidazole is also similar to metronidazole in that it has multiple drug–drug interactions and potentially may cause a disulfiram reaction.[22] Persons using this agent should be cautioned to avoid alcohol during treatment and for 3 days after completing treatment.

Recurrent Bacterial Vaginosis

Metronidazole (Flagyl) and clindamycin (Cleocin) have similar effectiveness, with cure rates averaging less than 65% to 70% after 1 month and recurrence rates nearing 50% after 6 months.[14,23] As many as 70% of women who have experienced an episode of BV will report a recurrence within 3 to 6 months. The CDC guidelines suggest retreating recurrent BV with the original therapy, using metronidazole gel (MetroGel) intravaginally weekly for 4 to 6 months, or monthly oral metronidazole (Flagyl) as noted in Table 31-2.[3] No studies have found a single regimen effective enough to be recommended for treatment of all women with recurrent BV.

Special Populations: Pregnancy, Lactation, and the Elderly

Although BV is associated with an increased risk for preterm birth, treatment of asymptomatic infections does not decrease the risk of preterm birth. Therefore BV is treated during pregnancy only if the woman is symptomatic. In years past, treatment with metronidazole (Flagyl) was discouraged during the first trimester of pregnancy for fear of teratogenicity. However, studies have failed to find teratogenic effects associated with either metronidazole or clindamycin (Cleocin) when used during the first trimester.[1,3] Limited data are available regarding the human safety of tinidazole (Tindamax), and some animal studies suggest tinidazole may have some toxic effects. Most clinicians choose to prescribe metronidazole (Flagyl) during pregnancy because a larger number of studies have evaluated this drug.[24]

Older studies found that intravaginal formulations of clindamycin given in the second half of pregnancy are not effective and perhaps are associated with an increased risk for low birth weight and neonatal infection. For this reason, vaginal preparations of clindamycin are not recommended for use during pregnancy, although the oral regimen is recommended.[3]

Small, if any, amounts of the vaginal formulations approved for treatment of women with BV have been found in breast milk, making that delivery method a good one for women requiring BV treatment who are breastfeeding. Most drugs orally consumed by a breastfeeding woman are excreted into the breast milk in small amounts, usually less than 5% of the maternal dose. Metronidazole (Flagyl), however, becomes concentrated in breast milk, with the relative infant dose being approximately 12.6% to 13.5% of the maternal dose. No reports of adverse outcomes have been found among the infants breastfed by women who received metronidazole, although some infants may reject the breast milk because of its metallic taste. The dose of metronidazole received by the infant is less than may be directly administered to the child in the event the child develops an infection for which metronidazole is the recommended treatment. For women who receive a single high dose of 2 g, because of the limited studies and the probability of neonatal gastric distress, it is recommended that they receive the medication after a feeding and then discard expressed breast milk for 12 to 24 hours—the "pump and dump" method.[25]

If the tinidazole (Tindamax) 2 g treatment is employed, it is recommended that the woman refrain from feeding the infant breast milk during treatment and for 3 days after therapy.[3] Clindamycin (Cleocin) is also detectable in breast milk, but the relative infant dose is 0.9% to 1.8% of the oral maternal dose; thus, this agent is safe to use by lactating women.[26]

The incidence of BV has been reported to increase with a woman's age.[27] However, there are no special considerations to modify treatment guidelines for the older woman.

Emerging Therapies: BV Prevention, Treatment, and Recurrence of Bacterial Vaginosis

A pilot study found that high doses of intravaginal administration of metronidazole (750 mg), with or without the use of intravaginal miconazole (Monistat), significantly improved cure rates by the fourth visit for women with recurrent BV (68.4% versus 33.3%; $P < 0.05$).[23] A separate multicenter trial demonstrated that a 1.3% dose of metronidazole given intravaginally for 1, 3, or 5 days showed similar effectiveness, safety, and tolerability as the standard metronidazole 0.75 mg dose.[28]

Other antibiotics, antiseptics, acidifying agents, prebiotics, and probiotics (the latter two as adjunctive therapies) have been investigated for treatment and prevention of recurrence of BV. Antiseptics such as chlorhexidine and povidone-iodine have been instilled in vaginal suppositories or pessaries. One double-blinded, placebo-controlled randomized clinical trial (RCT) found that 250 mg of ascorbic acid placed vaginally 6 days per month for 6 months reduced the rate of recurrence by half (from 32.4% to 16.2%; $P = 0.024$).[29] A Cochrane review concluded there was insufficient evidence to recommend probiotics for treatment of women with BV or as an adjunctive therapy.[30] However, a subsequent review acknowledged that while results of studies examining use of probiotics for prevention of recurrent BV had conflicting results, most identified favorable results and no adverse effects.[31] This review of the literature also suggested that addition of probiotics to the therapeutic regimen for a woman with recurrent BV is not harmful and may be of value, although more studies are needed to ascertain the precise level of effectiveness.[31]

In summary, BV remains a conundrum. Studies showing direct evidence of its etiology, treatments demonstrating better cure rates, and means to prevent recurrences continue to be needed.

Trichomoniasis

Trichomoniasis, also known as *Trichomonas* vaginitis (TV), is one of the most common sexually transmitted infections in the United States, with an annual incidence estimated of 3 to 5 million cases. The majority of women affected are between 15 and 24 years.[32] The estimated prevalence of TV is 3.1%, but distinct racial and ethnic disparities exist. The prevalence of TV among non-Hispanic black women is more than 10 times higher than that among non-Hispanic white and Mexican American women.[32]

Trichomoniasis is caused by infection with a single-cell, flagellated protozoan, *T. vaginalis*. This organism thrives only in a human host and infects the vagina, vulva, and urethra in women. Although TV is a sexually transmitted infection, it is not reportable to any state health department within the United States.[32]

Treatment of Women with Symptomatic Trichomoniasis

Trichomoniasis is exclusively transmitted sexually; there are no proven cases of transmission via fomites.[19] Studies estimate that anywhere from 10% to 85% of women are asymptomatic carriers of trichomoniasis—that is, they are infected with *T. vaginalis* but do not exhibit any symptoms.[19,33] This infection is associated with acquisition and transmission of HIV and other sexually transmitted infections, adverse outcomes of pregnancy, and pelvic inflammatory disease, especially among women infected with HIV.[19] Untreated infections may last for months or years without producing symptoms.

All current sexual partners of women with symptomatic trichomoniasis, including any partners within the previous 4 months (male and female), should be treated for trichomoniasis, regardless of testing results, and screened for other sexually transmitted infections.[3] Treatment regimens are the same for men and women. Women who are HIV-positive can be treated with the same regimen as those who are HIV-negative; however, in a randomized clinical trial, Kissinger et al. found a 500 mg, twice-daily regimen of metronidazole (Flagyl) for 7 days was more effective among women with HIV than a single 2 g dose.[34] Tinidazole (Tindamax) is a recent alternative to metronidazole but has similar effectiveness.[35] Recommended treatments for TV are listed in Table 31-3, and Box 31-2 presents a case study of a woman with trichomoniasis.

Metronidazole (Flagyl) is the pharmacotherapeutic agent most commonly used to treat trichomoniasis. Its mechanism of action against protozoa remains unclear, but the drug appears to be selective for anaerobic bacteria due to their ability to reduce metronidazole to its active form within the cell.[36] Once in active form, the reduced

Table 31-3 Recommended Treatment of a Woman with Trichomoniasis

Drug: Generic (Brand)	Dose	Duration
Uncomplicated TV		
Metronidazole (Flagyl)	2 g by mouth	Single dose
Tinidazole (Tindamax)	2 g by mouth	Single dose
Alternative Regimen		
Metronidazole (Flagyl)	500 mg by mouth 2 times/day	7 days
During Pregnancy (Symptomatic Women)		
Metronidazole (Flagyl)	2 g by mouth	Single dose
Recurrent Trichomoniasis (Reinfection)		
Metronidazole (Flagyl)	500 mg by mouth 2 times/day	7 days
Tinidazole (Tindamax)	2 g by mouth	Single dose
Treatment Failures Where Reinfection Has Been Excluded		
Metronidazole (Flagyl)	500 mg by mouth daily	7 days
Metronidazole (Flagyl)	2 g by mouth daily	5 days
Tinidazole (Tindamax)	2 g by mouth daily	5 days

Source: Data from Workowski KA, Berman S; Centers for Disease Control and Prevention. Sexually transmitted diseases treatment guidelines, 2010. *MMWR Recommend Rep.* 2010;59(RR-12):1-110.[3]

Box 31-2 Case Study: A Woman with Trichomoniasis

WF is a 25-year-old woman who reports burning and vaginal pruritus. Her last normal menstrual period was 3 weeks ago, and she uses condoms for birth control. A vaginal examination revealed a yellow-green discharge positive for flagellated protozoa upon microscopic visualization. There is no question that WF should be treated for trichomoniasis because she is symptomatic.

The most common treatment is 2 g of oral metronidazole (Flagyl). However, there are other issues to consider. Trichomoniasis is a sexually transmitted infection. When a sexually transmitted infection is diagnosed, it is imperative to screen for other sexually transmitted infections, including gonorrhea, chlamydia, HIV, syphilis, and hepatitis, depending on the woman's individual risks, local prevalence of disease, and the practice's protocols.

Because WF is not pregnant, she and her sexual partner(s) can begin treatment immediately. Metronidazole may cause a disulfiram effect if an individual ingests alcohol while taking the drug. Thus, WF should be advised to abstain from alcoholic beverages for 24 hours after completing her course of metronidazole. The most common side effects of metronidazole are gastrointestinal in nature, such as nausea, vomiting, and an unpleasant metallic taste.

Urethral infection with *Trichomonas* is found in 90% of women who report symptomatic vaginal symptoms.[33] Metronidazole vaginal gels are not effective for treatment of urethral infection; instead, the oral regimen is recommended as it will provide therapeutic levels sufficient to treat TV in both the vagina and the urethra.

WF's partner(s) should be treated with the same dose of metronidazole prescribed for WF. Providing a prescription for WF to take to her partner(s) without examination by a provider—a practice known as expedited therapy[3]—is both evidence based and widely recommended. WF should be counseled to avoid unprotected intercourse until both she and her partner(s) have completed treatment; otherwise, treated individuals may become reinfected.

No test of cure is needed unless WF's symptoms do not resolve within 1 to 2 weeks. In such a case, a subsequent examination is likely to find another condition that was previously obscured by her TV.

metronidazole binds to DNA and disrupts its structure, culminating in cell death. Metronidazole is readily concentrated in tissues and becomes highly lethal to *T. vaginalis*. Treatment with topical metronidazole gel is less efficacious than oral therapy for trichomoniasis, however, and is not recommended. Metronidazole gel does not result in therapeutic levels sufficient to eradicate urethral organisms. Therefore, the single 2-g oral dose of metronidazole is the CDC's recommended first-line therapy and is superior to a multiday treatment with the same agent. Cure rates are more than 90% to 95% after the single-dose treatment with metronidazole and 86% to 100% after treatment with tinidazole (Tindamax).[3]

If reinfection occurs, the CDC recommends metronidazole 500 mg orally twice daily for an additional 7 days. For those failing a second treatment, metronidazole or tinidazole can be taken daily for an additional 5 to 7 days.[3,19] If this protracted treatment fails, the provider should consider consulting the CDC.[3]

Treatment of Women with Asymptomatic Trichomoniasis

For some healthcare professionals, evidence-based recommendations not to screen or treat asymptomatic women with TV present an ethical dilemma. The evidence does not provide clear guidance for caring for women under these circumstances. Although TV is a sexually transmitted infection, it generally has not been associated with major adverse reproductive health outcomes. Nevertheless, some studies have suggested an association between trichomoniasis and having a child with an intellectual disability or attention disorder.[19] If more rigorous research confirms these associations, recommendations against screening for asymptomatic TV would benefit from reevaluation. Better and larger RCTs are needed to equip providers and women with stronger level evidence and updated guidelines.

Recurrent Trichomoniasis and Treatment Failure

Treatment recommendations for recurrent infection and treatment failure can be found in Table 31-3. Because nitroimidazoles are highly effective, it is important to distinguish recurrent infection from treatment failure. However, resistance is an emerging concern because there are few, if any, alternative therapies for TV.[19] If treatment failure is suspected, the provider should consult a specialist and consider susceptibility testing. Both consultation and susceptibility testing are available from the CDC.[3]

Special Populations: Pregnancy, Lactation, and the Elderly

The CDC currently recommends screening and treating women who are pregnant and report symptoms that suggest trichomoniasis. Metronidazole 2 g orally as one dose can be given at any time during pregnancy.[3] While TV has been associated with adverse pregnancy outcomes, there is no evidence to show that treatment with metronidazole during pregnancy reduces perinatal morbidity.[37] However, treatment will reduce symptoms, reduce the risk of sexual transmission, and result in cure for women with symptomatic disease. Two older studies found rates of preterm birth increased following treatment with metronidazole, but limitations of these trials prevent definitive conclusions from being drawn and causality cannot be assumed.[3,37,38] The safety of tinidazole during pregnancy has not been evaluated; consequently, this agent is not recommended for use during pregnancy.[3]

Women who are breastfeeding should ingest the oral medication after a feeding and then discard expressed breast milk for 12 to 24 hours.[25] If Tinidazole 2 g treatment is employed, expressed milk should be discarded during treatment and for 3 days after therapy.[39]

Because of liver-associated adverse drug effects, older women in particular should be carefully monitored when they take either metronidazole or tinidazole.

Alternative Therapies and Complemental Treatments for Women with Trichomoniasis

In past decades, several different douches were advocated to treat a woman with trichomoniasis, including a dedicated brand known as Trichotin that included a mild detergent used as a cleansing douche. Dilute betadine douches also were promoted by some providers.[40] Alternative therapies such as douching with a boric acid, vinegar solution, or other substances such as calendula, goldenseal, or echinacea, or insertion of garlic cloves into the vagina may relieve symptoms temporarily. However, because trichomonal organisms live not only in the vagina but also in the urethra and urogenital glands, systemic treatment is still needed to eradicate the organism.

Vulvovaginal Candidiasis

Candida albicans is a normal inhabitant of the vagina, but when found in large amounts it is the most common cause of **vulvovaginal candidiasis (VVC)**. VVC, which is also known as candida vaginitis, yeast vaginitis, and fungal infection, affects as many as 75% of women at least once during their lifetime.[41] While more than 90% of all VVC is caused by *C. albicans*, other species of *Candida*—such as *glabrata*, *tropicalis*, and *krusei*—have also been implicated. The latter species are more resistant to commonly used azole antifungal therapies.[1,3]

Research currently focuses on identification of the complex set of circumstances that facilitates symptomatic infection in women who otherwise tolerate low levels of *Candida* species without difficulty. The new focus involves host immune function, availability of estrogen, virulence of the specific organism, and an increase in vaginal pH as reflected by diminished levels of lactobacilli.[42] VVC is classified as uncomplicated or complicated depending on symptoms, frequency of occurrence, implicated organism, response to treatment, and general health of the host (e.g., immunocompromised health status).[3] The classification scheme for VVC is listed in Table 31-4 and is the basis for some treatments.

Treatment of Women with Uncomplicated Vulvovaginal Candidiasis

The majority of women with uncomplicated VVC have a vaginitis caused by *C. albicans*. They can be adequately treated with a short course of one of the topical azole drugs, such as butoconazole (Gynezole-1), clotrimazole (Gyne-Lotrimin), miconazole (Monistat), tioconazole (Monistat 1-Day), and terconazole (Terazol-3), as listed in Table 31-5.

Table 31-4 Classification of Vulvovaginal Candidiasis

	Uncomplicated Vulvovaginal Candidiasis	Complicated Vulvovaginal Candidiasis
Frequency of symptoms	Sporadic or infrequent episodes	Recurrent episodes (4 or more per year)
Severity of symptoms	Mild to moderate symptoms	Severe vulvovaginal symptoms
Causative agent	Causative agent most likely *C. albicans*	Suspected or culture-proven non-*albicans* etiology
Populations affected	Nonpregnant women without medical comorbidities	Women with uncontrolled diabetes, severe medical illness, immunosuppression, concurrent vaginal conditions, and/or pregnancy

Source: Data from Workowski KA, Berman S; Centers for Disease Control and Prevention. Sexually transmitted diseases treatment guidelines, 2010. *MMWR Recommend Rep.* 2010;59(RR-12):1-110.[3]

Table 31-5 Recommended Treatment for a Woman with Uncomplicated Vulvovaginal Candidiasis

Intravaginal Agents: Generic (Brand)	Dose	Duration
Butoconazole 2% cream (Gynazole-1)	5 g intravaginally at bedtime	3 days
Clotrimazole 1% cream (Gyne-Lotrimin cream, Mycelex-7)	5 g intravaginally at bedtime	7–14 days
Clotrimazole 2% cream (generic brands common in retail pharmacies)	5 g intravaginally at bedtime	3 days
Miconazole 2% cream (Monistat-7)	5 g intravaginally at bedtime	7 days
Miconazole 4% cream (Monistat-3)	5 g intravaginally at bedtime	3 days
Miconazole 100-mg suppository (Monistat-7)	1 suppository intravaginally at bedtime	7 days
Miconazole 200-mg suppository (Monistat-3)	1 suppository intravaginally at bedtime	3 days
Monistat 1200-mg suppository (Monistat-1)	1 suppository intravaginally at bedtime	Single dose
Tioconazole 6.5% ointment (Monistat 1-Day, Vagistat 1; Equate)	5 g intravaginally at bedtime	Single dose
Terconazole 0.4% cream (45 g) (Terazol-7)	5 g intravaginally at bedtime	7 days
Terconazole 0.8% cream (30 g) (Terazol-3)	5 g intravaginally at bedtime	3 days
Terconazole 80-mg suppository (Terazol-3)	1 suppository intravaginally at bedtime	3 days
Oral Agents		
Fluconazole (Diflucan)[a]	150-mg oral tablet	Single dose

[a] Prescription only.

Sources: Data from Angotti LB, Lambert LC, Soper DE. Vaginitis: making sense of over-the-counter treatment options. *Infect Dis Obstet Gynecol.* 2007;97424. doi:10.1155/2007/97424[43]; Workowski KA, Berman S; Centers for Disease Control and Prevention. Sexually transmitted diseases treatment guidelines, 2010. *MMWR Recommend Rep.* 2010;59(RR-12):1-110.[3]

To ensure that the selected regimen is effective, women should be familiar with the best method in which to insert the creams or suppositories. Box 31-3 lists information that can be of value for consumers who are learning how to use the medications.

All of the topical drugs for VVC work by interfering with synthesis of ergosterol which is an essential molecule in the fungal cell membrane. There is no evidence that any specific azole is more effective than others for treatment of *C. albicans* infection: All have cure rates between 80% and 90%.[41] Instead, cost, availability, and route of administration of the drug are the factors to consider when recommending one drug over another.[1,43] Treatment of partners is not warranted because uncomplicated VVC is not typically acquired through sexual transmission. However, at least one study suggests that in women who have recurrent episodes of VVC, the organisms may be transmitted through sexual contact.[43] Hormonal contraceptives have been identified as increasing a woman's risk for the development of VVC, but that finding is likely associated only with older high-dose, combined oral contraceptives; no such link between current contraceptive methods and VVC has been found.[44,45]

The widespread availability of several different over-the-counter products to treat *Candida* vaginitis ensures that women have multiple options for treatment.[43] While self-treatment may save an office visit, several studies show that women often misdiagnose their vaginal symptoms, thereby delaying accurate diagnosis and treatment.[46] At least one study using culture-proven diagnoses found only 33% of women who self-diagnosed VVC actually had the condition.[47] Therefore, in addition to knowing how to appropriately insert the medication, women should know when *not* to treat themselves. Box 31-4 lists suggested indications and contraindications for women to use when considering self-treatment.

Topical azoles may cause mild and self-limiting local skin reactions such as burning or irritation. Women using condoms and/or diaphragms and prescribed topical azoles should be informed that many vaginal preparations are oil based and may weaken the latex in their contraceptive device.

Box 31-3 Directions for Self-Administration of Vaginal Cream or Suppository

1. Load the applicator to the fill line with cream.
   Or
   Unwrap the suppository and place it in the applicator.
2. Lie down on your back with knees drawn up.
3. Gently insert the applicator high into the vagina and apply the medication as the applicator is withdrawn.
4. Discard the applicator if it is disposable, or wash it with soap and rinse well with water.
5. To keep the medication from getting on clothing, wear a mini-pad or panty liner.
6. Do not use tampons or douche.
7. Avoid intercourse until the course of therapy is completed.

Box 31-4 Indications and Contraindications for Self-Treatment of Vulvovaginal Candidiasis

Women should seek professional care for vaginal symptoms if they:

- Have a foul-smelling vaginal discharge
- Experience pain in lower abdomen, back, or shoulder
- Have diabetes, are pregnant, or have or suspect they have HIV infection
- Are febrile
- Do not experience relief or improvement within 3 days after self-treatment
- Have recurrence of symptoms within 2 months

Self-treatment of *Candida* infections is best reserved for women who:

- Are at least 12 years or older
- Have previously had an episode of vulvovaginal candidiasis diagnosed by a health professional

Another treatment option for women with VVC is an oral antifungal such as fluconazole (Diflucan). Fluconazole is available as a prescription-only formulation containing 150 mg given as a single dose and has cure rates comparable to vaginal preparations that require doses for 3 or 4 days.[3] Use of this fluconazole (Diflucan) may cause elevated liver enzymes, and laboratory studies of liver enzymes should be monitored if it is taken as long-term therapy.[2,14] Fluconazole may also cause nausea, headache, and abdominal pain.[3] The cost of generic fluconazole compares favorably with the over-the-counter azole cream or suppository therapies. This option is often preferred by women because it is a convenient, oral, single-dose therapy.

Other azoles that are not on the CDC's list of recommended VVC treatments include itraconazole (Sporanox) and ketoconazole (Nizoral). Itraconazole is manufactured in a capsule that is relatively large, making it difficult for some women to swallow. Ketoconazole has been available for years, but has been largely replaced by fluconazole (Diflucan) because fluconazole has less toxicity and better absorption.[48,49]

When used in high doses or for long periods of time, oral azoles are inhibitors of some of the important CYP450 enzymes and substrates for others. Azoles can precipitate dangerous drug–drug interactions, and it is essential to know which medications (prescription and nonprescription) a woman is using prior to prescribing an oral azole to avoid drug interactions. Some drug–azole combinations are contraindicated. Drug interactions with azoles are discussed in more detail in the *Antimicrobials* chapter.

Complicated Vulvovaginal Candidiasis

VVC is considered complicated if the woman has one of the following: (1) severe signs and symptoms; (2) a history of four or more episodes per year; (3) is diagnosed with a *Candida* species other than *C. albicans*, especially *C. glabrata*; or (4) if she is pregnant, immunosuppressed, debilitated for any reason, or if she has poorly controlled diabetes. Although it is unknown if one azole is better than another for treatment of complicated VVC, women with one of these four factors will require a longer duration of therapy. Recommended treatment options for complicated VVC are found in Table 31-6.

Treatment of Women with Severe Symptoms

Women with severe symptoms such as extensive vulvar erythema, edema, or fissures, are usually treated with fluconazole (Diflucan) 150 mg administered orally for 2 or 3 sequential doses each 72 hours apart. If the woman prefers topical therapy, a 7 to 10 day course is preferred over the usual 1- to 3-day course.

Treatment of Women with Non-albicans Vulvovaginal Candidiasis

Women with infections caused by *C. albicans* or *C. glabrata* usually respond favorably to the azole medications but often require longer than the 1- to 3-day period of therapy recommended for uncomplicated VVC. The optimal treatment of a woman with non-*albicans* VVC is unknown. The CDC recommendations for treatment are listed in Table 31-6.

Boric acid is an effective treatment for non-*albicans* species; it is taken in the form of a 600-mg suppository or capsule administered via the vagina once daily for 14 days.[50] One review of 14 studies, including 2 RCTs, concluded that use of intravaginal boric acid capsules for recurrent and chronic VVC symptoms is a safe, alternative option when conventional therapies fail and when non-*albicans* or azole-resistant strains have been identified.[50]

Women who have diabetes develop VVC present more often with *C. glabrata* infection than with *C. albicans* infection.[51] The participants in one study who had infections involving the *glabrata* strain responded more favorably to treatment with boric acid 600 mg suppositories

Table 31-6 Treatment of a Woman with Complicated forms of Vulvovaginal Candidiasis

Drug: Generic (Brand)	Dose	Length of Therapy
Recurrent or Severe VVC		
Topical azoles (e.g., Monistat)	Daily	7–14 days
Fluconazole (Diflucan)	100, 150, or 200 mg by mouth every 3 days	3 doses (days 1, 4, and 7)
Maintenance Therapy		
Fluconazole (Diflucan)	100, 150, or 200 mg by mouth	Weekly for 6 months
Clotrimazole (Gyne-Lotrimin)	500 mg intravaginally	Weekly for 6 months
Non-albicans VVC		
Amphotericin B cream 3%[a,b] (AmB)	intravaginally	7–14 days
Flucytosine 17%[a,b,c] (Ancobon)	5 g intravaginally	14 days
Boric acid capsules 600 mg[a]	1 capsule intravaginally	14 days

[a] Found in compounding pharmacies.
[b] Failure to respond to azole or boric acid preparations.
[c] May be used alone or in combination with amphotericin B.
Sources: Data from Pappas PG, Kauffman CA, Andes D, et al. Clinical practice guidelines for the management of candidiasis: 2009 update by the Infectious Diseases Society of America. *Clin Infectious Dis.* 2009;48(5):503-535[49]; Phillips AJ. Treatment of non-*albicans Candida* vaginitis with amphotericin B vaginal suppositories. *Am J Obstet Gynecol.* 2005;192(6):2009-2012[56]; Sobel JD, Chaim W, Nagappan V, Leaman D. Treatment of vaginitis caused by *Candida glabrata*: use of topical boric acid and flycytosine. *Am J Obstet Gynecol.* 2003;189(5):1297-1300[55]; Workowski KA, Berman S; Centers for Disease Control and Prevention. Sexually transmitted diseases treatment guidelines, 2010. *MMWR Recommend Rep.* 2010;59(RR-12):1-110.[3]

administered once daily for 14 days than did women who were treated with a single dose of oral fluconazole 150 mg (63.6% versus 28.6%, respectively; $P = .01$).[51] The long-term safety of intravaginal boric acid has not been evaluated, however, nor is there any evidence of its safety when used in pregnancy. At all times, when using intravaginal boric acid, women should be counseled to keep capsules away from children and pets because oral ingestion can be fatal.

Treatment of Women with Recurrent Vulvovaginal Candidiasis

VVC is termed recurrent if four or more symptomatic episodes occur per year.[3] Recurrent VVC affects fewer than 5% of women each year. Approximately 10% to 20% of recurrent VVC cases is caused by *C. albicans* or *C. glabrata*. Recurrent VVC is considered multifactorial in origin; all efforts to eliminate contributing factors should be undertaken and cultures obtained to identify the specific causative organism. Once symptoms resolve and a culture is negative, failure to initiate a maintenance regimen results in a relapse of symptoms within 3 months among 50% of women.[52] Maintenance regimens include once-weekly treatment with either clotrimazole (Gyne-Lotrimin) intravaginal suppositories or fluconazole (Diflucan). Even with a maintenance regimen, relapse is common. Two older studies showed some success with suppressing recurrence using depo-medroxyprogesterone acetate (Depo-Provera), yogurt, and antihistamines.[53,54] Older studies that examined treatment for male partners of women with recurrent VVC have not shown any benefit to this practice,[54] but treatment of male partners has not been evaluated in recent studies.

While the incidence of VVC among women with HIV is not known, rates of vaginal colonization of *Candida* are higher in HIV-positive women as compared to seronegative women.[3] Treatment for women with HIV need not differ from that of other women who may have complicated VVC and are HIV-negative. Optimal treatment for women with non-*albicans* VVC has not been established.

Special Populations: Pregnancy, Lactation, and the Elderly

VVC frequently occurs during pregnancy. In 2006, the CDC categorized VVC during pregnancy as "complicated," but the 2010 guidelines for treatment of sexually transmitted infections do not classify such infection in this way.[3] In 2013, the American College of Obstetricians and Gynecologists reaffirmed pregnancy as a complicated form of VVC.[1]

Currently, topical azoles are the only forms of treatment for VVC recommended for use by pregnant women.[1,3,49] Some teratogenicity was noted in animal studies when high doses of fluconazole (Diflucan) were used. No controlled studies of the effects of fluconazole in humans have been conducted, however, nor have teratogenic effects in the fetus or newborn been noted when fluconazole is used during pregnancy. When fluconazole is used in the first trimester, doses higher than 400 mg over extended periods of time have been suggested to be associated with malformations in humans, although use of a single lower dose (150 mg) has not demonstrated similar associations. Fluconazole is safe for breastfeeding women.[57]

The incidence of VVC has been found to decrease as women age, yet *Candida* infections have been reported to be the most important cause of opportunistic infections, which predominantly affect individuals older than 65 years.[27] Fortunately, the antifungals appropriate for reproductive-age women appear to be safe and appropriate for older women as well.[58]

Alternative Therapies and Complemental Therapies for Women with Vulvovaginal Candidiasis

Few, if any, recent studies have examined the effectiveness of alternative therapies for VVC. Older studies explored vinegar douches, vitamin C, garlic clove vaginal inserts, and oral ingestion or vaginal application of yogurt, goldenseal, and gentian violet. However, no large, randomized, controlled trials have been conducted. Several studies have evaluated use of *Lactobacillus* capsules and/or yogurt with mixed findings regarding cure rates.[59,60] Some strains of *Lactobacillus* have demonstrated the ability to colonize the vagina and prevent growth of *Candida* both in vitro and in some human studies; however, clinical trials have yielded mixed results.[60]

Gentian violet is a purple dye with antifungal properties that has been used to treat vaginal yeast infections as well as thrush in neonates for many years. It is perhaps the oldest known treatment for yeast infections, although studies on its effectiveness are lacking. Gentian violet is infrequently used today because azoles are more effective and less inconvenient. Gentian violet permanently stains a woman's clothes and often leaves stains on office examination tables.

Nonpharmacologic behaviors related to VVC prevention and treatment are aimed at activities to decrease moisture in the vaginal area, such as use of cotton underwear, loose-fitting pants, and avoidance of pantyhose. Decreasing use of unnecessary antibiotics and reducing intake of refined sugars in a woman's diet may diminish *Candida* colonization. The novel approach of sterilizing cotton underwear in a microwave oven was theorized as a method to decrease self-reinoculation many years ago and caused many women to adopt this intervention.[61] However, no RCTs have been published that have evaluated any of these common interventions.

The development of antifungal vaccines is currently being investigated using animal models; results seem promising, but no data are available regarding use in humans.[62] Other studies continue to explore host genetic factors, anti-*Candida* defense mechanisms, and genetic yeast factors that facilitate vaginal persistence.

Atrophic Vaginitis

Atrophic vaginitis is a symptomatic condition frequently found among women experiencing decreased estrogen production as a result of perimenopause, postmenopausal status, or lactation. It develops as a consequence of vulvovaginal atrophy; however, while the terms "atrophic vaginitis" and "vulvovaginal atrophy" are often used interchangeably, they are not necessarily the same. Some authors distinguish between an atrophic vagina, resulting from urogenital atrophy, and atrophic vaginitis, also resulting from urogenital atrophy and accompanied by inflammation.[63,64] Moreover, the new term "genitourinary syndrome of menopause" (GSM) has been recently suggested to replace the less accurate term of "atrophy."[65] Women who are breastfeeding also experience a drop in estrogen, and some may experience the same symptoms as postmenopausal woman. Some authorities term this condition "lactational vaginal atrophy," although most sources continue to use the term "vaginal atrophy."

Atrophic vaginitis is a local condition characterized by scant secretions, immature epithelial cells, elevated vaginal pH, and an increase in white blood cells. Symptoms include genital itching and burning as well as urinary frequency and pain. An estimated 10% to 40% of postmenopausal women have symptoms of atrophic vaginitis.[63,66] If left untreated, vulvovaginal atrophy is a progressive condition that can significantly interfere with quality of life. Very little has been published specifically about lactational atrophic vaginitis. A case study published in 2003 noted only three articles found in a Medline search dating back to 1966.[67]

Treatment of Women with Atrophic Vaginitis

Treatment for atrophic vaginitis will depend on the woman's preference, the severity of her symptoms, and the effectiveness and safety of treatments.[63] Nonprescription therapies include regular use of lubricants and moisturizing agents to decrease symptoms and discomfort. These agents may be water-, silicone-, or oil-based preparations. Low-dose vaginal estrogen therapy can replace the loss of estrogen in women with atrophic vaginitis and is administered either locally (vaginally) or orally. While oral estrogen can be used, vaginal estrogen is the preferred mode of delivery and is generally more effective that the oral route when vaginal symptoms are the primary concern.[63] The subject of atrophic vaginitis is discussed in more detail in the chapter *The Mature Woman.*

Special Populations: Pregnancy, Lactation, and the Elderly

The majority of women who report the symptoms associated with atrophic vaginitis are older women and, therefore, the general guidelines for treatment are appropriate for them.[68,69] Vaginal atrophy does not occur among pregnant women, but it can occur among breastfeeding women. Estrogen is the preferred treatment, and it can be administered topically or through hormonal contraceptives, including pills, rings, and patches for lactating women. However, aside from contraceptives, if estrogen alone is administered, ovulation may occur, prolactin levels subsequently decrease, and breast milk production may be diminished.

Desquamative Inflammatory Vaginitis

Desquamative inflammatory vaginitis (DIV) is a rare syndrome characterized by a profuse, noninfectious vaginal discharge, accompanied by vaginal irritation, erythema, burning, and dyspareunia. This condition is most commonly found among perimenopausal women. In DIV, the predominant lactobacilli flora of the vagina are replaced with gram-positive coccobacilli, usually group B *Streptococcus.*

The diagnosis of DIV is one of exclusion; that is, it is made only after more common conditions have been ruled out. Treatment includes either topical antibiotics or topical corticosteroids. Clindamycin cream 2% (Cleocin) is used intravaginally for both its anti-inflammatory and antimicrobial activities for 2 to 4 weeks; women are then reevaluated. Sobel reported results of a study of outcomes in 98 women diagnosed with DIV. Although improvement was reported in 86% of the women by 3 weeks, relapse was common, lending support to the perception of DIV as a chronic inflammatory process.[70] If women are concurrently diagnosed with vaginal estrogen deficiency, local estrogen therapy may aid in maintaining remission.[70] The noticeable difference between DIV and atrophic vaginitis is that DIV does not respond to estrogen therapy alone. Some authorities suggest that prescribers consider the addition of weekly oral fluconazole (Diflucan) or an intravaginal azole to minimize the occurrence of secondary *Candida* infection when using intravaginal antimicrobial agents or corticosteroids.[71]

Although some researchers have suggested that group B *Streptococcus* (GBS) could be the etiological agent for DIV, most scientists believe there is not a causal relationship between the two.[72] Vaginal colonization by GBS is common, and the vast majority of women with GBS and a vaginal discharge have another condition such as BV, TV, or VVC.

Special Populations: Pregnancy, Lactation, and the Elderly

Desquamative inflammatory vaginitis is primarily a condition among perimenopausal women, rather than pregnant or lactating women. Therefore, there are no special considerations for the latter two groups.

The Clinical Challenge

Although BV, VVC, and TV represent the most common causes of vaginal symptomatology, other conditions can cause vaginal discharge and can prove challenging to diagnose and treat. These conditions are less common, but may include DIV as well as vulvar dermatoses, eczema, irritant or contact dermatitis, lichen sclerosis, lichen planus, and vulvar aphthae.[71] Group A *Streptococcus* is a rare, but possible cause of a vaginal discharge.[73] Irritants such as spermicides, latex, sanitary pads, douches, soaps, perfumed products, and vaginal sprays; antifungal drugs; and barrier contraceptives may all cause irritation or allergic reactions. Multiple visits for a vaginal discharge wherein no abnormalities are apparent may suggest the woman is in an abusive situation.[74]

Conclusion

Vaginal discharge is not an innocuous event. Women seeking treatment of symptomatic vaginal conditions make approximately 10 million visits to healthcare providers per year. Usually the symptoms are caused by one of the three most common types of vaginitis: bacterial vaginosis, candidiasis, or trichomoniasis. Vaginal conditions can coexist with other ones or in conjunction with a sexually transmitted infection. Most of these infections respond readily to appropriate therapy. Careful history taking and accurate diagnoses are critical skills for guiding the selection of the most appropriate therapies.

Resources

Organization	Description	Website
Centers for Disease Control and Prevention	Guidelines for treatment of sexually transmitted infections, including vaginal conditions	www.cdc.gov/std/treatment/2010/
	Guidelines as a smartphone app (iOS and Android)	www.cdc.gov/std/std-tx-app.htm
	Facebook page with active discussion on wall	www.facebook.com/CDCSTD
	Twitter homepage	https://twitter.com/CDCSTD
	Self-study module on vaginitis for healthcare professionals	www2a.cdc.gov/stdtraining/self-study/vaginitis/default.htm
	Educational materials designed for clinical instructors to accompany information in self-study module	www2a.cdc.gov/stdtraining/ready-to-use/vaginitis.htm

References

1. Nyirjesy P. ACOG Clinical Practice Bulletin, No. 72, reaffirmed 2013: vaginitis. *Obstet Gynecol.* 2006;107(5):1195.
2. Mashburn J. Etiology, diagnosis, and management of vaginitis. *J Midwifery Womens Health.* 2006;51:423-430.
3. Workowski KA, Berman S; Centers for Disease Control and Prevention. Sexually transmitted diseases treatment guidelines, 2010. *MMWR Recommend Rep.* 2010;59(RR-12):1-110.
4. Edwards L. Dermatologic causes of vaginitis: a clinical review. *Dermatol Clin.* 2010;28(4):727-735.
5. Ma B, Forney LJ, Ravel J. Vaginal microbiome: rethinking health and disease. *Annu Rev Microbiol.* 2012;66:371-389.
6. Lazenby GB, Soper DE, Nolte FS. Correlation of leukorrhea and *Trichomonas vaginalis* infection. *J Clin Microbiol.* 2013;51(7):2323-2327.
7. Witkin SS, Mendes-Soares H, Linhares IM, Jayaram A, Ledger WJ, Forney LJ. Influence of vaginal bacteria and d- and l-lactic acid isomers on vaginal extracellular matrix metalloproteinase inducer: implications for protection against upper genital tract infections. *Molecul Biol.* 2013;4(4):e00460-13.
8. Fethers KA, Fairley CK, Hocking JS, Gurrin LC, Bradshaw CS. Sexual risk factors and bacterial vaginosis: a systematic review and meta-analysis. *Clin Infect Dis.* 2008;47(11):1426-1435.
9. Verstraelen H, Verhelst R. Bacterial vaginosis: an update on diagnosis and treatment. *Expert Rev Anti Infect Ther.* 2009;7(9):1109-1124.
10. Wolrath H, Forsum U, Larsson PG, Borén H. Analysis of bacterial vaginosis–related amines in vaginal fluid by gas chromatography and mass spectrometry. *J Clin Microbiol.* 2001;39(11):4026-4031.
11. Forsum U, Holst E, Larsson PG, Vasquez A, Jakobsson T, Mattsby-Baltzer I. Bacterial vaginosis: a microbiological and immunological enigma. *APMIS.* 2005;113(2):81-90.
12. van Ostrum N, De Sutter P, Meys J, Verstraelen H. Risks associated with bacterial vaginosis in infertility patients: a systematic review and meta-analysis. *Hum Reprod.* 2013;28(7):1809-1815.
13. Leitich H, Kiss H. Asymptomatic bacterial vaginosis and intermediate flora as risk factors for adverse pregnancy outcome. *Best Pract Res Clin Obstet Gynaecol.* 2007;21:375.
14. Brocklehurst P, Gordon A, Heatley E, Milan SJ. Antibiotics for treating bacterial vaginosis in pregnancy. *Cochrane Database Syst Rev.* 2013;1:CD000262. doi:10.1002/14651858.CD000262.pub4.
15. Oduyebo OO, Anorlu RI, Ogunsola FT. The effects of antimicrobial therapy on bacterial vaginosis in non-pregnant women. *Cochrane Database Syst Rev.* 2009;3:CD006055. doi:10.1002/14651858.CD006055.pub2.
16. Hanson JM, McGregor JA, Hillier SL, et al. Metronidazole for bacterial vaginosis: a comparison of vaginal gel vs. oral therapy. *J Reprod Med.* 2000;45(11):889-896.
17. Wilson J. Managing recurrent bacterial vaginosis. *Sex Transm Infect.* 2004;80:8-11.
18. Reichman O, Akins R, Sobel JD. Boric acid addition to suppressive antimicrobial therapy for recurrent bacterial vaginitis. *Sex Transm Dis.* 2006;36(11):732-734.
19. Meites E. Trichomoniasis: the "neglected" sexually transmitted disease. *Infect Dis Clin North Am.* 2013;27(4):755-764.
20. Fjeld H, Raknes G. Is combining metronidazole and alcohol really hazardous? *Tidsskr Nor Laegeforen.* 2014;134(17):1661-1663.
21. Visapää JP, Tillonen JS, Kaihovaara PS, Salaspuro MP. Lack of disulfiram-like reaction with metronidazole and ethanol. *Ann Pharmacother.* 2002;36(6):971-974.

22. Miljkovic V, Arsic B, Bojanic Z, et al. Interactions of metronidazole with other medicines: a brief review. *Pharmazie.* 2014;69(8):571-577.
23. Aguin TJ, Akins RA, Sobel JD. High-dose vaginal metronidazole for recurrent bacterial vaginosis: a pilot study. *J Low Genit Tract Dis.* 2014;18(2):156-161.
24. Briggs G, Freeman R. *Drugs in Pregnancy and Lactation.* 10th ed. Philadelphia, PA: Lippincott Williams & Wilkins; 2014.
25. American Academy of Pediatrics Committee on Drugs. The transfer of drugs and other chemicals into human milk. *Pediatrics.* 1994;93(1):137-150.
26. Mitrano JA, Spooner LM, Belliveau P. Excretion of antimicrobials used to treat methicillin-resistant *Staphylococcus aureus* infections during lactation: safety in breastfeeding infants. *Pharmacother.* 2009; 29(9):1103-1109.
27. Hoffmann JN, You HM, Hedberg EC, Jordan JA, McClintock MK. Prevalence of bacterial vaginosis and *Candida* among postmenopausal women in the United States. *J Gerontol B Psychol Sci Soc Sci.* 2014;69(suppl 2):S205-S214.
28. Chavoustie SE, Jacobs M, Reisman HA, et al. Metronidazole vaginal gel 1.3% in the treatment of bacterial vaginosis: a dose-ranging study. *J Low Genit Tract.* 2015;19(2):129-134.
29. Krasnopolsky VN, Prilepskaya VN, Polatti F, et al. Efficacy of vitamin C vaginal tablets as prophylaxis for recurrent bacterial vaginosis: a randomized, double-blind, placebo-controlled clinical trial. *J Clin Med Res.* 2013;5(4):309-315.
30. Senok AC, Verstraelen H, Temmerman M, Botta GA. Probiotics for the treatment of bacterial vaginosis. *Cochrane Database Syst Rev.* 2009;4:CD006289. doi: 10.1002/14651858.CD006289.pub2.
31. Homayouni A, Bastani P, Ziyadi S, et al. Effects of probiotics on the recurrence of bacterial vaginosis: a review. *J Low Genit Tract Dis.* 2013;18(1):79-86.
32. Sutton M, Sternberg M, Koumans EH, McQuillan G, Berman S, Markowitz L. The prevalence of *Trichomonas vaginalis* infection among reproductive-age women in the United States, 2001–2004. *Clin Infect Dis.* 2007;45(10):1319-1326.
33. Sherrard J, Donders G, White D, Jensen JS, European IUSTI. European (IUSTI/WHO) guideline on the management of vaginal discharge, 2011. *Int J STD AIDS.* 2011;22(8):421-429.
34. Kissinger P, Mena L, Levison J, et al. A randomized treatment trial: single versus 7-day dose of metronidazole for the treatment of *Trichomonas vaginalis* among HIV-infected women. *J AIDS.* 2010; 55(5):565-571.
35. Johnson GL. Tinidazole (Tindamax) for trichomoniasis and bacterial vaginosis. *Am Fam Physician.* 2009; 79(2):102-105.
36. Schwebke JR, Burgess D. Trichomoniasis. *Clin Microbiol Rev.* 2004;17(4):794-803.
37. Klebanoff MA, Carey JC, Hauth JC, et al.; National Institute of Child Health and Human Development Network of Maternal–Fetal Medicine Units. Failure of metronidazole to prevent preterm delivery among pregnant women with asymptomatic *Trichomonas vaginalis* infection. *N Engl J Med.* 2001;345(7):487-493.
38. Kigozi GG, Brahmbhatt H, Wabwire-Mangen F, et al. Treatment of *Trichomonas* in pregnancy and adverse outcomes of pregnancy: a subanalysis of a randomized trial in Rakai, Uganda. *Am J Obstet Gynecol.* 2003;189(5):1398-1400.
39. Lactmed. http://toxnet.nlm.nih.gov/cgi-bin/sis/search2/f?./temp/~T1TIs3:1. Accessed October 29, 2014.
40. Ratzan JJ. Monilial and trichomonal vaginitis: topical treatment with povidone-iodine preparations. *Calif Med.* 1969;110(1):24-27.
41. Sobel JD. Vulvovaginal candidiasis. *Lancet.* 2007; 369(9577):1961-1971.
42. Peters BM, Yano J, Noverr MC, Fidel PL Jr. *Candida* vaginitis: when opportunism knocks, the host responds. *PLoS Pathog.* 2014;10(4):e1003965.
43. Angotti LB, Lambert LC, Soper DE. Vaginitis: making sense of over-the-counter treatment options. *Infect Dis Obstet Gynecol.* 2007;97424. doi:10.1155/2007/97424.
44. Reed BD, Zazove P, Pierson CL, Gorenflo DW, Horrocks J. *Candida* transmission and sexual behaviors as risks for a repeat episode of *Candida* vulvovaginitis. *J Womens Health.* 2003;12(10): 979-989.
45. Güzel AB, Küçükgöz-Güleç U, Aydin M, Gümral R, Kalkanci A, Ilkit M. *Candida* vaginitis during contraceptive use: the influence of methods, antifungal susceptibility and virulence patterns. *J Obstet Gynaecol.* 2013;33(8):850-856.
46. Hoffstetter SE, Barr S, LeFevre C, Leong FC, Leet T. Self-reported yeast symptoms compared with clinical wet mount analysis and vaginal yeast culture in a specialty clinic setting. *J Reprod Med.* 2008;53(6):402-406.
47. Ferris D, Nyirjesy P, Sobel JD, Soper D, Pavlectic A, Litaker MS. Over-the-counter antifungal drug

misuse associated with patient-diagnosed vulvovaginal candidiasis. *Obstet Gynecol.* 2002;99(3):419-425.

48. Moudgal V, Sobel J. Antifungals to treat *Candida albicans. Exp Opin Pharmacotherapy.* 2010; 11(12): 2037-2048.
49. Pappas PG, Kauffman CA, Andes D, et al. Clinical practice guidelines for the management of candidiasis: 2009 update by the Infectious Diseases Society of America. *Clin Infectious Dis.* 2009;48(5):503-535.
50. Iavuzzo C, Gkegkes ID, Zarkada IM, Falagas ME. Boric acid for recurrent vulvovaginal candidiasis: the clinical evidence. *J Womens Health.* 2011;20(8): 1245-1255.
51. Ray D, Goswami R, Banerjee U, et al. Prevalence of *Candida glabrata* and its response to boric acid vaginal suppositories in comparison with oral fluconazole in patients with diabetes and vulvovaginal candidiasis. *Diab Care.* 2007;30(2):312-317.
52. Carvalho LP, Bacellar O, Neves N, de Jesus AR, Carvalho EM. Downregulation of IFN-gamma production in patients with recurrent vaginal candidiasis. *J Allergy Clin Immunol.* 2002;109(1):102-105.
53. Dinnerstein GJ. Depo-Provera in the treatment of recurrent vulvovaginal candidiasis. *J Reprod Med.* 1986;31(9):801-803.
54. Hilton E, Isenberg HD, Alperstein P, France K, Borenstein MT. Ingestion of yogurt containing *Lactobacillus acidophilus* as prophylaxis for candidal vaginitis. *Ann Intern Med.* 1992;116(5):353-357.
55. Sobel JD, Chaim W, Nagappan V, Leaman D. Treatment of vaginitis caused by *Candida glabrata*: use of topical boric acid and flycytosine. *Am J Obstet Gynecol.* 2003;189(5):1297-1300.
56. Phillips AJ. Treatment of non-*albicans Candida* vaginitis with amphotericin B vaginal suppositories. *Am J Obstet Gynecol.* 2005;192(6):2009-2012.
57. Spencer JP, Gonzalez LS III, Barnhart DJ. Medications in the breast-feeding mother. *Am Fam Phys.* 2001;64(1):119-126.
58. Flevari A, Theodorakopoulou M, Velegraki A, Armaganidis A, Dimopoulos G. Treatment of invasive candidiasis in the elderly: a review. *Clin Interv Aging.* 2013;8:1199-1208.
59. Watson C, Calabretto H. Comprehensive review of conventional and non-conventional methods of management of recurrent vulvovaginal candidiasis. *Aust NZ J Obstet Gynecol.* 2007;47(4):262-272.
60. Falagas ME, Betsi GI, Athanasiou S. Probiotics for prevention of recurrent vulvovaginal candidiasis: a review. *J Antimicrob Chemother.* 2006;58(2): 266-272.
61. Friedrich EG Jr, Phillips LE. Microwave sterilization of *Candida* on underwear fabric: a preliminary report. *J Reprod Med.* 1988;33(5):421-422.
62. De Bernardis F, Amacker M, Arancia S, et al. A virosomal vaccine against candidal vaginitis: immunogenicity, efficacy and safety profile in animal models. *Vaccine.* 2012;30(30):4490-4498.
63. North American Menopause Society (NAMS), 2013 Symptomatic Vaginal Atrophy Advisory Panel. Management of symptomatic vulvovaginal atrophy: 2013 position statement of the North American Menopause Society. *Menopause.* 2013;20(9):888-902.
64. Edwards L, Goldbaum BE. Chronic vulvar irritation, itching, and pain: what is the diagnosis? *OBG Management.* 2104;26(6):30-37.
65. Portman DJ, Gass ML; Vulvovaginal Atrophy Terminology Consensus Conference Panel. Genitourinary syndrome of menopause: new terminology for vulvovaginal atrophy from the International Society for the Study of Women's Sexual Health and the North American Menopause Society. *Maturitas.* 2014;79(3):349-354.
66. Bond SM, Horton LS. Management of postmenopausal vaginal symptoms in women. *J Gerontol Nurs.* 2010;36(7):3-7.
67. Palmer AE, Likis FE. Lactational atrophic vaginitis. *J Midwifery Womens Health.* 2003;48(4):282-284.
68. Suckling JA, Kennedy R, Lethaby A, Roberts H. Local oestrogen for vaginal atrophy in postmenopausal women. *Cochrane Database Syst Rev.* 2006;4:CD001500. doi:10.1002/14651858.CD001500.pub2.
69. Simon JA, Lin VH, Radovich C, Bachman GA; Ospemifene Study Group. One-year long-term safety extension study of ospemifene for the treatment of vulvar and vaginal atrophy in postmenopausal women with a uterus. *Menopause.* 2013;20(4): 418-427.
70. Sobel J. Prognosis and treatment of desquamative inflammatory vaginitis. *Obstet Gynecol.* 2011;117(4):850-855.
71. Edwards L. Dermatologic causes of vaginitis: a clinical review. *Dermatol Clin.* 2010;28(4):727-735.

72. Leclair CM, Hart AE, Goetsch MF, Carpentier H, Jensen JT. Group B *Streptococcus* prevalence in a non-obstetric population. *J Low Genit Tract Dis.* 2010;14(3):162-166.
73. Verstraelen H, Verhelst R, Vaneechoutte M, Temmerman M. Group A streptococcal vaginitis: an unrecognized cause of vaginal symptoms in adult women. *Arch Gynecol Obstet.* 2011;284(1):95-98.
74. Ellsberg M, Jansen HA, Heise L, et al.; WHO Multi-country Study on Women's Health and Domestic Violence against Women Study Team. Intimate partner violence and women's physical and mental health in the WHO Multi-country Study on Women's Health and Domestic Violence: an observational study. *Lancet.* 2008;371(9619):1165-1172.

32 Vulvar Disorders

Marianne (Teri) Stone-Godena

Chapter Glossary

Allodynia Light touch.

Behçet's syndrome Syndrome of unknown etiology characterized by recurrent painful genital ulcerations that lead to scarring.

Desiccant Drying agent.

Extramammary Paget's disease Cutaneous adenocarcinoma that is classified based on source of the primary lesion.

Folliculitis Inflammation of hair follicles that occurs primarily where hairs are subjected to trauma, such as the buttocks, perineal area, thighs, and inguinal area.

Hidradenitis suppurativa Rare disease characterized by chronic, painful, inflamed, suppurative lesions of the apocrine glands that may be manifested by furuncles on the vulva. Also known as Verneuil's disease or acne inverse.

Inflammatory dermatosis Contact dermatitis of the genital skin characterized by lesions that may include simple erythema, edema, vesicles, or scaling.

Lichen planus Inflammatory condition that includes lesions and papules on mucous membranes such as the vulva. Although the etiology is unknown, the condition may be of autoimmune origin.

Lichen sclerosus Relatively rare condition of unknown etiology, but which is manifested by dermatological lesions that often result in scarring on and around the vulva.

Molluscum contagiosum Condition caused by a benign poxvirus and clinically expressed by genital lesions.

Psoriasis Skin condition characterized by inflamed skin patches and excessive skin production that can occur over various areas of the body, including the vulva.

Squamous cell hyperplasia Skin condition that can occur on the vulva and is characterized by thickened skin secondary to an itch–scratch–itch cycle. Also known as lichen simplex chronicus.

Vulvar intraepithelial neoplasia (VIN) Intraepithelial lesion of the vulva that has various degrees of atypia. The basement membrane is normal, so the lesion is not invasive.

Vulvodynia Condition characterized by symptoms of pain or burning in the vulva.

Introduction

Some women experience conditions affecting the vulva that have a readily identifiable etiology and well-known evidence-based treatments; other vulvar conditions are not easily categorized or treated, which makes it challenging to identify appropriate treatment strategies. Although most of the conditions discussed in this chapter are a manifestation of a disease affecting other parts of the body, such as psoriasis, lichen planus, and Behçet's syndrome, some are specific to the vulva, such as vulvodynia. When diseases that can affect multiple organs are identified here, only treatments for the vulvar conditions are addressed. Specific sexually transmitted lesions such as genital herpes, warts caused by human papillomavirus, and pediculosis are reviewed in the *Sexually Transmitted Infections* chapter. Seborrheic dermatitis and **psoriasis** are addressed in the *Dermatology* chapter.

Folliculitis

Folliculitis is inflammation of hair follicles occurring primarily on portions of the body where hairs are subjected to trauma, such as the scalp, neck, and face as well as the buttocks, perineal area, and thighs and groin. The pathogen most frequently associated with folliculitis is the bacterium *Staphylococcus aureus*. Another less common form of the disorder, often termed hot tub folliculitis, is caused by *Pseudomonas aeruginosa*, which is found in inadequately chlorinated warm water. Persons who have been on suppressive antibiotics for other conditions are especially susceptible to fungal folliculitis. Sterile folliculitis can occur following occlusion of an area or chemical irritation, although it is rare. Sterile folliculitis is diagnosed in the absence of any microorganisms found in the fluid around the hair follicle.[1,2]

Folliculitis affects persons of all age groups and ethnicities. Practices that damage hair follicles encourage the development of the disorder. For example, shaving, waxing, plucking, electrolysis, and wearing tight clothes abrade hair follicles and cause microscopic breaks in integrity of the skin at the base of the hair, which then facilitates development of folliculitis. Common substances like sweat, cocoa butter, or makeup, as well as more uncommon agents such as machine oils, tar, and creosote, which are components of some medications used to treat psoriasis, can also irritate or block hair follicles. Changes in skin flora following long-term use of antibiotics or steroid creams may predispose individuals to develop folliculitis. More virulent bacteria or fungi may spread to nearby hair follicles through altered skin integrity in a vulnerable area.

Once injured, follicles are more likely to become infected by bacteria entering the break in the skin as the hair regrows. The ensuing lesions appear as red papules or pimples with a hair in the center of each one. Some lesions may be pustular, in which case they may cause itching or burning. If the infection involves the deep part of the follicle, it results in a painful furuncle. Recurrent folliculitis in the same follicle can result in scarring or hair loss.[1]

Treatment of Women with Folliculitis

Treatment of mild folliculitis includes keeping the area clean and dry with an expectation that lesions generally will heal spontaneously within approximately 2 weeks. Burow's solution (5% aluminum subacetate) may help relieve itching. A common treatment uses self-made compresses composed of warm water with varying amounts of white vinegar, with the proportions usually ranging from 1 tablespoon of vinegar to several cups of water to a ratio of 1:3 of vinegar to water. No studies support the effectiveness of vinegar for this indication, although it has been used as an antipruritic agent since Roman times.

If the infection is more severe or recurrent, antibiotic or antifungal creams or systemic antibiotics may be used. Mupirocin 2% (Bactroban), an antibiotic ointment, often is applied topically. As a general rule, it is advisable to verify that topical treatments do not contain alcohol. Ointments rarely include alcohol, but some creams may contain this irritant. Table 32-1 lists treatments for folliculitis.

Table 32-1 Treatments for Women with Folliculitis

Drug: Generic (Brand)	Adult Dose	Contraindications	Clinical Considerations	Selected Drug–Drug Interactions
Burow's solution	Apply for 5–10 minutes, 3–6 times/day	None	Used to decrease itching; available over the counter.	No interactions known.
Cephalexin (Keflex)	250–500 mg PO 4 times/day for 10–14 days[a]	Hypersensitivity, penicillin allergy		Increases nephrotoxicity of aminoglycosides. Increased effectiveness of metformin (Glucophage).
Ciprofloxacin (Cipro)	250–750 mg PO every 12 hours for 10–14 days[a]	Hypersensitivity	Need increased water consumption.	Many drug interactions. Ciprofloxacin is a strong inhibitor of CYP1A2.
Clindamycin (Cleocin)[b]	150–300 mg/dose PO every 6–8 hours for 10–14 days[a] Topical: apply 2% lotion sparingly over affected area	Documented hypersensitivity, regional enteritis, ulcerative colitis, hepatic impairment, antibiotic-associated colitis	Adjust dose if severe hepatic dysfunction. Associated with possibly fatal colitis from overgrowth of *Clostridium difficile*. Topical agent can cause dryness and burning.	Antidiarrheals may delay absorption. Clindamycin (Cleocin) and erythromycin (E-Mycin) may antagonize each other. May prolong neuromuscular blockade associated with use of tubocurarine.

Dicloxacillin (Dynapen)	250–500 mg PO 4 times/day for 14–21 days[a]	Hypersensitivity, penicillin allergy		Decreases effectiveness of oral contraceptives and anticoagulants. Probenecid and disulfiram may increase dicloxacillin blood levels.
Erythromycin (E-Mycin, EES, Ery-Tab) Topical erythromycin (Emgel, Erycette)	250 mg erythromycin stearate/base (or 400 mg ethylsuccinate) every 6 hours PO, or 500 mg every 12 hours Alternatively, 333 mg PO every 8 hours; may increase to 4 g/day for 10–14 days[a] Topical: apply at bedtime or 2 times/day until clear	Hypersensitivity, megaloblastic anemia	Use with caution in persons with liver disease; estolate formulation may cause cholestatic jaundice; gastrointestinal side effects are common. Discontinue if nausea, vomiting, malaise, abdominal colic, or fever occurs.	Many drug interactions. Erythromycin is an inhibitor of CYP3A4.
Mupirocin (Bactroban)	2% applied topically 3 or 4 times/day for 14 days	Hypersensitivity	Concern that chronic use may result in drug resistance.	No major interactions known.
Trimethoprim–sulfamethoxazole (Bactrim, Septra)	160 mg TMP/800 mg SMZ PO every 12 hours for 10–14 days	Hypersensitivity, megaloblastic anemia; third-trimester pregnancy; G6PD deficiency	Discontinue if rash or sign of adverse reaction. Obtain complete blood counts frequently; discontinue if hematologic changes occur. Use with caution in persons with folate deficiency or renal or hepatic impairment.	Concomitant use of warfarin (Coumadin) may increase prothrombin time. Blood levels of dapsone, phenytoin (Dilantin), and methotrexate (Rheumatrex) may be increased. Effectiveness of tricyclic antidepressants may be decreased. Potentiates the effects of oral hypoglycemic agents.

Abbreviations: G6PD = glucose-6-posphate dehydrogenase; SMZ = sulfamethoxazole; TMP = trimethoprim.
[a] Duration of therapy depends on the severity of infection.
[b] Effective against *Staphylococcus* and *Streptococcus*.

Because the nares are a known source of *S. aureus*, some authorities recommend applying mupirocin to the nares 2 times per day during treatment of the perineum in an attempt to eliminate the carrier state. Mupirocin as a sole treatment for perineal carriage of *S. aureus* is not effective, but it has been recommended as a concurrent treatment with other agents, although the effectiveness of this strategy is not clear.[3] The systemic drug of choice for treatment of a woman with *S. aureus* infection is dicloxacillin (Dynapen), an agent that is prescribed for 14 to 21 days depending on the severity of the infection. For a woman who has a penicillin allergy without cross-sensitivity to cephalosporins, a first-generation cephalosporin may be employed. When a true penicillin allergy is known or when the *Staphylococcus* species is methicillin resistant, clindamycin (Cleocin) or 2 double-strength trimethoprim–sulfamethoxazole (Bactrim, Septra) tablets may be taken twice a day for 7 to 14 days if the individual weighs less than 80 kg; for those women with body weights of 80 kg or greater, double-strength trimethoprim–sulfamethoxazole may be taken 3 times daily.[1] Although only one randomized controlled trial (RCT) has demonstrated the effectiveness of trimethoprim–sulfamethoxazole for treating folliculitis, a large body of anecdotal evidence, case studies, and small, open-label studies support the use of this agent.[4,5]

Prevention of folliculitis commonly consists of employing good hand washing technique, wearing loose clothing, avoiding oils on the skin, and avoiding public hot tubs and other risky behaviors.[6–8] Folliculitis occurs more frequently among obese individuals, thus weight loss may be associated with a decrease in incidence.

Special Populations: Pregnancy, Lactation, and the Elderly

The drugs dicloxacillin (Dynapen), cephalexin (Keflex), clindamycin (Cleocin), and erythromycin (E-Mycin) are all safe for use by women who are pregnant or breastfeeding. Mupirocin is a topical ointment that is safe to use during pregnancy and lactation, although the data on its use in humans are limited. Data are also limited regarding the use of ciprofloxacin (Cipro), but it appears to pose a low risk for pregnant women and little, if any, significant risk to a nursing newborn, especially if a short course of maternal therapy is used.[9,10]

Caution should be exercised when prescribing sulfa-based drugs such as trimethoprim–sulfamethoxazole (Septra, Bactrim) during the third trimester, because ingestion of sulfonamides close to the time of birth has been associated with newborn jaundice and hemolytic anemia. For the same reason, these drugs should be avoided in the neonatal period if the woman is breastfeeding, although they are safe for older infants.[9,10] No restrictions or special considerations exist for the older woman with regard to treatments for folliculitis.

Lichen Sclerosus

Lichen sclerosus of the vulva is a chronic, progressive disease of unknown etiology and is one of the more common vulvar dermatoses. It has a higher incidence among Caucasians and is found in clusters in families, which suggests a genetic predisposition for developing this disorder might exist. The overall prevalence of lichen sclerosus among women is 2%. Its distribution is bimodal, with 15% of cases occurring among prepubescent children and the remainder being found among postmenopausal women. Lichen sclerosus is found more often among females; indeed, the female-to-male ratio is 6:1. Penile lichen sclerosus, although very rare, is found almost exclusively in uncircumcised males.

Extracellular matrix glycoprotein antibodies (ECM-1) have been noted in 75% to 80% of lichen sclerosus lesions, and as many as 20% of persons with lichen sclerosus have a concomitant thyroid dysfunction.[11,12] Thus, current research is focused on determining whether this condition has an autoimmune etiology.

Lesions of lichen sclerosus can be found anywhere on the vulva, but not in the vagina. These lesions are usually symmetrical and white, with rough, thin, parchment paper-like crinkled patches usually termed plaques. Inflammation and altered fibroblast function in the papillary dermis lead to fibrosis of the upper dermis and cause epidermal atrophy. Changes in the appearance of the labial, perineal, and perianal areas, accompanied by introital narrowing, may be termed *keyhole, hourglass,* or *figure of 8*. The atrophy leads to fissures, ulcers, submucosal hemorrhages, and pigmentation changes. Affected areas may be either depigmented or hyperpigmented. In addition, because 5% of women who have had lichen sclerosus can develop squamous cell carcinoma, the diagnosis of lichen sclerosus requires a biopsy.[13] Table 32-2 provides a list of pharmacologic treatments for women with this condition.

Table 32-2 Treatments for Women with Lichen Sclerosus and Squamous Cell Hyperplasia

Drug: Generic (Brand)	Adult Dose	Contraindications	Clinical Considerations	Selected Drug–Drug Interactions
Clobetasol propionate 0.05% (Temovate)	Cream or lotion: apply thin layer once daily for 1 month, then use a pulse dose for 1 month, consisting of 2 consecutive days of the week, then off 5 days Maximum dose is 50 g/week	Hypersensitivity	Reversible HPA-axis suppression, Cushing's syndrome, hyperglycemia, or glycosuria can occur following systemic absorption. Glucocorticoid insufficiency can occur after withdrawal of treatment. Do not apply to skin with decreased circulation or over a large surface area. Do not use with occlusive dressings.	No major interactions known.
Pimecrolimus (Elidel)	0.1% ointment: apply to affected areas 2 times/day for 12 weeks	Hypersensitivity; immunocompromise	Use only if other agents fail. An FDA-mandated black box warning states that pimecrolimus is associated with a risk of cancer in animal studies.	Many significant drug–drug interactions. Drugs that are CYP3A4 inhibitors may significantly decrease the metabolism of pimecrolimus.
Triamcinolone (Kenalog, Aristocort)	0.1% ointment: apply thin film 2–3 times/day until a favorable response occurs, or 1 mL injected intralesionally with bupivacaine once every 3–6 months	Hypersensitivity or concomitant fungal infection	Prolonged use can cause Cushing's syndrome from systemic absorption. Avoid more than one 40-mg injection weekly.	No major interactions known with topical formulation.
Adjunct Treatments for Pruritus				
Amitriptyline (Elavil)	10–40 mg at bedtime; increase weekly to maximum 150 mg	Pregnancy; recent myocardial infarction		Potentiates effects of alcohol and MAO inhibitors.

Diphenhydramine (Benadryl)	25–50 mg PO at bedtime	Hypersensitivity	Do not operate machinery or drive. May cause constipation or dry mouth.	Increases anticholinergic effects of MAO inhibitors.
Doxepin, systemic (Silenor)	25–75 mg PO at bedtime	Hypersensitivity; narrow-angle glaucoma, urinary retention, use of MAO inhibitors within 14 days	Label carries an FDA-mandated black box warning about increased suicidal ideation in adolescents and young adults with major depressive disorder. Do not operate machinery or drive. Do not use longer than 8 days. Can cause anticholinergic effects, CNS depression, anxiety, orthostatic hypotension, and pupillary dilation. Use with caution in persons with cardiovascular disease, diabetes, hepatic impairment, respiratory disease, or seizure disorder.	Many major drug–drug interactions are associated with the oral formulation. Increases serum concentrations of CYP2D6 substrates. Potentiates effects of MAO inhibitors and should not be used concomitantly. See the *Mental Health* chapter for discussion of drug–drug interactions of tricyclic antidepressants.
Doxepin 5% cream (Zonalon)	Apply thin film to affected area at bedtime or up to 3 times/day; do not use more than 8 days			

Abbreviations: CNS = central nervous system; HPA = hypothalamic–pituitary–adrenal; MAO = monoamine oxidase.

Treatment of Women with Lichen Sclerosus

Treatment of women with lichen sclerosus usually includes ultrapotent topical steroids such as clobetasol (Temovate). No large-scale RCTs have been published providing evidence that application of any specific corticosteroid 1 to 2 times daily is the most effective regimen, or documenting that one drug is superior to another.[13] A vulvovaginal disorders clinic at the University of Michigan reports use of clobetasol (Temovate) as a treatment for lichen sclerosus, as illustrated in the case study found in Box 32-1.[14]

The value of systemic long-term steroids after the initial 3 months of therapy is controversial. Some researchers recommend using clobetasol (Temovate) on an as-needed basis; for mild cases, a medium-potency steroid such as triamcinolone (Kenalog, Aristocort) may be prescribed. The Cochrane Collaboration reviewed seven small RCTs involving six treatments in 2011 and concluded that clobetasol

Box 32-1 Case Study: A Woman with Lichen Sclerosus

BT is a 58-year-old woman who reports that approximately 3 months ago she became involved with a new male sexual partner. Over the next several weeks, she noted that intercourse was increasingly uncomfortable. She attributed the dyspareunia to vaginal dryness secondary to her postmenopausal state and began using lubricants. However, the topical agents were not helpful and the dyspareunia continued. In the last few weeks, she began experiencing mild burning and increasing itching of her vulva.

BT's past obstetric history includes two healthy, full-term pregnancies and births. She currently takes a multiple vitamin, low-dose aspirin because of a family history of cardiovascular disease, and levothyroxine (Synthroid) for mild hypothyroidism, which was diagnosed last year. She has never used estrogen therapy. She and her partner are using condoms for sexually transmitted infection (STI) protection.

Upon physical examination, this woman's vulva is marked by a pale, almost white, patch of skin around the introitus. Some areas of redness on the edges are apparent, with irritation suggestive of scratching dry skin. BT has lichen sclerosus. She also has a thyroid dysfunction, which is relatively common among women with lichen sclerosus. A biopsy could be performed for confirmation, although she may also be treated empirically based on the physical examination findings.

Given that BT's condition is mild, one potential option is prescription of clobetasol (Temovate) to be used as needed once or twice a day on her vulva. A 15- or 30-g tube of medication should be sufficient, as it should be applied sparingly. Oral diphenhydramine hydrochloride (Benadryl) can be recommended at bedtime for its antihistamine and sedative effects. Relief is likely to be gradual. A follow-up visit in 2 to 3 months should enable the provider to assess whether the therapy has been successful. BT should be advised that the condition, even if resolved with the initial therapy, may reoccur but is not cancerous nor it is likely to be transmitted to her sexual partner.

and pimecrolimus (Elidel) provided similar results and had the most evidence to support their use.[15] The *Dermatology* chapter provides more information about steroids used in the clinical management of skin conditions.

Hormones have been used for lichen sclerosus treatment in the past, but neither testosterone nor progesterone has been found to be superior to placebos in RCTs.[16] On the assumption that lichen sclerosus is immune moderated, some researchers have found success with the use of topical immunomodulators, especially pimecrolimus (Elidel), which inhibits the action of interleukin-2 (IL-2) by stimulating T-helper cells.[17] The FDA issued a public health advisory in 2005 regarding a potential cancer risk from use of pimecrolimus ointment, advising that this medication be used only when other treatments fail or cannot be tolerated. Some clinicians combine pimecrolimus and clobetasol (Temovate) in a pulsatile fashion, such as 2 weeks of using one medication, followed by 2 weeks of using the other drug.

Based on the hypothesis that cyclosporine (Sandimmune), an immunomodulator, might be as effective for treatment of lichen sclerosus as it is for treatment of psoriasis, two small, open-label trials investigated the use of oral cyclosporine for treatment of severe lichen sclerosus.[18] The 7 participants all experienced improvements in their lesions within 4 weeks, and all achieved clearance by 12 weeks. Three individuals experienced minor side effects, none of which led to discontinuation of the drug. Larger studies needed to confirm these findings are in progress. However, when compared to standard steroid treatments, none of the alternatives has been reported to work as quickly or as effectively.

When lichen sclerosus causes significant vulvar discomfort, a sedative may be used for the first 2 weeks of treatment until the effect of the steroids is noted. Oral antihistamines, doxepin hydrochloride topical cream 5% (Zonalon, Prudoxin), and antidepressants such as doxepin (Silenor) or amitriptyline (Elavil) may be prescribed if pruritus is severe.[13]

When pharmacologic treatments fail or when a stenotic introitus or deep fissuring is present, a perineoplasty may offer relief.[19] Emollients such as Aquaphor, which contains petroleum as an active ingredient, may be useful in keeping tissues soft.

Special Populations: Pregnancy, Lactation, and the Elderly

Although lichen sclerosus is most common among postmenopausal women, it may occasionally affect reproductive-age women, including those who are pregnant. All topical steroids, emollients, and immunomodulators are considered safe for use in pregnancy and during lactation.[9,10] Use of tricyclic antidepressants in pregnant or breastfeeding women is more controversial; additional information on this topic can be found in the *Mental Health* chapter. In particular, little information exists about the effects of doxepin during pregnancy or lactation, suggesting that, if this agent is needed, it should be limited to the topical form. The majority of women with lichen sclerosus are older adults, and the treatments identified are appropriate for individuals in that age group.

Squamous Cell Hyperplasia

Squamous cell hyperplasia, sometimes known as lichen simplex chronicus, is not a distinct disease entity, but rather a skin change resulting from an itch–scratch–itch cycle. By the time squamous cell hyperplasia develops, the original trigger—whether it was lichen sclerosus, eczema, candidal infection, psoriasis, chemical irritants, or allergens—may no longer be discernible. Lesions appear similar to lichen sclerosus in the early stages but without the loss of skin folds or shrinkage. As the disorder progresses, squamous cell hyperplasia causes thickening of the epidermis. Burning, extreme itching, pain, and tenderness are hallmarks of this condition. Classically, the lesions are red or pink, raised, acanthotic (thickened), and leathery; they may also be asymmetrical. Lesions should be biopsied to rule out invasive squamous cell cancer. If atypia is found on biopsy, it usually is the result of a human papillomavirus (HPV) infection and is classified as **vulvar intraepithelial neoplasia (VIN)**.[20] The peak incidence of VIN occurs among women in their sexual maturity; this condition is rarely found among pubertal or young women.[21]

Treatment of Women with Squamous Cell Hyperplasia

Treatment of squamous cell hyperplasia begins with removal of the source of the itching and interruption of the itch–scratch–itch cycle. Irritants such as laundry detergents, soap with additives, and perfumes should be identified and eliminated. Infection, if present, needs to be treated with an appropriate anti-infective agent. The oral route of antibiotic delivery is more effective than topical application of antibiotics, but can result in worsening of symptoms if fungal overgrowth results. Therefore, when treating with antibiotics, the provider should periodically add an antifungal agent as a prophylaxis agent. No single antifungal treatment has shown to be superior compared to another. Suggestions include using a 100-mg dose of oral fluconazole (Diflucan), a single-dose vaginal preparation every 3 days, a 3-day vaginal preparation, or a 150-mg dose of oral fluconazole every 7 days.

Mild to moderate disease can be treated with short-term medium-potency steroids such as triamcinolone (Kenalog, Aristacort) used as an ointment or intralesional injections given for 2 to 4 weeks.[21] Some authors recommend steroids with concomitant use of crotamiton (Eurax) as an antipruritic therapy.[14] For severe disease, an ultrapotent steroid such as clobetasol (Temovate) can be applied topically for 2 to 4 weeks, then replaced with triamcinolone (Kenalog, Aristocort).[14]

Systemic sedating antihistamines such as diphenhydramine (Benadryl), hydroxyzine (Atarax), and amitriptyline (Elavil) have achieved some success in the treatment of several disorders in which pruritus is a presenting issue.[14] Medications used to treat women with squamous cell hyperplasia are listed in Table 32-2.

Special Populations: Pregnancy, Lactation, and the Elderly

Squamous cell hyperplasia of the vulva is rare during pregnancy.[22] As topical steroids, emollients, and immunomodulators are considered safe for use in pregnancy and during lactation, they are the preferred agents treating squamous cell hyperplasia during pregnancy. The tricyclic antidepressants, such as doxepin (Silenor) and amitriptyline, have many adverse effects and should be avoided if possible, although amitriptyline can be used during pregnancy if other agents are not available. Diphenhydramine (Benadryl) is considered safe for women during pregnancy and lactation, although prolonged or high doses of this drug may cause a decrease in milk supply if used by breastfeeding women.[9,10]

No modifications of the usual treatments for squamous cell hyperplasia are needed for older women.

Lichen Planus

Lichen planus, an acute or chronic inflammatory lesion of the skin and mucous membranes, is of unknown etiology but is likely to be an autoimmune disease. Rarely found in children or the elderly, its peak incidence is among women 30 to 60 years, suggesting a role for hormones in the disease.[18]

The lesions of lichen planus are erosive and can resemble lichen sclerosus, HPV infection, syphilis, chancroid, Behçet's syndrome, or pemphigus. These lesions may range from white papules or plaques to homogenously white epithelium or erosions surrounded by white epithelium (lacy pattern); they are found on the genitals, in the mouth, and on the scalp. Whereas lichen sclerosus is not found in the vagina, lichen planus lesions begin in the vestibule and can obliterate the vagina.[22] Lichen planus can cause scarring, leading to obliteration of the vagina, labia minora, and the clitoral hood. Hair loss and pruritus may be present, and contact bleeding and dyspareunia are common. Diagnosis is confirmed via biopsy.[20]

Treatment of Women with Lichen Planus

No treatments for lichen planus have been evaluated in RCTs; instead, many drugs are used on an off-label basis for this condition. The first-line treatment is an ultrapotent topical steroid. For extensive disease, oral steroids such as prednisone (Deltasone) may be necessary until skin healing begins, at which time topical steroids should be used. Drugs commonly used to treat women with this condition are listed in Table 32-3.

Emollients, such as petroleum jelly, mineral oil, and olive oil, may have some therapeutic value in keeping tissues soft. If use of topical steroids is planned, the initial drug should be an ultrapotent one such as clobetasol (Temovate); it may be used for 2 weeks and then tapered to a medium-potency steroid such as topical or intralesional triamcinolone acetonide (Kenalog, Aristocort).[24] In observational studies, hydrocortisone suppositories in the form of Anusol HC 25 mg have been shown to be effective for treatment of vaginal lichen planus.[23] Some authorities recommend continuing the treatment indefinitely using 1 to 3 suppositories per week, whereas others have noted no further improvement after an initial 4 months of such therapy.[23,25] For recalcitrant lichen planus, tacrolimus 0.1% (Protopic) can be applied externally as an ointment twice a day, and tacrolimus 0.1% vaginal suppositories can be made by a compounding pharmacist by mixing 2 mg of tacrolimus with 2 g of an inert base.[25] This suppository can be used nightly for 2 months. Some authors recommend using vaginal dilators during treatment to decrease the risk of scarring.[26] When this therapy is used, the vaginal dilator can be lubricated with a mild- to medium-potency steroid such as hydrocortisone.

Table 32-3 Treatments for Women with Lichen Planus

Drug: Generic (Brand)	Adult Dose	Contraindications	Clinical Considerations	Selected Drug–Drug Interactions
Clobetasol propionate 0.05% (Temovate)	Apply thin layer once daily for 1 month; maximum dose is 50 g/week	Hypersensitivity	Reversible HPA-axis suppression, Cushing's syndrome, hyperglycemia, or glycosuria can occur following systemic absorption. Glucocorticoid insufficiency can occur after withdrawal of treatment. Do not apply to skin with decreased circulation or over a large surface area. Do not use with occlusive dressings.	No major interactions known.
Dapsone (Avlosulfon)	50–100 mg daily PO	Hypersensitivity, G6PD deficiency	Screen for G6PD deficiency prior to using dapsone.	Many drug–drug interactions: blood dyscrasia with folic acid antagonists; decreased effectiveness with rifampin (Rifadin); increased risk of methemoglobinemia with local anesthetics.
Hydrocortisone (Anusol HC)	Half of a 25-mg (2.5%) suppository vaginally 2 times/day for 2 months, then once daily for 1 month	Hypersensitivity, serious infections, fungal infections, varicella	Do not use with occlusive dressings.	Barbiturates decrease effect of hydrocortisone suppository. Anticoagulants, live vaccines, and tacrolimus (Protopic) effects may be decreased.
Methotrexate (Rheumatrex)	7.5–25 mg/week PO/SC	Hypersensitivity, alcoholism, hepatic insufficiency, immunodeficiency syndromes, blood dyscrasias, leukopenia, thrombocytopenia, significant anemia, renal insufficiency	Photosensitivity reaction, hepatotoxicity, fibrosis, cirrhosis, bone marrow suppression. Monitor complete blood counts monthly and discontinue if any significant drop occurs. Monitor liver and renal function every 1–3 months during therapy.	Many drug–drug interactions: Aminoglycosides and charcoal decrease absorption. Folic acid decreases response. Probenecid, salicylates, procarbazine (Matulane), and sulfonamides, including TMP-SMZ (Bactrim, Septra), increase effects. Etretinate (Tegison) may cause hepatotoxicity.
Prednisone (Deltasone)	30–60 mg/day PO for 4–6 weeks, followed by gradual taper	Hypersensitivity	Adrenal crisis can occur following abrupt discontinuation. Hyperglycemia, edema, osteonecrosis, myopathy, peptic ulcer disease, hypokalemia, osteoporosis, psychosis, myasthenia gravis, growth suppression, and infections may occur.	Acetaminophen, alcohol, NSAIDs, amphotericin B, carbonic anhydrase inhibitors, and antacids decrease absorption. Other drug–drug interactions: anticoagulants, tricyclic antidepressants, antidiabetic agents, antithyroid hormones, estrogens, digoxin (Lanoxin), diuretics, ephedrine, folic acid, immunosuppressants, and potassium supplements.
Tacrolimus (Protopic)	0.1% ointment: apply to affected areas 2 times/day for 2–6 weeks	Hypersensitivity Ointments can lead to maceration in skin folds Not recommended for immunocompromised persons	None known.	No major interactions known with topical formulation.

Abbreviations: CBC = complete blood count; G6PD = glucose-6-phosphate dehydrogenase; HPA = hypothalamic–pituitary–adrenal; NSAIDs = nonsteroidal anti-inflammatory drugs; TMP-SMZ = trimethoprim–sulfamethoxazole.

Alternative treatments include dapsone (Avlosulfon), an antibacterial commonly used in the treatment of Hansen's disease, as well as antimetabolites such as methotrexate (Rheumatrex), cyclosporine (Neoral, Sandimmune), cyclophosphamide (Neosar, Cytoxan), and azathioprine (Imuran), which are used in the treatment of psoriasis and Behçet's syndrome.[23] These drugs are more expensive and entail greater risks; therefore, they are generally reserved for use by a specialist in vulvar diseases. Retinoids have been reported to be effective in the treatment of oral lesions but have not been associated with improvement of vulvovaginal disease.[27]

Special Populations: Pregnancy, Lactation, and the Elderly

Retinoids and methotrexate (Rheumatrex) are known teratogens and, therefore, are contraindicated for use in pregnancy. Given the lack of associated improvement and increased risk, these agents have no place in the treatment of vulvar lichen planus.[23] Topical agents such as tacrolimus (Protopic) and clobetasol (Temovate) are considered safe for pregnant and lactating women. Studies of prednisone and other systemic steroids reveal contradictory information in animal models, although no reports of teratogenicity has been found among humans. Use of dapsone (Avlosulfon) administered orally in pregnancy has not been associated with birth defects.[9,10]

Regarding breastfeeding, high doses of prednisone may cause a decrease in milk supply. Dapsone rarely has been associated with an increased risk of neonatal hemolytic anemia, especially if the newborn has glucose-6-phosphate dehydrogenase (G6PD) deficiency. Methotrexate is contraindicated for women who are breastfeeding.[9,10] No special considerations have been reported for the agents commonly used for treatment of older women with lichen planus.

Hidradenitis Suppurativa

Hidradenitis suppurativa, also known as Verneuil's disease or acne inversa, affects 1% to 4% of the population. It is a disease for which there is no consensus about its name, pathogenesis, prevalence, or treatment.[28] Perhaps because it resembles other lesions, the average time from onset to diagnosis is 8 years.[29] This condition is characterized by chronic, painful, inflamed, suppurative lesions of the apocrine glands. The lesions arise when a defect in the follicular epithelium of a hair follicle is aggravated by friction, sweat, heat, stress, tight clothing, or hormonal changes. Boil-like, often malodorous, nodular lesions form, with sinus tracts emerging between them and the glands' surface. Inflammation, infection, and extension to the subcutaneous tissue follow. Healing is associated with scarring.

Obesity is not an etiologic agent for hidradenitis suppurativa, but has been found to be an aggravating factor.[28,29] Approximately 38% of all persons with this disorder report a family history, suggesting genetics may be involved.[30] The disease affects women more often than men by a ratio of 4:1 and occurs almost exclusively between puberty and age 40 years, lending support to a hormonally mediated etiology, although the precise link remains unclear. Flares are more common in women with shorter menstrual cycles and longer menstrual flow, but also have been noted to begin with the onset of combined oral contraceptive use.[31] Complications of hidradenitis suppurativa include local or systemic infection, anemia from chronic infection, arthritis, lymphedema, fistulae, and frustration and depression.[32]

Diagnosis of hidradenitis suppurativa is based on clinical presentation. The disease is present in discrete portions of the anatomy—the axillae, the inframammary, and the genito-anal area, which includes genitofemoral creases, gluteal folds, perianal area, and mons pubis. Hidradenitis suppurativa is chronic and recurring, and progresses through three stages, as noted in Table 32-4.

Table 32-4 Treatments for Women with Hidradenitis Suppurativa According to Stage of the Disorder

Stage and Description	Nonpharmacologic Treatment	Pharmacologic Treatment
Stage 1: Single or multiple nodular lesions form without sinus tracts or scars	Hydrotherapy; warm compresses; stress management; weight loss	
Stage 2: Recurrent single or multiple lesions in widely spread areas form with tracts, and fibrosis	Hydrotherapy; warm compresses; stress management; weight loss	Antibiotics for infections (culture directed): • Dicloxacillin (Dynapen) 250–500 mg 4 times/day for 10–14 days based on severity • Doxycycline (Vibramycin) 100 mg PO 2 times/day for 7–10 days based on severity • Clindamycin (Cleocin) topical: apply sparingly to area 2 times/day for 7–10 days Zinc gluconate 90 mg daily Clobetasol (Dermovate, Temovate): apply sparingly to area daily for 14 days NSAIDs as needed for discomfort Anti-tissue necrosing factor-α as infliximab (Remicade): 2 infusions at 5 mg/kg Antiandrogens in the form of drospirenone (Yasmin): 1 tablet daily
Stage 3: Lesions form in multiple, scattered, broad areas with multiple tracts and scars	Warm compresses; exposure to light and air	Antibiotics for infections (culture directed) as listed for stage 2

Abbreviations: NSAIDs = nonsteroidal anti-inflammatory drugs.

No single pharmaceutical agent is the most effective treatment for hidradenitis suppurativa. Antibiotics are used routinely, even though many lesions are bacteria free and tend to heal in the same amount of time whether antibiotics are used or are not used.[31] In general, treatment is tailored to the severity of the lesions. Stage 1 lesions often are managed with nonpharmacologic measures. In one study, 45% of those individuals with hidradenitis suppurativa reported heat, exercise, and sweat aggravated their symptoms. However, hydrotherapy, in the forms of warm, moist compresses and swimming, relieved the symptoms for approximately one third of those afflicted.[32] Stage 2 lesions require medical or surgical treatment. Stage 3 lesions are most appropriately managed with an invasive intervention such as wide local excision with healing by secondary intention.[33] Radiotherapy and cryotherapy are being investigated as treatment options as well.[34,35]

Some association appears to exist between acne and hidradenitis suppurativa, so the antibiotics used in the treatment of individuals with acne are often used in the treatment of women with hidradenitis suppurativa.[34] While systemic antibiotics are commonly used, the only RCT of such agents found that topical clindamycin (Cleocin) was not statistically different from systemic tetracycline (Sumycin) in its effectiveness as a treatment of axillary hidradenitis suppurativa.[36]

A variety of organisms have been isolated from hidradenitis suppurativa lesions, including *Staphylococcus*, *Escherichia coli*, and beta-hemolytic *Streptococcus*. Axillary hidradenitis suppurativa is more commonly infected with *Staphylococcus* and is better treated with antistaphylococcal agents such as dicloxacillin (Dynapen) and clindamycin. For perineal hidradenitis suppurativa, broad-spectrum coverage is needed, and doxycycline (Vibramycin, Adoxa) and minocycline (Minocin) are commonly used antibiotics for this purpose.[36]

Zinc salts have also been used in the treatment of individuals with dermatoses. These salts activate natural killer cells and stimulate phagocytosis by granulocytes. In France, a small pilot study was conducted with individuals who were primarily in stage 2 of hidradenitis suppurativa. The participants were treated initially with 90 mg of zinc gluconate orally per day for 4 months. As their symptoms abated, the dose was reduced by 15 mg every 2 months. Success was defined as 6 months of no new or recurrent lesions, with total follow-up lasting for 2 years. Eight of the 22 participants experienced complete remission, and 14 experienced partial remission. One person discontinued treatment due to nausea and vomiting, while three others had gastrointestinal side effects but continued the program. The dose of zinc was higher than that routinely used in the treatment of dermatoses.[37] Although the size of this study precludes generalization of its results to a larger or different population, zinc supplements might be an attractive, inexpensive option; they require further exploration before final conclusions can be drawn about their utility.

Because of the association between hidradenitis suppurativa and hormonal changes, antiandrogen medications have been suggested as potential treatments. Because combined oral contraceptives may help ameliorate symptoms, some oral contraceptives containing drospirenone have been used for treatment of hidradenitis suppurativa. Drospirenone can increase the risk of stroke, especially in women who smoke, so use of oral contraceptives is limited to women who desire contraception and do not have any contraindications to use of specific agents. In case reports, two individuals were reported to improve with the use of finasteride (Proscar), but another, larger series demonstrated no improvement following use of this agent.[38] Most studies have found that isotretinoin (Accutane) works well for individuals with acne but not for persons with hidradenitis suppurativa.[39] Research is currently being conducted to assess the effectiveness of corticosteroids and immunomodulators. Although topical and injectable triamcinolone (Kenalog) is being investigated, the lack of large clinical trials precludes this drug from consideration as a first-line treatment for hidradenitis suppurativa. ACTH, azathioprine (Imuran), and cyclosporine (Neoral, Sandimmune) have also been used experimentally for this condition, with some preliminary favorable results.[36,40]

Hidradenitis suppurativa often accompanies Crohn's disease. A growing body of evidence suggests that hidradenitis suppurativa may be an autoimmune disease itself. Given this understanding, drugs used for other autoimmune disorders are being investigated for use with hidradenitis suppurativa. The most promising research is in the area of antitumor necrosis factor (TNFα) drugs. Etanercept (Enbrel) and infliximab (Remicade) are FDA-approved drugs for rheumatoid arthritis and Crohn's disease and are currently being studied in the United States and Europe for use in treating hidradenitis suppurativa. Although the number of participants in these studies has been small and the enrollees in the trials have not been randomized, the initial results appear promising.[41,42]

Even with the variety of drugs available for treatment of hidradenitis suppurativa, 24% of participants in one study reported that none of the interventions was helpful.[33] For many individuals, even with successful treatment of lesions, new lesions often develop, resulting in a cycle of exacerbation–remission–exacerbation.

Counseling is a critical adjunct to providing medical or surgical treatment.[42] Women need to understand that hidradenitis suppurativa is a chronic condition that is not associated with poor hygiene.

Special Populations: Pregnancy, Lactation, and the Elderly

Some of the agents used to treat hidradenitis suppurative are known teratogens and should not be used by women of reproductive age. Isotretinoin (Accutane) causes multiple congenital anomalies and is only administered under strict policies that document use of contraception. Doxycycline (Vibramycin) and minocycline (Minocin) are tetracycline derivatives and known teratogens associated with staining of fetal teeth and bone. Among the drugs that are considered safe for use by women during pregnancy and lactation are dicloxacillin (Dynapen), clindamycin (Cleocin), and infliximab (Remicade). Oral contraceptives are not used during pregnancy, but inadvertent use in the first trimester has not been associated with fetal teratogenicity or toxicity.

Doxycycline and minocycline should be used with caution by women who are breastfeeding, and only for short courses when no other options are available. The breast milk itself facilitates production of insoluble salts, which inhibit transfer of a clinically relevant amount of these drugs into breast milk. Hormonal contraceptives are considered safe for lactating women, although some concerns exist that early postpartum use may decrease production of breast milk. Both finasteride (Proscar) and isotretinoin (Accutane) may pose potential toxicity concerns in the nursing dyad; although data on this topic are sparse, these drugs are rarely recommended for use by breastfeeding women.[9,10] No special considerations of note have been found regarding treatment of older women with hidradenitis suppurativa.

Inflammatory Dermatosis

Inflammatory dermatosis, or contact dermatitis of the genital skin, can be initiated by friction from tight clothes, physical activities such as bicycle riding, chemical irritation from urine or stool, perfumed personal hygiene products, and excessive washing, especially with harsh soaps.[43] Diagnosis is usually made by history and physical examination. Lesions may vary from simple erythema and edema to the presence of vesicles or bullae; in case of severe disease, lichenification (scale formation) or erosion with exudates and crusting may be present.[44]

Treatment begins with removal of the source of irritation. If urinary incontinence is the presumed source, it should be managed with treatment based on severity and type of incontinence, as discussed in detail in the chapter *Lower Urinary Tract Disorders*. The vulva and anus should be rinsed with plain water after each episode of toileting, and the area given an opportunity to thoroughly dry. If adult diapers or other occlusive clothing are used, they should be changed frequently. Zinc oxide ointment, ointment with vitamins A and D, or petroleum jelly will help provide a protective barrier to the inflammatory agent.[43] Application of Burow's solution may provide symptomatic relief.[44] A mild steroid such as triamcinolone acetonide cream (Kenalog) will decrease inflammation. Soaps coming in contact with the genital area should be free of perfumes and additives. Underwear should be loose, all cotton, and washed in hot water and dried using high heat.

Special Populations: Pregnancy, Lactation, and the Elderly

Most of the pharmacologic agents used to treat women with inflammatory dermatosis are topical. All topical steroids, emollients, and immunomodulators are considered safe for use in pregnancy and during lactation.[9,10]

Women of any age can experience inflammatory dermatosis, but the elderly are particularly vulnerable to this condition. After menopause, the vaginal mucosa becomes thinner and the tissue is less elastic and easily traumatized. Women who may have difficulty with removing waste products from the skin when toileting, such as older persons who are obese or those with limited mobility, are particularly prone to inflammatory dermatosis. However, there is no evidence regarding implications of drug therapy for the older woman.

Behçet's Syndrome

Behçet's syndrome is named after a Turkish dermatologist, Hulusi Behçet, who in 1937 described a syndrome of recurrent oral aphthous ulcers, genital ulcerations, and uveitis leading to blindness. Although the cause of this syndrome is unknown, it has become recognized as a multisystemic inflammatory disease characterized by painful ulcerations with erythematous borders and yellow bases, beginning first in the oral cavity but affecting many parts of the body, especially the uvea of the eye and the genital area. Rarely found among individuals of Western European or African descent, this syndrome most commonly affects those of

Eastern Mediterranean or Asian origin.[45,46] The mouth and genital ulcers associated with Behçet's syndrome are generally painful and recur in crops of many shallow ulcers that appear at the same time. The ulcers range in size from a few millimeters to 20 millimeters in diameter.

Many sets of diagnostic criteria for Behçet's syndrome have been proposed since the disorder was first recognized. The criteria used most commonly since 1990 are the ones set forth by the International Study Group (ISG). The specificity of the ISG criteria is high, but the sensitivity is low. In 2006, the International Criteria for Behçet's Disease (ICBD) were developed; they retain the five criteria proposed by the ISG group and add vascular manifestations as the sixth criterion.

The ICBD assigns a numerical weight to each of the criteria. Oral, cutaneous, and vascular lesions and pathergy phenomena each receive one point. Ocular and genital lesions are each assigned a weight of 2. A score of 3 is necessary for a diagnosis or classification of Behçet's syndrome.[46] Table 32-5 compares the ISG and ICBD standards for diagnosis of the syndrome.

Table 32-5 Criteria for Diagnosis of Behçet's Syndrome

International Study Group (ISG) Criteria[40]	International Criteria for Behçet's Disease (ICBD)[41]

Recurrent oral ulcerations (≥ 3 episodes in a 12-month period) plus two of any of the following:
• Recurrent genital ulcerations
• Eye lesions:
  ◦ Anterior uveitis
  ◦ Posterior uveitis
• Cells in the vitreous
• Retinal vasculitis
• Skin lesions:
  ◦ Erythema nodosum
  ◦ Pseudo-folliculitis
  ◦ Papulopustular lesions
• Acneiform nodules (in a postadolescent not taking corticosteroids)
• Positive pathergy test (The pathergy test includes piercing the skin of the forearm with a blunt, sterile needle. The test is positive if, after 24–48 hours, a small pustule develops.)
	Recurrent oral ulcerations (≥ 3 episodes in a 12-month period) plus:
	• Recurrent genital ulcerations
	• Eye lesions:
	  ◦ Anterior uveitis
	  ◦ Posterior uveitis
	• Cells in the vitreous
	• Retinal vasculitis
	• Skin lesions:
	  ◦ Erythema nodosum
	  ◦ Pseudo-folliculitis
	  ◦ Papulopustular lesions
	• Acneiform nodules (in a postadolescent not taking corticosteroids)
	• Positive pathergy test (The pathergy test includes piercing the skin of the forearm with a blunt, sterile needle. The test is positive if, after 24–48 hours, a small pustule develops.)
	• Vascular manifestations: superficial phlebitis, deep vein thrombosis, large vein, thrombosis, arterial thrombosis, and aneurysm

Sources: Data from Davatchi F, Chams-Davatchi C, Ghodsi Z, et al. Diagnostic value of pathergy test in Behçet's disease according to the change in incidence over the time. *Clin Rheum.* 2011;30(9):1151-1155[47]; Dohil M, Prendiville JS. Treatment of molluscum contagiosum with oral cimetidine: clinical experience on 13 patients. *Pediatr Dermatol.* 1996;13(4):310-312[48]; Haslund P, Lee RA, Jemec G. Treatment of hidradenitis suppurativa with tumour necrosis factor-alpha inhibitors. *Acta Derm Venereol.* 2009;89(6):595-600.[41]

Treatment of Women with Behçet's Syndrome

Drugs used for treatment of women with Behçet's syndrome can be found in Table 32-6.

Colchicine (Colcrys) is an anti-inflammatory drug originally derived from the autumn crocus, *Colchicum autumnale*. Colchicine is most frequently used as an FDA-approved agent to treat individuals with gout, but it is also effective for treatment of genital lesions in individuals with Behçet's syndrome. A double-blind trial of colchicine administered to 116 persons with Behçet's syndrome found members of the treated group had statistically significant improvement compared to the untreated group ($P = 0.004$).[49]

Topical anesthetics are generally ineffective for Behçet's syndrome.[50] Mild- to moderate-strength topical steroid gels and creams and intralesional triamcinolone often are prescribed for small lesions. For larger lesions, systemic steroids (e.g., prednisone) are more effective.[51]

Recent studies suggest that thalidomide (Thalomid) may be of benefit for certain individuals with Behçet's syndrome by treating and preventing ulcerations of the mouth and genitals. Side effects of thalidomide include fever, sweating, acne, nerve injury (neuropathy), and sedation.

Antimetabolites and interferon should be reserved for persons whose condition does not respond following a course of prednisone. A dermatologist or gynecologist with extensive experience with the drugs should manage the treatment program.[52] Some individuals with mild lesions have noted improvement with the use of an herbal remedy called Canker Rid, which is a by-product of honeybee products. There have been no randomized trials of this product, and caution should be used by individuals with diabetes and those with bee allergies.

Special Populations: Pregnancy, Lactation, and the Elderly

Thalidomide (Thalomid) is a well-known teratogen and should be not be used by women who are of reproductive age. [9,10,53] In addition, this drug should be prescribed only by a specialist familiar with its use. Data about prednisone and other systemic steroids used during pregnancy reveal contradictory information in animal models, although no reports of teratogenicity have emerged among humans

Table 32-6 Treatments for Women with Behçet's Syndrome

Drug: Generic (Brand)	Adult Dose	Contraindications	Clinical Considerations	Selected Drug–Drug Interactions
Azathioprine (Imuran)	100–150 mg/ 1 time/day PO	Hypersensitivity, pregnancy and lactation, low levels of serum TPMT	Use with caution in persons with liver and renal impairment; check TPMT level prior to therapy. Monitor liver, renal, and hematologic functions.	Toxicity with allopurinol. Leucopenia with ACE inhibitors. Increases methotrexate (Rheumatrex, Trexall) metabolites. Decreases effects of anticoagulants, neuromuscular blockers, and cyclosporine (Neoral).
Colchicine (Colcrys)	1–2 mg per day in 3–4 divided doses/day	Hypersensitivity, renal or hepatic disease	Gastrointestinal discomfort at higher doses. Alopecia at higher doses.	None known.
Cyclosporine (Sandimmune, Neoral)	5 mg/kg/day PO based on ideal body weight	Hypersensitivity, uncontrolled hypertension, malignancies, abnormal renal function, concomitant use of methotrexate, other immunosuppressive agents, coal tar or radiation therapy	An FDA black box warning states that use of cyclosporine increases risk of opportunistic infections, neoplasia, systemic hypertension, and nephropathy. Only providers experienced in immunosuppressive therapy should prescribe this drug. Renal function should be monitored. May cause gingival hyperplasia.	Many major drug–drug interactions. Carbamazepine (Tegretol), phenytoin (Dilantin), isoniazid (INH), rifampin (Rifadin), and phenobarbital (Luminal) have decreased drug concentrations. Azithromycin (Zithromax), azoles, nicardipine (Cardene), erythromycin (E-Mycin), verapamil (Calan), grapefruit juice, diltiazem (Cardizem), aminoglycosides, acyclovir (Zovirax), amphotericin B (Fungizone), and clarithromycin (Biaxin) have increased toxicity. Concomitant use of lovastatin (Mevacor) is associated with acute renal failure, rhabdomyolysis, myositis, and myalgias.
Prednisone (Deltasone, Sterapred)	15 mg/day, with tapering to 10 mg/day after 1 week and discontinuation over a 2- to 3-week period	Hypersensitivity	Adrenal crisis with abrupt discontinuation. Hyperglycemia, edema, osteonecrosis, myopathy, peptic ulcer disease, hypokalemia, osteoporosis, psychosis, myasthenia gravis, growth suppression, and infections may occur.	Acetaminophen (Tylenol), alcohol, NSAIDs, amphotericin B (Fungizone), carbonic anhydrase inhibitors, and antacids decrease absorption. Anticoagulants, tricyclic antidepressants, antidiabetic agents, antithyroid hormones, estrogens, digitalis (Lanoxin), diuretics, ephedrine, folic acid, immunosuppressants, potassium supplements, and ritodrine (Yutopar) are associated with pulmonary edema.

Abbreviations: ACE = angiotensin-converting enzyme; NSAIDs = nonsteroidal anti-inflammatory drugs; TPMT = thiopurine methyltransferase.

and systemic steroids are considered safe for use while breastfeeding. Colchicine (Colcrys) has not been studied among humans, but no case reports have been published suggesting it confers an increased risk of miscarriage, stillbirth, or congenital anomalies. Teratogenicity has been reported when high doses of the drug are administered to hamsters. Colchicine can be found in breast milk, but there are no reports of adverse effects among infants who breastfeed, although some concerns have been cited regarding potential gastrointestinal cell renewal. Some data suggest azathioprine (Imuran) causes immunosuppression during pregnancy, but the benefits usually outweigh the risks and this drug is unlikely to be toxic during breastfeeding. Cyclosporine has limited data regarding use in pregnancy but it is unlikely to be teratogenic. Nevertheless, although it is considered compatible with breastfeeding, some concern has been expressed about a theoretical interference with the cellular metabolism of the nursling. Canker Rid is a botanical agent composed of propolis, bee pollen, and nectar, among other ingredients. No data exist regarding the safety of this agent in pregnancy or lactation, although its administration through the topical route likely prevents major transfer, if any, of the drug.

Molluscum Contagiosum

Molluscum contagiosum is a viral disease caused by a benign poxvirus. Although it more frequently affects children, a person in any age group can acquire this disorder. Since the late 1980s, the incidence of molluscum contagiosum has increased, primarily within the sexually active population and HIV-immunocompromised individuals.[54]

The virus that causes molluscum contagiosum is communicable through direct contact with someone who has the lesion or contact with a surface that has been in contact with mature lesions, such as a towel, exercise mats, or equipment.[4] The lesions have a predilection for skin already inflamed by psoriasis or eczema. They proceed through three stages of development and are often found on flexor surfaces. Among adult women, the genital area is most commonly affected. Initially lesions are often described as tiny goose bumps (cutis anserina), often 20 or more concentrated in a 3-cm diameter. However, within a few days to weeks, the lesions evolve into mole-like lesions, which are usually pale, 2 to 6 mm in diameter, and umbilicated. The final stage occurs after several weeks, when the lesions appear similar to pimples about to erupt.[54] The core of the lesion contains a white, waxy substance.

Diagnosis is usually made by examination of the characteristic lesions, but DNA analysis can be performed if the diagnosis is unclear. Within each cluster of lesions, there are usually 1 or 2 dominant lesions that appear to control the growth of other lesions. Eliminating the dominant lesion seems to be the key to curing the disorder. Molluscum contagiosum is self-limiting and not associated with cancer or long-term morbidity. Individual lesions usually resolve within 2 months, but full resolution decrease may take as long as 2 years due to auto-inoculation; consequently, treatment is recommended.[55]

Treatment of Women with Molluscum Contagiosum

No FDA-approved medications exist for treatment of individuals with molluscum contagiosum, but several drugs have traditionally been used for this indication. Some of these treatments emerged from treatments of condylomata acuminata, including podophyllin derivatives, trichloroacetic acid 85%, cantharidin solution, and the antiviral topical cream imiquimod (Aldara) 5%, as shown in Table 32-7.

No one treatment regimen for molluscum contagiosum has been found to be most effective. Hanna et al. reviewed four common treatments used for molluscum contagiosum in children: curettage, cantharidin, imiquimod (Aldara), and a mixture of salicylic acid.[55] Curettage is considered the most effective treatment but has the significant drawback of needing anesthesia and being time consuming. In terms of the medical treatments, cantharidin (Cantharone) had the lowest rate of side effects (19%), but more than 20% of individuals required three or more visits to to effect a cure.[55] Imiquimod was considered a safe alternative with a relatively low side-effect rate (23%); most individuals required only one or two visits to their healthcare providers for cure. The most significant drawback to the imiquimod (Aldara) regimen was its cost. Imiquimod 5% cream is a potent topical immunomodulatory agent that is FDA approved for the treatment of condylomata acuminatum. It works by inducing high levels of interferon alpha (IFN-α) and other cytokines locally. This agent has been used for more than a decade to treat molluscum contagiosum. Well tolerated, imiquimod has no known systemic or toxic effects, although application-site irritation is common.

Table 32-7 Treatments for Women with Molluscum Contagiosum

Drug: Generic (Brand)	Adult Dose	Contraindications	Clinical Considerations	Selected Drug–Drug Interactions
Cantharidin solution (Cantharone)	Single application 1 time/month	Hypersensitivity	Use sparingly	None known
Imiquimod (Aldara)	Apply to lesions 3 times/week	Hypersensitivity		None known
Podophyllin (Podocon)	Apply to lesion 1 time/week; leave on lesion for 30–40 minutes after first application, then 1–4 hours following subsequent applications if no adverse reactions occur		Contraindicated during pregnancy, during lactation, or with concurrent use of steroids; local skin reactions often occur	None known
Podophyllotoxin (Podofilox, Condylox)	0.5% topical gel: Apply 2 times/day for 3 days, discontinue for 4 days, then repeat for a maximum 4 cycles	Hypersensitivity	Contraindicated during pregnancy, during lactation, or with concurrent use of steroids; local skin reactions often occur	None known
Tretinoin (Retin-A)	Apply nightly	Hypersensitivity	Use sparingly	Toxicity with benzoyl peroxide, salicylic acid, spices, and lime
Trichloroacetic acid	Apply to lesions sparingly, repeat in 1–2 weeks	Hypersensitivity	Use sparingly; avoid sun	None known

Podophyllin (Pododerm) is a caustic **desiccant**. A 25% suspension of podophyllin in a tincture of benzoin or alcohol may be applied to molluscum contagiosum once a week. Podophyllotoxin is derived from the roots and rhizomes of *Podophyllum* (mandrake), a member of the juniper family found throughout North America. Its precise mechanism of action is unknown, but the alcoholate drug is cytotoxic, causing tissue necrosis by arresting cellular division in metaphase and antiproliferative effects by preventing DNA synthesis; these processes lead to cell failure and erosion of tissue. Some of the listed side effects for this medication include severe erosive damage in adjacent normal skin that may cause scarring and systemic effects such as peripheral neuropathy, renal damage, adynamic ileus, leucopenia, and thrombocytopenia. This treatment should be applied only by a health professional. Podophyllotoxin (Podofilox, Condylox) is a more stable form of podophyllin. This self-applied agent is composed of only the biologically active portion of the compound. The treatment consists of application of 0.05 mL of 5% cream or gel in lactate-buffered ethanol twice a day for 3 days.

Cantharidin (Cantharone, Cantharone Plus), a 0.9% solution of collodion and acetone, is a blister-inducing agent. A synthetic version of a substance produced by several insect species to protect their eggs, cantharidin has a long history of use in Eastern and folk medicine. Its precise mechanism of action is unclear, but it involves intraepithelial blistering and lysis of the skin.[54] Applied in the same fashion as podophyllin, carefully and sparingly, to the dome of the lesion, the cantharidin solution is left in place for at least 6 hours before washing and applying a bandage. The bandage should be removed after 24 hours. Cantharidin should be tested on a single lesion before treating large numbers of lesions. This treatment is repeated every week until the lesions clear, which usually requires one to three treatments.[54]

Trichloroacetic acid—or, less commonly, bichloroacetic acid—may be administered to eliminate molluscum contagiosum by destroying proteins in the cells. It is applied by healthcare providers in the same fashion as podophyllin, weekly for three applications. Trichloroacetic acid is most commonly used prior to prescribing home treatment with imiquimod (Aldara).

All of the burning or blistering agents work best on moist tissues but still can burn healthy surrounding tissues, so a waterproof barrier such as petroleum jelly should be applied to the adjacent tissues before such agents are administered in order to protect the nearby healthy tissue. If burning is intolerable after application, sodium bicarbonate should be available to be applied immediately to the tissues to inactivate the burning.

Cimetidine (Tagamet) is a histamine-2 receptor antagonist used in the treatment of ulcers and heartburn. It is known to stimulate T-lymphocyte production, which is important in controlling viral infections. One uncontrolled study found resolution of lesions in 9 of 13 participants with molluscum contagiosum who received this medication. In this study, the dose was 40 mg/kg/day orally in two divided doses, given for 2 months.[56] The authors recommended further placebo-controlled, double-blind studies be completed to determine the effectiveness of cimetidine in treating molluscum contagiosum. Because cimetidine interacts with many systemic medications, anyone who uses this agent should have all other medications routinely reviewed.

Tretinoin (Retin-A) 0.05–0.1% cream has also been used on an off-label basis in the treatment of molluscum contagiosum. Erythema at the site of removed lesions is a common side effect.

Special Populations: Pregnancy, Lactation, and the Elderly

Trichloroacetic acid and cimetidine (Tagamet) are considered safe for use during pregnancy and lactation. Limited data are available regarding the use of imiquimod (Aldara), but this medication generally is considered to be of low risk during pregnancy and lactation. Similarly, few data have been published about the effects of cantharidin (Cantharone); however, because agents such as trichloroacetic acid are known to be safe, use of cantharidin is not recommended.

Podophyllin contains two mutagens, quercetin and kaempferol. Podophyllin and a similar agent, podophyllotoxin, have been reported to be teratogens, although the evidence regarding this designation is controversial. However, their manufacturers have stated that these agents are contraindicated during pregnancy and lactation.[9] As a known teratogen, tretinoin (Retin-A) should be reserved for those women who are not at risk for pregnancy, such as women who are postmenopausal or using a highly effective form of birth control.[9,10]

Extramammary Paget's Disease

Extramammary Paget's disease is a type of cutaneous adenocarcinoma that may be classified based on the source of the primary lesion. Approximately 75% to 90% of cases are histologically diagnosed as adenocarcinoma in situ. A rare form of cancer, Paget's disease accounts for only 1% to 2% of vulvar cancers.[57] The pathogenesis of Paget's disease remains controversial. Histologically, the lesions from mammary and extramammary Paget's disease are identical, and the physical examination should include an evaluation of the breasts and other areas rich in apocrine glands. Although the disease can involve areas other than the vulva, this chapter focuses on extramammary Paget's disease of the vulva.

A disease of senescence, the peak incidence of extramammary Paget's disease occurs among Caucasian females who are in their 60s.[58] Symptoms include intense pruritus, irritation, a weeping or bleeding lesion, and (rarely) pain. Lesions can appear well defined, moist, and white (macerated) or reddish tan and scaling.[59] These manifestations may be infiltrated, eroded, or similar to an ulcerated plaque. The differential diagnosis for extramammary Paget's disease includes psoriasis, contact dermatitis, fungal infections, lichen sclerosus, intraepithelial neoplasia, and melanoma.[1] There is no pharmacologic treatment for Paget's disease.

Vulvodynia

Vulvodynia is the term used when a woman has pain or burning in the vulva of more than 3 months' duration, which cannot be explained by any specific, clinically identifiable disorder.[60] Vulvodynia may be generalized or focal, unilateral or bilateral, constant or sporadic, provoked or nonprovoked. Dyspareunia may or may not be a feature, but intercourse can trigger pain. **Allodynia** (light touch) is a hallmark of this disorder (Figure 32-1). Women may report wearing tight pants, sitting for prolonged periods, or even the movement of pubic hair as provoking pain. Some women have symptoms of a urinary tract infection with a sterile urine culture. Others report hyperalgesia, an increased response to a stimulus that is normally painful. This disorder is thought to occur in as many as 16% of women at some time during their lifespan.[61]

Vulvodynia is a diagnosis of exclusion and is usually established through history, although laboratory testing including biopsy may be performed to exclude other causes. One theory of vulvar pain is that an abnormal pain arc develops between the spinal cord and the brain.[62] Trauma (chemicals, injury, or disease) is thought to initiate a pain response, and after the trauma is removed, the pain receptors continue to respond as if the trauma is ongoing.[62] Another theory is that the pain is nociceptive from repeated, long-term trauma.[63,64] According to this theory, the cells themselves develop an abnormal pain response. A third theory relates to estrogen: Estrogen is thought to affect sensory perception, and alteration in estrogen levels may be associated with vulvodynia.[65] This etiology might explain why dysesthetic or essential vulvodynia begins at approximately the same time that menopause occurs.

Primary vestibulodynia occurs with first intercourse, first tampon insertion, or other initial contact of pressure or friction against the vestibule. Secondary vestibulodynia occurs after a pain-free interval.[60] Secondary vestibulodynia has a peak incidence in women in their mid-30s.[61] Triggers may include a prolonged bout with a vaginal infection or childbirth, even if the birth is by the cesarean route. Provoked vestibulodynia—a subset of vulvodynia limited to the vulvar vestibule—often occurs during a woman's reproductive years. Some women spontaneously develop pain without a readily observable trigger. Because the etiology is unknown, diagnosis can take as long as 5 years and treatments are largely based on anecdotal evidence, small series of cases, or expert opinion.[61]

Treatment of Women with Vulvodynia

As with squamous cell hyperplasia, breaking the itch–scratch–itch cycle is the first step in treatment of vulvodynia. Lidocaine (Xylocaine) application has been theorized to be therapeutic by desensitizing the nerve fibers. Application of topical anesthetics prior to intercourse or

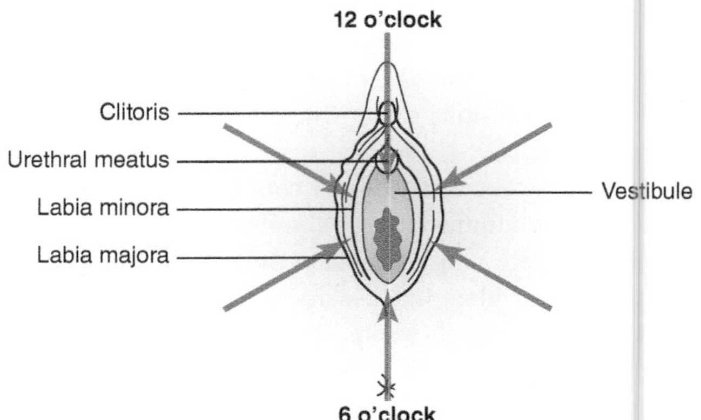
12 o'clock
Clitoris
Urethral meatus
Labia minora
Labia majora
Vestibule
6 o'clock
Apply gentle pressure with a cotton-tipped swab to sites around the introitus moving from 1 o'clock through 12 o'clock positions. Ask the woman to rate the severity of pain she experiences at each application of pressure with the swab. Pain is typically most severe in the posterior vestibule between the 5 and 7 o'clock positions

Figure 32-1 Cotton-tip application to elicit allodynia.

vaginal examinations allows penetration without pain. When applied only to the vestibule, anesthetics do not alter vaginal or clitoral sensation. Used nightly, lidocaine ointment (Topicaine) has been associated with gradually diminishing pain in some women.[66]

Eutectic mixture of local anesthetics (EMLA) is another intervention. The term EMLA is both the generic and brand name for a combination of 2.5% lidocaine and 2.5% prilocaine with eutectic properties, meaning the presence of a melting point lower than either constituent alone. While EMLA has been demonstrated to be as effective as lidocaine in dermatologic surgery, the disadvantage of this drug is that it is only available by prescription and is significantly more expensive than an equivalent amount of lidocaine alone. Lidocaine provides relief within 15 minutes and requires no occlusive dressing, whereas EMLA takes from 45 to 90 minutes to achieve its peak effect and requires an occlusive dressing. The prilocaine in EMLA has been associated with methemoglobinemia, albeit rarely.[14]

A newer drug, LMX 4 (Lidoderm, Lmx4), is a 4% lidocaine solution that is reported to have a similar pain relief profile and a cost equivalent to EMLA, but that requires less time to act and no occlusive dressing. LMX 4 is limited in that its half-life is only 50% of that of EMLA.[14]

The muscles enervating the vulva in women with vulvodynia have been shown to be hypertonic. Botulinum toxin (Botox) has been used successfully to paralyze these muscles, breaking the pain response.[67]

Tricyclic antidepressants are among the best-researched treatments for neurogenic pain, as noted in Table 32-8. Their precise mechanism of action is unknown. The amount of medication needed for pain relief is less

Table 32-8 Treatments for Women with Vulvodynia[a]

Drug: Generic (Brand)	Initial Dose	Continuing Dose	Side Effects/ Adverse Effects	Clinical Considerations
Tricyclic Antidepressants				
Amitriptyline	25 mg PO at bedtime for 7 nights, then increase every 3–4 nights until symptoms improve	150 mg at bedtime is maximum dose; average needed is 60 mg at bedtime	SE: Dry mouth, constipation, weight gain, sedation, urinary retention, blurred vision, confusion AE: seizure, stroke, myocardial infarction, arrhythmia, agranulocytosis, thrombocytopenia	May take 2–3 weeks to obtain full effect. Most sources advise avoidance of alcohol because the drug enhances the effects of alcohol. Use gradual tapering when discontinuing. Multiple drug–drug interactions
Desipramine (Norpramin)	10 mg PO at bedtime for 5 days then increase dose by 10 mg every 5 days until symptoms improve	150 mg at bedtime is maximum dose		See amitriptyline. Less sedating than amitriptyline.
Nortriptyline (Aventyl)	10 mg PO at bedtime for 3–4 nights, then increase every 3–4 nights until symptoms improve	50–150 mg at bedtime; average needed is 60 mg at bedtime		See amitriptyline. Less sedating than amitriptyline.
Anticonvulsants				
Gabapentin (Neurontin)	300 mg at night for 3 nights, then 300 mg 2 times/day for 3 days; increase by 300 mg every 3 days until symptoms improve	Maximum of 1200 mg 3 times daily; average needed is 1500 mg daily in divided doses	SE: Somnolence, fatigue, nausea, drowsiness, dizziness, anorgasmia, weight gain AE: Leukopenia	May take 2–3 weeks to obtain full effect. Does not have anticholinergic effects associated with the tricyclic antidepressants.
Selective Norepinephrine Reuptake Inhibitors				
Duloxetine (Cymbalta)	20–30 mg PO daily; increase to 60 mg/day	Maximum dose is 120 mg per day in divided doses	SE: Headache, nausea, somnolence, weight loss, constipation, anxiety vision changes AE: Seizures, suicidal ideation, depression	Off-label use for treating vulvodynia.
Venlafaxine (Effexor XR)	37.5 mg PO daily A.M. Increase to 75 mg in 1–2 weeks.	Maximum dose is 150 mg daily Do not discontinue abruptly	SE: Headache, nausea, somnolence, weight loss, constipation, anxiety vision changes, hypertension, insomnia AE: Seizures, suicidal ideation, depression	Off-label use for treating vulvodynia. May take 2–3 weeks to obtain full effect. Many drug–drug interactions.

(continues)

Table 32-8 Treatments for Women with Vulvodynia[a] (*continued*)

Drug: Generic (Brand)	Initial Dose	Continuing Dose	Side Effects/ Adverse Effects	Clinical Considerations
Topical Agents				
Compound cream: amitriptyline 2%/ baclofen 2% in water washable base	0.5 mL applied to affected area 1–3 times/day		SE: contact dermatitis, and other side effects associated with amitriptyline	This is one example of several compound topical agents. Designed to lower the incidence of side effects associated with oral dosing. Effectiveness has not been tested in randomized trials.
Compounded cream of gabapentin 2–4%	Apply small amount to affected area once daily		SE: Irritation, erythema, rash	Few side effects, well tolerated and appears moderately effective in small, uncontrolled studies.
EMLA	Pea-sized amount to painful area	Increase to amount needed for comfort	SE: Redness, burning	Requires 30 minutes to work.
Estradiol vaginal cream 0.01% (Estrace)	2–4 g daily	Gradually taper off after 2 weeks of therapy	SE: Vaginal spotting, breast changes headache fluid retention. However, side effects are rare	For menopausal women with vaginal atrophy. No major drug interactions for topical use.
Lidocaine 5%	Pea-sized amount to painful area	Increase to amount needed for comfort	SE: Prolonged use may cause drying of tissue	Store away from light and moisture.
LMX 4% (Lidocaine 4%)	Pea-sized amount to painful area	Increase to amount needed for comfort	SE: Redness, burning	Requires 15 minutes to work.
Injectable Agents				
Triamcinolone in bupivacaine	2 mL of a 3 mg/mL solution with 1 mL bupivacaine 0.25–0.5%	May increase to 3 mL of triamcinolone	SE: Mild burning with injection	No major drug interactions.

Abbreviations: EMLA = eutectic mixture of lidocaine and prilocaine; LMX 4 = topical lidocaine.

[a] Drugs in this table represent commonly used treatments that were originally developed for other purposes; vulvodynia therapy represents an off-label use.

Sources: Modified from Clinical Effectiveness Group, British Association of Sexual Health and HIV. 2014 UK national guidelines on the management of vulvar conditions. http://www.bashh.org/documents/2014_vulval_guidelines%20Final.pdf. Accessed November 20, 2014[66]; Haefner HK, Colins ME, Davis GD, et al. The vulvodynia guideline. *J Low Gen Tract Dis*. 2005;9(1):40-51[14]; Margesson LJ. Contact dermatitis of the vulva. *Dermatol Ther*. 2004;17(1):20-27[43]; Seehusen DA, Baird DC, Bode DV. Dyspareunia in women. *Am Fam Physician*. 2014;1;90(7):465-470[70]; Stone-Godena M. Vulvar pain syndromes: vestibulodynia. *J Midwifery Womens Health*. 2006;51(6):502-509.[60]

than the amount used for the treatment of depression, and fewer side effects are observed with this regimen. Amitriptyline begins with a dose of 25 mg at bedtime for 1 week, with the dose then gradually increasing until symptoms improve.[68] Nortriptyline (Aventyl) is usually prescribed as 10 mg at bedtime for 3 to 4 days, with a gradual increase in dose every 3 to 4 days until symptoms improve. Most researchers recommend maintaining the therapeutic dose for 6 months before considering tapering this medication.[61] When discontinuing nortriptyline, decrease the dose by half every 3 to 4 days. Tricyclic antidepressants should be prescribed by a provider skilled in their use.

In 2008, Boardman et al. published the results of a study of 51 women with vulvodynia who were treated for a minimum of 8 weeks with a topical formulation of the anticonvulsant gabapentin (Neurontin).[69] In this study, 80% of the women reported at least a 50% improvement in pain scores and an increase in sexual function; 14% of the subjects discontinued the treatment regimen. Topical gabapentin was well tolerated.

Other treatments for vulvodynia reviewed in the literature without consensus or strong evidence to recommend them include other antiseizure medications, yoga, hypnotherapy, pelvic muscle physical therapy, and psychotherapy.[14] As with any vulvar disorder, hygiene measures provide comfort and imbue a woman with some control over her condition. A healthy diet provides support to the immune system, and emotional support encourages the woman to continue to explore treatment options until she finds an effective one for her.

Special Populations: Pregnancy, Lactation, and the Elderly

Tricyclic antidepressants are not associated with congenital anomalies; however, women who take these drugs during pregnancy may have an increased risk for preterm birth, low birth weight, and neonatal withdrawal symptoms. In general, tricyclic antidepressants should not be used by breastfeeding women. If a tricyclic antidepressant is considered necessary, nortriptyline appears to have the fewest side effects. Use of nortriptyline by breastfeeding women is controversial with some authorities suggesting it is not associated with adverse effects on the infant and others who recommend that it not be used during lactation. Additional information about antidepressants can be found in the *Mental Health* chapter. The off-label use of gabapentin (Neurontin) presents a challenge for pregnant or breastfeeding women. There are limited data on the effects of gabapentin during pregnancy and animal studies have reported teratogenic effects. Few data exist to support its use during lactation, although gabapentin generally is considered compatible with breastfeeding.[9,10] No special considerations exist for treatment of vulvodynia among older women.

Conclusion

Millions of women suffer with vulvar pain or lesions. Such conditions are both a private and public health issue. While some lesions are easily identified, many lack clear etiology or definitive treatment. Frustration with finding answers has caused some women to either abandon hope for relief or to lose productive hours of their lives seeking relief. Access to qualified providers and well-documented methods of relief is critical to health. It is incumbent upon women's health providers to foster optimism in the women in their care and to continue to lobby for research toward finding causes and cures of the various pain syndromes.

Resources

Organization	Description	Website
General Pain Diaries		
Pain diaries are used by consumers to track symptoms of pain from any source; they provide clinicians with information to aid in diagnosis and treatment. Many pain diary apps are available for free or for a modest cost.		
Chronic Pain Tracker	Offers a summary report to download or to forward to a provider	http://chronicpaintracker.com/
WebMD Pain Coach	Track symptoms, take quizzes, access pain-management tips and educational material	www.webmd.com/webmdpaincoachapp
My Pain Diary	Drop-down lists that can be customized; includes a section on level of disability and duration	https://itunes.apple.com/us/app/my-pain-diary-chronic-pain/id338627856?mt=8
Manage My Pain Lite	Creates reports specific for healthcare providers	https://play.google.com/store/apps/details?id=com.lcs.mmp.lite&hl=en
General Obstetrics/Gynecology		
American Congress of Obstetrics and Gynecology	Includes the most frequently used clinical guidelines in the delivery of health care for women, such as one specific to vulvar lesions for healthcare professionals	https://itunes.apple.com/us/app/american-congress-obstetricians/id616323665?mt=8

References

1. Hammock LA, Barrett TL. Inflammatory dermatoses of the vulva. *J Cutan Path.* 2005;32(9):604-611.
2. Yo Y, Cheng AS, Wang L, Dunne WM, Bayliss SJ. Hot tub folliculitis or hot hand foot syndrome caused by *Pseudomonas aeruginosa. J Am Acad Derm.* 2007; 57(4):596-600.
3. Wertheim HFL, Verveer J, Boelens HA, van Belkum A, Verbrugh HA, Vos MC. Effect of mupirocin treatment on nasal, pharyngeal and perineal carriage of *Staphylococcus aureus* in healthy adults. *Antimicrob Agents Chemother*. 2005;49(4):1465-1467.
4. Stevens DL, Bisno AL, Chambers HF, et al. Practice guidelines for the diagnosis and management of skin and soft-tissue infections. *Clin Infect Dis.* 2005; 41: 1373-1380.
5. Liu C, Bayer A, Cosgrove SE, et al. Clinical practice guidelines by the Infectious Diseases Society of America for the treatment of methicillin-resistant *Staphylococcus aureus* infections in adults and children. *Clin Infect Dis.* 2011;52(3):e18-e55.
6. Birnie AJ, Bath-Hextall FJ, Ravenscroft JC, Williams HC. Interventions to reduce *Staphylococcus aureus* in the management of atopic eczema. *Cochrane Database Syst Rev.* 2008;3:CD003871. doi:10.1002/14651858.CD003871.pub2.
7. Aiello AE, Larson EL, Levy SB. Consumer antibacterial soaps: effective or just risky? *Clin Infect Dis.* 2007; 45(suppl 2):S137-S147.
8. Bergstrom KG. Update on antibacterial soaps: the FDA takes a second look at triclosans. *J Drugs Dermatol.* 2014;13(4):501-503.

9. Briggs G, Freeman R. *Drugs in Pregnancy and Lactation.* 10th ed. Philadelphia, PA: Lippincott Williams & Wilkins; 2014.
10. Lactmed: A Toxnet Database. Drugs and lactation. http://toxnet.nlm.nih.gov/newtoxnet/lactmed.htm. Accessed November 15, 2014.
11. Cooper SM, Ali I, Baldo M, Wojnarowska F. The association of lichen sclerosus and erosive lichen planus of the vulva with autoimmune disease: a case-controlled study. *Arch Dermatol.* 2008;144(11);1432-1435.
12. Chan I, Oyama N, Neill SM, Wojnarowska F, Black MM, McGrath JA. Characterization of IgG autoantibodies to extracellular matrix protein 1 in lichen sclerosus. *Clin Exp Dermatol.* 2004;29(5):499-505.
13. Neill SM, Lewis FM, Tatnall, FM Cox, NH; British Association of Dermatologists. British Association of Dermatologists' guidelines for the management of lichen sclerosus 2010. *Br J Dermatol.* 2010; 163(4): 672-682.
14. Haefner HK, Colins ME, Davis GD, et al. The vulvodynia guideline. *J Low Gen Tract Dis.* 2005;9(1):40-51.
15. Chi CC, Kirtschig G, Baldo M, Brackenbury F, Lewis F, Wojnarowska F. Topical interventions for genital lichen sclerosus. *Cochrane Database Syst Rev.* 2011;12:CD008240. doi:10.1002/14651858.CD008240.pub2.
16. Fistarol SK, Itin PH. Diagnosis and treatment of lichen sclerosus: an update. *Am J Clin Dermatol.* 2013; 14(1):27-47.
17. Goldstein AT, Creasey A, Pfau R, Phillips D, Burrows LJ. A double-blind, randomized controlled trial of clobetasol versus pimecrolimus in patients with vulvar lichen sclerosus. *J Am Acad Dermatol.* 2011; 64(6): e99-e104.
18. Bulbul Baskan E, Turan H, Tunali S, Toker SC, Saricaoglu H. Open label trial of cyclosporine for vulvar lichen sclerosus. *J Am Acad Dermatol.* 2007; 57(2):276-278.
19. Rouzier R, Haddad B, Deyrolle C, Pelisse M, Moyal-Barracco M, Paniel BJ. Perineoplasty for the treatment of introital stenosis related to vulvar lichen sclerosus. *Am J Obstet Gynecol.* 2002;186(1):49-52.
20. Jiménez-Ayala M, Jiménez-Ayala B. Terminology for vulvar cytology based on the Bethesda system. *Acta Cytol.* 2002;46(2):645-650.
21. Ayhan A, Guvendag Guven ES, Guven S, Sakinci M, Kucukali T. Medical treatment of vulvar squamous cell hyperplasia. *Int J Gynaecol Obstet.* 2006; 95(3): 278-283.
22. Simpson RC, Thomas KS, Leighton P, Murphy R. Diagnostic criteria for erosive lichen planus affecting the vulva an electronic Delphi consensus exercise. *Br J Dermatol.* 2013;169(2):337-343.
23. Bradford J, Fischer G. Management of vulvovaginal lichen planus: a new approach. *J Low Genit Tract Dis.* 2013;17(1):28-32.
24. Shepherd J, Taheri A, Feldman S. Once daily topical treatment for psoriasis: calcipotriene + betamethasone, 2 compound topical formulation. *Clin Cosmet Investig Dermatol.* 2014;7:19-22.
25. Byrd JA, Davis M, Rogers R III. Recalcitrant symptomatic vulvar lichen planus response to tacrolimus. *Acta Derm.* 2004;140(6):715-720.
26. International Society for the Study of Vulvovaginal Diseases, Patient Education Committee. Vulvar lichen planus. 2010. http://issvd.org/wordpress/wp-content/uploads/2012/04/VULVARLICHENPLANUS2010.pdf. Accessed May 22, 2014.
27. Moyal-Barracco M, Wendling J. Vulvar dermatosis. *Best Pract Res Clin Obstet Gynaecol.* 2014;28(7): 946-958.
28. Pascoe VL, Kimball AB. Hidradenitis suppurativa: current progress and future questions. *JAMA Dermatol.* 2014;150(2):1263-1264.
29. Revuz J. Medical treatments of hidradenitis suppurativa: a new paradigm. *Dermatology.* 2007;215(2):95-96.
30. Von der Werth JM, Williams HC, Raeburn JA. The clinical genetics of hidradenitis suppurativa revisited. *Br J Dermatol.* 2000;142(5):947-953.
31. Yazdanyar S, Jemec G. Hidradenitis suppurativa: a review of cause and treatment. *Curr Opin Infect Dis.* 2011;24(2):118-123.
32. Kerdel FA. Current and emerging nonsurgical treatment options for hidradenitis suppurativa. *Semin Cutan Med Surg.* 2014;33(3 suppl):S57-S59.
33. Alharbi Z, Kauczok J, Pallua N. A review of wide surgical excision of hidradenitis suppurativa. *BMC Dermatol.* 2012;12:9. http://www.biomedcentral.com/1471-5945/12/9. Accessed May 22, 2014.
34. Shah N. Hidradenitis suppurativa: a treatment challenge. *Am Fam Physician.* 2005;72(8):1547-1552.
35. Bong JL, Shalders K, Saihan E. Treatment of persistent painful nodules of hidradenitis suppurativa with cryotherapy. *Clin Exp Dermatol.* 2003;28(3): 241-244.
36. Jemec GBE, Revuz J, Lyeden J, eds. *Hidradenitis suppurativa 2006.* Chapter 21. http://elib.fk.uwks.ac.id/asset/archieve/e-book/KULIT%20KELAMIN%

20-%20DERMATOLOGY/Hidradenitis%20Supurativa .pdf. Accessed May 18, 2014.

37. Brocard A, Knol A, Khammari A, Dréno B. Verneuil's disease and zinc: a new therapeutic approach—a pilot study. *Dermatology.* 2007;214(4):325-327.
38. Farrell AM, Randall VA, Vafaee T, Dawber RP. Finasteride as a therapy for hidradenitis suppurativa. *Br J Dermatol.* 1999;141(6):1138-1139.
39. Boer J, van Gemert MJ. Long-term results of isotretinoin in the treatment of 68 patients with hidradenitis suppurativa. *J Am Acad Dermatol.* 1999;40(1):73-76.
40. Rose RF, Goodfield MJD, Clark SM. Treatment of recalcitrant hidradenitis suppurativa with oral cyclosporin. *Clin Exp Dermatol.* 2006;31(1):154-155.
41. Haslund P, Lee RA, Jemec G. Treatment of hidradenitis suppurativa with tumour necrosis factor-alpha inhibitors. *Acta Derm Venereol.* 2009;89(6):595-600.
42. Wolkenstein P, Loundou A, Barrau K, Auquier P, Revuz J. Quality of life impairment in hidradenitis suppurativa: a study of 61 cases. *J Am Acad Dermatol.* 2007;56(4):621-623.
43. Margesson LJ. Contact dermatitis of the vulva. *Dermatol Ther.* 2004;17(1):20-27.
44. Bauer A, Rodiger C, Greif C, Kaatz M, Elsner P. Vulvar dermatoses: irritant and allergic contact dermatitis of the vulva. *Dermatology.* 2005;210(2):143-149.
45. International Study Group for Behçet's Disease. Evaluation of diagnostic ("classification") criteria in Behçet's disease: towards internationally agreed criteria. *Rheumatology.* 1992;31(5):299-308.
46. Davatchi F. Diagnosis and classification criteria for Behçet's disease. Pathology Research International; 2011. http://www.hindawi.com/journals/pri/2012/607921/. Accessed November 15, 2014.
47. Davatchi F, Chams-Davatchi C, Ghodsi Z, et al. Diagnostic value of pathergy test in Behçet's disease according to the change in incidence over the time. *Clin Rheum.* 2011;30(9):1151-1155.
48. Dohil M, Prendiville JS. Treatment of molluscum contagiosum with oral cimetidine: clinical experience on 13 patients. *Pediatr Dermatol.* 1996;13(4):310-312.
49. Yurdakul S, Mat C, Tüzün Y, et al. A double-blind trial of colchicine in Behçet's syndrome. *Arthritis Rheum.* 2001;44(11):2686.
50. Alpsoy E. Behçet's disease: treatment of mucocutaneous lesions. *Clin Exp Rheumatol.* 2005;23(4):532-539.
51. Mat C, Yurdakul S, Uysal S, et al. A double-blind trial of depot corticosteroids in Behçet's syndrome. *Rheumatology (Oxf).* 2006;45(3):348-352.
52. Anandarajah A. The American College of Rheumatology, annual scientific meeting: advances in the treatment of connective tissue diseases. *Fut Rheumatol.* 2007;2:379-384.
53. Hamuryudan V, Mat C, Saip S, et al. Thalidomide in the treatment of the mucocutaneous lesions of the Behçet syndrome: a randomized, double-blind, placebo-controlled trial. *Ann Intern Med.* 1998; 128(6):443.
54. Habif TP. *Clinical Dermatology.* 5th ed. St. Louis, MO: Mosby; 2010:242-245.
55. Hanna D, Hatami A, Powell J, et al. A prospective randomized trial comparing the efficacy and adverse effects of four recognized treatments of molluscum contagiosum in children. *Pediatr Dermatol.* 2006; 23(6):574-579.
56. Dohil M, Prendiville JS. Treatment of molluscum contagiosum with oral cimetidine: clinical experience on 13 patients. *Pediatr Dermatol.* 1996;13(4): 310-312.
57. Parker LP, Parker JR, Bodurka-Bevers D, et al. Paget's disease of the vulva: pathology, pattern of involvement, and prognosis. *Gynecol Oncol.* 2000;77(1):183-189.
58. Piura B, Rabinovich A, Dgani R. Extramammary Paget's disease of the vulva: report of five cases and review of the literature. *Eur J Gynaecol Oncol.* 1999; 20(2):98-101.
59. Mehta NJ, Torno R, Sorra T. Extramammary Paget's disease. *South Med J.* 2000;93(7):713-715.
60. Stone-Godena M. Vulvar pain syndromes: vestibulodynia. *J Midwifery Womens Health.* 2006;51(6): 502-509.
61. Harlow BL, Stewart BG. A population-based assessment of chronic unexplained vulvar pain: have we underestimated the prevalence of vulvodynia? *J Am Med Womens Assoc.* 2003;58(2):82-88.
62. Stein C, Clark JD, Oh U, et al. Peripheral mechanisms of pain and analgesia. *Brain Res Rev.* 2009;60(1):90-113.
63. Apkarian AV, Bushnell MC, Treede RD, Zubieta JK. Human brain mechanisms of pain perception and regulation in health and disease. *Eur J Pain.* 2005; 9(4):463-484.
64. Dworkin RH, Backonja M, Rowbotham MC, et al. Advances in neuropathic pain: diagnosis, mechanisms and treatment recommendations. *Arch Neurol.* 2003; 60(11):1524-1534.
65. Smith PG. Effects of estrogen on peripheral pain pathways. In: *Vulvodynia: Toward Understanding a Pain Syndrome.* Bethesda, MD: National Institute of

Child Health and Human Development; April 14–15, 2003:27-28.

66. Clinical Effectiveness Group, British Association of Sexual Health and HIV. 2014 UK national guidelines on the management of vulvar conditions. http://www.bashh.org/documents/2014_vulval_guidelines%20Final.pdf. Accessed November 20, 2014.
67. Gunter J, Brewer A, Tawfik O. Botulinum toxin A for vulvodynia: a case report. *J Pain.* 2004;5(4):238-240.
68. Reed BD, Caron AM, Gorenflo DW, Haefner HK. Treatment of vulvodynia with tricyclic antidepressants: efficacy and associated factors. *J Low Genit Tract Dis.* 2006;10(4):245-251.
69. Boardman LA, Cooper AS, Blais LR, Raker CA. Topical gabapentin in the treatment of localized and generalized vulvodynia. *Obstet Gynecol.* 2008;112(3):579-585.
70. Seehusen DA, Baird DC, Bode DV. Dyspareunia in women. *Am Fam Physician.* 2014;1;90(7):465-470.

33 Sexual Dysfunction

Jennifer G. Hensley, Mary C. Brucker

Chapter Glossary

Aphrodisiac Agent that is said to cause sexual desire.

Arousal disorders Persistent or recurring inability to attain or maintain adequate sexual excitement, causing personal distress. It may be experienced as lack of subjective excitement or lack of genital (lubrication/swelling) or other somatic responses.

Desire disorder Disorder that is most commonly subcategorized as a hypoactive sexual desire disorder.

Female sexual dysfunction Sexual dysfunction that includes both dysfunction and marked distress. Also called female sexual disorder.

Hypoactive sexual desire disorder Persistent or recurring deficiency (or absence) of sexual fantasies/thoughts and/or receptivity to sexual activity that causes personal distress.

Orgasmic disorders Persistent or recurrent difficulties, delays in, or absences of attaining orgasm following sufficient sexual stimulation and arousal that causes personal distress; it may be either a primary or secondary condition.

Pain disorders Female sexual pain disorders that include one of the following: dyspareunia, vaginismus, or noncoital pain.

Introduction

Humans are sexual beings. Sex is necessary for propagation of the species, but it is also an integral component of health and well-being across the lifespan. In the United States, discussion of sexuality has often been shrouded in taboo, with many women being reticent to express their sexual concerns. However, as the so-called baby boomers of the sexual revolution age, they are more likely to be healthier than their parents were at a similar age. And, unlike their parents, they are more likely to have high expectations for continued satisfying sexual activity.

The sexual conditions for which women most frequently seek help include decreased sexual desire, difficulty with orgasm, and dyspareunia. To identify the appropriate pharmacologic intervention, the provider must understand the normal sexual response across the lifespan.

Sexology in the United States

In the United States, sexuality and sexual expression were rarely discussed publicly until the twentieth century. Sexology, or the scientific study of sexuality, is associated with Alfred Kinsey, who, when teaching a marriage course for women at Indiana University, found the students had many unanswered questions about sexual relations. Kinsey created a research team, conducted thousands of interviews with persons of both genders about sex, and published the results of his study. In 1947, his team evolved into the Institute for Sex Research with the mission of advancing sexual health and knowledge worldwide; it remains in operation today (as the Kinsey Institute for Research in Sex, Gender, and Reproduction) studying sexology.[1]

In 1966, William H. Masters and Virginia E. Johnson explored the physiology of what they characterized as the normal sexual response.[2] Their research received widespread publicity by the media. Masters and Johnson identified four phases of the sexual response that occur in a linear progression: excitement, plateau, orgasm,

Table 33-1 Masters and Johnson Classic Model for Female Sexual Response: EPOR

Excitement (Arousal)	Plateau	Orgasm	Resolution
Initial arousal	Full arousal, preorgasm		Postorgasm
Vaginal lubrication Inner two-thirds of vagina expands Cervix and uterus pulled forward Labia majora become flatter and move outward in nulliparas women Labia majora increase in size in parous women Labia minora enlarge Clitoral gland become swollen Nipples become erect and breasts slightly increase in size Increased sexual tension above unaroused state Some increase in heart rate, respiratory rate, blood pressure, and muscle tension Blood flow to genitals increases Vasocongestion of skin, called "sex flush," occurs in 50–75% of women	The outer one-third of the vagina swells and the opening narrows by one-third; referred to as the "orgasmic platform" Inner two-thirds of vagina expands as uterus is elevated; called tenting Clitoris withdraws into the clitoral hood Labia minora engorge and enlarge Labia minora change color due to vasocongestion; change precedes orgasm Areola and breasts enlarge Further increase in heart rate, respiratory rate, and blood pressure Blotchy skin pattern may be seen as sex flush Increased muscle tension	Discharge of accumulated sexual intensity as rhythmic muscular contractions of the uterus, outer one-third of the vagina, anal sphincter, and clitoris Probable release of female ejaculate from Bartholin's glands; this remains unclear Heart rate, respiratory rate, and blood pressure at highest values Other muscles such as buttocks or feet may involuntarily contract	If continued sexual stimulation and interest, multiorgasmic response is possible Alternatively, may return to unaroused state Muscles relax and vasocongestion dissipates with loss of orgasmic platform; uterus returns to resting state; vagina shortens in width and length; clitoris returns to normal size and position Breasts decrease in size; areola and nipples flatten Breathing, heart rate, and blood pressure return to normal

Source: Modified from Masters WH, Johnson VE. *Human Sexual Response*. Boston, MA: Little, Brown; 1966.[2]

and resolution (EPOR). This classic model, which is summarized in Table 33-1, continues to be recognized today. Some current models include an additional initial phase of desire or libido, which refers to the urges or fantasies of sexual activity that occur just prior to the excitement/arousal stage.

As the complexity of sexual response in the female has become better understood, other models have emerged that incorporate more information about psychological (e.g., seduction), emotional (e.g., desire), and cognitive factors.[3,4] Sexual response of the woman specifically is addressed in more detail in some models.[5] For example, Basson's model incorporates psychologic and biologic factors such as emotional intimacy, sexual stimuli, and satisfaction with relationships, and clarifies the subjective importance of a woman's arousability (Figure 33-1).[6] Although no single model explains what is the normal sexual response and its myriad associated factors, collectively these models provide a basis for diagnosing and treating female sexual dysfunction.

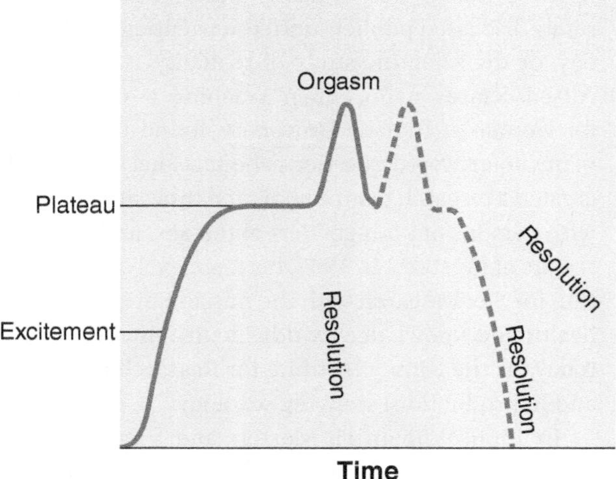

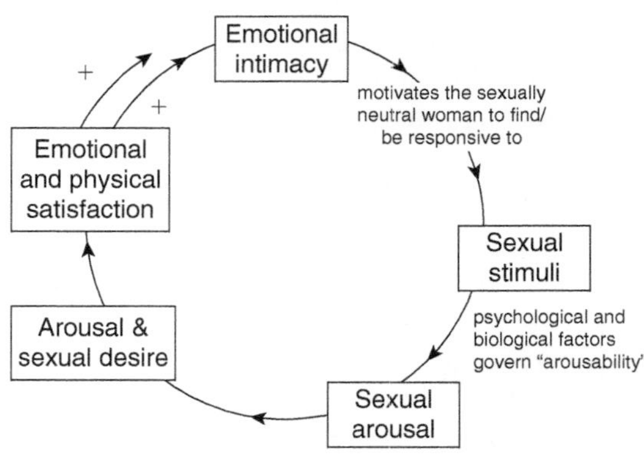

Figure 33-1 Traditional linear sex response cycle of Masters and Johnson alongside circular intimacy-based female sex response cycle.

Source: Data from Masters WH, Johnson VE. *Human Sexual Response*. Boston: Little, Brown; 1966[2]; Basson R. Women's sexual dysfunction: revised and expanded definitions. *CMAJ*. 2005;172(10):1327-1333.[6]

While Masters and Johnson were conducting their studies in the 1960s and 1970s, a sexual revolution occurred in the United States, reflecting liberalization of discussion of sexuality, sexual expression, and feminism thought, along with the advent of oral contraception. The last allowed sexual intercourse to be disentangled from procreation. In the years since the studies by Masters and Johnson were conducted, much additional information has been published about the physiology of sexuality.[7]

Sexual Physiology in Women

The mean age of menarche is 12 to 13 years, or 2 to 2.5 years after pubertal changes begin.[8] Prior to puberty and menarche, it is normal for female infants to touch and stimulate their genitals and for toddlers to exhibit curiosity about differences between sexes.[9,10] Sexual arousal is believed to occur secondary to classical conditioning (i.e., through stimulus/response association).[9] That is, positive experiences reinforce the value of the arousal, whereas negative responses do not. Masturbatory activities in childhood, alone or with peers, are common.[10] Adolescents may actively engage in sexual experimentation, which can lead to untoward consequences such as sexually transmitted infections or unintended pregnancies.[11] Many factors, including biology, family, culture, and society, play into adolescents' determinants of their sexual identities.[11]

Adult women actively engage in sexual activities for procreation, intimacy, and physiologic release. Sexual pleasure may be attained alone, with men or other women, or various combinations. As normal aging occurs, the body responds more slowly to the release of hormones, neurotransmitters, and chemical messengers that affect vasocongestion and neuromuscular tension. This can lead to a disruption in the sexual response beginning early in perimenopause and persisting postmenopausally.

Postmenopausal women continue to have interest in their sexuality and sexual expression, but might experience decreased desire and/or arousal or dyspareunia.[12] The menopausal decrease in estrogen results in urogenital atrophy, decreases in the side of the uterus and vagina, less vaginal lubrication, and decline in the erotic sensitivity of the nipple, clitoris, and vulvar tissue. The menopausal decrease in testosterone results in loss or lowering of libido. Thus, menopausal changes in sexual function include declines in sexual frequency, sexual responsiveness, lower libido, and possibly dyspareunia.

Two basic physiologic reactions occur during the sexual response: *vasocongestion*, as blood engorges the genitals and breasts, and *neuromuscular tension*, as energy builds up in the nerves and muscles.[2] The total response, however, is multifactorial, responding to neurotransmitters and hormones at both the central and peripheral levels. Estrogen, testosterone, progesterone, and oxytocin act centrally to incite sexual desire/arousal. Neurotransmitters and cellular messengers such as dopamine, norepinephrine, melanocortins, nitric oxide, vasoactive intestinal peptide, and cyclic guanosine monophosphate act peripherally to enhance sexual desire and excitement via vasocongestion and neuromuscular tension, whereas prolactin acts as a central inhibitor, and serotonin as a peripheral inhibitor.[13] Prolactin levels are high during breastfeeding and can lead to a decrease in sexual desire/arousal. High serotonin levels interfere with vasocongestion, and a decrease in sexual arousal/orgasm is often a noted side effect of selective serotonin reuptake inhibitor use. Figure 33-2 and

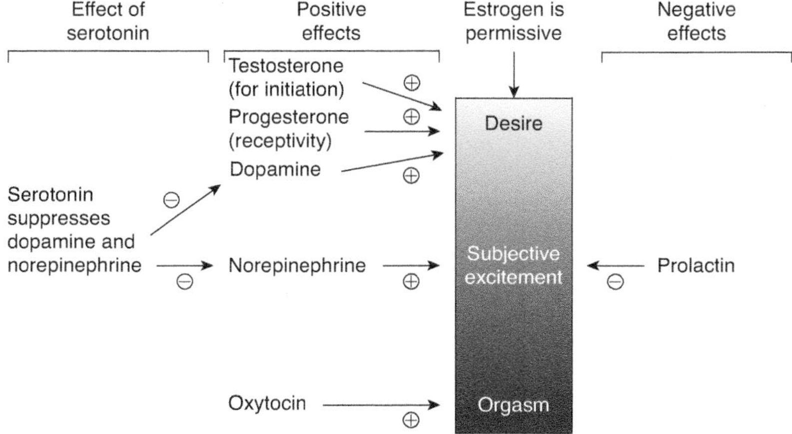

Figure 33-2 Central effect of sex hormones on the female sexual response.

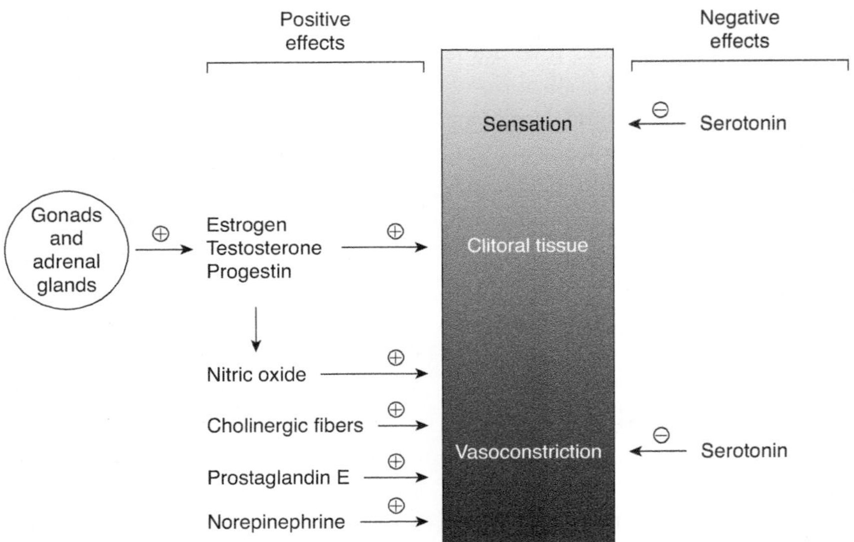

Figure 33-3 Peripheral effects on sexual function.

Source: Modified from Clayton A. Epidemiology and neurobiology of female sexual dysfunction. *J Sex Med.* 2007;4(suppl 4):260-268.[14]

Figure 33-3 illustrate the excitatory and inhibitory effects of these neurotransmitters.[14]

Female Sexual Dysfunction

Each woman is unique, and there is little consensus as to what defines "normal" in terms of female sexual function.[15] Multiple factors—such as age, physical health, emotional status, influence of past and present relationships, sexual expectations, religious/cultural background, and individual beliefs—affect sexual health, as illustrated in Figure 33-4. Thus, it is clear that sexuality differs both among individuals and within the individual herself based on age, partner, and other contexts. Because of the difficulty in defining "normal" sexuality, it should come as no surprise that it is equally difficult to define **female sexual dysfunction**. However, because taboos about discussing sex remain,

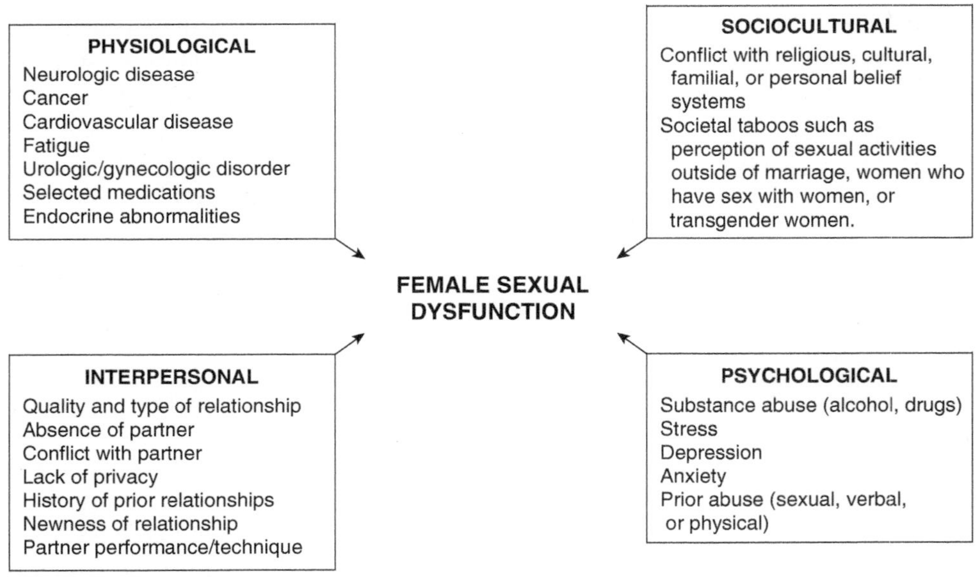

Figure 33-4 Factors affecting female sexual dysfunction.

it can be assumed that the number of women with sexual problems is likely to be underreported. In 2014, a protocol was published for an upcoming systematic review designed to clarify the prevalence of female sexual dysfunction and factors associated with this disorder.[16]

Unlike hypertension or hypercholesterolemia, for which an exact laboratory test is available to confirm the diagnosis, female sexual dysfunction is self-described or self-diagnosed. The ability to self-diagnose may be empowering to women, but it may have other implications as well. For example, some women may believe the popular media images and messages that suggest a woman should always be ready to respond sexually and be sexy. Some authorities have suggested that female sexual dysfunction does not exist as a distinct condition, but rather is the direct result of the "medicalization of sex."[17] Consequently, some researchers prefer the term "female sexual problem" to the terms "female sexual dysfunction" and "female sexual disorder."[18]

Categories of Female Sexual Dysfunction

In 2013, the American Psychiatric Association's *Diagnostic and Statistical Manual of Mental Disorders*, fifth edition (*DSM-5*) was released, combining some diagnoses for female sexual dysfunction into several categories, such as **arousal disorders**, **desire disorders** such as **hypoactive sexual desire disorder**, **orgasmic disorders**, and **pain disorders**. Most of these categories were in the previous edition of *Diagnostic and Statistical Manual of Mental Disorders* (*DSM-4*), although some were combined or eliminated in the fifth ediation.[19-21] Table 33-2 provides a comparison between the categories found in the two editions. Terminology from *DSM-4* is still in common use, although it will almost certainly be replaced in the future with the new categorizations.

DSM-5 Criteria for Female Sexual Dysfunction

Categories of female sexual dysfunctions now include the three listed in Table 33-2, substance/medication-induced sexual dysfunction, other specified sexual dysfunction, and other unspecified sexual dysfunction. It should be noted that the symptoms reported by a woman can encompass more than one *DSM-5* category. To distinguish transient sexual dysfunctions from more persistent conditions, the new criteria require the dysfunction to be present for at least 6 months, with the exception of drug- or substance-induced dysfunction. Sexual dysfunction symptoms must cause personal distress, and be quantified as mild, moderate, or severe. Each dysfunction must be categorized as lifelong or acquired, and generalized or situational. Symptoms must be present 75% to 100% of the time. The category of other unspecified sexual dysfunction includes symptoms that produce personal distress, but do not meet the full criteria for other categories.[19] The phenomenon of gender incongruence is not discussed in this chapter. Because the *DSM-5* classifications are relatively new, most research studies published to date have not used them.

Female sexual interest/arousal disorder includes desire disorders or low libido. *Libido* is a term that is difficult to define because sexual desire is personal, and a normal level is not only elusive but likely impossible to codify. Women with an interest or arousal disorder lack normal sexual fantasies, thoughts, and/or receptivity. Arousal disorders usually include the inability to attain or maintain sexual excitement. Orgasmic disorders include difficulty, delay, or absence of attaining orgasm. Genitopelvic pain/penetration disorder includes dyspareunia, vaginismus, and other pelvic/genital pain. In general, the symptoms most frequently reported in conjunction with female sexual dysfunction include low libido/lack of interest in sex, inability to orgasm, and problems with vaginal lubrication.

Table 33-2 Female Sexual Dysfunction Categories: *DSM-4-TR* and *DSM-5*

DSM Edition	Female Sexual Dysfunction Disorder					
DSM-4-TR	Sexual aversion disorder	Hypoactive sexual desire disorder (low libido)	Arousal disorder	Female orgasmic disorder	Dyspareunia	Vaginismus
DSM-5	*Eliminated due to rarity*	Female sexual interest/ arousal disorder		Female orgasmic disorder	Genitopelvic pain/ penetration disorder	

Source: Data from American Psychiatric Association. Sexual dysfunctions. In: *Diagnostic and Statistical Manual of Mental Disorders*. 5th ed. Arlington, VA: American Psychiatric Association; 2013[19]; American Psychiatric Association. *Diagnostic and Statistical Manual for Mental Disorders*. 4th ed., text rev. Washington, DC: American Psychiatric Press; 2000.[20]

Acquired hypoactive sexual desire disorder can develop as a result of surgical menopause.

Medical Conditions Associated with Female Sexual Dysfunction

Although it is unclear how many women have female sexual dysfunction, symptoms appear to increase with age, poor health, and depression. Table 33-3 lists some health conditions that can be associated with female sexual disorder.

Drugs Associated with Female Sexual Dysfunction

Certain pharmacologic agents can induce female sexual dysfunction. Table 33-4 lists some of the drugs commonly used that are associated with development of female sexual dysfunction.

Antidepressants and Sexual Depression

Antidepressants are among the most commonly prescribed pharmaceuticals in the United States.[24] Medications that inhibit reuptake of the neurotransmitters serotonin and norepinephrine, such as selective serotonin reuptake inhibitors (SSRIs) and serotonin–norepinephrine reuptake inhibitors (SNRIs), are used for treatment of individuals with depression. Women who are successfully treated with antidepressants may begin to feel better, only to experience decreased desire and arousal, and have difficulty with orgasm. Sexual dysfunction while taking SSRIs varies from a small percentage up to 80% and appears to be dose dependent.[25-27] Conversely, SNRIs may have sexual side effects, but perhaps not as many as the SSRIs.[27,28] Choice of antidepressant should be based on the woman's symptomology, not solely sexual satisfaction concerns.

SSRIs are theorized to interfere with the normal sexual response via serotoninergic, dopaminergic, and anticholinergic pathways, as well as through mechanisms that utilize nitric oxide and prolactin (Figures 33-2 and 33-3). Serotonin is known to have an inhibitory effect on sexual arousal, whereas dopamine has an excitatory effect. More available serotonin in the neural synapse and less available dopamine leads to decreased desire, decreased arousal, and difficulty achieving orgasm. Elevated levels of serotonin and decreased dopamine also trigger increased production of prolactin, which further inhibits dopamine. Higher serotonin levels, along with the anticholinergic effects of SSRIs, may impede the vasocongestive phase of the sexual response by blocking the release of acetylcholine, which is necessary for local vasodilation of the clitoral veins, and by inhibiting nitric oxide, a potent vasodilator.[26]

Table 33-3 Selected Medical Conditions Associated with Female Sexual Dysfunction

Condition	Sexual Function Affected
Depression	Desire
Diabetes	Arousal and orgasm
Thyroid disease	Desire
Cardiovascular conditions	Arousal
Neurologic disorders	Arousal and orgasm
Androgen insufficiency	Desire
Estrogen deficiency	Arousal

Sources: Data from Basson R, Schultz WW. Sexual sequelae of general medical disorders. *Lancet*. 2007;369(9559):409-424;[22] Kingsberg SA, Janata JW. Female sexual disorders: assessment, diagnosis, and treatment. *Urol Clin North Am*. 2007;34(4):497-506.[23]

Table 33-4 Selected Drugs Associated with Female Sexual Dysfunction

Drug Class	Example Medication(s) Generic (Brand)	Area of Sexual Dysfunction
Antidepressants and mood stabilizers	Serotonin/norepinephrine reuptake inhibitors; selective serotonin reuptake inhibitors	Desire, arousal, and orgasm
Antidepressants and mood stabilizers	Tricyclic antidepressants	Desire and arousal
Antidepressants and mood stabilizers	Antipsychotics	Arousal
Antidepressants and mood stabilizers	Monoamine oxidase inhibitors	Desire and orgasm
Antidepressants and mood stabilizers	Benzodiazepines	Desire, arousal, and orgasm
Antiepileptics	Carbamazepine (Tegretol)	Desire
Antiepileptics	Phenytoin (Dilantin)	Desire
Antihypertensives	Angiotensin-converting enzyme inhibitors	Desire
Antihypertensives	Beta blockers	Desire and arousal
Antihypertensives	Alpha blockers	Desire or arousal
Antihypertensives	Diuretics	Desire
Antihypertensives	Calcium channel blockers	Desire
Cardiovascular agents	Lipid-lowering agents	Desire
Cardiovascular agents	Digoxin (Lanoxin)	Desire
Chemotherapy	Platinum-based agents	Desire and arousal

Sources: Data from Basson R, Schultz WW. Sexual sequelae of general medical disorders. *Lancet*. 2007;369(9559):409-424;[22] Kingsberg SA, Janata JW. Female sexual disorders: assessment, diagnosis, and treatment. *Urol Clin North Am*. 2007;34(4):497-506.[23]

Treatment for Women with Female Sexual Dysfunction

Treatment for persons with female sexual dysfunction primarily starts with nonpharmacologic therapies such as office-based counseling, psychotherapy, couples treatment, pain management, and attention to comorbid conditions. Office-based education about normal sexual function and the heterogeneity of normal function should always be an initial intervention as many women are not aware of how varied normal sexual function is within the general population.

Although the FDA has approved a clitoral suction device that stimulates blood flow to the clitoris, effectiveness of this device does not appear to be better than use of vibrators or other manual stimulation techniques. Pharmacologic therapies are tailored to the specific sexual dysfunction diagnosis.

To date, few studies of female sexual dysfunction pharmacologic therapies have accounted for powerful confounding variables such as past relationships, history of sexual experiences, current relational status with partner(s), concomitant male sexual dysfunction, gender identity, environment, and medical disorders. Therefore, the following data on medications should be considered within the context of these limitations. The International Society for the Study of Women's Sexual Health has strongly advocated for recognition of a woman's concerns by customizing the use of a variety of treatment options.[27]

Treatment of Women with Arousal and Orgasmic Sexual Dysfunction

There are no FDA-approved medications that are designed specifically for treatment of low sexual desire in women or primary orgasmic dysfunction. Thus, this section focuses primarily on agents used for two populations: (1) women with antidepressant-associated sexual dysfunction and, (2) peri and postmenopausal women who have secondary arousal or orgasmic dysfunction. Although not FDA approved for women with sexual dysfunction, the phosphodiesterase type 5 inhibitor (PDE5I) known as sildenafil citrate (Viagra) has been explored for use among women with arousal and orgasmic disorders secondary to antidepressant use.[29,30] Estrogen products are used to treat menopausal symptoms that interfere with sexual dysfunction such as urogenital atrophy and hot flashes. Testosterone in combination with estrogen therapy is commonly prescribed for postmenopausal women but is used off-label and has side effects that are unacceptable for some women. Ospemifene (Osphena), discussed later in this chapter, is approved for treatment of women with dyspareunia, which can contribute to low desire.

Treatment of Women with Antidepressant-Associated Sexual Dysfunction

Antidepressant use is associated with reduced libido and anorgasmia and may worsen preexisting sexual dysfunction, although the frequency varies with different SSRIs. The initial approach for treating antidepressant-associated sexual dysfunction is to switch to a non-SSRI agent. In particular, bupropion (Wellbutrin) is not associated with sexual dysfunction as often as are SSRI medications. If the woman prefers continuing with an SSRI, switching to one that is less likely to induce sexual dysfunction may be beneficial. The side effect details of SSRI use are reviewed in the *Mental Health* chapter. Switching classes of antidepressants may be beneficial if tolerated in terms of the depressive symptoms experienced by women.[30] As many antidepressants have long half-lives, some women may benefit from a drug holiday so that they may have satisfying sexual intimacy. With this practice, the antidepressant usually is stopped on Friday and restarted on Sunday. Collaboration with the woman's mental health provider and the woman herself is recommended if this course is undertaken.

Sildenafil

Sildenafil (Viagra), which is FDA approved for male erectile dysfunction, acts by allowing smooth muscle relaxation and vasocongestion of the genitalia—one of the two necessary physiologic reactions for a full sexual response leading to orgasm (the other necessary reaction is neuromuscular tension).[2,29] At the cellular level, activation of the nitric oxide–cyclic guanosine monophosphatase pathway (cGMP) is necessary for a woman to experience smooth muscle relaxation, vasodilation, and engorgement of the clitoris. Nitric oxide activates guanylate cyclase, which increases levels of cGMP. Phosphodiesterase type 5 breaks down cGMP, thereby decreasing the effect of nitric oxide on vasodilation. Sildenafil, as an inhibitor of phosphodiesterase type 5, increases cGMP, allowing nitric oxide to vasodilate smooth muscle, which then leads to clitoral engorgement. Sildenafil was first proposed as a treatment for persons with angina pectoralis; its vasodilating effect on genitalia was an incidental finding.[31,32]

Thus, there is biologic plausibility for the use of sildenafil in women because of its effect on vasocongestion. However, most of the studies assessing sildenafil for female sexual dysfunction either are case reports, included only a small number of participants, or involve animal research.[33–35] The bulk of this evidence has not shown that sildenafil is more effective than placebo in improving the frequency of enjoyable sexual events.[35]

Sildenafil (Viagra) does appear to improve sexual function in both premenopausal and postmenopausal women who have SSRI-associated sexual dysfunction and may be beneficial for women with diabetes or multiple sclerosis. The primary benefit appears to be in improving problems with delayed orgasm. Sildenafil appears less effective in improving low libido. In 2008, Nurnberg et al. investigated the use of sildenafil in women with antidepressant–associated female sexual dysfunction. This randomized controlled trial was relatively small ($n = 49$) and relatively short (8 weeks), with a 22% attrition rate in each group. Sildenafil was dosed at 25 mg, 50 mg, or 100 mg by mouth 1 hour prior to attempting sexual arousal. The group taking sildenafil reported less sexual dysfunction (relative risk [RR], 0.8; 95% CI, 0.6–1.0; $P = 0.001$).[31]

Side Effects and Adverse Effects of Sildenafil

The most common side effects of sildenafil include flushing, headache, nasal congestion, dyspepsia, and transient visual disturbances.[31] Decreases in blood pressure secondary to vasodilator effects can occur. Individuals on antihypertensive therapy may be more susceptible to this effect.

Adverse effects are rare but quite serious. The FDA has a black box warning for all PDE5Is on the market that includes the possibility of a sudden decrease in or loss of hearing or eyesight; this effect may be permanent.

Drug–Drug Interactions and Contraindications to Sildenafil

Contraindications to the use of sildenafil (Viagra) include heart disease, use of nitrates, liver or kidney disease, and peptic ulcer disease. Sildenafil is associated with several drug–drug interactions some of which are contraindications to use. Providers should check a drug interaction table before prescribing this agent. Example drugs that interact with sildenafil include: alpha blockers, antifungals, bosentan (Tracleer) (for pulmonary hypertension), CYP3A4 inhibitors such as grapefruit or high-fat meals, fluoxetine (Prozac), etravirine (Intelence), HMG-CoA reductase inhibitors, macrolide antibiotics, protease inhibitors, sapropterin (Kuvan), organic nitrates, alcohol, and St. John's wort.

Flibanserin

Flibanserin is a 5-HT_{1A} receptor agonist and a 5-HT_{2A} receptor antagonist. This agent may help to restore an imbalance between the inhibitory/excitatory hormones and neurochemicals that regulate the sexual response for the woman with hypoactive sexual desire disorder.[36] In 2010, after flibanserin's developer failed to provide adequate data on the endpoint measurement (i.e., sexual desire), the FDA voted not to approve this medication. A new drug application was resubmitted in 2013 and at the time of this writing is under review.

Treatment of Perimenopausal and Postmenopausal Women with Female Sexual Dysfunction

Women who report sexual dysfunction during perimenopause or after the menopausal transition have a few options for treatment in addition to common topical treatments such as vaginal lubricants. Estrogen therapy and testosterone are the two primary pharmacologic treatments in use.

Estrogen Therapy

Estrogen therapy, administered via one of several routes (oral, transdermal, injection), may be offered to women who experience troublesome menopausal symptoms, albeit with the current recommendation of use for the shortest amount of time necessary.[37] Women who have an intact uterus and who take estrogen will need a progestin as well to prevent endometrial hyperplasia. It is important to note that systemic estrogen therapy with or without progestin has not been shown to improve sexual desire directly in the randomized trials within the Women's Health Initiative and there are adverse effects. However, improvement in some of the more troublesome menopausal symptoms such as hot flashes, night sweats, and fatigue, can result in improvement in sexual function. Vaginal application of estrogen is very effective in treating symptoms associated with urogenital atrophy and dyspareunia and is often recommended first for women who do not have an indication for systemic estrogen therapy.[39]

A 2013 Cochrane systematic review examined 27 randomized controlled studies ($n = 16{,}393$ women) to primarily assess the effect of hormone therapy versus placebo on a composite score for sexual function in symptomatic perimenopausal and postmenopausal women.[38] Secondary outcomes included scores on individual domains for arousal and sexual interest, orgasm, and pain. Trials included hormone therapy compared to placebo or no intervention. Hormone therapy included one of four regimens: (1) estrogen alone, (2) estrogens with progestogens, (3) synthetic steroids, or (4) selective estrogen receptor modulators. Data were analyzed in the form of standardized mean difference and relative risk. A standardized mean difference

Table 33-5 Comparison of Hormone Therapy to Placebo: Effects on Sexual Satisfaction and Function in Perimenopausal and Postmenopausal Women

Hormone Therapy	Effect on Sexual Satisfaction and Function	Estrogen vs Control SMD (95% CI); P
Estrogens alone	Small to moderate benefit	0.38 (0.23–0.54); $P < 0.00001$
Estrogens and progestogens	Small to moderate benefit	0.42 (0.19–0.64); $P = 0.0003$
SERMs (EAA)	Not statistically significant	0.23 (−0.04 to 0.50); $P = 0.09$
Synthetic steroids	Small to moderate benefit	0.13 (0.00–0.26); $P = 0.5$

Abbreviations: SMD = standardized mean deviation; SERMs = selective estrogen receptor modulators.
Source: Modified from Nastri CO, Lara LA, Ferriani RA, Rosa-E-Silva AC, Figueiredo JB, Martins WP. Hormone therapy for sexual function in perimenopausal and postmenopausal women. *Cochrane Database Syst Rev.* 2013;6:CD009672. doi:10.1002/14651858.CD009672.pub2.[38]

between 0.2 and 0.5 was considered a small effect; between 0.5 and 0.8, a moderate effect; and greater than 0.8, a large effect. Estrogen alone or in combination with a progestogen was found to be the best therapy to improve sexual function, although all the findings were associated with a small to moderate benefit at best and appeared to be most beneficial in improving pain scores. The evidence for use of synthetic steroids and selective estrogen receptor modulators is weak and requires more research. (Table 33-5). More details about use of estrogen and progesterone, including contraindications and current preparations with dosing, is found in the chapter *The Mature Woman*.

Testosterone for Mature Women with Sexual Desire/Arousal Dysfunction

Testosterone in combination with estrogen therapy is commonly prescribed for treating perimenopausal and menopausal sexual dysfunction, although this is an off-label use.[39,40] Overall, testosterone therapy is associated with improvements in number arousal, sexual desire, the number of sexual events, frequency of orgasm, and a reduction in personal distress.[39]

A Cochrane systematic review examined 35 trials (n = 4768 women) in which various formulations of testosterone were used with estrogen or estrogen/progesterone therapy in postmenopausal women with sexual desire or arousal dysfunction. Despite limitations in the studies, testosterone appeared to improve sexual function in postmenopausal women as evidenced by several specific reports including the composite sexual function score (mean difference, 0.41; 95% CI, 0.19–0.63). The review noted an increased risk of androgenic side effects such as hirsutism, acne, and reduction of high-density lipoprotein (HDL) cholesterol, but there were no statistical differences in discontinuation of treatment modalities between the groups of women who used testosterone and the women who did not.[40] Unanswered questions include side/adverse effects of long-term use and existence of any association with cardiovascular health or breast cancer.

As observed in several other hormone trials, the route of administration may influence a woman's treatment with testosterone. Although transdermal administration of testosterone improves libido and increases sexual activity in women with sexual dysfunction associated with natural or surgical menopause, such preparations are not FDA approved for this indication.[41] The pharmaceutical company BioSante, however, has announced positive safety data from its ongoing Phase 3 trials of LibiGel (testosterone); LibiGel is a topical testosterone gel that is absorbed through the skin and delivers testosterone to the bloodstream over time.

Side Effects, Adverse Effects, and Contraindications

Of note, testosterone therapy has not been studied on a long-term basis as a treatment for women with female sexual dysfunction; to date, studies have evaluated its use for no more than 26 weeks. Side effects of testosterone include acne, hirsutism, unfavorable changes in HDL levels, clitoromegaly, deepening of the voice, emotionality, uterine bleeding, and breast tenderness.[42] Topical testosterone is preferred over oral testosterone to avoid the first pass through the liver and untoward androgenic side effects. In spite of avoiding first-pass effect, women with liver disease should not use testosterone.

Clinical Use of Testosterone Products

The testosterone dose that appears more effective for postmenopausal women who are taking estrogen concurrently is 300 mcg per day.[41] Most of the agents available in the United States are formulated for men. Women need smaller doses and therefore agents marketed for men should be used with caution. Women should not use oral agents because they are associated with negative effects on lipids and liver function tests.[39] Testosterone patches and gels that are formulated for men such as Androderm and Androgel also have supraphysiologic doses for women. Because cutting patches is not recommended, these agents should not be used. In addition, the FDA has issued a warning about adverse effects in children who were secondarily exposed to testosterone applied to the skin of an adult that the child had direct contact with. In March of 2015, the FDA required a black box warning be applied to all testosterone products that warns that these products are associated with an increased risk of heart attack and stroke.[42]

At this time, the best option for women who want to use testosterone therapy is a topical compounded formulation of 1% testosterone cream (0.5 grams daily) applied to the skin of abdomen, arms, or legs. A 300-mcg patch is available in Europe but not available in the United States at this time.

Treatments for Women with Sexual Pain Disorders

Dyspareunia affects 8% to 22% of women at some point during their life.[44] The etymology of the word dyspareunia is "bad or difficult mating." Dyspareunia can affect women of all ages. Painful intercourse is a symptom of many conditions. It can be primary as pain at first intercourse, or secondary, which develops after having pain-free intercourse. Dyspareunia can occur just before, during, or after sexual intercourse. In addition, dyspareunia can occur with each sexual contact or it may be situational and occur with some partners but not others. There are a multitude of etiologies that range from anatomic or physiologic disorders to complex psychological factors. Common conditions that cause dyspareunia include urinary tract infections, vulvar disorders such as lichen sclerosus, vaginal atrophy, pelvic or menstrual disorders, infection, or vulvodynia just to mention a few.

Sexual pain disorders have been classified into three categories: (1) Dyspareunia that is recurrent or persistent genital pain associated with sexual intercourse; (2) Vaginismus that is recurrent or persistent involuntary spasm of the musculature of the outer third of the vagina; and (3) Noncoital sexual pain disorders that are recurrent or persistent genital pain induced by noncoital sexual stimulation.[45]

In general, treatment of women with dyspareunia is directed toward the underlying cause. Nonpharmacologic treatments for vaginismus can be highly successful.[46] Dyspareunia that is secondary to vulvar conditions falls into the third category and is addressed in the *Vulvar Disorders* chapter. Pelvic or menstrual conditions that cause dyspareunia are reviewed in the *Pelvic and Menstrual Disorders* chapter. The chapter *The Mature Woman* reviews the physiology of menopausal urogenital atrophy and use of estrogen therapy in more detail. This chapter presents an overview of pharmacologic treatments that are approved for the specific purpose of relieving dyspareunia.

Pathophysiology of Dyspareunia

The vulva, vestibule, urethra, and bladder have a common embryologic origin, all have estrogen receptors, and they have common neurologic pathways. This anatomical origin may explain why pain in one site is often accompanied by pain in one of the other sites.[43] The complex interactions between neuroanatomic, endocrine, and emotional factors that contribute to dyspareunia are beyond the scope of this chapter. The reader is referred to recent reviews for more detailed information.[44]

Treatments for Women with Dyspareunia: Ospemifene

The only FDA-approved pharmacologic agent that is specifically for treatment of women with menopausal-related dyspareunia is ospemifene (Osphena). Ospemifene is a selective estrogen receptor modulator (SERM). This drug activates estrogen pathways in some tissues and suppresses estrogen agonist action in others. Ospemifene increases the estrogen effects on the vagina thereby decreasing vaginal dryness and improving some aspects of urogenital atrophy.

The dose of ospemifene is 60 mg once per day PO. The most common side effects are hot flashes, vaginal discharge, and excessive sweating. Ospemifene stimulates the endometrium and therefore, women who have an intact uterus must watch for signs of endometrial cancer. The drug has a black box warning because of increased risks for deep vein thrombosis, thrombotic strokes, and endometrial cancer.

Herbal Aphrodisiacs for Female Sexual Dysfunction

For centuries, potent sexual effects have been attributed to various botanical and herbal combinations. In fiction, be it books, television, or film, women surreptitiously receive these agents in a drink or food and subsequently become overwhelmed with sexual desire. Actually, aphrodisiacs are more myth than reality.

The word **aphrodisiac** is derived from Aphrodite, the Greek goddess of love. Most so-called aphrodisiacs are targeted at men, particularly those with erectile dysfunction. Preparations containing tiger penis and rhinoceros horn are two commonly mentioned—albeit ineffective—treatments. Oysters, which are rich in zinc, have been suggested to be aphrodisiacs perhaps because zinc deficiency is related to male impotency.

Box 33-1 Gone But Not Forgotten: Spanish Fly

The powder of the Spanish fly has been suggested to be a powerful aphrodisiac, able to drive men and women wild with sexual desire. In reality, the "fly" is a beetle in the genus *Cantharis*, sometimes called a *cantharide*. Cantharides irritate a male's urethra, with subsequent inflammation causing penile erection. There is no indication that Spanish fly preparations affect sexual desire for either gender, and they can have significant toxic effects, especially on the kidneys. Spanish fly is illegal in the United States, although some herbal agents using a similar name may contain pepper, ginseng, or similar ingredients.

The Internet contains advertisements for a large number of aphrodisiacs specifically for women. Most of these agents are focused on increasing desire. Scents with pheromones, lubricants with warming sensations, chocolate food items, and a large variety of supplements are sold to women. However, no large, randomized, controlled trials support any of these products' use. Box 33-1 describes the classic aphrodisiac, Spanish fly.

Special Populations

Pregnancy and Postpartum

Sexual expression is unique to every woman, and every pregnancy is unique. No consensus exists regarding "normal" sexuality in pregnancy. However, a pregnant woman has a changing hormonal milieu and often is challenged with issues such as gestational nausea as well as a need to modify positions for intercourse as the abdomen enlarges. Women in the postpartum period may report discomfort, particularly if they have experienced an episiotomy or cesarean birth. Evidence suggests that there generally is a decrease in arousal and orgasms beginning after the first 3 months' gestation, which then resolves by 6 months postpartum.[47] Because these symptoms are relatively transitory, the usual treatment for pregnant women is education, support, and palliative treatments such as lubricants if needed.

Lactation

Postpartum women who are nursing their children often experience vaginal atrophy, similar to that observed among mature women. First-line treatments include education, support, and palliative treatments such as lubricants if needed. Rarely topical estrogen products can be used.

Elderly

Female sexual dysfunction is likely to be more common among perimenopausal and postmenopausal women. Treatments for these women may involve drugs, as discussed previously for such symptoms as dyspareunia, low libido, and/or arousal/orgasmic disorders.

Conclusion

The female sexual response is complex and not defined by physiology alone. Cultural mores have changed over the last 50 years, such that women today may be more likely to seek care when variations in sexual function occur. Because of the complexity of sexuality, no simple therapies exist for women with various sexual issues. Nevertheless, some targeted treatments may ameliorate specific symptoms and enable women to enjoy a satisfactory sex life.

Resources

Organization	Description	Website
Sexuality Information and Education Council of the United States (SIECUS)	National organization with both Facebook and Twitter social media options. Materials for providers and consumers about sexuality.	www.siecus.org
North American Menopause Society (NAMS)	Professional organization dedicated to issues surrounding menopause, including symptoms associated with sexual dysfunction. Some materials are free; others are limited to members of NAMS. A free consumer app, "MenoPro," features information for consumer as well as the ability to keep notes regarding bothersome symptoms so as to discuss them with the healthcare provider. NAMS's professional journal, *Menopause*, also is available as an app.	www.menopause.org
Apps		
Multiple apps exist focusing on sexology and sexual dysfunction, although most of the latter deal with male erectile disorders. Some apps are free; others are available at a modest cost. However, most are independent as opposed to being sponsored by national or federal groups. Check iTunes and Google Play, among other sources.		

References

1. Kinsey Institute. Mission statement. http://www.indiana.edu/~kinsey/resources/sexology.html. Accessed June 9, 2014.
2. Masters WH, Johnson VE. *Human Sexual Response.* Boston, MA: Little, Brown; 1966.
3. Kaplan HS. *The New Sex Therapy.* New York: Brunner-Routledge; 1976.
4. Stuart E, Thatcher A. *Christian Perspectives on Sexuality and Gender.* Grand Rapids, MI: Wm. B. Eerdmans Publishing; 1996.
5. Whipple B, Brash-McGreer K. Management of female sexual dysfunction. In: Sipski ML, Alexander CJ, eds. *Sexual Function in People with Disability and Chronic Illness: A Health Professional's Guide.* Gaithersburg, MD: Aspen; 1997:509-534.
6. Basson R. Women's sexual dysfunction: revised and expanded definitions. *CMAJ.* 2005;172(10):1327-1333.
7. Association of Reproductive Health Professionals. *ARHP Clinical Proceedings: Women's Sexual Health in Midlife and Beyond.* Washington, DC: Association of Reproductive Health Professionals, May 2005:1-25.
8. Biro FM, Huang B, Crawford PB, et al. Pubertal correlates in black and white girls. *J Pediatr.* 2006;148(2):234.
9. Erickson EH. *Identity: Youth and Crisis.* New York: Norton; 1968:30.
10. Abel GG, Coffey L, Osborn CA. Sexual arousal patterns: normal and deviant. *Psychiatr Clin North Am.* 2008;31(4):643-655.
11. Kellogg ND. Clinical report: the evaluation of sexual behaviors in children. *Pediatrics.* 2009;124(3):992-998.
12. Wang V, Depp CA, Ceglowski J, Thompson WK, Rock D, Jeste DV. Sexual health and function in later life: a population-based study of 606 older adults with a partner. *Am J Geriatr Psychiatry.* 2015;23(3):227-233.
13. Salonia A, Giraldi A, Chivers ML, et al. Physiology of women's sexual function: basic knowledge and new findings. *J Sex Med.* 2010;7(8):2637-2660.
14. Clayton A. Epidemiology and neurobiology of female sexual dysfunction. *J Sex Med.* 2007;4(suppl 4):260-268.
15. Rosen RC, Barsky JL. Normal sexual response in women. *Obstet Gynecol Clin North Am.* 2006;33(4):515-526.
16. McCool ME, Theurich MA, Apfelbacher C. Prevalence and predictors of female sexual dysfunction: a protocol for a systematic review. *Syst Rev.* 2014;3:75.
17. Graham CA. Medicalization of women's sexual problems: a different story? *J Sex Marital Ther.* 2007;33(5):443-447.
18. Wood JM, Koch PB, Mansfield PK. Women's sexual desire: a feminist critique. *J Sex Res.* 2006;43(3):236-244.
19. American Psychiatric Association. Sexual dysfunctions. In: *Diagnostic and Statistical Manual of Mental Disorders.* 5th ed. Arlington, VA: American Psychiatric Association; 2013.
20. American Psychiatric Association. *Diagnostic and Statistical Manual for Mental Disorders.* 4th ed., text rev. Washington, DC: American Psychiatric Press; 2000.
21. Binik YM, PhD, Brotto LA, et al. Response of the *DSM-V* sexual dysfunctions subworkgroup to commentaries published in *JSM. J Sex Med.* 2010;7(7):2382-2387.
22. Basson R, Schultz WW. Sexual sequelae of general medical disorders. *Lancet.* 2007;369(9559):409-424.
23. Kingsberg SA, Janata JW. Female sexual disorders: assessment, diagnosis, and treatment. *Urol Clin North Am.* 2007;34(4):497-506.
24. Kessler RC, Ormel J, Petukhova M, et al. Development of lifetime comorbidity in the World Health Organization world mental health surveys. *Arch Gen Psychiatry.* 2011;68(1):90-100.
25. Montejo-González AL, Liorca G, Izquierdo JA, et al. SSRI-induced sexual dysfunction: fluoxetine, paroxetine, sertraline, and fluvoxamine in a prospective, multicenter, and descriptive clinical study of 344 patients. *J Sex Marital Ther.* 1997;23(3):176-194.
26. Rosen RC, Lane RM, Menz M. Effects of SSRIs on sexual function: a critical review. *J Clin Psychopharm.* 1999;19(1):67-85.
27. O'Donnell JM, Shelton RC. Drug therapy of depression and anxiety disorders. In: Brunton LL, Chabner BA, Knollmann BC, eds. *Goodman & Gilman's the Pharmacological Basis of Therapeutics.* 12th ed. New York: McGraw-Hill; 2011:397-417.
28. Dolberg OT, Klag E, Gross Y, Schreiber S. Relief of serotonin selective reuptake inhibitor induced sexual dysfunction with low-dose mianserin in patients with traumatic brain injury. *Psychopharmacology.* 2002;161(4):404-407.
29. Berman JR, Berman LA, Toler SM, Gill J, Haughie S; Sildenafil Study Group. Safety and efficacy of sildenafil citrate for the treatment of female sexual arousal disorder: a double-blind, placebo controlled study. *J Urol.* 2003;170(6 pt 1):2333-2338.

30. Taylor MJ, Rudkin L, Bullemor-Day P, Lubin J, Chukwujekwu C, Hawton K. Strategies for managing sexual dysfunction induced by antidepressant medication. *Cochrane Database Syst Rev*. 2013;5:CD003382. doi:10.1002/14651858.CD003382.pub3.
31. Nurnberg HG, Hensley PL, Heiman JR, Croft HA, Debattista C, Paine S. Sildenafil treatment of women with antidepressant-associated sexual dysfunction. *JAMA*. 2008;300(4):395-404.
32. Cavalcanti Al, Bagnoli VR, Fonseca AM, et al. Effect of sildenafil on clitoral blood flow and sexual response in postmenopausal women with orgasmic dysfunction. *Int J Gynecol Obstet*. 2008;102(2):115-119.
33. Laan E, van Lunsen RH, Riley A, Scott E, Boolell M. The enhancement of vaginal vasocongestion by sildenafil in healthy premenopausal women. *J Womens Health Gend Based Med*. 2002;11(4):357-365.
34. Angulo J, Cuevas P, Cuevas B, Bischoff E, Sáenz de Tejada I. Vardenafil enhances clitoral and vaginal blood flow responses to pelvic nerve stimulation in female dogs. *Int J Impot Res*. 2003;15(2):137-141.
35. Basson R, McInnes R, Smith MD, Hodgson G, Koppiker N. Efficacy and safety of sildenafil citrate in women with sexual dysfunction associated with female sexual arousal disorder. *J Womens Health Gend Based Med*. 2002; 11(4):367-377.
36. Reviriego C. Flibanserin for female sexual dysfunction. *Drugs Today (Barc)*. 2014;50(8):549-556.
37. Stuenkel CA, Gass MLS, Manson JE, et al. A decade after the Women's Health Initiative: the experts do agree. *Menopause*. 2012;19(8):846-847.
38. Nastri CO, Lara LA, Ferriani RA, Rosa-E-Silva AC, Figueiredo JB, Martins WP. Hormone therapy for sexual function in perimenopausal and postmenopausal women. *Cochrane Database Syst Rev*. 2013;6: CD009672. doi:10.1002/14651858.CD009672.pub2.
39. Tan O, Bradshaw K, Carr BR. Management of vulvovaginal atrophy-related sexual dysfunction in postmenopausal women: an up-to-date review. *Menopause* 2012;19:109.
40. Kingsberg SA, Woodard T. Female sexual dysfunction: Focus on low desire. *Obstet Gynecol*. 2015; 125(2): 477-486.
41. Somboonporn W, Bell RJ, Davis SR. Testosterone for peri and postmenopausal women. *Cochrane Database Syst Rev*. 2010;4:CD004509. doi:10.1002/14651858. CD004509.pub2.
42. Shifren JL, Davis SR, Moreau M, et al. Testosterone patch for the treatment of hypoactive sexual desire disorder in naturally menopausal women: results from the INTIMATE NM1 Study. *Menopause*. 2006; 13(5):770-779.
43. FDA Drug safety communication: FDA cautions about using testosterone products for low testosterone due to aging; requires labeling change to inform of possible increased risk of heart attack and stroke with use. Available from http://www.fda.gov/Drugs/DrugSafety/ucm436259.htm. Accessed March 15, 2015.
44. Braunstein GD. Safety of testosterone treatment in postmenopausal women. *Fertil Steril*. 2007;88(1):1-17.
45. Wesselmann U, Burnett AL, Heinberg LJ. The urogenital and rectal pain syndromes. *Pain*. 1997; 73(3): 269-294.
46. Steege JF, Zolnoun DA. Evaluation and treatment of dyspareunia. *Obstet Gynecol*. 2009;113(5): 1124-1136.
47. Basson R, Berman J, Burnett A, et al. Report of the international consensus development conference on female sexual dysfunction: definitions and classifications. *J Urol*. 2000;163(3):888-893.
48. Pacik PT. Understanding and treating vaginismus: A multimodal approach. *Int URogyn J Pelvic Floor Dysfunction*. 2014;25(12):1613-1620.
49. Yeniel AO, Petri E. Pregnancy, childbirth, and sexual function: perceptions and facts. *Int Urogynecol J*. 2014;25(1):5-14.

34

The Mature Woman

Ivy M. Alexander

Based on the chapter by Nancy A. Carroll, Susan E. Davis Doughty, Mary Ellen Rousseau, and Mary C. Brucker in the first edition of Pharmacology for Women's Health

With acknowledgment to Sharon M. Bond for additional content on vaginal conditions

Chapter Glossary

Bioidentical hormone therapy (BHT) Hormone products that are molecularly identical to the hormones naturally present in the body.

Bisphosphonates Medications that reduce bone resorption by decreasing osteoclast activity.

Estradiol (E_2) Most biologically active human estrogen in reproductive-age women; it is ovarian in origin and can be a component of estrogen therapy. Also called 17 β-estradiol.

Estrogen agonists/antagonists (EAAs) Newer term for selective estrogen receptor modulators (SERMs). EAAs usually preserve bone by acting as a weak estrogen in some tissues and as an estrogen blocker in others.

Estrogen therapy (ET) Use of estrogen alone, without a progestin, for treatment of women with menopause-related symptoms.

Estrone (E_1) Dominant circulating estrogen in postmenopause; it is derived primarily from aromatization of androstenedione. Estrone is used in bioidentical hormone therapy.

Hormone replacement therapy (HRT) Older term that has been largely replaced by "hormone therapy." The use of "replacement" implies action not congruent with hormone therapy.

Hormone therapy (HT) Broad term for use of hormones to treat women with menopause-related symptoms. It may include estrogen alone; estrogen with a progestin; testosterone alone; estrogen with testosterone; or estrogen, progestin, and testosterone.

Phytoestrogens Botanical products including isoflavones and lignans that are occasionally used for treatment of women with menopausal symptoms with or without hormones.

Progestin Drug class whose members interact with progesterone receptors; it includes both synthetic agents and natural progesterone. Controversy exists regarding terminology, with some authorities using the term "progestin" for the synthetic agent and reserving use of the term "progesterone" for natural agents. A few others employ the label "progestogen" as a broad term encompassing both synthetic and natural agents.

Selective estrogen receptor modulators (SERMs) Older term for estrogen agonist/antagonists (EAAs).

Selective progesterone receptor modulators (SPRMs) Drug class that includes progesterone agonists and antagonists. These agents have progesterone effects in some tissues and block progesterone effects in others.

Introduction

Until the twentieth century, few women lived long enough to reach menopause or develop the chronic diseases that often accompany aging. For millennia, women died long before menopause, often from communicable diseases and complications from reproduction—a situation that continues to be seen today in several developing nations. A baby girl born in the United States in 1900 had an average life expectancy of 48.3 years,[1] whereas her counterpart born in 2012 has a life expectancy of 81 years and should not just reach menopause, but actually spend the last third of her life in the postmenopausal period.[2] This increase in life expectancy has evolved due to several factors, such as improved nutrition and sanitation, as well as increased knowledge about healthy habits and risky behaviors. Individuals older than age 65 represent the fastest-growing segment of the population today in the United States. By the year 2040, senior citizens are expected to account for 21% of the U.S. population.[3]

Medication use has also had positive influences on life expectancy. Compared to men, women are more likely to live longer, and most older adults regularly take medications for prophylactic reasons (e.g., aspirin to prevent a second cardiac event) or to treat chronic diseases (e.g., antihypertensive agents for hypertension). Frequently, individuals use medications for both reasons, and occasionally they add agents to treat acute conditions such as coughs and infections. In general, prescribing for older women requires balancing the safety and effectiveness evidence derived from clinical trials conducted with younger subjects, knowledge of the physiology of the elderly, practical considerations, and the desire of the individual.[4]

Many mature women simultaneously use multiple agents, including prescription and over-the-counter pharmaceuticals as well as dietary supplements. In a study of community-based individuals, women who were older than 65 years had the highest overall prevalence of drug use, with 12% taking at least 10 medications and 23% reporting taking at least five prescription drugs.[5] Women in nursing homes are estimated to use even more medications due to chronic health conditions. However, polypharmacy greatly increases the risk for drug–drug interactions,[6] especially when multiple prescribers are involved. Indeed, a woman may be prescribed medications by providers who are unaware that she is already taking different agents, with a resulting increased risk of adverse effects and drug–drug interactions. Other women may experience difficulty as they move from home to assisted living facilities to hospitals and finally to skilled nursing homes. Different sites and providers associated with these locales suggest higher risks of medication errors. Conversely, some drugs may be underused among the elderly, although factors associated with this phenomenon have not been well studied.[7,8] For example, vaccines for influenza and pneumococcal infections are recommended, yet often not obtained by individual women. Older women who sustain a fracture frequently go untreated for osteoporosis. Antidepressants can be either overused or underused among older women, even though depression is often reported among this age group.

Pharmacology and Aging

The physiology of aging presents special considerations for prescribing drugs, which are compounded because of the increased likelihood of polypharmacy in older women. Pharmacokinetics and pharmacodynamics can be profoundly influenced by the physiologic changes that occur as a woman ages.[9]

Absorption

Drugs that depend on an acidic environment for absorption, such as ketoconazole (Nizoral), cefuroxime (Ceftin), various antiviral agents, and calcium carbonate, have decreased effectiveness in the age-related higher pH of the stomach; this condition is due to atrophy of the parietal cells. Older individuals also tend to have a slowed rate of gastric emptying, reduced blood flow to the small intestine, and decreased surface area of the intestine. All of these factors may further decrease absorption of drugs. Fortunately, factors involved in drug absorption rarely are clinically important, especially considering that most modern drugs have wide therapeutic indices.

Distribution

The volume of distribution of drugs is also affected over time. With aging, muscle often is replaced with fat. The increased amount of fat allows for a larger volume of distribution of lipophilic agents and may extend the half-life of these drugs, thereby slowing their elimination. Extracellular and intracellular spaces have less body water, which results in higher concentration of some water-soluble drugs in both blood and tissues. Serum albumin levels also decrease; however, the clinical significance of lower serum albumin concentrations is unclear.

Metabolism

Changes in the liver are of major significance in aging women. Hepatic mass and blood flow decrease with age, and some agents show reduced hepatic metabolism and clearance rates. Due to the marked variability in metabolic changes, individual titration may be required, even for some pharmaceuticals used as maintenance doses. Among agents with reported reduced hepatic metabolism in older adults are acetaminophen (Tylenol); anti-inflammatory drugs such as naproxen (Aleve); cardiovascular drugs such as nifedipine (Procardia), propranolol (Inderal), and verapamil (Calan); estrogen; and psychoactive drugs such as diazepam (Valium).

Excretion

Similar to hepatic changes, renal mass, tubular function, and renal blood flow also decrease as a woman ages. As early as age 30, some women experience a drop in creatinine clearance, even though creatinine levels may remain in the normal range. Various agents have been found to have reduced renal elimination because of these factors. These drugs include antibiotics such as ciprofloxacin (Cipro), gentamicin (Garamycin), and nitrofurantoin (Macrobid); cardiovascular agents such as captopril (Capoten), digoxin (Lanoxin), and lisinopril (Zestril, Prinivil); diuretics such as furosemide (Lasix) and hydrochlorothiazide (Maxzide, Dyazide); as well as other agents such as cimetidine (Tagamet), lithium (Eskalith, Lithobid), and methotrexate (Trexall, Rheumatrex). Because of these risks, it is suggested that elderly individuals have regular assessment of renal function and that drug use be reviewed at every point of contact with a provider.

Pharmacodynamics

Compared to younger women, mature women may experience unpredictable larger or smaller drug concentrations at the site of action. The changes in effects on cellular and organ function may be due to a variety of factors, most prominently pathophysiology of organ systems. Some individuals become more sensitive to certain agents as they age, including morphine, warfarin (Coumadin), and angiotensin-converting enzyme (ACE) inhibitors. Production of active metabolites (e.g., benzodiazepines) among the elderly may be an additional factor in causing increased sedation.

Drug–Drug Interactions

Polypharmacy presents an important risk for adverse drug–drug interactions in this population. Nevertheless, women should not be denied appropriate therapy simply because of their age. A good rule of thumb is that mature women—indeed, all women—should be best treated when necessary, with the lowest effective doses, and monitored regularly for therapeutic and adverse effects.

Many of the chapters in this text focus on drugs for specific conditions and address use of those agents among the elderly. The reader is directed to the chapter of interest for specific drugs. Age-specific conditions associated with women such as menopause and osteoporosis are discussed in this chapter.

Transition to Menopause

Meno is derived from the Greek word meaning "month," and *pause* is derived from the Greek word meaning "pause or halt." Thus, *menopause* is the technical term for the point in time when menses and fertility cease. All healthy women make the transition to postmenopause, but each will experience this physiologic passage in a unique way. The shift from the reproductive phase of life begins in a woman's mid- to late 40s and continues for several years. The average age of natural menopause, approximately 51.5 years,[10,11] has remained constant for the last several hundred years despite reduction in age of menarche and improvements in nutrition and health care.

The Study of Women's Health Across the Nation (SWAN) is a multicenter, multiethnic research project that has been ongoing for more than a decade among more than 3000 U.S. women 45–57 years. One report from that federally funded study indicates that women report poorer physical functioning in general during this period than they felt prior to the perimenopausal time frame. Studies are ongoing to explore if a relationship exists between these perceptions and the physiological hormonal changes that occur in connection with menopause.[12]

An individual woman's experience during this time period will be influenced by her beliefs regarding aging as well as her lifestyle, culture, and menopause-related symptoms. Most women experience some symptoms (e.g., vasomotor symptoms, mood changes, sleep disturbances, vulvovaginal problems, low libido); however, the symptoms are not always considered bothersome. A classic study of more than 8000 women in the United Kingdom conducted by Porter et al. found that 57% reported one or more of the 15 common menopausal symptoms, but only 22% of them characterized the symptom(s) as problematic.[13] In 2012, another study in the United Kingdom reported that among 695 women reporting symptoms, 10% noted severe psychological issues and 25% had early or late vasomotor symptoms that they characterized as severe.[14] In large part, a woman's tolerance for symptoms may be influenced by whether she is experiencing normal life stressors such as parenting adolescents, caring for her own parents or those of a spouse, working outside the home, and any number of other responsibilities. Similar menopause-related symptoms can be perceived by one woman as just one more part of life, while for another woman those same symptoms can be severe and negatively influence her quality of life.

Stages in the Reproductive Cycle

In 2011, a multidisciplinary, international workshop was held to update the 2001 Stages of Reproductive Aging Workshop (STRAW) framework.[15] The STRAW + 10 framework

Final menstrual period (FMP)

Stages:	25	24	23	22	21	0	11	12
Terminology:	Reproductive			Menopausal transition		Postmenopause		
	Early	Peak	Late	Early	Late*	Early*		Late
				Perimenopause				
Duration of stage:	Variable			Variable		(a) 1 yr	(b) 4 yrs	Until demise
Menstrual cycles:	Variable to regular	Regular		Variable cycle length (.7 days different from normal)	$ 2 skipped cycles and an interval of amenorrhea ($ 60 days)	Amen 3 12 months	None	
Endocrine:	Normal FSH		↑ FSH	↑ FSH		↑ FSH		

Recommended staging system.
* Stages most likely to be characterized by vasomotor symptoms, follicle-stimulating hormone (FSH) increase, and amenorrhea. Stage 11 is subdivided into segment "a" for first 12 months after FMP and "b" for next 4 years.

Figure 34-1 Stages of Reproductive Aging Workshop + 10 (STRAW +10).

Source: Modified from Harlow SD, Gass M, Hall JE, et al. Executive summary of the Stages of Reproductive Aging Workshop + 10: addressing the unfinished agenda of staging reproductive aging. *Menopause.* 2012;19(4):387-395.[15]

is useful for describing the transition to postmenopause and identifies a continuum of seven stages (two with substages)—five occur before menopause and two after (Figure 34-1). This framework also is useful to standardize information about treatments of women with menopausal symptoms.

Not all women progress linearly through the various stages identified by STRAW + 10. Some women may skip a stage entirely, whereas others may slip in and out of adjacent categories.

The stages are primarily identified through menstrual cycle characteristics. Supporting evidence has been obtained through measurement of serum follicle-stimulating hormone (FSH), inhibin B, and anti-Müllerian hormone (AMH) levels; ultrasound-derived antral follicle counts (AFC); and woman-reported menopause-related symptoms. STRAW + 10 includes FSH and inhibin B because the assays used to determine these levels now have fairly high international standardization. AMH, which reflects the number of ovarian follicles, and AFC have limited roles in determining reproductive stage; rather, they are primarily used as markers for infertility and it is recognized that they lack standardization.

The STRAW criteria can be used for women with an intact uterus and who menstruate with regularity. They are not applicable to women who have had endometrial ablation or who experience induced or spontaneous early menopause.

The first three stages of STRAW + 10 occur during the reproductive years. These stages are divided into early reproductive, or –5 (cycles are variable to regular, and FSH levels indicate ovarian responsiveness); peak reproductive, or –4 (regular cycles and FSH indicative of responsive ovaries); and late reproductive, or –3b (regular cycles with normal to low FSH) and –3a (subtle cycle changes in length and/or flow with variable FSH levels).[15]

The menopausal transition begins at stage –2, continues through stage –1, and ends with stage 0 or the final menstrual period (FMP).[12] The FMP is considered the date of menopause, which is identified 12 months afterward, making menopause a retrospective diagnosis. *Perimenopause* encompasses stages –2, –1, and +1a (the first year following the FMP). In stage –2, the *early transition,* cycle interval shortens by 7 days or more in 10 or more cycles and FSH is highly variable. Amenorrhea of 60 days or more and extremely variable/elevated FSH levels define stage –1, the *late transition.* Vasomotor symptoms are also likely during stage –1. *Early postmenopause* encompasses stages +1a, +1b, and +1c. Stage +1a and +1b each last approximately 1 year and are characterized by highly variable FHS and estrogen levels; vasomotor symptoms are highly likely. Stage +1a encompasses the year following the FMP and the final year of perimenopause. Stage +1c lasts approximately 3 to 6 years and is characterized by stabilizing FSH levels. *Late postmenopause*, stage +2, encompasses the rest of a woman's life and is characterized by long-term effects of low estrogen such as urogenital atrophy.[15]

This section focuses on the early and late menopausal transition stages, −2 and −1, leading to the FMP. Pharmacologic management of women with menopause-related symptoms may involve the use of hormones. Therefore, a brief review of the reproductive hormones and hormone receptors follows. Additional information can be found in the *Steroid Hormones* chapter.

Hormones in Flux: An Overview of Estrogen and Progesterone for the Mature Woman

Changes in the central nervous system control of the ovaries and accelerated ovarian follicular atresia precede menopause. The remaining follicles tend to be resistant to FSH. In response to the reduced number and increased resistance of follicles, the pituitary increases secretion of FSH in an attempt to promote ovulation. An FSH level of 40 mIU or greater is considered to be in the postmenopausal range, and repeatedly elevated results can indicate that a woman has reached postmenopause.[11] However, because fluctuations in endogenous hormones as well as hormonal therapy can interfere with the clinical usefulness of FSH testing, the best marker for menopause is 12 months of consecutive, natural amenorrhea.[11,16]

Initially, ovarian follicular development may be sustained. On occasion, more than one follicle can be recruited per cycle, which stimulates ovarian production of estrogen and causes elevated levels of 17 β-estradiol, also called **estradiol (E_2)**.[16] In addition to thickening the endometrium, increased E_2 secretion may lead to uterine fibroid growth and menorrhagia, as well as symptoms of breast tenderness, bloating, and irritability.

Later in the transition, the remaining ovarian follicles become increasingly resistant to FSH and luteinizing hormone (LH). Ovulation usually is erratic, and the levels of E_2 can fluctuate widely. When estrogen levels are low because of the failure of follicular development, ovulation may not occur, resulting in lack of a corpus luteum. Without a corpus luteum, there is inadequate progesterone to allow the endometrial lining to be converted to secretory tissue. Although irregular or unpredictable bleeding is often a normal part of the perimenopause transition, it should be assessed while considering the risk of endometrial polyps and endometrial hyperplasia, which is associated with an increased risk for uterine cancer. Irregular bleeding is the most frequently reported sign of the transition to menopause.[15,17]

As follicles become increasingly unresponsive to FSH, E_2 levels decline and women continue to experience irregular bleeding, ultimately culminating in permanent amenorrhea. Vasomotor symptoms and vaginal dryness may precede or coincide with the last menstrual period.[10,15,17] **Estrone (E_1)**, by default, becomes the dominant circulating estrogen derived primarily from aromatization of androstenedione. Obese women may have higher levels of estrone, with adipose tissue as a primary source of this hormone.[14]

Women in the perimenopausal and postmenopausal stages continue to produce ovarian androgens, albeit not in the same amounts as in earlier years. Although androgens often are thought of as male hormones, they may positively affect female libido, body habitus, muscle development, energy, and sense of well-being. Because they are precursors of estrogen, androgens have an important role for postmenopausal women. Androgens are produced in the ovary, adrenal glands, and peripherally by substrate conversion to become the weakest estrogen, estrone.

The adrenal androgens, dehydroepiandrosterone (DHEA) and androstenedione, decline with age regardless of menopausal status. Testosterone levels of ovarian origin do not change appreciably during the menopausal transition, but later decline slowly over time.[14] This relationship demonstrates the appreciable role that postmenopausal ovaries continue to play in women past their menopause. At any point, only 1% to 2% of testosterone is unbound and, therefore, metabolically active. The remainder is tightly attached to sex hormone-binding globulin (SHBG). Oral estrogens have been shown to increase SHBG, causing a decline in bioavailable testosterone.[17]

Hormone Receptors

Proteins found in the fluid within the cell, or the cytosol, bind to sex hormones and transfer the hormone into the cell nucleus. Two estrogen receptors have been identified: ER-α and ER-β. Concentrations of these receptors vary in different tissues, with more ER-α receptors being found in the reproductive tissue and liver, and more ER-β receptors being present in bone, blood vessels, and lungs.[18] Both types of receptors are found in the ovary and central nervous system and are discussed in more detail in the *Steroid Hormones* chapter. Estrogen receptors bind to a variety of substances, or ligands, which vary in their affinity for ER-α and ER-β. Both estrogen receptors bind to 17 β-estradiol, but the weaker phytoestrogens found in some plants and foods seem to have a higher affinity for ER-β.[19]

The response to ligand binding to an estrogen receptor is complex and initiates a series of steps that involve coactivators or corepressors. This phenomenon is the origin of the term **selective estrogen receptor modulators (SERMs)**, a class of drugs today known as **estrogen agonists/antagonists (EAAs)**. These agents can cause an antagonist effect in one tissue, yet stimulate an agonist effect in different tissue when bound to the estrogen receptor (as discussed in the *Steroid Hormones* chapter). For example, the drug tamoxifen (Nolvadex) is an antagonist in breast tissue, where it is associated with decreased risk of breast cancer, and a partial agonist in uterine tissue, where it is associated with an increased risk of endometrial cancer.

Progesterone receptors (PRs) are subtyped in a similar fashion to the estrogen receptors. PR-α and PR-β are found in most tissues, with PR-α dominant in the ovary and uterus and PR-β prevailing in the breast. **Selective progesterone receptor modulators (SPRMs)** are currently being evaluated for clinical effectiveness.[16]

Hormone Therapy for Primary Prevention of Chronic Conditions: Panacea or Poison?

As the menopausal transition evolves (from stage −2 to stage −1), more women note vasomotor symptoms (hot flashes), vaginal dryness, genitourinary symptoms such as dyspareunia or pruritus, and sleep disturbances, although the relationship between these symptoms and menopause is not always clear.[11,17] Each of these conditions is addressed later in this chapter. It is difficult to discuss care of the perimenopausal or postmenopausal woman without first discussing clinical use of hormones, however, especially because these drugs may be prescribed for multiple reasons, including as a general panacea.

Estrogen therapy was first advocated in the 1960s for treatment of women with menopausal symptoms and then rapidly moved into a role of antiaging remedy as discussed in Box 34-1.[20,21] Later, the finding that unopposed estrogen could be carcinogenic caused a rapid decrease in use of the agent. However, when progesterone was added to the regimen to counteract estrogen's effects on the uterine endometrium, the formulations prescribed were commonly termed **hormone replacement therapy (HRT)** and regained popularity. In 2001, approximately 90 million prescriptions for conjugated estrogens Premarin or Prempro, the two most commonly used formulations, were written.[22]

Today, the word *replacement* is falling into disuse because hormone formulations of estrogen and progesterone do not replace hormones to the same levels found premenopausally. Consequently, the term **hormone therapy (HT)** currently is preferred to designate all combinations of hormone therapy used for menopause-related symptoms, including **estrogen therapy (ET)**, estrogen with **progestin** therapy (EPT), and estrogen with testosterone therapy (ETT). In this chapter, HT, ET, and EPT will be used to indicate the specific regimen employed. Although the term *hormone* may refer to a wide variety of agents including thyroid and growth hormones, for the sake of simplicity in this chapter, it is used to refer to estrogens, progesterones, and androgens.

Box 34-1 Estrogen-Deficient State: Gone But Not Forgotten

Estrogen products for the treatment of women with menopause-related symptoms were first approved by the Food and Drug Administration (FDA) in 1941 and became popular in the 1960s following the publication of Robert Wilson's book, *Feminine Forever*.[21] Wilson, a gynecologist, described menopause as an estrogen-deficient state and promoted the use of estrogen for treatment of women with multiple symptoms, some of which were likely to be secondary to aging and not specific to menopause. Wilson's work was widely disseminated and pharmaceutical companies marketed the products before the 1962 amendments to the Food Drug and Cosmetics Act required demonstrated safety of medications. By 1975, however, it had become clear that unopposed estrogen therapy was associated with a significantly increased risk for endometrial hyperplasia and endometrial cancer (fivefold increased risk after 3 years of therapy).[22] Until it was discovered that the addition of a progestin could decrease the endometrial risks, hormonal use fell into disfavor.

State of the Science: Hormone Therapy Research

After the concern about endometrial carcinoma abated, EPT became popular at the same time that more women were entering menopause. Much as combination oral contraceptives had been found to provide noncontraceptive benefits, estrogen was touted as having additional benefits—on the heart in particular—and research on these purported effects ensued. Observational studies and the Postmenopausal Estrogen/Progestin Interventions (PEPI) trial initially suggested positive cardioprotective effects associated with HT.[23–26] Other studies demonstrated possible protective effects for bone health, dementia, and colon cancer.[27–30] Still others presented contradictory evidence regarding the risks of or protection from breast cancer.[31] To address the questions related to HT, over the last two decades multiple trials have explored the risks and benefits of these agents' use for indications in addition to treatment of women with menopausal symptoms. Table 34-1 summarizes selected major trials that evaluated effects of HT on heart disease and breast cancer in postmenopausal women.

Table 34-1 Selected Research Studies Evaluating Effects of Hormone Therapy on Heart Disease and Breast Cancer Among Postmenopausal Women

Trial Name	Year Initiated	Type of Study	Participants	Main Purpose	Major Findings
Postmenopausal Estrogen/Progestin Interventions (PEPI)[26]	1991	RCT	875 postmenopausal; 32% previous hysterectomy	Effects of HT on CHD risk factors	Studied ET (CEE) and EPT (CEE plus 2.5 mg MPA, 10 mg MPA, or 200 mg micronized progesterone) versus placebo. Found increased HDL, decreased LDL, and fibrinogen. Micronized progesterone had less blunting of estrogen lipid benefit than MPA. No effect on BP.
Heart and Estrogen/Progestin Replacement Study (HERS,[32] HERS II[33])	1993	RCT	2763 postmenopausal with established CHD	Secondary cardiac protection	Studied EPT (CEE/MPA) versus placebo. Found increased risk of CHD events, 2–3 times increased risk of DVT, and increased gallbladder disease.
Women's Health Initiative Estrogen and Progesterone Therapy Arm (WHI EPT)[34,35]	1993	RCT	16,608 postmenopausal age 50–79; mean age 63; most 10 years after FMP	Primary cardiac protection	Studied EPT (CEE/MPA) versus placebo. Found increased risk of CHD, VTE, CVA, and breast cancer; decreased risk of colon cancer and hip fracture. Only VTE was statistically significant after analysis corrections.
Women's Health Initiative Estrogen Therapy Arm (WHI ET)[36]	1993	RCT	10,739 postmenopausal; mean age 62; all without uterus	Primary cardiac protection	Studied ET (CEE) versus placebo. Found increased risk of CVA; decreased risk of hip fracture. No difference for CHD, breast cancer, colon cancer, or VTE. No differences were statistically significant after analysis corrections.
Estrogen in the Prevention of Atherosclerosis Trial (EPAT)[37]	1994	RCT	222 postmenopausal; mean age 62	Progression of atherosclerosis	Studied ET (17 β-estradiol) versus placebo. Found less atherosclerosis progression with ET. No difference in progression versus placebo if also taking lipid-lowering medication.
Million Woman Study (MWS), United Kingdom[38–40]	1996	Observational	1,084,110 aged 50–64	EPT, ET influence on risk of various conditions	Studied ET and EPT through reports by more than 1 million women older than age 50 (approximately 25% of this U.K. age cohort). ET users were 30% more likely and EPT users were 100% more likely than nonusers to have breast cancer. Prior users had no increased risk. Higher mortality was observed if the women had breast cancer. Risk was much higher with EPT than with ET. Lower risk for breast cancer was found if women started HT 5 years or more after FMP. This study is ongoing, with additional research being published on various conditions such as HT and gallbladder risk.

(continues)

Table 34-1 Selected Research Studies Evaluating Effects of Hormone Therapy on Heart Disease and Breast Cancer Among Postmenopausal Women *(continued)*

Trial Name	Year Initiated	Type of Study	Participants	Main Purpose	Major Findings
Papworth HRT Atherosclerosis (PHASE)[41]	1997	RCT	255 postmenopausal women with known heart disease; 5 years from FMP; mean age 63.6	CHD event (secondary cardiac prevention)	Studied transdermal ET/EPT versus placebo. Failed to find statistical differences between groups in regard to CHD.
Kronos Early Estrogen Prevention Study (KEEPS)[42]	2005	RCT	727 postmenopausal; within 6 months to 36 months from FMP; mean age 52	Progression of atherosclerosis	Studied oral CEE and transdermal 17 β-estradiol versus placebo. Enrollment began in 2005 but studies are ongoing. Found improved HDL, LDL, C-reactive protein, and sex hormone-binding globulin levels with CEE and 17 β-estradiol. No reports on number of cardiac events. Reduced insulin resistance with 17 β-estradiol. No difference in carotid artery intima-media thickness, coronary artery calcium score, and interlukin-6.

Abbreviations: BP = blood pressure; CEE = conjugated equine estrogens; CHD = coronary heart disease; CVA = cerebrovascular accident; DVT = deep vein thrombosis; EPT = estrogen plus progestin therapy; ET = estrogen therapy; FMP = final menstrual period; HDL = high-density lipoprotein; HT = hormone therapy; LDL = low-density lipoprotein; MI = myocardial infarction; MPA = medroxyprogesterone acetate; RCT = randomized controlled trial; VTE = venous thromboembolism.

Sources: Data from Anderson GL, Limacher M, Assaf AR, et al.; Women's Health Initiative Steering Committee. Effects of conjugated equine estrogen in postmenopausal women with hysterectomy: the Women's Health Initiative randomized controlled trial. *JAMA.* 2004;291(14):1701-1712[36]; Beral V; Million Women Study Collaborators. Breast cancer and hormone-replacement therapy in the Million Women Study. *Lancet.* 2003;362(9382):419-427[38]; Beral V, Reeves G, Bull D, Green J; Million Women Study Collaborators. Breast cancer risk in relation to the interval between menopause and starting hormone therapy. *J Natl Cancer Inst.* 2011;103(4):296-305[40]; Clarke SC, Kelleher J, Lloyd-Jones H, Slack M, Schofiel PM. A study of hormone replacement therapy in postmenopausal women with ischaemic heart disease: the Papworth HRT atherosclerosis study. *BJOG.* 2002;109(9):1056-1062[41]; Grady D, Herrington D, Bittner V, et al. Cardiovascular disease outcomes during 6.8 years of hormone therapy: Heart and Estrogen/Progestin Replacement Study follow-up (HERS II). *JAMA.* 2002;288(1):49-57[33]; Hodis HN, Mack WJ, Lobo RA, et al.; Estrogen in the Prevention of Atherosclerosis Trial Research Group. Estrogen in the prevention of atherosclerosis: a randomized, double-blind, placebo controlled trial. *Ann Intern Med.* 2001;135(11):939-953[37]; Hulley S, Grady D, Bush T, et al. Randomized trial of estrogen plus progestin for secondary prevention of coronary heart disease in postmenopausal women. Heart and Estrogen/Progestin Replacement Study (HERS) Research Group. *JAMA.* 1998;280(7):605-613[32]; Manson JE, Hsia J, Johnson KC, et al.; WHI Investigators. Estrogen plus progestin and the risk of coronary heart disease. *N Engl J Med.* 2003;349(6):523-634[35]; Harman SM, Black DM, Naftolin F, et al. Arterial imaging outcomes and cardiovascular risk factors in recently menopausal women: a randomized trial. *Ann Intern Med.* 2014;161(4):249-260[42]; Reeves GK, Beral V, Green J, Gathani T, Bull D; Million Women Study Collaborators. Hormonal therapy for menopause and breast cancer risk by histological type: a cohort study and meta-analysis. *Lancet Oncol.* 2006;7(11):910-918[39]; Rossouw JE, Anderson GL, Prentice RL, et al. Risks and benefits of estrogen plus progestin in healthy postmenopausal women: principal results from the Women's Health Initiative randomized controlled trial. *JAMA.* 2002;288(3):321-333[34]; Writing Group for PEPI. Effects of estrogen or estrogen/progestin regimens on heart disease risk factors in postmenopausal women. The Postmenopausal Estrogen/Progestin Interventions (PEPI) trial. *JAMA.* 1995;273(3):199-208.[26]

Heart Disease and Hormones: Protective or Problematic?

By the mid-1990s, many clinicians were prescribing HT to ward off heart disease in asymptomatic postmenopausal women. In 1996, the United States Preventive Services Task Force (USPSTF) recommended that clinicians counsel women to consider HT use for cardioprevention.[43] However, when approached for approval of an on-label indication, the FDA requested randomized controlled trials (RCTs) to prospectively evaluate the effects of HT on cardiovascular disease in women. As a result, the Women's Health Initiative (WHI) study and the Heart and Estrogen/Progestin Replacement Study (HERS) was designed using a method similar to statin trials to evaluate effects of HT on women with and without known coronary heart disease (CHD).[32,34,36]

The HERS participants were postmenopausal women with a history of established CHD. Results released in 1998 showed that use of EPT during the first year of the trial increased CHD events among women receiving conjugated equine estrogens (CEE) 0.625 mg and medroxyprogesterone (MPA) 2.5 mg in a single pill (treatment) versus women taking placebo (control) (relative hazard [RH], 1.52; 95% confidence interval [CI], 1.01–2.29). Over the next 3 years, fewer CHD events were observed among women in the treatment group, which resulted in no significant differences between the groups over the 4.1 years of follow-up.[32] Women in the treatment group did have lower lipid levels. HERS was extended in HERS II to evaluate the effects of EPT over 2.7 additional years, which demonstrated no added benefits in use of this therapy.[33] The researchers concluded that use of EPT did not prevent cardiac events in women who already had CHD disease.

Some experts questioned whether using a different formulation or route of administration for EPT would change the results from those obtained in the HERS/HERS II investigations. The Papworth PHASE RCT evaluated effects of a patch with 17 ß-estradiol 2.5 mg (or 17 ß-estradiol 3 mg with an addition of norethindrone 4 mg for half of the month for women with a uterus) among women with CHD. Similar to the HERS investigations, this study found an increased number of events after 2.5 years of follow-up, although the result was not statistically significant. In any case, the authors concluded that ET/EPT should not be used for secondary prevention of CHD.[41]

The WHI was a large, 15-year research project with multiple aims, including hormone trials specifically investigating women and risks/protection of those agents associated with cardiovascular, osteoporosis, and breast cancer. Study participants were postmenopausal women without established CHD at the initiation of the study. Groups included women taking placebos, using estrogen alone, or using estrogen plus progestin; two specific trials focused on the effects of HT on CHD prevention over 8.5 years.

The EPT arm included women with an intact uterus randomized into treatment (CEE 0.625 mg and MPA 2.5 mg in a single pill daily) or control (placebo) groups. In 2002, the treatment arm was stopped after a mean of 5.2 years follow-up because the global index—a preset statistical limit—indicated that risks (coronary events, stroke, pulmonary embolism, and breast cancer) were outweighing benefits (reduced colon cancer and osteoporosis-related fracture) and it was statistically impossible for these factors to demonstrate benefits. Later, full analyses were conducted with data corrections, and the only statistically significant risk was found for venous thromboembolic events.[34,35] Therefore, similar to the results obtained in studies of women with history of CHD, there was no statistical association between HT use and cardioprotection, causing the then common prescription of hormones for women without CHD for cardiac prophylaxis to be questioned.

Widespread media coverage of the WHI results publicized the risks before the data corrections were made, and the popular press paid special attention to the increased risk of breast cancer. The media did not emphasize the lack of cardiac prevention with the agents, although that finding was likely the one with the most influence on clinical practice. In addition, when corrections were made, the press paid little attention to the revised results. Table 34-2 provides an overview of the WHI EPT study, including initial statistical findings and their adjusted corrections.

Over the final 3 years of additional observation, it also was noted that mortality rates were not different among the WHI groups.[44] Also, after statistical adjustments were made, WHI associations remained. The statistical significance of the link between venous thromboembolism (VTE) and HT, while correct, can be somewhat misleading. For example, when the incidence of VTE was considered, it was calculated that the absolute risk for women using EPT versus women using a placebo meant among 10,000 women, 8 additional women would be affected by the condition over a 1-year period. Similar single-digit findings were calculated for the other factors, but as mentioned, the specific factors themselves were not found to be statistically significant.

The WHI ET arm included postmenopausal women without a uterus and also was discontinued early, in 2004, after 6.8 years of follow-up. The cause of the early termination was the increased risk of cerebrovascular accidents (CVA)/stroke found among women in the treatment group (CEE 0.625 mg orally daily) versus the control group

Table 34-2 Summary of Women's Health Initiative Study Estrogen Plus Progestin Therapy Results

	Outcome Measure	Hazard Ratio (Risk Difference)	95% Confidence Interval for EPT versus Placebo (Initial Calculation without Corrections)	95% Confidence Interval for EPT versus Placebo (Adjusted Calculation with Corrections)
Potential risks	Invasive breast cancer	1.26 (increase 26%)	1.00–1.59 (NS)	0.83–1.92 (NS)
	Coronary heart disease	1.29 (increase 29%)	1.02–1.63	0.85–1.97 (NS)
	Cerebrovascular accident/stroke	1.41 (increase 41%)	1.07–1.85	0.86–2.31 (NS)
	VTE	2.11 (increase 211%)	1.58–2.52	1.26–3.55
Potential benefits	Hip fractures	0.66 (decrease 34%)	0.45–0.98	0.33–1.33 (NS)
	Colorectal cancer	0.63 (decrease 38%)	0.43–0.92	0.32–1.34 (NS)

Abbreviations: EPT = estrogen plus progestin therapy; NS = not significant; VTE = venous thromboembolism.

Table 34-3 Summary of Women's Health Initiative Study Estrogen Therapy Results

	Outcome Measure	Hazard Ratio (Risk Difference)	95% Confidence Interval for ET versus Placebo (Initial Calculation without Corrections)	95% Confidence Interval for ET versus Placebo (Adjusted Calculation with Corrections)
Potential risks	Cerebrovascular accident/stroke	1.39 (increase 39%)	1.10–1.77	0.97–1.99 (NS)
	VTE	1.33 (increase 33%)	0.99–1.79 (NS)	0.86–2.08 (NS)
	Colorectal cancer	1.08 (increase 0.08%)	0.75–1.55 (NS)	0.63–1.86 (NS)
Potential benefits	Invasive breast cancer	0.77 (decrease 23%)	0.59–1.01 (NS)	0.57–1.06 (NS)
	Coronary heart disease	0.91 (decrease 9%)	0.75–1.12 (NS)	0.7–1.15 (NS)
	Hip fractures	0.61 (decrease 39%)	0.41–0.91	0.33–1.11 (NS)

Abbreviations: ET = estrogen therapy; NS = not significant; VTE = venous thromboembolism.

(placebo), as noted in Table 34-3.[36] This arm showed a protective effect in women taking ET against hip fracture but no differences in prevention of CHD, breast cancer, pulmonary embolism, or colon cancer. However, after adjustments for corrections, none of the factors was found to be statistically significant.[36]

Following the WHI initial results, experts questioned whether timing of hormone initiation might influence potential cardiac protection or other benefits/risks. The average participant in the WHI was 63 years, more than a full decade past typical FMP. Follow-up analyses with a subgroup of WHI participants in both the EPT and ET arms, however, showed that those women aged 50 to 59 years and those who had experienced menopause within the past 10 years did not demonstrate a statistically significant change in the risks or benefits for CHD or stroke.[45]

Another major question raised was whether using different formulations of estrogen or routes of administration would have made a difference in the CHD results.[32,33] This line of questioning prompted the Kronos Early Estrogen Prevention Study (KEEPS), which included postmenopausal women within 6 to 36 months of their FMP.[42] Women were randomized to take either placebo, oral CEE 0.45 mg, or transdermal 17 β-estradiol 50 mcg daily with oral micronized progesterone 200 mg daily for 12 days out of each month. Preliminary results after 4 years have indicated improvements in low- and high-density lipoprotein cholesterol, and increases in C-reactive protein, sex hormone-binding globulin, and triglycerides among women randomized to CEE. Those in the 17 β-estradiol group had reduced insulin resistance, although information about cardiac events has not been reported. Women with a coronary artery calcification (CAC) score at baseline (who accounted for fewer than 13% of participants) were more likely to progress than those without such a score, and progression was slower in both treatment groups than for placebo.[42] The effects on carotid artery intima-media thickness were not significant.

The KEEPS data have been reported at several large meetings, and publications have addressed specific aspects of the findings. These data support WHI data that suggested early use of oral micronized with CEE or 17 β-estradiol may provide some protective effect against CHD development—in this case, CAC. However, additional research is needed to elucidate the ongoing effects of HT use on heart disease in postmenopausal women and nuances of choosing different hormones and formulations.

Cancer and Hormones: Reality or Public Scare?

Estrogen is said to be a known carcinogen because of the correlation between unopposed estrogen and endometrial cancer. However, its exact relationship with other cancers remains more elusive. As discussed in the section regarding the state of the science and reflected in the WHI results, research studies have demonstrated inconsistent results in regard to breast cancer among women who take EPT or ET.[31,35,36,44] In the first 2 years of the EPT arm of the WHI, breast cancer incidence among treated women was lower than among women on placebo. The incidence rose over the 5.6 years of follow-up in women on EPT, but then fell back to baseline within 3 to 5 years of discontinuing EPT.[46] The women who were diagnosed with breast cancer while taking EPT in the WHI were more likely to have invasive breast cancer (node-positive) (hazard ratio [HR], 1.78; 95% CI, 1.23–2.58) and possibly a higher mortality rate, though the statistical findings were nonsignificant. Among women in the ET arm, breast cancer incidence was lower among women taking ET than among those taking placebo. Early in the follow-up, this was a nonsignificant trend; after 10.7 years of follow-up, however, it was found to be a statistically significant benefit (HR, 0.77; 95% CI, 0.62–0.95).[47]

Therefore, in contrast to the popular belief that estrogen is an etiologic agent for breast cancer, this finding raised questions about the role of progestins in breast cancer.[10]

The results from the observational Million Women Study (MWS) were congruent with this finding. The MWS identified an increased risk for six types of breast cancer among users versus nonusers of EPT and ET,[38,40] with a higher risk among EPT users. National data in the United States and Canada both demonstrate a decrease in breast cancer incidence that coincides with the decline in HT prescribing that occurred after the WHI results were released. Despite HT prescription rates remaining low, the incidence of breast cancer has leveled off in the United States and has begun to rise again in Canada.[48–50] These epidemiological data argue against a causative relationship of ET and EPT on breast cancer incidence. Rather, taking HT may stimulate preexisting malignant breast cell proliferation.[51] Importantly, and supporting this potential explanation, later data analyses in the WHI ET arm indicated that women with a low risk for breast cancer at baseline did not experience any increase in incidence during the trial.[47]

Use of hormones among women who are breast cancer survivors has also been evaluated in regard to recurrence. Some observational studies have reported no increase in incidence of recurrence with HT use.[52] However, an RCT involving survivors who were experiencing vasomotor symptoms was ended after 2 years of follow-up due to increased incidence of recurrence in women taking HT versus placebo.[53] The North American Menopause Society (NAMS), the International Menopause Society (IMS), and the Global Consensus Statement on Menopause HT note the lack of definitive data shedding light on this issue and do not support the use of HT at this time among women who are breast cancer survivors.[54,55]

As with breast cancer, results from observational studies and meta-analyses evaluating HT and ovarian cancer are contradictory.[56–59] The Million Woman Study identified an increase in incidence of ovarian cancer and mortality while using EPT and ET, which returned to baseline when HT was discontinued.[59] The only RCT to evaluate this relationship to date has been the WHI EPT study, in which researchers noted a small increase in ovarian cancer among women using EPT versus placebo, though it was not statistically significant.[60]

Hormone Trials and Other Factors

Although most of the hormone trials to date have focused on cardiac health or breast cancers, large trials such as the WHI and the Study of Women's Health Across the Nation have provided a wealth of information about use of hormones by mid-life and older women. A Cochrane review published in 2012 analyzed 23 double-blinded RCTs and found that HT was not protective against dementia, cognitive decline, or decrease in the risk of colorectal cancers, nor was it indicated for primary or secondary prevention of cardiovascular disease.[61] However, there was little risk found for healthy women who use HT for short-term treatment of women with menopausal symptoms.

Hormone Therapy

Indications for Initiating Hormones

Hormone therapy, whether it is ET or EPT, provides the most effective relief for menopause-related hot flashes, night sweats, sleep problems related to hot flashes, and vaginal discomforts.[10,11] Women who are bothered by these symptoms usually seek advice from a healthcare practitioner. A stepped approach to treating women with symptoms is recommended, including lifestyle changes first, followed by consideration of complementary and alternative medicine therapies and hormone therapy.[10,54] Once a woman starts HT, relief often is afforded within days for hot flashes, though it can take as long as 6 weeks for full benefits of the treatment to become apparent. Vaginal conditions may be associated with sexual problems, both of which are likely to be relieved with hormonal use, although improvement of vaginal problems may take longer. A clear discussion of individualized risks and benefits is important to help every woman make an informed decision about how to proceed with pharmacologic management.

Known Risks and Benefits

The case for and against the use of HT has become increasingly controversial as more data have emerged. After the WHI results were released, multiple organizations (e.g., NAMS, National Association of Nurse Practitioners in Women's Health), the FDA, and the USPSTF agreed that the use of HT was appropriate for treating women with menopause-related, moderate to severe vasomotor symptoms and vaginal atrophy, but not for the purpose of preventing heart disease or osteoporosis.[62–65] Currently, the FDA has approved use of HT for menopause-related, moderate to severe vasomotor symptoms and vulvar/vaginal atrophy, as well as prevention of postmenopausal osteoporosis.[65] However, before using hormones for prevention of osteoporosis, other options should be considered because

Table 34-4 Potential Risks and Benefits of the Use of Hormones

Potential Risks	Potential Benefits
Stroke Venous thromboembolism Breast cancer[a] Endometrial cancer[b] Ovarian cancer[a]	Relief of vasomotor symptoms Relief of vulvovaginal atrophy Reduced risk of osteoporosis and osteoporosis-related fractures Reduced risk of colorectal cancer Reduced risk of coronary heart disease potentially among healthy women in early postmenopause (STRAW stages +1a, +1b, +1c)[a] Reduced risk of dementia[a] Reduced risk of diabetes mellitus

[a] Controversial among research findings.
[b] Among women with an intact uterus treated with estrogen alone; risk mediated with use of progestin or bazedoxifene.
Sources: Data from Alexander IM. The history of hormone therapy use and recent controversy related to heart disease and breast cancer arising from prevention trial outcomes. *J Midwifery Womens Health*. 2012;57:547-557[20]; de Villiers TJ, Gass ML, Haines CJ, et al. Global consensus statement on menopausal hormone therapy. *Climacteric*. 2013;16(2):203-204[55]; de Villiers TJ, Pines A, Panay N, et al.; International Menopause Society. Updated 2013 International Menopause Society recommendations on menopause hormone therapy and preventive strategies for midlife health. *Climacteric*. 2013;16(3):316-337[54]; Harlow SD, Gass M, Hall JE, et al. Executive summary of the Stages of Reproductive Aging Workshop + 10: addressing the unfinished agenda of staging reproductive aging. *Menopause*. 2012;19(4):387-395[15]; Jane FM, Davis SR. A practitioner's toolkit for managing the menopause. *Climacteric*. 2014;17(5):564-579[11]; North American Menopause Society (NAMS), 2012 Hormone Therapy Position Statement Advisory Panel. The 2012 hormone therapy position statement of the North American Menopause Society. *Menopause*. 2012;19(3):257-271.[10]

of the risk profile associated with these agents. The same recommendations have been made by NAMS, IMS, and the USPSTF.[10,55,66] Table 34-4 summarizes the benefits and risks associated with the use of hormones and can be used to augment health education as women consider their choices.

Contraindications for Initiation or Continuation of Hormones

Important cautions and contraindications exist to the use of hormones, as listed in Table 34-5. Contraindications usually can be identified with a thorough health history, complete physical exam, and screening mammography. Use of HT should be avoided in women with known or suspected breast cancer because of a lack of clear research findings on the purported HT–breast cancer relationship and because many breast cancers are hormone dependent. Ovarian and endometrial cancers also may be hormonally dependent, which precludes the use of steroidal hormones for women with these diseases. Known heart disease, including coronary heart disease, stroke, and history of thromboembolic disease, is a contraindication as well. In addition, hormones are contraindicated for women with a history of biliary tract disease or liver disease. Estrogen is metabolized through the liver, and if there is compromised liver function, serum estrogen levels can become dangerously high.

Use of a Risk Profile

Discussing the benefit of symptom relief and weighing that against any potential risks is important in the woman's decision to use HT. Assessing for contraindications and cautions (Table 34-5) and carefully determining personal risk for breast cancer and heart disease (Table 34-6) assists in identifying those women who have a lower likelihood of developing potential risks when they use hormones, although not every factor has an equal association. Understanding the absolute risks for heart disease and breast cancer identified in research and considering her own personal health history can assist a woman in determining which treatment option she might consider. As with use of any medication, it is important to provide and document informed decision making prior to initiating HT.

Table 34-5 Contraindications and Cautions for Hormone Therapy Use

Contraindications and Cautions for Estrogen Use	Contraindications and Cautions for Progestin Use
Gallbladder disease History of coronary heart disease or stroke History of or active thromboembolic disease History of uterine or ovarian cancer Known, suspected, or history of breast cancer Known, suspected, or history of estrogen-dependent neoplasia Pregnancy Undiagnosed abnormal genital bleeding	History of coronary heart disease or stroke History of or active thromboembolic disease Known, suspected, or history of cancer of the breast Known, suspected, or history of progestin-dependent neoplasia Liver dysfunction or disease Pregnancy Undiagnosed abnormal genital bleeding

Sources: Data from Alexander IM. The history of hormone therapy use and recent controversy related to heart disease and breast cancer arising from prevention trial outcomes. *J Midwifery Womens Health*. 2012;57:547-557[20]; de Villiers TJ, Gass ML, Haines CJ, et al. Global consensus statement on menopausal hormone therapy. *Climacteric*. 2013;16(2):203-204[55]; de Villiers TJ, Pines A, Panay N, et al.; International Menopause Society. Updated 2013 International Menopause Society recommendations on menopause hormone therapy and preventive strategies for midlife health. *Climacteric*. 2013;16(3):316-337[54]; Harlow SD, Gass M, Hall JE, et al. Executive summary of the Stages of Reproductive Aging Workshop + 10: addressing the unfinished agenda of staging reproductive aging. *Menopause*. 2012;19(4):387-395[15]; Jane FM, Davis SR. A practitioner's toolkit for managing the menopause. *Climacteric*. 2014;17(5):564-579[11]; North American Menopause Society (NAMS), 2012 Hormone Therapy Position Statement Advisory Panel. The 2012 hormone therapy position statement of the North American Menopause Society. *Menopause*. 2012;19(3):257-271.[10]

Table 34-6 Risk Profile to Consider Prior to Initiating Hormone Therapy

Cardiovascular Risks	Breast Cancer Risks
Active smoking	Active smoking
Age older than 50; postmenopausal	Alcohol use in excess of 2 drinks per day
CRP elevated	Atypia diagnosed by breast biopsy
Diabetes	Breast density increased
Elevated waist-to-hip ratio	Female gender
First-degree relative with MI before age 50	First pregnancy after 30
HDL cholesterol < 50 mg/dL	First-degree relative with diagnosis
HDL-to-LDL cholesterol ratio greater than 2.1	Increases with aging
Hypertension	Lack of exercise/obesity
LDL cholesterol > 130 mg/dL	Low-vegetable and -fruit diet
Obesity	Menarche before 12
Sedentary lifestyle	Menopause after 53
Triglycerides > 150 mg/dL	Nulliparous
	Radiation exposure

Abbreviations: CRP = C-reactive protein; HDL = high-density lipoprotein; LDL = low-density lipoprotein; MI = myocardial infarction.
Sources: Data from Alexander IM. The history of hormone therapy use and recent controversy related to heart disease and breast cancer arising from prevention trial outcomes. *J Midwifery Womens Health.* 2012;57:547-557[20]; de Villiers TJ, Pines A, Panay N, et al.; International Menopause Society. Updated 2013 International Menopause Society recommendations on menopause hormone therapy and preventive strategies for midlife health. *Climacteric.* 2013;16(3):316-337[54]; de Villiers TJ, Gass ML, Haines CJ, et al. Global consensus statement on menopausal hormone therapy. *Climacteric.* 2013;16(2):203-204[55]; Harlow SD, Gass M, Hall JE, et al. Executive summary of the Stages of Reproductive Aging Workshop + 10: addressing the unfinished agenda of staging reproductive aging. *Menopause.* 2012;19(4):387-395[15]; Jane FM, Davis SR. A practitioner's toolkit for managing the menopause. *Climacteric.* 2014;17(5):564-579[11]; North American Menopause Society (NAMS), 2012 Hormone Therapy Position Statement Advisory Panel. The 2012 hormone therapy position statement of the North American Menopause Society. *Menopause.* 2012;19(3):257-271.[10]

Formulations and Route

A number of HT options are available for women with menopause-related symptoms. Therapy is available as ET, EPT, and in a combination of CEE with bazedoxifene (BZD). BZD is a third-generation EEA (previously labeled SERM) that stimulates some estrogen receptors and blocks others. This selective effect allows BZD to provide protection against osteoporosis while simultaneously guarding against endometrial hyperplasia and endometrial cancer. The CEE with BZD (CEE/BZD) combination has proved effective in reducing vasomotor symptoms related to menopause, preventing endometrial hyperplasia, and preventing postmenopausal osteoporosis.[67] A progestin is not needed when a woman with an intact uterus uses CEE/BZD. Therefore, the CEE/BZD combination eliminates the potential progestin-related side effects as well as concerns about any role that progestins may play in breast cancer growth.

Table 34-7 provides doses and routes of administration for various FDA-approved HT products. All formulations are equally effective in treating menopause-related symptoms and preserving bone density, although not all formulations have FDA approval for osteoporosis prevention. Some women prefer synthetic hormones or hormones from plant products rather than CEE. CEE is available by brand only—namely, as Premarin, an equine-based product derived from pregnant mare urine.

Table 34-7 FDA-Approved Medications for Treating Women with Menopausal Symptoms

Drug: Generic (Brand)	Dose	Indications for Postmenopausal Women
Estrogen (Oral)		
Conjugated equine estrogens (Premarin)[a]	0.3 mg, 0.45 mg, 0.625 mg, 0.9 mg, 1.25 mg PO daily	VMS, VVA, osteoporosis prevention
Esterified estrogens (Menest)[a]	0.3 mg, 0.625 mg, 1.25 mg, 2.5 mg PO daily	VMS, VVA
17 β-Estradiol micronized (Estrace)*	0.5 mg, 1 mg, 2 mg PO daily	VMS, VVA, osteoporosis prevention
Estropipate (generic)[a]	0.625 mg (0.75), 1.25 mg (1.5), 2.5 mg (3.0) PO daily	VMS, VVA, osteoporosis prevention
Synthetic conjugated estrogens, A (Cenestin)[a]	0.3 mg, 0.45 mg, 0.625 mg, 0.9 mg, 1.25 mg PO daily	VMS, VVA, osteoporosis prevention
Synthetic conjugated estrogens, B (Enjuvia)[a]	0.3 mg, 0.45 mg, 0.625 mg, 0.9 mg, 1.25 mg PO daily	VMS, VVA, osteoporosis prevention
Estrogen (Transdermal) (Doses in mg E_2/day)		
17 β-Estradiol emulsion (Estrasorb)[a]	0.05 mg/2 packets; apply mixture daily	VMS
17 β-Estradiol gel (Divigel)[a]	0.03 mg, 0.25 mg, 0.5 mg, 1.0 mg/packet; apply gel daily	VMS
17 β-Estradiol gel (EstroGel)[a]	0.75 mg/pump; apply gel daily	VMS, VVA
17 β-Estradiol gel (Elestrin)[a]	0.125 mg/pump, 0.375 mg/2 pumps; apply gel daily	VMS
17 β-Estradiol patch (Alora)[a]	0.025 mg, 0.05 mg, 0.075 mg, 0.1 mg per day; apply patch twice weekly	VMS, VVA, osteoporosis prevention

(continues)

Table 34-7 FDA-Approved Medications for Treating Women with Menopausal Symptoms (*continued*)

Drug: Generic (Brand)	Dose	Indications for Postmenopausal Women
Estrogen (Transdermal) (Doses in mg E_2/day) (continued)		
17 β-Estradiol patch (Climara)[a]	0.003 mg, 0.009 mg, 0.027 mg per day; apply patch weekly	VMS, VVA
17 β-Estradiol patch (Menostar)[a]	0.014 mg per day; apply patch weekly	Osteoporosis prevention
17 β-Estradiol patch (Minivelle)[a]	0.0375 mg, 0.05 mg, 0.075 mg, 0.1 mg per day; apply patch twice weekly	VMS, VVA, osteoporosis prevention
17 β-Estradiol patch (Vivelle-Dot)[a]	0.025 mg, 0.0375 mg, 0.05 mg, 0.075 mg, 0.1 mg per day; apply patch twice weekly	VMS, VVA, osteoporosis prevention
17 β-Estradiol transdermal spray (Evamist)[a]	1.53 mg; spray daily at first, adjust based on symptoms	VMS
Estrogen (Vaginal)		
Estradiol cream (Estrace Vaginal)	2–4 g/day, reduce cream to 1 g 2–3 times weekly (0.1%)	VVA
Estradiol ring (Estring)	7.5 mcg/24 hours; replace ring every 3 months (2 mg)	VVA
Estradiol acetate (Femring)[a]	0.05 mg daily, 0.1 mg daily; replace ring every 3 months	VMS, VVA
Estradiol (Vagifem)	10 mcg; insert tablet daily at first, adjust based on symptoms	VVA
Conjugated equine estrogens cream (Premarin Vaginal)	0.5–2 g daily for 2 weeks, then adjust amount of cream based on symptoms (0.625 mg/g)	VVA
Progestin (Oral)		
Medroxyprogesterone acetate (Provera)	2.5 mg/day, or 5–10 mg PO daily for 10–14 days every 4 weeks	Postmenopausal endometrial hyperplasia prevention
Progesterone micronized (Prometrium)	100 mg, 200 mg; 200 mg PO at bedtime daily for 12 days every 4 weeks	Postmenopausal endometrial hyperplasia prevention
Combined Estrogen and Bazedoxifene (Oral)		
Conjugated equine estrogens and bazedoxifene (Duavee)	0.45 mg/20 mg PO daily	VMS, osteoporosis prevention
Combined Estrogen and Progestin (Oral)		
Conjugated equine estrogens/ medroxyprogesterone (Premphase)	Continuous cyclic 0.625 mg PO daily for 14 days, then 0.625 mg/5 mg for 14 days, repeating cycle	VMS, VVA, osteoporosis prevention
Conjugated equine estrogens/ medroxyprogesterone (Prempro)	Continuous combined 0.3 mg/1.5 mg; 0.45 mg/1.5 mg; 0.625 mg/2.5 mg; 0.625 mg/5 mg PO daily	VMS, VVA, osteoporosis prevention
17 β-Estradiol/ drospirenone (Angeliq)	Continuous combined 0.5 mg/0.25 mg; 1.0 mg/0.5 mg PO daily	VMS, VVA
17 β-Estradiol/ norethindrone acetate (Activella)	Continuous combined 0.5mg/0.1mg; 1.0mg/0.5mg PO daily	VMS, VVA, osteoporosis prevention
17 β-Estradiol/ norgestimate (Prefest)	Pulsed continuous combined 1.0 mg/0 mg PO daily for 3 days, then 1.0 mg/ 0.09 mg for 3 days, repeating cycle	VMS, VVA, osteoporosis prevention
Ethinyl estradiol/ norethindrone acetate (Femhrt)	Continuous combined 2.5 mcg/0.5 mg; 5 mcg/1 mg PO daily	VMS, osteoporosis prevention
Combined Estrogen and Progestin (Transdermal)		
Estradiol/ levonorgestrel (Climara Pro)	0.45 mg/0.015 mg daily patch; apply twice weekly	VMS, osteoporosis prevention
17 β-Estradiol/ norethindrone acetate (CombiPatch)	0.05 mg/0.14 mg daily patch, 0.05 mg/ 0.25 mg daily	VMS, VVA
Estrogen + Androgen (Oral)		
Esterified estrogens/ methyl testosterone (generic)[a]	0.625 mg/1.25 mg, 1.25 mg/2.5 mg PO daily	VMS
Selective Estrogen Receptor Modulator (Oral)		
Ospemifene (Osphena)	60 mg PO daily	Dyspareunia (related to VVA)
Selective Serotonin Reuptake Inhibitor (Oral)		
Paroxetine (Brisdelle)	7.5 mg PO at bedtime daily	VMS

Dose Comparisons	
Estrogens	**Low Dose**
Conjugated estrogens oral	0.3–0.45 mg
17 β-Estradiol oral	0.5–1.0 mg
17 β-Estradiol transdermal	25–37.5 mcg
Progestins	
Drospirenone	0.5 mg
Medroxyprogesterone acetate	2.5–5 mg
Norethindrone acetate	0.5–1.25 mg
Norgestimate	0.09 mg
Progesterone micronized	100 mg

Abbreviations: VMS = vasomotor symptoms; VVA = vulvovaginal atrophy.

[a] Requires use of progestin if the woman has a uterus.

Sources: Data from Jane FM, Davis SR. A practitioner's toolkit for managing the menopause. *Climacteric.* 2014;17(5):564-579[11]; North American Menopause Society (NAMS). Hormone therapy tables. http://www.menopause.org/docs/default-source/2014/nams-ht-tables.pdf. Accessed July 31, 2014.[65]

Few clinically significant differences have been found among estrogens. Despite this fact, if a specific formulation is not working well, it can be beneficial to change to a different one or to change to a different route of administration, as pharmacokinetics differs by route.

The oral route often is preferred because today's women tend to be comfortable taking pills. Estrogen taken orally has a greater effect on the liver secondary to the first-pass effect, which delivers high concentrations via the portal circulation; consequently, oral formulations require higher doses than drugs provided by the transdermal route. Estrogen stimulates hepatic production of sex hormone-binding globulin, triglycerides, high-density lipoprotein, and clotting factors, which are, therefore, increased in women who take oral formulations. Non-oral hormones offer the advantages of elimination of the first-pass hepatic effect, thereby diminishing the peaks and nadirs of the drug's concentration; maintenance of more stable serum hormone levels; prevention of the gastrointestinal tract conversion of more potent estradiol to the weaker estrone as well as other gastrointestinal side effects; and use of lower doses.[10] Due to differences in effects, such as lower rates of deep vein thrombosis, myocardial infarction, and stroke as well as reductions in triglyceride levels,[10,11] transdermal and vaginal preparations are preferred in certain clinical situations, such as for women with hypertension, hypertriglyceridemia, and increased risk for cholelithiasis (Box 34-2).

Box 34-2 Potential Indications for Non-oral Routes for Hormone Therapy

- Cigarette smoker/nicotine dependent
- Decreased libido
- Depression
- Elevated triglyceride levels
- Gallbladder disease
- Gastrointestinal dysfunction
- Hypertension
- Migraines sensitive to hormones
- Obese
- Symptoms not responding to oral therapy or increasing doses needed
- Type 2 diabetes
- Woman prefers a nondaily regimen such as a transdermal patch

Note: Skin redness or pruritus at the transdermal patch sites is an indication to switch to a transdermal gel.

Sources: Data from Jane FM, Davis SR. A practitioner's toolkit for managing the menopause. *Climacteric.* 2014;17(5):564-579[11]; North American Menopause Society (NAMS), 2012 Hormone Therapy Position Statement Advisory Panel. The 2012 hormone therapy position statement of the North American Menopause Society. *Menopause.* 2012;19(3):257-271.[10]

Dosing Considerations

The general recommendation is to use the lowest dose of hormones possible that is effective in reducing symptoms.[10] Estrogen doses are usually based on self-reported symptom relief; on rare occasions (e.g., early menopause, refractory symptoms), serum evaluation is useful. The following are approximate equivalent daily doses: conjugated equine estrogen (0.3–0.625 mg) = micronized 17 β-estradiol (0.5–1 mg) = transdermal estradiol (14–100 mcg).[68]

When a woman is taking exogenous estrogen, serum estradiol levels of 60–120 pg/mL are considered to be in a therapeutic range and reflect adequate dosing. However, symptom reports tend to be more accurate clinically than serum estradiol levels. For example, CEE—the most frequently used estrogen—is primarily converted to estrone in the liver. Thus, serum estradiol is an inadequate marker of CEE levels. In general, if vasomotor symptoms have improved, the medication is considered effective and the dose adequate.

Serum progestin levels have not been studied. However, in practice, formulations containing progestins are used to counteract possible endometrial hyperplasia in women who have an intact uterus. In this setting, unexplained uterine bleeding or withdrawal bleeding prior to day 7 after onset of progestin therapy use may suggest inadequate progestin therapy, and further evaluation is warranted to rule out endometrial hyperplasia. Comparable progestin choices to offset the estrogen effect on the endometrium include MPA at 2.5 mg daily or 5 mg for 10 to 12 days per month, micronized progesterone at 100 mg daily or 200 mg for 10 to 12 days per month, norethindrone at 0.35 mg daily or 5 mg for 10 to 12 days per month, or levonorgestrel at 0.075 mg daily. Use of a progestin to counteract endometrial hyperplasia among women who use topical estrogen agents varies in clinical practice.[10,11,69]

Box 34-3 To Treat or Not to Treat: Are Progestins Needed with Vaginal Topical Estrogens?

For women who use estrogen therapy or hormone therapy post hysterectomy, a progestin is unnecessary because there is no risk of endometrial hyperplasia or cancer. In contrast, when a woman with an intact uterus takes systemic estrogen orally or transdermally, a progestin or bazedoxifene is added to counter the risk of abnormal endometrial growth.[10,11,71] However, it is controversial as to whether progestin is needed when a woman uses a vaginal topical estrogen (e.g., creams and rings for vaginal atrophy). The North American Menopause Society states that a progestin is likely not needed for women using low-dose local estrogen for vaginal atrophy.[10] However, the American Association of Clinical Endocrinologists cautions that even local vaginal estrogen can produce increased systemic estrogen serum levels.[69] Local vaginal estrogen preparations carry an FDA black box warning describing the possibility of endometrial cancer with their use and noting that adding a progestin may reduce this risk. Until there is clear evidence, professionals must use their clinical judgment and partner with women in deciding whether to use progestins with local vaginal ET.

An example of a clinical quandary in this area can be found in Box 34-3.

Topical progestins have not been proved effective in reducing the risk of estrogen-induced endometrial hyperplasia. In contrast, intrauterine progestins, delivered via an intrauterine contraceptive device (IUD), have demonstrated effectiveness.[70] This route of administration can reduce progestin-related side effects and frequently results in amenorrhea. Although the use of a progestin (levonorgestrel)-containing IUD (LNG IUD; e.g., Mirena) to counter estrogen-induced endometrial hyperplasia is evidence-based practice, it is not yet FDA approved.[10,11]

Prescription Regimens

Many different options are available when prescribing HT. There are varied doses, modes of administration, and types of estrogens or progesterone. The use of lower HT doses is associated with as much as a 50% reduction in irregular bleeding and breast tenderness, which are common side effects that can be obstacles to the use of hormones. Some women strongly prefer a specific route of therapy or type of estrogen or progestin, and their desires are an important component in selecting a pharmaceutical agent and regimen.

Systemic ET can be prescribed to women without a uterus because there is no risk of endometrial hyperplasia or cancer. Routes of administration include oral, transdermal (spray, gel, patch), or vaginal (systemic ring), as noted in Table 34-7. Oral ET is taken daily for symptom management. When daily continuous oral therapy is not needed for symptom management, some clinicians will prescribe ET in an off-label regimen of every other day. Systemic EPT or CEE/BZD can be prescribed to women with an intact uterus. As with ET, the estrogen in oral EPT or CEE/BZD is taken every day for symptom management. When daily oral dosing is not needed, the ET can usually either be tapered to a lower dose or may be able to be discontinued (as discussed later in the section on duration and discontinuation of HT).

A progestin or BZD is needed for women with an intact uterus to protect against the possibility of estrogen-induced endometrial hyperplasia.[10,11,54,71] BZD is taken daily in a combination single pill with CEE. Progestins are FDA approved for daily use or for intermittent use on 10 to 14 days of each month depending on the product being used (as described in Table 34-7).[10] The progestin is taken by the woman for a finite period; when it is completed for the month, the woman usually will have a withdrawal bleed similar to that experienced with oral contraceptive pills (as discussed in the *Contraception* chapter). This agent causes regular shedding of the endometrial tissue and eliminates any opportunity for hyperplasia or malignancy to develop. Women who take a progestin on a daily basis (e.g., CEE with MPA) or who have an LNG IUD in situ are less likely to experience bleeding after they have been on the regimen for several months. Initially, there may be spotting or breakthrough bleeding due to the exogenous estrogen effect. After several months on the regimen, however, the continuous progestin effect usually causes amenorrhea and the endometrium tends to become ischemic. Women who take progestin intermittently and experience bleeding outside of the withdrawal period or who use a progestin continuously and have bleeding after the initial few months of use need to be evaluated for endometrial hyperplasia or malignancy with ultrasound and/or endometrial biopsy.

Vaginal bleeding is a major reason why women discontinue hormones. Unscheduled bleeding is bothersome for some women; others may even prefer to avoid scheduled bleeding. For women who prefer no bleeding at all, use of daily progestin may achieve amenorrhea following a few months of breakthrough bleeding. Adequate teaching about what to expect depending on how the hormones are taken is essential. Abnormal bleeding, whether between periods or simply unpredicted, necessitates careful monitoring of the endometrium with ultrasound or endometrial biopsy.

Some women experience bothersome side effects with MPA, the most commonly prescribed progestin. MPA can cause cyclic weight gain, decreased libido, headache, bloating, and feelings of depression. In those situations, other oral options include micronized progesterone (Prometrium), norethindrone acetate (Aygestin), norgestimate (combined with 17 β-estradiol in Prefest), and drospirenone (combined with 17 β-estradiol in Angeliq), which may be better tolerated. A combined EPT transdermal patch or use of an LNG IUD also may be less problematic. Because of progestin's side effects, some women choose not to take this hormone at all or to take it less frequently. Various regimens are used, ranging from every other month, to every 3 to 4 months, to every 6 months, to annually. Table 34-8 differentiates among continuous-cyclic, sequential, and long-cycle administration. Although not FDA approved, these regimens are evidence-based practices and provide some endometrial protection, although women should understand that they represent off-label indications.[72] Women who choose not to take any progestin should have annual endometrial biopsies to monitor for endometrial hyperplasia and malignancy. Data are lacking on the effectiveness, safety, and cost of this approach.

Table 34-8 Current Oral Estrogen Plus Progestin Therapy Regimens[a]

Regimen	Estrogen	Progestin
Continuous-cyclic (sequential)	Daily	10–14 days every month
Continuous-cyclic (sequential) long-cycle	Daily	14 days every 2–6 months
Continuous-combined	Daily	Daily
Pulsed-continuous-combined (pulsed-progestin; continuous-estrogen)	Daily	Repeating cycle of 3 days on, 3 days off

[a] EPT prescriptions include a daily estrogen to avoid the symptoms that may arise during the week off the hormone. Women who do not need daily estrogen for symptom management may be candidates for a lower dose or therapy discontinuation.

Sources: Data from Jane FM, Davis SR. A practitioner's toolkit for managing the menopause. *Climacteric.* 2014;17(5):564-579[11]; North American Menopause Society (NAMS), 2012 Hormone Therapy Position Statement Advisory Panel. The 2012 hormone therapy position statement of the North American Menopause Society. *Menopause.* 2012;19(3):257-271.10

Several different regimens are available for oral EPT. If a woman is in early postmenopause or in STRAW stage +1a, within 6 to 12 months after her last menstrual period, she is more likely to have erratic spotting for as long as 6 months if placed on a continuous-combined regimen, followed by amenorrhea. Many women do well on a continuous-cyclic regimen of daily estrogen, adding progestin for the first 12 days of the month.[52] With this approach, most women will usually experience a withdrawal bleed after the combined estrogen/progestin dose days (after calendar day 12), which becomes shorter and lighter over time. Cyclic (estrogen days 1–25, progestin days 15–25) and cyclic combined (estrogen and progestin days 1–25) regimens were popular when EPT was used for chronic disease prevention. These regimens include one week off estrogen, during which a withdrawal bleed occurs, similar to the bleeding pattern with standard combined oral contraceptive pills. The cyclic and cyclic-combined regimens are no longer used because women who do not have breakthrough symptoms during a week off estrogen likely do not need HT.

Currently used oral EPT regimens include continuous-cyclic, continuous-combined, and pulsed-continuous-combined options. The pulsed-continuous-combined regimen includes intermittent progestin therapy, which may decrease the incidence of erratic spotting and side effects that can accompany continuous progestin exposure. Pulsed therapy may also reduce the potential risk for breast cancer that was associated with continuous progestin use in the WHI.[34] Women taking continuous-combined or pulsed-continuous-combined EPT who continue to have bleeding past the first 3 to 6 months should have endometrial evaluation with ultrasound and/or biopsy.[11]

Progestins

Progestins have been used both with and without estrogen to reduce the incidence of vasomotor symptoms (Box 34-4). As demonstrated in the WHI, progestins may contribute to increased cancer risk.[34] Therefore, the use of these hormones alone for management of a woman's vasomotor symptoms is an off-label indication, but may be considered if the risk–benefit ratio supports its use. Among women with a history of breast cancer or endometrial cancer, there are no data demonstrating safety of progestin-only regimens.

Mammographic density is increased with progestin use, which has been linked with a higher breast cancer risk and makes mammogram data more difficult to

Box 34-4 Every Woman Has a Story

MM is a 51-year-old woman whose last normal menses was 9 months ago, but she reports experiencing irregular menses most of her life. She presents for help coping with hot flashes. These symptoms occur both day and night, and she finds that they interfere with work and her relationships. MM has a copper intrauterine device (ParaGard IUD) in situ, a contraceptive method she has used regularly since the birth of her child many years ago. Her vital signs and basic laboratory findings (including blood glucose and thyroid-stimulating hormone [TSH] values) are normal, and her body mass index (BMI) is 34. MM has been a lacto-ovarian vegetarian for the last 4 years.

MM is a perimenopausal woman with significant symptoms that are interfering with her activities of daily living. Her history of irregular menses, one pregnancy, and high BMI places her at risk for long periods of unopposed estrogen. By taking EPT, she can obtain relief from the vasomotor symptomatology as well as protection from potential endometrial hyperplasia.

After a discussion of her personal risks and benefits in relation to HT, MM chooses to take Femhrt, a synthetic product that is administered as a continuous regimen and combines estrogen and progestin, with the intention of using this hormone product for the shortest period possible. General health education for MM includes suggestions of nonpharmacologic interventions such as wearing natural fibers for clothing, discussion of achieving and maintaining a healthy weight, and encouraging regular exercise and screening tests including mammograms and colonoscopy. MM should also be encouraged to continue using the ParaGard IUD until she reaches menopause since she is still potentially fertile.

interpret. Medroxyprogesterone acetate (MPA, Provera, Depo-Provera) has demonstrated effectiveness in providing hot flash relief.[73] Oral MPA (Provera) is taken daily in a dose of 20 mg by mouth. Injected MPA (Depo-Provera) is injected intramuscularly at doses of 150 mg monthly or 400 to 500 mg every 3 months. Megestrol acetate (Megace), which is primarily used to treat metastatic breast cancer, is another oral progestin that has demonstrated effectiveness for vasomotor symptom relief at a dose of 20 mg by mouth daily. Megestrol acetate is not recommended for women with diabetes or thromboembolic disease. Progestin-alone therapy can take as many as 4 weeks to achieve symptom relief. Common side effects of progestins include irregular bleeding, weight gain, bloating, fluid retention, depression, sexual dysfunction, and headache.[11]

Side Effects/Adverse Effects of Hormones

Estrogen use can have both nuisance and serious side effects. Nuisance side effects may include vaginal bleeding or spotting, nausea, headache/migraine, mood changes, glucose intolerance, and libido changes. Serious reactions may include breast, ovarian, and endometrial cancers, as well as cholestatic jaundice, gallbladder disease, pancreatitis, hypertension, and depression.[16]

Progestins are associated with menstrual irregularities, amenorrhea, breast tenderness, weight changes, headache, fluid retention, and abdominal distention.[16] Because of these side effects, some women self-discontinue the agent while continuing use of estrogen—which puts them at risk for endometrial hyperplasia and cancer. Progestin products also are associated with adverse reactions such as thromboembolism, hypertension, breast cancer, depression, and cholestatic jaundice.[16] Different formulations of progestins may be better tolerated by some women, so changing to a different formulation or delivery system (e.g., change to a transdermal or IUD product if using an oral formulation) can be beneficial for some women experiencing side effects.

Hormonal Influences on Laboratory Testing

Use of HT can confound diagnosis or monitoring of certain health conditions because of hormones' effects on common laboratory tests. Some of these changes are related to the hepatic changes associated with estrogen, whereas others occur for unknown reasons.

Drug–Drug Interactions

Oral estrogen can interfere with many drugs.[16] For example, estrogen increases liver metabolism of several drugs, thereby decreasing their blood levels. Examples include lamotrigine (Lamictal), carbamazepine (Tegretol), nevirapine (Viramune), phenytoin (Dilantin), phenobarbital (Luminal), primidone (Mysoline), rifampin (Rifadin), aromatase inhibitors, and ursodiol (Actigall). Estrogen also increases the incidence of hyperglycemia when it is taken with diazoxide (Proglycem), thiazolidinediones (e.g., exenatide or Byetta), and other hypoglycemic agents including metformin (Glucophage). Estrogens decrease blood levels of omega-3 acids, thereby minimizing their antihyperlipidemia effect. In contrast, hepatic metabolism of aripiprazole (Abilify), dasatinib (Sprycel), and lapatinib (Tykerb) is inhibited with concomitant estrogen, which can increase the risk of toxicity. Erythromycin, fluvoxamine (Luvox), and telithromycin (Ketek) can increase estrogen blood levels. Griseofulvin (Fulvicin), oxcarbazepine (Trileptal), rifampin (Rifadin), and rifapentine (Priftin) may decrease estrogen levels when taken concurrently.[16]

Fewer drugs interfere with the action of progestins. Agents such as aprepitant (Emend), bexarotene (Targretin), bosentan (Tracleer), carbamazepine (Tegretol), griseofulvin (Grifulvin V), oxcarbazepine (Trileptal), phenytoin (Dilantin), rifabutin (Mycobutin), and rifampin (Rifadin) may result in decreased progestin levels and, therefore, decreased effectiveness.

Duration and Discontinuation

To minimize risks of conditions such as breast cancer, NAMS supports the use of EPT for approximately 3 to 5 years.[10] As the risk profile is different for ET, NAMS suggests that use of such therapy for 7 years or longer may be appropriate. IMS and other sources suggest HT use is safe for at least 5 years in women younger than 60 and potentially longer for women with a low risk profile.[11,54] Despite the potential risks associated with HT use, women who continue to have distressing symptoms beyond the usual 5 to 7 years after menopause may wish to continue HT for years. The need for ongoing HT use should be reevaluated regularly and the lowest possible dose used. The decision to continue HT should be individualized based on the risk–benefit ratio discussed between the woman and her provider and the belief that continuation is necessary to contribute to quality of life.[10,54] For women who experience early menopause, NAMS, IMS, and others recommend continuing HT until the usual age of menopause (approximately 51 years).[10,11,54]

Adherence to hormone regimens can be low. Some women start therapy but then discontinue it due to concerns about safety, annoying side effects, cost, or other personal beliefs and reasons. Some women never fill their prescription. Today, HT is focused on treatment of women with bothersome symptoms; therefore, it is not critical for a woman to fill or continue therapy. What is critical is for estrogen use to be balanced with progestin use or to have careful endometrial monitoring for a woman with an intact uterus.

Bioidentical Hormone Therapy

Bioidentical hormone therapy (BHT) refers to products that have the same molecular structure as hormones produced in the body. The appeal of BHT is that some women think it is more "natural" and may carry a lower side effect profile because the hormones are like those that the body naturally produces. BHT agents are divided into two kinds.

The first type includes the BHT products that are produced by pharmaceutical companies and approved by the FDA. These agents are the ones in common use. Examples include estradiol (Estrace) and micronized progesterone.

The second type of BHT is compounded BHT. These drugs are made for women by selected pharmacists who mix various hormones into a personalized preparation. Compounded BHT is usually composed of various amounts of estradiol, estrone, estriol, and natural progesterone. In 2008, the FDA notified compounding pharmacies that claims of increased safety and superior protection of compounded BHT against conditions such as Alzheimer's disease are unfounded based on science. The FDA also warned against continued use of estriol because the safety and effectiveness of this agent are unknown.[74] Estriol is not FDA approved and does not have proven safety data to support its use as HT. These FDA statements created a furor among the compounding pharmacies, which accused the FDA of being subject to undue influence from the pharmaceutical companies that manufacture commercial hormone formulations.

Compounded hormones are individualized in amount or route of delivery, such as a sublingual troche or tablet, oral capsules, and transdermal gels, creams, and patches. Most products combine all three estrogens: estradiol, estrone, and estriol. Doses tend to be smaller or different than those available through regular prescriptions. Other compounded products may include DHEA and testosterone. Many compounding pharmacies offer hormone saliva testing to quantify the amount of hormones in the body and determine appropriate doses. There is little evidence to support this practice, and saliva hormone testing is not approved by the FDA.

Topical progesterone in nonprescription form is synthesized by a chemical process using plants such as soybeans and wild yam, a Mexican herb. The end product is nearly identical to endogenous progesterone, but research has failed to demonstrate that it provides any protection for the endometrial lining. Diosgenin, the precursor of progesterone found in these plants, cannot be converted to progesterone in the body when ingested; rather, it must be converted through a manufacturing process.

Therefore, eating soybeans or Mexican yams will not provide endometrial protection.

Using a compounding pharmacy to prepare oral progesterone can be beneficial for a woman with a peanut allergy who cannot take micronized progesterone in peanut oil. In such situations, it is essential to work with an accredited compounding pharmacy and, as with any off-label medication use, to provide full disclosure to the woman regarding the risks, benefits, and implications of using products that do not have FDA approval so she can make an informed decision whether to use the compounded product.

Many FDA-approved products on the market are synthetic hormones that do not have a bioidentical agent available. These drugs include CEE or conjugated estrogens. The effectiveness of BHT for the treatment of women with menopausal symptoms is controversial, and a 2013 review by Whelan et al. has called it into question.[75]

Complementary and Alternative Therapies

The use of complementary and alternative medicine (CAM) therapies among perimenopausal and postmenopausal women is increasing, with as many as 91% of women reporting use in some studies.[76] Women have reported using CAM for menopause-related vasomotor symptoms, sleep disturbances, mood changes, night sweats, vaginal dryness, reduced energy, and muscle and/or joint pain. CAM is used because many women may think it helps their symptoms, is more natural and has fewer side effects than prescriptions, and will promote overall health and quality of life. Other reasons for CAM use include preventing disease and a recommendation from a family member, friend, or clinician. Women are more likely to obtain CAM information from family and friends and often do not disclose CAM use to their clinicians due to negative experiences with their clinicians and lack of knowledge among providers.[76] Because of the large number of women who use CAM and the self-described lack of disclosure by women, it is incumbent upon clinicians to become knowledgeable about various CAM options and to discuss this information with women.

One reason why clinicians have limited knowledge regarding the safety and effectiveness of CAM is the lack of high-quality research on these therapies. Few high-quality RCTs have been conducted for CAM, and the studies that have been carried out often suffer in quality due to the small treatment groups, lack of a control group, and short duration. This leaves providers with a difficult task when caring for women who use CAM as well as a limited ability to confidently include CAM in their management plans.

Despite the lack of quality data, various CAM therapies are commonly used to allay menopause-related symptoms. The *Complementary and Alternative Therapies* chapter addresses CAM for various menopause-related symptoms in more detail. The most commonly used botanical products for menopause-related symptoms[77–80] are addressed briefly in the following section and listed in Table 34-9. Several other CAM therapies, such as relaxation techniques, hypnosis, cognitive-behavioral therapy, paced breathing, and acupuncture, have been shown to reduce vasomotor symptoms and improve sleep but discussion of them is beyond the scope of this chapter.

Black Cohosh

Cimicifuga racemosa, or black cohosh, has a long history of use as a remedy for women's health ailments and is the most commonly taken herbal for menopause-related symptoms. Indigenous to North America, the dried rhizome and root are taken in doses of 40 to 200 mg daily through standardized extract drops or oral tablet (e.g., Remifemin, Estroven). The most common dose is 40 mg daily taken as a single dose or 20 mg twice daily. Black cohosh was initially thought to have estrogen-like properties; however, the exact mechanism of action is unclear.[81,82]

Hepatotoxicity was reported in several women using black cohosh. This condition may have been caused by contaminants, particularly because a meta-analysis in 2011 demonstrated no toxicity effects found among five RCTs.[83]

A 2012 Cochrane review included 16 randomized controlled trials, involving 2027 women, that were conducted to evaluate the effectiveness of black cohosh for vasomotor symptoms, menopause symptom scores, vulvovaginal symptoms, and adverse effects.[84] Among the studies evaluated, black cohosh was compared against placebo, red clover, fluoxetine, and HT. The meta-analysis found no significant difference between black cohosh versus placebo for hot flashes or menopause symptoms scores. Other therapies either did not show statistically significant differences or had too few studies for adequate comparison. Although some small studies have demonstrated effectiveness and many women report relief when taking black cohosh, the Cochrane review concluded that there is not enough evidence to support use of black cohosh for menopause-related symptoms.[84] Additional research is needed.

Table 34-9 Complementary and Alternative Therapies Commonly Used for Menopausal Symptom Relief

Product	Usual Dose[a]	Purpose in Menopause	Clinical Considerations
Black cohosh (*Cimicifuga racemosa*)	20 mg PO 2 times daily (proprietary standardized extract)	Vasomotor symptoms	Multiple products and formulations are available. Research evidence is conflicting regarding effects on menopause-related symptoms. Safety for use lasting more than 6 months is not established. Product labels frequently recommend much higher doses. Can potentiate antihypertensive agents. Wide variations in product ingredients, extraction processes, and purity. Side effects are rare—usually intestinal upset, headache, dizziness, hypotension, or painful extremities; more common with higher doses. Has been associated with liver toxicity, use with caution if the woman is taking statins, CYP450-active drugs, or liver-toxic drugs.
Chastetree berry (*Vitex agnus castus*)	Effective dose unknown; hard to find standardized extract	Menstrual irregularity	More popular in Europe than the United States; approved in Germany for premenstrual syndrome (PMS), mastalgia, and menopause symptoms. Often found in combination products. Research has evaluated chastetree berry only in mixed products; does not show benefit for menopause-related symptoms. May be helpful for menstrual irregularities. Side effects are rare—usually headache, intestinal upset.
Dong quai (*Angelica sinensis*)	2 capsules PO 2–3 times daily, usually in combination products	Gynecologic conditions	Widely used in Asia. Research found no benefit for menopause symptoms. May be beneficial when used in combination with other botanicals (e.g., chasteberry, black cohosh, chamomilla, milk thistle, ginseng)— often in Chinese herb combination products (*Chinese Materia Medica* advises against giving it alone). A "heating" herb, it can cause a red face, hot flashes, sweating, irritability, or insomnia. Contains coumarin derivatives; contraindicated in those persons taking warfarin. Can cause photosensitivity and hypotension.
Evening primrose oil (*Oenothera biennis*)	3–4 g PO daily in divided doses	Hot flashes, mastalgia	Oil has omega-6 fatty acids and is used for rheumatoid arthritis, atopic dermatitis, mastalgia, and menopause-related and menstrual-related symptoms. Research showed no difference from placebo for hot flashes and sweating. Potentiates risk for seizure if taken by persons with seizure disorder, with phenothiazines, and with other medications that lower the seizure threshold. Side effects include diarrhea and nausea.
Ginkgo (*Ginkgo biloba*)	40–80 mg PO of standardized extract 3 times/day	Memory changes	Used mainly for cognition and memory. Research showed no difference from placebo for mood, sleep disturbances, menopause-related symptoms, memory, or sustained attention; improvement in mental flexibility was noted. Memory changes are often related to sleep disturbances, menopausal sleep disturbances frequently related to vasomotor symptoms, or other life stressors. Side effects include gastrointestinal distress and hypotension; chronic use has been linked with subarachnoid hemorrhage, subdural hematoma, and increased bleeding times.
Ginseng (*Panax ginseng*)	1–2 g root PO daily in divided doses	General "tonic"; improved mood, fatigue	Used to increase energy and treat menopause-related symptoms and sexual dysfunction. Research showed no benefit on menopausal symptoms, but some benefits on well-being, general health, and depression. Can cause uterine bleeding and mastalgia. Contraindicated in women with breast cancer, and with use of monoamine oxidase inhibitors, stimulants, or anticoagulants; may potentiate digoxin and other drugs (multiple drug interactions). Side effects include rash, nervousness, insomnia, and hypertension.
Hops (*Humulus lupulu*)	100 mcg 8-prenylnaringenin daily PO as dried herb or topically as gel	Hot flashes, sweats, palpitations, irritability, insomnia	Traditionally used as a mild hypnotic for sleep disturbances, headache, and gynecologic disorders. Research showed a benefit in hot flash relief in 2 small trials. Hops gel in combination with supplements showed relief of vaginal dryness.
Kava (*Piper methysticum*)	150–300 mg PO of root extract daily in divided doses	Irritability, insomnia	Used for sedative and analgesic effects. Research supports use for reducing anxiety. One study showed a decrease in hot flashes, anxiety, and depression, and improved well-being; a second study showed no difference. Banned in several countries due to hepatotoxicity; thus, it is not recommended. Contraindicated in persons with depression. Side effects include gastrointestinal discomfort, impaired reflexes and motor function, weight loss, hepatotoxicity, and rash.

(*continues*)

Table 34-9 Complementary and Alternative Therapies Commonly Used for Menopausal Symptom Relief (*continued*)

Product	Usual Dose[a]	Purpose in Menopause	Clinical Considerations
St. John's wort (*Hypericum perforatum*)	300 mg 3 times daily (standardized extract)	Vasomotor symptoms, irritability, depression	Used for depression and menopause-related symptom relief. Research showed improved sleep and menopause-related quality of life, but no benefit for hot flashes. Often combined with black cohosh for menopause symptom treatment. Interferes with metabolism of many medications that are metabolized in the liver (CYP450; e.g., estrogen, digoxin, theophylline); reduces International Normalized Ratio (INR) levels. Should not be used concomitantly with antidepressants, monoamine oxidase inhibitors, or immunosuppressants. Side effects include photosensitivity, rash, constipation, cramping, dry mouth, fatigue, dizziness, restlessness, and insomnia.
Valerian root (*Valeriana officinalis*)	300–600 mg aqueous extract PO 0.5–1 hour before bed (insomnia); 150–300 mg PO aqueous extract each morning and 300–400 mg PO each evening (anxiety)	Sedative, antianxiety drug	Used for insomnia with intermittent dosing; used for anxiety with chronic dosing. Research showed improvement in sleep and depression/mood scales (generally, not specific to postmenopause). Side effects include headache, uneasiness, excitability, arrhythmias, morning sedation, gastrointestinal upset, and cardiac function disorders (with long-term use).
Wild yam (*Dioscorea villosa*)	Unknown	Menopausal symptoms	Some products claim that creams are converted in situ to progesterone; however, the human body cannot convert topical or ingested wild yam into progesterone. Research showed no benefit on menopausal symptoms and no change in serum progesterone levels.

[a] Doses vary and differ according to formulation (e.g., tincture, liquid extract, drops, essential oil).

Sources: Modified from Alexander IM, Andrist LC. Menopause. In: Schuiling KD, Likis FE, eds. *Women's Gynecologic Health*. 2nd ed. Burlington, MA: Jones & Bartlett Learning; 2013:285-328.[86]

Phytoestrogens

Similar to black cohosh, **phytoestrogens** are widely used by women for menopause-related symptom management. Also similar to black cohosh, data supporting their effectiveness are minimal and contradictory. Phytoestrogens are plant-based compounds and include isoflavones (found in legumes such as chickpeas, clover, soybeans, and lentils), lignans (found in rye, linseed flax, legumes, and millet), and coumestrans (found in sprouts, sunflower seeds, and red clover). They are chemically similar to estrogen and can exert both estrogenic and antiestrogenic properties depending on their concentration and the concentration of endogenous sex hormones.

Isoflavones are the most commonly used phytoestrogen. More than 1000 types of isoflavones exist, though only two are used most frequently for menopausal symptoms: genistein and daidzein. Genistein and daidzein are found in soybeans, soy products, and red clover. Foods often have most of the phytochemicals removed during the processes to promote taste and obtain color-free preparations.

A 2012 meta-analysis that included 17 RCTs reported that ingesting synthesized or extracted soy isoflavones (54 mg daily dose on average) reduced hot flash frequency and severity statistically significantly more than placebo.[85] Supplements that provided more than 18.8 mg of genistein were twice as effective in reducing hot flashes than products with less genistein. As soy products vary in composition and concentration, it is important to carefully evaluate each supplement individually prior to recommending its use. The meta-analysis noted that the majority of studies were small and that larger, more rigorous studies are needed.

Perimenopause and Fertility

The ability to conceive declines 10 to 15 years before the FMP. By the age of 45 years, among women who are able to conceive, there is a 50% increase in spontaneous abortions, chromosomal abnormalities, and pregnancy complications such as premature labor. If a mature woman desires to become pregnant, and a cycle-day 3 FSH level is elevated, (stage −3b or −3a, late reproductive on the STRAW scale), she should consider seeking early assistance to enhance fertility. Additional information about infertility treatments can be found in the *Pelvic and Menstrual Disorders* chapter.

The perimenopausal woman who does not desire pregnancy should know that unplanned pregnancy is still possible until the FMP is established, in other words, 12 months after this event. Perimenopausal women constitute the group with the second highest rate of unplanned pregnancy. Most healthy perimenopausal woman can use any of the contraceptive methods. In well-screened women, these options include traditional or extended regimens of hormonal methods such as low-dose combination estrogen–progestin oral contraceptives, progestin-only oral contraceptives (POPs), injectables, implants, transdermal or ring-delivery products, and IUDs. However, products containing estrogen are not advised for women who smoke or those who have a history of deep vein thrombosis or other major cardiovascular risk factors.[16] All options should be explained, as the best contraceptive method for a healthy perimenopausal woman is the one she chooses and is able to use successfully.

Common Menopausal Symptoms: Abnormal Uterine Bleeding and Vasomotor Symptoms

Multiple hormone trials have investigated the safety of HT using a variety of health indicators. However, it is also important to explore the effectiveness of these agents for women with menopausal symptoms. The two most commonly reported symptoms are abnormal uterine bleeding and vasomotor symptoms.

Abnormal Uterine Bleeding

The most frequently reported symptom during perimenopause is irregular uterine bleeding. The flow may be heavier or lighter, or prolonged or shortened; there may be spotting between menses; and the interval between cycles may change. Abnormal uterine bleeding (AUB) includes any type of bleeding that is outside of normal parameters in frequency, duration, or amount. AUB may be treated with a variety of pharmacologic agents that may or may not offer contraceptive effects, such as contraceptive agents (estrogen with progestin or progestin alone), noncontraceptive progestin agents, LNG IUD, and nonsteroidal anti-inflammatory drugs.

When evaluating a midlife woman with AUB, it is first important to determine if she has the potential for pregnancy. Once pregnancy is ruled out, the next assessment usually is in line with the Federation Internationale de Gynecologie et d'Obstetrique (FIGO) system.[87] During perimenopause and menopause, the most common etiologies of abnormal uterine bleeding include endometrial polyps, endometrial hyperplasia, leiomyomas, and (rarely) coagulopathies or carcinoma. Other possibilities to consider in a differential diagnosis include thyroid disease and liver dysfunction.

Any bleeding that occurs at or after 1 year following the FMP (not caused by EPT withdrawal) is presumed to be endometrial cancer until proven otherwise. Therefore it requires evaluation, including a pelvic examination; uterine/endometrial assessment, including a possible biopsy, pelvic ultrasound, or hysteroscopy; and hormonal testing including thyroid, pituitary, and adrenal evaluation.

Abnormal uterine bleeding is reviewed in detail the *Pelvic and Menstrual Disorders* chapter.

Vasomotor Symptoms

During the perimenopausal period, vasomotor symptoms—also called hot flashes or hot flushes and night sweats—are the second most frequently reported symptoms after AUB. Vasomotor symptoms increase during perimenopause and are most frequent and intense in the first 2 years after the FMP.[16] Approximately 75% of women experience hot flashes, with almost 50% experiencing moderate to severe hot flashes in the first 2 years following the FMP. Hot flash frequency and severity may decline with time, yet some women, especially those with severe symptoms, will continue to have significant symptoms for many more years.[88] Climate, diet, lifestyle, weight, and race may play a role in hot flash experiences. Ninety percent or more of women have hot flashes after bilateral oophorectomy or surgical induction of menopause.

Physiology of Vasomotor Symptoms

Hot flashes occur when estrogen is reduced, but the exact causative mechanism is poorly understood. The most prevalent explanation is that hot flashes occur when lowered estrogen levels disrupt the hypothalamic thermoregulatory process. Reduced estrogen levels cause decreased concentrations of circulating serotonin, increased concentrations of circulating norepinephrine, and decreased concentrations of estrogen, which collectively lead to a narrowing of the thermo-neutral zone. Temperatures above this neutral threshold cause sweating, and those below cause shivering.[89]

Nonpharmacologic Treatments for Vasomotor Symptoms

Some women manage their vasomotor symptoms during perimenopause with environmental and lifestyle changes,

Box 34-5 Behavioral Strategies for Managing Hot Flashes

- Avoid personally perceived hot flash triggers, such as caffeine, hot beverages or foods, sugar, and alcohol.
- Dress in layers.
- Engage in regular exercise to help maintain a healthy weight, promote better sleep, and help with thermal regulation.
- Maintain a cool ambient room temperature, especially in the bedroom.
- Maintain a normal weight.
- Pace respiration during a hot flash (slow, deep, abdominal breathing).
- Practice regular relaxation activities such as supported by music, massage, meditation, or yoga to help lessen stress and anxiety, which are positively associated with hot flashes.
- Use a fan to circulate air and avoid "hot spots."
- Wear clothing that allows air flow (e.g., cotton, linen, wicking fabrics).

Sources: Data from Alexander IM, Andrist LC. Menopause. In: Schuiling KD, Likis FE, eds. *Women's Gynecologic Health.* 2nd ed. Burlington, MA: Jones & Bartlett Learning; 2013:285-328[86]; Jane FM, Davis SR. A practitioner's toolkit for managing the menopause. *Climacteric.* 2014;17(5):564-579[11]; North American Menopause Society (NAMS). *Menopause Practice: A Clinician's Guide.* 4th ed. Mayfield Heights OH: North American Menopause Society; 2010.[17]

although data about the effectiveness of these modalities tend to be anecdotal. Box 34-5 lists some suggested strategies.

Pharmacologic Nonhormonal Treatments for Vasomotor Symptoms

When hot flashes annoy a woman to the degree that she requests treatment, estrogen-containing pharmaceuticals are the most effective and most commonly prescribed agents, using the dosages and regimens discussed earlier in this chapter.[10,11] For women who cannot or prefer not to take hormones, nonhormonal drugs may be considered (Table 34-10). Most of these nonhormonal drugs are prescribed based on anecdotal evidence; paroxetine (Brisdelle), however, has received formal FDA approval for treating women with menopause-related vasomotor symptoms.[90] Brisdelle is available as a lower dose (7.5-mg tablet) than Paxil (10-mg tablet), although both are brand names of paroxetine; however, they contain different salts—the former having mesylate and the latter hydrochloride. The FDA advisory panel voted against Brisdelle receiving FDA approval for this indication, but few nonhormonal treatments for women with hot flashes are available and it was approved in 2013.[91] Some providers advocate use of generic paroxetine for women with menopause-related vasomotor symptoms because of its lower cost, or use of other antidepressants on an off-label basis.

Selective Serotonin Reuptake Inhibitors and Selective Norepinephrine Reuptake Inhibitors

Selective serotonin reuptake inhibitors (SSRIs) and selective norepinephrine reuptake inhibitors (SNRIs) have been shown to decrease hot flashes in women. This is likely the result of alterations of central serotonin or norepinephrine concentrations that accompany menopause. Several agents have been studied, most often in breast cancer survivors. Paroxetine, dosed at 7.5 mg taken orally at bedtime, was studied in women who are not breast cancer survivors; in this population, it demonstrated a significant decrease in hot flashes versus placebo.[90] Other SSRIs and SNRIs such as escitalopram (Lexapro), venlafaxine (Effexor), fluoxetine (Prozac), sertraline (Zoloft), and citalopram (Celexa) have also demonstrated effectiveness in decreasing vasomotor symptoms.[73,92] Desvenlafaxine (Pristiq) is a novel SNRI that has also demonstrated modest effectiveness in this indication.[93] Overall, venlafaxine, escitalopram, and paroxetine appear to have the strongest evidence supporting their use.[73,92]

Vasomotor symptom relief usually is accomplished within the first week of starting SSRIs and SNRIs, but any mood benefits may not be observed for 6 to 8 weeks.[16] Side effects of nausea or sexual dysfunction may become a deterrent to use, although nausea will subside within 2 weeks if the medication is taken with food and sexual side effects were not reported with 7.5 mg paroxetine. If drowsiness occurs, bedtime dosing is encouraged. Use of SSRIs and SNRIs may be related to low bone density and fracture, a risk often found among mature women.[16] To minimize side effects, use of the lowest applicable dose is suggested for 1 week, with the dose then being increased if necessary. Abrupt cessation of SSRIs and SNRIs may cause anxiety and headache, so women should taper off their dose for a period of at least 2 weeks.

Table 34-10 Pharmacologic Nonhormonal Treatments for Vasomotor Symptoms

Drug: Generic (Brand)	Drug Category	Dose	Clinical Considerations
Citalopram (Celexa)	SSRI	10 mg, 20 mg, 40 mg PO daily	Side effects include nausea, somnolence, sweating, and tremor. Avoid in women with recent myocardial infarction or congestive heart failure. Avoid abrupt withdrawal.
Clonidine (Catapres)	Antihypertensive	0.05 mg PO 2 times daily to 0.1 mg PO 2 times daily	Side effects include hypotension, bradycardia, arrhythmias at high doses, dry mouth, dizziness, constipation, and sedation.
Clonidine (Catapres)	Antihypertensive	0.1 mg patch 2 times daily	Gradual tapering is necessary to avoid nervousness, headache, agitation, confusion, and abrupt hypertension.
Desvenlafaxine (Pristiq)	SNRI	50 mg, 100 mg PO extended release daily	Side effects include nausea, dizziness, insomnia, constipation, and fatigue. Use with caution in women with renal or liver failure.
Escitalopram (Lexapro)	SSRI	5 mg, 10 mg, 20 mg PO daily	Side effects include nausea, insomnia, diarrhea, somnolence, sweating, and fatigue. Use with caution in women with renal or liver failure.
Fluoxetine (Prozac)	SSRI	10 mg, 20 mg, 40 mg PO daily	Side effects include reduced orgasm and/or libido, nausea, insomnia, diarrhea, and anxiety. Use with caution in women with diabetes or liver failure.
Gabapentin (Neurontin)	Antiepileptic drug	100 mg, 300 mg, 400 mg, 600 mg, 800 mg PO daily to start (100 mg daily if older than age 65), up to 900 mg	Side effects include dizziness, somnolence, fatigue, and nausea. Use with caution in women with renal failure, depression, or alcohol use. Bedtime administration is recommended to minimize drowsiness during waking hours. Antacids reduce bioavailability.
Methyldopa (Aldomet)	Cardiovascular agents/antiadrenergic agents, centrally acting	250–500 mg PO up to 2 times daily	Not recommended for persons with hepatitis, cirrhosis, or impaired liver function, or those taking monoamine oxidase inhibitors. Rare association with hemolytic anemia, leucopenia, thrombocytopenia, sedation, headache, and hyperprolactinemia.
Paroxetine (Paxil, Brisdelle)	SSRI	12.5–25 mg PO daily (Paxil) 7.5 mg PO at bedtime (Brisdelle)	Side effects include headache, fatigue, and nausea. Use with caution in women with alcohol use, seizure disorder, or depression. Potential drug–drug interaction with tamoxifen (Nolvadex). Paroxetine inhibits CYP2D6, which converts tamoxifen to its active metabolite. Brisdelle is the only SSRI with FDA approval for treating women with vasomotor symptoms.
Sertraline (Zoloft)	SSRI	50 mg PO daily	Side effects include weight gain, blurred vision, nausea, headache, insomnia, and somnolence. Use with caution in women with seizure disorder, alcohol use, or hyponatremia.
Venlafaxine (generic, Effexor XR)	SSRI	37.5 mg, 75 mg, 150 mg ER PO daily	Side effects include nausea, headache, somnolence, dizziness, constipation, and sweating. Use with caution in women with hypertension, anorexia, or renal or liver failure.

Abbreviations: SNRI = serotonin norepinephrine reuptake inhibitor; SSRI = selective serotonin reuptake inhibitor.
Sources: Data from Alexander IM, Andrist LC. Menopause. In: Schuiling KD, Likis FE, eds. *Women's Gynecologic Health.* 2nd ed. Burlington, MA: Jones & Bartlett Learning; 2013:285-328[86]; Shams T, Firwana B, Habib F, et al. SSRIs for hot flashes: a systematic review and meta-analysis of randomized trials . *J Gen Intern Med.* 2014;29(1):204-213[92]; Thacker HL. Assessing risks and benefits of nonhormonal treatments for vasomotor symptoms in perimenopausal and postmenopausal women. *J Womens Health.* 2011;20(7):1007-1016.[73]

Gabapentin

Gabapentin (Neurontin) is an antiepileptic drug that has demonstrated effectiveness similar to SSRIs/SNRIs in relieving hot flashes. Its mechanism of action is unknown. For a woman to manage her vasomotor symptoms, the dose is started as low as 100 mg at bedtime and increased to as much as 900 mg at bedtime. Although this medication is effective, its somnolence side effects can inhibit its acceptance by women.[73]

Clonidine

Clonidine (Catapres) is an alpha-adrenergic antihypertensive drug that has demonstrated some effectiveness in hot flash relief. Its use is limited due to its significant side effects of hypotension, bradycardia, arrhythmias, constipation, insomnia, and dizziness.[73]

Common Conditions Associated with Aging

Aging presents additional concerns specific to women. Other chapters in this text address pharmacology and the elderly in relationship to the identified topic. However, for the mature woman, certain disorders, like osteoporosis, are best addressed in this chapter.

Bone Health and Aging

Osteoporosis can be a clinical challenge because most women are asymptomatic until a fracture occurs. Bone loss, including osteoporosis and low bone mass (previously known as osteopenia), is estimated to affect more than 53 million Americans.[94] The clinical concern with osteoporosis and low bone mass is fracture, which is associated with significant morbidity and mortality. Approximately 50% of all White women will experience an osteoporosis-related fracture, and fracture risk increases with age. In the year following a hip fracture, there is excess mortality of as much as 36%. Approximately 20% of women who experience such injuries enter long-term care, and only approximately 40% regain their pre-fracture independence.[94] Although often thought of as a concern for older postmenopausal women, the roots of osteoporosis begin in childhood when bone is developing.

Peak bone mass is achieved in the late 20s to mid-30s. Achieving a high peak bone mass requires normal levels of circulating hormones (e.g., estrogen, progesterone, testosterone, growth hormone), gastrointestinal absorption, and endocrinologic function; intake of needed nutrients such as calcium, vitamin D, and protein; and physical activity during childhood and adolescence.

Between approximately 30 and 35 years, women begin to slowly lose bone. This loss occurs when the bone remodeling process of resorption exceeds that of bone formation. The remodeling process constantly breaks down older bone tissue in response to microtrauma and replaces it with new bone so that it does not become too brittle. Osteocytes control the formation and resorption of this tissue by managing osteoclast and osteoclast activity. Osteoclasts resorb bone by creating microscopic holes in the bone surface, a process that takes weeks. Osteoblasts then line the holes created by osteocytes and secrete and mineralize osteoid tissue to form new bone, a process that takes months.

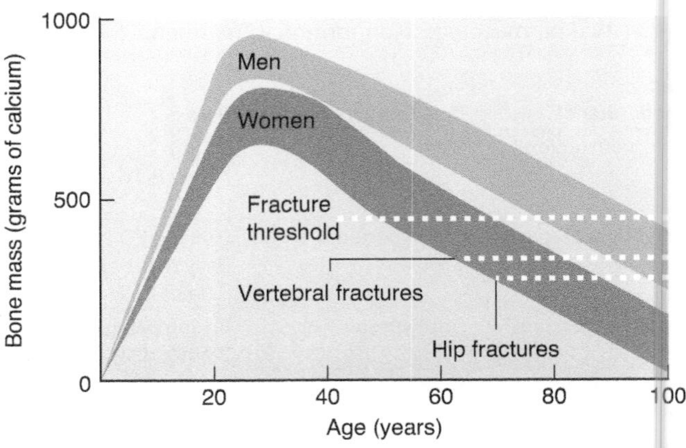

Bone mass density builds until a woman's late 20s, and then declines at a slow rate until menopause. These are times to prepare for menopause by having the highest possible bone mass density by ensuring adequate calcium and vitamin D intake and participating in weight-bearing exercise. For the 6 or 7 years following menopause, bone loss declines most rapidly, as seen above. Women then continue to lose bone mass for the rest of their lives at a slower rate.

Figure 34-2 Changes in bone mass density (BMD) in women and men over time.

During perimenopause, the process of resorption exceeds that of formation, resulting in a more rapid decline in bone density (Figure 34-2).[95] Bone is lost at a rate of approximately 5% to 7% per year during the first 5 years after menopause. Bone loss then slows to approximately the same rate of loss as seen in men, 0.5% to 1.0% per year. This process can result in low bone mass or osteoporosis and explains why women are at higher risk than men for this condition.

Genetics is also an important factor in bone loss. Osteoporosis rates are higher among Whites than among African Americans, with persons of Asian and other racial heritages in between the two. This ethnic association does not mean that African American individuals cannot be at risk for fracture. Indeed, a Black woman who has developed osteoporosis has the same increased risk for fracture as a White woman with osteoporosis.[94]

Bone Mineral Density

Osteoporosis or low bone mass is present when bone strength is compromised, resulting in an increased risk for fracture. Bone strength is related to both bone density and bone quality. While bone quality is difficult to measure, bone mineral density (BMD) can be measured using dual-energy X-ray absorptiometry (DXA). DXA results are used as surrogate markers for identifying the risk for fracture.

DXA results are reported as *T*-scores and *Z*-scores. The *T*-score is a standard deviation calculated above or below the mean score for a sex-matched cohort of young adults. A *T*-score of −1.0 to −2.5 identifies low bone mass, whereas a score of −2.5 or lower identifies osteoporosis.[94] The *Z*-score is a standard deviation calculated above or below the mean score for a gender- and age-matched cohort; a low score suggests possible osteoporosis secondary to a disease process or medications causing extra bone loss. *T*-scores are the most commonly used metrics in testing BMD.

Fractures

Many risk factors for fracture are not related entirely to BMD. As noted earlier, age, gender, and race play a role. Other factors, such as smoking, nutrition, fall risks, and use of drugs such as glucocorticoids, are also potential risk factors for bone loss and fracture.

The World Health Organization's FRAX algorithm (available via the Internet and included on many DXA result reports) was developed to help quantify fracture risk.[96] A 10-year probability for hip and any major osteoporosis-related fracture is calculated through this algorithm, based on the 12 risk factors listed in Box 34-6.

Box 34-6 Risk Factors Included in FRAX Calculation

- Age
- Alcohol (3 or more units per day)
- Body mass index
- Femoral neck BMD (*T*-score or the unit specific to the DXA machine used)
- Gender
- Glucocorticoid therapy (current use or prednisone ≥ 5 mg daily for over any 3-month period)
- Parental history of hip fracture
- Personal history of low-trauma fracture
- Race
- Rheumatoid arthritis
- Secondary osteoporosis
- Smoking currently

Source: Modified from Kanis JA on behalf of the World Health Organization Scientific Group. *Assessment of Osteoporosis at the Primary Health Care Level*. Technical Report. Sheffield, UK: World Health Organization Collaborating Center for Metabolic Bone Diseases, University of Sheffield, UK; 2007. http://www.iofbonehealth.org/sites/default/files/WHO_Technical_Report-2007.pdf.[96]

The FRAX score is applicable to postmenopausal women with low bone mass (*T*-score of −1.0 to −2.5) who have not previously taken medication for osteoporosis. Women who have not taken osteoporosis medications for 1 to 2 years can be considered untreated.[97] The FRAX algorithm is used to assist clinicians in determining when treatment would be cost-effective. In the United States, treatment of a woman with a FRAX score of 3% or higher at the hip or 20% or higher for any major osteoporosis-related fracture is considered cost-effective.[98]

Nonpharmacologic Treatments

Treatment of women with osteoporosis or low bone mass is a multifactorial process. Nonpharmacologic approaches are important both for women with normal BMD to prevent bone loss and for those who already have low bone mass. These measures include adequate dietary calcium and vitamin D; smoking cessation; regular weight-bearing exercises; moderation of alcohol intake; and lifestyle changes to avoid falls. Box 34-7 presents a case study involving a postmenopausal woman with bone health issues.

Pharmacologic Treatment of Women with Osteoporosis

In addition to nonpharmacologic and lifestyle approaches to bone health, pharmacologic therapy is recommended for women with osteoporosis (*T*-score of −2.5 or lower) and select women with low bone mass (*T*-score of −1.0 to −2.5). The National Osteoporosis Foundation (NOF) recommends FDA-approved pharmacotherapy in persons older than age 50 who have any of the conditions listed in Box 34-8.[94]

The goal of treatment for osteoporosis is fracture prevention, and multiple effective treatment options are available. Medications are available in oral, subcutaneous, and intravenous methods of administration and can be taken on varied schedules. Regular—at least yearly—review of the management plan, including nonpharmacologic and pharmacologic approaches, may help the woman continue use of the agents.[94] Drugs are generally selected based on a woman's preference and presence of any existing contraindications. Effectiveness for all approved medication has been established, though few data are available comparing one formulation against another.

Table 34-11 summarizes prescribing information and effectiveness data for FDA-approved therapies for postmenopausal osteoporosis. Prior to initiating pharmacologic therapy, a woman must have a full clinical evaluation, including comprehensive history, physical examination, and selected laboratory testing. Laboratory testing is

Box 34-7 Fact or Fiction? A Woman Can Never Be Too Rich or Too Thin

AM is a 59-year-old woman who experienced menopause at age 53. She has three children ranging in age from 17 to 35 years. AM reports normal menses during her reproductive years. Her current BMI is 21, and she engages in regular exercise three times per week. Her mother had a hip fracture at age 67 subsequent to a fall and never regained full mobility.

AM has not used any hormone therapy. She is generally healthy and takes no regular medications. She reports drinking two glasses of nonfat milk daily and eating a balanced diet. She enjoys a glass of wine occasionally with friends and does not smoke.

AM is at risk for osteoporosis as suggested by her age, low BMI, and mother's hip fracture. She had not previously had a DXA scan, so a FRAX score without BMD was calculated. It indicated that her major osteoporosis-related fracture risk was 14% (greater than 9.5%, the score for a 65-year-old woman without additional risk factors). A DXA was then ordered.[99] AM's DXA *T*-score was found to be −1.4.

To treat her low bone mass, AM was encouraged to assure daily intake of calcium 1200 mg and vitamin D 800 mg to 1000 mg, preferably through her diet but using supplements if needed. Increasing her weight to a BMI of 22 or greater by building lean muscle through strength training that includes resistance and weight-bearing exercise is also important.

AM is scheduled to return in 1 year for a repeat DXA. Ideally, her BMD will stabilize. If it goes down and her FRAX score for major fracture increases to 20% or greater or her hip score reaches 3%, medications should be considered.

important to identify potential contraindications for use, such as hypocalcemia, as well as potentially correctable underlying causes of bone loss.[94]

Health Education and Important Side Effects/Adverse Effects

Health education is critical when initiating any type of pharmacotherapy. Notably, when starting a medication for bone loss, women need to know the signs of osteonecrosis of the jaw (ONJ) as well as low-trauma femoral fracture.

ONJ is a rare adverse effect seen with **bisphosphonates** and very rarely with denosumab. It occurs when a woman who taking one of these medications and who has not had radiation to the jaw develops exposed bone in the mouth that persists for 8 weeks or more.[112] ONJ is more common in women being treated with high-dose bisphosphonates for bone malignancies and who have invasive dental procedures (e.g., periodontal procedures, implant placement, tooth extraction). The risk for ONJ increases with the length of bisphosphonate use. Overall, the risk for ONJ in women taking bisphosphonates for bone loss is less than 1%. Women should have an oral exam prior to initiating bisphosphonate or denosumab therapy and complete any invasive dental procedures if possible. The best prevention against ONJ is to continue regular dental visits and practice excellent personal oral care.[112]

Low-trauma femoral fracture is another unusual adverse effect on which women need education. This type of fracture is also seen with use of bisphosphonates and very rarely with use of denosumab. This kind of fracture has an unusual morphology and occurs with little to no trauma. Many women who develop low-trauma femoral fracture will experience groin or thigh pain prior to the atypical fracture. Women with groin or thigh pain should be carefully evaluated to determine if a stress fracture is present. Bilateral femoral X rays are ordered, followed by magnetic resonance imaging (MRI) or radionuclide bone scan if needed. If treated early, the full fracture may be avoided.[94]

Box 34-8 Indications for Treatment of Women with Osteoporosis Agents

- Hip or vertebral fracture (regardless of DXA *T*-score)
- *T*-score of −2.5 or less at lumbar spine, total hip, or femoral neck
- Low bone mass with FRAX 10-year major osteoporosis fracture probability of 20% or greater or hip fracture probability of 3% or greater

Table 34-11 FDA-Approved Pharmacotherapy Options for Treatment of a Woman with Low Bone Mass and Osteoporosis

Class	Drug: Generic (Brand)	Indication and Doses	Data on Effectiveness	Method of Action	Comments
Bisphosphonate	Alendronate (Fosamax, Binosto)	PMO prevention: 5 mg PO daily; 35 mg PO weekly PMO treatment: 10 mg PO daily, 70 mg PO weekly, 70 mg effervescent PO weekly	50% decrease spine and hip fractures over 3 years in those with prior vertebral fractures or osteoporosis at hip 48% decrease vertebral fractures among women without prior vertebral fractures	Bisphosphonates inhibit osteoclast activity and may have a beneficial effect on osteoblast activity. They reside in the bone tissue and are thought to exert effects for many years after discontinuation.	First-line agents. Contraindicated if estimated GFR < 30–35 mL/minute. Take with 8 oz plain water. Take prior to food, drink, or other drugs. Wait 30 minutes (60 minutes for ibandronate) until consuming any food or drink or lying down. Binostro is taken in 4 oz of room-temperature water on an empty stomach first thing in the morning. Use with caution in women with upper gastrointestinal disease; clinically associated with esophagitis, dysphagia, and ulceration. Effects may last for years after discontinuation. Consider discontinuation after 3–5 years in low-risk women. IV forms are not associated with gastrointestinal effects and do not require timing around food, water, or medications. Check serum creatinine prior to administration of IV ibandronate. Hydrate well and consider acetaminophen on a pretreatment basis prior to use of zolendronic acid to reduce acute-phase reactions (fever, headache, malaise, arthralgias). ONJ is possible with long-term use. Atypical, low-trauma femur fracture occurs in rare instances.
	Alendronate with D (Fosamax Plus D)	PMO treatment: 70 mg/2800 IU PO weekly			
	Ibandronate (Boniva)	PMO prevention and treatment: 150 mg PO monthly PMO treatment: 150 mg PO monthly, 3 mg IV every 3 months	50% decrease vertebral fractures over 3 years Nonvertebral fractures not documented		
	Risedronate (Actonel, Atelvia)	PMO prevention and treatment: 5 mg PO daily, 35 mg PO weekly, 35 mg delayed release PO weekly, 75 mg PO 2 consecutive days monthly, 150 mg PO monthly	41-49% decrease vertebral fractures over 3 years 39% decrease nonvertebral fractures over 3 years		
	Risedronate with calcium (Actonel with Calcium)	PMO prevention and treatment: 35 mg PO weekly with 500 mg calcium carbonate on days not taking active pill			
	Zoledronic acid (Reclast)	PMO prevention: 5 mg IV over 125 minutes every 2 years PMO treatment: 5 mg IV over 15 minutes yearly	70% decrease vertebral fractures over 3 years 25% decrease nonvertebral fractures over 3 years		
Calcitonin	Calcitonin (Miacalcin, Fortical)	PMO treatment in women 5 years post menopause when other agents are ineffective: 200 IU intranasal spray daily, alternate nostrils; 100 u SC/IM daily	30% decrease in vertebral fractures in those women with prior vertebral fractures Has not been shown to reduce nonvertebral fractures	Calcitonin inhibits osteoclast activity and thereby decreases resorption.	Intranasal use is associated with epistaxis, rhinitis, and allergic reactions. May increase risk of malignancy (type not specified).[121] Has been used off-label for pain relief following vertebral fractures.
Estrogen	Conjugated equine estrogens, 17 β-estradiol with or without progestin	PMO prevention	34% decrease of vertebral fractures 23% decrease of other osteoporotic fractures	Estrogens promote osteoblast activity and assist with maintaining balance in bone remodeling processes.	Take with or without food. Also reduces menopause-related vasomotor symptoms and vulvovaginal atrophy. Use lowest effective dose for shortest period of time. Not used for osteoporosis prevention unless also needed for relief of menopause-related symptoms. May increase risk for coronary heart disease, stroke, venous thromboembolic events, and cholelithiasis.
Estrogen agonist/antagonist	Raloxifene (Evista)	PMO prevention and treatment: 60 mg PO daily	30% decrease vertebral fractures in those women with prior vertebral fractures over 3 years 55% decrease vertebral fractures in those women without prior vertebral fractures over 3 years	Raloxifene exerts estrogenic actions on bone to assist in maintaining balance in bone remodeling processes.	First-line agent. Take with or without food. Also approved for breast cancer prevention. May cause hot flashes and leg cramps. May increase risk for venous thromboembolism. Do not combine with estrogen.

(continues)

Table 34-11 FDA-Approved Pharmacotherapy Options for Treatment of a Woman with Low Bone Mass and Osteoporosis (*continued*)

Class	Drug: Generic (Brand)	Indication and Doses	Data on Effectiveness	Method of Action	Comments
Tissue-selective estrogen complex	Conjugated estrogens/ bazedoxifene (Duavee)	PMO prevention: 0.45 mg/20 mg daily	1.51% decrease lumbar spine BMD after 12 months 1.21% decrease total hip BMD after 12 months	Bazedoxifene exerts estrogenic actions on bone to assist in maintaining balance in bone remodeling processes.	For use in women with a uterus. Take with or without food. Also reduces menopause-related vasomotor symptoms and vulvovaginal atrophy. Use lowest effective dose for shortest period of time. Not used for osteoporosis prevention unless also needed for relief of menopause-related symptoms. May increase risk for coronary heart disease, stroke, venous thromboembolic events, and cholelithiasis.
Parathyroid hormone	PTH(1-34), teriparatide (Forteo)	PMO treatment: 20 mcg SC daily (woman self-administers)	65% decrease vertebral fractures after 18 months 53% decrease nonvertebral low-trauma fractures after 18 months	PTH is an anabolic agent that activates osteoblasts when administered in intermittent doses. Daily injections stimulate new bone formation.	Second-line agent; use if first-line agents are ineffective. Duration of therapy no more than 18–24 months. Most effective when used sequentially after bisphosphonate. A first-line agent is prescribed to maintain BMD after PTH therapy. Can cause leg cramps, dizziness, and nausea. Not to be taken by women at high risk for osteosarcoma, hypercalcemia, bone metastases, or bone malignancy history.
RANKL inhibitor	Denosumab (Prolia)	PMO treatment for women at high risk of fractures: 60 mg SC every 6 ms, administered by healthcare professional	68% decrease vertebral fractures over 3 years 48% decrease hip fractures over 3 years 20% decrease nonvertebral fractures over 3 years	Denosumab binds to RANKL. RANKL is needed to mature pre-osteoclasts into osteoclasts for the bone resorption process.	Bone loss can be rapid after discontinuation. Can cause skin rash and skin infection. Rare occurrence of ONJ. Atypical, low-trauma femur fracture occurs in rare instances.

Abbreviations: BMD = bone mineral density; ONJ = osteonecrosis of the jaw; PMO = postmenopausal osteoporosis; PTH = parathyroid hormone; RANKL = receptor activator of nuclear factor kappa-B ligand.

Sources: Data from Black DM, Cummings SR, Karpf DB, et al. Randomised trial of effect of alendronate on risk of fracture in women with existing vertebral fractures. Fracture Intervention Trial Research Study Group. *Lancet.* 1996;348(9041):1535-1541[100]; Black DM, Reid IR, Boonen S, et al. The effect of 3 versus 6 years of zoledronic acid treatment of osteoporosis: a randomized extension to the HORIZON-Pivotal Fracture Trial (PFT) [erratum, *J Bone Miner Res.* 2012;27(12):2612]. *J Bone Miner Res.* 2012;27(2):243-254[101]; Boonen S, Adachi JD, Man Z, et al. Treatment with denosumab reduces the incidence of new vertebral and hip fractures in postmenopausal women at high risk. *J Clin Endocrinol Metab.* 2011;96(6):1727-1736[102]; Chesnut CH III, Silverman S, Andriano K, et al. A randomized trial of nasal spray salmon calcitonin in postmenopausal women with established osteoporosis: the prevent recurrence of osteoporotic fractures study. PROOF Study Group. *Am J Med.* 2000;109:(4):267-276[103]; Chesnut CH III, Skag A, Christiansen C, et al.; Oral Ibandronate Osteoporosis Vertebral Fracture Trial in North American and Europe. Effects of oral ibandronate administered daily or intermittently on fracture risk in postmenopausal osteoporosis. *J Bone Miner Res.* 2004;19(8):1241-1249[104]; Cummings SR, Black DM, Thompson DE, et al. Effect of alendronate on risk of fracture in women with low bone density but without vertebral fractures: results from the Fracture Intervention Trial. *JAMA.* 1998;280(24):2077-2082[105];Delmas PD, Ensrud KE, Adachi JD, et al.; Multiple Outcomes of Raloxifene Evaluation Investigators. Efficacy of raloxifene on vertebral fracture risk reduction in postmenopusal women with osteoporosis: four-year results from a randomized clinical trial. *J Clin Endocrinol Metab.* 2001;87(8):3609-3617[106]; Harris ST, Watts NB, Genant HK, et al. Effects of risedronate treatment on vertebral and nonvertebral fractures in women with postmenopausal osteoporosis: a randomized controlled trial. Vertebral Efficacy with Risedronate Therapy (VERT) Study Group. *JAMA.* 1999;282(14):1344-1352[107]; Hodsman AB, Hanley DA, Ettinger MP, et al. Efficacy and safety of human parathyroid hormone-(1-84) in increasing bone mineral density in postmenopausal osteoporosis. *J Clin Endocrinol Metab.* 2003;88(11):5212-5220[108]; National Osteoporosis Foundation (NOF). *2014 Guide to Prevention and Treatment of Osteoporosis.* Washington, DC: National Osteoporosis Foundation; 2014. www .nof.org/hcp/clinicians-guide. Accessed August 4, 2014[94]; Overman RA, Borse M, Gourlay ML. Salmon calcitonin use and associated cancer risk. *Ann Pharmacother.* 2013;47(12):1675-1684[109]; Rossouw JE, Anderson GL, Prentice RL, et al. Risks and benefits of estrogen plus progestin in healthy postmenopausal women: principal results from the Women's Health Initiative randomized controlled trial. *JAMA.* 2002;288(3):321-333[34]; Silverman SL, Christiansen C, Genant HK, et al. Efficacy of bazedoxifene in reducing new vertebral fracture risk in postmenopausal women with osteoporosis: results from a 3-year, randomized, placebo-, and active-controlled clinical trial. *J Bone Miner Res.* 2008;23(12):1923-1934[110]; U.S. Preventive Services Task Force. Screening for osteoporosis: U.S. Preventive Services Task Force recommendation statement. *Ann Intern Med.* 2011;154(5):356-364. http://www.uspreventiveservicestaskforce.org/uspstf10/osteoporosis/osteors.htm.[111]

Follow-up and Discontinuing Pharmacotherapy

NOF recommends repeating the DXA every 2 years or more often if needed until the BMD stabilizes.[94] Women who achieve a significantly improved BMD with therapy may be able to discontinue pharmacotherapy temporarily. Although the optimal duration of therapy has not been clearly established, several medications now have the recommendation to evaluate for discontinuation after 3 to 5 years (e.g., bisphosphonates, raloxifene).

If a woman discontinues pharmacotherapy, it is imperative that she continues with nonpharmacologic management. Her BMD should be reevaluated regularly, usually every 2 years.[94] If her BMD levels fall again, she can be reevaluated for resuming pharmacotherapy. If the BMD is in the low bone mass range and she has been off pharmacotherapy for 1 to 2 years, a FRAX calculation can be done to assist with guiding the decision to resume pharmacotherapy.[94]

Aging and Cognitive Function, Mood, and Depression

Many midlife women experience labile moods, anxiety, and depression. Cognitive changes such as forgetfulness, difficulty concentrating, and word finding are also frequently described.[113–115] Whether these changes are related to normal aging processes, menopause-related hormonal changes, sleep difficulties, or some combination of these factors is unclear. Cognitive and mood symptoms may also be related to medication side effects and can be heightened with increased stress.

Treatment of Women with Mood Changes and Depressive Symptoms

Women who describe dysphoric symptoms need to have a full history and physical examination to determine the etiology. Depression may recur in a small subset of postmenopausal women who experienced postpartum depression or have a prior history of depressive disorder. Women who experienced menopause surgically may have an increased risk for depression and may benefit from ET.

Potential drug side effects and sleep disturbances must also be considered. For example, MPA use has been associated with labile mood and dysphoria. Use of a different progestin may reduce or eliminate these symptoms. If sleep disruptions are present, improving sleep may positively affect mood. Antidepressants used to minimize vasomotor symptoms may have an added benefit by treating mood disorders.[10] More information can be found in the *Mental Health* chapter.

Treatment of Women with Cognition Deficits

Women who describe cognitive changes need to have a full history and physical examination to determine the seriousness of the changes. Reproductive hormones and cortisol influence brain function; however, the effect of hormones on concentration, memory, and other cognitive functions is not well understood. Sleep disruptions have been associated with transient cognitive changes and, as with mood alterations, may improve when sleep is restored. Word finding and quick-recall memory problems can occur intermittently at varied times among both women and men at midlife and is usually not serious. Permanent memory loss or the inability to complete usual tasks at home and work can be serious, however, and may require referral for an in-depth neurologic evaluation.

Dementia risk may be reduced through various modalities. Maintaining physical and mental activity and a healthy diet high in vitamin E may provide some protection. Multiple dietary supplements (e.g., gingko biloba, B-complex vitamins, omega-3 fatty acids) are advertised as preventing cognitive decline and dementia; however, data supporting these claims are sparse and contradictory. The longitudinal Study of Women's Health Across the Nation (SWAN)[113] demonstrated a protective effect among women who used oral contraceptives or HT prior to their FMP, but deleterious effects were identified when HT was started after the FMP in the SWAN study and the WHI Memory Study (WHIMS).[116] NAMS and IMS do not recommend the use of HT for dementia or cognition protection.[10,54]

Headaches Among Midlife and Older Women

During perimenopause, women may note that headaches increase in frequency and intensity, especially among individuals who have a history of menstrual-related headaches. Extended-release estrogen/progestin monophasic pills or patches may reduce or eliminate menstrual-related headaches in perimenopausal women. Although there is not a clear association between headaches and menopause, some data suggest that progestins, especially MPA, may precipitate or aggravate a headache. For these women, micronized progesterone may be better tolerated. The chapter *The Central Nervous System* provides information about acute and preventive therapy for headaches.

Sleep Disturbances and Women

Wakefulness, which may begin in perimenopause, is a common postmenopausal symptom. Approximately 50% of women report experiencing sleep disturbances at midlife.[117] Sleep disturbances may be attributed to nocturnal hot flashes, wakefulness related to anxiety or stress, nocturia, and other chronic conditions (e.g., restless leg syndrome, arthritis, fibromyalgia), as well as to age- and hormone-related changes in sleep architecture. These factors result in extended sleep latency, longer transitions from one sleep stage to the next, and reduced time in deep sleep stages (3, 4, and rapid-eye movement [REM]). Sleep disturbances affect different women in different ways and may present as difficulty falling asleep, periods of nocturnal wakefulness, and early awakening resulting in poor-quality, nonrestorative sleep. Sleep disturbances increase the risk for stroke, cardiovascular disease, hypertension, and motor vehicle accidents. They are also associated with weight gain, insulin resistance, depression, and reduced libido as well as difficulty with cognitive functioning in recall, concentration, and problem solving.[117]

Treatment of Women with Sleep Disturbances

The first step to treating women with sleep disorders is recognition that a problem exists. Careful clinical evaluation is needed to determine if there is an underlying cause such as restless leg syndrome, sleep apnea, or hot flashes. If a woman is waking because of hot flashes and sweats, amelioration of her vasomotor symptoms may restore sleep. Although not prescribed solely for sleep disturbances, estrogen has been shown to reduce sleep latency and improve sleep quality.[118] Certain medications that a woman is taking for other reasons may be taken at bedtime to promote sleep—for example, gabapentin or micronized progesterone may have soporific effects. If a sleep disturbance does not have an underlying etiology, lifestyle changes are the first-line therapy. Behavioral therapies and many mind–body therapies can be beneficial as well.[117]

Pharmacologic Treatment of Women with Sleep Disturbances

If behavioral and mind–body therapies are ineffective, medication therapy to help with difficulty falling or staying asleep may be successful. Several medication classes can be used for a short period of time to break a cycle of insomnia or sleep disturbance, but should not be continued routinely.[114] FDA-approved medications for insomnia include non-benzodiazepine ligands (new-generation hypnotics), doxepin (Silenor), ramelteon (Rozerem), and some benzodiazepines. Other prescription and over-the counter drugs are also used for insomnia due to their soporific side effects (e.g., antihistamines, Trazodone). Melatonin (available in varied over-the-counter formulations) has evidence-based support for use in treating circadian rhythm phase disturbances.[114] Consideration is needed for potential drug–drug interactions and side effects such as parasomnias and morning fatigue ("hangover" effect). These considerations are especially important in aging women who are at increased risk for polypharmacy, falls, and motor vehicle accidents. Medications with a longer half-life may provide assistance for middle-of-the-night or early waking; however, these agents also have an increased potential for morning fatigue if taken during the night. Conversely, zolpidem has the shortest half-life and potentially can be dosed during the night when early awakening occurs with a lower risk for morning fatigue.[114] Table 34-12 lists selected medications used for sleep disturbances in midlife women.

Sexual Desire and Functioning

Decreased sexual desire is a common concern among perimenopausal and postmenopausal women. Although low libido among women is generally accepted to be related to low androgen levels, "testosterone deficiency" has not been standardized for women and androgen levels (free and total testosterone, and androstenedione) do not correlate with sexual function in women.[115] Nevertheless, testosterone supplementation, both with estrogen and alone, in postmenopausal women has been demonstrated to increase sexual desire, satisfaction, and frequency and to reduce distress, although most studies do not use standardized criteria, especially to determine androgen deficiency.[119–121]

A comprehensive sexual history is essential to determine which type of sexual problem is being experienced and whether the woman might benefit from available therapies. Potential physical, psychological, and social factors amenable to intervention need to be addressed, including depression, anxiety, and fatigue; response to stress; relationship issues; and sexual dysfunction in the partner. Drugs that might affect sexual function must also be taken into consideration. For example, lipid-lowering medications can reduce libido, and oral estrogen therapy reduces bioavailable androgen by increasing SHBG, which binds free testosterone and may decrease libido.

Pharmacologic Treatment of Women with Sexual Dysfunction

Testosterone is used on an off-label basis with evidence-based practice in small doses to treat low libido in postmenopausal women. Formulations include testosterone creams and gels that are FDA approved for use in men and custom compounded preparations of micronized testosterone in oral, transdermal, or intramuscular pellet

Table 34-12 Selected Medications Used to Treat Women with Sleep Disturbances

Prescription Drugs	
Name and Dose	**Half-life**
Sedatives and Hypnotics *(May break a cycle of insomnia; use as a last resort for a short period of time.)*	
Short-Acting Non-benzodiazepines *(Fewer withdrawal effects, lower addictive tendency, and less decrease in effectiveness with time than benzodiazepines. May cause memory loss if awakened or inadequate time in bed for sleep.)*	
Eszopiclone (Lunesta) 1 mg, 2 mg, 3 mg	6 hours
Zolpidem (Ambien) 5 mg,10 mg; (Ambien CR) 6.25 mg, 12.5 mg	2.5–3 hours
Zaleplon (Sonata) 5 mg, 10 mg	1–3 hours
Benzodiazepines *(To be used no more than 3 times per week to minimize tolerance and dependence. Next-day sedation and rebound insomnia with discontinuation may occur. High-fat meals delay effects.)*	
Alprazolam (Xanax) 0.25 mg, 0.5 mg, 1 mg, 2 mg; (Xanax XR) 0.5 mg, 1 mg, 2 mg, 3 mg; avoid with glaucoma	11–16 hours
Diazepam (Valium) 2 mg, 5 mg, 10 mg; avoid with glaucoma	30–60 hours
Flurazepam (generic) 15 mg, 30 mg	40–250 hours
Lorazepam (Ativan) 0.5 mg, 1 mg, 2 mg	14 hours
Temazepam (Restoril) 7.5 mg, 15 mg, 22.5 mg, 30 mg	8–9 hours
Other Drugs	
Ramelteon (Rozerem) 8 mg; a synthetic melatonin receptor agonist	1–2.5 hours
Trazodone (generic) 50 mg, 100 mg, 150 mg, 300 mg; antidepressant used off-label as a sleep aid at doses of 25–50 mg	3–6 hours
Nonprescription Drugs	
Diphenhydramine (e.g., Benadryl): Combination medications have diphenhydramine HCl as a sleep aid along with the analgesic acetaminophen (Tylenol PM) or ibuprofen (Advil PM) Acetaminophen combinations combined with 3 or more alcoholic drinks daily may cause liver damage Daily use may cause rebound wakefulness	3.5–9 hours
Botanicals *(Lack scientific data to support effectiveness.)*	
Chamomile	
Hops	
Lavender	
Lemon balm	
Passion flower	
Valerian	
Melatonin, Serotonin *(Beneficial for sleep-phase disorders.)*	

Source: Modified from Proctor A, Bianchi MT. Clinical pharmacology in sleep medicine. *ISRN Pharmacol.* 2012;2012(914168):1-14. http://dx.doi.org/10.5402/2012/914168. Accessed August 4, 2014.[114]

forms. Topical gels and creams are applied to the genital area (vulva, clitoral, mons pubis). Topical preparations may stimulate dark hair growth on any skin surface, so the mons pubis is an optimal site for application. Lipid levels and liver function studies are monitored prior to and during use. Serum free testosterone levels should be maintained below the upper limit for premenopausal women. It may require 6 to 8 weeks for effects to be apparent. Side effects with appropriate doses are rare. If high doses are used, a woman may experience acne, fluid retention, lipid derangement, and masculinization (e.g., excess body hair, deepened voice, cliteromegaly). Testosterone should be avoided in perimenopausal and postmenopausal women with preexisting acne, or who are pregnant or lactating.[11]

Only one testosterone formulation has received FDA approval as a treatment for postmenopausal women with moderate to severe vasomotor symptoms, although this product is also used off label for low libido. Available as a generic, it comes in a combination tablet with esterified estrogens (EE) and methyl testosterone (MT) in two strengths: 0.625 mg EE with 1.25 MT or 1.25 mg EE with 2.5 mg MT. Women who have an intact uterus need endometrial protection with a progestin or endometrial monitoring when taking EE with MT. Some clinicians are using this preparation less frequently because the estrogen dose in EE with MT is higher than most low doses used today. Additional information about testosterone and sexual dysfunction can be found in the *Sexual Dysfunction* chapter.

Vaginal and Vulvar Symptoms

As estrogen levels change after menopause, the lining of the vagina becomes thinner, pale, and less elastic with flattened rugae. Vaginal fluid becomes scant and yellow, with an absence of lactobacilli and a more alkaline pH. These changes increase the likelihood of symptomatic vaginitis, which is discussed in the *Vaginal Conditions* chapter. Sexual activity may be painful and cause vaginal spotting from microabrasions, which in turn increase the likelihood of acquiring sexually transmitted infections. Vulvodynia, which can also cause postmenopausal dyspareunia, is discussed in the *Vulvar Disorders* chapter. Vaginal atrophy will develop over time in all postmenopausal women. Bothersome atrophy symptoms will benefit from excellent perineal hygiene (use gentle cleansers externally only, avoid fragrances, wear breathable fabrics) with the use of lubricants and moisturizers, and local estrogen may also be needed.

Treatment of Women with Vulvovaginal Symptoms

Nonprescription water-based lubricants (e.g., Astro-glide, K-Y Jelly, Gyne-Moistrin) may be helpful for dryness during sexual activity. Women should be counseled to avoid non-water-based products (e.g., Vaseline, baby oil, butter, coconut butter, fish oils) because they can irritate the sensitive mucous membranes around and inside the vagina and may damage condoms. It is important to discuss sexual activity with women and to remind women that regular stimulation from sexual activity promotes blood flow to the vagina, protects the vagina to some degree from atrophy, and supports improved sexual response.

Vaginal moisturizers can reduce vaginal irritation not related to intercourse. Lubricants are still usually needed during sexual activity even when a vaginal moisturizer is used.

Vaginal symptoms that are not fully relieved with moisturizers and lubricants will usually be relieved with HT. Both systemic HT and local vaginal estrogen therapy are effective. Estrogen therapy promotes revascularization of the vaginal epithelium and restores the normal pH of the vagina. Non-oral routes are also more advantageous than oral delivery, because local therapy avoids the first pass through the liver, helps to maintain steady blood levels, and decreases the incidence of gastrointestinal side effects. Low-dose vaginal therapy has a more benign risk profile than oral therapy because blood levels of the active ingredients are lower, yet still effective. A Cochrane review noted no increase in women's risk for venous thromboembolism when using vaginal estrogen, but there are no studies in women at high risk for VTE.[122] Most studies indicate that the risk of endometrial cancer in women using low-dose vaginal estrogen is low, but long-term studies are lacking. For women whose risk for breast cancer is unknown, studies are unclear about risk of subsequent breast cancer development and low-dose vaginal estrogen use. Contraindications to vaginal estrogen include women with undiagnosed vaginal bleeding. Use by women with current or past endometrial or breast cancer is controversial.[123]

Local therapy is used for women who essentially have only vulvovaginal symptoms.[10] Local therapy will begin to provide relief within a few days, whereas systemic therapy may take weeks to become effective. For this reason, both may be used initially for a woman who needs systemic therapy and is also experiencing significant vulvovaginal symptoms. The local therapy will provide relief for the vulvovaginal symptoms quickly and can be tapered off and discontinued once the systemic therapy has reached full effect. NAMS suggests that systemic progestin therapy is not needed when local estrogen alone is used; however, this recommendation is controversial.[10]

Ospemifene (Osphena) is an estrogen agonist/antagonist with FDA approval for treating women with moderate to severe menopause-related dyspareunia, which often occurs as a result of vulvovaginal atrophy or atrophic vaginitis. A small one-year study of effectiveness and safety demonstrated improvement in women's symptoms and no cases of VTE, endometrial hyperplasia, or cancer.[124] As previously mentioned, ospemifene works by activating estrogen pathways in some tissues and blocking estrogen pathways in others. This agent has agonistic effects on the endometrium, thereby reducing the risk of endometrial hyperplasia or cancer.

Conclusion

The transition to postmenopause can be smooth or may be accompanied by bothersome symptoms. For those women who experience moderate to severe symptoms, several therapies are available.

Many women identify midlife as a time for reflecting on their health and life accomplishments. This provides an opportunity for clinicians to discuss health-promoting behaviors with women that will reduce risks for conditions such as heart disease, diabetes, bone loss, and cardiovascular disease; health-promoting behaviors can also reduce menopause-related symptoms such as hot flashes and sleep disturbances.

Some of the changes women experience at midlife have more to do with aging, such as decreased skin resilience and turgor, bone loss, or weight gain, than with menopause per se. Other significant changes may include relationships, as this may the time when children are leaving home or returning—some of whom are doing well and others who are not. Relationships with partners may need to be renegotiated whether or not children are involved. Midlife presents a perfect opportunity for clinicians to encourage women to take time to reinvest in themselves as individual women because it is likely that they live for many more years.

Resources

Organization	Description	Website
Centers for Disease Control and Prevention and National Institute of Aging	Federal site with consumer and provider general information about menopause and aging. The majority of the information is available in both English and Spanish.	www.cdc.gov/reproductivehealth/womensrh/ www.nia.nih.gov/health/publication/menopause
National Osteoporosis Foundation	Organization dedicated to issues concerning osteoporosis. Includes webpages called "Bone Source" for healthcare providers with current literature available for downloading.	http://nof.org/
North American Menopause Society (NAMS)	Professional organization dedicated to issues surrounding menopause. Some materials are free; others are limited to members of NAMS. The free consumer app "MenoPro" features information for consumers as well as ability to keep notes about bothersome symptoms so as to discuss them with the healthcare provider. *Menopause*, NAMS's professional journal, is also available as an app.	www.menopause.org/

Apps

Multiple apps exist, such as "Menopause Tracking," that help a woman keep a diary of bothersome symptoms. Some are free while others are available at a modest cost. However, most are independent, as opposed to NAMS's "MenoPro" app. Check iTunes and Google Play, among others.

References

1. Centers for Disease Control and Prevention. National vital statistics, health, United States 2011 web updates. http://www.cdc.gov/nchs/data/hus/2011/022.pdf. Accessed July 7, 2014.
2. World Bank. Data tables: life expectancy at birth, female. 2014. http://data.worldbank.org/indicator/SP.DYN.LE00.FE.IN?order=wbapi_data_value_2012+wbapi_data_value+wbapi_data_value-last&sort=desc. Accessed July 7, 2014.
3. Administration on Aging, Administration for Community Living, Department of Health and Human Services. A profile of older Americans: 2012. http://www.aoa.gov/Aging_Statistics/Profile/2012/docs/2012profile.pdf.
4. Wooten JM. Pharmacotherapy considerations in elderly adults. *So Med J.* 2012;105(8):437-445.
5. Kaufman DW, Kelly JP, Rosenberg L, Anderson TE, Mitchell AA. Recent patterns of medication use in the ambulatory adult population of the United States: the Slone survey. *JAMA.* 2002;287(3):337-344.
6. Qato DM, Alexander GC, Conti RM, Johnson M, Schumm P, Lindau ST. Use of prescription and over-the-counter medications and dietary supplements among older adults in the United States. *JAMA.* 2008;300(24):2867-2878.
7. Piau A, Hein C, Nourhashemi F, Sebbagh M, Legrain S. Definition and issue of medications underuse in frail elderly patients. *Geriatr Psychol Neuropsych.* 2012;10(2):129-135.
8. Siris ES, Modi A, Tang J, Gandi S, Sen S. Substantial under-treatment among women diagnosed with osteoporosis in a U.S. managed-care population: a retrospective analysis. *Curr Med Res Opin.* 2014;30(1):123-130.
9. Fontenot HB, Fantasia HC. Women's health, pharmacology, and aging. *JOGNN.* 2014;43(2):224-225.
10. North American Menopause Society (NAMS), 2012 Hormone Therapy Position Statement Advisory Panel. The 2012 hormone therapy position statement of the North American Menopause Society. *Menopause.* 2012;19(3):257-271.
11. Jane FM, Davis SR. A practitioner's toolkit for managing the menopause. *Climacteric.* 2014;17(5):564-579.
12. El Khoudary SR, McClure CK, VoPham T. Longitudinal assessment of the menopausal transition, endogenous sex hormones, and perception of physical functioning: the Study of Women's Health Across the Nation. *J Gerontol A Biol Sci Med Sci.* 2014;69(8):1011-1017.

13. Porter M, Penney GC, Russell D, Russell E, Templeton A. A population based survey of women's experience of the menopause. *Br J Obstet Gynaecol.* 1996; 103(10):1025-1028.
14. Mishra GD, Kuh D. Health symptoms during midlife in relation to menopausal transition: British prospective cohort study. *BMJ.* 2012;344:e402.
15. Harlow SD, Gass M, Hall JE, et al. Executive summary of the Stages of Reproductive Aging Workshop + 10: addressing the unfinished agenda of staging reproductive aging. *Menopause.* 2012;19(4):387-395.
16. Fritz MA, Speroff L. *Clinical Gynecologic and Endocrinology and Infertility.* 8th ed. Philadelphia, PA: Lippincott Williams & Wilkins, 2010: 673-748.
17. North American Menopause Society (NAMS). *Menopause Practice: A Clinician's Guide.* 4th ed. Mayfield Heights OH: North American Menopause Society; 2010.
18. Babiker FA, De Windt LJ, van Eickels M, Grohe C, Meyer R, Doevendans PA. Estrogenic hormone action in the heart: regulatory network and function. *Cardiovasc Res.* 2002;53(3):709-719.
19. Htun H, Holth LT, Walker D, Davie JR, Hager GL. Direct visualization of the human estrogen receptor alpha reveals a role for ligand in the nuclear distribution of the receptor. *Mol Biol Cell.* 1999;10(2): 471-486.
20. Alexander IM. The history of hormone therapy use and recent controversy related to heart disease and breast cancer arising from prevention trial outcomes. *J Midwifery Womens Health.* 2012;57:547-557.
21. Wilson R. *Feminine Forever.* New York: Evans; 1996.
22. Mack TM, Pike MC, Henderson BE, et al. Estrogens and endometrial cancer in a retirement community. *N Engl J Med.* 1976;294(23):1262-1267.
23. Smith DC, Prentice R, Thompson DJ, Herrmann WL. Association of exogenous estrogen and endometrial carcinoma. *N Engl J Med.* 1975;293(23):1164-1167.
24. Bush TL, Barrett-Connor E, Cowan LD, et al. Cardiovascular mortality and noncontraceptive use of estrogen in women: results from the Lipid Research Clinics Program Follow-up Study. *Circulation.* 1987; 75(6):1102-1109.
25. Stampfer MJ, Colditz GA, Willett WC, et al. Postmenopausal estrogen therapy and cardiovascular disease: ten-year follow-up from the Nurses' Health Study. *N Engl J Med.* 1991;325(11):756-762.
26. Writing Group for PEPI. Effects of estrogen or estrogen/progestin regimens on heart disease risk factors in postmenopausal women. The Postmenopausal Estrogen/Progestin Interventions (PEPI) trial. *JAMA.* 1995;273(3):199-208.
27. Weiss NS, Ure CL, Ballard JH, Williams AR, Daling JR. Decreased risk of fractures of the hip and lower forearm with postmenopausal use of estrogen. *N Engl J Med.* 1980;303(21):1195-1198.
28. Baldereschi M, Di Carlo A, Lepore V, et al. Estrogen-replacement therapy and Alzheimer's disease in the Italian Longitudinal Study on Aging. *Neurology.* 1998; 50(4):996-1002.
29. Tang MX, Jacobs D, Stern Y, et al. Effect of oestrogen during menopause on risk and age at onset of Alzheimer's disease. *Lancet.* 1996;348(9025):429-432.
30. Jacobs EJ, White E, Weiss NS. Exogenous hormones, reproductive history, and colon cancer (Seattle, Washington, USA). *Cancer Causes Control.* 1994; 5(4): 359-366.
31. Bush TL, Whiteman M, Flaws JA. Hormone replacement therapy and breast cancer: a qualitative review. *Obstet Gynecol.* 2001;98(3):498-508.
32. Hulley S, Grady D, Bush T, et al. Randomized trial of estrogen plus progestin for secondary prevention of coronary heart disease in postmenopausal women. Heart and Estrogen/Progestin Replacement Study (HERS) Research Group. *JAMA.* 1998;280(7):605-613.
33. Grady D, Herrington D, Bittner V, et al. Cardiovascular disease outcomes during 6.8 years of hormone therapy: Heart and Estrogen/Progestin Replacement Study follow-up (HERS II). *JAMA.* 2002;288(1):49-57.
34. Rossouw JE, Anderson GL, Prentice RL, et al. Risks and benefits of estrogen plus progestin in healthy postmenopausal women: principal results from the Women's Health Initiative randomized controlled trial. *JAMA.* 2002;288(3):321-333.
35. Manson JE, Hsia J, Johnson KC, et al.; WHI Investigators. Estrogen plus progestin and the risk of coronary heart disease. *N Engl J Med.* 2003;349(6):523-634.
36. Anderson GL, Limacher M, Assaf AR, et al.; Women's Health Initiative Steering Committee. Effects of conjugated equine estrogen in postmenopausal women with hysterectomy: the Women's Health Initiative randomized controlled trial. *JAMA.* 2004;291(14):1701-1712.
37. Hodis HN, Mack WJ, Lobo RA, et al.; Estrogen in the Prevention of Atherosclerosis Trial Research Group. Estrogen in the prevention of atherosclerosis: a randomized, double-blind, placebo controlled trial. *Ann Intern Med.* 2001;135(11):939-953.
38. Beral V; Million Women Study Collaborators. Breast cancer and hormone-replacement therapy in the Million Women Study. *Lancet.* 2003;362(9382):419-427.

39. Reeves GK, Beral V, Green J, Gathani T, Bull D; Million Women Study Collaborators. Hormonal therapy for menopause and breast cancer risk by histological type: a cohort study and meta-analysis. *Lancet Oncol.* 2006;7(11):910-918.
40. Beral V, Reeves G, Bull D, Green J; Million Women Study Collaborators. Breast cancer risk in relation to the interval between menopause and starting hormone therapy. *J Natl Cancer Inst.* 2011;103(4):296-305.
41. Clarke SC, Kelleher J, Lloyd-Jones H, Slack M, Schofiel PM. A study of hormone replacement therapy in postmenopausal women with ischaemic heart disease: the Papworth HRT atherosclerosis study. *BJOG.* 2002; 109(9):1056-1062.
42. Harman SM, Black DM, Naftolin F, et al. Arterial imaging outcomes and cardiovascular risk factors in recently menopausal women: a randomized trial. *Ann Intern Med.* 2014;161(4):249-260.
43. U.S. Preventive Service Task Force. *Guide to Preventive Services.* Rockville, MD: Agency for Healthcare Research and Quality; 1996.
44. Heiss G, Wallace R, Anderson GL, et al.; WHI Investigators. Health risks and benefits 3 years after stopping randomized treatment with estrogen and progestin. *JAMA.* 2008;299(9):1036-1045.
45. Rossouw JE, Prentice RL, Manson JE, et al. Postmenopausal hormone therapy and risk of cardiovascular disease by age and years since menopause. *JAMA.* 2007;297(13):1465-1477.
46. Chlebowski RT, Kuller LH, Prentice RL, et al.; WHI Investigators. Breast cancer after use of estrogen plus progestin in postmenopausal women. *N Engl J Med.* 2009;360(6):573-587.
47. LaCroix AZ, Chlebowski RT, Manson JE, et al.; WHI Investigators. Health outcomes after stopping conjugated equine estrogens among postmenopausal women with prior hysterectomy: a randomized controlled trial. *JAMA.* 2011;305(13):1305-1314.
48. Jemal A, Ward E, Thun MJ. Recent trends in breast cancer incidence rates by age and tumor characteristics among U.S. women. *Breast Cancer Res.* 2007; 9(3):R28.
49. Glass AG, Lacey JV Jr, Carreon JD, Hoover RN. Breast cancer incidence, 1980-2006: combined roles of menopausal hormone therapy, screening mammography, and estrogen receptor status. *J Natl Cancer Inst.* 2007;99(15):1152-1161.
50. De P, Neutel CI, Olivotto I, Morrison H. Breast cancer incidence and hormone replacement therapy in Canada. *J Natl Cancer Inst.* 2010;102(19):1489-1495.
51. Alexander IM. Hormone therapy and incidence of breast cancer. *Climacteric.* 2011;14(2):299-300.
52. Col NF, Kim JA, Chlebowski RT. Menopausal hormone therapy after breast cancer: a meta-analysis and critical appraisal of the evidence. *Breast Cancer Res.* 2005;7:R535-R540.
53. Holmberg L, Iversen OE, Rudenstam CM, et al.; HABITS Study Group. Increased risk of recurrence after hormone replacement therapy in breast cancer survivors. *J Natl Cancer Inst.* 2008;100(7): 475-482.
54. de Villiers TJ, Pines A, Panay N, et al.; International Menopause Society. Updated 2013 International Menopause Society recommendations on menopause hormone therapy and preventive strategies for midlife health. *Climacteric.* 2013;16(3):316-337.
55. de Villiers TJ, Gass ML, Haines CJ, et al. Global consensus statement on menopausal hormone therapy. *Climacteric.* 2013;16(2):203-204.
56. Sit AS, Modugno F, Weissfeld JL, Berga SL, Ness RB. Hormone replacement therapy formulations and risk of epithelial ovarian carcinoma. *Gynecol Oncol.* 2002;86(2):118-123.
57. Greiser CM, Greiser EM, Dören M. Menopausal hormone therapy and risk of ovarian cancer: systematic review and meta-analysis. *Hum Reprod Update.* 2007;13:453-463.
58. Zhou B, Sun Q, Cong R, et al. Hormone replacement therapy and ovarian cancer risk: a meta-analysis. *Gynecol Oncol.* 2008;108(3):641-651.
59. Beral V; Million Women Study Collaborators. Ovarian cancer and hormone replacement therapy in the Million Women Study. *Lancet.* 2007;369(9574): 1703-1710.
60. Anderson GL, Judd HL, Kaunitz AM, et al.; WHI Investigators. Effects of estrogen plus progestin on gynecologic cancers and associated diagnostic procedures: the Women's Health Initiative randomized trial. *JAMA.* 2003;290(13):1739-1748.
61. Marjoribanks J, Farquhar C, Roberts H, Lethaby A. Long term hormone therapy for perimenopausal and postmenopausal women. *Cochrane Database Syst Rev.* 2012;7:CD004143. doi:10.1002/14651858. CD004143.pub4.
62. North American Menopause Society (NAMS). Recommendations for estrogen and progestogen use in peri- and postmenopausal women: October 2004 position statement of the North American Menopause Society. *Menopause.* 2004;11(6 pt 1): 589-600.

63. U.S. Preventive Services Task Force. Hormone therapy for the prevention of chronic conditions in postmenopausal women: recommendation statement. 2005. http://www.ahrq.gov/clinic/uspstf05/ht/htpostmenrs.pdf. Accessed August 7, 2014.
64. U.S. Department of Health and Human Services. Guidance for industry noncontraceptive estrogen drug products for the treatment of vasomotor symptoms and vulvar and vaginal atrophy symptoms: recommended prescribing information for health care providers and patient labeling. 2011. http://www.fda.gov/downloads/Drugs/GuidanceCompliance RegulatoryInformation/Guidances/ucm075090.pdf. Accessed August 7, 2014.
65. North American Menopause Society (NAMS). Hormone therapy tables. http://www.menopause.org/docs/default-source/2014/nams-ht-tables.pdf. Accessed July 31, 2014.
66. Moyer VA; U.S. Preventive Services Task Force. Menopausal hormone therapy for the primary prevention of chronic conditions: U.S. Preventive Services Task Force recommendation statement. *Ann Intern Med.* 2013;158(1):47-54.
67. Kharode Y, Bodine PVN, Miller CP, Lyttle CR, Komm BS. The pairing of a selective estrogen receptor modulator, bazedoxifene, with conjugated estrogens as a new paradigm for the treatment of menopausal symptoms and osteoporosis prevention. *Endocrinol.* 2008;149(12):6084-6091.
68. Goodman MP. Are all estrogens created equal? A review of oral vs. transdermal therapy. *J Womens Health (Larchmt).* 2012;21(2):161-169.
69. Goodman NF, Cobin RH, Ginzberg SB, Katz IA, Woode DE; American Association of Clinical Endocrinologists. American Association of Clinical Endocrinologists medical guidelines for clinical practice for the diagnosis and treatment of menopause. *Endocr Pract.* 2011;17(suppl 6):1-25.
70. Somboonporn W, Panna S, Temtanakitpaisan T, Kaewrudee S, Soontrapa S. Effects of the levonorgestrel-releasing intrauterine system plus estrogen therapy in perimenopausal and postmenopausal women: systematic review and meta-analysis. *Menopause.* 2011;18(10):1060-1066.
71. Furness S, Roberts H, Marjoribanks J, Lethaby A, Hickey M, Farquhar C. Hormone therapy in postmenopausal women and risk of endometrial hyperplasia. *Cochrane Database Syst Rev.* 2004;3:CD000402.
72. Jaakkola S, Lyytinen H, Pukkala E, Ylikorkala O. Endometrial cancer in postmenopausal women using estradiol-progestin therapy. *Obstet Gynecol.* 2009; 114(6):1197-1204.
73. Thacker HL. Assessing risks and benefits of nonhormonal treatments for vasomotor symptoms in perimenopausal and postmenopausal women. *J Womens Health.* 2011;20(7):1007-1016.
74. U.S. Food and Drug Administration (FDA). FDA takes action against compounded menopause hormone therapy drugs. 2008. http://www.fda.gov/newsevents/newsroom/pressannouncements/2008/ucm116832.htm. Accessed August 1, 2014.
75. Whelan AM, Jurgens TM, Trinacty M. Bioidentical progesterone cream for menopause-related vasomotor symptoms: is it effective? *Ann Pharmacother.* 2013;47(1):112-116.
76. Peng W, Adams J, Sibbritt DW, Frawley JE. Critical review of complementary and alternative medicine use in menopause: focus on prevalence, motivation, decision-making, and communication. *Menopause.* 2014;21(5):536-548.
77. Gold EB, Bair Y, Zhang G, et al. Cross-sectional analysis of specific complementary and alternative medicine (CAM) use by racial/ethnic group and menopausal status: the Study of Women's Health Across the Nation (SWAN). *Menopause.* 2007;14(4):612-623.
78. Taylor M. Complementary and alternative medicine preparations used to treat symptoms of menopause. *Menopausal Med.* 2012;20(1):S1-S8.
79. Depypre HT, Comhaire FH. Herbal preparations for the menopause: beyond isoflavones and black cohosh. *Maturitas.* 2014;77(2):191-194.
80. Hudson T. Botanicals for managing menopause-related symptoms: state of the science. *Integrative Med.* 2010;8(6):30-37.
81. Bolle P, Mastrangelo S, Perrone F, Evandri MG. Estrogen-like effect of a *Cimicifuga racemosa* extract sub-fraction as assessed by in vivo, ex vivo and in vitro assays. *J Steroid Biochem Mol Biol.* 2007;107(3-5): 262-269.
82. Rice S, Amon A, Whitehead SA. Ethanolic extracts of black cohosh (*Actaea racemosa*) inhibit growth and oestradiol synthesis from oestrone sulphate in breast cancer cells. *Maturitas.* 2007;56(4):359-367.
83. Naser B, Schnitker J, Minkin MJ, de Arriba SG, Nolte KU, Osmers R. Suspected black cohosh hepatotoxicity: no evidence by meta-analysis of randomized

controlled clinical trials for isopropanolic black cohosh extract. *Menopause.* 2011;18(4):366-375.

84. Leach MJ, Moore V. Black cohosh (*Cimicifuga* spp.) for menopausal symptoms. *Cochrane Database Syst Rev.* 2012;9:CD007244.
85. Taku K, Melby MK, Kronenberg F, Kurzer MS, Messina M. Extracted or synthesized soybean isoflavones reduce menopausal hot flash frequency and severity: systematic review and meta-analysis of randomized controlled trials. *Menopause.* 2012;19(7):776-790.
86. Alexander IM, Andrist LC. Menopause. In: Schuiling KD, Likis FE, eds. *Women's Gynecologic Health.* 2nd ed. Burlington, MA: Jones & Bartlett Learning; 2013:285-328.
87. Munro MG, Critchley HOD, Fraser IS; FIGO Menstrual Disorder Working Group. The FIGO classification of causes of abnormal uterine bleeding in the reproductive years. *Fert Steril.* 2011;95(7):2204-2208.
88. Freeman EW, Sammel MD, Sanders RJ. Risk of long-term hot flashes after natural menopause: evidence from the Penn Ovarian Aging Study cohort. *Menopause.* 2014;21(9):1-9.
89. Freedman RR. Pathophysiology and treatments of hot flashes. *Semin Reprod Med.* 2005;23(2):117-125.
90. Orleans RJ, Li L, Kim M-J, et al. FDA approval of paroxetine for menopausal hot flashes. *N Engl J Med.* 2014;370(19):1777-1779.
91. Slaton RM, Champion MN, Palmore KB. A review of paroxetine for the treatment of vasomotor symptoms. *J Pharm Pract.* 2015;28(3):266-274.
92. Shams T, Firwana B, Habib F, et al. SSRIs for hot flashes: a systematic review and meta-analysis of randomized trials . *J Gen Intern Med.* 2014;29(1):204-213.
93. Archer DF, Dupont CM, Constantine GD, Pickar JH, Olivier S; Study 319 Investigators. Desvenlafaxine for the treatment of vasomotor symptoms associated with menopause: a double-blind, randomized, placebo-controlled trial of efficacy and safety. *Am J Obstet Gynecol.* 2009;200(3):238.
94. National Osteoporosis Foundation (NOF). *2014 Guide to Prevention and Treatment of Osteoporosis.* Washington, DC: National Osteoporosis Foundation; 2014. www.nof.org/hcp/clinicians-guide. Accessed August 4, 2014.
95. Edlin G, Golanty E. *Health and Wellness.* 11th ed. Burlington, MA: Jones & Bartlett Learning; 2014.
96. Kanis JA on behalf of the World Health Organization Scientific Group. *Assessment of Osteoporosis at the Primary Health Care Level.* Technical Report. Sheffield, UK: World Health Organization Collaborating Center for Metabolic Bone Diseases, University of Sheffield, UK; 2007. http://www.iofbonehealth.org/sites/default/files/WHO_Technical_Report-2007.pdf.
97. National Osteoporosis Foundation, International Society for Clinical Densitometry. Recommendations to DXA manufacturers for FRAX® implementation. http://www.nof.org/files/nof/public/content/resource/862/files/392.pdf. Accessed August 6, 2014.
98. Dawson-Hughes B, Tosteson AN, Melton LJ III, et al.; National Osteoporosis Foundation Guide Committee. Implications of absolute fracture risk assessment for osteoporosis practice guidelines in the U.S.A. *Osteoporos Int.* 2008;19(4):449-458.
99. Gold DT, Alexander IM, Ettinger MP. How can osteoporosis patients benefit more from their therapy? Adherence issues with Bisphosphonate therapy. *Ann Pharmacother.* 2006;40(6):1143-1150.
100. Black DM, Cummings SR, Karpf DB, et al. Randomised trial of effect of alendronate on risk of fracture in women with existing vertebral fractures. Fracture Intervention Trial Research Study Group. *Lancet.* 1996;348(9041):1535-1541.
101. Black DM, Reid IR, Boonen S, et al. The effect of 3 versus 6 years of zoledronic acid treatment of osteoporosis: a randomized extension to the HORIZON-Pivotal Fracture Trial (PFT) [erratum, *J Bone Miner Res.* 2012;27(12):2612]. *J Bone Miner Res.* 2012;27(2):243-254.
102. Boonen S, Adachi JD, Man Z, et al. Treatment with denosumab reduces the incidence of new vertebral and hip fractures in postmenopausal women at high risk. *J Clin Endocrinol Metab.* 2011;96(6):1727-1736.
103. Chesnut CH III, Silverman S, Andriano K, et al. A randomized trial of nasal spray salmon calcitonin in postmenopausal women with established osteoporosis: the prevent recurrence of osteoporotic fractures study. PROOF Study Group. *Am J Med.* 2000;109:(4):267-276.
104. Chesnut CH III, Skag A, Christiansen C, et al.; Oral Ibandronate Osteoporosis Vertebral Fracture Trial in North America and Europe. Effects of oral ibandronate administered daily or intermittently on fracture risk in postmenopausal osteoporosis. *J Bone Miner Res.* 2004;19(8):1241-1249.
105. Cummings SR, Black DM, Thompson DE, et al. Effect of alendronate on risk of fracture in women with low

bone density but without vertebral fractures: results from the Fracture Intervention Trial. *JAMA.* 1998; 280(24):2077-2082.

106. Delmas PD, Ensrud KE, Adachi JD, et al.; Multiple Outcomes of Raloxifene Evaluation Investigators. Efficacy of raloxifene on vertebral fracture risk reduction in postmenopusal women with osteoporosis: four-year results from a randomized clinical trial. *J Clin Endocrinol Metab.* 2001;87(8):3609-3617.
107. Harris ST, Watts NB, Genant HK, et al. Effects of risedronate treatment on vertebral and nonvertebral fractures in women with postmenopausal osteoporosis: a randomized controlled trial. Vertebral Efficacy with Risedronate Therapy (VERT) Study Group. *JAMA.* 1999;282(14):1344-1352.
108. Hodsman AB, Hanley DA, Ettinger MP, et al. Efficacy and safety of human parathyroid hormone-(1-84) in increasing bone mineral density in postmenopausal osteoporosis. *J Clin Endocrinol Metab.* 2003; 88(11):5212-5220.
109. Overman RA, Borse M, Gourlay ML. Salmon calcitonin use and associated cancer risk. *Ann Pharmacother.* 2013;47(12):1675-1684.
110. Silverman SL, Christiansen C, Genant HK, et al. Efficacy of bazedoxifene in reducing new vertebral fracture risk in postmenopausal women with osteoporosis: results from a 3-year, randomized, placebo-, and active-controlled clinical trial. *J Bone Miner Res.* 2008;23(12):1923-1934.
111. U.S. Preventive Services Task Force. Screening for osteoporosis: U.S. Preventive Services Task Force recommendation statement. *Ann Intern Med.* 2011;154(5):356-364. http://www.uspreventiveservicestaskforce.org/uspstf10/osteoporosis/osteors.htm.
112. Ruggerio SL, Dodson TB, Fantasia J, et al. Medication-related osteonecrosis of the jaw: 2014 update. American Association of Oral and Maxillofacial Surgeons; 2014. http://www.aaoms.org/docs/position_papers/mronj_position_paper.pdf?pdf=MRONJ-Position-Paper. Accessed August 6, 2014.
113. Greendale GA, Wight RG, Huang MH, et al. Menopause-associated symptoms and cognitive performance: results from the Study of Women's Health Across the Nation. *Am J Epidemiol.* 2010;171(11): 1214-1224.
114. Proctor A, Bianchi MT. Clinical pharmacology in sleep medicine. *ISRN Pharmacol.* 2012;2012(914168): 1-14.http://dx.doi.org/10.5402/2012/914168.Accessed August 4, 2014.
115. Davis SR, Davison SL, Donath S, Bell R. Relationships between circulating androgen levels and self-reported sexual function in women. *JAMA.* 2005;294(1): 91-96.
116. Shumaker S, Legault C, Rapp S, et al.; WHIMS Investigators. Estrogen plus progestin and the incidence of dementia and mild cognitive impairment in postmenopausal women: the Women's Health Initiative Memory Study: a randomized controlled trial. *JAMA.* 2003;289(20):2651-2662.
117. Frame KO, Alexander IM. Mind–body therapies for sleep disturbances in women at midlife. *J Hol Nurs.* 2013;31(4):276-284.
118. Antonijevic IA, Stalla GK, Steiger A. Modulation of the sleep electroencephalogram by estrogen replacement in postmenopausal women. *Am J Obstet Gynecol.* 2000;182(2):277-282.
119. Elraiyah T, Sonbol MB, Wang Z, et al. Clinical review: the benefits and harms of systemic testosterone therapy in postmenopausal women with normal adrenal function: a systematic review and meta-analysis. *J Clin Endocrinol Metab.* 2014;99(10):3543-3550.
120. Simon J, Braunstein G , Nachtigall L, et al. Testosterone patch increases sexual activity and desire in surgically menopausal women with hypoactive sexual desire disorder. *J Clin Endocrinol Metab.* 2005;90(9): 5226-5233.
121. Panay N, Al-Azzawi F, Bouchard C , et al. Testosterone treatment of HSDD in naturally menopausal women: the ADORE study. *Climacteric.* 2010;13(2):121-131.
122. Suckling JA, Kennedy R, Lethaby A, Roberts H. Local oestrogen for vaginal atrophy in postmenopausal women. *Cochrane Database Syst Rev.* 2006;4: CD001500. doi:10.1002/14651858.CD001500.pub2.
123. North American Menopause Society (NAMS), 2013 Symptomatic Vaginal Atrophy Advisory Panel. Management of symptomatic vulvovaginal atrophy: 2013 position statement of the North American Menopause Society. *Menopause.* 2013;20(9): 888-902.
124. Simon JA, Lin VH, Radovich C, Bachman GA. The Ospemifene Study Group: one-year long-term safety extension study of ospemifene for the treatment of vulvar and vaginal atrophy in postmenopausal women with a uterus. *Menopause.* 2013;20(4):418-427.

VI
Pregnancy and Lactation

The last section of this book reviews pharmacology and pharmacotherapeutics as they pertain to women during pregnancy and breastfeeding. It would be ideal if all women were healthy throughout the childbearing cycle so that no drugs were necessary. However, some drugs, such as folic acid, are recommended as preventive measures. Other agents are used to treat common conditions such as anemia and various infections. In the presence of chronic conditions such as asthma or diabetes, some medications are essential to maintain maternal and/or child health. Others are used to treat a medical emergency such as postpartum hemorrhage.

The *Pregnancy* chapter reviews the pharmacologic management of a wide variety of conditions in the context of pregnancy. The pharmacotherapeutic challenge of considering two individuals—the woman and her fetus—simultaneously is addressed at length.

The *Labor* chapter discusses various conditions that may occur during the intrapartum period, including preterm labor and infections. Pain management for women in labor is reviewed as well.

The *Postpartum* chapter acknowledges that healthy women rarely need drugs after giving birth. However, those conditions that are best treated pharmacologically are presented.

There is no controversy over the admonition that "breast is best," but some breastfeeding women have conditions that also are best treated with drugs. The *Breastfeeding* chapter provides a discussion of the challenges involved in choosing the best treatments for the mother–newborn dyad while promoting the continuation of breastfeeding.

The last chapter, *The Newborn*, reviews pharmacotherapeutics used to treat common conditions that affect neonates in the first days and weeks following birth. Topics include how the unique newborn physiology affects pharmacokinetics, drugs used for newborn prophylaxis, newborn eye prophylaxis, immunizations, and drugs used to treat newborn infection.

35 Pregnancy

Nicole T. Lassiter, Laura E. Manns-James

Chapter Glossary

Erythroblastosis fetalis Alloimmune condition that develops in the fetus when maternal immunoglobulin G antibodies cross the placenta and attack fetal red blood cells causing fetal anemia. The presence of a large number of erythroblasts or immature red blood cells in the fetal circulation is the basis of the name.

Fetotoxin Agent that produces toxic effects in a fetus that result abnormal size, growth, or development of specific organ(s).

Ion trapping Presence of a higher concentration of a chemical on one side of a cell membrane against a concentration gradient that would normally equalize concentrations. This occurs when the ion is altered on one side of the membrane in a way that prevents its transport across the membrane.

Placental barrier Layer of placental tissue that separates maternal and fetal circulations. Because it is not an actual barrier, this term is somewhat misleading.

Teratogenis Any agent that irreversibly alters the growth, structure, or function of a developing embryo or fetus. This term generally refers to structural abnormalities.

Introduction

Approximately one in two women reports use of at least one prescription drug during pregnancy, and more than 90% of pregnant women report using at least one prescription medication during the first trimester.[1] The drugs most commonly used by pregnant women include analgesics, antibiotics, antiemetics, and antidepressants.[1]

When a pregnant woman uses a medication, the usual considerations of safety and effectiveness extend to include the fetus as well as the woman. The public often assumes that the studies performed prior to a drug's approval by the U.S. Food and Drug Administration (FDA) focus on all adverse effects of a drug, including those that affect a fetus. Unfortunately, this is not true. Data sufficient to determine the safety of most medications used during pregnancy do not exist. In fact, such information is not available for more than 91% of the FDA-approved medications on the market since 1980.[2,3] The majority of adverse effects of drugs are actually discovered after a medication has been on the market and used by large numbers of individuals, including pregnant women.

This chapter reviews the basics of how drugs cause birth defects and other adverse outcomes in the fetus/neonate, as well as physiologic changes of pregnancy that affect pharmacokinetics, and pharmacotherapeutic considerations for treating common conditions that affect pregnant women. Pregnancy considerations related to conditions that also occur outside of pregnancy, such as depression, thyroid disorders, and epilepsy, may be primarily addressed in other chapters. Similarly, most doses and drug–drug interactions are addressed in the chapter that focuses specifically on a drug class. Thus this chapter should be read in conjunction with others to obtain full information about the medications discussed.

Teratogenic and Fetotoxic Effects of Drugs

One of the earliest observations was that timing of exposure is a determinant of the effect a drug has on the developing fetus. Based on this observation, researchers developed the concept of a critical period to identify the time when the fetus is more sensitive to environmental influences.[4] This concept aided subsequent research.

Today, it is understood that because adverse effects occur at different times during pregnancy, they can be classified into three categories:

- Embryocidal—that is, leading to fetal death.
- Teratogenic—that is, leading to irreversible changes in structure or function. Teratogenic effects include structural abnormalities, developmental impairment, or late carcinogenesis. Thalidomide, alcohol, and diethylstilbesterol (DES) are examples of **teratogenis**.
- Fetotoxic—that is, altering growth or development in the second and third trimesters. Nicotine is an example of a **fetotoxin**; it does not cause birth defects, but can cause intrauterine growth restriction.

Sometimes the difference between the terms fetotoxic and teratogenic are not appreciated and the term teratogenic is used colloquially when fetotoxic is appropriate. In addition, some drugs, such as ethanol, can be both teratogenic and fetotoxic. Ethanol can cause the structural and functional abnormalities of fetal alcohol syndrome and the developmental alterations of alcohol-related neurodevelopmental disorder.

Teratogens may be chemical, physical, infectious, or environmental in nature.[3] The background risk for all congenital malformations is approximately 3% to 4%,[5] yet only 2% to 3% of all congenital malformations are attributable to drug exposure.[6] The criteria used to determine that a drug is a teratogen are listed in Box 35-1.[7] Relatively few drugs are categorically teratogenic, and the list of drugs within this category has remained remarkably consistent and amazingly short for the last several decades, despite the explosion of the number of drugs used in clinical practice. Table 35-1 presents a selected list of known teratogenic and/or fetotoxic drugs.[8–12]

In the late 1970s, the embryologist Wilson identified six principles of teratology, summarized in Table 35-2.[13] These principles remain relevant today.[14] Wilson noted the importance of host susceptibility in his first principle, which explains why not all fetuses have the same reaction to a specific teratogen. His second principle provided credence for the concept of the critical period.

Based on the critical period concept, fetal development is divided into three stages (Figure 35-1).[15] The *preimplantation* period occurs immediately after fertilization and before implantation. An exposure to a teratogen at this point in gestation likely has an "all-or-nothing" effect on the developing embryo—that is, the embryo will either die or survive, and if the embryo survives, no adverse effects will occur. *Organogenesis* occurs at 3 to 8 weeks post fertilization. It is the period of maximum vulnerability to teratogenic drugs during which major congenital anomalies, miscarriage, or more mild but permanent defects can occur.

Box 35-1 Criteria for Proof of Human Teratogenicity[a]

1. Proven exposure to the agent at critical time(s) in prenatal development (e.g., prescriptions, personal health records, dates).
2. Consistent findings by two or more epidemiologic studies of high quality:
   a. Control of confounding factors
   b. Sufficient numbers
   c. Exclusion of positive and negative bias factors
   d. Prospective studies, if possible
   e. Relative risk of 6 or more
3. Careful delineation of the clinical cases. A specific defect or syndrome, if present, is very helpful.
4. Rare environmental exposure associated with rare defect—usually three or more cases (e.g., oral anticoagulants and nasal hypoplasia, methimazole [Tapazole] and scalp defects).
5. Teratogenicity in experimental animals is important but not essential.
6. The association is biologically plausible.
7. Proof in an experimental system that the agent acts in an unaltered state. This is important information for prevention.

[a] Items 1–3 or 1, 3, and 4 are essential criteria.

Sources: Reproduced from Shephard TH. "Proof" of human teratogenicity [letter]. *Teratology.* 1994;50:97-98.[7]

Table 35-1 Drugs That Are Teratogenic or Fetotoxic

Drug: Category or Name (Brand Name)	Teratogenic or Fetotoxic Effects	Comments
Aminoglycosides: Gentamycin (Garamycin) Streptomycin	Neonatal ototoxicity	Streptomycin in the high doses used to treat tuberculosis has a clear risk of fetal ototoxicity. The risk associated with gentamycin may be smaller but this drug is still not recommended for use in pregnancy.
Aminopterin	Multiple anomalies	Chemotherapeutic drug that is a folic acid antagonist.
Amiodarone (Cordarone)	Contains iodine and can cause transient fetal hypothyroidism	Can interfere with fetal thyroid function in the second and third trimesters.
Androgens and testosterone derivatives: Danocrine (Danazol)	Virilization of females Advanced genital development of males Before 9 weeks' gestation, labioscrotal fusion is the common teratogenic effect	Dose dependent and based on critical period. Brief exposure rarely is significant.
Angiotensin II receptor blockers: Losartan (Cozaar)	Prolonged renal failure and hypotension in the newborn Decreased skull ossification Renal tubular agenesis	All trimesters are considered critical periods.
Angiotensin-converting enzyme (ACE) inhibitors: Captopril (Capoten) Enalapril (Vasotec) Lisinopril (Prinivil)	Intrauterine growth restriction Oligohydramnios Renal failure Decreased skull ossification Renal tubular dysgenesis	Growth restriction is approximately 25%, with fetal morbidity of approximately 30%. Risk of effects increases in the second and third trimesters (probably due to decreased uteroplacental flow).
Anticonvulsants: Carbamazepine (Tegretol) Phenytoin (Dilantin) Trimethadione (Tridione) Valproate (Depacon) Valproic acid (Depakene)	1% risk of neural tube defect, cardiovascular defects, developmental delays, intrauterine growth restriction Reduced intelligence associated with use of valproic acid or valproate Phenytoin is specifically associated with cardiac defects and cleft palate	All trimesters are considered critical periods. Risk of neural tube defects is increased, especially when anticonvulsants are used with other antiepileptic drugs. Risk of neural tube defects is decreased with increased folic acid supplementation. Polytherapy with more than one anticonvulsant increases risk. Newer anticonvulsants such as gabapentin (Neurontin) do not appear to have a risk of congenital anomalies.
Antithyroid drugs: Methimazole Propylthiouracil (PTU)	Fetal and neonatal goiter, fetal hypothyroidism, and aplasia cutis associated with methimazole but not propylthiouracil	All trimesters are considered critical periods. Women who need to take antithyroid drugs will generally be counseled to take propylthiouracil. The risk of fetal goiter is approximately 1–5%.
Aspirin	More than 150 mg/day associated with prolonged gestation, prolonged labor, bleeding complications in the neonate, premature closure of the ductus arteriosis, intrauterine growth restriction	All trimesters are considered critical periods. Although low-dose aspirin may be of benefit for women with a risk of preeclampsia, antiphospholipid syndrome, or lupus; normal adult doses should be avoided.
Benzodiazepines: Alprazolam (Xanax) Chlordiazepoxide (Librium) Diazepam (Valium)	Increased risk of neonatal withdrawal Some studies show increased risk of oral clefts with first-trimester exposure to diazepam	Early data on oral cleft association are controversial. Benzodiazepines are highly lipophilic and have a long half-life in the fetus/neonate.
Chemotherapeutic drugs: Cyclophosphamide (Cytoxan) Methotrexate (Rheumatrex)	Multiple congenital anomalies, growth restriction	The first trimester is the most critical period, but these agents can adversely affect the fetus throughout gestation. If a woman needs one of these drugs, refer her for consultation with perinatologist and oncologist. Methotrexate may be used to treat a woman with an ectopic pregnancy.
Chloramphenicol	Gray baby syndrome in neonate 2–9 days after therapy is administered	Oral chloramphenicol contraindicated throughout pregnancy.
Corticosteroids: Methylprednisone (Medrol)	Possible increase in risk of oral and cleft defects	Critical period is first trimester only and relationship has not been definitively proven. Because the risk is low, oral corticosteroids are used in the first trimester to treat hyperemesis gravidarum and other health conditions. No known risk is associated with topical use in second and third trimesters.
Diazepam (Valium)	Neonatal symptoms: central nervous system depression, poor suck, hypotonia, sedation, apneic spells "Floppy infant" syndrome, neonatal withdrawal	

(*continues*)

Table 35-1 Drugs That Are Teratogenic or Fetotoxic (*continued*)

Drug: Category or Name (Brand Name)	Teratogenic or Fetotoxic Effects	Comments
Diethylstilbestrol (DES)	Clear cell adenocarcinoma Vaginal adenosis Cervical and uterine abnormalities	First trimester is the most critical period.
Ergot alkaloids: Ergotamine (Cafergot)	Spontaneous abortion Moebius syndrome Intestinal atresia Cerebral developmental abnormalities Low birth weight Preterm birth	All trimesters are considered critical periods.
Fluconazole (Diflucan)	Brachycephaly Abnormal facies Abnormal calvarial development Cleft palate Congenital heart disease	Chronic high-dose exposure during the first trimester only. These effects are not seen following a single 150-mg dose for treatment of woman with vaginal candidiasis.
Folic acid antagonists: Carbamazepine (Tegretol) Methotrexate (Rheumatrex) Phenobarbital (Solfoton) Phenytoin (Dilantin) Primidone (Mysoline) Trimethoprim (Trimpex)	Spontaneous abortion Neural tube defects Cardiovascular defects Urinary tract defects	Drugs in many different categories are folic acid antagonists. Some suggest that risk can be decreased with folic acid supplementation. Methotrexate may be used to treat a woman with an ectopic pregnancy. Trimethoprim is a component of trimethoprim–sulfamethoxazole (Septra), which is commonly used to treat urinary tract infections. Contraindicated in the first and third trimesters.
Iodine/iodides	Transient hypothyroidism in some newborns Development of fetal goiter	All trimesters are considered critical periods. Significant absorption occurs following maternal topical, vaginal, or perineal use.
Isotretinoin (Accutane)	Central nervous system (CNS) abnormalities Craniofacial anomalies Conotruncal cardiovascular malformations Thymic defects Branchial-arch mesenchymal-tissue defects Miscellaneous anomalies	Oral isotretinoin is contraindicated in pregnancy. Topical preparations are unlikely to have serious teratogenic effects but remain contraindicated because other agents can be used.
Lindane (Kwell)	Single case of stillbirth reported	All trimesters are considered critical periods. Lindane should be given to pregnant women only if there are no alternatives. Over-the-counter topical treatments for head lice are safe to use in pregnancy.
Lithium (Lithobid)	Cardiac defects Epstein's anomaly	Absolute risk is small but alternative drugs recommended if possible.
Methadone	Neonatal dependence/withdrawal	Women who use methadone during pregnancy will need careful management in the third trimester to mitigate neonatal withdrawal.
Mifepristone (Mifeprex, RU-486)	Antiprogestogen; used as an abortifacient Human data limited	Primarily used for abortion in combination with misoprostol.
Misoprostol (Cytotec)	Abortion Moebius sequence (brain stem ischemia, vascular disruption) for misoprostol	Potent uterostimulant capable of initiating uterine contractions at all gestational weeks.
Mycophenolate (CellCept)	Miscarriage Major malformations of the face, limbs, and organs	Immunosuppressive agent used to prevent rejection of organ transplant.
Nonsteroidal anti-inflammatory drugs (NSAIDs): Ibuprofen (Advil) Naproxen (Aleve)	Miscarriage in first trimester Theorized premature closure of the ductus arteriosus Necrotizing enterocolitis	Contraindicated in general, but especially in third trimester.
Opioids	Neural tube defects Cardiac defects Gastroschisis	Findings of teratogenicity from retrospective population-based studies need further research to confirm them. In 2015, FDA released a safety alert counseling pregnant women to avoid opioids when possible.

Penicillamine (Cuprimine)	Cutis laxa Other congenital malformations	First trimester is the most critical period.
Phenytoin (Dilantin)	Fetal hydantoin syndrome: distinct facial abnormalities, anomalies of the digits, hypoplasia and ossification of the distal phalanges Orofacial clefts; impaired development (physical and mental) and congenital heart defects Data suggest transplacental carcinogenicity	First trimester is the most critical period.
Pseudoephedrine (Sudafed)	Gastroschisis	An association between pseudoephedrine use and gastroschisis has been identified in case-control studies. Prospective studies are needed to determine if this finding is etiologic.
Selective serotonin reuptake inhibitors (SSRIs): Fluoxetine (Prozac) Paroxetine (Paxil) Sertraline (Zoloft)	Paroxetine increases risk of cardiac defects 1.5- to 2-fold. Fluoxetine also has been suggested to have similar effects but sertraline has not been found to have major risks of teratogenic effects. Exposure in third trimester associated with neonatal withdrawal. Persistent pulmonary hypertension noted in case reports.	Overall, absolute risk of teratogenic and fetotoxic effects is low. Antidepressants should not be discontinued during pregnancy. If initiating antidepressant therapy during pregnancy, general advice is to use sertraline and particularly avoid paroxetine. Up-to-date information regarding this controversial area can be found on the CDC website as listed in the Resources table.
Statins: Atorvastatin (Lipitor) Lovastatin (Mevacor)	Interfere with cholesterol production Primarily theoretical adverse effects on the fetus	Contraindicated throughout pregnancy.
Streptomycin and kanamycin	Hearing loss Eighth nerve damage	No ototoxicity has been found with gentamicin or vancomycin.
Sulfonamides: Sulfamethoxazole (Bactrim, Septra)	Hyperbilirubinemia in neonate	Third trimester is the most critical period.
Tamoxifen (Nolvadex)	Increased risk of spontaneous abortion or loss	All trimesters are considered critical periods.
Tetracyclines: Tetracycline (Terramycin) Doxycycline (Adoxa)	Abnormalities of teeth discoloration	After the first trimester is the critical period. Discoloration of permanent teeth is possible if exposure is after 24 weeks' gestation. No well-controlled studies of doxycycline, but case-controlled studies suggest it is not associated with teratogenic risk. Recommend that doxycycline be used only if it is the only effective agent.
Thalidomide	Limb deficiencies Cardiac and gastrointestinal abnormalities	First trimester is the most critical period with 20–30% risk (very potent). Used for years before teratogenic effects became obvious. Back on market for treatment of women with oral lesions in human immunodeficiency virus (HIV) infection, Hansen's disease, tuberculosis, and multiple myeloma. STEPS (System for Thalidomide Education and Prescribing Safety) available online from the drug's manufacturer, Celgene.
Tricyclic antidepressants: Clomipramine (Anafranil)	Neonatal lethargy, hypotonia, cyanosis, and hypothermia	Generally not recommended during pregnancy unless these antidepressants are the only effective agents.
Trimethoprim	Theoretic risk of neural tube defects, oral clefts, cardiovascular defects, and hypospadias Trimethoprim is a folate antagonist	First trimester is the most critical period.
Valproic acid	Spina bifida: 1–2% incidence Increases other congenital malformations 3-fold Evidence of developmental delay	First trimester is the most critical period.
Vitamin A	Avoid doses greater than 8000 IU/day; doses ≥ 10,000 mg/day are teratogenic Marked deficiency may also cause malformations	All trimesters are considered critical periods.
Warfarin (Coumarin)	Bone defects Growth restriction CNS defects Developmental delays	First trimester is the most critical period, especially during 6–9 gestational weeks with 15–25% risk when anticoagulants that impair vitamin K are used. Later use in pregnancy is associated with abruption, CNS defects, stillbirth, and hemorrhage of the fetus/newborn.

Table 35-2 Wilson's Six Principles of Teratology

1	Susceptibility to teratogenesis depends on the genotype of the conceptus and the manner in which it interacts with environmental factors.
2	Susceptibility to teratogenic agents varies with the developmental stage at the time of exposure.
3	Teratogenic agents act in specific ways (mechanisms) on developing cells and tissues to initiate abnormal embryogenesis (pathogenesis).
4	The final manifestations of abnormal development are death, malformation, growth retardation, and functional disorder.
5	The access of adverse environmental influences to developing tissues depends on the nature of the influences (agent).
6	Manifestations of deviant development increase in degree as the dosage increases from the no-effect level to the totally lethal level.

Source: Modified from Wilson J. Current status of teratology, general principles and mechanisms derived from animal studies. In: Wilson J, Fraser F, eds. *Handbook of Teratology*. 4 vols. New York: Plenum Press; 1977:47-74.[13]

This critical gestational period is often complete by the time a woman discovers she is pregnant or has an initial prenatal visit. The *fetal* period begins the ninth week post fertilization and continues throughout the rest of the pregnancy. The primary organ that continues to differentiate during the fetal period is the brain. Obvious birth defects are unusual at this time; however, fetotoxic effects may occur.

Wilson's third principle notes that drugs have specific mechanisms that induce teratogenic consequences. A 2010 review of drugs in pregnancy identified the mechanisms of most teratogens as involving folate antagonism, neural crest cell disruption, endocrine disruption of sex hormones, oxidative stress, vascular disruption, or specific receptor- or enzyme-mediated reactions.[16] Current research into these mechanisms is being conducted to see if changing the chemical design of drugs might ameliorate or prevent their teratogenic effects.

Wilson's last two principles address the potency and type of teratogen. Dose is a critical determinant of fetal effect. Many drugs have a threshold below which no fetal harm occurs. Conversely, high doses of a potent teratogen have the potential for more severe result

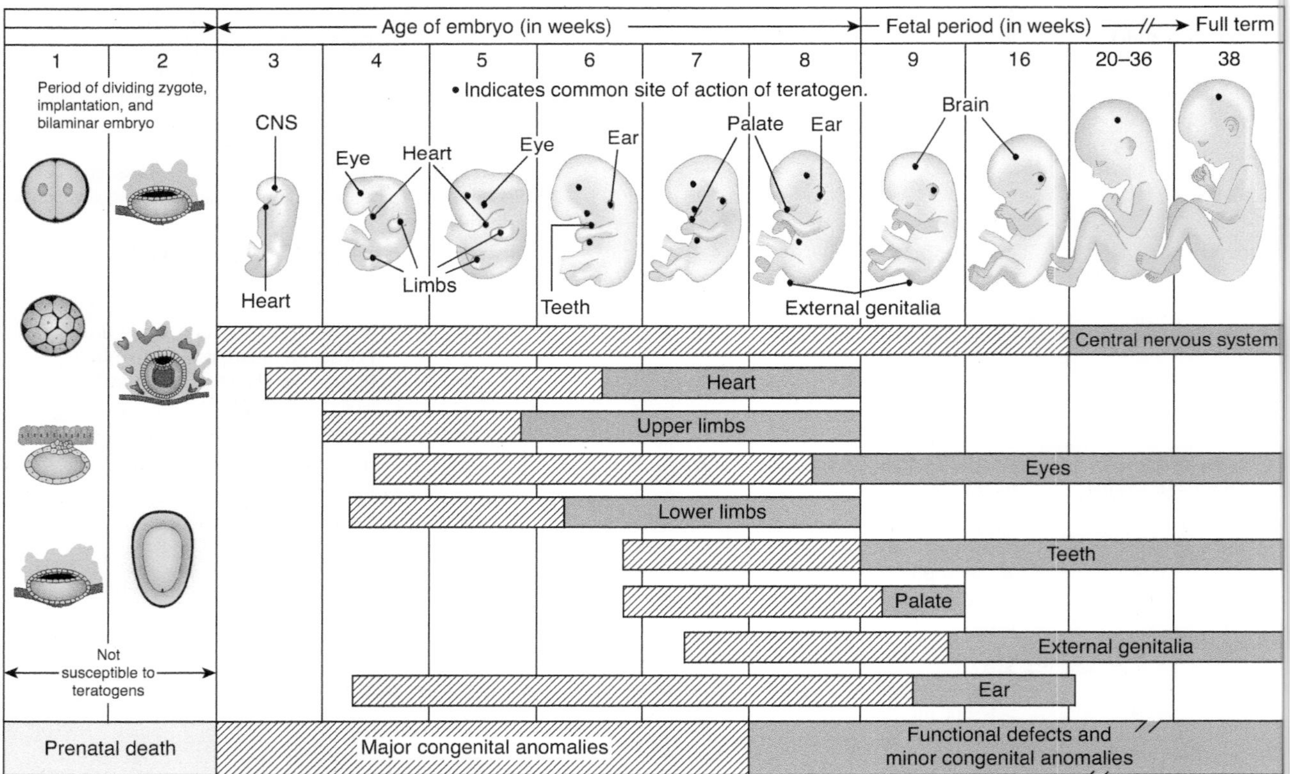

Figure 35-1 Critical periods in human development.

Source: Modified from Moore KL, Persaud TVN. *The Developing Human: Clinically Oriented Embryology*. 8th ed. Philadelphia, PA: Elsevier; 2007.[15]

Table 35-3 Pharmacokinetic Changes in Pregnancy

Pharmacokinetic Process	Changes During Pregnancy
Absorption	• Decreased with gestational nausea and vomiting resulting in decreased plasma drug concentrations. • Gastric pH is increased, which can affect the bioavailability of drugs that are dependent on low pH for absorption or change to an active agent. • Longer intestinal transport time (30–50% increase in gastric emptying time) may facilitate absorption of hydrophilic drugs. No change in absorption of lipophilic drugs.
Distribution	• Maternal plasma volume expands approximately 50%. • Increased volume of distribution occurs as the fetal compartment develops; this may result in lower serum levels and requirements for larger loading doses of hydrophilic drugs. • Reduction in plasma proteins (especially albumin) may result in higher levels of free metabolically active drug. • Plasma levels of steroid hormones such as estradiol and progesterone increase in the latter half of pregnancy; these steroids compete for protein-binding sites on albumin and other plasma proteins. Steroid hormones may also displace drugs already bound to plasma proteins. The overall effect is more free drug fraction. • As maternal albumin levels decrease, the fetus produces endogenous plasma proteins. This can lead to a concentration gradient favoring increased transport of free drug from mother to fetus. This purported mechanism explains why diazepam (Valium) can be found in higher concentrations in the fetus than in the mother.
Metabolism	• Blood flow through the liver during pregnancy is not changed to a large degree, so first-pass effects are not significantly altered. • Hepatic CYP450 enzyme systems are affected by rising levels of estrogen and progesterone, leading to slower metabolism of some drugs (e.g., caffeine) and faster metabolism of others. CYP3A4 and CYP2D6 activity is increased during pregnancy, whereas CYP1A2 is downregulated. • Lower albumin levels mean more unbound drug, with the potential for periods of more rapid clearance.
Excretion/clearance	• Excretion via the lungs is more rapid secondary to an increased respiratory rate. Absorption of inhaled medications may be increased. • Renal blood flow and glomerular filtration rate increase by 50% and peak at 34 weeks' gestation, inducing shorter half-lives of those medications undergoing renal clearance. • Drugs such as nicotine, fluoxetine (Prozac), and citalopram (Celexa) may be excreted so easily that decreased therapeutic effectiveness may ensue. Lower levels of selective serotonin reuptake inhibitors may require higher or more frequent doses to achieve therapeutic benefits in the third trimester.

Sources: Data from Costantine MM. Physiologic and pharmacokinetic changes in pregnancy. *Front Pharmacol.* 2014;5:65[18]; Gedeon C, Koren G. Designing pregnancy centered medications: drugs which do not cross the human placenta. *Placenta.* 2006;27:861-868.[19]

Pharmacokinetic Changes During Pregnancy

In 1941 the first teratogenic agent was recognized; this was not a drug but rather the infection rubella. Prior to this discovery, the placenta was viewed as a protective barrier that kept the fetus from being exposed to harmful agents.[17] It is now known that the placenta is a permeable barrier and that most drugs and their metabolites cross the placenta, particularly those that are lipophilic and those with low plasma protein binding.

The physiologic changes of pregnancy have a significant impact on the pharmacokinetics of most medications.[18] Almost all organ systems are affected by pregnancy-related anatomic and physiologic changes, some of which begin in very early gestation. These changes are reviewed elsewhere for the interested reader.[18,19] Pharmacokinetic changes in distribution, absorption, metabolism, and excretion are summarized in Table 35-3.

Drug Transport in the Placenta

Once a substance reaches the intervillous space in the placenta, contact is made with the fetal placental villi and **placental barrier**. The substance must then traverse the several biologic layers that make up the placental barrier: (1) the syncytiotrophoblast membrane; (2) the syncytiotrophoblast cell; (3) the syncytiotrophoblast basal membrane; (4) the connective tissue of the cytotrophoblast villus; and (5) the endothelial cells that line the fetal vessels. This barrier thins as the pregnancy progresses and by the third trimester, the cytotrophoblast villus tissue becomes discontinuous so the two separate circulations are closer to each other.

The placenta also has several enzyme systems that metabolize selected drugs, and the placental cells express P-glycoprotein, which actively pumps some substrates away from the fetus. Drugs known to be substrates for P-glycoprotein have lower concentrations in the fetal circulation than in the maternal circulation.[20]

Most substances move into the fetal compartment via diffusion. Molecules can also be transported via facilitated diffusion, active transport, or pinocytosis (Figure 35-2). Drugs that have a molecular weight of less than 500 daltons, those that are lipophilic (e.g., antibiotics and anesthetics), and those that are un-ionized readily diffuse across the placental cell membrane barriers.[5] Larger drugs gain access to the fetal compartment more slowly via pinocytosis, and a few drugs with molecular weights of more than 1000 daltons (e.g., heparin, insulin, oxytocin, thyroid supplements, glyburide, and interferon) do not cross into the fetal compartment in any appreciable amount.

The Fetal Compartment

The fetal liver has a degree of capacity to metabolize drugs by approximately 8 to 10 weeks post conception. At term, the fetal liver has approximately 30% to 60% of the CYP450 activity of an adult.[20]

Concentration gradients between maternal and fetal blood affect rates of diffusion, as does a slight difference between maternal and fetal pH. As a result of this pH gradient, weak basic drugs such as opiates may become concentrated in the fetal compartment. The slightly acidotic

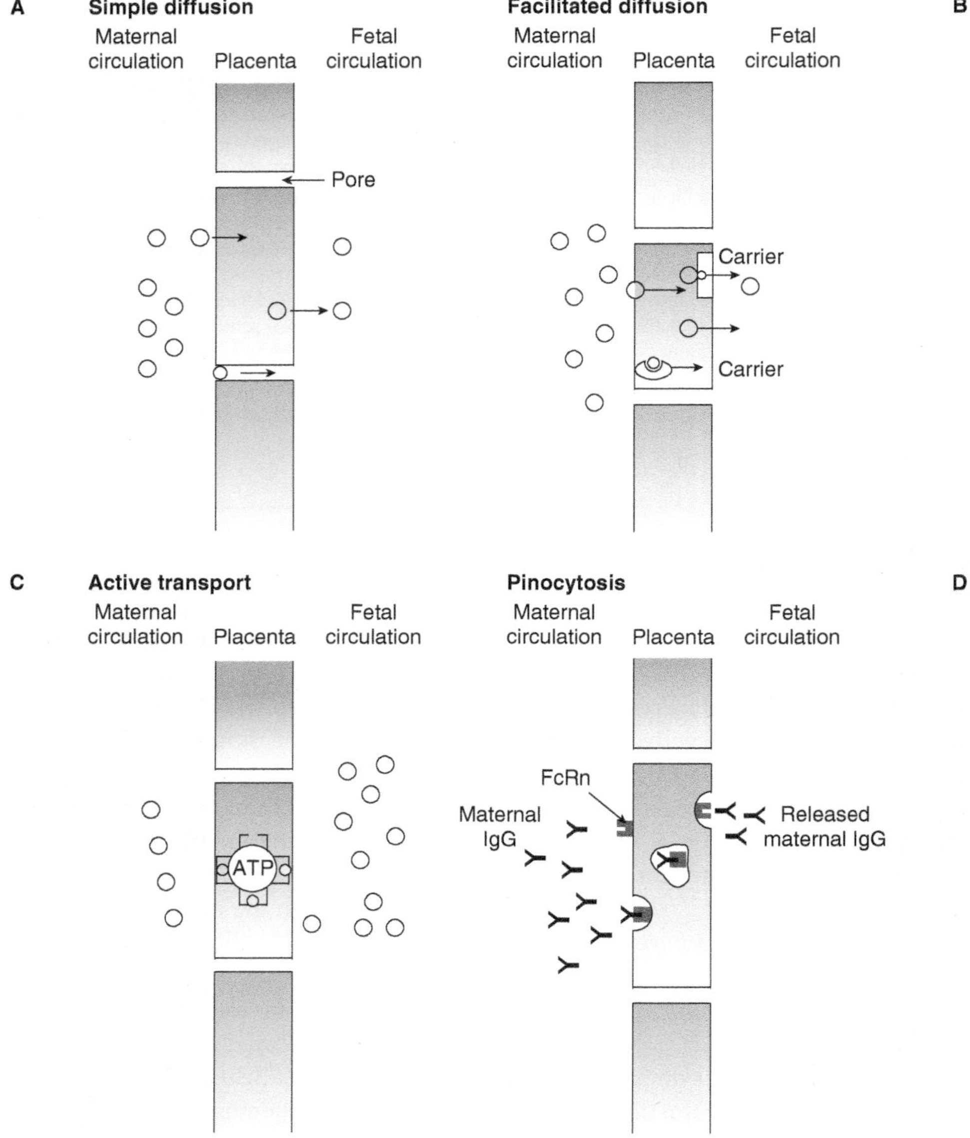

Figure 35-2 Methods of transporting molecules across the placenta.

environment in the fetal circulation encourages their ionization, which changes their shape and makes return to the more basic maternal blood more difficult, a phenomenon known as **ion trapping**.

Once a drug is in the fetal compartment, distribution is influenced by the stage of gestation. Prior to skin keratinization at 20 weeks' gestation, amniotic fluid acts as extracellular fluid, with drugs diffusing readily across the fetal skin. As fetal development continues, skin permeability decreases significantly, and drugs that enter the fetus must be excreted rather than simply diffused into the amniotic fluid. Drugs that enter the fetal circulation via the umbilical vein can be either metabolized within the liver via the first-pass effect or shunted across the ductus venosus directly to the heart and general circulation. Both the placenta and the fetal liver are capable of some drug metabolism. Ultimately, fetal concentrations of most drugs achieve steady-state levels that range between 50% and 100% of the maternal concentration.

Pregnancy Risks Associated with Medication Use: Overview

Prior to gaining FDA approval to market a drug for a specific indication, the FDA requires completion of animal studies that assess for adverse fetal effects of drugs. However, adverse effects or lack thereof identified in these studies cannot be reliably translated to humans. The subsequent preapproval human clinical trials evaluating the safety and effectiveness of drugs most often do not include pregnant women,[21] because including such women in the research usually is considered unethical or unsafe.[22] For those preapproval studies that *do* involve pregnant women, the numbers of participants are often too small to detect any fetal risks.[21]

Drug Labeling: FDA Pregnancy Categories

In 1963, the limb deformities caused by prenatal use of thalidomide were made public. In response to this new understanding of the possible teratogenic effects of drugs, the FDA developed a pregnancy labeling system that classifies drugs into lettered safety categories.[23] This system was put into place and used extensively until 2014.

The letter system, however, had some significant problems. It was generally assumed that the risk categories—A, B, C, D, and X—progressively ranked an increasing risk of adverse effects, and that drugs in the same category shared the same risk level. But, neither assumption was true. Furthermore, the categories did not incorporate information about the severity of the risk, threshold dose, or timing of the adverse effect.[24]

After many years of criticism and calls for revision, in 2008 the FDA proposed that the letter-based system be replaced by a narrative text. This new system was adopted in late 2014[25] and is described in detail in the *Modern Pharmacology* chapter.

Drug Safety for Pregnant Women

Safe prescribing for a pregnant woman begins with an accurate diagnosis of the condition that requires pharmacologic intervention. The goal is to use the lowest effective dose of the drug known to be the safest for the shortest period of time. If several different drugs are equally effective, the one that has been used for the longest period of time and has the most data supporting its safety should be chosen.[21] Additional principles for prescribing in pregnancy include avoiding drugs during the first trimester when possible, choosing topical instead of oral formulations if both are equally effective, and using medications only if the benefit outweighs the risk of the untreated disorder.

Women may already be taking a medication for a preexisting condition when they become pregnant. These drugs should not be discontinued unless there is a high suspicion or known risk of maternal or fetal harm. Some drugs, such as antiepileptic agents, have a risk of harming the fetus but may need to be continued during pregnancy to maintain the woman's health. Women who become pregnant while taking one of these agents should be referred to specialist for in-depth counseling. The following sections of this chapter review the pharmacotherapeutics used by women during pregnancy.

Vitamin and Mineral Supplementation During Pregnancy

Supplemental multivitamins, folic acid, and iron are commonly recommended for pregnant women. The evidence for folic acid supplements is strong, whereas the evidence for routine use of multivitamins with iron is controversial. This chapter presents a brief review of folic acid, iron, and vitamin D. The benefits, risks, and pharmacotherapeutic considerations associated with vitamin use are also covered in more detail in the *Vitamins and Minerals* chapter.

Folic Acid

Folate is required to support the increase in red cell volume that occurs during pregnancy. Folate is absorbed better following ingestion of a supplement than when it is consumed in food sources. Low maternal folate levels are associated with an increased risk of neural tube defects in the fetus.

In 2010, an updated Cochrane systematic review reaffirmed that folic acid supplementation, either alone or with other vitamin/mineral supplements, is an effective intervention to prevent open neural tube defects (relative risk [RR], 0.28; 95% confidence interval [CI], 0.15–0.52).[26] Folic acid supplementation does not decrease the risk of miscarriage or other birth defects such as cleft palate or cardiovascular defects. An additional Cochrane review assessed the effect of folic acid supplementation on hematologic parameters and pregnancy outcomes.[27] The authors of this review did not find that folic acid supplementation improves pregnancy outcomes such as preterm birth or stillbirth. Folic acid supplementation has been found to decrease the incidence of megaloblastic anemia.[27]

In 1998, the Institute of Medicine recommended that women capable of becoming pregnancy consume 400 mcg per day of folic acid via supplement or diet or a combination of both to prevent open neural tube defects. The Centers for Disease Control and Prevention (CDC) also recommends that all women between the ages of 15 and 45 years take the same amount of folic acid every day. This recommendation is based on the fact that approximately half of all pregnancies are unplanned; neural tube defects occur in the first few weeks following conception before woman are usually aware of pregnancy. The current recommendation by the U.S. Preventive Services Task Force (USPSTF) is that all women planning a pregnancy or who are capable of becoming pregnant take 400 to 800 mcg of folic acid every day.[28]

Women with a History of a Pregnancy Complicated by a Neural Tube Defect

For women who have experienced a previous pregnancy complicated by an open neural tube defect, the American College of Obstetricians and Gynecologists recommends 4 mg of folic acid daily for at one month prior to conception and through the first 3 months of pregnancy.[29] This recommendation, also from the CDC, was based on findings from the Medical Research Council Vitamin Study Research Group that those women with a previous pregnancy affected by a neural tube defect who took 4 mg folic acid daily had a 72% reduction in their risk of having an affected fetus in the subsequent pregnancy (RR, 0.28; 95% CI, 0.12–0.71).[30]

Women with Other Risks for a Pregnancy Complicated by a Neural Tube Defect

Additional risk factors for a neural tube defect include having a previous child with an orofacial cleft, family history of neural tube defects or known genetic mutations in folate-related enzymes, antiepileptic drug use, epilepsy, insulin-dependent diabetes, medically diagnosed obesity, and use of antifolate drugs. However, it is not yet clear that high-dose folic acid supplementation will reduce the incidence of neural tube defects in women with many of these risk factors. Therefore, the USPSTF recommends that these women take the standard 400 to 800 mcg per day dose routinely during the childbearing years and during pregnancy. By contrast, the American College of Obstetricians and Gynecologists recommends the higher 4 mg dose per day for women at high risk of bearing a child with neural tube defect.[29]

Risks of Folate Supplementation

A theoretical concern exists that folic acid supplementation could mask vitamin B_{12} deficiency anemia and allow the neurologic abnormalities associated with vitamin B_{12} deficiency to become permanent. Although there is no evidence that the incidence of vitamin B_{12} deficiency increases in women who take folic acid, daily doses exceeding 1 mg are not encouraged for routine supplementation and require prescription.

Iron

Iron needs approximately double during pregnancy secondary to the fetus's need for iron and the large increase in maternal blood volume.[31] This extra demand can exhaust iron stores in women who have normal stores prior to becoming pregnant. Women who have hemoglobin values less than 9.5 g/dL before or during the second trimester have an increased incidence of preterm birth and low-birth-weight infants.[32]

Absorption of iron by a woman in late pregnancy is approximately six times higher than during the nonpregnant state, and an average of 5.6 mg of iron per day crosses the placenta.[31] Nonetheless, for many women it is difficult to obtain enough iron from dietary sources, and iron supplementation is sometimes recommended. The CDC recommends that pregnant women who are anemic take 60–120 mg of elemental iron orally each day; if the anemia does not respond after 4 weeks of such treatment, further evaluation is advised to assess iron stores and look for causes of anemia other than iron deficiency. A Cochrane review found that intermittent (2 to 3 times per week) oral administration of iron has similar outcomes for mothers and infants, as does daily administration, with fewer side effects.[33]

Routine iron supplementation for all women during pregnancy is controversial. Since 1998, the CDC has recommended that all women receive, as primary prevention, 30 mg per day of oral iron supplements starting at the first prenatal visit.[34] In contrast, the USPSTF has concluded that the evidence is insufficient to recommend routine iron supplementation for women with normal hemoglobin levels. However, a recent Cochrane review found that routine iron supplementation, with or without folic acid, for both anemic and non-anemic women is associated with a decreased prevalence of low birth weight (average RR, 0.81; 95% CI, 0.68–0.97) and preterm birth (less than 37 weeks' gestation; RR, 0.88; 95% CI, 0.77–1.01).[32]

The various iron preparations of ferrous or ferric salts contain differing amounts of elemental iron. The ferrous salts are more bioavailable compared to the ferric salts.

Side effects of oral iron supplementation are primarily gastrointestinal and related to the dose of elemental iron. The products containing higher amounts of elemental iron generally induce more gastrointestinal side effects. Constipation, abdominal pain, nausea, and vomiting are the side effects most frequently reported.[33] Women taking ferrous fumarate and intermediate-release ferrous sulfate report uncomfortable side effects most often (56.3% and 53.7%, respectively). Slow-release ferrous sulfate is not recommended because iron is absorbed in the proximal portion of the small intestine of the stomach and the slow-release formulations do not dissolve quickly enough to become bioavailable in that site. Iron administered as ferrous fumarate within a multivitamin preparation and as the amino acid iron chelate ferric bisglycinate (Ferro Chel) have the fewest side effects (23.7% and 21.2%, respectively) and lower rates of discontinuation (0.0% and 6.1%, respectively, due to side effects alone). Unfortunately, ferric bisglycinate also contains the smallest amount of elemental iron.[35]

Parenteral iron therapy should be reserved only for those persons with documented severe iron-deficiency anemia in pregnancy who cannot tolerate any form of oral iron. Although parenteral iron improves hemoglobin levels more quickly than does oral supplements, potential harms include anaphylaxis, thrombosis, tissue staining, and significant pain. More information on parenteral forms of iron can be found in the *Hematology* chapter.

Iron supplementation for the iron-replete woman is not without risks. Increased rates of preeclampsia, low birth weight, and prematurity are associated with high hemoglobin levels (greater than 13.0 g/dL at term), and daily iron supplementation may increase oxidative stress.[31]

Calcium

Next to iron, calcium is the nutrient most difficult to obtain in sufficient amounts from the typical diet in the United States. The woman's calcium stores can be depleted as the fetus accumulates 25 to 30 g of calcium over the course of pregnancy. The fetal calcium needs are met through extraction of calcium from maternal bone, and at 35 weeks' gestation, the fetus obtains approximately 350 mg per day. The Institute of Medicine recommends women obtain 1300 mg of calcium per day during pregnancy and lactation, via either diet or supplements.

An inverse relationship between dietary intake of calcium and the incidence of hypertensive disorders was first noted in 1980 in epidemiologic studies. Several randomized trials and a meta-analysis were then conducted to evaluate the effect of calcium supplementation.[36] Calcium supplementation with at least 1 g per day lowered the risk of preeclampsia by half (RR, 0.45; 95% CI, 0.31–0.65), particularly in women at high risk for this condition (RR, 0.22; 95% CI, 0.12–0.42; 5 trials, n = 587) and in women with low baseline calcium intake (RR, 0.36; 95% CI, 0.20–0.65; 8 trials, n = 10,678).[36] Women with an adequate dietary intake of calcium had a reduction in their risk of preeclampsia of 38%, but this reduction was not statistically significant.[37] This meta-analysis found a positive association between high-dose calcium supplementation (greater than 1 g/day) and HELLP syndrome (RR, 2.67; 95% CI, 1.05–6.82; 2 trials; n = 12,901). Thus calcium supplementation for the purpose of lowering the incidence of hypertensive disorders is not recommended until more data verifying this relationship become available.

Calcium may be formulated in several ways, with these versions containing various amounts of elemental calcium.[37] Calcium carbonate may be either produced in a laboratory (refined) or mined from limestone derived from fossilized oyster shell (natural source). Dolomite is calcium magnesium carbonate in mineral form. Calcium phosphate or hydroxyapatite is produced from powdered bone (bone meal). Calcium is also bound to organic chelates to produce calcium gluconate, calcium lactate, and amino acid calcium products.

Inevitably, calcium supplements contain some lead because these elements have the same charge density.[38] Calcium receptors in the body preferentially bind with lead, making lead levels in calcium supplements a potential concern. A study of calcium supplements available in the United States found that most supplements taken at levels recommended in pregnancy would not approach the provisional tolerable daily lead levels, and many had no detectable lead.[39] However, clinicians working internationally should be aware that national brands produced in other countries may contain more significantly more lead than those produced by multinational companies.

The most common adverse effects of calcium supplements are bloating, excess gas, and constipation, and these occur most often with calcium carbonate preparations. Changing to a different calcium preparation such as calcium gluconate and increasing fluid intake usually relieve these symptoms. Calcium citrate may be better absorbed and cause fewer gastrointestinal side effects than other calcium preparations, but it is often formulated to provide less elemental calcium per tablet.[38] Higher percentages of calcium are absorbed from supplements lower in elemental calcium; therefore, supplements containing 500 mg or less of elemental calcium are preferred. Taking calcium supplements with a meal generally increases the absorption of the calcium. In contrast, intake of some foods (e.g., wheat bran, spinach, and rhubarb) may decrease absorption. Calcium can interfere with absorption of iron and zinc, so it should be taken separately from other multiple micronutrient or iron supplements in pregnancy.

Vitamin D

Research into the physiologic functions of the essential pro-hormone vitamin D, or calciferol, has grown exponentially in recent years. While vitamin D was once believed to have a role primarily in calcium and bone metabolism, it has been recognized for some time that hormone receptors for vitamin D are present in most body tissues, including the placenta.[41] Vitamin D deficiency in pregnancy may cause rickets in the newborn. Vitamin D deficiency and insufficiency have been associated with a number of adverse perinatal outcomes, including preeclampsia, preterm labor, preterm birth, perinatal infections, small-for-gestational-age infants, and gestational diabetes in some, but not all, observational studies.

Current evidence from randomized trials and meta-analyses does not support routine supplementation of vitamin D during pregnancy.[41] While supplementation does effectively raise vitamin D levels in women who take supplements, there is no clear and established benefit for perinatal outcomes of pregnant women who are not deficient in vitamin D. Additionally, excessive vitamin D, even though rarely associated with oral supplements, can be harmful. Vitamin D is fat soluble, and hypervitaminosis D can, through hypercalcemia, cause symptoms including gastrointestinal symptoms, drowsiness, bone pain, and cardiac arrhythmias.[42]

Therefore, although routine vitamin D screening during pregnancy is not recommended, clinicians may consider measuring vitamin D for women whom they consider to be at increased risk for deficiency. If deficiency is found, supplementation of 1000 to 2000 IU per day is recommended.[43] The controversy regarding the definitions of vitamin D insufficiency and deficiency is discussed in more detail in the *Vitamins and Minerals* chapter.

Multivitamins and Micronutrients

Because the large doses of some vitamins found within multivitamins can be harmful, women should not exceed the recommended number of tablets or capsules per day in an effort to increase their intake of a single micronutrient. Excess vitamin A is teratogenic, but no human studies have determined the level of exposure required for teratogenesis. Conversely, doses of less than 10,000 mg per day are known to be safe. Theoretically, excessive vitamin E may interfere with platelet aggregation and leukocyte function.[44]

Deficiencies of some vitamins and elements—particularly zinc, selenium, calcium, vitamin A, folic acid, iodine, iron, magnesium, selenium, and copper—have been linked with various pregnancy and neonatal complications, especially in developing countries where nutritional deficiencies are more prevalent and severe. Some evidence indicates that supplementation with multiple micronutrients decreases the number of low-birth-weight infants and small-for-gestational-age infants when compared to placebo. A Cochrane analysis found that multi-micronutrient supplements were associated with slightly reduced risk for both of these conditions compared with supplements containing solely iron and folate; however, there was insufficient evidence to recommend advocating to replace the current recommendation for use of iron and folate with a new recommendation that pregnant women take micronutrient supplements.[44]

Therapies Used to Treat Common Gestational Discomforts

Most pregnant women experience some uncomfortable physiologic changes. The need for relief when these conditions interfere with the woman's ability to maintain her normal daily activities must be balanced against the risks involved in drug therapy for these conditions. Many of the women with common discomforts of pregnancy do not need pharmacologic agents. For those women with conditions that are amenable to pharmacologic treatment, choosing the lowest effective dose of the safest medical therapy for the shortest duration is a useful approach, and whenever appropriate, promoting nonpharmacologic comfort measures prior to prescribing a pharmacologic agent is preferred.

Back and Pelvic Pain

Lower back pain and pelvic pain are the most common musculoskeletal discomforts during pregnancy, especially during the second and third trimesters.[45] Some women who experience lower back pain have concomitant sciatica. Approximately 20% of women experience pelvic pain during pregnancy.[46]

In the past several years, various nonpharmacologic modalities to treat both lower back pain and pelvic pain have been assessed in randomized controlled trials (RCTs) and systemic reviews, including strengthening and stabilizing maneuvers, abdominal and pelvic support materials, acupuncture, massage, spinal and osteopathic manipulation, and various combinations of these measures.[45,46] While the evidence is limited and somewhat conflicting overall, exercise and acupuncture appear to be most effective in relieving such pain.[46] Ideally, treatment will include a multidisciplinary approach, with input from specialties such as physical therapists being sought as needed.

The only over-the-counter analgesic that is commonly used in pregnancy is acetaminophen (Tylenol), but it is generally not effective for treating pregnancy-related back pain. Severe pain can be treated with opiate analgesia if needed.[45,46] Muscle relaxants are not used in pregnancy, so there is no single pharmacologic treatment other than analgesics. Limited information is available regarding the use of cyclobenzaprine (Flexeril) for this indication, but one case study introduced the possibility of a direct correlation between late pregnancy use of cyclobenzaprine and early ductal closure and persistent pulmonary hypertension in the newborn. The proposed etiology was the prostaglandin inhibitory mechanism of action of cyclobenzaprine.[46]

Constipation

Due to the physiologic and anatomic changes that occur in the gastrointestinal tract of the pregnant woman, constipation is a common discomfort for many women during pregnancy. Causes include slowed intestinal motility due to increased circulating progesterone; decreased motilin levels; reduced activity due to nausea, vomiting, and fatigue; iron and prenatal vitamin supplementation; and increasing pressure on the intestines from the growing uterus.[47] A first-line approach to management includes lifestyle changes such as increasing fluids and fiber; regular, moderate exercise; and promotion of good bowel habits. Regular supplementation with bran (2–6 spoonfuls per meal, coupled with sufficient liquid to prevent bloating) is highly effective.[48] However, pharmacologic intervention may be needed for adequate relief.

Laxatives are the second-line treatment. While data are insufficient to guarantee these medications' effectiveness or safety during pregnancy, systemic absorption is likely minimal and existing studies are reassuring.[49] The bulk-forming laxatives such as psyllium, methylcellulose, and polycarbophil are not associated with increased risk of fetal malformations; therefore, they are considered the first choice and are appropriate for long-term use.[49] When taken with sufficient water (1–2 glasses), stool weight and fecal water will increase while colonic transit time will decrease. Surface-active agents such as stool softeners (docusate sodium) may also be helpful at this time.[48]

While considered the most effective agents, simulant laxatives are associated with more adverse effects such as abdominal pain and diarrhea; consequently, they are indicated only for short-term use for intractable cases that are unresponsive to bulk or osmotic laxatives.[44,49] Enemas and strong cathartic agents are contraindicated during pregnancy. Women should be cautioned that bowel dependence may be associated with any laxative.

Headaches

Women experience tension headaches, migraines, and cluster headaches more frequently than men. The incidence of tension headaches does not change during pregnancy, and the treatment is the same as treatment in nonpregnant women. More information about tension headaches and cluster headaches can be found in the chapter *The Central Nervous System*.

Migraines

As many as 18% of women experience migraines, an incidence three times greater than that in men.[50] Among other triggers, fluctuations of the female sex hormones during the reproductive years influence migraine frequency and severity. While the severity of migraine increases sharply with the onset of menarche, most women experience relief during pregnancy, especially women who have migraines *without* aura.[51] The MIGRA study—the largest prospective study of migraines during pregnancy ($n = 2126$)—followed women with headaches during pregnancy and the puerperium. This study found that 50% to 75% of women with migraines experienced either a reduction in severity of these headaches or a complete cessation during pregnancy, especially after the first trimester,—and that new onset of headache is uncommon in pregnancy. Nonetheless, symptoms worsen for some women, and a small minority of women will experience migraine for the first time during pregnancy. Most women with new migraine onset at this time experience aura.[52]

No matter which pattern is apparent, migraine during pregnancy requires further evaluation. Specifically, the clinician must differentiate among various etiologies such as primary headache disorder, potential secondary headache disorder due to underlying disease such as preeclampsia, or headache secondary to a condition that may emulate migraine.[51] Studies indicate that women who have migraines during pregnancy are likely at increased risk for vascular events such as preeclampsia, gestational hypertension, and thromboembolic events.[53]

Pharmacologic treatment may be necessary if avoidance of triggers and healthy lifestyle changes are not effective. Pharmacologic therapy is available for both acute and preventive treatment. First-line treatment for acute migraine attacks in pregnancy begins with 650 mg of acetaminophen (Tylenol).[51] If single agents are not effective in relieving the pain, combination agents containing acetaminophen 300 mg/caffeine 40 mg/butalbitol50 mg (Fioricet) is often prescribed for treatment of migraines but has some limitations on its use during pregnancy. Butalbital and codeine should not be taken more than four or five days per month to prevent medication-overuse headache, and these drugs should not be used close to the time of birth because both can cause neonatal withdrawal. Caffeine is a common ingredient in many nonspecific short-term therapies and is usually present as 40 to 50 mg per tablet. Studies indicate caffeine used as an adjuvant medication at a dose of 100 mg or more provides analgesic relief for acute pain,[54] and intake of less than 300 mg per day is considered safe during pregnancy.[50] Acetaminophen should be limited to no more than 4000 mg per day to avoid hepatotoxicity.

The NSAIDs are also considered effective second-line therapies when added to other migraine medications, but should be used only during the second trimester. NSAIDs are associated with birth defects if used in the first trimester; when taken in the third trimester, they can cause oligohydramnios or potential premature closure of the patent ductus arteriosus.

Ergot alkaloids such as caffeine–ergotamine (Cafergot, Wigraine), dihydroergotamine (DHE, Migranal), ergotamine (Ergomar), and methysergide (Sansert) are contraindicated during pregnancy due to their teratogenic, abortifacient, or fetotoxic effects.[50,51]

The triptans are selective serotonin receptor agonists used for both treatment and prevention of migraines. These agents selectively constrict brain vessels and are most effective when taken at the first onset of symptoms.[50,51] Triptans are contraindicated in women with cardiovascular disease because they are potent vasoconstrictors.[50] Traditionally, the triptans have been contraindicated in pregnancy secondary to a theoretic concern that they might constrict utero-placental vessels or cause increased uterotonic activity. Manufacturer pregnancy registries for sumatriptan (Imitrex), naratriptan (Amerge) and the combination formulation of sumatriptan/naratriptan (Treximet) over the period from 1996 to 2012, revealed no reports of teratogenic effects,[55] yet use of these agents in clinical practice remains rare due to the limited data.[56]

Sumatriptan (Imitrex) is the most widely studied of the triptans, and is becoming more frequently used in pregnancy for women with severe, frequent migraine headaches. Large studies and pregnancy registries suggest its use is not associated with an overall increased risk of congenital malformations or teratogenesis; however, women who use triptans late in pregnancy appear to have a small but statistically significant increased risk of uterine atony (adjusted odds ratio [aOR], 1.4; 95% CI, 1.1–1.8) and increased blood loss (aOR, 1.3; 95% CI, 1.1–1.5).[57] Sumatriptan has also been associated with low birth weight and preterm birth in a large population-based study,[58] although no etiologic connection has been identified. Independent studies are needed to confirm the current findings. Although prescribers must remain cautious, current data are reassuring regarding initiation or continuation of a triptan when necessary, especially sumatriptan.[58]

Opioids are considered third-line therapies during pregnancy, after both simple analgesics and medications specific to migraine.[59] At times, opioids may provide relief from acute attacks, yet adverse effects such as early headache recurrence, central sensitization, sedation, nausea, dizziness, and complications related to addiction history make this option less useful.[60]

Preventive agents for migraines that are intractable, frequent, or associated with emesis and dehydration may be needed. While not without risk, possible options include beta blockers, calcium-channel blockers, and antidepressants such as amitriptyline. The nausea and vomiting that often accompany migraine may be treated by the same agents recommended as treatments for the nausea and vomiting of early pregnancy.[50]

Alternative therapies such as butterbur, magnesium, riboflavin, feverfew, and coenzyme Q-10 have all been studied as therapies for migraines; however, only magnesium is considered safe in pregnancy.[61] Magnesium may be used either alone or in combination with some migraine medications to increase therapeutic effectiveness and reduce aura.[61]

Heartburn and Gastroesophageal Reflux Disease

Due to both the hormonal and structural changes of pregnancy, many pregnant women experience heartburn, which is the result of an increased pressure in the abdomen and decreased lower esophageal sphincter tone.[62] Symptoms are usually worse after meals and at bedtime. For some women, lifestyle changes may be useful, such as elevating the head of the bed; eating smaller, more frequent meals; avoiding food for at least 3 hours before sleep; and avoiding food triggers.[62,63] Other women will need medication to control their symptoms.

Data are limited on both the safety and the effectiveness of pharmacologic interventions for heartburn relief. As a consequence, management includes a step-up approach that begins with antacids, then introduction of histamine-2 (H_2)-receptor antagonists, followed by proton pump inhibitors for women with the most severe, intractable symptoms.[64]

Antacids neutralize stomach acid and provide protection to the mucosal gastrointestinal tract. Most are easily obtained as over-the-counter products and provide quick, short-term relief.[65] Most tablet and liquid antacids contain magnesium hydroxide, calcium carbonate, or aluminum salts, and all are considered safe during pregnancy when taken in the recommended dosages.[62] Magnesium can induce diarrhea, and calcium can induce constipation and muscle cramps. Serious adverse effects are rare, but can be severe if the usual doses are exceeded. Antacids containing sodium bicarbonate (e.g., Alka-Seltzer) may cause maternal or fetal metabolic alkalosis and fluid overload, and should be avoided in pregnancy.[62] Low gastric pH enhances the absorption of iron; therefore, antacids should be taken separately from vitamin or iron supplements. Those antacids containing aspirin, such as bismuth subsalicylate (Pepto-Bismol), should not be used during pregnancy. Specific information about antacids can be found in the *Gastrointestinal Conditions* chapter.

When symptoms persist, the next step after antacids is the H_2-receptor antagonists such as cimetidine (Tagamet), famotidine (Pepcid), nizatidine (Axid), and ranitidine (Zantac). These agents act by reducing gastric acid secretion. The H_2-receptor antagonists may be particularly effective for nocturnal symptoms because of the theoretical reduction in the nighttime histamine surge and resultant gastric acid secretion.[65] Because cimetidine has multiple drug interactions, it is not recommended in pregnancy. Conversely, ranitidine is often a first-line recommendation, as it is the only H_2-receptor antagonist for which studies show effectiveness during pregnancy.[64]

The proton pump inhibitors act by inhibiting acid-producing stomach enzymes, thereby providing healing properties for erosive esophagitis.[65,65] Lansoprazole (Prevacid), rabeprazole (Aciphex), esomeprazole (Nexium), and pantoprazole (Protonix) are all considered safe for use during pregnancy.[66,67] Omeprazole (Prilosec), however, has been associated with embryonic and fetal mortality in animal studies. However, a large study of human data from Denmark that published in 2010 reviewed more than 840,000 births and found no significant associations between any of the proton pump inhibitors and birth and defects, including omeprazole, the most commonly prescribed proton pump inhibitor in the study.[66] In addition, a 2009 meta-analysis of human studies found no association between first-trimester proton pump inhibitor use and an increased risk of spontaneous abortion, preterm delivery, or any major congenital birth defects.[67] Even so, the proton pump inhibitors generally are reserved for appropriate implementation according to the stepwise approach, and only for severe cases of gastroesophageal reflux disease.

Past therapies to improve gastric motility and emptying, such as metoclopramide (Reglan), are no longer recommended due to their limited benefits and numerous side effects.[65]

Peptic Ulcer Disease

Peptic ulcer disease has no known effect on fetal outcomes, but may complicate a woman's pregnancy. It is also unknown if fetal outcomes differ depending on whether the mother is treated for peptic ulcer disease during pregnancy.[68] While data on this subject are limited, one large population-based study found a 1.18-fold increased risk of low birth weight (95% CI, 1.01–1.30), a 1.20-fold increased risk of preterm delivery (95% CI, 1.02–1.41) and a 1.25-fold (95% CI, 1.11–1.41)higher risk for small-for-gestational-age babies in women with peptic ulcer disease.[68] This study, however, was not able to identify an improvement in neonatal outcomes with medication treatment during pregnancy.[68]

Nonetheless, women with peptic ulcer disease usually require treatment. Management of peptic ulcer disease involves lifestyle changes such as smoking cessation, diet, and rest, followed by four levels of medication: antacids, H_2-receptor antagonists, proton pump inhibitors, and *Helicobacter pylori* treatments including cytoprotective agents.[69] The first three groups of medications are considered safe if used during pregnancy.

H. pylori treatment during pregnancy depends on accurate diagnosis of this infection, and the benefits of such treatment are debatable: Some experts recommend treating this condition during pregnancy, while others recommend waiting until the postpartum period. Medication regimens for *H. pylori* eradication consist of proton pump inhibitors and two antibiotics administered over a 1- to 2-week period.[70] The antibiotics included in this regimen must be confirmed as safe for use during pregnancy.

Cytotec (Misoprostol), a synthetic prostaglandin E_1 analogue, is FDA approved for both prevention and treatment of gastrointestinal ulcers and peptic ulcer disease that is secondary to NSAID use. However, this drug is contraindicated for this use during pregnancy because it causes uterine contractions.

Sucralfate (Carafate) is also used in the treatment of gastroesophageal reflux disease and peptic ulcer disease. Consisting of a sucrose sulfate salt and aluminum hydroxide, sucralfate provides mucosal protection via several mechanisms, including acting as a physical barrier and reducing exposure to acid, pepsin, and bile acids. No teratogenicity has been found in animal studies, and human use of sucralfate is generally considered safe secondary to minimal absorption.[62]

Hemorrhoids

Hemorrhoids are quite common, and they occur more often during pregnancy and the puerperium.[48] Symptoms range from mild to severe and acute to chronic, and include itching, pain, and bleeding. While recovery may be spontaneous, symptoms typically persist throughout the postpartum period. Addressing constipation is an important first step and includes management approaches such as fiber supplementation, increased liquid intake, and stool softeners.

Topical hemorrhoidal preparations provide short-term relief, and include witch hazel compresses (Tucks), anesthetics, glucocorticoids, phlebotonics, and warm sitz baths. Delivery systems include sprays, emollient creams, and suppositories. Products containing epinephrine or phenylephrine should be avoided for women with hypertension.[49] Information on prescribing many of these agents is provided in the *Gastrointestinal Conditions* chapter.

Insomnia

Insomnia may be a result of common discomforts in pregnancy or may occur secondary to an underlying sleep disorder. The three most common sleep disorders are habitual snoring, obstructive sleep apnea, and upper airway resistance syndrome. Restless leg syndrome and primary insomnia can also occur more often among women who are pregnant compared to those who are not. Hormonal and anatomic changes likely contribute to sleep disturbance in pregnant women. For example, weight gain and the gravid uterus displace the diaphragm upward, creating reduced lung capacity and breathing difficulty, while estrogen-related changes lead to increased edema of the mucous membranes and nasal passages, which also increases breathing difficulties due to congestion.[71]

Evidence correlates sleep disturbance with pro-inflammatory markers, an increased incidence of hypertension, diabetes, preeclampsia, a prolonged and more painful labor, preterm birth, and cesarean birth. Maternal–fetal outcomes may improve with better recognition and treatment of disordered sleep.[71]

Treatment depends on the particular disorder. For discomfort during pregnancy, sleep hygiene education, fluid restriction prior to bedtime, pillows, and warm packs may help, along with traditional remedies such as warm milk and chamomile tea. Research indicates massage, yoga, acupuncture, and exercise may also be helpful.[71]

For breathing-related sleep disorders, there are no drugs for use during pregnancy. Mild obstructive sleep apnea may be relieved by avoiding excessive weight gain in pregnancy, lateral positioning, and raising the head of the bed to sleep.[72] Oral appliances work best in the supine position, which is not recommended during pregnancy.[71] The sedative-hypnotic drugs most commonly prescribed in the nonpregnant population are largely contraindicated during pregnancy.

A common practice in the general population is to employ over-the-counter antihistamines or antihistamines combined with analgesics as sleep aids. Many of these pharmaceuticals are considered safe during pregnancy (e.g., first-generation antihistamines), yet are associated with central nervous system depression and drowsiness.[71] Diphenhydramine (Benadryl), hydroxyzine (Vistaril), and doxylamine (Unisom SleepTabs) may be used on a short-term basis to improve rest. Zolpidem (Ambien) has limited data on its use in pregnancy; if used at all, it should be considered second-line therapy. Other sleep medications such as ramelteon (Rozerem), a melatonin receptor agonist, are contraindicated due to unknown effects on pregnancy and the fetus. Information on the safety and effectiveness of melatonin itself is likewise limited.

Leg Cramps and Restless Leg Syndrome

Many women experience leg cramps during pregnancy, and some have or develop restless leg syndrome. Occurring primarily at night, both can significantly disrupt sleep, and are considered potential diagnostic sleep disorders by the American Academy of Sleep Medicine. Muscle cramps in the legs occur in as many as 30% of pregnant women—most commonly in the third trimester—may be intensely painful, and most often affect the foot or calf.[73] The etiology is unknown. Although limited, studies suggest 350 mg of magnesium at bedtime may reduce nightly leg cramps.[73]

Restless leg syndrome is a sensory motor syndrome that primarily involves the lower extremities. Women often have difficulty describing the nerve-like sensations that occur with this disorder. The symptoms most often reported are difficulty falling asleep and maintaining sleep, fatigue, daytime sleepiness, and reduced functioning.[73] Restless leg syndrome can be associated with iron deficiency or ferritin or folate deficiency and malabsorption.[71] If iron-deficiency anemia is the cause, iron supplementation with vitamin C may relieve symptoms. Drugs such as dopamine antagonists may also cause restless leg syndrome; therefore, a first step is reviewing the woman's current medication regimen and changing current drugs to those that have a different mechanism of action.

Some medications that are effective for treating restless leg syndrome are not used during pregnancy because of related toxicity or teratogenicity. For example, little is known about the pregnancy effects of dopamine precursors and agonists such as pramipexole ropinirole, so they are not recommended for use.[74] Other medication classes such as opioids, anticonvulsants, and benzodiazepines are also largely contraindicated in pregnancy; however, off-label use of some of these agents may be considered for severe symptoms. Short-term use of zolpidem (Ambien) is one option,[71] but even this commonly prescribed medication may be associated with adverse pregnancy outcomes.[72]

Nausea and Vomiting

Nausea and vomiting of pregnancy (NVP) commonly begins at approximately 4 to 9 weeks' gestation, is often most bothersome between 10 and 15 weeks' gestation, and usually resolves by 20 weeks' gestation, if not sooner. It is one of the most common pregnancy conditions for which pharmacotherapeutics are used. Approximately 70% to 85% of women experience nausea in early pregnancy, and 50% vomit.[75] A few women experience NVP throughout gestation. The etiology of this condition is unknown, although there is a positive relationship between high levels of human chorionic gonadotropin (hCG) and increasing severity of nausea and vomiting.

Several different neurotransmitters may stimulate the chemoreceptor trigger zone within the brain that initiates vomiting. The chemoreceptor trigger zone has receptors for histamine, dopamine, and serotonin, plus receptors for opioids and benzodiazepines. This variety of target neurotransmitters is beneficial because drugs in several different classes can be used as antiemetics. Current evidence suggests that women experiencing both heartburn and NVP should be treated for both; treatment of heartburn may reduce nausea and vomiting symptoms. In addition, antacids containing magnesium or calcium may improve nutrition if a woman is vomiting.[76]

Complementary Therapies for Nausea and Vomiting of Pregnancy

Herbal remedies used by pregnant women to alleviate nausea and vomiting include ginger, peppermint, chamomile, and lemon oil.[77] Randomized controlled studies have found that ginger is more effective than placebo in reducing both nausea and vomiting and is equivalent in effectiveness to pyridoxine (vitamin B_6).[76] The safe, effective dose of ginger has been shown to be approximately 1 g or more per day in 3 or 4 divided doses of dried, powdered rhizome or ginger syrup containing 250 mg ginger administered orally. At this dose, no significant adverse effects have been observed other than mild sedation, heartburn, or intolerance of treatment. Peppermint tea may be effective, is widely used, and is likely a reasonable treatment, although no data on its effectiveness or safety in humans are available.

Pharmacologic Therapies for Nausea and Vomiting of Pregnancy

Medications useful for treating NVP include (1) first-generation, sedating antihistamine-anticholinergics such as doxylamine (Unisom SleepTabs), diphenhydramine (Benadryl), and meclizine (e.g., Antivert, Bonine); (2) dopamine antagonists, metoclopramide (Reglan), and phenothiazines such as promethazine (Phenergan) and prochlorperazine (Compazine); and (3) serotonin antagonists such as ondansetron (Zofran). Table 35-4 shows a protocol for managing nausea and vomiting, and doses of the antiemetic drugs used are listed in Table 35-5.[77]

There is no evidence to determine when to begin pharmacologic therapy for NVP, as a woman's quality of life can be negatively affected even by infrequent retching and vomiting. Women with mild nausea may find sufficient relief from nonpharmacologic interventions such as small, frequent meals, avoiding triggers, and discontinuing prenatal vitamins. Sea-Bands, ginger capsules, and vitamin B_6 all have some effectiveness for minimizing nausea.[77]

For women with moderate nausea, no vomiting, and no evidence of dehydration, pyridoxine (vitamin B_6) at doses of 10 to 25 mg by mouth taken three times per day significantly improves nausea, and higher doses are more effective than lower doses.[77] There are no adverse effects associated with these doses of pyridoxine, and it is usually the first-line pharmacologic agent recommended.

An over-the-counter formulation of doxylamine (Unisom tablets) can be added to pyridoxine to create the same formulation that constituted Bendectin, a brand no longer available in the United States. Bendectin, perhaps the first well-known litogen, was withdrawn from the U.S. market in 1983. After the product was removed, hospitalizations due to hyperemesis tripled in the United States while remaining stable in elsewhere in the world where the drug combination was still available. In 2013, a sustained-release tablet containing pyridoxine 10 mg and doxylamine 10 mg was approved; it is sold under the brand name Diclegis. Evidence shows that Diclegis is safe and effective.[78]

Finding the right combination of medication for a woman with moderate to severe nausea and vomiting is often a matter of trial and error. The first-generation antihistamines are antiemetics, but they can cause drowsiness and, albeit more rarely, confusion, blurred vision, dry mouth, or urinary retention. High doses can induce complications of asthma or narrow-angle glaucoma due to these medications' anticholinergic properties. The

Table 35-4 Treatment Options for Nausea and Vomiting During Pregnancy

1. Mild nausea without vomiting or with occasional vomiting:

a. Discontinue prenatal vitamins with iron; replace with folic acid supplement
b. Pyridoxine (vitamin B_6) 25–50 mg PO 3 times/day
c. Ginger root powder, capsules, or extract up to 250 mg PO 4 times/day
d. P6 acupressure (Sea-Bands)
e. Lifestyle counseling

2. Mild to moderate nausea with mild vomiting but no dehydration:

- Pyridoxine 25 mg PO 2–3 times/day and doxylamine (Unisom Night Time Sleep Aid) 12.5 mg PO 2 times/day or at bedtime only (1/2 tablet) *or*
- 10 mg of doxylamine combined with 10 mg of pyridoxine (Diclegis) up to 4 tabs daily; adjust schedule and dose according to symptom severity

If insufficient, *add* one of the following (if vomiting frequently, take 30–45 minutes before taking Diclegis):

- Promethazine (Phenergan) 12.5–25 mg every 4–6 hours *or*
- Dimenhydrinate (Dramamine)[a] 50–100 mg every 4–6 hours PO or PR, up to 200 mg/day

If still insufficient, *add* one of the following:

- Metoclopramide (Reglan) 5–10 mg every 8 hours PO or IM
- Chlorpromazine (Thorazine) 10–25 mg every 4–6 hours PO or IM, or 50–100 mg every 6–8 hours PR
- Prochlorperazine (Compazine) 5–10 mg every 6–8 hours PO or IM
- Promethazine (Phenergan) 12.5–25 mg every 4–6 hours PO, IM, or PR
- Ondansetron (Zofran) 4–8 mg every 6–8 hours PO

3. Nausea and vomiting with dehydration, ketonuria, unable to orally rehydrate:

a. Start IV fluids for rehydration
b. 1 ampule multivitamin supplement in first liter and daily thereafter (until able to tolerate oral medications) or 100 mg thiamine IV once daily
c. Dimenhydrinate (Dramamine)[a] 50 mg IV (in 50 mL saline over 20 min) every 4–6 hours

If insufficient, *add* one of the following:

- Promethazine (Phenergan) 12.5–25 mg IV every 4–6 hours *or*
- Chlorpromazine (Thorazine) 25–50 mg IV every 4–6 hours *or*
- Prochlorperazine (Compazine) 5–10 mg IV every 6–8 hours *or*
- Metoclopramide (Reglan) 5–10 mg IV every 8 hours

4. If insufficient, consider consultation and adding one of the following:

- Methylprednisolone (Solu-Medrol) 15–20 mg IV every 8 hours *or* 1 mg/hour continuously up to 24 hours (preferred after the 10th week of pregnancy due to possible increased risks for oral clefts) *or*
- Ondansetron 8 mg over 15 minutes every 12 hours or 1 mg/hour continuously up to 24 hours (Avoid single IV doses larger than 16 mg due to increased risk for QT prolongation; see FDA black box warning.)

5. For intractable vomiting, refer to obstetric specialist

[a] In the United States diphenhydramine (Benadryl) is used more often than dimenhydrinate (Dramamine).

Source: Data from Koren G, Phelan ST. Nausea and vomiting of pregnancy monograph. Association of Professors of Gynecology and Obstetrics Educational Series on Women's Health Issues; 2013. http://www.nationalperinatal.org/Resources/APGO%20Educational%20Series%202011.pdf. Accessed May 28, 2014.[75]

Table 35-5 Doses of Antiemetics Used to Treat Nausea and Vomiting in Pregnancy

Drug: Generic (Brand)	Dose	Clinical Considerations
Combination Product		
Pyridoxine hydrochloride (10 mg) with doxylamine succinate (10 mg) (Diclegis), delayed-release tablets	2 tablets PO at bedtime, with addition of 1 tablet in the morning and 1 tablet in the afternoon as needed. Maximum 8–12 tablets per day if increased BMI.	May cause drowsiness; anticholinergics
Antihistamines (H_1 Antagonists)		
Dimenhydrinate (Dramamine)	50–100 mg every 4–6 hours PO/PR[a]	May cause drowsiness Can be used to offset anxiety caused by metoclopramide (Reglan) or phenothiazines
Diphenhydramine (Benadryl)	50–100 mg every 4–6 hours PO/IM/IV	May cause drowsiness Can be used to offset anxiety caused by metoclopramide or phenothiazines
Doxylamine (Unisom Sleep-Tabs)	12.5 mg PO 2 times/day or 12.5 mg in the morning and 25 mg in the evening	Active ingredient in Diclegis
Phenothiazines (Central D_2 Antagonists)		
Prochlorperazine (Compazine)	5–10 mg every 6–8 hours PO/IM/IV 25-mg rectal suppository 2 times/day Maximum dose: 40 mg/day	Sedation, anticholinergic effects, dry mouth, dystonic reaction Hypotension if rapidly administered via IV route
Promethazine (Phenergan)	12.5–25 mg every 4–6 hours PO/IM/IV/PR	Sedation, anticholinergic effects, dry mouth, dystonic reaction Hypotension if rapidly administered via IV route
Benzamides (Central and Peripheral D_2 Antagonists)		
Metoclopramide (Reglan)	5–10 mg every 8 hours PO/IM/IV	Agitation, anxiety, acute dystonic reactions Give 50 mg diphenhydramine before IV dose to prevent extrapyramidal symptoms
Serotonin Antagonists		
Ondansetron (Zofran)	4–8 mg PO every 6–8 hours 4–8 mg over 15 minutes IV every 12 hours May be given as 1 mg/hour continuously for 24 hours	Headache Concern for potential cardiac arrhythmia: black box warning regarding QT prolongation for IV single doses greater than 16 mg
Butyrophenones		
Droperidol[b] (Inapsine)	0.625–2.5 mg IV over 15 minutes, then 1.25 mg as needed, or 2.5 mg IM Can be given IV continuously at 1–1.25 mg/hours	Dystonic reaction, prolonged QT syndrome Give 50 mg diphenhydramine before dose to prevent dystonic reaction Reserve for women who have failed other regimens although there is no evidence it is superior to promethazine

[a] Maximum dose is 200 mg/day if taken concomitantly with doxylamine, 400 mg/day if taken as a single agent.
[b] To be used only following consultation with medical specialist and if other medications have failed to resolve symptoms, secondary to risk for prolonged QT syndrome.

phenothiazines are effective antiemetics, but they are also dopamine antagonists; as such, they may induce excessive sedation, and rarely oculogyric crisis. These agents can also rarely induce an acute dystonic condition called extrapyramidal symptoms that involves deviation of the eyes upward, involuntary contractions of the muscles of the face, neck, trunk or pelvis, and unusual gait.[79]

Metoclopramide (Reglan) has both central and peripheral mechanisms of action. A dopamine antagonist and a serotonin antagonist in the chemoreceptor vomiting center in the central nervous system, metoclopramide is also a promotility agent in the gastrointestinal tract. A large case-control study supported its safe use in early pregnancy.[80] Metoclopramide is usually well tolerated but does cross the blood–brain barrier and can induce extrapyramidal effects. A 2010 FDA black box warning states that metoclopramide (Reglan) may cause potentially irreversible tardive dyskinesia, particularly with high cumulative exposure and when used for longer than 12 weeks. Metoclopramide does not cause sedation, however, and is being used more in the outpatient setting because it is better tolerated than the antihistamines and phenothiazines.

The most expensive, yet anecdotally effective, drug is the serotonin antagonist ondansetron (Zofran). Ondansetron is used via an off-label basis for nausea and vomiting in pregnancy, yet there is a relative paucity of evidence that substantiates the safety or effectiveness of this drug. Most authorities suggest reserving its use for situations in which other agents have been insufficient to control symptoms.

Hyperemesis

Severe nausea and vomiting of pregnancy that begins in the first trimester and causes dehydration, ketonuria, and weight loss of 5% or more usually is termed hyperemesis gravidarum. A diagnosis of exclusion, hyperemesis can involve electrolyte disturbance, biochemical (though not clinical) hyperthyroidism, and elevated liver enzymes. Some studies have suggested there may be genetic tendencies toward developing hyperemesis. There is also an association in the literature between *Helicobacter pylori* infection and hyperemesis. It is not yet known whether treatment of active *H. pylori* infections might improve hyperemesis.

The cornerstones of hyperemesis management are fluids, electrolytes, vitamin replacement, and antiemetic therapy that is usually initiated intravenously. When any of the dopamine antagonists is given intravenously, the risk of inducing extrapyramidal effects is significant; therefore when these agents are used, 50 mg of diphenhydramine (Benadryl) may be concomitantly administered intravenously with the dopamine antagonist.[81]

Rarely, severe thiamine deficiency due to prolonged periods of vomiting will cause Wernicke's encephalopathy, a condition manifested by changes in level of consciousness, confusion, ataxia, diplopia, abnormal ocular movements, and permanent neurologic sequelae. Wernicke's encephalopathy may be triggered by rapid initiation of intravenous glucose or dextrose, which increases thiamine requirements, so it is essential to replace thiamine prior to initiating intravenous solutions containing glucose in women with severe nausea and vomiting or hyperemesis.[75] Thiamine at 100 mg daily intravenously is recommended.

Systemic steroid therapy has been used with some success to treat women with hyperemesis that is unresponsive to other antiemetic therapy.[82] Prednisone or prednisolone (Millipred) is used for this indication because these steroids are metabolized quickly by the placenta, whereas dexamethasone (Decadron) readily crosses the placenta and can suppress fetal adrenal function.[52] To date, the effectiveness of corticosteroids over other agents has not been conclusively demonstrated, however, and these hormones are not without risk.[83] Systemic corticosteroids have been associated with a small increased risk for fetal orofacial clefting. When possible, corticosteroids should be reserved for situations in which other agents have failed, and limited to later than 10 weeks' gestation to reduce the risk of fetal teratogenic effects.[75]

Ptyalism

Ptyalism, defined as excessive salivation, can accompany severe nausea and vomiting in pregnancy or occasionally occur independently.[84] Its etiology in pregnancy remains unknown, and there has been no real success in use of drugs for symptom relief. Women report that attempting to swallow the saliva increases nausea, and many prefer privately to spit the saliva out into a receptacle; thus, the condition can contribute to social isolation. In the 1940s, belladonna, atropine, and hexamethonium were used to treat the condition. In more modern times, glucose solutions (e.g., Emetrol), lozenges, candies, fluids, chewing gum, and lifestyle changes such as eating smaller, more frequent meals have all been tried but with little evidence of benefit. Effective treatment of nausea and vomiting may help. More research is indicated to address this frustrating condition.

Urinary Tract Infections

Urinary tract infection (UTI) is the most common bacterial infection experienced by pregnant women. UTIs occur more frequently in pregnancy secondary to ureteral dilatation and increased urinary stasis, also enhancing the risk of ascending infection. Approximately 2% to 10% of pregnant women have asymptomatic bacteriuria, and 2% to 4% develop pyelonephritis.[85] If asymptomatic bacteruria is not treated, 15% to 45% of women will develop pyelonephritis.[85] All UTIs increase the risk for preterm labor.[86]

The most common bacteria that cause UTIs include *Enterobacteriaceae, Escherichia coli, Proteus, Klebsiella, Enterobacter, Pseudomonas, Citrobacter*, group B *Streptococcus*, and *Staphylococcus saprophyticus*.[87] *E. coli* susceptibility to antibiotics has high regional variance. Resistance rates are higher than 20% in all regions of the United States for ampicillin (Amoxil), and numbers are similar for trimethoprim with or without sulfamethoxazole. Fluoroquinolone- resistant *E. coli* generally accounts for fewer than 10% of UTIs, but its numbers are increasing. Nitrofurantoin (Macrobid) maintains good in vitro activity in most areas.[88]

Table 35-6 summarizes the antibiotics commonly used to treat urinary tract infections during pregnancy. All antibiotics to which the offending organism is not resistant are effective. A Cochrane review found insufficient evidence for recommending any specific antimicrobial agent or

Table 35-6 Antibiotics Used to Treat Urinary Tract Infections During Pregnancy

Antibiotic: Generic (Brand)	Dose	Clinical Considerations	Contraindications
Asymptomatic Bacteriuria			
Amoxicillin (Amoxil)	250–500 mg PO 3 times/day for 3–7 days	20% resistance overall, but wide geographic variation Must have susceptibilities before prescribing a beta-lactam Used to treat GBS without urine culture sensitivities	Allergy to penicillin
Amoxicillin–clavulanic acid (Augmentin)	250/125 mg PO 4 times/day for 3–7 days	20% resistance overall, but wide geographic variation Must have susceptibilities before prescribing a beta-lactam Used to treat GBS without urine culture sensitivities	Allergy to penicillin
Cephalexin (Keflex)	500 mg PO 4 times/day for 5-10days	Widely used in many regions	Cross-sensitivity if significant allergy to penicillin exists
Clindamycin (Cleocin)	300 mg PO 2 times/day for 3–7 days	Used for treatment of GBS bacteriuria in women who are allergic to penicillin	
Trimethoprim–sulfamethoxazole DS (Bactrim DS, Septra DS)	160/800 mg PO 2 times/day for 3–7 days	Folate antagonist Adverse effects include fever, rash, photosensitivity, nausea and vomiting, neutropenia, and Stevens-Johnson syndrome	Contraindicated in first trimester and also in third trimester for women with G6PD deficiency Allergy to sulfa
Uncomplicated Urinary Tract Infection (Cystitis)			
Amoxicillin (Amoxil)	500 mg PO 4 times/day for 7 days	20% resistance overall, but wide geographic variation Used to treat GBS without urine culture sensitivities	Allergy to penicillin
Amoxicillin–clavulanic acid (Augmentin)	250/125 mg PO 4 times/day for 7 days	20% resistance overall, but wide geographic variation Used to treat GBS without urine culture sensitivities	Allergy to penicillin
Cephalexin (Keflex)	500 mg PO 4 times/day for 7 days	First line for gram-positive organisms Ineffective for eradicating gram-negative organisms in vaginal reservoir	Cross-sensitivity if significant allergy to penicillin exists
Ciprofloxacin (Cipro)	250 mg PO 2 times/day for 3 days	Recommended if other agents are not available secondary to concern for increasing fluoroquinolone resistance	Hypersensitivity to fluoroquinolones
Nitrofurantoin (Macrodantin)	100 mg PO 4 times/day for 7 days	Urinary antiseptic; concentrates in urine Ineffective for pyelonephritis	Contraindicated for persons with G6PD deficiency Controversy regarding use near term to avoid hemolytic anemia in an infant with G6PD deficiency Generally considered safe for first trimester use, though ACOG recommends using other agents first (ACOG Committee opinion #494)
Nitrofurantoin (Macrobid) sustained release	100 mg PO 2 times/day for 7 days	Urinary antiseptic; concentrates in urine Ineffective for pyelonephritis	Contraindicated for women with G6PD deficiency Controversy regarding use near term to avoid hemolytic anemia in an infant with G6PD deficiency Generally considered safe for first trimester use, though ACOG recommends using other agents first
Trimethoprim–sulfamethoxazole (Bactrim DS, Septra DS)	160/800 mg PO 2 times/day for 7 days	Folate antagonist with theoretic increased risk of neural tube defects	Contraindicated in first trimester and also in third trimester for persons with G6PD deficiency and allergy to sulfa

(*continues*)

Table 35-6 Antibiotics Used to Treat Urinary Tract Infections During Pregnancy (*continued*)

Antibiotic: Generic (Brand)	Dose	Clinical Considerations	Contraindications
Pyelonephritis			
Aztreonam (Azactam)	1 g IV every 8–12 hours	Hospitalization until afebrile × 48 hours, then conversion to oral antibiotics, followed by discharge if woman remains afebrile	May be used for women allergic to beta-lactam antibiotics
Cefazolin (Ancef)[a,b]	1–2 g IV every 6–8 hours		Cross-sensitivity if significant allergy to penicillin exists
Ceftriaxone (Rocephin)[c]	1–2 g IV or IM every 24 hours until afebrile		Cross-sensitivity if significant allergy to penicillin exists
Cefuroxime (Ceftin)[b]	0.75–1.5 g IV every 8 hours		Cross-sensitivity if significant allergy to penicillin exists
Gentamicin (Garamycin)[b]	2 mg/kg loading dose, followed by 1.7 mg/kg IV every 8 hours		Potential ototoxicity; monitor serum concentrations and adjust dosing as needed
Suppression Therapy			
Cephalexin (Keflex)	125–250 mg PO daily	To be used for remainder of pregnancy with monthly cultures to verify suppression of microorganism Suggested use for 4–6 weeks postpartum for pyelonephritis	
Nitrofurantoin (Macrodantin)	100 mg PO at bedtime	To be used for remainder of pregnancy with monthly cultures to verify suppression of microorganism Suggested use for 4–6 weeks postpartum for pyelonephritis	Contraindicated for women with G6PD deficiency Controversy regarding use near term
Postcoital Prophylaxis			
Cephalexin (Keflex)	125–250 mg PO once daily	To be used for remainder of pregnancy to verify suppression of microorganism	
Nitrofurantoin (Macrodantin)	50–100 mg PO at bedtime	To be used for remainder of pregnancy to verify suppression of microorganism	Contraindicated for women with G6PD deficiency Controversy regarding use near term
Other			
Phenazopyridine (Pyridium, Uristat, Azo-Stat)	200 mg PO 3 times/day as needed for dysuria	May turn urine and contact lenses orange	

Abbreviations: ACOG = American College of Obstetricians and Gynecologists; G6PD = glucose-6-phosphate dehydrogenase; GBS = group B *Streptococcus*.
[a] May use with or without gentamicin 2 mg/kg intravenous loading dose, then 1.7 mg/kg every 8 hours for duration of therapy.
[b] Conversion to oral agents once afebrile: cephalexin (e.g., Keflex, Keftab) 500 mg PO 3 or 4 times/day for total therapy of 14 days, or cefuroxime 250 mg twice daily for total therapy of 14 days.
[c] If the woman is pregnant at 24 weeks' or less gestation, healthy, and able to comply with therapeutic plan, outpatient therapy can be instituted following hydration, antipyretics, the first intramuscular or intravenous dose of ceftriaxone followed by a second injection 24 hours later, then conversion to oral agents if she is afebrile.

regimen for treatment of uncomplicated symptomatic UTI in pregnancy.[89]

Medications for UTIs

Trimethoprim–sulfamethoxazole, which is often abbreviated as TMP/SMX, (Bactrim, Septra) is a sulfonamide that inhibits folate metabolism. Although research findings are mixed, at least one controlled, retrospective study found that exposure to this combination therapy in the first trimester was associated with an increased risk of cardiovascular defects (RR, 3.4; 95% CI, 1.8–6.4) and oral clefting (RR, 2.6; 95% CI, 1.1–6.1).[90] Women in this study who took folic acid supplements were less likely to have an affected infant; the cardiovascular defect relative risk was 1.5 (95% CI, 0.6–3.8) compared with 7.7 (95% CI, 2.8–21.7) among women who did not take such supplements. Despite these findings, the recommendation to supplement with folic acid when TMP/SMX is used has not been adopted in clinical practice. TMP/SMX used near term may also increase the risk of hyperbilirubinemia in the neonate due to competition with albumin binding.[87]

Nitrofurantoin concentrates solely in urine and is an effective therapy for uncomplicated cystitis. However, this agent can increase the risk for hemolytic anemia in individuals who have glucose-6-phosphate dehydrogenase (G6PD) deficiency. The National Birth Defects Prevention Study found an association between use of nitrofuran derivatives or sulfonamides and multiple categories of birth defects; however, this study was subject to recall bias and anti-infective prescriptions were not confirmed via medical records review.[91] A subsequent large population-based case-control study in Israel, which used medical records to confirm which drugs were dispensed, found no increased risk for malformations with use of nitrofurantoin (aOR, 0.85; 95% CI, 0.67–1.08).[92] Because of these conflicting findings, it is recommended that sulfonamides and nitrofurantoin be used in the first trimester only when other agents are not effective or appropriate.

The urinary pain reliever phenazopyridine (Uristat, Azo-Stat), which is available over the counter, has not been associated with congenital anomalies. Another over-the-counter product, sodium salicylate and methenamine (Cystex), contains an aspirin derivative and is not recommended for use in pregnancy, although methenamine has not been shown to be associated with birth defects. The urinary anesthetic phenazopyridine (Pyridium) is safe for use in pregnancy.

Duration of Treatment

The optimal length of treatment for asymptomatic bacteriuria has not been determined. A Cochrane review reported that while some evidence supports the effectiveness of single-dose treatment, treatment failures are more common if single-dose regimens are used.[85] Asymptomatic bacteriuria caused by group B *Streptococcus* (GBS) should be treated with an antibiotic to which the organism is sensitive, and the pregnant woman should receive intrapartum prophylaxis.[93] Additional information about intrapartum antibiotic prophylaxis for GBS can be found in the *Labor* chapter.

Cystitis is generally treated for 7 days. Some authors suggest a 3-day course is sufficient, although this recommendation has not been universally adopted in practice as yet. The standard 7-day course is generally recommended. Suppressive therapy can be prescribed either as a single postcoital dose or daily therapy regimen.

Pyelonephritis

Pyelonephritis has traditionally been treated with an initial hospitalization for hydration, monitoring for preterm labor, and initiation of intravenous antibiotic therapy. Parenteral first-generation cephalosporin agents such as cefazolin (Ancef), with or without gentamicin, cefuroxime (Ceftin), and ceftriaxone (Rocephin), are appropriate first-line agents, and cephalexin (Keflex) may be used as oral continuation therapy for susceptible organisms. Ampicillin is no longer a first-line drug for pyelonephritis. Intravenous antibiotics are used until the woman has been afebrile for 48 hours, after which time oral therapy is initiated for 10 to 14 days.

Outpatient therapy is beginning to replace hospitalization in selected women who are in the first or early second trimester of pregnancy, generally healthy, and able to comply with therapy. If an outpatient regimen is chosen, ceftriaxone (Rocephin) is administered intravenously or intramuscularly once every 24 hours until the woman is afebrile, followed by an oral agent for 10 to 12 days. Women who have experienced acute pyelonephritis in pregnancy have a 6% to 8% chance of recurrence before giving birth; therefore it is recommended that daily prophylaxis with nitrofurantoin (Macrobid) or cephalexin be maintained until 4 to 6 weeks postpartum.[94]

Pharmacologic Prevention of Perinatal Complications

Some medications are prescribed during pregnancy to help prevent premature birth or neonatal infections. Examples include antiviral suppression to prevent herpes, and progesterone for women at high risk for preterm birth. Women may also experience some other conditions during pregnancy that are associated with preterm birth and susceptible to pharmacologic intervention, yet no improvements in perinatal outcomes are seen despite successful treatment. This section reviews preventive therapies used during pregnancy.

Herpes Infections

Herpes simplex virus infections of the genital area can be caused by either herpes simplex virus type 1 (HSV-1) or type 2 (HSV-2). HSV-2 almost always occurs as a genital pathogen, but HSV-1 can manifest in either the genital area or the circumoral region.[95] HSV-1 is becoming a more common genital pathogen, with one-third to one-half of all neonatal herpes infections now caused by this virus.[96] Neonatal herpes is usually acquired via vertical transmission during labor and birth. To lower this risk, antiviral suppression is commonly prescribed at 36 weeks' gestation

Table 35-7 Antiviral Therapy for Genital Herpes in Pregnancy

Drug: Generic (Brand)	Suppression to Prevent Outbreak at Birth	Recurrent Episodes	Primary Episode	Disseminated Disease
Acyclovir (Zovirax)	400 mg PO 3 times/day until birth starting at 36 weeks' gestation	400 mg PO 3 times/day or 800 mg PO 2 times/day for 5 days	400 mg PO 3 times/day for 7–10 days (or longer if healing is incomplete at 10 days)	5–10 mg/kg IV every 8 hours for 2–7 days, then oral therapy for primary infection to complete 10 days of therapy in total
Valacyclovir (Valtrex)	500 mg PO 2 times/day until birth starting at 36 weeks' gestation	500 mg PO 2 times/day for 3 days or 1 g PO once daily for 5 days	1 g PO 2 times/day for 7–10 days (or longer if healing is incomplete at 10 days)	N/A

to prevent the woman from developing a herpes outbreak near the time of birth.

Treatment of a woman with genital herpes during pregnancy consists of oral acyclovir (Zovirax) or valacyclovir (Valtrex) (Table 35-7).[96] Valacyclovir is associated with consistently higher serum concentrations and is dosed only twice a day. Both drugs are safe for use during pregnancy. Published data about use of famciclovir in pregnancy are limited.[96]

Preterm Birth Prevention

Preterm birth is the primary cause of perinatal morbidity and mortality in the United States. Although treatment for premature infants has vastly improved, prevention of preterm labor and treatment of women with preterm labor are still problematic and often not very successful. This area of pharmacotherapeutics in maternal-fetal care is the subject of much current research.

Preterm Birth and Vaginal Infection

Two common vaginal conditions, trichomoniasis vaginalis and bacterial vaginosis, have been associated with an increased risk for premature birth.[97] The evidence for trichomoniasis as a factor in premature birth is somewhat mixed,[98] but the evidence for bacterial vaginosis is strong. Considering these correlations, antimicrobial treatment seems an intuitively sound preventive strategy. However, evidence to date does not support screening for either bacterial vaginosis or trichomoniasis in asymptomatic women. Both of these conditions represent a disturbance in the vaginal microbiome—due to either a single sexually transmitted organism (*Trichomonas*) or an imbalance of microflora favoring anaerobic bacteria—and it is likely that among some women, inflammatory cytokines triggered by these microbiome shifts do trigger preterm labor. However, the introduction of anti-infective agents does not interrupt this pathway, and in some cases may exacerbate it.[99]

A Cochrane review of metronidazole use in pregnant women with trichomoniasis vaginalis found that while metronidazole (Flagyl) was effective in eradicating the pathogenic organism, it was associated with a slight increase in the odds of preterm birth (RR, 1.78; 95% CI, 1.19–2.66).[98] Similarly, a Cochrane review revealed no benefits from screening and subsequent treatment of bacterial vaginosis in terms of preventing preterm birth. Even if a woman has a history of preterm birth, screening for asymptomatic bacterial vaginosis is not recommended as there is insufficient evidence of benefit and some evidence of harm from this approach.[97]

Treatment with antimicrobials effectively resolves symptomatic bacterial vaginosis and trichomoniasis, and pregnant women experiencing symptoms should be offered treatment. The CDC's 2010 treatment guidelines for sexually transmitted diseases are available to guide therapy.

Progestational Agents for Prevention of Preterm Birth

Progestogens have gained support as effective preventive measures for preterm birth in women with a singleton pregnancy and either a history of spontaneous preterm birth at less than 37 weeks' gestational age or a short cervix (less than 20 mm in length). A Cochrane review indicates that treatment with antenatal progesterone or 17 alpha-hydroxyprogesterone caproate (17-OHPC) lengthened gestation and reduced perinatal/neonatal morbidity and mortality when it is provided to women with either of the two aforementioned risk factors.[100] The optimal dose and route of administration for these formulations have not been established.

A separate systematic review and meta-analysis conducted on behalf of the Agency for Healthcare Research and Quality concluded that evidence to support the use of progestogens in women with other risk factors for preterm birth is insufficient to guide care.[101] Current recommendations for prevention of preterm birth are summarized in Table 35-8.

Table 35-8 Drugs Used for Prevention of Preterm Birth in Women with a Singleton Pregnancy

Clinical Factor	Recommendation	Regimen
History of spontaneous preterm birth	17 alpha-hydroxyprogesterone caproate (17-OHPC)	250 mg IM weekly from 16–24 weeks' through 36 weeks' gestation (or until delivery)
No history of spontaneous preterm birth, but cervical length ≤ 2 cm by transvaginal ultrasound at or before 24 weeks' gestation	Vaginal progesterone supplementation	Progesterone gel, 90 mg daily per vagina *or* micronized progesterone gel capsules (200 mg), 1 per vagina daily until 34–37 weeks' gestation

17-OHPC, which is a synthetic progestogen, is generally well tolerated. It appears to be safe, although a few studies suggest a possibly increased risk of gestational diabetes among women who used it; insufficient evidence currently exists to determine whether this association is causal or circumstantial. The most common side effect is a local skin reaction at the injection site. While 17-OHPC may be compounded, the FDA recognizes the brand-name formulation (Makena). Vaginal progesterone gel has long been regarded as safe for use in pregnancy.

Prevention of Preeclampsia

Although multiple preventive therapies for preeclampsia have been evaluated in large randomized controlled trials, only a few have shown any clear benefit. Calcium is associated with some success in preventing preeclampsia, particularly in women with high risk of this condition and among women with low baseline intake of calcium. Antiplatelet agents, particularly low-dose aspirin (60–80 mg), may have some benefit in preventing or delaying the onset of preeclampsia and preventing adverse perinatal outcomes.[102] It is currently recommended that those women at highest risk for preeclampsia initiate 60 to 80 mg per day of aspirin late in the first trimester.[102]

While there is no known harm associated with low-dose aspirin supplementation, substantial long-term evidence is not available.[103] Data for other preventive measures are inconclusive. The antioxidants vitamin C and E are not recommended either in low- or high-risk populations. Encouraging results in small trials have not been substantiated in larger trials; thus, sufficient data are not available to support this recommendation. Additional measures such as restricted salt intake and vitamin D supplementation also do not have sufficient evidence to support their use.

Prevention of Rh Isoimmunization

Historically, **erythroblastosis fetalis** and hemolytic disease of the newborn were common and often fatal events. With use of antenatal and postpartum prophylaxis, incidence of Rh alloimmunization has decreased from 1% to as little as 0.2%.[104] Box 35-2 tells the history of anti-D immune globulin (RhoGAM).

Routine prophylaxis with anti-D immune globulin is initiated at 28 weeks' gestation because the possibility of a transplacental hemorrhage large enough to cause maternal sensitization before that time is small.[104] Routine prophylaxis is also indicated within 72 hours post birth. Additional sensitizing events requiring prophylaxis include therapeutic or spontaneous abortion, ectopic pregnancy, antepartum hemorrhage, external cephalic version, and in utero procedures such as amniocentesis and chorionic villus sampling (CVS). For first-trimester events, 50 mcg of anti-D immune globulin is adequate for exposures as much as 2.5 mL of fetal red blood cells (RBCs); however, 300 mcg is recommended following first-trimester abortion.

Synthetic anti-D immune globulin (RhoGAM) is a human γ-globulin concentrate derived from pooled donor blood; it has a high titer of antibodies to red blood cell Rh D antigens. Various formulations of the anti-D immunoglobulin blood product are available in IM and IV forms in the United States. While both routes of administration are considered equally efficacious, sufficient data do not exist to support use of one over the other, although IM is used most commonly.

In the United States, the standard dose of anti-D immune globulin is 300 mcg administered intramuscularly, which prevents the development of antibodies for an exposure of as much as 30 mL of Rh D-positive blood or 15 mL of fetal RBCs. While the exact mechanism of action is unknown, the passive anti-D immunity created by the anti-D immune globulin allows clearance of anti-D–coated fetal RBCs from the maternal circulation before the RBCs are destroyed, thereby inhibiting development of the maternal immune process.[104] This process does not appear to have any maternal side effects. Moreover, while small amounts of passive anti-D immune globulin may reach the fetus, there are no known adverse fetal side effects from this treatment.[104]

After prenatal administration of anti-D immune globulin, a low serum anti-D antibody titer of 1:4 or less normally develops, reflecting the presence of the injected anti-D antibodies. Thus, the woman will have a weakly positive indirect Coombs test for approximately 12 weeks after anti-D immune globulin is given.

Box 35-2 The Story of RhoGAM

In 1939, while studying the blood of rhesus monkeys, Landsteiner discovered the Rhesus factor antigen. His work was considered one of the great successes of modern obstetric care, and he was awarded the Nobel Prize in Medicine for his discovery, which set the stage for better understanding hemolytic disease of the fetus and newborn. It took another 28 years to develop an agent, anti-D immune globulin (RhoGAM), that would prevent Rh immunization. The first clinical trials to test the effectiveness of anti-D immune globulin exclusively involved male inmate participants at Sing Sing Prison in Ossining, New York, who had the Rh-negative blood type. The trials were successful, and in 1968 anti-D immune globulin was introduced for the prevention of Rh isoimmunization.

There are five main rhesus antigens—D, C/c, and E/e—and two genes that encode for these antigens, although the term *Rhesus factor* or *Rh factor* usually refers only to the D antigen because the D antigen triggers the immune response. If an Rh-negative woman is pregnant with an Rh-positive fetus and is exposed to a sufficient number of those fetal red blood cells (RBCs), her body will produce anti-D antibodies against the Rh-positive (fetal) RBCs. In contrast to red blood cells that are large and do not commonly cross the placenta in either direction, anti-D antibodies are small immunoglobulin G (IgG) molecules that can easily cross and destroy Rh-positive fetal RBCs.

The first exposure to significant quantities of fetal blood usually occurs with a "silent" or "occult" event such as a small feto-maternal hemorrhage at birth. This is most likely to occur when the placenta separates directly after the birth. Subsequently, anti-D antibodies develop in the woman and remain present in her sera. In a subsequent pregnancy with an Rh-positive fetus, those antibodies can cross the placenta and cause hemolytic disease of the fetus or newborn (HDFN), which, depending on the severity, may lead to anemia, hydrops fetalis, jaundice, kernicterus, or death.

Some theoretic risks associated with RhoGAM do exist. The source for anti-D immune globulin is pooled human plasma; therefore, contamination with known or unknown blood-borne infections such as human immunodeficiency virus, hepatitis B and C, and parvovirus B19 is theoretically possible; however, no transmission from any U.S.-licensed product has ever been noted.[104] Since 1985, anti-D immune globulin has undergone a fractionation process that removes any viral particles. The risk for transmission of viral infections is considered minimal to absent.

Therapies for Medical and Pregnancy-Related Complications

Women can have chronic disorders that require pharmacotherapeutic drugs prior to pregnancy. In some cases, no changes in drug regimen are required. In others, however, the physiologic changes of pregnancy alter the course of the disorder or the pharmacokinetics of the drugs, or both. In these cases, pharmacologic management is adjusted and monitored by expert clinicians. In addition, a few conditions require pharmacologic treatment and appear only during pregnancy, such as gestational diabetes, gestational hypertension, pruritic urticarial papules and plaques of pregnancy (PUPPP), and intrahepatic cholestasis. This section reviews chronic disorders and pregnancy-specific conditions that require changes in pharmacologic management.

Diabetes

Type 1 diabetes, in which the body fails to produce sufficient insulin, most often predates pregnancy. With this condition, insulin therapy is required throughout gestation. Type 2 diabetes, in which the body develops resistance to endogenous insulin and relative insulin deficiency, is becoming more common in women of childbearing age. Gestational diabetes (GDM), which is diabetes that is first diagnosed during pregnancy, is the most common diabetic condition in pregnancy; it involves both insulin resistance and relative insulin deficiency.

Type 1 Diabetes

Diabetes that predates pregnancy has been associated with increased risks for congenital anomalies, spontaneous abortion, prenatal morbidity and mortality, and neonatal morbidity. Risks for the aforementioned complications increase concomitantly with higher maternal glucose levels.[105] For many years, pharmacologic treatment for type 1 diabetes, both prior to and during pregnancy, has involved the exclusive use of exogenous human insulin (Humulin, Novolin), which remains the treatment of choice for this condition.

Recent developments in synthetic insulin analogues have been promising, and these medications are being used more frequently. The most widely studied insulin analogue for use during pregnancy is insulin lispro (Humalog), a synthetic molecule similar to human insulin. Cord blood studies have found that like human exogenous insulin, insulin lispro crosses the placenta only minimally and may, in fact, be transferred less extensively than human insulin.[106] The advantages of this agent include increased absorption after subcutaneous injection, enabling a faster onset of action for improved postprandial blood glucose control, and reduced late hypoglycemia. Insulin lispro is associated with lower hemoglobin A_{1c} levels, lower rates of pregnancy loss, and higher satisfaction from women using it compared with human insulin.[107] A newer insulin analogue, insulin aspart (NovoLog), has been minimally studied during pregnancy and cannot yet be recommended for use. Insulin glargine (Lantus), a long-acting insulin analogue, has also not been studied for use in pregnancy; further studies are needed to determine its safety and effectiveness.

Type 2 Diabetes

Women who have type 2 diabetes are usually switched from an oral agent to insulin during pregnancy because use of insulin allows for tighter control of blood glucose levels and the teratogenic or fetotoxic effects of oral agents are unknown. Oral hypoglycemic agents such as metformin (Fortamet, Glucophage), sulfonylurea glyburide (DiaBeta, Micronase), and acarbose (Precose) have been studied in recent years and appear to be safe for use during pregnancy. These agents are beginning to be used by specialists who care for women with diabetes during pregnancy. Sulfonylurea drugs are contraindicated during pregnancy, however, because they cross the placenta and can induce fetal hyperinsulinemia.

Gestational Diabetes

Gestational diabetes mellitus (GDM) is diabetes that manifests or is first diagnosed during pregnancy, usually during screening at approximately 24–26 weeks' gestation. Diabetes that is discovered in very early pregnancy is likely to be either type 1 or type 2 and may be termed preexisting diabetes to differentiate it from gestational diabetes. GDM is commensurate with type 2 diabetes because it is a form of "carbohydrate intolerance" that may manifest as mild or severe. Treatment includes diet and exercise and/or medication. One of the most common disorders of pregnancy, its incidence depends on individual characteristics and varying diagnostic criteria. Prevalence is increasing worldwide, due to increasing rates of obesity and sedentary lifestyle.[108]

Pregnancy itself is a state of insulin resistance that increases with advancing gestational age. The hormones of pregnancy, such as progesterone, cortisol, prolactin, and human placental lactogen, decrease the effectiveness of insulin and increase insulin resistance. In a nondiabetic individual, this endocrinologic shift is inherently protective for the fetus and ensures adequate nutritional delivery to the feto-placental unit; however, in diabetes, either an inadequate amount of insulin is available or insulin effectiveness is decreased, resulting in hyperglycemia. Excessive amounts of glucose are present not only within the woman, but also in the placenta and her fetus.

Gestational diabetes is associated with an increased risk of complications, for both members of the maternal–fetal dyad. Fetal risks include macrosomia and birth injury. After birth, the infant is at increased risk of respiratory distress syndrome, neonatal hypoglycemia, hyperbilirubinemia, and polycythemia. A woman with GDM is at increased risk for polyhydramnios, operative delivery, cesarean birth, and preeclampsia. Unless severe, GDM is initially managed with diet and exercise. If these lifestyle changes are insufficient to maintain consistent normoglycemia, pharmacotherapy is indicated.

Traditionally, insulin has been the drug of choice for treating gestational diabetes. The insulin molecule does not cross the placenta or crosses it very minimally, so it does not cause adverse fetal effects.[108] However, insulin must be parenterally delivered. The dose of insulin is calculated based on the woman's weight. Total daily insulin is based on a ratio of 0.5–0.7 unit per kilogram of the mother's weight. Combining intermediate- and short-acting insulin yields the best result for most women. Two insulin doses are given daily, with two-thirds of the total insulin being administered in the morning to cover energy needs of the active day and one-third being taken at night. If a woman works at night, the proportions of the dose would be reversed so that two-thirds is given at night. If daytime were the primary time of activity, the morning dose would contain one-third of the total dose of the short-acting insulin and two-thirds of the dose of intermediate-acting insulin. The evening dose is reversed, with two-thirds of short-acting insulin serving to cover dinner and basal needs during the night and one-third of the intermediate-acting insulin covering the activity of the evening. Insulin needs may increase during the second and early third trimesters and then decrease at the end of pregnancy when the insulin resistance secondary to placental hormones decreases.

Two oral antidiabetic agents, sulfonylurea glyburide and metformin, have become increasingly popular as alternatives to insulin,[109] albeit on an off-label basis, as neither is FDA approved for this indication.[110] Human studies confirm both oral agents cross the placenta and, therefore, are associated with fetal exposure.[110]

The first-generation sulfonylureas are associated with fetal hyperinsulinemia and are contraindicated in pregnancy. The second-generation sulfonylurea glyburide does cross the placenta, but adverse fetal effects have not been reported. This agent appears to be as effective as insulin with regard to maternal and neonatal outcomes. The recommended starting dose is 2.5 to 5 mg daily or twice daily, and the maximum dose is 20 mg per day. Plasma levels peak within 4 hours of administration and the half-life is approximately 10 hours. The main side effect of glyburide is hypoglycemia.

Metformin (Glucophage) also appears to have effectiveness that is equal to insulin. Its doses range from 500 to 2500 mg per day. The dose is usually increased in increments of 500 to 850 mg until blood glucose levels are stable. The peak plasma level occurs in 4 hours and the half-life is approximately 6 hours. Unlike glyburide (Micronase), metformin does not cause maternal hypoglycemia or neonatal hyperinsulinemia, although women using metformin are more likely to need supplemental insulin as compared to women who use glyburide.

While use of oral antihyperglycemic agents has increased in the past several years, available data on their safety and effectiveness during pregnancy remain somewhat controversial and inconclusive.[110] Current evidence indicates glycemic control and maternal and neonatal safety are comparable to the results achieved with insulin therapy, and oral agents are associated with high acceptability and compliance by women. Even so, until studies on long-term outcomes are available, women starting oral antihyperglycemic agents during pregnancy need counseling about placental transfer and possible risks.

Hypertensive Disorders of Pregnancy

Hypertensive disorders of pregnancy complicate as many as 10% of pregnancies worldwide and are a leading cause of maternal and perinatal morbidity and mortality. For the fetus, hypertension in pregnancy increases the risk for prematurity, growth restriction, and hypertension later in life. Women who have hypertension during pregnancy are at increased risk for pulmonary edema, myocardial infarction, stroke, and renal failure. There is a positive relationship between the severity of hypertension and an increased risk for adverse outcomes. In addition, medications used to treat hypertension may have fetotoxic effects. Thus the management of these disorders is complex, and women who have severe hypertension during pregnancy require care by specialists.

This section reviews the drugs that are available for treatment of hypertension during pregnancy when medication is needed in the outpatient setting. For medications used to treat these disorders when a woman is admitted to the hospital, clinicians are directed to the most recent guidelines for details of management of hypertensive disorders in pregnancy, as the treatment approach for a woman may vary depending on multiple individual factors.[102]

The hypertensive disorders that may occur during pregnancy include chronic hypertension, chronic hypertension with superimposed preeclampsia, gestational hypertension, and preeclampsia–eclampsia.[102] Treatment goals for hypertension during pregnancy are threefold: (1) prevention of acute maternal complications; (2) support in continuing a healthy pregnancy for as long as possible; and (3) reduction of fetal risks associated with hypertension and vascular disease, including those related to side effects of antihypertensive medications. There is no evidence to support a specific target blood pressure at which to initiate pharmacologic therapy, nor is any one medication recommended as most effective. Pharmacologic therapies are not used to treat gestational hypertension or mild/moderate preeclampsia in the prenatal outpatient setting. In contrast, antihypertensive medications are recommended for the woman who presents with a blood pressure that is higher than 160 mm Hg systolic and 95 mm Hg diastolic or for the woman who is already taking an antihypertensive medication at the onset of pregnancy.

All antihypertensive medications cross the placenta. Certain classes of medications used to treat hypertension are known to be fetotoxic, others have not been found to affect the embryo or fetus, and others are equivocal in terms of their safety data for pregnancy. For example, angiotensin-converting enzyme (ACE) inhibitors and angiotensin receptor blockers (ARBs) have known fetotoxic effects including growth restriction. The antihypertensive agents considered safe and most frequently prescribed for pregnant women include methyldopa (Aldomet), labetalol (Trandate), and nifedipine (Procardia). Table 35-9 lists the medications used to treat hypertensive disorders during pregnancy.

Table 35-9 Antihypertensive Medications Used During Pregnancy

Drug: Generic (Brand)	Class	Dose	Clinical Considerations
Labetalol (Trandate)	Alpha- and beta-agonist blocker	100 mg PO 2 times/day Increase by 100 mg 2 times/day every 2–3 days as needed Usual dose: 200–2400 mg/day in divided doses	More rapid onset of action compared to methyldopa Possible bronchoconstriction; avoid in persons with asthma or cardiac compromise Possible increased risk for low-birth-weight infant with use of labetalol Side effects: lethargy, sleep disturbances
Methyldopa (Aldomet)	Centrally acting $alpha_2$-agonist	500–3000 mg PO per day in 2–3 divided doses Increase every 2 days as needed Usual dose: 250–1000 mg/day in divided doses	Mild antihypertensive with slow onset of action (6–8 hours); may not be effective for severe hypertension Full effect may take 2–3 days to be evident Childhood safety data up to 7 years after birth Side effects: sedation at high doses Rare adverse effects: hepatic dysfunction, hemolytic anemia
Nifedipine ER (Procardia)	Calcium-channel blocker	30–120 mg PO once daily Increase every 1–2 weeks as needed Usual dose: 30–90 mg/day	Slow-release form is used because immediate-acting form can cause a rapid drop in blood pressure; do not use sublingual form or immediate-acting form No adverse effects on uterine or umbilical blood flow

Source: American College of Obstetricians and Gynecologists; Task Force on Hypertension in Pregnancy. Hypertension in pregnancy. *Obstet Gynecol.* 2013;122(5):1122-1131.[102]

Angiotensin-Converting Enzyme Inhibitors and Angiotensin Receptor Blockers

Angiotensin-converting enzyme (ACE) inhibitors, angiotensin receptor blockers (ARBs), renin inhibitors, and mineralocorticoid antagonists are contraindicated for use during pregnancy. These drugs can cause fetal renal abnormalities and cardiac anomalies.[111]

Methyldopa, Labetalol, and Nifedipine

Methyldopa (Aldomet) is a nonselective $alpha_2$-adrenergic agonist. It has been extensively studied in pregnancy and is probably the most commonly used antihypertensive medication due to the availability of data on its safety in childhood and its long-term effects.

Labetalol (Trandate) is an alpha- and beta-adrenergic blocker that may protect uterine and umbilical blood flow better than does methyldopa. Labetalol is more effective for severe hypertension than mild hypertension.

Although data are more limited on the use of calcium-channel blockers to treat hypertension during pregnancy, nifedipine (Procardia) appears to be safe for this indication. This drug is increasingly used as a second agent if methyldopa or labetalol is not acceptable.

Intrahepatic Cholestasis of Pregnancy

Intrahepatic cholestasis of pregnancy is a pregnancy-specific liver disorder that occurs in the third trimester, and tends to resolve within several days to 2–3 weeks after birth. Intrahepatic cholestasis is associated with severe adverse outcomes such as preterm birth, meconium-stained amniotic fluid, and stillbirth.[113] The pathophysiology of this condition is poorly understood, but may include a combination of genetic, endocrinologic, and environmental factors. The incidence varies from less than 1 in 1000 pregnancies in Central and Western Europe and North America, to 5% to 15 % in Araucanian Indians in Chile and Bolivia.[113]

Intrahepatic cholestasis of pregnancy involves a buildup of bile acids in the liver and deposition of bile salts in the skin, which causes severe pruritus (without an accompanying rash). Itching occurs mostly on the palms of the hands and soles of the feet, although it may become generalized. Occasionally, jaundice, steatorrhea, and fat malabsorption causing vitamin K deficiency may occur.[114] Bile salt values of 40 mmol/L or more are associated with sudden intrauterine fetal demise (1–2%), preterm birth (19–60%), and nonreassuring fetal heart patterns in labor (22–33%).[115] Thus management of this disorder often includes early induction of labor in an attempt to avoid stillbirth. Specialist care is needed for women with intrahepatic cholestasis.

Various pharmacotherapeutic attempts have been used to reduce symptoms and improve perinatal outcomes, although no specific recommendations or guidelines have been developed that suggest using one intervention over the others. Table 35-10 summarizes the drugs used to treat intrahepatic cholestasis. Ursodeoxycholic acid (ursodiol; Urso, Actigall) appears most promising and is the drug most often used for this condition.[113]

Ursodeoxycholic acid is a hydrophilic bile acid, first found in traditional Chinese medicine in 618 AD when it

Table 35-10 Drugs Used to Treat Intrahepatic Cholestasis of Pregnancy

Drug: Generic (Brand)	Dose	Formulation	Mechanism of Action
Cholestyramine (Questran)[a]	8–16 g/day in divided doses	4 g cholestyramine contained in 9-g powder packet	Bile acid sequestrant that binds bile acids in the gut to facilitate excretion
Diphenhydramine (Benadryl)	25–50 mg PO every 6–8 hours Maximum dose: 300 mg/day	25- or 50-mg tablets	Antihistamine treats itching but does not treat disorder
Hydroxyzine (Vistaril)	25–50 mg PO/day	25- or 50-mg tablets	Antihistamine treats itching but does not treat disorder
Ursodeoxycholic acid (ursodiol; Urso, Actigall)	15 mg/kg/day PO in divided doses Usual dose: 900 mg per day in divided doses	300-mg capsules 250- or 500-mg tablets	Natural water-soluble bile acid interferes with the nonsoluble bile acids that injure cell membranes, thereby decreasing release of pruritic agents
Vitamin K	10 mg PO/day	5-mg tablet	Fat-soluble vitamin that plays a role in the clotting cascade used to replace vitamin K as cholesteramine interferes with absorption of fat-soluble vitamins

[a] Cholestyramine is not as effective as ursodeoxycholic acid in reducing pruritus. Women treated with cholestyramine should be given supplemental fat-soluble vitamins and vitamin K 10 mg/day.

was derived from dried powdered black bear's bile. This agent detoxifies bile acids and improves their solubility, thereby increasing bile flow. Ursodiol improves pruritus and leads to resolution of abnormal liver function tests. It is not clear if use of this medication can prevent sudden stillbirth, however, so early delivery is still the primary approach to prevent adverse fetal effects.

The most effective dose of ursodiol remains to be determined, although 500 mg twice daily is a commonly prescribed dose. This medication should be taken with food and should not be taken concomitantly with aluminum-based antacids or the bile acid sequestrant cholestyramine, as these agents can result in lower plasma levels of ursodiol.

Cholestyramine (Questran) is an anion exchange resin that binds to bile acids, thereby interfering with their enterohepatic circulation. It is less effective than ursodiol in reducing pruritus, but is often used in conjunction with ursodiol. Relief of pruritus may not occur until several days following initiation of regular dosing. Side effects include constipation, bloating, and gastrointestinal distress. Cholestyramine is frequently not well tolerated by users.

Cholestasis reduces absorption of fat-soluble vitamins, which can lead to vitamin K deficiency. In addition, cholestyramine can increase steatorrhea and cause vitamin K deficiency. Therefore supplemental vitamin K at 10 mg per day is recommended if this drug is prescribed, and some women need supplemental vitamin K even if they are not taking cholestyramine. Cholestyramine must be given on a staggered schedule with ursodiol to prevent a lessening of the ursodiol plasma levels.

While data are not available to support their use, topical emollients and antihistamines may provide some symptom relief. These agents include hydroxyzine (Vistaril) and diphenhydramine (Benadryl). For this indication, the sedating effects of antihistamines may play a bigger role in relief of pruritus than their effects on histamine production.[113]

Pruritic Urticarial Papules and Plaques of Pregnancy

A benign, self-limited, inflammatory condition unique to pregnancy, pruritic urticarial papules and plaques of pregnancy (PUPPP) is the most common dermatosis of pregnancy.[116] PUPPP is more common in primiparous women, who are usually affected at the end of pregnancy. Typically, this condition is characterized by pruritic urticarial papules, which present first within the striae of the pregnant abdomen, characteristically sparing the umbilicus, and eventually converge into plaques with an erythematous base. A small minority of women will present with just erythematous patches. Lesions may spread to the buttocks and thighs, and in most women, this is the extent of skin involvement.[117] The condition resolves spontaneously after birth.

Symptom relief is the treatment goal, as this condition poses no known risk to the woman or her fetus. Topical corticosteroids and first-generation antihistamines are the mainstay treatments.[116,117] Topical steroids are usually successful, and low-, medium-, and high-potency formulations may be used. Often, relief is obtained within 24 to 72 hours.

Caution should be used when applying high-potency steroids to avoid non-intact skin and durations of treatment beyond 2 weeks, as considerable systemic absorption may occur. This risk is higher with ointments than with creams or lotions. Other topical treatments include bland emollients (e.g., calamine), oatmeal (Aveeno), or antipruritic lotions with menthol (e.g., Sarna).

For some time, there has been concern regarding a possible correlation between first-trimester use of any corticosteroid preparation and orofacial clefts in the fetus; however, most studies have been confounded by inadequate statistical power and combinations of different corticosteroids with varying doses and varying routes of administration. More studies are needed to determine if an association exists. Prolonged use of steroids may increase the risk of preterm birth, fetal growth restriction, and maternal hypertension, diabetes, and osteoporosis; however, the underlying disorders for which prolonged corticosteroids are used may also have an independent effect on adverse outcomes.

In summary, although an association between topical corticosteroids and oral clefting has not been proven or disproven, short-term courses of topical steroids appear safe. The placenta deactivates steroids to some extent after the first trimester and subsequent fetal exposure is low. PUPPP rarely appears before the onset of the third trimester. When treating it, the lowest-potency corticosteroid that is effective should be used. Women who have a severe case of PUPPP may be prescribed a short course of systemic steroids such as oral prednisolone (starting dose of 40 to 60 mg daily and tapered over several days).

Thyroid Disorders

To meet the increased metabolic needs of the woman and fetus, thyroid physiology and function change during pregnancy. These changes alter interpretation of the thyroid function tests. Thus, diagnosis and management of thyroid disorders require an understanding of normal thyroid function during pregnancy. Pharmacologic management of thyroid disorders in pregnancy is reviewed in more detail in the *Thyroid Disorders* chapter. This section presents a brief summary of its components.

Overt clinical hypothyroidism is associated with spontaneous abortion, stillbirth, preeclampsia, placental abruption, and low birth weight. In addition, there is some association between hypothyroidism during pregnancy and subsequent cognitive impairment in the child.[118] Levothyroxine is safe for the woman and her fetus and is the drug of choice to treat thyroid disorders. Such treatment can prevent the adverse effects of untreated hypothyroidism.

Subclinical hypothyroidism, however, is the subject of current controversy. Some evidence exists that placental abruption, preterm birth, neonatal intensive care admission, and neonatal respiratory distress are more common in women with subclinical hypothyroidism compared with euthyroid women. Nevertheless, universal screening for and treatment of subclinical hypothyroidism have not been shown to reduce the incidence of these complications.[119] Until more data are available that document advantages from undertaking such therapy, it is recommended that women with subclinical hypothyroidism not be treated.

Overt hyperthyroidism, most commonly caused by Graves' disease, occurs in approximately 2 in 1000 pregnant women and is a more complex disorder to treat during pregnancy. Hyperthyroidism is associated with pregnancy loss, thyroid storm, preterm birth, preeclampsia, intrauterine growth restriction, and maternal congestive heart failure. The fetus can develop *thyrotoxicosis*, which may arise secondary to the disease or to the medications used to treat the disease. Thioamide drugs, including methimazole (Tapazole) and propylthiouracil, which is often abbreviated as PTU, (Propyl-Thyracil) are available to treat hyperthyroidism in pregnancy; radio-ablative techniques are contraindicated and surgery is reserved for failure of medical management.

The agent of choice in pregnancy has traditionally been propylthiouracil, based on the belief that propylthiouracil transfers into the fetal compartment in small amounts than does methimazole. More recently, it has been shown that both agents cross the placenta equally effectively and both can cause fetal hypothyroidism. There is an association between methimazole use and certain congenital anomalies such as aplasia cutis and esophageal atresia. However, propylthiouracil can induce liver dysfunction in women who use it. The current recommendation is to use propylthiouracil in the first trimester and then switch to methimazole for the duration of the pregnancy.[120]

Initiation of pharmacologic therapies for hypothyroidism or hyperthyroidism in pregnancy should involve consultation with a specialist.

Venous Thromboembolism

Deep vein thrombosis (DVT) results from occlusive blood clot formation in a deep vein. The most morbid complication of DVT is pulmonary embolism (PE), which can occur if the thrombus lodges in the lung. Venous thromboembolism refers to both DVT and PE. While rare, VTE is a major cause of maternal morbidity and mortality,[121] and PE is the leading cause of maternal death. Approximately 80% of pregnancy-associated VTE manifests as DVT, and 20% as PE.[122]

The normal physiologic, anatomic, and hemodynamic changes that occur during pregnancy result in an increased risk for VTE that extends into the postpartum period. These changes include smooth muscle relaxation resulting in increased venous prominence, vasodilation, blood volume expansion, decreased venous circulation, blood stasis, and valvular incompetence. The enlarged uterus also increases compression of the iliac veins and the inferior vena cava, resulting in increased venous pressure. Hypercoagulability and alterations in all three aspects of Virchow's triad (hypercoagulation, venous stasis, and vessel wall injuries) are also major contributors to the increased risk for VTE in pregnancy.

Women who have an a priori increased risk for VTE may require preventive measures and prophylaxis during pregnancy. Risk factors include a personal or family history of VTE and inherited or acquired thrombophilias.[122] Those thrombophilias of particular concern are factor V Leiden (homozygosity), prothrombin gene mutation (homozygosity), and antiphospholipid syndrome (APS). The American College of Obstetricians and Gynecologists[122] and the American College of Chest Physicians[123] have established criteria for who should be offered prophylactic anticoagulation during pregnancy.

Heparin is the mainstay anticoagulation therapy during pregnancy, whether it is used for prevention or for treatment. Warfarin (Coumadin) is the treatment of choice for long-term management for VTE in nonpregnant women, but this agent is contraindicated in pregnancy secondary to its known teratogenic effects.[123] The older version of unfractionated heparin has largely been replaced with the newer low-molecular-weight heparin due to its greater ease of use and better safety profile.[123] Although quality evidence on this relationship is lacking, low-molecular-weight heparin may be associated with less bleeding than unfractionated heparin. In addition, low-molecular-weight heparin has a longer half-life, higher bioavailability, and better predictability than the older version; thus it has become the heparin of choice for use in pregnancy.

The usual initial doses of low-molecular-weight heparin are listed in Table 35-11.[121–125] Doses are adjusted based on response and weight gain during pregnancy and generally divided into prophylactic, intermediate, and therapeutic regimens. Intermediate doses include the increased dose that may be needed as pregnancy advances. Specialists care for pregnant women who need anticoagulant therapy.

Table 35-11 Low-Molecular-Weight Heparin for Treatment of Deep Vein Thrombosis in Pregnancy

Drug: Generic (Brand)	DVT Prophylaxis	DVT Treatment
Dalteparin (Fragmin)	5000 units SQ once daily	200 units/kg/day
Enoxaparin (Lovenox)	40 mg SQ once daily	1 mg/kg/12 hours

Abbreviation: DVT = deep vein thrombosis.
Sources: Data from American College of Obstetricians and Gynecologists, Women's Health Care Physicians. ACOG Practice Bulletin No. 138: inherited thrombophilias in pregnancy. *Obstet Gynecol.* 2013;122:706[122]; Bates SM, Greer IA, Middeldorp S, et al. VTE, thrombophilia, antithrombotic therapy, and pregnancy: antithrombotic therapy and prevention of thrombosis, 9th ed: American College of Chest Physicians evidence-based clinical practice guidelines. *Chest.* 2012;141 (2 suppl):e691-e736[123]; Che Yaakob CA, Dzarr AA, Ismail AA, Zuky Nik Lah NA, Ho JJ. Anticoagulant therapy for deep vein thrombosis (DVT) in pregnancy. *Cochrane Database Syst Rev.* 2010;6:CD007801.[125]

Neither form of heparin crosses the placental barrier in any significant amount; therefore, fetal safety is largely confirmed and heparin is not associated with any teratogenic or fetotoxic effects.[121–125] Conversely, adverse effects for the woman may include heparin-induced thrombocytopenia (low platelets), bleeding and hemorrhage, allergic reactions, and osteoporosis if this medication is used on a long-term basis. These complications can occur at any of the doses that are used.

Complementary and Alternative Medicine in Pregnancy

Women often seek effective, safe remedies for physiologic discomforts in pregnancy, and look for herbal or homeopathic remedies in the belief that these agents are safer than pharmacologic doses of drugs. Although herbal remedies are frequently used by pregnant women, data regarding their use remain for the most part experiential, and some data suggest that specific agents might be harmful. Table 35-12 lists selected herbs that are commonly recommended for use in pregnancy and summarizes the safety information available for them.[126–128]

Table 35-12 Selected Herbal Agents Used in Pregnancy

Herbal Agent	Alternative Names	Indication	Effectiveness and Safety Data
Alfalfa	*Medicago sativa*, lucerne, medicago, phytoestrogen, purple medick	Source of vitamins K, A, C, and E and the minerals calcium, potassium, phosphorus, and iron; Anecdotally used prenatally to decrease risk of PPH	Contains isoflavonoids with estrogenic effects and large amounts of vitamin K. Effectiveness: Undetermined. Safety: Possibly unsafe.
Arnica	*Arnica montana*, *Arnica flos*, arnica flower, leopard's bane, mountain tobacco, wolf's bane	Topical: anecdotally used to decrease inflammation associated with bruises, sprains, and aches Oral: abortifacient	May inhibit human platelet function. Can cause contact dermatitis and mucous membrane irritation. Effectiveness: Undetermined. Safety: Likely unsafe (oral or topical).
Basil	*Ocimum basilicum*, common basil, garden basil, sweet basil, St. Joseph wort	Promotion of circulation before and after childbirth, morning sickness	Effectiveness: Undetermined. Safety: Likely safe when leaves, stems, and flowers used as a spice. Possibly unsafe when used in larger amounts due to estragole in essential oil, which may have mutagenic effects. May cause hypoglycemia.
Black cohosh	*Actaea racemosa*, *Cimicifuga racemosa*, baneberry, black snakeroot, bugbane, bugwort, cimicifuga, rattlesnake root, squaw root	Uterotonic or uterotropic	Estrogen-like effects. Effectiveness: No clinical evidence of effectiveness for labor induction. Safety: May cause liver disease. May inhibit cytochrome CYP2D6, causing drug interactions. Possibly unsafe when used prior to term; may increase miscarriage risk. Case reports of hepatotoxicity.
Blue cohosh	*Caulophyllum thalictroides*, blue ginseng, caulophyllum, papoose root, squaw root, yellow ginseng	Uterotonic or uterotropic	Can induce labor. Constricts coronary arteries and may decrease oxygenation to the heart. Safety: Unsafe. Constituents may be teratogenic. When used near term, may cause life-threatening neonatal cardiovascular events.
Chamomile	*Matricaria recutita*, blue chamomile, German chamomile, Hungarian chamomile, true chamomile, wild chamomile, sweet false chamomile	Anxiety, digestive problems, insomnia, restlessness, afterpains postpartum	May compete with estrogen receptors. Effectiveness: Unknown. Safety: Insufficient reliable information available.
Cranberry		Prevention or treatment of urinary tract infections	Effectiveness: Not effective. Safety: Probably safe but insufficient data; gastrointestinal upset a common side effect.
Dandelion	*Taraxacum officinale*, blowball, common dandelion, cankerwort, lion's tooth, swine snout, wild endive	Reduction of anemia, swelling, and as a nutritional supplement	Effectiveness: Unknown. Safety: Insufficient information available. Avoid using in amounts greater than in food. May lower fluoroquinolone levels.
Echinacea	*Echinacea angustifolia*, coneflower, black Sampson, comb flower, red sunflower, scurvy root, snakeroot, Indian head	Immunostimulant, treatment for the common cold, treatment for genital herpes simplex virus and vaginal *Candida* infections	Effectiveness: Possibly effective to prevent recurrent vaginal yeast and for the common cold. Safety: Possibly safe when used orally, in the short term. No association with congenital malformations. Increases caffeine concentrations by 30% in nonpregnant population. Inhibits CYPA12 enzymes.
Evening primrose oil	*Oenothera biennis*, EPO, *cis*-linoleic acid, fever plant, gamma-linolenic acid (GLA), linoleic acid	Cervical ripening, prevention of preeclampsia, prevention of post-date pregnancy, shortening of labor	Effectiveness: Not effective. Safety: Possibly unsafe when used orally. May increase risk for prolonged rupture of membranes, increased use of oxytocin, and arrest of descent. Associated with increased rates of vacuum extraction.
Ginger	*Zingiber officinale*, African ginger, black ginger, Indian ginger, Jamaican ginger, race ginger, ardraka	Morning sickness	Appears to block intestinal serotonin receptors. Effectiveness: Good evidence that ginger is as effective as vitamin B_6 or diphenhydramine (Benadryl). Safety: No adverse effects reported in studies of ginger used for nausea during pregnancy. Theoretic risk of increased bleeding, as ginger inhibits platelet function and blood coagulation.

(*continues*)

Table 35-12 Selected Herbal Agents Used in Pregnancy (*continued*)

Herbal Agent	Alternative Names	Indication	Effectiveness and Safety Data
Red raspberry	*Rubus idaeus*, raspberry, raspberry ketone, rubus	Morning sickness, prevention of miscarriage, facilitation of labor and birth, uterotonic or uterotropic	Effectiveness: No evidence of effectiveness. Does not seem to decrease need for analgesia. A few studies found it shortened the second stage of labor and decreased the rate of operative delivery. Safety: Safe when used orally in amounts common in foods. Probably safe when used orally in medicinal doses in late pregnancy.

Sources: Data from Dante G, Neri I, Fachinetti F. Herbal therapies in pregnancy: what works? *Curr Opin Obstet Gynecol.* 2014;26:83-91[126]; Dugoua JJ. Herbal medicines and pregnancy. *J Popul Ther Clin Pharmacol.* 2010;17(3):e370-e378[127]; Holst L, Wright D, Haavik S, Nordeng H. Safety and efficacy of herbal remedies in obstetrics: review and clinical implications. *Midwifery.* 2011;27:80-86.[128]

Conclusion

Pregnancy is a unique state in the human lifespan due to the coexistence of two individuals in one physiologic system and can be a challenge for the prescribing clinician. As pregnancy is predominantly a normal, healthy stage of the female lifespan, no pharmacologic treatment may be needed at this time, particularly for a well-nourished woman. When drugs are prescribed, the imperative to avoid unnecessary medications must be balanced with conditions requiring treatment to best support the health or well-being of the woman and her fetus. The key is to provide individualized pharmacologic care that focuses on the preexisting health needs of each woman, the evolving development of the fetus, and the challenges that pregnancy itself may pose. In a few situations, several pharmacologic agents may be necessary, requiring close consultation between the primary provider and other specialists. The rewards of these ongoing, careful calculations are profound as the provider works collaboratively with the woman to achieve the best possible perinatal outcome.

Resources

Organization	Description	Website
Food and Drug Administration	New pregnancy labeling rules effective June 15, 2015.	www.fda.gov/Drugs/DevelopmentApproval Process/Development Resources/Labeling/ucm093307.htm?source=govdelivery&utm_medium=email&utm_source=govdelivery
Food and Drug Administration	Full list of pregnancy registries that are maintained to assemble data about pregnancy exposure to specific drugs.	www.fda.gov/womens/regsistries
Centers for Disease Control and Prevention	Treating for Two: Safer Medication Use in Pregnancy Initiative: This effort aims to prevent birth defects and improve maternal health by providing clinicians with the necessary tools and information on medication use in pregnancy to make informed clinical decisions regarding safe medication use for both pregnant and reproductive-age women. The initiative will include a formal review process and evaluation of the evidence regarding medication-associated embryonic, fetal, and perinatal risks such as, preterm birth, fetal death, structural birth defects, poor fetal growth, and severe adverse maternal events and other adverse outcomes (e.g., developmental disabilities, neurocognitive effects, behavioral effects). Participants include experts from academia, professional organizations, and federal agencies.	www.cdc.gov/ncbddd/birthdefects/documents/ncbddd_birth-defects_medicationuseonepager_cdcrole.pdf
Teratogen Information Sources		
Organization of Teratology Information Specialists (OTIS)	A nonprofit, evidence-based organization providing information for healthcare professionals, mothers, and general public regarding medication exposures during pregnancy and lactation.	www.mothertobaby.org

Motherisk	Canadian-based clinical research and teaching program based at the University of Toronto, Ontario, providing research, counseling, and recommendations to the public and to health providers on medication safety, chemicals, maternal disease, and health topics in pregnancy and lactation. Free. Includes helplines, updates, articles, and more.	www.motherisk.org
Teratogen Information System (TERIS)	Fee-based subscription online database for providers and healthcare professionals. Summaries based on published clinical and experimental data. Housed in the University of Washington's Department of Pediatrics.	http://depts.washington.edu/terisdb/terisweb/index.html
Reprotox	Online database focusing on environmental hazards to human reproduction and development. Available by subscription.	www.reprotox.org

References

1. Mitchell AA, Gilboa SM, Werler MM, et al. Medication use during pregnancy, with particular focus on prescription drugs: 1976–2008. *Am J Obstet Gynecol.* 2011;205(1):51.e1-51.e8.
2. Lo WY, Friedman JM. Teratogenicity of recently introduced medications in human pregnancy. *Obstet Gynecol.* 2002;100:465-473.
3. Adam MP, Polifka JE, Friedman JM. Evolving knowledge of the teratogenicity of medications in human pregnancy. *Am J Med Genet C Semin Med Genet.* 2011;157:175-182.
4. Stockard CR. Developmental rate and structural expression: an experimental study of twins, "double monsters," and single deformities and their interaction among embryonic organs during their origins and development. *Am J Anatomy.* 1921;28;115-275.
5. Thorpe PG, Gilboa SM, Hernandez-Diaz S. Medications in the first trimester of pregnancy: most common exposures and critical gaps in understanding fetal risk. *Pharmacoepidemiol Drug Saf.* 2013;22(9):1013-1018.
6. Koren G. Fetal risks of maternal pharmacotherapy, identifying signals. *Handb Exp Pharmacol.* 2011; 205;285-294.
7. Shephard TH. "Proof" of human teratogenicity [letter]. *Teratology.* 1994;50:97-98.
8. Koren G. Fetal risks of maternal pharmacotherapy, identifying signals. *Handb Exp Pharmacol.* 2011; 205:285-294.
9. Buhimschi CS, Weiner CP. Medications in pregnancy and lactation. Part 1. Teratology. *Obstet Gynecol.* 2009; 113:166-188.
10. Buhimschi CS, Weiner CP. Medications in pregnancy and lactation. Part 2. Drugs with minimal or unknown human teratogenic effect. *Obstet Gynecol.* 2009;113;417-432.
11. Stephansson O, Kieler H, Haglund B, et al. Selective serotonin reuptake inhibitors during pregnancy and risk of stillbirth and infant mortality. *JAMA.* 2013; 309:48.
12. Malm H, Artama M, Gissler M, Ritvanen A. Selective serotonin reuptake inhibitors and risk for major congenital anomalies. *Obstet Gynecol.* 2011;118:111.
13. Wilson J. Current status of teratology, general principles and mechanisms derived from animal studies. In: Wilson J, Fraser F, eds. *Handbook of Teratology.* 4 vols. New York: Plenum Press; 1977:47-74.
14. Friedman JM. The principles of teratology: are they still true? *Birth Defects Res A Clin Mol Terato.* 2010; 88(10):766-768.
15. Moore KL, Persaud TVN. *The Developing Human: Clinically Oriented Embryology*. 8th ed. Philadelphia, PA: Elsevier; 2007.
16. van Gelder MMHJ, van Rooij IALM, Miller R, Zielhuis GA, de Jong-van den Berg LTW, Roeleveld N. Teratogenic mechanisms of medical drugs. *Hum Reprod Update.* 2010;16(4):378-394.
17. Larimore WL, Petrie KA. Drug use in pregnancy and lactation. *Prim Care.* 2000;27:35-42.
18. Costantine MM. Physiologic and pharmacokinetic changes in pregnancy. *Front Pharmacol.* 2014;5:65.
19. Gedeon C, Koren G. Designing pregnancy centered medications: drugs which do not cross the human placenta. *Placenta.* 2006;27:861-868.
20. Tracy TS, Venkataramanan R, Glover DD, Caritis SN. National Institute for Child Health and Human Development Network of Maternal–Fetal Medicine Units. Temporal changes in drug metabolism (CYP1A2, CYP2D6 and CYP3A activity) during pregnancy. *Am J Obstet Gynecol.* 2005;192(2):633-639.

21. Hansen WF, Peacock AE, Yankowitz J. Safe prescribing practices in pregnancy and lactation. *J Midwifery Womens Health*. 2002;47(6):409-421.
22. van Gelder MM, de Jong-van den Berg LT, Roeleveld N. Drugs associated with teratogenic mechanisms. Part II: a literature review of the evidence on human risks. *Hum Reprod.* 2014;29(1):168-183.
23. Food and Drug Administration. Pregnancy labeling. *Fed Register*. 1979;44(124):37464-37465.
24. Ramoz LL, Patel-Shori NM. Recent changes in pregnancy and lactation labeling: retirement of risk categories. *Pharmacotherapy*. 2014;34(4):389-395.
25. Food and Drug Administration. *Fed Register.* 2014;79(233). http://www.gpo.gov/fdsys/pkg/FR-2014-12-04/pdf/2014-28241.pdf. Accessed December 5, 2014.
26. De-Regil LM, Fernández-Gaxiola AC, Dowswell T, Peña-Rosas JP. Effects and safety of periconceptional folate supplementation for preventing birth defects. *Cochrane Database Syst Rev.* 2010;10:CD007950.
27. Lassi ZS, Salam RA, Haider BA, Bhutta ZA. Folic acid supplementation during pregnancy for maternal health and pregnancy outcomes. *Cochrane Database Syst Rev.* 2013;3:CD006896.
28. U.S. Preventive Services Task Force. *Folic Acid to Prevent Neural Tube Defects: Recommendation Statement.* Rockville, MD: U.S. Preventive Services Task Force, Agency for Healthcare Research and Quality; May 2009. http://www.uspreventiveservicestaskforce.org/uspstf09/folicacid/folicacidrs.htm. Accessed April 16, 2014.
29. American College of Obstetricians and Gynecologists. ACOG Practice Bulletin No. 44: neural tube defects. *Obstet Gynecol.* 2003;83(1):123-133. Reaffirmed 2013.
30. Prevention of neural tube defects: results of the Medical Research Counsel Vitamin Study Research Group. *Lancet.* 1991;338(8760):131-137.
31. Cao C, O'Brien KO. Pregnancy and iron homeostasis: an update. *Nutr Rev*. 2013:71(1):35-51.
32. Peña-Rosas JP, De-Regil LM, Dowswell T, Viteri FE. Daily oral iron supplementation during pregnancy. *Cochrane Database Syst Rev.* 2012;12:CD004736.
33. Reveiz L, Gyte GML, Cuervo LG, Casasbuenas A. Treatments for iron-deficiency anaemia in pregnancy. *Cochrane Database Syst Rev*. 2011;10:CD003094.
34. Centers for Disease Control and Prevention. Recommendations to prevent and control iron deficiency in the United States. *MMWR*. 1998;47:1-29.
35. Melamed N, Ben-Haroush A, Kaplan B, Yogev Y. Iron supplementation in pregnancy: does the preparation matter? *Arch Gynecol Obstet.* 2007;276:601-604.
36. Hofmeyr GJ, Lawrie TA, Atallah ÁN, Duley L, Torloni MR. Calcium supplementation during pregnancy for preventing hypertensive disorders and related problems. *Cochrane Database Syst Rev.* 2014;6: CD001059.
37. Bourgoin BP, Evans DR, Cornett JR, Lingard SM, Quattrone AJ. Lead content in 70 brands of dietary calcium supplements. *Am J Public Health.* 1993;83:1155-1160.
38. Rehman S, Adnan M, Khalid N, Shaheen L. Calcium supplements: an additional source of lead contamination. *Biol Trace Elem Res.* 2011;143:178-187.
39. Ross EA, Szabo NJ, Tebbett IR. Lead content of calcium supplements. *JAMA*. 2000;284(11):1425-1429.
40. Christakos S, Hewison M, Gardner DG, et al. Vitamin D: beyond bone. *Ann NY Acad Sci*. 2013;1287:45-58.
41. De-Regil LM, Palacios C, Ansary A, Kulier R, Peña-Rosas JP. Vitamin D supplementation for women during pregnancy. *Cochrane Database Syst Rev.* 2012;2:CD008873.
42. Alshahrani F, Aljohani N. Vitamin D: sufficiency, deficiency and toxicity. *Nutrients.* 2013;5(9):3605-3616.
43. American College of Obstetricians and Gynecologists. ACOG Committee Opinion No. 495: vitamin D: screening and supplementation in pregnancy. *Obstet Gynecol.* 2011;118(1):197-198.
44. Haider BA, Bhutta ZA. Multiple-micronutrient supplementation for women during pregnancy. *Cochrane Database Syst Rev*. 2012;11:CD004905.
45. Pennick V, Liddle SD. Interventions for preventing and treating pelvic and back pain in pregnancy. *Cochrane Database Syst Rev*. 2013;8:CD001139.
46. Moreira A, Barbin C, Martinez H, Aly A, Fonseca R. Maternal use of cyclobenzaprine (Flexeril) may induce ductal closure and persistent pulmonary hypertension in neonates. *J Matern Fetal Neonatal Med.* 2014;27(11):1177-1179.
47. Longo SA, Moore RC, Canzoneri BJ, Robichaux A. Gastrointestinal conditions during pregnancy. *Clin Colon Rectal Surg.* 2010;23(2):80-89.
48. Avsar AF, Keskin HL. Haemorrhoids during pregnancy. *J Obstet Gynaecol.* 2010;30(3):231-237.
49. Trottier M, Erebara A, Bozzo P. Treating constipation during pregnancy. *Can Fam Physician.* 2012;58(8):836-838.
50. Moloney MF, Johnson CJ. Migraine headaches: diagnosis and management. *J Midwifery Womens Health.* 2011;56(3):282-292.
51. David PS, Kling JM, Starline AJ. Migraine in pregnancy and lactation. *Curr Neurol Neurosci Rep.* 2014;14(4):439.

52. Kvisvik EV, Stovner LJ, Helde G, Bovim G, Linde M. Headache and migraine during pregnancy and puerperium: the MIGRA-study. *J Headache Pain.* 2011; 12(4):443-451.
53. Allais G, Gabellari IC, Borgogno P, De Lorenzo C, Benedetto C. The risks of women with migraine during pregnancy. *Neurol Sci.* 2010;31(suppl 1):S59-S61.
54. Derry CJ, Derry S, Moore RA. Caffeine as an analgesic adjuvant for acute pain in adults. *Cochrane Database Syst Rev.* 2012;3:CD009281.
55. GlaxoSmithKline. *Sumatriptan/Naratriptan/Treximet Pregnancy Registry: Interim Report.* Wilmington, NC: Kendle International; May 2012. http://pregnancyregistry.gsk.com/documents/SumNarTrex_InterimReport_2012.pdf. Accessed June 15, 2014.
56. Nezvalova-Henriksen K, Spigset O, Nordeng H. Triptan safety during pregnancy: a Norwegian population registry study. *Eur J Epidemiol.* 2013;28(9):759-769.
57. Nezvalova-Henriksen K, Spigset O, Nordeng H. Triptan exposure during pregnancy and the risk of major congenital malformations and adverse pregnancy outcomes: results from the Norwegian mother and child cohort study. *Headache.* 2010;50:563-75. Errata in *Headache.* 2012;52(8):1319-1320.
58. Kallen B, Nilsson E, Otterblad Olausson P. Delivery outcome after maternal use of drugs for migraine: a register study in Sweden. *Drug Saf.* 2011;34(8):691-703.
59. Finocchi C, Viani E. Opioids can be useful in the treatment of headache. *Neurol Sci.* 2013;34(suppl 1):S119-S124.
60. Kelley NE, Tepper DE. Rescue therapy for acute migraine. Part 3: opioids, NSAIDs, steroids, and post-discharge medications. *Headache.* 2012;52(3):467-482.
61. Airola G, Allais G, Castagnoli Gabellari I, Rolando S, Mana O, Benedetto C. Non-pharmacological management of migraine during pregnancy. *Neurol Sci.* 2010;31(suppl 1):S63-S65.
62. Ali RA, Egan LJ. Gastroesophageal reflux disease in pregnancy. *Best Pract Res Clin Gastroenterol.* 2007;21(5):793-806.
63. Gerson LB. Treatment of gastroesophageal reflux disease during pregnancy. *Gastroenterol Hepatol.* 2012;8(11):763-776.
64. Neilson JP. Interventions for heartburn in pregnancy. *Cochrane Database Syst Rev.* 2008;4:CD007065. Reissued 2013.
65. Wang Y, Wen-Hung H, Wang SSW, et al. Current pharmacological management of gastroesophageal reflux disease. *Gastroenterol Res Pract.* 2013;2013:983653.
66. Pasternak B, Hviid A. Use of proton-pump inhibitors in early pregnancy and the risk of birth defects. *N Engl J Med.* 2010;363:2114-2123.
67. Gill SK, O'Brien L, Einarson TR, Koren G. The safety of proton pump inhibitors. *Am J Gastroenterol.* 2009; 104(6):1541-1545.
68. Chen Y-H, Lin H-C, Lou H-Y. Increased risk of low birthweight, infants small for gestational age, and preterm delivery for women with peptic ulcer. *Am J Obstet Gynecol.* 2010;202:164.e1-164.e8.
69. Bánhidy F, Dakhlaoui A, Puhó EH, Czeizel AE. Peptic ulcer disease with related drug treatment in pregnant women and congenital abnormalities in their offspring. *Congenit Anom.* 2011;51(1):26-33.
70. Cardaropoli S, Rolfo A, Todros T. *Helicobacter pylori* and pregnancy-related disorders. *World J Gastroenterol.* 2014;20(3):654-664.
71. Nodine PM, Matthews EE. Common sleep disorders: management strategies and pregnancy outcomes. *J Midwifery Womens Health.* 2013;58(4):368-377.
72. Jones CR. Diagnostic and management approach to common sleep disorders during pregnancy. *Clin Obstet Gynecol.* 2013;56(2):360-371.
73. Hensley JG. Leg cramps and restless legs syndrome during pregnancy. *J Midwifery Womens Health.* 2009; 54:211-218.
74. Bhardwaj A, Nagandla K. Musculoskeletal symptoms and orthopaedic complications in pregnancy: pathophysiology, diagnostic approaches and modern management. *Postgrad Med J.* 2014;90(1066): 450-460.
75. Koren G, Phelan ST. Nausea and vomiting of pregnancy monograph. Association of Professors of Gynecology and Obstetrics Educational Series on Women's Health Issues; 2013. http://www.nationalperinatal.org/Resources/APGO%20Educational%20Series%202011.pdf. Accessed May 28, 2014.
76. Dante G, Pedrielli G, Annessi E, Facchinetti F. Herb remedies during pregnancy: a systematic review of controlled clinical trials. *J Matern Fetal Neonatal Med.* 2013;26(3):306-312.
77. Matthews A, Haas DM, O'Mathúna DP, Dowswell T, Doyle M. Interventions for nausea and vomiting in early pregnancy. *Cochrane Database Syst Rev.* 2014; 3:CD007575.
78. Clark SM, Costantine MM, Hankins GDV. Review of NVP and HG and early pharmacotherapeutic intervention. *Obstet Gynecol Int.* 2013;2013:1-8.
79. Jarvis S, Nelson-Piercy C. Management of nausea and vomiting in pregnancy. *BMJ.* 2011;342:d3606.

80. Pasternak B, Svanström H, Mølgaard-Nielsen D, Melbye M, Hviid A. Metoclopramide in pregnancy and risk of major congenital malformations and fetal death. *JAMA.* 2013;310(15):1601-1611.
81. Vinson DR, Drotts DL. Diphenhydramine for the prevention of akathisia induced by prochlorperazine: a randomized, controlled trial. *Ann Emerg Med.* 2001;37(2):125-131.
82. Bondok RS, El Sharnouby NM, Eid HE, Abd Elmaksoud AM. Pulsed steroid therapy is an effective treatment for intractable hyperemesis gravidarum. *Crit Care Med.* 2006;34:2781-2783.
83. Tan PC, Omar SZ. Contemporary approaches to hyperemesis during pregnancy. *Curr Opin Obstet Gynecol.* 2011;23(2):87-93.
84. Cardwell MS. Eating disorders during pregnancy. *Obstet Gynecol Surv.* 2013;68(4):312-323.
85. Widmer M, Gülmezoglu AM, Mignini L, Roganti A. Duration of treatment for asymptomatic bacteriuria in pregnancy. *Cochrane Database Syst Rev.* 2011;12:CD000491.
86. Cunnington M, Kortsalioudaki C, Heath P. Genitourinary pathogens and preterm birth. *Curr Opin Infect Dis.* 2013; 26(3):219-230.
87. O'Dell K. Pharmacologic management of asymptomatic bacteriuria and urinary tract infections in women. *J Midwifery Womens Health.* 2011;56(3): 248-265.
88. Gupta K, Hooton TM, Naber KG, et al. International clinical practice guidelines for the treatment of acute uncomplicated cystitis and pyelonephritis in women: a 2010 update by the Infectious Diseases Society of America and the European Society for Microbiology and Infectious Diseases. *Clin Infect Dis.* 2011;52(5):e103-e120.
89. Vazquez JC, Abalos E. Treatments for symptomatic urinary tract infections during pregnancy. *Cochrane Database Syst Rev.* 2011;1:CD002256.
90. Hernandez-Diaz S, Werler MM, Walker AM, Mitchell AA. Folic acid antagonists during pregnancy and the risk of birth defects. *N Engl J Med.* 2000;343:1608-1614.
91. American College of Obstetricians and Gynecologists. ACOG Committee Opinion No. 494: sulfonamides, nitrofurantoin, and risk of birth defects. *Obstet Gynecol.* 2011;117(6):1484-1485.
92. Goldberg O, Koren G, Landau D, Lunenfeld E, Matok I, Levy A. Exposure to nitrofurantoin during the first trimester of pregnancy and the risk for major malformations. *J Clin Pharmacol.* 2013;53(9):991-995.
93. Centers for Disease Control and Prevention. Prevention of perinatal group B streptococcal disease: revised guidelines from CDC, 2010. *MMWR.* 2010;59:1-32. http://www.cdc.gov/mmwr/preview/mmwrhtml/rr5910a1.htm. Accessed June 26, 2014.
94. Jolley JA, Wing DA. Pyelonephritis in pregnancy: an update on treatment options for optimal outcomes. *Drugs.* 2010;70(13):1643-1655.
95. American College of Obstetricians and Gynecologists. ACOG Practice Bulletin No. 82: management of herpes in pregnancy. *Obstet Gynecol.* 2007;109:1489-1498. Reaffirmed 2012.
96. Kang S-H, Chua-Gocheco A, Bozzo P, Einarson A. Safety of antiviral medication for the treatment of herpes during pregnancy. *Can Fam Physician.* 2011;57: 427-428.
97. Brocklehurst P, Gordon A, Heatley E, Milan SJ. Antibiotics for treating bacterial vaginosis in pregnancy. *Cochrane Database Syst Rev.* 2013;1:CD000262.
98. Gülmezoglu AM, Azhar M. Interventions for trichomoniasis in pregnancy. *Cochrane Database Syst Rev.* 2011;5:CD000220.
99. Manns-James J. Bacterial vaginosis and preterm birth. *J Midwifery Womens Health.* 2011;56(6):575-583.
100. Dodd JM, Jones L, Flenady V, Cincotta R, Crowther CA. Prenatal administration of progesterone for preventing preterm birth in women considered to be at risk of preterm birth. *Cochrane Database Syst Rev.* 2013;7:CD004947.
101. Likis FE, Velez Edwards DR, Andrews JC, et al. Progestogens for preterm birth prevention: a systematic review and meta-analysis. *Obstet Gynecol.* 2012;120(4):897-907.
102. American College of Obstetricians and Gynecologists; Task Force on Hypertension in Pregnancy. Hypertension in pregnancy. *Obstet Gynecol.* 2013;122(5):1122-1131.
103. Henderson JT, Whitlock EP, O'Connor E, Senger CA, Thompson JH, Rowland MG. Low-dose aspirin for prevention of morbidity and mortality from preeclampsia: a systematic evidence review for the U.S Preventive Services Task Force. *Ann Intern Med.* 2014;160(10):695-703.
104. Crowther CA, Middleton P, McBain RD. Anti-D administration in pregnancy for preventing Rhesus alloimmunization. *Cochrane Database Syst Rev.* 2013;2:CD000020.
105. Hiersch L, Yogev Y. Management of diabetes and pregnancy: when to start and what pharmacological

agent to choose. *Best Pract Res Clin Obstet Gynecol.* 2015;29(2):225-236.

106. Homko CJ, Reece EA. Insulins and oral hypoglycemic agents in pregnancy. *J Matern Fetal Neonatal Med.* 2006;19(11):679-686.
107. Bhattacharyya A, Brown S, Hughes S, Vice PA. Insulin lispro and regular insulin in pregnancy. *QJM.* 2001; 94(5):255-260.
108. Nicholson W, Baptiste-Roberts K. Oral hypoglycaemic agents during pregnancy: the evidence for effectiveness and safety. *Best Pract Res Clin Obstet Gynaecol.* 2011;25(1):51-63.
109. Tieu J, Coat S, Hague W, Middleton P. Oral anti-diabetic agents for women with pre-existing diabetes mellitus/impaired glucose tolerance or previous gestational diabetes mellitus. *Cochrane Database Syst Rev.* 2010;10:CD007724.
110. Castillo WC, Boggess K, Sturmer T, Brookhart MA, Benjamin DK, Funk MJ. Trends in glyburide compared with insulin use for gestational diabetes treatment in the United States, 2000–2011. *Obstet Gynecol.* 2014;123(6):1177-1184.
111. Cooper WO, Hernandes-Diaz S, Arbogast PG, et al. Major congenital malformations after first trimester exposure to ACE inhibitors. *N Engl J Med.* 2006; 354: 2443-2451.
112. Yakoob MY, Bateman MT, Ho E, et al. The risk of congenital malformations associated with exposure to beta blockers early in pregnancy: a meta-analysis. *Hypertension.* 2013;62:375-381.
113. Gurung V, Stokes M, Middleton P, Milan SJ, Hague W, Thornton JG. Interventions for treating cholestasis in pregnancy. *Cochrane Database Syst Rev.* 2013; 6:CD000493.
114. Bruce K, Watson S. Management of intrahepatic cholestasis of pregnancy: a case report. *J Midwifery Womens Health.* 2007;52:67-72.
115. Glantz A, Marschall H-U, Lammert F, Mattsson L-A. Intrahepatic cholestasis of pregnancy: a randomized controlled trial comparing dexamethasone and ursodeoxycholic acid. *Hepatology.* 2005;42: 1399-1405.
116. Lehrhoff S, Pomeranz MK. Specific dermatoses of pregnancy and their treatment. *Dermatol Ther.* 2013; 26(4):274-284.
117. Bergman H, Melamed N, Koren G. Pruritus in pregnancy: treatment of dermatoses unique to pregnancy. *Can Fam Physician.* 2013;59(12):1290-1294.
118. Reid SM, Middleton P, Cossich MC, Crowther CA. Interventions for clinical and subclinical hypothyroidism in pregnancy. *Cochrane Database Syst Rev.* 2010;7:CD007752.
119. Vila L, Velasco I, Gonzalez S, et al. On the need for universal thyroid screening in pregnant women. *Euro J Endocrinol.* 2013:170(1):R17-R31.
120. Stagnaro-Green A, Abalovich M, Alexander E, et al.; American Thyroid Association Taskforce on Thyroid Disease During Pregnancy and Postpartum. Guidelines of the American Thyroid Association for the diagnosis and management of thyroid disease during pregnancy and postpartum. *Thyroid.* 2011;21(10):1081-1125.
121. Bain E, Wilson A, Tooher R, Gates S, Davis LJ, Middleton P. Prophylaxis for venous thromboembolic disease in pregnancy and the early postnatal period. *Cochrane Database Syst Rev.* 2014;2:CD001689.
122. American College of Obstetricians and Gynecologists, Women's Health Care Physicians. ACOG Practice Bulletin No. 138: inherited thrombophilias in pregnancy. *Obstet Gynecol.* 2013;122:706.
123. Bates SM, Greer IA, Middeldorp S, et al. VTE, thrombophilia, antithrombotic therapy, and pregnancy: antithrombotic therapy and prevention of thrombosis, 9th ed: American College of Chest Physicians evidence-based clinical practice guidelines. *Chest.* 2012;141(2 suppl):e691-e736.
124. Armstrong EM, Bellone JM, Hornsby LB, Treadway S, Phillippe HM. Pregnancy-related venous thromboembolism. *J Pharm Pract.* 2014;27(3):243-252.
125. Che Yaakob CA, Dzarr AA, Ismail AA, Zuky Nik Lah NA, Ho JJ. Anticoagulant therapy for deep vein thrombosis (DVT) in pregnancy. *Cochrane Database Syst Rev.* 2010;6:CD007801.
126. Dante G, Neri I, Fachinetti F. Herbal therapies in pregnancy: what works? *Curr Opin Obstet Gynecol.* 2014;26:83-91.
127. Dugoua JJ. Herbal medicines and pregnancy. *J Popul Ther Clin Pharmacol.* 2010;17(3):e370-e378.
128. Holst L, Wright D, Haavik S, Nordeng H. Safety and efficacy of herbal remedies in obstetrics: review and clinical implications. *Midwifery.* 2011;27:80-86.

36 Labor

Nancy K. Lowe, Maria Openshaw, Tekoa L. King

Chapter Glossary

Actin Double-helix protein strand that provides the scaffold to which myosin binds to create a muscle contraction.

Beta-sympathomimetics Drugs that mimic the effects of catecholamines, such as epinephrine and norepinephrine; also called beta agonists. Drugs in this category have traditionally been used as tocolytics.

Corticotropin-releasing hormone Hormone synthesized by the placenta, decidua, amnion, and myometrium, which plays a role in both maintaining uterine quiescence during pregnancy and determining the time of onset of labor.

Intrathecal Synonym for intraspinal. The intrathecal space is the space in the spinal cord where the spinal fluid resides.

Myosin Primary contractile protein in muscle, which is composed of two heavy chains, two light chains, and a globular head that protrudes from the filament. The myosin head binds to actin, which forms a cross-bridge and leads to a structural change that results in shortening or muscle contraction.

Myosin light-chain kinase (MLCK) Kinase is an enzyme that modifies a protein by adding a phosphate group to the protein. MLCK phosphorylates the myosin light chain, which converts myosin from an active state to an inactive state. This agent is able to make this structural change to myosin only after forming a bond with calmodulin. In turn, the MLCK–calmodulin complex appears when intracellular calcium is present.

Oxytocin Peptide hormone that is made in the hypothalamus and released by the pituitary. One of its many functions is stimulating an increase in intracellular calcium in myometrial cells, which initiates muscle contraction during labor.

Tocolytics Drugs used to suppress or inhibit labor, especially when preterm. From Greek word *tocos*, which means "for childbirth," and *lytic*, which means "capable of dissolving."

Introduction

The focus of this chapter is on drugs that may be used during labor and birth. The majority of these drugs are those used to inhibit, induce, or stimulate uterine contractions. Therefore, an understanding of the physiology of uterine function during labor and birth is necessary to safely prescribe many of the drugs and will be reviewed first.

A section of this chapter discusses pharmacotherapeutic options for relieving pain during labor, birth, and operative delivery. The remainder of the chapter reviews drugs used to treat common complications of parturition as well as those used for prophylactic purposes. These agents include drugs used to manage preterm labor; to induce and augment labor; and to prevent and treat complications including infections, preeclampsia and eclampsia, and acute postpartum hemorrhage.

Drug therapy during parturition, whether prophylactic or therapeutic, is always approached cautiously. All pharmacologic agents have significant risks of both maternal and fetal adverse effects despite their potential to prevent, treat, or ameliorate some adverse processes or outcomes that may be associated with labor and birth. Appropriate clinical judgment requires a healthy respect for the integrity of the maternal–fetal unit, the vulnerability of both, the physiology of parturition, and a healthy scrutiny of drugs to verify that potential benefits outweigh potential risks.

Overview of the Physiology of Parturition

Biologically, parturition is the process of producing offspring and includes all of its attendant physiologic mechanisms, particularly those that lead to the eventual maternal expulsion of the fetus. Although almost all maternal organ systems are involved in the physiology of reproduction, the uterus is the primary focus of parturition physiology. The uterus is remarkable in that it has the ability to accommodate itself to the presence of the growing fetus through hyperplasia and hypertrophy accompanied by myometrial quiescence, and then to expel the fetus on cue through the processes of labor and birth including maternal bearing-down efforts.

The uterine phases of parturition are designated as phases 0 through 3.[1] These phases correspond to stages of contractile activity of the myometrium: quiescence (phase 0), activation (phase 1), stimulation (phase 2), and involution (phase 3).[2]

The majority of pregnancy, designated as parturition phase 0, is characterized by extensive uterine growth and inhibition of myometrial activity through the actions of a host of endogenous substances including, but not limited to, progesterone, prostacyclin, relaxin, parathyroid hormone–related peptide, brain natriuretic peptide, nitric oxide, calcitonin gene–related peptide, adrenomedullin, and vasoactive intestinal peptide.[3,4] Generally, these endocrine and paracrine substances inhibit myometrial contraction by promoting potassium (K^+) conductance, inhibiting calcium (Ca^{2+}) release from intracellular stores, or reducing **myosin light-chain kinase (MLCK)** activity, thereby suppressing the connectivity between myocytes and muscle bundles.[5] Contemporary hypotheses contend that substances produced by the fetal membranes, such as brain natriuretic peptide acting through paracrine mechanisms are key to myometrial quiescence throughout phase 0.[2] Although the cervix normally remains rigid and unyielding during this phase,[4] it softens dramatically in early pregnancy due to increased vascularity and edema, hypertrophy of the cervical stroma, and hypertrophy and hyperplasia of the cervical glands. Throughout phase 0, a slow, progressive process of collagen reorganization occurs in the cervix.[6]

During phase 1 of parturition, the myometrium is activated in preparation for labor and birth, and the uterine cervix ripens to allow eventual dilatation and fetal passage. Myometrial activation occurs through the release of the pregnancy's inhibitory effects on the myometrium and the upregulation of a group of contraction-associated proteins, or labor genes, that act within the uterus to enable the myometrium to exert strong synchronous contractions.[3,7] Contraction-associated proteins can be categorized into three groups: (1) those that facilitate the interaction between **actin** and **myosin** molecules in the myocyte to cause myometrial contraction; (2) those that lower the depolarization threshold of myocytes to increase the excitability of the myometrium (oxytocin and prostaglandin F receptors); and (3) those that provide the intercellular connectivity of myocytes necessary for synchronous uterine contractions (gap junctions created by multimers of connexin-43).[3,7–9]

Phase 2 of parturition corresponds to the clinical stages of labor. This stimulation phase is characterized by synchronous and progressively more intense uterine contractions that effect cervical effacement and dilatation, fetal descent, and, in concert with the active bearing-down efforts of the mother, eventual birth of the fetus and placenta.[4] The strong contractions during phase 2 are stimulated by endogenous uterotonins such as prostaglandins and oxytocin.

Finally, parturition phase 3 is the period of postpartum uterine involution characterized by tonic uterine contractions influenced by neuroendocrine-released oxytocin in response to suckling of the infant at the mother's breast.

As described by Young,[10] these uterine phases occur over months (phase 0), to days (phase 1 involving upregulation of the contractile proteins), to hours (phase 2, the process of labor and birth), to minutes (phase 3 with the transition from phasic to tonic contraction).

Mechanisms of Initiation and Progression of Labor

The precise trigger that causes the onset of labor remains elusive, with a complex interaction of fetal and maternal neuronal, hormonal, and immune pathways likely being involved. However, considerable research evidence has implicated fetal control of the timing of the beginning of labor through maturation and activation of the fetal hypothalamic–pituitary–adrenal (HPA) axis associated with increased **corticotropin-releasing hormone** synthesis by the placenta.[3,11] Another factor proposed with the timing of human birth is the placental expression of the gene for corticotropin-releasing hormone production, suggesting a placental "clock" as the determining factor, although this hypothesis remains to be proven.[12] Contemporary understanding suggests that powerful positive feed-forward systems in both mother and fetus stimulate a rapidly increasing rate of placenta corticotropin-releasing hormone production in late gestation.[7,8,12,13]

The key feature of the progression from phase 0 to phase 1 of parturition is myometrial activation. This activation process is most likely precipitated by interactions of the fetal genome with maternal tissue, including increased placental corticotropin-releasing hormone production, through two mechanisms: (1) a growth pathway stimulating activation through uterine stretch; and (2) an endocrine/paracrine pathway characterized by increasing activity of the fetal HPA axis and production of fetal cortisol.[4,14] Increased placental production of corticotropin-releasing hormone drives increased fetal cortisol production, fetal pulmonary maturation, release of pro-inflammatory amniotic fluid proteins and phospholipids, and myometrial receptor expression. Placental corticotropin-releasing hormone also drives increasing maternal cortisol production and estrogen synthesis via corticotropin stimulation of the maternal adrenal glands. The production of both fetal and maternal cortisol stimulates a continued increase in placental corticotropin-releasing hormone production. Close to labor, local myometrial receptors change from forms favoring relaxation to those favoring contraction. These factors combine through a number of interlinked pro-inflammatory activating pathways to precipitate labor and birth in a robust fashion.[11]

Physiology of Cervical Ripening and Dilatation

Fibrous connective tissue dominates in the cervix. This tissue is composed of an extracellular matrix (collagen, elastin, and proteoglycans) and a cellular portion (smooth muscle and fibroblasts, epithelium, and blood vessels).[15] Cervical changes occur during the final 3 to 4 weeks of pregnancy in response to local and hormonal agents that create a bioactive catabolic environment, which in turn causes extensive remodeling of the extracellular matrix.[6,16] This process, often termed "ripening," results in a cervix that is soft, thin, and easily stretched.[6]

Although the precise mechanisms are not completely understood, cervical ripening is characterized by the dispersal and disorganization of collagen fibrils, an increase in collagen solubility, and increased quantities of glycosaminoglycans and noncollagenous proteins binding large amounts of water.[6] When labor commences, recruitment of extracellular matrix metalloproteases and leukocytes occurs in the cervix. This phenomenon is associated with a sharp rise in the cervical concentration of hyaluronic acid, causing the tissue to swell, the cervix to become more distensible, and the collagen framework to further weaken; collectively, these changes allow gradual passive cervical dilatation during labor.[6,16,17] Dilatation occurs in response to these biochemical changes, contraction-produced mechanical traction forces, and pressure exerted by the fetal presenting part during uterine contractions.[3] As the cervix continues to efface during labor, the internal os is taken up laterally, becoming indistinguishable from the lower uterine segment—a phenomenon that suggests the internal os may be the location of maximal cervical softening.

Physiology of Uterine Activity

Similar to other smooth muscle, the myometrium can exert substantial force with relatively little energy expenditure, can generate force in any direction within the cell, and exhibits significantly greater shortening than striated skeletal muscle. Uterine growth, initially due to myometrial hyperplasia, primarily results from extensive and remarkable myometrial hypertrophy in response to hormonal (e.g., progesterone and estrogen) and mechanical influences. This hypertrophy is associated with increases in oxytocin receptor proteins and the number of myocytes expressing oxytocin receptors as gestation advances toward term.[10]

Control of Myometrial Activity

The electrical activity of the myometrium changes during pregnancy, from a pattern of irregular spikes to the eventual regular activity of phasic uterine contractions during labor.[3] Although agonists such as oxytocin and prostaglandins are powerful modulators of uterine contraction, uterine smooth muscle is myogenic and able to contract without neuronal or hormonal input.[18,19] The uterine source of the phasic contractions remains unidentified. Potential mechanisms that may initiate and propagate uterine contractions include the following:

- Specialized myometrial cells within a heterogeneous population of smooth muscle cells acting as pacemakers
- Specialized interstitial cells acting as electrical pacemakers similar to Cajal cells in the gastrointestinal tract
- An electrical syncytium created by gap junctions that link myocyte to myocyte
- A metabolic syncytium allowing a group of cells to act as a local pacemaker
- A hydrodynamic-stretch activation mechanism that facilitates organ-level communication and myocyte recruitment to create a coordinated uterine contraction[10]

Mechanisms of Myometrial Contraction

Contraction of the uterine smooth muscle is structurally dependent upon the interaction between actin and myosin that is regulated by the calcium-sensitive enzyme known as myosin light-chain kinase.[3] Actin is a polymerized double-helical strand comprising the thin filaments. Myosin consists of the thick filaments of smooth muscle and is a hexamer of two myosin heavy-chain subunits and two pairs of myosin light-chain subunits molecularly arranged as a double-helix tail (two spirally wrapped heavy chains) with a double head at one end (two light chains to each free head). The myosin head, which is termed the "myosin motor," contains the actin-binding region and the ATP hydrolysis site that provides the needed energy for force generation.[18]

Depolarization of the myometrial cell membrane opens the voltage-sensitive calcium channels, allowing extracellular calcium ion influx and the release of calcium ions

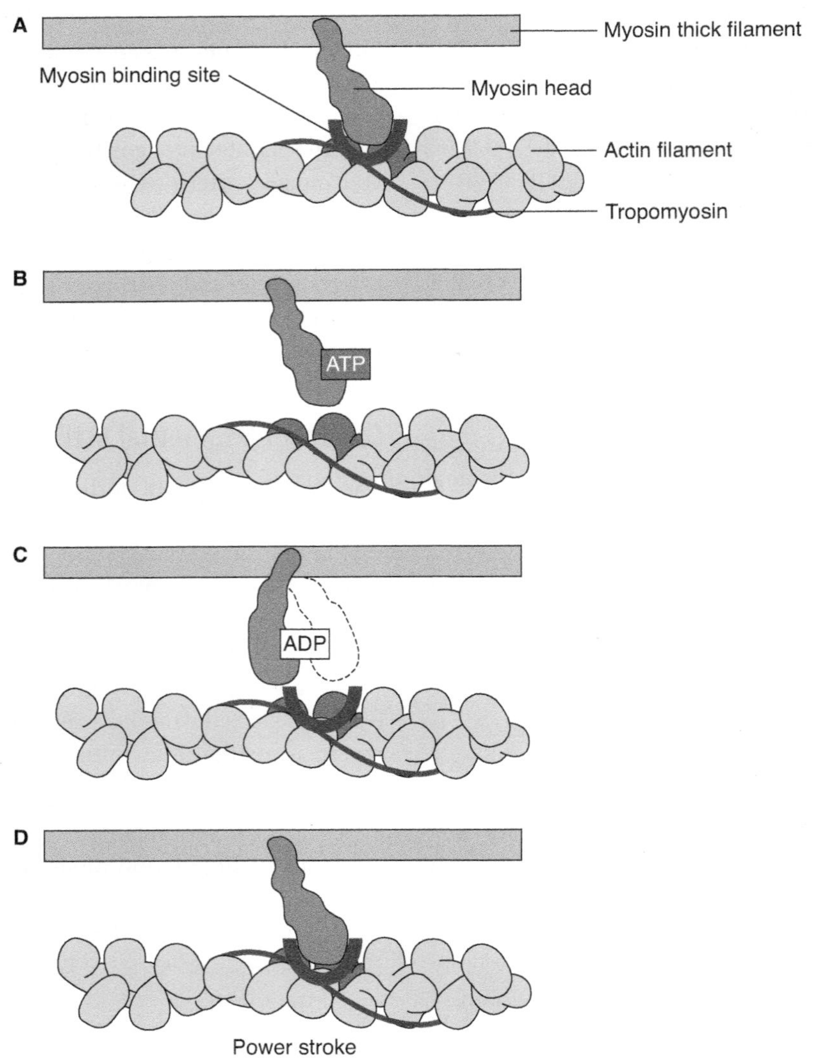

Figure 36-1 Uterine muscle contraction.

(A) Attached: At the start of the cycle, the myosin head is attached to the myosin binding site on the actin filament. **(B) Recharging:** A molecule of ATP binds to a large cleft at the back of the myosin head, which causes a slight change in the conformation of the myosin binding site that reduces the affinity the myosin head has for the myosin binding site. **(C) Cocked:** The cleft on the myosin head closes around the ATP, which causes a large shape change so that the head is displaced along the actin filament by a distance of approximately 5 nm. **(D) Force generating:** As ATP is hydrolyzed to ADP, the myosin head once again binds tightly to the next myosin binding site on the actin filament. In this process, the myosin head essentially ratchets along the actin filament, creating the muscle contraction.

from sarcoplasmic reticulum stores within the cell.[18] The binding of intracellular calcium to calmodulin forms a calcium–calmodulin complex that activates the essential enzyme MLCK, which in turn phosphorylates the regulatory myosin light chains to initiate binding with actin. The functional structural complex formed, which is known as actinomycin, converts the chemical energy of adenosine triphosphate (ATP) into the mechanical energy of contraction (Figure 36-1).[20] When the thin filaments exert tension along the longitudinal direction of the cell, muscle shortening or contraction occurs.[18] The frequency of myometrial action potentials is associated with the *frequency* of contractions, the number of spikes in the action potential with the *force* of contractions, and the duration of the action potentials with the *duration* of contractions.[3] From an organ-level perspective, uterine contractions of labor are characterized by a descending propagation of the contractile wave from the uterine fundus toward the lower uterine segment, and a longer duration and greater strength of contraction in the fundus. These characteristics serve to pull the cervix upward toward the fundus and push the fetus downward toward the cervix, producing cervical dilatation, fetal descent, and, in combination with maternal efforts, eventual birth.

Clinically, childbirth is divided into three stages. The first stage of labor is the time from the onset of regular, painful contractions and ongoing cervical dilatation until such dilatation is complete. This stage is often subdivided into the latent phase of labor and active labor. The second stage of labor commences when the cervix is fully dilated and ends with the birth of the infant. The third stage of labor begins at birth and ends when the placenta is expelled.

Treatments for Women in Preterm Labor

Current knowledge regarding uterine physiology forms the basis of drug therapy for women in preterm labor. The diagnosis of preterm labor is one of the most challenging clinical problems in the care of pregnant women. Preterm births are those that occur between 20 0/7 weeks' and 36 6/7 weeks' gestation. Preterm birth is the single most important contributor to infant morbidity and mortality, with 35.2% of infant deaths in 2010 being related to prematurity.[21] The American College of Obstetricians and Gynecologists (ACOG) estimates that preterm labor precedes half of all preterm births and notes that preterm labor is the most common cause of hospitalization during pregnancy.[23]

The complex etiology of preterm labor and birth is reflected in its epidemiologic risk factors, which include history of spontaneous preterm birth, multiple gestation, bleeding in pregnancy, genitourinary tract infection, African American race, young maternal age (less than 18 years), low maternal body mass index, cigarette smoking and substance use, uterine anomaly, and the use of assisted reproductive technology. Additionally, spontaneous preterm birth is correlated with psychosocial stressors including low socioeconomic status and low educational attainment, personal stress, and late entry to prenatal care. While there is no single pathogenic pathway to spontaneous preterm birth, proposed etiologies include activation of the maternal–fetal HPA axis, intrauterine infection and inflammation, decidual hemorrhage, and pathologic uterine distention.[24] At this time, historical risk factors are the most common screening factors used to identify women who are at increased risk of having a preterm birth. For women who have a history of preterm birth or preterm premature rupture of membranes, prophylactic therapy using injections of 17 alpha-hydroxyprogesterone caproate (17P, Makena) has been shown to decrease the incidence of a subsequent preterm birth. The pharmacotherapeutic considerations surrounding use 17 alpha-hydroxy-progesterone caproate are reviewed in the *Pregnancy* chapter.

Tocolysis

Tocolysis is the use of drugs to inhibit myometrial contractions (Box 36-1). Once the decision to attempt to stop preterm labor contractions via drug therapy has been made, the provider can choose one of several **tocolytics**. The primary goals of tocolytic therapy are to arrest labor and delay birth long enough to initiate prophylactic corticosteroid therapy for stimulation of fetal lung maturity, arrange for maternal–fetal transport to a perinatal tertiary care hospital if needed, and prolong pregnancy if the underlying etiology is self-limiting (e.g., pyelonephritis). The use of currently available tocolytics remains controversial because, overall, these drugs have not demonstrated success in improving perinatal outcomes. The primary problem may be that tocolytics simply attempt to stop the uterus from contracting, rather than treating the specific cause of the preterm labor.[24]

The four categories of drugs that have been used for tocolysis are calcium-channel blockers, beta-sympathomimetics, magnesium sulfate, and cyclooxygenase (COX)

Box 36-1 Gone But Not Forgotten: Pharmacologic Use of Alcohol as a Tocolytic

In the 1970s, alcohol was a commonly accepted treatment to inhibit labor. Women at term who were having prodromal labor or simply frequent Braxton-Hicks contractions were often counseled to have a therapeutic drink of alcohol to relax the uterus. For women with symptoms of preterm labor that included early or advanced cervical dilatation, alcohol was often recommended as a tocolytic. When used as a tocolytic for preterm labor, alcohol was administered intravenously. Women experienced similar effects as occur with oral ingestion, including intoxication, nausea and vomiting, and potential alcohol poisoning, followed by hangovers when the alcohol was discontinued. Overall, the use of alcohol as a tocolytic was a less than satisfying method for women and providers alike. Alcohol as a tocolytic fell into disuse, and today most women would be astounded if their providers even suggested a glass of wine as a treatment for prodromal labor.

inhibitors. Meta-analyses of the effects of tocolytic agents have found that cyclooxygenase inhibitors (odds ratio [OR], 5.39; 95% confidence interval [CI], 2.14–12.34) and magnesium sulfate (OR, 2.76; 95% CI, 1.58–4.94) are the most likely to delay birth for 48 hours, followed by calcium-channel blockers (OR, 2.71; 95% CI, 1.17–5.91) and beta-sympathomimetics (OR, 2.41; 95% CI, 1.27–4.55).[25] The differences in effectiveness are relatively small, but each tocolytic has a unique profile with regard to side effects, safety, contraindications, and gestational age effects. Therefore, the selection of a particular tocolytic may be individualized and based more on side-effect profile than on effectiveness. Contraindications to tocolysis are listed in Table 36-1. The pharmacologic properties, maternal side effects, and fetal side effects of tocolytics used in the United States are presented in Table 36-2. In addition, the reader is referred to the discussion by Simhan et al. for a review of tocolytic drug clinical protocols.[26]

Tocolytic therapy is discontinued when contractions have ceased or occur less frequently than four per hour without any accompanying cervical change. There is no evidence that continued tocolysis after acute management prolongs pregnancy or reduces the rate of preterm birth.[25,26]

Table 36-1 Contraindications to Tocolysis

Maternal	Fetal
Cardiac disease	Chorioamnionitis
Chorioamnionitis	Gestational age > 36 weeks
Hemorrhage with hemodynamic instability	Intrauterine fetal demise
Intolerant to tocolytics	Intrauterine fetal growth restriction
Maternal contraindication to a tocolytic drug	Lethal fetal anomaly
Placental abruption	Nonreassuring fetal status
Preterm contractions without cervical change	
Severe preeclampsia or eclampsia	

Beta-Sympathomimetics

Beta-sympathomimetics, also known as beta-adrenergic receptor agonists or beta agonists, have been prescribed for the treatment of women in preterm labor for more than 30 years and were once the most frequently used tocolytic agents. Beta$_2$-adrenoreceptor agonist tocolytics, such as the commonly used terbutaline (Brethine), produce smooth muscle relaxation by increasing intracellular production of cyclic adenosine monophosphate (cAMP); the greater concentration of cAMP results in inactivation of MLCK, thereby inhibiting the interaction of actin and myosin.[25,27]

In 1998, the Food and Drug Administration (FDA) issued an advisory regarding the subcutaneous infusion of terbutaline, warning that its effectiveness and safety had not been established and alerting practitioners that "the continuous administration of subcutaneous terbutaline sulfate has not been demonstrated to be effective and is potentially dangerous."[28] Since this advisory was issued, the use of terbutaline as a tocolytic has waned in the United States.

Current uses of terbutaline in the intrapartum period include as single-dose therapy for the initiation of acute tocolysis and to stop uterine tachysystole if fetal heart rate decelerations are present. This drug is used as part of intrauterine fetal rescue and resuscitation in the event of uterine tachysystole and nonreassuring fetal heart rate patterns during labor.

Maternal and fetal cardiovascular and metabolic physiology can be dramatically affected by terbutaline due to the ubiquitous presence of beta-adrenergic receptors in multiple organs, cross-reactivity of β_1 and β_2 receptors, and the free passage of the drug across the placenta that results in fetal serum concentrations equivalent to maternal concentrations.[27,29] The peak serum concentration is reached 20 to

Table 36-2 Tocolytic Treatment of Preterm Labor

Drug: Generic (Brand)	Dose	Maternal Side Effects/ Adverse Effects	Fetal Side Effects/ Adverse Effects	Contraindications	Clinical Considerations
Beta-Sympathomimetics					
Terbutaline (Brethine)	SQ: 0.25 mg; may consider repeating every 20–40 minutes until tocolysis is achieved (maximum of 4 doses), then every 2–4 hours if maternal heart rate < 120 beats/minute IV: 2.5–5 mcg/minute, increased by 2.5–5 mcg/ minute to maximum infusion of 25 mcg/ minute	SE: Flushing, tachycardia, palpitations, hypotension, hyperglycemia, hypokalemia, nervousness, nausea, or vomiting AE: Arrhythmia, chest pain, myocardial ischemia, shortness of breath, pulmonary edema, adult respiratory distress syndrome	SE: Tachycardia, hyperinsulinemia AE: Fetal hyperglycemia, neonatal hypoglycemia, hypocalcemia, hypotension, ileus	Known or suspected cardiac disease, hyperthyroidism, or convulsive disorders	Diabetes is not a contraindication if blood glucose levels are monitored and stable. Use with caution in women with a risk for hemorrhage, such as placental previa. FDA black box warning indicates this drug should not be used for prevention of PTL or for treatment of more than 48 hours secondary to the risk of maternal cardiac problems and/or death. Monitor fluid intake and urine output, and for signs of pulmonary edema.
Calcium-Channel Blockers					
Nifedipine (Procardia)	Loading dose: 30 mg PO; repeated every 20 minutes if contractions persist, until maximum of 3 doses (30 mg); then 10–20 mg orally every 4–6 hours	SE: Transient hypotension, tachycardia, headache, flushing, dizziness, nausea, palpitations, edema	None known	Cardiovascular disease or hemodynamic instability. Do not combine with beta-sympathomimetic drugs.	Not used concomitantly with magnesium sulfate or beta-sympathomimetics
Cyclooxygenase Inhibitors					
Indomethacin (Indocin)	Loading dose: 50 mg orally or 50–100 mg by rectal suppository; then 25–50 mg orally every 6 hours, for 48–72 hours	SE: Gastritis, nausea AE: Impairment of renal function, increased postpartum hemorrhage, hypertension	AE: Oligohydramnios, bronchopulmonary dysplasia, premature constriction of ductus arteriosus, necrotizing enterocolitis, intraventricular hemorrhage	Presence of fetal growth restriction or oligohydramnios History of asthma, urticaria, or allergic-type reactions to aspirin or other nonsteroidal anti-inflammatory drugs	Safe for use between 24 and 32 weeks' gestation
Magnesium Sulfate					
Magnesium sulfate	Loading dose: 4–6 g intravenously over 30 minutes; then 1–4 g/ hour by continuous IV infusion titrated beginning at 2 g/hour and increasing by 1 g/hour until maximum of 4 g for 24 hours Should not be used for more than 5–7 days	SE: Flushing, nausea and vomiting, diplopia, blurred vision, headache, lethargy AE: Ileus, hypocalcemia, muscle weakness, pulmonary edema, cardiac arrest	AE: Hypotonia, lethargy, bone demineralization	Women with myasthenia gravis, myocardial compromise, cardiac conduction defects, or poor renal function	Meta-analysis suggests magnesium sulfate is not effective as a tocolytic, and it is no longer recommended for use as a tocolytic. Recommended for fetal neuroprotection.

Abbreviations: AE = adverse effects; PTL = preterm labor; SE = side effects.
Sources: Data from American College of Obstetricians and Gynecologists. Practice Bulletin No. 130: prediction and prevention of preterm birth. *Obstet Gynecol.* 2012;120:964-973[23]; Simhan HN, Caritis SN. Prevention of preterm delivery. *N Engl J Med.* 2007;357:477-487.[24]

30 minutes after subcutaneous injection of terbutaline, and the serum half-life is estimated at 3 hours. These estimates have not been confirmed in pregnant women.

Calcium-Channel Blockers

Calcium-channel blockers promote uterine relaxation by decreasing the influx of calcium ions into myometrial cells through the voltage-dependent calcium channels as well as the release of intracellular calcium to inhibit MLCK activity and hence myometrial contraction.[24] Because these drugs are nonspecific, the same effect is seen in cardiac, vascular, and nonvascular smooth muscle.

Nifedipine (Procardia) has been the calcium-channel blocker most widely studied as a tocolytic agent, as it has less effect on the cardiac conduction apparatus than older drugs such as verapamil (Isoptin, Covera-HS). Nifedipine has an onset of action of less than 20 minutes after oral administration and 1 to 5 minutes after sublingual administration. Its half-life is approximately 1.3 hours.[30]

Calcium-channel blockers are preferred tocolytic agents because of their ease of administration and their favorable side-effect profile compared to beta agonists and magnesium sulfate. A review of the safety of these drugs as tocolytics concluded that they should not be combined with intravenously administered beta agonists due to an increased risk of pulmonary edema, and should not be used in the presence of maternal cardiovascular compromise or multiple gestations. The mother's blood pressure should be monitored frequently for the development of hypotension during the administration of immediate-release tablets, and women should be cautioned not to chew these tablets.[31] Lyell and colleagues suggested that hydrating women with 500 mL of lactated Ringer's solution intravenously prior to nifedipine administration may ameliorate the risk of significant hypotension.[32] A meta-analysis reported that, for acute tocolysis, nifedipine was superior to beta agonists in terms of safety and effectiveness and was superior to magnesium in terms of safety, although it proved ineffective as maintenance tocolytic.[33]

Cyclooxygenase Inhibitors

Cyclooxygenase is the enzyme responsible for the formation of specific prostaglandins. Several isoforms of cyclooxygenase exist. The COX-1 and COX-2 enzymes are necessary for the biosynthesis of prostaglandins critical in parturition. The nonspecific COX inhibitor indomethacin (Indocin), a nonsteroidal anti-inflammatory drug (NSAID), is the most commonly used tocolytic in this drug class and has been the subject of a number of small clinical trials. Indomethacin (Indocin) inhibits uterine contractions by reducing the synthesis of prostaglandins. Although a Cochrane review found that indomethacin is effective when compared to placebo in terms of reducing the incidence of preterm birth, the authors of another review found insufficient evidence to support the safety of indomethacin tocolysis in relation to neonatal outcomes.[34]

The potential for serious adverse fetal effects, such as constriction of the ductus arteriosus, neonatal pulmonary hypertension, intraventricular hemorrhage, and oligohydramnios, has led to recommendations that indomethacin (Indocin) tocolysis not be used after 32 weeks' gestation, in women who have growth-restricted fetuses, or in the presence of oligohydramnios.[34] Peak serum levels of indomethacin are reached within 2 hours of administration, and the drug has a mean half-life of approximately 4.5 hours.

Magnesium Sulfate

Magnesium sulfate has been shown to be ineffective as a tocolytic agent and does not reduce the likelihood of birth within 48 hours, birth within 7 days, or subsequent preterm birth.[35] Despite the lack of evidence regarding effectiveness, magnesium sulfate remains a popular tocolytic in the United States. This drug has long been used for women at risk of eclampsia as discussed later in the chapter and most providers are comfortable with the agent. The theoretical underpinning for the use of magnesium sulfate as a tocolytic is potential inhibition of myometrial contractility by hyperpolarizing the plasma membrane and competing with intracellular calcium to inhibit MLCK activity, although its precise mechanism of action as a tocolytic is unknown.

Additionally, magnesium sulfate is a high-alert medication that must be administered under strict protocols.[36] Because magnesium is exclusively excreted by the kidneys, adequate renal function, as evidenced by urine output that is 100 mL per hour or more, is essential for safe administration of this agent. Acute magnesium toxicity is evidenced by a sudden decline in blood pressure and respiratory paralysis. Frequent monitoring of maternal respiratory effort and patellar deep tendon reflexes is essential for the early recognition of overdose. In the event of respiratory arrest, 10 to 20 mL of a 5% solution of calcium gluconate is an effective antidote.

While magnesium sulfate is falling out of favor as a tocolytic agent, evidence has shown a role for this medication as a neuroprotective agent that works to prevent cerebral palsy in the preterm fetus. A Cochrane review found that magnesium sulfate therapy given to women at risk for preterm birth reduces the incidence of cerebral palsy by more than 30%, (relative risk [RR], 0.68; 95% CI, 0.54–0.87; five trials; 6145 infants) and the drug does not adversely impact neonatal mortality or major maternal complications.[37] Current protocols advocate the use of magnesium sulfate for fetal neuroprotection among pregnant women with preterm prelabor rupture of membranes, preterm labor, or an indication for preterm delivery and who are between 23 0/7 and 31 6/7 weeks' gestation.[38] Institutional protocols vary with regard to the gestational age at which magnesium may be started. Magnesium for neuroprotection can be given simultaneously with tocolytics during the first 48 hours after the advent of preterm labor, while still allowing for corticosteroid administration to accelerate fetal pulmonary maturation.[38] The most effective dose and duration of treatment have not been determined, but treatment with magnesium sulfate for more than 5 to 7 days could have adverse effects on fetal bones and is not recommended.[39] Retreatment is also not recommended.

Corticosteroid Prophylaxis

There is widespread agreement that the most beneficial medical treatment for women at high risk for preterm birth is the antenatal administration of corticosteroids to accelerate fetal pulmonary maturation. Corticosteroid medications, such as betamethasone (Celestone) and dexamethasone (Decadron), enhance fetal lung maturity by stimulating surfactant synthesis, increasing compliance of pulmonary tissues, and reducing vascular capillaries. A single course of steroids for all women at risk of giving birth before 34 weeks' gestation has been the standard of care since 1994.[40] Antenatal corticosteroid administration is associated with significant reductions in neonatal death, respiratory distress syndrome, intraventricular hemorrhage, necrotizing enterocolitis, and early systemic infections in the neonate, without increasing maternal risk of death, chorioamnionitis, or puerperal sepsis.[41] Further, antenatal corticosteroid administration is effective in reducing neonatal morbidity and mortality for women with premature rupture of membranes and pregnancy-related hypertension syndromes. The two commonly used regimens for this purpose are detailed in Table 36-3.

Table 36-3 Corticosteroid Prophylaxis to Promote Fetal Maturation in Preterm Labor

Drug: Generic (Brand)	Dose
Betamethasone (Celestone)	12 mg intramuscular (6 mg each of betamethasone acetate and betamethasone sodium phosphate) 2 doses given 24 hours apart
Dexamethasone (Decadron)	6 mg intramuscular Every 12 hours for 4 doses

Women at risk of preterm birth between 24 and 34 weeks' gestation are candidates for corticosteroid treatment. Studies have not shown improved respiratory outcomes for infants born after 34 weeks when their mothers receive such therapy.[42] The evidence regarding the effectiveness of corticosteroids in multiple gestations, growth-restricted fetuses, and very early preterm fetuses prior to 24 weeks remains unclear.[43]

Maternal side effects of corticosteroids include maternal glucose intolerance with transient hyperglycemia among women without diabetes and increased insulin requirements among women with diabetes. Corticosteroids also predispose pregnant women to develop pulmonary edema—a risk that is higher if beta-adrenergic drugs are used for tocolysis simultaneously, or among women who have a multiple gestation.

Fetal side effects from corticosteroid therapy tend to be somewhat unusual, demonstrating a biphasic presentation. The initial response is often a mild elevation in heart rate. On days 2 and 3 after the first dose, the fetal heart rate often exhibits decreased variability. The longest research studies have followed children exposed to corticosteroids prenatally from birth to the age of 30 years.[44] No known long-term effects have been reported concerning children who were given one antenatal dose of corticosteroids with regard to cognition, behavior, or neurodevelopmental outcomes. However, because cortisol is the primary end product of the hypothalamic–pituitary axis, potential long-term effects on cortisol production and regulation of the stress response are possible and the subject of current investigation.

Current evidence suggests that the benefits of prenatal corticosteroids are optimal if 48 hours or more has elapsed between the initial dose and birth. However, in the setting of clinical chorioamnionitis, delivery should be expedited and not delayed to complete the corticosteroid therapy. Further, while the duration of corticosteroid effect is unclear, the benefits appear to decline after 7 days, and repeat dosing may be considered *if a significant risk of preterm birth remains.* Although repeat doses of corticosteroids are believed to reduce the occurrence and severity of neonatal lung disease and the risk of serious health problems in the first few weeks of life, critics have questioned the data analyses on which these recommendations have been based, and repeat doses are associated with reduced birth weight and head circumference at birth.[45] Current ACOG guidelines indicate that a second "rescue" course may be given if a woman is likely to deliver before 34 weeks' gestation and more than 7 days has elapsed since the first steroid administration, but state that no more than two courses should be given in total.[23]

Although betamethasone has gained popularity as the drug of choice due to the belief that it offers more benefits and a lower risk profile, a double-blinded trial reported that betamethasone and dexamethasone were equivalent in reducing the rates of most major neonatal morbidities and mortality. Dexamethasone was superior in reducing the rate of intraventricular hemorrhage, with a reported absolute risk reduction of approximately 11.3% (95% CI, 2.7–11.9%).[46] It should also be noted that dexamethasone is more widely available globally and generally has a lower cost than betamethasone.

Induction and Augmentation of Labor

Induction of labor involves artificially stimulating the uterus to contract in a rhythmic manner prior to the onset of spontaneous labor with the goal of a vaginal birth. Induction of labor is one of the most common procedures in the United States. After having more than doubled over the past two decades, induction rates may have plateaued, decreasing in 2012 to 23.3% of singleton pregnancies, from the 2010 peak rate of 23.8%.[47]

Campaigns by professional groups such as ACOG, Association of Women's Health, Obstetric, and Neonatal Nurses (AWHONN), and the March of Dimes are discouraging early and elective induction. Induction of labor should be considered a therapeutic option only when the benefits of birth outweigh the risks of continuing the pregnancy for the woman or her fetus and there is no contraindication to vaginal birth. Indications for induction of labor and contraindications to the procedure as identified by ACOG and other organizations are listed in Table 36-4.[48]

Induction of labor is associated with an approximately twofold increased overall risk of operative birth via cesarean section among nulliparous women[49] Analysis, however, has shown that induction of labor is associated with a lower risk of cesarean section birth among women at more than 41 weeks of gestation.[50] Thus the decision to electively induce labor must be one that is carefully considered with the woman.

Induction of labor using drugs has two components: (1) cervical ripening; and (2) induction of contractions. Drugs used to induce either cervical ripening or induction of contractions are listed in Table 36-5.

Prostaglandins for Cervical Ripening

In 1930, two American gynecologists, Kurzok and Lieb, discovered that strips of human uterine muscle would relax when exposed to semen. A few years later, Von Euler identified the active material in semen and named it *prostaglandin*. Prostaglandins are local or paracrine endocrine agents that exert their effect locally and are then metabolized locally. This is a challenging issue from a pharmacologic standpoint because it is difficult to make a prostaglandin formulation that works when given orally or systemically. Prostaglandin receptors are always present in myometrial tissue, which is why prostaglandins can be used to induce labor throughout pregnancy, whereas

Table 36-4 Indications, Contraindications, and Special Considerations to Induction of Labor

Indications for Labor Induction	Contraindications to Labor Induction	Clinical Situations Requiring Special Attention and Vigilance[a]
Abruptio placentae	Active genital herpes infection	One or more previous low-transverse cesarean births
Chorioamnionitis	Category III fetal heart rate tracing	Breech presentation; funic presentation
Fetal demise	Invasive cervical cancer	"Logistic" or psychosocial factors
Gestational hypertension	Placenta previa	Multifetal pregnancy
Preeclampsia, eclampsia, HELLP syndrome[b]	Previous myomectomy involving the endometrial cavity	Polyhydramnios
Premature rupture of membranes	Previous transfundal uterine surgery (classical uterine incision)	Presenting part above the pelvic inlet
Post-term pregnancy	Prior uterine rupture	Prior stillbirth
Maternal medical conditions (e.g., diabetes mellitus, renal disease, chronic pulmonary disease, chronic hypertension, cholestasis of pregnancy)	Transverse fetal lie	Severe hypertension
Fetal compromise (e.g., severe fetal growth restriction, isoimmunization, nonreassuring fetal status)	Umbilical cord prolapse	Abnormal fetal heart rate patterns not necessitating emergent delivery

[a] These situations are not absolute contraindications to induction.

[b] HELLP syndrome is characterized by hemolysis, elevated liver enzymes, and low platelet count.

Source: Data from American College of Obstetricians and Gynecologists. Practice Bulletin 107: induction of labor. *Obstet Gynecol.* 2009;114:386-397.[48]

Table 36-5 Drugs for Induction or Augmentation of Labor

Drug: Generic (Brand)	Dose and Route	Contraindications	Side Effects/ Adverse Effects	Clinical Considerations
Cervical Ripening Prostaglandin Agents[a]				
Dinoprostone; prostaglandin E_2 (Prepidil, Cervidil)	Cervical gel (Prepidil): 0.5 mg (in 2.5-mL syringe) inserted into the endocervix May repeat in 6–12 hours Maximum of 3 doses (1.5 mg) in 24 hours	Any contraindication to induction of labor Contraindicated if abnormal fetal heart rate pattern present	Uterine tachysystole and fetal heart rate decelerations	Woman should remain recumbent for 30 minutes to prevent leakage. Oxytocin may be initiated 6 or more hours after insertion. Electronically monitor uterine activity and fetal heart rate prior to and for 2 hours after insertion. Disadvantage is that it cannot be easily removed in the event of uterine tachysystole or abnormal fetal heart rate pattern.
	Vaginal insert (Cervidil): 10-mg slow release at 0.3 mg/hour Remains in place until active labor begins or for 12 hours		Uterine tachysystole and fetal heart rate decelerations	Oxytocin may be initiated 30 or more minutes after insert removal. Electronically monitor uterine activity and fetal heart rate prior to and after placement for 15 or more minutes after insert removal.
Misoprostol; prostaglandin E_1 (Cytotec)	25–50 mcg intravaginally; 100-mcg oral tablet is divided into four 25-mcg pieces or two 50-mcg pieces (alternatively, a 200-mcg oral tablet is divided into four 50-mcg pieces) 50-mcg tablet orally; may repeat every 4 hours, with maximum of 6 doses 20–25 mcg oral solution; may repeat every 2 hours, until maximum of 12 doses (41)	Any contraindication to induction of labor Contraindicated for women with history of prior cesarean birth or uterine surgery	Uterine tachysystole and fetal heart rate decelerations	Electronically monitor uterine activity and fetal heart rate prior to and after placement for 2–4 hours. Oxytocin may be initiated 4 or more hours after the last dose of misoprostol. Disadvantage is that it cannot be easily removed in the event of uterine tachysystole or abnormal fetal heart rate pattern.
Induction or Augmentation Agent				
Oxytocin (Pitocin)	10 units in 500–1000 mL of normal saline or lactated Ringer's (some use 60 units in 1000 mL or 30 units in 500 mL) *Low-dose regimen:* 0.5–2.0 mU/minute, increased by 1–2 mU/minute at 30- to 60-minute intervals *High-dose regimen:* 6 mU/minute, increased by 3–6 mU/minute at 15- to 40- minute intervals Maximum dose 20–40 mU/minute	Any contraindication to induction of labor	Hyponatremia due to the antidiuretic effect of oxytocin. Symptoms do not usually appear until the plasma sodium level < 125 mEq/L. Hypotension if rapid infusion occurs.	Administer via infusion pump to provide continuous, precise dose control via piggyback to nonmedicated intravenous infusion line. Continuous electronic monitoring of uterine activity and fetal heart rate required. Never administer in an electrolyte-free solution.

[a] May also lead to uterine contractions and the induction of labor.

oxytocin is dependent upon the upregulation of receptors in myometrial tissue just before and during labor to exert its uterotonic effects.

For women with an unfavorable cervix (total Bishop score < 6) for whom induction of labor is indicated, pharmacologic methods of cervical ripening include administration of synthetic prostaglandin E_1 (misoprostol) or prostaglandin E_2 (dinoprostone) (Table 36-5). Unlike prostaglandin $F_{2\alpha}$ (Hemabate), these drugs are not contraindicated in the presence of maternal asthma.

Cervical ripening agents may be used following or in combination with a number of nonpharmacologic mechanical cervical ripening methods, such as stripping the fetal membranes during a vaginal examination, use of hygroscopic endocervical dilators, or placement of a balloon catheter ("Foley bulb") above the internal cervical os.

The most frequent complication of prostaglandin administration is uterine tachysystole; hence attentive monitoring of uterine activity and fetal status during administration is essential. It is important to note that only dinoprostone is approved by the FDA for use as a cervical ripening agent, although ACOG acknowledges the apparent safety and effectiveness of misoprostol for this purpose.[48] For women with a favorable Bishop score

(6 or greater), most induction methods will stimulate the onset of uterine contractions. Due to the increased risk of uterine rupture in women who have experienced a prior cesarean birth, the use of prostaglandins is contraindicated for women planning a vaginal birth after cesarean (VBAC).

Misoprostol is the least expensive agent for cervical ripening and has traditionally been given vaginally, although it can also be administered orally. According to a Cochrane review, orally administered misoprostol is as effective a cervical ripening agent as vaginal misoprostol and results in fewer cesarean section births than dinoprostone or oxytocin.[51] Oral misoprostol may be selected as an agent for women with ruptured membranes, particularly because oral administration eliminates the need for a vaginal examination and thereby reduces the risk for ascending uterine infections.[52]

Oxytocin for Induction of Labor

In 1909, Dale discovered **oxytocin** as a substance from the posterior pituitary. He named oxytocin using the Greek words *tokos* (meaning "to give birth") and *oxus* (meaning "quick"). Fifty years later, the biochemist du Vigneaud succeeded in synthesizing oxytocin; he won the Nobel Prize in Chemistry for his discovery. Today, induction of uterine contractions is usually accomplished via intravenous administration of synthetic oxytocin. Oxytocin causes uterine contractions sufficient to induce birth, but it is not effective in ripening the cervix—a necessary precursor to active labor. Consequently, this agent is best used for induction when the cervix is favorable.

Although reports of the biologic half-life of oxytocin vary widely, it is now generally agreed that the half-life is between 6 and 10 minutes and that continuous intravenous oxytocin infusion is associated with a linear increase in plasma oxytocin concentration, reaching a steady state in approximately 40 minutes.[53–55]

Oxytocin (Pitocin) is a powerful drug that may quickly hyperstimulate the uterus. Clark et al. noted that oxytocin is "the drug most commonly associated with preventable adverse perinatal outcomes."[55] This agent is designated by the Institute for Safe Medicine Practices as a "high alert" medication.[36] The most frequent adverse effect of oxytocin, uterine tachysystole, is defined as more than 5 uterine contractions in 10 minutes, averaged over a 30-minute period.[56] Uteroplacental perfusion may be compromised in these situations, leading to fetal heart rate decelerations or bradycardia and subsequent neonatal acidemia. Frequent assessment of uterine activity and fetal well-being is required during the administration of oxytocin. Although institutional policies often dictate continuous electronic fetal monitoring (EFM) during oxytocin administration, there are no data that indicate EFM is essential to adequate ongoing fetal assessment or the monitoring of uterine response.

Oxytocin (Pitocin) is administered via an electronic infusion pump to carefully control the titration of the dose. This intravenous infusion pump should be connected via a secondary intravenous line that is piggybacked into the primary intravenous line in close proximity to the catheter's entrance into the woman's skin. These measures improve safety by decreasing the amount of oxytocin that will be administered if the infusion must be suddenly discontinued due to uterine tachysystole or fetal compromise and by protecting the integrity of the primary intravenous line.

Unfortunately, neither the optimal oxytocin administration regimen nor the maximum dose has been established through research or agreed-upon expert opinion, although the two most common approaches are low-dose and high-dose regimens, as presented in Table 36-5 and Table 36-6. Advocates of high-dose oxytocin regimens note that labor tends to be more rapid and failure of induction is less common than with low doses, whereas advocates of low-dose oxytocin regimens emphasize the finding that tachysystole and abnormal fetal heart rate patterns are less common with this approach, while the progress of labor is similar. Clark et al. recommended that oxytocin should be "aggressively titrated to the lowest dose compatible with sustained levels of appropriate uterine activity"—that is, the safest dose is the lowest dose that produces adequate uterine contractions.[55] Other unresolved safety concerns include how duration of infusion is related to outcomes, whether there is a maximum dose of oxytocin that should not be exceeded, whether oxytocin should be administered in a pulsatile rather than continuous infusion to more closely

Table 36-6 Oxytocin Protocol: Four Steps to Improving Safety

Step 1: Dilution	10 units of oxytocin in 1000 mL of normal saline (2.5 units of oxytocin in 250 mL of normal saline) Resultant concentration is 10 mU/mL
Step 2: Initial dose	0.5–2 mU/minute
Step 3: Incremental increase	Increase by 2 mU/minute every 30–40 minutes until adequate labor is achieved
Step 4: Maximum dose	16–40 mU/minute

Sources: Data from American College of Obstetricians and Gynecologists. Practice Bulletin 107: induction of labor. *Obstet Gynecol.* 2009;114: 386-397[48]; Clark SL, Simpson KR, Knox GE, Garite TJ. Oxytocin: new perspectives on an old drug. *Am J Obstet Gynecol.* 2009;200(1): 35.e1-35.e6[55]; Hayes EJ, Weinstein L. Improving patient safety and uniformity of care by a standardized regimen for the use of oxytocin. *Am J Obstet Gynecol.* 2008;198(622):e1-e7.[53]

mimic the physiologic pattern, and how epidural anesthesia is related to the dosing of oxytocin.

Despite these questions, institutional standardization of the dilution and dosing regimen for intravenous oxytocin remains an important strategy to improve safety. Hayes and Weinstein have proposed a four-step approach of dilution, initial dose, incremental increase, and maximum dose for the safe administration of oxytocin (Table 36-6).[53]

Because of the antidiuretic properties of oxytocin and the physiologic maternal adaptations to pregnancy and labor, water intoxication, a form of hyponatremia, is one of the most severe adverse effects of oxytocin administration, albeit a relatively rare event.[58] The risk of this complication can be reduced by administering oxytocin only in isotonic intravenous solutions such as lactated Ringer's solution, avoiding high doses of oxytocin for prolonged periods of time, and limiting large-volume boluses of intravenous fluids. In addition, maternal intake and output should be monitored closely. Central nervous system, gastrointestinal, and musculoskeletal system symptoms of water intoxication usually do not appear until the serum sodium levels fall below 125 mEq/L. Mild symptoms may include apathy, lethargy, headache, nausea and vomiting, muscle cramps, and diminished deep tendon reflexes. More severe symptoms are confusion and disorientation to seizures, coma, tentorial herniation, and death.[58] The clinician must remember that the fetus or newborn of a woman with hyponatremia also is at significant risk of water intoxication.

Oxytocin for Augmentation of Labor

Pharmacologic augmentation of labor is also accomplished with intravenous synthetic oxytocin administration. The use of oxytocin for this purpose has increased dramatically over the past 20 years with the concomitant increase in the use of epidural analgesia during labor. Oxytocin protocols for augmentation of labor are typically similar to those for induction, and are described in Table 36-5. Nonpharmacologic methods of augmentation include manual- or breast-pump–induced nipple stimulation to induce the endogenous release of oxytocin.

Drug augmentation of labor is a decision based on the clinical evaluation of the adequacy of uterine activity to promote cervical dilatation and the pace of cervical dilatation. Dystocia or abnormal labor is commonly categorized as protraction (slower-than-normal progress) or arrest disorders (cessation of labor progress). While the *diagnosis* of dystocia may be iatrogenic in origin, the etiology of true dystocia may be the result of one or more abnormalities of the cervix, uterus, maternal pelvis, or fetus. Although it is beyond the scope of this chapter to review the critical aspects of this important clinical evaluation, the clinician must be cognizant of this fundamental responsibility in the diagnosis and management of dystocia.

Complementary and Alternative Methods Used for Cervical Ripening and Labor Induction

Several herbs have putative uterotonic effects and are used to induce labor. Black cohosh and blue cohosh are reviewed in the *Complementary and Alternative Therapies* chapter. However, neither blue cohosh nor black cohosh has proven benefit for this indication.[59–61] Moreover, case reports describe perinatal stroke and myocardial infarction associated with ingestion of black and blue cohosh; thus, these preparations should be avoided.[59–61] Homeopathic doses of these agents appear to be safe, but again, no proven benefit has been reported to date.

Red raspberry leaves have been recommended as a means to alter general uterine tone during labor. Red raspberry leaves have no effect on initiating or augmenting labor but appear to be safe.

Evening primrose is another herb that may be used to induce labor. It has been evaluated in one small retrospective study and does not appear to shorten gestation.

Castor oil is a stimulant laxative that is contraindicated in pregnancy because it can cause uterine contractions, but has been used to induce labor at term. Its purported mechanism of action is irritation of the gastrointestinal tract, which subsequently stimulates the uterus to contract; however, some evidence indicates that ricinoleic acid, the active component of castor oil, actually enters the systemic circulation and has a direct effect on the uterus, causing colic-like, uncoordinated contractions. Ricinoleic acid can transfer to the fetus and is theorized to cause meconium passage. In addition, castor oil consistently causes nausea and diarrhea. Overall, this agent's lack of proven effectiveness in combination with its unpleasant side effects and theoretic adverse effects result in the recommendation to not use castor oil for induction.

Analgesia and Anesthesia During Labor

Relief for the pain of labor has been desired since antiquity. Prior to the 1700s, pain and suffering were seen as signs of sin; endurance, therefore, was the only recourse women had. During the Age of Enlightenment, pain became viewed as a natural phenomenon that could potentially be controlled. Since then, methods of abrogating the pain of labor have been an ongoing preoccupation of childbearing women, anesthesia providers, and clinicians who care for women in labor.

When drugs are used to treat labor pain, they are evaluated from four perspectives: (1) the effectiveness of pain relief; (2) side effects or adverse effects for the woman; (3) side effects or adverse effects for the fetus; and (4) side effects or adverse effects on the progress of labor. Strategies for ameliorating labor pain can be divided into three general categories: (1) those that remove or diminish the painful stimuli, such as regional anesthesia; (2) those that provide sensory stimulation that competes with and inhibits painful awareness, such as transcutaneous electric nerve stimulation (TENS), intradermal water injections, and acupressure; and (3) techniques that modify the individual's reaction and perception of pain such as hypnosis, prepared childbirth, and the use of doulas. Opioids have two of these effects, in that they both diminish painful stimuli and modify the perception of pain.[62,63]

The nonpharmacologic methods have varied evidence for their safety and effectiveness. This topic has been extensively reviewed elsewhere and will not be discussed in this chapter. The interested reader is referred to the published systematic reviews.[62–64]

Physiology of Labor Pain

Labor pain is complex and affected by many physiologic and psychologic variables. To simplify this process, one can identify three general types of pain that women experience in labor: abdominal pain, contraction-related back pain, and continuous low back pain. All women experience abdominal pain. A seminal survey of a small group of multipara and primipara women conducted by Melzack and Schaffelberg in the 1980s found that 74% experienced contraction-related back pain, and 33% had continuous low back pain.[65]

Pain during the first stage of labor is secondary to cervical dilatation and developing ischemia within the uterine muscle. These pain signals are transferred to the spinal cord via C and A-delta afferent nerve fibers that enter the spinal cord between L1 and T10. The pain, which is usually of a dull, cramping, visceral nature, may radiate to the lower back or legs. Pain during the second stage of labor is attributable to pelvic floor distention, is transmitted to the spinal cord via the pudendal nerve, and enters the spinal cord at the level of S4 through S2. This pain is usually sharp and somatic. The affected fibers enter the spinal cord through the dorsal horn, and then cross the spinal cord to enter the ascending nerve bundles in the spinothalamic tract. These nerves terminate in the cortex of the brain.[66]

Although it is often assumed that labor pain becomes more severe as labor progresses, women report marked variability in the intensity of labor pain. Some women experience more pain in the active phase of the first stage of labor, whereas others report the second stage of labor as being the most painful. There is both inter-individual and intra-individual variability in the intensity of pain experienced throughout the course of labor. Genetic differences in how one metabolizes opioids may also affect a woman's experience.

Sedatives and Hypnotics

Barbiturates, phenothiazines, and benzodiazepines all have sedative-hypnotic effects (Table 36-7). Barbiturates are contraindicated for laboring women because they are highly lipophilic and cross the placental barrier easily and quickly. The half-life of barbiturates is long, so a single dose given in early labor can cause decreased motor tone and difficulty breastfeeding in the neonate for as long as 48 to 72 hours after birth. Benzodiazepines are contraindicated because they have some amnesic effects and are associated with neonatal depression.

The phenothiazines listed in Table 36-7 are primarily used to augment pain relief during the latent phase of labor and to mitigate the effects of morphine when it is given to stop prodromal uncoordinated contractions. A combination of promethazine (Phenergan) and morphine, given either intramuscularly or intravenously, is one

Table 36-7 Sedative-Hypnotics for Prolonged Latent Phase of Labor

Drug: Generic (Brand)	Dose	Clinical Considerations
Promethazine (Phenergan)	50 mg IV or IM	Associated with a reduction in FHR variability but no effect on labor progress and association
Hydroxyzine hydrochloride (Vistaril)	50–100 mg IM	Painful IM injection; cannot be given IV No effect on labor progress Associated with neonatal depression
Prochlorperazine (Compazine)	25 mg PR or 5–10 mg IV or IM or 5–10 mg PO	Given with morphine sulfate for sleep during prolonged latent phase

Abbreviation: FHR = fetal heart rate.

standard regimen. Hydroxyzine (Vistaril), which is actually an antihistamine, can also be used; unlike promethazine, however, it cannot be given intravenously and must be administered orally or intramuscularly. Neither promethazine nor hydroxyzine has known adverse effects on the fetus/newborn or the progress of labor.

The actual effect of phenothiazines on pain is controversial, however. Sedatives such as phenothiazines have a known mild analgesic effect when administered alone. However, when given one drug that decreases anxiety (phenothiazine) and another drug that inhibits pain (opioid), the woman will exhibit less pain behavior and may be tranquil, which can lead caregivers to conclude that the sedative potentiates the pain relief of the opioid. However, sedation can prevent a woman from communicating her actual level of pain. Although the pain relief potentiation theory may be biologically plausible, it has not been evaluated in a well-constructed study. The use of this combination may be beneficial in certain situations, such as during latent labor or as preoperative medication, but sedative-hypnotics in combination with opioids should not be used to treat moderate or severe pain.

Opioids

Opioids are the only agents used systemically to mitigate the pain of active labor (Table 36-8). Even though these medications have actually been used for centuries, opioids produce incomplete analgesia and have significant side effects of clinical import.[67]

The opioids are categorized based on their effect on the various opioid receptors, as reviewed in the *Analgesia and Anesthesia* chapter. Meperidine (Demerol), fentanyl (Sublimaze), and morphine are pure mu agonists, whereas butorphanol (Stadol) and nalbuphine (Nubain) are mixed agonist/antagonists. The action of these drugs on their respective opioid receptors accounts for their clinical effect. For example, when an agonist binds to the mu opioid receptor, the result is slowed gastrointestinal motility, nausea and vomiting, respiratory depression, analgesia, sedation, and euphoria. Agonists that bind to the kappa receptor elicit sedation and analgesia but no nausea or vomiting. The agonists/antagonists cause less nausea and vomiting and less sedation secondary to mu receptor antagonism, but continue to provide analgesia secondary to the kappa agonist effect.

Table 36-8 Opioid Doses for Management of Pain During Active Labor

Drug: Generic (Brand)	IM Dose (Dose/Peak/Duration)	IV Dose (Dose/Peak/Duration)	Agonist Effect	Maternal Side Effects	Fetal/Neonatal Effects
Butorphanol (Stadol)	2 mg/30–60 minutes/ 3–4 hours	1–2 mg/30 minutes/2–4 hours	Kappa and sigma agonist	Ceiling effect	Transient pseudo-sinusoidal FHR pattern
Fentanyl (Sublimaze)	50–100 mcg/ 1–2 hours/1–2 hours Maximum dose: usually 500–600 mcg	50–100 mcg/ 3–5 minutes/ 1–2 hours Maximum dose: usually 500–600 mcg	Pure agonist at mu receptor,[a] kappa receptor,[b] sigma receptor,[c] and delta receptor[d]	Short acting; less effective than morphine or meperidine (Demerol) but very few side effects noted	None reported
Meperidine (Demerol)	75 mg/40–50 minutes/ 2–4 hours	75–80 mg/5 minutes/2–4 hours	Pure agonist at mu and kappa receptors	Nausea and vomiting, urinary retention, respiratory depression, sedation	Respiratory depression 1–4 hours after dose; effect is independent of dose Neonatal developmental depression 20–60 hours after last dose
Morphine[e]	10 mg/1–2 hours/ 2–4 hours	2.5–5 mg/ 20 minutes/ 2–4 hours	Pure agonist at mu and kappa receptors	Pruritus, nausea and vomiting, urinary retention, respiratory depression	Decreased FHR variability Cumulative effect on respiratory depression
Nalbuphine (Nubain)	10–20 mg/ 30–60 minutes/ 2–4 hours	10–20 mg/ 30 minutes/ 2–4 hours	Mu antagonist and kappa partial agonist	Ceiling effect	Transient pseudo-sinusoidal FHR pattern

Abbreviation: FHR = fetal heart rate.

[a] Mu-receptor stimulation causes slowed gastrointestinal motility, nausea and vomiting, respiratory depression, spinal and supraspinal analgesia, sedation, urinary retention, pruritus, and euphoria.

[b] Kappa-receptor stimulation causes sedation, spinal analgesia, and miosis.

[c] Sigma-receptor stimulation causes dysphoria, hallucination, and mydriasis.

[d] Delta-receptor stimulation causes spinal and supraspinal analgesia.

[e] Morphine can cause more pruritus and urinary retention when administered epidurally or intrathecally compared to when it is administered orally. Maternal respiratory depression can be a late effect following epidurally administered morphine sulfate secondary to slow uptake into the central nervous system.

All opioids are lipophilic and cross the placental barrier easily. These drugs all reach equilibrium between maternal and fetal circulations. Opioids are weak bases and subject to ion trapping in a fetus with acidemia, an effect that is important to remember if newborn resuscitation is needed.

In general, the opioids do not affect labor progress in the active phase.[67] Morphine is used to halt contractions in women who are experiencing a prolonged latent phase of labor, with the putative mechanism being termination of uncoordinated contraction activity. If the woman is actually in the active phase of labor when morphine is given, labor will progress unimpeded.

Meperidine

Meperidine (Demerol) has been the most frequently used opioid for treating labor pain worldwide. In decades, however, this agent has been studied extensively and has fallen out of favor, for good reasons. Indeed, it can now be stated definitively that meperidine should not be used to treat women in the active phase of labor. Most importantly, this drug does not appear to provide sufficient pain relief. When women are queried about their satisfaction with meperidine, more than half report that it did not mitigate labor pain effectively.[67]

The half-life of meperidine in the fetus is between 13 and 26 hours, so neonatal depression can occur several hours after birth when this agent is given to a woman in labor. In addition, meperidine has active metabolites that are the presumed etiology of the altered neurobehavioral tests in the newborn observed for as long as 3 days after birth. Thus the acute newborn effects appear related to the dose of meperidine given in labor, and the delayed newborn effects most likely occur secondary to the active metabolite normeperidine. The list of negative clinical outcomes in the newborn from use of this opioid include lower Apgar scores, difficulty establishing breastfeeding, and decreased neonatal alertness.[67]

Fentanyl and Morphine

The two mu opioid receptor antagonists most often used for laboring women in the United States today are fentanyl (Sublimaze) and morphine. Fentanyl is given intravenously or subcutaneously several times as needed. It can also be used as a continuous intravenous drip in a patient-controlled intravenous setup. Fentanyl is often placed in the epidural space along with local anesthetics to augment the effects of regional analgesia.

Morphine administered intramuscularly or intravenously is used to treat the prolonged latent phase of labor. This opioid can also be placed in the epidural catheter as an adjunct for pain relief following a cesarean birth or extensive perineal laceration.

Butorphanol and Nalbuphine

Butorphanol (Stadol) and nalbuphine (Nubain) exhibit antagonism to the mu receptor and kappa agonists. They are typically used in settings where epidural analgesia is not available or desired. The primary clinical consideration to remember when using these agents is that they are contraindicated for use by women who have a history of drug abuse or addiction, because the mu antagonism can elicit immediate withdrawal symptoms in this population.

Naloxone

Naloxone (Narcan) is the opioid antagonist used to reverse the respiratory depression effect of opioids, especially useful when treating an affected newborn. This drug is an antagonist to all of the opioid receptors. Naloxone can be given intravenously or intramuscularly and comes in three formulations: 0.02 mg/mL, 0.4 mg/mL, and 1 mg/mL. The dose is 0.01 mg/kg of body weight. The effect following an intravenous dose should be evident in 1 to 2 minutes, with the peak effect occurring in 5 to 15 minutes. The onset of action following an intramuscular dose is 2 to 5 minutes, and the peak effect appears in 5 to 15 minutes.[68]

Naloxone (Narcan) should be administered within the confines of a clinical protocol that dictates the required supervision and assessment of vital signs; it should not be used routinely.[68] If the dose is insufficient, respiratory depression can reoccur when the naloxone dissipates. If more than one dose is needed, the infant should be monitored closely.

Naloxone is also used to counter the intense maternal pruritus associated with intrathecal morphine. When this agent is required, the analgesic effect of the morphine is blocked, such that the woman will need additional systemic analgesia. Because naloxone will induce withdrawal effects in a person who is opioid dependent, it is contraindicated for individuals with a history of opioid abuse.

Regional Analgesia

Epidural analgesia is the most popular form of regional analgesia for managing labor pain in the United States today. Other regional techniques include spinal anesthesia for cesarean section, pudendal block for perineal laceration repair, and, rarely, paracervical block to relieve the pain of the late first stage or second stage of labor. Epidural and spinal analgesia are initiated and managed by anesthesia personnel; however, a general understanding of the technique and thorough understanding of the effects are important for all clinicians who care for women in labor. Pudendal blocks are less complicated and usually are initiated by a physician or midwife. Paracervical blocks are infrequently used secondary to their association with fetal bradycardia and are not reviewed here.

Various local anesthetics are used in regional blocks. All of them have the same basic mechanism of actions, which are reviewed in detail in the *Analgesia and Anesthesia* chapter.

Anatomy of the Epidural Space

The epidural space surrounds the meninges—that is, the dural and subarachnoid membranes, which in turn surround the spinal cord. This space is bounded posteriorly by the ligamentum flavum and is commonly described as divided into an anterior space in the front and dorso-lateral spaces on the sides of the spinal cord. The anterior epidural space is very narrow because of the proximity of the dura. This space is widest posteriorly, and the width varies with the vertebral level, ranging from 1–1.5 mm at C5 to 5–6 mm at L2. The anterior space or portion is frequently divided by membranes or connective tissue (Figure 36-2).[69]

Several anatomic structures are found within the epidural space. For example, nerve root ganglia traverse the epidural space, but are blocked when local anesthetics are placed in the area. Fat extends throughout the epidural space. Fat has great affinity for drugs with high lipid solubility such as bupivacaine; in turn, uptake of drug into fat competes with vascular and neural uptake. Large, valveless veins that communicate with the occipital venous systems within the cranium superiorly and the uterine and iliac veins inferiorly are also present in the epidural space. Drugs placed in the epidural space will diffuse into the maternal circulation via the epidural vessels in a quantity that depends on their lipid solubility and concentration.

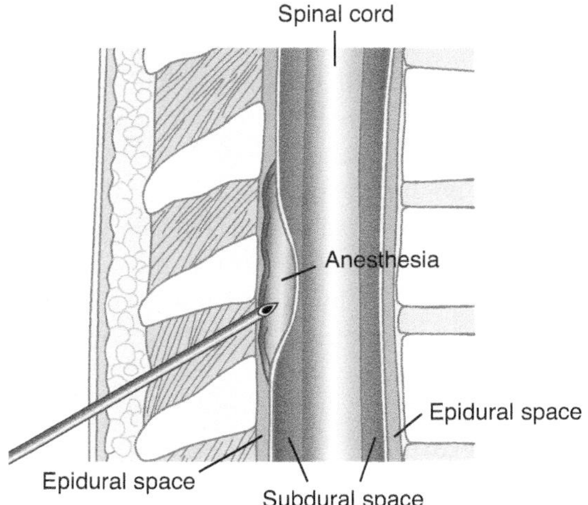

Figure 36-2 Epidural analgesia technique for placement of anesthetic drug.

Epidural Analgesia

Epidural analgesia is categorized by the route of drug administration and the type of medication used. The delivery technique can be an intermittent bolus, continuous infusion, or patient-controlled epidural anesthesia (PCEA). A newer technique, referred to as combined spinal–epidural (CSE), utilizes an initial intrathecal injection of fentanyl (Sublimaze) to provide immediate pain relief followed by a regular epidural placement later.

Local anesthetics placed in the epidural space inhibit infusion of sodium ions into the neural cell, which effectively blocks nerve transmission. This block affects all nerves that the local anesthetic touches, resulting in both a sensory and a motor block. The sensory and motor blocks can vary from minimal to complete, depending on the dose and concentration of anesthetic injected.

Epidural analgesia is associated with many side effects and a few rare adverse effects. These effects can be subdivided into (1) those that are secondary to the technique of anesthetic placement; (2) maternal and fetal effects; and (3) effects on labor progress. The technique is generally quite safe, and adverse effects that are caused by epidural catheter placement are exceedingly rare. Inadvertent dural puncture can cause a spinal headache that appears in the first 24 hours after birth. Misplacement and injection of epidural doses into the **intrathecal** space can cause a high spinal and maternal respiratory depression. Systemic toxicity reactions can occur if the anesthetic is inadvertently injected into the circulation instead of the epidural space (Table 36-9).[70] Epidural abscess and hematoma are also possible, albeit adverse, outcomes of catheter placement.

The effects of regional analgesia on the woman and her fetus as well as the effects on the progress of labor have been the subject of both controversy and extensive review. Readers who care for women in labor are referred to several summary analyses that address these controversies.[70–73] The systematic review by Mayberry et al. summarizes the evidence for managing common side effects of regional analgesia.[73]

Table 36-9 Signs of Toxicity Following Epidural Injection

Placement of Anesthetic	Signs and Symptoms of Toxicity
Intrathecal	Rapid cephalad spread of anesthesia Profound hypotension Respiratory depression Loss of consciousness
Intravascular	Tinnitus Dizziness Metallic taste in the mouth Disorientation Seizures Cardiac dysrhythmias Cardiac arrest

Source: Reproduced from Trout KK, Eschkevari L. Support for women in labor. In: King TL, Brucker MC, Kriebs J, et al., eds. *Varney's Midwifery*. Burlington, MA: Jones & Bartlett Learning; 2015:883-915.[70]

Pudendal Block

A pudendal block involves placement of 10 to 15 mL of 1% lidocaine (Xylocaine) transvaginally, just behind the ischial spines bilaterally. This placement effectively blocks transmission of the afferent fibers in the pudendal nerve, which initiates anesthesia of the perineum. Pudendal blocks are most often used for repair of perineal lacerations or for anesthesia during second stage of labor. Their primary adverse effect is an inadvertent intravascular injection that can be minimized by careful positioning of the needle and aspiration prior to injection.

Inhalent Analgesia

Today, the sole inhaled analgesic used by laboring women is nitrous oxide.[74] This gas is safe and effective and has minimal side effects or adverse effects.[74] The nitrous oxide is mixed in a 50/50 mixture with oxygen. The woman holds the mask over her face and breathes the gas mixture intermittently during contractions. Self-administration allows the women to control the amount of drug inhaled. Should she become disoriented, her hand will drop the mask, discontinuing the drug. This agent is an analgesic, not an anesthetic and its primary effect is one of mild euphoria.

The onset of action occurs in approximately 50 seconds and the drug is rapidly cleared from the woman's lungs after she stops inhalation. At birth, the newborn also can rapidly clear any of the agent within one or two breaths. Nitrous oxide had been used several decades ago in the United States but fell into disfavor as epidurals became popular. This analgesic has continued to be commonly used among laboring women in other countries and still is a staple in the U.S. dental care. Today it is reemerging as an option for pain relief in labor, especially because newer machines have effective scavenging units that minimize any dispersion of the gas into the environment, a concern that existed when using the older units.

Anti-infectives During Parturition

Women in labor are at increased risk for several infectious disorders, and some infections may be transmitted to the fetus during the labor and birth process. Consequently, standard protocols that address chemoprophylaxis for these infections are recommended.

Group B *Streptococcus:* Antibiotic Prophylaxis in Labor

Systematic efforts to prevent early-onset neonatal sepsis secondary to group B *Streptococcus* (GBS) infection via intrapartum antibiotic prophylaxis began in the 1990s, when the condition emerged as the leading infectious cause of neonatal morbidity and mortality. Although the majority of women with GBS colonization of the genital tract are asymptomatic, this organism is responsible for both early-newborn-onset (first week of life) infections and late-onset (more than 1 week to approximately 3 months of age) infant infections. GBS infection in infants appears most commonly as septicemia or pneumonia, and less commonly as meningitis, osteomyelitis, or septic arthritis.[75]

The CDC monitors GBS infections and publishes national guidelines for intrapartum prophylaxis.[75] These guidelines are based on the central principle of universal screening of all pregnant women for vaginal and rectal GBS colonization at 35 to 37 weeks' gestation. Figure 36-3 depicts the CDC recommendations for intrapartum antibiotic prophylaxis regimens to prevent perinatal GBS disease, and Box 36-2 presents a case study that illustrates the management of women who may be allergic to penicillin.[75,76] It is important to remember that the antibiotics recommended for GBS prophylaxis are not the recommended treatment for chorioamnionitis, which is discussed separately in this chapter.

Infective Endocarditis

The recommendations for antibiotic prophylaxis for prevention of infective endocarditis have changed in years, principally because most cases of infective endocarditis are the result of randomly occurring bacteremias acquired

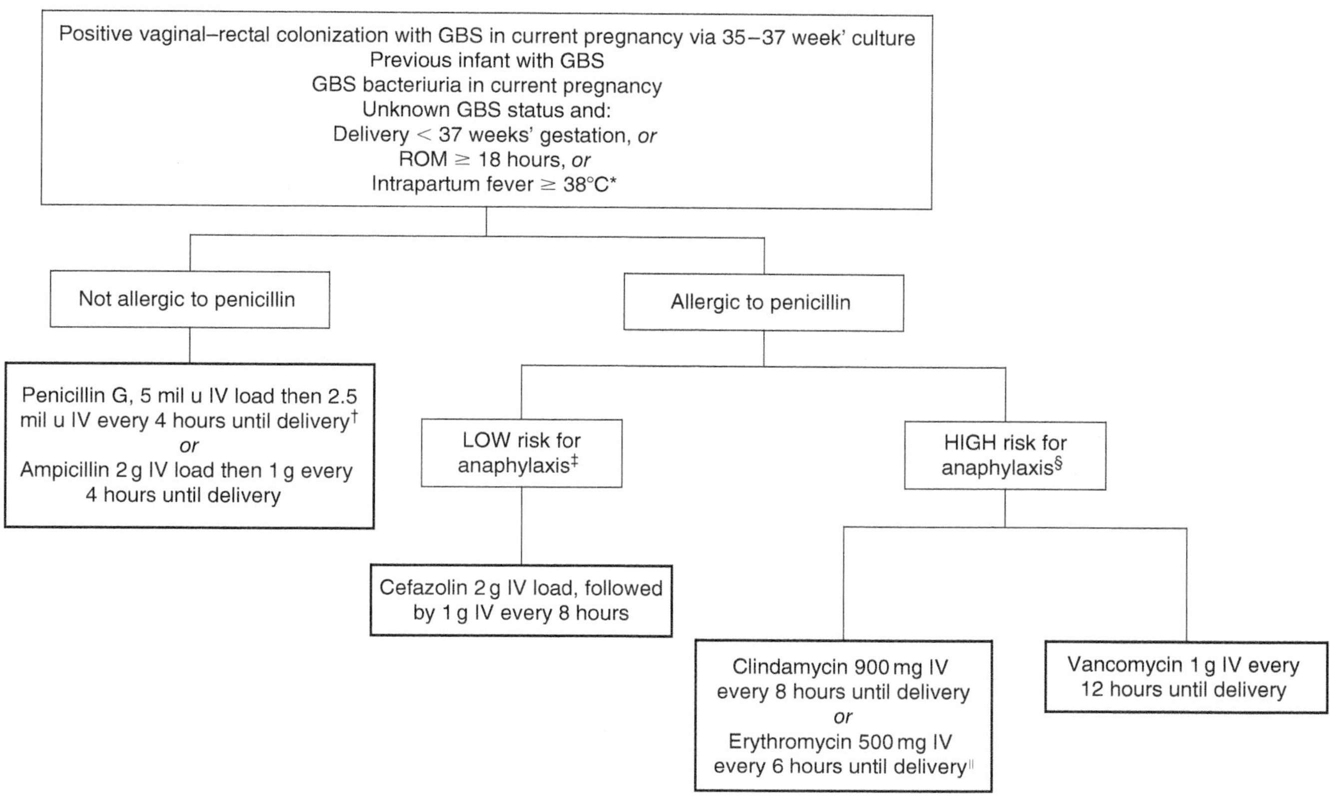

GBS = group B streptococcus; ROM = rupture of membranes.

* Broad-spectrum agents that include an agent effective against GBS should be used for treatment of chorioamnionitis.

† It is anticipated that the recommended dose of penicillin will change to 6 million units loading dose and 3 million units for ongoing doses until delivery in 2010. Readers should check the Centers for Disease Control and Prevention website for the most recent recommendations for the dose of penicillin.

‡ Persons with a history of rash only.

§ Persons who have experienced an immediate hypersensitivity reaction.

‖ Resistance to erythromycin is often associated with resistance to clindamycin. If a strain is resistant to either antibiotic, it may have inducible resistance to the other.

Figure 36-3 Antibiotic regimen for group B *Streptococcus* prophylaxis in labor.

Source: Modified from Centers for Disease Control and Prevention. Prevention of perinatal group B streptococcal disease: a revised guideline from CDC, 2010. *MMWR Recomm Rep*. 2010;59(RR-10):1-36.[75]

from routine daily activities rather than being attributable to invasive procedures. Routine antibiotic prophylaxis is not recommended for women undergoing vaginal or cesarean birth in the absence of infection. However, the current guidelines from the American Heart Association and ACOG suggest that prophylaxis can be considered for women who have a high risk of adverse cardiac outcomes and are having vaginal births. Examples of high-risk conditions include women with prosthetic cardiac valves or valve repair material, a history of cyanotic cardiac disease, or both.[77,78]

Antiretroviral Prophylaxis in Human Immunodeficiency Virus–Infected Women

The risk of perinatal transmission of human immunodeficiency virus type 1 (HIV-1) may be substantially reduced through a multifaceted approach described in the national perinatal guidelines.[79] Universal HIV screening is recommended upon the initiation of prenatal care. For women found to be infected with HIV, combined prenatal, intrapartum, and infant prophylaxis with antiretroviral drugs should be offered. Combination therapy, consisting of three or four

Box 36-2 Intrapartum Antibiotic Prophylaxis for GBS

LN is a 22-year-old primigravida at a gestation of 37 weeks and 2 days with a negative past health history and a healthy pregnancy. LN reports she is allergic to penicillin. When queried about her allergy during a prenatal visit, she stated that she got a nonpruritic rash subsequent to taking ampicillin (Principen) as a child and has not had subsequent exposures to penicillin.

LN's allergy is most likely the classic "ampicillin rash," which is actually an allergic reaction to impurities in the drug. This is not a Type 1 hypersensitivity reaction that puts her at risk for anaphylaxis or angioedema. Because the incidence of cross-reactivity between penicillin and cephalosporins is low and she does not have a history of a true penicillin allergy, a cephalosporin is the best choice for GBS prophylaxis when she is in labor if her vaginal/rectal culture is positive for GBS.

The culture is obtained at this visit. LN's practitioner does not request sensitivities. This professional could order these lab tests to determine if this particular GBS isolate is sensitive to erythromycin (E-Mycin) or clindamycin (Cleocin), but obtaining sensitivities in this situation would be an unnecessary step that adds to the cost of LN's care.

LN's culture was positive for GBS. She came to the in-hospital birth center in active labor at a gestation of 40 weeks and 4 days. An intravenous catheter was placed in LN's left forearm, a bag containing 1000 mL of lactated Ringer's (LR) solution was hung, and 2 g of cefazolin (Ancef) was administered as a loading dose, followed by 1 g 6 hours later for asymptomatic GBS prophylaxis. LN's labor progressed normally, and she gave birth to a healthy male infant.

medications, should be selected based on teratogenicity as well as comorbidities, convenience of dosing, adverse effects, resistance testing, and the woman's desire. Acceptable combination regimens are described in the national perinatal guidelines. Viral loads and CD4 cell counts should be routinely monitored to ensure effective suppression of the virus, and the importance of adhering to the prescribed regimens should be emphasized to the woman.

HIV-infected women whose viral load has been consistently 1000 copies or less in late pregnancy do not require intrapartum prophylaxis. The oral antiviral drug regimen used prenatally should be continued, however. For women with HIV, RNA levels of more than 1000 copies/mL or unknown viral load at term, scheduled cesarean section birth at 38 weeks' gestation is recommended following 3 hours of preoperative intravenous zidovudine (Retrovir) prophylaxis. Intrapartum zidovudine prophylaxis is typically given at a 2 mg/kg IV loading dose for 1 hour and then continuously at 1 mg/kg per hour for the following 2 hours.

Because of the rapid evolution of HIV management recommendations, practitioners should consult the AIDS information website of the National Institutes of Health on a regular basis to obtain the most current information.[79]

Complications in the Intrapartum Period

Chorioamnionitis

Chorioamnionitis (i.e., intra-amniotic infection, amnionitis, intrapartum infection, amniotic fluid infection) is an inflammation or infection of the placenta, amniotic fluid, and fetal membranes.[80,81] This condition may be a clinical, histologic, or subclinical diagnosis. Independent risk factors for clinical chorioamnionitis include nulliparity, long labor, prolonged rupture of membranes, multiple vaginal examinations during labor, internal fetal monitoring, and long duration of monitoring.[82] Clinical chorioamnionitis occurs in 1% to 2% of term births and as many as 15% of preterm births.[80] Generally an ascending polymicrobial infection, this condition is manifested by maternal fever, maternal or fetal tachycardia, foul-smelling amniotic fluid, uterine tenderness, and leukocytosis, which is defined as more than 15,000 cells with a left shift.

Clinical chorioamnionitis is highly associated with preterm birth before 30 weeks' gestation and preterm premature rupture of the membranes.[83] At term, dysfunctional labor—particularly decreased uterine contractility that may be unresponsive to oxytocin augmentation—and an increased incidence of cesarean section are common occurrences following the development of chorioamnionitis. Neonatal risks include higher incidence of respiratory distress syndrome, intraventricular hemorrhage, and periventricular leukomalacia in preterm infants, and higher incidence of neonatal sepsis, hypoxic–ischemic encephalopathy, and cerebral palsy among both preterm and term infants.[84]

Clinical chorioamnionitis is treated with broad-spectrum intravenous antibiotics and antipyretics.[84] The antibiotic therapy is designed to cover a wide range of gram-positive and gram-negative organisms and both anaerobic and aerobic organisms. Table 36-10 lists common antibiotic regimens that combine a beta-lactam and aminoglycoside for the treatment of clinical chorioamnionitis. If a cesarean section birth occurs, coverage for anaerobic bacteria such as clindamycin (Cleocin) or metronidazole (Flagyl) should be provided as well. Although antibiotics may be continued postpartum until the woman is afebrile and asymptomatic for 24 hours, a single postpartum intravenous administration of each drug at its next scheduled dose is equally effective.[85]

Table 36-10 Antibiotic Regimens for the Intrapartum Treatment of Intra-amniotic Infection

Drug: Generic (Brand)	Dose
Combination Therapies	
Ampicillin (Principen) and gentamicin (Garamycin)	2 g ampicillin every 6 hours and 2 mg/kg loading dose, *plus* 1.5 mg/kg gentamicin every 8 hours or single dose of 5 mg/kg gentamicin once daily
Penicillin plus gentamycin	Aqueous penicillin G, 5 M units IV every 6 hours, *plus* Single dose of 5 mg/kg gentamicin once daily
Single-Agent Therapies	
Ampicillin–sulbactam (Unasyn)	3 g IV every 6 hours
Ticarcillin–clavulanic acid (Timentin)	3.1 g IV every 4 hours
Cefoxitin (Mefoxin)	2 g IV every 6 hours
Cefotetan (Cefotan)	2 g IV every 12 hours
Cefuroxime (Ceftin)	1.5 g IV every 8 hours
Penicillin Allergic with History of Anaphylaxis	
Vancomycin (Vanocin)	500 mg every 6 hours
Penicillin Allergic without History of Anaphylaxis	
Cefuroxime (Ceftin)	1.5 g IV every 8 hours
Cefazolin (Ancef) and gentamycin	1 g IV every 8 hours 2 mg/kg loading dose followed by 1.5 mg/kg every 8 hours
Penicillin Allergic without History of Anaphylaxis and GBS-Positive with Culture Sensitivities Available	
Erythromycin (E-Mycin)	1 g every 6 hours
Clindamycin (Cleocin)	900 mg every 8 hours
Add One of These Agents If Cesarean Section Performed[a]	
Clindamycin (Cleocin)	900 mg every 8 hours or single dose 900 mg at cord clamping
Metronidazole (Flagyl)	500 mg every 6 hours at cord clamping

[a] Not needed with penicillin-allergic regimens.

Source: Reproduced from Fahey JO. Clinical management of intraamniotic infection and chorioamnionitis: a review of the literature. *J Midwifery Womens Health.* 2008;53:227-235.[82]

Preeclampsia/Eclampsia

The hypertensive disorders of pregnancy include (1) preeclampsia/eclampsia; (2) chronic hypertension; (3) chronic hypertension with superimposed preeclampsia; and (4) gestational hypertension.[86] Prenatal management of chronic hypertension and preeclampsia is reviewed in the *Pregnancy* chapter. Gestational hypertension does not generally require pharmacologic therapy. This section reviews the intrapartum management of preeclampsia/eclampsia and chronic hypertension with superimposed preeclampsia.

Preeclampsia/eclampsia is a disorder unique to pregnancy. This multi-organ, progressive condition is characterized by hypertension and proteinuria that occurs after 20 weeks' gestation. Cure is obtained only after birth and delivery of the placenta, although some women will continue to exhibit new-onset symptoms in the first few days after birth. Complications of preeclampsia include severe adverse sequela such as placental abruption, liver rupture, disseminated intravascular coagulation, stroke, and eclampsia.

Eclampsia is diagnosed if new-onset grand mal seizures or unexplained coma occurs in a woman with signs and symptoms of preeclampsia.[86] This condition affects approximately 2% to 3% of women who have severe preeclampsia if they are not treated with magnesium sulfate, and approximately 0.6% of women who have preeclampsia without severe features.[87] Management of eclampsia includes measures to prevent maternal injury and support respiratory and cardiovascular functions, followed by medical therapy to prevent recurrent convulsions and reduce blood pressure to a safe range without inducing hypotension.

Treatment of preeclampsia during the intrapartum period is aimed at preventing convulsions, reducing blood pressure, maintaining renal and uterine perfusion, and facilitating birth. The overall management of women with this disorder has many components, and the interested reader is referred to clinical texts for a thorough review.

Intravenous magnesium sulfate is administered to prevent initial or recurrent seizures by potentially changing the seizure threshold, and antihypertensives are used as needed to reduce the maternal blood pressure to a safe range.

Magnesium Sulfate for Seizure Prophylaxis

The mechanism of action for the anticonvulsant effect of magnesium sulfate has not been clearly determined. This is the same drug used for neuroprotection of the fetus when preterm labor occurs. For treatment of a woman at risk of eclampsia, the magnesium sulfate regimen consists of a loading dose of 4 to 6 g administered over 15 to 20 minutes, followed by 1 to 3 g per hour administered intravenously. The therapy is usually continued for 24 hours postpartum but may be extended to 48 hours if ongoing seizure prophylaxis is believed necessary. Immediate common side effects of magnesium sulfate include flushing, a feeling of warmth, and a lowering of blood pressure. Nausea, vomiting, visual disturbances, and palpitations may occur. Magnesium sulfate crosses the placenta easily, and fetal side effects include a mild decrease in the baseline fetal heart rate and a decrease in fetal heart rate variability.

Magnesium is contraindicated for women with myasthenia gravis. Because it has tocolytic properties, the risk of postpartum hemorrhage is slightly higher in women who are administered magnesium sulfate during labor.

The therapeutic range for magnesium sulfate seizure prophylaxis is between 4.8 and 9.6 mg/dL. Magnesium is excreted renally, and unless the woman has renal compromise, magnesium toxicity is rare. Toxicity is related to the magnesium concentration. The first sign is loss of patellar reflexes, which occurs at approximately 8 to 12 mg/dL (7 to 10 mEq/L). Respiratory paralysis occurs at 12 to 16 mg/dL (10 to 13 mEq/L), and cardiac conduction is altered at concentrations higher than 18 mg/dL (15 mEq/L). Absence of deep tendon reflexes may be an unreliable sign in women with epidural analgesia/anesthesia. At the first sign of toxicity, 1 g of calcium gluconate (10 mL of a 10% solution) should be given intravenously over 3 minutes. Calcium gluconate should be readily available, labeled, and kept at the bedside ready for use during magnesium sulfate administration.

Antihypertensive Therapy

Severe hypertension is treated with an antihypertensive agent to prevent cardiovascular complications such as stroke, renal injury, or congestive heart failure. Hydralazine, labetalol, and nifedipine are the antihypertensive agents most often used in the intrapartum setting. The recommended doses of these three agents are presented in Table 36-11.[88–90] A Cochrane review failed to identify clear evidence to recommend one of these antihypertensives over the others.[88] To provide adequate cerebral and uteroplacental perfusion, blood pressure targets should be between 140 and 160 mm Hg systolic and between 90 and 105 mm Hg diastolic.

Corticosteroids

If a woman develops severe preeclampsia before 34 weeks' gestation, administration of corticosteroids to facilitate maturation of the fetal lung is recommended.

Table 36-11 Antihypertensive Agents Used to Treat Severe Preeclampsia During Labor

Drug: Generic (Brand)	Dose	Onset and Peak Action	Clinical Considerations
First-Line Agents			
Hydralazine	5–10 mg IV every 15–20 minutes until target blood pressure is established	Onset: 5–20 minutes Peak: 15–30 minutes	Mechanism of action: Dilates arteries. May cause tachycardia Side effects: Headache, hypotension, fetal heart rate bradycardia
Labetalol	20 mg IV bolus given over 2 minutes, followed by 40 mg IV given over 2 minutes If not effective in 10 minutes, then 80 mg IV given over 2 minutes every 10 minutes until target blood pressure is established	Onset: 2–5 minutes Peak: 5 minutes	Mechanism of action: Combined alpha- and beta-blocking agent that dilates arterioles and lowers heart rate Side effects: Contraindications include asthma, cocaine, and amphetamine use
Second-Line Agents			
Nifedipine	10 mg PO	Onset: 5–20 minutes Peak: 30–60 minutes	Mechanism of action: Calcium-channel blocker

Sources: Data from Brown CL, Garovic VD. Drug treatment of hypertension in pregnancy. *Drugs*. 2014;74(3):283-296;[90] Duley L, Meher S, Jones L. Drugs for the treatment of very high blood pressure during pregnancy. *Cochrane Database Syst Rev*. 2013;7:CD001449[88]; Druzin ML, Shields LE, Peterson NL, et al. *Preeclampsia Toolkit: Improving Health Care Response to Preeclampsia (California Maternal Quality Care Collaborative Toolkit to Transform Maternity Care)*. Developed under contract #11-10006 with the California Department of Public Health; Maternal, Child and Adolescent Health Division; Published by the California Maternal Quality Care Collaborative. November 2013.[89]

Treatments for Eclampsia

The initial treatment for a woman with eclamptic seizures is a loading dose of magnesium sulfate. If the seizure does not immediately resolve, an anticonvulsant medication can be administered. The drugs and doses for treating eclampsia are listed in Table 36-12.

Postpartum Hemorrhage

Postpartum hemorrhage (PPH) is defined as more than 500 mL blood loss following a vaginal birth or more than 1000 mL during a cesarean birth. The clinical challenge is that estimation of blood loss often is incorrect, leading many authorities to advocate that blood loss be measured, not estimated. Another challenge is that nearly half of women are thought to lose in excess of 500 mL during a normal vaginal birth.

However, using the historical definition of PPH, it is estimated that the condition occurs in approximately 1% to 5% of women immediately after giving birth.[91] Uterine atony is the most common cause of postpartum hemorrhage, but other etiologies include genital tract trauma, abnormal placentation, retained products, and coagulopathies.

Postpartum hemorrhage is more common in women with a hyperdistended uterus (e.g., macrosomia, multiple gestation, or polyhydramnios), a prolonged or very rapid labor, chorioamnionitis, or a history of previous PPH. Women also are more likely to experience a postpartum hemorrhage if they have received oxytocin for induction or augmentation of labor, magnesium sulfate during labor, or general anesthesia for birth.

Pharmacologic therapy is one component of the overall management in both prevention and treatment of postpartum hemorrhage. Table 36-13 reviews the first- and second-line drug therapies commonly used to treat postpartum hemorrhage in the United States.[92–94]

Table 36-12 Drugs for Treating Eclampsia

Drug: Generic (Brand)	Dose
Magnesium sulfate	4–6 g loading dose followed by 1–2 g/hour continuous IV infusion Contraindicated if pulmonary edema, myasthenia gravis, or renal failure is present
Lorazepam (Ativan)	2–4 mg IV; may repeat once after 10–15 minutes to maximum dose of 8 mg in 12 hours
Diazepam (Valium)	5–10 mg IV every 5–10 minutes, to maximum dose of 30 mg
Phenytoin (Dilantin)	15–20 mg/kg IV; may repeat at 10 mg/kg IV after 20 minutes

Sources: Data from American College of Obstetricians and Gynecologists. Practice Bulletin No. 76: postpartum hemorrhage. *Obstet Gynecol.* 2006; 108:1039-1047[92]; Brown CL, Garovic VD. Drug treatment of hypertension in pregnancy. *Drugs.* 2014;74(3):283-296[90]; Druzin ML, Shields LE, Peterson NL, et al. *Preeclampsia Toolkit: Improving Health Care Response to Preeclampsia* (*California Maternal Quality Care Collaborative Toolkit to Transform Maternity Care*). Developed under contract #11-10006 with the California Department of Public Health; Maternal, Child and Adolescent Health Division; published by the California Maternal Quality Care Collaborative; November 2013.[89]

Prevention of Postpartum Hemorrhage

Active management of the third stage of labor comprises a package of care practices that include administration of oxytocin (Pitocin), early cord clamping, and controlled cord traction. Active management of the third stage has been proven to decrease the incidence of postpartum hemorrhage and is widely promoted throughout the world.[95] More analyses of such care have found that administration of oxytocin is the most important and most effective component of the three care practices.[96] Women treated with oxytocin prophylactically have a significant decrease in the incidence of postpartum hemorrhage, defined as a blood loss more than 500 mL (RR, 0.53; 95% CI, 0.38–0.74; n = 4203 women), and need for additional uterotonic drugs (RR, 0.56; 95% CI, 0.36–0.87, n = 3174 women).[97]

Several effective protocols are available. For example, oxytocin can be given intravenously as 10 to 40 U diluted in 500 mL or 1000 mL of fluid administered at a rate of 125 mL to 250 mL per hour or intramuscularly as 10 U. Oxytocin (Pitocin) should never be given intravenously as an undiluted bolus, as this practice can cause a profound hypotensive reaction. Doses higher than 10 U in 500 mL of fluid administered over 1 hour do not appear to be more effective than lower doses for preventing postpartum hemorrhage, although it is common to administer 20 or 40 U in 500 mL of fluid if active bleeding is encountered.[98]

Women who have received oxytocin prior to birth for induction or augmentation of labor may be less responsive to postpartum oxytocin due to saturation of the myometrial oxytocin receptors. The primary side effect of oxytocin is uterine cramping. The only clinically significant adverse effect is hyponatremia, which is more likely to occur when large doses are given during the treatment of postpartum hemorrhage. Oxytocin increases the tone and intensity of uterine contractions when given in small doses and is believed to cause uterine tetany when administered in larger doses.[99]

Other uterotonics, such as ergonovine maleate, methylergonovine (Methergine), or the prostaglandin analogue misoprostol (Cytotec), have been considered for prevention

Table 36-13 Uterotonic Treatment of Immediate Postpartum Hemorrhage Due to Uterine Atony

Drug: Generic (Brand)	Dose and Route	Contraindications	Side Effects	Clinical Considerations
First-Line Therapy				
Oxytocin (Pitocin)	10–80 U IV in 250 or 500 mL of normal saline or lactated Ringer's solution *or* 10 U IM	Hypersensitivity	Cramping Large doses can cause hyponatremia	Onset of action: 2–3 minutes Effective in 15–30 minutes Duration of action: 2–3 hours if given IM Rapid infusion of an undiluted bolus can cause hypotension and cardiac collapse
Second-Line Therapies				
Methylergonovine maleate (Methergine)	0.2 mg IM May repeat in 5 minutes Thereafter every 2–4 hours	Hypertension, preeclampsia Do not give intravenously secondary to risk of sudden vasospasm and hypertensive or cerebrovascular accident	Cramping Nausea, vomiting Hypertension, seizure, headache	It is recommended that the woman's blood pressure be taken prior to administration Onset of action: 2–5 minutes Peak plasma concentration: 20–30 minutes Plasma half-life: 3–4 hours Women with coronary artery disease may have increased risk for myocardial infarction FDA black box warning to avoid breastfeeding for first 12 hours of newborn's life
Carboprost tromethamine or 15 methyl prostaglandin F_{2a} analogue (Hemabate)	250 mcg IM May repeat every 15–90 minutes, up to 8 doses	Asthma or active cardiac, pulmonary, renal, or hepatic disease	Nausea, vomiting, diarrhea, bronchospasm, hypertension Pyrexia is common	FDA black box warning to use recommended doses only and in a hospital setting as well as avoiding breastfeeding for first 12 hours of newborn's life Peak serum concentration: 30 minutes
Dinoprostone or (Prostin E_2)	20 mg vaginal or rectal suppository May repeat every 2 hours	Hypotension, cardiac disease	Nausea, vomiting and diarrhea Pyrexia is common	FDA black box warning to use recommended doses only and in a hospital setting Onset of action: 10 minutes
Misoprostol (Cytotec)	600–800 mcg sublingually or 800–1000 mcg per rectum; 1 dose		Nausea, vomiting, diarrhea, abdominal pain Pyrexia can occur with higher doses	Onset of action: 3–5 minutes Peak concentration: 30 minutes following sublingual administration and 40–60 minutes following rectal administration

Sources: Data from American College of Obstetricians and Gynecologists. Practice Bulletin No. 76: postpartum hemorrhage. *Obstet Gynecol.* 2006;108:1039-1047[92]; Lyndon A, Lagrew D, Shields L, Melsop K, Bingham B, Main E, eds. *Improving Health Care Response (Maternity Care).* Developed under contract #08-85012 with the California Department of Public Health; Maternal, Child and Adolescent Health Division; published by the California Maternal Quality Care Collaborative. https://www.cmqcc.org/ob_hemorrhage Accessed March 3, 2015[94]; Tang OS, Gemzell-Danielsson K, Ho PC. Misoprostol: pharmacokinetic profiles, effects on the uterus and side effects. *Int J Gynaecol Obstet.* 2007;99(suppl 2):S160.[93]

of postpartum hemorrhage. Ergonovine maleate is not used in the United States. Although ergonovine maleate and methylergonovine are slightly better than oxytocin at preventing postpartum hemorrhage, both are associated with more uncomfortable side effects, such as pain and hypertension.[100] Misoprostol does not appear to confer any advantage with regard to lower incidence of postpartum hemorrhage.[101] Thus, oxytocin remains the preferred uterotonic for prevention of severe postpartum hemorrhage in the United States and most developed nations. Misoprostol is recommended for use in low-income settings because it is inexpensive, is stable at room temperature, and can be administered orally, sublingually, or rectally.

Treatment of Postpartum Hemorrhage

Management of postpartum hemorrhage that occurs secondary to uterine atony includes administration of intravenous fluids, drug therapy with a uterotonic agent, and emptying the bladder. In addition, preparation for possible blood transfusion, uterine tamponade procedures, or surgical intervention is initiated. Several uterotonics can be employed in the treatment of an immediate postpartum hemorrhage.

Oxytocin

Oxytocin (Pitocin) is widely accepted as the first line therapy for treating immediate postpartum hemorrhage secondary to uterine atony. Oxytocin is routinely administered as 10 U diluted in 240 mL, 500 mL, or 1000 mL of normal saline and administered intravenously at a rate of 125 mL per hour or 250 mL per hour. The dose is often increased to 40 U if active bleeding is present. The onset of action of oxytocin when administered this way is 3 to 4 minutes. The half-life is 15 minutes, and the duration of action depends on how long the infusion is maintained.[92]

Methylergonovine Maleate

Methylergonovine maleate (Methergine), a semi-synthetic ergot alkaloid, is often the second drug choice if postpartum hemorrhage continues despite treatment with oxytocin. Ergot alkaloids are alpha-adrenergic agonists and initiate contraction of vascular smooth muscle in both arteries and veins. Contraction of uterine muscle is evidenced as an increase in force and frequency such that the contraction becomes tetanic.

Side effects of methylergonovine maleate when given in a few doses immediately postpartum are rare. This drug is contraindicated in the presence of maternal hypertension because its vasoconstrictive action may cause sudden severe hypertension. Rare reports of myocardial infarction have been cited in conjunction with overdose toxicity. The hypertensive effect of methylergonovine maleate may be exaggerated in women who have received other vasoactive agents during labor, such as ephedrine for treatment of hypotension following epidural initiation. Methylergonovine maleate plasma levels may be higher in women who are taking CYP3A4-inhibiting agents, such as macrolide antibiotics, azole antifungals, or protease inhibitors.[94]

The product labeling recommends that women wait 12 hours to breastfeed after being given methylergonovine maleate and to discard breast milk during this period. However, this recommendation is based on reports of adverse effects in infants (tachycardia, vomiting, diarrhea) whose mothers were taking methylergonovine maleate for prolonged periods of time.

Prostaglandins: Misoprostol, Prostaglandin $F_{2\alpha}$, and Dinoprostone

Three prostaglandins—PGF_{a2} (Carboprost [Hemabate]), PGE_2 (Dinoprostone [Prostin E_2]), and misoprostol (Cytotec), which is a PGE_1 analogue—can be used to treat postpartum hemorrhage. Each of these agents has both advantages and disadvantages. The American College of Obstetricians and Gynecologists does not recommend one prostaglandin versus another.[92]

PGF_{a2} is FDA approved for treatment of postpartum hemorrhage that has not resolved with uterine massage and oxytocin. Because this agent has significant side effects and contraindications, misoprostol is often used instead. PGF_{a2} is contraindicated for women with asthma due to the risk of bronchial spasm.

Misoprostol (Cytotec) is frequently chosen as second-line therapy instead of methylergonovine maleate because it can be used in women who have hypertension and can be administered orally, sublingually, or rectally. Although use of misoprostol for treatment of postpartum hemorrhage is an off-label indication, this agent is increasingly being adopted given its ease of use and effectiveness. Delivery of misoprostol by the oral and sublingual routes offers a faster onset of action, but administration by the rectal route provides for a longer duration of action.[99] Randomized trials that have compared misoprostol to oxytocin or other prostaglandins as a second-line agent after oxytocin have found that misoprostol works as well as a second administration of oxytocin.[103,104] However, misoprostol causes shivering and fever in a dose-dependent manner. Adverse effects include a fever higher than 40°C. Misoprostol is converted to a prostaglandin F analogue. Therefore, if PGF_{a2} has been unsuccessful in treating a woman with a postpartum hemorrhage, misoprostol is not likely to be more effective.[94]

PGE_2 can be used as a substitute for misoprostol, but its side-effect profile is similar to that of PGF_{a2} and its use for this indication is also on an off-label basis. PGE_2 is not a potent bronchoconstrictor, so it is safe for use by women who have a history of asthma.

Conclusion

Few drugs are used for women during parturition. Pregnant women in developed nations are generally healthy, and providers are cautious about exposing a pregnant woman and her fetus to adverse drug effects. Nevertheless, the drugs that are used for this population can be life saving, and clinicians caring for women during labor and birth often need to make complicated judgments quickly; thus, a thorough knowledge of the drugs discussed in this chapter is an important component of clinical acumen and clinical practice.

Resources

Organization	Description	Website
California Maternal Quality Care Collaborative (CMQCC)	Obstetric Hemorrhage Toolkit; free resources for managing postpartum hemorrhage and establishing a massive transfusion protocol	www.cmqcc.org/ob_hemorrhage
Centers for Disease Control and Prevention (CDC)	GBS App provides all the algorithms for management of GBS prophylaxis in the antepartum and intrapartum setting	www.cdc.gov/groupbstrep/guidelines/prevention-app.html

References

1. Challis JRG. Mechanism of parturition and preterm labor. *Obstet Gynecol Surv.* 2000;55(10):650-660.
2. Carvajal JA. The role of brain natriuretic peptide in maintaining myometrial quiescence during pregnancy. *Experi Physiol.* 2014;99:489-494.
3. Norwitz ER, Mahendroo M, Lye SJ. Biology of parturition. In: Creasy RK, Resnik R, Iams JD, Lockwood CJ, Moore TR, Greene MF, eds. *Creasy and Resnik's Maternal–Fetal Medicine: Principles and Practice.* Philadelphia, PA: Elsevier; 2014:66-79.
4. Gibb W, Lye SJ, Challis JRG. Parturition. In: Neill JD, Plant TM, Phfaff DW, et al., eds. *Knobil and Neill's Physiology of Reproduction.* Vol. 2. Amsterdam: Elsevier; 2006:2925-2974.
5. Arrowsmith S, Kendrick A, Hanley JA, Noble K, Wray S. Myometrial physiology: time to translate? *Experi Physiol.* 2014;99:495-402.
6. Word RA, Li X-H, Hnat M, Carrick K. Dynamics of cervical remodeling during pregnancy and parturition: mechanisms and current concepts. *Semin Reprod Med.* 2007;25;69-80.
7. Smith R. Parturition. *N Engl J Med.* 2007;356:271-283.
8. Challis JRG, Bloomfield FH, Bocking AD, et al. Fetal signals and parturition. *J Obstet Gynecol Res.* 2005;31:492-499.
9. Blanks AM, Hymygol A, Thornton S. Regulation of oxytocin receptors and oxytocin receptor signaling. *Semin Reprod Med.* 2007;25:52-59.
10. Young RC. Myocytes, myometrium and uterine contractions. *Ann N Y Acad Sci.* 2007;1101:72-84.
11. Golightly E, Jabbour HN, Norman JE. Endocrine immune interactions in human parturition. *Mol Cellul Endocrinol.* 2011;335:52-59.
12. Petraglia F, Imperatore A, Challis JRG. Neuroendocrine mechanisms in pregnancy and parturition. *Endocrinol Rev.* 2010;31:783-816.
13. Smith R, Paul J, Maiti K, Tolosa J, Madsen G. Recent advances in understanding the endocrinology of human birth. *Trends Endocrinol Metab.* 2012;23: 516-523.
14. Beshay VE, Carr BH, Bainey WE. The human fetal adrenal gland, corticotropin-releasing hormone, and parturition. *Semin Reprod Med.* 2007;25:14-20.
15. Ludmir J, Sehdev HM. Anatomy and physiology of the uterine cervix. *Clin Obstet Gynecol.* 2000; 43:433-439.
16. Bauer ME, Mazza E, Nava A, et al. In vivo characterization of the mechanics of human uterine cervices. *Ann N Y Acad Sci.* 2007;1101:186-202.
17. Bauer M, Mazza E, Nava A, et al. In vivo characterization of the mechanics of human uterine cervices. *Ann N Y Acad Sci.* 2007;1101:186-202.
18. Aguilar HN, Mitchell BF. Physiological pathways and molecular mechanisms regulating uterine contractility. *Hum Reprod Update.* 2010;16:725-744.
19. Wray S, Kupittayanant S. The physiological basis of uterine contractility: a short review. *Experi Physiol.* 2001;86(2):239-246.
20. Bernal AL. Mechanisms of labour: biochemical aspects. *BJOG.*2003;110(suppl 20):39-45.
21. Mathews TJ, DacDorman MF. Infant mortality statistics from the 2010 period linked birth/infant death data set. *Natl Vital Stat Rep.* 2013;62(8):1-26.
22. Hamilton BE, Martin JA, Osterman MJK, Curtain SC. Births: preliminary data for 2013. *Natl Vital Stat Rep.* 2014;63(2):1-18.
23. American College of Obstetricians and Gynecologists. Practice Bulletin No. 130: prediction and prevention of preterm birth. *Obstet Gynecol.* 2012;120:964-973.
24. Simhan HN, Caritis SN. Prevention of preterm delivery. *N Engl J Med.* 2007;357:477-487.
25. Haas DM, Caldwell DM, Kirkpatrick P, McIntosh JJ, Welton NL. Tocolytic therapy for preterm delivery; systematic review and network meta-analysis. *BMJ.* 2012;345:e6226.
26. Simhan HN, Iams JD, Romero R. Preterm birth. In: Gabbe SG, Niebyl RJ, Simpson JL, eds. *Obstetrics: Normal and Problem Pregnancies.* 6th ed. Philadelphia, PA: Elsevier; 2012:627-659.
27. Lam F, Gill P. Beta-agonist tocolytic therapy. *Obstet Gynecol Clin North Am.* 2005;32:457-484.
28. Food and Drug Administration. Warning on use of terbutaline sulfate for preterm labor. *JAMA.* 1998; 279:9.
29. Caritis S. Adverse effects of tocolytic therapy. *BJOG.* 2005;112(suppl 1):74-78.
30. Oei SG. Calcium channel blockers for tocolysis: a review of their role and safety following reports of serious adverse events. *Eur J Obstet Gynecol.* 2006;126:137-145.
31. Papatsonis DNM, Lok CAR, Bos JM, van Geijn HP, Dekker GA. Calcium channel blockers in the management of preterm labor and hypertension in pregnancy. *Eur J Obstet Gynecol Reprod Biol.* 2001;97: 122-140.

32. Lyell DJ, Pullen K, Campbell L, et al. Magnesium sulfate compared with nifedipine for acute tocolysis of preterm labor: a randomized controlled trial. *Obstet Gynecol.* 2007;110:61-67.
33. Conde-Agudelo A, Romero R, Kusanovic JP. Nifedipine in the management of preterm labor: a systematic review and metaanalysis. *Am J Obstet Gynecol.* 2011;204(134):e1-e20.
34. Loe SM, Sanchez-Ramos L, Kaunitz AM. Assessing the neonatal safety of indomethacin tocolysis: a systematic review with meta-analysis. *Obstet Gynecol.* 2005;106:173-179.
35. Abramovici A, Cantu J, Jenkins SM. Tocolytic therapy for acute preterm labor. *Obstet Gynecol Clin North Am.* 2012;39:77-87.
36. Institute for Safe Medication Practices. ISMP's list of high-alert medications. 2012. https://www.ismp.org/tools/institutionalhighAlert.asp. Accessed July 18, 2014.
37. Doyle LW, Crowther CA, Middleton P, Marret S, Rouse D. Magnesium sulphate for women at risk of preterm birth for neuroprotection of the fetus. *Cochrane Database Syst Rev.* 2009;1:CD004661.
38. Reeves SA, Gibbs RS, Clark SL. Magnesium for fetal neuroprotection. *Am J Obstet Gynecol.* 2011;204(202):e1-e4.
39. FDA recommends against prolonged use of magnesium sulfate to stop pre-term labor due to bone changes in exposed babies. http://www.fda.gov.ucsf.idm.oclc.org/downloads/Drugs/DrugSafety/UCM353335.pdf. Accessed on May 30, 2013.
40. National Institutes of Health. Consensus development statement: effect of corticosteroids for fetal maturation on perinatal outcomes. *Am J Obstet Gynecol.* 1995;183(246):252.
41. Roberts D, Dalziel SR. Antenatal corticosteroids for accelerating fetal lung maturation for women at risk of preterm birth. *Cochrane Database Syst Rev.* 2006;3:CD004454.
42. Gyamfi-Bannerman C, Gilbert S, Landon MD, et al. Effect of antenatal corticosteroids on respiratory morbidity in singletons after late-preterm birth. *Obstet Gynecol.* 2012;119(3):555-559.
43. Bonanno C, Wapner RJ. Antenatal corticosteroids in the management of preterm birth: are we back where we started? *Obstet Gynecol Clin North Am.* 2012;39:47-63.
44. Dalziel SR, Lim VK, Lambert A, et al. Antenatal exposure to betamethasone: psychological functioning and health related quality of life 31 years after inclusion in randomised controlled trial. *BMJ.* 2005;331:665.
45. Crowther CA, McKinlay CJD, Middleton P, Harding JE. Repeat doses of prenatal corticosteroids for women at risk of preterm birth for preventing neonatal health outcomes. *Cochrane Database Syst Rev.* 2011;6:CD003935.
46. Elimian A, Garry D, Figueroa R, Spitzer A, Wiencek V, Quirk JG. Antenatal betamethasone compared with dexamethasone (Betacode trial): a randomized controlled trial. *Obstet Gynecol.* 2007;110:26-30.
47. Osterman MJK. *Recent Declines in Induction of Labor by Gestational Age.* NCHS Data Brief, No. 155. Hyattsville, MD: National Center for Health Statistics; 2014.
48. American College of Obstetricians and Gynecologists. Practice Bulletin 107: induction of labor. *Obstet Gynecol.* 2009;114:386-397.
49. Lowe NK. A review of factors associated with dystocia and cesarean section in nulliparous women. *J Midwifery Womens Health.* 2006;52:216-218.
50. Caughey AB, Sundaram V, Kaimal AJ, et al. Systematic review: elective induction of labor versus expectant management. *Ann Intern Med.* 2009;151(4):252-263.
51. Alfirevic Z, Aflaifel N, Weeks A. Oral misoprostol for induction of labor. *Cochrane Database Syst Rev.* 2014;6:CD001338.
52. Radoff KA. Orally administered misoprostol for induction of labor with prelabor rupture of membranes at term. *J Midwifery Womens Health.* 2014;59(3):254-263.
53. Hayes EJ, Weinstein L. Improving patient safety and uniformity of care by a standardized regimen for the use of oxytocin. *Am J Obstet Gynecol.* 2008;198(622):e1-e7.
54. Arias F. Pharmacology of oxytocin and prostaglandins. *Clin Obstet Gynecol.* 2000;43:455-468.
55. Clark SL, Simpson KR, Knox GE, Garite TJ. Oxytocin: new perspectives on an old drug. *Am J Obstet Gynecol.* 2009;200(1):35.e1-35.e6.
56. Macones GA, Hankins GDV, Spong CY, Hauth J, Moore T. The 2008 National Institute of Child Health and Human Development workshop report on electronic fetal monitoring. *Obstet Gynecol.* 2008;112:661-666.
57. Smith JG, Merrill DC. Oxytocin for induction of labor. *Clin Obstet Gynecol.* 2006;49:594-608.
58. Ophir E, Solt I, Odeh M, Bornstein J. Water intoxication: a dangerous condition in labor and delivery rooms. *Obstet Gynecol Surv.* 2007;62:731-738.

59. Dugoua JJ, Perri D, Seely D, Mills E, Koren G. Safety and efficacy of blue cohosh (*Caulophyllum thalictroides*) during pregnancy and lactation. *Can J Clin Pharmacol*. 2008;15:e66-e73.
60. Finkle RF, Zarlengo KM. Blue cohosh and perinatal stroke. *New Engl J Med*. 2004;351:302.
61. Dugoua JJ, Seely D, Perri D, Koren G, Mills E. Safety and efficacy of black cohosh (*Cimicifuga racemosa*) during pregnancy and lactation. *Can J Clin Pharmacol* 2008;15:e257-e261.
62. Chaillet N, Belaid L, Crochetiere C, et al. Nonpharmacologic approaches for pain management during labor compared with usual care: a meta-analysis. *Birth*. 2014;41(2):122-137.
63. Simkin P, Bolding A. Update on nonpharmacologic approaches to relieve labor pain and prevent suffering. *J Midwifery Womens Health*. 2004; 49(6):489-505.
64. Jones L, Othman M, Dowswell T, et al. Pain management for women in labour: an overview of systematic reviews. *Cochrane Database Syst Rev*. 2012;3:CD009234.
65. Melzack R, Schaffelberg D. Low-back pain during labor. *Am J Obstet Gynecol*. 1987;156(4):901-905.
66. Trout KK. The neuromatrix theory of pain: implications for selected nonpharmacologic methods of pain relief for labor. *J Midwifery Womens Health*. 2004;49(6):482-488.
67. Bricker L, Lavender T. Parenteral opioids for labor pain: a systematic review. *Am J Obstet Gynecol*. 2002;186:S94-S109.
68. Guinsburg R, Wyckoff MH. Naloxone during neonatal resuscitation: acknowledging the unknown. *Clin Perinatol*. 2006;22:121-132.
69. Eltzschig HK, Lieberman ES, Camann WR. Regional anesthesia and analgesia for labor and delivery. *N Engl J Med*. 2003;348(4):319-332.
70. Trout KK, Eschkevari L. Support for women in labor. In: King TL, Brucker MC, Kriebs J, et al., eds. *Varney's Midwifery*. Burlington, MA: Jones & Bartlett Learning; 2015:883-915.
71. Curtin WM, Katzam PJ, Florescue H, Metlay LA, Ural SH. Intrapartum fever, epidural analgesia, and histologic chorioamnionitis. *J Perinatol*. 2015. 35(6):396-400.
72. Anim-Somuah M, Smyth RMD, Jones L. Epidural versus non-epidural or no analgesia in labour. *Cochrane Database Syst* Rev. 2011;12:CD000331.
73. Mayberry LJ, Clemmens D, De A. Epidural analgesia side effects, co-interventions, and care of women during labor: a systematic review. *Am J Obstet Gynecol* 2002;186:S81-S94.
74. Likis FE, Andrews JC, Collins MR, Lewis RM, et al. Nitrous oxide for the management of labor pain: a systematic review. *Anesth Analg*. 2014;118(1):153-167.
75. Centers for Disease Control and Prevention. Prevention of perinatal group B streptococcal disease: a revised guideline from CDC, 2010. *MMWR Recomm Rep*. 2010;59(RR-10):1-36.
76. Jolivet RR. Early-onset neonatal group B streptococcal infection: 2002 guidelines for prevention. *J Midwifery Womens Health*. 2002;47:435-466.
77. American College of Obstetricians and Gynecologists. Practice Bulletin No. 120: use of prophylactic antibiotics in labor and delivery. *Obstet Gynecol*. 2011; 117(6):1472-1483.
78. Nishimura RA, Carabello BA, Faxon DP, et al. ACC/AHA 2008 guideline update on valvular heart disease: focused update on infective endocarditis. *Circulation*. 2008;118:887-896.
79. Panel on Treatment of HIV-Infected Pregnant Women and Prevention of Perinatal Transmission. Recommendations for use of antiretroviral drugs in pregnant HIV-1–infected women for maternal health and interventions to reduce perinatal HIV transmission in the United States. 2014. http://aidsinfo.nih.gov/content files/lvguidelines/perinatalgl.pdf. Accessed July 12, 2014.
80. Edwards RK. Chorioamnionitis and labor. *Obstet Gynecol Clin North Am*. 2005;32:287-296.
81. Tita AT, Andrews WW. Diagnosis and management of clinical chorioamnionitis. *Clin Perinatol*. 2010; 37(2):339-354.
82. Fahey JO. Clinical management of intraamniotic infection and chorioamnionitis: a review of the literature. *J Midwifery Womens Health*. 2008;53:227-235.
83. Chapman E, Reveiz L, Illanes E, Bonfill Cosp X. Antibiotic regimens for management of intra-amniotic infection. *Cochrane Database Syst Rev*. 2014;12:CD010976.
84. Shatrov JG, Birch SC, Lam LT, et al. Chorioamnionitis and cerebral palsy: a meta-analysis. *Obstet Gynecol*. 2010;116:387.
85. Hermansen MC, Hermansen HM. Perinatal infections and cerebral palsy. *Clin Perinatol*. 2006;33:315-333.
86. American College of Obstetricians and Gynecologists, Task Force on Hypertension in Pregnancy. Hypertension in pregnancy: report of the American College of Obstetricians and Gynecologists' Task Force on Hypertension in Pregnancy. *Obstet Gynecol*. 2013;122:1122.

87. Sibai BM. Magnesium sulfate prophylaxis in preeclampsia: lessons learned from recent trials. *Am J Obstet Gynecol.* 2004;190:1520.
88. Duley L, Meher S, Jones L. Drugs for the treatment of very high blood pressure during pregnancy. *Cochrane Database Syst Rev.* 2013;7:CD001449.
89. Druzin ML, Shields LE, Peterson NL, et al. *Preeclampsia Toolkit: Improving Health Care Response to Preeclampsia (California Maternal Quality Care Collaborative Toolkit to Transform Maternity Care).* Developed under contract #11-10006 with the California Department of Public Health; Maternal, Child and Adolescent Health Division; published by the California Maternal Quality Care Collaborative; November 2013.
90. Brown CL, Garovic VD. Drug treatment of hypertension in pregnancy. *Drugs.* 2014;74(3):283-296.
91. Callaghan WM, Kuklina EV, Berg CJ. Trends in postpartum hemorrhage: United States, 1994–2006. *Am J Obstet Gynecol.* 2010;202:353.e1.
92. American College of Obstetricians and Gynecologists. Practice Bulletin No. 76: postpartum hemorrhage. *Obstet Gynecol.* 2006;108:1039-1047.
93. Tang OS, Gemzell-Danielsson K, Ho PC. Misoprostol: pharmacokinetic profiles, effects on the uterus and side effects. *Int J Gynaecol Obstet.* 2007;99(suppl 2):S160.
94. Lyndon A, Lagrew D, Shields L, Melsop K, Bingham B, Main E, eds. *Improving Health Care Response (Maternity Care).* Developed under contract #08-85012 with the California Department of Public Health; Maternal, Child and Adolescent Health Division; published by the California Maternal Quality Care Collaborative. https://www.cmqcc.org/ob_hemorrhage. Accessed March 3, 2015.
95. Dahlke JD, Mendez-Figueroa H, Maggio L, et al. Prevention and management of postpartum hemorrhage: a comparison of four national guidelines. *Am J Obstet Gynecol.* 2015;213(1):1-76.
96. Du Y, Ye M, Zheng F. Active management of the third stage of labor with and without controlled cord traction: a systematic review and meta-analysis of randomized controlled trials. *Acta Obstet Gynecol Scand.* 2014;93:626.
97. Westhoff G, Cotter AM, Tolosa JE. Prophylactic oxytocin for the third stage of labour to prevent postpartum haemorrhage. *Cochrane Database Syst Rev.* 2013; 10:CD001808.
98. Tita AT, Szychowski JM, Rouse DJ, et al. Higher-dose oxytocin and hemorrhage after vaginal delivery: a randomized controlled trial. *Obstet Gynecol.* 2012;119:293.
99. Gizzo S, Patrelli ST, Gangi SD, et al. Which uterotonic is better to prevent postpartum hemorrhage? Latest news in terms of clinical efficacy, side effects, and contraindications: a systematic review. *Reprod Sci.* 2012;20(9):1011-1019.
100. Liabsuetrakul T, Choobun T, Peeyananjarassri K, Islam QM. Prophylactic use of ergot alkaloids in the third stage of labour. *Cochrane Database Syst Rev.* 2007;2:CD005456.
101. Tunçalp Ö, Hofmeyr GJ, Gülmezoglu AM. Prostaglandins for preventing postpartum haemorrhage. *Cochrane Database Syst Rev.* 2012;8:CD000494.
102. Hofmeyr GJ, Walraven G, Gulmezoglu AM, Maholwana B, Alfirevic Z, Villar J. Misoprostol to treat postpartum haemorrhage: a systematic review. *BJOG.* 2005;112:547-553.
103. Winikoff B, Dabash R, Durocher J, et al. Treatment of post-partum haemorrhage with sublingual misoprostol versus oxytocin in women not exposed to oxytocin during labour: a double-blind, randomised, non-inferiority trial. *Lancet.* 2010;375(9710):210-216.
104. Blum J, Winikoff B, Raghavan S, et al. Treatment of post-partum haemorrhage with sublingual misoprostol versus oxytocin in women receiving prophylactic oxytocin: a double-blind, randomised, non-inferiority trial. *Lancet.* 2010;375(9710):217-223.

37 Postpartum

Mary Ann Rhode

Chapter Glossary

Cocooning Immunization of family members and close contacts of newborns to prevent infection of infants 1 year and younger. Most commonly used to prevent pertussis of infant.

Kleihauer-Betke Laboratory test used to ascertain how much fetal hemoglobin is in the maternal circulation. Usually performed after birth on women who are Rh(D)-negative to determine required dose of Rho(D) immune globulin (RhoGAM).

Multimodal analgesia Approach to analgesia that uses concurrent administration of different classes of analgesics, each of which relieves pain by a different mechanism. Also known as balanced analgesia.

Preemptive analgesia Analgesia administered prior to surgery and as a means to reduce postoperative pain and postoperative use of analgesia, especially opiates.

Rosette test Qualitative laboratory test that detects D-antigen-positive red blood cells in maternal circulation. If rosette test is positive, Kleihauer-Betke test can be performed to determine amount of fetal hemoglobin present in maternal circulation. If negative, one ampule or 300 mcg Rho(D) immune globulin should be adequate.

Introduction

The postpartum period or puerperium is a unique part of a woman's life, during which the most commonly occurring situations rarely require pharmacologic intervention. During the postpartum period, nonpharmacologic comfort measures often work well and minimize or eliminate the need for drugs; women who are not heavily medicated have more opportunities to accomplish essential tasks of the postpartum. Nevertheless, when they have pain or discomforts that are unrelieved by such interventions, women who are appropriately medicated have more energy to care for their infants. Negotiating the fine line between under-medication and over-reliance on drugs requires careful assessment and appropriate management by care providers. A closer look at agents commonly used in the postpartum period, many of which are over-the-counter agents, facilitates the delivery of individualized care.

Postpartum is an area that cries out for more rigorous, modern evidence, especially evidence that supports or refutes routine interventions, including pharmacologic agents. Many of the research studies that provide the rationale for today's interventions were conducted decades ago. This chapter discusses pharmaceuticals used during the management of the woman during the immediate postpartum period and through the first few weeks after giving birth.

Physiologic Changes During the Postpartum Period

The postpartum period is a time of rapid physiologic changes, several of which may potentially influence pharmacology. During this 6- to 8-week period, women experience involution of the uterus, lactogenesis, and multiple endocrine changes as the body returns to a nonpregnant state.[1] Gastrointestinal motility is slowed in the immediate postpartum period. Cardiac output initially increases as blood circulated through the placenta shifts back to the systemic circulation, but then slowly declines until it reaches a nonpregnant state at approximately 2 weeks postpartum. By the 10th postpartum day, the circulating blood volume has returned to the normal prepregnant volume secondary to urinary diuresis. The bladder has increased volume and occasionally decreased sensitivity that can result in urinary retention. Anatomic changes of pregnancy such as dilation of ureters may take several months to resolve.

Considerations Prior to Prescribing Drugs in the Postpartum Period

Puerperal changes, although dramatic, rarely require modifications in dosing or choice of drugs. Instead, treatment of postpartum symptoms should be designed to be therapeutic and to minimize side effects, especially those that can limit the woman's ability to care for her newborn. Fortunately, most commonly used pharmacologic agents have wide therapeutic ranges, although drugs used to treat some conditions such as diabetes and hypothyroidism may require changes in dosing. In addition, prescribing drugs to lactating women requires careful assessment of the advisability of the drug chosen and the amount of drug that is transferred to the newborn via breast milk. Lactation and drug use are discussed in more detail in the *Breastfeeding* chapter. All of these variables beg for true individualization of care in a healthcare environment that, for the most part, often views this part of a woman's life as "routine."

Pharmaceutical Agents Specific to the Postpartum Period

Immunobiologics

Vaccines and immune globulins are two types of immunobiologics that may be prescribed for women in the immediate postpartum period. A relatively small number of these agents are regularly administered in the postpartum period (Table 37-1). They are used when there is a specific indication based on documentation of the woman's nonimmune status, potential for exposure, or imminent international travel.

Both killed and attenuated vaccines are compatible with breastfeeding. In contrast, live vaccines such as the smallpox vaccine and the nasal influenza vaccine should not be given to breastfeeding women or to household contacts of breastfeeding women. Specific data regarding the effects of most vaccines by breastfeeding women are generally unavailable. In some settings, postpartum women are an identified population group whose own vaccination can address public health recommendations for specific immunizations. For example, the pertussis vaccine cannot be given to newborns, yet newborns can experience significant morbidity if they come in contact with this virus. Immunization of close family members provides a cocoon or **cocooning** effect for neonatal protection in such a case. The immunobiologics most commonly offered to postpartum women are the rubella vaccine for women who are rubella nonimmune, Rho(D) immune globulin (RhoGAM) for women who are Rh negative, and the tetanus, diphtheria, and pertussis (Tdap) vaccine.

Rho(D) Immune Globulin (Human)

Rho(D) immune globulin (RhoGAM) administered within 72 hours after birth reduces the incidence of Rh sensitization from 12% to 13% to 1% to 2%,[5] as illustrated in Figure 37-1. If Rho(D) immune globulin also is administered at 28 weeks' gestation, the incidence is reduced even

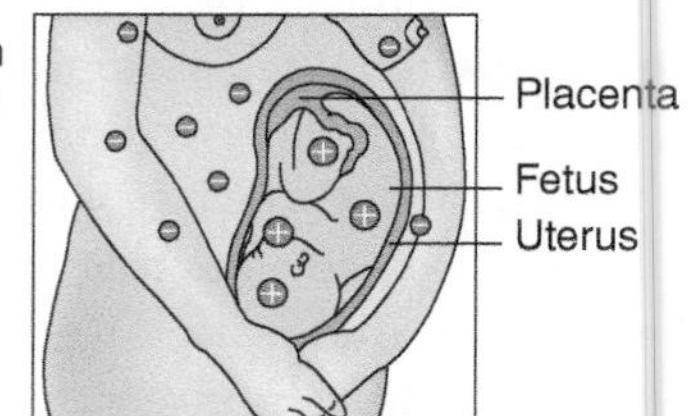

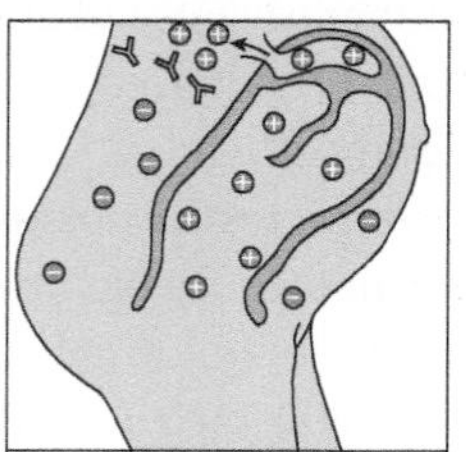

A pregnant woman with Rh negative blood with a fetus with Rh positive blood. No maternal antibodies are present at this time.

Initiation of isoimmunization process when fetal blood gets into the maternal circulation during the birth of the fetus or placenta.

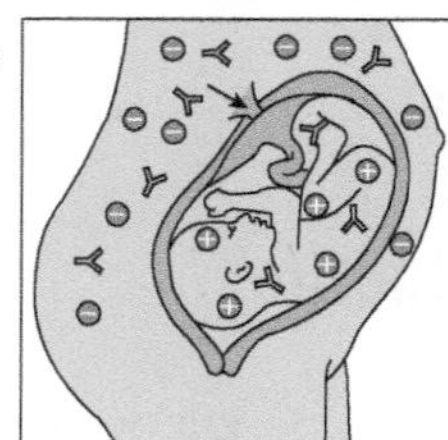

In the next pregnancy, if the fetus is RH+, the woman who is isoimmunized has RH+ antibodies that will cross the placenta and attack the fetus's RH+ blood cells.

Figure 37-1 Rh isoimmunization.

Table 37-1 Immunobiologics Commonly Administered in the Postpartum Period[a]

Immunobiologic	Indication	Type	Route/Dose	Clinical Considerations
Rubella	Nonimmune or equivocal rubella status	Live, attenuated virus vaccine	Single subcutaneous dose	Virus or virus antigen may be found in breast milk, but no reported adverse effects or symptoms of clinical disease in infants have been found. Side effects include mild fever, transient lymphadenopathy, transient rash (lasting 7–10 days), arthralgias, or transient arthritis (commencing 1–3 weeks after vaccination and lasting 1–3 weeks).
Rho(D) immune globulin (human) (RhoGAM)	Nonsensitized Rh-negative mother with Rh-positive newborn or a newborn who tests weakly D-positive	Immune globulin	IM; usual dose is 300 mcg, which will suppress an immune response to ≤15 mL Rh(D)-positive red blood cells	Given within 72 hours postpartum. Available in prefilled, single-dose syringes. Contraindicated if Rho(D)-positive or Du-positive, or previously sensitized to Rho(D) or Du antigens.
Tdap: Tetanus toxoid, diphtheria toxoid, acellular pertussis vaccine booster (Adacel)	Postpartum women who have not previously received Tdap	Combination toxoid and vaccine	Single IM dose 0.5 mL	May be given concurrently with hepatitis B and trivalent inactivated influenza vaccine. 2-year interval between last tetanus vaccination and Tdap is recommended unless there is an ensuing pregnancy, in which case revaccination is recommended.
Pneumococcal polysaccharide vaccine (PPSV23)	Postpartum women, 19 years or older, who have asthma or who smoke or with certain chronic medical conditions	Inactive	0.5 mL IM or subcutaneous	
Hepatitis B vaccine (Energix-B, Recombivax HB)	Preexposure or postexposure for those at risk or if required for school or work	Noninfectious, purified surface antigen vaccine	19 years or older: 20 mcg/1.0 mL IM given as a three-dose series at 0, 1, and 6 months	If a series has been started, it is not necessary to start the series over if all doses are not administered on schedule. Just resume the series. First dose of series is recommended for newborns prior to hospital discharge.
Trivalent inactivated influenza vaccine	Influenza season, nonvaccinated mother	Inactivated virus vaccine	Single IM dose	Vaccination for unvaccinated mothers during influenza season (October to March). Recommended prior to discharge if woman gave birth in hospital or birth center.

[a] Since administration of all immunobiologics may cause hypersensitivity in some individuals, 20 minutes of observation after administration is advised.

Sources: Data from Tingle AJ, Chantler JK, Pot KH, Paty DW, Ford DK. Postpartum rubella immunization: association with development of prolonged arthritis, neurological sequelae, and chronic rubella viremia. *J Infect Dis.* 1985;152(3):606-612[2]; Centers for Disease Control and Prevention. ACIP provisional updated recommendations on use of tetanus toxoid, reduced diphtheria toxoid and acellular pertussis vaccine (Tdap) for pregnant women. *ACIP Recommendations.* December 6, 2012:1[3]; Centers for Disease Control and Prevention. Advisory committee on immunization practices recommended immunization schedule for adults aged 19 years or older—United States, 2015. *MMWR.* 2015;64(4):91-92.[4]

further, to 0.1% to 0.2%.[6] Information regarding the effectiveness of Rho(D) immune globulin administered beyond 72 hours after birth is limited, but the vaccine should be administered beyond the 72-hour window when necessary because this time frame was initially based on the limits of the original clinical trial; thus this biologic may be effective in some recipients after the 72-hour period.[7] One of the rare studies conducted on this topic reported no isoimmunization in approximately 50% of subjects when Rho(D) immune globulin was given 13 days after exposure.[8]

Prior to postpartum administration, testing to detect fetal–maternal hemorrhage in excess of that covered by a single dose of the globulin is required by the American Association of Blood Banks. Several tests may be performed for this purpose. The **rosette test** is a qualitative test that can detect a fetal–maternal hemorrhage of approximately 10 mL of fetal blood in the maternal serum. The rosette test may not be reliable if the newborn is weak D-positive, however. If this test is positive or if the newborn is weak D-positive, quantitative tests must be done to determine the correct dose. These tests include the enzyme-linked antiglobulin test (ELAT) and flow cytometry hemoglobin F (HbF) assay, although they may not detect fetal–maternal hemorrhage if the fetus is weak D-positive. Alternatively, the **Kleihauer-Betke** acid-elution test may be used in all instances. Testing for fetal–maternal hemorrhage is recommended for women who have received an antepartum dose of Rho(D) immune globulin within 3 weeks of giving birth who otherwise do not need a postpartum dose. It is possible for a large-enough number of Rh-positive fetal red blood cells to cross the placenta into the maternal circulation late in pregnancy to cause a positive antiglobulin test for weak D (Du). Rho(D) immune globulin should be administered in the absence of documented maternal Rh status.

Because Rho(D) immune globulin is derived from human blood, the origin of this agent may pose a problem for some individuals, such as those who refuse to receive blood because of religious convictions. Not all women ascribing to the Jehovah's Witnesses religion will refuse blood products. A study of 61 women who stated that they were Jehovah's Witnesses revealed that 50.1% would not accept any type of blood, but the rest would.[9] Therefore, each woman, regardless of stated religion, should be approached individually and provided with full information. In cases where women will refuse anti-D serum on the basis of religious beliefs, those convictions should be honored.

Rubella Vaccine

Theoretically, concurrent administration of Rho(D) immune globulin might potentially interfere with the development of antibodies to live vaccines, such as the rubella vaccine. However, little evidence exists to support this theory. Therefore, when indicated, the rubella vaccination should be administered to women receiving Rho(D) immunoglobulin. Whenever two vaccinations are given at the same time, it is recommended that the vaccinations be given in separate anatomic sites. When possible, rubella immunity should be verified at 3 months postpartum. Traditional postpartum practice requires administration of the rubella vaccine just prior to discharge from a hospital setting to avoid a febrile response that could be confused with puerperal morbidity, but evidence-based support for this practice is lacking. In 2001, the Centers for Disease Control and Prevention (CDC) revised its recommendations to state that women who receive a rubella vaccine should be counseled to avoid pregnancy for 28 days—not 3 months, as previously recommended.[10]

Tdap Vaccine

Tdap (Adacel) administration in the postpartum period has been receiving increased attention due to the rising incidence of adult pertussis. Research has identified the mother as the source in 32% of infant pertussis infection cases, and cases of adult pertussis are increasing.[11,12] Administration of Tdap between 27 and 36 weeks' gestation during every pregnancy is now recommended by the CDC.

Vitamin Supplementation

Women who have been taking prenatal vitamins during pregnancy will often ask how long they should continue those vitamins on a postpartum basis. Although it is uncommon in developed countries for a woman's diet to be deficient enough to lower vitamin levels in her breast milk, lactating women generally are encouraged to continue prenatal vitamins as long as they are breastfeeding, even though evidence of any improved health benefits from this practice is limited. In general, initiation of vitamin supplementation during the postpartum period is recommended only for women who have restricted diets or health conditions wherein vitamins are part of the therapeutic regimen.[13]

Postpartum Contraception

Ideally, desired methods of contraception postpartum, if any, should have been discussed prior to the infant's birth. Some women, however, will remain uncertain about which contraceptives are available or undecided about their choice during the postpartum period. Those women will need a review of available methods, including the risks and benefits of each option relative to their needs and lifestyle.

Resumption of sexual intercourse and, therefore, risk of pregnancy are subject to the personal desires of the woman and her partner, as well as cultural mores, especially given that evidence-based recommendations are lacking. Ovulation occurs approximately 10 weeks postpartum in bottle-feeding women. Although the first menses tends to be anovulatory, a woman cannot depend on that event as a contraceptive alert. Therefore, for women desiring a method of postpartum contraception, it is recommended that a method be started during the third week postpartum for partially breastfeeding and bottle-feeding women. Women who are breastfeeding exclusively and who are amenorrheic are eligible to use the lactational amenorrheic method (LAM); it is a highly effective contraceptive option

Table 37-2 U.S. Medical Eligibility Criteria for Postpartum Contraception

Condition	Subcondition	Combined Pill, Patch, Ring	POP	Injection	Implant	LNG—IUD	Copper-IUD
Postpartum (see also Breastfeeding)	(a) < 21 days	4[a]	1[d]	1	1		
	(b) 21 days to 42 days						
	(i) with other risk factors for VTE	3[b]	1	1	1		
	(ii) without other risk factors for VTE	2[c]	1	1	1		
	(c) > 42 days	1	1	1	1		
Postpartum (in breastfeeding or non-breastfeeding women, including those post cesarean section)	(a) < 10 minutes after delivery of the placenta					2	1
	(b) 10 minutes after delivery of the placenta to < 4 weeks					2	2
	(c) ≥ 4 weeks					1	1
	(d) Puerperal sepsis					4	4

Abbreviations: LNG—IUD = levonorgestrel—intrauterine device; POP = progestin-only pill; VTE = venous thromboembolism.
[a] Category 1: No restriction; method can be used.
[b] Category 2: Advantages generally outweigh theoretical or proven risks.
[c] Category 3: Theoretical or proven risks generally outweigh advantages.
[d] Category 4: Unacceptable health risk; method not to be used.
Source: Reproduced from Centers for Disease Control and Prevention. U.S. medical eligibility criteria for contraceptive use, 2010. *MMWR.* 2010;59(RR-4). http://www.cdc.gov/mmwr/preview/mmwrhtml/rr5904a1.htm. Accessed August 30, 2014.[14]

for these women for as long as 6 months if the LAM-required components are consistently in place.

Although general information about contraception is discussed in depth in the *Contraception* chapter, the postpartum period presents some specific considerations, including lactation and a continuation of an increased risk of thromboembolic events. Recognizing the uniqueness of the postpartum period, in 2010, the CDC published evidence-based recommendations for the use of contraceptive methods during the postpartum period.[14] Table 37-2 lists these recommendations for hormonal contraceptives for women who are postpartum, including differences based on whether they are breastfeeding.

Breastfeeding women who use combined oral contraceptives breastfeed for a mean of 3.7 months versus 4.6 months for control subjects, although this finding is not known to be causal. A contraceptive method that will not interfere with milk production, such as the progestin-only pill, depot-medroxyprogesterone acetate (Depo-Provera), single-rod contraceptive implant (Nexplanon), or a barrier method can be encouraged for the breastfeeding woman. Women also can be educated regarding other nonhormonal methods such as LAM.

In large part because of drug interactions, CDC issued separate contraceptive recommendations for all women who are at high risk for human immunodeficiency virus (HIV) infection in 2012.[15] These recommendations may be of value for this specific group of women during the postpartum period.

Pain and Other Discomforts During the Puerperium

Women can experience pain from several different anatomic sites in the early postpartum period. Pain associated with changes in the gastrointestinal system, breasts, muscles and even pain from a full bladder all require different treatments. When analgesia is necessary, many options are available and may be used selectively in conjunction with complementary alternative therapies. Most of these agents are compatible with breastfeeding.

Postoperative Pain

In the United States, approximately one of every three neonates is now born via cesarean section. There is wide variation in the intensity of postoperative incision pain experienced by women, and traditionally opiate pain medications are among the first-line drugs to be used for this indication. Intravenous administration of analgesia has largely replaced administration by the intramuscular route. Changes in obstetric practice, such as allowing early intake of oral fluids and solids after cesarean section, have also led some to question the primary reliance on traditional post-cesarean parenteral pain management strategies that limit a woman's movement and that can result in higher rates of nausea, vomiting, pruritus, urinary retention, constipation, and respiratory depression. In the postpartum period, several different analgesics and different modalities for delivery are used.

Common Analgesics

The analgesics most commonly used to treat a woman with postpartum pain include acetaminophen (e.g., Tylenol), ibuprofen (e.g., Advil), combinations of acetaminophen with oxycodone (e.g., Percocet), hydrocodone (Vicodin) or codeine, plus ketorolac (e.g., Toradol) and morphine for severe pain (Table 37-3). Women should be counseled that 4000 mg of acetaminophen daily is the maximum recommended dosage. Many women may not recognize that Tylenol and acetaminophen are the same medication or appreciate that acetaminophen often is an ingredient in other brands advertised for pain and colds. For this reason, it is important to counsel women about the ubiquitous nature of these agents and potential risks prior to taking them.

Codeine and codeine combinations should not be used by women who may be ultra-rapid metabolizers of codeine, especially those who have chosen to breastfeed, due potential accumulation of high doses of morphine in the neonate. Additional information about this genetic variation can be found in the *Pharmacogenetics* chapter. Morphine—the primary metabolite of codeine—accumulates in breast milk in slightly higher levels than in maternal plasma.[16,17] In contrast, hydrocodone and oxycodone combination products are widely used for postpartum pain and are generally considered safe.[18] However, prolonged or frequent doses of these medications can lead to neonatal sedation in a breastfeeding scenario.

Aspirin or aspirin combinations should not be prescribed for breastfeeding women due to a theoretic risk that the newborn will develop Reye syndrome or metabolic acidosis from salicylate poisoning.[19] More information about the non-opioid and opioid medications commonly used in the postpartum period may be found in the *Analgesia and Anesthesia* chapter.

Preemptive Analgesia

Preemptive analgesia refers to analgesia administered prior to surgery or an anticipated painful experience. This technique is being investigated as a means to reduce postoperative pain and postoperative opiate use via inhibition of central sensitization and the pain-processing system.[24] Local anesthetics and opioids both can be used for preemptive analgesia prior to a cesarean birth. Studies on epidural placement of local anesthetics on a preincision basis have been conflicting, so use of this technique is not widespread.

Multimodal Analgesia

Multimodal analgesia, or balanced analgesic regimens (i.e., the concurrent administration of different classes of analgesics), has been found to be more effective than use of single agents.[25,26] Because each class of analgesics relieves pain via a different mechanism, members of each class potentiate each other when administered together. NSAID use, such as ketorolac (Toradol), is associated with a 30% to 50% opiate-sparing effect for either systemic- or neuraxial-administered opiates.[27]

Scheduled Dosing

Scheduled dosing may also be more effective than as-needed dosing, especially for individuals who have severe pain. Several authors mention administration of medications at fixed intervals to postoperative women as a strategy that results in increased maternal satisfaction.[28] Use of scheduled dosing for women after vaginal birth has not been well studied, however, and more research is needed.

Relatively new devices that continuously infuse local anesthetic (bupivacaine or ropivacaine) directly into the incision site (e.g., On Q Pain Buster Post-op Relief System) can take advantage of both scheduled dosing and a multimodal analgesic regimen. Although no significant difference in pain scores between groups using a continuous local anesthetic infusion system infusing either bupivacaine or normal saline was noted in a randomized trial, women in the bupivacaine group used less postoperative morphine.[29] A small, randomized clinical trial (RCT) of women post-cesarean section compared standard care with continuous infusion of ropivacaine (Naropin) into the incision. The investigators found that the women in the ropivacaine-treatment group had significantly reduced pain due to movement and reduced need for additional analgesics ($P < 0.01$).[30]

Neuraxial Morphine Installation

Single-dose preservative-free morphine sulfate (Duramorph) placed into the neuraxial space is used widely by anesthesia providers immediately after cesarean birth, as part of a multimodal approach to pain relief. Neuraxial morphine provides pain relief for long periods without loss of motor, sensory, or sympathetic function.

Table 37-3 Analgesics Commonly Used in the Postpartum Period

Drug: Generic (Brand)	Formulations	Indication and Dose	Recommendations for Lactation	Clinical Considerations
NSAIDs				
Acetaminophen (Tylenol)	325 mg, 500 mg	Mild to moderate pain 500 mg every 4–6 hours with maximum 4 g/day	Compatible with breastfeeding	Total acetaminophen daily dose should not exceed 4000 mg/day. Toxic metabolite, *N*-acetyl-*p*-benzoquinone-imine, present only in acute overdose or when maximum dose is exceeded over a prolonged period of time.
Ibuprofen (Motrin, Advil)	200, 400, 600 mg	Mild to moderate pain 600 mg every 6 hours	Compatible with breastfeeding	
Ketorolac tromethamine (Toradol)	15, 30, 60 mg for IM dose 10 mg for oral dose	Short-term treatment for postoperative pain 60 mg IM × 1 dose	Compatible with breastfeeding	Can reduce opiate use by 25–45% and lower side effects attributable to opiate medications. Switch to alternative analgesics as soon as possible. Side effects include gastrointestinal ulcerations, bleeding, perforation, and postoperative bleeding. Use with caution if the woman has impaired maternal renal function or hypertension including preeclampsia.
Codeine Combination Products				
Acetaminophen (Tylenol)/codeine	Tylenol with codeine No. 2: 300 mg acetaminophen/ 15 mg codeine Tylenol with codeine No. 3: 300 mg acetaminophen/30 mg codeine Tylenol No. 4: 300 mg acetaminophen/60 mg codeine	Moderate pain relief Tylenol No. 3 every 4–6 hours	Compatible with breastfeeding	Potential for abnormally high levels or active metabolite in breast milk of ultra-rapid metabolizers of codeine. Women should watch for increased sleepiness, difficulty breastfeeding or breathing, or decreased tone in newborn.
Hydrocodone bitartrate and acetaminophen (Vicodin, Lortab, Lorcet)	Vicodin 5 mg/500 mg Lortab 2.5/500, 5/500, 7.5/500 Lorcet Plus 7.5 mg/650 mg Lorcet 10/650	Moderate pain 1–2 tablets every 4–6 hours	No human data	Anecdotal information suggests probable compatibility with breastfeeding.
Oxycodone/ acetaminophen (Percocet, Magnacet)	Percocet: 2.5/325 mg, 5/325 mg, 7.5/325 mg Magnacet: 5/400, 5/400; 7.5/400 mg	Moderate pain 1–2 tablets every 4–6 hours Maximum dose of acetaminophen is 3250 mg/day	Limited human data	Anecdotal information suggests probable compatibility with breastfeeding, although monitoring for neonatal sedation is suggested.
Morphine				
Meperidine (Demerol)	50, 100 mg/mL	Severe pain 50–100 mg IM every 1–3 hours	Compatible with breastfeeding	Use in breastfeeding women with caution because of reports of neonatal sedation. Meperidine has active metabolites.
Morphine sulfate, opiate agonist analgesic	Several formulations for IV administration	Severe pain 5–10 mg IM or IV	Compatible with breastfeeding	Additional opioids or sedatives should not be used. All administration routes have the potential to result in clinically significant amounts of opiate in breast milk.

Abbreviations: OTC = over the counter; PCA = patient-controlled analgesia; PCEA = patient-controlled epidural analgesia.

Sources: Koren G, Cairns J, Chitayat D, Gaedigk A, Leeder SJ. Pharmacogenetics of morphine poisoning in a breastfed neonate of a codeine-prescribed mother. *Lancet.* 2006;368(9536):704[20]; Windle ML, Booker LA, Rayburn WF. Postpartum pain after vaginal delivery: a review of comparative analgesic trials. *J Reprod Med.* 1989;34(11):891-895[21]; Clark JH, Wilson WG. A 16-day-old breast-fed infant with metabolic acidosis caused by salicylate. *Clin Pediatr (Phila).* 1981;20(1):53-54[19]; Anderson PO, Sauberan JB, Lane JR, Rossi SS. Hydrocodone excretion into breast milk: the first 2 reported cases. *Breastfeeding Med.* 2007;2(1):10-14[22]; Pavy TJG, Paech MJ, Evans SF. The effect of intravenous ketorolac on opioid requirement and pain after cesarean delivery. *Anesth Analg.* 2001;92(4):1010-1014[23]; Montgomery A, Hale T. Academy of Breastfeeding Medicine Clinical Protocol No. 15: analgesia and anesthesia for the breastfeeding mother. *Breastfeed Med.* 2012;7(6):548-553.[18]

Generalized pruritus and urinary retention are common side effects of this treatment. Women who receive neuraxial morphine need a Foley catheter to effectively drain the bladder for the first 12 to 24 hours after birth. Side effects, in general, respond to naloxone (Narcan) administration, which should be readily available whenever this technique is used. However, naloxone will reverse the pain-relieving effect in addition to resolving side effects, so it is used only when pruritus is markedly uncomfortable for a woman. The neuraxial route produces negligible maternal plasma levels of morphine and is compatible with breastfeeding.

Neuraxial administration of morphine can cause acute respiratory depression or respiratory arrest, or delayed respiratory depression for up to 24 hours, so this analgesic approach requires observation by personnel skilled in resuscitation. Women who have a depleted blood volume or who are administered other drugs such as phenothiazines or general anesthetics have an increased risk of developing significant hypotension. Dysphoric reactions and toxic psychoses have been reported following use of morphine sulfate.

A study comparing scheduled oral oxycodone–acetaminophen (Percocet) versus neuraxial installation of morphine after planned cesarean section found that women who received the oral pain medication reported less pain and nausea than women who had patient-controlled analgesia. No statistical difference was noted in emesis, oral fluid intake, or ambulation.[31]

Management of Postoperative Pain for Women on Methadone

Women who are on methadone maintenance are a unique subset of individuals who require extra help in controlling post-cesarean pain. These women can require as much as 70% more opiate medication following cesarean section when compared to the medication requirements of women who are not on methadone. Unfortunately, these women may be the least likely to receive adequate pain relief based on misconceptions of care providers regarding their pain relief needs.[32] The usual daily oral methadone dose should be resumed as soon as possible after birth. Opioid antagonists or mixed antagonists/agonists should not be administered to women who are on methadone maintenance because these agents can trigger withdrawal symptoms.

Afterpains or Afterbirth Pains

Approximately 50% of primiparas and 86% of multiparas experience uterine cramping or afterpains (sometimes termed afterbirth pains), with multiparas describing afterpains as more severe.[33,34] Cramping during breastfeeding also increases as parity increases.[34] In this situation, administration of an analgesic prior to nursing can be useful and is perhaps an interesting example of preemptive analgesia. Uterine cramping is theorized to be due to release of prostaglandin, a myometrial stimulant. This discomfort rarely lasts more than 2 or 3 days after delivery. Afterpains are often subjectively felt as back pain, a fact that can be confusing to women.[35] Common alternative methods for relief of afterpains, such as emptying the bladder, applying heat, and lying prone, can provide relief in as many as 40% of women.[34] Nonsteroidal anti-inflammatory drugs are particularly effective in reducing afterpains due to their antiprostaglandin properties.[21]

On occasion, afterpains can be iatrogenic. In the past, 0.2 mg of methylergonovine (Methergine) was routinely administered every 4 hours for 6 doses to minimize bleeding. Women commonly reported afterpains after administration of the pills. This practice was discontinued when research demonstrated that blood loss with the methylergonovine regimen was not statistically different from blood loss in untreated women.

Gas Pains

Thomas et al., in an era in which early ambulation was not common, studied the effects of several regimens, including various combinations of low-gas-producing foods, simethicone, rocking, and bisacodyl suppositories for relief of gas pains.[36] Rocking for 60 minutes or more per day (possibly the equivalent of contemporary early ambulation) reduced gas pains. Simethicone use combined with rocking was no more effective than simethicone alone. Bisacodyl suppositories used independently were even less effective.[36] Early movement and ambulation remains the best treatment to avoid, as well as treat, gas pains.

Perineal Lacerations

The goal of treatment of perineal lacerations is to facilitate healing, increase maternal comfort, and decrease edema. Most practices traditionally employed for postpartum perineal care are not evidence based, and few have been found to increase the rate of perineal healing. Use of both nonpharmacologic and pharmacologic methods in tandem has been found to be more effective than use of either modality alone.[37,38]

Nonpharmacologic Treatments

Ice is rarely categorized as a pharmacologic agent, but it is frequently used as a treatment during the immediate postpartum period. Cold packs, either commercially made or handmade, may be applied to the perineum immediately postpartum. Compared to no treatment, ice has been associated with decreased discomfort, most likely by minimizing edema and reducing inflammation, decreasing capillary permeability, and reducing nerve conduction velocity.[37] When used, it should be employed only for the first 24 to 48 hours, should never be placed in direct contact with the skin, and is most effective in cooling gel pads.[37] Conversely, the immediate use of heat postpartally is inadvisable because it has been found to enhance maternal discomfort.[38]

Herbal Sitz Bath Additives

Herbal and botanical agents are types of pharmaceutical agents discussed in the *Complementary and Alternative Therapies* chapter. During the immediate postpartum period, many over-the-counter herbal preparations are advertised for use either in sitz baths, for irrigation of the perineum, or as perineal compresses. Botanicals such as calendula, comfrey, yarrow, rosemary, lavender, sage, uva ursi, garlic, myrrh, and shepherd's purse all have been proposed for use either individually or in combination with other herbs because of their proposed astringent, antiseptic, or anti-inflammatory effects. RCTs of lavender oil, salt, and a chlorhexidine gluconate/cetrimide (Savlon) concentrate found no statistically significant differences in pain relief associated with the use of these additives.[39] Although future studies may find that sitz bath additives are effective, their appeal may simply reflect the fact that they provide a more esthetically pleasing postpartum experience.

Ointments, Compresses, Anesthetic Sprays, and Suppositories

A variety of topical agents, such as ointments, compresses using various solutions, and anesthetic sprays, have been used over the years as methods to provide relief from perineal discomfort or pain. Most of these preparations either have not been studied or are justified based on older, less rigorous research.[40,41] An RCT comparing witch hazel (a botanical derived from *Hamamelis virginiana*) compresses, ice, and pramoxine/hydrocortisone foam (Epifoam) found no difference in pain relief among the three treatments and no difference in timing of resumption of intercourse, wound healing, or resolution of perineal pain.[42] Similarly, a randomized, double-blind, placebo-controlled trial that compared pain relief among women using 5% lidocaine ointment to that among women using a placebo found no significant difference in outcomes.[43] In summary, a Cochrane review of eight RCTs concluded that evidence for effectiveness of topically applied local anesthetics used to treat perineal pain is not compelling.[44]

Another Cochrane review of the use of NSAID rectal suppositories found 2 RCTs that compared analgesic rectal suppositories with placebo. The women who received NSAID suppositories were less likely to experience pain in the first 24 hours after birth (relative risk [RR], 0.37; 95% confidence interval [CI], 0.10–1.38; 2 trials, 150 women) and requested less supplemental analgesia (RR, 0.31; 95% CI, 0.17–0.54; 1 trial, 89 women) than those in the placebo group.[45] However, suppository use has not been widely adopted in the United States, and it would be inappropriate to extrapolate the findings from these small studies to other methods of drug delivery. The use of sulfonamide vaginal creams, dimethyl sulfoxide (DMSO), and proteolytic enzymes from the papaya plant (which are consumed orally) also have been proposed, but evidence is lacking about the value of these agents in reducing postpartum perineal pain and their effects on perineal healing.

Compresses may be made from solutions such as magnesium sulfate solution (Epsom salts) by soaking sterile gauze pads in the chosen solution. Witch hazel compresses are marketed under several brand names, with Tucks being the most common. Witch hazel is an astringent and an anti-inflammatory agent whose main active ingredient is tannin. Today's commercially prepared witch hazel removes the tannin and relies on the 14% alcohol content for the astringent action. Although anecdotal reports advocate the use of witch hazel, there is little or no research on its effectiveness.

Arnica (*Arnica montana*) is a botanical that has been suggested as a means of reducing postoperative pain, muscle aches, bruising, hemorrhoids, and edema. This agent is available as a homeopathic preparation and as an herbal product. When used as a homeopathic agent, the oral preparation contains a minute amount of natural product in keeping with the homeopathic principles of exposure to small amounts of agents. Research exploring the effectiveness of homeopathic arnica is inconclusive.[46] Herbal arnica, which is available commercially as a cream or an ointment, is more potent but there is a paucity of evidence about the effectiveness of this topical version. Little information is available about the amounts of arnica absorbed when used topically, so questions about the use of this product by women who are breastfeeding are not settled. Topical use in high concentrations or for prolonged periods of time may cause blistering or scarring; therefore, use on broken skin or mucous membranes such as perineal lacerations or episiotomies is not recommended.

Hemorrhoids

Postpartum women are predisposed to hemorrhoid development due to pressure during vaginal birth, constipation, relaxation of the smooth muscles in vein walls, and impaired blood return, secondary to increased pressure from the pregnant uterus, and due to trauma sustained during birth. Nonpharmacologic methods to control hemorrhoid pain include many of the aforementioned interventions as well as digitally reinserting hemorrhoids into the rectum and various surgical interventions. Prevention or correction of constipation[47] via increased fluid and fiber intake, advocating the use of a side-lying position, and proper toileting habits and positions that minimize pressure on the hemorrhoids during defecation are useful. A meta-analysis of seven controlled trials found that increasing dietary fiber significantly reduced episodes of bleeding from hemorrhoids (RR, 0.50; 95% CI, 0.28–0.68).[48]

Moderate to severe hemorrhoid pain may require oral analgesia and topical analgesics with added corticosteroids to reduce pain, inflammation, and itching. Topical corticosteroids decrease inflammation by suppressing the migration of polymorphonuclear leukocytes and reversal of increased capillary permeability. Other over-the-counter preparations have not been shown to be effective in larger studies, but are reported as useful by many women. Typically, these topical medications contain substances that have a vasoconstrictive or protective effect. Such agents are not designed for long-term use, and in the absence of thrombosed hemorrhoids or rectal fissures, hemorrhoid pain will decrease over time, even without treatment. Common agents used to treat hemorrhoids and additional information regarding treatment of hemorrhoids can be found in the *Gastrointestinal Conditions* chapter.

Constipation

Constipation is a common postpartum condition that occurs secondary to lax abdominal muscles, hormonal effects on the intestine during pregnancy, inadequate fluid and fiber intake, decreased physical activity, decreased anal sensitivity, use of perinatal opiate analgesia, and avoidance of bowel movements due to real or anticipated perineal pain. Gastroenterologists recommend first asking a woman to self-define the term "constipation" when this condition is reported, as it may be useful to help distinguish between decreased frequency of bowel movements and hardened stools for a day or two, which is a common consequence of minimal solid food intake during labor. Reassurance that sutures, if present, are sturdy and reviewing comfort measures can be helpful. Women should be encouraged to increase fluids and choose high-fiber foods for a few weeks after birth. After the initial postpartum recovery period, regular exercise should also be encouraged to correct or prevent constipation. These measures are preferable to laxative use, and healthcare providers should offer information to women that will promote healthy lifestyle decisions for themselves and their families. More information about laxative preparations can be found in the *Gastrointestinal Conditions* chapter.

Of special note during the puerperium is the use of emollients or stool softeners. Docusate sodium (Colace) is an over-the-counter medication. Docusate sodium capsules are administered orally and dissolve in the stomach; rectal administration is also possible, but rare, as the medication may be administered with a saline or oil retention enema. As a relatively large, water-soluble, anionic molecule, docusate sodium passes unaltered through the gastrointestinal tract and is absorbed in small amounts from the duodenum and jejunum; it is then excreted in bile. The various docusate salts are indicated for women in whom straining is contraindicated, rather than for their laxative effect. They are commonly ordered for women who have sustained third- or fourth-degree lacerations so that they can avoid putting pressure on their sutures, although there is no clear evidence for this intervention.

The pharmacokinetic parameters of docusate sodium have not been determined and its exact mechanism of action is unknown, but research indicates two possible explanations for this medication's effects. First, docusate decreases surface tension, allowing water and lipids to penetrate and soften feces. Second, water and electrolyte secretion is stimulated in the colon, which may account for most of the laxative effect noted. Increased concentrations of cyclic adenosine monophosphate (cAMP) are found in mucosal cells of the colon after administration of docusate. This finding suggests involvement of G-protein–based second messenger receptors. Via a second messenger system, the permeability of mucosal cells is altered and active ion secretion is stimulated, which produces increased fluid within the colon.

The dosing range for docusate is 50 to 360 mg each day, with the precise dose being tailored to the severity of the condition and therapeutic response. If stool softeners are indicated, higher doses may be needed at first. A response can be expected in 1 to 3 days. Women should be cautioned against overuse of this product, as it has been associated with neonatal hypomagnesaemia.[49] Theoretically, stool softeners may improve absorption of many oral medications. For this reason, some clinicians avoid concurrent administration of these products with oral drugs with narrow therapeutic indices such as theophylline (Theo-Dur) and lithium (Lithobid).

Because the expected response time to therapy is fairly long, the few doses of docusate routinely given to women who do not have extensive lacerations or other indications may be of little use, unnecessarily contributing to hospital costs and giving the false impression that laxative use is always necessary after having a baby. Ultimately, education of women about nonpharmacologic measures to avoid constipation—such as ambulation, a high-fiber diet, and adequate fluid intake—is more likely to be efficacious for many women.

Anal Fissures

Some women experience anal fissures for the first time in their lives during the postpartum period. Such a condition is commonly associated with rectal bleeding, anal itching, and pain with defecation (dyschezia). Nitroglycerin ointment is commonly used to relieve pain and allow healing of anal fissures. The mechanism of action is to reduce internal anal tone and increase anodermal blood flow[50]—the same mechanism of action suggested as underlying the successful use of warm baths for treatment of hemorrhoid pain.[48] Because a reduction in anal tone and an increase in anodermal blood flow can reduce pressure in seriously engorged external hemorrhoids, some surgeons have used nitroglycerin ointment for individuals with intractable hemorrhoid pain, in an attempt to avoid surgery. Use of nitroglycerin ointment in this manner is anecdotal at this time, but the application site (either intra-anal or perianal) and the rationale are comparable to those cited for treatment of persons with anal fissures. A 0.5% nitroglycerin ointment is compounded using 2% nitroglycerin ointment (commercially available) and a lanolin ointment. The compounded ointment is lightly applied to the external hemorrhoid up to 3 times daily with a gloved hand, to avoid absorption through the fingers. If successful, relief will be rapid and surgery may be postponed. Hypotension or headaches are possible side effects, but are not commonly noted with controlled dosing. Research is indicated for this promising addition to the treatment options for intractable hemorrhoidal pain.[50,51]

Urinary Retention

Postpartum urinary retention (PUR) is a possible complication of the postpartum period (Box 37-1).[52] Risk factors include second stage greater than 4 hours, epidural anesthesia, operative vaginal delivery, episiotomy, nulliparity, and obesity.[53,54] The incidence of this condition is difficult to ascertain, as there has been no single standardized definition of PUR; hence reported incidence rates vary from 0.05% to 51.7%.[55] Interventions include encouragement of voiding and possible catheterization. There is no evidence supporting pharmaceutical treatments including anti-infectives or antimuscarinics, except for analgesics if a woman with PUR experiences associated pain.

Box 37-1 A Case of Severe Afterpains

FR is a multiparous woman (G4 P4004) with postpartum abdominal pain. She had ibuprofen ordered, but says it is not even "touching her pain." She had an uneventful labor and birth with no perineal lacerations 12 hours prior to this examination.

In talking to FR, she reported that the abdominal pain was constant and steadily increasing since she gave birth. It was somewhat exacerbated by breastfeeding. She denied any perineal pain. She ate a regular diet and reported no nausea. She denied any excessive vaginal bleeding or clots. Her breasts were soft and her nipples were not red. Her uterus was palpated at three fingerbreadths above the umbilicus, and a soft mass was palpated above the symphysis pubis. FR reported she had not voided since delivery.

Upon catheterization, 2200 cc of clear yellow urine was obtained.[56] The uterus was then one fingerbreadth below the umbilicus, and the mother reported her abdominal pain had disappeared. Medicating FR with an opiate would likely not have relieved her pain.

Vaginal Dryness

Due to their altered hormonal status during breastfeeding, many women experience some vaginal dryness with intercourse after giving birth, similar to the atrophic vaginitis experienced by postmenopausal women. Timing of first intercourse postpartally should be based on the comfort of the woman. There is no evidence for the long-held recommendation of abstinence of 6 weeks, although many providers suggest factors to consider in addition to maternal comfort include resolution of lochia and initiation of contraception if desired. For the majority of women, use of a water-based lubricant will alleviate vaginal dryness, especially with first intercourse. Over-the-counter treatments include water-based lubricants such as Astroglide, K-Y Jelly, Gyne-Motrin, and Duragel. Vaginal suppositories also may be used. Conversely, women should avoid non-water-based products such as petroleum jelly (Vaseline) or A&D ointment because they can be irritating to vaginal mucosa and also weaken the integrity of male condoms. Vaginal moisturizers such as Liquibeads, Replens, and Silken Secret may decrease vaginal dryness. In severe cases, a short-term, 1- to 3-week course of an estrogen vaginal cream (e.g., Premarin or Estrace) may be needed to control symptoms, although a more rapid return of ovulation and decreased milk production are possible with estrogen use.[57]

Backache

Approximately 25% of women have persistent pregnancy-related lumbopelvic pain after giving birth, and 5% of women have lumbopelvic pain that is serious enough to require healthcare intervention.[35] Two types of back pain must be differentiated in such women. Pelvic girdle pain is pregnancy-associated pain that is felt between the posterior iliac crest and gluteal fold near the sacroiliac crests and/or pain over the symphysis. This condition is generally more severe during pregnancy, but regresses postpartum. The putative etiology is excessive mobility of the pelvic joints. NSAIDs may be of value in alleviating this pain, although palliative care often is recommended because the pain will spontaneously resolve.

The other type of back pain, lumbar or low back pain, may be exacerbated during pregnancy; if it persists, however, it tends to worsen during the postpartum period. Factors associated with persistent lumbopelvic pain include presence of back pain before pregnancy, presence of back pain during pregnancy, physically heavy work, and multiple pregnancies.[35] Treatment of women with lumbopelvic pain is an area in which both alternative methods and short-term use of medications can be helpful. Specifically, physical therapy and acupuncture have documented effectiveness. Pelvic-stabilizing exercises and pelvic belts are frequently recommended. Pharmacologically, NSAIDs are efficacious for relieving discomfort from low back pain. Muscle relaxants are not commonly used because limited human data are available regarding the use of muscle relaxants by lactating women. In addition, spasmolytics such as diazepam (Valium) can cause sedation, which may be dangerous for a woman who is caring for a newborn.

Local discomfort at the site of placement of continuous lumbar epidural anesthesia is also common, simply due to the local anesthetic injection and pressure on tissues when palpating for correct placement. A brief explanation of the cause of this discomfort and the duration of the local tenderness usually is sufficient to reassure new mothers. As with any injury, heat may be applied after 24 to 48 hours to promote healing.

Anemia

The two most common reasons for anemia in the postpartum period are preexisting iron-deficiency anemia and acute blood loss at the time the woman gives birth. It is important to distinguish between the two. Women with chronic iron-deficiency anemia may be in any of three stages of iron deficiency: iron depletion (iron stores are low but hemoglobin levels are adequate), iron deficiency without anemia (low serum iron and transferrin saturation), or iron-deficiency anemia with low hemoglobin levels.[58] Examination of the initial prenatal hemoglobin/hematocrit values, the values obtained during late second trimester, and the values obtained on admission in labor can provide a picture of the severity and duration of anemia. The need for postpartum iron supplementation can be identified based on these values, even before knowing the amount of blood loss after delivery (Table 37-4).

A woman with high prenatal hemoglobin/hematocrit values, presumably adequate iron stores, and a large blood loss may recover well without additional iron supplementation or with a shorter course of supplementation than a woman who had iron-deficiency anemia prior to birth. Multiparous women—particularly those with short

Table 37-4 Examples of Varying Needs for Postpartum Iron Supplementation After Vaginal Birth

Woman's Gravidity/Parity[a]	G2 P1001 Hgb/Hct	G5 P4004 Hgb/Hct	G1 P0000 Hgb/Hct	G1 P0000 Hgb/Hct	G3 P1011 Hgb/Hct	G3 P2002 Hgb/Hct
Initial prenatal hematocrit/ hemoglobin	40.4/13.9	32.4/10.9	41.4/14.4	39.5/13.0	32.3/10.2	26.7/8.9
Antepartum ferritin/transferrin saturation values	Not indicated	Not indicated	Not indicated	Not indicated	Not indicated	Decreased ferritin, increased transferrin
Prenatal hematocrit/ hemoglobin at 26–28 weeks	38.8/13.0	30.8/10	39.1/14.3	38.1/13.2	30.8/10	27.8/9
Admission hematocrit/ hemoglobin	41.6/14.0	32.1/10.9	41.0/14.0	39.0/13.4	29.3/9.7	29.1/9.7
Estimated blood loss greater than 500 mL?	No	No	Yes	Yes	Yes	No
Postpartum orthostatic symptoms present?	No	No	No	Yes	Yes	No
Postpartum hematocrit/ hemoglobin	Not indicated, unlikely to change management plan	Not indicated, unlikely to change management plan	34.3/10.8	27.9/9.3	20.3/6.9	Not indicated, unlikely to change management plan
Postpartum iron supplementation?	Not needed	Yes, correct preexisting chronic anemia	Acute anemia without evidence of preexisting iron deficiency; iron in prenatal vitamins and diet may be sufficient to correct anemia	Yes, correct significant acute anemia	Yes, correct both chronic and acute anemia; blood transfusion may be considered if severe orthostatic symptoms persist	Yes, continue iron supplementation started antepartum to correct chronic but improving iron-deficiency anemia; monitor for improvement

[a] Parity at time of first prenatal visit.

intervals between pregnancies—are more likely to have depleted iron stores, as are women with multiple fetuses, wherein the demand for iron during pregnancy is higher than normal. Women who have declined to take iron preparations during pregnancy due to gastrointestinal side effects should be reminded that both vitamins and iron are often better tolerated in the nonpregnant state.

Postpartum blood tests for anemia can be misleading. Absolute levels may vary according to the woman's level of hydration, the amount of blood loss, preexisting hemoglobin levels, altitude (higher normal values at higher altitudes), and timing of the blood draw after birth. Based on Nelson's findings, postpartum hematocrit measurements are recommended to be obtained no sooner than 16 hours after birth unless clinically necessary.[59] In addition, postpartum hematocrit levels are not reliable markers for the need for postpartum iron supplements and correlate poorly with postpartum serum ferritin levels. When necessary, differential diagnosis of anemia should wait until blood parameters return to normal nonpregnant values 1 to 3 weeks after the birth.

The usual recommended dose to ensure the maximal rate of hemoglobin regeneration is 150 to 200 mg of elemental iron daily, taken in divided doses to minimize side effects. Iron absorption can vary greatly among individual women. As a woman recovers from anemia, the rate of change in her hemoglobin levels slows. Rebuilding iron stores is a slow process that may take up to a year, with various sources recommending from 3 to 12 months of therapy after hematocrit/hemoglobin levels return to normal. Further research to determine reliable indicators for postpartum iron supplementation and best dose schedules to enhance compliance would be beneficial.

Consumption of orange juice, meat, poultry, and fish enhances dietary iron absorption, whereas intake of cereals, tea, red wine, and milk inhibits it.[58,60] Iron is best absorbed between meals, but ferrous supplements may need to be taken with food to minimize gastric upset.

Many different formulations of iron are available. Iron can cause numerous bothersome gastrointestinal side effects, such as heartburn, nausea, abdominal cramps, constipation, and diarrhea. The most common side effect is constipation. In one double-blind study, in which ferrous sulfate, ferrous gluconate, ferrous fumarate, and placebo were given in identical-appearing tablets, there were no significant differences in the gastrointestinal symptoms observed with the various iron salts.[58,60]

Several strategies to improve a woman's ingestion of ferrous supplements are available. Generally, ferrous sulfate (325-mg tablets with 65 mg of elemental iron) has the lowest cost, but this formulation is often the least tolerated. However, side effects may be diminished by encouraging women to start the medication incrementally—for example, one tablet every 3 days for a week, increasing to one tablet every 2 days for a week, and finally one tablet or more daily. Different types of iron preparations may be tried if one type is not tolerated. Lowering the dose may also decrease side effects. Enteric-coated or prolonged-release preparations are not recommended because the reduction in side effects is accompanied by less absorption. Combination products may increase costs, side effects, or both. Because iron preparations are primarily over-the-counter medications, it is important to assess the woman's ability to pay for these supplements. Writing a prescription for an over-the-counter medication can incur a charge for filling the prescription and necessitate a copayment that may exceed the actual over-the-counter cost.

Postpartum Infections

The most common infections during the postpartum period include mastitis, urinary tract infections, and endometritis. Such infections frequently present with a febrile episode. Since 1935, postpartum febrile morbidity has been defined by the United States Joint Commission on Maternal Welfare as an oral temperature of 38.0°C (100.4°F) on any 2 of the first 10 days postpartum or 38.7°C (101.6°F) or higher during the first 24 hours after giving birth. Isolated, single fever spikes (38.7°C or higher) that occur during the first 24 hours are common and do not require treatment.[61,62] Fever in the postpartum period is most likely to be associated with the previously mentioned conditions but also can occur secondary to surgical-site infection (cesarean surgical incision, episiotomy/dehiscence, or perineal lacerations) and, more rarely, pelvic abscess. Treatment of these more uncommon conditions is dictated by cultures and agents specific to the etiology. Causes unrelated to pregnancy, such as appendicitis or viral syndrome, are also possible.

Mastitis

Mastitis, or inflammation of the breast(s), refers to a spectrum of conditions that develop most commonly between 2 and 3 weeks postpartum. However, mastitis can occur anytime from 5 days to 1 year postpartum. The most common etiologic organism is *Staphylococcus aureus*, although other organisms include group A and B streptococci, *Haemophilus influenzae*, and *Haemophilus parainfluenzae*. Increased fluids, bed rest, frequent breastfeeding, moist heat applications, and non-opioid analgesics usually are instituted at the first signs of mastitis. Antibiotics are indicated if fever is present or if no improvement is seen in afebrile women after 12 to 24 hours.

Treatment options for the various stages and types of mastitis are listed in Table 37-5.[63] Antibiotic treatment for less than 10 to 14 days is associated with recurrent mastitis. Vitamin E–rich sunflower,[64] Echinacea,[65] and vitamin C supplements[66] have also been mentioned as being helpful in prevention or treatment of mastitis, although scientific evidence of their effectiveness is lacking.

Urinary Tract Infection

Asymptomatic bacteriuria is present among as many as 17% of women on the first postpartum day, with spontaneous resolution occurring in approximately 75% by the third postpartum day.[68] Symptomatic urinary tract infections are the most common cause of postpartum febrile illness in the postpartum period. Risks include previous urinary tract infection, catheterization, multiple vaginal exams during labor, and trauma to the bladder or urethra during labor and birth.[1]

The choice of therapeutic agent is based on the specific organism involved, but because women have an increased risk for developing pyelonephritis during this time, empirical treatment generally is begun before urine culture results are available. The pathogens found in postpartum women are the same pathogens that cause urinary tract infections in pregnancy and in nonpregnant women; therefore, a 3-day course of trimethoprim–sulfamethoxazole (Bactrim, Septra) is the antibiotic regimen of choice unless the woman has an allergy to sulfa or resides in an area where there is known significant resistance to trimethoprim–sulfamethoxazole. This agent causes eradication of pathogens and cure in approximately 94% of women with urinary tract infections.[68] If trimethoprim–sulfamethoxazole is contraindicated, a 3-day course of ciprofloxacin (Cipro) or a 7-day course of nitrofurantoin (Macrodantin, Macrobid) can be substituted.

Table 37-5 Pharmacologic Treatments for Mastitis

Disorder	Antibiotics	Antifungal[a]	Other Therapy
Blocked duct/ nipple blebs	Mupirocin 2% ointment (not cream) if blocked pore (bleb) opened.	Only if recurrent or persistent, then culture the nipple/areola, bleb (if present), and milk. Fluconazole: (Diflucan) 200–400 mg × 1 dose followed by 100–200 mg daily for 2–3 weeks or until blocked duct has resolved for 1 week. Consider undiagnosed maternal IgA deficiency.	If no improvement within 24–48 hours, then order therapeutic ultrasound 2 watts/ cm^2, continuous, for 5 minutes once a day to the affected region. It may be repeated once the next day. Lecithin, 1 tablespoon per day or 1200 mg 3–4 times per day, can be used to prevent or treat recurrences. If recurrent, have the mother limit her intake of saturated fats and increase rest. Lecithin can also be rubbed into a bleb to soften it.
Noninfectious mastitis	If symptoms do not resolve within 12–24 hours, treat for infectious mastitis.	None	Hot compresses, massage of affected area, frequent milk removal on affected side.
Infectious mastitis	Dicloxacillin (Dynapen) 500 mg 4 times/ day for 10–14 days or cephalexin (Keflex) 500 mg 4 times/day for 10–14 days. If penicillin allergic, use clindamycin 300 mg 4 times/day or erythromycin 250 mg or 500 mg 4 times/day for 10–14 days.	If indicated based on cultures or the development of burning breast pain.	As noted for noninfectious mastitis. Cultures of milk and nipple are indicated for maternal acute illness, failure to respond to treatment, high suspicion of MRSA, and bilateral mastitis. The infant may need to be treated concurrently, particularly if group A or B *Streptococcus* is suspected.
Recurrent mastitis	Culture and treat as appropriate for 14–30 days.	Culture and treat as appropriate for 14–30 days.	Low-dose erythromycin or clindamycin may be given on a daily or weekly basis. Consider cultures and treatment with nasal mupirocin (Bactroban) if *S. aureus* carrier state is suspected.
Ductal infections	Culture and treat for at least 14 days. Can empirically start treatment with clindamycin 300 mg 4 times/day or sulfamethoxazole–trimethoprim (Bactrim) double strength 2 times/day.	Treat with antifungals if any signs of yeast on infant. First line: Fluconazole (Diflucan) 200–400 mg as one dose, followed by 100–200 mg daily for 2–3 weeks or until symptoms have resolved for 1 week. Ketoconazole (Nizoral) may also be used.	Sterilize any object that comes in contact with maternal breast, breast milk, or infant mouth (e.g., pumping parts, bottles, pacifiers, toys). Consider other family members as carriers if yeast is recurrent.
Nipple infections	Mupirocin 2% ointment (not cream): 15 g or polymyxin B sulfate (Bacitracin). If no improvement, culture and treat based on sensitivity results or treat empirically for yeast. Apply mupirocin or polymyxin after each nursing or pumping session.	Nystatin (Nilstat) Neonate: 100,000 units/mL. Place 1 mL in cup, then swab inside of infant's mouth 4 times/day. Use 2 mL 4 times/day for older infants. Have infant drink what is left. Maternal: May treat topically with nystatin suspension or with cream. Apply cream or suspension after each nursing. Allow suspension to air dry or, if using cream, rub in small amount. Gentian violet 1% in 10% alcohol can be applied to the infant's mouth with a cotton swab before feeding so the nipple will be coated during the feeding. Use daily for 4–7 days. Apply clotrimazole cream (Gyne-Lotrimin) after each feeding/pumping session and rub in well.	The topical treatment known as Dr. Newman's "All-Purpose Nipple Ointment" (APNO) will treat bacterial and yeast infections. APNO is compounded and contains mupirocin 2% ointment (not cream) 15 g. Betamethasone 0.1% ointment (not cream): 15 g. Add miconazole powder to formulate a final concentration of 2% miconazole. If miconazole is unavailable, substitute clotrimazole powder added so the final concentration is 2% clotrimazole. Sparingly apply APNO after each feeding and use until nipple soreness has dissipated.
Abscess (puerperal)	Outpatient: Dicloxacillin (Dynapen) 500 mg PO 4 times/day for 10–14 days or clindamycin (Cleocin) 300 mg PO 4 times/ day. Inpatient: Nafcillin or oxacillin 2.0 g every 4 hours IV or cefazolin 1.0 g every 6 hours IV or vancomycin 1.0 g every 12 hours IV.	If indicated based on cultures or the development of burning breast pain.	I and D (incision and drainage) or use ultrasound-guided needle for aspiration. Send aspirate or discharge for culture. Infants may continue nursing on affected side unless the area of incision involves the areola. May want to treat the infant concurrently if *S. aureus* or streptococcal disease is present.

Abbreviation: MRSA = methicillin-resistant *Staphylococcus aureus*.

[a] If *Candida* is suspected or diagnosed, the mother and the infant must be treated concurrently even if one is asymptomatic.

Source: Reprinted with permission from Betzhold CM. An update on the recognition and management of lactational breast inflammation. *J Midwifery Womens Health*. 2007;52(6):595-605.[63]

Trimethoprim–sulfamethoxazole should not be given to breastfeeding women whose infants have hyperbilirubinemia or who have known glucose-6-phosphate dehydrogenase (G6PD) deficiency. Because even a small amount of nitrofurantoin can cause a hemolytic reaction, it should not be prescribed to individuals who have a risk for G6PD deficiency. Trimethoprim–sulfamethoxazole and nitrofurantoin are considered compatible with breastfeeding by the American Academy of Pediatrics. Ciprofloxacin is also considered compatible with breastfeeding by the American Academy of Pediatrics, albeit not the first choice. Fluoroquinolone use during lactation has been controversial because juvenile animal studies have found an association between fluoroquinolones and cartilage damage.

Pyelonephritis is usually treated with hospitalization and ciprofloxacin (Cipro) or a combination of ampicillin (Principen) and gentamicin (Garamycin) administered intravenously until the fever and acute symptoms have subsided.

Endometritis

Postpartum endometritis is a polymicrobial infection involving several gram-positive or gram-negative aerobes and anaerobes. Many risk factors for endometritis exist, with cesarean birth—especially cesarean birth after labor—being the most prominent. The onset of this infection can occur either early (within 48 hours) or late (up to 6 weeks) in the postpartum period. Antibiotic treatment is initiated on the basis of fever and clinical symptoms such as uterine tenderness, foul-smelling lochia, chills, and lower abdominal pain. At present, a treatment regimen of clindamycin (Cleocin), 900 mg every 8 hours, and gentamicin (Garamycin), 1.5 mg/kg every 8 hours for women with normal renal function, administered intravenously is considered the gold standard and is often the control regimen for clinical trials of other treatment regimens.[69] Fever should resolve within 48–72 hours of treatment, and the antibiotics should be discontinued once the woman has been afebrile for 24 hours if she had a vaginal birth and after 48 hours if she had a cesarean section. Oral antibiotic therapy after intravenous therapy is not indicated.[69]

Postpartum Mood Disturbances

Puerperal changes often are discussed solely from a physiologic point of view. However, it is increasingly apparent that the psychological health of a woman can be at risk during this period of time. The vast majority of new mothers experience some degree of sadness and moodiness in the first 10 days after giving birth, and the incidence of postpartum depression is significant. A thorough discussion of treatments for postpartum mood disorders can be found in the *Mental Health* chapter.

Restarting Medications for Selected Chronic Health Conditions

Women with chronic conditions such as epilepsy, thyroid disease, hypertension, depression, thromboembolic disease, and diabetes will usually be counseled during pregnancy about appropriate use of usual medications during labor and after birth. In the postpartum period, it is rare that a previously used medication is contraindicated. However, several studies have shown significantly lower breastfeeding rates in women with chronic health conditions, presumably because their care providers were not aware of recommendations for medication use during lactation or the woman was fearful of problems with her newborn in spite of reassurance.[70,71] An overview of information concerning continued use of selected medications in postpartum women with coincidental health conditions is provided in Table 37-6.

Table 37-6 Postpartum Considerations for Medications to Treat Women with Selected Chronic Health Conditions

Commonly Used Medications Generic (Brand)	Clinical Considerations Regarding Transition to Postpartum Use/Precautions/Use in Breastfeeding
Diabetes	
Alpha-glucosidase inhibitors: Acarbose (Precose)	Low bioavailability, large molecular size, and water soluble. Unlikely to be excreted into breast milk in clinically significant amounts.
Biguanides: Metformin (Glucophage)	Nonsignificant amounts in breast milk. Compatible with breastfeeding.
Insulin	Insulin requirements are significantly lower in the first postpartum week compared with preconception requirements and remain significantly lower over the first 2 postpartum months. Not secreted in breast milk. Safe for breastfeeding, and breastfeeding should be encouraged to assist a rapid return to lower blood sugar levels.

Sulfonylureas: Tolbutamide (Orinase) Glyburide (Micronase) Glipizide (Glucotrol)	Tolbutamide is compatible with breastfeeding. Other sulfonylureas are less well studied. Glyburide and glipizide are highly protein bound and unlikely to pass into breast milk.[71]
Thiazolidinediones: Rosiglitazone (Avandia) Pioglitazone (Actos)	No studies have been done to date that have evaluated the passage of thiazolidinediones into breast milk. Thiazolidinediones are associated with risk for lactic acidosis and hepatotoxicity.
Epilepsy	
Sedative drugs: Phenobarbitol (Luminal) Mysoline (Primidone) Benzodiazepines: Carbamazepine (Tegretol) Diazepam (Valium) Lorazepam (Ativan) Alprazolam (Xanax) Oxcarbazepine (Trileptal) Phenytoin (Dilantin) Lamotrigine (Lamictal) Valproate (Depakote) Topiramate (Topamax) Gabapentin (Neurontin)	The best antiepileptic drug (AED) is the one that effectively controls seizures prior to pregnancy, using monotherapy and the lowest possible drug dose. However, the higher teratogenicity associated with valproate makes it less desirable for use. Changing drugs at any time, either antepartum or postpartum, exposes the fetus or newborn to an additional drug and should be avoided when possible. Hormonal contraceptive failure may occur with AEDs that are inducers of the hepatic cytochrome P450 system, such as carbamazepine, phenytoin, phenobarbital, primidone, topiramate, and oxcarbazepine. If AED dose has been changed during pregnancy, consider a return to the prepregnancy dose during the first few weeks postpartum. AEDs are not contraindicated during breastfeeding. Carbamazepine and phenytoin are preferred choices for women who are breastfeeding. The sedative AEDs may cause infant irritability, sleepiness, and failure to thrive, so the infant needs to be monitored closely if sedative AEDs are prescribed. Phenobarbital, primidone, and benzodiazepines are found in neonatal plasma for several days; infants of mothers receiving these medications prior to birth should be monitored for sedation and possibly neonatal withdrawal syndrome. Although valproate is considered compatible with breastfeeding, there is a potential for fatal hepatotoxicity in breastfed children younger than 2 years. Primidone should be avoided with breastfeeding.
Hypertension	
Beta blockers: Propranolol (Inderal) Metoprolol (Lopressor) Labetalol (Normodyne)	Listed medications have lowest transfer into breast milk. Atenolol (Tenormin), nadolol (Corgard), and sotalol (Betapace) are excreted in higher amounts that can lead to hypotension, bradycardia, and tachypnea in infants.
Thiazide diuretics	Excreted in small amounts into breast milk. Do not suppress lactation.
Angiotensin-converting enzyme (ACE) inhibitors	Use with caution in first few weeks postpartum in breastfeeding women due to possible effects on the neonate's kidneys.
Hyperthyroidism	
Beta blockers: Propranolol (Inderal)	Beta blockers are used to mitigate moderate to severe acute symptoms, and then use is decreased as symptoms resolve due to reports of occasional cases of neonatal growth restriction when prescribed for breastfeeding women. Thyroid storm precipitated by labor, infection, preeclampsia, or cesarean section is rare.
Methimazole (Tapazole)	Probable association with fetal developmental abnormalities such as choanal or esophageal atresia.
Thionamides: Propylthiouracil (PTU) (preferred)	Compatible with breastfeeding.
Radioactive iodine	Contraindicated in pregnancy and breastfeeding.
Hypothyroidism	
Levothyroxine	Most women will need the dose reduced to prepregnancy levels after delivery; measure serum TSH 4–6 weeks later.
Thromboembolic Disease	
Unfractionated heparin	Safe for use in lactation due to its high molecular weight, which means the molecule does not transfer into milk easily. Any heparin transferred into breast milk would be destroyed in the intestines of the baby.
Warfarin (Coumadin)	Considered safe in pregnancy. Possibly associated with prolonged prothrombin time in some infants. Infants should be monitored for signs and symptoms of bleeding.

Sources: Data from Abalovich M, Amino N, Barbour LA, et al. Management of thyroid dysfunction during pregnancy and postpartum: an Endocrine Society clinical practice guideline. *J Clin Endocrinol Metab.* 2007;92(8 suppl):S1-S47[71]; Kaplan MM. Management of thyroxine therapy during pregnancy. *Endocr Pract.* 1996;2(4):281-286[72]; Kuhnz W, Koch S, Helge H, Nau H. Primidone and phenobarbital during lactation period in epileptic women: total and free drug serum levels in the nursed infants and their effects on neonatal behavior. *Dev Pharmacol Ther.* 1988;11(3):147-154[73]; Saez- de-Ibarra L, Gaspar R, Obesso A, Herranz L. Glycaemic behaviour during lactation: postpartum practical guidelines for women with type 1 diabetes. *Practical Diabetes Int.* 2003;20(3):271-275[70]; Spencer JP, Gonzalez LS, Barnhart DJ. Medications in the breast-feeding mother. *Am Fam Physician.* 2001;64(1):119-126[69]; Tran TA, Leppik IE, Blesi K, Sathanandan ST, Remmel R. Lamotrigine clearance during pregnancy. *Neurology.* 2002;59:251.[74]

Conclusion

While most providers are sympathetic to the needs of new mothers, this relatively brief period in a woman's life cycle has not attracted the same interest and scientific inquiry as other life phases. Disease states, pregnancy, and labor have been more pressing or perhaps more interesting subjects for research. Far too many postpartum practices are in place simply because of tradition. While more research is now being conducted, there is much room for improvement in postpartum care. For the most part, women have done well, perhaps because the postpartum period is a normal event, designed to be uncomplicated. Women may do even better when evidence-based practice guides more of the pharmaceutical and nonpharmaceutical care they receive after having a baby, leaving them free to be mothers.

Resources

Organization	Description	Website
American Academy of Pediatrics and American Congress of Obstetricians and Gynecologists	*Guidelines for Perinatal* Care; updated frequently and provides professionals with general guidelines for care, including postpartum	http://reader.aappublications.org/guidelines-for-perinatal-care-7th-edition/4

Apps

An app for the U.S. Medical Eligibility Criteria, including the postpartum recommendations, can be found on iTunes and available from http://www.cdc.gov/reproductivehealth/unintendedpregnancy/usmec.htm.
Multiple consumer-oriented apps exist, including apps to help women keep track of when to take medications. These apps are available in iOS and android formats.
The Edinburgh Postpartum Depression Scale also can be found as one of several apps.

References

1. Fahey JO. Anatomy and physiology of postpartum. In: King TL, Brucker MC, Kriebs JM, Fahey JO, Gegor CL, Varney H, eds. *Varney's Midwifery.* 5th ed. Burlington, MA: Jones & Bartlett Learning; 2015:1101-1110.
2. Tingle AJ, Chantler JK, Pot KH, Paty DW, Ford DK. Postpartum rubella immunization: association with development of prolonged arthritis, neurological sequelae, and chronic rubella viremia. *J Infect Dis.* 1985;152(3):606-612.
3. Centers for Disease Control and Prevention. ACIP provisional updated recommendations on use of tetanus toxoid, reduced diphtheria toxoid and acellular pertussis vaccine (Tdap) for pregnant women. *ACIP Recommendations.* December 6, 2012:1.
4. Centers for Disease Control and Prevention. Advisory committee on immunization practices recommended immunization schedule for adults aged 19 years or older—United States, 2015. *MMWR.* 2015; 64(4):91-92.
5. Freda VJ, Gorman JG, Pollack W, Bowe E. Prevention of Rh hemolytic disease: ten years' clinical experience with Rh immune globulin. *N Engl J Med.* 1975;29(19):1014-1016.
6. Bowman JM, Chown B, Lewis M, Pollock JM. Rh isoimmunization during pregnancy: antenatal prophylaxis. *Can Med Assoc J.* 1978;118(6):623-627.
7. Samson D, Mollison PL. Effect on primary Rh immunization of delayed administration of anti-Rh. *Immunology.* 1975;28(2):349-357.
8. Hogan LS. Weak D effect on estimating fetal–maternal hemorrhage: a case study. *Clin Lab Sci.* 1998;11(4): 204-205.
9. Gyamfi C, Berkowitz RL. Responses by pregnant Jehovah's Witnesses on health care proxies. *Obstet Gynecol.* 2004;104(3):541-544.
10. Centers for Disease Control and Prevention. Revised ACIP recommendation for avoiding pregnancy after receiving a rubella-containing vaccine. *MMWR.* 2001;50(49):1117.
11. Lloyd KL. Protecting pregnant women, newborns, and families from pertussis. *J Midwifery Womens Health.* 2013:58(3):288-296.
12. McIntyre P, Wood N. Pertussis in early infancy: disease burden and preventive strategies. *Curr Opin Infect Dis.* 2009;22(3):215-223.
13. Weiss R, Fogelman Y, Bennett M. Severe vitamin B_{12} deficiency in an infant associated with a maternal deficiency and a strict vegetarian diet. *J Pediatr Hematol Oncol.* 2004;26(4):270-271.
14. Centers for Disease Control and Prevention. U.S. medical eligibility criteria for contraceptive use, 2010. *MMWR.* 2010;59(RR-4). http://www.cdc.gov/mmwr/preview/mmwrhtml/rr5904a1.htm. Accessed August 30, 2014.
15. Centers for Disease Control and Prevention. Update to CDC's U.S. medical eligibility criteria for

contraceptive use, 2012: revised recommendations for the use of hormonal contraception among women at high risk for HIV infection or infected with HIV. *MMWR.* 2012;61(24):449-452.

16. Madadi P, Ross CJ, Haydon MR, et al. Pharmacogenetics of neonatal opioid toxicity following maternal use of codeine during breastfeeding. *Clin Pharmacol Ther.* 2009;85(1):31-35.
17. U.S. Food and Drug Administration. Public health advisory: use of codeine by some breastfeeding mothers may lead to life-threatening side effects in nursing babies. http://www.fda.gov/Safety/MedWatch/SafetyInformation/SafetyAlertsforHumanMedicalProducts/ucm152107.htm. Accessed July 30, 2014.
18. Montgomery A, Hale T. Academy of Breastfeeding Medicine Clinical Protocol No. 15: analgesia and anesthesia for the breastfeeding mother. *Breastfeed Med.* 2012;7(6):548-553.
19. Clark JH, Wilson WG. A 16-day-old breast-fed infant with metabolic acidosis caused by salicylate. *Clin Pediatr (Phila).* 1981;20(1):53-54.
20. Koren G, Cairns J, Chitayat D, Gaedigk A, Leeder SJ. Pharmacogenetics of morphine poisoning in a breastfed neonate of a codeine-prescribed mother. *Lancet.* 2006;368(9536):704.
21. Windle ML, Booker LA, Rayburn WF. Postpartum pain after vaginal delivery: a review of comparative analgesic trials. *J Reprod Med.* 1989;34(11):891-895.
22. Anderson PO, Sauberan JB, Lane JR, Rossi SS. Hydrocodone excretion into breast milk: the first 2 reported cases. *Breastfeeding Med.* 2007;2(1):10-14.
23. Pavy TJG, Paech MJ, Evans SF. The effect of intravenous ketorolac on opioid requirement and pain after cesarean delivery. *Anesth Analg.* 2001;92(4):1010-1014.
24. Ke RW. A preemptive strike against surgical pain. *Contem Ob Gyn.* 2001;46(1):65-70.
25. Rosaeg OP, Lui AC, Cicutti NJ, Bragg PR, Crossan ML, Krepski B. Peri-operative multimodal pain therapy for caesarean section: analgesia and fitness for discharge. *Can J Anaesth.* 1997;44(8):803-809.
26. Pasero C. Multimodal balanced analgesia in the PACU. *J Perinaesthesia Nurs.* 2003;18(4):265-268.
27. Lowder JL, Shackelford DP, Holbert D, Beste TM. A randomized, controlled trial to compare ketorolac tromethamine versus placebo after cesarean section to reduce pain and narcotic usage. *Am J Obstet Gynecol.* 2003;189(6):1559-1562.
28. World Health Organization. *Cancer pain relief.* Geneva, Switzerland: WHO; 1986:51.
29. Fredman B, Shapiro A, Zohar E, et al. The analgesic efficacy of patient-controlled ropivacaine instillation after cesarean delivery. *Anesth Analg.* 2000;91(6):1436-1440.
30. Givens VA, Lipscomb GH, Meyer NL. A randomized trial of postoperative wound irrigation with local anesthetic for pain after cesarean delivery. *Am J Obstet Gynecol.* 2002;186(6):1188-1191.
31. Davis KM, Esposito MA, Meyer BA. Oral analgesia compared with intravenous patient-controlled analgesia for pain after cesarean delivery: a randomized controlled trial. *Am J Obstet Gynecol.* 2006;194(4):967-971.
32. Meyer M, Wagner K, Benvenuto A, Plante D, Howard D. Intrapartum and postpartum analgesia for women maintained on methadone during pregnancy. *Obstet Gynecol.* 2007;110(2 pt 1):261-266.
33. Murray A, Holdcroft A. Incidence and intensity of postpartum lower abdominal pain. *Br Med J.* 1989;298(6688):1619.
34. Holdcroft A, Snidvongs S, Cason A, Doré CJ Berkley KJ. Pain and uterine contractions during breast feeding in the immediate post-partum period increase with parity. *Pain.* 2003;104(3):589-596.
35. Gutke A, Ostgaard HC, Oberg B. Predicting persistent pregnancy-related low back pain. *Spine.* 2008;33(12):E386-E393.
36. Thomas L, Ptak H, Giddings LS, et al. The effects of rocking, diet modifications, and antiflatulent medication on postcesarean section gas pain. *J Perinatal Neonatal Nurs.* 1990;4(3):12-24.
37. East CE, Begg L, Henshall NE, Marchant PR, Wallace K. Local cooling for relieving pain from perineal trauma sustained during childbirth. *Cochrane Database Syst Rev.* 2012;5:CD006304. doi:10.1002/14651858.CD006304.pub3.
38. Hubb AJ, Orr KL, Stockdale CK. Puerperal vulvar edema and hematoma complicated by overuse of cold therapy: a report of two cases. *Am Soc Colposcopy Cervical Pathol.* 2014;19(2):1-4.
39. Dale A, Cornwell S. The role of lavender oil in relieving perineal discomfort following childbirth: a blind randomized clinical trial. *J Adv Nurs.* 1994;19(1):89-96.
40. Meyer H. Postpartum care of the perineum: the use of a topical anesthetic spray. *J La State Med Soc.* 1964;116(6):221-222.
41. Moore W, James DK. A random trial of three topical analgesic agents in the treatment of episiotomy pain following instrumental vaginal delivery. *J Obstet Gynaecol.* 1989;10(1):35-39.

42. Bouis PJ, Martinez LA, Hambrick TL. Epifoam (hydrocortisone acetate) in the treatment of postepisiotomy patients. *Curr Ther Res.* 1981;30(6):912-916.
43. Minassian VA, Jazayeri A, Prien SD, Timmons RL, Stumbo K. Randomized trial of lidocaine ointment versus placebo for the treatment of postpartum perineal pain. *Obstet Gynecol.* 2002;100(6):1239-1243.
44. Hedayati H, Parsons J, Crowther CA. Topically applied anaesthetics for treating perineal pain after childbirth. *Cochrane Database Syst Rev.* 2005;2:CD004223. doi:10.1002/14651858.CD004223.pub2.
45. Hedayati H, Parsons J, Crowther CA. Rectal analgesia for pain from perineal trauma following childbirth. *Cochrane Database Syst Rev.* 2003;3:CD003931. doi:10.1002/14651858.CD003931.
46. Stevinson C, Devaraj VS, Fountain-Barber A, Hawkins S, Ernst E. Homeopathic arnica for prevention of pain and bruising: randomized placebo-controlled trial in hand surgery. *J R Soc Med.* 2003;96(2):60-65.
47. Alonso-Coello P, Guyatt GH, Heels-Ansdell D, et al. Laxatives for the treatment of hemorrhoids. *Cochrane Database Syst Rev.* 2005;4:CD004649. doi:10.1002/14651858.CD004649.pub2.
48. Shafik A. Role of warm-water bath in the anorectal conditions: the "thermosphincteric reflex." *J Clin Gastroenterol.* 1993;16(4):304-308.
49. Schindler AM. Isolated neonatal hypomagnesaemia associated with maternal overuse of stool softener. *Lancet.* 1984;2(8406):822.
50. Torrabadella L, Salgado G. Controlled dose delivery in topical treatment of anal fissure: pilot study of a new paradigm. *Dis Colon Rectum.* 2005;49(6):865-868.
51. Jimenez ER, Whitney-Caglia L. Treatment of chronic lower extremity wound pain with nitroglycerin ointment. *J Wound Ostomy Continence Nurs.* 2012; 39(6):649-652.
52. Yip SK, Sahota D, Pang MW, Day L. Postpartum urinary retention. *Obstet Gynecol.* 2005;106(3): 602-606.
53. Handler SJ, Cheng YW, Knight S, Lyell D, Caughery AB. What factors are associated with postpartum urinary retention? *Am J Obstet Gynecol.* 2011; 204(1 suppl):S79.
54. Mulder FE, Schoffelmeer RA, Limpens J, et al. Risk factors for postpartum urinary retention: a systematic review and meta-analysis. *Obstet Anesth Dig.* 2014;34(1):14.
55. Salemnic Y, Gold R, Toov JH, et al. Prevalence, obstetric risk factors and natural history of asymptomatic postpartum urinary retention after first vaginal delivery: a prospective study of 200 primipara women. *J Urol.* 2012;187(4S):e788.
56. Dodds P, Hans AL. Distended urinary bladder drainage practices among hospital nurses. *Appl Nurs Res.* 1990;3(2):68-69.
57. Wisniewski PM, Wilkinson EG. Postpartum vaginal atrophy. *Am J Obstet Gynecol.* 1991;165(4 pt 2): 1249-1254.
58. Buetler E. Disorders of iron metabolism. In: Kaushanshky K, Lichtman MA, Buetler E, Kipps TJ, Seligsohn U, Prchal JT, eds. *Williams Hematology.* 8th ed. New York: McGraw-Hill Medical; 2010: 565-606.
59. Nelson GH, Donnell S, Griffin G, Nelson RM. Timing of postpartum hematocrit determinations. *Southern Med J.* 1980;73(9):1202-1204.
60. Goodnough LT, Nemeth E. Iron deficiency and related disorders. In: Greer JP, Arber DA, Glader B, et al., eds. *Wintrobe's Clinical Hematology.* 13th ed. Philadelphia, PA: Lippincott Williams & Wilkins; 2014: 617-642.
61. Filker R, Monif G. The significance of temperature during the first 24 hours postpartum. *Obstet Gynecol.* 1979;53(3):358-361.
62. Mantha VR, Vallejo MC, Ramesh V, Phelps AL, Ramanthan S. The incidence of maternal fever during labor with intermittent than with continuous epidural analgesia: a randomized controlled trial. *Int J Obstet Anesth.* 2008;17(2):123-129.
63. Betzhold CM. An update on the recognition and management of lactational breast inflammation. *J Midwifery Womens Health.* 2007;52(6):595-605.
64. Filteau SM, Lietz G, Mulokozi G, Bilotta S, Henry CJ, Tomkins AM. Milk cytokines and subclinical breast inflammation in Tanzanian women: effect of dietary red palm oil or sunflower oil supplementation. *Immunology.* 1999;97(4):595-600.
65. Binns SE. Light-mediated antifungal activity of Echinacea extracts. *Plant Med.* 2000;66(3):241-244.
66. Kettle C, Dowswell T, Ismail KMK. Continuous and interrupted suturing techniques for repair of episiotomy or second-degree tears. *Cochrane Database Syst Rev.* 2012;11:CD000947. doi:10.1002/14651858.CD000947.pub3.
67. Marraro RV, Harris RE. Incidence and spontaneous resolution of postpartum bacteriuria. *Am J Obstet Gynecol.* 1977;128(7):722-723.

68. Karsnitz DB. Puerperal infections of the genital tract: a clinical review. *J Midwifery Womens Health.* 2013;58(6):632-642.
69. Spencer JP, Gonzalez LS, Barnhart DJ. Medications in the breast-feeding mother. *Am Fam Physician.* 2001;64(1):119-126.
70. Saez-de-Ibarra L, Gaspar R, Obesso A, Herranz L. Glycaemic behaviour during lactation: postpartum practical guidelines for women with type 1 diabetes. *Practical Diabetes Int.* 2003;20(3):271-275.
71. Abalovich M, Amino N, Barbour LA, et al. Management of thyroid dysfunction during pregnancy and postpartum: an Endocrine Society clinical practice guideline. *J Clin Endocrinol Metab.* 2007;92 (8 suppl):S1-S47.
72. Kaplan MM. Management of thyroxine therapy during pregnancy. *Endocr Pract.* 1996;2(4): 281-286.
73. Kuhnz W, Koch S, Helge H, Nau H. Primidone and phenobarbital during lactation period in epileptic women: total and free drug serum levels in the nursed infants and their effects on neonatal behavior. *Dev Pharmacol Ther.* 1988;11(3):147-154.
74. Tran TA, Leppik IE, Blesi K, Sathanandan ST, Remmel R. Lamotrigine clearance during pregnancy. *Neurology.* 2002;59:251.

38 Breastfeeding

Teresa E. Baker, Thomas W. Hale

Chapter Glossary

Absolute infant dose (AID) Estimate of the drug concentration in milk (per milliliter), which is calculated by multiplying the volume of breast milk ingested per day by either the maximum or the average concentration of drug in breast milk per day.

Colostrum Liquid produced and secreted by lactocytes prior to lactogenesis. Colostrum has limited fat but large amounts of the maternal immunoglobulins necessary for stimulating the infant's immune system.

Dopamine agonist Drug whose actions mimic dopamine. Dopamine agonists are prolactin antagonists and inhibit milk production.

Dopamine antagonists Drugs that inhibit dopamine by preventing the usual effect dopamine has in maintaining prolactin storage within the lactotrophs in the pituitary gland. When dopamine is inhibited, prolactin is released from the pituitary.

Galactagogue Drug that induces milk production.

Human *ether-a-go-go*-related gene (HERG) Gene that encodes for the potassium ion channel that repolarizes the current in the cardiac action potential. Many drugs can bind to this channel and alter its function, thereby resulting in a prolonged QT interval.

Lactocytes Secretory epithelial cells within the alveoli of the breast. The lactocytes produce and secrete breast milk.

Lactogenesis I Stage of mammary gland development in which the lactocytes have the ability to produce and secrete colostrum. This stage ends when lactogenesis II starts.

Lactogenesis II Onset of breast milk secretion, which occurs about 40 hours after birth.

Milk/plasma (M/P) Ratio of the concentration of a drug in breast milk to the concentration of the same drug in maternal plasma. This ratio quantifies the amount of drug that is transferred into the breast milk based on the amount that is bioavailable in the maternal plasma.

Relative infant dose (RID) Estimate of the weight-normalized infant dose of a drug relative to the mother's dose of the same drug.

Introduction

Breast milk is the infant's first and perfect choice for protection against infectious disease during the first year of life.[1] Not only is breast milk perfectly suited for the infant's gastrointestinal tract, but numerous growth factors in breast milk enhance the growth and maturation of the infant's relatively permeable gastrointestinal tract. Breast milk components also modify the infant's gastrointestinal (GI) bacterial environment so that it is best suited for the gastrointestinal tract of the infant. This is done by enhancing the growth of bifidus bacterium and reducing the growth of hazardous bacteria.

The benefits from breastfeeding extend to the mother as well. Women who breastfeed have enhanced weight loss and a major reduction in breast cancer risk compared to women who do not breastfeed. Numerous studies now suggest that the longer a woman breastfeeds, the greater the reduction in her risk of breast cancer.[2] While recent studies have clearly suggested that the number of women who choose to breastfeed is rising (approximately

76% of new mothers currently initiate breastfeeding in the United States), it is known that many women are advised to discontinue breastfeeding when they are prescribed other medications.

While the drugs used early postnatally primarily include analgesics, methylergonovine (Methergine), antihypertensives, and sedatives, many other new mothers are now taking antidepressants, antipsychotics, anticonvulsants, antibiotics, steroids, and medications from other drug categories. Hence, the number of medications to which a nursing infant may be exposed appears to be increasing. This chapter describes the physiology and anatomy of the breast, reviews the biochemistry of milk production, details the transfer of medications into breast milk, and discusses the implications of this transfer for the infant.

Although the American Academy of Pediatrics[1] and others[3] have published compendia that provide data about the relative safety of many medications, some newer medications have not yet been studied, and some background on the pharmacokinetics of drug entry into breast milk is in order. Therefore, this chapter identifies methods that clinicians can use to properly evaluate the safety of medications used by breastfeeding women, and how to evaluate medications for which data are lacking. Recommending that a woman discontinue breastfeeding due to medication exposure is almost never required and should be done only as a last resort.

The Alveolar Subunit and Breast Milk Production

Whereas the anatomy of the human breast is to some degree well understood, many biologic principles of human milk synthesis remain poorly understood. Figure 38-1 depicts the anatomy of the breast, including the ductal system. Milk ducts start in the extensive lobular alveolar clusters, and terminate at the nipple, as illustrated in Figure 38-2. Each alveolus is lined with a single layer of polarized secretory epithelial cells called **lactocytes** that are uniquely capable of synthesizing milk. The layer of lactocytes is itself surrounded by a basketlike network of specialized smooth muscle cells called the *myoepithelial cells*. These specialized smooth muscle cells have receptors for oxytocin. When the myoepithelial cells are stimulated by the release of oxytocin from the pituitary, they contract and milk is forced out of the alveoli and into the terminal ductal system near the nipple.

During pregnancy, the size and number of the alveolar complexes increase significantly due to the high levels of maternal estrogen, progesterone, placental lactogen, prolactin, and oxytocin, all of which act directly on the mammary gland to bring about developmental changes.[4] Lactocytes, however, remain small in size and poorly functional, largely due to high circulating levels of progesterone.

In the early postpartum period, the initial fluid secreted by the lactocytes is called **colostrum**; the stage featuring production of colostrum is referred to as **lactogenesis I**. Colostrum has limited fat and small volume, averaging less than 60 mL the first few days. During this early postnatal stage of development, large intercellular gaps exist between lactocytes, such that numerous components from the maternal plasma compartment are able to leak into colostrum. These components include immunoglobulins (IgG, IgA, IgM, and IgE), macrophages, lymphocytes, and leukocytes, among others.

Colostrum is believed to be critical for maturation of the newborn's GI tract because it provides numerous growth factors, such as IGF-1, and maternal antibodies

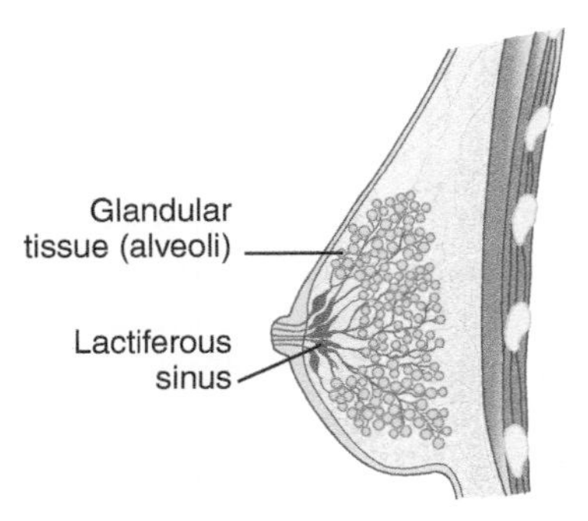

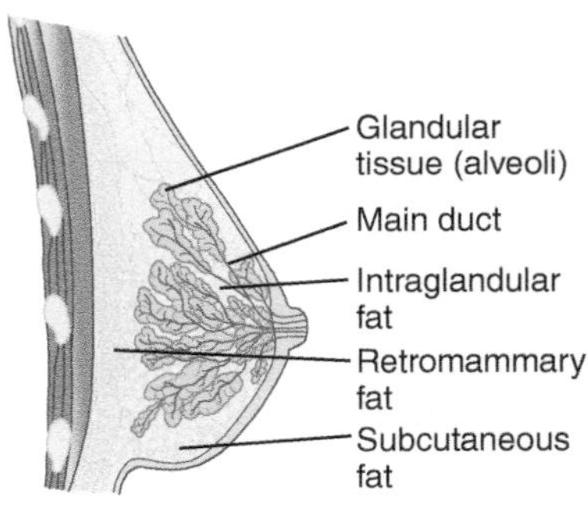

Figure 38-1 A schematic drawing of the anatomy of the human breast.

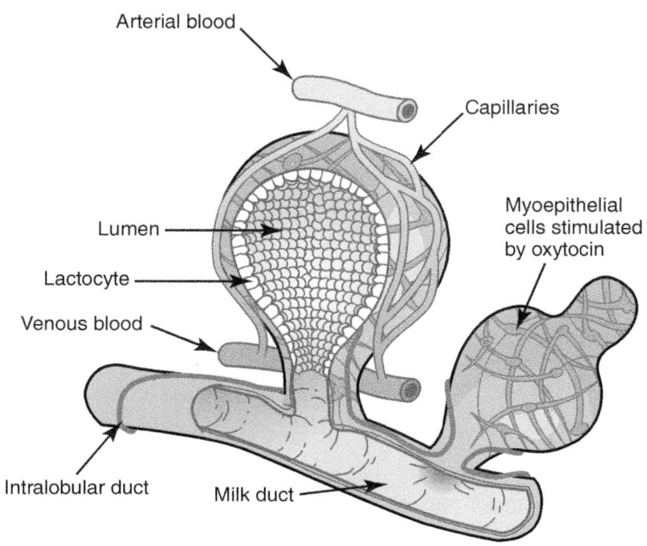

Figure 38-2 Structure of the alveolar subunit with blood supply and milk-creating lactocytes.

that suppress hazardous bacterial growth and promote beneficial bacterial colonization.

After delivery of the placenta, maternal estrogen and progesterone levels drop to below prepregnancy levels. Approximately 40 hours after delivery of the placenta, plasma progesterone levels are at a nadir, and copious milk production ensues (secretory activation or **lactogenesis II**). During lactogenesis II prolactin stimulates the lactocytes to produce milk, and the lactocytes connect to one another via an apical junctional complex that inhibits direct paracellular exchange of substances from the maternal compartment into the breast milk compartment. This tight cell-to-cell junction persists until lactation ceases, whereupon the lactocytes begin to involute and shrink in size.

Prolactin is the driving force behind milk synthesis. Much of the physiology and release of prolactin production by the pituitary is understood. Less well known is how prolactin actually stimulates or supports milk synthesis by the lactocytes in the breast. Thus, when evaluating drug use in breastfeeding women, one must always first evaluate the effect the drug may have on prolactin and milk production.

Drugs That Inhibit Milk Production

Because weight gain and development of a breastfeeding infant are directly linked to milk production and milk volume, even modest changes in milk supply can have profound effects on the child. Thus, the use of various medications that inhibit or stimulate prolactin levels will have significant effects on milk synthesis. Box 38-1 lists commonly used medications that may inhibit milk production.

Estrogen and Progesterone

Drugs that can suppress prolactin release include the estrogens and the progestins.

Historically, large doses estrogen were used to suppress lactation in women who did not choose to breastfeed. It has long been thought that contraceptive doses of estrogens suppress milk production and could also adversely affect infant growth and development if passed into the breast milk. However, estrogen doses of greater than 30 mcg per day are needed to suppress lactation; the dose in current contraceptive formulations, therefore, is likely to be lower than that needed for lactation suppression. Studies that have compared milk production and infant growth in women who used hormonal contraception and women who did not use oral contraception have produced conflicting results.[5] In addition, the quality of these studies has not been sufficiently high to permit researchers to draw clinically helpful conclusions.[5] Given the possibility of adverse effects associated with estrogen use during lactation and the importance of breastfeeding for the infant, both the World Health Organization (WHO)[6] and the Centers for Disease Control and Prevention (CDC)[7] have established medical eligibility criteria for contraception that addresses

Box 38-1 Drugs That May Inhibit Breast Milk Production

Generic (Brand)

Alcohol in large amounts
Bromocriptine (Parlodel)
Cabergoline (Dostinex)
Estrogen-containing contraceptives
Ergotamine (Cafergot)
Progestins
Pseudoephedrine (Sudafed)
Testosterone
Tamoxifen and other estrogen-receptor blockers
Bupropion (Wellbutrin)[a]

[a] The risk to a newborn from exposure to bupropion via breast milk is theoretical.

Table 38-1 Medical Eligibility Criteria for Contraceptive Use by Breastfeeding Women

Risk Category	World Health Organization	U.S. Medical Eligibility Criteria
Estrogen-Containing Contraceptive Products		
Category 4	< 6 weeks postpartum	< 21 days postpartum
Category 3	≥ 6 weeks postpartum and 6 months postpartum	21–42 days postpartum if risk factors for VTE are present
Category 2	≥ 6 weeks postpartum	21–42 days postpartum if risk factors for VTE are not present
Category 1		> 42 days postpartum
Progestin-Only Contraceptive Products		
Category 3	< 6 weeks postpartum	NA
Category 2	NA	< 1 month postpartum
Category 1	≥ 6 weeks postpartum	> 6 weeks postpartum

Abbreviation: VTE = venous thromboembolism.
Category 1: A condition for which there is no restriction for the use of the contraceptive method.
Category 2: A condition for which the advantages of using the method generally outweigh the theoretical or proven risks.
Category 3: A condition for which the theoretical or proven risks usually outweigh the advantages of using the method.
Category 4: A condition that represents an unacceptable health risk if the contraceptive method is used.

Sources: Data from Update to CDC's U.S. Medical Eligibility Criteria for Contraceptive Use, 2010: revised recommendations for the use of contraceptive methods during the postpartum period. *MMWR.* July 30, 2011. http://www.cdc.gov/mmwr/preview/ mmwrhtml/mm6026a3.htm#tab1. Accessed July 30, 2011[7]; World Health Organization Medical Eligibility Criteria, 4th ed. 2009. http://whqlibdoc.who.int/publications/2010/9789241563888_eng.pdf.[6]

use of estrogen-containing contraceptive products by breastfeeding women. The WHO criteria were designed as broad global recommendations and the U.S. criteria address the population of reproductive age women who reside in the United States (Table 38-1).

As progesterone is the primary inhibitor of lactation during gestation, progestins used early postnatally (in the first 48 hours after delivery) could also theoretically impede the activation of the lactocytes by prolactin. Research conducted to date has not yielded strong evidence supporting this effect. Use of progestin-only contraceptives is classified into U.S. Medical Eligibility Criteria (MEC) Category 2 (i.e., the advantages of the using the contraceptive method outweigh the theoretical risks associated with the method) during the first month postpartum and Category 1 (i.e., there is no restriction for use of the contraceptive method) thereafter for breastfeeding women. However, even when initiated after 6 weeks postpartum, some women report a reduction in milk synthesis when using progestin-only contraceptives. Because hormonal agents such as estrogen or progesterone may theoretically decrease milk production, women should be informed of the possible risk during prenatal and/or postpartum contraception counseling.

Bromocriptine (Parlodel)

Bromocriptine (Parlodel) is a **dopamine agonist** and a prolactin antagonist. In the past, this agent was used to reduce engorgement and inhibit milk production in women who chose not to breastfeed. However, it was found to be associated with numerous cases of cardiac dysrhythmias, stroke, intracranial bleeding, cerebral edema, convulsions, and myocardial infarction; thus bromocriptine is no longer approved for lactation suppression.[8]

Cabergoline (Dostinex)

A drug occasionally used to treat Parkinson's disease or hyperprolactinemia, cabergoline (Dostinex), is also a dopamine agonist. It, too, suppresses milk production but may also have adverse cardiac effects. Lactating women should avoid cabergoline.

Pseudoephedrine (Sudafed)

In one study published in 2003, the nasal decongestant pseudoephedrine (Sudafed) was shown to suppress milk production.[9] Studies of this agent are still preliminary, but women who choose to breastfeed should be cautious when using pseudoephedrine, particularly if they are at late-stage lactation (> 8 months) or have a poor milk supply.

Drugs That Stimulate Milk Production

The majority of women who produce insufficient milk do so as a result of infrequent emptying of the breasts, engorgement, poor infant latch, or other factors that can usually be rectified in the early postpartum period. In many of these women, milk production may be recovered by proper management, and in some instances the use of various **galactagogues**, including some **dopamine antagonists**.

Milk production is a complex process, much of which remains poorly understood. During pregnancy, breast tissue should enlarge significantly under the influence of progesterone and estrogen. These hormones stimulate growth and development of the ductal and alveolar system in the breast. Lack of breast tissue growth may foreshadow lack of full development of lactogenesis II. Other etiologies of failed lactogenesis II include thyroid dysfunction, pituitary disorders, retained placental tissue, and gestational ovarian theca lutein cysts.[10]

Following birth, gestational prolactin levels initially are quite high (as high as 400 ng/mL), but over the next 6 months, these levels drop significantly (to approximately 80 ng/mL), even though milk production levels are virtually unchanged.[11] Thus, as long as the levels of prolactin are slightly higher than baseline (at least 50–70 ng/mL), most women can produce large quantities of milk. However, as prolactin levels drop to near prepregnancy (10–20 ng/mL) levels, the production of milk suffers.

In women who have low prolactin levels, dopamine antagonist medications that inhibit dopamine receptors in the hypothalamus, such as metoclopramide (Reglan) or domperidone (Motilium), can be used as galactagogues. Prolactin is stored in the lactotrophs of the pituitary under the inhibitory influence of dopamine. If dopamine production is blocked, then prolactin is released from the lactotrophs and enters the plasma compartment. Dopamine-receptor antagonists dramatically stimulate maternal prolactin levels and, therefore, milk production, but only in those women with low prolactin levels (< 50 ng/mL). Other dopamine antagonists, such as risperidone (Risperdal), chlorpromazine (Thorazine), and other phenothiazine neuroleptics, are all well-known agents that stimulate milk production, even in males (resulting in clinical gynecomastia). The two drugs most commonly used to stimulate milk production in breastfeeding women are metoclopramide (Reglan)[12,13] and domperidone (Motilium); however, the latter agent is not available in the United States.

Metoclopramide (Reglan)

Metoclopramide (Reglan) can, in some cases, induce milk production as much as 100%, by stimulating the release of prolactin.[12,13] However, it is difficult to predict which women will respond to this drug with elevated milk synthesis. Theory would suggest this agent would be most useful for women whose prolactin levels were originally high but have dropped.

The prolactin-stimulating effect of metoclopramide is dose related. The standard dose required for effectiveness is 10–15 mg given orally 3 times per day for a maximum dosage of 30–45 mg per day.[13] Milk production normally responds quickly, with the woman noticing significant increases of milk volume within 24–48 hours. The dose of metoclopramide present in milk is small, approximately 45 mcg/L, in the early puerperium.[14] This dose is far less than the clinical dose administered directly to infants (800 mcg/kg/day) for other conditions.

Side Effects/Adverse Effects

While milk synthesis may rebound efficiently, metoclopramide does cross the blood–brain barrier. In turn, a drug-induced depression can occur in women who take metoclopramide for more than 3 weeks. Other adverse effects include extrapyramidal symptoms, gastric cramping, and tardive dyskinesia. Although one must be alert to the possibility of these adverse effects, their occurrence is rare. Currently, metoclopramide is recommended for a duration of a maximum of 1 month with a 3- to 4-week slow weaning when it is discontinued.

Domperidone (Motilium)

Domperidone (Motilium) is a dopamine antagonist used outside the United States that stimulates prolactin levels. It is possibly safer than metoclopramide because it does not penetrate the blood–brain barrier. However, domperidone was banned by the Food and Drug Administration (FDA) secondary to reports of cardiac arrhythmia and sudden death among individuals with cancer.[13,14] Numerous studies have found that domperidone stimulates milk production quite well.[14,15] Levels of domperidone in milk are extraordinarily low, secondary to its significant first-pass metabolism and high protein binding.[14] Two recent dosing studies have shown that higher maternal doses are not necessary. The plasma levels of prolactin in women who take 10 mg twice daily are no different than those in women who take 20 mg twice daily, although milk production was slightly higher in the groups taking 20 mg doses.[16] Hence, doses higher than 20 mg twice daily should be avoided, as they may increase the risk of cardiac arrhythmia.

Side Effects/Adverse Effects

Unfortunately, domperidone is an antagonist to the **human *ether-a-go-go*-related gene (HERG)** potassium channel receptor. Because the HERG potassium channel repolarizes the cardiac action potential, use of domperidone may cause minor arrhythmias. While the FDA has issued a black box warning that recommends domperidone not be used to stimulate milk production, the world community outside of the United States has largely ignored this warning, and domperidone remains the preferred galactagogue in other countries.

Because a woman's milk supply depends on an elevated prolactin level, the precipitous withdrawal of a galactagogue may result in a significant loss of milk supply. A slow taper of the drug is generally recommended over several weeks to a month to prevent loss of milk supply.

Passage of Drugs Across the Alveolar Epithelium into Breast Milk

The passage of drugs, protein, and lipids across the apical membrane of the breast alveolar cell and into breast milk is affected by many factors, including lipid solubility, molecular weight of the drug, pH differentials, and protein binding. Most drugs move from the maternal compartment into the breast milk compartment via simple diffusion across a concentration gradient. Diffusion and paracellular diffusion for drug entry into milk are illustrated in Figure 38-3.[17] Drug transfer into breast milk is largely a result of equilibrium forces between the maternal plasma and the milk compartment. As maternal plasma levels of a drug rise, the medication is subsequently forced over into the milk compartment. While influx transporters exist for a few drugs (e.g., ranitidine [Zantac], nitrofurantoin [Macrobid], acyclovir [Zovirax], and iodine), most drugs enter breast milk by simple diffuse across the alveolar bilayer membranes from an area of higher concentration (maternal plasma) to an area of lower concentration (milk). Subsequently, the drugs maintain a close equilibrium with the plasma compartment, diffusing into and out of milk largely as a function of the maternal plasma level.

Molecular Weight of the Drug

The passive diffusion of medication across the lipid bilayer that forms the lactocyte cell wall is largely determined by the molecular weight of the compound. The lower the molecular weight (< 500 daltons), the more likely the drug is to transfer into breast milk. Drugs larger than 800 daltons seldom reach clinically relevant levels in milk. Any drug larger than 1000 daltons is unlikely to enter breast milk in clinically relevant amounts. Very large molecules, such as heparin (12,000–15,000 daltons), are largely excluded from breast milk. It is now apparent that many IgG preparations, such as infliximab (Remicade) and etanercept (Enbrel), are virtually excluded from the milk compartment as well. Likewise, high-molecular-weight products like beta interferons minimally transfer into breast milk.[18] In contrast, a medication such as lithium (Lithobid), which has no protein binding and a low molecular weight of 6.94 daltons, readily enters the milk compartment and can achieve high levels in breast milk.

Lipid Solubility of the Drug

The lipid content of milk is high, ranging from 2.3% in foremilk to as high as 8% in hindmilk. The lipophilicity of a drug is measured by its octanol: water partition coefficient ($\log_{10}P$). The more lipid soluble a drug, the better able it is to penetrate through the lipid bilayer of the cell membrane of the lactocytes and become concentrated in the milk compartment. Such drugs are often those that readily

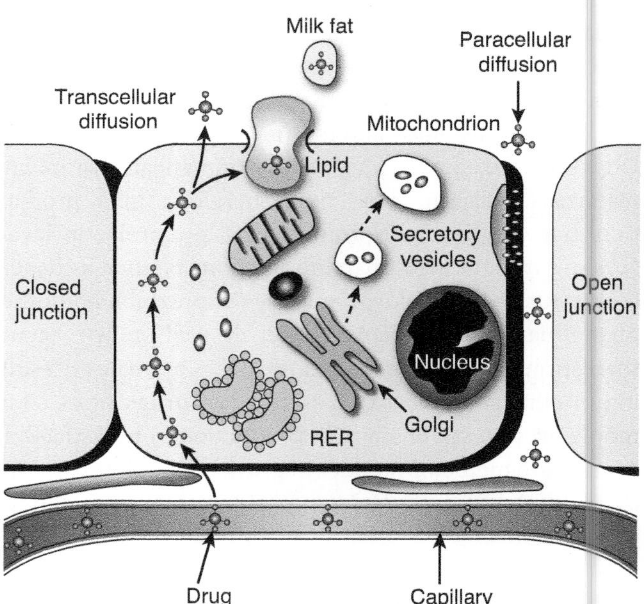

Figure 38-3 Diagrammatic representation of the various pathways for drug transfer into the breast milk compartment.

Source: Reprinted with permission from Hale TW, Hartmann PE, eds. *Textbook of Human Lactation*. Amarillo, TX: Hale; 2007.[17]

penetrate the blood–brain barrier and reach high levels in the central nervous system (CNS); the antidepressant mirtazapine (Remeron) is a classic example. The concentration of mirtazapine in hindmilk (high lipid content) is 2.3 times higher than that in foremilk (low lipid content). Thus, if a drug is active in the CNS, it may attain high levels in breast milk as well.

Milk pH and Drug pK_a

The pK_a of a drug is a unique physicochemical property that controls its ionization state when the drug is in solution. If the pH of the solution in which the drug exists is the same as its pK_a, then 50% of the drug exists in an ionized form and 50% exists in a non-ionized form. As the pH of the solution changes, the state of ionization changes as well. If the drug is relatively un-ionized at a pH of 7.4 in the plasma, once it enters the breast milk (pH = 7.2), it may become more ionized and, then become trapped in the milk compartment. In general, drugs with a pK_a higher than 7.4 may become significantly trapped in the milk compartment.[19]

Protein Binding

Most drugs travel in plasma bound to albumin or other plasma proteins. Those with high binding affinity have difficulty diffusing out of the plasma compartment. Thus, only the free drug is available to transfer into peripheral compartments. This is especially true with respect to breast milk. Drugs with high maternal protein binding concentrate in low levels in breast milk. For example, warfarin sodium (Coumadin), which is 99% bound, is virtually excluded from breast milk. Other highly protein-bound drugs, such as celecoxib (Celebrex), are found in low levels in milk.[20] Conversely, drugs that do not engage in protein binding, such as lithium (Lithobid), are found in higher levels in milk.

Bioavailability of Drugs in Mother and Infant

An infant's exposure to medications used by the breastfeeding mother is a function of the dose administered to the mother, the bioavailability of the drug in the mother, and the amount transferred into breast milk. The bioavailability of a medication refers to the proportion of a dose that reaches the systemic circulation after it is administered. Classically, this term is used when referring to drugs administered by all routes except the intravenous route, because bioavailability is 100% when a medication is administered intravenously. Drugs administered orally are absorbed into the portal circulation of the gut and then pass through the liver prior to their delivery to the general circulation. The liver can sequester and metabolize a drug, thereby eliminating its systemic effect. This is particularly true of opiates (e.g., morphine), which are largely eliminated from the circulation during their first pass through the liver.

While little is known about the oral absorption or bioavailability of medications in infants, there are apparently many similarities to what occurs in adults, particularly after the first month of life.[21,22] In neonates, gastric emptying time is delayed and intestinal absorption is irregular. Slower intestinal absorption can be advantageous, as this would tend to keep plasma concentrations of medications lower in the infant.[22] Medications presented to the infant via breast milk can, in rare instances, produce gastrointestinal symptoms of diarrhea or constipation. For example, diarrhea has been reported in some infants who were exposed to antibiotics or 5-aminosalicylic acid products. Most medications must be systemically absorbed into the infant's plasma compartment to produce untoward effects. Usually, those medications with poor oral bioavailability in adults are also poorly absorbed in infants.

Thus, for breastfeeding women, medications that have poor oral bioavailability are recommended when possible, as such choices ultimately reduce the infant's exposure to the medication. Table 38-2 lists a number of medications that are poorly bioavailable and are ideal for breastfeeding women.

Milk/Plasma Ratio

The ratio of the concentration of drugs in breast milk to the concentration in maternal plasma is known as the **milk/plasma (M/P)** ratio (Figure 38-4). The M/P ratio is primarily used to quantify the extent of drug transfer into milk. Clinically, it has no or little role unless one knows the absolute level of drug in the maternal plasma compartment at the time the M/P ratio is measured. Ultimately, the concentration of a drug in milk (C_{milk}) determines the extent of infant exposure, which in turn can be used to assess safety. Thus, one should avoid the use of M/P ratios unless they are exceedingly low. With the exception of iodine, most other drugs with high M/P ratios often fail to attain clinically relevant doses via breast milk.

$$\text{M/P Ratio} = \frac{C_{milk}}{C_{plasma}}$$

Figure 38-4 Milk/plasma ratio formula.

Table 38-2 Maternal Medications That Are Safe for the Breastfed Infant Secondary to Decreased Bioavailability

Drug: Generic (Brand)	Molecular Weight (Daltons)	Oral Bioavailability in Adults	Clinical Considerations
Albuterol and related inhaled beta-adrenergic agonists	239	Insignificant	Systemic absorption minimal; inactivated by first-pass uptake in liver. Administered via inhalation.
Budesonide (Rhinocort)	430	10.7% orally	Poor oral absorption. High first-pass uptake in liver.
Ceftriaxone (Rocephin)	555	Not absorbed orally	Administered intravenously.
Etanercept (Enbrel)	51,235	Not absorbed	Decomposed in gut by proteases. Administered subcutaneously.
Fluticasone (Flonase)	500	< 0.5%	Administered via inhalation; systemic absorption minimal.
Gentamicin (Garamycin) and related aminoglycosides	478	Insignificant	First-pass hepatic inactivation. Intravenous only.
Heparin	12,000–15,000	Not absorbed	Unabsorbed; decomposed in GI tract.
Infliximab (Remicade)	144,190	Not absorbed	Decomposed by gut proteases. Only available intravenously.
Interferon-α and interferon-β	22,500–28,000	Minimally absorbed orally	Decomposed by gut pH and protease enzymes. Administered subcutaneously.
Lansoprazole (Prevacid)	369	80% (enteric coated)	Unstable at low pH. Extensive metabolism by hepatic enzymes.
Omeprazole (Prilosec)	345	30–40% (enteric coated)	Unstable at low pH. Half-life is about 1–1.2 hours.
Pantoprazole (Protonix)	405	77% (enteric coated)	Unstable at low pH. Rapidly metabolized by hepatic enzymes.

Active Transport of Medications into and out of Breast Milk

While most drugs transfer into milk largely as a function of equilibrium forces between the maternal plasma and milk compartment, there are a few drugs that are transported by various transporters. These drugs include nitrofurantoin (Macrodantin, Macrobid),[23] acyclovir (Zovirax),[24] ranitidine (Zantac),[25] and iodine.[26,27] While these drugs may become concentrated in milk, with the exception of iodine they normally do not attain ranges that have a clinical effect. Iodine, however, is transported so extensively that clinically hazardous ranges have been noted.[26]

Active transport out of the breast milk compartment could also potentially occur. For example, P-glycoprotein is extensively expressed in intestinal epithelium, the blood–brain barrier, hepatocytes, and renal tubules. This efflux transporter actively transports drugs out of cells and has been found in both apical and basolateral epithelial membranes. Metformin (Glucophage) provides an example of a drug that is transported via this mechanism. Assuming a passive diffusion model, theoretic calculations of the transfer of metformin into breast milk would suggest an M/P ratio of 2.93.[28,29] However, the clinically observed M/P ratios in three studies were reported to be much lower (0.63, 0.35, and 0.46, respectively) and a flat milk concentration–time profile was noted.[29–32] The lower observed M/P ratios may indicate an active efflux transporter, pumping metformin out of milk and back into the plasma compartment.[31] Apparently, metformin is a substrate for the OCT1 and OCT2 organic cation transporters. The OCT1 efflux transporter is also expressed in human mammary gland epithelium.[32]

Calculation of Infant Dose

Ultimately, the evaluation of risk to an infant depends on the dose of medication that the infant receives.[33] There are two ways of calculating this dose: the **absolute infant dose (AID)** and the **relative infant dose (RID)**.[34]

Absolute Infant Dose

The AID (Figure 38-5) is an estimate of the drug concentration in milk (per milliliter) multiplied by the volume of milk received each day, where C_{max} is equal to the maximum concentration of drug in milk or where $C_{average}$ is the average concentration of drug in milk throughout the dosing period.

$$\text{AID} = \text{Drug concentration in milk } (C_{max} \text{ or } C_{average}) \times \text{Volume of milk received per day}$$

Figure 38-5 Absolute infant dose.

$$RID = \frac{\text{Dose infant}\left(\frac{mg/kg}{day}\right)}{\text{Dose mother}\left(\frac{mg/kg}{day}\right)}$$

Dose infant = dose in infant/day
Dose mother = dose in mother/day

Figure 38-6 Relative infant dose.

This method assumes that the volume of milk received each day is known—an element that is its weakest point. Many sources use a value of 150 cc/kg per day as an estimate of daily milk delivery to an infant. The use of C_{max} almost always leads to an overestimate of the actual infant dose. When $C_{average}$ is available, it is more clinically accurate.

Relative Infant Dose

The relative infant dose (Figure 38-6) provides an estimate of the weight-normalized dose relative to the mother's dose. This measurement is the most useful method for assessing drug safety for breastfeeding women and their infants, and it is commonly used in many reviews and textbooks in this field.

This method provides the clinician with a good estimate of how much of the mother's dose (as a percentage) of the drug is actually transferred to the infant daily on a dose-per-weight basis. The relative infant dose tells the clinician what percent of the mother's dose is potentially transferred to the infant during a particular dosing interval. Interpretation of the relative risk in this method depends on a notional safe level of concern. This level of concern was suggested by Bennett in 1966 to be a cutoff value of 10% of the mother's dose.[35] Doses higher than 10% of the maternal dose were considered more risky; thus, infant exposure of less than 10% of the maternal dose is considered relatively safe. Although this level has been widely accepted, it has not been the subject of rigorous research and the actual level of concern depends on the relative toxicity of the specific drug. Medications that are extremely hazardous would require much lower values than the 10% level (e.g., methotrexate [Rheumatrex], other anticancer agents). Figure 38-7 provides an algorithm for risk–benefit analysis in assessing drug use in breastfeeding mothers.

Predisposing Infant Factors

The ability of an infant to adjust and maintain homeostasis when exposed to varying quantities of drug is largely a function of the infant's metabolic status. All infants should be categorized as being at low, moderate, or potentially high risk for exposure to the medication of interest. Infants at low risk are generally older infants (6–18 months) who can metabolize and handle drugs efficiently. Moderate-risk infants are those 4 months or younger who suffer from

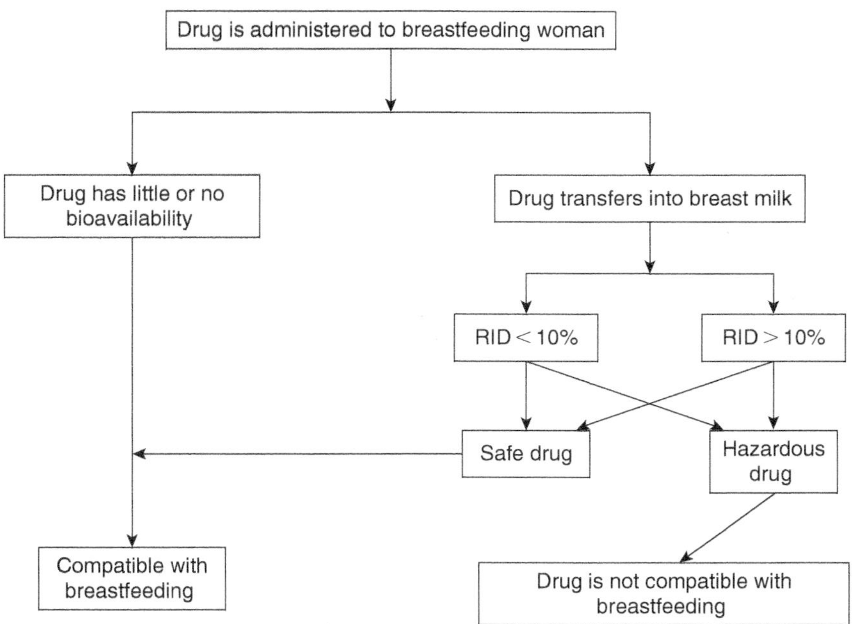

Figure 38-7 Algorithm for risk–benefit analysis commonly used to assess drug use in breastfeeding women.

various metabolic problems, such as complications from the birth, apnea, gastrointestinal abnormalities, hepatitis, or other metabolic problems. Infants at higher risk are newborn or premature infants, infants who are unstable, or infants with poor renal output.

Risk–Benefit Analysis

Unfortunately, infants have little to gain from exposure to medication via breast milk, but they do have much to gain from continued breastfeeding. The ultimate evaluation of the safety of drugs in breast milk, therefore, depends on three major factors: (1) the amount of medication present in the breast milk; (2) the oral bioavailability of the medication in the infant; and (3) the ability of the infant to metabolize and excrete the medication if absorbed. Even though numerous studies have reviewed the levels of drugs in breast milk and their bioavailability, the ability of the specific infant to metabolize most medications is highly variable and requires close evaluation by the attending clinician. Techniques used to reduce infant exposure to drugs used by a breastfeeding woman include brief interruption of breastfeeding, using alternative and safer drugs, postponing treatment until the infant is less sensitive, or, in rare cases, using donor breast milk or hydrolyzed formulas while pumping and discarding her own milk. Each case must be individually assessed, taking into account the importance of medication therapy, the timing of therapy, the choice of medications, the ability of the infant to tolerate the medication, and the overall toxicity of the drug itself.

The following sections of this chapter describe the transfer into breast milk of common drugs within specific drug classes.

Analgesics

Analgesics are the most commonly used medications by breastfeeding women and are most frequently used in the early postpartum period. Table 38-3 provides the relative infant dose and compatibility of most analgesics and anti-inflammatory drugs.

Aspirin

Aspirin levels in milk are generally quite low, approximately 2.5% to 10.8% of the maternal dose. Used briefly and in low doses, aspirin probably poses little risk to a breastfed infant. Unfortunately, the relative risk of Reye syndrome remains unknown as a function of the dose of aspirin or even the age of infant. Most cases of Reye syndrome occur among adolescents using therapeutic doses of aspirin (650 mg or higher). Current practice suggests low-dose (81 mg) aspirin is likely to be compatible with breastfeeding. Aspirin is almost completely metabolized to salicylic acid within 2 hours of administration. Because aspirin, and not salicylic acid, has been associated with Reye syndrome, a brief waiting period of 2 hours to breastfeed following administration of aspirin would likely remove any risk.

Acetaminophen (Tylenol)

Published levels of acetaminophen (Tylenol) in milk vary enormously but are generally less than 8.8% of the maternal dose. Acetaminophen is safe to administer to infants and young children. There is little or no concern about the use of this medication by breastfeeding women.

Nonsteroidal Anti-inflammatory Drugs

Numerous NSAIDs are available and many of them have been studied in breastfeeding women. Ibuprofen (Advil) and ketorolac (Toradol) are perhaps the two most preferred options in this drug family. Ibuprofen is an ideal analgesic for breastfeeding women, as levels in breast milk are quite low. Approximately 0.38% of the maternal dose is

Table 38-3 Relative Infant Doses of Various Analgesic and Anti-inflammatory Drugs in Breast Milk

Drug: Generic (Brand)	Relative Infant Dose	Lactation Risk Category
Acetaminophen (Tylenol)	8.8–24.2%	Compatible
Aspirin	< 2.5–10.8%	Compatible in low doses (82 mg); prolonged use may be associated with Reye syndrome so other analgesics are preferred
Celecoxib (Celebrex)	0.3–0.7%	Compatible
Codeine	8.1%	Possibly/ hazardous
Fentanyl (Sublimaze)	2.9–5%	Probably compatible
Hydrocodone (Vicodin, Lortab, Norco)	2.4–3.7%	Probably compatible
Hydromorphone (Dilaudid)	0.7%	Probably compatible
Ibuprofen (Advil)	0.1–0.7%	Compatible
Indomethacin (Indocin)	1.2%	Probably compatible
Ketorolac (Toradol)	0.14–0.2%	Compatible
Morphine	9–35%	Probably compatible
Naproxen (Aleve, Naprosyn)	3.3%	Probably compatible; possibly hazardous if used for prolonged period
Oxycodone (Percocet)	1.5–3.5%	Probably compatible

transferred daily to the infant, which is equivalent to 0.2% of the infant dose.[36]

Ketorolac (Toradol) is a popular NSAID that is controversial. While this drug may cause bleeding problems in some postpartum women owing to its inhibition of platelet aggregation, its documented levels in breast milk are almost insignificant. In a study of 10 lactating women who received 10 mg of ketorolac orally 4 times daily, milk levels of ketorolac were not detectable in four of the subjects.[37] In the six remaining women, the concentration of ketorolac in milk 2 hours after a dose ranged from 5.2–7.3 mcg/L on day 1 to 5.9–7.9 mcg/L on day 2. For most women, the breast milk level never exceeded 5 mcg/L. The relative infant dose would be 0.2% of the daily maternal dose. This study used oral administration, which is subject to the first-pass effect, thus, intramuscular or intravenous dosing may result in higher breast milk levels. Even so, ketorolac should still be considered a safe analgesic for breastfeeding women.

Recent studies of celecoxib (Celebrex) suggest that this agent is a safe analgesic for breastfeeding women. Knoppert estimates that the daily intake in an infant is approximately 20 mcg/kg per day.[38] In a study of women receiving 200 mg celecoxib daily, the drug levels in breast milk averaged 66 mcg/L.[20] Using these data, the relative infant dose was 0.3% to 0.7% of the maternal dose. Plasma levels of celecoxib in two infants studied were undetectable (< 10 ng/mL).

Morphine and Congeners

The data on morphine and breast milk levels are highly variable. Some studies show morphine levels are relatively high, whereas others have found them to be relatively low. An even more important factor with morphine is its poor oral bioavailability: Less than 25% is orally absorbed due to a high first-pass effect in the liver. Baka et al. assessed the concentration of morphine in breast milk following use of intravenous morphine for managing pain post cesarean section and found the milk to plasma ratio of morphine was always less than 1 in breast milk.[39] Given its rather limited transfer into breast milk, morphine is considered compatible with breastfeeding so long as the maternal doses remain low to moderate and the infant is stable.

Codeine and hydrocodone are the opioid analgesics most commonly used to treat pain in breastfeeding women. Codeine is a prodrug that is metabolized into morphine, which is the active ingredient. Thus, the rate of metabolism in an individual affects the effectiveness of pain relief. In addition, codeine is metabolized by CYP2D6, which is expressed in varying degrees secondary to several different polymorphisms.[40] Older pharmacokinetic studies of codeine transfer into human breast milk had conflicting results; however, one infant death has been reported following maternal use of codeine (60 mg every 12 hours, subsequently reduced to 30 mg every 12 hours from days 2 to 14).[41] In this case, the morphine levels in the mother were apparently elevated, as CYP2D6 genotyping of the mother suggested that she was an ultra-rapid genotype. Subsequent analyses have confirmed there is a risk for infant sedation that is related to the maternal CYP2D6 polymorphism status.[42-45] In 2007, the FDA issued a Public Health Advisory that reviewed the rare but potentially fatal side effect of neonatal death from morphine overdose obtained via breast milk.[46] In most cases, codeine taken for a limited period of time at usual doses is safe for a healthy full-term newborn or healthy breastfed infant.

While codeine is probably acceptable in most situations, hydrocodone (Vicodin, Vicoprofen, Norco, Lorcet, Lortab) may be a safer alternative for a breastfeeding woman. Approximately 5% to 6% of hydrocodone is metabolized into an active metabolite, hydromorphone, which has a 5- to 6-fold higher potency than hydrocodone. Persons with polymorphisms that make them nonmetabolizers or poor metabolizers are frequently encountered, as 7% of the population falls into one of these categories. Rapid metabolizers are rare—fewer than 6 per 1000 population. Ultimately, each infant should be closely monitored for symptoms of overdose, which may include somnolence, apnea, and poor feeding.

Antibiotics and Antifungals

After analgesics, the next most commonly used class of medications used by breastfeeding women are antibiotics. Levels and relative infant doses of these medications are provided in Table 38-4. Numerous reviews of the transfer of antibiotics into breast milk are available for the interested reader.[47-49]

Penicillins

Most penicillins are small molecules with molecular weights in the range of 300–500 daltons. Cephalosporins are slightly larger but not significantly so. Virtually all of the penicillins and cephalosporins have been studied and are known to occur only trace levels in breast milk.[50-55]

Tetracyclines

The transfer of the tetracycline antibiotics, such as tetracycline and oxytetracycline (Terramycin), into breast

Table 38-4 Relative Infant Doses of Various Antibiotics in Breast Milk

Drug: Generic (Brand)	Relative Infant Dose	Clinical Considerations
Amoxicillin (Amoxil)	1.0%	Compatible. Observe infant for diarrhea or thrush.
Azithromycin (Zithromax)	5.8%	Compatible. Observe infant for diarrhea or thrush.
Cefotaxime (Claforan)	0.34%	Compatible. Observe infant for diarrhea or thrush.
Cephalexin (Keflex)	0.5–1.5%	Compatible. Observe infant for diarrhea or thrush.
Ciprofloxacin (Cipro)	2.1–6.3%	Compatible. One case of pseudomembranous colitis reported. Observe for diarrhea or *Candida* overgrowth.
Clarithromycin (Biaxin)	2.1%	Compatible. Observe infant for diarrhea or diaper rash.
Clindamycin (Cleocin)	0.9–1.8%	Compatible. One case of pseudomembranous colitis reported. Observe infant for diarrhea or *Candida* overgrowth.
Dicloxacillin (Dynapen)	0.6–1.4%	Compatible. Observe infant for diarrhea or *Candida* diaper rash.
Doxycycline (Adoxa, Vibramycin)	4.2–13.3%	Compatible for short-term use (< 3 weeks). Avoid chronic dosing. Observe infant for diarrhea or *Candida* overgrowth.
Erythromycin (E-Mycin)	1.4–1.7%	Compatible. Postnatal use is associated with infantile hypertrophic pyloric stenosis. Observe for diarrhea or thrush.
Metronidazole (Flagyl)	12.6–13.5%	Moderate transfer. No adverse effects reported in exposed infants. Dose via milk is less than the therapeutic dose. May impose bitter taste to milk. For 2-g single oral dose, discard milk for 12–24 hours.
Tetracycline (Achromycin, Sumycin)	0.6%	Compatible for short-term use. Oral absorption low. Observe infant for diarrhea or *Candida* overgrowth.
Vancomycin (Vanocin)	6.6%	Compatible. Poor oral bioavailability. Dose via milk is subclinical.

milk is very low. When they are mixed with calcium salts, the bioavailability of these drugs is significantly reduced, so it is unlikely an infant would absorb the small levels present in breast milk. However, doxycycline (Vibramycin, Adoxa) is less influenced by milk components and its absorption is delayed, but not blocked; thus absorption of doxycycline may be significant over time.[54] Short-term use of these compounds is considered safe and is suitable for treatment of many syndromes. Long-term use, such as for acne, is not recommended for breastfeeding women due to the possibility of dental staining in the infant and reduced linear growth rate.

Fluoroquinolones

Use of fluoroquinolones during lactation is somewhat controversial. This class of antibiotic has not been approved for use in infants and children secondary to the findings of animal reproduction studies in which fluoroquinolones were associated with fetal arthropathy. Although the dose received via breast milk is low, pseudomembranous colitis has been reported in one breastfed infant whose mother was taking ciprofloxacin.[56] In one group of infants exposed to fluoroquinolones for as long as 20 days, a greenish discoloration of the infants' teeth was noted at 12–23 months of age.[57] However, ciprofloxacin (Cipro) use in pediatrics has increased in recent years,[58] and numerous studies now indicate that there is little risk from ciprofloxacin exposure. Calcium reputedly may compromise the bioavailability of ciprofloxacin; hence breast milk calcium may suppress the oral bioavailability in an infant. Ciprofloxacin ophthalmic products are poorly absorbed and the dose is low, so these products may be used by breastfeeding women.

Metronidazole (Flagyl)

The use of the antiprotozoal metronidazole (Flagyl) among breastfeeding women has also been controversial[59,60] (Box 38-2). Older data suggested it was potentially mutagenic in rodents, although this outcome has never been documented in humans. Topical and vaginal preparations of metronidazole are safe for use during breastfeeding due to the limited absorption that occurs via these routes of administration. Following oral doses of 1200 mg per day, the maximum concentration in breast milk has been reported to average 15.5 mg/L.[61] Although the relative infant dose of metronidazole is moderate, approximating 13% of the maternal dose, metronidazole is virtually nontoxic, and no untoward effects have been reported in infants. A slight metallic taste of the milk has been reported, potentially prompting some infants to reject the breast milk due to this taste. Large oral doses (2-g oral dose administered as one dose), which are commonly prescribed for treatment of vaginal trichomoniasis, should be followed by a brief interruption of breastfeeding for perhaps 12–24 hours. In those instances where the 2-g dose cannot be used, a regimen of 500 mg twice daily for 5 days is suitable. Following the use of intravenous metronidazole, a short withholding period of a few hours (2–3 hours) to avoid the peak is advised to avoid even higher breast milk levels of this drug.

Macrolides

Erythromycin (E-Mycin) should be avoided by breastfeeding women if possible. Following a case report of hypertrophic pyloric stenosis in an infant, several population-based studies have assessed this relationship with conflicting results.[63–65]

Erythromycin levels in milk are quite low. Following a dose of 500 mg erythromycin, breast milk levels varied from 1.0 to 1.6 mg/L at 2, 4, and 6 hours.[66] Azithromycin (Zithromax) transfer to breast milk is difficult to determine as this antibiotic has a long half-life and may accumulate in breast milk. If a macrolide antibiotic is required, erythromycin is the preferred choice.[67]

Box 38-2 A Mother's Concerns

A 23-year-old woman is successfully breastfeeding her 12-week-old daughter. She seeks care for vaginal discomfort and subsequently is diagnosed with bacterial vaginosis. This woman has been scrupulous about her diet and avoidance of any medications because of concern about untoward effects on her child.

The first choice for treatment of symptomatic bacterial vaginosis is metronidazole (Flagyl) 500 mg taken twice daily for 7 days. Some clinicians, however, are hesitant to prescribe metronidazole because of unproven myths about its mutagenicity. Other providers note that the relative infant dose is 9% to 13%, which is a moderate relative infant dose level. In addition, no untoward effects have been reported among breastfeeding infants at the recommended dose. Thus, the usual treatment offered to nonpregnant individuals is reasonable for this breastfeeding dyad.

Because this woman has expressed concerns about drugs and breastfeeding, it may be best to prescribe an alternative treatment—that is, metronidazole gel (MetroGel). This topical treatment is effective for bacterial vaginosis, and essentially there is no transfer of the drug into milk following vaginal application of the topical gel.

Regardless of the route of administration for metronidazole, breastfeeding should not be discontinued. For women with conditions (e.g., *Trichomonas vaginalis* infection) for which metronidazole is usually indicated in a large oral dose (2-g single dose), a brief interruption of breastfeeding of 12–24 hours is typically suggested, especially because the milk may have a metallic taste during this period, causing the infant to reject it.

Antifungals

Nystatin (Mycostatin) is virtually unabsorbed orally, so its transfer into breast milk is almost nil. Fluconazole (Diflucan) transfers significantly into breast milk, leading to a relative infant dose of 16%.[68] This is a subclinical level in infants, and less than the dose commonly prescribed directly for infants for treatment of thrush. Thus, although it is higher than the 10% safety range, fluconazole is considered safe for breastfeeding women.

Sulfonamides

Sulfamethoxazole is frequently used in combination with trimethoprim (sulfamethoxazole–trimethoprim [Bactrim]) for various infections, now including methicillin-resistant *Staphylococcus aureus* (MRSA). If a breastfeeding women takes the usual dose of 160 mg trimethoprim/800 mg sulfamethoxazole per day, the infant will receive 1.97 mg/L of trimethoprim and 4.71 mg/L of sulfamethoxazole.[69] The relative infant doses of sulfamethoxazole and trimethoprim are 2.32% to 2.95%[69] and 3.9% to 9%, respectively. These doses are still far lower than typical clinical doses used to treat infants. However, sulfonamides have the theoretic risk of displacing bilirubin from albumin-binding sites, thereby causing jaundice. For this reason, the American Academy of Pediatrics recommends that sulfonamides be used with caution by mothers of infants who have hyperbilirubinemia, glucose-6-phosphate dehydrogenase deficiency, illness, or those who are premature.[28]

Anticonvulsants

The anticonvulsants are a heterogeneous group with regard to safety for breastfeeding infants. Many women take a combination of two anticonvulsants, and the resulting drug–drug interactions will affect drug transfer to breast milk. Most anticonvulsants are found in low levels in breast milk; because the infant's ability to metabolize these drugs is immature, however, a newborn can accumulate enough active drug to have a clinical effect. For example, phenobarbital (Luminal) has a very long half-life, and over time it can reach high levels in the infant.

Phenobarbitol, ethosuximide (Zarontin), lamotrigine (Lamictal), zonisamide (Zonegran), and primidone (Mysoline) should not be used or be used with caution if needed.[70] Phenytoin (Dilantin), carbamazepine (Tegretol), and valproate (Depakote) are safer anticonvulsants, as the relative infant dose for these agents is approximately 3% to 5%.[71] Some case reports have noted adverse events associated with carbamazepine and valproate. Specifically, carbamazepine has been associated with hepatic dysfunction in a breastfed infant, and valproate has been associated with thrombocytopenia.[70]

Antiemetics

The use of phenothiazine analogues for treating nausea and vomiting in breastfeeding women should be avoided if possible. Chlorpromazine (Thorazine) may cause infant sedation, and its long-term effects in children are unknown. Of note, chlorpromazine can cause galactorrhea and was historically used to induce lactation. In contrast, promethazine (Phenergan) may inhibit prolactin and milk production, but breast milk levels have not been determined given the rapid metabolism of this drug. Occasional short-term use of this agent for treatment of nausea and vomiting does not appear to be harmful for a woman with established lactation, but other antiemetics are still preferred. The effects of infant exposure to ondansetron (Zofran) are unknown, although the drug should be expected to appear in breast milk based on its molecular weight.

Antihypertensives

Antihypertensives are commonly used postnatally. Fortunately, only drugs within the family of beta-adrenergic blockers present a risk to breastfed infants, and then only specific agents within this family. Excretion of beta blockers into breast milk is largely a function of protein binding; that is, those drugs that do not extensively bind to protein in maternal plasma can concentrate in breast milk. Atenolol (Tenormin) and acebutolol (Sectral) have been associated with cyanosis, bradycardia, and hypotension in case reports in breastfed infants. Preferred beta blockers include propranolol (Inderal) and metoprolol (Lopressor), both of which have lower M/P ratios, accumulate to minimal levels in breast milk, and have no untoward effects as yet reported in breastfeeding infants.[72] Hydralazine (Apresoline) and methyldopa (Aldomet) have been used for years by breastfeeding mothers without complications; studies suggest their levels in breast milk are low. Calcium-channel blockers have been studied extensively and tend to produce low levels in breast milk, particularly verapamil (Isoptin, Covera-HS) and nifedipine (Procardia). Both of these agents have been used extensively in breastfeeding women without complications. Nifedipine (Procardia) levels in breast milk are less than 0.01 mg/kg per day, a particularly low level.[73]

Angiotensin-converting enzyme (ACE) inhibitors have been extensively studied in breastfeeding women and have the lowest M/P ratios of the general class of antihypertensives.[70] Captopril (Capoten) and enalapril (Vasotec)—but not nadolol (Corgard)—are preferred ACE inhibitors in breastfeeding women, as their levels in breast milk are quite low.[74] Because these drugs can cause severe nephrotoxicity when used in the last trimester of pregnancy, they should be used cautiously by women with very premature infants, at least until the infant is at the gestational age of a full-term infant.

Diuretics, including hydrochlorothiazide and furosemide (Lasix), have not been studied extensively in breastfeeding women but are presumed to be compatible with breastfeeding if doses are low. A large diuresis could inhibit milk production.

Thyroid and Antithyroid Medications

The transfer of levothyroxine into breast milk is negligible, so treatment of hypothyroidism with oral thyroid supplement is safe for lactating women.[75] Liothyronine (Synthroid, L-Thyroxine) levels in breast milk are reportedly slightly higher than levothyroxine levels, but are still too low to affect thyroid function in the neonate.[76]

With regard to treatment of hyperthyroid states, propylthiouracil (PTU) and methimazole (Tapazole) have been extensively studied in breastfeeding women. Propylthiouracil levels in breast milk are generally the lowest of these agents—at least 10 times less than the maternal plasma levels. The absolute infant dose would be approximately 0.1 mg/kg per day or 1.8% of the maternal dose. In at least two studies, no changes in infant thyroid function have been reported with use of either drug. Historically, propylthiouracil was recommended for breastfeeding women because it accumulated in lower doses in breast milk. However, recent reports associating propylthiouracil with liver injury have caused a reevaluation of this medication.[77] In 2009, the FDA released a warning about possible propylthiouracil-induced liver failure[78]; as a consequence, methimazole is now considered the first choice for breastfeeding women. The relative infant dose of propylthiouracil is approximately 1.8% and the relative infant dose of methimazole is 2.3%.[79]

Psychotherapeutic Agents

The postnatal period is associated with numerous psychiatric disorders, including depression, generalized anxiety disorder, and psychosis. It is estimated that the prevalence of major depression during pregnancy and postpartum ranges from 5.5% to 33%.[80] Using medications in the early postpartum period has always been controversial. However, untreated depression is also associated with multiple adverse outcomes for both women and their children.[81] Unfortunately, it is not clear that pharmacologic treatment of depression mitigates adverse outcomes, and pharmacologic treatments may be associated with adverse outcomes as well.[81] Thus the cost–benefit relationship for treatment has not been determined.[82]

Although a burgeoning literature has addressed the neonatal effects of in utero exposure to antidepressant medications, this chapter focuses on effects during breastfeeding only. Additional information about prenatal exposure can be found in the *Mental Health* chapter. Given that many breastfeeding women are using antidepressant drugs, it behooves clinicians to keep up-to-date with recommendations regarding their use.

Table 38-5 lists the various antidepressants and their relative infant doses.

Anxiolytics: Sedatives and Hypnotics

Breast milk levels of diazepam (Valium), lorazepam (Ativan), midazolam (Versed), and other benzodiazepines are not excessive, but these agents should be used with caution by lactating women.[70] Diazepam has a long half-life and an active metabolite that concentrates in breast milk. Indeed, some reports cite infant lethargy and sedation as outcomes following maternal use of this drug despite the fact that the relative infant dose for diazepam is less than 14% of the maternal dose and approximately 5% of the therapeutic pediatric dose.[83] Although a single dose of diazepam for seizure control or sedation prior to a procedure is considered safe, its long-term use is not recommended in breastfeeding women. If a sedative is required, the analogues with a shorter half-life, such as lorazepam (Ativan) and midazolam (Versed), are preferred. The relative infant doses of lorazepam (2.6%) and midazolam (< 0.6%) are quite low, and sedation in breastfeeding infants is unlikely.[83]

Tricyclic Antidepressants

Almost all of the current antidepressants have been studied in breastfeeding women, and most studies suggest that the levels of these agents in breast milk are low. Nevertheless, compliance is often poor with the tricyclic antidepressants secondary to troublesome side effects such as anticholinergic symptoms, xerostomia, blurred vision, and sedation. Amitriptyline (Elavil) is metabolized to nortriptyline and, therefore, has an active metabolite. The relative infant dose of amitriptyline (Elavil) is less than 1.9% to 2.8% of the maternal dose.[84] Studies thus far have been unable to detect the transfer of this medication into the infant's plasma. Doxepin (Sinequan) should be avoided due to case reports of hypotonia, poor suckling, vomiting, and jaundice.[85] Desipramine (Norpramin) levels in breast milk

Table 38-5 Relative Infant Doses of Various Antidepressants in Breast Milk

Drug: Generic (Brand)	Relative Infant Dose	Clinical Considerations
Amitriptyline (Elavil)	1.9–2.8%	Compatible; observe for sedation in infant.
Bupropion (Wellbutrin)	0.2–2%	Compatible; do not use in patients subject to seizures. Observe for possible milk suppression.
Citalopram (Celexa)	3.56–5.37%	Caution; somnolence reported in some newborns.
Desipramine (Norpramin)	0.3–0.9%	Compatible; observe for sedation in infant.
Doxepin (Sinequan)	1.2–3%	Unsafe; respiratory arrest and sedation reported.
Escitalopram (Lexapro)	5.2–7.9%	Compatible; observe for sedation in infant.
Fluvoxamine (Luvox)	0.8–1.38%	
Fluoxetine (Prozac)	1.6–14.6%	Compatible; avoid high maternal dose early postpartum.
Paroxetine (Paxil)	1.2–2.8%	Compatible for infant; avoid use in adolescents.
Sertraline (Zoloft)	0.4–2.2%	Compatible; preferred SSRI.
St. John's wort	No data	Compatible; recent data suggest transfer to milk is minimal. No untoward effects noted.
Venlafaxine (Effexor)	6.8–8.1%	Probably safe; no side effects noted in one study, but relative infant dose is somewhat high.

are minimal. One study of desipramine suggests that a 300 mg per day regimen results in a relative infant dose of approximately 1%.[86] Nortriptyline is the recommended drug in this category for initiating treatment as it has the best safety record.

Selective Serotonin Reuptake Inhibitors

The selective serotonin reuptake inhibitors (SSRIs) are presently the mainstay of pharmacologic treatment for depression, primarily because they are effective and have minimal toxicity in overdoses. The most often studied drug in breastfeeding mothers in the beginning of the twenty-first century has been the SSRI antidepressants.

Neonatal withdrawal symptoms have been reported in infants exposed to SSRIs during pregnancy. These symptoms, which occur early in the postnatal period, consist of poor adaptation, irritability, jitteriness, and poor gaze control in neonates. The drugs most commonly involved are paroxetine (Paxil)[87] and fluoxetine (Prozac).[88]

Clinical studies of breastfeeding women taking sertraline (Zoloft), fluvoxamine (Luvox), and paroxetine suggest that the transfer of these medications into breast milk is low and uptake by the infant is even lower. Thus far, no untoward effects have been reported following the use of these three agents in breastfeeding mothers. Sertraline and paroxetine are the preferred first line drugs in this class for initiation of therapy given their safety records.

Fluoxetine (Prozac) has an active metabolite and transfers into breast milk in relatively higher concentrations, equivalent to 1.6% to 14.6% of the maternal dose.[89] In reality, the risk of untoward effects is probably small, and women who cannot tolerate other SSRIs should be maintained on fluoxetine while breastfeeding (Box 38-3).

Citalopram (Celexa) and its new congener, escitalopram (Lexapro), transfer into breast milk to a moderate extent. In a study of seven women receiving an average of 0.41 mg/kg per day of citalopram, the average milk level was 97 mcg/L for citalopram and 36 mcg/L for its metabolite (RID = 3.7%).[90] Low concentrations of citalopram and its metabolite were noted in the infants' plasma (2 and 2.3 mcg/L, respectively). While no untoward effects have been noted in the published studies, two cases of somnolence have been reported to the manufacturer and at least four other anecdotal cases have been reported to this author. Citalopram should be used cautiously by women with premature infants or those subject to apnea. By comparison, in a recent study of eight breastfeeding women taking an average of 10 mg per day of escitalopram (Lexapro), the total relative infant dose of this drug and its metabolite was reported to be 5.3%.[91] The drug and its metabolite were undetectable in most of the infants tested. No adverse events in the infants have been reported.

In summary, the SSRIs with the best breastfeeding profile are sertraline (Zoloft), paroxetine (Paxil), and fluvoxamine (Luvox).[84] Fluoxetine (Prozac), citalopram (Celexa), and escitalopram (Lexapro) are generally contraindicated because they have long half-lives and high relative infant doses.[84] That said, women should not be switched from one SSRI to another during pregnancy or breastfeeding if they are doing well using the original medication, secondary to the risk that the new antidepressant might not work, such that the woman will lapse into depression.

Serotonin Norepinephrine Reuptake Inhibitors

The serotonin norepinephrine reuptake inhibitors (SNRIs) inhibit reuptake of both serotonin and norepinephrine in contrast to the SSRIs, which inhibit the reuptake of serotonin only. Although fewer studies have examined SNRIs than have addressed SSRIs in breastfeeding dyads, those investigations that have been carried out have reported similar findings. SNRIs do transfer to breast milk in differing amounts; there are case reports of mild side effects in infants, and the neurodevelopmental effects following long-term use are unknown. To date, however, no data have been published that suggest they produce untoward neurobehavioral effects in any infants. Consequently, if the woman is stable using an SNRI, we recommend that she be maintained on the SNRI throughout breastfeeding.

Antipsychotics

The literature on the older antipsychotics and their transfer into breast milk is poor. These data seem to suggest that low levels of the phenothiazines, such as chlorpromazine (Thorazine), transfer into milk, and infant sedation has been reported. Because of their association with neonatal apnea and sedation, the older phenothiazines should be avoided by breastfeeding women.[28] The transfer of haloperidol (Haldol) into breast milk is reported to be minimal (RID ≤ 0.2% to 12%),[92] but this agent has been categorized as a drug to use with caution and under medical supervision.[28]

A number of reports suggest that the newer atypical antipsychotics may be a better choice of therapy for breastfeeding women. Risperidone (Risperdal) levels are reportedly quite low in breast milk, with an estimated relative infant dose of 2.8% to 9.1%, and without any reported sedation in the breastfed infants.[93] In several studies of

Box 38-3 A Case of Postpartum Depression

FL had her first baby 5 weeks ago and is breastfeeding her son. FL is feeling increasingly anxious about caring for her baby alone because her parents are returning to their home out of state soon. She reports that she is unable to sleep: "My thoughts just keep running in my head all night." She presents for a visit requesting "sleeping medicine that will not hurt the baby."

FL has a history of depression for which she took fluoxetine (Prozac) until a year ago. She weaned herself from this medication slowly over a few months prior to trying to get pregnant. The rest of her medical history is negative. She has never been hospitalized for a psychiatric disorder. She is not taking any other medications.

FL's speech is quite rapid and she sounds very anxious. She does not want to take an antidepressant medication and continues to suggest she "just needs something to help me sleep when I am not nursing the baby." She denies suicidal ideation or abnormal thoughts about the baby and exhibits appropriate concern for her baby during the visit.

FL's anxiety and insomnia may be symptoms of postpartum depression, bipolar disorder, or an anxiety disorder. The serotonin reuptake inhibitors, which include fluoxetine (Prozac), have been studied in breastfeeding women and infants, and although they all transfer into breast milk to a small extent, there are no reports of harm to the breastfeeding infant. Because postpartum depression can be harmful to the woman, infant, and family, treatment is recommended. However, acute anxiety can also be a symptom of bipolar disorder, which can be made worse if the woman is taking an SSRI, so an accurate diagnosis is essential.

FL agrees to an acute visit with a provider who specializes in women's health, and an appointment is made for her in 2 days. After consultation with the professional, FL is prescribed lorazepam (Ativan) for the next 2 nights with the caveat that FL's partner must be with her and the baby at all times. The provider also recommends initiating sertraline (Zoloft), as FL does not have a history of bipolar disorder or manic episodes that could be symptomatic of bipolar disorder. FL agrees to return for future care, but requests fluoxetine because she is familiar with it.

The clinician tells FL that fluoxetine is not recommended for breastfeeding women because it has a long half-life and clinically effective doses have been detected in infants of breastfeeding mothers. Additional health education includes the fact that sertraline takes several days to weeks to become completely effective, so medications that help FL deal with her symptoms in the short term may be a good idea. FL is told that the drugs in the sedative/hypnotic family that are used to aid sleep, such as lorazepam, are safe for use for a short time: Although the medication transfers to breast milk, the dose is slightly less than 9% and sedation has rarely been noted in newborns exposed to these drugs.

Finally, the clinician recommends that FL get 5 to 7 hours of uninterrupted sleep each night to help ameliorate her symptoms. She is encouraged to pump her milk in the day so the infant can be fed by her partner at night for at least a few nights.

olanzapine (Zyprexa), the relative infant dose ranged from 0.3% to 2.2%,[94,95] but no untoward effects were noted in any of the infants.

Mood Stabilizers

Women who have bipolar disorder are at higher risk for developing postpartum depression and psychosis. Thus medication can be an important component of therapy for this population. Lithium (Lithobid) is contraindicated for breastfeeding women because it concentrates in breast milk and can reach toxic levels in the infant.[96] Valproate (Depakote) and carbamazepine (Tegretol) are considered compatible with breastfeeding.[70,96] As noted in the section on anticonvulsants, carbamazepine has been associated with hepatotoxicity, and valproate has been associated with thrombocytopenia.

Clinical Implications

The reader may wonder where to find a simple rating scale to use as a guide in identifying drugs that are safe for

Box 38-4 Major Concepts in Using Drugs in Breastfeeding Mothers

- Avoid the unnecessary use of medications, including most herbal drugs.
- Some radioisotopes may require brief interruptions and discarding of pumped breast milk.
- Select drugs with the lowest relative infant dose.
- Select drugs with shorter half-lives, and avoid drugs with a long half-life if possible.
- Select drugs with poor oral bioavailability to reduce their absorption in infants.
- Select drugs for which there are published milk studies.
- Check the infant's medications for drug–drug interactions.
- Evaluate the age, stability, and condition of the infant to determine if the infant can handle exposure to the medication.
- Premature infants may be more susceptible to adverse effects of medications. Their clearance mechanisms have not matured.
- CNS-active drugs always penetrate breast milk to some degree; an increased level of concern is recommended when such medications are prescribed.
- Most drugs can be safely used by breastfeeding women, but a risk-versus-benefit assessment is always required prior to use.
- A relative infant dose of less than 10% is generally considered compatible with breastfeeding.

breastfeeding women. Although no single source exists, several rating scales have been developed. Box 38-4 lists some basic principles that may aid clinicians. Several detailed texts are also available, which can help the reader in selecting appropriate drugs for breastfeeding dyads.[3,17,97–99] Each of these texts utilizes a slightly different set of recommendation categories, but cross-comparisons for specific drugs reveal no significant differences in the actual recommendations, as all of them use peer-reviewed research for the basis of their recommendations. In addition, the Specialized Information Services of the National Institutes of Health sponsors a searchable peer-reviewed referenced database, known as LactMed, that summarizes the fetal and infant risks for most, if not all, commonly prescribed medications.[99]

Food and Drug Administration Categories

In 2014, the FDA issued a final rule for new standards for labeling information about the use of medications during pregnancy. Contrary to the older labeling using letters to identify safety of drugs in pregnancy, the new labeling includes more narrative detail as well as a specific subsection on lactation. The lactation subsection includes three subheadings: risk summary; clinical considerations; and data. This rule goes into effect in 2015 for new products, but labeling older products are anticipated to be phased in gradually.

Lactation Risk Categories

Perhaps the most commonly used scale is a relatively simple one, progressing from a category of drugs that are

Table 38-6 Lactation Risk Categories

Category	Description
L1—Compatible	Drug that has been taken by a large number of breastfeeding women without any observed increase in adverse effects in the infant. Controlled studies in breastfeeding women fail to demonstrate a risk to the infant, and the possibility of harm to the breastfeeding infant is remote; *or* the product is not orally bioavailable in an infant.
L2—Probably Compatible	Drug that has been studied in a limited number of breastfeeding women without an increase in adverse effects in the infant *and/or* the evidence of a demonstrated risk that is likely to follow use of this medication in a breastfeeding woman is weak.
L3—Probably Compatible	There are no controlled studies in breastfeeding women; however, untoward effects in a breastfed infant are possible *or* controlled studies show only minimal nonthreatening adverse effects. Drugs should be given only if the potential benefit justifies the potential risk to the infant. (New medications that have absolutely no published data are automatically placed in this category, regardless of how safe they may be.)
L4—Possibly Hazardous	There is positive evidence of risk to a breastfed infant or to breast milk production, but the benefits from use in breastfeeding women may be acceptable despite the risk to the infant (e.g., if the drug is needed in a life-threatening situation or for a serious disease for which safer drugs cannot be used or are ineffective.)
L5—No Data: Hazardous	Studies in breastfeeding women have demonstrated that there is significant and documented risk to the infant based on human experience *or* it is a medication that has a high risk of causing significant damage to an infant. The risk of using the drug in breastfeeding women clearly outweighs any possible benefit from breastfeeding. The drug is contraindicated for women who are breastfeeding an infant.

Source: Modified from Hale TW, Rowe H. *Medications and Mothers' Milk.* Amarillo, TX: Hale; 2014.[3]

contraindicated, to a category that is termed *safest*. The elegance of this simple scale enables clinicians to use the system easily. However, any system is limited because new studies are constantly emerging, as are new drugs that have not been well studied for use by the breastfeeding woman and her infant. Table 38-6 shows the lactation risk categories.[3]

Finally, when information about the transfer of a specific drug into breast milk is not available, a reasonable assessment can be made by assessing the molecular size, solubility, pH, protein binding, peak plasma time, half-life, and activity of metabolites.

Conclusion

All medications transfer into breast milk to some degree. However, few agents actually produce clinically relevant levels in infants. Ultimately, the most important information about a drug is its relative infant dose. Such data give the prescriber an accurate estimate of just how much medication the infant will receive daily. If this level is low relative to the normal infant dose, then the medication is probably safe to use in breastfeeding dyads.

In each case, before prescribing a medication to a breastfeeding woman, the clinician must first perform a relative risk–benefit analysis for the individual infant. Infant factors that must be assessed include prematurity, weakness, apnea, contraindicated medications, and other factors that would reduce the ability of the infant to tolerate even low levels of maternal medications. The infant has nothing to gain from exposure to medications via breast milk, so reducing or eliminating exposure should be the desired outcome. However, in most instances, the exposure to medication is generally subclinical. In such cases, the relative risk of avoiding breast milk far exceeds the risk of taking the medication. Formula-fed infants are known to have higher rates of gastrointestinal syndromes, upper respiratory tract infections, obesity, and numerous other syndromes; thus, it is often riskier to use formula than a mother's own milk.

Often, the amount of medication delivered to the infant via breast milk is substantially less than 4% of the maternal dose, and the amount the infant actually absorbs orally is even less. In healthy infants, this amount is often easily tolerated without untoward effects. In contrast, as the relative infant dose rises above 7% to 10% and the toxicity of the medication increases, clinicians should be more cautious in recommending continued breastfeeding if the medication is required.

All healthcare providers are advised to carefully choose those medications with lower relative infant doses and fewer side effects in infants when prescribing medications to breastfeeding women. Almost invariably, a suitable drug can be chosen so that a woman can continue to breastfeed her infant safely.

Resources

Organization	Description	Website
Motherisk	Service of the Hospital for Sick Children in Toronto. This site has a wealth of reviews on current drug topics of interest for breastfeeding. Motherisk counselors are available for phone contact (1-877-439-2744) during the week.	www.motherisk.org/prof/breastfeeding.jsp
National Institutes of Health	Database (Lactmed) that summarizes information on drugs and other chemicals to which breastfeeding women can be exposed. Reviews studies of pharmacokinetics; recommends alternatives where appropriate. Data are well-referenced. App available.	http://toxnet.nlm.nih.gov/newtoxnet/lactmed.htm
Organization of Teratology Information Specialists (OTIS)	MotherToBaby service of OTIS provides fact sheets and counseling about medications and other exposures.	www.mothertobaby.org/fact sheets-s13037

References

1. American Academy of Pediatrics. Breastfeeding and the use of breast milk. *Pediatrics.* 2012;129(3):e827-e841.
2. Collaborative Group on Hormonal Factors in Breast Cancer. Breast cancer and breastfeeding: collaborative reanalysis of individual data from 47 epidemiological studies in 30 countries, including 50,302 women with breast cancer and 96,973 women without the disease. *Lancet.* 2002;360(9328):187-195.
3. Hale TW, Rowe H. *Medications and Mothers' Milk.* Amarillo, TX: Hale; 2014.
4. Neville MC, McFadden TB, Forsyth I. Hormonal regulation of mammary differentiation and milk secretion. *J Mammary Gland Biol Neoplasia.* 2002;7(1):49-66.
5. Truitt ST, Fraser AB, Grimes DA, Gallo MF, Schulz KF. Combined hormonal versus nonhormonal versus

progestin-only contraception in lactation. *Cochrane Database Syst Rev.* 2003;2:CD003988. PubMed PMID: 12804497.

6. World Health Organization Medical Eligibility Criteria, 4th ed. 2009. http://whqlibdoc.who.int/publications/2010/9789241563888_eng.pdf.
7. Update to CDC's U.S. Medical Eligibility Criteria for Contraceptive Use, 2010: revised recommendations for the use of contraceptive methods during the postpartum period. *MMWR.* July 30, 2011. http://www.cdc.gov/mmwr/preview/mmwrhtml/mm6026a3.htm#tab1. Accessed July 30, 2011.
8. Iffy L, O'Donnell J, Correia J, Hopp L. Severe cardiac dysrhythmia in patients using bromocriptine postpartum. *Am J Ther.* 1998;5(2):111-115.
9. Aljazaf K, Hale TW, Ilett KF, et al. Pseudoephedrine: effects on milk production in women and estimation of infant exposure via breastmilk. *Br J Clin Pharmacol.* 2003;56(1):18-24.
10. Arbour MW, Kessler JL. Mammary hypoplasia: not every breast can produce sufficient milk. *J Midwifery Womens Health.* 2013;58(4):457-461.
11. Cox DB, Owens RA, Hartmann PE. Blood and milk prolactin and the rate of milk synthesis in women. *Exp Physiol.* 1996;81(6):1007-1020.
12. Academy of Breastfeeding Medicine Protocol Committee. ABM Clinical Protocol #9: use of galactagogues in initiating or augmenting the rate of maternal milk secretion (first revision January 2011). *Breastfeed Med.* 2011;6:41-49.
13. Betzold CM. Galactogogues. *J Midwifery Womens Health.* 2004;49(2):151-154.
14. Zuppa AA, Sindico P, Orchi C, Carducci C, Cardiello V, Romagnoli C. Safety and efficacy of galactagogues: substances that induce, maintain and increase breast milk production. *J Pharm Pharm Sci.* 2010;13(2):162-174.
15. Osadchy A, Moretti ME, Koren G. Effect of domperidone on insufficient lactation in puerperal women: a systematic review and meta-analysis of randomized controlled trials. *Obstet Gynecol Int.* 2012; 2012:642893.
16. Knoppert DC, Page A, Warren J, et al. The effect of two different domperidone doses on maternal milk production. *J Hum Lact.* 2013;29(1):38-44.
17. Hale TW, Hartmann PE, eds. *Textbook of Human Lactation.* Amarillo, TX: Hale; 2007.
18. Hale TW, Siddiqui AA, Baker TE. Transfer of interferon β-1a into human breastmilk. *Breastfeed Med.* 2012;7(2):123-125.
19. Hale TW, Ilett KF. *Drug Therapy and Breastfeeding: From Theory to Clinical Practice.* London: Parthenon Press; 2002.
20. Hale TW, McDonald R, Boger J. Transfer of celecoxib into breast milk. *J Hum Lact.* 2004;20(4):397-403.
21. Alcorn J, McNamara PJ. Pharmacokinetics in the newborn. *Adv Drug Deliv Rev.* 2003;55(5):667-686.
22. Dotta A, Chukhlantseva N. Ontogeny and drug metabolism in newborns. *J Matern Fetal Neonatal Med.* 2012;25(suppl 4):83-84.
23. Gerk PM, Kuhn RJ, Desai NS, McNamara PJ. Active transport of nitrofurantoin into breast milk. *Pharmacotherapy.* 2001;21(6):669-675.
24. Lau RJ, Emery MG, Galinsky RE. Unexpected accumulation of acyclovir in breast milk with estimation of infant exposure. *Obstet Gynecol.* 1987;69(3 pt 2): 468-471.
25. Kearns GL, McConnell RF Jr, Trang JM, Kluza RB. Appearance of ranitidine in breast milk following multiple dosing. *Clin Pharm.* 1985;4(3):322-324.
26. Delange F, Chanoine JP, Abrassart C, Bourdoux P. Topical iodine, breastfeeding, and neonatal hypothyroidism. *Arch Dis Child.* 1988;63(1):106-107.
27. Postellon DC, Aronow R. Iodine in mother's milk. *JAMA.* 1982;247(4):463.
28. Eyal S, Easterling TR, Carr D, et al. Pharmacokinetics of metformin during pregnancy. *Drug Metab Dispos.* 2010;38(5):833-840.
29. Hale TW, Kristensen JH, Hackett LP, Kohan R, Ilett KF. Transfer of metformin into breast milk. *Diabetologia.* 2002;45(11):1509-1514.
30. Gardiner SJ, Kirkpatrick CMJ, Begg EJ, Zhang M, Moore MP, Saville DJ. Transfer of metformin into breast milk. *Clin Pharmacol Ther.* 2003;73(1):71-77.
31. Briggs GG, Ambrose PJ, Nageotte MP, Padilla G, Wan S. Excretion of metformin into breast milk and the effect on nursing infants. *Obstet Gynecol.* 2005;105(6):1437-1441.
32. Alcorn J, Lu X, Moscow JA, McNamara PJ. Transporter gene expression in lactating and nonlactating human mammary epithelial cells using real-time reverse transcription–polymerase chain reaction. *J Pharmacol Exp Ther.* 2002;303(2):487-496.
33. Ilett KF, Kristensen JH. Drug use and breastfeeding. *Expert Opin Drug Saf.* 2005;4(4):745-768.
34. Begg EJ, Duffull SB, Hackett LP, Ilett KF. Studying drugs in breast milk: time to unify the approach. *J Hum Lact.* 2002;18(4):323-332.
35. Bennett PN. *Drugs and Human Lactation.* Amsterdam: Elsevier; 1996.

36. Rigourd V, de Villepin B, Amirouche A, et al. Ibuprofen concentrations in human mature milk—first data about pharmacokinetics study in breast milk with AOR-10127 "Antalait" study. *Ther Drug Moni.* 2014 Oct;36(5):590-6.
37. Wischnik A, Manth SM, Lloyd J, et al. The excretion of ketorolac tromethamine into breast milk after multiple oral dosing. *Eur J Clin Pharmacol.* 1989;36(5): 521-524.
38. Knoppert DC, Stempak D, Baruchel S, Koren G. Celecoxib in breast milk: a case report. *Pharmacotherapy.* 2003;23(1):97-100.
39. Baka NE, Bayoumeu F, Boutroy MJ, Laxenaire MC. Colostrum morphine concentrations during postcesarean intravenous patient-controlled analgesia. *Anesth Analg.* 2002;94(1):184-187.
40. Sindrup SH, Brosen K. The pharmacogenetics of codeine hypoalgesia. *Pharmacogenetics.* 1995;5(6): 335-346.
41. Koren G, Cairns J, Chitayat D, Gaedigk A, Leeder SJ. Pharmacogenetics of morphine poisoning in a breastfed neonate of a codeine-prescribed mother. *Lancet.* 2006;368(9536):704.
42. Hendrickson RG, McKewn NJ. Is maternal opioid use hazardous to breastfed infants? *Clin Toxicol (Phila).* 2012;50(1):1-14.
43. Madidi P, Ross CJD, Hayden MR, et al. Pharmacogenetics of neonatal opioid toxicity following maternal use of codeine during breastfeeding: a case control study. *Clin Pharmacol Ther.* 2009;85(1): 31-35.
44. Findlay JW, DeAngelis RL, Kearney MF, Welch RM, Findlay JM. Analgesic drugs in breast milk and plasma. *Clin Pharmacol Ther.* 1981;29(5):625-633.
45. Berlin CM, Paul IM, Vesell ES. Safety issues of maternal drug therapy during breastfeeding. *Clin Pharmacol Ther.* 2009;85(1):20-22.
46. FDA Public Health Advisory. Use of codeine by some breastfeeding mothers may lead to life-threatening side effects in nursing babies. May 7, 2007. http://www.fda.gov/cder/drug/advisory/codeine.htm. Accessed January 20, 2009.
47. Kristensen JH, Ilett K. Antibiotic, antifungal, antiviral and antiretroviral drugs. In: Hale TW, Hartmann PE, eds. *Textbook of Human Lactation.* Amarillo, TX: Hale; 2007:513-521.
48. Nahum GG, Uhl K, Kennedy DL. Antibiotic use in pregnancy and lactation: what is and is not known about teratogenic and toxic risks. *Obstet Gynecol.* 2006;107(5):1120-1138.
49. Mathew JL. Effect of maternal antibiotics on breastfeeding infants. *Postgrad Med J.* 2004;80(942):196-200.
50. Blanco JD, Jorgensen JH, Castaneda YS, Crawford SA. Ceftazidime levels in human breast milk. *Antimicrob Agents Chemother.* 1983;23(3):479-480.
51. Kafetzis DA, Siafas CA, Georgakopoulos PA, Papadatos CJ. Passage of cephalosporins and amoxicillin into the breast milk. *Acta Paediatr Scand.* 1981;70(3):285-288.
52. Matsuda S. Transfer of antibiotics into maternal milk. *Biol Res Pregnancy Perinatol.* 1984;5(2):57-60.
53. Shyu WC, Shah VR, Campbell DA, et al. Excretion of cefprozil into human breast milk. *Antimicrob Agents Chemother.* 1992;36(5):938-941.
54. Chung AM, Reed MD, Blumer JL. Antibiotics and breastfeeding: a critical review of the literature. *Paediatr Drugs.* 2002;4(12):817-832.
55. Bourget P, Quinquis-Desmaris V, Fernandez H. Ceftriaxone distribution and protein binding between maternal blood and milk postpartum. *Ann Pharmacother.* 1993;27(3):294-297.
56. Harmon T, Burkhart G, Applebaum H. Perforated pseudomembranous colitis in the breastfed infant. *J Pediatr Surg.* 1992;27(6):744-746.
57. Lumbiganon P, Pengsaa K, Sookpranee T. Ciprofloxacin in neonates and its possible adverse effect on the teeth. *Pediatr Infect Dis J.* 1991;10(8):619-620.
58. Ghaffer F, McCraken GH. Quinolones in pediatrics. In: Hoper DC, Rubenstein E, eds. *Quinolone Antimicrobial Agents.* Washington, DC: ASM Press; 2003:343-354.
59. Schwebke JR. Metronidazole: utilization in the obstetric and gynecologic patient. *Sex Transm Dis.* 1995; 22(6):370-376.
60. Einarson A, Ho E, Koren G. Can we use metronidazole during pregnancy and breastfeeding? Putting an end to the controversy. *Can Fam Physician.* 2000; 46:1053-1054.
61. Passmore CM, McElnay JC, Rainey EA, D'Arcy PF. Metronidazole excretion in breast milk and its effect on the suckling neonate. *Br J Clin Pharmacol.* 1988; 26(1):45-51.
62. Sørensen HT, Skriver MV, Pedersen L, Larsen H, Ebbesen F, Schønheyder HC. Risk of infantile hypertrophic pyloric stenosis after maternal postnatal use of macrolides. *Scand J Infect Dis.* 2003;35(2):104-106.
63. Lund M, Pasternak B, Davidsen RB, et al. Use of macrolides in mother and child and risk of infantile hypertrophic pyloric stenosis: nationwide cohort study. *BMJ.* 2014;348:g1908.

64. Cooper WO, Ray WA, Griffin MR. Prenatal prescription of macrolide antibiotics and infantile hypertrophic pyloric stenosis. *Obstet Gynecol.* 2002; 100(1):101-106.
65. Hauben M, Amsden GW. The association of erythromycin and infantile hypertrophic pyloric stenosis: causal or coincidental? *Drug Saf.* 2002;25(13): 929-942.
66. Matsuda S. Transfer of antibiotics into maternal milk. *Biol Res Pregnancy Perinatol.* 1984;5(2):57-60.
67. Kelsey JJ, Moser LR, Jennings JC, Munger MA. Presence of azithromycin breast milk concentrations: a case report. *Am J Obstet Gynecol.* 1994;170(5 pt 1): 1375-1376.
68. Force RW. Fluconazole concentrations in breast milk. *Pediatr Infect Dis J.* 1995;14(3):235-236.
69. Chung AM, Reed MD, Blumer JL. Antibiotics and breast-feeding: a critical review of the literature. *Paediatr Drugs.* 2002;4(12):817-837.
70. Ito S. Drug therapy for breastfeeding women. *N Engl J Med.* 2000;343(2):118-126.
71. Harden CL, Pennell PB, Koppel BS, et al. Practice parameter update: management issues for women with epilepsy—focus on pregnancy (an evidence-based review): vitamin K, folic acid, blood levels, and breastfeeding: report of the Quality Standards Subcommittee and Therapeutics and Technology Assessment Subcommittee of the American Academy of Neurology and American Epilepsy Society. *Neurology.* 2009;73(2):142-1429.
72. Beardmore KS, Morris JM, Gallery ED. Excretion of antihypertensive medication into human breast milk: a systematic review. *Hypertens Pregnancy.* 2002;21(1):85-95.
73. Penny WJ, Lewis MJ. Nifedipine is excreted in breast milk. *Eur J Clin Pharmacol.* 1989;36(4):427-428.
74. Shannon ME, Malecha SE, Cha AJ. Angiotensin converting enzyme inhibitors (ACEIs) and angiotensin II receptor blockers (ARBs) and lactation: an update. *J Hum Lact.* 2000;16(2):152-155.
75. Mizuta H, Amino N, Ichihara K, et al. Thyroid hormones in breast milk and their influence on thyroid function of breast-fed babies. *Pediatr Res.* 1983;17(6):468-471.
76. Varma SK, Collins M, Row A, Haller WS, Varma K. Thyroxine, tri-iodothyronine, and reverse tri-iodothyronine concentrations in breast milk. *J Pediatr.* 1978;93(5):803-806.
77. Karras S, Krassas GE. Breastfeeding and antithyroid drugs: a view from within. *Eur Thyroid J.* 2012; 1(1):30-33.
78. U.S. Food and Drug Administration. Propylthiouracil (PTU)-induced liver failure. *FDA Alert* June 3, 2009. http://www.fda.gov/Drugs/DrugSafety/PostmarketDrugSafetyInformationforPatientsandProviders/ucm209023.htm. Accessed September 1, 2014.
79. Rylance GW, Woods CG, Donnelly MC, Oliver JS, Alexander WD. Carbimazole and breastfeeding. *Lancet.* 1987;1(8538):928.
80. Le Strat Y, Dubertret C, Le Foll B. Prevalence and correlates of major depressive episode in pregnant and postpartum women in the United States. *J Affect Disord.* 2011;135(1-3):128-138.
81. McDonagh M, Matthews A, Phillipi C, et al. *Antidepressant treatment of depression during pregnancy and the postpartum period.* Evidence Report/Technology Assessment No. 216. (Prepared by the Pacific Northwest Evidence-Based Practice Center under Contract No. 290-2007-10057-I.) AHRQ Publication No. 14-E003-EF. Rockville, MD: Agency for Healthcare Research and Quality; July 2014. http://www.effectivehealthcare.ahrq.gov/reports/final.cfm.
82. McDonagh MS, Matthews A, Phillipi C, et al. Depression drug treatment outcomes in pregnancy and the postpartum period: a systematic review and meta-analysis. *Obstet Gynecol.* 2014;124(3):526-534.
83. Hagg S, Spigset O. Anticonvulsant use during lactation. *Drug Saf.* 2000;22(6):425-440.
84. Fortinguerra F, Clavenna A, Bonati M. Psychotropic drug use during breastfeeding: a review of the evidence. *Pediatrics.* 2009;124(4):e547-e556.
85. Frey OR, Scheidt P, von Brenndorff AI. Adverse effects in a newborn infant breast-fed by a mother treated with doxepin. *Ann Pharmacother.* 1999;33(6):690-693.
86. Stancer HC, Reed KL. Desipramine and 2-hydroxydesipramine in human breast milk and the nursing infant's serum. *Am J Psychiatry.* 1986; 143(12): 1597-1600.
87. Knoppert DC, Nimkar R, Principi T, Yuen D. Paroxetine toxicity in a newborn after in utero exposure: clinical symptoms correlate with serum levels. *Ther Drug Monit.* 2006;28(1):5-7.
88. Moses-Kolko EL, Bogen D, Perel J, et al. Neonatal signs after late in utero exposure to serotonin reuptake inhibitors: literature review and implications for clinical applications. *JAMA.* 2005;293(19): 2372-2383.
89. Kristensen JH, Ilett KF, Hackett LP, Yapp P, Paech M, Begg EJ. Distribution and excretion of fluoxetine and norfluoxetine in breast milk. *Br J Clin Pharmacol.* 1999;48(4):521-527.

90. Rampono J, Kristensen JH, Hackett LP, Paech M, Kohan R, Ilett KF. Citalopram and demethylcitalopram in breast milk: distribution, excretion and effects in breast fed infants. *Br J Clin Pharmacol.* 2000;50(3):263-268.
91. Rampono J, Hackett LP, Kristensen JH, Kohan R, Page-Sharp M, Ilett KF. Transfer of escitalopram and its metabolite demethylescitalopram into breastmilk. *Br J Clin Pharmacol.* 2006;62(3):316-322.
92. Ohkubo T, Shimoyama R, Sugawara K. Measurement of haloperidol in human breast milk by high-performance liquid chromatography. *J Pharm Sci.* 1992;81(9):947-949.
93. Ilett KF, Hackett LP, Kristensen JH, Vaddadi KS, Gardiner SJ, Begg EJ. Transfer of risperidone and 9-hydroxyrisperidone into breast milk. *Ann Pharmacother.* 2004;38(2):273-276.
94. Croke S, Buist A, Hackett LP, Ilett KF, Norman TR, Burrows GD. Olanzapine excretion in human breast milk: estimation of infant exposure. *Int J Neuropsychopharmacol.* 2002;5(3):243-247.
95. Gardiner SJ, Kristensen JH, Begg EJ, et al. Transfer of olanzapine into breast milk, calculation of infant drug dose, and effect on breast-fed infants. *Am J Psychiatry.* 2003;160(8):1428-1431.
96. Chaudron LH. When and how to use mood stabilizers during breastfeeding. *Prim Care Update Ob Gyn.* 2000;7(3):113-117.
97. Briggs GG, Freeman RK, Yaffee SJ. *Drugs in Pregnancy and Lactation.* 8th ed. Philadelphia: Lippincott Williams & Wilkins; 2008.
98. Lawrence RA, Lawrence R. *Breastfeeding: A Guide for the Medical Profession.* 6th ed. St. Louis, MO: Mosby; 2005.
99. Drugs and Lactation Database (LactMed). A peer-reviewed and fully referenced database of drugs to which breastfeeding mothers may be exposed. [Among the data included are maternal and infant levels of drugs, possible effects on breastfed infants and on lactation, and alternate drugs to consider.] http://toxnet.nlm.nih.gov/cgi-bin/sis/htmlgen?LACT. Accessed June 26, 2009.

39 The Newborn

Cheryl A. Carlson, Mary C. Brucker

Based on the chapter by Judy Wright Lott in the first edition of Pharmacology for Women's Health

Chapter Glossary

Hyperoxia Excessive oxygenation; antonym to *hypoxia*.

Omphalitis Infection of the umbilical cord; one of the most common neonatal infections.

Ophthalmia neonatorum Neonatal conjunctivitis usually due to gonococcal or chlamydial infection.

Vitamin K–deficiency bleeding (VKDB) Most common form of hemorrhagic disease of the newborn.

Introduction

Few women's healthcare professionals also provide direct neonatal care. However, when a clinician cares for a woman who has had a newborn, a basic knowledge about infants and their health is needed to provide anticipatory guidance and good health education.

Newborns are not miniature adults; they have unique physiologic attributes that influence treatments when needed. Identifying the appropriate drugs for neonates present special challenges. This chapter provides an overview of the pharmacologic principles that underlie safe and effective drug therapy for term newborns, including common prophylaxis, health maintenance, and recognition and initial treatment for selected newborn problems.

The Unique Newborn

Principles that govern medication—selection, administration, and monitoring—are generally the same for newborns as for individuals of other ages; however, the relative immaturity of the neonate's organ systems has a significant impact on the way the newborn body responds to drugs. A general discussion of pharmacologic principles, pharmacokinetics, and pharmacotherapeutics can be found in the chapter *Principles of Pharmacology.*

However, the neonate is physiologically different when compared to children and adults. These differences affect the specific dosage forms and dosing regimens used in newborns.[1] Variables that influence the action of a specific drug may include gestational and postnatal age, classification of appropriate gestational age and birth weight (e.g., small for gestational age), overall condition, presence of underlying disease, development and function of organ systems, and polypharmacy.

Pharmacokinetics and The Newborn

The uniqueness of the neonate's physiology regarding absorption, protein binding, distribution, metabolism, and excretion must be taken into consideration in the design of drug regimens.

Absorption

Enteral, intramuscular, and topical routes of administration require absorption from the site to be effective. Intramuscular administration of medications is not as efficient as intravenous administration of the same drugs. Neonates have decreased muscle mass and tone, which may lead to unpredictable and incomplete absorption from the intramuscular route. In addition, decreased blood flow to specific organs can decrease absorption of drugs administered intramuscularly in many disease states that affect neonates.[2] Decreased or erratic absorption can delay the therapeutic response, cause a delay in peak concentration, and result in a longer duration of action.

Topical administration depends on skin integrity, blood flow, and subcutaneous fat for absorption.[3] Increased skin-to-body surface area and decreased integrity of the skin barrier can predispose the neonate to toxicity from topical medications that are typically considered benign when administered to adults. Drugs such as hydrocortisone and antifungal creams, for example, may be absorbed through the skin in levels that lead to adverse systemic effects. Conversely, the diminished skin barrier may allow for unique dosing of some medications that takes advantage of this physiologic difference to promote drug absorption. For example, a topical anesthetic, eutectic mixture of local anesthetic (EMLA), has been used for local pain relief in term newborns, although it has been associated with methemoglobinemia in preterm newborns.

Intravascular administration generally is the preferred route in newborns because the drug is delivered directly into the circulatory system bypassing gastrointestinal absorption, which varies because of the neonate's slower gastric emptying time, the lower level of microbial colonization, and the immaturity of the pancreas and biliary system. With intravascular administration, therapeutic effects are often immediate, although any adverse effects also may become apparent rapidly.

Distribution

Protein binding is an important consideration for the newborn. Once in the circulation, medications may remain as free drugs in the plasma or bind to a variety of plasma proteins, although the majority bind to albumin. Serum albumin concentrations are lower; there are also fewer protein binding sites available in neonates and infants. Newborns have higher levels of maternal estrogen and bilirubin in their circulation that can compete with administered drugs for the albumin binding sites. As a result, for a specific serum concentration, there is more free or active drug available for pharmacologic action in the newborn than in an adult.

A clinical disorder experienced by the newborn can further affect protein binding. In particular, hepatic or renal failure results in altered protein binding. Neonatal albumin levels are important considerations when establishing dosage and monitoring regimens. For example, a newborn with hyperbilirubinemia may have an altered response to a medication because of the excess bilirubin bound to albumin, which decreases the number of albumin binding sites available to the medication. Conversely, when fewer binding sites than normal are available, administration of medications that bind to albumin may in turn displace bilirubin from albumin thereby increasing the bilirubin levels, resulting in an icteric newborn.[4]

Metabolism and Elimination

Delayed neonatal maturation affects metabolism and the newborn's ability to eliminate some medications, such as morphine. In an adult, morphine is rapidly metabolized to morphine-6-glucuronide, an active metabolite and more potent compound than morphine. However, in the newborn, this metabolism of morphine does not occur, so the newborn may need a higher dose (mg/kg) of morphine than adults for adequate analgesia. Methylation, reduction, and sulfation are well developed at birth, but the other drug metabolism pathways do not develop fully until 1 to 3 months post birth.[1,3,5]

As is true in the adult, metabolism can be affected by drug-drug interactions. Medications that induce CYP450 enzymes, such as phenobarbital, can increase liver enzyme activity in the neonate and cause increased clearance of other drugs that are metabolized by the enzyme that is induced, such as opioids. Conversely, medications that inhibit CYP450 enzymes may cause slower clearance of other medications.[4,6]

Organ function is especially important if most of the elimination of the medication occurs in one organ system. For example, a neonate with renal failure will have decreased clearance of gentamicin (Garamycin) because gentamicin is primarily excreted via the kidneys. Finally, the rate of excretion of drugs may vary based on the relative immaturity of the neonatal kidney. The neonatal kidney has a high resistance to blood flow, incomplete glomerular and tubular development, and a short loop of Henle. In addition, the kidney receives a low fraction of cardiac output. These variables can result in higher peak concentrations or longer duration of action of some medications by decreasing the rate of the drug's elimination.

Pharmacogenetics

Similar to adults, newborns can have variants of the metabolizing enzymes such as CYP450. One of the best known of these enzymes, CYP3A4, exists during fetal life in the form of CYP3A7. The amount of this variant decreases after birth and within the first few months of life is replaced by the adult form. However, this transition is not predictable, which makes dosing of any agent known to have a drug interaction with this enzyme more challenging. For this reason, newborns who are administered multiple agents should be monitored for potential drug–drug reactions. Among the drugs most commonly associated with such reactions are macrolide antibiotics, azole antifungals, rifampin (Rifadin), and phenobarbital.[7] Additional information about drug–drug reactions can be found in the *Principles of Pharmacology* and *Drug Toxicity* chapters.

Exposure to Drugs via the Placenta and via Breast Milk

Two other important variables need to be considered in the pharmacology of the neonate—the effects of fetal exposure to drugs and newborn exposure through human milk. Any medication or substance given to a pregnant woman can cross the placenta, though fetal exposure may or may not produce any degree of effect. Several factors affect the untoward effects of drugs on the fetus, including the drug's molecular weight, protein binding, lipid solubility, and ionization; maternal serum concentrations; and placental integrity. For example, intrapartum administration of opioids may result in any several symptoms, such as neonatal central nervous system sedation, lethargy, or difficulty nursing.

Transfer of substances from human milk to the neonate is an often-overlooked source of drug actions in the neonate. In addition to pharmacokinetics, other factors influencing this transfer include the time of medication administration relative to the time of nursing, the dose of the medication, the length of nursing, and the total volume of human milk ingested.[8] More information about drugs and the nursling can be found in the *Breastfeeding* chapter.

Drugs for Prophylaxis Used in the Neonatal Period

Following a term birth, the newborn is generally in one of the healthiest periods of life, and thus does not require drug therapy. However, it is incumbent upon the healthcare provider to adequately and appropriately assess the newborn, offer appropriate prophylactic medications, diagnose any problematic conditions, and work with parents so that drug therapy can be initiated as needed.

Prophylaxis Against Ophthalmia Neonatorum

Ophthalmia neonatorum conjunctivitis can occur in a newborn when a woman infected with *Neisseria gonorrhea* or *Chlamydia trachomatis* gives birth vaginally and the newborn is exposed to the organism at the time of birth. These microorganisms are the most common cause of acute ophthalmic disease in newborns.[9] Symptoms of chlamydial conjunctivitis most often appear 5 to 12 days after birth and include redness, swelling of the eyelids, and pustular discharge. Gonococcal conjunctivitis is seen usually at about 2 to 4 days of life, and is characterized by redness, thick pustular discharge, and swelling. Ophthalmia neonatorum can cause corneal ulceration, endophthalmitis, and blindness. Since the introduction of routine eye prophylaxis for all newborns, the incidence of neonatal conjunctivitis and blindness has dramatically decreased.

Historically, the first drug used for prophylactic eye treatment was 1% silver nitrate solution. Side effects of this solution included chemical conjunctivitis accompanied by edema, redness, and watery discharge. The post-treatment appearance of the newborn could be distressing to parents. In addition, silver nitrate is ineffective against *Chlamydia trachomatis.* Today, silver nitrate has largely been replaced in this indication due to the availability of agents that have a broader spectrum of action and fewer side effects.[10] Effective agents for eye prophylaxis include 0.5% erythromycin (EES) ointment, 1% tetracycline ointment, or 1.5 to 2.5% povidone-iodine solution.[9–12] However, erythromycin ophthalmic ointment (0.5%) is the only Centers for Disease Control and Prevention (CDC)–recommended therapy for prophylaxis of ophthalmia neonatorum available in the United States.[13]

The majority of states in the United States mandate eye prophylaxis be administered to all neonates. Some, but not all, states require that the eye care be performed within the first hour of life, although there is little pharmacologic evidence regarding timing of such therapy. Most parents do not object to this drug treatment, although some will be concerned that their newborn may not be able to engage well at their first interaction due to a degree of temporary blurry vision following placement of the ointment. Many providers and facilities delay eye therapy until the newborn is stable, in skin-to-skin contact with the mother, and breastfeeding.[14]

Although eye prophylaxis is performed routinely in the United States, the agents used are not effective against every type of microorganism. If a newborn develops signs of conjunctivitis, the infant should be promptly evaluated to determine the cause. Therapy will be determined based on the microorganism.

Prophylaxis Against Vitamin K Deficiency

Hemostasis depends on an adequate supply of clotting factors, which are primarily produced by the liver. The prothrombin complex specifically requires the action of vitamin K, which is synthesized by bacteria in the human colon. Vitamin K–dependent clotting factor levels in the cord blood of a term fetus are 30% to 70% of adult levels. In addition, a significant drop in these levels occurs at birth, due to poor placental transfer of maternal vitamin K, immature liver function, and delayed synthesis of vitamin K by bacteria in the neonatal bowel. Vitamin K–dependent clotting factors gradually rise but do not reach adult levels until the child is approximately 9 months old.

Hemorrhage due to a deficiency of vitamin K–dependent clotting factors during the neonatal period is classified as **vitamin K-deficiency bleeding (VKDB)**. Full-term newborns have approximately 30% to 60% of the adult function of vitamin K–dependent coagulation activity.[15]

Three syndromes of vitamin K–deficiency bleeding are distinguished: early VKDB, which has an onset within the first 24 hours of life; classic VKDB, which is the most common type and has an onset between 2 and 7 days of life; and late VKDB, which may present between 3 weeks and 8 months of life.[16,17] Early-onset VKD usually presents with a cephalohematoma, intracranial bleeding, or intra-abdominal bleeding.[17] Intracranial hemorrhage is seen in 20% to 25% of affected neonates[18] and often is associated with intrauterine exposure to drugs that interfere with vitamin K, such as anticonvulsants, anticoagulants, or antibiotics taken by the woman during pregnancy. A newborn with classic VKDB presents with generalized cutaneous, umbilical, gastrointestinal, or circumcision bleeding. This form of VKDB usually is found among neonates who did not receive vitamin K prophylaxis at birth. Late-onset VKDB may be associated with exclusively breastfed infants who did not receive vitamin K prophylaxis at birth. In rare cases, it can be seen in newborns with chronic diseases that impair absorption of fat-soluble vitamins, such as liver disease, galactosemia, celiac disease, and chronic diarrhea.[19] Late-onset VKDB also can be associated with intracranial hemorrhage.[20]

Administration of Vitamin K

The recommended intramuscular dose is 1 mg administered intramuscularly. This dose was adopted without the benefit of research that determined the best dose and it is a massive dose compared to the newborn's daily requirement of 5–10 mcg per day. Plasma concentrations of vitamin K following the intramuscular dose exceed endogenous levels by a factor of 10,000. Despite the dose being very large, it is effective and no significant side effects or adverse effects have been documented.

Several different factors are associated with the timing of vitamin K administration. The United States Preventive Task Force, the American Academy of Pediatrics, and the United Kingdom Department of Health, among others, recommend administration of vitamin K to all newborns but do not specify the time frame in which the medication should be administered. The Canadian Paediatric Society recommends that administration occur within 6 hours of birth. Some U.S. states mandate administration within an hour of birth, and some statutes do not allow parents to decline, although some institutions will accept such a request on the grounds they cannot intervene for a non-life-threatening condition without appropriate parental consent.[21]

Controversies Relating to Prophylaxis for VKDB

Because VKDB rarely is seen today, parents may be unaware of the risks. Overall, the number of newborns who do not receive vitamin K prophylaxis is rising.[22–24] Reasons given for not accepting vitamin K prophylaxis include a concern about vitamin K being associated with subsequent development of leukemia, a desire to avoid the intramuscular injection, and general concern about introducing synthetic substances into the newborn's system.

Oral versus Intramuscular Administration

Another part of the controversy concerns the necessity of an intramuscular dose. Some parents refuse the intramuscular administration and request that vitamin K instead be given orally. Vitamin K has been administered orally in Europe. Studies that have compared the effectiveness have found that vitamin K administered intramuscularly is more effective than the oral administration of vitamin K for all types of VKDB. Single oral doses are protective against early-onset VKDB, and classic VKDB in healthy term exclusively breastfed infants, but prevention of late-onset VKDB requires multiple oral doses. Oral prophylaxis failures of 1.2 to 1.8 per 100,000 live births have been reported for late-onset VKDB. As a result, the late-onset doses range from 25 mcg daily for 13 weeks; to 2 mg with first feeding, followed by 2 mg between days 2 and 7 of life; to 1 mg weekly for 3 months in countries that use oral dosing. The American Academy of Pediatrics recommends one intramuscular injection of 1 mg because there are virtually no prophylaxis failures following this regimen.

Vitamin K and Childhood Cancer

Older studies regarding adverse effects of intramuscular vitamin K noted a small increased risk for developing leukemia in children who received such a dose of vitamin K at birth. In contrast, a subsequent case controlled study from the United Kingdom of more than 7000 children failed to find any relationship between vitamin K and leukemia.[26]

Immunizations

Although the immune system begins developing in early gestation, the immune system of the newborn is immature compared to that of older children and adults. The fetus receives the benefits of transplacental diffusion of maternal antibodies during gestation. After birth, once the circulating antibodies from the mother are no longer available, the newborn becomes more susceptible to communicable infections. Vaccines that protect against communicable diseases have resulted in reductions in the incidence of once-common diseases such as diphtheria, polio, varicella (chickenpox), rubella (German measles), and pertussis (whooping cough).[27,28] Table 39-1 summarizes the recommended vaccination schedule for children from birth through 15 months of age. Note that

Table 39-1 Recommended Immunization Schedule for Persons Aged 0–18 Months, United States, 2015

These recommendations must be read with the footnotes that follow. For those who fall behind or start late, see the catch-up schedule.

	Age								
Vaccine	**Birth**	**1 Month**	**2 Months**	**4 Months**	**6 Months**	**9 Months**	**12 Months**	**15 Months**	**18 Months**
Hepatitis B[a] (HepB)	1st dose	2nd dose			3rd dose				
Rotavirus[b] (RV)			1st dose	2nd dose	See footnote b				
Diphtheria, tetanus, pertussis[c] (DTap)			1st dose	2nd dose	3rd dose			4th dose	
Haemophilus influenzae type b[d] (Hib)			1st dose	2nd dose	See footnote d		3rd or 4th dose See footnote d		
Pneumococcal conjugate[e] (PCV13)			1st dose	2nd dose	3rd dose		4th dose		
Inactivated poliovirus[f] (IPV)			1st dose	2nd dose	3rd dose				
Influenza[g] (IIV, LAIV) 2 doses for some, see footnote g					Influenza (Yearly)				
Measles, mumps, rubella[h] (MMR)					See full schedule		1st dose		
Varicella[i] (VAR)							1st dose		
Hepatitis A[j] (HepA)							2-dose series See footnote j		
Meningococcal[k] (Hib-MenCY ≥ 6 weeks; MenACWY-D ≥ 9 months; ≥ MenACWY-CRM ≥ 2 months)				See full schedule					

Range of recommended ages for all children	Range of recommended ages for catch-up immunization	Range of recommended ages for certain high-risk groups	Not routinely recommended

This schedule includes recommendations in effect as of January 1, 2015. Any dose not administered at the recommended age should be administered at a subsequent visit, when indicated and feasible. The use of a combination vaccine generally is preferred over separate injections of its equivalent component vaccines. Vaccination providers should consult the relevant Advisory Committee on Immunization Practices (ACIP) statement for detailed recommendations, available online at http://www.cdc.gov/vaccines/hcp/acip-recs/index.html. Clinically significant adverse events that follow vaccination should be reported to the Vaccine Adverse Event Reporting System (VAERS) online (http://www.vaers.hhs.gov) or by telephone (800-822-7967). Suspected cases of vaccine-preventable diseases should be reported to the state or local health department. Additional information, including precautions and contraindications for vaccination, is available from CDC online (http://www.cdc.gov/vaccines/recs/vac-admin/contraindications.htm) or by telephone (800-CDC-INFO [800-232-4636]).

This schedule is approved by the Advisory Committee on Immunization Practices (http//www.cdc.gov/vaccines/acip), the American Academy of Pediatrics (http://www.aap.org), the American Academy of Family Physicians (http://www.aafp.org), and the American College of Obstetricians and Gynecologists (http://www.acog.org).

(continues)

Table 39-1 Recommended Immunization Schedule for Persons Aged 0–18 Months, United States, 2015 (*continued*)

a. Hepatitis B (HepB) vaccine. (*Minimum age: birth*)
Routine vaccination:
At birth:
- Administer monovalent HepB vaccine to all newborns before hospital discharge.
- For infants born to hepatitis B surface antigen (HBsAg)-positive mothers, administer HepB vaccine and 0.5 mL of hepatitis B immune globulin (HBIG) within 12 hours of birth. These infants should be tested for HBsAg and antibody to HBsAg (anti-HBs) 1 to 2 months after completion of the HepB series at age 9 through 18 months (preferably at the next well-child visit).
- If mother's HBsAg status is unknown, within 12 hours of birth administer HepB vaccine regardless of birth weight. For infants weighing less than 2000 grams, administer HBIG in addition to HepB vaccine within 12 hours of birth. Determine mother's HBsAg status as soon as possible and, if mother is HBsAg-positive, also administer HBIG for infants weighing 2000 grams or more as soon as possible, but no later than age 7 days.

Doses following the birth dose:
- The second dose should be administered at age 1 or 2 months. Monovalent HepB vaccine should be used for doses administered before age 6 weeks.
- Infants who did not receive a birth dose should receive 3 doses of a HepB-containing vaccine on a schedule of 0, 1 to 2 months, and 6 months starting as soon as feasible. See catch-up schedule.
- Administer the second dose 1 to 2 months after the first dose (minimum interval of 4 weeks), administer the third dose at least 8 weeks after the second dose AND at least 16 weeks after the **first** dose. The final (third or fourth) dose in the HepB vaccine series should be administered **no earlier than age 24 weeks**.
- Administration of a total of 4 doses of HepB vaccine is permitted when a combination vaccine containing HepB is administered after the birth dose.

b. Rotavirus (RV) vaccines. (*Minimum age: 6 weeks for both RV1 [Rotarix] and RV5 [RotaTeq]*)
Routine vaccination:
Administer a series of RV vaccine to all infants as follows:
1. If Rotarix is used, administer a 2-dose series at 2 and 4 months of age.
2. If RotaTeq is used, administer a 3-dose series at ages 2, 4, and 6 months.
3. If any dose in the series was RotaTeq or vaccine product is unknown for any dose in the series, a total of 3 doses of RV vaccine should be administered.

c. Diphtheria and tetanus toxoids and acellular pertussis (DTaP) vaccine. (*Minimum age: 6 weeks. Exception: DTaP-IPV [Kinrix]: 4 years*)
Routine vaccination:
- Administer a 5-dose series of DTaP vaccine at ages 2, 4, 6, 15 through 18 months, and 4 through 6 years. The fourth dose may be administered as early as age 12 months, provided at least 6 months have elapsed since the third dose. However, the fourth dose of DTaP need not be repeated if it was administered at least 4 months after the third dose of DTaP.

d. *Haemophilus influenzae* type b (Hib) conjugate vaccine. (*Minimum age: 6 weeks for PRP-T [ACTHIB, DTaP-IPV/Hib (Pentacel) and Hib-MenCY (MenHibrix)], PRP-OMP [PedvaxHIB or COMVAX], 12 months for PRP-T [Hiberix]*)
Routine vaccination:
- Administer a 2- or 3-dose Hib vaccine primary series and a booster dose (dose 3 or 4 depending on vaccine used in primary series) at age 12 through 15 months to complete a full Hib vaccine series.
- The primary series with ActHIB, MenHibrix, or Pentacel consists of 3 doses and should be administered at 2, 4, and 6 months of age. The primary series with PedvaxHib or COMVAX consists of 2 doses and should be administered at 2 and 4 months of age; a dose at age 6 months is not indicated.
- One booster dose (dose 3 or 4 depending on vaccine used in primary series) of any Hib vaccine should be administered at age 12 through 15 months. An exception is Hiberix vaccine. Hiberix should only be used for the booster (final) dose in children aged 12 months through 4 years who have received at least 1 prior dose of Hib-containing vaccine.
- For recommendations on the use of MenHibrix in patients at increased risk for meningococcal disease, please refer to the meningococcal vaccine footnotes and also to *MMWR* February 28, 2014 / 63(RR01);1-13, available at http://www.cdc.gov/mmwr/PDF/rr/rr6301.pdf.

** Patients who have not received a primary series and booster dose or at least 1 dose of Hib vaccine after 14 months of age are considered unimmunized.*

e. Pneumococcal vaccines. (*Minimum age: 6 weeks for PCV13, 2 years for PPSV23*)
Routine vaccination with PCV13:
- Administer a 4-dose series of PCV13 vaccine at ages 2, 4, and 6 months and at age 12 through 15 months.
- For children aged 14 through 59 months who have received an age-appropriate series of 7-valent PCV (PCV7), administer a single supplemental dose of 13-valent PCV (PCV13).

f. Inactivated poliovirus vaccine (IPV). (*Minimum age: 6 weeks*)
Routine vaccination:
- Administer a 4-dose series of IPV at ages 2, 4, 6 through 18 months, and 4 through 6 years. The final dose in the series should be administered on or after the fourth birthday and at least 6 months after the previous dose.

g. Influenza vaccines. (*Minimum age: 6 months for inactivated influenza vaccine [IIV], 2 years for live, attenuated influenza vaccine [LAIV]*)
Routine vaccination:
- Administer influenza vaccine annually to all children beginning at age 6 months. For most healthy, nonpregnant persons aged 2 through 49 years, either LAIV or IIV may be used. However, LAIV should NOT be administered to some persons, including 1) persons who have experienced severe allergic reactions to LAIV, any of its components, or to a previous dose of any other influenza vaccine; 2) children 2 through 17 years receiving aspirin or aspirin-containing products; 3) persons who are allergic to eggs; 4) pregnant women; 5) immunosuppressed persons; 6) children 2 through 4 years of age with asthma or who had wheezing in the past 12 months; or 7) persons who have taken influenza antiviral medications in the previous 48 hours. For all other contraindications and precautions to use of LAIV, see *MMWR* August 15, 2014 / 63(32);691-697 [40 pages] available at http://www.cdc.gov/mmwr/pdf/wk/mm6332.pdf.

For children aged 6 months through 8 years:
- For the 2014-15 season, administer 2 doses (separated by at least 4 weeks) to children who are receiving influenza vaccine for the first time. Some children in this age group who have been vaccinated previously will also need 2 doses. For additional guidance, follow dosing guidelines in the 2014-15 ACIP influenza vaccine recommendations, *MMWR* August 15, 2014 / 63(32);691-697 [40 pages] available at http://www.cdc.gov/mmwr/pdf/wk/mm6332.pdf.
- For the 2015–16 season, follow dosing guidelines in the 2015 ACIP influenza vaccine recommendations.

h. Measles, mumps, and rubella (MMR) vaccine. (*Minimum age: 12 months for routine vaccination*)
Routine vaccination:
- Administer a 2-dose series of MMR vaccine at ages 12 through 15 months and 4 through 6 years. The second dose may be administered before age 4 years, provided at least 4 weeks have elapsed since the first dose.
- Administer 1 dose of MMR vaccine to infants aged 6 through 11 months before departure from the United States for international travel. These children should be revaccinated with 2 doses of MMR vaccine, the first at age 12 through 15 months (12 months if the child remains in an area where disease risk is high), and the second dose at least 4 weeks later.
- Administer 2 doses of MMR vaccine to children aged 12 months and older before departure from the United States for international travel. The first dose should be administered on or after age 12 months and the second dose at least 4 weeks later.

i. Varicella (VAR) vaccine. (*Minimum age: 12 months*)
Routine vaccination:
- Administer a 2-dose series of VAR vaccine at ages 12 through 15 months and 4 through 6 years. The second dose may be administered before age 4 years, provided at least 3 months have elapsed since the first dose. If the second dose was administered at least 4 weeks after the first dose, it can be accepted as valid.

j. Hepatitis A (HepA) vaccine. (*Minimum age: 12 months*)
Routine vaccination:
- Initiate the 2-dose HepA vaccine series at 12 through 23 months; separate the 2 doses by 6 to 18 months.
- Children who have received 1 dose of HepA vaccine before age 24 months should receive a second dose 6 to 18 months after the first dose.
- For any person aged 2 years and older who has not already received the HepA vaccine series, 2 doses of HepA vaccine separated by 6 to 18 months may be administered if immunity against hepatitis A virus infection is desired.

k. Meningococcal conjugate vaccines. (*Minimum age: 6 weeks for Hib-MenCY [MenHibrix], 9 months for MenACWY-D [Menactra], 2 months for MenACWY-CRM [Menveo]*)
Routine vaccination:
- Administer a single dose of Menactra or Menveo vaccine at age 11 through 12 years, with a booster dose at age 16 years.
- Adolescents aged 11 through 18 years with human immunodeficiency virus (HIV) infection should receive a 2-dose primary series of Menactra or Menveo with at least 8 weeks between doses.
- For children aged 2 months through 18 years with high-risk conditions, see full schedule.

For other catch-up recommendations for these persons, and complete information on use of meningococcal vaccines, including guidance related to vaccination of persons at increased risk of infection, see MMWR March 22, 2013 / 62(RR02);1-22, available at http://www.cdc.gov/mmwr/pdf/rr/rr6202.pdf.

Source: Data from the Centers for Disease Control and Prevention. Recommended immunization schedule for persons age 0 through 18 years, United States, 2015. http://www.cdc.gov/vaccines/schedules/hcp/imz/child-adolescent.html. Accessed January 26, 2015.[29]

immunization schedules are frequently modified as new information emerges.

One vaccine is recommended for newborns.[29] Hepatitis B virus (HBV), a small, double-shelled virus in the family Hepadnaviridae, is the most common cause of chronic viremia. There are potentially more than 350 million persons with chronic HBV worldwide. HBV infection causes acute and chronic hepatitis, cirrhosis of the liver, and approximately 80% of hepatocellular carcinomas. The virus can be transmitted through the placenta to the fetus from an infected mother; in some cases, the mother may not know she has HBV (Box 39-1). Newborns who become infected with hepatitis B virus have a 90% chance of developing chronic hepatitis B virus infection with all its serious potential sequelae, including up to a 25% risk of death from cirrhosis or liver cancer. Thus, the high prevalence of HBV in women of childbearing age, the high transmission rate, and the severe consequences of HBV make the HepB vaccine for newborns cost-effective.

HepB vaccine is administered intramuscularly as a dose of 0.5 mL of vaccine (10 mcg), in a series of three injections. This vaccine has been given routinely in the United States since 1991, and the reported incidence of HBV has decreased by 95% in children and by 75% among all age groups. The second and third doses are given at age 1–2 months and age 6 months, respectively. Healthcare providers must be aware that thimerosal-free HepB vaccine has been available since 1999; there is no need to delay vaccination for any newborn.[30] Thimerosal is discussed in more detail in the *Immunizations* chapter. Delayed administration of the first dose by even a few weeks puts the newborn at risk for developing HBV infection later in infancy.[31,32]

Newborns born to mothers who have chronic hepatitis B (HBsAg positive) should receive hepatitis B immunoglobulin (0.5 mL) intramuscularly in addition to the HepB vaccine after physiologic stabilization of the newborn and preferably within 12 hours of birth. Approximately 19,000 women with chronic hepatitis B virus infection give birth in the United States each year. Postexposure prophylaxis administered within 12 hours after birth will prevent HBV infection in 90% of these neonates.[33] The hepatitis immune globulin can be administered at the same time as the HepB vaccine, albeit at a separate site.[34]

One additional vaccination, palivizumab (Synagis), a monoclonal antibody produced by recombinant DNA is recommended for newborns who have a high risk for developing respiratory syncytial virus. Preterm newborns who have chronic lung disease and neonates with congenital heart defects need to be evaluated for appropriateness of this vaccine.[35–38]

Box 39-1 Case Study: Why Does My Newborn Need a Vaccine for Hepatitis?

KM is 24 hours postpartum. The pediatric staff at the hospital where she gave birth have asked for permission to give her baby the first vaccine to protect against hepatitis B. KM states she understands that hepatitis B is a sexually transmitted disease but she knows she is not a chronic carrier of the hepatitis antigen. Therefore, she does not think her baby needs this vaccine as a newborn. In addition, she is worried about preservatives in the vaccine that might harm her baby.

Hepatitis B can be transmitted across the placenta as well as through contact with body fluids. If the mother has acquired hepatitis B since her initial prenatal lab samples were drawn, she and her newborn are at risk for developing serious complications—newborns who get infected with hepatitis B have a 90% chance of developing chronic infection. The healthcare provider gave this information to KM so she could make an informed consent or informed refusal.

Additionally, the healthcare provider told KM that the three-shot series, which is given in the first 6 months of life, will protect her baby if she is exposed to body fluids of a person—for example, a family member—who knowingly or unknowingly has hepatitis B. The healthcare provider also reassured KM that the vaccines used for newborns do not contain thimerosal, a mercury-containing preservative.

Protection against hepatitis B appears to be lifelong after completing the vaccination series, and booster doses are not necessary. Approximately 3% to 9% of newborns or children have some signs of pain at the injection site for a day or two after the injection, and 0.4% to 6% of newborns and/or children who receive the vaccine will get a slight fever (37.7°C or lower). The incidence of anaphylaxis is less than 1 in 600,000, and the incidence of hypersensitivity reaction is theoretic, but no cases have been reported.

Treatment of Newborns with Common Disorders

Hypoglycemia

Normal serum glucose ranges for the late preterm and term newborn remain controversial. Asymptomatic neonates at term may have glucose concentrations as low as 30 mg/dL in the first few hours of life. The definition of hypoglycemia that has been generally accepted is less than 47 mg/dL, but there is a lack of good evidence to support this number.[39] In any case, untreated hypoglycemia can lead to neurologic sequelae,[40] although the exact glucose concentration and length of time of the hypoglycemia that causes these long-term complications have not been clearly defined. Newborns at risk for hypoglycemia, such as those whose mothers have diabetes; newborns at the extremes of size, either small or large; newborns who are preterm or postmature should be screened until glucose homeostasis is stable. Any newborn who exhibits clinical signs of hypoglycemia, such as jitteriness, irritability, poor feeding, cyanosis, tachypnea, lethargy, and eye-rolling, also requires glucose monitoring.[41] These clinical manifestations are not specific to hypoglycemia and may require further evaluation.

The recommendations for asymptomatic, at-risk neonates are to check the initial blood glucose after the first feeding, which should take place within the first hour of life, and then to check blood glucose prior to feeding the newborn every 2 to 3 hours for the next 24 hours.[39] A blood glucose level greater than or equal to 45 mg/dL is acceptable. An initial level less than 25 mg/dL in the first 4 hours of life or less than 35 mg/dL from 4 to 24 hours after birth indicates the need to feed the neonate and repeat the glucose in 1 hour. If the follow-up glucose is greater than 40–45 mg/dL, the newborn should continue to be monitored with blood glucose screens until stable. However, in some situations, increasing regular feeding may be inadequate.

If the glucose level remains 35 mg/dL or less, intravenous glucose administration is indicated.[39] Intravenous glucose is given as an initial bolus of dextrose 10% 200 mg/kg (2 mL/kg), followed by a continuous infusion of IV glucose at an infusion rate of 5–6 mg/kg/min ($D_{10}W$ at 80 mL/kg/day). This therapy will need to be closely monitored and may need to be increased to maintain serum glucose levels higher than 45 mg/dL. Such newborns require frequent monitoring and additional evaluation to determine the cause of the hypoglycemia.

Infection

The incidence of infection in the term newborn in the United States has remained stable at approximately 2% to 4% since the 1980s.[42] Infection in the newborn period is associated with serious morbidity and mortality. Fifty percent of neonatal deaths in the first 24 hours after birth are caused by infection. Early recognition and implementation of appropriate antimicrobial agents can significantly improve the prognosis.

Neonatal Sepsis

The incidence of culture-proven neonatal sepsis in the United States is 1 to 2 per 1000 live births. Newborn sepsis is categorized as early-onset neonatal sepsis or late-onset neonatal sepsis. Early-onset neonatal sepsis usually occurs secondary to ascending infection from organisms that are in the vagina. Late-onset neonatal sepsis is usually attributed to infection acquired in the hospital or home.[43]

In early-onset infection, the microorganisms most commonly implicated are *Escherichia coli* and group B *Streptococcus* (GBS).[44] The CDC and the American Academy of Pediatrics (AAP) Committee on Fetus and Newborn (COFN) have published recommendations to guide the caregiver on the risk factors, treatment, and length of treatment for those newborns at risk for early-onset sepsis as it relates to maternal antibiotic treatment, GBS exposure, and chorioamnionitis.

In 2011, the AAP published an updated algorithm providing additional recommendations to the 2010 CDC guidelines regarding GBS.[45] This algorithm provides recommendations for neonates at risk for early-onset sepsis, including guidance on timing of laboratory evaluations and length of observation or treatment. Depending on the risk factors, including gestational age, duration of rupture of membranes, and duration of maternal antibiotics prior to birth, a neonate may require close observation or a limited laboratory evaluation. A newborn at high risk for infection, due to clinical manifestations of infection or maternal chorioamnionitis, should have a full sepsis evaluation with blood culture and complete blood count (CBC) with differential.

Initial antibiotic therapy is initiated with a combination of ampicillin and an aminoglycoside, usually gentamicin. These antibiotics have a synergistic activity against GBS and *Listeria monocytogenes*. Third-generation cephalosporins have been used instead of gentamicin, but there have been reports of resistance with their routine use and the development of candidiasis.[46]

Initial therapy depends on the clinical presentation and hemodynamic stability of the newborn. For those neonates who are hemodynamically stable, initiation of therapy with a semisynthetic penicillin, such as nafcillin, along with an aminoglycoside is often used. If the newborn is clinically unstable, vancomycin (Vanocin) and piperacillin/tazobactam (Zosyn) may be the drugs of choice. With culture results, the selection of antimicrobial agents is based on identification of the microorganism, the sensitivity of the organism to the drug, and the neonate's response to therapy.

Gram-positive organisms generally respond to broad-spectrum antibiotics, such as beta-lactamase penicillins, penicillin analogues, and first-generation cephalosporins (beta-lactamases). Gram-negative microorganisms are treated with aminoglycosides and cephalosporins.[42,47–49] Tests must be conducted to determine the specific sensitivity of a microorganism to the antimicrobial agent selected to ensure that the appropriate agent is prescribed.

Gram-positive cocci generally respond to penicillin, unless the microorganism produces beta-lactamase (or penicillinase). *Staphylococcus aureus* is a beta-lactamase–producing microorganism and, therefore, is not responsive to penicillin. A group of semisynthetic penicillins with added side chains are used to treat *S. aureus* sepsis, including methicillin, nafcillin, oxacillin, dicloxacillin, and cloxacillin. First-generation cephalosporins, such as cefazolin (Ancef), cephalexin (Keflex), and cephalothin (Keflin), are also resistant to beta-lactamase.[50–52]

Staphylococcus epidermidis and *S. aureus* strains may be resistant to penicillin, semisynthetic penicillins, and cephalosporins. Methicillin-resistant *S. aureus* (MRSA) is unresponsive to the semisynthetic penicillins; with this infection, vancomycin is the drug of choice.[53] Vancomycin (Vanocin) may also be used for treatment of the neonate with *S. epidermidis* infection and infection related to foreign bodies or invasive procedures. The emergence of resistant strains to available antimicrobial agents is an increasing problem.[54]

Third-generation cephalosporins treat gram-negative cocci that are penicillin and methicillin resistant. Aminoglycosides or third-generation cephalosporins are the drugs of choice for gram-negative enteric rods. Some gram-negative rods are classified according to their lactose fermentation ability. The lactose fermenters, *E. coli* and *Klebsiella*, are sensitive to aminoglycosides and third-generation cephalosporins. *Shigella* and *Salmonella* are non-lactose fermenters that respond well to ampicillin and third-generation cephalosporins.[47,55–58]

Haemophilus influenzae is usually sensitive to ampicillin and third-generation cephalosporins, although some strains are ampicillin resistant. *Pseudomonas* requires combination therapy of an aminoglycoside and an anti-*Pseudomonas* penicillin such as azlocillin, carbenicillin, imipenem, mezlocillin, piperacillin, or ticarcillin. Two anaerobic microorganisms, *Bacteroides fragilis* (gram negative) and *Clostridium* (gram positive), are sometimes the cause of newborn infection. *B. fragilis* is susceptible to metronidazole (Flagyl), clindamycin (Cleocin), and some of the newer beta-lactamases, such as imipenem and ampicillin with sulbactam (Unasyn). *Clostridium* is usually susceptible to penicillin.[43]

A combination of ampicillin or penicillin and gentamicin is useful for antibacterial action against *Streptococcus*, *Listeria monocytogenes*, and gram-negative enteric rods. This combination of antimicrobial agents has a synergistic effect (in vitro), increasing the efficacy of these drugs compared to when they are used alone. Additional therapy or selection of other agents is necessary if staphylococcal infection is suspected, if *Pseudomonas* or *Bacteroides* (most often iatrogenically acquired) is present, if there is an outbreak of resistant organisms, or if prolonged ampicillin and gentamicin therapy has been used.

Candida Infections

Oral thrush or monilia is caused by an overgrowth of the fungus *Candida albicans* in the mouth. It most often occurs among newborns or infants whose mothers have infections secondary to a *Candida* organism or among those who received antimicrobial agents that destroyed the normal flora. Thrush appears as white or yellowish raised spots on the tongue or sides of the mouth. It is treated with an oral antifungal agent such as nystatin suspension (Mycostatin) or fluconazole (Diflucan)[59] (Box 39-2). Gentian violet is an old-fashioned remedy that can be used, but has several disadvantages. Specifically, this agent is not as effective as nystatin, it stains clothing, and it can cause mucosal ulcerations under rare circumstances, so it is not recommended unless a family desires to avoid other antifungal medications.[60]

C. albicans infection may also present as a diaper rash, particularly in neonates with oral thrush. The diaper rash appears as superficial blisters that are usually nontender. The lesions may group together and coalesce to form a large area with smaller satellite blisters at the edges. These satellite lesions are characteristic of candidal infection. Treatment includes topical application of nystatin ointment, which may be combined with oral administration of fluconazole

Box 39-2 A Case of Thrush

CT is being seen for a 6-week postpartum visit and asks her provider to check for a yeast infection on her nipples. She is breastfeeding her daughter and has developed breast pain while feeding her. She is also worried about the baby's diaper rash. CT had an uncomplicated vaginal birth and has not had any problems breastfeeding. She says the baby latches well, nurses for an average of 20 to 30 minutes during each nursing episode, and is gaining weight. This is her third child; CT breastfed her first two children for several months each. She denies stabbing pain in her breasts and says the pain is localized to the nipples and areolae.

Infection with *Candida albicans* is common in infants and can also colonize the nipples and areolae of breastfeeding women; therefore, examination of both the mother and the infant in this breastfeeding dyad is important. Interestingly, little correlation exists between the strains of *Candida* found in the oral cavity of an infant and the vagina of that child's mother. Infants can develop thrush without known exposure, but cross-contamination between an infant and a mother's breast does occur.

On exam, CT is afebrile. She has bright red areolae that look shiny and have some flaking but no cracks. The rest of the breast exam is benign. Her daughter has white patches inside both cheeks that cannot be wiped away, and she has a diaper rash that is distinctive for a bright shiny red appearance without cracking or bleeding.

The presumptive diagnosis is *C. albicans* infection of the nipple and corresponding *C. albicans* infection in the infant's mouth (thrush) and perianal area. CT asks her provider if there is a natural treatment she can use so she doesn't have to give the baby any drugs.

CT's provider describes the use of gentian violet, which would be painted on the inside of the baby's mouth and on the woman's nipples. Gentian violet is effective but stains clothing, and there are no studies of its use for treating diaper rash.

The provider suggests nystatin (Mycostatin) and CT agrees to use it. CT is given the following prescriptions:

- Nystatin oral suspension 100,000 units; 1 mL is to be placed in each cheek inside the baby's mouth 4 times per day for 5 days. CT is instructed not to feed the infant for 5 to 10 minutes after the dose is administered.
- Nystatin ointment 100,000 units/g. A 30-g tube is ordered and CT is instructed to apply a small amount to the infant's diaper area and to her nipples twice a day for 7 to 10 days as needed.

In addition, the provider advises CT to wash pacifiers, to keep diapers off so the baby's bottom is exposed to the air when sleeping, and to avoid wearing bras and nipple pads so all areas that are infected are exposed to dry air whenever possible. She is also advised to wash her hands well after applying the nystatin ointment to her nipples and to her baby. Perhaps most importantly, the provider encourages and supports the woman in continuing to breastfeed her daughter.

to reduce the intestinal content of *C. albicans*, which may lower the risk of invasive candidiasis in the neonate.[61]

Systemic *C. albicans* infection is becoming more prevalent in neonatal intensive care units (NICUs) and is one of the most common causes of late-onset sepsis.[34] Factors that increase the risk of this infection include indwelling intravenous or arterial catheters, prolonged or indiscriminate use of antibacterial agents, use of third-generation cephalosporins, total parenteral nutrition, mechanical ventilation, long hospitalization, and previous colonization with *Candida*. The treatment of a systemic infection requires intravenous therapy with an antifungal agent, such as amphotericin B (Fungizone), for a prolonged period of time.[62] New drugs are under development for treatment of fungal infections in neonates; however, data are lacking on the efficacy of these agents in neonates and children.[63]

Omphalitis or Umbilical Cord Infections

Omphalitis is an infection of the umbilical cord. It rarely occurs in developed countries, although the exact incidence is not known because for hospital-born neonates, this infection typically occurs after discharge. Omphalitis is generally localized, but rarely can spread directly into the bloodstream due to delayed obliteration of the umbilical vessels, causing severe systemic infection. Signs of omphalitis include erythema, edema, discharge, foul smell, bleeding from the cord, and failure of the cord to dry out. This infection should be treated with systemic antimicrobial agents based on the most likely causative microorganism. First-line agents include intravenous treatment with ampicillin and gentamicin.

There is no evidence that application of topical agents such as isopropyl alcohol, povidone-iodine, chlorhexidine, or dyes prevents the incidence of omphalitis in developed countries. Conversely, application of these agents and routine daily care with isopropyl alcohol may prolong the time needed for cord drying and separation. Therefore, prophylactic treatment of the umbilical stump with topical agents is no longer recommended.[64] In developing countries, application of chlorhexidine appears to be effective against omphalitis, and there is some evidence that application of breast milk also may reduce infection.[64–67]

Seizures

Seizures are the most common sign of a neurologic disorder during the neonatal period; the incidence ranges from 1 to 5 per 1000 live births.[68] The first month of life is one of the highest-risk periods for seizures. Seizures in the newborn are generally triggered by an acute disorder, such as hypoxic-ischemic encephalopathy, congenital malformation, stroke, or infection. They are a sign of an acute disturbance within the brain and are caused by excessive, synchronous electrical discharges or depolarization, producing stereotypic, repetitive behaviors. Uncontrolled seizures can increase the damage to the central nervous system, and neonatal seizures may be associated with lifelong epilepsy.[69]

Seizures can be classified as subtle, tonic, clonic, or myoclonic, with subtle seizure being the most common and sometimes misdiagnosed as an episode of hypoglycemia-caused jitteriness. Expression of seizures in the newborn include abnormal movement or alterations in tone in the trunk and extremities; abnormal facial, oral, and tongue movements; abnormal eye movements; and changes in respiratory effort.

A prolonged generalized seizure that causes cyanosis, significant changes in heart rate, or apnea that does not respond to adequate ventilation and perfusion therapy should be treated with anticonvulsant medication. The first-line anticonvulsant used in the newborn period is phenobarbital, at a dosage of 20 mg/kg given intravenously for a maximum of 40 mg/kg as a loading dose, followed by 3–5 mg/kg per day administered in a divided dose given once every 12 hours.[70] Intravenous phenobarbital reaches the brain rapidly and has a rapid onset of action. This agent is metabolized by the liver and eliminated by the kidneys. Therapeutic levels vary but generally are in the range of 40 to 60 mcg/mL. Subsequent management may include levetiracetam (Keppra), phenytoin (Dilantin), lidocaine, and midazolam (Versed) under the direction of a pediatric neurologist.

Neonatal Stroke

Myoclonic or multifocal seizures, especially followed by coma, absence of neonatal reflexes, and irregularities of vital signs, may indicate a perineal (neonatal) stroke. Timing of these seizures can range from a few hours of life to a week after birth and may result in lifelong disability, including cerebral palsy and learning disabilities.[71,72] No standard treatment regimen exists, although some authorities suggest administering magnesium sulfate based on evidence that antepartum administration may provide neuroprotection and decrease the incidence of cerebral palsy in preterm infants.[73] Other interventions under investigation include antithrombotic agents, umbilical stem cells, and hypothermia.[74]

Resuscitation of the Newborn

Oxygen: Too Little or Too Much?

Healthcare professionals who regularly provide care for newborns should be knowledgeable and certified to perform neonatal resuscitation, including ordering and administering drugs for resuscitation. Among the drugs most commonly used in such situations is oxygen—an agent that often is not thought of as a drug.

Oxygen has been widely used in newborn resuscitation and in the care of newborns with respiratory distress. Most providers have been concerned about hypoxia, but recently issues of high levels of oxygen or **hyperoxia** of the newborn have emerged. With advances in research and technology, the effects of hyperoxia on the brain, retinal vessels, and lung tissue have been identified. In the mid-twentieth century, an association was found between administration of oxygen to preterm neonates and development of vision loss and blindness. Originally known as retrolental fibroplasia, this disease is now termed retinopathy of prematurity.

At the time the association was discovered, 100% oxygen was freely used without adequate monitoring of arterial oxygen content. In the 1960s, the association between oxygen toxicity and the development of bronchopulmonary dysplasia was identified.

Increased amounts of oxygen can lead to the formation of oxygen free radicals or reactive oxygen species within the body. There is a delicate balance that the body works to maintain to prevent damage from oxidative stress. Antioxidants present both within and outside the cells serve as the body's defense against the oxygen free radicals. Due to the immaturity of the premature neonate's organ systems, however, such a newborn has diminished ability to deal with oxidative stress due to a deficiency of antioxidants.

Damage to the brain has been associated with high oxygen concentrations, as has damage to the retinas and lungs. Hyperoxia can lead to toxicity in the developing neonatal brain, though it is not clear which level or duration of time leads to the damaging effects. Retinal damage is found most commonly among newborns younger than 32 weeks' gestation. Hyperoxia or severe fluctuations in arterial oxygen content may damage the still developing retinal vessels in the premature newborn. Oxidative stress causes harm to the alveolar–capillary membrane in the lungs and, in conjunction with an increase in inflammatory mediators, damages the newborn lungs, leading to pulmonary edema and fibrosis.

In 2010, the American Heart Association's *Guidelines for Neonatal Resuscitation* were revised in terms of the recommendations for oxygen use during newborn resuscitation. The guidelines cite two meta-analyses of several randomized controlled trials of resuscitation of newborns with either 100% oxygen or room air, which demonstrated an increase in survival among those neonates resuscitated with room air.[75] In addition, it was discovered that resuscitation with 100% oxygen reduces time to first spontaneous breath, lowers the Apgar score, and decreases the neonate's heart rate.[76] Current recommendations for neonatal resuscitation are to begin with 21% oxygen (also known as room air) for term newborns and then adjust oxygen administration based on oxygen saturation measurements.

Further research is needed to help define preventive measures to prevent hyperoxic damage and the effects of inflammation. The use of antioxidants for use in newborns is under study as a means to prevent injury from oxidative stress.

Other Drugs for Resuscitation

Table 39-2 provides a general overview of the agents recommended in the Neonatal Resuscitation Program (NRP) developed by the American Academy of Pediatrics and the American Heart Association.[77] Performance of appropriate resuscitation requires a sophisticated interplay

Table 39-2 Drugs for Resuscitation of a Newborn

Drug	Indication/Rationale	Route	Dose	Comments
Epinephrine 1:10,000	Cardiac simulant	Umbilical vein	0.1–0.3 mg/kg IV	Rapid administration. Follow with 0.5–1 mL normal saline flush.
		Intratracheal tube (ET tube [ETT])	0.5–1.0 ml/kg in ETT	Rapid administration. Follow with positive-pressure ventilation. Usually administered while obtaining IV access.
Normal saline (first choice) or Ringer's lactate, O-negative blood, or red packed cells	Volume expander	Umbilical vein	10 mL/kg	Administer over 5–10 minutes by syringe or infusion pump.
Sodium bicarbonate 4.2% solution	Buffers to counter metabolic acidosis	Umbilical vein or other large vein with good return	0.5 mEq/mL	Slow administration to avoid side effects, including cerebral hemorrhage. Contraindicated if inadequate ventilation. Contraindicated by ETT route.
Naloxone (Narcan)	Opioid antagonist	IV route (first choice) May give IM but onset delayed	0.1 mg/kg	Prepare 1 mL in 1-mL syringe and administer rapidly. Contraindicated for neonate born to woman suspected of addiction to opioids or on methadone program because of increased risk of newborn seizures.

Source: Modified from American Academy of Pediatrics, American Heart Association. *Textbook of Neonatal Resuscitation*. Elk Grove Village, IL: Academy of Pediatrics; 2011.[77]

among cognitive knowledge, clinical observations, and psychomotor skills. Fortunately, few newborns will require pharmaceutical interventions. Readers are directed to the NRP program for detailed discussion of how these drugs fit into the context of neonatal resuscitation. Simple knowledge of the agents themselves alone is insufficient for performing appropriate resuscitation

Conclusion

The relative immaturity of the newborn's organ systems affects the pharmacokinetics and pharmacodynamics of pharmacologic agents used in the neonatal period. The selection and administration of drugs for the newborn should be based on a thorough physical examination, careful maternal and neonatal history, and knowledge of the unique physiologic function of the newborn organ systems. Additionally, evaluation of the therapeutic effects of the drug and identification of adverse effects are critical. Some medications will require the measurement of serum drug levels to identify therapeutic or potentially toxic levels.

Resources

Organization	Description	Website
American Academy of Pediatrics	Professional organization for pediatricians. Partner with American Heart Association for Neonatal Resuscitation Program.	www.aap.org
National Association of Neonatal Nurses	Professional organization for nurses and nurse practitioners in neonatology. Provides guidelines for practice. Particularly focused on intensive care.	www.nann.org
Apps		
Prevent GBS	App to help providers manage the treatment of pregnant women so as to eradicate GBS.	www.cdc.gov/groupbstrep/guidelines/prevention-app.html
Micomedix Neofax Essentials	Multiple apps exist for care of the neonate, especially drug therapy for sick infants/newborns in a NICU. Downloading and paying for this app includes the annual fee for updating information during the year. Other apps are more limited, such as drug calculators, and usually are free.	For iPhone/iPad: https://itunes.apple.com/us/app/micromedex neofax-essentials/id460060130?mt=8 Other options also may be available.

References

1. Allegaert K, van den Anker JN. Clinical pharmacology in neonates: small size, huge variability. *Neonatology.* 2014;105(4):344-349.
2. Richter WF, Jacobsen B. Subcutaneous absorption of biotherapeutics: knowns and unknowns. *Drug Metab Dispos.* 2014;42(11):1881-1889.
3. Allegaert K, Fanos V, van den Anker JN, Laër S. Perinatal pharmacology. *Biomed Res Int.* 2014; 2014:101620.
4. Hansen TW. Mechanisms of bilirubin toxicity: clinical implications. *Clin Perinatol.* 2002;29(4):765-778.
5. McMillin GA, Wood KE, Strathmann FG, Krasowski MD. Patterns of drugs and drug metabolites observed in meconium: what do they mean? *Ther Drug Monit.* January 6, 2015. [Epub ahead of print].
6. Allegaert K1, van den Anker JN, Naulaers G, de Hoon J. Determinants of drug metabolism in early neonatal life. *Curr Clin Pharmacol.* 2007;2(1):23-29.
7. Ward RM, Kern SE, Lugo RA. Pharmacokinetics, pharmacodynamics, and pharmacogenetics. In: Gleason CA, Devaskar SU, eds. *Avery's Diseases of the Newborn.* 9th ed. Philadelphia: Elsevier/Saunders; 2012:417-428.
8. Schirm E, Tobi H, de Jong-van den Berg LT. Identifying parents in pharmacy data: a tool for the continuous monitoring of drug exposure to unborn children. *J Clin Epidemiol.* 2004;57:737-741.
9. Matinzadeh ZK, Beiragdar F, Kavemanesh Z, Abolgasemi H, Amirsalari S. Efficacy of topical ophthalmic prophylaxis in prevention of ophthalmia neonatorum. *Trop Doct.* 2007;37:47-49.
10. Chen CJ, Starr CE. Epidemiology of gram-negative conjunctivitis in neonatal intensive care unit patients. *Am J Ophthalmol.* 2008;145:966-970.
11. Richter R, Below H, Kadow I, et al. Effect of topical 1.25% povidone-iodine eyedrops used for prophylaxis of ophthalmia neonatorum on renal iodine excretion and thyroid-stimulating hormone level. *J Pediatr.* 2006;148:401-403.
12. Simon JW. Povidone-iodine prophylaxis of ophthalmia neonatorum. *Br J Ophthalmol.* 2003;87:1437.
13. CDC guidance on shortage of erythromycin (0.5%) ophthalmic ointment: update March 2010. http://www.fda.gov/Drugs/DrugSafety/DrugShortages/ucm050793.htm. Accessed November 11, 2015.
14. Sobel HL, Silvestre MA, Mantaring JB III, Oliveros YE, Nyunt-U S. Immediate newborn care practices

delay thermoregulation and breastfeeding initiation. *Acta Paediatr.* 2011;100(8):1127-1133.

15. Autret-Leca E, Jonville-Bera AP. Vitamin K in neonates: how to administer, when and to whom. *Paediatr Drugs.* 2001;3:1-8.
16. Lippi G, Franchini M. Vitamin K in neonates: facts and myths. *Blood Transfus.* 2011;9(1):4-9.
17. Shearer, MJ. Vitamin K deficiency bleeding (VKDB) in early infancy. *Blood Rev.* 2009;23:49-59.
18. Volpe, JJ. Teratogenic effects of drugs and passive addiction. In: *Neurology of the Newborn.* 5th ed. Philadelphia: Elsevier; 2008:1009-1054.
19. Zengin E, Sarper N, Turker G, Corapcioglu F, Etus V. Late hemorrhagic disease of the newborn. *Ann Trop Paediatr.* 2006;26:225-231.
20. Elalfy MS, Elagouza IA, Ibrahim FA, AbdElmessieh SK, Gadallah M. Intracranial haemorrhage is linked to late onset vitamin K deficiency in infants aged 2–24 weeks. *Acta Paediatr.* 2014;103(6):3273-3276.
21. Tulchinsky TH, Patton MM, Randolph LA, et al. Mandating vitamin K prophylaxis for newborns in New York State. *Am J Public Health.* 1993;83(8):1166-1168.
22. Schulte R, Jordan LC, Morad A, Naftel RP, Wellons JC III, Sidonio R. Rise in late onset vitamin K deficiency bleeding in young infants because of omission or refusal of prophylaxis at birth. *Pediatr Neurol.* 2014; 50(6):564-568.
23. Block SL. Playing newborn intracranial roulette: parental refusal of vitamin K injection. *Pediatr Ann.* 2014;43(2):53-59.
24. Volpe J. Commentary: Intracranial hemorrhage in early infancy: renewed importance of vitamin K deficiency. *Pediatr Neurol.* 2014;50:545-546.
25. Ipema HJ. Use of oral vitamin K for prevention of late vitamin K deficiency bleeding in neonates when injectable vitamin K is not available. *Ann Pharmacother.* 2012;46(6):879-883.
26. Fear NT, Roman E, Ansell P, Simpson J, Day N, Eden OB; United Kingdom Childhood Cancer Study. Vitamin K and childhood cancer: a report from the United Kingdom Childhood Cancer Study. *Br J Cancer.* 2003;89(7):1228-1231.
27. Hviid A. Postlicensure epidemiology of childhood vaccination: the Danish experience. *Expert Rev Vaccines.* 2006;5:641-649.
28. Marshall GS, Happe LE, Lunacsek OE, et al. Use of combination vaccines is associated with improved coverage rates. *Pediatr Infect Dis J.* 2007;26:496-500.
29. Centers for Disease Control and Prevention. Recommended immunization schedule for persons age 0 through 18 years, United States, 2015. http://www.cdc.gov/vaccines/schedules/hcp/imz/child-adolescent.html. Accessed January 26, 2015.
30. Marques RC, Dorea JG, Manzatto AG, Bastos WR, Bernardi JV, Malm O. Time of perinatal immunization, thimerosal exposure and neurodevelopment at 6 months in breastfed infants. *Acta Paediatr.* 2007; 96:864-868.
31. Chang MH. Hepatitis B virus infection. *Semin Fetal Neonatal Med.* 2007;12:160-167.
32. Cohn AC, Broder KR, Pickering LK. Immunizations in the United States: a rite of passage. *Pediatr Clin North Am.* 2005;52:669, 93, v.
33. Lee C, Gong Y, Brok J, Boxall EH, Gluud C. Hepatitis B immunisation for newborn infants of hepatitis B surface antigen-positive mothers. *Cochrane Database Syst Rev.* 2006;2:CD004790. doi:10.1002/14651858.CD004790.pub2.
34. Chapman RL. Prevention and treatment of *Candida* infections in neonates. *Semin Perinatol.* 2007; 31:39-46.
35. Elhassan NO, Sorbero ME, Hall CB, Stevens TP, Dick AW. Cost-effectiveness analysis of palivizumab in premature infants without chronic lung disease. *Arch Pediatr Adolesc Med.* 2006;160:1070-1076.
36. Grimaldi M, Gouyon B, Sagot P, et al. Palivizumab efficacy in preterm infants with gestational age < or = 30 weeks without bronchopulmonary dysplasia. *Pediatr Pulmonol.* 2007;42:189-192.
37. Simoes EA, Groothuis JR, Carbonell-Estrany X, et al. Palivizumab prophylaxis, respiratory syncytial virus, and subsequent recurrent wheezing. *J Pediatr.* 2007; 151:34-42.
38. Ventre K, Randolph A. Ribavirin for respiratory syncytial virus infection of the lower respiratory tract in infants and young children. *Cochrane Database Syst Rev.* 2010;5:CD000181. doi:10.1002/14651858.CD000181.pub4.
39. Committee on Fetus and Newborn of the American Academy of Pediatrics, Adamkin DH. Postnatal glucose homeostasis in late-preterm and term infants. *Pediatrics.* 2011;127(3):575-579.
40. Lang TF, Hussain K. Pediatric hypoglycemia. *Adv Clin Chem.* 2014;63:211-245.
41. Zhou W, Yu J, Wu Y, Zhang H. Hypoglycemia incidence and risk factors assessment in hospitalized neonates. *J Matern Fetal Neonatal Med.* 2015;28(4):422-425.
42. Du Pont-Thibodeau G, Joyal JS, Lacroix J. Management of neonatal sepsis in term newborns. *F1000 Prime Rep.* 2014;6:67.

43. Brady MT, Polin RA. Prevention and management of infants with suspected or proven neonatal sepsis. *Pediatrics.* 2013;132(1):166-168.
44. American College of Obstetricians and Gynecologists Committee on Obstetric Practice. ACOG Committee Opinion No. 485: prevention of early-onset group B streptococcal disease in newborns. *Obstet Gynecol.* 2011;117(4):1019-1027.
45. Committee on Infectious Diseases, Committee on Fetus and Newborn; Baker CJ, Byington CL, Polin RA. Policy statement: recommendations for the prevention of perinatal group B streptococcal (GBS) disease. *Pediatrics.* 2011;128(3):611-616. doi:10.1542/peds.2011-1466.
46. Polin RA, Committee on Fetus and Newborn. Management of neonates with suspected or proven early-onset bacterial sepsis. *Pediatrics.* 2012;129(5):1006-1015.
47. Lima-Rogel V, Medina-Rojas EL, Del Carmen Milan-Segovia R, et al. Population pharmacokinetics of cefepime in neonates with severe nosocomial infections. *J Clin Pharm Ther.* 2008;33:295-306.
48. Murphy JE. Prediction of gentamicin peak and trough concentrations from six extended-interval dosing protocols for neonates. *Am J Health Syst Pharm.* 2005;62:823-827.
49. Pong AL, Bradley JS. Guidelines for the selection of antibacterial therapy in children. *Pediatr Clin North Am.* 2005;52:869, 94, viii.
50. Marschall J, Muhlemann K. Duration of methicillin-resistant *Staphylococcus aureus* carriage, according to risk factors for acquisition. *Infect Control Hosp Epidemiol.* 2006;27:1206-1212.
51. Baltimore RS. Consequences of prophylaxis for group B streptococcal infections of the neonate. *Semin Perinatol.* 2007;31:33-38.
52. Tzialla C, Borghesi A, Stronati M. Neonatal antibiotic prophylaxis for the prevention of early- and late-onset group B streptococcal sepsis. *J Perinat Med.* 2007;35:252, 253; author reply 254.
53. Bond CA, Raehl CL. Clinical and economic outcomes of pharmacist-managed aminoglycoside or vancomycin therapy. *Am J Health Syst Pharm.* 2005;62:1596-1605.
54. Fanos V, Cuzzolin L, Atzei A, Testa M. Antibiotics and antifungals in neonatal intensive care units: a review. *J Chemother.* 2007;19:5-20.
55. Boyle EM, Brookes I, Nye K, Watkinson M, Riordan FA. "Random" gentamicin concentrations do not predict trough levels in neonates receiving once daily fixed dose regimens. *BMC Pediatr.* 2006;6:8.
56. Clark RH, Bloom BT, Spitzer AR, Gerstmann DR. Empiric use of ampicillin and cefotaxime, compared with ampicillin and gentamicin, for neonates at risk for sepsis is associated with an increased risk of neonatal death. *Pediatrics.* 2006;117:67-74.
57. Dellagrammaticas HD, Christodoulou C, Megaloyanni E, Papadimitriou M, Kapetanakis J, Kourakis G. Treatment of gram-negative bacterial meningitis in term neonates with third-generation cephalosporins plus amikacin. *Biol Neonate.* 2000;77:139-146.
58. Schrag SJ, Hadler JL, Arnold KE, Martell-Cleary P, Reingold A, Schuchat A. Risk factors for invasive, early-onset *Escherichia coli* infections in the era of widespread intrapartum antibiotic use. *Pediatrics.* 2006;118:570-576.
59. Moorhead AM, Amir LH, O'Brien PW, Wong S. A prospective study of fluconazole treatment for breast and nipple thrush. *Breastfeed Rev.* 2011;19(3):25-29.
60. Su CW, Gaskie S, Jamieson B, Triezenberg D. Clinical inquiries: what is the best treatment for oral thrush in healthy infants? *J Fam Pract.* 2008;57(7):484-485.
61. Ozturk MA, Gunes T, Koklu E, Cetin N, Koc N. Oral nystatin prophylaxis to prevent invasive candidiasis in neonatal intensive care unit. *Mycoses.* 2006;49:484-492.
62. Cetin H, Yalaz M, Akisu M, Hilmioglu S, Metin D, Kultursay N. The efficacy of two different lipid-based amphotericin B in neonatal *Candida* septicemia. *Pediatr Int.* 2005;47:676-680.
63. Smolinski KN, Shah SS, Honig PJ, Yan AC. Neonatal cutaneous fungal infections. *Curr Opin Pediatr.* 2005;17:486-493.
64. Imdad A, Bautista RMM, Senen KAA, Uy MEV, Mantaring JB III, Bhutta ZA. Umbilical cord antiseptics for preventing sepsis and death among newborns. *Cochrane Database Syst Rev.* 2013;5:CD008635. doi:10.1002/14651858.CD008635.pub2.
65. Imdad A, Mullany LC, Baqui AH, et al. The effect of umbilical cord cleansing with chlorhexidine on omphalitis and neonatal mortality in community settings in developing countries: a meta-analysis. *BMC Public Health.* 2013;13(suppl 3):S15.
66. Zupan J, Garner P, Omari AAA. Topical umbilical cord care at birth. *Cochrane Database Syst Rev.* 2004;3:CD001057. doi:10.1002/14651858.CD001057.pub2.
67. Golshan M, Hossein N. Impact of ethanol, dry care and human milk on the time for umbilical cord separation. *J Pak Med Assoc.* 2013;63(9):1117-1119.

68. Clancy RR. Summary proceedings from the neurology group on neonatal seizures. *Pediatrics.* 2006;117:S23-S27.
69. Pisani F, Facini C, Pavlidis E, Spagnoli C, Boylan G. Epilepsy after neonatal seizures: literature review. *Eur J Paediatr Neurol.* 2015;19(1):6-14.
70. Slaughter LA, Patel AD, Slaughter JL. Pharmacological treatment of neonatal seizures: a systematic review. *J Child Neurol.* 2013;28(3):351-364.
71. Lynch JK. Epidemiology and classification of perinatal stroke. *Semin Fetal Neonatal Med.* 2009;14:245-249.
72. Rutherford MA, Ramenghi LA, Cowan FM. Neonatal stroke. *Arch Dis Child Fetal Neonatal.* 2011; 20:377-384.
73. Doyle LW, Crowther CA, Middleton P, Marret S. Antenatal magnesium sulfate and neurologic outcome in preterm infants: a systematic review. *Obstet Gynecol.* 2009;113(6):1327-1333.
74. Kirton A, deVeber G. Paediatric stroke: pressing issues and promising directions. *Lancet Neurol.* 2015;14(1):92-102.
75. Kattwinkel J, Perlman JM, Aziz K, et al.; American Heart Association. Neonatal resuscitation: 2010 American Heart Association guidelines for cardiopulmonary resuscitation and emergency cardiovascular care. *Pediatrics.* 2010;126(5):e1400-e1413.
76. Saugstad OD. Oxygen toxicity. In: Donn SM, Sinha SK, eds. *Manual of Neonatal Respiratory Care.* 3rd ed. New York: Springer; 2012:55-61.
77. American Academy of Pediatrics, American Heart Association. *Textbook of Neonatal Resuscitation.* Elk Grove Village, IL: Academy of Pediatrics; 2011.

APPENDIX
Glossary of Abbreviations

Abbreviation	Expanded Form
ac	before meals (abbreviation no longer recommended)
ad lib	use freely
AM	morning, before noon
amt	amount
bid	twice daily (abbreviation no longer recommended)
cap, caps	capsule
cc	cubic centimeter
cf	with food (abbreviation no longer recommended)
CR	controlled release
d/c	discontinue
disp	dispense
DS	double strength
dL	deciliter
elix	elixir
ER	extended release
et	and
g	gram
gr	grain
gtt(s)	drop, drops
h, hr, hrs	hour, hours
hs	at bedtime (abbreviation no longer recommended)
IM	intramuscular injection
IP	Intraperitoneal (abbreviation no longer recommended)
IU	International Units
IV	intravenous
LA	long acting
L	liter
m	meter (often reported as squared)
max	maximum
mcg	microgram (also abbreviated in some sources as *μg*)
mEq	milliequivalent
mg	milligram
mL	milliliter
ng	nanogram
od	once per day (abbreviation no longer recommended)
oz	ounce
per	by or through
pc	after meals (abbreviation no longer recommended)
pH	hydrogen ion concentration
PM	evening or afternoon
PO	by mouth or orally
PR	by rectum
prn	as needed; from Latin *pro re nata*
q	Every (abbreviation no longer recommended)
qd	every day (abbreviation no longer recommended)
qhs	every night at bedtime (abbreviation no longer recommended)
qid	four times daily (abbreviation no longer recommended)
SC	subcutaneous (may also be abbreviated as subc, subq, or SQ)
sig	write on label
SL	sublingually, under the tongue
SR	slow release
sol	solution
supp	suppository
susp	suspension
tab	tablet
tbsp	tablespoon
troche	lozenge
tsp	teaspoon
tid	three times a day (abbreviation no longer recommended)
U	units
U.S.P.	United States Pharmacopeia
vag	vaginally
XL, XT	extended release

Index

Note: Page numbers in bold indicate in-depth discussion or dosage information for specific drugs. Brand names are capitalized; generic names are lowercase, *f, b, t* indicate materials in figures, boxes and tables respectively

A

B

C

D

E

F

G

H

I

J

K

L

M

N

O

P

Q

R

S

T

U

V

W

X

Y

Z